12-02

2003 EDITION

PDR®

NURSE'S DRUG HANDBOOK™

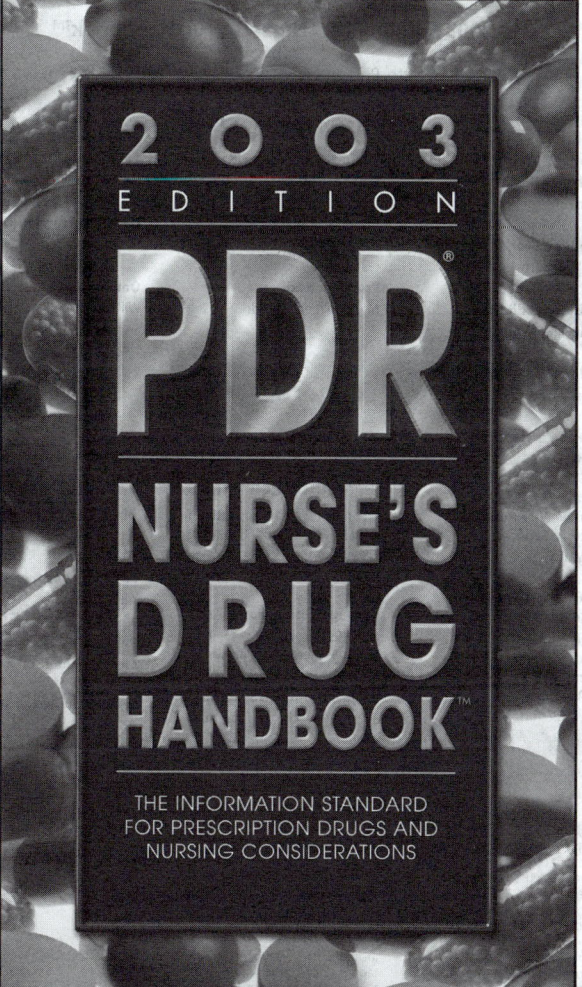

George R. Spratto, PhD
Dean and Professor of Pharmacology,
School of Pharmacy,
West Virginia University
Morgantown, West Virginia

Adrienne L. Woods, MSN, ARNP, FNP-C
Family Nurse Practitioner,
Primary Care at the
Department of Veterans Affairs Medical and Regional Office Center,
Wilmington, Delaware

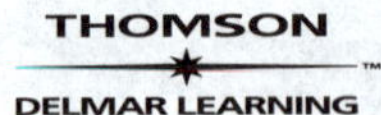

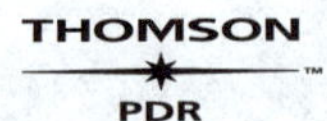

2003 Edition PDR® Nurse's Drug Handbook™

by

George R. Spratto, PhD and Adrienne L. Woods, MSN, ARNP, FNP-C

Printed in the United States
1 2 3 4 5 XXX 05 06 05 04 03

For more information contact Delmar Learning, Executive Woods, 5 Maxwell Drive, Clifton Park, NY 12065-2919

Or find us on the World Wide Web at http://www.delmar.com

ISBN: 0-7668-6382-4

Table of Contents

Notice to the Reader

The monographs in this edition of the PDR® Nurse's Drug Handbook™ are the work of two distinguished authors: George R. Spratto, PhD, Dean and Professor of Pharmacology of the School of Pharmacy at West Virginia University, Morgantown, West Virginia, and Adrienne L. Woods, MSN, ARNP, FNP-C, Family Nurse Practitioner, Primary Care, at the Department of Veterans Affairs Medical and Regional Office Center, Wilmington, Delaware.

The publisher and the authors do not warrant or guarantee any of the products described herein or perform any independent analysis in connection with any of the product information contained herein. The publisher and the authors do not assume and expressly disclaim any obligation to obtain and include information other than that provided by the manufacturer.

The reader is expressly warned to consider and adopt all safety precautions that might be indicated by the activities described herein and to avoid all potential hazards. By following the instructions contained herein, the reader willingly assumes all risks in connection with such instructions.

The publisher and the authors make no representations or warranties of any kind, including but not limited to the warranties of fitness for a particular purpose or merchantability nor are any such representations implied with respect to the material set forth herein, and the publisher and the authors take no responsibility with respect to such material. The publisher and the authors shall not be liable for any special, consequential, or exemplary damages resulting, in whole or in part, from the reader's use of, or reliance upon, this material.

The authors and publisher have made a conscientious effort to ensure that the drug information and recommended dosages in this book are accurate and in accord with accepted standards at the time of publication. However, pharmacology and therapeutics are rapidly changing sciences, so readers are advised, before administering any drug, to check the package insert provided by the manufacturer for the recommended dose, for any contraindications for administration, and for any added warnings and precautions. This recommendation is especially important for new, infrequently used, or highly toxic drugs.

Preface

The PDR® Nurse's Drug Handbook™ is a trusted resource used by nursing students, practicing nurses, and other health care professionals. Each annual edition provides updates affecting thousands of bits of information and introduces monographs of drugs recently approved by the FDA and marketed by the drug manufacturers. Drug information changes rapidly, including the introduction of new drugs, new uses for established drugs, revised and new administration routes (dosage forms), newly identified side effects and drug interactions, and changes in dosing and use recommendations based on feedback from professionals and consumers. Health care professionals depend on this handbook to provide the latest information on drug therapy, guidelines for monitoring efficacy of the therapy, and recommendations for teaching the client and family about important aspects of the drug therapy.

Organization of Content

Chapter 1 includes general information on important therapeutic or chemical classes of drugs. The classes are listed alphabetically. Consult the Table of Contents for a concise listing of the therapeutic/chemical classes included in Chapter 1. Each class begins with a list of drugs for which a monograph appears in Chapter 2. The information provided in the class applies to all drugs listed for the class. Information that is specific to one of the drugs listed is included in the drug monograph in Chapter 2. For a complete picture of a specific drug, consult the class information in Chapter 1 as well as the appropriate monograph in Chapter 2.

Chapter 2 contains individual drug monographs in alphabetical order by generic name. The purpose and meaning of each of the components of a monograph are described under *Using the Drug Monographs* below.

The **Visual Identification Guide** is a color insert of drug products organized alphabetically by generic name. More than two hundred photographs of tablets, capsules, and other solid dosage forms are provided. These images cover leading brands. All items are reproduced in actual size and color. For products with distinguishing features on both sides, the front view is supplemented with a picture of the back view. Each product is labeled with its brand name and the name of the manufacturer.

The **appendices** provide additional information to assist in administering drugs and monitoring drug therapy. Appendix 1 contains brief monographs of drugs approved by the FDA too late to be included in Chapter 2. Most of these drugs will be developed as full monographs for the next edition of the handbook. New appendices provide listings of drug regimens for specific conditions, such as arthritis, diabetes, and hypertension; chemotherapy protocols for the treatment of neoplasms are also new to this edition.

Two indexes are found in the back of the handbook. The **IV index** lists IV drugs by generic name. The **general index** is extensively cross-referenced: each generic drug name entry includes the major trade name(s) entry in parentheses and each trade name entry is followed by the generic drug name in parentheses. Each page of the general index contains a key identifying boldface as the generic drug name, italics as the therapeutic drug class, regular type as the trade name, and capitals as the combination drug name.

Using the Drug Monographs

The following components are described in the order in which they appear in the monographs. All components may not appear in each monograph but are represented where appropriate and when information is available. Refer also to the sample monograph with explanatory notes for the purpose and use of each component.

Drug Name: The generic drug name is the first item in the name block (in color at the beginning of each monograph).

Phonetic Pronunciation: pronunciation guide for generic name to assist in mastering often complex names

Pregnancy Category: Lists the FDA pregnancy category (A, B, C, D, or X) assigned to the drug (pregnancy categories are defined in the appendices).

Classification: Defines the type of drug or the class under which the drug is listed. A classification or descriptor is provided for each drug name in Chapter 2. If the drug class is new and only one drug is available in the class at the time of printing the handbook, the classification will not appear in Chapter 1. It will be added at a later date as more drugs in the class reach the market.

Trade Name: Trade names are identified as Rx (prescription) or OTC (over the counter, no prescription required). If numerous forms of the drug are available, the trade names are identified by form. Trade names available only in Canada are identified as Canadian.

Controlled Substance: If the drug is controlled by the U. S. Federal Controlled Substances Act, the schedule in which the drug is placed follows the trade name listing (C-I, C-II, C-III, C-IV, C-V). See the appendices for a listing of controlled substances in both the United States and Canada.

Combination Drug: This heading at the top of the name block indicates that the drug is a combination of two or more drugs in the same product. Additional combination drugs are listed in the appendix on *Commonly Used Combination Drugs*.

The following components may appear in the body of a drug monograph.

Cross Reference: "See also …" directs the reader to the classification entry in Chapter 1 that matches the classification of the drug being reviewed. General information about the drugs in the class is provided in Chapter 1. Information specific to a drug appears in the monograph in Chapter 2. Consult the class information in Chapter 1 for a complete picture of the drug.

General Statement: This appears in a few drug monographs but is more common in the class entries in Chapter 1. Information about the drug class and/or anything specific or unusual about a group of drugs is presented. Information may also be presented about the disease(s) or condition(s) for which the drugs are indicated.

Content: For combination drugs, provides the generic name and amount of each drug in the combination product.

Action/Kinetics: The action portion describes the proposed mechanism(s) by which a drug achieves its therapeutic effect. Not all mechanisms of action are known, and some are self-evident, as when a hormone is administered as a replacement. The kinetics portion lists critical information, if known, about the rate of drug absorption, distribution, time for peak plasma levels or peak effect, minimum effective serum or plasma level, biological half-life, duration of action, metabolism, and excretion route(s). Metabolism and excretion routes may be important for clients with systemic liver disease, kidney disease, or both.

The half-life (the time required for half the drug to be excreted or removed from the blood, serum, or plasma - **t½**) is important in determining how often a drug is to be administered and how long the client is to be assessed for side effects. Therapeutic levels indicate the desired concentration, in serum or plasma, for the drug to exert its beneficial effect and are helpful in predicting the onset of side effects or the lack of effect. Drug therapy is often monitored in this manner (e. g., antibiotics, theophylline, phenytoin, amiodarone). See the appendices for a listing of commonly accepted therapeutic drug levels.

Uses: Approved therapeutic uses for the drug are listed. Some investigational uses are also listed for selected drugs.
Contraindications: Disease states or conditions in which the drug should not be used are noted. The safe use of many of the newer pharmacologic agents during pregnancy, lactation, or childhood has not been established. As a general rule, the use of drugs during pregnancy is contraindicated unless the benefits of drug therapy are determined to far outweigh the potential risks.
Special Concerns: Covers considerations for use with pediatric, geriatric, pregnant, or lactating clients. Situations and disease states when the drug should be used with caution are also listed.
Side Effects: Undesired or bothersome effects the client *may* experience while taking a particular agent are described. Side effects are listed by the body organ or system affected and are usually presented with the most common side effects in descending order of incidence. Nearly all potential side effects are listed. In any given clinical situation, however, a client may experience no side effects, one or two side effects, or several side effects. If potentially life-threatening, the side effect is highlighted.
OD **Overdose Management:** When appropriate, this section provides a list of the symptoms observed following an overdose (*Symptoms*) as well as treatment approaches and/or antidotes for the overdose (*Treatment*).
Drug Interactions: Alphabetical listing of drugs and herbals that may interact with the drug under discussion. The study of drug interactions is an important area of pharmacology that changes constantly as a result of new drugs introduced, clinical feedback, use of herbals, and increased client usage. Because of the significant increase in the use of herbal products, interactions of medications with herbals are included in this section if known or suspected. These interactions are designated by the icon [add H icon]. The listing of drug/drug and drug/herbal interactions is far from complete; therefore, listings in this handbook are to be considered *only* as general cautionary guidelines.

Drug interactions may result from a number of different mechanisms: (1) additive or inhibitory effects; (2) increased or decreased metabolism of the drug; (3) increased or decreased rate of elimination; (4) decreased absorption from the GI tract; (5) competition for or displacement from receptor sites or plasma protein binding sites. Such interactions may manifest themselves in a variety of ways; however, an attempt has been made throughout the handbook to describe these interactions whenever possible as an increase (↑) or a decrease (↓) in the effect of the drug, and a reason for the change. It is important to realize that any side effects that accompany the administration of a particular agent may be increased as a result of a drug or herbal interaction.

Drug/herbal interactions are often listed for classes of drugs. Thus, the drug/herbal interaction is likely to occur for all drugs in a particular class. Refer to Chapter 1.
Laboratory Test Considerations: The manner in which a drug may affect laboratory test values is presented. Some of the effects are caused by the therapeutic or toxic effects of the drugs; others result from interference with the testing method itself. The laboratory considerations are described as increased (↑) or false positive (+) values and as decreased (↓) or false negative (-) values. Also included, when available, are drug-induced changes in blood or urine levels of endogenous substances (e.g., glucose, electrolytes, and so on).
How Supplied: The various dosage forms available for the drug and amounts of the drug in each of the dosage forms is presented. Such information is important as one dosage form may be more appropriate for a client than another. This information also allows the user to ensure the appropriate dosage form and strength is being administered.
Dosage: The dosage form and route of administration is followed by the disease state or condition (in italics) for which the dosage is recommended. This is

followed by the adult and pediatric doses, when available. The listed dosage is to be considered as a general guideline; the exact amount of the drug to be given is determined by the provider. However, one should question orders when dosages differ markedly from the accepted norm.

Nursing Considerations: The guidelines provided in this section are designed to help the practitioner in applying the nursing process to pharmacotherapeutics to ensure safe practice. In each monograph the following sections are provided when applicable.

- ❑ Administration/Storage: guidelines for preparing medications for administration, administering the medication, and storage and disposal of the medication. Guidelines for administration by IV are indicated by an icon **IV**.
- ❑ Assessment: guidelines for monitoring/assessing client before, during, and after prescribed drug therapy.
- ❑ Interventions: guidelines for specific nursing actions related to the drug being administered.
- ❑ Client/Family Teaching: guidelines to promote education, active participation, understanding, and adherence to drug therapy by the client and/or family members. Precautions about the drug therapy are also noted for communication to the client/family.
- ❑ Outcomes/Evaluate: guidelines identify desired outcomes of the drug therapy and client response. These will help determine the effectiveness and positive therapeutic outcome of the prescribed drug therapy.

Notes on Assessment and Interventions. The following tasks are critical in assessing the client for drug therapy and for planning the interventions needed to undertake the therapy.

- ❑ Gather physical data and client history
- ❑ Assess specific physiologic functions likely to be affected by the drug therapy
- ❑ Determine specific laboratory tests needed to monitor the course of the drug therapy
- ❑ Identify sensitivities/interactions and conditions that may preclude a particular drug therapy
- ❑ Document specific indications for therapy and describe symptom characteristics related to this condition
- ❑ Know the physiologic, pharmacologic, and psychologic effects of the drug and how these may affect the client and impact the nursing process
- ❑ Know adverse reactions that can arise as a result of drug therapy and be prepared with appropriate nursing interventions
- ❑ Monitor the client for side effects and document/report them to the provider. Severe side effects generally require dosage modification or discontinuation of the drug.
- ❑ Ensure client safety when receiving drug therapy

When taking the nursing history, place emphasis on the client's ability to read and to follow directions. Language barriers must be identified and appropriate written translations should be provided to promote adherence to the drug therapy. In addition, client lifestyle, culture, income, availability of health insurance, and access to transportation are important factors that may affect adherence with therapy and follow-up care.

The assessment should include the potential for the client being/becoming pregnant, and if a mother is breast feeding her infant.

The age and orientation level of the client, whether learned from personal observation or from discussion with close friends or family members, can be critical in determining potential relationships between drug therapy and/or drug interactions.

Including these factors in the nursing assessment will assist all members of the health care team to determine the type of pharmacotherapy, drug delivery system, and monitoring and follow-up plan best suited to a particular client to promote the highest level of adherence

Notes on Client/Family Teaching. Specific information for the client is provided for each drug. Client/family teaching assists the client/family to recognize side effects and avoid potentially dangerous situations, and alleviates anxiety associated with starting and maintaining drug therapy.

Details on administration are included to enhance client understanding and adherence. Side effects that require medical intervention are included, as are recommendations for minimizing the side effects for certain medications (e.g., take medication with food to decrease GI upset, or take at bedtime to minimize daytime sedative effects).

The proper education of clients is one of the most challenging aspects of nursing. The instructions must be tailored to the needs, awareness, and sophistication of each client. For example, clients who take medication to lower blood pressure should assume responsibility for taking their own blood pressure or having it taken and recorded.

Clients should carry identification listing the drugs currently prescribed. They should know what they are taking and why, and develop a mechanism to remind themselves to take their medication as prescribed. Clients should carry this drug list with them whenever they go for a checkup or seek medical care. The drug list may also be shared with the pharmacist if there is a question concerning drugs prescribed; if the client is considering taking an over-the-counter medication, or if the client has to change pharmacies.

The records, especially blood pressure readings, should be shared with the health care provider to ensure accurate evaluation of the response to the prescribed drug therapy. This may also alert the provider to any drug/food/herbal consumption by the client that they did not prescribe, were not aware of, or that may interfere with (i. e., potentiate or antagonize) the current pharmacologic regimen. The provider may also encourage the client to call with any questions or concerns about the drug therapy.

Remember: the components described previously are covered for all drugs or drug classes. When drugs are presented as a group (as in Chapter 1), the information for each component is given only once for the group. Check each component for information relevant to all drugs covered in the class. Note that many of the drug monographs in Chapter 2 are cross-referenced to the general information in Chapter 1. Critical information or information relevant to a specific drug is provided in the individual drug monograph in Chapter 2 under appropriate headings, such as *Additional Contraindications, Additional Side Effects, or Additional Nursing Considerations*. These are **in addition to** and **not instead of** the entry in Chapter 1, which is referenced and must be consulted.

Please join us on the web at www.nursespdr.com for a searchable drug database, links to pharmaceutical company and related sites, drug headlines, and a drug archive.

Also Available from Medical Economics

Although you'll find virtually all major prescription drugs covered in this one compact handbook, nurses know that the pursuit of wellness is no longer limited to traditional medications. Today, more and more patients routinely use nutritional supplements to fight chronic illness, improve health, and maintain fitness. To keep you abreast of this increasingly complex field of healthcare, PDR now publishes *PDR® for Nutritional Supplements™*, a compendium of the latest consensus on over 200 popular supplement products, including an array of amino acids, co-factors, fatty acids, probiotics, phytoestrogens, phytosterols, over-the-counter hormones, hormonal precursors, and much more. Focused on the scientific evidence (or lack of evidence) for each supplement's claims, this unique new reference offers you today's most detailed, informed, and objective overview of this burgeoning new area in the field of self-treatment. To protect your clients from bogus remedies and steer them towards truly beneficial products, this book is a must.

As additional armament in the battle to maintain truly safe and effective self-medication, PDR also offers a dramatically expanded second edition of the best-selling *PDR® for Herbal Medicines™*, the nation's most comprehensive guide to botanical agents. With over 1,000 pages, this authoritative compendium provides healthcare professionals with an unparalleled fund of facts about the physical characteristics, chemical composition, and physiological effects of 700 medicinal herbs, along with their accepted indications, contraindications, drug interactions, side effects, overdose, and dosage. Also included are specifics on hundreds of leading commercial preparations, indices of traditional Asian and homeopathic indications, and a Safety Guide that lists herbs to be avoided during pregnancy and nursing, and herbs to be used only under professional supervision.

Although botanical products are not officially regulated or monitored in the United States, *PDR® for Herbal Medicines* provides you the closest analog to FDA-approved labeling—the findings of the German Regulatory Authority's herbal watchdog agency, Commission E—augmented with exhaustive literature reviews from the PhytoPharm U.S. Institute for Phytopharmaceuticals. These reports represent the most accurate, impartial, and reliable assessment of a botanical agent's safety and effectiveness currently available in medicine.

Now, when clients pepper you with questions about the latest "herb du jour," *PDR for Herbal Medicines* can provide you with a rational basis for response. It tells which botanicals to encourage—and which to avoid. It clearly distinguishes between valid indications and specious claims, warns of conflicting conditions and drugs, and provides you with an exhaustive bibliography of the relevant clinical literature on each medicinal plant. It is a truly indispensable reference in an era when more and more patients are experimenting with the host of exotic—and sometimes dangerous—herbal remedies that have recently gained growing popularity.

New Pocket and Electronic Reference Options: For the many times when all you need is quick confirmation of dosage, PDR now offers the ultra-miniaturized *PDR Pharmacopoeia™ Pocket Edition*. Only slightly larger than an index card, and a quarter of an inch thick, it fits easily into any pocket, while providing you with FDA-approved dosing recommendations for over 1,500 drugs.

Unlike other condensed drug references, this new handbook is drawn almost exclusively from the FDA-approved drug labeling published in *Physicians' Desk Reference*, so you can rely on it for authoritative, official dosage guidelines. Its tabular presentation makes lookups a breeze. And to expedite comparisons, it lists drugs by major category and specific indication. At $9.95 a copy, it's a tool you really can't afford to be without.

If portability is your goal, PDR has two other intriguing new options for you. Now you can get the essential facts on six key topics for every fully-described prescription drug in *PDR* and *PDR for Ophthalmic Medicines* and load it into your Palm®, Visor™, Pocket PC®, or other handheld personal digital assistant. Or if you prefer, you can get a brand new Franklin eBookman unit loaded with the same information.

Whatever handheld device you use, you'll get crucial information on these six topics: Indications and Usage, Contraindications, Warnings, Adverse Reactions, How Supplied, and Dosage and Administration. (These topics are also available on a traditional *Pocket PDR*® DataCard.) No matter how you choose to view it, you'll have a complete databank of prescribing information at your fingertips wherever you go!

For more information on this or any other member of the growing family of *PDR* products and services, please call, toll-free, 1-800-232-7379 or fax 201-722-2680.

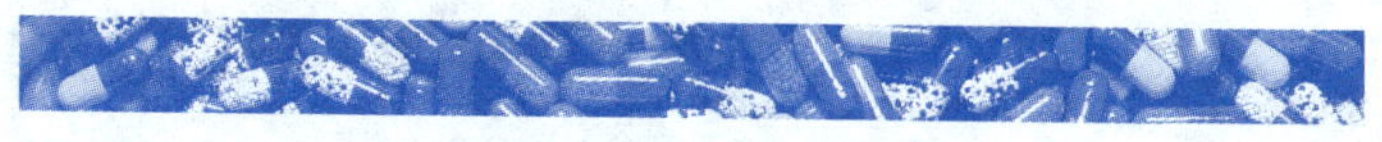

Acknowledgments

We would like to extend our thanks to the Delmar team who work so diligently to ensure that the manuscript process flows smoothly and to try to keep us on track. Team members include Matthew Kane, Mary Colleen Liburdi, Linda Helfrich, Laurie Davis, and Marjorie Bruce. Team members Marge Bruce, Mary Colleen Liburdi, and Linda Helfrich deserve a special note of thanks and appreciation; their hard work and dedication to the project, as well as their understanding of the difficulty in meeting deadlines, is an inspiration for us to keep working. Thanks are also expressed to Dave Hillman and Datapage Technologies for their work in continuing to establish and refine our database.

George Spratto extends appreciation to his colleagues at West Virginia University. Special thanks are extended to Diane Casdorph of the Drug Information Center, School of Pharmacy, West Virginia University, who assisted in researching information on new drugs. Greatest appreciation and love go to my wife, Lynne, sons, Chris and Gregg, daughter-in-law Kim, granddaughter, Alexandra, and grandson, Dominic, who continue to be supportive and maintain a high level of excitement for the project.

Adrienne Woods would like to extend her appreciation to her colleagues at the VA and to Sally Marshall, who knows the sacrifice. Also, to my husband, Howard, the best father, and friend, I have ever known, for his patience, love and understanding. To my children, Katy and Nate, for enduring hectic schedules and a few missed soccer, baseball, and basketball games. Finally, to Peanut butter, Fudge and Oreo for their patience and affection.

QUICK REFERENCE GUIDE TO A DRUG MONOGRAPH

Here is a quick guide to reading and understanding the drug monographs found in Chapter 2.

Cyclosporine

(sye-kloh-**SPOR**-een)

PREGNANCY CATEGORY: C

CLASSIFICATION(S):

Immunosuppressant

Rx: Cyclosporine Softgel Capsules, Gengraf, Neoral , Sandimmune

✱**Rx:** Sandimmune I.V.

ACTION/KINETICS

Thought to act by inhibiting the immunocompetent lymphocytes in the G_0 or G_1 phase of the cell cycle. T-lymphocytes are specifically inhibited; both the T-helper cell and the T-suppressor cell may be affected. Also in-

1. **GENERIC NAME OF DRUG**
2. **PHONETIC PRONUNCIATION** of generic name
3. **PREGNANCY CATEGORY** assigned by the FDA. Defined in Appendix 3.
4. **CLASSIFICATION:** Defines the type of drug or the class under which the drug is listed.
5. **TRADE NAMES** by which a drug is marketed. If numerous forms of the drug are available, the trade names are identified by form. **Rx** denotes prescription drugs. **OTC** denotes over-the-counter, nonprescription drugs **CANADIAN** trade names are indicated by a maple leaf. (✱)
6. **CONTROLLED SUBSTANCE:** If the drug is controlled by the U. S. Federal Controlled Substances Act, the schedule in which the drug is placed follows the trade name listing. Controlled substance schedules are placed after Rx drugs. (ex: **C-II**) **CROSS REFERENCE** (for selected drugs): "See also ..." directs the reader to the classification entry in Chapter 1 that gives a complete picture of the drug.
7. **ACTION/KINETICS:** Critical information about the rate of drug absorption, distribution, time for peak plasma levels or peak effect, minimum effective serum or plasma level, duration of action, metabolism, and excretion route(s). Metabolism and excretion routes may be important for clients with systemic liver disease, kidney disease, or both.

tines. **Peak plasma levels:** 3.5 hr. Food may both delay and impair drug absorption. **t½:** Approximately 19 hr for adults and 7 hr in children. Metabolized by the liver; inactive metab

8 MAXIMUM PLASMA LEVELS archieved at therapeutic doses.

9 BIOLOGICAL HALF-LIFE, the time required for half the drug to be excreted or removed from the blood, serum, or plasma.

USES
(1) Prophylaxis of rejection in kidney, liver, and heart allogeneic transplants.

10 APPROVED THERAPEUTIC USES Some investigational uses are also listed for selected drugs.

CONTRAINDICATIONS
Hypersensitivity to cyclosporine or polyoxyethylated castor oil. Lactation. Use of potassium-sparing diuretics. Neoral in psoriasis or rheumatoid ar-

11 CONTRAINDICATIONS: Disease states or conditions in which the drug should not be used are noted.

SPECIAL CONCERNS
Use with caution in clients with impaired renal or hepatic function. Safety and efficacy have not been established in children. Clients with malabsorption may not achieve therapeutic levels following PO use.
SIDE EFFECTS
GI: N&V, diarrhea, gum hyperplasia, anorexia, gastritis, hiccoughs, peptic ulcer, abdominal discomfort, UGI

12 SPECIAL CONCERNS Considerations for use with pediatric, geriatric, pregnant, or lactating clients. Situations and disease states when the drug should be used with caution are also listed.

13 SIDE EFFECTS listed by the body organ or system affected. Usually presented with the most common side effects first in descending order of incidence. If potentially life-threatening, the side effect is highlighted.

LABORATORY TEST CONSIDERATIONS
↑ Serum creatinine, potassium, BUN, total bilirubin, alkaline phosphatase. Possibly ↑ cholesterol, LDL, and apolipoprotein B. Hyperglycemia/kalemia/uricemia.
OD OVERDOSE MANAGEMENT
Symptoms: Transient hepatotoxicity and nephrotoxicity. *Treatment:* Induction of vomiting (up to 2 hr after ingestion). General supportive measures.
DRUG INTERACTIONS

14 LABORATORY TEST CONSIDERATIONS: The manner in which the drug may affect laboratory test values is presented as increased values (↑), false positive values (+) decreased values (↓) or false negative values (-). Also included, when available, are drug-induced changes in blood or urine levels of endogenous substances.

15 OVERDOSE MANAGEMENT: Symptoms observed following an overdose and treatment approaches and/or antidotes for the overdose.

16 DRUG INTERACTIONS Alphabetical listing of drugs and herbals that may interact with the drug. ↑ increase, ↓ decrease, → leading to.

H *Echinacea* / Do not give with cyclosporine
Erythromycin / ↑ Cyclosporine plasma level R/T ↓ liver breakdown and ↓ biliary excretion → possible nephrotoxicity

17 **HERBALS:** Because of the significant increase in the use of herbal products, interactions with herbals are included if known or suspected.

HOW SUPPLIED
Capsule, Soft Gelatin: 25 mg, 50 mg, 100 mg; *Capsule, Soft Gelatin for Microemulsion:* 25 mg 100 mg; *Injection:* 50 mg/mL; *Oral Solution:* 100 mg/mL; *Oral Solution for Microemulsion:* 100 mg/mL

18 **HOW SUPPLIED:** Dosage forms and amounts of the drug in each of the dosage forms. One dosage form may be more appropriate for a client than another. This information also allows the user to ensure the appropriate dosage form and strength is being administered.

DOSAGE
- **CAPSULES, ORAL SOLUTION**
  Allogenic transplants.

Adults and children, initial: A single 15 mg/kg dose given 4–12 hr before transplantation; there is a trend to use

19 **DOSAGE:** The dosage form and route of administration is followed by the disease state or condition (in italics) for which the dosage is recommended. This is followed by the adult and pediatric doses, when available.

NURSING CONSIDERATIONS

ADMINISTRATION/STORAGE

1. Sandimmune and Neoral are not bioequivalent and should not be used interchangeably without the supervi-

20 **NURSING CONSIDERATIONS:** Guidelines to help the practitioner in applying the nursing process to pharmacotherapeutics to ensure safe practice.

21 **ADMINISTRATION/STORAGE:** Guidelines for preparing medications for administration, administering the medication, and proper storage and disposal of the medication.

IV 7. Dilute IV concentrate 1 mL (50 mg) in 20–100 mL 0.9% NaCl or D5% injection; give infusion slowly over 2–6 hr. Do not refrigerate once cyclo-

22 **GUIDESLINES FOR ADMINISTRATION BY IV**

ASSESSMENT

1. Document indications for therapy; note any previous treatments. List drugs prescribed and note any potential interactions. Anticipate concomi-

23 **ASSESSMENT:** Guidelines for monitoring/assessing client before, during, and after prescribed drug therapy.

CLIENT/FAMILY TEACHING

1. Review importance of following the written guidelines for medication therapy explicitly. Drug must be tak-

24 **CLIENT/FAMILY TEACHING:** Guidelines to promote education, active participation, understanding, and adherence to drug therapy by the client and/or family members. Precautions about drug therapy are also noted for communication to the client/family.

OUTCOMES/EVALUATE

- Prevention of transplant rejection; improved organ function
- Cyclosporine trough levels (100–200 ng/mL)

25 **OUTCOMES/EVALUATE:** Desired outcomes of the drug therapy and client response.

INTERVENTIONS (FOR SELECTED DRUGS): Guidelines for specific nursing actions related to the drug being administered.

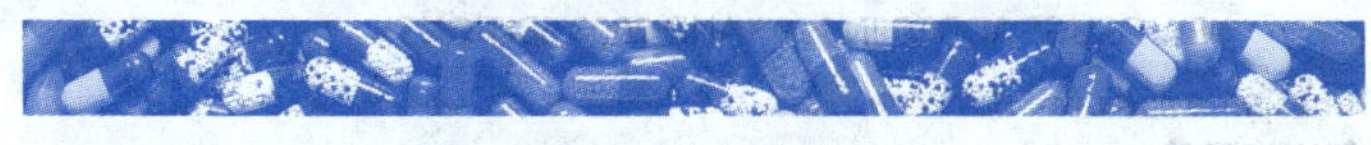

NEW DRUGS ADDED IN 2002 AND 2003 EDITIONS

Note: Drug names in boldface are new to the 2003 edition

alemtuzumab
almotriptan maleate
anakinra
argatroban
balsalazide disodium
BCG, intravesical
bexarotene
bimatoprost
bosentan
botulinum toxin, Type A
botulinum toxin, Type B
butenafine hydrochloride
caspofungin acetate
cefditoren pivoxil
cetrorelix acetate
cevimeline hydrochloride
choriogonadotropin alfa
cisatracuriun besylate
colesevelam hydrochloride
darbepoetin alfa
desloratadine
dexmethylphenidate hydrochloride
drotrecogin alfa (activated)
ertapenem sodium for injection
esomeprazole
fondaparinux sodium
formoterol fumarate
frovatriptan
gemtuzumab ozogamicin
imatinib mesylate
insulin aspart
insulin glargine
levobetaxolol hydrochloride
linezolid
meloxicam
mifepristone
nestiride
norelgestromin/ethinyl estradiol transdermal system
pantoprazole sodium
pimecrolimus
rivastigmine tartrate
tenecteplase
tenofovir disoproxil fumarate

tinzaparin sodium
travoprost
triptorelin pamoate
unoprostone isopropyl ophthalmic solution
valdecoxib
valganciclovir hydrochloride
verteporfin for injection
zoledronic acid for injection
zonisamide

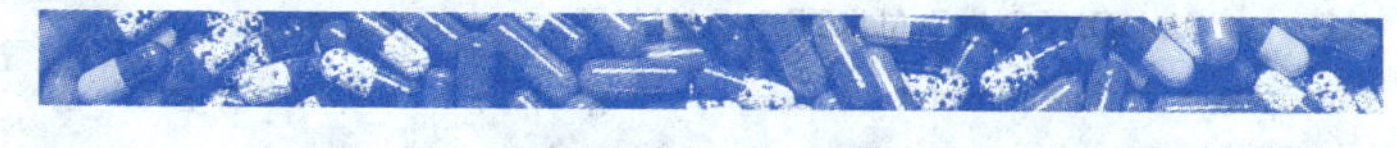

Common Sound-Alike Drug Names

The following is a list of common sound-alike drug names; trade names are capitalized. In parentheses next to each drug name is the pharmacological classification/use for the drug.

Accupril (ACE inhibitor)	Accutane (antiacne drug)
acetazolamide (antiglaucoma drug)	acetohexamide (oral antidiabetic drug)
Aciphex (proton pump inhibitor)	Accupril (ACE inhibitor)
Aciphex (proton pump inhibitor)	Aricept (drug for Alzheimer's disease)
Adriamycin (antineoplastic)	Aredia (bone growth regulator)
albuterol (sympathomimetic)	atenolol (beta-blocker)
Aldomet (antihypertensive)	Aldoril (antihypertensive)
Alkeran (antineoplastic)	Leukeran (antineoplastic) Myleran (antineoplastic)
allopurinol (antigout drug)	Apresoline (antihypertensive)
alprazolam (anti-anxiety agent)	lorazepam (anti-anxiety agent)
Ambien (sedative-hypnotic)	Amen (progestin)
amiloride (diuretic)	amlodipine (calcium channel blocker)
amiodarone (antiarrhythmic)	amrinone (inotropic agent)
amitriptyline (antidepressant)	nortriptyline (antidepressant)
Apresazide (antihypertensive)	Apresoline (antihypertensive)
Arlidin (peripheral vasodilator)	Aralen (antimalarial)
Artane (cholinergic blocking agent)	Altace (ACE inhibitor)
asparaginase (antineoplastic agent)	pegaspargase (antineoplastic agent)
Atarax (antianxiety agent)	Ativan (antianxiety agent)
atenolol (beta-blocker)	timolol (beta-blocker)
Atrovent (cholinergic blocking agent)	Alupent (sympathomimetic)
Avandia (oral hypoglycemic)	Coumadin (anticoagulant)
Avandia (oral hypoglycemic)	Prandin (oral hypoglycemic)
bacitracin (antibacterial)	Bactroban (anti-infective, topical)
Benylin (expectorant)	Ventolin (sympathomimetic)
Brevital (barbiturate)	Brevibloc (beta-adrenergic blocker)
Bumex (diuretic)	Buprenex (narcotic analgesic)
Cafergot (analgesic)	Carafate (antiulcer drug)
calciferol (Vitamin D)	calcitriol (Vitamin D)

carboplatin (antineoplastic agent)	cisplatin (antineoplastic agent)
Cardene (calcium channel blocker)	Cardizem (calcium channel blocker)
Cataflam (NSAID)	Catapres (antihypertensive)
Catapres (antihypertensive)	Combipres (antihypertensive)
cefotaxime (cephalosporin)	cefoxitin (cephalosporin)
cefuroxime (cephalosporin)	deferoxamine (iron chelator)
Celebrex (NSAID)	Cerebyx (anticonvulsant)
Celebrex (NSAID)	Celera (antidepressant)
Cerebyx (anticonvulsant)	Celera (antidepressant)
chlorpromazine (antipsychotic)	chlorpropamide (oral antidiabetic)
chlorpromazine (antipsychotic)	prochlorperazine (antipsychotic)
chlorpromazine (antipsychotic)	promethazine (antihistamine)
Clinoril (NSAID)	Clozaril (antipsychotic)
clomipramine (antidepressant)	clomiphene (ovarian stimulant)
clonidine (antihypertensive)	Klonopin (anticonvulsant)
Cozaar (antihypertensive)	Zocor (antihyperlipidemic)
cyclobenzaprine (skeletal muscle relaxant)	cyproheptadine (antihistamine)
cyclophosphamide (antineoplastic)	cyclosporine (immunosuppressant)
cyclosporine (immunosuppressant)	cycloserine (antineoplastic)
Cytovene (antiviral drug)	Cytosar (antineoplastic)
Cytoxan (antineoplastic)	Cytotec (prostaglandin derivative)
Cytoxan (antineoplastic)	Cytosar (antineoplastic)
Dantrium (skeletal muscle relaxant)	danazol (gonadotropin inhibitor)
Darvocet-N (analgesic)	Darvon-N (analgesic)
daunorubicin (antineoplastic)	doxorubicin (antineoplastic)
desipramine (antidepressant)	diphenhydramine (antihistamine)
DiaBeta (oral hypoglycemic)	Zebeta (beta-adrenergic blocker)
digitoxin (cardiac glycoside)	digoxin (cardiac glycoside)
diphenhydramine (antihistamine)	dimenhydrinate (antihistamine)
dopamine (sympathomimetic)	dobutamine (sympathomimetic)
Edecrin (diuretic)	Eulexin (antineoplastic)
enalapril (ACE inhibitor)	Anafranil (antidepressant)
enalapril (ACE inhibitor)	Eldepryl (antiparkinson agent)
Eryc (erythromycin base)	Ery-Tab (erythromycin base)
etidronate (bone growth regulator)	etretinate (antipsoriatic)
etomidate (general anesthetic)	etidronate (bone growth regulator)
Fioricet (analgesic)	Fiorinal (analgesic)
flurbiprofen (NSAID)	fenoprofen (NSAID)
folinic acid (leucovorin calcium)	folic acid (vitamin B complex)
Gantrisin (sulfonamide)	Gantanol (sulfonamide)
glipizide (oral hypoglycemic)	glyburide (oral hypoglycemic)
glyburide (oral hypoglycemic)	Glucotrol (oral hypoglycemic)

Hycodan (cough preparation)	Hycomine (cough preparation)
hydralazine (antihypertensive)	hydroxyzine (antianxiety agent)
hydrocodone (narcotic analgesic)	hydrocortisone (corticosteroid)
hydromorphone (narcotic analgesic)	morphine (narcotic analgesic)
Hydropres (antihypertensive)	Diupres (antihypertensive)
Hytone (topical corticosteroid)	Vytone (topical corticosteroid)
imipramine (antidepressant)	Norpramin (antidepressant)
Inderal (beta-adrenergic blocker)	Inderide (antihypertensive)
Inderal (beta-adrenergic blocker)	Isordil (coronary vasodilator)
Indocin (NSAID)	Minocin (antibiotic)
Lamictal (anticonvulsant)	Lamisil (antifungal)
Lanoxin (cardiac glycoside)	Lasix (diuretic)
Lantus (insulin product)	Lente insulin (insulin product)
Lioresal (muscle relaxant)	lisinopril (ACE inhibitor)
Lithostat (lithium carbonate)	Lithobid (lithium carbonate)
Lithotabs (lithium carbonate)	Lithobid (lithium carbonate)
Lodine (NSAID)	codeine (narcotic analgesic)
Lopid (antihyperlipidemic)	Lorabid (beta-lactam antibiotic)
lovastatin (antihyperlipidemic)	Lotensin (ACE inhibitor)
metolazone (thiazide diuretic)	methotrexate (antineoplastic)
metolazone (thiazide diuretic)	metoclopramide (GI stimulant)
metoprolol (beta-adrenergic blocker)	misoprostol (prostaglandin derivative)
Monopril (ACE inhibitor)	minoxidil (antihypertensive)
nelfinavir (antiviral)	nevirapine (antiviral)
Norlutate (progestin)	Norlutin (progestin)
Norvasc (calcium channel blocker)	Navane (antipsychotic)
Ocufen (NSAID)	Ocuflox (fluoroquinolone antibiotic)
Orinase (oral hypoglycemic)	Ornade (upper respiratory product)
Percocet (narcotic analgesic)	Percodan (narcotic analgesic)
paroxetine (antidepressant)	paclitaxel (antineoplastic)
Paxil (antidepressant)	paclitaxel (antineoplastic)
Paxil (antidepressant)	Taxol (antineoplastic)
penicillamine (heavy metal antagonist)	penicillin (antibiotic)
pindolol (beta-adrenergic blocker)	Parlodel (inhibitor of prolactin secretion)
Platinol (antineoplastic)	Paraplatin (antineoplastic)
Pravachol (antihyperlipidemic)	Prevacid (GI drug)
Pravachol (antihyperlipidemic)	propranolol (beta-adrenergic blocker)
prednisolone (corticosteroid)	prednisone (corticosteroid)
Prilosec (inhibitor of gastric acid secretion)	Prozac (antidepressant)
Prinivil (ACE inhibitor)	Prilosec (GE drug)

Prinivil (ACE inhibitor)	Proventil (sympathomimetic)
Procanbid (antiarrhythmic)	Procan SR (antiarrhythmic)
propranolol (beta-adrenergic blocker)	Propulsid (GI drug)
Provera (progestin)	Premarin (estrogen)
Prozac (antidepressant)	Proscar (androgen hormone inhibitor)
quinidine (antiarrhythmic)	clonidine (antihypertensive)
quinidine (antiarrhythmic)	Quinamm (antimalarial)
quinine (antimalarial)	quinidine (antiarrhythmic)
Regroton (antihypertensive)	Hygroton (diuretic)
Retrovir (drug for HIV)	ritonavir (drug for HIV)
Rifamate (antituberculous drug)	rifampin (antituberculous drug)
Rimantadine (antiviral)	flutamide (antineoplastic)
Soriatane (antipsoriasis)	Loxitane (antipsychotic)
Stadol (narcotic analgesic)	Haldol (antipsychotic)
Tegretol (anticonvulsant)	Tequin (antibacterial)
terbinafine (antifungal agent)	terfenadine (antihistamine)
terbutaline (sympathomimetic)	tolbutamide (oral hypoglycemic)
tolazamide (oral hypoglycemic)	tolbutamide (oral hypoglycemic)
torsemide (loop diuretic)	furosemide (loop diuretic)
trifluoperazine (antipsychotic)	trihexyphenidyl (antiparkinson drug)
Trimox (amoxicillin product)	Diamox (carbonic anhydrase inhibitor)
Vancenase (corticosteroid)	Vanceril (corticosteroid)
Vasosulf (sulfonamide/ decongestant)	Velosef (cephalosporin)
Versed (benzodiazepine sedative)	Vistaril (antianxiety agent)
Versed (benzodiazepine sedative)	VePesid (antineoplastic)
Xanax (antianxiety agent)	Zantac (H_2 histamine blocker)
Xenical (antiobesity)	Xeloda (antineoplastic)
Zantac (H_2 histamine blocker)	Zyrtec (H_1 antihistamine)
Zebeta (beta-blocker)	DiaBeta (oral hypoglycemic)
Zinacef (cephalosporin)	Zithromax (macrolide antibiotic)
Zocor (antihyperlipidemic)	Zoloft (antidepressant)
Zofran (antiemetic)	Zantac (H_2 histamine blocker)
Zosyn (penicillin antibiotic)	Zofran (antiemetic)
Zovirax (antiviral)	Zyvox (antibiotic)
Zyvox (antibiotic)	Vioxx (COX-2 inhibitor)

NOTE: Xydis is a technology consisting of a freeze-dried wafer that dissolves almost instantly on the tongue or contact with saliva. The name of the technology has been confused because it is written on prescriptions as if it were a drug name.

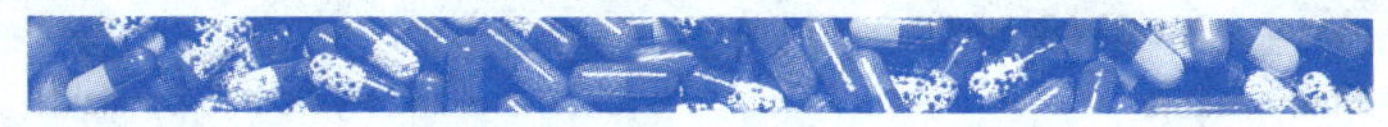

Drugs Archived on the Web

The drugs listed here were removed from the PDR® Nurse's Drug Handbook™ to make room for new drugs. The monograph for each of the drugs listed can be found in its entirety on the World Wide Web at www.nursespdr.com

Acetohexamide

Albendazole

Alglucerase

Aminophylline

Amitriptyline and Perphenazine

Amlodipine and Benazepril hydrochloride

Auranofin

Aurothioglucose suspension

Benzonatate

Bisoprolol fumarate and Hydrochlorothiazide

Buclizine hydrochloride

Butalbital and Acetaminophen

Carprofen

Cefmetazole sodium

Cefonicid sodium

Codeine phosphate and Guaifenesin

Cyclizine hydrochloride

Darvocet-N50 and Darvocet-N100

Darvon compound 65

Dextrothyroxine sodium

Diclofenac sodium and Misoprostol

Diethylpropion hydrochloride

Diethylstilbestrol diphosphate

Digitoxin

Donnatal capsules, elixir, tablets

Dorzolamide hydrochloride/Timolol maleate

Econazole nitrate

Eflornithine hydrochloride

Empirin with Codeine

Equagesic

Etretinate

Fiorinal

Gallium nitrate

Gold sodium thiomalate

Gonadorelin acetate

Hyaluronidase

Hycodan syrup and tablets

Hydroxychloroquine sulfate

Imiglucerase

Ipratropium bromide/Albuterol

sulfate

Levocarnitine

Librax

Lisinopril and Hydrochlorothiazide

Loratidine and Pseudoephedrine sulfate

Losartan potassium and Hydrochlorothiazide

Maprotiline hydrochloride

Mecamylamine hydrochloride

Methimazole

Methyldopa and Hydrochlorothiazide

Microfibrillar Collagen Hemostat

Oxamniquine

Oxycodone and Aspirin

Pediazole

Pentazocine hydrochloride/Naloxone hydrochloride

Pentobarbital

Percoset

Phenaphen-650 with Codeine Tablets

Phendimetrazine tartrate

Phenergan VC with Codeine Syrup

Phenergan with Codeine Syrup

Phenergan with Dextromethorphan Syrup

Phenoxybenzamine hydrochloride

Phosphorated carbohydrate solution

Pilocarpine and Epinephrine

Procyclidine hydrochloride

Propiomazine hydrochloride

Propranolol and Hydrochlorothiazide

Protriptyline hydrochloride

Quazepam

Riboflavin

Rifampin, Isoniazid and Pyrazinamide

Secobarbital Sodium

Selegiline hydrochloride

Soma Compound

Spironolactone and Hydrochlorothiazide

Streptomycin sulfate

Strontium-89 chloride

Sulconazole nitrate

Thyrotropin

Triamterene and Hydrochlorothiazide capsules

Tylenol with Codeine elixir or tablets

Tylox

Uracil Mustard

Urofollitropin for injection

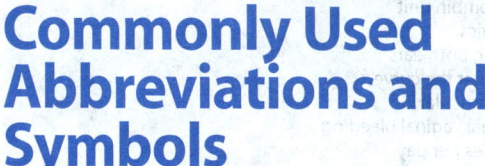

Commonly Used Abbreviations and Symbols

aa, A	of each
ABG	arterial blood gas
a.c.	before meals
ACE	angiotensin-converting enzyme
ACLS	advanced cardiac life support
ACS	acute coronary syndrome
ACTH	adrenocorticotropic hormone
ad	to, up to
a.d.	right ear
ADA	adenosine deaminase
ADD	attention deficit disorder
ADH	antidiuretic hormone
ADHD	attention deficit hyperactivity disorder
ADL	activities of daily living
ad lib	as desired, at pleasure
ADP	adenosine diphosphate
AF	atrial fibrillation
AFB	acid fast bacillus
AHF	antihemophilic factor
AIDS	acquired immune deficiency syndrome
a.l.	left ear
ALL	acute lymphocytic leukemia
ALS	amyotrophic lateral sclerosis
ALT	alanine aminotransferase
a.m., A.M.	morning
AMI	acute myocardial infarction
AML	acute myelogenous leukemia
AMP	adenosine monophosphate
ANA	antinuclear antibody
ANC	absolute neutrophil count
ANS	autonomic nervous system
APL	acute promyelocytic leukemia
APTT	activated partial thromboplastin time
aq	water
aq dist.	distilled water
ARBS	angiotensin receptor blockade agents
ARC	AIDS-related complex
ARDS	adult respiratory distress syndrome
ASA	aspirin (acetylsalicylic acid)
ASAP	as soon as possible
ASHD	arteriosclerotic heart disease
AST	aspartate aminotransferase
ATC	around the clock
ATP	adenosine triphosphate

ATS/CDC	American Thoracic Society/Centers for Disease Prevention and Control
ATU	antithrombin unit
ATX	antibiotics
a.u.	each ear, both ears
AUC	area under the curve
AV	atrioventricular
AVB	abnormal vaginal bleeding
b.i.d.	two times per day
b.i.n.	two times per night
BMR	basal metabolic rate
BP	blood pressure
BPD	bronchopulmonary dysplasia
BPH	benign prostatic hypertrophy
BK	below the knee
bpm	beats per minute
BS	blood sugar, bowel sounds
BSA	body surface area
BSE	breast self-exam
BSP	Bromsulphalein
BUN	blood urea nitrogen
C	Celsius/Centigrade
CABG	coronary artery bypass graft
C&DB	cough and deep breathe
CAD	coronary artery disease pneumonia
CAP	community-acquired
caps, Caps	capsule(s)
CBC	complete blood count
CCB	calcium channel blocker
CCR	creatinine clearance
CD4	helper T4 lymphocyte cells
CDC	Centers for Disease Control and Prevention
C&DB	cough and deep breathe
CF	cystic fibrosis
CFU	colony forming units
CHB	complete heart block
CHF	congestive heart failure
CHO	carbohydrate
CIS	carcinoma *in situ*
CJD	Creutzfeldt-Jakob disease
CLL	chronic lymphocytic leukemia
CLS	capillary leak syndrome
cm	centimeter
CML	chronic myelocytic leukemia
CMV	cytomegalovirus
CN	cranial nerve
CNS	central nervous system
CO	cardiac output
COMT	catechol-o-methyltransferase
COPD	chronic obstructive pulmonary disease
CP	cardiopulmonary
CPAP	continuous positive airway pressure
CPB	cardiopulmonary bypass
CPK	creatine phosphokinase
CPR	cardiopulmonary resuscitation
CRF	chronic renal failure

C&S	culture and sensitivity
CSF	cerebrospinal fluid
CSID	congenital sucrase-isomaltase deficiency
CT	computerized tomography
CTS	carpal tunnel syndrome
CTZ	chemoreceptor trigger zone
CV	cardiovascular
CVA	cerebrovascular accident
CVD	cardiovascular disease
CVP	central venous pressure
CXR	chest X ray
dATP	deoxyadenosine triphosphate
DBP	diastolic BP
dc	discontinue
ddATP	dideoxyadenosine triphosphate
DEA	Drug Enforcement Agency
DI	diabetes insipidus
DIC	disseminated intravascular coagulation
dil.	dilute
dL	deciliter (one-tenth of a liter)
DM	diabetes mellitus
DMARD	disease-modifying antirheumatic drug
DNA	deoxyribonucleic acid
DOE	dyspnea on exertion
DPT	diphtheria, pertussis, tetanus
dr.	dram (0.0625 ounce)
DTR	deep tendon reflex
DVT	deep vein thrombosis
EC	enteric-coated
ECB	extracorporeal cardiopulmonary bypass
ECG, EKG	electrocardiogram, electrocardiograph
EDTA	ethylenediaminetetraacetic acid
EEG	electroencephalogram
EENT	eye, ear, nose, and throat
Ef	ejection fraction
e.g.	for example
elix	elixir
emuls.	emulsion
ENL	erythema nodosum leprosum
ENT	ear, nose, throat
EPS	electrophysiologic studies, extrapyramidal symptoms
ER	extended release
ESR	erythrocyte sedimentation rate
ESRD	end-stage renal disease
ET	endotracheal
ET-1	Endothelin-1 (neurohormone)
ETOH	alcohol
ext.	extract
F	Fahrenheit, fluoride
FBS	fasting blood sugar
FDA	Food and Drug Administration
FEV	forced expiratory volume
FFP	fresh frozen plasma
FOB	fecal occult blood
FS	finger stick
FSH	follicle-stimulating hormone

F/U	follow-up
FVC	forced vital capacity
fx	fracture
g, gm	gram (1,000 mg)
GABA	gamma-aminobutyric acid
G-CSF	granulocyte colony-stimulating factor
GERD	gastroesophageal reflux disease
GFR	glomerular filtration rate
GGT	gamma-glutamyl transferase: syn. gamma-glutamyl transpeptidase
GH	growth hormone
gi, GI	gastrointestinal
GnRH	gonadotropin-releasing hormone
GP	glycoprotein
G6PD	glucose-6-phosphate dehydrogenase
gr	grain
gtt	a drop, drops
GU	genitourinary
h, hr	hour
HA, HAL	hyperalimentation
HbAlc	hemoglobin A1c
HCG	human chorionic gonadotropin
HCP	health-care provider
HCV	hepatitis C virus
HDL	high density lipoprotein
HFN	high flow nebulizer
Hg	mercury
H&H	hematocrit and hemoglobin
HIT	heparin-induced thrombocytopenia
HIV	human immunodeficiency virus
HMG-CoA	3-hydroxy-3-methyl-glutaryl-coenzyme A
HOB	head of bed
HR	heart rate
h.s.	at bedtime
HSE	herpes simplex encephalitis
HSV	herpes simplex virus
ht	height
5-HT	5-hydroxytryptamine
HTN	hypertension
IA	intra-arterial
IBD	inflammatory bowel disease
IBW	ideal body weight
ICP	intracranial pressure
ICU	intensive care unit
IDDM	insulin dependent diabetes mellitus
Ig	immunoglobulin
im, IM	intramuscular
IMV	intermittent mandatory ventilation
inh	inhalation
INR	international normalized ratio
I&O	intake and output
IOP	intraocular pressure
IPPB	intermittent positive pressure breathing
ITP	idiopathic thrombocytopenia purpura
IU	international units
IUNL	institutional upper limit of normal

iv, IV	intravenous
IVPB	IV piggyback, a secondary IV line
JVD	jugular venous distention
kg	kilogram (2.2 lb)
KIU	kallikrein inhibitor units
KVO	keep vein open
l, L	liter (1,000 mL)
L	left
lb	pound
LDH	lactic dehydrogenase
LDL	low density lipoprotein
LFTs	liver function tests
LH	luteinizing hormone
LHRH	luteinizing hormone-releasing hormone
LOC	level of consciousness
LV	left ventricular
LVEF	left ventricular ejection fraction
LVFP	left ventricular function pressure
M	mix
m2, M2	square meter
m	meter
MAC	Mycobacterium avium complex
MAO	monoamine oxidase
MAP	mean arterial pressure
max	maximum
mcg	microgram
MCH	mean corpuscular hemoglobin
mCi	millicurie
mcL	microliter
mcm	micrometer
MDI	metered-dose inhaler
mEq	milliequivalent
mg	milligram
MI	myocardial infarction
MIC	minimum inhibitory concentration
min	minute, minim
mist, mixt	mixture
mL	milliliter
mm3	cubic millimeter
MRI	magnetic resonance imaging
MS	multiple sclerosis
MU	million units
MUGA	multigated radionuclide angiography
NaCl	sodium chloride
ng	nanogram
NG	nasogastric
NGT	nasogastric tube
NIDDM	non-insulin dependent diabetes mellitus
NKA	no known allergies
NKDA	no known drug allergies
noct	at night, during the night
non rep	do not repeat
NPN	nonprotein nitrogen
NPO	nothing by mouth
NR	do not refill (e.g., a prescription)
NSAID	nonsteroidal anti-inflammatory drug

NSR	normal sinus rhythm
NSS	normal saline solution
NYHA	New York Heart Association
N&V	nausea and vomiting
O2	oxygen
OC	oral contraceptive
o.d.	once a day
O.D.	right eye
OH	orthostatic hypotension
OOB	out of bed
OR	operating room
os	mouth
O.S.	left eye
O2 sat	oxygen saturation
OTC	over the counter
O.U.	each eye, both eyes
oz	ounce
PA	pulmonary artery
PABA	para-aminobenzoic acid
PAC	premature atrial contraction
PAF	paroxysmal atrial fibrillation
PAS	amino salicylate
PAWP	pulmonary artery wedge pressure
PBI	protein-bound iodine
p.c.	after meals
PCA	patient-controlled analgesia
PCI	percutaneous coronary intervention
PCN	penicillin
PCP	Pneumocystis carinii pneumonia
PCWP	pulmonary capillary wedge pressure
PDE	phosphodiesterase
PE	pulmonary embolus
PEEP	positive end expiratory pressure
per	by, through
PFTs	pulmonary function tests
pH	hydrogen ion concentration
PID	pelvic inflammatory disease
PMH	past medical history
PMI	point of maximal intensity
PMS	premenstrual syndrome
PND	paroxysmal nocturnal dyspnea
po, p.o., PO	by mouth
PPAR	peroxisome proliferator-activated receptor
PPD	purified protein derivative
PR	by rectum
p.r.n., PRN	when needed or necessary
PSA	prostatic specific antigen
PSP	phenolsulfonphthalein
PSVT	paroxysmal supraventricular tachycardia
PT	prothrombin time
PTCA	percutaneous transluminal coronary angioplasty
PTH	parathyroid hormone
PTSD	post traumatic stress disorder
PTT	partial thromboplastin time
PUD	peptic ulcer disease
PUVA	psoralen and ulraviolet A

PVC	premature ventricular contraction; polyvinyl chloride
PVD	peripheral vascular disease
PVR	peripheral vascular resistance
q.d.	every day
q.h.	every hour
q2hr	every two hours
q3hr	every three hours
q4hr	every four hours
q6hr	every six hours
q8hr	every eight hours
qhs	every night
q.i.d.	four times a day
qmo	every month
q.o.d.	every other day
q.s.	as much as needed, quantity sufficient
RA	right atrium; rheumatoid arthritis
RBC	red blood cell
RDA	recommended daily allowance
RDS	respiratory distress syndrome
REM	rapid eye movement
Rept.	let it be repeated
RICE	rest, ice, compression and elevation
RNA	ribonucleic acid
R/O	rule out
ROM	range of motion
ROS	review of systems
RRMS	relapsing-remitting multiple sclerosis
R/T	related to
RV	right ventricular
RUQ	right upper quadrant
Rx	symbol for a prescription
SA	sinoatrial; sustained-action
SAH	subarachnoid hemorrhage
SBE	subacute bacterial endocarditis
SBP	systolic BP
sc, SC, SQ	subcutaneous
SCID	severe combined immunodeficiency disease
SGOT	serum glutamic-oxaloacetic transaminase
SGPT	serum glutamic-pyruvic transaminase
S., Sig.	mark on the label
SI	sacroiliac
SIADH	syndrome inappropriate antidiuretic hormone
SIMV	synchronized intermittent mandatory ventilation
SL	sublingual
SLE	systemic lupus erythematosus
SOB	shortness of breath
sol	solution
sp	spirits
SR	sustained-release
ss	one-half
SSRI	selective serotonin reuptake inhibitor
SSS	sick sinus syndrome
S&S	signs and symptoms
stat	immediately, first dose
STD	sexually transmitted disease
SV	stroke volume

SVT	supraventricular tachycardia
syr	syrup
sz	seizure
t1/2	halflife
tab	tablet
TB	tuberculosis
TCA	tricyclic antidepressant
TENS	transcutaneous electric nerve stimulation
THR	total hip replacement
TIA	transient ischemic attack
TIBC	total iron binding capacity
t.i.d.	three times per day
t.i.n.	three times per night
TKR	total knee replacement
TNF	tumor necrosis factor
T.O.	telephone order
TPN	total parenteral nutrition
TSH	thyroid stimulating hormone
TUR	transurethral resection
TURP	transurethral resection of the prostate
μ	micron
μCi	microcurie
μg	microgram
μL	microliter
μm	micrometer
U	unit
U/A	urinalysis
UGI	upper gastrointestinal
ULN	upper limit of normal
ung	ointment
UO	urine output
URI, URTI	upper respiratory infection
US	ultrasound
USP	U. S. Pharmacopeia
ut dict	as directed
UTI	urinary tract infection
UV	ultraviolet
UVB	ultraviolet B (portion of ultraviolet radiation spectrum)
VAD	venous access device
VF	ventricular fibrillation
vin	wine
vit	vitamin
VLDL	very low density lipoprotein
VMA	vanillylmandelic acid
V.O.	verbal order
VS	vital signs
VT	ventricular tachycardia
WBC	white blood cell
WHO	World Health Organization
wt	weight
XRT	radiation therapy
&	and
>	greater than
<	less than
≠	increased, higher

Ø	decreased, lower
-	negative, minus
/	per
%	percent
+	positive, plus
x	times, frequency

chapter 1

Therapeutic Drug Classifications

ALKYLATING AGENTS

SEE ALSO THE FOLLOWING INDIVIDUAL ENTRIES:

Busulfan
Carboplatin for Injection
Carmustine
Chlorambucil
Cisplatin
Cyclophosphamide
Dacarbazine
Ifosfamide
Lomustine
Mechlorethamine hydrochloride
Melphalan
Mesna
Streptozocin
Thiotepa

ACTION/KINETICS

Alkylating agents donate an alkyl group (carbonium ion) to biologically important macromolecules, such as DNA. The molecule is inactivated bringing *cell division* to a halt. This cytotoxic activity affects replication of cancerous cells and other cells, especially in rapidly proliferating tissues, such as the bone marrow, intestinal epithelium, and hair follicles. The toxic effects are usually cell-cycle nonspecific and become apparent when the cell enters the S phase and cell division is blocked at the G_2 phase (premitotic phase), resulting in cells having a double complement of DNA.

Resistance of cancer cells to alkylating agents usually develops slowly and gradually. Resistance seems to be the sum total of several minor adaptations, including decreased permeability of the cells, increased production of noncancer receptors (nucleophilic substances), and increased efficiency of the DNA repair system.

NURSING CONSIDERATIONS

SEE *NURSING CONSIDERATIONS* FOR INDIVIDUAL AGENTS AND *ANTINEOPLASTIC AGENTS.*

ASSESSMENT

1. Note indications for therapy; ensure that client is well hydrated and restrict dosage within 4 weeks after full XRT or chemotherapy to prevent critical bone marrow depression.
2. Schedule lab work to assess hematopoietic function weekly during therapy.
3. Review list of side effects and identify ways to cope, i.e. N&V, loss of appetite; small frequent meals, dividing dose, and consuming 10-12 glasses of fluid per day. Infertility; have eggs/sperm harvested prior to therapy. Birth defects; practice reliable contraception.
4. Advise to report any unusual bleeding/bruising, fever, chills, sore throat, cough, sob, yellowing of skin/eyes, flank or stomach pain, or changes in bladder/bowel function.

OUTCOMES/EVALUATE

Clinical/radiographic evidence of tumor regression and disease stabilization

ALPHA-1-ADRENERGIC BLOCKING AGENTS

SEE ALSO THE FOLLOWING INDIVIDUAL ENTRIES:

Doxazosin mesylate
Prazosin hydrochloride
Tamsulosin hydrochloride
Terazosin

ACTION/KINETICS

Selectively block postsynaptic alpha-1-adrenergic receptors. Results in dilation of both arterioles and veins leading to a decrease in supine and standing BP. Diastolic BP is affected the most. Prazosin and terazosin do not produce reflex tachycardia. Terazosin also relaxes smooth muscle in the bladder neck and prostate, making it useful to treat BPH. Have many undesirable effects which, although not toxic, limit their use. Always start treatment at low doses and increase gradually.

USES

Alone or in combination with diuretics or beta-adrenergic blocking agents to treat hypertension. Doxazocin and terazosin are used to treat BPH. *Investigational:* Prazosin is used for refractory CHF, management of Raynaud's vasospasm, and to treat BPH. Doxazosin, along with digoxin and diuretics, is used to treat CHF.

CONTRAINDICATIONS

Hypersensitivity to these drugs (i.e., quinazolines).

SPECIAL CONCERNS

The first few doses may cause postural hypotension and syncope with sudden loss of consciousness. Use with caution in lactation, with impaired hepatic function, or if receiving drugs known to influence hepatic metabolism. Safety and efficacy have not been established in children.

SIDE EFFECTS

The following side effects are common to alpha-1-adrenergic blockers. See individual drugs as well.

CV: Palpitations, postural hypotension, hypotension, tachycardia, chest pain, arrhythmia. **GI:** N&V, dry mouth, diarrhea, constipation, abdominal discomfort or pain, flatulence. **CNS:** Dizziness, depression, decreased libido, sexual dysfunction, nervousness, paresthesia, somnolence, anxiety, insomnia, asthenia, drowsiness. **Musculoskeletal:** Pain in the shoulder, neck, or back; gout, arthritis, joint pain, arthralgia. **Respiratory:** Dyspnea, nasal congestion, sinusitis, bronchitis, ***bronchospasm,*** cold symptoms, epistaxis, increased cough, flu symptoms, pharyngitis, rhinitis. **Ophthalmic:** Blurred vision, abnormal vision, reddened sclera, conjunctivitis. **GU:** Impotence, urinary frequency, incontinence. **Miscellaneous:** Tinnitus, vertigo, pruritus, sweating, alopecia, lichen planus, headache, edema, weight gain, facial edema, fever.

OD OVERDOSE MANAGEMENT

Symptoms: Extension of the side effects, especially on BP. *Treatment:* Keep supine to restore BP and normalize heart rate. Shock may be treated with volume expanders or vasopressors; support renal function.

DRUG INTERACTIONS

Alpha-1 blockers ↓ the antihypertensive effect of clonidine.

LABORATORY TEST CONSIDERATIONS

↑ Urinary VMA.

DOSAGE

See individual agents.

NURSING CONSIDERATIONS

ADMINISTRATION/STORAGE

Take the first dose of prazosin and terazosin at bedtime to prevent dizziness.

ASSESSMENT

1. Note any history of PUD; drug should be used cautiously.
2. Document indications for therapy, onset, and characteristics of symptoms.
3. Monitor electrolytes, ECG, and VS. Base titration on standing BP due to postural effects.
4. Assess for heart or lung disease and note currently prescribed therapy. Some agents may cause vasospasm with Prinzmetal or vasospastic angina.

5. Use cautiously in older clients due to possibility of orthostatic hypotension. They may tolerate a slower, more gradual increase in dosage (i.e., terazosin 1 mg/day for 7 days followed by 2 mg/day for 7 days, etc., until desired response).

CLIENT/FAMILY TEACHING

1. May take with milk or meals to minimize GI upset.
2. Take first dose at bedtime to minimize syncope and hypotensive effects. Do not drive or undertake hazardous tasks for 12–24 hr after the first dose and after increasing dose or following an interruption of dosage.
3. Avoid symptoms of orthostatic hypotension by rising slowly from a sitting or lying position and waiting until symptoms subside.
4. Keep record of BP and weight. Report any weight gain or ankle swelling; without a diuretic, one may experience retention of salt and water due to vasodilation.
5. Dizziness, lassitude, headache, and palpitations may occur as well as transient apprehension, fear, anxiety, and/or palpitations. Report if persistent so dosage may be adjusted.
6. Report for yearly DRE and PSA to ensure lesion free.
7. Review life-style changes needed for BP control; i.e., dietary restrictions of fat and sodium; weight reduction; regular physical exercise; decreased use of alcohol; stress reduction; and smoking cessation. For BPH control: no fluid intake 4 hr before bedtime, empty bladder before going to sleep; avoid caffeine and alcohol in the evening, and if no improvement report to provider.
8. Avoid excess caffeine and OTC agents (especially cold remedies).
9. Do not stop abruptly. Will have to retitrate up to effective dose if stopped.

OUTCOMES/EVALUATE

- ↓ BP
- ↓ Nocturia, urgency/frequency

SEE ALSO *BETA-ADRENERGIC BLOCKING AGENTS*.

AMINOGLYCOSIDES

SEE ALSO THE FOLLOWING INDIVIDUAL ENTRIES:

Amikacin sulfate
Gentamicin sulfate
Kanamycin sulfate
Neomycin sulfate
Paromomycin sulfate
Tobramycin sulfate

ACTION/KINETICS

Broad-spectrum antibiotics believed to inhibit protein synthesis by binding irreversibly to ribosomes (30S subunit), thereby interfering with an initiation complex between messenger RNA and the 30S subunit. This leads to production of nonfunctional proteins; polyribosomes are split apart and are unable to synthesize protein. Usually bactericidal due to disruption of the bacterial cytoplasmic membrane. Poorly absorbed from the GI tract; usually administered parenterally (exceptions: some enteric infections of the GI tract and prior to surgery). Also absorbed from the peritoneum, bronchial tree, wounds, denuded skin, and joints. Distributed in the extracellular fluid and cross the placental barrier, but not the blood-brain barrier. Penetration of the CSF is increased when the meninges are inflamed.

Rapidly absorbed after IM injection. **Peak plasma levels, after IM:** Usually ½–2 hr. Measurable levels persist for 8–12 hr after a single administration. **t½:** 2–3 hr (increases sharply in impaired kidney function). Ranges of t½ from 24 to 110 hr have been observed. Excreted mainly unchanged in urine. Resistance develops slowly.

USES

Are powerful antibiotics that induce serious side effects—**do not use for minor infections**. Gram-negative bacteria causing bone and joint infections, septicemia (including neonatal sepsis), skin and soft tissue infections (including those from burns), respiratory tract infections, postoperative infections, intra-abdominal infections (including peritonitis), UTIs. In combination with clindamycin for mixed aerobic-anaerobic infections. Also, see individual drugs.

Used for gram-positive bacteria only when other less toxic drugs are either ineffective or contraindicated. Use in CNS *Pseudomonas* infections such as meningitis or ventriculitis is questionable.

CONTRAINDICATIONS

Hypersensitivity to aminoglycosides, long-term therapy (except streptomycin for tuberculosis).

SPECIAL CONCERNS

Use with extreme caution with impaired renal function or preexisting hearing impairment. Safe use in pregnancy and during lactation not established. Assess premature infants, neonates, and older clients closely; they are particularly sensitive to toxic effects. Considerable cross-allergenicity occurs among the aminoglycosides.

SIDE EFFECTS

Ototoxicity: Both auditory and vestibular damage have been noted. The risk is increased with poor renal function and in the elderly. Auditory symptoms include tinnitus and hearing impairment, while vestibular symptoms include dizziness, nystagmus, vertigo, and ataxia. **Renal Impairment:** May be characterized by cylindruria, oliguria, proteinuria, azotemia, hematuria, increase or decrease in frequency of urination; in-creased BUN, NPN, or creatinine; and increased thirst. **Neurotoxicity:** Neuromuscular blockade, headache, tremor, lethargy, paresthesia, peripheral neuritis (numbness, tingling, or burning of face/mouth), arachnoiditis, encephalopathy, acute OBS. CNS depression, characterized by stupor, flaccidity, and rarely, ***coma, and respiratory depression in infants.*** Optic neuritis with blurred vision or loss of vision. **GI:** N&V, diarrhea, increased salivation, anorexia, weight loss. **Allergic:** Rash, urticaria, pruritus, burning, fever, stomatitis, eosinophilia. Rarely, ***agranulocytosis and anaphylaxis.*** Cross-allergy among aminoglycosides has been observed. **Miscellaneous:** Joint pain, ***laryngeal edema, pulmonary fibrosis,*** superinfection.

OD OVERDOSE MANAGEMENT

Symptoms: Extension of side effects. *Treatment:* Undertake hemodialysis (preferred) or peritoneal dialysis.

DRUG INTERACTIONS

Bumetanide / ↑ Risk of ototoxicity
Capreomycin / ↑ Muscle relaxation
Cephalosporins / ↑ Risk of renal toxicity
Ciprofloxacin HCl / Additive antibacterial activity
Cisplatin / Additive renal toxicity
Colistimethate / ↑ Muscle relaxation
Digoxin / Possible ↑ or ↓ effect
Ethacrynic acid / ↑ Risk of ototoxicity
Furosemide / ↑ Risk of ototoxicity
Methoxyflurane / ↑ Risk of renal toxicity
Penicillins / ↓ Effect of aminoglycosides
Polymyxins / ↑ Muscle relaxation
Skeletal muscle relaxants (surgical) / ↑ Muscle relaxation
Vancomycin / Additive ototoxicity and renal toxicity
Vitamin A / ↓ Effect R/T ↓ absorption from GI tract

LABORATORY TEST CONSIDERATIONS

↑ BUN, BSP retention, creatinine, AST, ALT, bilirubin. ↓ Cholesterol values.

NURSING CONSIDERATIONS

SEE ALSO *GENERAL NURSING CONSIDERATIONS* FOR *ALL ANTI-INFECTIVES.*

ADMINISTRATION/STORAGE

1. Check expiration date.
2. Warn if drug being administered stings or causes a burning sensation.
3. During IM administration
• Inject deep into muscle mass to minimize transient pain.
• Use a Z track method for thin, elderly clients.
• Rotate/document injection sites.

IV 4. With IV administration
• Dilute with compatible solution.
• Infuse at the rate ordered to prevent excessive serum concentrations.

5. Administer for only 7–10 days. Avoid repeating course of therapy unless serious infection present that doesn't respond to other antibiotics.
6. Administer ATC to maintain therapeutic drug levels.

ASSESSMENT

1. Assess for allergic reactions; note any knowledge/history of sensitivity to anti-infectives.
2. Weigh/calculate BMI to ensure correct dosage.
3. Determine baseline liver, renal, auditory, and vestibular function; assess for nephrotoxicity. Obtain C&S prior to therapy.
4. Assess for presence and source(s) of infection. Document fever, culture/lab reports, and wound characteristics (i.e., color, odor, drainage, temperature).

INTERVENTIONS

1. Monitor VS and I&O; increase fluids to prevent renal tubule irritation.
2. Monitor drug levels; (e.g., Amikacin levels > 30 mcg/mL are considered toxic.)
3. With vestibular dysfunction protect by supervised ambulation and side rails; note (potential for) fall hazard.
4. Assess for ototoxicity with pretreatment audiograms. Hearing loss is a dose-related side effect of drug therapy most commonly associated with amikacin, kanamycin, neomycin, or paromomycin. Tinnitus, dizziness, and loss of balance are also signs of vestibular injury and more commonly seen with gentamicin and streptomycin. Deafness may occur several weeks after discontinuing drug.
5. Do not administer concurrently or sequentially with a topical or systemic nephrotoxic or ototoxic drug (e.g., potent diuretics such as ethacrynic acid or furosemide) unless provider designates benefits outweigh risks.
6. Observe for neuromuscular blockade with muscular weakness leading to apnea, when administered with a muscle relaxant or after anesthesia. Have calcium gluconate or neostigmine available to reverse blockade.
7. Note cells or casts in the urine, oliguria, proteinuria, lowered specific gravity, increasing BUN/creatinine, all of which indicate altered renal function.

CLIENT/FAMILY TEACHING

1. Review goals of therapy and prescribed method of administration.
2. Take as prescribed, ATC, until prescription is completed.
3. Follow a well-balanced diet and consume at least 2–3 L/day of fluids. If N&V or loss of appetite, try small frequent meals and frequent mouth care.
4. Report symptoms of superinfection (black, furry tongue; loose, foul-smelling stools; vaginal itching) or other adverse effects.
5. Report alterations in hearing, vision, and/or ambulation. Use safety measures to prevent injury. Note lack of response after 3 days of therapy.

OUTCOMES/EVALUATE

- Negative culture reports
- Resolution of infection with ↓ WBCs, ↓ fever, ↓ drainage; symptomatic improvement

AMPHETAMINES AND DERIVATIVES

SEE ALSO THE FOLLOWING INDIVIDUAL ENTRIES:

Amphetamine sulfate
Dexmenthylphenidate
Dextroamphetamine sulfate
Phenylpropanolamine hydrochloride (OTC products removed from market)

ACTION/KINETICS

Thought to act on the cerebral cortex and reticular activating system (including the medullary, respiratory, and vasomotor centers) by releasing norepinephrine from central adrenergic neurons. High doses cause release of dopamine from the mesolimbic system. The stimulatory effect on the CNS causes an increase in motor activity and mental alertness, a mood-elevating effect, a slight euphoric effect, and an anorexigenic effect. The anorexigenic effect is thought to be produced by direct stimulation of the satiety center in the lateral hypothalamic feeding center of the brain. Peripheral effects are mediated by alpha- and beta-adrenergic receptors and include increases in both systolic and diastolic BP and respiratory stimulation. Readily absorbed from the GI tract and distributed throughout most tissues, with the highest concentrations in the brain and CSF. Duration of anorexia (PO): 3–6 hr. Metabolized in liver and excreted by kidneys. Excreted slowly (5–7 days); cumulative effects may occur with continued administration.

Psychic stimulation is often followed by a rebound effect manifested as fatigue. Tolerance will develop to all drugs of this class. There is a relatively wide margin of safety between the therapeutic and toxic doses of amphetamines. However, both acute and chronic toxicity can occur.

USES

See individual drugs.

CONTRAINDICATIONS

Hyperthyroidism, advanced arteriosclerosis, nephritis, diabetes mellitus, hypertension, narrow-angle glaucoma, angina pectoris, CV disease, and individuals with hypersensitivity to these drugs. Use in emotionally unstable persons susceptible to drug abuse and in agitated states. Psychotic children. Lactation. Appetite suppressants in children less than 12 years of age. Within 14 days of MAO inhibitors.

SPECIAL CONCERNS

Use with caution in clients suffering from hyperexcitability states; in elderly, debilitated, or asthenic clients; and in clients with psychopathic personality traits or a history of homicidal or suicidal tendencies.

SIDE EFFECTS

CNS: Nervousness, dizziness, depression, headache, insomnia, euphoria, symptoms of excitation. Rarely, psychoses. In children, manifestation of vocal and motor tics and Tourette's syndrome. **GI:** N&V, cramps, diarrhea, dry mouth, constipation, metallic taste, anorexia. **CV:** Arrhythmias, palpitations, dyspnea, pulmonary hypertension, peripheral hyper- or hypotension, precordial pain, fainting. **Dermatologic:** Symptoms of allergy including rash, urticaria, erythema, burning. Pallor. **GU:** Urinary frequency, dysuria. **Ophthalmologic:** Blurred vision, mydriasis. **Hematologic:** ***Agranulocytosis,*** leukopenia. **Endocrine:** Menstrual irregularities, gynecomastia, impotence, and changes in libido. **Miscellaneous:** Alopecia, increased motor activity, fever, sweating, chills, muscle pain, chest pain. Long-term use results in psychic dependence, as well as a high degree of tolerance.

OD OVERDOSE MANAGEMENT

Symptoms of Acute Overdose (Toxicity): Restlessness, irritability, insomnia, tremor, hyperreflexia, rhabdomyolysis, rapid respiration, ***hyperpyrexia,*** assaultiveness, hallucinations, panic states, sweating, mydriasis, flushing, hyperactivity, confusion, hypertension or hypotension, extrasystoles, tachypnea, fever, delirium, self-injury, arrhythmias, ***seizures, coma, circulatory collapse, death. Death usually results from CV collapse or convulsions.*** *Symptoms of Chronic Toxicity:* Chronic use/abuse is characterized by emotional lability, loss of appetite, severe dermatoses, hyperactivity, insomnia, irritability, somnolence, mental impairment, occupational deterioration, a tendency to withdraw from social contact, teeth grinding, continuous chewing, and ulcers of the tongue and lips. Prolonged use of high doses can elicit symptoms of paranoid schizophrenia, including auditory and visual hallucinations and paranoid ideation.

Treatment of Acute Toxicity (Overdosage):

• Symptomatic treatment. After oral ingestion, induce emesis or perform gastric lavage, followed by use of activated charcoal. Acidification of the urine increases the rate of excretion. Give fluids until urine flow is 3–6 mL/kg/hr; furosemide or mannitol may be beneficial.

• Maintain adequate circulation and respiration.

• Treat CNS stimulation with chlorpromazine and psychotic symptoms with haloperidol. Treat hyperactivity with diazepam or a barbiturate. Reduce stimuli and maintain in a quiet, dim environment. Treat clients who have ingested an overdose of long-acting products for toxicity until all symptoms of overdosage have disappeared.

• IV phentolamine may be used for hypertension, whereas hypotension may be reversed by IV fluids and possibly vasopressors (used with caution).

DRUG INTERACTIONS

Acetazolamide / ↑ Effect of amphetamine by ↑ renal tubular reabsorption
Ammonium chloride / ↓ Effect of amphetamine by ↓ renal tubular reabsorption
Anesthetics, general / ↑ Risk of cardiac arrhythmias
Antihypertensives / ↓ Effect
Ascorbic acid / ↓ Effect of amphetamine by ↓ renal tubular reabsorption
Furazolidone / ↑ Toxicity of anorexiants due to MAO activity of furazolidone
Guanethidine / ↓ Effect by displacement from its site of action
Haloperidol / ↓ Effect of amphetamine by ↓ uptake of drug at its site of action
Insulin / Altered requirements
MAO inhibitors / All peripheral, metabolic, cardiac, and central effects of amphetamine are potentiated for up to 2 weeks after termination of MAO inhibitor therapy (symptoms include hypertensive crisis with possible intracranial hemorrhage, hyperthermia, convulsions, coma); death may occur. ↓ Effect of amphetamine by ↓ uptake of drug into its site of action
Methyldopa / ↓ Hypotensive effect by ↑ sympathomimetic activity
Phenothiazines / ↓ Effect of amphetamine by ↓ uptake of drug at its site of action
Sodium bicarbonate / ↑ Effect of amphetamine by ↑ renal tubular reabsorption
Thiazide diuretics / ↑ Effect of amphetamine by ↑ renal tubular reabsorption
Tricyclic antidepressants / ↓ Effect of amphetamines

LABORATORY TEST CONSIDERATIONS

↑ BUN and creatinine (both are transient and reversible). ↑ Liver enzymes, serum bilirubin, uric acid, blood glucose. Small ↑ in serum potassium.

DOSAGE

See individual drugs. Many compounds are timed-release preparations.

NURSING CONSIDERATIONS

ADMINISTRATION/STORAGE

1. If prescribed to suppress appetite, administer 30 min before anticipated meal time.
2. Use a small initial dose; then increase gradually as necessary.
3. Unless otherwise ordered, give last dose of day at least 6 hr before bedtime.

ASSESSMENT

1. Identify meds currently taking, indications, and effectiveness.
2. Note physical conditions that would preclude using drugs in this category i.e. ASHD, hyperthyroidism, DM, glaucoma.
3. Note age and if debilitated.
4. Monitor electrolytes, ECG, weight, VS, and CBC.
5. Under the Controlled Substances Act; follow appropriate policy for dispensing/handling to restrict availability and discourage abuse.

INTERVENTIONS

1. If agitated or complains of sleeplessness, reduce dosage of drug.
2. If receiving MAO inhibitors or received them 7–14 days before amphetamine therapy, assess for hyper-

tensive crisis. Monitor and report fever, marked sweating, excitation, delirium, tremors, or twitching; pad side rails and have suction available.
3. Monitor VS. Assess for arrhythmias, tachycardia, or hypertension. CV changes with psychotic syndrome may indicate toxicity.
4. If somnolent or appears mentally or physically impaired, stop the drug. Observe for signs of psychologic dependence and drug tolerance.
5. Monitor heighth to assess for growth inhibition.

CLIENT/FAMILY TEACHING

1. When anorexiants are used for weight reduction, their effect lasts only 4–6 weeks; use is short term. Follow an established dietary and exercise regimen to maintain weight loss and attend a behavioral modification weight control program.
2. Take only as prescribed, 1 hr before meals and last dose 6 hr before bedtime to ensure adequate rest. Abrupt withdrawal may cause adverse symptoms.
3. Diets high in fiber, fruit, and fluids assist to reduce drugs' constipating effects. See dietitian to discuss weight control and/or reducing diets when weight loss is the goal.
4. Record food intake and weight daily the first week and then at least once a week. May become anorexic; report any persistent, severe weight loss so therapy can be adjusted.
5. Report any changes in attention span and ability to concentrate.
6. Take only as directed; do not share meds. Report S&S of tolerance.
7. May cause a false sense of euphoria and well being and mask extreme fatigue. These may impair judgment and ability to perform potentially hazardous tasks, such as operating a machine or an automobile. Using amphetamines to treat fatigue is inappropriate because rebound effects may be severe.
8. Seek medical assistance if experiencing extreme fatigue and depression once drug is discontinued. Periodic "drug holidays" may be ordered to assess progress and prevent dependence.
9. Avoid OTC medications and ingesting large amounts of caffeine in any form. Read labels for the detection of caffeine since this contributes to CV side effects.
10. Manage dry mouth by frequent rinsing, chewing sugarless gum, or sucking sugarless hard candies.
11. Store safely out of child's reach.

OUTCOMES/EVALUATE

- ↑ Attention span/concentration
- Weight reduction
- ↓ Episodes of narcolepsy

ANGIOTENSIN II RECEPTOR ANTAGONISTS

SEE ALSO THE FOLLOWING INDIVDIUAL ENTRIES:

Candesartan cilexetil
Irbesartan
Losartan potassium
Telmisartan
Valsartan

ACTION/KINETICS

Angiotensin II, a potent vasoconstrictor, is the primary vasoactive hormone of the renin-angiotensin system; it is involved in the pathophysiology of hypertension. Angiotensin II increases systemic vascular resistance, causes sodium and water retention, and leads to increased HR and vasoconstriction. The angiotensin II receptor antagonists competitively block the angiotensin AT_1 receptor located in vascular smooth muscle and the adrenal glands, thus blocking the vasoconstrictor and aldosterone-secreting effects of angiotensin II. Thus, BP is reduced. No significant effects on HR with minimal orthostatic hypotension and no significant effect on potassium levels. Do not inhibit angiotensin converting enzyme (ACE).

USES

Alone or in combination with other drugs to treat hypertension. *Investigational:* Treatment of heart failure. Can be combined with ACE inhibitors to reduced morbidity and mortality in clients with moderate to severe CHF.

CONTRAINDICATIONS

Lactation.

DOSAGE

See individual drugs.

NURSING CONSIDERATIONS

ASSESSMENT

1. Document indications for therapy, characteristics of S&S, and other agents trialed.
2. Ensure adequate hydration to prevent severe hypotensive episode.
3. Not for use during pregnancy or lactation.
4. Observe infants exposed to an Angiotension II inhibitor in utero for hypotension, oliguria, fetal defects, and ↑ K.
5. Monitor CBC, lytes and renal function.

CLIENT/FAMILY TEACHING

1. Take only as directed usually once daily. May take with or without food.
2. Advise surgeon that ARB is being taken; blockage of renin-angiotensin system following surgery may cause problems.
3. Avoid activities that may lead to a reduction in fluid volume i.e., excessive perspiration, vomiting, diarrhea, dehydration may all lead to hypotension.
4. Do not skip or double up on medications. Dizziness may occur; avoid activites that require mental alertness until drug effects realized.
5. Continue regular exercise, dietary restrictions, including low salt, tobacco/ETOH cessation and life style changes necessary to ensure lowered BP.
6. Practice reliable contraception. Stop drug and report if pregnancy suspected. Do not nurse while on this drug.
7. Record BP regularly at different times of day for provider review. Continue regular medical followup and lab studies as scheduled; report any unusual side effects. Symptomatic hypotension may occur in those who are intravascularly volume-depleted. Fetal and neonatal morbidity and death are possible if given to pregnant women. Safety and efficacy have not been determined in children less than 18 years of age.

OUTCOMES/EVALUATE

- Control of BP
- Improvement in S&S of CHF

ANGIOTENSIN-CONVERTING ENZYME (ACE) INHIBITORS

SEE ALSO THE FOLLOWING INDIVIDUAL ENTRIES:

Benazepril hydrochloride
Captopril
Enalapril maleate
Fosinopril sodium
Lisinopril
Moexipril hydrochloride
Quinapril hydrochloride
Ramipril
Trandolapril

ACTION/KINETICS

Believed to act by suppressing the renin-angiotensin-aldosterone system. Renin, synthesized by the kidneys, produces angiotensin I, an inactive decapeptide derived from plasma globulin substrate. Angiotensin I is converted to angiotensin II by ACE. Angiotensin II is a potent vasoconstrictor that also stimulates secretion of aldosterone from the adrenal cortex, resulting in sodium and fluid retention. The ACE inhibitors prevent the conversion of angiotensin I to angiotensin II. This results in a decrease in plasma angiotensin II and subsequently a decrease in peripheral resistance and decreased aldosterone secretion (leading to fluid loss) and therefore a decrease in BP. There may be either no change or an increase in CO. Several weeks of therapy may be required to achieve the maximum effect to reduce BP. Standing and supine BPs are lowered to about the same extent. Are also antihypertensive in low renin hypertensive clients. ACE inhibitors are additive with thiazide diuretics in lowering blood pressure; however, β-blockers and captopril have less than additive effects when used with ACE inhibitors.

USES

Alone or in combination with other antihypertensive agents (especially thiazide diuretics) for the treatment of hypertension. Can be used as first-line therapy in hypertensive African Americans with or at risk for renal dysfunction. Some are effective in CHF as adjunctive therapy or to treat LV dysfunction. See also individual drug entries. *Investigational:* Reduce mortality following MI.

CONTRAINDICATIONS

History of angioedema due to previous treatment with an ACE inhibitor. Use of fosinopril, ramipril, or trandolapril in lactation.

SPECIAL CONCERNS

Use during the second and third trimesters of pregnancy can result in injury and even death to the developing fetus. May cause a profound drop in BP following the first dose; initiate therapy under close medical supervision. Use with caution in renal disease (especially renal artery stenosis) as increases in BUN and serum creatinine have occurred. Use with caution in clients with aortic stenosis due to possible decreased coronary perfusion following vasodilator use. Most are used with caution during lactation. Geriatric clients may show a greater sensitivity to the hypotensive effects of ACE inhibitors although these drugs may preserve or improve renal function and reverse LV hypertrophy. For most ACE inhibitors, safety and effectiveness have not been determined in children. Compliance in taking the medication and inadequate dosage is a problem with ACE inhibitors.

SIDE EFFECTS

See individual entries. Side effects common to most ACE inhibitors include the following. **GI:** Abdominal pain, N&V, diarrhea, constipation, dry mouth. **CNS:** Sleep disturbances, insomnia, headache, dizziness, fatigue, nervousness, par-esthesias. **CV:** Hypotension (especially following the first dose), palpitations, angina pectoris, ***MI,*** orthostatic hypotension, chest pain. **Hepatic:** Rarely, cholestatic jaundice progressing to ***hepatic necrosis and death.*** **Miscellaneous:** Chronic cough, dyspnea, increased sweating, diaphoresis, pruritus, rash, impotence, syncope, asthenia, arthralgia, myalgia. ***Angioedema*** of the face, lips, tongue, glottis, larynx, extremities, and mucous membranes. ***Anaphylaxis.***

OD OVERDOSE MANAGEMENT

Symptoms: Hypotension is the most common. *Treatment:* Supportive measures. The treatment of choice to restore BP is volume expansion with an IV infusion of NSS. Certain of the ACE inhibitors (captopril, enalaprilat, lisinopril, trandolaprilat) may be removed by hemodialysis.

DRUG INTERACTIONS

Allopurinol / ↑ Risk of hypersensitivity reactions

Anesthetics / ↑ Risk of hypotension if used with anesthetics that also cause hypotension

Antacids / Possible ↓ bioavailability of ACE inhibitors

Capsaicin / May cause or worsen cough associated with ACE inhibitor use

Digoxin / ↑ Plasma digoxin levels

Indomethacin / ↓ Hypotensive effects of ACE inhibitors, especially in low renin or volume-dependent hypertensive clients

Lithium / ↑ Serum lithium levels → ↑ risk of toxicity

Phenothiazines / ↑ Effect of ACE inhibitors

Potassium-sparing diuretics / ↑ Serum potassium levels

Potassium supplements / ↑ Serum potassium levels

Thiazide diuretics / Additive effect to ↓ BP

LABORATORY TEST CONSIDERATIONS

↑ BUN and creatinine (both are transient and reversible). ↑ Liver enzymes, serum bilirubin, uric acid, blood glucose. Small ↑ in serum potassium.

DOSAGE

See individual drugs.

NURSING CONSIDERATIONS

ADMINISTRATION/STORAGE

Do not interrupt or discontinue ACE inhibitor therapy without consulting provider.

ASSESSMENT

1. Note any previous therapy with ACE inhibitors or antihypertensive agents and the outcome.
2. Monitor VS (BP—both arms while lying, standing, and sitting), electrolytes, CBC, and renal and LFTs; check urine for protein if negative on urinalysis check for microalbuminuria esp. in diabetics.
3. Document hereditary angioedema (especially if caused by a deficiency of C1 esterase inhibitor). Report any evidence of angioedema (swelling of face, lips, extremities, tongue, mucous membranes, glottis, or larynx) esp. after first dose (but may also be delayed response). Relieve S&S with antihistamines. If involves laryngeal edema, observe for airway obstruction. *Stop* drug; use epinephrine (1:1000 SC).
4. Monitor VS, I&O, weight, serum potassium, and renal function studies. Those hypovolemic due to diuretics, GI fluid loss, or salt restriction may exhibit severe hypotension after initial doses; supervise ambulation until drug response evident.
5. Assess for neutropenia (esp. with captopril); precludes drug therapy.
6. If undergoing surgery or general anesthesia with drugs that cause hypotension, ACE inhibitors will block angiotensin II formation; correct hypotension by volume expansion.
7. Document weight, risk factors, and medical problems. Identify lifestyle changes needed to achieve and maintain lowered BP. Assess motivation and ensure that a trial of "good behavior" with dietary modifications and regular exercise for 3–6 months has been done unless BP stage >2.

CLIENT/FAMILY TEACHING

1. Take 1 hr before or 2 hr after meals and only as directed.
2. Review prescribed dietary guidelines; do not use potassium or salt substitutes containing potassium.
3. Medication controls but does not cure hypertension; take as prescribed despite feeling better and do not stop abruptly.
4. Take BP readings at various times during the day and record to prevent treating "white collar" readings.
5. Do not perform activities that require mental alertness until drug effects realized; initially may cause dizziness, fainting, or lightheadedness.
6. Rise slowly from a lying position and dangle feet before standing; avoid sudden position changes to minimize postural effects.
7. Practice birth control; report if pregnancy suspected. Do not nurse on drug therapy.
8. Report adverse side effects:
- Nonproductive, persistent, chronic cough
- Sore throat, fever, swelling of hands or feet, irregular heartbeat, chest pains, difficulty breathing, or hoarseness
- Excessive perspiration, dehydration, vomiting, and diarrhea
- Itching, joint pain, fever, or skin rash

9. Report edema and weight gain of more than 3 lb/day or 5 lb/week.
10. With diabetes (with or without hypertension), ACE inhibitors have been shown to reduce proteinuria and slow progression of renal disease.
11. Avoid OTC meds, especially cold remedies.
12. NSAIDs and aspirin may impair the hypotensive effects of ACE inhibitors while antacids may decrease bioavailability.
13. Avoid excessive amounts of caffeine (e.g., tea, coffee, cola).
14. Advise surgeon that ACE is being taken; angiotensin II formation sub-

sequent to compensatory renin release during surgery will be blocked; may reverse hypotension with volume expansion.
15. Avoid activities that may lead to a reduction in fluid volume i.e., excessive perspiration, vomiting, diarrhea, dehydration may all lead to hypotension.
16. Regular exercise, proper diet, weight loss, stress management, and adequate rest in conjunction with medications are needed in the overall management of hypertension. Additional interventions such as discontinuing alcohol/tobacco products, and reducing salt intake may also assist in BP control.

OUTCOMES/EVALUATE

- ↓ BP
- Improvement in S&S of CHF
- ↓ Proteinuria/renal damage
- ↓ Morbidity post-AMI

ANTIANGINAL DRUGS—NITRATES/NITRITES

SEE ALSO BETA-ADRENERGIC BLOCKING AGENTS, CALCIUM CHANNEL BLOCKING DRUGS, AND THE FOLLOWING INDIVIDUAL ENTRIES:

Isosorbide dinitrate chewable tablets
Isosorbide mononitrate
Nitroglycerin IV
Nitroglycerin sublingual
Nitroglycerin sustained release capsules and tablets
Nitroglycerin topical ointment
Nitroglycerin transdermal system
Nitroglycerin translingual spray

ACTION/KINETICS

Nitrates relax vascular smooth muscle by stimulating production of intracellular cyclic guanosine monophosphate. Dilation of postcapillary vessels decreases venous return to the heart due to pooling of blood; thus, LV end-diastolic pressure (preload) is reduced. Relaxation of arterioles results in a decreased systemic vascular resistance and arterial pressure (afterload). The oxygen requirements of the myocardium are reduced and there is more efficient redistribution of blood flow through collateral channels in myocardial tissue. Diastolic, systolic, and mean BP are decreased. Also, elevated central venous and pulmonary capillary wedge pressures, pulmonary vascular resistance, and systemic vascular resistance are reduced. Reflex tachycardia may occur due to the overall decrease in BP. Cardiac index may increase, decrease, or remain the same; those with elevated left ventricular filling pressure and systemic vascular resistance values with a depressed cardiac index are likely to see improvement of the cardiac index. The onset and duration depend on the product and route of administration (sublingual, topical, transdermal, parenteral, oral, and buccal). **Onset:** 1 to 3 min for IV, sublingual, translingual, and transmucosal nitroglycerin or sublingual isosorbide dinitrate; 20 to 60 min for sustained-release, topical, and transdermal nitroglycerin or oral isosorbide dinitrate or mononitrate; and up to 4 hr for sustained-release isosorbide dinitrate. **Duration of action:** 3 to 5 min for IV nitro-glycerin; 30 to 60 min for sublingual or translingual nitroglycerin; several hours for transmucosal, sustained-release, or topical nitroglycerin and all isosorbide dinitrate products; and up to 24 hr for transdermal nitroglycerin.

USES

Treatment and prophylaxis of acute angina pectoris (use sublingual, transmucosal, or translingual nitroglycerin). Nitrates are first-line therapy for unstable angina. Prophylaxis of chronic angina pectoris (topical, transdermal, translingual, transmucosal, or oral sustained-release nitroglycerin; isosorbide dinitrate and mononitrate; erythrityl tetranitrate; pentaerythritol tetranitrate). IV nitroglycerin is used to decrease BP in surgical procedures resulting in hypertension, as well as an adjunct in treating hypertension or CHF associated with MI. *Investigational:* Nitroglycerin ointment has been used as an adjunct in treating Raynaud's disease. Also, isosorbide dinitrate with prostaglandin E_1 for peripheral vascular disease. Sublingual and topical nitroglycerin and oral nitrates have been used to decrease cardiac workload in clients with acute MI and in CHF.

CONTRAINDICATIONS

Sensitivity to nitrites, which may result in severe hypotensive reactions, MI, or tolerance to nitrites. Severe anemia, cerebral hemorrhage, recent head trauma, postural hypotension, closed angle glaucoma, impaired hepatic function, hypertrophic cardiomyopathy, hypotension, recent MI. PO dosage forms should not be used in clients with GI hypermotility or with malabsorption syndrome. IV nitroglycerin should not be used in clients with hypotension, uncorrected hypovolemia, inadequate cerebral circulation, constrictive pericarditis, increased ICP, or pericardial tamponade.

SPECIAL CONCERNS

Use with caution during lactation and in glaucoma. Tolerance to the antianginal and vascular effects may occur. Safety and efficacy have not been determined during lactation and in children.

SIDE EFFECTS

CNS: Headaches (most common) which may be severe and persistent, restlessness, dizziness, weakness, apprehension, vertigo, anxiety, insomnia, confusion, nightmares, hypoesthesia, hypokinesia, dyscoordination. **CV:** Postural hypotension (common) with or without paradoxical bradycardia and increased angina, tachycardia, palpitations, syncope, rebound hypertension, crescendo angina, retrosternal discomfort, ***CV collapse,*** atrial fibrillation, PVCs, ***arrhythmias.*** **GI:** N&V, dyspepsia, diarrhea, dry mouth, abdominal pain, involuntary passing of feces and urine, tenesmus, tooth disorder. **Dermatologic:** Crusty skin lesions, pruritus, rash, exfoliative dermatitis, cutaneous vasodilation with flushing. **GU:** Urinary frequency, impotence, dysuria. **Respiratory:** URTI, bronchitis, pneumonia. **Allergic:** Itching, wheezing, tracheobronchitis. **Miscellaneous:** Perspiration, muscle twitching, methemoglobinemia, cold sweating, blurred vision, diplopia, ***hemolytic anemia,*** arthralgia, edema, malaise, neck stiffness, increased appetite, rigors.

• **TOPICAL**

Peripheral edema, contact dermatitis.

Tolerance can occur following chronic use. Nitrites convert hemoglobin to methemoglobin, which impairs the oxygen-carrying capacity of the blood, resulting in ***anemic hypoxia.*** This interaction is dangerous in clients with preexisting anemia.

OD OVERDOSE MANAGEMENT

Symptoms (Toxicity): Severe toxicity is rarely encountered with therapeutic use. Symptoms include hypotension, flushing, tachycardia, headache, palpitations, vertigo, perspiring skin followed by cold and cyanotic skin, visual disturbances, syncope, nausea, dizziness, diaphoresis, initial hyperpnea, dyspnea and slow breathing, slow pulse, ***heart block,*** vomiting with the possibility of bloody diarrhea and colic, anorexia, and increased ICP with symptoms of confusion, moderate fever, and paralysis. Tissue hypoxia (due to methemoglobinemia) may result in ***cyanosis, metabolic acidosis, coma, seizures, and death due to CV collapse.***

Treatment (Toxicity):

• Induction of emesis or gastric lavage followed by activated charcoal (nitrates are usually rapidly absorbed from the stomach). Gastric lavage may be used if the drug has been recently ingested.

• Maintain in a recumbent shock position and keep warm. Give oxygen and artificial respiration if required.

• Monitor methemoglobin levels.

• Elevate legs and administer IV fluids to treat severe hypotension and reflex tachycardia. Phenylephrine or methoxamine may also be helpful.

• Do not use epinephrine and similar drugs as they are ineffective in reversing severe hypotension.

DRUG INTERACTIONS

Acetylcholine / Effects ↓ when used with nitrates
Alcohol, ethyl / Hypotension and CV collapse due to vasodilator effect of both agents
Antihypertensive drugs / Additive hypotension
Aspirin / ↑ Serum levels and effects of nitrates
Beta-adrenergic blocking drugs / Additive hypotension
Calcium channel blocking drugs / Additive hypotension, including significant orthostatic hypotension
Dihydroergotamine / ↑ Effect R/T ↑ bioavailability or antagonism resulting in ↓ antianginal effects
Heparin / Possible ↓ effect
Narcotics / Additive hypotensive effect
Phenothiazines / Additive hypotension
Sympathomimetics / ↓ Effect of nitrates; also, nitrates may ↓ effect of sympathomimetics resulting in hypotension

LABORATORY TEST CONSIDERATIONS

↑ Urinary catecholamines. False negative ↓ in serum cholesterol.

DOSAGE

See individual agents.

NURSING CONSIDERATIONS

ADMINISTRATION/STORAGE

Store tablets and capsules tightly closed in their original container. Avoid exposure to air, heat, and moisture.

ASSESSMENT

1. Note any sensitivity to nitrites.
2. Document location, intensity, duration, extension, and any precipitating factors (i.e., activity, stress) surrounding anginal pain. Use a pain-rating scale to rate pain.
3. If history of anemia, administer with extreme caution.
4. Nitrates are contraindicated with elevated intracranial pressure and viagra.
5. Note any changes in ECG or elevated cardiac panel. Document results of echocardiogram, stress test, and/or catheterization.

INTERVENTIONS

1. Determine experience with self-administered medications; note if SL tablets ordered for bedside.
2. While hospitalized, note drug required to keep angina under control. Record:
   • Frequency given
   • Duration and intensity of pain (use a pain-rating scale; rate pain initially and 5 min after administration) and if relief is partial or complete
   • Time it takes for relief to occur
   • Any side effects
3. Report when consumed so effectiveness can be determined and usage monitored.
4. Monitor VS. Assess for sensitivity to hypotensive effects (N&V, pallor, restlessness, and CV collapse).
5. Monitor for hypotension when on additional drugs; adjust as needed. Supervise activities/ ambulation until drug effects realized.
6. Assess for signs of tolerance, which occur following chronic use but may begin several days after starting treatment; manifested by absence of response to the usual dose. (Nitrites may be discontinued temporarily until tolerance is lost, and then reinstituted. During interim, other vasodilators may be used.)
7. Observe for N&V, drowsiness, headache, or visual disturbances with long-term therapy (prolonged effects which require a change in drug).
8. Note change in activity and response to drug therapy. Determine if less discomfort experienced when performing regular activity.

CLIENT/FAMILY TEACHING

1. Take oral nitrates on an empty stomach with a glass of water. The drug decreases myocardial oxygen demand and reduces workload of the heart.
2. To prevent postural hypotension, use inhalation products or take SL tabs while sitting or lying down.

Make position changes slowly and rise only after dangling feet for several minutes.
3. Elderly clients should sit or lie down when taking nitroglycerin; may become dizzy and fall.
4. Do not change from one brand to another due to differences in effectiveness between different companies.
5. Always carry SL tablets for use in aborting an attack. Check expiration date; replace when needed or every 6 mo. A burning sensation under the tongue attests to drug potency.
6. Carry SL tablets in a *glass* bottle, tightly capped. Keep in original container as heat, moisture, and air cause deterioration. Do not use plastic containers; drug deteriorates in plastic; avoid child-proof caps as client must get to the tablets quickly.
7. If pain is not relieved in 5 min by first SL tablet, take up to 2 more tablets at 5-min intervals. If pain has not subsided 5 min after third tablet, client should be taken to the emergency room; *do not* drive; call 911.
8. Take SL tabs 5–15 min prior to any situation likely to cause pain (e.g., climbing stairs, sexual intercourse, exposure to cold weather).
9. Record attacks; report any increase in the frequency/intensity of attacks and loss of effectiveness.
10. Schedule frequent rest periods, pace activities, and avoid stressful situations. Use Tylenol for headaches.
11. Follow instructions on how to apply topical nitroglycerin. Remove at bedtime and apply upon arising; a nitrate-free period of 8 hr may reduce/prevent nitrate tolerance.
12. Avoid alcohol; nitrite syncope, a severe shock-like state, may occur.
13. Inhalation products are flammable; do not use under situations where they might ignite.
14. Do not smoke. Review risks and life-style changes necessary to prevent further CAD (i.e., weight control, dietary changes, ↓ salt intake, modified regular exercise program, no alcohol/tobacco, and stress reduction).
15. Have family or significant other learn CPR; survival rate is greatly increased when CPR is initiated immediately.
16. Carry ID with prescribed drugs. Know what you are taking and why.

OUTCOMES/EVALUATE

- ↓ Myocardial oxygen requirements; ↑ activity tolerance
- Improved myocardial perfusion
- Relief of coronary artery spasm

ANTIARRHYTHMIC DRUGS

SEE ALSO THE FOLLOWING INDIVIDUAL ENTRIES:

Adenosine
Amiodarone hydrochloride
Bretylium tosylate
Calcium Channel Blocking Agents
Digoxin
Diltiazem hydrochloride
Disopyramide phosphate
Dofetilide
Flecainide acetate
Ibutilide fumarate
Lidocaine hydrochloride
Moricizine hydrochloride
Phenytoin
Phenytoin sodium
Procainamide hydrochloride
Propafenone hydrochloride
Propranolol hydrochloride
Quinidine gluconate
Quinidine polygalacturonate
Quinidine sulfate
Tocainide hydrochloride
Verapamil

GENERAL STATEMENT

Examples of cardiac arrhythmias are *premature ventricular beats, ventricular tachycardia, atrial flutter, atrial fibrillation, ventricular fibrillation,* and *atrioventricular heart block*. The various antiarrhythmic drugs are classified according to both their mechanism of action and their effects on the action potential of cardiac cells. Importantly, one drug in a particular class may be more effective and safer in an individual client. The antiarrhythmic drugs are classified as follows:

1. Class I. Decrease the rate of entry of sodium during cardiac membrane depolarization, decrease the rate of rise of phase O of the cardiac membrane action potential, prolong the effective refractory period of fast-response fibers, and require that a more negative membrane potential be reached before the membrane becomes excitable (and thus can propagate to other membranes). Class I drugs are further listed in subgroups (according to their effects on action potential duration) as follows:

• Class IA: Depress phase O and prolong the duration of the action potential. Examples: Disopyramide, procainamide, and quinidine.

• Class IB: Slightly depress phase O and are thought to shorten the action potential. Examples: Lidocaine, mexiletine, phenytoin, and tocainide.

• Class IC: Slight effect on repolarization but marked depression of phase O of the action potential. Significant slowing of conduction. Examples: Flecainide, indecainide, and propafenone.

NOTE: Moricizine is classified as a Class I agent but it has characteristics of agents in groups IA, B, and C.

2. Class II. Competitively block beta-adrenergic receptors and depress phase 4 depolarization. Examples: Acebutolol, esmolol, and propranolol.

3. Class III. Prolong the duration of the membrane action potential (relative refractory period) without changing the phase of depolarization or the resting membrane potential. Examples: Amiodarone, bretylium, dofetilide, ibutilide, and sotalol.

4. Class IV. Diltiazem and verapamil, calcium channel blockers that slow conduction velocity and increase the refractoriness of the AV node.

Adenosine and digoxin are also used to treat arrhythmias. Adenosine slows conduction time through the AV node and can interrupt the reentry pathways through the AV node. Digoxin causes a decrease in maximal diastolic potential and duration of the action potential; it also increases the slope of phase 4 depolarization.

SPECIAL CONCERNS

Monitor serum levels of antiarrhythmic drugs since some drugs can cause toxic side effects which can be confused with the purpose for which the drug is used. For example, toxicity from quinidine can result in cardiac arrhythmias. Antiarrhythmic drugs may cause new or worsening of arrhythmias, ranging from an increase in frequency of PVCs to severe ventricular tachycardia, ventricular fibrillation, or tachycardia that is more sustained and rapid. Such situations (called proarrhythmic effect) may make it difficult to distinguish the proarrhythmic effect from the underlying rhythm disorder.

DRUG INTERACTIONS

H *Aloe* / Chronic aloe use → ↑ serum potassium loss causing ↑ effect of antiarrhythmics

H *Buckthorn bark/berry* / Chronic buckthorn use → ↑ serum potassium loss causing ↑ effect of antiarrhythmics

H *Cascara sagrada bark* Chronic cascara use → ↑ serum potassium loss causing ↑ effect of antiarrhythmics

H *Rhubarb root* / Chronic rhubarb use → ↑ serum potassium loss causing ↑ effect of antiarrhythmics

H *Senna pod/leaf* / Chronic senna use → ↑ serum potassium loss causing ↑ effect of antiarrhythmics

NURSING CONSIDERATIONS

ASSESSMENT

1. Note drug sensitivity and any previous experiences with these drugs.
2. Assess extent of palpitations, fluttering sensations, chest pains, fainting episodes, or missed beats; obtain ECG documenting arrhythmia.
3. Assess heart sounds and VS. Use cardiac monitor if administering drugs by IV route; monitor for rhythm changes.

4. Monitor BP and pulse. A HR < 50 bpm or > 120 should be avoided. Obtain written parameters for BP and pulse ranges.
5. Monitor BS, electrolytes, drug levels, liver and renal function studies. Ensure that serum pH, electrolytes, pO_2 and/or O_2 saturations are WNL.
6. Assess life-style related to cigarettes and caffeine use, alcohol consumption, and lack of regular exercise. Certain foods, emotional stress, and other environmental factors may also trigger arrhythmias; identify and eliminate before instituting drugs.

CLIENT/FAMILY TEACHING

1. Drugs work by controlling the irregular heart beats so the heart can pump more efficiently.
2. Take as ordered; If a dose is missed, do not double up.
3. Record BP and pulse for review.
4. Avoid OTC products. Eliminate caffeine, cigarettes, and alcohol; alters drug absorption and may precipitate arrhythmias.
5. Keep follow-up visits so that therapy can be adjusted and evaluated.
6. Report concerns/fears or problems R/T sexual activity and side effects of drug therapy.
7. Always carry list of prescribed meds and condition being treated. Keep all F/U appointments to evaluate drug response.
8. Family/significant other should learn CPR; survival rates are greatly increased when initiated immediately.

OUTCOMES/EVALUATE

- ECG evidence of arrhythmia control; restoration of stable cardiac rhythm
- Serum drug concentrations within therapeutic range

ANTICONVULSANTS

SEE ALSO THE FOLLOWING INDIVIDUAL ENTRIES:

Acetazolamide
Acetazolamide sodium
Carbamazepine
Clonazepam
Clorazepate dipotassium
Diazepam
Ethosuximide
Felbamate
Fosphenytoin sodium
Gabapentin
Lamotrigine
Levetiracetam
Magnesium sulfate
Methsuximide
Oxcarbazepine
Phenobarbital
Phenobarbital sodium
Phensuximide
Phenytoin
Phenytoin sodium extended
Phenytoin sodium parenteral
Phenytoin sodium prompt
Primidone
Tiagabine hydrochloride
Topiramate
Valproic acid/divalproex sodium
Zonisamide

GENERAL STATEMENT

Therapeutic agents cannot cure convulsive disorders, but do control seizures without impairing the normal functions of the CNS. This is often accomplished by selective depression of hyperactive areas of the brain responsible for the convulsions. Therefore, these drugs are taken at all times (prophylactically) to prevent the occurrence of the seizures. There are several different types of epileptic disorders; consult the International Classification of Epileptic Seizures. No single drug can control all types of epilepsy; thus, accurate diagnosis is important. Drugs effective against one type of epilepsy may not be effective against another. Therapy begins with a small dose of the drug, which is continuously increased until either the seizures disappear or drug toxicity occurs. Monotherapy is preferred but if a certain drug decreases the frequency of seizures but does not completely prevent them, another drug can be added to the dosage regimen and administered concomitantly with the first. Failure of therapy most often results from the administration of doses too small to have a therapeutic effect or from failure to use two or more drugs together. With appropriate diagnosis and selection of drugs, four out of five cases of epilepsy can be controlled adequately, but it may take the provider some time to find the best drug or combination of drugs with which to treat the client.

DOSAGE

Dosage is highly individualized. However, trauma or emotional stress may necessitate an increase in drug dosage requirements (e.g., if the client requires surgery and starts having seizures). For details, see individual agents.

NURSING CONSIDERATIONS

ADMINISTRATION/STORAGE

1. Shake oral suspensions thoroughly before pouring to ensure uniform mixing.
2. Drug therapy must be individualized according to client needs.
3. Do not discontinue abruptly unless provider approved. To avoid severe, prolonged convulsions, withdraw over a period of days or weeks.
4. If there is reason to substitute one anticonvulsant drug for another, withdraw the first drug at the same time the dosage of the second drug is being increased.
5. Be prepared, in case of acute oral toxicity, to assist with inducing emesis (provided the client is not comatose) and with gastric lavage, along with other supportive measures such as administration of fluids and oxygen.

ASSESSMENT

1. Check medical history for hypersensitivity to anticonvulsant drugs. Note derivatives to avoid.
2. Assess orientation to time and place, affect, reflexes, and VS.
3. Document seizure classification (partial or generalized). Determine the frequency/severity of seizures, noting location, duration, consciousness, type, frequency and any precipitating factors, presence of an aura, and any other characteristics. Note EEG, CT/MRI results.
4. Assess skin, eyes, and mucous membranes.
5. Determine if pregnant; may cause fetal abnormalities.
6. Monitor CBC, glucose, uric acid, urinalysis, renal and LFTs.
7. Determine why receiving therapy and when. If no seizures for over 1 year with prophylactic therapy, may try gradual drug discontinuation.

INTERVENTIONS

1. With IV administration, monitor closely for respiratory depression and CV collapse.
2. Note any evidence of CNS side effects, such as blurred vision, dimmed vision, slurred speech, nystagmus, or confusion; supervise ambulation until resolved.
3. Observe for muscle twitching, loss of muscle tone, episodes of bizarre behavior, and/or subsequent amnesia.
4. With phenytoin, check Ca levels; contributes to bone demineralization which can result in osteomalacia in adults and rickets in children. Risk increases with inactivity.
5. Administer vitamin K to pregnant women 1 month before delivery to prevent postpartum hemorrhage/bleeding in the newborn and mother.

CLIENT/FAMILY TEACHING

1. Take drug as prescribed. Do not increase, decrease, or discontinue without approval; seizures may result.
2. May initially cause a decrease in mental alertness, drowsiness, headache, vertigo, and ataxia. CNS symptoms are dose-related and should subside with continued therapy; avoid hazardous tasks until symptoms resolve.
3. Lessen GI distress by taking with large amounts of fluids or with food.
4. Dosage may require adjusting if undergoing physical trauma or emotional distress.
5. Vitamin D may be prescribed to prevent hypocalcemia (4,000 units of vitamin D weekly); folic acid may prevent megaloblastic anemia.
6. Avoid alcohol and any other CNS depressants.
7. Increase fluid intake and include fruit and other foods with roughage and bulk in the diet.

8. With gingival hyperplasia, intensify oral hygiene, routinely use dental floss, soft tooth brush, massage gums, and obtain dental exams.
9. If slurred speech develops, try to consciously slow speech patterns to avoid the problem.
10. Avoid situations/exposures that result in fever and low glucose and sodium levels; may lower seizure threshold.
11. Report if rash, fever, severe headaches, stomatitis, rhinitis, urethritis, or balanitis (inflammation of the glans penis) occur; S&S of hypersensitivity; requires change in drug.
12. Report sore throat, easy bruising, bleeding, or nosebleeds; signs of hematologic toxicity.
13. Report jaundice, dark urine, anorexia, and abdominal pain; may indicate liver toxicity. To detect for hepatitis, hepatocellular degeneration, and fatal hepatocellular necrosis include LFTs.
14. Practice reliable birth control; may harm fetus. If nursing, observe infant for signs of toxicity.
15. Carry ID with the type of seizures and prescribed therapy. Family should learn CPR and how to protect client during a seizure.
16. Identify support groups (Epilepsy Foundation; National Head Injury Group) that may assist to understand and cope with disorder.

OUTCOMES/EVALUATE

• ↓ Frequency of seizures; improved seizure control
• Serum drug levels within desired range

ANTIDEPRESSANTS, TRICYCLIC

SEE ALSO THE FOLLOWING INDIVIDUAL ENTRIES:

Amitriptyline hydrochloride
Amoxapine
Desipramine hydrochloride
Doxepin hydrochloride
Imipramine hydrochloride
Imipramine pamoate
Nortriptyline hydrochloride
Trimipramine maleate

GENERAL STATEMENT

Drugs with antidepressant effects include the tricyclic antidepressants (TCAs), selective serotonin reuptake inhibitors (SSRIs) i.e., fluoxetine, fluvoxamine, paroxetine, sertraline; and monoamine oxidase inhibitors (MAOIs) i.e., phenelzine, tranylcypromine.

ACTION/KINETICS

It is now believed that antidepressant drugs cause adaptive changes in the serotonin and norepinephrine receptor systems, resulting in changes in the sensitivities of both presynaptic and postsynaptic receptor sites. These effects may increase the sensitivity of postsynaptic α-1 adrenergic and serotonin receptors and decrease the sensitivity of presynaptic receptor sites. The overall effect is a reregulation of the abnormal receptor neurotransmitter relationship.

The tricyclic antidepressants are chemically related to the phenothiazines; thus, they exhibit many of the same pharmacologic effects (e.g., anticholinergic, antiserotonin, sedative, antihistaminic, and hypotensive). The TCAs are less effective for depressed clients in the presence of organic brain damage or schizophrenia. Also, they can induce mania; note when given to clients with manic-depressive psychoses. Well absorbed from the GI tract; significant first-pass effect. All have a long serum half-life. Up to 46 days may be required to reach steady plasma levels and maximum therapeutic effects may not be noted for 24 weeks. Because of the long half-life, single daily dosage may suffice. More than 90% bound to plasma protein. Partially metabolized in the liver; some are metabolized to active compounds. Excreted primarily in the urine.

USES

Endogenous and reactive depressions. Drugs with significant sedative effects may be useful in depression associated with anxiety and sleep disturbances. Preferred over MAO inhibitors because they are less toxic. See also individual drugs.

CONTRAINDICATIONS

Severely impaired liver function. Use during acute recovery phase from MI. Concomitant use with MAO inhibitors.

SPECIAL CONCERNS

Use with caution during lactation and with epilepsy (seizure threshold is lowered), CV diseases (possibility of conduction defects, arrhythmias, CHF, sinus tachycardia, MI, strokes, tachycardia), glaucoma, BPH, suicidal tendencies, a history of urinary retention, and the elderly. Use during pregnancy only when benefits clearly outweigh risks. Generally not recommended for children less than 12 years of age. Geriatric clients may be more sensitive to the anticholinergic and sedative side effects. Electroconvulsive therapy may increase the hazards of therapy.

SIDE EFFECTS

Most frequent side effects are sedation and atropine-like reactions. **CNS:** Agitation, akathisa, EEG pattern alterations, ataxia, anxiety, coma, confusion, disorientation, disturbed concentration, dizziness, drowsiness, dysarthria, exacerbation of psychosis, excitement, excessive appetite, extrapyaramidal symptoms (including tardive dyskinesia), fatigue, hallucinations, delusions, headache, hyperthermia, hypomania, incoordination, insomnia, mania, nervousness, neuroleptic malignant syndrome, numbness, panic, nightmares, paresthesias of extremities, peripheral neuropathy, tremors, seizures, restlessness, weakness, tingling. **Anticholinergic:** Dry mouth, blurred vision, increased IOP, disturbed accommodation, mydriasis, constipation, paralytic ileus, urinary retention, delayed micturition, urinary tract dilation, hyperpyrexia. **GI:** N&V, abdominal pain or cramps, anorexia, aphthous stomatitis, constipation, diarrhea, epigastric distress, black tongue, dysphagia, increased pancreatic enzymes, flatulence, indigestion, GI disorder, parotid swelling, stomatitis, taste disturbance, peculiar taste, ulcerative stomatitis, hepatitis (rare), jaundice. **CV:** Arrhythmias, ECG changes, flushing, change in AV conduction, ***heart block, stroke, sudden death,*** hot flushes, hypertension, hypotension, orthostatic hypotension, palpitations, CHF, PVCs, syncope, tachycardia. **Dermatologic:** Skin rashes, urticaria, flushing, pruritus, petechie, photosensitivity, edema. **GU:** Testicular swelling and gynecomastia in males, increase or decrease in libido, impotence, menstrual irregularities and galactorrhea in females, breast enlargement, impotence, painful ejaculation, nocturia, urinary frequency. **Hematologic:** Agranulocytosis, aplastic anemia, leukopenia, thrombocytopenia, purpura, eosino-philia. **Hypersensitivity:** Drug fever, edema (generalized or of face/tongue), itching, petechiae, photosensitivity, pruritus, rash, urticaria, vasculitis. **Metabolic:** Increase or decrease in blood sugar, inappropriate ADH secretion. **Miscellaneous:** Sweating, alopecia, fever, hyperthermia, proneness to falling, weight gain or loss, nasal congestion, abnormal lacrimation, tinnitus, chills, worsening of asthma.

High dosage increases the frequency of seizures in epileptic clients and may cause epileptiform attacks in normal subjects.

OD OVERDOSE MANAGEMENT

Symptoms: CNS symptoms include agitation, confusion, hallucinations, hyperactive reflexes, choreoathetosis, ***seizures, coma.*** Anticholinergic symptoms include dilated pupils, dry mouth, flushing, and ***hyperpyrexia.*** CV toxicity includes depressed myocardial contractility, decreased HR, decreased coronary blood flow, tachycardia, intraventricular block, ***complete AV block, re-entry ventricular arrhythmias, PVCs, ventricular tachycardia or fibrillation, sudden cardiac arrest, hypotension, pulmonary edema.*** *Treatment:* Admit client to hospital and monitor ECG closely for 3 to 5 days.

• Empty stomach in alert clients by inducing vomiting followed by gastric lavage and charcoal administration **after insertion of cuffed ET tube.** Maintain respiration and avoid the use of respiratory stimulants.
• Normal or half-normal saline to prevent water intoxication.
• To reverse the CV effects (e.g., hypotension and cardiac dysrhythmias), give hypertonic sodium bicarbonate. The usual dose is 0.52 mEq/kg by IV bolus followed by IV infusion to maintain the blood at pH 7.5. If hypotension is not reversed by bicarbonate, vasopressors (e.g., dopamine) and fluid expansion may be needed. If the cardiac dysrhythmias do not respond to bicarbonate, lidocaine or phenytoin may be used.
• Isoproterenol may be effective in controlling bradyarrhythmias and torsades de pointes ventricular tachycardia. Use propranolol, 0.1 mg/kg IV (up to 0.25 mg by IV bolus), to treat life-threatening ventricular arrhythmias in children.
• Treat shock and metabolic acidosis with IV fluids, oxygen, bicarbonate, and corticosteroids.
• Control hyperpyrexia by external means (ice pack, cool baths, spongings).
• To reduce possibility of convulsions, minimize external stimulation. If necessary, use diazepam or phenytoin to control convulsions. Avoid barbiturates if MAO inhibitors have been used recently.

DRUG INTERACTIONS

Acetazolamide / ↑ Effect of tricyclics by ↑ renal tubular reabsorption
Alcohol, ethyl / Concomitant use may lead to ↑ GI complications and ↓ performance on motor skill tests–death has been reported
Ammonium chloride / ↓ Effect of tricyclics by ↓ renal tubular reabsorption of the drug
Anticholinergic drugs / Additive anticholinergic side effects
Anticoagulants, oral / ↑ Hypoprothrombinemia R/T ↓ liver breakdown
Anticonvulsants / TCAs may ↑ incidence of epileptic seizures
Antihistamines / Additive anticholinergic side effects
Ascorbic acid / ↓ TCA effects by ↓ renal tubular drug reabsorption
Barbiturates / Additive depressant effects; also, may ↑ liver breakdown of antidepressants
H *Belladonna leaf/root* / Additive anticholinergic effects
Benzodiazepines / TCAs ↑ effect of benzodiazepines
Beta-adrenergic blocking agents / TCAs ↓ effect of the blocking agents
Carbamazepine / ↓ Serum TCA levels; ↑ serum carbamazepine levels → ↑ pharmacologic/toxic effects
Charcoal / ↓ Absorption of TCAs → ↓ effectiveness (or toxicity)
Chlordiazepoxide / Concomitant use may cause additive sedative effects and/or additive atropine-like side effects
Cimetidine / ↑ Effect of TCAs (especially serious anticholinergic symptoms) R/T ↓ liver breakdown
Clonidine / Dangerous ↑ BP and hypertensive crisis
Diazepam / Concomitant use may cause additive sedative effects and/or additive atropine-like side effects
Dicumarol / TCAs may ↑ the t½ of dicumarol → ↑ anticoagulation effects
Disulfiram / ↑ Levels of TCAs; also, possibility of acute organic brain syndrome
Ephedrine / TCAs ↓ effects of ephedrine by preventing uptake at its site of action
Estrogens / Depending on the dose, estrogens may ↑ or ↓ the effects of TCAs
Ethchlorvynol / Combination may result in transient delirium
H *Evening primrose oil* / May worsen temporal lobe epilepsy or schizophrenia when taken with TCAs
Fluoxetine / ↑ Pharmacologic and toxic effects of TCAs (effect may persist for several weeks after fluoxetine discontinued)

Furazolidone / Toxic psychoses possible
Glutethimide / Additive anticholinergic side effects
Grepafloxacin / ↑ Risk of life-threatening cardiac arrhythmias, including torsade de pointes
Guanethidine / TCAs ↓ antihypertensive effect of guanethidine by preventing uptake at its site of action
Haloperidol / ↑ TCA effects R/T ↓ liver breakdown
H *Henbane leaf* / ↑ Anticholinergic effects
Histamine H-2 antagonists / ↑ Serum TCA levels
H *Kava Kava* / Additive effects
Levodopa / ↓ Effect of levodopa R/T ↓ absorption
MAO inhibitors / Concomitant use may result in hyperpyretic crisis, excitation, hyperthermia, delirium, tremors, DIC, severe convulsions, coma, flushing, confusion, tachycardia, tachypnea, headache, mydriasis, and death although combinations have been used successfully
Meperidine / TCAs enhance narcotic-induced respiratory depression; also, additive anticholinergic side effects
Methyldopa / TCAs may block hypotensive effects of methyldopa
Methylphenidate / ↑ TCA effects R/T ↓ liver breakdown
Narcotic analgesics / TCAs enhance narcotic-induced respiratory depression; also, additive anticholinergic effects
Oral contraceptives / ↑ TCA plasma levels R/T ↓ liver breakdown
Oxazepam / Concomitant use may cause additive sedative effects and/or atropine-like side effects
Phenothiazines / Additive anticholinergic side effects; also, phenothiazines ↑ TCA effects R/T ↓ liver breakdown
Procainamide / Additive cardiac effects
Quinidine / Additive cardiac effects
Quinolone antibiotics / ↑ Risk of life-threatening cardiac arrhythmias, including torsade de pointes
Rifamycins / ↓ Serum TCA levels
H *Scopolia root* / ↑ TCA effects
Selective serotonin reuptake inhibitors / ↑ Pharmacologic/toxic effects of TCAs; symptoms may persist for at least 5 weeks
Sodium bicarbonate / ↑ TCA effects by ↑ renal tubular drug reabsorption
Sparfloxacin / ↑ Risk of life-threatening cardiac arrhythmias, including torsade de pointes
Sympathomimetics / Potentiation of sympathomimetic effects→ hypertension or cardiac arrhythmias
Tobacco (smoking) / ↓ Serum TCA levels R/T ↑ liver breakdown
Thyroid preparations / Mutually potentiating effects observed
Valproic acid / ↑ Plasma TCA levels → ↑ side effects
Vasodilators / Additive hypotensive effect

LABORATORY TEST CONSIDERATIONS

↑ Alkaline phosphatase, transaminase, prolactin, bilirubin; ↑ or ↓ blood glucose. False + or ↑ urinary catecholamines. Altered LFTs.

DOSAGE

See individual drugs.

Dosage levels vary greatly in effectiveness from one client to another; therefore, carefully individualize dosage regimens.

NURSING CONSIDERATIONS

ADMINISTRATION/STORAGE

1. In adolescents and elderly clients, use a lower initial dosage than in adults; gradually increase the dose as required.
2. Individualize dose according to age, weight, physical and mental condition, and response to the therapy.
3. For maintenance therapy, a single daily dose may suffice.
4. Dose usually administered at bedtime, so any anticholinergic and/or sedative effects will not impact ADL.
5. To reduce incidence of sedation and anticholinergic effects, start with small doses and then gradually increase to desired dosage levels.

ASSESSMENT

1. Document indications for therapy, behavioral manifestations, symptom onset, and causative factors.
2. Assess for dysphoric mood, suicide ideations, and excessive appetite/weight changes.
3. Note sleep disturbances, lethargy, apathy, impaired thought processes, or lack of responses.
4. List drugs currently prescribed; some that may intensify depressive reactions include antihypertensives (i.e., reserpine, methyldopa, beta blockers), antiparkinsonians, hormones, steroids, anticancer agents, and antituberculins (cycloserine) as well as barbiturates and alcohol.
5. Monitor CBC, renal and LFTs.
6. Record ECG, assess heart sounds, note any CAD, and evaluate neurologic functioning. Assess for tachycardia and increase in anginal attacks; may precede MI or stroke.
7. Note eye exam; report visual changes, headaches, halos, eye pain, dilated pupils, or nausea. May need med change, esp. with glaucoma.
8. Monitor I&O; Check for abdominal distention, urinary retention, and absence of bowel sounds (as in paralytic ileus).
9. Differentiate type of depression based on diagnostic features related to reactive, major depressive, or bipolar affective disorders. Review symptoms to determine if affective, somatic, psychomotor, or psychological.

INTERVENTIONS

1. Note S&S of allergic response, i.e., rash, alopecia, and eosinophilia.
2. Sore throat, fever, easy bruising, unusual bleeding, presence of petechiae or purpura may be S&S of blood dyscrasias. Check for evidence of agranulocytosis, among elderly women and during the second month of drug therapy.
3. With hyperthyroidism, assess for arrhythmias precipitated by TCAs.
4. Assess for adverse endocrine disturbances such as increased or decreased libido, gynecomastia, testicular swelling, and impotence.
5. Report symptoms of cholestatic jaundice and biliary tract obstruction such as high fever, yellowing of the skin, mucous membranes and sclera, pruritus, and upper abdominal pain.
6. TCAs may alter blood sugar levels and require adjustment of hypoglycemic agent.
7. Report if receiving electroshock therapy; hazardous combination.
8. Discontinue several days prior to surgery; may adversely affect BP.
9. Withdraw slowly to avoid any withdrawal symptoms.
10. Assess for epileptiform seizures precipitated by the drug.

CLIENT/FAMILY TEACHING

1. GI complaints of anorexia, N&V, epigastric distress, diarrhea, blackened tongue, or a peculiar taste require a dosage adjustment. Take with or immediately following meals to reduce gastric irritation.
2. Take sedating meds at bedtime to minimize daytime sedation; take those that cause insomnia in the a.m. or upon arising.
3. Avoid other drugs and alcohol during and for 2 weeks following TCA therapy.
4. Use caution when performing tasks requiring mental alertness or physical coordination; may cause drowsiness or ataxia.
5. Rise slowly from a supine position; do not remain standing in one place for any length of time. If feeling faint, lie down to minimize orthostatic hypotension.
6. Increase oral hygiene, take frequent sips of water, suck on hard candy, or chew sugarless gum to maintain a moist mouth. A high-fiber diet, increased fluid intake, exercise, and stool softeners may prevent constipation.
7. May affect carbohydrate metabolism; an adjustment of hypoglycemic agent and diet may be indicated.
8. If photosensitive, stay out of the sun; wear protective clothing, sunglasses, and a sunscreen.
9. May alter libido or reproductive function.

10. Practice reliable birth control; report if pregnancy suspected.
11. Report any alterations in perceptions, i.e., hallucinations, blurred vision, or excessive stimulations. Watch those recovering from depression for suicidal tendencies; remove firearms from the home.
12. May take 24 weeks to realize a maximum clinical response; stay on the treatment regimen.
13. Will see provider more often the first 2–3 weeks; scripts will be for only small amounts to ensure compliance and to prevent an overdose; excess consumption can be lethal. Obtain number to call for help.
14. Do not stop abruptly, may experience withdrawl S&S.
15. Review when and how to take meds, reportable side effects and importance of regular participation in psychotherapy programs when prescribed.

OUTCOMES/EVALUATE

• Understand illness and need for counselling, drug therapy/medical supervision
• ↓ Depression evidenced by improved appetite, renewed interest in outside activities, ↑ socialization, improved sleeping patterns, ↑ energy
• ↓ Anxiety; improved coping skills
• ↓ Chronic Pain

ANTIDIABETIC AGENTS: HYPOGLYCEMIC AGENTS

SEE ALSO *ANTIDIABETIC AGENTS: INSULINS*. SEE ALSO THE FOLLOWING INDIVIDUAL ENTRIES:

Acarbose
Glimepiride
Glipizide
Glyburide
Metformin hydrochloride
Miglitol
Pioglitazone hydrochloride
Rosiglitazone maleate
Tolazamide
Tolbutamide
Tolbutamide sodium

GENERAL STATEMENT

The American Diabetes Association has developed standards for treating clients with diabetes. If followed, these standards will enable clients to decrease their blood glucose levels closer to normal; this will reduce the risk of complications, including blindness, kidney disease, heart disease, and amputations. The goals of these standards include establishing specific targets for control of blood glucose (usually between 80 and 120 mg/dL before meals and between 100 and 140 mg/dL at bedtime) and increased emphasis on educating clients for self-management of their disease. Targets for BP and lipid levels are also provided. If the guidelines are followed, it is estimated that the risk of development or progression of retinopathy, nephropathy, and neuropathy can be reduced by 50%–75% in clients with insulin-dependent (type I) diabetes. The guidelines suggest the following treatment modalities:

• Frequent monitoring of blood glucose.
• Regular exercise.
• Close attention to meal planning; consult a registered dietitian.
• For type I diabetics, either continuous SC insulin infusion or multiple daily insulin injections; for type II diabetics, consider insulin administration in certain situations, although dietary modification, exercise, and weight reduction are the cornerstone of treatment.
• Instruction in the prevention and treatment of hypoglycemia and other complications (both acute and chronic) of diabetes.
• Development of a process for ongoing support and continuing education for the client.
• Routine assessment of treatment goals.

ACTION/KINETICS

Oral hypoglycemic drugs are classified as either first or second generation. *Generation* refers to structural changes in the basic molecule. Second-generation oral hypoglycemic drugs are more lipophilic and, as such, have greater hypoglycemic potency. Also, second-generation drugs are bound to plasma protein by covalent bonds, whereas first-generation drugs are bound to plasma protein by ionic bonds. The implication is that the second-generation drugs are potentially less susceptible to displacement from plasma protein by drugs such as salicylates and oral anticoagulants.

The oral hypoglycemics bind to plasma membranes of functional beta cells in the pancreas causing a decrease in potassium permeability and membrane depolarization. This leads to an increase in intracellular calcium and subsequent release from insulin-containing secretory granules. The sulfonylureas enhance betacell response rather than change the sensitivity of beta-cells to glucose. To be effective, the client must have some ability for endogenous insulin production. Differences in oral hypoglycemic drugs are mainly in their pharmacokinetic properties and duration of action. Sulfonylureas are well absorbed after PO use.

USES

Non-insulin-dependent diabetes mellitus (type II) that does not respond to diet management and exercise alone. Concurrent use of insulin and an oral hypoglycemic for type II diabetics who are difficult to control with diet and sulfonylurea therapy alone. One method used is the BIDS system: bedtime insulin (usually NPH) with daytime (morning only or morning and evening) oral hypoglycemic.

Guidelines for oral hypoglycemic therapy include onset of diabetes generally in clients over 40 years of age (but is being noted more in children that are overweight and inactive, with poor dietary habits), duration of diabetes less than 5 years, absence of ketoacidosis, client is obese or has normal body weight, fasting serum glucose of 200 mg/dL or less, elevated glucose tolerance test, normal or high C-Peptide, and hepatic and renal function is normal.

CONTRAINDICATIONS

Stress before and during surgery, ketosis, severe trauma, fever, infections, pregnancy, diabetes complicated by recurrent episodes of ketoacidosis or coma; juvenile, growth-onset, insulin-dependent, or brittle diabetes; impaired endocrine, renal, or liver function. Use in diabetics who can be controlled by diet alone. Relapse may occur with the sulfonylureas in undernourished clients. Long-acting products in geriatric clients.

SPECIAL CONCERNS

Use with caution in debilitated and malnourished clients, during lactation since hypoglycemia may occur in the infant, and in those with impaired renal or hepatic function. Safety and effectiveness in children have not been established. Geriatric clients may be more sensitive to oral hypoglycemics and hypoglycemia may be more difficult to recognize in these clients. Use of sulfonylureas has been associated with an increased risk of CV mortality compared to treatment with either diet alone or diet plus insulin. There may be loss of blood glucose control if the client experiences stress such as infection, fever, surgery, or trauma or develops Syndrome X (insulin resistance or metabolic syndrome).

SIDE EFFECTS

Hypoglycemia is the most common side effect. **GI:** Nausea, heartburn, epigastric fullness, diarrhea, GI pain, constipation, dyspepsia, gastralgia, vomiting, proctocolitis, hunger, flatulence. **CNS:** Fatigue, dizziness, drowsiness, nervousness, asthenia, insomnia, tremor, anxiety, depession, chills, hypesthesia, hypertonia, somnolence, confusion, abnormal gait, decreased libido, migraine, anorexia, myalgia, arthralgia, weakness, paresthesia, dizziness, weakness, vertigo, malaise, head-ache.. **Hepatic:** Cholestatic jaundice, aggravation of hepatic porphyria, hepatitis. **Dermatologic:** Skin rashes, urticaria, erythema multiforme, pruritus, eczema, photophobia, morbilliform or maculopapular eruptions, rash, sweating, lichenoid reactions, porphyria cutanea tardia. **Hematologic:** Thrombocytopenia, leukopenia, ***agranulocytosis, aplastic anemia,*** pancytopenia, eosinophilia, ***hemolytic anemia.*** **Endocrine:** Inappropriate secretion of ADH resulting in excessive water retention, hyponatremia, low serum osmolality, and high urine osmolality. **CV:** Arrhythmia, flushing, hypertension, vasculitis. **Ophthalmic:** Eye pain, blurred vision, conjunctivitis, retinal hemorrhage. **Miscellaneous:** Tinnitus, disulfiram-like reaction if taken with alcohol, rhinitis, polyuria, trace blood in stool, thirst, edema, pharyngitis, dysuria, dyspnea, leg cramps, syncope, resistance to drug action develops in a small percentage of clients.

OD OVERDOSE MANAGEMENT

Symptoms: Hypoglycemia. The following symptoms of hypoglycemia are listed in their general order of appearance: tingling of lips and tongue, hunger, nausea, decreased cerebral function (lethargy, yawning, confusion, agitation, nervousness), increased sympathetic activity (tachycardia, sweating, tremor), seizures, stupor, coma. *Treatment:* Mild hypoglycemia is treated with PO glucose and adjusting the dose of the drug or meal patterns. Severe hypoglycemia requires hospitalization. Concentrated (50%) dextrose is given by rapid IV and is followed by continuous infusion of 10% dextrose at a rate that will maintain blood glucose above 100 mg/dL. Client should be monitored for at least 24–48 hr as hypoglycemia may recur (clients with chlorpropamide toxicity should be monitored for 3–5 days due to the long duration of action of this drug).

DRUG INTERACTIONS

Alcohol / Possible Antabuse-like syndrome, especially flushing of face and SOB. Also, ↓ effect of oral hypoglycemic R/T to ↑ liver breakdown
Androgens/anabolic steroids / ↑ Hypoglycemic effect
Anticoagulants, oral / ↑ Oral hypoglycemic effects by ↓ liver breakdown and ↓ plasma protein binding
Azole antifungals ↑ Oral hypoglycemic effect
Beta-adrenergic blocking agents / ↓ Hypoglycemic effect; also, symptoms of hypoglycemia may be masked
H *Bilberry* / Possible potentiation of antidiabetic agents
Calcium channel blockers / ↓ Hypoglycemic effect
Charcoal / ↓ Hypoglycemic effect R/T ↓ GI tract absorption
Chloramphenicol / ↑ Effect R/T ↓ liver breakdown and ↓ renal excretion
Cholestyramine / ↓ Hypoglycemic effect
Clofibrate / ↑ Hypoglycemic effect R/T ↓ plasma protein binding
Corticosteroids / ↓ Hypoglcylemic effect
Diazoxide / ↓ Effects of both drugs
Digitoxin / ↑ Digitoxin serum levels
Estrogens / ↓ Hypoglycemic effect
Fenfluramine / ↑ Hypoglycemic effect
Fluconazole / ↑ Hypoglycemic effect
Gemfibrozil / ↑ Hypoglycemic effect
H *Ginseng* / ↑ Hypoglycemic effect
Histamine H_2 antagonists / ↑ Hypoglycemic effect R/T ↓ liver breakdown
Histamine H-2 angatonists / ↑ Hypoglycemic effect
Hydantoins / ↓ Effect of sulfonylureas R/T ↓ insulin release
Isoniazid / ↓ Hypoglycemic effect
Itraconazole / Possible hypoglycemia; monitor BG
Magnesium salts / ↑ Hypoglycemic effect
MAO inhibitors / ↑ Hypoglycemic effect R/T ↓ liver breakdown
Methyldopa / ↑ Hypoglycemic effect R/T ↓ liver breakdown
Niacin,Nicotinic acid / ↓ Hypoglycemic effect
NSAIDs / ↑ Hypoglycemic effect of oral antidiabetics
Oral contraceptives / ↓ Hypoglycemic effect
Phenothiazines / ↓ Hypoglycemic effect
Probenecid / ↑ Hypoglycemic effect

Rifampin / ↓ Effect of sulfonylureas R/T ↑ liver breakdown
Salicylates / ↑ Effect of oral hypoglycemics by ↓ plasma protein binding
Sulfinpyrazone / ↑ Hypoglycemic effect
Sulfonamides / ↑ Effect of oral hypoglycemics by ↓ plasma protein binding and ↓ liver breakdown
Sympathomimetics / ↓ Hypoglcyemic effect
Thiazides / ↓ Hypoglycemic effect
Tricyclic antidepressants / ↑ Hypoglycemic effect
Urinary acidifiers / ↑ Hypoglycemic effect R/T ↓ renal excretion
Urinary alkalinizers / ↓ Hypoglycemic effect R/T ↑ renal excretion

LABORATORY TEST CONSIDERATIONS

↑ BUN, serum creatinine, AST, LDH, alkaline phosphatase. Elevated LFTs. Hyponatremia.

DOSAGE

PO. See individual preparations. Adjust dosage according to needs of client. Exercise, weight loss, and diet are of primary importance in the control of diabetes.

NURSING CONSIDERATIONS

SEE ALSO *NURSING CONSIDERATIONS* FOR *INSULINS*.

ADMINISTRATION/STORAGE

1. To decrease the incidence of gastric upset, take PO drugs with food.
2. If ketonuria, acidosis, increased glycosuria, or serious side effects occur, withdraw the med.
3. Transfer from insulin:
• If receiving 20 units or less of insulin daily, initiate oral hypoglycemic therapy and discontinue insulin abruptly.
• For clients receiving 20–40 units of insulin daily, initiate oral hypoglycemic therapy and reduce insulin dose by 25%–50%. Discontinue insulin gradually, using the absence of glucose in the urine as a guide. With glyburide, insulin may be discontinued abruptly.
• For clients receiving more than 40 units of insulin daily, initiate PO therapy and reduce insulin by 20%. Discontinue insulin gradually, using glucose in the urine or finger sticks as a guide. It may be advisable to hospitalize clients on such high doses of insulin while they are being transferred to oral hypoglycemic agents.
4. Transfer from one oral hypoglycemic agent to another:
• Except for chlorpropamide, no transition period is necessary. When transferring from chlorpropamide, use caution for 1–2 weeks due to the long drug half-life.
• Mild symptoms of hyperglycemia may appear during the transfer period. Perform finger sticks and test urine for ketones regularly (1–3 times daily) during the transfer period. Positive results must be reported.
5. Be prepared to treat if client develops severe hypoglycemia.
6. Review prescribed drugs to ensure none interact.
7. Type II diabetics who do not respond to the sulfonylureas are said to be *primary failures*. Responses to the sulfonylureas during the initial months of therapy followed by failure to respond are referred to as *secondary failures*. A glucophage trial or combination therapy with insulin and/or up to three oral agents may be useful in these clients.

ASSESSMENT

1. Obtain a thorough nursing history.
2. If unsure type of diabetes may differentiate I and II with C-Peptide levels. Many younger children that are obese and inactive are developing type II diabetes at a very early age.
3. Document any stress. Clients about to undergo surgical procedures, who have suffered severe trauma, who have a fever and infection, or who are pregnant should generally not be placed on oral hypoglycemic agents.
4. Assess mental functions to determine if able to understand the complexities of the transfer process and when and how to take prescribed agents.

5. Note if taking oral contraceptives; effectiveness is lessened by oral hypoglycemic agents.
6. Note any previous experience with sulfonylureas and the outcome. Determine metformin and/or thiazolidinedione trial and the outcome; elderly do better with a slower metformin titration (i.e., increase dose weekly or increase by ½ tablet instead of a whole tablet).
7. Diabetics benefit from ACE and ASA therapy.
8. Assess for syndrome of insulin resistance i.e., obesity, HTN, ASHD, dyslipidemia, hyperinsulinumia and Type II DM.
9. Monitor VS, ECG, cholesterol panel, electrolytes, CBC, HbA1c, and urine for microalbuminuria.

CLIENT/FAMILY TEACHING

1. Record blood sugar (and if directed urine for ketones) at different times during the day and night for provider review. (Urine testing is not an accurate reflection of true serum glucose levels and should not be used to modify treatment.)
2. With hypoglycemic episodes, check finger stick at the time of the reaction. Then drink 4 oz of juice (fast-acting CHO), followed by a longer acting CHO (approximately 10 g) such as half a meat sandwich or several peanut butter crackers, and recheck finger stick in 15 min. If glucose is less than 100, repeat the process, i.e., juice and a CHO and another finger stick. Report if this occurs often.
3. Medication helps to control high BS but does not cure diabetes; therapy is usually long term.
4. Must adhere to prescribed diet if drug is to be effective; most secondary failures are due to poor dietary compliance; see dietitian as needed.
5. Regular exercise, diet, and weight control/loss are imperative.
6. Insulin may be necessary if complications occur. Review administration of insulin and how to rotate sites. Do not change brands of insulin or syringes. Review equipment, methods of storage and discarding used syringes.
7. Report illness or if unusual itching, skin rash, jaundice, dark urine, fever, sore throat, nausea/vomiting, or diarrhea occurs.
8. With thyroid scan advise lab as sulfonylureas interfere with the uptake of radioactive iodine.
9. Avoid alcohol; a disulfuram-like reaction may occur.
10. Do not take any OTC meds without approval.
11. Need close medical supervision for the first 6 weeks and periodic lab tests; oral agents may cause blood dyscrasias, acidosis or liver dysfunction.
12. Carry ID, a list of prescribed drugs, juice, and hard candy (such as Lifesavers) or a fast-acting CHO (candy bar) at all times.

OUTCOMES/EVALUATE

- Knowledge/control of diabetes; adherence with drug/diet therapy
- ↓ Hypo/hyperglycemic episodes
- HbA1c within desired range < 7
- Prevention of target organ damage

ANTIDIABETIC AGENTS: INSULINS

SEE ALSO *ANTIDIABETIC AGENTS: HYPOGLYCEMIC AGENTS.* SEE ALSO THE FOLLOWING INDIVIDUAL ENTRIES:

Insulin aspart
Insulin glargine
Insulin injection
Insulin injection concentrated
Insulin lispro injection
Insulin zinc suspension (Lente)
Insulin zinc suspension, Extended (Ultralente)

GENERAL STATEMENT

Insulin preparations with different times of onset, peak activity, and duration of action have been developed. Such products are prepared by precipitating insulin in the presence of zinc chloride to form zinc insulin crystals and/or by combining insulin with a protein such as protamine. Based on these modifications, insulin products are classified as fast-acting, intermediate-acting, and long-acting.

These preparations permit the provider to select the preparation best suited to the life-style of the client.

RAPID-ACTING INSULIN: Insulin injection (Regular Insulin, Crystalline Zinc Insulin, Unmodified Insulin)

INTERMEDIATE-ACTING INSULIN
1. Insulin zinc suspension (Lente)

LONG-ACTING INSULIN: Insulin zinc suspension extended (Ultralente)

NOTE: Insulin preparations with various times of onset and duration of action are often mixed to obtain optimum control in diabetic clients.

ACTION/KINETICS

Following combination with insulin receptors on cell plasma membranes, insulin facilitates the transport of glucose into cardiac and skeletal muscle and adipose tissue. It also increases synthesis of glycogen in the liver. Insulin stimulates protein synthesis and lipogenesis and inhibits lipolysis and release of free fatty acids from fat cells.This latter effect prevents or reverses the ketoacidosis sometimes observed in the type I diabetic. Insulin also causes intracellular shifts in magnesium and potassium.

Since insulin is a protein, it is destroyed in the GI tract. Thus, it must be administered SC so that it is readily absorbed into the bloodstream and distributed throughout the extracellular fluid. Metabolized mainly by the liver.

USES

Human insulins are being used almost exclusively. Replacement therapy in type I diabetes. Diabetic ketoacidosis or diabetic coma (use regular insulin). Insulin is also indicated in type II diabetes when other measures have failed (e.g., diet, exercise, weight reduction) or with surgery, trauma, infection, fever, endocrine dysfunction, pregnancy, gangrene, Raynaud's disease, kidney or liver dysfunction.

Regular insulin is used in IV HA solutions, in IV dextrose to treat severe hyperkalemia, and IV as a provocative test for growth hormone secretion.

Insulin and oral hypoglycemic drugs have been used in type II diabetics who are difficult to control with diet and PO therapy alone.

DIET

The dietary control of diabetes is as important as medication with appropriate drugs. The role of the nurse and dietitian in teaching the client how to eat properly cannot be underestimated. They must teach the client how to calculate exchange values of various foods. Food lists and food-exchange values published by the American Diabetes Association and the American Dietetic Association are valuable teaching aids.

Diabetic clients should adhere to a regular meal schedule. The frequency of meals and the overall caloric intake vary with the type of drug taken and individual client needs. Close attention to meal frequency and meal planning is imperative and a registered dietitian should be consulted. Diabetic children may be on a less restricted diet, adjusting the insulin dosage according to blood and urine glucose readings. Children with negative urine glucose tend to become hypoglycemic rapidly with exercise or decrease in appetite, and many providers allow for glucose spilling.

CONTRAINDICATIONS

Hypersensitivity to insulin.

SPECIAL CONCERNS

Pregnant diabetic clients often manifest decreased insulin requirements during the first half of pregnancy and increased requirements during the latter half. Lactation may decrease insulin requirements.

SIDE EFFECTS

Hypoglycemia: Due to insulin overdose, delayed or decreased food intake, too much exercise in relationship to insulin dose, or when transferring from one preparation to another. Even carefully controlled clients occasionally develop signs of insulin overdosage characterized by one or more of the following: hunger, weakness, fatigue, nervousness, pallor or flushing, profuse sweating, headache, palpitations, numbness of mouth, tingling in the fingers, tremors, blurred and double vision, hypothermia, excess yawning, mental confusion, incoordination, tachycardia, loss of sensitivity, and loss of consciousness. Level of awareness is markedly diminished after an attack.

Symptoms of hypoglycemia may mimic those of psychic disturbances. Severe prolonged hypoglycemia may cause brain damage, and in the elderly, may mimic stroke. **Allergic:** Urticaria, angioedema, lymphadenopathy, bullae, anaphylaxis. Occurs mostly following intermittent insulin therapy or IV administration of large doses to insulin-resistant clients. Antihistamines or corticosteroids may be used to treat these symptoms. Clients who are highly allergic to insulin and cannot be treated with oral hypoglycemics may respond to human insulin products. **At site of injection:** Swelling, stinging, redness, itching, warmth. These symptoms often disappear with continued use. Lipoatrophy or hypertrophy of subcutaneous fat tissue (minimize by rotating site of injection). **Insulin resistance:** Usual cause is obesity. Acute resistance may occur following infections, trauma, surgery, emotional disturbances, or other endocrine disorders. **Ophthalmologic:** Blurred vision, transient presbyopia. Occurs mainly during initiation of therapy or in clients who have been uncontrolled for a long period of time.

Hypokalemia.

Hyperglycemic rebound (Somogyi effect): Usually in clients who receive chronic overdosage.

DIFFERENTIATION BETWEEN DIABETIC COMA AND HYPOGLYCEMIC REACTION (INSULIN SHOCK)

Coma in diabetes may be caused by uncontrolled diabetes (high sugar content in blood or urine, ketoacidosis) or by too much insulin (insulin shock, hypoglycemia).

Diabetic coma and insulin shock can be differentiated in the following manner:

HYPERGLYCEMIA (DIABETIC COMA) (Diabetic Coma)

Onset / Gradual (days)
Medication / Insufficient insulin
Food intake / Normal or excess
Overall appearance / Extremely ill
Skin / Dry and flushed
Infection / Frequent
Fever / Frequent
Mouth / Dry
Thirst / Intense
Hunger / Absent
Vomiting / Common
Abdominal pain / Frequent
Respiration / Increased, air hunger
Breath / Acetone odor
BP / Low
Pulse / Weak and rapid
Vision / Dim
Tremor / Absent
Convulsions / None
Urine sugar / High
Ketone bodies / High (type I only)
Blood sugar / High

HYPOGLYCEMIA (INSULIN SHOCK) (Insulin Shock)

Onset / Sudden (24–48 hr)
Medication / Excess insulin
Food intake / Probably too little
Overall appearance / Very weak
Skin / Moist and pale
Infection / Absent
Fever / Absent
Mouth / Drooling
Thirst / Absent
Hunger / Occasional
Vomiting / Absent
Abdominal pain / Rare
Respiration / Normal
Breath / Normal
BP / Normal
Pulse / Full and bounding
Vision / Diplopia
Tremor / Frequent
Convulsions / In late stages
Urine sugar / Absent in second specimen
Ketone bodies / Absent in second specimen
Blood sugar / Less than 60 mg/100 mL

Source: Adapted with permission from *The Merck Manual*, 11th ed.

Diabetic coma is usually precipitated by the client's failure to take insulin. Hypoglycemia is often precipitated by the client's unpredictable response, excess exertion, stress due to illness or surgery, errors in calculating dosage, or failure to eat.

TREATMENT OF DIABETIC COMA OR SEVERE ACIDOSIS: Administer 30–60 units regular insulin. This is followed by doses of 20 units or more q 30 min. To avoid a hypoglycemic state, 1 g dextrose is administered for each unit of insulin given. Treatment is often supplemented by electrolytes and fluids. Urine samples are collected for analysis, and VS are monitored as ordered.

TREATMENT OF HYPOGLYCEMIA (INSULIN SHOCK): Mild hypoglycemia can be relieved by PO administration of CHO such as orange juice, candy, or a lump of sugar. If comatose, adults may be given 10–30 mL of 50% dextrose solution IV; children should receive 0.5–1 mL/kg of 50% dextrose solution. Epinephrine, hydrocortisone, or glucagon may be used in severe cases to cause an increase in blood glucose.

DRUG INTERACTIONS

ACE Inhibitors / ↑ Hypoglycemic effect of insulin
Acetazolamide / ↓ Hypoglycemic effect of insulin
AIDS Antiviral drugs / ↓ Hypoglycemic effect of insulin
Albuterol / ↓ Hypoglycemic effect of insulin
Alcohol, ethyl / ↑ Hypoglycemia → low blood sugar and shock
Anabolic steroids / ↑ Hypoglycemic effect of insulin
Asparaginase / ↓ Hypoglycemic effect of insulin
Beta-adrenergic blocking agents / ↑ Hypoglycemic effect of insulin
Calcitonin / ↓ Hypoglycemic effect of insulin
Calcium / ↑ Hypoglycemic effect of insulin
Chloroquine / ↑ Hypoglycemic effect of insulin
Chlorthalidone / ↓ Hypoglycemic effect of antidiabetics
Clofibrate / ↑ Hypoglycemic effects of insulin
Clonidine / ↑ Hypoglycemic effect of insulin
Contraceptives, oral / ↑ Dosage of antidiabetic due to impairment of glucose tolerance; / ↓ Hypoglycemic effect of insulin
Corticosteroids / ↓ Effect of insulin due to corticosteroid-inducedhyperglycemia
Cyclophosphamide / ↓ Hypoglycemic effect of insulin
Danazol / ↓ Hypoglycemic effect of insulin
Dextrothyroxine / ↓ Effect of insulin due to dextrothyroxine-induced hyperglycemia
Diazoxide / Diazoxide-induced hyperglycemia ↓ diabetic control
Digitalis glycosides / Use with caution, as insulin affects serum potassium levels
Diltiazen / ↓ Effect of insulin
Disopyramide / ↑ Hypoglycemic effect of insulin
Diuretics / ↓ Hypoglycemic effect of insulin
Dobutamine / ↓ Effect of insulin
Epinephrine / ↓ Effect of insulin due to epinephrine-induced hyperglycemia
Estrogens / ↓ Effect of insulin due to impairment of glucose tolerance
Ethacrynic acid / ↓ Hypoglycemic effect of antidiabetics
Fenfluramine / Additive hypoglycemic effects
Fluoxetine / ↑ Hypoglycemic effect of insulin
Furosemide / ↓ Hypoglycemic effect of antidiabetics
H *Ginseng* / Possible additive hypoglycemic effects
Glucagon / Glucagon-induced hyperglycemia ↓ effect of antidiabetics
Guanethidine / ↑ Hypoglycemic effect of insulin
Isoniazid / ↓ Hypoglycemic effect of insulin
Lithium carbonate / ↑ or ↓ Hypoglycemic effect of insulin

MAO inhibitors / MAO inhibitors ↑ and prolong hypoglycemic effect of antidiabetics
Mebendazole / ↑ Hypoglycemic effect of insulin
Morphine sulfate / ↓ Hypoglyemic effect of insulin
Niacin ↓ Hypoglyemic effect of insulin
Nicotine ↓ Hypoglyemic effect of insulin
Octreotide / ↑ Hypoglycemic effect of insulin
Oxytetracycline / ↑ Effect of insulin
Pentamidine / ↑ Hypoglycemic effect of insulin; may be followed by hyperglycemia
Phenothiazines / ↑ Dosage of antidiabetic due to phenothiazine-induced hyperglycemia
Phenytoin / Phenytoin-induced hyperglycemia ↓ diabetic control
Propoxyphene / ↑ Hypoglycemic effect of insulin
Propranolol / Inhibits rebound of blood glucose after insulin-induced hypoglycemia
H *Psyllium seed/Blonde psyllium seed husk* / Possible need to ↓ insulin dose
Pyridoxine / ↑ Hypoglycemic effect of insulin
Salicylates / ↑ Effect of hypoglycemic effect of insulin
Somatropin ↓ Hypoglyemic effect of insulin
Sulfinpyrazone / ↑ Hypoglycemic effect of insulin
Sulfonamide / ↑ Hypoglycemic effect of insulin
Terbutaline ↓ Hypoglyemic effect of insulin
Tetracyclines / May ↑ hypoglycemic effect of insulin
Thiazide diuretics / ↓ Hypoglycemic effect of antidiabetics
Thyroid preparations / ↓ Effect of antidiabetic due to thyroid-induced hyperglycemia
Triamterene / ↓ Hypoglycemic effect of antidiabetic

LABORATORY TEST CONSIDERATIONS

Alters liver function tests and thyroid function tests. False + Coombs' test, ↑ serum protein, ↓ serum amino acids, calcium, cholesterol, potassium, and urine amino acids.

DOSAGE

Dosage highly individualized. Usually administered SC. Insulin injection (regular insulin) is the **only** preparation that may be administered IV. Give IV only for clients with severe ketoacidosis or diabetic coma. Dosage for insulin is always expressed in USP units.

Dosage is established and monitored by blood glucose (often using glucose monitoring machines in the home), urine glucose, and acetone tests. Furthermore, since requirements may change with time, dosage must be checked at regular intervals. It may be advisable to hospitalize some clients while their daily insulin and caloric requirements are being established. The main goal is to control the blood sugar and send the client home to fine tune as generally the home environment is more reliable for determining drug requirements.

In pregnancy, insulin requirements may increase suddenly during the last trimester. After delivery, requirements may suddenly drop to prepregnancy levels. To prevent the development of hypoglycemia, insulin is often discontinued on the day of delivery and glucose is administered IV.

The various insulin preparations can be mixed to obtain the combination best suited for the individual client. However, mixing must be done according to the directions received from the physician/provider and/or pharmacist.

NURSING CONSIDERATIONS

Also includes general applications for all clients with diabetes controlled by medication (whether it be insulin or an oral hypoglycemic agent).

ADMINISTRATION/STORAGE

1. Read product information and any important notes inserted into the insulin package.

2. Discard open vials not used for several weeks or whose expiration date has passed.
3. Refrigerate stock supply of insulin but avoid freezing. Freezing destroys the manner in which insulin is suspended in the formulation.
4. Store vial in a cool place, avoiding extremes of temperature or exposure to sunlight.
5. Use the following guidelines with respect to mixing the various insulins:
• Regular insulin may be mixed with NPH or Lente insulins. However, to avoid transfer of the longer-acting insulin into the regular insulin vial, withdraw regular insulin into the syringe first.
• Give a mixture of regular insulin with NPH or Lente insulin within 15 min of mixing due to binding of regular insulin by excess protamine and/or zinc in the longer-acting preparations.
• Lente or Ultralente insulins may be mixed with each other in any proportion; however, do not mix these with NPH insulins.
• When used in an insulin infusion pump, insulin may be mixed in any proportion with either 0.9% NaCl injection or water for injection. Due to stability changes, use such mixtures within 24 hr of their preparation. Buffered insulin is usually the form prescribed and utilized in pumps.
6. Store compatible insulin mixtures for no longer than 1 month at room temperature or 3 months at 2–8°C (36–46°F); bacterial contamination may occur.
7. To ensure a constant amount of precipitate in each dose, invert the vial several times to mix before withdrawing the material. Avoid vigorous shaking and frothing of the material. (Regular and globin insulin are the only two insulins that do not have a precipitate.)
8. Discard any vial in which the precipitate is clumped or granular in appearance or which has formed a solid deposit of particles on the side of the vial.
9. To prevent dosage error, do not alter the order of mixing insulins or change the model or brand of syringe or needle.
10. Administer at a 90° angle with a 28- or 29-gauge needle. Syringes come in 0.3-cc (30-U), 0.5-cc (50-U) and 1-cc (100-U) sizes. Get the smallest syringe with the smallest needles to enhance dosage validity (e.g., if client is prescribed less than 30 U insulin, advise to obtain the 0.3-cc syringe).
11. Provide an automatic injector for clients fearful of injections.
12. Assist visually impaired clients to obtain information and devices for self-administration by consulting their local diabetes association or by writing to the American Diabetes Association, 149 Madison Avenue, New York, NY 10016 (telephone: 212-725-4925), for their buyer's guide, which lists numerous available products for diabetics. Clients may also contact The Lighthouse, Inc., 800 Second Avenue, New York, NY 10017 (telephone: 212-808-0077) for additional information on visual impairments.
13. Lipoatrophy may occur. This may appear as mild dimpling of the skin or as deep pits in young girls and women and lipodystrophy, appearing as well-developed muscle on the anterior and lateral thighs of young boys and men. To prevent, rotate injection sites.
• Make a chart indicating the injection sites (see Figure 1).
• Allow 3–4 cm between sites.
• Do not inject in the same site for at least 1–2 weeks.
• Avoid injecting within 1 cm around the umbilicus because of the high vascularity in this area.
• Avoid injections around the waistline because of the sensitive nerve supply to this area and the potential for fabric irritation.
• Use insulin at room temperature to prevent lipodystrophy.
14. Rotation of injection sites may lead to differences in blood levels of insulin. The abdomen is considered the

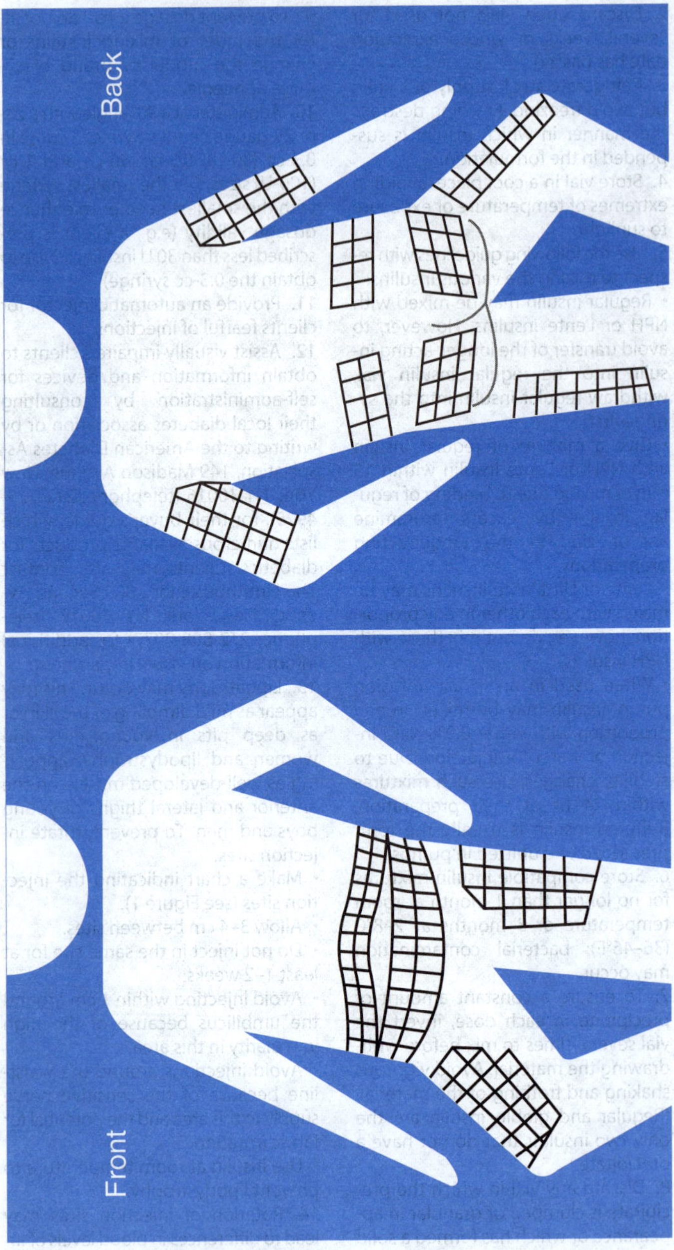

Back

Front

best site due to constant insulin peak times with better gradual absorption. Apply gentle pressure after injection but do not massage since this may alter rate of absorption.
15. If insulin has been refrigerated, allow it to remain at room temperature for at least 1 hr before using.
16. If breakfast is delayed for lab tests, check for dosage adjustment.

ASSESSMENT

1. Obtain a thorough history and physical exam. Note any first-degree relatives with disease.
2. Assess for S&S of hyperglycemia: thirst, polydypsia, polyuria, drowsiness, blurred vision, loss of appetite, fruity odor to the breath, and flushed dry skin.
3. Assess for S&S of hypoglycemia: drowsiness, chills, confusion, anxiety, cold sweats, cool pale skin, excessive hunger, nausea, headache, irritability, shakiness, rapid pulse, and unusual weakness or tiredness.
4. Determine when first noticed changes in physical condition and what these changes were.
5. Weigh to determine amount of agent needed.
6. Monitor electrolytes, lipid profile, thyroid studies, BS, phosphate, Mg, CBC, HbA1c, and urinalysis. Assess for microalbuminuria.
7. Assess psychologic state, including disease acceptance, readiness to learn, support system, evidence of depression, or need for counseling.
8. During physical exam assess DTRs; check extremities (use monofilament) to assess sensation and for evidence of neuropathy. Review proper foot care with each visit.
9. Consider ACE therapy to prevent/preserve renal function and inhibit organ damage and ASA for CAD protection.
10. Assess injection sites, monitor VS, plot growth and weight every 3–4 months.
11. Schedule yearly eye exams if over 12 yrs; or younger if > 5 yrs with the disease.

INTERVENTIONS

1. For a *hyperglycemic reaction:*
- Have regular insulin available.
- Obtain BS or finger stick.
- Monitor after giving insulin for further signs of hyperglycemia such as SOB, facial flushing, air hunger, and acetone breath.

2. Assess for S&S of *hypoglycemia,* such as easy fatigue, hunger, headache, cold, clammy, drowsiness, nausea, lassitude, and tremulousness. Most likely to occur before meals, during or after exercise, and at insulin peak action times (i.e., 3 a.m. with evening dosing).
- Weakness, sweating, tremors, and/or nervousness may occur later.
- Excessive restlessness and profuse sweating at night.
- Obtain BS or finger stick; promptly give 4 oz of juice and a CHO, if conscious.
- If conscious and taking long-acting insulin, also give a slowly digestible CHO, such as bread with corn syrup or honey. Give additional CHO such as crackers and milk for the next 2 hr.

Figure 1 Each injection area is divided into squares; each square is an injection site. Start in a corner of an injection area and move down or across the injection sites in order. Jumping from site to site will make it more difficult to remember where the last shot was administered. Keep track of the rotation pattern to assist in maintaining site rotation. A grid may be developed from this figure and numbered to keep track of injections. Systematically use all the sites in one area before moving to another (for example, use all the sites in both arms before moving to the legs). This will help keep the blood sugar more even from day to day. An important consideration when choosing injection sites is that insulin is absorbed into the bloodstream faster from some areas than from others; it enters the bloodstream most quickly from the abdomen (stomach), a little more slowly from the arms, even more slowly from the legs, and most slowly from the buttocks. (Courtesy Eli Lilly & Company.)

• If unconscious, apply honey or Karo syrup to the buccal membrane or give glucagon.
• If hospitalized, minimally responsive or unconscious, give 10%–20% IV dextrose solution.
3. A Somogyi effect is often mistaken as client not following the prescribed therapy. This occurs when hypoglycemia triggers the release of epinephrine and glucocorticoids, which stimulates glycogenesis and results in a higher a.m. BS level. Reduction in bedtime insulin dosage is necessary to stabilize. If treated for hypoglycemia, check 3 a.m. BS; if normal and then BS rises between 3 a.m. and 7 a.m., this is related to growth hormone release—termed the Dawn Phenomenon. To control, give long-acting insulin at bedtime instead of at dinnertime.
4. Juveniles with type I diabetes demand closer attention and observation for infection or emotional disturbances and hypoglycemia. They are more susceptible to insulin shock and have a more limited response to glucagon. Determine if managed with intensive or conventional insulin therapy; adjust for hypoglycemia unawareness (when client passes out due to loss of catecholamine response). Assess for insulin pump placement for better control.
5. For the newly diagnosed elderly client, start insulin doses low and gradually increase.
6. The usual dose of NPH insulin is 0.8–1.5 U/kg; give two-thirds of dose in a.m. and one-third of dose in p.m. If using regular insulin, try 1:2 in a.m. and 1:1 in p.m. with NPH.
7. Identify BS goals, i.e., young child 80–150 mg/dL premeal and 100–150 mg/dL at bedtime; adolescent 70–150 mg/dL premeal and 100–150 mg/dL at bedtime; adult 70–150 mg/dL premeal and 100–150 mg/dL at bedtime and adjust as symptoms and condition dictate.

CLIENT/FAMILY TEACHING

1. Medications assist to control diabetes but do not cure it. Type I diabetes is usually early onset and the pancreas makes little or no insulin; individuals with type I diabetes must take insulin injections or they will die. Type II diabetes is usually later onset and the pancreas still makes insulin, but the body cannot use it (termed insulin resistance); individuals with type II diabetes can use either oral hypoglycemic agents or insulin to lower their blood sugar or a combination of different oral agents and to help them utilize their own insulin better. Elevated C-Peptide lab test may help with differentation between type I and type II.
2. In type I diabetics, urine ketones indicate that there is not enough insulin present to get the body's sugar into the cells so it is burning body fat as an alternative and producing ketones as waste products; may lead to ketoacidosis, a life-threatening condition. Test urine for ketones with a "dip-and-read" product when:
• Finger sticks > 240 mg/dL
• Pregnant
• Experiencing severe stress
• Vomiting or sick to stomach
• Sick with flu/cold or virus infection
• Experiencing symptoms of hyperglycemia (unusual fatigue, vision difficulty, increased thirst and/or hunger, polydipsia, unusually tired or sleepy, stomach pain, increased nausea, fruity odor to breath, rapid respirations, weight loss without altering food intake or activity patterns)
3. Perform finger sticks to monitor glucose levels. Review instructions for technique, calibration, operation, and device maintenance. Bring in periodically to double check machine accuracy and to review data bank to ensure values coincide with client log. Some general principles may be followed.
• Rotate sites.
• Cleanse area with soap and water or alcohol prior to stabbing.
• Use a lancet and lancet device to access sample
• Stab finger outside, by nail, where the capillaries are abundant and let a bead of blood form.
• Wipe off with a cotton ball.

• Let blood bead re-form and apply to the test strip.
• Use proper test strips for designated machine; check expiration date
• Follow specific guidelines for the device in use.
4. Regimens are specific to the individual, based on age, severity of diabetes, weight, any other medical problems they have, as well as the philosophy of the health care team.
5. Take insulin 30 min before a meal (exception is Humalog, which can be taken at meal time). Administer at a 90° angle with a 28- or 29-gauge needle. Syringes come in 0.3-cc (30-U), 0.5-cc (50-U) and 1-cc (100-U) sizes. Purchase the smallest syringe with the smallest needles to enhance dosage validity (e.g., if prescribed less than 30 U insulin, obtain the 0.3-cc syringe). May reuse disposable insulin syringes; based on comfort and perceived dullness.
6. Use a chart as in figure 1 to document and rotate injection sites to avoid lipohypertrophy of injection sites (lumps from scar tissue after many injections). Avoid these areas due to unreliable absorption.
• For self-injection, may brace the arm against a hard surface such as the wall or a chair.
• Cleanse the area thoroughly with alcohol, allow to dry, then, depending on the condition of the skin, either pinch between the thumb and forefingers of one hand, or spread the skin using the thumb and fingers of one hand.
• Insert into the subcutaneous tissue and aspirate to be sure needle is not in a blood vessel.
• Inject insulin and withdraw the needle.
7. Review use and care of equipment, proper storage and disposal of needles and syringes, and provision and storage of drug.
8. *Always* check expiration dates; have an extra vial and equipment on hand for traveling, away from home, or when detained or hospitalized.
9. Have regular insulin for emergency use.
10. Must balance food, insulin, and exercise. Exercise increases the utilization of CHO and increases CHO needs. Have snacks available; 5–8 Lifesavers, juice, or hard candy helps counteract hypoglycemia.
11. Adhere to prescribed diet, weight control, and ingestion of food relative to the peak action of insulin being used. Record weekly weights; reduce intake of animal fats and salt; select a variety of foods to meet starch and sugar, protein, and fat requirements (usual recommendation, CHO 50%; protein 20%; fat 30%). Consume the kinds of fiber that help lower BS and fat levels (breads, cereals, and crackers made from whole grains, such as whole wheat and brown rice, fresh vegetables and fruits, dried beans, and peas), low cholesterol and polyunsaturated and monosaturated fats.
12. Confer with dietitian for assistance in shopping, food selection/exchanges, diet, and meal planning. Consume premeal snacks in the a.m., midday, and at bedtime.
13. If ill and omit a meal because of fever, nausea, or vomiting, replace solid foods that contain starch and sugar, such as bread and fruit, with liquids that contain sugar (fruit juice, regular sodas) and follow designated sliding scale for "sick days." Do not omit insulin or hypoglycemic agents unless instructed. Perform finger sticks q 4 hr, and with type I, also test urine for ketones; report if moderate or high.
14. Blurred vision may occur at beginning of insulin therapy; should subside in 6–8 weeks. The effect is caused by fluctuation of blood glucose levels, which produce osmotic changes in the lens of the eye and within the ocular fluids. If it does not clear up in 8 weeks, consult eye doctor.
15. May experience allergic responses: itching, redness, swelling, stinging, or warmth may occur at the injection site and usually disappears after a

few weeks of therapy. Report as purified or human insulins are used for local allergy and lipohypertrophy at injection site.

16. Failure to take insulin will result in ketoacidosis. Adjust insulin based on BS and guidelines for insulin administration during sick days. Identify soft foods and liquids to consume for sick days (i.e., regular soda, apple juice, clear broth, cream soups, puddings, apple sauce, popsicle, ice cream).

17. If ill, notify provider; to prevent coma, maintain adequate hydration by drinking 1 cup or more of noncaloric fluids such as coffee, tea, water, or broth every hour. Test finger sticks and urine more; identify when to go to the emergency room.

18. If there is no insulin/equipment to administer, decrease food intake by one-third and drink plenty of noncaloric fluids. Obtain supplies as soon as possible and return to prescribed diet and insulin dosage.

19. Follow good hygienic practices to prevent infection. Bathe daily with mild soap and lukewarm water. Use lotion to prevent skin dryness. Avoid injury from punctures. Avoid scratches; wear gloves when working with the hands. Always protect feet and wear shoes. Use sunscreen and protective clothing to avoid sunburn, and dress appropriately for the weather; prevent frostbite.

20. Establish a daily routine of checking and caring for the feet (use a mirror if unable to bend over). Wear comfortable shoes (leather or canvas) and stockings (no garters or elastic tops) and do exercises. Clip toenails (straight across); do not undertake any self-treatment for ingrown toenails, corns, warts, or calluses. Do not use any heat treatments, hot water bottles, or heating pads, and do not smoke, as this decreases blood flow to the feet. Obtain annual foot screen.

21. Hyperglycemia compounds risk for tooth and gum problems; brush after meals, floss, and see dentist regularly.

22. Diabetes can damage the small blood vessels to the eye; obtain yearly eye exams. Eye damage has no symptoms in the early, treatable stage. Report blurred or double vision, narrowed visual fields, increased difficulty seeing in dim light, pressure or pain in the eye, or seeing dark spots.

23. May experience decreased sensation in feet, legs, and hands; use care when handling hot or cold items, wear shoes to protect feet, and dress appropriately for the weather.

24. Carry ID noting "diabetic" and list of meds, who to notify and what to do if unable to respond.

25. Avoid alcohol; causes hypoglycemia. Excessive intake may require a reduction of insulin; also causes a disulfiram-type reaction with oral hypoglycemic agents.

26. Carry all medications, syringes, glucagon, and blood testing equipment in carry-on luggage when traveling. Always carry diabetes ID. Keep to the usual meal, exercise, and medication routines as closely as possible. Carry food and fast-acting sugar in the event meals are delayed. Request meds for vomiting/diarrhea and plan ahead for mealtimes when crossing two or more time zones. Protect insulin and test strips from extremes in heat or cold (keeping between 15 and 30°C or 59 and 86°F).

27. Use only the insulin prescribed; check for correct species (human, beef, pork, or mixed beef-pork), brand name (Lispro, Humulin, Iletin I, Iletin II, etc.), and type (Regular, Lente, NPH, etc.).

28. Check vials before each dose is taken. Regular and Buffered Regular insulin (for pumps) should be clear and colorless, whereas other forms may be cloudy except for the new longest acting form.

29. Two kinds of insulin can be mixed in the same syringe:

- Regular insulin can be mixed with any other insulin.
- Lente forms can be mixed with other Lente insulins but cannot be mixed

with other insulins except regular insulin.
• Do not mix the fast acting lispro with other agents
• A single form of insulin in a syringe can be stable for weeks or a month.
• Except for the commercially prepared mixtures, mixtures of insulin are not stable and should be administered within 5 min of preparation.
• When mixed, regular (unmodified) insulin should always be drawn up in the syringe first.

30. Impotence may be caused by damaged nerves and reduced blood flow related to diabetes; see urologist to find cause and best treatment.
31. Silent heart attacks may occur. Identify risk factors and alter life-style to prevent CAD (i.e., regular exercise, low-fat, low-salt, low-cholesterol diet, no tobacco or alcohol, stress/weight reduction).
32. Identify local diabetic educator and support groups to assist in understanding and coping with this disease. The American Diabetes Association, 1660 Duke Street, Alexandria, VA 22314 (telephone: 703-549-1500 or 1-800-ADA-DISC) and local diabetes support groups offer additional information and support.

OUTCOMES/EVALUATE

• Understanding/control of DM
• Positive lifestyle changes
• BS, HbA1c, renal and LFTs WNL
• Healthy skin at injection sites
• Prevent target organ damage

ANTIEMETICS

SEE ALSO THE FOLLOWING INDIVIDUAL ENTRIES:

Dimenhydrinate
Diphenhydramine hydrochloride
Dronabinol
Granisetron hydrochloride
Hydroxyzine hydrochloride
Hydroxyzine pamoate
Meclizine hydrochloride
Ondansetron hydrochloride
Prochlorperazine
Prochlorperazine edisylate
Prochlorperazine maleate
Scopolamine hydrobromide
Trimethobenzamide hydrochloride

GENERAL STATEMENT

Nausea and vomiting can be caused by a variety of conditions, such as infections, drugs, radiation, motion, organic disease, or psychologic factors. The underlying cause of the symptoms must be elicited before emesis is corrected. Many drugs used for other conditions, such as the antihistamines, phenothiazines, barbiturates, and scopolamine, have antiemetic properties and can be used. However, CNS depression make their routine use undesirable.

DRUG INTERACTIONS

Because of their antiemetic and antinauseant activity, the antiemetics may mask overdosage caused by other drugs.

NURSING CONSIDERATIONS

ASSESSMENT

1. Determine if nausea is an unusual occurrence or a recurring phenomenon; establish onset, duration, and associated factors such as vertigo, chemotherapy, or illness. Note past use of antiemetics and response.
2. Ensure no intestinal obstruction, drug overdose, or increased ICP.
3. Determine physiologic mechanism triggering N&V. Generally, if centrally mediated to the CTZ, would see nausea without vomiting, whereas if the vomiting center were triggered directly, then may see retching with vomiting.
4. Assess for other effects; antiemetics may mask signs of underlying pathology or overdosage of other drugs.
5. Monitor I&O; observe for dehydration. Offer liquids and advance to regular foods as tolerated.

CLIENT/FAMILY TEACHING

1. Drug may cause dizziness/drowsiness; avoid driving or other hazardous tasks til drug effects evaluated.
2. Practice measures to decrease

nausea such as ice chips, sips of water, nongreasy foods, removal of noxious stimuli (odors or materials), and frequent oral hygiene. Advance diet only as tolerated.
3. Dangle legs before standing, rise slowly to prevent symptoms of orthostatic hypotension (↓ BP, ↑ dizziness).
4. Report any unresponsive N&V or abdominal pain.
5. Avoid alcohol and any other nonprescribed CNS depressants.

OUTCOMES/EVALUATE

- Control of N&V; prevention of dehydration
- Improved nutritional status with weight gain/ ↑ caloric intake

ANTIHISTAMINES (H_1 BLOCKERS)

SEE ALSO THE FOLLOWING INDIVIDUAL ENTRIES:

FIRST GENERATION:
Brompheniramine maleate
Chlorpheniramine maleate
Cyproheptadine hydrochloride
Diphenhydramine hydrochloride
Hydroxyzine hydrochloride
Hydroxyzine pamoate
Meclizine hydrochloride
Promethazine hydrochloride

SECOND GENERATION:
Cetirizine hydrochloride
Desloratadine
Fexofenadine hydrochloride
Loratidine

OPHTHALMIC ANTIHISTAMINES:
Emedastine difumarate
Levocabastine hydrochloride
Olopatadine hydrochloride

ACTION/KINETICS

Compete with histamine at H_1 histamine receptors (reversible competitive inhibition), thus preventing or reversing the effects of histamine. First-generation antihistamines bind to central and peripheral H_1 receptors and can cause CNS depression or stimulation. Second-generation antihistamines are selective for peripheral H_1 receptors and cause less sedation. Antihistamines do not prevent the release of histamine, antibody production, or antigen-antibody interactions. Antihistamines prevent or reduce increased capillary permeability (i.e., decrease edema, itching) and bronchospasms. Allergic reactions unrelated to histamine release are not affected by antihistamines. Certain of the first-generation antihistamines also have anticholinergic, antiemetic, antipruritic, or antiserotonin effects. Clients unresponsive to a certain antihistamine may regain sensitivity by switching to a different antihistamine.

From a chemical point of view, the antihistamines can be divided into the following classes.

FIRST GENERATION:

1. **Alkylamines.** Among the most potent antihistamines. Minimal sedation, moderate anticholinergic effects, and no antiemetic effects. Paradoxical excitation may also occur. Examples: Brompheniramine, chlorpheniramine, dexchlorpheniramine.
2. **Ethanolamine Derivatives.** Moderate to high sedative, anticholinergic, and antiemetic effects. Low incidence of GI side effects. Examples: Clemastine, diphenhydramine.
3. **Phenothiazines.** High antihistaminic, sedative, and anticholinergic effects; very high antiemetic effect. Example: Promethazine.
4. **Piperazine.** High antihistaminic, sedative, and antiemetic effects; moderate anticholinergic effects. Example: Hydroxyzine.
5. **Piperidines.** Moderate antihistaminic and anticholinergic effects; low to moderate sedation; no antiemetic effects. Examples: Azatadine, cyproheptadine, phenindamine.

SECOND GENERATION:

1. **Phthalazinone.** High antihistaminic effect; low to no sedative and anticholinergic effects; no antiemetic effect. Example: Azelastine.
2. **Piperazine.** Moderate to high antihistamine effect; low to no sedation or anticholinergic effects; no antiemetic activity. Example: Cetirizine.
2. **Piperidines.** Moderate to high antihistamine activity; low to no seda-

tion and anticholinergic activity; no antiemetic action. Examples: Desloratadine, fexofenadine, loratidine.

The kinetics of most first-generation antihistamines are similar. **Onset:** 15–30 min; **peak:** 1–2 hr; **duration:** 4–6 hr (piperidines have a longer duration). Many antihistamines are available as timed-release preparations. Most first-generation antihistamines are metabolized by the liver and excreted in the urine. The pharmacokinetics of the second-generation antihistamines vary; consult individual drugs.

USES

PO: Treatment of vasomotor, perennial, or seasonal allergic rhinitis and allergic conjunctivitis. Treatment of angioedema, urticarial transfusion reactions, urticaria, pruritus. Atopic dermatitis, contact dermatitis, pruritus ani, pruritus vulvae, insect bites. Sneezing and rhinorrhea due to the common cold. Treatment of anaphylaxis, parkinsonism, drug-induced extrapyramidal reactions, vertigo. Prophylaxis and treatment of motion sickness, including N&V. Nighttime sleep aid.

Parenteral: Relief of allergic reactions due to blood or plasma. As an adjunct to epinephrine in treating anaphylaxis. Uncomplication allergic conditions when PO therapy is not possible.

SEE ALSO THE INDIVIDUAL DRUGS.

CONTRAINDICATIONS

First-generation antihistamines. Hypersensitivity to the drug, narrow-angle glaucoma, symptomatic prostatic hypertrophy, stenosing peptic ulcer, and pyloroduodenal or bladder neck obstruction. Use with MAO inhibitors. Pregnancy or possibility thereof (some agents), lactation, premature and newborn infants. The phenothiazine-type antihistamines are contraindicated in CNS depression from any cause, bone marrow depression, jaundice, dehydrated or acutely ill children, and in comatose clients. Use to treat lower respiratory tract symptoms such as asthma.

Second-generation antihistamines. Hypersensitivity to specific or chemically-related antihistamines.

SPECIAL CONCERNS

Administer with caution to clients with convulsive disorders and in respiratory disease. May diminish mental alertness in children and may occasionally cause excitation; larger doses may cause hallucinations, convulsions, and death in infants and children. Use in geriatric clients may result in dizziness, excessive sedation, syncope, toxic confusional states, and hypotension.

SIDE EFFECTS

CNS: Sedation ranging from mild drowsiness to deep sleep. Dizziness, incoordination, faintness, fatigue, confusion, lassitude, restlessnesss, excitation, nervousness, tremor, ***tonic-clonic seizures,*** headache, irritability, insomnia, euphoria, paresthesias, oculogyric crisis, torticollis, catatonic-like states, hallucinations, disorientation, tongue protrusion (usually with IV use or overdosage), disturbing dreams, nightmares, pseudoschizophrenia, weakness, diplopia, vertigo, hysteria, neuritis, paradoxical excitation, epileptiform seizures in clients with focal lesions. Extrapyramidal reactions include opisthotonus, dystonia, akathisia, dyskinesia, and parkinsonism. **CV:** Postural hypotension, palpitations, bradycardia, tachycardia, reflex tachycardia, extrasystoles, increased or decreased BP, ECG changes (including blunting of T waves and prolongation of the Q-T interval), ***cardiac arrest.*** **GI:** Epigastric distress, anorexia, increased appetite and weight gain, N&V, diarrhea, constipation, change in bowel habits, stomatitis. **GU:** Urinary frequency, dysuria, urinary retention, gynecomastia, inhibition of ejaculation, decreased libido, impotence, early menses, induction of lactation. **Hematologic:** Hypoplastic anemia, ***aplastic anemia, hemolytic anemia,*** thrombocytopenia, leukopenia, pancytopenia, ***agranulocytosis,*** thrombocytopenic purpura. **Respiratory:**

Thickening of bronchial secretions, wheezing, nasal stuffiness, chest tightness, sore throat, ***respiratory depression;*** dry mouth, nose, and throat. **Ophthalmic:** Blurred vision, diplopia. **Miscellaneous:** Tinnitus, photosensitivity, acute labyrinthitis, obstructive jaundice, erythema, high or prolonged glucose tolerance curves, glycosuria, elevated spinal fluid proteins, increased plasma cholesterol, increased perspiration, chills; tingling, heaviness, and weakness of the hands.

• **TOPICAL**

Prolonged use may result in local irritation and allergic contact dermatitis.

OD OVERDOSE MANAGEMENT

Symptoms (Acute Toxicity): Although antihistamines have a wide therapeutic range, overdosage can nevertheless be fatal. Children are particularly susceptible. Early toxic effects may be seen within 30–120 min and include drowsiness, dizziness, blurred vision, tinnitus, ataxia, and hypotension. Symptoms range from CNS depression (sedation, ***coma,*** decreased mental alertness) to ***CV collapse*** and CNS stimulation (insomnia, hallucinations, tremors, or ***seizures***). Also, ***profound hypotension, respiratory depression, coma, and death*** may occur. Anticholinergic effects include flushing, dry mouth, hypotension, fever, ***hyperthermia*** (especially in children), and fixed, dilated pupils. Body temperature may be as high as 107°F. In children, symptoms include hallucinations, toxic psychosis, delirum tremens, ataxia, incoordination, muscle twitching, excitement, athetosis, ***hyperthermia, seizures,*** and hyperreflexia followed by postictal depression and ***cardiorespiratory arrest.*** *Treatment:*

• Treat symptoms and provide supportive care.

• Vomiting is induced with syrup of ipecac (do not use for phenothiazine overdosage) followed by activated charcoal and a cathartic. If vomiting has not been induced within 3 hr of ingestion, gastric lavage can be undertaken.

• Hypotension can be treated with a vasopressor such as norepinephrine, dopamine, or phenylephrine (do not use epinephrine).

• For convulsions, use only short-acting depressants (e.g., diazepam). IV physostigmine can be used to treat centrally mediated convulsions.

• Ice packs and a cool sponge bath are effective in reducing fever in children.

• Take precautions to protect against aspiration, especially in infants and children.

• Severe cases of overdose can be treated by hemoperfusion.

DRUG INTERACTIONS

Also see *Drug Interactions* for *Phenothiazines.*

Alcohol, ethyl / See *CNS depressants*

Antidepressants, tricyclic / Additive anticholinergic side effects

CNS depressants, antianxiety agents, barbiturates, narcotics, phenothiazines, procarbazine, sedative-hypnotics / Potentiation or addition of CNS depressant effects. Concomitant use may lead to drowsiness, lethargy, stupor, respiratory depression, coma, and possibly death

H *Henbane leaf* / Enhanced anticholinergic effects

Heparin / Antihistamines may ↓ the anticoagulant effects

MAO inhibitors / Intensification and prolongation of anticholinergic side effects; use with phenothiazine antihistamine → hypotension and extrapyramidal reactions

LABORATORY TEST CONSIDERATIONS

Discontinue antihistamines 4 days before skin testing to avoid false – result.

DOSAGE

Usually PO. Parenteral administration is seldom used because of irritating nature of drugs. Topical usage is also limited because antihistamines often cause hypersensitivity reactions. When given for motion sickness, antihistamines are usually given 30–60 min before anticipated travel. See individual drugs.

NURSING CONSIDERATIONS

ADMINISTRATION/STORAGE

1. Inject IM preparations deep into the muscle; irritating to tissues.
2. Swallow sustained-release preparations whole. May break scored tablets before swallowing. If difficulty swallowing capsules, may open and put contents into soft food for ingestion.
3. Do not apply topical preparations to raw, blistered, or oozing areas of the skin.
4. Do not apply to the eyes, around the genitalia, or to mucous membranes.

ASSESSMENT

1. Note any drug sensitivity; document known allergens and all meds prescribed.
2. Document type, onset, and characteristics of symptoms; note triggers.
3. Avoid with any ulcers, glaucoma, or pregnancy.
4. Stop antihistamines 2–4 days prior to skin testing to avoid false negative results.
5. Document VS, CV status, lung sounds and characteristics of secretions.
6. Describe extent and characteristics of any rash, if present.

CLIENT/FAMILY TEACHING

1. Take med before or at the onset of symptoms; cannot reverse reactions but may prevent them.
2. Do not drive or operate equipment until drug effects realized or drowsiness worn off. Sedative effects may disappear after several days or may not occur at all.
3. PO preparations may cause gastric irritation; administer with meals, milk, or a snack.
4. Report sore throat, fever, unexplained bruising, bleeding, or petechiae; may cause blood dyscrasia.
5. May cause sensitivity to sun or ultraviolet light; avoid long exposures, use sunscreen, sunglasses, and protective clothing when exposed.
6. For motion sickness, take 30 min before travel time.
7. Reduce symptoms of dry mouth by frequent rinsing, good oral hygiene, and sugarless gum or candies.
8. Severe CNS depression is a symptom of overdosage. Report dizziness or weakness; avoid other CNS depressants.
9. Ensure adequate hydration. If bronchial secretions are thick, increase fluids to decrease secretion viscosity; avoid milk temporarily. If urinating problems, go prior to taking the drug.
10. Exercise regularly; consume 2 L fluids/day and fruits, fruit juices, and dietary fiber to prevent constipation. Stool softeners as needed.
11. Recurrent reactions may be referred to an allergist. Protect self from undue exposure and create an allergen-free living area.
12. Raises BP, use with high BP only if medically supervised.
13. Avoid alcohol or OTC agents.
14. Children may manifest excitation rather than sedation.
15. Clinical effectiveness may diminish with continued usage; switching to another class may restore drug effectiveness.
16. Family/significant other should learn CPR; survival is greatly increased when CPR is initiated immediately.

OUTCOMES/EVALUATE

- ↓ Frequency/intensity of allergic manifestations; ↓ itching/swelling
- Prevention of motion sickness
- Effective nighttime sedation

ANTIHYPERLIPIDEMIC AGENTS—HMG-COA REDUCTASE INHIBITORS

SEE ALSO THE FOLLOWING INDIVIDUAL ENTRIES:

Atorvastatin calcium
Fluvastatin sodium
Lovastatin

Pravastatin sodium
Simvastatin

GENERAL STATEMENT

The National Cholesterol Education Program Expert Panel on Detection, Evaluation, and Treatment of High Blood Cholesterol in Adults has developed guidelines for the treatment of high cholesterol and LDL in adults. Cholesterol levels less than 200 mg/dL are desirable. Cholesterol levels between 200 and 239 mg/dL are considered borderline-high while levels greater than 240 mg/dL are considered high. With respect to LDL, the following goals have been established: All people should be at 160 mg/dL or below; levels of130 mg/dL are considered desirable in individuals with two or more risk factors (cigarette smoking, hypertension, HDL below 40 mg/dL, or family history of premature CAD). HDL above 60 mg/dL is a negative risk factor, i.e., its presence removes one of the previous risk factors from the total count. The LDL goal for those clients with diabetes and/or existing CAD is 100 mg/dL or lower. Depending on the levels of cholesterol and LDL and the number of risk factors present for CAD, the provider will develop a treatment regimen.

ACTION/KINETICS

The HMG-CoA reductase inhibitors competitively inhibit HMG-CoA reductase; this enzyme catalyzes the early rate-limiting step in the synthesis of cholesterol. HMG-CoA reductase inhibitors increase HDL cholesterol and decrease LDL cholesterol, total cholesterol, apolipoprotein B, VLDL cholesterol, and plasma triglycerides. The mechanism to lower LDL cholesterol may be due to both a decrease in VLDL cholesterol levels and induction of the LDL receptor, leading to reduced production or increased catabolism of LDL cholesterol. The maximum therapeutic response is seen in 4–6 weeks.

USES

See individual drugs. Uses include primary hypercholesterolemia, mixed dyslipidemia, hypertriglycidemia, prevention of coronary events, and prevention of CV events. *Investigational:* Treatment of osteoporosis. Lower risk of developing type 2 diabetes and stroke when taken to reduce cholesterol.

CONTRAINDICATIONS

Active liver disease or unexplained persistent elevated liver function tests. Pregnancy, lactation. Use in children.

SPECIAL CONCERNS

Use with caution in those who ingest large quantities of alcohol or who have a history of liver disease. May cause photosensitivity. Safety and efficacy have not been established in children less than 18 years of age.

SIDE EFFECTS

The following side effects are common to most HMG-CoA reductase inhibitors. Also see individual drugs.

GI: N&V, diarrhea, constipation, abdominal cramps or pain, flatulence, dyspepsia, heartburn. **CNS:** Headache, dizziness, dysfunction of certain cranial nerves (e.g., alteration of taste, facial paresis, impairment of extraocular movement), tremor, vertigo, memory loss, paresthesia, anxiety, insomnia, depression. **Musculoskeletal:** Localized pain, myalgia, muscle cramps or pain, myopathy, rhabdomyolysis, arthralgia. **Respiratory:** URI, rhinitis, cough. **Ophthalmic:** Progression of cataracts (lens opacities), ophthalmoplegia. **Hypersensitivity:** ***Anaphylaxis, angio-edema,*** vasculitis, purpura, thrombocytopenia, leukopenia, ***hemolytic anemia,*** lupus erythematosus-like syndrome, polymyalgia rheumatica, positive ANA, ESR increase, arthritis, arthralgia, eosinophilia, urticaria, photosensitivity, fever, chills, flushing, malaise, dyspnea, ***toxic dermal necrolysis, Stevens-Johnson syndrome.*** **Miscellaneous:** Rash, pruritus, cardiac chest pain, fatigue, influenza, alopecia, edema, dryness of skin and mucous membranes, changes to hair and nails, skin discoloration.

DRUG INTERACTIONS

See also individual drugs.

Antifungals, azole / ↑ Levels of HMG-CoA inhibitors R/T ↓ metabolism

Clarithromycin / ↑ Levels of HMG-CoA inhibitors R/T ↓ metabolism
Cyclosporine / ↑ Risk of severe myopathy or rhabdomyolysis
Digoxin / Slight ↑ in digoxin levels
Erythromycin / ↑ Risk of severe myopathy or rhabdomyolysis
Gemfibrozil / Possibility of severe myopathy or rhabdomyolysis
Itraconazole / ↑ Levels of HMG-CoA inhibitors
Niacin/Nicotinic acid / Possibility of myopathy or severe rhabdomyolysis
Propranolol / ↓ Antihyperlipidemic activity
Protease inhibitors / ↑ Levels of HMG-CoA inhibitors R/T ↓ metabolism
Warfarin / ↑ Anticoagulant effect of warfarin.

LABORATORY TEST CONSIDERATIONS

↑ AST, ALT, CPK, alkaline phosphatase, bilirubin. Abnormal thyroid function tests.

DOSAGE

See individual drugs.

NURSING CONSIDERATIONS

ADMINISTRATION/STORAGE

Lovastatin should be taken with meals; cerivastatin, fluvastatin, pravastatin, and simavastatin may be taken without regard to meals.

ASSESSMENT

1. Review life-style, risk factors, attempts to control with diet, exercise, and weight reduction.
2. Note any alcohol abuse or liver disease.
3. Review PMH, ROS, and physical exam; document risk factors.
4. Monitor LFTs as recommended. Transaminase levels 3 times normal may precipitate severe hepatic toxicity. If CK elevated, assess renal function as rhabdomyolsis with myoglobinuria could cause renal shutdown. Stop drug therapy.
5. Note nutritional analysis by dietician; assess cholesterol profile (HDL, LDL, cholesterol, and triglycerides) after 3–6 months of exercise and diet therapy if risk factors do not require immediate drug therapy. With diabetes and coronary heart disease a more aggressive drug approach should be instituted in addition to diet therapy with goals of reducing LDL below 100 or ratio below 3.

CLIENT/FAMILY TEACHING

1. Take only as directed.
2. May cause photosensitivity; avoid prolonged sun or UV light exposure. Use sunscreens, sunglasses, and protective clothing when exposed.
3. Report any pain in skeletal muscles or unexplained muscle pain, tenderness, or weakness promptly, especially with fever or malaise.
4. Stop drug with any major trauma, surgery, or serious illness.
5. Continue life-style modifications that include low-fat, low-cholesterol, and low-sodium diets, weight reduction with obese clients, smoking cessation, reduction of alcohol consumption, HRT with menopause, and regular aerobic exercise in the overall goal of cholesterol reduction.
6. May use niaspan (SR form of niacin) with careful monitoring. Use a fibrate cautiously; monitor LFTs and assess for muscle pain.
7. Avoid OTC agents.
8. Report regularly for labs to prevent liver toxicity and to assess drug response.

OUTCOMES/EVALUATE

- ↓ LDL, triglycerides, and total cholesterol levels; ↓ risk of CAD and death

ANTIHYPERTENSIVE AGENTS

SEE ALSO THE FOLLOWING DRUG CLASSES AND INDIVIDUAL DRUGS:

Agents Acting Directly on Vascular Smooth Muscle

Diazoxide IV
Nitroprusside sodium

Alpha-1-Adrenergic Blocking Agents

Doxazosin mesylate
Prazosin hydrochloride
Terazosin

Angiotensin-II Receptor Blockers

Candesartan cilexetil
Eprosartan mesylate
Irbesartan
Losartan potassium
Valsartan

Angiotensin-Converting Enzyme Inhibitors

Benazepril hydrochloride
Captopril
Enalapril maleate
Fosinopril sodium
Lisinopril
Moexipril hydrochloride
Perindopril erbumine
Quinapril hydrochloride
Ramipril
Trandolopril

Beta-Adrenergic Blocking Agents

Calcium Channel Blocking Agents

Amlodipine
Bepridil hydrochloride
Diltiazem hydrochloride
Felodipine
Isradipine
Nicardipine hydrochloride
Nifedipine
Nimodipine
Nisoldipine
Verapamil

Centrally-Acting Agents

Clonidine hydrochloride
Guanabenz acetate
Guanfacine hydrochloride
Methyldopa
Methyldopate hydrochloride

Combination Drugs Used for Hypertension

See Table in Appendix

Miscellaneous Agents

Bosentan
Carvedilol
Epoprostenol sodium
Labetalol hydrochloride
Minoxidil, oral

Peripherally-Acting Agents

Guanadrel sulfate
Phentolamine mesylate

GENERAL STATEMENT

The Sixth Report of the Joint National Committee on Prevention, Detection, Evaluation and Treatment of High Blood Pressure classifies BP for adults aged 18 and over as follows: Optimal as <120/<80 mm Hg, Normal as <130/<85 mm Hg, High Normal as 130–139/85–89 mm Hg, Stage 1 Hypertension as 140–159/90–99 mm Hg, Stage 2 Hypertension as 160–179/100–109 mm Hg, and Stage 3 Hypertension as 180 or greater/110 or greater mm Hg. Drug therapy is recommended depending on the BP and whether certain risk factors (e.g., smoking, dyslipidemia, diabetes, age, gender, target organ damage, clinical CV disease) are present. Life-style modification is an important component of treating hypertension, including weight reduction, reduction of sodium intake, regular exercise, cessation of smoking, and moderate alcohol intake.

The goal of antihypertensive therapy is a BP of <140/90 mm Hg, except in hypertensive diabetics where the goal is <130/80 mm Hg and those with renal insufficiency where the goal is <130/85 mm Hg. Genreally speaking, the primary agents for initial monotherapy to treat uncomplicated hypertension are diuretics and beta-adrenergic blocking agents. Alternative drugs include ACE inhibitors, alpha-1-blocking agents, alpha-beta blocking agents, and calcium channel blockers. Treatment recommendations for clients with high BP and diabetes are as follows: (1) Begin therapy with ACE inhibitors. Increase doses as needed to the moderate or high-dose range, depending on side effects. (2) If target BP is not reached, add diuretics or calcium channel blockers. (3) Switch to a single-dose, multi-drug combination of an ACE inhibitor/diuretic or an ACE inhibitor/calcium channel blocker after BP is controlled.

DRUG INTERACTIONS

H *Black cohosh* / May potentiate antihypertensive drugs

H *Garlic* / May potentiate antihypertensive drugs
H *Hawthorn* / Cardioactive, hypotensive, and coronary vasodilator action of hawthorn may affect antihypertensive effect; monitor.

NURSING CONSIDERATIONS

ASSESSMENT

1. Note any family history of hypertension, stroke, CVD, CHD, MI, dyslipidemia, and diabetes.
2. Determine baseline BP before starting antihypertensive therapy. To ensure accuracy of baseline readings, take BP in both (bared and supported) arms (lying, standing, and sitting) 2 min apart (30 min after last cigarette or caffeine consumption) at least three times during one visit and on two subsequent visits. Document BMI (body mass index), or height, weight and risk factors.
3. Ascertain life-style modifications (weight reduction, ↓ alcohol intake, regular exercise, reduced sodium/fat intake, and smoking cessation) needed to achieve lowered BP. Offer a trial following these modifications and reassess in 3–6 mo before starting therapy unless BP in severe range or > 2 risk factors.
4. Monitor ECG, chem-7, CBC, uric acid, urinalysis, cholesterol panel, and lfts; always check for proteinuria.
5. Note funduscopic and neurologic exam findings.
6. Assess for thyroid enlargement and presence of target organ damage. If difficult to control, assess for renal artery stenosis or secondary causes of HTN and refer for 24-hr ambulatory BP monitoring.

CLIENT/FAMILY TEACHING

1. Drugs control but do not cure hypertension. Take meds despite feeling fine and do not stop abruptly; may cause rebound hypertension. Drugs only provide protection/control of BP for the day in which they are taken. They must be taken daily as prescribed to ensure control.
2. There are generally no S&S of high blood pressure. When S&S become evident is when organ damage has already occurred.
3. Keep a record of BP readings; helps identify "white coat syndrome."
4. Adhere to a low-sodium, low-fat diet; see dietitian as needed for education, meal planning, and food selections.
5. Weakness, dizziness, and fainting may occur with rapid changes of position from supine to standing (postural hypotension). Rise slowly from a lying or sitting position and dangle legs for several minutes before standing to minimize orthostatic effects. Exercising in hot weather may enhance these effects.
6. If dose missed, do not double up or take two doses close together.
7. Have yearly eye exams to detect early retinal changes from ↑ BP.
8. Avoid agents that may lower BP (e.g., alcohol, barbiturates, CNS depressants) or that could elevate BP (e.g., OTC cold remedies, oral contraceptives, steroids, NSAIDs, appetite suppressants, tricyclic antidepressants, MAO inhibitors). Sympathomimetic amines in products used to treat asthma, colds, and allergies must be used with extreme caution
9. Avoid excessive amounts of caffeine (tea, coffee, chocolate, or colas).
10. Notify provider if sexual dysfunction occurs as med can usually be changed to minimize symptoms or other options for sexual dysfunction explored.
11. Identify holistic interventions/life-style modifications necessary for BP control: dietary restrictions of fat and sodium (2–3 g/day), weight reduction, ↓ alcohol (i.e., less than 24 oz beer or less than 8 oz of wine or less than 2 oz of 100-proof whiskey per day), tobacco cessation, ↑ physical activity, regular exercise programs, proper rest, and methods to reduce and deal with stress.

OUTCOMES/EVALUATE

- Understanding of disease/compliance with prescribed therapy
- ↓ BP (SBP < 140 and DBP < 85 mm Hg)

• Control/prevent target organ damage, stroke, and death

ANTI-INFECTIVE DRUGS

SEE ALSO THE FOLLOWING INDIVIDUAL DRUGS AND DRUG CLASSES:

Amebicides and Trichomonacides
Aminoglycosides
4-Aminoquinolines
Anthelmintics
Antimalarials
Antiviral Drugs
Aztreonam for injection
Bacitracin
Becaplermin
Butenafine hydrochloride
Cephalosporins
Chloramphenicol
Clindamycin hydrochloride
Clindamycin palmitate hydrochloride
Clindamycin phosphate
Drotrecogin alfa
Ertapenem for injection
Erythromycins
Fluoroquinolones
Fosfomycin tromethamine
Imipenem-Cilastatin sodium
Lincomycin hydrochloride
Linezolid
Loracarbef
Macrolides
Meropenem
Mupirocin
Mupirocin calcium
Penicillins
Pentamidine isethionate
Quinupristin/Dalfopristin
Spectinomycin hydrochloride
Sulfonamides
Tetracyclines
Trovafloxacin mesylate injection
Vancomycin hydrochloride

GENERAL STATEMENT

The following general guidelines apply to the use of most anti-infective drugs:

1. Anti-infective drugs can be divided into those that are *bacteriostatic*, that is, arrest the multiplication and further development of the infectious agent, or *bactericidal*, that is, kill and thus eradicate all living microorganisms. Both time of administration and length of therapy may be affected by this difference.
2. Some anti-infectives halt the growth of or eradicate many different microorganisms and are termed *broad-spectrum antibiotics*. Others affect only certain specific organisms and are termed *narrow-spectrum antibiotics*.
3. Some of the anti-infectives elicit a hypersensitivity reaction in some persons. Penicillins cause more severe and more frequent hypersensitivity reactions than any other drug.
4. Because of differences in susceptibility of infectious agents to anti-infectives, the sensitivity of the microorganism to the drug ordered should be determined before treatment is initiated. Several sensitivity tests are commonly used for this purpose.
5. Certain anti-infective agents have marked side effects, some of the more serious of which are neurotoxicity, including ototoxicity, and nephrotoxicity. Care must be taken not to administer two anti-infectives with similar side effects concomitantly, or to administer these drugs to clients in whom the side effects might be damaging (e.g., a nephrotoxic drug to a client suffering from kidney disease). The choice of anti-infective also depends on its distribution in the body (i.e., whether it passes the blood-brain barrier).
6. Anti-infective drugs can also eradicate the normal intestinal flora necessary for proper digestion, synthesis of vitamin K, and control of fungi that may gain access to the GI tract (superinfection).

ACTION/KINETICS

The mechanism of action of the anti-infectives varies. The following modes of action have been identified.* Note

*Chambers, H.F., Sande, M.A.: Antimicrobial agents. In *Goodman and Gilman's The Pharmacological Basis of Therapeutics*, 9th ed. Edited by Hardman, J.G., Limbud, L.E., New York, McGraw-Hill, 1996, p. 1029.

the considerable overlap among these mechanisms:
1. Inhibition of synthesis of or activation of enzymes that disrupt bacterial cell walls leading to loss of viability and possibly cell lysis (e.g., penicillins, cephalosporins, cycloserine, bacitracin, vancomycin, miconazole, ketoconazole, clotrimazole).
2. Direct effect on the microbial cell membrane to affect permeability and leading to leakage of intracellular components (e.g., polymyxin, colistimethate, nystatin, amphotericin).
3. Effect on the function of 30S and 50S bacterial ribosomes to cause a reversible inhibition of protein synthesis (e.g., chloramphenicol, tetracyclines, erythromycin, clindamycin).
4. Bind to the 30S ribosomal subunit that alters protein synthesis and leads to cell death (e.g., aminoglycosides).
5. Effect on nucleic acid metabolism which inhibits DNA-dependent RNA polymerase (e.g., rifampin) or inhibition of gyrase (e.g., fluoroquinolones).
6. Antimetabolites that block specific metabolic steps essential to the life of the microorganism (e.g., trimethoprim, sulfonamides).
7. Bind to viral enzymes that are essential for DNA synthesis leading to a halt of viral replication (e.g., acyclovir, ganciclovir, vidarabine, zidovudine).

USES

See individual drugs. The choice of the anti-infective depends on the nature of the illness to be treated, the sensitivity of the infecting agent, and the client's previous experience with the drug. Hypersensitivity and allergic reactions may preclude the use of the agent of choice.

CONTRAINDICATIONS

Hypersensitivity or allergies to the drug.

SIDE EFFECTS

The antibiotics and anti-infective agents have few direct toxic effects. Kidney and liver damage, deafness, and blood dyscrasias are occasionally observed.

The following undesirable manifestations, however, occur frequently: 1. Suppresion of the normal flora of the body, which in turn keeps certain pathogenic microorganisms, such as *Candida albicans, Proteus,* or *Pseudomonas,* from causing infections. If the flora is altered, superinfections (monilial vaginitis, enteritis, UTIs), which necessitate the discontinuation of therapy or the use of other antibiotics, can result. 2. Incomplete eradication of an infectious organism. Casual use of anti-infectives favors the emergence of *resistant* strains insensitive to a particular drug. To minimize the chances for the development of resistant strains, anti-infectives are usually given at specified doses for a prescribed length of time after acute symptoms have subsided.

OD OVERDOSE MANAGEMENT

Treatment: Discontinue the drug and treat symptomatically. Supportive measures should be instituted as needed. Hemodialysis may be used although its effectiveness is questionable, depending on the drug and the status of the client (i.e., more effective in impaired renal function).

LABORATORY TEST CONSIDERATIONS

The bacteriologic sensitivity of the infectious organism to the anti-infective (especially the antibiotic) should be tested by the lab before initiation of therapy and during treatment.

NURSING CONSIDERATIONS

GENERAL NURSING CONSIDERATIONS FOR ALL ANTI-INFECTIVES

ADMINISTRATION/STORAGE

1. Check expiration date.
2. Store according to recommended storage method.
3. Mark date and time of reconstitution, your initials, and the solution strength. Mark expiration date; store under appropriate conditions.
4. Complete infusion (or as ordered) before the drug loses potency; check drug info.

ASSESSMENT

1. Document onset and characteristics of symptoms, location and source of infection (if known).
2. Note any unusual reaction/sensitivity with any anti-infectives (usually penicillin).
3. Obtain cultures before administering empiric therapy. Use correct procedure for obtaining, storing, and transporting specimens.
4. Monitor CBC, renal and LFTs.

INTERVENTIONS

1. Conspicuously mark allergy in red on the chart, medication record, ID band, care plan, pharmacy record, and bed. Insert on electronic record; note if observed or reported by client.
2. Assess for hives, rashes, or difficulty breathing, which may indicate a hypersensitivity or allergic response.
3. Monitor VS, I&O; ensure adequate hydration.
4. If drug mainly excreted by the kidneys, reduce dose with renal dysfunction. Nephrotoxic drugs are usually contraindicated with renal dysfunction because toxic drug levels are rapidly attained.
5. Verify orders when two or more anti-infectives are ordered for the same client, especially if they have similar side effects, such as nephrotoxicity and/or neurotoxicity. Electronic entry prevents confusion.
6. Assess for superinfections, particularly of fungal origin, characterized by black furred tongue, nausea, and/or diarrhea. *Prevent superinfections by:*
   - Limiting exposure to persons suffering from an active infectious process
   - Rotating IV site q 72 hr; changing IV tubing q 24–48 hr
   - Providing/emphasizing good hygiene
   - Washing hands carefully before and after contact with client
7. Schedule administration throughout 24-hr period to maintain therapeutic drug levels. Administration schedule is determined by the drug half-life (t½), severity of infection, evidence of organ dysfunction, and client's need for sleep. Assess drug levels (peak and trough) to determine dosing and to assess adequacy of levels.

CLIENT/FAMILY TEACHING

1. Take meds at prescribed intervals; use only under supervision.
2. Do not share with friends or family members. Prevent recurrence by completing entire prescription, despite feeling well. This ensures that the organism is eradicated and diminishes the emergence of drug-resistant bacterial strains. Incomplete therapy and indiscriminate use may render client unresponsive to the antibiotic with the next infection.
3. Report any unusual bruising or bleeding, e.g., bleeding gums, blood in stool, urine, or other secretions; S&S of allergic reactions, including rash, fever, itching, and hives or superinfections such as pain, swelling, redness, drainage, perineal itching, diarrhea, rash, or a change in S&S.
4. Discard any unused drug after therapy completed.
5. Take antipyretics as prescribed ATC for fever reduction as needed.

OUTCOMES/EVALUATE

- Prevention/resolution of infection
- ↓ Fever, WBCs; ↑ appetite
- Negative culture reports
- Therapeutic serum drug levels

ANTINEOPLASTIC AGENTS

SEE ALSO THE FOLLOWING INDIVIDUAL ENTRIES:

Aldesleukin
Alemtuzumab
Altretamine
Amifostine
Anastrozole
Asparaginase
BCG Intravesical
Bicalutamide
Bleomycin sulfate
Busulfan
Capecitabine
Carboplatin for injection
Carmustine
Chlorambucil

Cisplatin
Cladribine injection
Cyclophosphamide
Cytarabine
Cytarabine liposomal
Dacarbazine
Dactinomycin
Daunorubicin hydrochloride
Daunorubicin citrate liposomal
Denileukin diftitox
Docetaxel
Doxorubicin hydrochloride conventional
Doxorubicin hydrochloride liposomal
Epirubicin hydrochloride
Estramustine phosphate sodium
Etoposide
Exemestane
Floxuridine
Fludarabine phosphate
Fluorouracil
Flutamide
Gemcitabine hydrochloride
Gemtuzumab ozogamicin
Goserelin acetate
Hydroxyurea
Idrarubicin hydrochloride
Ifosfamide
Imatinib mesylate
Interferon Alfa-n3
Interferon Alfa-2a Recombinant
Interferon Alfa-2b Recombinant
Irinotecan hydrochloride
Letrozole
Leuprolide acetate
Lomustine
Mechlorethamine hydrochloride
Megestrol acetate
Melphalan
Mercaptopurine
Mesna
Methotrexate
Methotrexate sodium
Mitomycin
Mitotane
Mitoxantrone hydrochloride
Nilutamide
Paclitaxel
Pegaspargase
Pentostatin
Plicamycin
Porfimer sodium
Procarbazine hydrochloride
Rituximab
Streptozocin
Tamoxifen
Temozolomide
Teniposide
Testolactone
Thioguanine
Thiotepa
Topotecan hydrochloride
Toremifene citrate
Trastuzumab
Triptorelin pamoate
Valrubicin
Vinblastine sulfate
Vincristine sulfate
Vinorelbine tartrate

GENERAL STATEMENT

The choice of the chemotherapeutic agent(s) depends both on the cell type of the tumor and on its site of growth. All antineoplastic agents are cytotoxic (i.e., cell poisons) and therefore interfere with normal as well as neoplastic cells. However, neoplastic cells are more active and multiply more rapidly than normal cells and are thus more affected by the antineoplastic agents. Normal, rapidly growing tissue cells, such as those of the bone marrow, the GI mucosal epithelium, and hair follicles, are particularly susceptible to antineoplastic agents. The margin between the dose of antineoplastic drug needed to destroy the neoplastic cells and that needed to cause bone marrow damage, for example, is narrow. Since WBCs or platelets show the effect of an overdose more rapidly than do erythrocytes, the platelet and WBC counts are often used as a guide to dosage. If a blood or marrow test indicates a precipitous fall in the WBC or platelet count, the antineoplastic agent may have to be discontinued or the dosage modified significantly. Drugs are frequently withheld when the WBC count falls below $2,000/mm^3$ and the platelet count falls below $100,000/mm^3$. With the advent of granulocyte colony-stimulating factors, providers may now utilize this to support large dosing on an aggressive cancer, thus preventing postponement of therapy until recovery of the client's hematologic parameters. Sometimes the effect of the antineoplastic drugs on the bone marrow is cumulative, with the depression of WBCs and platelets occurring weeks or months after initiation of therapy.

GI tract toxicity is manifested by development of oral ulcers, intestinal bleeding, nausea, vomiting, loss of appetite, and diarrhea. Finally, alopecia often results from antineoplastic drug therapy.

ACTION/KINETICS

During division, cells go through a number of stages during which they may be susceptible to various chemotherapeutic agents (see *Action/Kinetics* of various agents). The various cell stages are described in Figure 2.

USES

Most of the drugs discussed in this section are used exclusively for neoplastic disease. A few are used on an experimental basis for some of the rheumatic diseases.

CONTRAINDICATIONS

Hypersensitivity to drug. Some antineoplastic agents may be contraindicated for a period of 4 weeks after radiation therapy or chemotherapy with similar drugs. During first trimester of pregnancy.

SPECIAL CONCERNS

Use with caution, and at reduced dosages, in clients with preexisting bone marrow depression, malignant infiltration of bone marrow or kidney, liver dysfunction, or previous recent chemotherapy usage. The safe use of these drugs during pregnancy has not been established.

SIDE EFFECTS

Bone marrow depression (leukopenia, thrombocytopenia, ***agranulocytosis,*** anemia) is the major danger of antineoplastic therapy. ***Bone marrow depression can sometimes be irreversible.*** *It is mandatory that the client have frequent total blood counts and periodic bone marrow examinations. Precipitous falls must be reported to a physician.* Other side effects include: **GI:** N&V (may be severe), anorexia, diarrhea (may be hemorrhagic), stomatitis, mucositis, enteritis, abdominal cramps, intestinal ulcers. **Hepatic:** Hepatic toxicity including jaundice and changes in liver enzymes. **Dermatologic:** Dermatitis, erythema, various dermatoses including maculopapular rash, alopecia (reversible), pruritus, staining of vein path with some drugs, urticaria, cheilosis. **Immunologic:** Immunosuppression with increased susceptibility to viral, bacterial, or fungal infections. **CNS:** Depression, lethargy, confusion, dizziness, headache, fatigue, malaise, fever, weakness. **GU:** ***Acute renal failure,*** reproductive abnormalities including amenorrhea and azoospermia. *NOTE:* Alkylating agents, in particular, may be both carcinogenic and mutagenic.

NURSING CONSIDERATIONS

GENERAL NURSING CONSIDERATIONS FOR ANTINEOPLASTIC AGENTS

ADMINISTRATION/STORAGE

1. Antineoplastic drugs should be prepared only by trained personnel; avoid if pregnant.
2. Cytotoxic exposure may be through inhalation, ingestion, and absorption during preparation; prepare under a laminar flow (biologic) hood.
   - If not available, prepare in a separate room in a work area away from cooling or heating vents and away from other people. Cover work table area with a disposable plastic liner.
   - Use latex gloves to protect the skin when reconstituting; do not use gloves made of PVC since these are permeable to some cytotoxic drugs. Good handwashing before and after preparation is essential. Prevent drug contact with skin or mucous membranes; document occurrence and wash area immediately with copious amounts of water.
   - Wear disposable, nonpermeable gown with closed front and knit cuffs completely covering wrists.

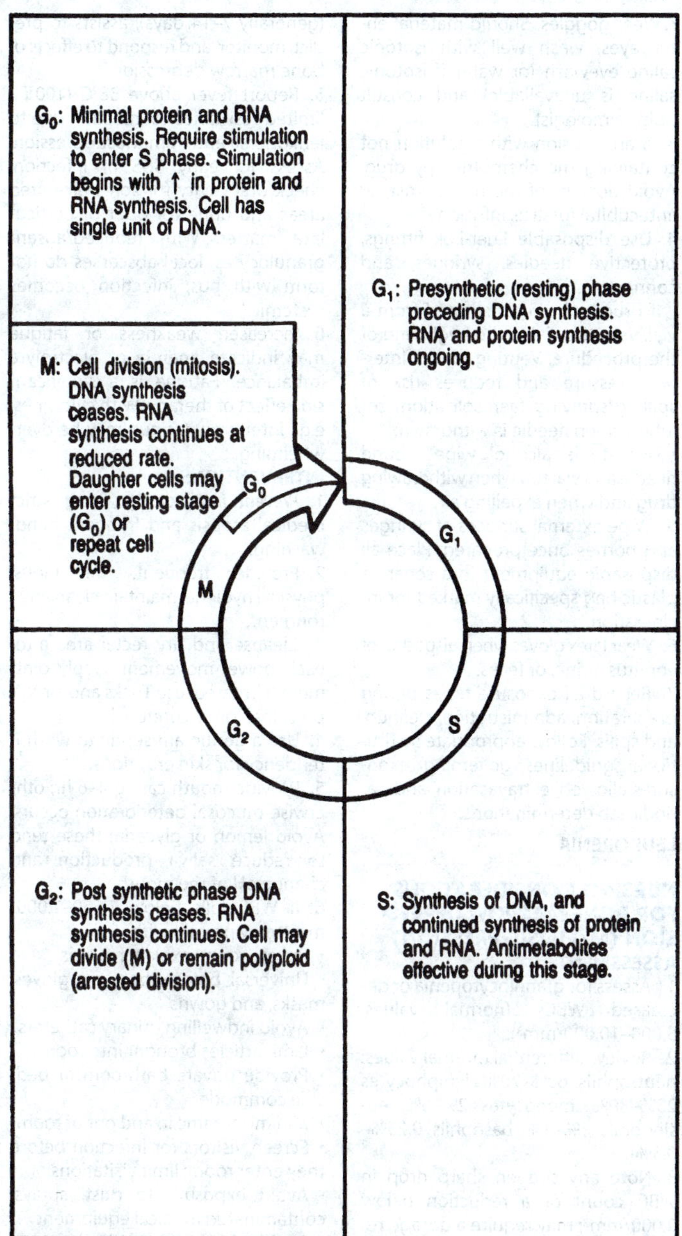

G_0: Minimal protein and RNA synthesis. Require stimulation to enter S phase. Stimulation begins with ↑ in protein and RNA synthesis. Cell has single unit of DNA.
G_1: Presynthetic (resting) phase preceding DNA synthesis. RNA and protein synthesis ongoing.
M: Cell division (mitosis). DNA synthesis ceases. RNA synthesis continues at reduced rate. Daughter cells may enter resting stage (G_0) or repeat cell cycle.
G_0
G_1
M
S
G_2
G_2: Post synthetic phase DNA synthesis ceases. RNA synthesis continues. Cell may divide (M) or remain polyploid (arrested division).
S: Synthesis of DNA, and continued synthesis of protein and RNA. Antimetabolites effective during this stage.

Figure 2 Cell stages.

• Wear goggles. Should material enter eyes, wash well with isotonic saline eyewash (or water if isotonic saline is unavailable) and consult ophthalmologist.
3. Start infusion with a solution not containing the chemotherapy drug. Avoid dorsum of the hand, wrist, or antecubital fossa as infusion site.
4. Use disposable Luer-Lok fittings, protective needles, syringes, and connectors.
• If drug to be reconstituted from a vial, vent the vial at the beginning of the procedure. Venting lowers internal pressure and reduces risk of spilling/spraying (aerosolization) solution when needle is withdrawn.
• Use sterile alcohol wipe around needle and vial top when withdrawing drug and when expelling air.
5. Wipe external surfaces of syringes and bottles once prepared. Place all disposable equipment in a separate plastic bag specifically marked for incineration.
6. Wear latex gloves when disposing of vomitus, urine, or feces.
7. Record all exposure times during preparation, administration, cleanup, and spills. Follow appropriate institutional guidelines governing exposures allowed, extravasation, and periodic lab determinations.

LEUKOPENIA

NURSING CONSIDERATIONS FOR BONE MARROW DEPRESSION (MYELOSUPPRESSION)

ASSESSMENT

1. Assess for granulocytopenia or decreased WBCs (normal values: 5,000–10,000/mm^3).
2. Review differential (normal values: neutrophils 60%–70%, lymphocytes 25%–30%, monocytes 2%–6%, eosinophils 1%–3%, basophils 0.25%–0.5%).
3. Note any sudden sharp drop in WBC count or a reduction below 2,000/mm^3; may require a dosage reduction or withdrawal of drug.
4. Determine nadir (time the blood count reaches its lowest point after chemotherapy) for prescribed agent (generally 7–14 days); assists to predict, monitor, and respond to effects of bone marrow depression.
5. Report fever above 38°C (100°F); limited resistance to infection due to leukopenia and immunosuppression. Assess for early S&S of infection: check oral cavity for sores/ulcerated areas and urine for odor or particulate matter. With reduced/absent granulocytes, local abscesses do not form with pus; infection becomes systemic.
6. Increased weakness or fatigue may indicate anemia or electrolyte imbalance. Fatigue is a significant side effect of therapy. With cytobines, e.g., interferon, fatigue may be overwhelming.

INTERVENTIONS

1. *Prevent infection by* using strict medical asepsis and frequent handwashing.
2. Provide frequent, meticulous, physical hygiene; maintain clean environment.
3. Cleanse and dry rectal area after each bowel movement. Apply ointment if irritated; use Tucks and/or Nupercainal for discomfort.
4. Use a gentle antiseptic to wash if tendency for skin eruptions.
5. Provide mouth care q 4–6 hr; otherwise mucosal deterioration occurs. Avoid lemon or glycerin; these tend to reduce saliva production and change pH of the mouth.
6. If WBC falls below 1,500–2,000/mm^3, may protect with:
• Private room; explain reasons
• Universal precautions; use gloves, masks, and gowns
• Avoid indwelling urinary catheters
• Limit articles brought into room
• Provide private bathroom or bedside commode
• Minimize traffic in and out of room
• Screen visitors for infection before they enter room; limit visitations
• Avoid exposure to dust, sprays, contaminated medical equipment
• Avoid deodorants; blocks sebaceous gland secretion
• Keep fresh fruits, vegetables, cut flowers, and any source of stagnant

water (water pitcher, humidifiers, flower vases) away from client
• Review/stress kitchen hygiene and food safety at home
• Dogs, cats, birds, and other pets may carry infection; avoid contact
• Assess orders for granulocyte colony-stimulating factors and ensure availability
7. Prevent nosocomial infections from invasive procedures by:
• Washing hands before and after any contact
• Cleansing skin with antiseptic before procedure
• Changing IV tubing q 24 hr
• Changing IV site q 48 hr, if no implanted device or other designated catheter for long-term use
• Practice strict asepsis with all treatments and dressing changes

NAUSEA & VOMITING; ANOREXIA

NURSING CONSIDERATIONS FOR GI TOXICITY

ASSESSMENT

1. N&V may be due to either a CNS effect on the chemoreceptor trigger zone or direct irritation to the GI tract. With radiation therapy, N&V may be attributed to the accumulation of toxic waste products of cell destruction and localized damage to the lining of the throat, stomach, and intestine.
2. Anticipatory N&V is a conditioned response of unknown origin prior to chemotherapy which does respond to premedication.
3. Determine if refusing food or fluids or experiencing anorexia.
4. Monitor nutritional status and weights.
5. Examine the frequency, character, and amount of vomitus. List antiemetics prescribed and results.

INTERVENTIONS

1. *To prevent N&V:*
• Antiemetics 30–60 min before or just after drug therapy.
• Therapy on empty stomach, with meals, or at bedtime
• Antiemetic suppository
• Ice chips at onset of nausea
• Avoid carbonated beverages
• Ingest dry carbohydrates such as toast/dry crackers before any activity
• Wait for N&V to pass before serving food
• Small, nutritious snacks; plan meal schedules to coincide with best tolerance time
• Cold foods and salads with little cooking aroma to minimize N&V
• Nourishing foods client likes
• Consume a high-protein diet
• Freeze and serve dietary supplements like ice cream; ↑ palatability
• Avoid foods with overpowering aroma
• Chew foods well
• Good oral hygiene before and after meals (try 1 tsp baking soda in a glass of warm water)
• Eat favorite foods
• Eat meals with others, preferably at a table. Sharing encourages eating.
2. Antiemetics that have different actions/pharmacokinetics may be administered concurrently in an effort to control severe N&V.
3. *To treat N&V:*
• Administer antiemetic(s). Report all vomiting; a change in therapy or need for electrolyte correction.
• Give other meds after meals
• Offer simple foods: rice, toast, noodles, bananas, scrambled eggs, mashed potatoes, custards, ice cream
• Offer salty foods (pretzels, crackers)
• Avoid solid and liquid foods at the same meal
• Eliminate any room odors; avoiding malodorous foods (e.g., cabbage, sauerkraut, etc.)
• Keep as comfortable, clean, and free from odor as possible
• Try another or concurrent antiemetic agents
• Correct electrolytes; provide hyperalimentation prn
• Screen visitors/calls until client ready
4. *For anorexia:*
• Provide small, frequent meals q 2 or 3 hr on schedule
• Maximize caloric intake by offering nutrient-dense snacks and drinks (yogurt, cheese and crackers, peanut

butter and jelly sandwiches, cereal, dried fruit, fruit nectars, and instant breakfast drink mixes)
• Make nutrient-dense supplements with whole milk
• Suggest a walk or activity before eating to boost appetite
• Concentrate on obtaining favorite foods

5. *To increase caloric intake and protein consumption:*
• Add high-calorie foods such as mayonnaise, butter, and gravy to foods
• Use whole milk in puddings, cream soups, custards
• Make double-strength milk — add powdered milk to whole milk for gravies, hot cereals, mashed potatoes, eggs, casseroles, baked things, etc.
• Add whipped cream to frosting and desserts
• Offer milkshakes, nectar, and eggnog when thirsty
• Offer peanut butter on crackers, bagels with cream cheese, trail mix, and nuts and seeds for snacks
• Cut up meats and cheeses and add to salads, soups, scrambled eggs, etc.

NURSING CONSIDERATIONS FOR NEUROTOXICITY

ASSESSMENT

1. Be aware of agents causing or having the potential to cause neurotoxic effects; further administration once symptoms have become prominent may be life threatening.
2. Report symptoms of minor neuropathies, i.e., tingling in hands and feet; loss of deep tendon reflexes. Use a monofilament to measure progressive loss of sensation.
3. Report serious neuropathies, i.e., weakness of hands, ataxia, loss of coordination, foot drop, wrist drop, or paralytic ileus.

INTERVENTIONS

1. *To prevent functional loss due to neurotoxicity:*
• Identify neuropathies early so drug regimen can be adjusted
• Practice/teach seizure precautions

2. *To treat neuropathies:*
• Use safety measures with functional losses
• Maintain good body alignment by frequent and anatomically correct repositioning; ROM exercises.
• Provide stool softeners/laxatives as needed
• Identify causative agent and stop

NURSING CONSIDERATIONS FOR OTOTOXICITY

ASSESSMENT

Assess for hearing difficulties before initiating therapy.

INTERVENTIONS

1. Report tinnitus or new onset hearing impairment.
2. Perform audiometry testing p.r.n. during therapy.

NURSING CONSIDERATIONS FOR HEPATOTOXICITY

ASSESSMENT

1. Obtain/assess the following LFTs:
• Total serum bilirubin (normal values: 0.1–1.0 mg/dL); elevations may indicate liver disease or increased rate of RBC hemolysis.
• AST (normal: 8–33 units/L). Elevations indicative of changes in liver, skeletal muscles, lungs, pancreas, and heart. Hepatitis produces striking elevations in the AST.
• ALT (normal: 8–20 units/L). Elevations may precede hepatic necrosis.
• LDH (normal: 70–250 units/L). Elevations may indicate hepatitis, pulmonary infarction, and CHF.

2. Assess for liver involvement, i.e., abdominal pain, high fever, diarrhea, and yellowing of skin/sclera.
3. Screen for sources of liver destruction i.e alcohol ingestion, heavy acetaminophen use, hepatitis B or C.

INTERVENTIONS

1. Prevent further hepatotoxicity by reporting LFT elevations and signs of liver involvement so drug regimen can be changed.
2. Assist with the treatment for hepatotoxicity by providing supportive nursing care for pain, fever, diarrhea, and jaundice associated symptoms.

NURSING CONSIDERATIONS FOR RENAL TOXICITY

ASSESSMENT

1. Assess the following renal function tests:
• Protein (normal urine: negative)
• BUN (normal: 5–20 mg/dL)
• Serum uric acid (normal: men, 3.5–7.0 mg/dL; women, 2.4–6.0 mg/dL)
• C_{CR} (normal: women, 0.8–1.7 g/24 hr; men, 1.0–1.9 g/24 hr)
• Quantitative uric acid (normal: 250–750 mg/day)
2. Report stomach pain, swelling of feet or lower legs, shakiness, unusual body movement, or stomatitis.

INTERVENTIONS

1. Monitor I&O.
2. Limit hyperuricemia with extra fluids to speed excretion of uric acid and to decrease hazard of crystal and urate stone formation. Administer uricosuric agents (i.e., probenecid) or antigout agents (i.e., allopurinol, colchicine) to lower uric acid levels.
3. Test pH and alkalinize urine.

NURSING CONSIDERATIONS FOR IMMUNOSUPPRESSION

ASSESSMENT

1. Assess for the presence of fever, chills, or sore throat.
2. Note any changes in CBC.

INTERVENTIONS

1. To treat immunosuppression:
• Prevent infection as noted under bone marrow depression
• Delay active immunization for several months after therapy is completed; may experience a hypo- or hyperactive response
• Avoid contact with children who have recently taken the oral polio vaccine
• Avoid crowds and persons with known infections
• May be administered granulocyte colony-stimulating factor
2. Review food safety (e.g., storage, handling, washing, cook meats thoroughly, avoid raw eggs) and stress importance of kitchen hygiene when preparing meals at home.

NURSING CONSIDERATIONS FOR GU ALTERATIONS

ASSESSMENT

1. Assess for altered GU function. Most S&S, such as amenorrhea, cease after med is discontinued.
2. Review risks; sterility may be a permanent result of therapy.

CLIENT/FAMILY TEACHING

1. Certain drugs may render individuals sterile. Advise that egg/sperm harvesting may be performed prior to therapy to accommodate future pregnancies.
2. To prevent teratogenesis, teach client and partner to use reliable contraceptive measures to avoid pregnancy, both during and for several months after therapy.
3. Report any change in elimination patterns, new onset incontinence or sexual dysfunction.

NURSING CONSIDERATIONS FOR ALOPECIA

CLIENT/FAMILY TEACHING

1. Hair loss is a normal occurrence during chemotherapy. Treatment disrupts the mitotic activity of the hair follicle which weakens the hair shaft which causes it to break off. This includes all hair, i.e., eyebrows, body, and pubic hair.
2. Alopecia may occur within 2–3 weeks after the initial treatment. Assist to understand, be prepared for, and expect this as normal with chemotherapy. People respond differently; some may lose hair with a certain agent, others may not.
3. Reinforce that hair will grow back but may be of a different texture or color. It should start to grow in again about 8 weeks after therapy is completed.
4. If receiving more than 4,500 rad to the cranium, hair loss may be permanent.
5. To manage alopecia:
• Shop for a wig before hair loss begins
• Wear a bandana or hat to cover head, and take special care to protect the bare head from sun exposure

• Shave head, if hair starts to fall out in large clumps, and use a wig or scarf until scalp hair regrows
• Wear a night cap at bedtime so hair that falls out during the night will be collected in one place and not all over the bed in the morning.
• Encourage expression of feelings related to changes in self-image

NURSING CONSIDERATIONS FOR ALTERATIONS IN SKIN

ASSESSMENT

1. Document skin turgor and integrity.
2. Slight changes in skin color may occur during therapy.

INTERVENTIONS

1. Maintain cleanliness of skin through bathing with oilated soaps and frequent linen changes.
2. Prevent dryness and replenish skin moisture with emollient lotions.
3. Prevent excessive exposure to sun or artificial ultraviolet light; use sunscreen and protective clothing when exposed.
4. Use a special mattress or bed to redistribute weight on bony prominences and to minimize pressure and friction on pressure points.
5. Establish and document a schedule for repositioning, massaging, and assessing skin condition.
6. Ensure adequate nutritional intake.
7. Refer for assistance with makeup application.
8. With itching, attempt to stop scratching as this may impair skin integrity. Administer antihistamines, corticosteroids, nonirritating moisturizers, and cool/ice compresses as needed.

NURSING CONSIDERATIONS DURING INITIATION OF CHEMOTHERAPY

ASSESSMENT

1. Identify condition requiring therapy and any previous radiation, surgery, or chemotherapy treatments.
2. Assess emotional status; note any hypersensitivity to drugs or foods.
3. Determine nutritional status; note height, weight, and VS; doses are based on BSA (m^2).
4. Examine oral mucosa for any abnormalities or problems.
5. Monitor bone marrow function (CBC with differential), platelets, liver and renal function.
6. Note prescribed route of administration: oral, IV, IM, or directly at the tumor site (intracavity, intrapleural, intrathecal, intravesical, intraperitoneal, intra-arterial, or topical).
7. Depending on the route, length of therapy, frequency of access, venous integrity, and client preference, determine access device.
8. Rate pain using a pain rating scale. Assess pain control regimen to ensure pain is controlled.
9. Premedicate (antiemetic, antihistamine, and/or anti-inflammatory) 30–60 min before therapy and as needed.

INTERVENTIONS

1. Monitor VS, I&O.
2. Report any pain, redness, or edema near injection site during or after treatment. If extravasation occurs, stop infusion and follow institutional protocol for minimizing effects. General guidelines for managing an extravasation include:
   • Document/report.
   • Aspirate drug through cannula with small syringe (tuberculin size).
   • Administer antidote as indicated.
   • Remove needle and apply ice (heat if vinca alkaloids).
   • Assess until site is healed.
3. Chart antineoplastic drugs on the medication administration record (MAR) and according to the established protocol.
   • Record therapy on the MAR:
   • Day 1: first day of the first dose.
   • Number each day after that in sequence, even though may not receive drug daily.
   • Indicate when nadir (the time of most severe physiologic depression) is likely to occur so that possible complications, such as infection and bleeding, can be anticipated and treated early; note recovery time.

• When repeating drug regimen, the first day of therapy is charted as day 1.
4. Establish interventions to promote client adherence. Keep informed and interpret complicated terminology/therapy; support client/family and help distinguish/understand unconventional emotions/anger.
5. Identify references, information centers, and support groups to assist in coping with illness, understanding complex therapy, and emotional upset within the family unit.

CLIENT/FAMILY TEACHING

1. Comply with all aspects of the therapeutic regimen.
2. Ensure reliable contraception. Determine if egg/sperm harvesting indicated in young persons desiring a family.
3. Review information/literature R/T condition requiring treatment. The American Cancer Society provides many free booklets on cancers, chemotherapy, and how to deal with the side effects of treatments. Go to the library, internet, local cancer society, and provider with unanswered questions. May also call 1-800-4-CANCER, the Cancer Information Service at the National Cancer Institute, or access sites through the Internet
4. Review drug side effects that may occur and a means for coping with these problems.
5. Identify community support groups that assist to cope with illness.
6. Identify who to call to report adverse side effects or to request clarification of instructions.
7. When antineoplastic agents are prepared and administered in the home, advise families how to dispose of urine, feces, vomitus, and equipment and how to handle spills.

THROMBOCYTOPENIA

ASSESSMENT

1. Obtain platelet count (normal values: 150,000–400,000/mm^3). If below 50,000/mm^3 monitor closely.
2. Inspect skin for petechiae/bruising; assess all orifices for bleeding.
3. May hemorrhage spontaneously, transfuse if platelets <20,000.

INTERVENTIONS

1. Minimize SC or IM injections; apply pressure for 3–5 min to prevent leakage or hematoma.
2. Do not apply BP cuff or other tourniquet for excessive periods.
3. Avoid rectal temps and constipation; test all urine, GI secretions, and stool for occult blood.
4. Use safety precautions to avoid falls.
5. *Control bleeding*
• With epistaxis: pinch nose for 10 min and apply pressure to upper lip to stop; in severe cases, small sponges saturated with neosynephrine ¼% gently inserted into nare, or nasal packing, may be needed.
• With transfusions, monitor VS before and 15 min after transfusion started and after completed. Assess for histoincompatibility, indicated by chills, fever, and urticaria. Stop transfusion, provide supportive care, and follow appropriate institutional protocol for transfusion reaction.
6. Advise to *prevent bleeding* by:
• Not picking or forcefully blowing their nose
• Avoiding contact sports and any activities that may cause injury
• Reporting any severe frontal headaches
• Using an electric razor for shaving rather than a blade
• Using a soft-bristled toothbrush or massaging gums with fingers or a cotton ball and avoiding dental floss to limit irritation
• Avoiding rectal irritation by contact with enemas, suppositories, or thermometers
• Using a water-based lubricant before intercourse
• Consuming plenty of fluids, increasing activity, and taking stool softeners to prevent constipation
• Rearranging furniture so that area for ambulation is unimpeded and also to prevent bumping into furniture at night when getting out of bed to go to the bathroom

• Having a night light to permit visualization during the night
• Wearing shoes or slippers when ambulating

ANEMIA

ASSESSMENT

1. Monitor CBC, reticulocyte count, MCV and hemoglobin (normal values: men, 13.5–18.0 g/dL blood; women, 11.5–15.5 g/dL blood), and hematocrit (normal values: men, 40%–52%; women, 35%–46%), and iron panel.
2. Assess for pallor, lethargy, dizziness, increased SOB/ ↑ fatigue.

INTERVENTIONS

1. *Minimize anemia by:*
• Providing nutritious tolerable diet
• Taking vitamins/iron supplements
2. *Assist with treatment of anemia by:*
• Administering diet high in iron
• Giving vitamins with minerals
• Administering blood transfusions
• Spacing/scheduling activities to permit frequent rest periods
• Positioning to facilitate ventilation; teaching breathing/relaxation techniques and administering oxygen
• Controlling room temperature for comfort/providing emotional support

BOWEL DYSFUNCTION (DIARRHEA/ ABDOMINAL CRAMPING)

ASSESSMENT

1. Note frequency and severity of cramping caused by hypermotility.
2. Document frequency, color, consistency, and amount of diarrhea; indicates tissue destruction. C&S stool.
3. Assess for dehydration and acidosis indicating electrolyte imbalance; monitor I&O.

INTERVENTIONS

1. *To prevent diarrhea/abdominal cramping:*
• Provide small, frequent meals on a schedule
• I• dentify factors that aggravate/increase incidence
• Use constipating foods, i.e., hard cheeses
2. *To treat diarrhea:*
• Administer antidiarrheal and narcotic agent (i.e., codeine, tincture of opium, imodium, or lomotil). Report S&S as a change in therapy or electrolyte correction may be needed.
• Increase fluids/avoid dehydration
• Provide foods to correct sodium and potassium losses, e.g., bananas, potatoes, fish and meat, apricot nectar, tomato juice, and sports drinks with "electrolytes"
• Avoid high-fiber foods that contain "insoluble fiber," such as wheat bran, brown rice, popcorn
• Administer bulk-forming agents (i.e., metamucil)
• Offer "soluble-fiber" foods, i.e., white rice, oatmeal, applesauce, mashed potatoes, and pears
• Avoid fried/greasy foods
• Avoid excessive sweets; may aggravate diarrhea due to sorbitol, found in many gums and candies
• Use alumimum-containing antacids
• Avoid gas-forming foods, such as broccoli, corn, onion, garlic, lentils, and kidney beans
• Consider lactose-free products or Lact-Aid, which facilitates digestion of lactose
• Restrict oral intake to rest the bowel if necessary
• Provide good skin care, especially to perianal area to prevent skin breakdown. Apply A&D ointment for perianal tenderness. Change gown and bed linens frequently; use special mattresses and room deodorizers as needed.
3. *To prevent constipation:*
• Provide a high-fiber diet
• Give stool softeners and bulk-forming agents
• Increase fluid intake
• Increase activity levels
• Monitor frequency, consistency, and amount of stool
4. *To prevent obstruction:*
• Aggressively manage constipation
• Assess for early S&S such as abdominal pain, N&V, and diminished or absent bowel sounds
• Keep NPO, using NG suction to relieve before referring for surgical intervention.

STOMATITIS (MUCOSAL ULCERATION)

ASSESSMENT

1. Assess for mouth dryness, erythema, soreness, painful swallowing, and white patchy areas of oral mucosa.
2. Symptom onset usually 5 days to 2 weeks after starting therapy; assess regularly.

INTERVENTIONS

1. *To prevent stomatitis:*
• Assess oral cavity t.i.d. and report bleeding gums or burning sensation when acid liquids such as fruit juice are ingested
• Set up a regular schedule for oral preventive care
• Provide good mouth care
• Apply lubricant (Vaseline) to lips t.i.d.
2. *To treat stomatitis:*
• Provide good oral care
• Apply topical viscous anesthetic, such as benzocaine 20%, or a swish and gargle anesthetic dyclonine hydrochloride 0.5%, or a swish, swallow/discard agent such as lidocaine 2% (Xylocaine), before meals or as needed to anesthetize oral mucosa. May swallow lidocaine after swishing it around oral cavity but encourage to expectorate it.
• Puncture a vitamin E capsule and apply to painful lesions to promote healing
• Offer "Magic Mouthwash," which consists of 4 g (approx. ⅛ teaspoon) baking soda, 30mL viscous xylocaine, 30mL benedryl elixir, and 30mL Maalox (optional) in 1 L NSS; swish and spit out q 1–2 hr as needed
• Provide allopurinol mouthwash for fluorouracil-related stomatitis; or try sucking ice chips ½ hr before and during treatment
• Offer small, frequent meals of bland foods at medium temperatures
• Administer nystatin solution or clotrimazole troches orally for fungal infections
3. Administer medications (antifungals, antivirals) to prevent general infections.
4. Systemic antifungals may be required. If no relief investigate alternative therapies i.e, neupogen etc. Do NOT let client continue to suffer as this is very painful and impairs recovery.

ANTIPARKINSON AGENTS

SEE ALSO THE FOLLOWING INDIVIDUAL ENTRIES:

DOPAMINERGIC AGENTS:
Amantadine hydrochloride
Bromocriptine mesylate
Carbidopa
Carbidopa/Levodopa
Entacapone
Levodopa
Pergolide mesylate
Pramipexole
Ropinirole hydrochloride
Tolcapone

ANTICHOLINERGIC DRUGS:
Benztropine mesylate
Biperiden hydrochloride
Diphenhydramine hydrochloride
Trihexyphenidyl hydrochloride

GENERAL STATEMENT

Parkinson's disease is a progressive disorder of the nervous system, affecting mostly people over the age of 50. Parkinsonism is a frequent side effect of certain antipsychotic drugs, including prochlorperazine, chlorpromazine, and reserpine. Drug-induced symptoms usually disappear when the responsible agent is discontinued. The cause of Parkinson's disease is unknown; however, it is associated with a depletion of the neurotransmitter dopamine in the nervous system. Treatment focuses on administration of domapinergic agents and/or anticholinergic drugs. Administration of levodopa—the precursor of dopamine—relieves symptoms in 75–80% of the clients. Most of the newer antiparkinson drugs must be given with levodopa. Anticholinergic agents also have a beneficial effect by reducing tremors and rigidity and improving mobility, muscular coordination, and motor performance. They are often administered together with levodopa. Certain antihistamines, notably diphenhydramine (Benadryl), are also useful in the treatment of parkinsonism. Clients suffering from Parkinson's disease need emotional support and encouragement because the debilitating nature of the disorder often causes depression. Comprehensive treatment also includes physical therapy.

NURSING CONSIDERATIONS

SEE *NURSING CONSIDERATIONS* FOR INDIVIDUAL DRUGS.

ASSESSMENT

1. Document PMH, onset and characteristics of symptoms, and progression.
2. Determine if S&S drug induced with agents such as haldol or phenothiazines.
3. Assess for depression, behavioral changes, and suicide ideations.

CLIENT/FAMILY TEACHING

1. Parkinson's disease is a movement disorder of unknown origin; is usually progressive and leads to disability if untreated.
2. Drug therapy is aimed at restoring normal balances of cholinergic and dopaminergic influences in the brain (basal ganglia) to control tremor and permit ADL.
3. Take only as prescribed; some have many adverse side effects.
4. Close neurologic follow-up is imperative; some drugs may lose effectiveness and changes or additional therapy may be needed.

OUTCOMES/EVALUATE

- Improved motor function/mood
- ↓ Drooling, ↓ rigidity, ↓ tremors
- Improved gait, posture, and ↓ muscle spasms

ANTIPSYCHOTIC AGENTS, PHENOTHIAZINES

SEE ALSO THE FOLLOWING INDIVIDUAL ENTRIES:

Chlorpromazine hydrochloride
Fluphenazine decanoate
Fluphenazine enanthate
Fluphenazine hydrochloride
Perphenazine
Prochlorperazine
Prochlorperazine edisylate
Prochlorperazine maleate
Thioridazine hydrochloride
Trifluoperazine

GENERAL STATEMENT

Antipsychotic drugs do not cure mental illness, but they calm the intractable client, relieve the despondency of the severely depressed, activate the immobile and withdrawn, and make some more accessible to psychotherapy.

Most phenothiazines induce some sedation, especially during the initial phase of the treatment. Medicated clients can, however, be easily roused. In this manner, the phenothiazines differ markedly from the narcotic analgesics and sedative hypnotics. However, phenothiazines potentiate the analgesic properties of opiates and prolong the action of CNS depressant drugs. These drugs also cause sedation, decrease spontaneous motor activity, and many lower BP.

According to their detailed chemical structure, the phenothiazines belong to three subgroups:

1. **Aliphatic compounds.** Moderate to high sedative, anticholinergic, and orthostatic hypotensive effects. Moderate extrapyramidal symptoms. Often the first choice for clients in acute excitatory states. Examples: Chlorpromazine, promazine, triflupromazine.
2. **Piperazine compounds.** Act most selectively on the subcortical sites. Low to moderate sedative effects; low anticholinergic and orthostatic hypotensive effects; high incidence of extrapyramidal symptoms. Greatest antiemetic effects because they specifically depress the CTZ of the vomiting center. Examples: Fluphenazine, perphenazine, prochlorperazine, trifluoperazine.
3. **Piperidine compounds.** Low incidence of extrapyramidal effects; high sedative and anticholinergic effects; low to moderate orthostatic hy-

potensive effect. Examples: Mesoridazine, thioridazine.

ACTION/KINETICS

It has been postulated that excess amounts of dopamine in certain areas of the CNS cause psychoses. Phenothiazines are thought to act by blocking postsynaptic mesolimbic dopamine receptors, leading to a reduction in psychotic symptoms. Phenothiazines block both D_1 and D_2 dopamine receptors. The antiemetic effects are thought to be due to inhibition or blockade of dopamine (D_2) receptors in the chemoreceptor trigger zone in the medulla as well as by peripheral blockade of the vagus nerve in the GI tract. Relief of anxiety is manifested as a result of an indirect decrease in arousal and increased filtering of internal stimuli to the brain stem reticular system. Alpha-adrenergic blockade produces sedation. Phenothiazines also raise pain threshold and produce amnesia due to suppression of sensory impulses. In addition, these drugs produce anticholinergic and antihistaminic effects and depress the release of hypothalamic and hypophyseal hormones. Peripheral effects include anticholinergic and alpha-adrenergic blocking properties.

Peak plasma levels: 2–4 hr after PO administration. Widely distributed throughout the body. **t½ (average):** 10–20 hr. Most metabolized in the liver and excreted by the kidney.

USES

Psychoses, especially if excessive psychomotor activity manifested. Involutional, toxic, or senile psychoses. Used in combination with MAO inhibitors in depressed clients manifesting anxiety, agitation, or panic (use with caution). With lithium in acute manic phase of manic-depressive illness. As an adjunct in alcohol withdrawal to reduce anxiety, tension, depression, nausea, and/or vomiting. For severe behavioral problems in children, manifested by hyperexcitable and/or combative behavior; also, for short-term use in hyperactive children who exhibit excess motor activity and conduct disorders.

Prophylaxis and control of severe N&V due to cancer chemotherapy, radiation therapy, postoperatively. Intractable hiccoughs, intermittent porphyria, tetanus (as adjunct). As preoperative and/or postoperative medications. Some phenothiazines are antipruritics. See also individual drugs.

CONTRAINDICATIONS

Severe CNS depression, coma, clients with subcortical brain damage, bone marrow depression, lactation. In clients with a history of seizures and in those on anticonvulsant drugs. Geriatric or debilitated clients, hepatic or renal disease, CV disorders, glaucoma, prostatic hypertrophy. Contraindicated in children with chickenpox, CNS infections, measles, gastroenteritis, dehydration due to increased risk of extrapyramidal symptoms.

SPECIAL CONCERNS

Use with caution in clients exposed to extreme heat or cold and in those with asthma, emphysema, or acute respiratory tract infections. Use during pregnancy only when benefits outweigh risks. Children may be more sensitive to the neuromuscular or extrapyramidal effects (especially dystonias); those especially at risk include children with chickenpox, CNS infections, measles, dehydration, or gastroenteritis. Thus, generally, phenothiazines are not recommended for use in children less than 12 years of age. Geriatric clients often manifest higher plasma levels due to decreases in lean body mass, total body water, and albumin and an increase in total body fat. Also, geriatric clients may be more likely to manifest orthostatic hypotension, anticholinergic effects, sedative effects, and extrapyramidal side effects.

SIDE EFFECTS

CNS: Depression, drowsiness, dizziness, lethargy, fatigue. Extrapyramidal effects, Parkinson-like symptoms including shuffling gait or tic-like movements of head and face, tardive dyskinesia (see what follows), akathisia, dystonia. ***Seizures,*** especially in clients with a history thereof. ***Neuroleptic malignant syndrome (rare).*** **CV:** Orthostatic hypotension, increase or decrease in BP, tachycardia, fainting. **GI:** Dry mouth, anorexia, constipation, paralytic ileus, diarrhea. **Endocrine:** Breast engorgement, galactorrhea, gynecomastia, increased appetite, weight gain, hyper- or hypoglycemia, glycosuria. Delayed ejaculation, increased or decreased libido. **GU:** Menstrual irregularities, loss of bladder control, urinary difficulty. **Dermatologic:** Photosensitivity, pruritus, erythema, eczema, exfoliative dermatitis, pigment changes in skin (long-term use of high doses). **Hematologic:** ***Aplastic anemia,*** leukopenia, ***agranulocytosis,*** eosinophilia, thrombocytopenia. **Ophthalmologic:** Deposition of fine particulate matter in lens and cornea leading to blurred vision, changes in vision. **Respiratory:** ***Laryngospasm, bronchospasm, laryngeal edema,*** breathing difficulties. **Miscellaneous:** Fever, muscle stiffness, decreased sweating, muscle spasm of face, neck, or back, obstructive jaundice, nasal congestion, pale skin, mydriasis, systemic lupus-like syndrome.

Tardive dyskinesia has been observed with all classes of antipsychotic drugs, although the precise cause is not known. The syndrome is most commonly seen in older clients, especially women, and in individuals with organic brain syndrome. It is often aggravated or precipitated by the sudden discontinuance of antipsychotic drugs and may persist indefinitely after the drug is discontinued. Early signs of tardive dyskinesia include fine vermicular movements of the tongue and grimacing or tic-like movements of the head and neck. Although there is no known cure for the syndrome, it may not progress if the doșage of the drug is slowly reduced. Also, a few drug-free days may unmask the symptoms of tardive dyskinesia and help in early diagnosis.

OD OVERDOSE MANAGEMENT

Symptoms: CNS depression including deep sleep and ***coma,*** hypotension, extrapyramidal symptoms, agitation, restlessness, seizures, hypothermia, ***hyperthermia,*** autonomic symptoms, ***cardiac arrhythmias,*** ECG changes. *Treatment:* Emetics are not to be used as they are of little value and may cause a dystonic reaction of the head or neck that may result in aspiration of vomitus.

- Hypotension: Volume replacement; norepinephrine or phenylephrine may be used (do not use epinephrine).
- Ventricular arrhythmias: phenytoin, 1 mg/kg IV, not to exceed 50 mg/min; may be repeated q 5 min up to 10 mg/kg.
- Seizures or hyperactivity: Diazepam or pentobarbital.
- Extrapyramidal symptoms: Antiparkinson drugs, diphenhydramine, barbiturates.

DRUG INTERACTIONS

Alcohol, ethyl / Potentiation or addition of CNS depressant effects. Concomitant use may lead to drowsiness, lethargy, stupor, respiratory collapse, coma, or death
Aluminum salts (antacids) / ↓ Absorption from GI tract
Amphetamine / ↓ Drug effect by ↓ drug uptake to the action site
Anesthetics, general / See *Alcohol*
Antacids, oral / ↓ Effect of phenothiazines R/T ↓ GI tract absorption
Antianxiety drugs / See *Alcohol*
Anticholinergic drugs / Additive anticholinergic side effects and/or ↓ antipsychotic effect
Antidepressants, tricyclic / Additive anticholinergic side effects; also, ↑ TCA serum levels
Barbiturate anesthetics / ↑ Chance of tremor, involuntary muscle activity, and hypotension
Barbiturates / See *Alcohol;* also, drugs may ↓ effect R/T ↑ liver breakdown
Bromocriptine / Phenothiazines ↓ effect
Charcoal / ↓ Effect of phenothiazines R/T ↓ GI tract absorption

CNS depressants / See *Alcohol;* also, ↓ effect of phenothiazines R/T ↑ liver breakdown
Colistimethate / Additive respiratory depression
Diazoxide / Additive hyperglycemic effect
H *Evening primrose oil* / May worsen temporal lobe epilepsy or schizophrenia when used with phenothiazines
H *Ginseng* / Do not use with antipsychotics
Guanethidine / ↓ Drug effect by ↓ drug uptake at action site
H *Henbane leaf* / Additive anticholinergic effects
Hydantoins / ↑ Risk of hydantoin toxicity
Lithium carbonate / ↑ Risk of extrapyramidal symptoms, disorientation, or unconsciousness
MAO inhibitors / ↑ Effect of phenothiazines R/T ↓ liver breakdown
Meperidine / ↑ Risk of hypotension and sedation
Metrizamide / ↑ Risk of seizures during subarachnoid administration of metrizamide
H *Milk thistle* / Helps prevent liver damage from phenothiazines
Narcotics / See *Alcohol*
Phenytoin / ↑ or ↓ Serum levels of phenytoin
Pimozide / Additive effect on QT interval; do not use together
Propranolol / ↑ Plasma levels of both drugs
Sedative-hypnotics, nonbarbiturate / See *Alcohol*

LABORATORY TEST CONSIDERATIONS

False +: Bile (urine dipstick), ferric chloride, pregnancy tests, urinary porphobilinogen, urinary steroids, urobilinogen (urine dipstick). False –: Inorganic phosphorus, urinary steroids. *Caused by pharmacologic effects:* ↑ Alkaline phosphatase, bilirubin, serum transaminases, serum cholesterol, urinary catecholamines. ↓ Glucose tolerance, serum uric acid, 5-HIAA, FSH, growth hormone, LH, vanillylmandelic acid.

DOSAGE

See individual drugs. Effective over a wide dosage range. Dosage is usually increased gradually to minimize side effects over 7 days until the minimal effective dose is attained. Dosage is increased more gradually in elderly or debilitated clients because they are more susceptible to the effects and side effects of drugs. After symptoms are controlled, dosage is gradually reduced to maintenance levels. It is usually desirable to keep chronically ill clients on maintenance levels indefinitely. Medication, especially in clients on high dosages, should not be discontinued abruptly.

NURSING CONSIDERATIONS

ADMINISTRATION/STORAGE

1. Do not interchange brands of PO form of drug or suppositories; may differ in bioavailability.
2. Do not use pink or markedly discolored solutions.
3. When preparing or administering parenteral solutions, nurse and client should avoid contact of drug with skin, eyes, and clothing to prevent contact dermatitis.
4. Do not mix antipsychotic drugs with other drugs in the same syringe.
5. Order a specific flow rate when administering parenteral solutions.
6. To lessen injection pain, dilute commercially available injectable solutions in saline or local anesthetic.
7. When administering IM, inject drug deeply into the muscle.
8. Massage area of injection site after IM administration to reduce pain.
9. Prevent extravasation of the IV solution.
10. Store solutions in a cool dry place in amber-colored containers.

ASSESSMENT

1. Take a complete medical and drug history; note any drug hypersensitivity or genetic predisposition. (These agents are referred to as neuroleptics in Europe.)
2. Determine any history of seizures; this class of drugs may lower seizure threshold.

3. Document indications for therapy. Assess baseline mental status, noting mood, behavior, and any depression.
4. If administering to children, note extent of hyperexcitability.
5. Assess child for chickenpox or measles.
6. Note any history of asthma or emphysema.
7. Monitor VS; assess BP in both arms in a reclining position, standing position, and sitting position, 2 min apart.
8. Monitor hematologic profile, liver and renal function studies, urinalysis, ECG, and ocular findings.

INTERVENTIONS

1. If administered IV, monitor flow rate and BP. Keep recumbent for at least 1 hr after IV completed, then slowly elevate HOB and observe for tachycardia, faintness, or dizziness; supervise ambulation.
2. If hospitalized, ensure that med has been swallowed. May give a liquid preparation to permit better control over drug taking and to improve compliance.
3. Measure I&O; report abdominal distention and urinary retention. May need to reduce dosage, add antispasmodics, or change therapy.
4. Note any changes in carbohydrate metabolism (e.g., glycosuria, weight loss, polyphagia, increased appetite, or excessive weight gain); may require a change in diet/drug therapy and can be significant with diabetes.
5. Some may develop a hypersensitivity reaction with fever, asthma, laryngeal edema, angioneurotic edema, and anaphylactic reaction. *Stop medication, notify provider, and treat symptomatically.*
6. The antiemetic effects of phenothiazines may mask other pathology such as toxicity to other drugs, intestinal obstruction, or brain lesions.
7. If receiving barbiturates to relieve anxiety, reduce barbiturate dose. If administered as an anticonvulsant, do not reduce dosage.
8. Discontinue drug gradually to minimize severe GI disturbances or tardive dyskinesia.

CLIENT/FAMILY TEACHING

1. May take with food or milk to minimize GI upset. Take as directed, may be weeks or months before the full effects will be noticed
2. Do not stop taking abruptly. Abrupt cessation of high doses of phenothiazines can cause N&V, tremors, sensations of warmth and cold, sweating, tachycardia, headache, and insomnia.
3. Report distress when in a hot or cold room; may affect heat-regulating mechanism.
   - Provide extra blankets if cold.
   - Bathe in tepid water if too warm.
   - Do *NOT* use heating pads or hot water bottles if feeling cold.
   - Avoid hot tubs, hot baths/showers; low BP may occur from vasodilation.
4. Report if excessively active or depressed. Spasms of face, neck, back, or tongue may be treated with antihistamines, or drug discontinuation.
5. Report S&S of blood dyscrasias: ↑ body temperature, weakness, easy bruising, or sore throat.
6. Take slow, deep breaths if respiratory S&S occur; may depress cough reflex.
7. May cause menstrual irregularity and false positive pregnancy tests; may develop engorged breasts and begin lactating. Keep accurate record of periods and report if pregnant.
8. Males may experience decreased libido and develop breast enlargement. Report so drug can be adjusted.
9. May develop photosensitivity reactions; wear protective clothing, sunglasses, sunscreen and avoid sunbathing.
10. Drug may discolor the urine pink or reddish brown. With long-term therapy may develop a yellow-brown skin reaction that may turn grayish purple.
11. Avoid driving a car or operating heavy machinery or engaging in any activities that require mental alertness until effects realized; consult provider prior to resuming.
12. Long-term therapy may affect vision; schedule regular ophthalmic ex-

ams. Report blurred vision and avoid driving.

13. Report evidence of early cholestatic jaundice, such as high fever, upper abdominal pain, nausea, diarrhea, itching, and rash.

14. Withhold drug and report if yellowing of the sclera, skin, or mucous membranes occurs; may indicate biliary obstruction.

15. To prevent dry mouth, rinse mouth frequently, increase fluid intake, chew sugarless gum, and suck on sugarless hard candies.

16. Increase fluids and bulk in diet to minimize constipation; may need laxatives. Report any urinary retention or persistent constipation.

17. Rise slowly from a lying or sitting position; dangle legs before standing to avoid orthostatic symptoms.

18. Avoid alcohol, OTC drugs, and any other CNS depressants without approval.

19. When working with the elderly, be particularly observant for symptoms of tardive dyskinesia. May exhibit puffing of the cheeks or tongue; may develop chewing movements and involuntary movements of the extremities and trunk.

20. If administering to a child, note neuromuscular reactions, especially if dehydrated or has an acute infection making more susceptible to side effects.

21. Report for periodic labs and follow-up care to evaluate and adjust drug dosage.

OUTCOMES/EVALUATE

- ↓ Excitable, withdrawn, agitated, or paranoid behaviors
- Orientation to time and place, and an understanding of illness
- Adherence to prescribed drug regimen
- Relief of N&V

ANTIVIRAL DRUGS

SEE ALSO THE FOLLOWING INDIVIDUAL ENTRIES:

Abacavir sulfate
Acyclovir
Amantadine hydrochloride
Amprenavir
Cidofovir
Delavirdine mesylate
Didanosine
Efavirenz
Famciclovir
Fomivirsen sodium
Foscarnet sodium
Ganciclovir sodium
Idoxuridine
Indinavir sulfate
Lamivudine
Lamivudine/Zidovudine
Nelfinavir mesylate
Nevirapine
Oseltamivir phosphate
Penciclovir
Ribavirin
Rimantidine hydrochloride
Ritonavir
Saquinavir mesylate
Stavudine
Tenofovir disoproxil fumarate
Trifluridine
Valacyclovir hydrochloride
Valganciclovir hydrochloride
Vidarabine
Zalcitabine
Zanimivir
Zidovudine

ACTION/KINETICS

To maintain their growth and reproduce, viruses must enter living cells. Thus, it is difficult to find a drug that is specific for the virus and that does not interfere with the function of the host cell. However, there are enzymes and replicative mechanisms that are unique to viruses and an increasing number of drugs with specific antiviral activity have been developed. The antiviral drugs currently marketed act by one of the following mechanisms:

1. Inhibition of enzymes required for DNA synthesis. Example: Idoxuridine.
2. Inhibition of viral nucleic acid synthesis by interacting directly with herpes virus DNA polymerase or HIV reverse transcriptase. Example: Foscarnet.
3. Inhibition of viral DNA or protein synthesis. Examples: Acyclovir, cidofovir, famciclovir, fomivirsen, ganci-

clovir, penciclovir, trifluridine, valacyclovir, vidarabine.

4. Prevent penetration of the virus into cells by inhibiting uncoating of the RNA virus. Examples: Amantadine, rimantadine.

5. Protease inhibitors resulting in release of immature, noninfectious viral particles. Examples: Indinavir, nelfinavir, ritonavir, saquinavir.

6. Reverse transcriptase inhibitors (nucleoside and non-nucleoside) resulting in inhibition of replication of the virus. Examples of nucleoside inhibitors: Abacavir, didanosine, lamivudine, stavudine, zalcitabine, zidovudine. Examples of non-nucleoside inhibitors: Efavirenz, delavirdine, nevirapine. It is often necessary to combine two antiviral drugs that have the same or different mechanisms of action in order to treat HIV infections and to minimize development of resistant viruses. For example, regimens of choice include two nucleosides and one protease inhibitor or two nucleosides and one non-nucleoside.

USES

HIV infection. Guidelines suggest five different combinations as initial therapy: (1) one protease inhibitor plus two nucleoside reverse transcriptase inhibitors; (2) two nucleoside reverse transcriptase inhibitors and a nonnucleoside reverse transcriptase inhibitor; (3) two protease inhibitors with or without nucleoside reverse transcriptase inhibitors; (4) a nucleoside reverse transcriptase inhibitor, a nonnucleoside reverse transcriptase inhibitor, and a protease inhibitors; or, (5) three nucleoside reverse transcriptase inhibitors.

NURSING CONSIDERATIONS

SEE *GENERAL NURSING CONSIDERATIONS* FOR *ALL ANTI-INFECTIVES*.

ASSESSMENT

1. Document indications for therapy, type/onset of symptoms, and exposure characteristics.

2. Monitor CBC, renal and LFTs; also viral loads/T cells as indicated.

3. List other agents prescribed to ensure none interact unfavorably.

4. Note underlying medical conditions that may preclude drug therapy.

5. Assess support systems and client adherance potential.

CLIENT/FAMILY TEACHING

1. Review method and frequency for drug administration. Stress importance of adherance to multi drug regimens and how to take exactly as directed; do not share meds.

2. Identify specific measures to decrease/halt disease spread.

3. Maintain adequate nutrition; consume 2–3 L/day of fluids to prevent crystalluria.

4. Report any rashes or unusual drug side effects.

5. Report if symptoms do not improve or worsen after specified time.

6. Close medical supervision/follow-up required during therapy.

OUTCOMES/EVALUATE

- Prophylaxis of viral infections
- Reduction in length and severity of symptoms of viral infections

BETA-ADRENERGIC BLOCKING AGENTS

SEE ALSO ALPHA-1-ADRENERGIC BLOCKING AGENTS AND THE FOLLOWING INDIVIDUAL AGENTS:

Acebutolol hydrochloride
Atenolol
Betaxolol hydrochloride
Bisoprolol fumarate
Carteolol hydrochloride
Esmolol hydrochloride
Levobunolol hydrochloride
Metipranolol hydrochloride
Metoprolol succinate
Metoprolol tartrate
Nadolol
Penbutolol sulfate
Pindolol
Propranolol hydrochloride
Sotalol hydrochloride
Timolol maleate

ACTION/KINETICS

Combine reversibly with beta-adrenergic receptors to block the response to sympathetic nerve impulses, circulating catecholamines, or adrenergic drugs. Beta-adrenergic receptors are classified as beta-1 (predominantly in the cardiac muscle) and beta-2 (mainly in the bronchi and vascular musculature). Blockade of beta-1 receptors decreases HR, myocardial contractility, and CO; in addition, AV conduction is slowed. These effects lead to a decrease in BP, as well as a reversal of cardiac arrhythmias. Blockade of beta-2 receptors increases airway resistance in the bronchioles and inhibits the vasodilating effects of catecholamines on peripheral blood vessels. The various beta-blocking agents differ in their ability to block beta-1 and beta-2 receptors (see individual drugs); also, certain of these agents have intrinsic sympathomimetic action.

Certain of these drugs (betaxolol, carteolol, levobunolol, metipranolol, and timolol) are used for glaucoma. Act by reducing production of aqueous humor; metipranolol and timolol may also increase outflow of aqueous humor. Drugs have little or no effect on the pupil size or on accommodation.

USES

See individual drugs. Depending on the drug uses include hypertension, angina pectoris, MI, migraine, and several other uses. Should be part of the standard therapy for CHF. Are important in clients who have survived a first MI.

CONTRAINDICATIONS

Sinus bradycardia, second- and third-degree AV block, cardiogenic shock, CHF unless secondary to tachyarrhythmia treatable with beta blockers, overt cardiac failure. Most are contraindicated in chronic bronchitis, bronchial asthma or history thereof, bronchospasm, emphysema, severe COPD.

SPECIAL CONCERNS

Use with caution in diabetes, thyrotoxicosis, cerebrovascular insufficiency, and impaired hepatic and renal function. Withdrawing beta blockers before major surgery is controversial. Safe use during pregnancy and lactation and in children has not been established. May be absorbed systemically when used for glaucoma; thus, there is the potential for an additive effect with beta blockers used systemically. Certain of the products for use in glaucoma contain sulfites, which may result in an allergic reaction. Also, see individual agents.

SIDE EFFECTS

CV: Bradycardia, hypotension (especially following IV use), CHF, cold extremities, claudication, worsening of angina, strokes, edema, syncope, arrhythmias, chest pain, peripheral ischemia, flushing, SOB, sinoatrial block, pulmonary edema, vasodilation, increased HR, palpitations, conduction disturbances, ***first-, second-, and third-degree heart block,*** worsening of AV block, thrombosis of renal or mesenteric arteries, precipitation or worsening of Raynaud's phenomenon. Sudden withdrawal of large doses may cause angina, ventricular tachycardia, ***fatal MI, sudden death,*** or ***circulatory collapse.*** **GI:** N&V, diarrhea, flatulence, dry mouth, constipation, anorexia, cramps, bloating, gastric pain, dyspepsia, distortion of taste, weight gain or loss, retroperitoneal fibrosis, ischemic colitis. **Hepatic:** Hepatomegaly, acute pancreatitis, elevated liver enzymes, liver damage (especially with chronic use of phenobarbital). **Respiratory:** Asthma-like symptoms, ***bronchospasms, bronchial obstruction, laryngospasm with respiratory distress,*** wheeziness, worsening of chronic obstructive lung disease, dyspnea, cough, nasal stuffiness, rhinitis, pharyngitis, rales. **CNS:** Dizziness, fatigue, lethargy, vivid dreams, depression, hallucinations, delirium, psychoses, paresthesias, insomnia, nervousness, nightmares, headache, vertigo, disorientation of time and place, hypoesthesia or hyperesthesia, decreased concentration, short-term memory loss, change in behavior, emotional lability, slurred speech, lightheadedness. In the elderly, paranoia, disorientation, and combativeness have occurred. **Hematologic:** ***Agranulocytosis,*** thrombocytopenia. **Allergic:** Fever, sore throat, respiratory distress, rash, pharyngitis, ***laryngospasm, anaphylaxis.*** **Skin:** Pruritus, rashes, increased skin pigmentation, sweating, dry skin, alopecia, skin irritation, psoriasis (reversible). **Musculoskeletal:** Joint and muscle pain, arthritis, arthralgia, back pain, muscle cramps, muscle weakness when used in clients with myasthenic symptoms. **GU:** Impotence, decreased libido, dysuria, UTI, nocturia, urinary retention or frequency, pollakiuria. **Ophthalmic:** Visual disturbances, eye irritation, dry or burning eyes, blurred vision, conjunctivitis. When used ophthalmically: keratitis, blepharoptosis, diplopia, ptosis, and visual disturbances including refractive changes. **Other:** Hyperglycemia or hypoglycemia, lupus-like syndrome, Peyronie's disease, tinnitus, increase in symptoms of myasthenia gravis, facial swelling, decreased exercise tolerance, rigors, speech disorders. **Systemic effects due to ophthalmic beta-1 and beta-2 blockers:** Headache, depression, arrhythmia, heart block, CVA, syncope, CHF, palpitation, cerebral ischemia, nausea, localized and generalized rash, bronchospasm (especially in those with preexisting bronchospastic disease), respiratory failure, masked symptoms of hypoglycemia in insulin-dependent diabetics, keratitis, visual disturbances (including refractive changes), blepharoptosis, ptosis, diplopia.

OD OVERDOSE MANAGEMENT

Symptoms: CV symptoms include bradycardia, hypotension, CHF, ***cardiogenic shock,*** intraventricular conduction disturbances, ***AV block, pulmonary edema, asystole,*** and tachycardia. Also, overdosage of pindolol may cause hypertension and overdosage of propranolol may result in systemic vascular resistance. CNS symptoms include respiratory depression, decreased consciousness, ***coma, and seizures.*** Miscellaneous symptoms include ***bronchospasm*** (especially in clients with obstructive pulmonary disease), hyperkalemia, and hypoglycemia.

- *Treatment:* To improve blood supply to the brain, place client in a supine position and raise the legs.
- Measure blood glucose and serum potassium. Monitor BP and ECG continuously.
- Provide general supportive treatment such as inducing emesis or gastric lavage and artificial respiration.
- *Seizures:* Give IV diazepam or phenytoin.
- *Excessive bradycardia:* If hypotensive, give atropine, 0.6 mg; if no response, give q 3 min for a total of 2–3 mg. Cautious administration of isoproterenol may be tried. Also, glucagon, 5–10 mg rapidly over 30 sec, followed by continuous IV infusion of 5 mg/hr may reverse bradycardia. Transvenous cardiac pacing may be needed for refractory cases.
- *Cardiac failure:* Digitalis, diuretic, and oxygen; if failure is refractory, IV aminophylline or glucagon may be helpful.
- *Hypotension:* Place client in Trendelenburg position. IV fluids unless pulmonary edema is present; also vasopressors such as norepinephrine (may be drug of choice), dobutamine, dopamine with monitoring of BP. If refractory, glucagon may be helpful. In intractable cardiogenic shock, intra-aortic balloon insertion may be required.
- *Premature ventricular contractions:* Lidocaine or phenytoin. Disopyramide, quinidine, and procainamide should be avoided as they depress myocardial function further.
- *Bronchospasms:* Give a beta-2-adrenergic agonist, epinephrine, or theophylline.
- *Heart block, second or third degree:* Isoproterenol or transvenous cardiac pacing.

DRUG INTERACTIONS

Aluminum salts / ↓ Bioavailability of certain beta-blockers → ↓ effect
Ampicillin / ↓ Bioavailability of certain beta-blockers → ↓ effect

Anesthetics, general / Additive depression of myocardium
Anticholinergic agents / Counteract bradycardia produced by beta-adrenergic blockers
Antihypertensives / Additive hypotensive effect
Barbiturates / ↓ Bioavailability of certain beta-blockers → ↓ effect
Benzodiazepines / ↑ Effect of certain benzodiazepines by lipophilic beta-blockers
Calcium channel blockers / ↑ Effect of certain beta-blockers
Calcium salts / ↓ Bioavailability of certain beta-blockers → ↓ effect
Chlorpromazine / Additive beta-adrenergic blocking action
Cholestyramine / ↓ Bioavailability of certain beta-blockers → ↓ effect
Cimetidine / ↑ Effect of beta blockers R/T ↓ liver breakdown
Clonidine / Paradoxical hypertension; also, ↑ severity of rebound hypertension
Colestipol / ↓ Bioavailability of certain beta-blockers → ↓ effect
Diphenhydramine / ↑ Plasma levels and CV effects of certain beta-blockers R/T ↓ metabolism
Disopyramide / ↑ Effect of both drugs
Epinephrine / Beta blockers prevent beta-adrenergic action of epinephrine but not alpha-adrenergic action → ↑ systolic and diastolic BP and ↓ HR
Ergot alkaloids / ↑ Risk of peripheral ischemia R/T ergot alkaloid-mediated vasoconstriction and peripheral effects of beta-blockers
Flecainide / Possible ↑ bioavailability of either drug → ↑ effects
Furosemide / ↑ Beta-adrenergic blockade
Haloperidol / ↑ Risk of hypotensive episodes
Hydralazine / ↑ Effect of both beta-blockers and hydralazine
Hydroxychloroquine / ↑ Plasma levels and CV effects of certain beta-blockers R/T ↓ metabolism
Indomethacin / ↓ Effect of beta blockers possibly due to inhibition of prostaglandin synthesis
Insulin / Beta blockers ↑ hypoglycemic effect of insulin
Lidocaine / ↑ Drug effect R/T ↓ liver breakdown
Methyldopa / Possible ↑ BP to alpha-adrenergic effect
Muscle relaxants, nondepolarizing / Beta-blockers may potentiate, counteract, or have no effect on action of nondepolarizing muscle relaxants
NSAIDs / ↓ Effect of beta blockers, possibly due to inhibition of prostaglandin synthesis
Ophthalmic beta blockers / Additive systemic beta-blocking effects if used with oral beta blockers
Oral contraceptives / ↑ Effect of beta blockers R/T ↓ liver breakdown
Phenformin / ↑ Hypoglycemia
Phenobarbital / ↓ Effect of beta blockers R/T ↑ liver breakdown
Phenothiazines / ↑ Effect of both drugs
Phenytoin / Additive depression of myocardium; also ↓ effect of beta blockers R/T ↑ liver breakdown
Prazosin / ↑ First-dose effect of prazosin (acute postural hypotension)
Propafenone / ↑ Plasma levels of certain beta-blockers R/T ↓ liver metabolism
Quinidine / ↑ Plasma levels of beta-blockers in extensive metabolizers → ↑ effects
Quinolone antibiotics / ↑ Bioavailability of beta-blockers metabolized by the cytochrome P450 system
Rifampin / ↓ Effect of beta blockers due to ↑ breakdown by liver
Ritodrine / Beta blockers ↓ effect of ritodrine
Salicylates / ↓ Effect of beta blockers, possibly due to inhibition of prostaglandin synthesis
Selective serotonin reuptake inhibitors / Possible excessive beta-blockade R/T ↓ metabolism
Succinylcholine / Beta blockers ↑ effects of succinylcholine
Sulfonylureas / ↓ Effect of sulfonylureas
Sympathomimetics / Reverse effects of beta blockers

Theophylline / Beta blockers reverse the effect of theophylline; also, beta blockers ↓ renal drug clearance
Thioamines / ↑ Effects of beta blockers
Thyroid hormones / Effects of certain beta-blockers may be ↓ when hypothyroid client is converted to euthyroid state
Tubocurarine / Beta blockers ↑ effects of tubocurarine
Verapamil / Possible side effects since both drugs ↓ myocardial contractility or AV conduction; bradycardia and asystole when beta blockers are used ophthalmically

LABORATORY TEST CONSIDERATIONS
↓ Serum glucose.

DOSAGE

See individual drugs.

NURSING CONSIDERATIONS

ADMINISTRATION/STORAGE

1. Sudden cessation of beta blockers may precipitate or worsen angina.
2. The lowering of intraocular pressure (IOP) may take a few weeks to stabilize when using betaxolol or timolol.
3. Due to diurnal variations in IOP, the response to b.i.d. therapy is best assessed by measuring IOP at different times during the day.
4. If IOP is not controlled using beta blockers, add additional drugs to the regimen, including pilocarpine, dipivefrin, or systemic carbonic anhydrase inhibitors.

ASSESSMENT

1. Note indications for therapy and characteristics of symptoms. List any history of depression; assess mental status.
2. Determine pulse and BP in both arms while lying, sitting, and standing.
3. Monitor EKG, glucose, CBC, electrolytes, renal and LFTs.
4. Note any history of asthma, diabetes, or impaired renal function.
5. With asthma, avoid nonselective beta antagonists due to beta-2 receptor blockade which may lead to increased airway resistance.
6. Review drugs currently prescribed to ensure none interact.

INTERVENTIONS

1. Monitor HR and BP; obtain written parameters for holding (e.g., for SBP < 90 or HR < 45).
2. When assessing respirations note rate and quality; may cause dyspnea and bronchospasm.
3. Monitor I&O and daily weights. Observe for increasing dyspnea, coughing, difficulty breathing, fatigue, or edema—symptoms of CHF, may require digitalization, diuretics, and/or drug discontinuation.
4. Complaints of cold S&S, easy fatigue, or feeling lightheaded may require a drug change.
5. With diabetics watch for S&S of hypoglycemia, such as hypotension or tachycardia; most mask these signs.
6. During IV administration, monitor EKG (may slow AV conduction and increase PR interval) and activities closely until drug effects evident.

CLIENT/FAMILY TEACHING

1. When prescribed for BP control, drug helps control hypertension but does not cure it. Must continue to take despite feeling better. With MI, drug is prescribed to decrease sudden death after heart attack.
2. Record BP and take pulse immediately prior to first dose each day so medication can be adjusted.
3. Review instructions when to call provider, i.e., if HR < 50 beats/min or SBP < 80 mm Hg.
4. Review life-style changes for BP control: regular exercise, low-fat and reduced-calorie diet, decreased salt and alcohol intake, smoking cessation, and relaxation techniques.
5. Always consult provider before interrupting therapy; abrupt withdrawal may precipitate angina, MI, or rebound hypertension. A 2-week taper is useful.
6. May cause blurred vision, dizziness, or drowsiness; avoid activities that require mental alertness until drug effects realized.
7. Rise from a sitting or lying position slowly and dangle legs before standing

to avoid symptoms of orthostatic hypotension. Elastic support hose may help decrease symptoms.
8. Dress warmly during cold weather. Diminished blood supply to extremities may cause cold sensitivity; check extremities for warmth.
9. Avoid excessive intake of alcohol, coffee, tea, or cola. Avoid OTC agents without approval.
10. If diabetic, monitor BS and report S&S of hypoglycemia.
11. Report any asthma-like symptoms, cough, or nasal stuffiness; may be symptoms of CHF.
12. Report any bothersome side effects or changes, especially new-onset depression.

OUTCOMES/EVALUATE

- ↓ BP; ↓ IOP
- ↓ Frequency/severity of anginal attacks; improved exercise tolerance
- ↓ Anxiety levels; ↓ tremors
- Migraine prophylaxis
- Control of cardiac arrhythmias

CALCIUM CHANNEL BLOCKING AGENTS

SEE ALSO THE FOLLOWING INDIVIDUAL ENTRIES:

Amlodipine
Bepridil hydrochloride
Diltiazem hydrochloride
Felodipine
Isradipine
Nicardipine hydrochloride
Nifedipine
Nimodipine
Nisoldipine
Verapamil

ACTION/KINETICS

For contraction of cardiac and smooth muscle to occur, extracellular calcium must move into the cell through openings called *calcium channels.* The calcium channel blocking agents (also called *slow channel blockers* or *calcium antagonists*) inhibit the influx of calcium through the cell membrane, resulting in a depression of automaticity and conduction velocity in both smooth and cardiac muscle. This leads to a depression of contraction in these tissues. Drugs in this class have different degrees of selectivity on vascular smooth muscle, myocardium, and conduction and pacemaker tissues. In the myocardium, these drugs dilate coronary vessels in both normal and ischemic tissues and inhibit spasms of coronary arteries. They also decrease total peripheral resistance, thus reducing energy and oxygen requirements of the heart. Also effective against certain cardiac arrhythmias by slowing AV conduction and prolonging repolarization. In addition, they depress the amplitude, rate of depolarization, and conduction in atria.

USES

See individual drugs. Depending on the drug, uses include angina pectoris (chronic stable, unstable, vasospastic), essential hypertension, arrhythmias, and other uses.

CONTRAINDICATIONS

Sick sinus syndrome, second- or third-degree AV block (except with a functioning pacemaker). Use of bepridil, diltiazem, or verapamil for hypotension (<90 mm Hg systolic pressure). Lactation.

SPECIAL CONCERNS

Abrupt withdrawal may result in increased frequency and duration of chest pain. Hypertensive clients treated with calcium channel blockers have a higher risk of heart attack than clients treated with diuretics or beta-adrenergic blockers. May also be an increased risk of heart attacks in diabetics (only nisoldipine studied). Safety and effectiveness of bepridil, diltiazem, felodipine, and isradipine have not been established in children.

SIDE EFFECTS

Side effects vary from one calcium channel blocker to another; refer to individual drugs.

OD OVERDOSE MANAGEMENT

Symptoms: Nausea, weakness, drowsiness, dizziness, slurred speech, confusion, marked and prolonged hypotension, bradycardia, junctional rhythms, ***second- or third-degree block.***

• *Treatment:* Treatment is supportive. Monitor cardiac and respiratory function.

• If client is seen soon after ingestion, emetics or gastric lavage should be considered followed by cathartics.

• *Hypotension:* IV calcium, dopamine, isoproterenol, metaraminol, norepinephrine. Also, provide IV fluids. Place client in Trendelenburg position.

• *Ventricular tachycardia:* IV procainamide or lidocaine; also, cardioversion may be necessary. Also, provide slow-drip IV fluids.

• *Bradycardia, asystole, AV block:* IV atropine sulfate (0.6–1 mg), calcium gluconate (10% solution), isoproterenol, norepinephrine; also, cardiac pacing may be indicated. Provide slow-drip IV fluids.

DRUG INTERACTIONS

Beta-adrenergic blocking agents / Beta blockers may cause depression of myocardial contractility and AV conduction

Cimetidine / ↑ Effect of CCBs R/T ↓ first-pass metabolism

H *Dong quai* / Possible additive effect

Fentanyl / Severe hypotension or ↑ fluid volume requirements

H *Ginger* / May alter effect of CCBs R/T ↑ calcium uptake by heart muscle

Itraconazole / Edema when used with amlodipine or nifedipine

Ranitidine / ↑ Effect of CCBs R/T ↓ first-pass metabolism

DOSAGE

See individual drugs.

NURSING CONSIDERATIONS

ASSESSMENT

1. Document indications for therapy, type and onset of symptoms. List other agents used and the outcome.
2. Note any experience with these agents and the response. List drugs prescribed to ensure none interact.
3. Assess and document CV and mental status. These drugs cause peripheral vasodilation. Any excessive hypotensive response and increased HR may precipitate angina.
4. Document VS, weight, ECG and BP in both arms while lying, sitting, and standing. Assess for CHF (weight gain, peripheral edema, dyspnea, rales, jugular vein distention).
5. Monitor BS, electrolytes, I&O, liver and renal function studies.

CLIENT/FAMILY TEACHING

1. These agents work by decreasing myocardial contractile force, which in turn decreases the myocardial oxygen requirements.
2. Take with meals to ↓ GI upset.
3. Review goals of therapy (e.g., ↓ DBP by 10 mm Hg, ↓ HR by 20 beats/min).
4. Record pulse and BP at least twice a week as well as weights; review instructions regarding when to hold meds and contact provider.
5. Do not perform activities that require mental alertness until drug effects realized.
6. Report side effects such as dizziness, vertigo, unusual flushing, facial warmth, edema, nausea, or persistent constipation; toxic drug effects
7. If postural hypotension occurs, change positions slowly, especially when standing from a reclining position. Sit down immediately if lightheadedness occurs. Move slowly from a lying to a sitting or standing position.
8. Avoid long periods of standing, excessive heat, hot showers or baths, and ingestion of alcohol; may exacerbate postural hypotension.
9. Report any swelling of the hands or feet, pronounced dizziness, or chest pain accompanied by diaphoresis, SOB, or severe headaches.
10. Review life-style changes for BP control, i.e., regular exercise, low-fat, low-cholesterol, reduced-calorie diet, decreased salt and alcohol consumption, smoking cessation, and stress reduction.

OUTCOMES/EVALUATE

• Control of hypertension; ↓ HR
• ↓ Frequency/intensity of angina
• Stable cardiac rhythm

CALCIUM SALTS

SEE ALSO THE FOLLOWING INDIVIDUAL ENTRIES:

Calcium carbonate
Calcium chloride
Calcium gluconate

ACTION/KINETICS

Calcium is essential for maintaining normal function of nerves, muscles, the skeletal system, and permeability of cell membranes and capillaries. The normal serum calcium concentration is 9–10.4 mg/dL (4.5–5.2 mEq/L). Hypocalcemia is characterized by muscular fibrillation, twitching, skeletal muscle spasms, leg cramps, tetanic spasms, cardiac arrhythmias, smooth muscle hyperexcitability, mental depression, and anxiety states. Excessive, chronic hypocalcemia is characterized by brittle, defective nails, poor dentition, and brittle hair. Calcium is well absorbed from the upper GI tract. However, severe low-calcium tetany is best treated by IV administration of calcium gluconate. The presence of vitamin D is necessary for maximum calcium utilization. The hormone of the parathyroid gland is necessary for the regulation of the calcium level.

USES

IV: Acute hypocalcemic tetany secondary to renal failure, hypoparathyroidism, premature delivery, maternal diabetes mellitus in infants, and poisoning due to magnesium, oxalic acid, radiophosphorus, carbon tetrachloride, fluoride, phosphate, strontium, and radium. To treat depletion of electrolytes. Also during cardiac resuscitation when epinephrine or isoproterenol has not improved myocardial contraction (may also be given into the ventricular cavity for this purpose). To reverse cardiotoxicity or hyperkalemia. **IM or IV:** Reduce spasms in renal, biliary, intestinal, or lead colic. To relieve muscle cramps due to insect bites and to decrease capillary permeability in various sensitivity reactions. **PO:** Osteoporosis, osteomalacia, chronic hypoparathyroidism, rickets, latent tetany, hypocalcemia secondary to use of anticonvulsant drugs. Myasthenia gravis, Eaton-Lambert syndrome, supplement for pregnant, postmenopausal, or nursing women. Also, prophylactically for primary osteoporosis. *Investigational:* As an infusion to diagnose Zollinger-Ellison syndrome and medullary thyroid carcinoma. To antagonize neuromuscular blockade due to aminoglycosides.

CONTRAINDICATIONS

Digitalized clients, sarcoidosis, renal or cardiac disease, ventricular fibrillation. Cancer clients with bone metastases. Renal calculi, hypophosphatemia, hypercalcemia.

SPECIAL CONCERNS

Calcium requirements decrease in geriatric clients; thus, dose may have to be adjusted. Also, low levels of active vitamin D metabolites may impair calcium absorption in older clients. Use with caution in cor pulmonale, respiratory acidosis, renal disease or failure, ventricular fibrillation, hypercalcemia.

SIDE EFFECTS

Following PO use: GI irritation, constipation. **Following IV use:** Venous irritation, tingling sensation, feeling of oppression or heat, chalky taste. Rapid IV administration may result in vasodilation, decreased BP and HR, ***cardiac arrhythmias,*** syncope, or ***cardiac arrest.*** **Following IM use:** Burning feeling, necrosis, tissue sloughing, cellulitis, soft tissue calcification. *NOTE:* If calcium is injected into the myocardium rather than into the ventricle, ***laceration of coronary arteries, cardiac tamponade, pneumothorax, and ventricular fibrillation*** may occur. **Symptoms due to excess calcium (hypercalcemia):** Lassitude, fatigue, GI symptoms (anorexia, N&V, abdominal pain, dry mouth, thirst), polyuria, depression of nervous and neuromuscular function (emotional disturbances, confusion, skeletal muscle weakness, and constipation), confusion, delirium, stupor,

coma, impairment of renal function (polyuria, polydipsia, and azotemia), renal calculi, arrhythmias, and bradycardia.

OD OVERDOSE MANAGEMENT

Symptoms: Systemic overloading from parenteral administration can result in an acute hypercalcemic syndrome with symptoms including markedly increased plasma calcium levels, lethargy, intractable N&V, weakness, ***coma, and sudden death.*** *Treatment:* Discontinue therapy and lower serum calcium levels by giving an IV infusion of sodium chloride plus a potent diuretic such as furosemide. Consider hemodialysis.

DRUG INTERACTIONS

Atenolol / ↓ Drug effect R/T ↓ bioavailability and plasma levels
Cephalocin / Incompatible with calcium salts
Corticosteroids / Interfere with absorption of calcium from GI tract
Digitalis / ↑ Digitalis arrhythmias and toxicity. Death has resulted from combination of digitalis and IV calcium salts
Iron salts / ↓ Absorption of iron from the GI tract
H *Lily-of-the-valley herb* / ↑ Effectiveness and side effects of calcium
Milk / Excess of either may cause hypercalcemia, renal insufficiency with azotemia, alkalosis, and ocular lesions
Norfloxacin / ↓ Drug bioavailability
H *Pheasant's eye herb* / ↑ Effectiveness and side effects of calcium
Sodium polystyrene sulfonate / Metabolic alkalosis and ↓ binding of resin to potassium with renal impairment
H *Squill* / ↑ Effectiveness and side effects of calcium
Tetracyclines / ↓ Drug effect R/T ↓ GI tract absorption
Thiazide diuretics / Hypercalcemia R/T to thiazide-induced renal tubular reabsorption of calcium and bone release of calcium
Thyroid hormones / ↓ GI absorption of thyroid hormones R/T calcium
Verapamil / Calcium antagonizes the effect of verapamil
Vitamin D / Enhances intestinal absorption of dietary calcium

DOSAGE

See individual agents.

NURSING CONSIDERATIONS

ADMINISTRATION/STORAGE

ORAL

1. Administer 1–1.5 hr after meals. Alkalis and large amounts of fat decrease the absorption of calcium.
2. If difficulty swallowing large tablets, obtain a calcium in water suspension. Because calcium goes into suspension six times more readily in hot water than in cold water, the solution can be prepared by diluting the medication with *hot* water. Cool solution before administering.

IV

1. Warm solutions to body temperature and give slowly (0.5–2 mL/min), stop if pain experienced.
2. Administer slowly, observing for bradycardia, hypotension, and cardiac arrhythmias.
3. Prevent leakage of salts into the tissues; extremely irritating.
4. Keep client recumbent for a short time following the injection.
5. Do not mix calcium salts with carbonates, phosphates, sulfates, or tartrates in parenteral admixtures.

IM

1. Rotate injection sites; calcium may cause tissue sloughing.
2. Do not administer IM calcium gluconate to children.

ASSESSMENT

1. Perform a thorough nursing history, noting indications for therapy and any underlying causes.
2. Note if receiving digitalis products; drug may be contraindicated.
3. Monitor calcium levels and renal function; assess for renal disease. Give Vitamin D; facilitates absorption.
4. With hypocalcemic tetany, protect client from injury.
5. Assess for S&S of hypercalcemia, i.e., fatigue and CNS depression.

CLIENT/FAMILY TEACHING

1. Calcium requirements are best met by dietary sources (including milk in the diet). Supplements need vitamin D to facilitate absorption.
2. Multivitamin and mineral preparations are expensive and do not contain sufficient calcium to meet daily requirements.
3. Consult a dietitian to assist with proper food selection and meal planning/preparation.
4. Review prescribed replacement regimen. Need follow-ups for dosage adjustments to prevent hypercalcemia and hypercalciuria.

OUTCOMES/EVALUATE

- Resolution of hypocalcemia
- Relief of muscle cramps
- Osteoporosis prophylaxis
- Serum calcium levels within desired range (8.8–10.4 mg/dL)

CEPHALOSPORINS

SEE ALSO THE FOLLOWING INDIVIDUAL ENTRIES:

Cefaclor
Cefadroxil monohydrate
Cefazolin sodium
Cefdinir
Cefditoren pivoxil
Cefepime hydrochloride
Cefixime oral
Cefoperazone sodium
Cefotaxime sodium
Cefotetan disodium
Cefoxitin sodium
Cefpodoxime proxetil
Cefprozil
Ceftazidime
Ceftibuten
Ceftizoxime sodium
Ceftriaxone sodium
Cefuroxime axetil
Cefuroxime sodium
Cephalexin hydrochloride monohydrate
Cephalexin monohydrate
Cephapirin sodium
Cephradine
Loracarbef

GENERAL STATEMENT

Cephalosporins are broad-spectrum antibiotics classified as first-, second-, and third-generation drugs. The difference among generations is based on pharmacokinetics and antibacterial spectra. Generally, third-generation cephalosporins have more activity against gram-negative organisms and resistant organisms and less activity against gram-positive organisms than first-generation drugs. Third-generation cephalosporins are also stable against beta-lactamases. Cephalosporins can be destroyed by cephalosporinase.

ACTION/KINETICS

The cephalosporins interfere with a final step in the formation of the bacterial cell wall (inhibition of mucopeptide biosynthesis), resulting in unstable cell membranes that undergo lysis (same mechanism of actions as penicillins). Also, cell division and growth are inhibited. The cephalosporins are most effective against young, rapidly dividing organisms and are considered bactericidal. Cephalosporins are widely distributed to most tissues and fluids. First- and second-generation drugs do not enter the CSF well but third-generation drugs enter inflamed meninges readily. Rapidly excreted by the kidneys.

USES

See individual drugs. A listing of the drugs in each generation follows:

First-Generation Cephalosporins: Cefadroxil, cefazolin, cephalexin, cephapirin, cephradine.

Second-Generation Cephalosporins: Cefaclor, cefmetazole, cefonicid, cefotetan, cefoxitin, cefprozil, cefuroxime, and loracarbef.

Third-Generation Cephalosporins: Cefdinir, cefepime, cefixime, cefoperazone, cefotaxime, cefpodoxime, ceftazidime, ceftibuten, ceftizoxime, ceftriaxone.

CONTRAINDICATIONS

Hypersensitivity to cephalosporins or related antibiotics.

SPECIAL CONCERNS

Safe use in pregnancy and lactation has not been established (pregnancy category: B). Use with caution in the presence of impaired renal or hepatic function, together with other nephrotoxic drugs, and in clients over 50 years of age. Perform C_{cr} on all clients with impaired renal function who receive cephalosporins. If hypersensitive to penicillin, may occasionally cross-react to cephalosporins.

SIDE EFFECTS

GI: N&V, diarrhea, abdominal cramps or pain, dyspepsia, glossitis, heartburn, sore mouth or tongue, dysgeusia, anorexia, flatulence, cholestasis. Pseudomembranous colitis. **Allergic:** Urticaria, rashes (maculopapular, morbilliform, or erythematous), pruritus (including anal and genital areas), fever, chills, erythema, ***angioedema,*** serum sickness, joint pain, exfoliative dermatitis, chest tightness, myalgia, erythema multiforme, edema, itching, numbness, chills, ***Stevens-Johnson syndrome, anaphylaxis.*** *NOTE:* Cross-allergy may be manifested between cephalosporins and penicillins. **Hematologic:** Leukopenia, leukocytosis, lymphocytosis, neutropenia (transient), eosinophilia, thrombocytopenia, thrombocythemia, ***agranulocytosis,*** granulocytopenia, bone marrow depression, ***hemolytic anemia,*** pancytopenia, decreased platelet function, ***aplastic anemia,*** hypoprothrombinemia (may lead to bleeding), thrombocytosis (transient). **CNS:** Headache, malaise, fatigue, vertigo, dizziness, lethargy, confusion, paresthesia, precipitation of ***seizures*** (especially in clients with impaired renal function). **Hepatic:** Hepatomegaly, hepatitis. Intrathecal use may result in hallucinations, nystagmus, or ***seizures.*** **Miscellaneous:** Superinfection including oral candidiasis and enterococcal infections, hypotension, sweating, flushing, dyspnea, interstitial pneumonitis. IV or IM use may result in local swelling, inflammation, cellulitis, paresthesia, burning, phlebitis, thrombophlebitis. IM use may also cause pain and induration, tenderness, increased temperature. Sterile abscesses have been observed following SC use. Nephrotoxicity (≠ BUN with and without ≠ serum creatinine) may occur in clients over 50 and in young children.

OD OVERDOSE MANAGEMENT

Symptoms: Parenteral use of large doses of cephalosporins may cause seizures, especially in clients with impaired renal function. *Treatment:* If seizures occur, discontinue the drug immediately and give anticonvulsant drugs. Hemodialysis may also be effective.

DRUG INTERACTIONS

Alcohol / Antabuse-like reaction if used with cefazolin, cefmetazole, cefoperazone, or cefotetan
Aminoglycosides / ↑ Risk of renal toxicity with certain cephalosporins
Antacids / ↓ Plasma levels of cefaclor, cefdinir, or cefpodoxime
Anticoagulants / ↑ Hypoprothrombinemic effects with cefazolin, cefmetazole, cefoperazone, or cefotetan
Colistimethate / ↑ Risk of renal toxicity
Colistin / ↑ Risk of renal toxicity
Ethacrynic acid / ↑ Risk of renal toxicity
Furosemide / ↑ Risk renal toxicity
H_2 antagonists / ↓ Plasma levels of cefpodoxime or cefuroxime
Polymyxin B / ↑ Risk renal toxicity
Probenecid / ↑ Effect of cephalosporins by ↓ excretion by kidneys
Vancomycin / ↑ Risk renal toxicity

LABORATORY TEST CONSIDERATIONS

False + for urinary glucose with Benedict's solution, Fehling's solution, or Clinitest tablets. Enzyme tests (Clinistix, Tes-Tape) are unaffected. False + Coombs' test and urinary 17-ketosteroids.

↑ AST, ALT, total bilirubin, GGTP, LDH, alkaline phosphatase.

DOSAGE

See individual drugs.

NURSING CONSIDERATIONS

SEE ALSO *GENERAL NURSING CONSIDERATIONS FOR ALL ANTI-INFECTIVES.*

ADMINISTRATION/STORAGE

1. Parenteral solutions infused too rapidly may cause pain and irritation; infuse over 30 min unless otherwise indicated and assess site.
2. Continue therapy for at least 2–3 days after symptoms of infection have disappeared.
3. For group A beta-hemolytic streptococcal infections, continue therapy for at least 10 days to prevent the development of glomerulonephritis or rheumatic fever.

ASSESSMENT

1. With hypersensitivity reactions to penicillin, assess for cross-sensitivity to cephalosporins.
2. Many agents in this group of antibiotics are quite expensive. Clients on fixed incomes with limited health benefits may not afford them.
3. Document indications for therapy and symptoms of infection; obtain baseline cultures.
4. Monitor CBC, BS, lytes, renal and LFTs. With renal impairment reduce dose; for dialysis clients, administer after treatment.
5. May cause false + Coombs' test.

INTERVENTIONS

1. The cephalosporins all have similar sounding and similarly spelled names. Use care when transcribing orders for administration and request clarification as needed.
2. Pseudomembranous colitis may occur. If diarrhea develops, report any fevers. Monitor VS, I&O, stool C&S, and electrolytes.
3. Persistent temperature elevations may be drug-induced fever.

CLIENT/FAMILY TEACHING

1. Oral meds should be taken on an empty stomach but, if GI upset occurs, may be administered with meals.
2. Report any S&S that may necessitate drug withdrawal such as vaginal itching/drainage, fever, or diarrhea.
3. Yogurt or buttermilk (4 oz) may be prescribed daily for diarrhea related to intestinal superinfections (to restore intestinal flora); consult provider.
4. Report signs of superinfection (black furry tongue, vaginal itching or discharge, and loose, foul-smelling stools). Nystatin may be ordered for secondary infections.
5. Immediately report any abnormal bleeding or bruising.
6. May cause false positive Coombs' test. Would be of concern if being cross-matched for blood transfusions or in newborns whose moms used cephalosporins during pregnancy.
7. Avoid alcohol and alcohol-containing products, as a disulfiram-type reaction may occur.

OUTCOMES/EVALUATE

- Negative C&S reports
- Resolution of infection
- Symptomatic improvement, i.e., ↓ WBCs, ↓ fever, improved appetite

CHOLINERGIC BLOCKING AGENTS

Atropine sulfate
Benztropine mesylate
Biperiden hydrochloride
Dicyclomine hydrochloride
Ipratropium bromide
Propantheline bromide
Scopolamine hydrobromide
Scopolamine transdermal therapeutic system
Trihexyphenidyl hydrochloride

ACTION/KINETICS

Cholinergic blocking agents prevent the neurotransmitter acetylcholine from combining with receptors on the postganglionic parasympathetic nerve terminal (muscarinic site). Effects include reduction of smooth muscle spasms, blockade of vagal impulses to the heart, decreased secretions (e.g., gastric, salivation, bronchial mucus, sweat glands), production of mydriasis and cycloplegia, and various CNS effects. In therapeutic doses, these drugs have little effect on transmission of nerve impulses across ganglia (nicotinic sites) or at the neuromuscular junction. Several anticholinergic drugs abolish or reduce the S&S of Parkinson's disease, such as tremors and rigidity, and result in some improvement in mobility, muscular coordination, and motor performance. These effects may be due to blockade of the effects of acetylcholine in the CNS.

USES

See individual drugs.

CONTRAINDICATIONS

Glaucoma, adhesions between iris and lens of the eye, tachycardia, myocardial ischemia, unstable CV state in acute hemorrhage, partial obstruction of the GI and biliary tracts, prostatic hypertrophy, renal disease, myasthenia gravis, hepatic disease, paralytic ileus, pyloroduodenal stenosis, pyloric obstruction, intestinal atony, ulcerative colitis, obstructive uropathy. Cardiac clients, especially when there is danger of tachycardia; older persons suffering from atherosclerosis or mental impairment. Lactation.

SPECIAL CONCERNS

Use with caution in pregnancy. Infants and young children are more susceptible to the toxic side effects of anticholinergic drugs. Use in children when the ambient temperature is high may cause a rapid increase in body temperature due to suppression of sweat glands. Geriatric clients are particularly likely to manifest anticholinergic side effects and CNS effects, including agitation, confusion, drowsiness, excitement, glaucoma, and impaired memory. Use with caution in hyperthyroidism, CHF, cardiac arrhythmias, hypertension, Down syndrome, asthma, spastic paralysis, blonde individuals, allergies, and chronic lung disease.

SIDE EFFECTS

These are desirable in some conditions and undesirable in others. Thus, the anticholinergics have an antisalivary effect that is useful in parkinsonism. This same effect is unpleasant when the drug is used for spastic conditions of the GI tract. Most side effects are dose-related and decrease when dosage decreases.

GI: N&V, dry mouth, dysphagia, constipation, heartburn, change in taste perception, bloated feeling, paralytic ileus, epigastric distress, acute suppurative parotitis, dilation of the colon, development of duodenal ulcer. **CNS:** Dizziness, drowsiness, nervousness, disorientation, headache, weakness, insomnia, fever (especially in children). Large doses may produce CNS stimulation including tremor and restlessness. **Anticholinergic psychoses:** ataxia, euphoria, confusion, disorientation, loss of short-term memory, decreased anxiety, fatigue, insomnia, hallucinations, dysarthria, agitation. **CV:** Palpitations, tachycardia, hypotension, postural hypotension. **GU:** Urinary retention or hesitancy, dysuria, impotence. **Ophthalmologic:** Blurred vision, dilated pupils, diplopia, increased intraocular tension, angle-closure glaucoma, photophobia, cycloplegia, precipitation of acute glaucoma. **Dermatologic:** Urticaria, skin rashes, other dermatoses. **Musculoskeletal:** Muscle weakness, muscle cramping. **Other:** ***Anaphylaxis,*** flushing, decreased sweating, nasal congestion, numbness of fingers, suppression of glandular secretions including lactation. Heat prostration (fever and heat stroke) in presence of high environmental temperatures due to decreased sweating.

OD OVERDOSE MANAGEMENT

Symptoms ("Belladonna Poisoning"): Infants and children are especially susceptible to the toxic effects of atropine and scopolamine. Poisoning (dose-dependent) is characterized by the following symptoms: dry mouth, burning sensation of the mouth, difficulty in swallowing and speaking, blurred vision, photophobia, dilated and sluggish pupils, rash, tachycardia, ***circulatory collapse, cardiac arrest,*** increased respiration, ***increased body temperature*** (up to 109°F, 42.7°C), restlessness, irritability, confusion, anxiety, ataxia, hyperactivity, combativeness, toxic psychosis, anhidrosis, muscle incoordination, dilated pupils, hot dry skin, dry mucous membranes, dysphagia, foul-smelling breath, decreased bowel sounds, ***respiratory depression and paralysis,*** tremors, ***seizures,*** hallucinations, and ***death.***

• *Treatment ("Belladonna Poisoning"):* Gastric lavage or induction of vomiting followed by activated charcoal. General supportive measures.

• Anticholinergic effects can be reversed by physostigmine (Eserine), 1–3 mg IV (effectiveness uncertain; thus use other agents if possible). Neostigmine methylsulfate, 0.5–2 mg IV, repeated as necessary.

• If there is excitation, diazepam, a short-acting barbiturate, IV sodium thiopental (2% solution), or chloral hydrate (100–200 mL of a 2% solution by rectal infusion) may be given.

• For fever, cool baths may be used. Keep client in a darkened room if photophobia is manifested.

• Artificial respiration should be instituted if there is paralysis of respiratory muscles.

DRUG INTERACTIONS

Amantadine / Additive anticholinergic side effects
Antacids / ↓ Absorption of anticholinergics from GI tract
Antidepressants, tricyclic / Additive anticholinergic side effects
Antihistamines / Additive anticholinergic side effects
Atenolol / Anticholinergics ↑ effects of atenolol
Benzodiazepines / Additive anticholinergic side effects
Corticosteroids / Additive ↑ intraocular pressure
Cyclopropane / ↑ Chance of ventricular arrhythmias
Digoxin / ↑ Drug effect R/T ↑ GI tract absorption
Disopyramide / Potentiation of anticholinergic side effects
Guanethidine / Reversal of inhibition of gastric acid secretion caused by anticholinergics
Haloperidol / Possible worsening of schizophrenic symptoms, ↓ haloperidol serum levels, and development of tardive dyskinesia
Histamine / Reversal of inhibition of gastric acid secretion caused by anticholinergics
Levodopa / Possible ↓ drug effect R/T ↑ breakdown of levodopa in stomach (due to delayed gastric emptying time)
MAO inhibitors / ↑ Effect of anticholinergics R/T ↓ liver breakdown
Meperidine / Additive anticholinergic side effects
Methylphenidate / Potentiation of anticholinergic side effects
Metoclopramide / Anticholinergics block action of metoclopramide
Nitrates, nitrites / Potentiation of anticholinergic side effects
Nitrofurantoin / ↑ Bioavailability of nitrofurantoin
Orphenadrine / Additive anticholinergic side effects
Phenothiazines / Additive anticholinergic side effects; also, ↓ phenothiazine effects
Primidone / Potentiation of anticholinergic side effects
Procainamide / Additive anticholinergic side effects
Quinidine / Additive anticholinergic side effects
Reserpine / Reversal of inhibition of gastric acid secretion caused by anticholinergics
Sympathomimetics / ↑ Bronchial relaxation
Thiazide diuretics / ↑ Bioavailability of thiazide diuretics
Thioxanthines / Potentiation of anticholinergic side effects

DOSAGE

See individual drugs.

NURSING CONSIDERATIONS

ADMINISTRATION/STORAGE

Dosage is often small. To prevent overdosage, check dose and measure exactly.

ASSESSMENT

1. Document indications for therapy; assess for asthma, glaucoma, or duodenal ulcer (contraindications for therapy).

2. Note any renal disease, cardiac problems, or hepatic disease.
3. Determine age; elderly clients, especially those with mental impairment or atherosclerosis, should not receive these drugs.
4. Assess for constipation and urinary retention and tolerance.

INTERVENTIONS

1. For complaints of a dry mouth, provide frequent mouth care and cold drinks, especially postoperatively. Sugarless hard candies and chewing gum may also be of some benefit.
2. Drugs such as atropine may suppress thermoregulatory sweating; counsel client concerning activity (especially in hot weather) and appropriate clothing. Also, children and infants may exhibit "atropine fever."

CLIENT/FAMILY TEACHING

1. Certain side effects are to be expected, such as dry mouth or blurred vision, and may have to be tolerated because of the overall beneficial effects of drug therapy. These should be reported so symptoms may be alleviated by reducing the dose or temporarily stopping drug.
2. With parkinsonism, do not withdraw abruptly. If the medication is changed, one drug should be withdrawn slowly and the other started in small doses.

CARDIOVASCULAR

ADDITIONAL NURSING CONSIDERATIONS RELATED TO PATHOLOGIC CONDITIONS FOR WHICH THE DRUG IS ADMINISTERED

ASSESSMENT

1. Monitor VS and ECG. Assess for any hemodynamic changes and intraventricular conduction blocks.
2. Note complaints of palpitations.

OCULAR

ASSESSMENT

1. Determine any experience with these drugs and results.
2. Document IOP; assess accommodation and pupillary response.

INTERVENTIONS

1. Note complaints of dizziness or blurred vision; assist with ambulation and institute safety measures.
2. Hold meds and report any complaints of eye pain after instillation.

CLIENT/FAMILY TEACHING

1. Review methods for instillation of drops or ointment and frequency.
2. Vision will be affected by the meds; temporary stinging and blurred vision will occur. Assess response and plan activities for safety.
3. Night vision may be impaired. Photophobia, which may occur, can be relieved by wearing dark glasses.
4. Report any marked changes in vision, eye irritation, or persistent headaches immediately.
5. With large doses, tears may diminish; may experience dry or "sandy" eyes.

GASTROINTESTINAL

CLIENT/FAMILY TEACHING

1. Take early enough before a meal (at least 20 min) so that it will be effective when needed.
2. Review printed information related to the prescribed diet; see dietitian for assistance in meal planning.
3. Gastric emptying times may be prolonged and intestinal transit time lengthened. Drug-induced intestinal paralysis is temporary and should resolve after 1–3 days of therapy.

GENITOURINARY

CLIENT/FAMILY TEACHING

1. Report any evidence of urinary retention; may be more pronounced in elderly men with BPH.
2. Monitor I&O. Report evidence of bladder distention and need for catheterization if no u.o. >8 hr.
3. Consult with the provider for medication adjustment if impotence occurs; may be drug-related.

CORTICOSTEROIDS

SEE ALSO THE FOLLOWING INDIVIDUAL ENTRIES:

Beclomethasone dipropionate
Betamethasone
Betamethasone dipropionate
Betamethasone sodium phosphate

Betamethasone sodium phosphate and Betamethasone acetate
Betamethasone valerate
Budesonide
Corticotropin injection
Corticotropin repository injection
Cortisone acetate
Cosyntropin
Dexamethasone
Dexamethasone acetate
Dexamethasone sodium phosphate
Fludrocortisone acetate
Flunisolide
Fluticasone propionate
Hydrocortisone
Hydrocortisone acetate
Hydrocortisone buteprate
Hydrocortisone butyrate
Hydrocortisone cypionate
Hydrocortisone sodium phosphate
Hydrocortisone sodium succinate
Hydrocortisone valerate
Loteprednol etabonate
Methylprednisolone
Methylprednisolone acetate
Methylprednisolone sodium succinate
Mometasone furoate monohydrate
Prednisolone
Prednisolone acetate
Prednisolone sodium phosphate
Prednisolone tebutate
Prednisone
Triamcinolone
Triamcinolone acetonide
Triamcinolone diacetate
Triamcinolone hexacetonide

ACTION/KINETICS

The hormones of the adrenal gland influence many metabolic pathways and all organ systems and are essential for survival. These processes include carbohydrate metabolism (e.g., glycogen deposition in the liver and conversion of glycogen to glucose), protein metabolism (e.g., gluconeogenesis, protein catabolism), fat metabolism (e.g., deposition of fatty tissue), and water and electrolyte balance (e.g., fluid retention, excretion of potassium, calcium, and phosphorus).

According to their chemical structure and chief physiologic effect, the corticosteroids fall into two subgroups, which have considerable functional overlap. First are those, like cortisone and hydrocortisone, that mainly regulate the metabolic pathways involving protein, carbohydrate, and fat. This group is often referred to as *glucocorticoids*. In the second group are those, like aldosterone and desoxycorticosterone, that are more specifically involved in electrolyte and water balance. These are often referred to as *mineralocorticoids*. Hormones, such as cortisone and hydrocortisone, although classified as glucocorticoids, possess significant mineralocorticoid activity. Therapeutically, a distinction must be made between physiologic doses used for replacement therapy and pharmacologic doses used to treat inflammatory and other disease states.

The hormones have a marked anti-inflammatory effect because of their ability to inhibit prostaglandin synthesis. These agents also inhibit accumulation of macrophages and leukocytes at sites of inflammation as well as inhibit phagocytosis and lysosomal enzyme release. They aid the organism in coping with various stressful situations (trauma, severe illness). The immunosuppressant effect is thought to be due to a reduction of the number of T lymphocytes, monocytes, and eosinophils. Corticosteroids also decrease binding of immunoglobulin to receptors on the cell surface and inhibit the synthesis and/or release of interleukins which, in turn, decrease T-lymphocyte blastogenesis and reduce the primary immune response.

USES

When used for anti-inflammatory or immunosuppressant therapy, the corticosteroid should possess minimal mineralocorticoid activity. Therapy with glucocorticoids is not curative and in many situations should be considered as adjunctive rather than primary therapy. The following list is not inclusive but provides examples of the physiologic and pharmacologic uses of corticosteroids.

1. **Replacement therapy.** Acute and chronic adrenal insufficiency, including Addison's disease. For replacement therapy, drugs must possess both glucocorticoid and mineralocorticoid effects.
2. **Rheumatic disorders,** including rheumatoid arthritis (including juveniles), other types of arthritis, ankylosing spondylitis, acute and subacute bursitis.
3. **Collagen diseases,** including SLE.
4. **Allergic diseases,** including control of severe allergic conditions as serum sickness, drug hypersensitivity reactions, anaphylaxis.
5. **Respiratory diseases,** including prophylaxis and treatment of chronic bronchial asthma, seasonal or perennial rhinitis. Regular use of inhaled steroids in children could be a lifesaving treatment.
6. **Ocular diseases,** including severe acute and chronic allergic and inflammatory conditions. Corneal injury.
7. **Dermatologic diseases,** including angioedema or urticaria, contact dermatitis, atopic dermatitis, severe erythema multiforme (Stevens-Johnson syndrome).
8. **Diseases of the intestinal tract,** including chronic ulcerative colitis, regional enteritis.
9. **Nervous system,** including acute exacerbations of multiple sclerosis, optic neuritis.
10. **Malignancies,** including leukemias and lymphomas in adults and acute leukemia in children.
11. **Nephrotic syndrome,** including that due to lupus erythematosus or of the idiopathic type.
12. **Hematologic diseases,** including acquired hemolytic anemia, RBC anemia, idiopathic and secondary thrombocytopenic purpura in adults, congenital hypoplastic anemia.
13. **Intra-articular or soft tissue administration,** including acute episodes of synovitis osteoarthritis, rheumatoid arthritis, acute gouty arthritis, bursitis.
14. **Intralesional administration,** including keloids, psoriatic plaques, discoid lupus erythematosus.

Lotions are considered best for weeping eruptions, especially in areas subject to chafing (axilla, feet, and groin). Creams are suitable for most inflammations; ointments are preferred for dry, scaly lesions.

CONTRAINDICATIONS

Suspected infection as these drugs may mask infections. Also peptic ulcer, psychoses, acute glomerulonephritis, herpes simplex infections of the eye, vaccinia or varicella, the exanthematous diseases, Cushing's syndrome, active tuberculosis, myasthenia gravis. Recent intestinal anastomoses, CHF or other cardiac disease, hypertension, systemic fungal infections, open-angle glaucoma. Also, hyperlipidemia, hyperthyroidism or hypothyroidism, osteoporosis, myasthenia gravis, tuberculosis. Lactation (if high doses are used). Inhalation products to relieve acute bronchospasms.

Topically in the eye for dendritic keratitis, vaccinia, chickenpox, other viral disease that may involve the conjunctiva or cornea, and tuberculosis and fungal or acute purulent infections of the eye. Topically in the ear in aural fungal infections and perforated eardrum. Topically in tuberculosis of the skin, herpes simplex, vaccinia, varicella, and infectious conditions in the absence of anti-infective agents.

Inhalation products for relief of acute bronchospasms, primary treatment of status asthmaticus, or other acute episodes of asthma.

SPECIAL CONCERNS

Use with caution in diabetes mellitus, hypertension, chronic nephritis, thrombophlebitis, convulsive disorders, infectious diseases, renal or hepatic insufficiency, pregnancy. Use of orally inhaled or intranasal products may inhibit the growth and development of children or adolescents,although this may only be temporary.

Pediatric clients are also at greater risk for developing cataracts, osteoporosis, avascular necrosis of the femoral heads, and glaucoma. Geriatric clients are more likely to develop hypertension and osteoporosis (especially postmenopausal women). Use inhalation products with caution in children less than 6 years of age.

SIDE EFFECTS

Small physiologic doses given as replacement therapy or short-term high-dosage therapy during emergencies rarely cause side effects. Prolonged therapy may cause a Cushing-like syndrome with atrophy of the adrenal cortex and subsequent adrenocortical insufficiency. A steroid withdrawal syndrome may occur following prolonged use; symptoms include anorexia, N&V, lethargy, headache, fever, joint pain, desquamation, myalgia, weight loss, hypotension.

• **SYSTEMIC**

Fluid and electrolyte: Edema, hypokalemic alkalosis, hypokalemia, hypocalcemia, hypotension or shock-like reaction, hypertension, CHF. **Musculoskeletal:** Muscle wasting, muscle pain or weakness, osteoporosis, spontaneous fractures including vertebral compression fractures and fractures of long bones, tendon rupture, aseptic necrosis of femoral and humeral heads. **GI:** N&V, anorexia or increased appetite, diarrhea or constipation, abdominal distention, pancreatitis, gastric irritation, ulcerative esophagitis. ***Development or exacerbation of peptic ulcers with the possibility of perforation and hemorrhage; perforation of the small and large bowel,*** especially in inflammatory bowel disease. **Endocrine:** Cushing's syndrome (e.g., central obesity, moonface, buffalo hump, enlargement of supraclavicular fat pads), amenorrhea, postmenopausal bleeding, menstrual irregularities, decreased glucose tolerance, hyperglycemia, glycosuria, increased insulin or sulfonylurea requirement in diabetics, development of diabetes mellitus, negative nitrogen balance due to protein catabolism, suppression of growth in children, secondary adrenocortical and pituitary unresponsiveness (especially during periods of stress). **CNS/Neurologic:** Headache, vertigo, insomnia, restlessness, increased motor activity, ischemic neuropathy, EEG abnormalities, ***seizures,*** pseudotumor cerebri. Also, euphoria, mood swings, depression, anxiety, personality changes, psychoses. **CV:** Thromboembolism, thrombophlebitis, ECG changes (due to potassium deficiency), fat embolism, necrotizing angiitis, cardiac arrhythmias, ***myocardial rupture following recent MI,*** syncopal episodes. **Dermatologic:** Impaired wound healing, skin atrophy and thinning, petechiae, ecchymoses, erythema, purpura, striae, hirsutism, urticaria, ***angioneurotic edema,*** acneiform eruptions, allergic dermatitis, lupus erythematosus-like lesions, suppression of skin test reactions, perineal irritation. **Ophthalmic:** Glaucoma, posterior subcapsular cataracts, increased intraocular pressure, exophthalmos. **Miscellaneous:** Hypercholesterolemia, atherosclerosis, aggravation or masking of infections, leukocytosis, increased or decreased motility and number of spermatozoa. **In children:** Suppression of linear growth; reversible pseudobrain tumor syndrome characterized by papilledema, oculomotor or abducens nerve paralysis, visual loss, or headache.

• **PARENTERAL USE**

Sterile abscesses, Charcot-like arthropathy, subcutaneous and cutaneous atrophy, burning or tingling (especially in the perineal area following IV use), scarring, inflammation, paresthesia, induration, hyperpigmentation or hypopigmentation, blindness when used intralesionally around the face and head (rare), transient or delayed pain or soreness, nystagmus, ataxia, muscle twitching, hiccoughs, ***anaphylaxis with or without circulatory collapse, cardiac arrest, bronchospasm,*** arachnoiditis after intrathecal use, foreign body granulomatous reactions.

- **INTRA-ARTICULAR**

Postinjection flare, Charcot-like arthropathy, tendon rupture, skin atrophy, facial flushing, osteonecrosis. Due to reduction in inflammation and pain, clients may overuse the joint.

- **INTRASPINAL**

Aseptic, bacterial, chemical, cryptococcal, or tubercular meningitis; adhesive arachnoiditis, conus medullaris syndrome.

- **INTRAOCULAR**

Increased ocular pressure, thereby inducing or aggravating simple glaucoma. Stinging, burning, dendritic keratitis (herpes simplex), corneal perforation (especially when the drugs are used for diseases that cause corneal thinning). Posterior subcapsular cataracts, especially in children. Exophthalmos, secondary fungal or viral eye infections.

- **TOPICAL USE**

When used over large areas, when the skin is broken, or with occlusive dressings, may cause atrophy of the epidermis, drying of the skin, or atrophy of the dermal collagen. When used on the face, diffuse thinning and homogenization of the collagen, epidermal thinning, and striae formation. Occasionally, sensitization reaction may occur, which necessitates discontinuation of the drug.

OD OVERDOSE MANAGEMENT

Symptoms (Continued Use of Large Doses)—Cushing's Syndrome: Acne, hypertension, moonface, striae, hirsutism, central obesity, ecchymoses, myopathy, sexual dysfunction, osteoporosis, diabetes, hyperlipidemia, increased susceptibility to infection, peptic ulcer, electrolyte and fluid imbalance. Acute toxicity or death is rare. *Treatment of Chronic Overdose:* Gradually taper the dose of the steroid and frequently monitor lab tests. During periods of stress, steroid supplementation is necessary. Dose should be reduced to the lowest one that will control the symptoms (or discontinue the steroid completely). Recovery of normal adrenal and pituitary function may take up to 9 months. Large, acute overdoses may be treated with gastric lavage, emesis, and general supportive measures.

DRUG INTERACTIONS

Acetaminophen / ↑ Risk of hepatotoxicity R/T ↑ rate of formation of hepatotoxic acetaminophen metabolite
Alcohol / ↑ Risk of GI ulceration or hemorrhage
H *Aloe* / Hypokalemia due to both drugs could potentiate the effect of digoxin
Amphotericin B / Corticosteroids ↑ K depletion caused by amphotericin B
Aminoglutethimide / ↓ Adrenal response to corticotropin
Anabolic steroids / ↑ Risk of edema
Antacids / ↓ Effect of corticosteroids R/T ↓ GI tract absorption
Antibiotics, broad-spectrum / Concomitant use may result in emergence of resistant strains, leading to severe infection
Anticholinergics / Combination ↑ IOP; aggravates glaucoma
Anticoagulants, oral / ↓ Effect of anticoagulants by ↓ hypoprothrombinemia; also ↑ risk of hemorrhage R/T vascular effects of corticosteroids
Anticholinesterases / Corticosteroids may ↓ effect of anticholinesterases when used in myasthenia gravis
Antidiabetic agents / Hyperglycemic effect of corticosteroids may necessitate ↑ antidiabetic dose
Asparaginase / ↑ Hyperglycemic drug effect and the risk of neuropathy and disturbances in erythropoiesis
Barbiturates / ↓ Effect of corticosteroids R/T ↑ liver breakdown
Bumetanide / Enhanced potassium loss R/T potassium-losing properties of both drugs
Carbonic anhydrase inhibitors / Corticosteroids ↑ K depletion caused by carbonic anhydrase inhibitors
Cholestyramine / ↓ Effect of corticosteroids R/T ↓ GI tract absorption
Colestipol / ↓ Effect of corticosteroids R/T ↓ GI tract absorption

Contraceptives, oral / Estrogen ↑ anti-inflammatory effect of hydrocortisone by ↓ liver breakdown
Cyclophosphoramide / ↑ Effect of cyclophosphoramide R/T ↓ liver breakdown
Cyclosporine / ↑ Effect of both drugs R/T ↓ liver breakdown
Digitalis glycosides / ↑ Chance of digitalis toxicity (arrhythmias) R/T hypokalemia
Ephedrine / ↓ Effect of corticosteroids R/T ↑ liver breakdown
Estrogens / ↑ Anti-inflammatory effect of hydrocortisone by ↓ liver breakdown
Ethacrynic acid / Enhanced potassium loss R/T potassium-losing properties of both drugs
Folic acid / Requirements may ↑
Furosemide / Enhanced potassium loss R/T potassium-losing properties of both drugs
H *Ginseng* / Possible additive effects; do not use together
Heparin / Ulcerogenic effects of corticosteroids may ↑ risk of hemorrhage
Immunosuppressant drugs / ↑ Risk of infection
Indomethacin / ↑ Chance of GI ulceration
Insulin / Hyperglycemic effect of corticosteroids may necessitate ↑ antidiabetic dose
Isoniazid / ↓ Effect of isoniazid R/T ↑ liver breakdown and ↑ excretion
Ketoconazole / ↑ Corticosteroid availability and ↓ clearance → possible toxicity
H *Licorice* / ↑ Levels of corticosteroids
H *Lily-of-the-valley* / ↑ Effectivness and side effects of chronic glucocorticoid therapy
Mexiletine / ↓ Effect of mexiletine R/T ↑ liver breakdown
Mitotane / ↓ Response of adrenal gland to corticotropin
Muscle relaxants, nondepolarizing / ↓ Effect of muscle relaxants
Neuromuscular blocking agents / ↑ Risk of prolonged respiratory depression or paralysis
NSAIDs / ↑ Risk of GI hemorrhage or ulceration
H *Pheasant's eye herb* / ↑ Effectivness and side effects of chronic glucocorticoid therapy
Phenobarbital / ↓ Effect of corticosteroids R/T ↑ liver breakdown
Phenytoin / ↓ Effect of corticosteroids R/T ↑ liver breakdown
Potassium supplements / ↓ Plasma levels of potassium
Rifampin / ↓ Effect of corticosteroids R/T ↑ liver breakdown
Ritodrine / ↑ Risk of maternal edema
Salicylates / Both are ulcerogenic; also, corticosteroids may ↓ blood salicylate levels
Somatrem, Somatropin / Glucocorticoids may inhibit effect of somatrem
H *Squill* / ↑ Effectivness and side effects of chronic glucocorticoid therapy
Streptozocin / ↑ Risk of hyperglycemia
Theophyllines / Corticosteroids ↑ effect of theophyllines
Thiazide diuretics / Enhanced potassium loss R/T potassium-losing properties of both drugs
Tricyclic antidepressants / ↑ Risk of mental disturbances
Vitamin A / Topical vitamin A can reverse impaired wound healing in clients receiving corticosteroids

LABORATORY TEST CONSIDERATIONS

↑ Urine glucose, serum cholesterol, serum amylase. ↓ Serum potassium, triiodothyronine, serum uric acid. Alteration of electrolyte balance.

NURSING CONSIDERATIONS

ADMINISTRATION OF ORAL CORTICOSTEROIDS

1. Administer PO forms of drug with food to minimize ulcerogenic effect.
2. At frequent intervals, reduce the dose gradually to determine if symptoms of the disease can be effectively controlled by smaller drug dose.
3. When treating clients with conditions such as asthma, ulcerative colitis, and rheumatoid arthritis, corticosteroids, given every other day, pro-

vide the beneficial effect of the steroid while minimizing pituitary-adrenal suppression. With this therapy, twice the usual daily dose of an intermediate-acting steroid is given every other morning.
4. Local administration of corticosteroids is preferred over systemic therapy to minimize systemic side effects.
5. Discontinue gradually if used chronically.
6. Use the lowest effective dose in children and monitor routinely to avoid reduced rate of growth.TOPICAL

ADMINISTRATION OF TOPICAL CORTICOSTEROIDS

1. Cleanse area before applying the medication.
2. Wear gloves, apply sparingly, and rub gently into the area.
3. When prescribed, apply an occlusive dressing (not to be used if an infection is present) to promote hydration of the stratum corneum and increase the absorption of the medication. The following are two methods of applying an occlusive type dressing:
• Apply a large amount of medication to the cleansed area. Cover with a thin, pliable, nonflammable plastic film, which is then sealed to the surrounding tissue with skin tape or held in place with gauze. Change the dressing q 3–4 days.
• Apply a small amount of medication to the area and cover with a damp cloth. Then cover with a thin, pliable, nonflammable plastic film and seal to the surrounding tissue with tape, or hold in place with gauze. Change dressing b.i.d.

ASSESSMENT(GENERAL)

1. Document indications for therapy, type, onset, and characteristics of symptoms; note underlying cause: adrenal or nonadrenal disorder.
2. Note mental status (i.e., mood, affect, aggression, behavioral changes, depression) and neuro function.
3. Check for any allergic reactions to corticosteroids or tartrazine.
4. Monitor ECG, electrolytes, BS, urinalysis, renal and LFTs.
5. Document VS and weight. Obtain CXR and PPD if therapy prolonged.
6. Note childhood illnesses and immunization status.
7. List medications taking and identify those that may interact with corticosteroids. These include antidiabetic agents, cardiac glycosides, oral contraceptives, anticoagulants, and drugs influenced by liver enzymes.
8. If female, determine if pregnant.
9. In conditions requiring long term therapy determine if other agents (e.g., methotrexate) can be used to spare long term harmful steroid effects.
10. With trigger point injections, determine if oral trial effective in reducing pain levels before referral.

INTERVENTIONS

TOPICAL CORTICOSTEROIDS

1. Assess for local sensitivity reaction at the site of application.
2. Absorption varies regionally with highest absorption in scrotal skin and lowest on the foot. Inflamed skin increases absorption several-fold.
3. Better action has been noted with the ointment bases than with the lotion or cream vehicles.
4. Observe for signs of infections since corticosteroids tend to mask. Avoid occlusive dressing when an infection is present. Document site of infection, nature of infection, and characteristics (e.g., redness, swelling, odor, or drainage).
5. With large occlusive dressing, take temperatures q 4 hr. Report if elevated and remove the dressing.
6. Assess for evidence of systemic absorption. Protracted use of large quantities of potent topical corticosteroids to large BSAs may precipitate iatrogenic Cushing's syndrome. Symptoms may include edema and transient inhibition of pituitary-adrenal cortical function as manifested by muscular pain, lassitude, depression, hypotension, and weight loss.
7. Advise when applying topical ointment, to wash hands and to wear

gloves or to apply with a sterile applicator (e.g., tongue blade).
8. Report erythema, telangiectases, purpura, bruising, pustules, and depressed shiny, wrinkled skin. Prolonged use of potent topical corticosteroids may increase incidence of systemic side effects.

ORAL CORTICOSTEROIDS

1. When first placed on corticosteroids, check BP b.i.d. until maintenance dose established.
2. Short-term oral therapy (e.g., 60 mg PO for 5 days) does not require divided doses or titration. With long-term therapy, monitor for symptoms of adrenal insufficiency, which include hypotension, confusion, restlessness, lethargy, weakness, N&V, anorexia, and weight loss; titrate dose to withdraw.
3. Evaluate for increased sodium and fluid retention. Monitor weight and observe for edema. If noted, adjust to low—sodium, high— potassium diet. Anticipate a small weight gain due to increased appetite, but sudden increases are probably due to edema. Edema occurs most frequently with cortisone or desoxycorticosterone acetate and less frequently with the synthetic agents.
4. Assess for SOB, distended neck veins, edema, and easy fatigue; S&S of CHF. Obtain a CXR and ECG.
5. Monitor serum glucose, electrolytes, and platelet counts with long-term therapy. Report any unusual bleeding, bruising, presence of petechiae, symptoms of diabetes, and any other skin changes.
6. Assess muscles for weakness and wasting; signs of a negative nitrogen balance.
7. Report changes in appearance, especially those resembling Cushing's syndrome (such as rounding of the face, hirsutism, presence of acne, and thinning of the hair and nails) so dosage can be adjusted.
8. With diabetes, may develop hyperglycemia necessitating a change in diet and insulin dosage.
9. Assess for signs of depression, lack of interest in personal appearance, insomnia or anorexia.
10. Discuss potential for menstrual difficulties and amenorrhea related to long-term therapy.
11. Observe for S&S of other illnesses as these drugs tend to mask the severity of most illnesses.
12. GI bleeding may occur; periodically test stools for occult blood and monitor hematologic profile.

CLIENT/FAMILY TEACHING

1. These agents generally work by inhibiting or decreasing the inflammatory response.
2. Take the oral medication with food and report any symptoms of gastric distress. To prevent gastric irritation, may use antacids and eat frequent small meals. If the symptoms persist, diagnostic X rays may be indicated. High doses of glucocorticoids stimulate the stomach to produce excess acid and pepsin and may cause peptic ulcers. Antacids 3–4 times/day may relieve epigastric distress.
3. Report changes in mood or affect.
4. Obtain weight daily at the same time, wearing clothing of approximately the same weight, and using the same scales. Consistent weight gain may reflect fluid retention; initiate caloric management to prevent obesity.
5. Identify foods high in potassium and low in sodium to prevent electrolyte disturbances. Supplement diet with potassium-rich foods such as citrus juices, collard greens, or bananas. Read labels of canned or processed foods and consult dietician for assistance in shopping and meal preparation.
6. Eat a diet high in protein to compensate for the loss due to protein breakdown from gluconeogenesis.
7. Exercise daily and consume foods high in calcium to decrease possibility of osteoporosis (due to catabolic bone effects). Consume adequate protein, calcium, and vitamin D to minimize bone loss. On-going bone

resorption with depressed bone formation is the cause of osteoporosis.
8. Avoid falls and accidents. Steroids may cause osteoporosis, which makes the bones more susceptible to fractures. Use a night light and a hand rail or other device for support if need to get up at night.
9. Corticosteroids can cause a loss of contraceptive action with oral contraceptives. Keep accurate menstrual records and consider alternative methods of birth control. May also have an adverse effect on sperm production and count.
10. Weight gain, acne, and excess hair growth may occur.
11. Need to gradually withdraw the medication when therapy has exceeded 7 consecutive days. This should proceed slowly so that the adrenal cortex will gradually be reactivated and take over the production of hormones. Sudden withdrawal may be life-threatening. Any sudden change will provoke symptoms of adrenal insufficiency.
12. With dosage reduction, flare-ups may occur; these are caused by the reduction.
13. With arthritis, do not overuse the joint once injected and painless. Permanent joint damage may result from overuse, because underlying pathology is still present.
14. With diabetes, monitor glucose levels frequently and report changes as insulin dose and diet may require adjustment.
15. Wounds may heal slowly because steroid therapy causes a delay in development of granulation tissue, increasing potential for infection. Observe any healing process for signs of infection and report any injury or postoperative separation of wound or suture line.
16. These drugs mask symptoms of infection and cause immunosuppression. Because antibody production is decreased by corticosteroids, clients are at risk for infection. Must maintain general hygiene and scrupulous cleanliness to avoid infection. Report if sore throat, cough, fever, malaise, or an injury that does not heal occurs. Avoid contact with persons with contagious diseases.
17. Delay any vaccinations, immunizations, or skin testing while receiving corticosteroid therapy because there is limited immune response.
18. Clients on long-term eye therapy are prone to developing cataracts, exophthalmus, and increased IOP. Schedule routine eye exams.
19. Avoid OTC meds, including aspirin and ibuprofen compounds, as well as alcohol, since these may aggravate gastric irritation and bleeding.
20. Carry ID, listing drugs and dosage, condition being treated, and who to contact in the event of an emergency.
21. Check child's height and weight regularly and graph; growth suppression may occur with corticosteroid therapy; not prevented by growth hormone administration.
22. Large doses of glucocorticoids in children may increase intracranial pressure (pseudotumor cerebri); report symptoms: vertigo, headache, and convulsions. These should disappear once therapy discontinued.

OUTCOMES/EVALUATE

- Effective wound healing
- Chronic pain control
- Suppression of inflammatory/immune responses or disease manifestation in allergic reactions, autoimmune diseases, organ transplants
- Serum cortisol levels within desired range in adrenal deficiency states (8 a.m. level 110–520 nmol/L)

DIURETICS, LOOP

SEE ALSO THE FOLLOWING INDIVIDUAL ENTRIES:

Bumetanide
Ethacrynate sodium
Ethacrynic acid
Furosemide
Torsemide

ACTION/KINETICS

Loop diuretics inhibit reabsorption of sodium and chloride in the proximal and distal tubules and the loop of

Henle. Metabolized in the liver and excreted primarily through the urine. Significantly bound to plasma protein.

USES

See individual drugs.

CONTRAINDICATIONS

Hypersensitivity to loop diruetics or to sulfonylureas. In hepatic coma or severe electrolyte depletion (until condition improves or is corrected). Lactation.

SPECIAL CONCERNS

Sudden alterations of electrolytes in hepatic cirrhosis and ascites may precipitate hepatic encephalopathy and coma. SLE may be activated or worsened. Ototoxicity is most common with rapid injection, in severe renal impairment, with doses several times the usual dose, and with concurrent use of other ototoxic drugs. The risk of hospitalization is doubled in geriatric clients who take diuretics and NSAIDs. Safety and efficacy of most loop diuretics have not been determined in children or infants.

SIDE EFFECTS

See individual drugs. Excessive diuresis may cause dehydration with the possibility of ***circulatory collapse and vascular thrombosis or embolism.*** Ototoxicity including tinnitus, hearing impairment, deafness (usually reversible), and vertigo with a sense of fullness are possible. Electrolyte imbalance, especially in clients with restricted salt intake. Photosensitivity. Changes include hypokalemia, hypomagnesemia, and hypocalcemia.

OD OVERDOSE MANAGEMENT

Symptoms: Acute profound water loss, volume and electrolyte depletion, dehydration, decreased blood volume, and ***circulatory collapse with possibility of fascicular thrombosis and embolism.*** *Treatment:* Replace fluid and electrolyte loss. Carefully monitor urine and plasma electrolyte levels. Emesis and gastric lavage may be useful. Supportive measures may include oxygen or artificial respiration.

DRUG INTERACTIONS

Aminoglycosides / ↑ Ototoxicity with hearing loss
Anticoagulants / ↑ Drug activity
Chloral hydrate / Transient diaphoresis, hot flashes, hypertension, tachycardia, weakness and nausea
Cisplatin / Additive ototoxicity
Digitalis glycosides / ↑ Risk of arrhythmias R/T diuretic-induced electrolyte disturbances
Lithium / ↑ Plasma levels of lithium → toxicity
Muscle relaxants, nondepolarizing / Effect of muscle relaxants either ↑ or ↓, depending on diuretic dose
Nonsteroidal anti-inflammatory drugs / ↓ Effect of loop diuretics
Probenecid / ↓ Effect of loop diuretics
Salicylates / Diuretic effect may be ↓ with cirrhosis and ascites
Sulfonylureas/ Loop diuretics may ↓ glucose tolerance
Theophyllines / Action of theophyllines may be ↑ or ↓
Thiamine / High doses of loop diuretics → thiamine deficiency
Thiazide diuretics / Additive effects with loop diuretics → profound diuresis and serious electrolyte abnormalities

DOSAGE

See individual drugs.

NURSING CONSIDERATIONS

SEE ALSO *DIURETICS, THIAZIDES.*

ASSESSMENT

1. Document indications for therapy. Note other agents prescribed and the outcome.
2. Monitor CBC, lytes, Mg, Ca, BS, uric acid, renal and LFTs.
3. Note any sensitivity to sulfonamides. May exhibit cross-reactivity with furosemide.
4. Determine presence of SLE; drug may worsen condition.
5. Assess auditory function carefully when large doses are anticipated or when used concurrently with other ototoxic agents. Ototoxicity is dose related and generally reversible.

INTERVENTIONS

1. Record weights I&O; keep bedpan or urinal within reach. Report absence/decrease in diuresis and note changes in lung sounds.
2. When ambulatory, check for edema in the extremities; if on bed rest, check for edema in the sacral area.
3. Monitor for serum electrolyte levels, pH, and the following *signs of electrolyte imbalance:*
   - *Hyponatremia* (low-salt syndrome)—characterized by muscle weakness, leg cramps, dryness of mouth, dizziness, and GI upset.
   - *Hypernatremia* (excessive sodium retention)—characterized by CNS disturbances, i.e., confusion, loss of sensorium, stupor, and coma. ↓ Skin turgor and postural hypotension not as prominent as with combined sodium and water deficits.
   - *Water intoxication* (caused by defective water diuresis)—characterized by lethargy, confusion, stupor, and coma. Neuromuscular hyperexcitability with ↑ reflexes, muscular twitching, and convulsions if acute.
   - *Metabolic acidosis*—characterized by weakness, headache, malaise, abdominal pain, and N&V. Hyperpnea occurs in severe metabolic acidosis. S&S of volume depletion: poor skin turgor, soft eyeballs, and dry tongue may be observed.
   - *Metabolic alkalosis*—characterized by irritability, neuromuscular hyperexcitability, tetany if severe.
   - *Hypokalemia (potassium deficiency)*—characterized by muscular weakness, peristalsis failure, postural hypotension, respiratory embarrassment, and cardiac arrhythmias.
   - *Hyperkalemia (excess potassium)*—characterized by early signs of irritability, nausea, intestinal colic, and diarrhea; and by later signs of weakness, flaccid paralysis, dyspnea, dysphagia, and arrhythmias.
4. With high doses monitor for hyperlipidemia and hyperuricemia; precipitating a gout attack.
5. With liver dysfunction, assess for electrolyte imbalances, which could cause stupor, coma, and death.
6. If receiving EC potassium tablets, assess for abdominal pain, distention, or GI bleeding; can cause small bowel ulceration. Check stool for intact tablets.
7. Diuretics potentiate the effects of antihypertensive agents; monitor BP.
8. May precipitate symptoms of diabetes with latent or mild diabetes. Test urine or perform finger sticks and monitor chemisty studies.
9. Hyper- or hypokalemia associated with diuretic therapy may potentiate the toxic effects of digitalis and precipitate arrhythmias.
10. Assess for sore throat, skin rash, and yellowing of the skin or sclera; may be blood dyscrasias.

CLIENT/FAMILY TEACHING

1. May cause frequent, copious voiding. Plan activities; take in the am to prevent sleep disruption.
2. Take with food or milk to decrease GI upset.
3. Weakness and/or dizziness may occur. Rise slowly from bed and sit down or lie down if evident. Use caution in driving a car or operating other hazardous machinery until drug effects apparent.
4. The use of alcohol, standing for prolonged periods, and exercise in hot weather may enhance/lower BP.
5. Ensure adequate fluids; monitor BP and weight. Report excessive weight loss, loss of skin turgor or if dizziness, nausea, muscle weakness, cramps, or tingling of the extremities occurs.
6. Wear protective clothing, sunscreens, and sunglasses to prevent photosensitivity reactions.
7. Include foods high in potassium, such as citrus, grape, cranberry, apple, pear, and apricot juices; bananas; meat, fish, or fowl; cereals; and tea and cola beverages. This is preferable to taking potassium chloride supplements but potassium supplements are usually prescribed with non-potassium-sparing diuretics. Unless conditions such as gastric ulcer or diabetes exists, drink a large glass of orange juice daily. Consult dietitian as needed, for assistance in selecting and preparing foods.

8. Avoid all OTC preparations without approval.

OUTCOMES/EVALUATE

• Symptomatic relief (↓ weight, ↓ swelling/edema, ↑ diuresis)

• Clinical improvement in S&S associated with CHF and renal failure

DIURETICS, THIAZIDES

SEE ALSO THE FOLLOWING INDIVIDUAL ENTRIES:

Chlorothiazide
Chlorothiazide sodium
Chlorthalidone
Hydrochlorothiazide
Indapamide

ACTION/KINETICS

Thiazides promote diuresis by decreasing the rate at which sodium and chloride are reabsorbed by the distal renal tubules of the kidney. By increasing the excretion of sodium and chloride, they force excretion of additional water. They also increase the excretion of potassium and, to a lesser extent, bicarbonate, as well as decrease the excretion of calcium and uric acid. Sodium and chloride are excreted in approximately equal amounts. Thiazides do not affect the glomerular filtration rate. Thiazides also have an antihypertensive effect which is attributed to direct dilation of the arterioles, as well as to a reduction in the total fluid volume of the body and altered sodium balance. The thiazide diuretics are related chemically to the sulfonamides. Although devoid of anti-infective activity, the thiazides can cause the same hypersensitivity reactions as the sulfonamides. A large fraction is excreted unchanged in urine.

USES

Edema, CHF, hypertension, pregnancy, and premenstrual tension. Thiazides are used for edema due to CHF, nephrosis, nephritis, renal failure, PMS, hepatic cirrhosis, corticosteroid or estrogen therapy. Hypertension. *Investigational:* Thiazides are used alone or in combination with allopurinol (or amiloride) for prophylaxis of calcium nephrolithiasis. Nephrogenic diabetes insipidus.

CONTRAINDICATIONS

Hypersensitivity to drug, anuria, renal decompensation. Impaired renal function and advanced hepatic cirrhosis. Do not use indiscriminately in clients with edema and toxemia of pregnancy, even though they may be therapeutically useful, because the thiazides may have adverse effects on the newborn (thrombocytopenia and jaundice).

SPECIAL CONCERNS

Geriatric clients may manifest an increased risk of hypotension and changes in electrolyte levels. The risk of hospitalization is doubled in geriatric clients who take diuretics and NSAIDs. Administer with caution to debilitated clients or to those with a history of hepatic coma or precoma, gout, diabetes mellitus, or during pregnancy and lactation. Particular care must be exercised when thiazides are administered concomitantly with drugs that also cause potassium loss, such as digitalis, corticosteroids, and some estrogens. Clients with advanced heart failure, renal disease, or hepatic cirrhosis are most likely to develop hypokalemia. May activate or worsen SLE.

SIDE EFFECTS

The following side effects may be observed with most thiazides. See also individual drugs. **Electrolyte imbalance:** Hypokalemia (most frequent) characterized by cardiac arrhythmias. Hyponatremia characterized by weakness, lethargy, epigastric distress, N&V. Hypokalemic alkalosis. **GI:** Anorexia, epigastric distress or irritation, N&V, cramping, bloating, abdominal pain, diarrhea, constipation, jaundice, pancreatitis. **CNS:** Dizziness, lightheadedness, headache, vertigo, xanthopsia, paresthesias, weakness, insomnia, restlessness. **CV:** Orthostatic hypotension, MIs in elderly clients with advanced arteriosclerosis, especially if the client is also receiving therapy with other antihypertensive agents. **Hematologic:** ***Agranulocytosis, aplastic or hypoplastic anemia, hemolytic anemia,*** leukopenia, thrombocytopenia. **Dermatologic:** Purpura, photosensitivity, photosensitivity dermatitis, rash, urticaria, necrotizing angiitis, vasculitis, cutaneous vasculitis. **Metabolic:** neutropenia, hemolytic anemia. **Endocrine:** Hyperglycemia, glycosuria, hyperuricemia. **Miscellaneous:** Blurred vision, impotence, reduced libido, fever, muscle cramps, muscle spasm, respiratory distress.

OD OVERDOSE MANAGEMENT

Symptoms: Symptoms of plasma volume depletion, including orthostatic hypotension, dizziness, drowsiness, syncope, electrolyte abnormalities, hemoconcentration, hemodynamic changes. Signs of potassium depletion, including confusion, dizziness, muscle weakness, and GI disturbances. Also, N&V, GI irritation, GI hypermotility, CNS effects, cardiac abnormalities, ***seizures, hypotension, decreased respiration, and coma.***

Treatment:

- Induce emesis or perform gastric lavage followed by activated charcoal. Undertake measures to prevent aspiration.
- Electrolyte balance, hydration, respiration, CV, and renal function must be maintained. Cathartics should be avoided, as use may enhance fluid loss.
- Although GI effects are usually of short duration, treatment may be required.

DRUG INTERACTIONS

Allopurinol / ↑ Risk of hypersensitivity reactions to allopurinol

H *Aloe* / Hypokalemia as both drugs could potentiate effects of digoxin

Amphotericin B / Enhanced loss of electrolytes, especially potassium

Anesthetics / Thiazides may ↑ effects of anesthetics

Anticholinergic agents / ↑ Effect of thiazides R/T ↑ amount absorbed from GI tract

Anticoagulants, oral / Anticoagulant effects may be decreased

Antidiabetic agents / Thiazides antagonize hypoglycemic drug effects

Antigout agents / Thiazides may ↑ uric acid levels; thus, ↑ dose of antigout drug may be necessary

Antihypertensive agents / Thiazides potentiate drug effects

Antineoplastic agents / Thiazides may prolong drug induced leukopenia

Calcium salts / Hypercalcemia R/T renal tubular reabsorption or bone release may be ↑ by exogenous calcium

Cholestyramine / ↓ Effect of thiazides R/T ↓ GI tract absorption

Colestipol / ↓ Effect of thiazides R/T ↓ GI tract absorption

Corticosteroids / Enhanced potassium loss R/T potassium-losing properties of both drugs

Diazoxide / Enhanced hypotensive effect. Also, ↑ hyperglycemic response

Digitalis glycosides / Thiazides produce ↑ potassium and magnesium loss with ↑ chance of digitalis-induced arrhythmias

Ethanol / Additive orthostatic hypotension

Fenfluramine / ↑ Antihypertensive effect of thiazides

Furosemide / Profound diuresis and electrolyte loss

Guanethidine / Additive hypotensive effect

Indomethacin / ↓ Effect of thiazides, possibly by inhibition of prostaglandins

Insulin / ↓ Effect R/T thiazide-induced hyperglycemia

H *Licorice root* / Potassium loss R/T thiazides and licorice → ↑ sensitivity to digitalis glycosides

Lithium / ↑ Risk of lithium toxicity R/T ↓ renal excretion; may be used together but use should be carefully monitored

Loop diuretics / Additive effect to cause profound diuresis and serious electrolyte losses

Methenamine / ↓ Effect of thiazides R/T alkalinization of urine by methenamine

Methyldopa / ↑ Risk of hemolytic anemia (rare)

Muscle relaxants, nondepolarizing / ↑ Effect of muscle relaxants R/T hypokalemia
Norepinephrine / Thiazides ↓ arterial response to norepinephrine
Quinidine / ↑ Effect of quinidine R/T ↑ renal tubular reabsorption
Reserpine / Additive hypotensive effect
Sulfonamides / ↑ Effect of thiazides R/T ↓ plasma protein binding
Sulfonylureas / ↓ Effect R/T thiazide-induced hyperglycemia
Tetracyclines / ↑ Risk of azotemia
Tubocurarine / ↑ Muscle relaxation and ↑ hypokalemia
Vasopressors (sympathomimetics) / Thiazides ↓ responsiveness of arterioles to vasopressors
Vitamin D / ↑ Effect of vitamin D R/T thiazide-induced hypercalcemia

LABORATORY TEST CONSIDERATIONS

Hypokalemia, hypercalcemia, hyponatremia, hypomagnesemia, hypochloremia, hypophosphatemia, hyperuricemia. ↑ BUN, creatinine, glucose in blood and urine. ↓ Serum PBI levels (no signs of thyroid disturbance). Initial ↑ total cholesterol, LDL cholesterol, and triglycerides.

DOSAGE

See individual drugs.

NURSING CONSIDERATIONS

ADMINISTRATION/STORAGE

1. Clients resistant to one type of thiazide may respond to another.
2. Liquid potassium preparations are bitter. Administer with fruit juice or milk to enhance palatability.
3. To minimize electrolyte imbalance, thiazides may be taken every other day or on a 3–5-day basis for treatment of edema.
4. To prevent excess hypotension, reduce dose of other antihypertensive agents when beginning therapy.

ASSESSMENT

1. Note any drug hypersensitivity. Document indications for therapy and any use of these drugs.
2. Monitor CBC, glucose, electrolytes, Ca, Mg, renal and LFTs.
3. Note any history of heart disease or gout; check uric acid levels.
4. Determine extent of edema; assess skin turgor, mucous membranes, extremities, and lung fields.
5. With cirrhosis, avoid K+ depletion and hepatic encephalopathy.

INTERVENTIONS

1. Stop drug at least 48 hr before surgery. Thiazide inhibits pressor effects of epinephrine.
2. Potassium supplements should be given only when dietary measures are inadequate. If required, use liquid preparations to avoid ulcerations that may be produced by potassium salts in the solid dosage form. Exceptions include slow-K forms (potassium salt imbedded in a wax matrix) and micro-K forms (microencapsulated potassium salt).

CLIENT/FAMILY TEACHING

1. Administer in the morning so that the major diuretic effect will occur before bedtime.
2. Take with food or milk if GI upset occurs.
3. Eat a diet high in potassium. Include orange juice, bananas, citrus fruits, broccoli, spinach, tomato juice, cucumbers, beets, dried fruits, or apricots. Avoid black licorice; may precipitate severe hypokalemia.
4. Rise slowly and dangle legs before standing to minimize orthostatic effects. Sit or lie down if feeling faint or dizzy.
5. With gout, avoid foods high in purines and continue antigout agents as prescribed.
6. With diabetes, monitor finger sticks more frequently; may need adjustment of insulin or oral hypoglycemic agent.
7. Avoid alcohol; causes severe hypotension.
8. Do not take any other medication (including OTC drugs for asthma, cough and colds, hay fever, weight control) unless approved.
9. Report any severe weight loss,

muscle weakness, cramps, dizziness, or fatigue.
10. Skin rashes may occur but severe symptoms R/T allergic reactions include acute pulmonary edema, acute pancreatitis, thrombocytopenia, cholestatic jaundice, and hemolytic anemia; report immediately.

OUTCOMES/EVALUATE

- Control of hypertension; ↓ BP
- ↑ Urine output; ↓ edema; ↓ weight
- Adequate tissue perfusion with warm dry skin and good pulses
- Normal electrolyte levels and fluid balance

ESTROGENS

SEE ALSO THE FOLLOWING INDIVIDUAL ENTRIES:

Esterified estrogens
Estradiol hemihydrate
Estradiol transdermal system
Estrogens conjugated, oral
Estrogens conjugated, parenteral
Estrogens conjugated, synthetic
Estrogens conjugated, vaginal
Estropipate
Oral Contraceptives

ACTION/KINETICS

The three primary estrogens in the human female are estradiol 17–β, estrone, and estriol, which are steroids. Nonsteroidal estrogens include diethylstilbestrol. Estrogens combine with receptors in the cytoplasm of the cell, resulting in an increase in protein synthesis. For example, estrogens are required for development of secondary sex characteristics, development and maintenance of the female genital system and breasts. They also produce effects in the pituitary and hypothalamus. In adult women, estrogens participate in bone maintenance by aiding the deposition of calcium in the protein matrix of bones. They increase elastic elements in the skin, tend to cause sodium and fluid retention, and produce an anabolic effect by enhancing the turnover of dietary nitrogen and other elements into protein. Furthermore, they tend to keep plasma cholesterol at relatively low levels. Natural estrogens have a significant first-pass effect; thus, they are given parenterally. Synthetic derivatives can be given PO and are rapidly absorbed, distributed, and excreted. Estrogens are metabolized in the liver and excreted in urine (major portion) and feces. When given transdermally, the skin metabolizes estradiol only to a small extent.

USES

Uses include hormone replacement therapy in postmenopausal women and as a component of combination oral contraceptives. See individual drugs. Estrogens are used both systemically and vaginally.

CONTRAINDICATIONS

Breast cancer, except in those clients being treated for metastatic disease. Cancer of the genital tract and other estrogen-dependent neoplasms. Undiagnosed abnormal genital bleeding. History of thrombophlebitis, thrombosis, or thromboembolic disorders associated with previous estrogen use (except when used to treat breast or prostatic cancer). Known or suspected pregnancy. Prolonged therapy in women who plan to become pregnant. Use during lactation. May be contraindicated in clients with blood dyscrasias, hepatic disease, or thyroid dysfunction.

SPECIAL CONCERNS

Use with caution, if at all, in those with asthma, epilepsy, migraine, cardiac failure, renal insufficiency, diseases involving calcium or phosphorous metabolism, or a family history of mammary or genital tract cancer. Increased risk of endometrial carcinoma in postmenopausal women. Hormone replacement therapy does not prevent MI or stroke in women with established CV disease and estrogen should not be used solely for CV effects. Safety and effectiveness have not been determined in children and should be used with caution in adolescents in whom bone growth is incomplete.

SIDE EFFECTS

• SYSTEMIC USE.

Side effects to estrogens are dose dependent.

CV: Potentially, the most serious side effects involve the CV system. ***Thromboembolism,*** thrombophlebitis, ***MI, pulmonary embolism,*** retinal thrombosis, ***mesenteric thrombosis, subarachnoid hemorrhage, postsurgical thromboembolism.*** Hypertension, edema, ***stroke.*** **GI:** N&V, abdominal cramps, bloating, cholestatic jaundice, colitis, acute pancreatitis, changes in appetite. **Dermatologic:** Most common are chloasma or melasma. Also, erythema multiforme, erythema nodosum, hemorrhagic eruptions, urticaria, dermatitis, photosensitivity. **Hepatic:** Cholestatic jaundice, aggravation of porphyria, benign (most common) or malignant liver tumors. **GU:** Breakthrough bleeding, spotting, changes in amount and/or duration of menstrual flow, amenorrhea during and after use, dysmenorrhea, premenstrual-like syndrome, change in cervical eversion and degree of cervical secretion, cystitis-like syndrome, hemolytic uremic syndrome, endometrial cystic hyperplasia, increased incidence of *Candida* vaginitis. **CNS:** Mental depression, dizziness, changes in libido, chorea, headache, aggravation of migraine headaches, fatigue, nervousness, ***convulsions***. **Ocular:** Steepening of corneal curvature resulting in intolerance of contact lenses. Optic neuritis or retinal thrombosis, resulting in sudden or gradual, partial or complete loss of vision, double vision, papilledema. **Hematologic:** Increase in prothrombin and blood coagulation factors VII, VIII, IX, and X. Decrease in antithrombin III. **Local:** Pain at injection site, sterile abscesses, postinjection flare, redness and irritation at site of application of transdermal system. **Miscellaneous:** Breast tenderness, enlargement, or secretions. Increased risk of gallbladder disease (with high doses). Premature closure of epiphyses in children. Increased frequency of benign or malignant tumors of the cervix, uterus, vagina, and other organs. Weight gain. Increased risk of congenital abnormalities. Hypercalcemia in clients with metastatic breast carcinoma. In males, estrogens may cause gynecomastia, loss of libido, decreased spermatogenesis, testicular atrophy, and feminization. Prolonged use of high doses may inhibit the function of the anterior pituitary. Estrogen therapy affects many laboratory tests.

• VAGINAL USE.

GU: Vaginal bleeding, vaginal discharge, endometrial withdrawal bleeding, serious bleeding in ovariectomized women with endometriosis. **Miscellaneous:** Breast tenderness.

DRUG INTERACTIONS

Anticoagulants, oral / ↓ Drug response by ↑ activity of certain clotting factors

Anticonvulsants / Estrogen-induced fluid retention may precipitate seizures. Also, contraceptive steroids ↑ drug effects by ↓ liver breakdown and ↓ plasma protein binding

Antidiabetic agents / Estrogens may impair glucose tolerance and thus change requirements for antidiabetic agent

Barbiturates / ↓ Effect of estrogen by ↑ liver breakdown

H *Black cohosh* / May interfere with estrogen effects

Corticosteroids / ↑ Pharmacologic and toxicologic effects of corticosteroids

H *Ginseng* / Additive effects; avoid concomitant use

Phenytoin / See *Anticonvulsants*

Rifampin / ↓ Effect of estrogen R/T ↑ liver breakdown

H *Saw palmetto* / ↓ Effect of hormones R/T antiestrogen effect

Succinylcholine / Estrogens may ↑ drug effects

Thyroxine / Possible ↑ need for thyroxine

Tricyclic antidepressants / Possible ↑ drug effects

LABORATORY TEST CONSIDERATIONS

Alter LFTs and thyroid function tests. False + urine glucose test. ↓ Serum cholesterol, total serum lipids, pregnanediol excretion, serum folate, antithrombin III, antifactor Xa. ↑ Serum triglyceride levels, thyroxine-binding globulin, sulfobromophthalein retention. ↑ PT, partial thromboplastin time, platelet aggregation time, platelet count, fibrinogen, plasminogen, norepinephrine-induced platelet aggregability, and factors II, VII, IX, X, XI, VII-X complex, II-VII-X complex, and β–thromboglobulin. Impaired glucose tolerance, reduced response to metyrapone.

DOSAGE

PO, IM, SC, vaginal, topical, or by implantation. The dosage of estrogens is highly individualized and is aimed at the minimal effective amount.

NURSING CONSIDERATIONS

ADMINISTRATION/STORAGE

1. Most PO administered estrogens are metabolized rapidly and must be administered daily.
2. Parenterally administered estrogens are released more slowly from aqueous suspensions or oily solutions; give slowly and deeply.
3. To avoid continuous stimulation of reproductive tissue, cyclic therapy consisting of 3 weeks on and 1 week off is usually recommended for most uses.
4. To reduce postpartum breast engorgement, give during the first few days after delivery.

ASSESSMENT

1. Document indications for therapy, type/onset of symptoms. List other agents prescribed and outcome.
2. Note any history of thromboembolic problems as estrogens enhance blood coagulability; note if smoker.
3. Assess mental status; note any history of depression, migraine headaches, or suicide attempts.
4. Determine any undiagnosed genital bleeding, liver disease, asthma, migraines, epilepsy, or cancer of the endometrium or breast (estrogen-dependent neoplasms), as these preclude drug therapy.
5. Monitor ECG, VS, BS, triglycerides, electrolytes, renal and LFTs.

CLIENT/FAMILY TEACHING

1. Review the dose, form, and frequency of prescribed agent.
2. Taking oral agents with meals or a light snack will prevent gastric irritation and may eliminate nausea. With once-a-day therapy, taking at bedtime may eliminate problems. Nausea, bloating, abdominal cramping, changes in appetite, and vomiting may occur and usually disappear with continued therapy.
3. Report any alterations in mental attitude: depression or withdrawal, insomnia or anorexia, or a lack of attention to personal appearance.
4. With cyclical therapy, take meds for 3 weeks and then omit for 1 week. Menstruation may then occur, but pregnancy will not because ovulation is suppressed. Keep a record of periods and problems, such as missed menses, unusual vaginal bleeding, spotting, or irregularity. Report if pregnancy suspected.
5. Breast tenderness, enlargement, or secretion may occur. Perform BSE monthly (usually 2 weeks after menses) and report changes.
6. Report immediately: leg pains, sudden onset of chest pain, dizziness, SOB, weakness of the arms or legs, or any numbness (S&S of thromboembolic problems).
7. Changes in the curvature of the cornea may make it difficult to wear contact lenses; consult eye dr.
8. Report any changes, such as hair loss or skin discoloration.
9. May alter glucose tolerance. Monitor sugars and report increases; antidiabetic dose may need to be changed.
10. Males may develop feminine characteristics or suffer from impotence; usually resolves once therapy completed.
11. Insert suppositories high into the vault. Apply vaginal preparations at bedtime. Wear a sanitary napkin and avoid the use of tampons. Store suppositories in the refrigerator.

12. Report if estrogen ointments cause systemic reactions.
13. If pregnant and planning to breast-feed, do not take estrogens. Consult provider for alternative forms of contraception; breast-feeding does not provide contraception.
14. *Do not smoke.* Attend formal smoking cessation programs.
15. Some potential risks, related to endometrial/breast cancer, have been associated with estrogen therapy. Close medical follow-up required.

OUTCOMES/EVALUATE

- Control of estrogen imbalance
- Effective contraceptive agent
- Slowing of postmenopausal osteoporosis; ↓ risk of ASHD
- Relief of menopausal S&S
- Control of tumor size/spread in metastatic breast and prostate cancer

FLUOROQUINOLONES

SEE ALSO THE FOLLOWING INDIVIDUAL ENTRIES:

Ciprofloxacin hydrochloride
Enoxacin
Gatifloxacin
Levofloxacin
Lomefloxacin hydrochloride
Moxifloxacin hydrochloride
Norfloxacin
Ofloxacin
Sparfloxacin
Trovafloxacin mesylate injection

ACTION/KINETICS

Synthetic, broad-spectrum antibacterial agents. The fluorine molecule confers increased activity against gram-negative organisms as well as broadens the spectrum against gram-positive organisms. Are bactericidal agents by interfering with DNA gyrase and topoisomerase IV. DNA gyrase is an enzyme needed for the replication, transcription, and repair of bacterial DNA. Topoisomerase IV plays a key role in the partitioning of chromosomal DNA during bacterial cell division. Food may delay the absorption of ciprofloxacin, lomefloxacin, and norfloxacin. Ciprofloxacin, levofloxacin, ofloxacin, and trovafloxacin may be given IV; all fluoroquinolones may be given PO.

USES

See individual drugs. Used for a large number of gram-positive and gram-negative infections.

CONTRAINDICATIONS

Hypersensitivity to the quinolone group of antibiotics, including cinoxacin and nalidixic acid. Tendinitis or tendon rupture associated with quinolone use. Clients receiving dispyramide and amiodarone or other drugs (e.g., quinidine, procainamide, sotalol) that prolong the QTc interval and which may cause torsade de pointes. Lactation. Use in children less than 18 years of age.

SPECIAL CONCERNS

Use lower doses in impaired renal function. There may be differences in CNS toxicity between the various fluoroquinolones. Use may increase the risk of Achilles and other tendon inflammation and rupture. Several fluoroquinolones cause phototoxicity. May exacerbate the signs of myasthenia gravis and lead to life-threatening weakness of the respiratory muscles.

SIDE EFFECTS

See individual drugs. The following side effects are common to each of the fluoroquinolone antibiotics. **GI:** N&V, diarrhea, abdominal pain or discomfort, dry or painful mouth, heartburn, dyspepsia, flatulence, constipation, pseudomembranous colitis. **CNS:** Headache, dizziness, malaise, lethargy, fatigue, drowsiness, somnolence, depression, insomnia, ***seizures,*** paresthesia. **Dermatologic:** Rash, photosensitivity, pruritus (except for ciprofloxacin). **Hypersensitivity reactions:** Facial or ***pharyngeal edema,*** dyspnea, urticaria, itching, tingling, loss of consciousness, ***CV collapse.*** **Other:** Visual disturbances and ophthalmologic abnormalities, hearing loss, superinfection, phototoxicity, eosinophilia, crystalluria, Achilles and other tendon inflammation and rupture. Fluoroquinolones, except norfloxacin, may also cause vaginitis, syncope, chills, and edema.

OD OVERDOSE MANAGEMENT

Symptoms: Extension of side effects. *Treatment:* For acute overdose, vomiting should be induced or gastric lavage performed. The client should be carefully observed and, if necessary, symptomatic and supportive treatment given. Hydration should be maintained. Hemodialysis or peritoneal dialysis may help to remove ciprofloxacin but not other fluoroquinolones.

DRUG INTERACTIONS

Antacids / ↓ Serum fluoroquinolone levels R/T ↓ GI tract absorption
Anticoagulants / ↑ Anticoagulant effects
Cimetidine / ↓ Elimination of fluoroquinolones
Cyclosporine / ↑ Risk of nephrotoxicity
Didanosine / ↓ Serum fluoroquinolone levels R/T ↓ GI tract absorption due to Mg and Al buffers present in didanosine tablets
Iron salts / ↓ Serum fluoroquinolone levels R/T ↓ GI tract absorption
NSAIDs / ↑ RIsk of CNS stimulation and seizures
Probenecid / ↑ Serum fluoroquinolone levels R/T ↓ renal clearance
Sucralfate / ↓ Serum fluoroquinolone levels R/T ↓ GI tract absorption
Theophylline / ↑ Theophylline plasma levels and ↑ drug toxicity R/T ↓ clearance
Zinc salts / ↓ Serum fluoroquinolone levels R/T ↓ GI tract absorption

LABORATORY TEST CONSIDERATIONS

↑ ALT, AST. See also individual drugs.

DOSAGE

See individual drugs.

NURSING CONSIDERATIONS

SEE ALSO *GENERAL NURSING CONSIDERATIONS FOR ALL ANTI-INFECTIVES.*

ASSESSMENT

1. Document type, onset, and characteristics of symptoms and culture results.
2. Note any previous experiences with these antibiotics. Discontinue at first sign of rash or other allergic manifestations. Hypersensitivity reactions may occur latently.
3. Assess for soft tissue/extremity injury; note instability, pain, swelling, erythema, and discharge.
4. Monitor VS, I&O, CBC, cultures, liver and renal function studies.
5. If receiving anticoagulants and theophyllines, monitor closely; quinolones can cause increased drug levels with toxic drug effects i.e., bleeding or seizures.

CLIENT/FAMILY TEACHING

1. Take only as directed.
2. Consume >2.5 L/day of fluids.
3. Do not take any mineral supplements (i.e., iron or zinc) or antacids containing magnesium or aluminum simultaneously or 4 hr before or 2 hr after dosing with fluoroquinolones.
4. Do not perform hazardous tasks until drug effects realized; may experience dizziness.
5. Report any bothersome symptoms; N&V and diarrhea are most frequently reported side effects.
6. Report symptoms of superinfection (furry tongue, vaginal or rectal itching, diarrhea).
7. Stop drug and report any new onset tendon pain or inflammation as tendon rupture may occur.
8. Hypersensivity reactions may occur, even after the first dose. Discontinue drug at the first sign of skin rash or other allergic reaction.
9. Wear protective clothing and sunscreens; avoid excessive sunlight or artificial ultraviolet light. Photosensitivity reactions may occur up to several weeks after stopping therapy.
10. New onset pain in extremities should be reported as drug may need to be changed.

OUTCOMES/EVALUATE

- Symptomatic improvement
- Resolution of infection (↓ WBCs, ↓ temperature, ↑ appetite)
- Negative culture reports

HEPARINS, LOW MOLECULAR WEIGHT

SEE ALSO THE FOLLOWING INDIVIDUAL ENTRIES:

Ardeparin sodium
Dalteparin sodium
Enoxaparin
Tinzaparin sodium

ACTION/KINETICS

Obtained by depolymerization of unfractioned porcine heparin. Are antithrombotic drugs. They enhance the inhibition of Factor Xa and thrombin by binding to and accelerating antithrombin II activity. They potentiate the inhibition of Factor Xa preferentially; slightly affect thrombin and clotting time or activated partial thromboplastin time.

USES

Prophylaxis or treatment of thromboembolic complications following surgery or ischemic complications of unstable angina and MI. See individual drugs for specific uses.

CONTRAINDICATIONS

Hypersensitivity to heparin, pork products, methylparaben, sulfites, or benzyl alcohol. Active major bleeding. Thrombocytopenia with positive in vitro tests for antiplatelet antibody in presence of a low molecular weight heparin. IM or IV use.

SPECIAL CONCERNS

Cannot be used interchangeably with each other or with unfractionated heparin. Use with extreme caution in those with a history of heparin-induced thrombocytopenia. Use with caution in clients with an increased risk of hemorrhage, including those with severe uncontrolled hypertension, bacterial endocarditis, congenital or acquired bleeding disorders, active ulceration and angiodysplastic GI disease, or hemorrhagic stroke or shortly after brain, spinal, or ophthalmologic surgery. Also, use with caution in clients with bleeding diathesis, severe liver or kidney disease, hypertensive or diabetic retinopathy, and recent GI bleeding. Use with caution during lactation. Increased risk of epidural or spinal hematoma, which can result in long-term or permanent paralysis, in clients who are on low molecular weight heparins and who require neuraxial anesthesia or spinal puncture. Safety and efficacy have not been determined in children.

Increased risk of epidural or spinal hematoma, which can result in long-term or permanent paralysis, in clients who are on low molecular weight heparins and who require neuraxial anesthesia or spinal puncture.

OD OVERDOSE MANAGEMENT

Symptoms: Hemorrhagic complications. *Treatment:* Slow IV protamine sulfate (1%) at a dose of 1 mg for every 100 anti-Xa IU of dalteparin and ardeparin or 1 mg for every 1 mg of enoxaparin. A second infusion of protamine sulfate, 0.5 mg per 100 anti-Xa IU of dalteparin or ardeparin or per 1 mg of enoxaparin may be given if the aPTT measured 2–4 hr after the first infusion of protamine sulfate remains prolonged. Take care not to give an overdose of protamine.

DRUG INTERACTIONS

Aspirin / ↑ Risk of bleeding
H *Bromelain* / ↑ Risk of bleeding
Dextran / ↑ Risk of bleeding
Dipyridamole / ↑ Risk of bleeding
H *Feverfew* / Possible additive antiplatelet effect
H *Garlic* / Possible additive antiplatelet effect
H *Ginger* / Possible additive antiplatelet effect
Ketorolac tromethamine / ↑ Risk of bleeding
NSAIDs / ↑ Risk of bleeding
Sulfinpyrazone / ↑ Risk of bleeding
Thrombolytics / ↑ Risk of bleeding
Ticlopidine / ↑ Risk of bleeding

LABORATORY TEST CONSIDERATIONS

↑ AST, ALT.

DOSAGE

See individual drugs.

NURSING CONSIDERATIONS

ASSESSMENT

1. Assess for any sensitivity to heparin, sulfite, methylparaben, or pork products.
2. Note any evidence of active bleeding, bleeding disorders, or thrombocytopenia.
3. Review list of special concerns that may preclude client receiving drugs.
4. Those who received spinal anesthesia or taps require special monitoring to assess for neuro S&S and spinal/epidural hematoma formation which may cause permanent paralysis.
5. Assess carefully for masked bleeding. Drug does not usually affect PT/PTT values yet client may be hemorrhaging. Monitor VS, I&O, mental status, H/H, U/A, lytes and renal and LFTs; routinely check all potential bleeding sites. Any unexplained fall in BP or HCT should lead to a search for a bleeding site.

CLIENT/FAMILY TEACHING

1. Review indications for therapy, self administration techniques, length/frequency of therapy, and site rotation.
2. Many clients are treated with low molecular weight heparins at home. Educate about SC injection techniques and recognizing signs of complications.
3. To minimize bruising do not rub site after administering.
4. Avoid aspirin and NSAIDs and all OTC agents.
5. Report any unusual effects i.e., bruising, bleeding, chest pain, acute SOB, itching, rash, or swelling. Keep followup appointments as scheduled.

OUTCOMES/EVALUATE

DVT prophylaxis; inhibition of blood coagulation

HERBS

GENERAL STATEMENT

Herbs are medicinal plants, also called botanicals or phytomedicines. Phytomedicines are medicinal products that contain plant material as their pharmacologically active component. They are often complex mixtures of compounds that generally do not exert a strong, immediate action. Consumers use herbal products as therapeutic agents for the treatment/cure of illness/disease symptoms and prophylactically to prevent disease and to maintain health and wellness. Consumer use of herbs and medicinal products over the past two decades has risen dramatically. These agents are found in retail pharmacies, grocery stores, health food shops, corner markets, and other large outlet stores as well as mail order and TV/Internet sales. Some major health insurance companies are including coverage for herbs under "alternative therapies" and many more are considering this coverage. Herbs are regulated as Dietary Supplements under the Dietary Supplement Health and Education Act of 1994. (DSHEA) Extracts are concentrated preparations of a liquid, powdered, or viscous consistency that are usually made from dried plant parts by maceration or percolation. Tincture is an alcoholic or hydroalcoholic soution prepared from botanicals. Plant juices are formed from the freshly harvested plant parts macerated in water and pressed. Herbal teas are potable infusions made from infusion (pour boiling water over the herb), decoction (cover herb with cold water and bring to a boil and simmer for 5-10 min), or cold maceration (place herb in tap water and let stand at room temperature for 6-8 hr). Always ask about herbs, vitamins, teas or other remedies that client may be using for a problem or to maintain health/wellness. Clients generally do not consider these as medicines and often fail to mention them during a drug history. Advise that these agents are not regulated by the FDA and may contain a variety of agents and some have been found to not contain any of the agent it portrays. Agents approved by the APA (American Pharmaceutical Association) should be those that the consumer purchases to ensure some degree of reliability.

TABLE 1: Commonly Used Herbal Products

The following table presents some of the commonly used herbal products. It is not intended to be an extensive listing of information for each product. Rather, the table contains important information regarding use(s), dose, side effects, and other information.

NAME(S)	USE(S)	DOSE	CONTRAINDICATIONS	SIDE EFFECTS	OTHER INFORMATION
Aloe gel, Aloe vera	Gel is used in cosmetics and topical products to heal wounds, burns, skin ulcers, frostbite, dry skin. Laxative.	Aloe vera powder, aqueous or aqueous-alcoholic extract in powder/liquid/tablets/capsule forms: 100–200 mg (internal use). Use smallest dose to maintain a soft stool.	Intestinal obstruction, Crohn's disease, ulcerative colitis, appendicitis, abdominal pain of unknown origin. Children under 12 years, pregnancy, lactation.	GI cramps. Long term use/abuse: Potassium deficiency, albuminuria, hematuria.	Should not be used for longer than 1–2 weeks without medical advice. Potassium deficiency can be increased by simultaneous use of thiazides, corticosteroids, and licorice.
Bilberry fruit/leaf, blueberry	*Fruit:* Nonspecific, acute diarrhea. Mild inflammation of the mucous membranes of the mouth and throat. Improve night vision. *Leaf:* Arthritis, gout, dermatitis, hemorrhoids, CV problems, and prevention/treatment of GI, kidney, and GU symptoms and diseases	**Fruit. External:** 10% decoction. **Internal:** 20–60 g/day of the fruit. **Leaf.** Used as a tea (1–2 teaspoons of the finely chopped leaf in 150 mL boiling water for 5–10 min.		Chronic use of the leaf may cause anemia, jaundice, "wasting," excitation, and disturbances of muscle contraction.	Has an astringent effect. Consult a provider if diarrhea lasts for more than 3–4 days. Avoid prolonged use of the tea.

continues

NAME(S)	USE(S)	DOSE	CONTRAINDICATIONS	SIDE EFFECTS	OTHER INFORMATION
Cascara sagrada bark	Laxative.	Capsules, fluid extract, syrup, tablets : 20–30 mg hydroxyanthracene derivatives/day, calculated as cascaroside A. May be used as a tea (2 g finely chopped bark in150 mL boiling water for 5–10 min). **Fluid extract:** 2–5 mL t.i.d. Use smallest dose to maintain a soft stool.	Intestinal obstruction, Crohn's disease, colitis, appendicitis, abdominal pain of unknown origin. Children under 12 years, pregnancy, lactation.	Abdominal cramps. Long term use/abuse: Potassium deficiency, albuminuria, hematuria, disturbed cardiac function.	Do not use for more than 1–2 weeks without medical advice. Potassium deficiency can be increased by concomitant use of thiazides, corticosteroids, and licorice root.
Cat's Claw	Diverticulitis, hemorrhoids, peptic ulcer disease, colitis, parasites, antihypertensive, hypocholesterolemic, AIDS (in combination with Zidovudine)	**Capsules:** 300 mg t.i.d.; **Timed-release capsules:** 1000 mg once daily; **Liquid concentrate:** Diluted in water and taken 1–3 times/day; **Bark:** Used for tea (1 g root bark in 150 mL boiling water for 5–10 min).	Diarrhea (high doses), hypotension.	May contribute to unusual bruising or bleeding gums.	Use with caution in those taking antihypertensives.
Chamomile, German Chamomile	Topical: Inflammation of the mouth, skin, respiratory tract (inhalation). Internal: GI antispasmodic and anti-inflammatory. Allegedly has sedative, hypnotic, analgesic, and immunostimulant effects.	**PO. Dried flower heads:** 2–8 g t.i.d. or 1 cup of tea t.i.d.–q.i.d. **Liquid extract (1:1 in 45% alcohol):** 1–4 mL t.i.d. **Topical.** Prepared tea use (4 tsp. of dried flower heads in 1.5 cups boiling water for 15 min; strain).	Anaphylaxis, dermatitis, other hypersensitivity reactions.		Cautious use in those allergic to ragweed, asters, chrysanthemums, or other members of the Asteraceae family. Do not confuse with Roman Chamomile.

Chondroitin Sulfate	Osteoarthritis, osteoporosis, ischemic heart disease, hyperlipidemia. Ophthalmic product (FDA-approved) for dry eyes, as a viscoelastic agent in cataract surgery, and to preserve corneas for transplantation.	**Osteoarthritis. PO:** 200–400 b.i.d.–t.i.d. or 1200 mg/day as a single dose.	Pregnancy, lactation.	Epigastric pain, nausea, allergic reactions.	Has also been used IM.
Comfrey	External: Wound healing, ulcers, bruises/sprains. Internal: Stomach ulcers, "blood purifier," prevention of kidney stones, rheumatic/pulmonary disorders.	Ointments/other topical products containing 5–20% comfrey. Do not exceed 100 mcg/day of pyrrolizidine alkaloids.	Pregnancy, lactation. Use on broken skin.	Hazardous to health due to hepatotoxic alkaloids; internal use not safe. Veno-occlusive disease.	Use for no more than 10 days; maximum use is 4–6 weeks/year.
Cranberry	Urinary tract infections, urinary deodorizer for incontient clients.	**PO. Juice:** 3 oz/day to prevent urinary infection and 12–32 oz/day to treat infection. **Capsules:** 6 capsules (equivalent to 3 oz juice)/day. Some recommend 300–400 mg of concentrated juice capsules b.i.d.		High doses can cause diarrhea and other GI symptoms.	Do not confuse with highbush cranberry.

continues

NAME(S)	USE(S)	DOSE	CONTRAINDICATIONS	SIDE EFFECTS	OTHER INFORMATION
Dong Quai	Menstrual cramps/irregularity, retarded flow, menopausal symptoms. Treatment of skin pigmentation and psoriasis.	**PO, women:** 3–4 g/day in divided doses with meals.	Pregnancy, lactation.	Severe photodermatitis and photosensitivity. Potentially carcinogenic and mutagenic.	May potentiate the effect of warfarin.
Echinacea	Topical: Minor infections, snake/spider bites, poorly healing wounds, chronic ulcers. Internal: Viral, bacterial, and *Candida* infections, including colds, flu, urogenital, and upper respiratory tract infections. Immunostimulant.	**Topical:** Use cream or liquid t.i.d. **Internal:** 0.5–1 mL of the fluid extract (1:1 in 45% alcohol) t.i.d. or 300 mg of the solid extract (6.5:1) t.i.d.	Pregnancy. Use with immunosuppressants or in those with chronic progressive systemic diseases (e.g., tuberculosis, leucosis, multiple sclerosis, collagenosis).	N&V. Hypersensitivity reaction in those allergic to sunflower seeds/flowers. Tingling of the tongue; fever (due to the freshly pressed juice).	Use with caution in those with AIDS, rheumatoid arthritis, lupus, or leukemia. May antagonize immunosuppressants. Not generally recommended for regular daily use as an ongoing preventive or for those with autoimmune disorders.
Evening primrose oil	Breast disorders, premenstrual syndrome, hypercholesterolemia, eczema, psoriasis, multiple sclerosis, lupus erythematosus, antihypertensive.	4 g/day (maximum), equivalent to 300–360 mg gamma-linolenic acid.		Indigestion, nausea, soft stools, headache. Reduces platelet aggregation (monitor bleeding times and PT in those on antiplatelet drugs or warfarin.	If used with phenothiazines or TCAs, may worsen temporal lobe epilepsy or schizophrenia.

Feverfew	Fever, arthritis. Prophylaxis for migraine headache.	Dry powdered leaf capsules/tablets: 300 mg 2–6 times/day. To prevent migraine, 50–100 mg of dried leaves/day have been used.	Pregnancy and in children less than 2 years.	Dizziness, lightheadedness, nausea, indigesion, bloating, gas, diarrhea or constipation, palpitations, heavy menstrual flow, contact dermatitis, rash. Aphthous ulcers due to chewing leaves. Reduces platelet aggregation (monitor bleeding times and PT in those on antiplatelet drugs or warfarin).	May take 4–6 months for beneficial effects. Rebound headache may occur if abruptly discontinued.
Garlic	Lower serum cholesterol and BP. Mild respiratory and GI tract infections. GI disturbances.	10 mg of allicin, a total of allicin potential of 4 mg/day, or 1 clove (4 g) of fresh garlic/day.	Topical use. Large doses in pregnancy and lactation.	Mouth and GI burning or irritation, heartburn, flatulence, N&V, diarrhea, changes in gut flora, allergic reactions, odor to skin/breath. May decrease blood sugar (monitor).	Reduces platelet aggregation (monitor bleeding times and PT in those on antiplatelet drugs or warfarin). May potentiate antihypertensives. To assure efficacy, monitor lipids for 3 months.
Ginger, Jamaica Ginger, African Ginger, Cochin Ginger	Prevent morning sickness, motion sickness. Treat arthritis, muscle pain, migraine headache.	Powdered ginger root. Prevent motion sickness: 1 g 30 min before travel followed by 500 mg q.i.d. Prevent morning sickness: 250 mg q.i.d. Arthritis: 125–1,000 mg q.i.d., not to exceed 4 g/day.	With gallstones, use only after consultation with provider. Large doses during lactation.	High doses: GI discomfort if taken on an empty stomach, CNS depression, and cardiac arrhythmias.	Inhibits platelet aggregation (monitor bleeding times and PT in those on antiplatelet drugs or warfarin). May alter effect of calcium channel blockers.

continues

NAME(S)	USE(S)	DOSE	CONTRAINDICATIONS	SIDE EFFECTS	OTHER INFORMATION
Ginkgo biloba	Short-term memory loss, headache, vertigo, tinnitus due to vascular insufficiency. Depression. Intermittent claudication. Early Alzheimer's disease, senility. Diabetic retinopathy. Asthma.	100–300 mg/day, to provide 10 mg ginsenosides.	Pregnancy, lactation.	GI discomfort, headache, allergic skin reactions, contact dermatitis, severe allergic reactions, restlessness, diarrhea. Inhibits platelet aggregation (monitor bleeding time and PT in those taking anticoagulants).	May take up to 12 weeks for beneficial effect to be seen. Cross allergy in those allergic to poison ivy, poison oak, poison sumac, mango rind, and cashew shell oil. May cause complications if taken with thiazide diuretics.
Ginseng root	Improve cognitive function/concentration, fatigue, stress, enhance immune function, menopausal symptoms, impotence/infertility, reduce cholesterol.	**PO:** 100–300 mg/day, to provide 10 mg ginsenosides.	Panax ginseng in newborns.	Breast tenderness, insomnia, diarrhea, skin eruptions, nervousness/excitation (decreases with use). Hypoglycemia (monitor diabetics). Decreased platelet adhesiveness (monitor bleeding times and PT in those taking anticoagulants).	May interfere with digoxin activity or monitoring. May potentiate insulin or other antidiabetic drugs. May antagonize effect of anticoagulants including warfarin. May cause complications if taken with phenelzine.

Goldenseal	External: Treatment of trachoma. Internal: Diarrhea due to *E. coli.*	**Topical mouthwash:** Use t.i.d.–q.i.d. Prepare by steeping 6 g of dried herb in 150 mL boiling water for 5–10 min; strain and allow to cool. **Internal, dried root or rhizome:** 0.5–1 g t.i.d. **Use as a tea:** Prepare by simmering 0.5–1 g of dried root or rhizome in 150 mL boiling water for 5–10 min; strain. **Liquid extract (1:1, 60% ethanol):** 0.3–1 mL t.i.d. **Tincture (1:10, 60% ethanol):** 2–4 mL t.i.d.	Pregnancy (likely unsafe), lactation. Hypertension, infectious or inflammatory GI disease.	Chronic use: Digestive disorders, constipation, excitation, hallucinations, delirium, decrease in B vitamin absorption.	May interfere with antacids, sucralfate, H-2 antagonists, proton pump inhibitors, antihypertensives. Additive effects with CNS depressants.
Grape Seed Extract, Muskat	Varicose veins, hypoxia secondary to atherosclerosis, myocardial or cerebral infarction.	**Capsules/Tablets, initial:** 75–300 mg/day for 3 weeks; **maintenance:** 40–80 mg/day. **Concentrate liquid:** 15 mL in one cup of hot or cold water.	In pregnancy/lactation, avoid amounts greater than in food.	None reported.	May increase the effect of warfarin.
Green Tea	Stomach disorders, vomiting, diarrhea, headaches, as a diuretic. Traditional use to promote health and prevent cancer (antioxidant effect). As a beverage.	No reliable information on safe and effective dose. As many as ten cups of tea/day are consumed by some.	Use in infants, lactation. Use in those with gastric/duodenal ulcers.	Hyperacidity, gastric irritation, decreased appetite, constipation, diarrhea, restlessness, irritability, insomnia, palpitations, vertigo.	Increased CNS stimulation when used with caffeine-containing products or ephedrine. Many possible drug interactions, including warfarin.

continues

NAME(S)	USE(S)	DOSE	CONTRAINDICATIONS	SIDE EFFECTS	OTHER INFORMATION
Hawthorn Flower, Fruit, Leaves	Heart failure, hypertension, arteriosclerosis, angina pectoris, Buerger's disease, paroxysmal tachycardia.	**Dried fruit:** 300–1,000 mg t.i.d. **Fruit fluid extract (1:1 in 25% alcohol):** 0.5–1 mL t.i.d. **Fruit tincture (1:5 in 45% alcohol):** 1–2 mL t.i.d.	Pregnancy, lactation. Use with cardiac glycoside-containing products.	Nausea, GI complaints, fatigue, hand rash, palpitations, headache, dizziness, sleeplessness, agitation, circulatory disturbances.	Additive effects when used with vasodilators or CNS depressants.
Kava Kava	Stress, nervous anxiety, insomnia, restlessness.	**Anxiolytic:** 45–70 mg kavalactones t.i.d. **Sedative:** 180–210 mg kavalactones 1 hr before bedtime.	Alcohol use. Endogenous depression. Safety/efficacy not known in pregnancy/lactation.	GI discomfort, allergic skin reactions. Chronic use: Yellow discoloration of skin, hair, nails.	Additive effects with CNS depressants. May affect motor reflexes and judgment. May worsen Parkinson symptoms. Do not use more than 3 months without medical advice.
Licorice, Glycyrrhiza, Licorice Root	Upper respiratory tract mucous membrane inflammation. Gastric/duodenal ulcers.	**Root:** 5–15 g/day, equivalent to 200–600 mg glycyrrhizin.	Cholestatic liver disorders, liver cirrhosis, hypokalemia, hypertonia, severe kidney impairment, pregnancy.	Chronic use/high doses: Sodium and water retention, potassium loss, hypertension, edema, hypokalemia.	Use with thiazides increases potassium loss; may increase digitalis sensitivity. Do not use more than 4–6 weeks without medical advice.
Melatonin	Insomnia, especially to overcome jet lag or shift-work disorder.	**PO:** 0.3–5 mg at bedtime for sleep disturbances. For jet lag, 5 mg at bedtime for one week beginning three days before the flight.	Use in depression, children, pregnancy, lactation.	Headache, transient depression, daytime fatigue/drowsiness, dizziness, abdominal cramps, irritability, reduced alertness, tiredness.	Additive effects with CNS depressants. Use with caution if driving or operating hazardous machinery.

Milk Thistle, Our Lady's Thistle	Liver cirrhosis, chronic hepatitis, gallstones, psoriasis, liver protectant from toxins (e.g., butyrophenones, phenothiazines, phenytoin, acetaminophen, alcohol, halothane, cisplatin).	**PO:** 200 mg t.i.d. standardized to provide at least 140 mg silymarin t.i.d. or 100–200 mg of phosphatidylcholine-bound silymarin b.i.d.		Loose stools (prevent by ingesting psyllium and oat bran), mild allergic reactions.	Possible cross allergy in those sensitive to ragweed, chrysanthemums, marigolds, daisies. Efficacy to treat liver disease and cirrhosis not clearly established.
Saw Palmetto	Benign prostatic hypertrophy.	**PO:** 160 mg standardized fat-soluble extract b.i.d. (containing 85–95% fatty acids and sterols). Or, 0.5–1 g of the dried berry or one cup of tea t.i.d. Prepare tea by simmering 0.5–1 g dried berry in 150 mL boiling water for 5–10 min; strain.	Pregnancy, use in breast cancer.	Headache, mild abdominal pain, nausea, dizziness.	May require 4–6 weeks for effect to be seen. May interfere with oral contraceptive or hormone therapy. No significant effect on serum prostate-specific antigen levels. Due to lack of evidence, the FDA has banned all OTC medicines to treat BPH.
Senna leaf	Laxative.	**PO:** 20–30 mg hydroxyanthracene derivatives/day calculated as sennoside B. Use lowest dose to maintain a soft stool.	Intestinal obstruction, Crohn's disease, colitis ulcerosa, appendicitis, abdominal pain of unknown origin. Children under 12 years. Pregnancy, lactation.	GI cramps, abdominal discomfort, colic. Chronic use/abuse: Potassium deficiency, albuminuria, hematuria, "sluggish" colon.	Loss of potassium may potentiate effect of cardiac glycosides, diuretics, and corticosteroids on heart function.

continues

NAME(S)	USE(S)	DOSE	CONTRAINDICATIONS	SIDE EFFECTS	OTHER INFORMATION
St. John's Wort	External: Herpes simplex I, minor wounds/burns. Internal: Mild to moderate depression, anxiety, antiviral (HIV, AIDS)	**External:** Apply oil or cream b.i.d.–t.i.d. **Internal:** 300 mg t.i.d., standardized to 0.3% hypericin extract.	Use with MAOIs, selective serotonin reuptake inhibitors, and tricyclics due to potentiation of effects. Pregnancy, lactation.	Photosensitivity in fair-skinned clients. GI symptoms, fatigue, delayed hypersensitivity. Serotonin syndrome. Possible hypertensive crisis if taken with tyramine-containing foods.	To prevent GI upset, take with food. May decrease effect of cyclosporine, digoxin, and indinavir due to increased metabolism. May cause bleeding irregularities if used with oral contraceptives.
Valerian	Insomnia, anxiety, stress.	**Insomnia:** 150–300 mg valerian extract (0.8% valeric acid) 30–45 min before bed. **Anxiety:** 150 mg q.i.d.	Pregnancy, lactation.	Morning drowsiness (rare), headache, excitability, cardiac disturbances, uneasy feeling.	Additive effect with CNS depressants. Do not confuse with Valium.
Yohimbe Bark	Impotence, as an aphrodisiac. Exhaustion.	Available as a prescription drug with no FDA-approved uses.	Liver and kidney dysfunction. Pregnancy, lactation.	Nervous excitation, tremor, sleeplessness, anxiety, increased BP, tachycardia, N&V.	The FDA has determined the active compound (yohimbine) to be unsafe and ineffective for OTC use. Possibility of hypertensive crisis when taken with caffeine, tyramine-containing foods, or ephedrine. Additive therapeutic/toxic effects if taken with MAOIs. Interference with drugs to treat hypertension.

HISTAMINE H_2 ANTAGONISTS

SEE ALSO THE FOLLOWING INDIVIDUAL ENTRIES:

Cimetidine
Famotidine
Nizatidine
Ranitidine bismuth citrate
Ranitidine hydrochloride

ACTION/KINETICS

Histamine H_2 antagonists are competitive blockers of histamine. As such they inhibit all phases of gastric acid secretion including that caused by histamine, gastrin, and muscarinic agents. Both fasting and nocturnal acid secretion are inhibited. In addition, the volume and hydrogen ion concentration of gastric juice are decreased. Cimetidine, famotidine, and ranitidine have no effect on gastric emptying; cimetidine and famitidine have no effect on lower esophageal pressure. Fasting or postprandial serum gastrin is not affected by famotidine, nizatidine, or ranitidine. Cimetidine is known to affect the cytochrome P-450 drug metabolizing system for other drugs. Ranitidine also affects the P-450 enzyme system, but its effect on elimination of other drugs is not significant. Neither famotidine nor nizatidine affects the P-450 enzyme system.

USES

See individual drugs. Also, these drugs are used as part of combination therapy to treat *Helicobacter pylori*–associated duodenal ulcer and maintenance therapy after healing of the active ulcer.

CONTRAINDICATIONS

Hypersensitivity. Use of cimetidine, famotidine, and nizatidine during lactation.

SPECIAL CONCERNS

Use with caution in impaired hepatic and renal function. Symptomatic response to these drugs does not preclude gastric malignancy. Use ranitidine with caution during lactation. Safety and effectiveness have not been established for use in children. Use of cimetidine in children less than 16 years of age unless benefits outweigh risks.

SIDE EFFECTS

The following side effects are common to all or most of the H_2-histamine antagonists. See individual drugs for complete listing.

GI: N&V, abdominal discomfort, diarrhea, constipation, hepatocellular effects. **CNS:** Headache, fatigue, somnolence, dizziness, confusion, hallucinations, insomnia. **Dermatologic:** Rash, urticaria, pruritus, alopecia (rare), erythema multiforme (rare). **Hematologic:** Rarely, thrombocytopenia, agranulocytosis, granulocytopenia. **Other:** Gynecomastia, impotence, loss of libido, arthralgia, bronchospasm, transient pain at injection site, cardiac arrhythmias following rapid IV use (rare), arthralgia (rare), ***anaphylaxis*** (rare).

OD OVERDOSE MANAGEMENT

Symptoms: No experience is available for deliberate overdose. *Treatment:* Induce vomiting or perform gastric lavage to remove any unabsorbed drug. Monitor the client and undertake supportive therapy.

DRUG INTERACTIONS

Itraconazole / ↓ Itraconazole plasma levels due to changes in gastric pH
Ketoconazole / ↑ Gastric pH may inhibit ketoconazole absorption.

DOSAGE

See individual drugs.

NURSING CONSIDERATIONS

ASSESSMENT

1. Document symptoms noting onset, duration, intensity, other characteristics and previous treatment.
2. Assess number of reflux occurrences. Chronic treatment usually initiated after two to three recurrences.
3. Monitor CBC, renal and LFTs.
4. Perform CNS assessment noting level of orientation.
5. Note results of radiographic/endoscopic procedures; document *H. pylori* results and if/when treated.

6. Determine gastric pH; maintain greater than 5.

CLIENT/FAMILY TEACHING

1. May take without regard to meals; with food prolongs drug effect.
2. Stagger doses of antacids i.e., 1 hr before or 1 hr after cimetidine or ranitidine.
3. Do not take maximum dose of OTC products for more than 2 weeks without medical supervision.
4. Take as prescribed; do not stop if pain subsides or if "feeling better" as drug is necessary to inhibit gastric acid secretion.
5. These agents reduce the secretion of gastric acid and are usually prescribed for 4–8 weeks initially to control symptoms and promote ulcer healing.
6. Avoid activities that require mental alertness until drug effects realized. Report any confusion or disorientation immediately.
7. Avoid alcohol, caffeine, aspirin-containing products (cough and cold products), and foods that may cause GI irritation, i.e., harsh spices, black pepper.
8. Stop 24–72 hr before skin testing begins; may cause false negative response in tests with allergen extracts.
9. Smoking may interfere with drug's action. Stop smoking and do not smoke after last dose of day.
10. Any blood-tinged emesis or dark tarry stools as well as dizziness or rash, bruising, fatigue, malaise, require immediate reporting.
11. Review GERD instructions i.e., ↑ HOB, avoid lying down after eating and dietary restrictions.
12. May cause painful swelling of breast tissue and impotence, report as these are reversible.
13. Report for all scheduled follow-up studies; a response to these agents does not preclude gastric malignancy.

OUTCOMES/EVALUATE

- Duodenal ulcer healing
- ↓ Gastric irritation/bleeding; ↓ abdominal pain/discomfort
- Gastric pH > 5
- Stabilization of H&H

LAXATIVES

SEE ALSO THE FOLLOWING INDIVIDUAL ENTRIES:

Docusate calcium
Docusate sodium
Magnesium sulfate
Psyllium hydrophilic muciloid

ACTION/KINETICS

Laxatives act locally, either by stimulating the smooth muscles of the bowel or by changing the bulk or consistency of the stools. Laxatives can be divided into five categories.

1. *Stimulant laxatives:* Substances that chemically stimulate the smooth muscles of the bowel to increase contractions. Examples: Bisacodyl, cascara, danthron, and senna.
2. *Saline laxatives:* Substances that increase the bulk of the stools by retaining water. Examples: Magnesium salts and sodium phosphate.
3. *Bulk-forming laxatives:* Nondigestible substances that pass through the stomach and then increase the bulk of the stools. Examples: Methylcellulose and psyllium.
4. *Emollient and lubricant laxatives:* Agents that soften hardened feces and facilitate their passage through the lower intestine. Examples: Docusate and mineral oil.
5. *Miscellaneous:* Includes glycerin suppositories and lactulose.

USES

See individual agents. Short-term treatment of constipation. Prophylaxis in clients who should not strain during defecation, i.e., following anorectal surgery or after MI (fecal softeners or lubricant laxatives). To evacuate the colon for rectal and bowel examinations (certain lubricant, saline, and stimulant laxatives). In conjunction with surgery or anthelmintic therapy. The underlying cause of constipation should be determined since a marked change in bowel habits may be a symptom of a pathologic condition.

CONTRAINDICATIONS

Severe abdominal pain that *might* be caused by appendicitis, enteritis, ulcerative colitis, diverticulitis, intestinal obstruction. Laxative use in these conditions may cause rupture of the abdomen or intestinal hemorrhage. Undiagnosed abdominal pain. Children under the age of 2. Castor oil is contraindicated during pregnancy as the irritant effects may result in premature labor.

SIDE EFFECTS

GI: Excess activity of the colon resulting in nausea, diarrhea, griping, or vomiting. Perianal irritation, bloating, flatulence. **Electrolyte Balance:** Dehydration, disturbance of the electrolyte balance. **Miscellaneous:** Dizziness, fainting, weakness, sweating, palpitations. **Bulk laxatives:** Obstruction in the esophagus, stomach, small intestine, or rectum. **Stimulant laxatives:** Chronic abuse may lead to malfunctioning colon. **Mineral Oil:** Large doses may cause anal seepage resulting in itching, irritation, hemorrhoids, and perianal discomfort. Chronic use of laxatives may cause laxative dependency and result in chronic constipation and other intestinal disorders because the client may start to depend on the psychologic effect and physical stimulus of the drug rather than on the body's own natural reflexes.

DRUG INTERACTIONS

Anticoagulants, oral / ↓ Absorption of vitamin K from GI tract induced by laxatives may ↑ effects of anticoagulants and result in bleeding
Digitalis / Cathartics may ↓ absorption of digitalis
Tetracyclines / Laxatives containing Al, Ca, or Mg may ↓ effect of tetracyclines R/T ↓ GI tract absorption

DOSAGE

See individual drugs.

NURSING CONSIDERATIONS

ADMINISTRATION/STORAGE

1. When administering a laxative, note the length of time it takes for the laxative to take effect and give it so that the result of the laxative will not interfere with the client's rest or digestion and absorption of nutrients.
2. Administer liquid laxatives at an agreeable temperature.
3. If laxative administered in a liquid, select one palatable to client.
4. If ordered to prepare for a diagnostic exam, check directions carefully to ensure accurate administration.

ASSESSMENT

1. Determine length of use and underlying causes; note type taking and effectiveness.
2. With abdominal pain and discomfort, note location and type of discomfort experiencing. R/O other intestinal disorders where laxatives should not be used.
3. Determine stool characteristics and frequency. Client's definition of constipation may determine if, in fact, constipation exists.
4. Note age, state of health, activity level, and general nutritional status.
5. Identify any special restriction or limitation due to illness; may include fluid/sodium restrictions.
6. List other drugs that may contribute to constipation (i.e., diuretics, anticholinergics, antihistamines, antidepressants, narcotic analgesics, iron products, and some antihypertensive agents, especially verapamil).
7. Identify recent life-style changes that may contribute to problem.

CLIENT/FAMILY TEACHING

1. Have a regular schedule for defecation; keep record of bowel function and response to all laxatives taken.
2. Laxatives reduce the amount of time other drugs remain in the intestine and may diminish effectiveness.
3. If taken in prep for a diagnostic study, review instructions. If unable to read, find someone to review directions to ensure an accurate test.
4. Review techniques that facilitate elimination; sitting with legs slightly elevated and leaning forward to increase abdominal pressure often encourages elimination. If ill at home, consider a commode at the bedside. This will promote better bowel function by encouraging client to move about and ensure privacy.
5. Bowel tone will be lost with long-

term use of laxatives; bowel movements do not have to occur daily. Use diet to achieve same purpose; two or three prunes a day are preferable to laxatives.
6. Frequent use of any type of enemas may cause damage to the rectum and small bowel as well as inhibit bowel tone and may cause electrolyte abnormalities.
7. Review importance of diet high in fiber foods (and juices such as prune) and daily exercise and benefits in maintaining proper bowel function. Include bulk foods and sufficient fluids in diet to enhance elimination. Consult dietitian for assistance in meal planning/preparation and food selections.
8. Report N&V, abdominal pain or if constipation persists because there could be a physiologic problem that requires attention.
9. If pregnant, consult with provider before taking any laxatives to treat constipation.
10. Nursing mothers should avoid laxatives unless prescribed as many are excreted in breast milk and can cause infant diarrhea.

OUTCOMES/EVALUATE

- Relief of constipation; evacuation of a soft, formed stool
- Effective colon prep for diagnostic procedures (no stool in bowel)

NARCOTIC ANALGESICS

SEE ALSO THE FOLLOWING INDIVIDUAL ENTRIES:

Alfentanil hydrochloride
Buprenorphine hydrochloride
Butorphanol tartrate
Codeine phosphate
Codeine sulfate
Dezocine
Fentanyl citrate
Fentanyl transmucosal system
Fentanyl transdermal system
Hydrocodone bitartrate and Acetaminophen
Hydromorphone hydrochloride
Levomethadyl acetate hydrochloride
Meperidine hydrochloride
Methadone hydrochloride
Morphine hydrochloride
Morphine sulfate
Nalbuphine hydrochloride
Oxycodone hydrochloride
Oxymorphone hydrochloride
Paregoric
Propoxyphene hydrochloride
Propoxyphene napsylate
Remifentanil hydrochloride
Sufentanil
Tramadol hydrochloride

ACTION/KINETICS

Narcotic analgesics are classified as agonists, mixed agonist-antagonists, or partial agonists depending on their activity at opiate receptors.The narcotic analgesics attach to specific receptors located in the CNS (cortex, brain stem, and spinal cord) resulting in various CNS effects. The mechanism is believed to involve decreased permeability of the cell membrane to sodium, which results in diminished transmission of pain impulses. Five categories of opioid receptors have been identified: mu, kappa, sigma, delta, and epsilon. Narcotic analgesics are believed to exert their activity at mu, kappa, and sigma receptors. Mu receptors are thought to mediate supraspinal analgesia, euphoria, and respiratory and physical depression. Pentazocine-like spinal analgesia, miosis, and sedation are mediated by kappa receptors while sigma receptors mediate dysphoria, hallucinations, as well as respiratory and vasomotor stimulation (caused by drugs with antagonist activity). In addition to an alteration of pain perception (analgesia), the drugs, especially at higher doses, induce euphoria, drowsiness, changes in mood, mental clouding, and deep sleep.

The narcotic analgesics also produce a large number of secondary pharmacological effects. These include: (1) Depressed tidal volume and respiratory rate due to decreased sensitivity of the respiratory center to carbon dioxide. Death by overdosage is almost always the result of respiratory arrest. (2) Nausea and emesis due to direct stimulation of the CTZ. (3) Depression of the cough reflex by a direct effect on the medullary cough center. (4) Orthostatic hypotension and fainting due to peripheral vasodilation (when client stands), reduced peripheral resistance, and inhibition of barorectors. Little effect on BP when the client is in a supine position. (5) Pruritus, flushing, and red eyes due to histamine release. (6) Decrease in gastric motility leading to prolonged gastric emptying time and possible esophageal reflux. (7) In the small intestine decrease in biliary, pancreatic, and intestinal secretions causing delays in digestion of food. Increase in resting tone and periodic spasms occur. (8) Decreased propulsive peristalsis in the large intestine with an increase in tone to spasm. Causes severe constipation. (9) Constriction of the sphincter of Oddi causing epigastric distress or biliary colic. (10) Increased smooth muscle tone in the urinary tract can cause spsams with urinary urgency and difficulty with urination. (11) Pupillary constriction caused by certain narcotic analgesics is a sign of use/dependence. See also individual agents.

USES

See individual drugs. Generally are used to treat pain due to various causes (e.g., MI, carcinoma, surgery, burns, postpartum), as preanesthetic medication, as adjuncts to anesthesia, acute vascular occlusion, diarrhea, and coughs. Methadone once used for heroin withdrawal has more recently been used in chronic pain control.

CONTRAINDICATIONS

Asthma, emphysema, kyphoscoliosis, severe obesity, convulsive states as in epilepsy, delirium tremens, tetanus and strychnine poisoning, diabetic acidosis, myxedema, Addison's disease, hepatic cirrhosis, and children under 6 months.

SPECIAL CONCERNS

Use with caution in clients with head injury or after head surgery because of morphine's capacity to elevate ICP and mask the pupillary response. Use with caution in the elderly, in the debilitated, in young children, in individuals with increased ICP, in obstetrics, and with clients in shock or during acute alcoholic intoxication.

Use morphine with extreme caution in pulmonary heart disease (cor pulmonale). Deaths following ordinary therapeutic doses have been reported. Use cautiously in prostatic hypertrophy, because it may precipitate acute urinary retention. Use cautiously in clients with reduced blood volume, such as in hemorrhaging clients who are more susceptible to the hypotensive effects of morphine.

Since the drugs depress the respiratory center, give early in labor, at least 2 hr before delivery, to reduce the danger of respiratory depression in the newborn. When given before surgery, give at least 1–2 hr preoperatively so that the danger of maximum depression of respiratory function will have passed before anesthesia is initiated. These drugs may need to be withheld prior to diagnostic procedures so that the physician can use pain to locate dysfunction.

SIDE EFFECTS

Respiratory: ***Respiratory depression, apnea.*** **CNS:** Dizziness, lightheadedness, sedation, lethargy, headache, euphoria, mental clouding, fainting. Idiosyncratic effects including excitement, restlessness, tremors, delirium, insomnia. **GI:** N&V, vomiting, constipation, increased pressure in biliary tract, dry mouth, anorexia. **CV:** Flushing, changes in HR and BP, circulatory collapse. **Allergic:** Skin rashes including pruritus and urticaria. Sweating, ***laryngospasm,*** edema. **Miscellaneous:** Urinary retention, oliguria, reduced libido, changes in body temperature. Narcotics cross the placental barrier and depress respiration of the fetus or newborn.

DEPENDENCE AND TOLERANCE

All drugs of this group are addictive. Psychologic and physical dependence and tolerance develop even when clients use clinical doses. Tolerance is characterized by the fact that the client requires shorter periods of time between doses or larger doses for relief of pain. Tolerance usually develops faster when the narcotic analgesic is administered regularly and when the dose is large.

OD OVERDOSE MANAGEMENT

Symptoms (Acute Toxicity): Severe toxicity is characterized by ***profound respiratory depression, apnea, deep sleep, stupor or coma, circulatory collapse, seizures, cardiopulmonary arrest, and death.*** Less severe toxicity results in symptoms including CNS depression, miosis, respiratory depression, deep sleep, flaccidity of skeletal muscles, hypotension, bradycardia, hypothermia, pulmonary edema, pneumonia, shock. The respiratory rate may be as low as 2–4 breaths/min. The client may be cyanotic. Urine output is decreased, the skin feels clammy, and body temperature decreases. If death occurs, it almost always results from ***respiratory depression.*** *Symptoms (Chronic Toxicity):* The problem of chronic dependence on narcotics occurs not only as a result of "street" use but is also found often among those who have easy access to narcotics (physicians, nurses, pharmacists). All the principal narcotic analgesics (morphine, opium, heroin, codeine, meperidine, and others) have, at times, been used for nontherapeutic purposes.

The nurse must be aware of the problem and be able to recognize signs of chronic dependence. These are constricted pupils, GI effects (constipation), skin infections, needle scars, abscesses, and itching, especially on the anterior surfaces of the body, where the client may inject the drug.

Withdrawal signs appear after drug is withheld for 4–12 hr. They are characterized by intense craving for the drug, insomnia, yawning, sneezing, vomiting, diarrhea, tremors, sweating, mental depression, muscular aches and pains, chills, and anxiety. Although the symptoms of narcotic withdrawal are uncomfortable, they are rarely life-threatening. This is in contrast to the withdrawal syndrome from depressants, where the life of the individual may be endangered because of the possibility of tonic-clonic seizures.

Treatment (Acute Overdose): Initial treatment is aimed at combating progressive respiratory depression by maintaining a patent airway and by artificial respiration. Gastric lavage and induced emesis are indicated in case of oral poisoning. The narcotic antagonist naloxone (Narcan), 0.4 mg IV, is effective in the treatment of acute overdosage. Respiratory stimulants (e.g., caffeine) should not be used to treat depression from the narcotic overdosage.

DRUG INTERACTIONS

Alcohol, ethyl / Potentiation or addition of CNS depressant effects; concomitant use may lead to drowsiness, lethargy, stupor, respiratory collapse, coma, or death

Anesthetics, general / See *Alcohol*

Antianxiety drugs / See *Alcohol*

Antidepressants, tricyclic / ↑ Narcotic-induced respiratory depression

Antihistamines / See *Alcohol*

Barbiturates / See *Alcohol*

Cimetidine / ↑ CNS toxicity (e.g., disorientation, confusion, respiratory depression, apnea, seizures)

CNS depressants / See *Alcohol*

MAO inhibitors / Possible potentiation of either MAO inhibitor (excitation, hypertension) or narcotic (hypotension, coma) effects; death has resulted

Methotrimeprazine / Potentiation of CNS depression

Narcotic analgesics, mixed agonist/antagonists (buprenorphine, butorphanol, dezocine, nalbuphine, pentazocine) / May precipitate withdrawal symptoms in dependent clients

Phenothiazines / See *Alcohol*

Sedative-hypnotics, nonbarbiturate / See *Alcohol*

Skeletal muscle relaxants (surgical) / ↑ Respiratory depression and ↑ muscle relaxation

LABORATORY TEST CONSIDERATIONS

Altered liver function tests. False + or ↑ urinary glucose test (Benedict's). ↑ Plasma amylase or lipase.

DOSAGE

See individual drugs.

NURSING CONSIDERATIONS

ADMINISTRATION/STORAGE

1. Review list of drugs with which narcotics interact and effects.
2. Request that orders be rewritten at timed intervals as required for continued administration.
3. Record amount of narcotic used on the narcotic inventory sheet, noting drug, date, time, dose, and to whom, or if the drug was wasted; include appropriate witness as necessary, addressing all requirements for documentation.

ASSESSMENT

1. Document indications for therapy, type and onset of symptoms; differentiate acute vs. chronic syndromes and rate pain levels.
2. Note any prior experience with narcotic analgesics or adverse reactions.
3. Identify clinical conditions that may precipitate pain syndromes, i.e., cancer, neuropathic, postherpetic neuralgia, or musculoskeletal injury.
4. Determine cause and document amount of pain or discomfort, its location, intensity, and duration, frequency of occurrence, and what drug has been effective in the past.
5. Use a pain rating scale (e.g., 0–10) to assess pain quantitatively so clients can accurately describe their level of pain and measure effectiveness of therapy.
6. Obtain baseline VS; generally, if the respiratory rate < 12/min or the SBP < 90 mm Hg, a narcotic should not be administered unless there is ventilatory support or specific written guidelines, with parameters for administration.
7. Note weight, age, and general body size. Too large a dosage for the client's weight and age can result in serious side effects.
8. Document amount of time elapsed between doses for relief from recurring pain.
9. Note precipitating factors as well as the impact of the pain on the client's ability to function. Assess carefully for adequate control of pain.
10. Document asthma or other conditions that alter respirations.
11. Determine if pregnant. Narcotics cross the placental barrier and depress fetal respirations.
12. Monitor CBC, electrolytes, liver and renal function studies.

INTERVENTIONS

1. Determine when to use supportive measures, such as relaxation techniques, repositioning, and reassurance to assist in relieving pain.
2. Explore source of pain; use non-narcotic analgesics when possible. Coadministration (as with NSAIDs) may increase analgesic effects and permit lower narcotic doses.
3. Administer when needed; *prolonging until the maximum amount of pain experienced reduces drugs' effectiveness.*
4. Monitor VS and mental status. During parenteral therapy:
   - Monitor for ↓ respirations.
   - Narcotics depress cough reflex. Turn q 2 hr; cough and deep breathe to prevent atelectasis. Splinting incisions and painful areas may assist in compliance. Administer narcotic at least 30–60 min prior to activities or painful procedures.
   - Monitor for hypotension.
   - Report if HR below 50 beats/min in the adult or 110 beats/min in infant.
   - Observe for decrease in BP, deep sleep, or constricted pupils.
   - Assess during meals to prevent choking and aspiration.
   - Monitor closely when administered as sedation for a procedure.
   - Note effects on mental status. One who has experienced pain, fear, or anxiety may become euphoric and excited. Note dizziness, drowsiness, pupil reactions, or hallucinations.

5. Report if N&V occurs; may need an antiemetic or change in therapy.
6. A snack or milk may decrease gastric irritation and lessen nausea when taken orally.
7. Monitor bowel function; narcotics, especially morphine, can have a depressant effect on the GI tract and may promote constipation. Increase fluid intake to 2.5–3 L/day; consume fruit juices, fruits, and fiber. Increase level and frequency of exercise. Take stool softeners as directed.
8. Narcotics may cause urinary retention. Monitor I&O; palpate abdomen for distention; empty bladder q 3–4 hr. Question about difficulty voiding, pain in the bladder area, sensation of not emptying the bladder, dysuria, or any unusual odors.
9. Note difficulty with vision. Check pupillary response to light; report if pupils remain constricted.
10. Monitor mental status. If bedridden, use side rails and safety measures; assist with ambulation, BR, and transfers.
11. Reassure that flushing and a feeling of warmth may occur with therapeutic doses.
12. May perspire profusely; be prepared to bathe; change clothes and linens frequently.
13. Assess for evidence of tolerance and addiction with ATC therapy.
14. With terminal diseases and chronic debilitating pain, dependence on drug therapy is not a consideration, whereas *adequate pain control is of the utmost concern.*

CLIENT/FAMILY TEACHING

1. Drug may become habit forming; explore alternative methods for pain control. With chronic debilitating pain, addiction is not a concern whereas functionality is of concern.
2. Take as prescribed before the pain becomes too severe.
3. Avoid alcohol in any form.
4. Do not take OTC drugs without approval. Many contain small amounts of alcohol and some may interact unfavorably with the prescribed drug.
5. For fecal impaction, use preventive actions, such as increased fluid intake, increased use of fruit and fruit juices, and a stool softener.
6. Drug can cause drowsiness and dizziness; use caution when operating a motor vehicle or performing other tasks that require mental alertness.
7. Rise slowly from a lying to sitting position and dangle before standing, to minimize orthostatic effects.
8. When used as sedation for outpatient procedures, someone must accompany client. Expect a recovery period (to assess for adverse effects) up to several hours before release.
9. Store all drugs in a safe place, out of the reach of children and away from the bedside to prevent accidental overdosage.
10. During prolonged usage, do not stop abruptly; withdrawal symptoms may occur.
11. Determine extent of relief achieved with each dosage (e.g., pain level decreased from a level 5 to a level 2, 20 min after administration of medication). Keep a record of narcotic use for breakthrough pain so that dose can be adjusted.
12. Review techniques to enhance pain relief such as relaxation techniques, splinting incision, supporting painful areas, and taking medication before strenuous activities and before pain becomes severe.
13. Identify appropriate support groups for assistance with understanding, accepting, and managing chronic pain. Seek locale of regional pain management center for nonresponders with chronic pain syndromes.
14. For those with terminal diseases, identify local support groups to provide contact with those experiencing similar symptoms and treatments and local hospice program.
15. For the elderly, blood levels of narcotic may be higher, resulting in longer periods of pain relief. Assess physical parameters and client complaints carefully before readministering narcotic for short-term pain control

on the prescribed as-needed frequency.

OUTCOMES/EVALUATE

- Control of pain without altered hemodynamics or impaired level of consciousness
- Reduction in pain level on pain rating scale
- Client comfort
- Absence of acute toxicity, tolerance, or addiction, during short-term therapy

NARCOTIC ANTAGONISTS

SEE ALSO THE FOLLOWING INDIVIDUAL ENTRIES:

Nalmefene hydrochloride
Naloxone hydrochloride
Naltrexone

ACTION/KINETICS

Narcotic antagonists competitively block the action of narcotic analgesics by displacing previously given narcotics from their receptor sites or by preventing narcotics from attaching to the opiate receptors, thereby preventing access by the analgesic. Not effective in reversing the respiratory depression induced by barbiturates, anesthetics, or other nonnarcotic agents. These drugs almost immediately induce withdrawal symptoms in narcotic addicts and are sometimes used to unmask dependence.

NURSING CONSIDERATIONS

ASSESSMENT

1. Determine etiology of respiratory depression. Narcotic antagonists do not relieve the toxicity of nonnarcotic CNS depressants.
2. Note mental status and VS.

INTERVENTIONS

1. Note agent being reversed. If narcotic is long acting or sustained release, repeated doses will be required in order to continue to counteract drug effects. Monitor VS and respirations closely after duration of action of antagonist; additional doses may be necessary.
2. Observe for appearance of withdrawal symptoms characterized by restlessness, crying out due to sudden loss of pain control, lacrimation, rhinorrhea, yawning, perspiration, vomiting, diarrhea, sweating, writhing, anxiety, pain, chills, and an intense craving for the drug.
3. Observe for symptoms of airway obstruction; if comatose, turn frequently and position on side to prevent aspiration.
4. Maintain a safe, protective environment. Use side rails, supervise ambulation, and use soft supports as needed.
5. If used to diagnose narcotic use or dependence, observe for initial dilation of the pupils, followed by constriction.
6. Anticipate readministration of smaller doses of narcotic (once depressant symptoms reversed) with terminal pain and conditions that warrant narcotic pain management.

OUTCOMES/EVALUATE

- Reversal of toxic effects of narcotic analgesic evidenced by ↑ level of consciousness and improved breathing patterns
- Confirmation of narcotic dependence evidenced by withdrawal symptoms

NEUROMUSCULAR BLOCKING AGENTS

SEE ALSO THE FOLLOWING INDIVIDUAL ENTRIES:

Atracurium besylate
Cisatracurium besylate
Doxacurium chloride
Mivacurium chloride
Pancuronium bromide
Pipecuronium bromide
Rocuronium bromide
Succinylcholine chloride
Tubocurarine chloride
Vecuronium bromide

ACTION/KINETICS

These drugs are categorized as competitive (nondepolarizing) and depolarizing agents, both of which act peripherally. Competitive agents include all of the above listed drugs *except* succinylcholine. They compete with acetylcholine for the receptor site in the muscle cells. The depolarizing agent—succinylcholine—initially excites skeletal muscle and then prevents the muscle from contracting by prolonging the time during which the receptors at the end plate cannot respond to acetylcholine (depolarization during refractory time).

The muscle paralysis caused by the neuromuscular blocking agents is sequential in the following order: heaviness of eyelids, difficulty in swallowing/talking, diplopia, progressive weakening of extremities and neck, followed by relaxation of the trunk and spine. The diaphragm (respiratory paralysis) is affected last. They do not affect consciousness, and their use, in the absence of adequate levels of general anesthesia, may be frightening to the client. After IV infusion, flaccid paralysis occurs within a few minutes with maximum effects within about 6 min. Maximal effects last 35–60 min and effective muscle paralysis may last for 25–90 min with complete recovery taking several hours. There is a narrow margin of safety between a therapeutically effective dose causing muscle relaxation and a toxic dose causing respiratory paralysis. **The neuromuscular blocking agents are always administered initially by a trained physician.** The nurse must be prepared to maintain and monitor respiration until the effect of the drug subsides.

USES

See individual agents. General uses include as an adjunct to general anesthesia to cause muscle relaxation; to reduce the intensity of skeletal muscle contractions in either drug-induced or electrically induced convulsions; to assist in the management of mechanical ventilation.

CONTRAINDICATIONS

Allergy or hypersensitivity to any of these drugs.

SPECIAL CONCERNS

Use with caution in myasthenia gravis; renal, hepatic, endocrine, or pulmonary impairment; respiratory depression; during lactation; and in elderly, pediatric, or debilitated clients. The action may be altered in clients by electrolyte imbalances (especially hyperkalemia), some carcinomas, body temperature, dehydration, renal disease, and in those taking digitalis.

SIDE EFFECTS

Respiratory paralysis. Severe and prolonged muscle relaxation.

CV: Cardiac arrhythmias, bradycardia, hypotension, cardiac arrest. These side effects are more frequent in neonates and premature infants. **GI:** Excessive salivation during light anesthesia. **Miscellaneous:** ***Bronchospasms, hyperthermia,*** hypersensitivity (rare). See also individual agents.

OD OVERDOSE MANAGEMENT

Symptoms: Decreased respiratory reserve, extended skeletal muscle weakness, prolonged apnea, low tidal volume, sudden release of histamine, ***CV collapse.*** *Treatment:* There are no known antidotes.

• Use a peripheral nerve stimulator to monitor and assess client's response to the neuromuscular blocking medication.

• Have anticholinesterase drugs, such as edrophonium, pyridostigmine, or neostigmine available to counteract respiratory depression due to paralysis of skeletal muscles. These drugs increase the body's production of acetylcholine. To minimize the muscarinic cholinergic side effects, give atropine.

• Correct BP, electrolyte imbalance, or circulating blood volume by fluid and electrolyte therapy. Vasopressors can be used to correct hypotension due to ganglionic blockade.

DRUG INTERACTIONS

The following drug interactions are for nondepolarizing skeletal muscle relaxants. See also succinylcholine.

Aminoglycoside antibiotics / Additive muscle relaxation, including prolonged respiratory depression
Amphotericin B / ↑ Muscle relaxation
Anesthetics, inhalation / Additive muscle relaxation
Carbamazepine / ↓ Duration or effect of muscle relaxants
Clindamycin / Additive muscle relaxation, including prolonged respiratory depression
Colistin / ↑ Muscle relaxation
Corticosteroids / ↓ Effect of muscle relaxants
Furosemide / ↑ or ↓ Effect of skeletal muscle relaxants (may be dose-related)
Hydantoins / ↓ Duration or effect of muscle relaxants
Ketamine / ↑ Muscle relaxation, including prolonged respiratory depression
Lincomycin / ↑ Muscle relaxation, including prolonged respiratory depression
Lithium / ↑ Recovery time of muscle relaxants → prolonged respiratory depression
Magnesium salts / ↑ Muscle relaxation, including prolonged respiratory depression
Methotrimeprazine / ↑ Muscle relaxation
Narcotic analgesics / ↑ Respiratory depression and ↑ muscle relaxation
Nitrates / ↑ Muscle relaxation, including prolonged respiratory depression
Phenothiazines / ↑ Muscle relaxation
Pipercillin / ↑ Muscle relaxation, including prolonged respiratory depression
Polymyxin B / ↑ Muscle relaxation
Procainamide / ↑ Muscle relaxation
Procaine / ↑ Muscle relaxation by ↓ plasma protein binding
Quinidine / ↑ Muscle relaxation
Ranitidine / Significant ↓ effect of muscle relaxants
Theophyllines / Reversal of effects of muscle relaxant (dose-dependent)
Thiazide diuretics / ↑ Muscle relaxation due to hypokalemia
Verapamil / ↑ Muscle relaxation, including prolonged respiratory depression

DOSAGE

See individual drugs.

NURSING CONSIDERATIONS

ASSESSMENT

1. Document indications for therapy, desired outcome, and anticipated length of use.
2. Note age and condition; elderly and debilitated clients should not receive drugs in this category.
3. Monitor CBC, electrolytes, CXR, ECG, liver and renal function studies.
4. Note other drugs receiving. Clients requiring neuromuscular blocking agents are often receiving other drugs that may have the effect of prolonging response to neuromuscular blocking agent.
5. Question client concerning changes in vision, ability to chew or move the fingers.
6. Note initial selective paralysis in the following sequence: levator muscles of the eyelids, mastication muscles, limb muscles, abdominal muscles, glottis muscles, intercostal muscles, and the diaphragm muscles; neuromuscular recovery occurs in the reverse order.

INTERVENTIONS

1. Administer in a closely monitored environment and generally only when intubated.
2. Prevent overdosage during infusions by frequent evaluations with a peripheral nerve stimulator or partial return of muscle function.
3. Monitor VS frequently and pulmonary status continuously. Monitor and ventilator alarms should be set and checked frequently.
4. Observe for excessive bronchial secretions or respiratory wheezing; suction to maintain patent airway.
5. Perform frequent neurovascular assessments. Prolonged use of neuromuscular blocking agents may

cause profound weakness and paralysis; may precipitate an acute myopathy.
6. Observe for drug interactions which may potentiate muscular relaxation and prove fatal.
7. Consciousness and pain thresholds are not affected by neuromuscular blocking agents; clients can still hear, feel, and see while receiving these agents. Avoid discussions that should not be overheard. Adequate anxiolytic therapy and analgesics should be administered for pain or fear with procedures.
8. Clients requiring prolonged ventilatory therapy should be adequately sedated with analgesics and benzodiazepines. Anxiety levels may be very high, but client cannot communicate this.
9. Administer eye drops and patches to protect corneas during prolonged therapy; explain why this is done (i.e., blink reflex suppressed).
10. Avoid corticosteroids during prolonged neuromuscular blockade unless benefits outweigh the risks.
11. Perform passive range of motion to prevent loss of function and contractures with prolonged therapy.

OUTCOMES/EVALUATE

- Skeletal muscle paralysis
- Insertion of ET tube/tolerance of mechanical ventilation
- Suppression of twitch response

NONSTEROIDAL ANTI-INFLAMMATORY DRUGS

SEE ALSO THE FOLLOWING INDIVIDUAL ENTRIES:

Celecoxib
Diclofenac potassium
Diclofenac sodium
Diflunisal
Etodolac
Fenoprofen calcium
Flurbiprofen
Flurbiprofen sodium
Ibuprofen
Indomethacin
Indomethacin sodium trihydrate
Ketoprofen
Ketorolac tromethamine
Meclofenamate sodium
Mefenamic acid
Meloxicam
Nabumetone
Naproxen
Naproxen sodium
Oxaprozin
Piroxicam
Rofecoxib
Sulindac
Tolmetin sodium
Valdecoxib

ACTION/KINETICS

The anti-inflammatory effect is likely due to inhibition of the enzyme cyclooxygenase (COX). There are two COX isoenzymes— COX-1 and COX-2. Depending on the NSAID, either COX-1 or COX-2 or both enzymes may be inhibited. Inhibition of cyclooxygenase results in decreased prostaglandin synthesis. Effective in reducing joint swelling, pain, and morning stiffness, as well as in increasing mobility in individuals with inflammatory disease. They do not alter the course of the disease, however. Their anti-inflammatory activity is comparable to that of aspirin. The analgesic activity is due, in part, to relief of inflammation. Other mechanisms that contribute to the anti-inflammatory effect include reduction of superoxide radicals, induction of apoptosis, inhibition of adhesion molecule expression, decreae of nitric oxide synthase, decrease of proinflammatory cytokine levels, modification of lymphocyte activity, and alteration of cellualr membrane functions. Rheumatoid factor production may also be inhibited. The antipyretic action occurs by decreasing prostaglandin synthesis in the hypothalamus, resulting in an increase in peripheral blood flow and heat loss as well as promoting sweating. NSAIDs also inhibit miosis induced by prostaglandins during the course of cataract surgery; thus, these drugs are useful for a number of ophthalmic inflammatory conditions.

The NSAIDs differ from one another

with respect to their rate of absorption, length of action, anti-inflammatory activity, and effect on the GI mucosa. Most are rapidly and completely absorbed from the GI tract; food delays the rate, but not the total amount, of drug absorbed. These drugs are metabolized in the kidney and are excreted through the urine, mainly as metabolites.

USES

See individual drugs. Generally are used to treat inflammatory disease, including rheumatoid arthritis, osteoarthritis, ankylosing spondylitis, gout, and other musculoskeletal diseases. Treatment of nonrheumatic inflammatory conditions including bursitis, acute painful shoulder, synovitis, tendinitis, or tenosynovitis. Mild to moderate pain including primary dysmenorrhea, episiotomy pain, strains and sprains, postextraction dental pain. Primary dysmenorrhea. Ophthalmically to inhibit intraoperative miosis, for postoperative inflammation after cataract surgery, and for relief of ocular itching due to seasonal allergic conjunctivitis.

CONTRAINDICATIONS

Most for children under 14 years of age. Lactation. Individuals in whom aspirin, NSAIDs, or iodides have caused hypersensitivity, including acute asthma, rhinitis, urticaria, nasal polyps, bronchospasm, angioedema or other symptoms of allergy or anaphylaxis.

SPECIAL CONCERNS

Clients intolerant to one of the NSAIDs may be intolerant to others in this group. Use with caution in clients with a history of GI disease, reduced renal function, in geriatric clients, in clients with intrinsic coagulation defects or those on anticoagulant therapy, in compromised cardiac function, in hypertension, in conditions predisposing to fluid retention, and in the presence of existing controlled infection. The risk of hospitalization is doubled in geriatric clients taking NSAIDs and diuretics. The safety and efficacy of most NSAIDs have not been determined in children or in functional class IV rheumatoid arthritis (i.e., clients incapacitated, bedridden, or confined to a wheelchair). Use during pregnancy increases the risk of pulmonary hypertension in newborns.

Products must carry a warning about the possibility of stomach bleeding in clients who consume three or more alcoholic drinks per day.

SIDE EFFECTS

GI (most common): Peptic or duodenal ulceration and GI bleeding, intestinal ulceration with obstruction and stenosis, reactivation of preexisting ulcers. Heartburn, dyspepsia, N&V, anorexia, diarrhea, constipation, increased or decreased appetite, indigestion, stomatitis, epigastric pain, abdominal cramps or pain, gastroenteritis, paralytic ileus, salivation, dry mouth, glossitis, pyrosis, icterus, rectal irritation, gingival ulcer, occult blood in stool, hematemesis, gastritis, proctitis, eructation, sore or dry mucous membranes, ulcerative colitis, rectal bleeding, melena, ***perforation and hemorrhage of esophagus, stomach, duodenum, small or large intestine.*** **CNS:** Dizziness, drowsiness, vertigo, headaches, nervousness, migraine, anxiety, mental confusion, aggravation of parkinsonism and epilepsy, lightheadedness, paresthesia, peripheral neuropathy, akathisia, excitation, tremor, ***seizures,*** myalgia, asthenia, malaise, insomnia, fatigue, drowsiness, confusion, emotional lability, depression, inability to concentrate, psychoses, hallucinations, depersonalization, amnesia, ***coma,*** syncope. **CV:** CHF, hypotension, hypertension, arrhythmias, peripheral edema and fluid retention, vasodilation, exacerbation of angiitis, palpitations, tachycardia, chest pain, sinus bradycardia, peripheral vascular disease, peripheral edema. **Respiratory:** ***Bronchospasm, laryngeal edema,*** rhinitis, dyspnea, pharyngitis, hemoptysis, SOB, eosinophilic pneumonitis. **Hematologic:** Bone marrow depression, neutropenia, leukopenia, pancytopenia, eosinophila, thrombocytopenia, granulocytopenia, ***agranulocytosis, aplastic anemia, hemolytic anemia,*** decreased H&H, hypocoagulability, epistaxis. **Ophthalmologic:** Amblyopia, visual disturbances, corneal deposits, retinal hemorrhage, scotomata, retinal pigmentation changes or degeneration, blurred vision, photophobia, diplopia, iritis, loss of color vision (reversible), optic neuritis, cataracts, swollen, dry, or irritated eyes. **Dermatologic:** Pruritus, skin eruptions, sweating, erythema, eczema, hyperpigmentation, ecchymoses, petechiae, rashes, urticaria, purpura, onycholysis, vesiculobullous eruptions, cutaneous vasculitis, ***toxic epidermal necrolysis, angioneurotic edema,*** erythema nodosum, ***Stevens-Johnson syndrome,*** exfoliative dermatitis, photosensitivity, alopecia, skin irritation, peeling, erythema multiforme, desquamation, skin discoloration. **GU:** Menometrorrhagia, menorrhagia, impotence, menstrual disorders, hematuria, cystitis, azotemia, nocturia, proteinuria, UTIs, polyuria, dysuria, urinary frequency, oliguria, pyuria, anuria, renal insufficiency, nephrosis, nephrotic syndrome, glomerular and interstitial nephritis, urinary casts, acute renal failure in clients with impaired renal function, renal papillary necrosis **Metabolic:** Hyperglycemia, hypoglycemia, glycosuria, hyperkalemia, hyponatremia, diabetes mellitus. **Other:** Tinnitus, hearing loss or disturbances, ear pain, deafness, metallic or bitter taste in mouth, thirst, chills, fever, flushing, jaundice, sweating, breast changes, gynecomastia, muscle cramps, dyspnea, involuntary muscle movements, muscle weakness, facial edema, pain, serum sickness, aseptic meningitis, hypersensitivity reactions including asthma, acute respiratory distress, ***shock-like syndrome, angioedema,*** angiitis, dyspnea, ***anaphylaxis.***

Following ophthalmic use: Transient burning and stinging upon installation, ocular irritation.

OD OVERDOSE MANAGEMENT

Symptoms: CNS symptoms include dizziness, drowsiness, mental confusion, lethargy, disorientation, intense headache, paresthesia, and ***seizures.*** GI symptoms include N&V, gastric irritation, and abdominal pain. Miscellaneous symptoms include tinnitus, sweating, blurred vision, increased serum creatinine and BUN, and acute renal failure. *Treatment:* There are no antidotes; treatment includes general supportive measures. Since the drugs are acidic, it may be beneficial to alkalinize the urine and induce diuresis to hasten excretion.

DRUG INTERACTIONS

Aminoglycosides / ↑ Aminoglycoside levels in premature infants due to ↓ glomerular filtration rate
Anticoagulants / Concomitant use results in ↑ PT
Aspirin / ↓ Effect of NSAIDs R/T ↓ blood levels; also, ↑ risk of adverse GI effects
Beta-adrenergic blocking agents / ↓ Antihypertensive effects
Cholestyramine / ↓ GI absorption of NSAIDs
Cimetidine / ↑ or ↓ Plasma levels of NSAIDs
Cyclosporine / ↑ Risk of nephrotoxicity
H *Gingko biloba* / Additive effect on platelet aggregation → ↑ risk of bleeding
H *Ginseng* / Avoid concomitant use or monitor carefully
Lithium / ↑ Serum lithium levels
Loop diuretics / ↓ Drug effects
Methotrexate / ↑ Risk of methotrexate toxicity (i.e., bone marrow suppression, nephrotoxicity, stomatitis)
Phenobarbital / ↓ Effect of NSAIDs R/T ↑ liver breakdown
Phenytoin / ↑ Phenytoin effects R/T ↓ plasma protein binding
Probenecid / ↑ Levels and possibly toxicity of NSAIDs
Salicylates / Plasma levels of NSAIDs may be ↓; also, ↑ risk of GI side effects
Sulfonamides / ↑ Drug effects R/T ↓ plasma protein binding

Sulfonylureas / ↑ Drug effects R/T ↓ plasma protein binding

DOSAGE

See individual drugs.

NURSING CONSIDERATIONS

ADMINISTRATION/STORAGE

1. Do not take alcohol or aspirin together with NSAIDs.
2. Should GI upset occur, take with food, milk, or antacids.
3. NSAIDs may have an additive analgesic effect when administered with narcotic analgesics, thus permitting lower narcotic dosages.
4. Clients who do not respond clinically to one NSAID may respond to another.

ASSESSMENT

1. Note allergic responses to aspirin or other anti-inflammatory agents.
2. Document location, intensity, characteristics, and type of pain experienced. Assess joint mobility and ROM.
3. Review indications and dosage prescribed. For anti-inflammatory effects, high doses are required whereas analgesia and pain relief may be achieved with much lower dosages. Metastatic bone pain responds effectively to NSAIDS but not well to narcotics.
4. Asthma or nasal polyps may be exacerbated by NSAIDs.
5. Children under 14 years of age generally should not receive drugs in this category.
6. Monitor CBC, liver and renal function studies; causes platelet inhibition which is reversible in 24–48 hr, whereas aspirin requires 4–5 days to reverse antiplatelet effects. Cox-1 NSAIDS may inhibit the cardioprotective effects of aspirin.

CLIENT/FAMILY TEACHING

1. Take NSAIDs with a full glass of water or milk, with meals, or with a prescribed antacid and remain upright 30 min following administration to reduce gastric irritation or ulcer formation.
2. Consume 2–3 L/day of water.
3. Report any changes in stool consistency or symptoms of GI irritation. Sustained GI effects may require stomach protectant.
4. Regular intake of drug needed to sustain anti-inflammatory effects. If not obtained, another NSAID may provide desired response.
5. Report any episodes of bleeding, eye symptoms, tinnitus, skin rashes, purpura, weight gain, edema, decreased urine output, fever, or increased joint pain.
6. Use caution in operating machinery or in driving a car; may cause dizziness or drowsiness.
7. Avoid alcohol, aspirin, acetaminophen, and any other OTC preparations; may cause GI bleeding.
8. If diabetic, be aware of hypoglycemic effect of NSAIDs on hypoglycemic agents; dosage of agent and NSAID may need to be adjusted.
9. Record weights periodically and report any significant changes. NSAIDs cause Na and water retention; avoid with CHF.
10. Notify all providers of meds being taken to avoid unfavorable drug interactions.

OUTCOMES/EVALUATE

- ↑ Joint mobility and ROM
- ↓ Discomfort and pain
- Improvement in symptoms

ORAL CONTRACEPTIVES: ESTROGEN-PROGESTERONE COMBINATIONS

SEE TABLE 2.

GENERAL STATEMENT

There are three types of combination (i.e., both an estrogen and progestin in each tablet) oral contraceptives: (1) monophasic—contain the same amount of estrogen and progestin in each tablet; (2) biphasic— usually contain the same amount of estrogen in each tablet but the progestin

TABLE 2 Injectable & Oral Contraceptive Preparations & Hormone Replacement Combinations Available in the United States

TRADE NAME	ESTROGEN	PROGESTIN
	ORAL MONOPHASIC PRODUCTS	
Alesse 21-Day and 28-Day	Ethinyl estradiol (20 mcg)	Levonorgestrel (0.1 mg)
Apri	Ethinyl estradiol (30 mcg)	Desogestrel (0.15 mg)
Aviane (28 Day)	Ethinyl estradiol (20 mcg)	Levonorgestrel (0.1 mg)
Brevicon 28-Day	Ethinyl estradiol (35 mcg)	Norethindrone (0.5 mg)
Demulen 1/35 21 Day and 28 Day	Ethinyl estradiol (35 mcg)	Ethynodiol diacetate (1 mg)
Demulen 1/50 21 Day and 28 Day	Ethinyl estradiol (50 mcg)	Ethynodiol diacetate (1 mg)
Desogen (28 day)	Ethinyl estradiol (30 mcg)	Desogestrel (0.15 mg)
Levlen 21 and 28	Ethinyl estradiol (30 mcg)	Levonorgestrel (0.15 mg)
Levlite 21 Day and 28 Day	Ethinyl estradiol (20 mcg)	Levonorgestrel (0.1 mg)
Levora 28 Day	Ethinyl estradiol (30 mcg)	Levonorgestrel (0.15 mg)
Loestrin 21 1/20 (21 Day)	Ethinyl estradiol (20 mcg)	Norethindrone acetate (1 mg)
Loestrin 21 1.5/30 (21 Day)	Ethinyl estradiol (30 mcg)	Norethindrone acetate (1.5 mg)
Loestrin Fe 1/20 (28 day)	Ethinyl estradiol (20 mcg)	Norethindrone acetate (1 mg)
Loestrin Fe 1.5/30 (28 day)	Ethinyl estradiol (30 mcg)	Norethindrone acetate (1.5 mg)
Lo/Ovral 21 Day	Ethinyl estradiol (30 mcg)	Norgestrel (0.3 mg)
Low-Ogestrel (28 Day)	Ethinyl estradiol (30 mcg)	Norgestrel (0.3 mg)
Microgestin Fe 1/20 (28 Day)	Ethinyl estradiol (20 mcg)	Norethindrone acetate (1 mg)
Microgestin Fe 1.5/30 (28 Day)	Ethinyl estradiol (30 mcg)	Norethindrone acetate (1.5 mg)
Modicon 28 Day	Ethinyl estradiol (35 mcg)	Norethindrone (0.5 mg)
Necon 0.5/35-21 Day and 28 Day	Ethinyl estradiol (35 mcg)	Norethindrone (0.5 mg)
Necon 1/35-21 Day and 28 Day	Ethinyl estradiol (35 mcg)	Norethindrone (1 mg)
Necon 1/50-21 Day and 28 Day	Mestranol (50 mcg)	Norethindrone (1 mg)

TRADE NAME	ESTROGEN	PROGESTIN
ORAL MONOPHASIC PRODUCTS		
Nordette 21 Day and 28 Day	Ethinyl estradiol (30 mcg)	Levonorgestrel (0.15 mg)
Norinyl 1 + 35 28-Day	Ethinyl estradiol (35 mcg)	Norethindrone (1 mg)
Norinyl 1 + 50 28-Day	Mestranol (50 mcg)	Norethindrone (1 mg)
Nortrel 1/35	Ethinyl estradiol (35 mcg)	Norethindrone (1 mg)
Nortrel 0.5/35	Ethinyl estradiol (35 mcg)	Norethindrone (0.5 mg)
Ogestrel (28 Day)	Ethinyl estradiol (50 mcg)	Norgestrel (0.5 mg)
Ortho-Cept 28 Day	Ethinyl estradiol (30 mcg)	Desogestrel (0.15 mg)
Ortho-Cyclen 28 Day	Ethinyl estradiol (35 mcg)	Norgestimate (0.25 mg)
Ortho Novum 1/35 28 Day	Ethinyl estradiol (35 mcg)	Norethindrone (1 mg)
Ortho Novum 1/50 28 Day	Mestranol (50 mcg)	Norethindrone (1 mg)
Ovcon-35 21 Day and 28 Day	Ethinyl estradiol (35 mcg)	Norethindrone (0.4 mg)
Ovcon-50 28 Day	Ethinyl estradiol (50 mcg)	Norethindrone (1 mg)
Ovral 28 Day	Ethinyl estradiol (50 mcg)	Norgestrel (0.5 mg)
Yasmin	Ethinyl estradiol (30 mcg)	Drospirenone (3 mg)
Zovia 1/35E 21 Day and 28 Day	Ethinyl estradiol (35 mcg)	Ethynodiol diacetate (1 mg)
Zovia 1/50E 21 Day and 28 Day	Ethinyl estradiol (50 mcg)	Ethynodiol diacetate (1 mg)
ORAL BIPHASIC PRODUCTS		
Jenest-28	Ethinyl estradiol (35 mcg in each tablet)	Norethindrone (7 tablets of 0.5 mg followed by 14 tablets of 1 mg)
Mircette	Ethinyl estradiol (20 mcg for Days 1 - 21; 10 mcg for Days 24 - 28)	Desogestrel (150 mg for Days 1 - 21)
Necon 10/11 21 Day and 28 Day	Ethinyl estradiol (35 mcg in each tablet)	Norethindrone (10 tablets of 0.5 mg followed by 11 tablets of 1 mg)
Ortho-Novum 10/11 28 Day	Ethinyl estradiol (35 mcg in each tablet)	Norethindrone (10 tablets of 0.5 mg followed by 11 tablets of 1 mg)

continues

TRADE NAME	ESTROGEN	PROGESTIN
ORAL TRIPHASIC PRODUCTS		
Cyclessa	Ethinyl estradiol (25 mcg in each tablet)	First 7 days: Desogestrel (1 mg) Next 7 days: Desogestrel (0.125 mg) Last 7 days: Desogestrel (0.15 mg)
Enpresse	First 6 days: Ethinyl estradiol (30 mcg) Next 5 days: Ethinyl estradiol (40 mcg) Last 10 days: Ethinyl estradiol (30 mcg)	Levonorgestrel (0.05 mg) Levonorgestrel (0.075 mg) Levonorgestrel (0.125 mg)
Estrostep 21	First 5 days: Ethinyl estradiol (20 mcg) Next 7 days: Ethinyl estradiol (30 mcg) Last 9 days: Ethinyl estradiol (35 mg)	Norethindrone (1 mg in each tablet)
Estrostep Fe (28 Day)	Same levels of ethinyl estradiol and norethindrone for the first 21 days. Days 21–28 contain 75 mg ferrous fumarate/tablet.	
Ortho-Novum 7/7/7 (28 day)	Ethinyl estradiol (35 mcg in each tablet)	Norethindrone (0.5 mg the first 7 days, 0.75 the next 7 days, and 1 mg the last 7 days)
Ortho-Tri-Cyclen (28 day)	Ethinyl estradiol (35 mcg in each tablet)	Norgestimate (0.18 mg the first 7 days, 0.215 mg the next 7 days, and 0.25 mg the last seven days)
Tri-Levlen (21 or 28 Days)	First 6 days: Ethinyl estradiol (30 mcg) Next 5 days: Ethinyl estradiol (40 mcg) Last 10 days: Ethinyl estradiol (30 mcg)	Levonogestrel (0.05 mg) Levonorgestrel (0.075 mg) Levonorgestrel (0.125 mg)
Tri-Norinyl (28 day)	Ethinyl estradiol (35 mcg in each tablet)	Norethindrone (0.5 mg the first 7 days, 1 mg the next 9 days, and 0.5 mg the last 5 days)
Triphasil (21 or 28 day)	First 6 days: Ethinyl estradiol (30 mcg) Next 5 days: Ethinyl estradiol (40 mcg) Last 10 days: Ethinyl estradiol (30 mcg)	Levonorgestrel (0.05 mg) Levonorgestrel (0.075 mg) Levonorgestrel (0.125 mg)
Trivora (28 day)	First 6 days: Ethinyl estradiol (30 mcg) Next 5 days: Ethinyl estradiol (40 mcg) Last 10 days: Ethinyl estradiol (30 mcg)	Levonorgestrel (0.05 mg) Levonorgestrel (0.075 mg) Levonorgestrel (0.125 mg)

TRADE NAME	ESTROGEN	PROGESTIN
ORAL TRIPHASIC PRODUCTS		
EMERGENCY CONTRACEPTIVE KIT		
Plan B	No estrogen	Levonorgestrel (0.75 mg)
A total of 2 tablets containing levonorgestrel.		
Preven	Ethinyl estradiol (50 mcg)	Levonorgestrel (0.25 mg)
A total of four tablets containing the above hormones		

TRADE NAME	CONTENTS	ADMINISTRATION
HORMONE REPLACEMENT COMBINATIONS		
Activella	Estradiol 17-b, 1 mg Norethindrone, 0.5 mg	One tablet daily. To treat vasomotor symptoms in menopause, vulvar and vaginal atrophy, prevention of osteoporosis
CombiPatch	Estradiol, 50 mcg Norethindrone acetate (0.14 mg or 0.25 mg)	One patch replaced twice weekly. To treat vasomotor symptoms due to menopause; treat hypoestrogenism due to hypogonadism, castration, or primary ovarian failure.
Femhrt	Ethinyl estradiol, 5 mcg Norethindrone acetate, 1 mg	One tablet daily. To treat vasomotor symptoms or prevent osteoporosis.
Ortho-Prefest	Estradiol 17-B, 1 mg Norgestimate, 0.09 mg	Single tablet of estradiol, 1 mg, for 3 days followed by a single tablet of estradiol, 1 mg, and norgestimate, 0.09 mg, for 3 days. Repeat regimen continuously without interruption. To treat vasomotor symptoms in menopause, vulvar and vaginal atrophy, prevention of osteoporosis.
INJECTABLE CONTRACEPTIVES		
Lunelle	Medroxyprogesterone, 25 mg Estradiol cypionate, 5 mg	Inject 0.5 mL IM once a month, in cycles not to exceed 33 days.

All combination oral contraceptives and hormone replacement combinations are Rx and Pregnancy category: X.

content is lower for the first part of the cycle and higher for the last part of the cycle; (3) triphasic—the estrogen content may be the same or may vary throughout the medication cycle; the progestin content may be the same or varies, depending on the part of the cycle. The purpose of the biphasic and triphasic products is to provide hormones in a manner similar to that occurring physiologically. This is said to decrease breakthrough bleeding during the medication cycle. The other type of oral contraceptive is the progestin-only ("mini-pill") product, which contains a small amount of a progestin in each tablet.

Also available are emergency contraceptive kits (Plan B or Preven) containing just four tablets of ethinyl estradiol and levonorgestrel (Preven) or just two tablets of levonorgestrel (Plan B). These products are intended to be used after unprotected intercourse or known or suspected contraceptive failure.

ACTION/KINETICS

The combination oral contraceptives act by inhibiting ovulation due to an inhibition (through negative-feedback mechanism) of LH and FSH, which are required for development of ova. These products also alter the cervical mucus so that it is not conducive to sperm penetration and render the endometrium less suitable for implantation of the blastocyst should fertilization occur.

The estrogen used in combination oral contraceptives is either ethinyl estradiol or mestranol. Ethinyl estradiol is rapidly absorbed; **peak levels:** 2 hr. Mestranol is demethylated to ethinyl estradiol in the liver. **t½:** 6–20 hr. Several different progestins are used in combination oral contraceptives; they are desogestrel, drospirenone, ethynodiol diacetate, levonorgestrel, norethindrone, norethindrone acetate, norgestimate, or norgestrel. Terminal t½'s for progestins varies over a wide range.

The progestin-only products inhibit ovulation in about 50% of users. However, these products also alter the cervical mucus, render the endometrium unsuitable for implantation, lower midcycle LH and FSH peaks, and slow the movement of the ovum through the fallopian tubes. These products contain either norethindrone or norgestrel. This method of contraception is less reliable than combination therapy.

Although oral contraceptives may be associated with serious side effects, a number of noncontraceptive health benefits have been confirmed. These include increased regularity of the menstrual cycle, decreased incidence of dysmenorrhea, decreased blood loss, decreased incidence of functional ovarian cysts and ectopic pregnancies, and decreased incidence of diseases such as fibroadenomas, fibrocystic disease, acute pelvic inflammatory disease, endometrial cancer, and ovarian cancer. OC use has also been associated with a reduction for colorectal cancer use and positive effects on bone mineral density.

USES

Contraception. Prevent pregnancy after unprotected intercourse or a known or suspected contraceptive failure. Ortho Tri-Cyclen: Moderate acne vulgaris in females aged 15 and older who have no contraindications to oral contraceptive therapy, have reached menarche, desire contraception, and who are unresponsive to topical antiacne drugs.

CONTRAINDICATIONS

Thrombophlebitis, history of deep-vein thrombophlebitis, thromboembolic disorders, cerebral vascular disease, CAD, MI, current or past angina, known or suspected breast cancer or estrogen-dependent neoplasm, endometrial carcinoma, hepatic adenoma or carcinoma, undiagnosed abnormal genital bleeding, known or suspected pregnancy, cholestatic jaundice of pregnancy, jaundice with prior tablet use, acute liver disease. Smoking. Lactation.

Note: Yasmin may cause hyperkalemia in high-risk clients. Do not use in clients with conditions that predispose to hyperkalemia (e.g., renal insufficiency, hepatic dysfunction, adrenal insufficiency).

SPECIAL CONCERNS

Cigarette smoking increases the risk of cardiovascular side effects from use of oral contraceptives. Low estrogen-containing oral contraceptives do not increase the risk of stroke in women. There is an increased risk of thromboembolism, stroke, MI, hypertension, hepatic neoplasia, and gallbladder disease. The risk of CV and circulatory disease in OC users is significantly increased in women 35 years and older with other risk factors (e.g., smoking, uncontrolled hypertension, hypercholesterolemia, obesity, diabetes).

Use with caution in clients with a history of hypertension, preexisting renal disease, hypertension-related diseases during pregnancy, familial tendency to hypertension or its consequences, a history of excessive weight gain or fluid retention during the menstrual cycle; these individuals are more likely to develop elevated BP. Use with caution in clients with asthma, epilepsy, migraine, diabetes, metabolic bone disease, renal or cardiac disease, and a history of mental depression. Use with drugs (e.g., barbiturates, hydantoins, rifampin) that increase the hepatic metabolism of oral contraceptives may result in breakthrough bleeding and an increased risk of pregnancy.

Progestin-only products do not appear to have any adverse effects on breastfeeding performance or on the health, growth, or development of the infant.

SIDE EFFECTS

The oral contraceptives have wide-ranging effects. These are particularly important, since the drugs may be given for several years to healthy women. Many authorities have voiced concern about the long-term safety of these agents. Some advise discontinuing therapy after 18–24 months of continuous use. The majority of side effects of oral contraceptives are due to the estrogen component. **CV:** ***MI, thrombophlebitis, venous thrombosis with or without embolism, pulmonary embolism, coronary thrombosis, cerebral thrombosis, arterial thromboembolism, mesenteric thrombosis, thrombotic and hemorrhagic strokes, postsurgical thromboembolism, subarachnoid hemorrhage, cerebral hemorrhage,*** elevated BP, hypertension. **CNS:** Onset or exacerbation of migraine head-aches, depression, headaches, dizziness. **GI:** N&V, bloating, diarrhea, abdominal cramps. **Ophthalmic:** Optic neuritis, retinal thrombosis, steepening of the corneal curvature, contact lens intolerance. **Hepatic:** ***Benign and malignant hepatic adenomas,*** focal nodular hyperplasia, ***hepatocellular carcinoma,*** gallbladder disease, cholestatic jaundice. **GU:** Breakthrough bleeding, spotting, amenorrhea during and after treatment, change in menstrual flow, change in cervical erosion and cervical secretions, ***invasive cervical cancer,*** bleeding irregularities (more common with progestin-only products), vaginal candidiasis, ***ectopic pregnancies in con-traceptive failures, increase in size of preexisting uterine fibroids,*** temporary infertility after discontinuation, breast tenderness, breast enlargement, breast secretion. **Miscellaneous:** Acute intermittent porphyria, photosensitivity, congenital anomalies, melasma, skin rash, edema, increase or decrease in weight, decreased carbohydrate tolerance, increased incidence of cervical *Chlamydia trachomatis,* decrease in the quantity and quality of breast milk.

DRUG INTERACTIONS

Acetaminophen / ↓ Effect of acetaminophen R/T ↑ liver metabolism
Acitretin / Acitretin interferes with effect of progestin-only products
Anticoagulants, oral / ↓ Effect of anticoagulants by ↑ levels of certain clotting factors (however, an ↑ effect of anticoagulants has also been noted in some clients)

Antidepressants, tricyclic / ↑ Effect of antidepressants R/T ↓ liver metabolism
Benzodiazepines / ↑ Effect of alprazolam, chlordiazepoxide, diazepam, and triazolam R/T ↓ in liver breakdown; ↓ Effect of lorazepam, oxazepam, and temazepam R/T ↑ liver breakdown
Beta-adrenergic blockers / ↑ Effect of beta blockers R/T ↓ liver metabolism
H *Black cohosh* Interferes with effect of oral contraceptives
Caffeine / ↑ Effect of caffeine R/T ↓ liver metabolism
Carbamazepine / ↓ Effect of oral contraceptives R/T ↑ liver metabolism
Corticosteroids / ↑ Effect of corticosteroids R/T ↓ liver metabolism
Dexamethasone ↓ Effect of oral contraceptives R/T ↑ liver metabolism
Ethosuximide / ↓ Effect of oral contraceptives R/T ↑ liver metabolism
Felbamate / ↓ Effect of oral contraceptives R/T ↑ liver metabolism
Griseofulvin / ↓ Effect of oral contraceptives R/T ↑ liver metabolism and altered enterohepatic absorption
Hypoglycemics / ↓ Effect of hypoglycemics R/T their effect on carbohydrate metabolism
Insulin / OCs may ↑ insulin requirements
Nevirapine / ↓ Effect of oral contraceptives R/T ↑ liver metabolism
Oxcarbazepine / ↓ Hormone levels due to ↑ liver metabolism
Penicillins, oral / ↓ Effect of oral contraceptives R/T altered enterohepatic absorption
Phenobarbital / ↓ Effect of oral contraceptives R/T ↑ liver metabolism
Phenytoin / ↓ Effect of oral contraceptives R/T ↑ liver metabolism
Primidone / ↓ Effect of oral contraceptives R/T ↑ liver metabolism
Protease inhibitors / ↓ Effect of oral contraceptives R/T ↑ liver metabolism
Pyridoxine / Comcomitant use may ↑ pyridoxine requirements
Rifabutin, Rifampin, Rifapentine / ↓ Effect of contraceptives R/T ↑ liver metabolism
Ritonavir / ↓ Effect of contraceptives R/T ↑ liver breakdown of ethinyl estradiol
H *Saw palmetto* / ↓ Oral contraceptive effect R/T antiestrogenic activity
Selegeline / ↑ Selegeline plasma levels R/T ↓ metabolism
H *St. John's wort* / ↑ Risk of menstrual bleeding due to ↑ liver metabolism of oral contraceptive hormones
Tetracyclines / ↓ Effect of contraceptives R/T altered enterohepatic absorption
Theophyllines / ↑ Effect of theophyllines R/T ↓ liver breakdown
Troleandomycin / ↑ Chance of jaundice
Warfarin / ↑ Risk of clotting

LABORATORY TEST CONSIDERATIONS

↑ Prothrombin, Factors VII, VIII, IX, X; fibrinogen; thyroid-binding globulin (causes ↑ total thyroid hormones as measured by PBI, T_4 by column or radioimmunoassay); corticosteroids; triglycerides and phospholipids; aldosterone; amylase; gamma-glutamyltranspeptidase; iron-binding capacity; sex hormone-binding globulins; transferrin; prolactin; renin activity; vitamin A.

↓ Antithrombin III; free T_3 resin uptake; response to metyrapone test; folate; glucose tolerance; albumin; cholinesterase; haptoglobin; tissue plasminogen activator; zinc, vitamin B12; sex-hormone-binding globulin. Progestin-only products ↓ thyroxine due to ↓ thyroid-binding globulin.

Some progestins may ↑ LDL and ↓ HDL.

DOSAGE

- **TABLETS**

Contraception.

See *Administration/Storage.* Use only low dose tablets; rarely is there a need for tablets containing more than 50 mcg of estrogen.

Emergency contraception.

Take the initial 1 (Plan B) or 2 (Preven) tablets as soon as possible but within

72 hr of unprotected intercourse. A second dose of 1 (Plan B) or 2 (Preven) tablets is taken 12 hr later.

Acne vulgaris.

Ortho Tri-Cyclen: Take 1 hormone-containing tablet daily for 21 days followed by 1 inert tablet daily for 7 days. After 28 tablets have been taken, a new course is started the next day.

NURSING CONSIDERATIONS

SEE ALSO *NURSING CONSIDERATIONS* FOR *ESTROGENS,* AND *PROGESTERONE AND PROGESTINS.*

ADMINISTRATION/STORAGE

1. For combination oral contraceptive products:

• *Sunday start.* If the product is to be started on Sunday, the first tablet should be taken the Sunday following the beginning of menses; if menses begins on Sunday, the first tablet should be taken that day.

• *21-Day regimen.* Count the first day of menstrual bleeding as Day 1. Take 1 tablet/day for 21 days. No tablets are taken for 7 days. Whether menstrual flow has stopped or not, a new 21-day course of therapy is started. This schedule is followed whether flow occurs as expected or whether spotting or breakthrough bleeding occurs during the cycle.

• *28-Day regimen.* To eliminate the necessity to count the days between cycles, many products contain 7 inert or iron-containing tablets. Hormone-containing tablets are taken for the first 21 days followed by 7 days of inert or iron-containing tablets, i.e., a tablet is taken every day.

• *Biphasic and Triphasic products.* The biphasic and triphasic products have varying amounts of estrogen and/or progestin, depending on the stage of the cycle; the client should understand fully how these preparations are to be taken and which tablets are to be taken at various times during the medication cycle. Often tablets are different shapes and/or colors to help with compliance.

2. *Progestin-only products.* The first tablet is taken on the first day of menses; thereafter, 1 tablet is taken daily every day of the year with no interruption between tablet packs.

3. Take tablets at approximately the same time each day.

4. Spotting or breakthrough bleeding may occur for the first 1–2 cycles; report if it continues past this time.

5. For the initial cycle, use an **additional** form of contraception the first week.

6. For emergency contraception:

• Preven also contains a pregnancy test which can be used prior to taking the tablets. If a positive pregnancy test is obtained, the client is not to take the tablets in the kit.

• If vomiting occurs within 1 hr of taking either dose of the medication, the provider should be contacted to discuss whether or not to repeat the dose or take an antinausea medication.

• Emergency contraception tablets are not to be used for ongoing pregnancy protection and are not to be used as a routine form of contraception by women.

7. If it is necessary to switch from combination therapy to progestin-only therapy, take the first progestin-only tablet the day after the last hormone-containing combination therapy tablet is finished. None of the 7 inactive tablets are to be taken. If switching from progestin-only to combination therapy, take the first hormone-containing combination therapy tablet on the first day of menses, even if the progestin-only pack is not finished. If switching to another brand of progestin-only products, start the new brand any time.

8. Non-nursing mothers may begin oral contraceptive therapy at the first postpartum exam (i.e., 4–6 weeks), regardless of whether spontaneous menstruation has occurred. Nursing mothers should not take oral contraceptives until the infant is weaned. Start no earlier than 4–6 weeks after a midtrimester pregnancy termination.

Immediate postpartum use increases the risk of thromboembolism.

ASSESSMENT

1. Document annual physical/internal exams, mammography, and Pap smears.
2. Determine any previous experience with these agents and results.
3. Note any family history of breast or uterine cancer or any existing medical condition that may preclude this drug therapy; note smoking history.
4. Note any abnormal vaginal bleeding. Assess contraceptive needs and check to ensure not pregnant.

CLIENT/FAMILY TEACHING

1. Take tablets exactly as prescribed to prevent pregnancy.
2. If 1 combination therapy tablet is missed, take as soon as remembered or take 2 tablets the next day. As an alternative, take 1 tablet, discard the other missed tablet, and continue as scheduled. Use another form of contraception until menses.
3. If 2 combination therapy tablets have been missed, take 2 tablets as soon as remembered with the next tablet at the usual time; or, take 2 tablets daily for the next 2 days and then resume the regular schedule. Use an additional form of contraception for the remainder of the cycle. If 2 hormone-containing tablets are missed in a row in the third week and the client is on a Sunday start regimen, take 1 tablet every day until Sunday. On Sunday, the rest of the pack is discarded and a new pack of tablets started that same day. If 2 hormone-containing tablets are missed in a row in the third week and the client is a Day 1 starter, discard the rest of the pack and a new pack is started on that day. Menses may not occur during this month; this is expected. If menses does not occur 2 months in a row, contact the provider as pregnancy is possible.
4. If 3 combination therapy tablets are missed and the client is a Sunday starter, she should keep taking 1 tablet/day until Sunday. On Sunday, the rest of the pack is discarded and a new pack started that same day. If the client is a Day 1 starter, the rest of the pack is discarded and a new pack started that same day. Menses may not occur during this month; this is expected. If menses does not occur 2 months in a row, contact the provider as pregnancy is possible. Pregnancy may occur during the 7 days after tablets are missed; thus, use another method of birth control as a back-up for those 7 days.
5. If the client is more than 3 hr late or misses 1 or more progestin-only tablets, she should take the missed tablet as soon as remembered. Then, take tablets at the regular time. A back-up method must be used every time she has intercourse for the 48 hr following the late or missed tablet.
6. Report any missed menstrual periods. If two consecutive periods missed, discontinue therapy until pregnancy ruled out.
7. Report if pain in the legs or chest, respiratory distress, unexplained cough, severe headaches, dizziness, or blurred vision occurs, stop therapy and notify provider immediately.
8. Headaches, dizziness, blurred vision, or partial loss of sight, should be reported immediately.
9. Oral contraceptives decrease the viscosity of cervical mucus, increasing the susceptibility to vaginal infections which are difficult to treat; good hygienic practice is essential.
10. Report if persistent nausea, edema, and skin eruptions develop and last beyond the four cycles, a dose adjustment or different combination may be needed.
11. Alterations in thought processes, depression, or fatigue should be reported; preparations with less progesterone may be needed.
12. Androgenic effects, such as weight gain, increased oiliness of the skin, acne, or hirsutism, may require a change in medication or dosage.
13. Do not take longer than 18 months without medical consultation. Report for yearly Pap smear and physical examination; perform regular BSE (1 week after or 2 weeks before menstrual cycle).

14. Practice another form of contraception if receiving ampicillin, anticonvulsants, phenylbutazone, rifampin, or tetracycline. These may cause intermittent bleeding and interactions could result in pregnancy.
15. Contraceptives interfere with the elimination of caffeine. Limit caffeine consumption to prevent insomnia, irritability, tremors, and cardiac irregularities.
16. If breast-feeding infant, another form of contraception should be used until lactation is well established.
17. **Do not smoke.** Attend formal smoking cessation program.
18. Oral contraceptives do not provide any protection against STDs; use appropriate barrier protection with intercourse.

OUTCOMES/EVALUATE

- Desired contraception; ↓ acne
- Menstrual regularity
- ↓ Blood loss with hormone imbalances

PENICILLINS

SEE ALSO THE FOLLOWING INDIVIDUAL ENTRIES:

Amoxicillin
Amoxicillin and Potassium clavulanate
Ampicillin oral
Ampicillin sodium, parenteral
Ampicillin sodium/Sulbactam sodium
Bacampicillin hydrochloride
Carbenicillin indanyl sodium
Cloxacillin sodium
Dicloxacillin sodium
Mezlocillin sodium
Nafcillin sodium
Oxacillin sodium
Penicillin G sodium for injection
Penicillin G benzathine and procaine combined, intramuscular
Penicillin G benzathine, intramuscular
Penicillin G potassium for injection
Penicillin G procaine, intramuscular
Penicillin V potassium
Piperacillin sodium
Piperacillin sodium and Tazobactam sodium
Ticarcillin disodium
Ticarcillin disodium and Clavulanate potassium

GENERAL STATEMENT

Penicillins may be classifed as: (1) Natural: Penicillin G, Penicillin V. (2) Aminopenicillins: Amoxicillin, Amoxicillin/potassium clavulanate, Ampicillin, Ampicillin/sulbactam, Bacampicillin. (3) Penicillinase-resistant: Cloxacillin, Dicloxacillin, Nafcillin, Oxacillin. (4) Extended spectrum: Carbenicillin, Mezlocillin, Piperacillin, Piperacillin/tazobactam sodium, Ticarcillin, Ticarcillin/potassium clavulanate.

ACTION/KINETICS

The bactericidal action of penicillins depends on their ability to bind penicillin-binding proteins (PBP-1 and PBP-3) in the cytoplasmic membranes of bacteria, thus inhibiting cell wall synthesis. Some penicillins act by acylation of membrane-bound transpeptidase enzymes, thereby preventing cross-linkage of peptidoglycan chains, which are necessary for bacterial cell wall strength and rigidity. Cell division and growth are inhibited and often lysis and elongation of susceptible bacteria occur. Penicillin is most effective against young, rapidly dividing organisms and has little effect on mature resting cells. Depending on the concentration of the drug at the site of infection and the susceptibility of the infectious microorganism, penicillin is either bacteriostatic or bactericidal. Penicillins are distributed throughout most of the body and pass the placental barrier. They also pass into synovial, pleural, pericardial, peritoneal, ascitic, and spinal fluids. Although normal meninges and the eyes are relatively impermeable to penicillins, they are better absorbed by inflamed meninges and eyes. **Peak serum levels, after PO:** 1 hr. **t½:** 30–110 min; protein binding:

20%–98% (see individual agents). Excreted largely unchanged by the urine as a result of glomerular filtration and active tubular secretion.

USES

See individual drugs. Effective against a variety of gram-positive, gram-negative, and anaerobic organisms.

CONTRAINDICATIONS

Hypersensitivity to penicillins, imipenem, β-lactamase inhibitors, and cephalosporins. PO use of penicillins during the acute stages of empyema, bacteremia, pneumonia, meningitis, pericarditis, and purulent or septic arthritis. Use with a history of amoxicillin/clavulanate–associated cholestatic jaundice or hepatic dysfunction. Lactation.

SPECIAL CONCERNS

Use of penicillins during lactation may lead to sensitization, diarrhea, candidiasis, and skin rash in the infant. Use with caution in clients with a history of asthma, hay fever, or urticaria. Clients with cystic fibrosis have a higher incidence of side effects with broad spectrum penicillins. Safety and effectiveness of carbenicillin, piperacillin, and the beta-lactamase inhibitor/penicillin combinations (e.g., amoxicillin/potassium clavulanate, ticarcillin/ potassium clavulanate) have not been determined in children less than 12 years of age. The incidence of resistant strains of staphylococci to penicillinase-resistant penicillins is increasing. Use of prolonged therapy may lead to superinfection (i.e., bacterial or fungal overgrowth of nonsusceptible organisms). Cystic fibrosis clients have a higher incidence of side effects if given extended spectrum penicillins.

SIDE EFFECTS

Penicillins are potent sensitizing agents; it is estimated that up to 10% of the US population is allergic to the antibiotic. Hypersensitivity reactions are reported to be on the increase in pediatric populations. Sensitivity reactions may be immediate (within 20 min) or delayed (as long as several days or weeks after initiation of therapy).
Allergic: Skin rashes (including maculopapular and exanthematous), exfoliative dermatitis, erythema multiforme (rarely, ***Stevens-Johnson syndrome***), hives, pruritus, wheezing, ***anaphylaxis,*** fever, eosinophilia, hypersensitivity myocarditis, ***angioedema,*** serum sickness, ***laryngeal edema, laryngospasm, prostration, angioneurotic edema, bronchospasm, hypotension, vascular collapse, death.*** **GI:** Diarrhea (may be severe), abdominal cramps or pain, N&V, bloating, flatulence, increased thirst, bitter/unpleasant taste, glossitis, gastritis, stomatitis, dry mouth, sore mouth or tongue, furry tongue, black "hairy" tongue, bloody diarrhea, rectal bleeding, enterocolitis, pseudomembranous colitis. **CNS:** Dizziness, insomnia, hyperactivity, fatigue, prolonged muscle relaxation. Neurotoxicity including lethargy, neuromuscular irritability, ***seizures,*** hallucinations following large IV doses (especially in clients with renal failure). **Hematologic:** Thrombocytopenia, leukopenia, ***agranulocytosis,*** anemia, thrombocytopenic purpura, ***hemolytic anemia,*** granulocytopenia, neutropenia, bone marrow depression. **Renal:** Oliguria, hematuria, hyaline casts, proteinuria, pyuria (all symptoms of interstitial nephritis), nephropathy. Electrolyte imbalance following IV use. **Miscellaneous:** Hepatotoxicity (cholestatic jaundice), superinfection, swelling of face and ankles, anorexia, hyperthermia, transient hepatitis, vaginitis, itchy eyes. IM injection may cause pain and induration at the injection site, ecchymosis, and hematomas. IV use may cause vein irritation, deep vein thrombosis, and thrombophlebitis.

OD OVERDOSE MANAGEMENT

Symptoms: Neuromuscular hyperexcitability, convulsive seizures. Massive IV doses may cause agitation, asterixis, hallucinations, confusion, stupor, multifocal myoclonus, seizures, coma, hyperkalemia, and encephalopathy. *Treatment (Severe Al-*

lergic or Anaphylactic Reactions): Administer epinephrine (0.3–0.5 mL of a 1:1,000 solution SC or IM, or 0.2–0.3 mL diluted in 10 mL saline, given slowly by IV). Corticosteroids should be on hand. In those instances where penicillin is the drug of choice, the physician may decide to use it even though the client is allergic, adding a medication to the regimen to control the allergic response.

DRUG INTERACTIONS

Aminoglycosides / Penicillins ↓ effect of aminoglycosides, although they are used together
Antacids / ↓ Effect of penicillins R/T ↓ GI tract absorption
Antibiotics, Chloramphenicol, Erythromycins, Tetracyclines / ↓ Effect of penicillins, although synergism has also been seen
Anticoagulants / ↑ Bleeding risk by prolonging bleeding time if used with parenteral penicillins
Aspirin / ↑ Effect of penicillins by ↓ plasma protein binding
Chloramphenicol / Either ↑ or ↓ effects
Erythromycins / Either ↑ or ↓ effects
Heparin / ↑ Risk of bleeding following parenteral penicillins
Oral contraceptives / ↓ Effect of oral contraceptives
Probenecid / ↑ Effect of penicillins by ↓ excretion
Tetracyclines / ↓ Effect of penicillins

LABORATORY TEST CONSIDERATIONS

↓ Hematocrit, hemoglobin, WBC lymphocytes, serum potassium, albumin, total proteins, uric acid. ↑ Basophils, lymphocytes, monocytes, platelets, serum alkaline phosphatase, serum sodium. ↑ AST, ALT, bilirubin, LDH following semisynthetic penicillins.

DOSAGE

See individual drugs. Penicillins are available in a variety of dosage forms for PO, parenteral, inhalation, and intrathecal administration. PO doses must be higher than IM or SC doses because a large fraction of penicillin given PO may be destroyed in the stomach.

NURSING CONSIDERATIONS

SEE ALSO *GENERAL NURSING CONSIDERATIONS* FOR *ALL ANTI-INFECTIVES*.

ADMINISTRATION/STORAGE

1. IM and IV administration of penicillin causes a great deal of local irritation; thus, inject slowly.
2. IM injections are made deeply into the gluteal muscle. IV injections are usually diluted with an IV infusion.

ASSESSMENT

Assess for allergic reactions; if reaction occurs, stop drug immediately. Allergic reactions are more likely to occur with a history of asthma, hay fever, urticaria, or allergy to cephalosporins.

INTERVENTIONS

1. Detain in an ambulatory care site for at least 20 min after administering to assess for anaphylaxis.
2. Long-acting types of penicillin are for IM use only; may cause emboli, CNS pathology, or cardiac pathology if administered IV.
3. Do not massage repository (long-acting) penicillin products after injection; rate of absorption should not be increased.
4. Rapid administration of IV penicillin may cause local irritation and may precipitate convulsions. With some agents, high-dose therapy may precipitate aplastic anemia.
5. The elderly may be more sensitive to the effects of penicillin than younger people. Calculate dose based on weight and height.
6. Most penicillins are excreted in breast milk and should be prescribed cautiously to nursing mothers.

CLIENT/FAMILY TEACHING

1. Review drugs prescribed, method and frequency of administration, side effects, and expected outcome/goals of therapy.
2. Stop medication and report any S&S of allergic reactions, i.e., rashes, fever, joint swelling, angioneurotic edema, intense itching, and respiratory distress (during therapy and in some cases 7–12 days after therapy).

3. Oral penicillins may cause GI upset. Take with a glass of water 1 hr before or 2 hr after meals to minimize binding to foods.
4. Return for repository penicillin injections as scheduled.
5. Complete the entire prescribed course of therapy, even if feeling well. Incomplete therapy will predispose client to development of resistant bacterial strains. With α-hemolytic *Streptococcus* infection, must take for a minimum of 10 days, and preferably 14 days, to prevent development of rheumatic fever or glomerulonephritis.
6. Report S&S of superinfections (furry tongue, vaginal or rectal itching, diarrhea).
7. Report if S&S do not improve or get worse after 48–72 hr of therapy.

OUTCOMES/EVALUATE

- Symptomatic improvement
- Resolution of infection (↓ fever, ↓ WBCs, ↑ appetite, negative cultures)

PROGESTERONE AND PROGESTINS

SEE ALSO THE FOLLOWING INDIVIDUAL ENTRIES:

Levonorgestrel implants
Medroxyprogesterone acetate
Megestrol acetate
Oral Contraceptives
Progesterone gel

ACTION/KINETICS

Progesterone is the primary endogenous progestin. Progesterone inhibits, through positive feedback, the secretion of pituitary gonadotropins; in turn, this prevents follicular maturation and ovulation or alternatively promotes it for the "primed" follicle. It is required to prepare the endometrium for implantation of the embryo. Once implanted, progesterone is required to maintain pregnancy. Progestins inhibit spontaneous uterine contractions; certain progestins may cause androgenic or anabolic effects. Progestins given PO are rapidly absorbed and quickly metabolized in the liver. **Peak levels, after PO:** 1–2 hr. **t½, after PO:** 2–3 hr during the first 6 hr after ingestion; thereafter, 8–9 hr. **After IM,** effective levels can be maintained for 3–6 months with a **t½** of about 10 weeks. **t½, elimination, gel:** 5–20 min. A major portion is excreted in the urine with a small amount in the bile and feces.

USES

Abnormal uterine bleeding, primary or secondary amenorrhea (used with an estrogen), endometriosis. Alone or with an estrogen for contraception. May also be used in combination with an estrogen for endometriosis and hypermenorrhea. Certain types of cancer. AIDS wasting syndrome (megestrol acetate). Infertility (progesterone gel). *NOTE:* Not to be used to prevent habitual abortion or to treat threatened abortion. *Investigational:* Medroxyprogesterone has been used to treat menopausal symptoms.

CONTRAINDICATIONS

Carcinoma of the breast or genital organs, thromboembolic disease, thrombophlebitis, vaginal bleeding of unknown origin, impaired liver function, cerebral hemorrhage or those with a history of such, missed abortion, as a diagnostic test for pregnancy. Pregnancy, especially during the first 4 months.

SPECIAL CONCERNS

Use with caution in case of asthma, epilepsy, depression, migraine, and cardiac or renal dysfunction.

SIDE EFFECTS

See also individual drugs. Occasionally noted with short-term dosage, frequently observed with prolonged high dosage. **CNS:** Depression, insomnia, somnolence. **GU:** Breakthrough bleeding, spotting, amenorrhea, changes in amount and/or duration of menstrual flow, changes in cervical secretions and cervical erosion, breast tenderness or secretions. **Dermatologic:** Allergic rashes with and without pruritus, acne, melasma, chloasma, photosensitivity, local reactions at the site of injection. *NOTE:* Progesterone is especially irritating at the site of injection, especially aqueous products. **Miscellaneous:** Weight gain or loss, cholestatic jaundice, masculinization of the female fetus, nausea, edema, precipitation of acute intermittent porphyria, pyrexia, hirsutism.

LABORATORY TEST CONSIDERATIONS

Progestins may affect laboratory test results of hepatic function, thyroid, pregnanediol determination, and endocrine function. ↑ Prothrombin and Factors VII, VIII, IX, and X. ↓ Glucose tolerance (especially in diabetic clients).

DOSAGE

See individual drugs. The usual schedule of administration for *functional uterine bleeding, amenorrhea, infertility, dysmenorrhea, premenstrual tension, and contraception* is days 5 through 25 of the menstrual cycle, with day 1 being the first day of menstrual flow.

NURSING CONSIDERATIONS

ASSESSMENT

1. Identify indications for therapy. Assess for any thrombophlebitis, pulmonary embolism, cardiac, liver, or renal dysfunction, cerebral hemorrhage, breast or genital cancers.
2. Monitor VS, ECG, weight, and labs.
3. Note any history of psychic depression or diabetes mellitus. Review family history.
4. Document last menstrual period and absence of pregnancy.

CLIENT/FAMILY TEACHING

1. To avoid gastric irritation and nausea, take with a light snack, in the evening. Take at the same time each day.
2. Gastric distress usually subsides after the first few cycles of the drug; report if these symptoms persist.
3. Report any symptoms of thrombic disorders such as pains in the legs, sudden onset of chest pain, SOB, and coughing.
4. Weigh twice weekly and report any unusual weight gain/edema.
5. Report any yellowing of the skin or sclera (jaundice) which may necessitate discontinuation of the medication, evaluation of LFTs, and possibly a dosage change.
6. Report any unusual bleeding.
7. Progestins may reactivate or worsen psychic depression. Report any mental status changes and the circumstance of the depression.
8. With diabetes, progesterone may alter glucose tolerance and the dosage of antidiabetic medication may need to be adjusted.
9. Report early symptoms of ophthalmic pathology, such as headaches, dizziness, blurred vision, or partial loss of vision, and get a thorough eye exam.
10. Stop smoking; enroll in a formal smoking cessation program.
11. With birth control, injections must be administered every 3 mo to ensure adequate protection.
12. Progestin-only oral contraceptives may be used as early as 3 weeks after delivery in women who partially breast feed and within 6 weeks after delivery in women who fully breast feed.

OUTCOMES/EVALUATE

- Control of abnormal menstrual bleeding; menstrual regularity
- Weight gain with AIDS clients
- Effective contraceptive agent
- Symptomatic improvement in menstrual pain and flow
- ↓ Size/resolution ovarian cyst(s)

PROTON PUMP INHIBITORS

SEE ALSO THE FOLLOWING INDIVIDUAL ENTRIES:

Lansoprazole
Omeprazole
Pantoprazole sodium
Rabeprazole sodium

ACTION/KINETICS

Act to suppress gastric acid secretion by specifically inhibiting the H+/K+ ATPase enzyme system at the secretory surface of gastric parietal cells. This enzyme is the "acid (proton) pump" within the gastric mucosa. Thus, these drugs are classified as proton pump inhibitors as they block the final step of acid production. Both basal and stimulated acid secretion are inhibited. These agents also increase serum pepsinogen levels and decrease pepsin activity.

USES

Treatment or symptomatic relief of gastric and duodenal ulcers, gastroesophageal reflux disease, pathological hypersecretory conditions, and as part of combination therapy to treat *Helicobacter pylori* infections.

CONTRAINDICATIONS

Lactation.

SPECIAL CONCERNS

Symptomatic relief does not preclude gastric malignancy. Safety and efficacy have not been determined in children.

SIDE EFFECTS

See individual drugs. Side effects common to most proton pump inhibitors follow. **CV:** Chest pain, angina, palpitation, hypertension, tachycardia. **CNS:** Anxiety, apathy, confusion, depression, halllucinations, aggravated hostility, nervousness, paresthesia. **Dermatologic:** Rash, urticaria, pruritus, alopecia. **GI:** Anorexia, fecal discoloration, dry mouth, flatulence, gastric fundic gland polyps. **GU:** Hematuria, glycosuria, gynecomastia. **Hematologic:** Anemia, hemolysis. **Metabolic:** Hypoglycemia, gout, weight gain. **Musculoskeletal:** Arthralgia, myalgia. **Miscellaneous:** Epistaxis, taste perversion, tinnitus, fever, malaise.

DRUG INTERACTIONS

See individual drugs. Because of the profound and long-lasting inhibition of gastric acid secretion, these drugs may interfere with absorption of drugs where gastric pH is an important factor in bioavailability (e.g., ampicillin, cyanocobalamin, digoxin, iron salts, ketoconazole).

LABORATORY TEST CONSIDERATIONS

↑ AST, ALT, alkaline phosphatase, bilirubin.

DOSAGE

See individual drugs.

NURSING CONSIDERATIONS

ADMINISTRATION/STORAGE

1. Take with meals.
2. Antacids may be used with proton pump inhibitors.
3. Swallow capsules or tablets whole; do not chew, crush, split, or open.

ASSESSMENT

1. Note indications for therapy, onset, characteristics of symptoms and other agents trialed.
2. Record abdominal assessments, xray (UGI, US, Ba enema), endoscopic findings and *H. pylori results*.
3. Assess LFTs; with some may reduce dose to qod with dysfunction to prevent drug accumulations.
4. List drugs prescribed to ensure none interact or require acidity for metabolism.
5. Determine if pregnant.
6. Identify what may contribute to symptoms i.e. tomato based dishes, peppermint, also consumption of alcohol and tobacco, lying down after eating etc.

CLIENT/FAMILY TEACHING

1. Take as directed with meals. Swallow tablets whole; do not open, crush, chew, or split tablets.
2. Report any unusual bleeding, acid reflux, abdominal pain, severe lightheadedness/diarrhea, rash, worsening of symptoms or lack of effectiveness.
3. Avoid alcohol, NSAIDs, and salicylates; may increase GI upset.
4. Do not perform activities that require mental alertness until drug effects realized.
5. Follow prescribed diet and activities to control S&S of GERD. Drug should be withdrawn once condition cleared/resolved.
6. Review drug associated side effects; report if diarrhea persists.
7. Report any changes in urinary elimination or pain and discomfort.
8. Generally these are for short-term use only as drug inhibits total gastric acid secretion. Side effects of prolonged therapy and suppression of acid secretion alter bacterial colonization and lead to hypochlorhydria

and hypergastrinemia which may cause an increased risk for gastric tumors.

9. Keep all scheduled visits to ensure accurate dosing and drug for symptom control.

OUTCOMES/EVALUATE

- ↓ Intraesophageal acid exposure
- Promotion of ulcer healing; relief of pain
- ↓ gastric acid production

SELECTIVE SEROTONIN REUPTAKE INHIBITORS

SEE ALSO THE FOLLOWING INDIVIDUAL ENTRIES:

Citalopram hydrobromide
Fluoxetine hydrochloride
Fluvoxamine maleate
Paroxetine hydrochloride
Sertraline hydrochloride

ACTION/KINETICS

Antidepressant effect probably due to inhibition of CNS neuronal reuptake of serotonin and to a lesser extent on norepinephrine and dopamine neuronal reuptake. Not related chemically to tricyclic, tetracyclic, or other antidepressants. Slight to no anticholinergic, sedative, or orthostatic hypotensive effects. All are extensively metabolized by the liver.

USES

See individual entries. Drugs may be used for one or more of the following: Depression, obsessive-compulsive disorder, panic disorder, or bulimia nervosa.

CONTRAINDICATIONS

Use in combination with a monoamine oxidase inhibitor (MAOI) or within 14 days of discontinuing a MAOI. Lactation.

SPECIAL CONCERNS

Use with caution in clients with severe hepatic impairment. Use during pregnancy only if clearly needed. Safety and efficacy have not been determined in children less than 18 years of age.

SIDE EFFECTS

See individual drugs. The following side effects have been observed with all selective serotonin reuptake inhibitors:

CNS: Insomnia, somnolence, tremor, anxiety, nervousness, dizziness, drowsiness, decreased libido, agitation, amnesia, emotional lability, activation of mania/hypomania, seizures, suicide. **GI:** N&V, diarrhea or loose stools, dyspepsia, dry mouth, GI bleeding, anorexia, flatulence, gastroenteritis, weight loss or gain. **Dermatologic:** Sweating, acne, photosensitivity. **Miscellaneous:** Hyponatremia, taste perversion.

DRUG INTERACTIONS

See individual drugs. The following drug interactions are possible with any of the selective serotonin reuptake inhibitors.

Aspirin / ↑ Risk of GI bleeding
MAO inhibitors / Serious (and possibly fatal) reactions, including hyperthermia, rigidity, myoclonus, autonomic instability, mental status changes
NSAIDs / ↑ Risk of GI bleeding
H *St. John's wort* / Possible mild serotonin syndrome
Sympathomimetics / ↑ Sympathomimetic effects and ↑ risk of serotonin syndrome
Tricyclic antidepressants / Possible ↑ TCA plasma levels
L-Tryptophan / Both central (headache, sweating, dizziness, agitation, restlessness) and peripheral (GI distress, N&V) toxicity is possible
Warfarin / Altered anticoagulant effects

DOSAGE

See individual drugs.

NURSING CONSIDERATIONS

ASSESSMENT

1. Document indications for therapy, behavioral manifestations, symptom onset, and contributing factors.

2. Assess for dysphoric mood, suicide ideations, and excessive appetite/weight changes.
3. Note sleep disturbances, lethargy, apathy, impaired thought processes, or lack of responses.
4. List drugs currently prescribed to ensure none interact.
5. Monitor ECG, CBC, renal and LFTs; not for use with liver dysfunction.
6. Differentiate type of depression based on diagnostic features related to reactive, major depressive, or bipolar affective disorders.

CLIENT/FAMILY TEACHING

1. May take with or without food as directed.
2. Avoid other unprescribed or OTC agents and alcohol during therapy.
3. Use caution when performing tasks requiring mental alertness or physical coordination until drug effects realized.
4. Increase oral hygiene, take frequent sips of water, suck on hard candy, or chew sugarless gum to maintain a moist mouth. A high-fiber diet, increased fluid intake, exercise, and stool softeners may prevent constipation.
5. May cause postural hypotension. Rise slowly from a sitting or standing position to minimize effects.
6. May alter libido and sexual function.
7. Practice reliable birth control; report if pregnancy suspected.
8. Report any alterations in perceptions, i.e., hallucinations, blurred vision, or excessive stimulations. Watch those recovering from depression for suicidal tendencies; remove firearms from the home.
9. May take 1-4 weeks to notice any change in emotional state; stay on the treatment regimen.
10. Will see provider more often the first 2–3 months; scripts will be for a small dosage to start and to prevent adverse side effects. Obtain number from provider to call for help.
11. Do not stop abruptly at higher dosages; may experience withdrawl S&S.
12. Review when and how to take meds, reportable side effects esp rash or S&S of liver dysfunction (yellow skin, RUQ abd. pain, itching, fatigue and change in stool color) and importance of regular participation in psychotherapy programs when prescribed.

OUTCOMES/EVALUATE

- Understand illness and need for counselling, drug therapy/medical supervision
- ↓ Depression evidenced by improved appetite, renewed interest in outside activities, ↑ socialization, improved sleeping patterns, ↑ energy
- ↓ Anxiety; improved coping skills

ANTIMIGRAINE DRUGS

SEE ALSO THE FOLLOWING INDIVIDUAL ENTRIES:

Almotriptan maleate
Frovatriptan succinate
Naratriptan hydrochloride
Rizatriptan benzoate
Sumatriptan succinate
Zolmitriptan

ACTION/KINETICS

These drugs are selective 5-HT_1 receptor agonists. This receptor is present on human basilar arteries and in the vasculature of the dura mater. It is believed that symptoms of migraine are due to local cranial vasodilation or to the release of vasoactive and proinflammatory peptides from sensory nerve endings in an activated trigeminal system. The selective 5-HT1 agonists combine with 5-HT1B/1D receptors on the extracerebral, intracranial blood vessels that become dilated during a migraine attack. Activation of the receptors causes cranial vessel vasoconstriction, inhibition of neuropeptide release, and reduced transmission in trigeminal pain pathways.

USES

Acute treatment of migraine with or without aura. Use only when a clear diagnosis of migraine has been determined. Drugs are not intended to prevent or reduce the number of migraine attacks. See individual drugs.

CONTRAINDICATIONS
IV use of injectable products (due to possibility of coronary vasospasm). Use in ischemic bowel disease, angina pectoris, history of MI, strokes, TIAs, documented silent ischemia, Prinzmetal's variant angina, in those with signs and symptoms of ischemic heart disease or cornary artery vasospasm, coronary artery disease (or in presence of risk factors for CAD), uncontrolled hypertension. Concurrent use (or within 24 hr of use) of ergotamine-containing products, dihydroergotamine, methysergide; also, MAO inhibitor therapy (or within 2 weeks of discontinuing an MAOI). Within 24 hr of another 5-HT_1 agonist. Use to manage hemiplegic or basilar migraine.

SPECIAL CONCERNS
Use with caution during lactation and in those with diseases that may alter the absorption, metabolism, or excretion of drugs. Safety and efficacy have not been determined in children.

SIDE EFFECTS
See individual drugs. Most common side effects include paresthesia, asthenia, nausea, dizziness, fatigue, pain, chest or neck tightness or heaviness, somnolence, warm sensation, dry mouth, headache, flushing, hot or cold sensation, chest pain. More serious side effects follow:
CV: ***Acute MI, life-threatening disturbances of cardiac rhythm, and death*** within a few hours following use. ***Cerebral hemorrhage, subarachnoid hemorrhage, stroke.*** Vasospastic reactions, including coronary artery vasospasm; peripheral vascular ischemia, colonic ischemia with abdominal pain and bloody diarrhea, hypertension, ***hypertensive crisis.*** **Respiratory:** Nasal and throat irriation, burning, numbness, paresthesia, discharge, pain, soreness (all after using nasal spray). *Hypersensitivity:* ***Severe anaphylaxis/anaphylactoid reactions.*** **Miscellaneous:** Chest, jaw, or neck tightness; pain, tightness, pressure, or heaviness over the precordium. Photosensitivity.

OD OVERDOSE MANAGEMENT
Symptoms: Seizure, tremor, inactivity, extremity erythema, reduced respiratory rate, cyanosis, ataxia, mydriasis, injection site reaction, paralysis. *Treatment:* There are no antidotes. Gastric lavage followed by activated charcoal in overdose. Institute standard supportive measures. If chest pain or other symptoms of angina occur, start ECG monitoring for evidence of ischemia; continue monitoring for 10 or more hours.

DRUG INTERACTIONS
Ergot alkaloids / ↑ Risk of vasospastic reactions; do not use within 24 hr of each other
5-HT_1 agonists / ↑ Risk of vasospastic reactions if two agonists are used within 24 hr of each other
MAO inhibitors / Do not use 5-HT1 agonists within 2 weeks following discontinuation of an MAO inhibitor
Sibutramine / Possible "serotonin syndrome," including symptoms of CNS irritability, motor weakness, shivering, myoclonus, and altered consciousness
Selective serotonin reuptake inhibitors / Possible weakness, hyperreflexia, incoordination

DOSAGE
See individual drugs.

NURSING CONSIDERATIONS

ADMINISTRATION/STORAGE
1. Take a single PO dose with fluids as soon as symptoms of migraine appear. A second dose may be taken if symptoms return, but no sooner than 2 or 4 hours (depending on the drug) following the first dose.
2. If there is no response to the first dose, do not take a second dose without consulting a provider.

ASSESSMENT
1. Note indications for therapy, onset, family history, characteristics of symptoms, and ensure not hemiplegic or basilar migraine type of headaches.

2. Review neurologic exam and CT/MRI results. A clear diagnosis of migraine should be made; the drug should not be given for headaches due to other neurologic events.
3. List drugs currently prescribed to ensure none interact.
4. Assess for any CAD, CABG, uncontrolled HTN, circulation problems, IBD, or history of CVA/TIAs. With increased CAD risk factors give first dose in the office and assess client for adverse effects or have men undergo a stress test and women a thallium stress test.
5. Determine EKG, renal and LFT's; evaluate for dysfunction. Monitor VS; expect transient increases in BP.
6. Some clients may benefit from riboflavin 200 mg /day and magnesium 400-800 mg per day until drug induced diarrhea.
7. Assess for agents that may cause headaches i.e. tetracycline, niacin, nitrates, mg sulfate, red wines, nutrasweet, caffeine, conjugated estrogens etc.

CLIENT/FAMILY TEACHING

1. Take exactly as directed; strictly for migraine headaches. Do not exceed dosage or dosing intervals, do not share meds with another person regardless of symptoms; do not use for other types of headaches.
2. Report any chest pain, SOB, chest tightness, or wheezing.
3. Use caution if driving or performing activities that require mental alertness; may cause dizziness or drowsiness.
4. Drug acts to shrink swollen blood vessels surrounding the brain that cause migraine headaches. Keep a headache diary and identify factors/foods/events that surround migraine headaches. Continue other remedies i.e. noise reduction, reduced lighting, bed rest, that assist to control S&S.
5. Review package insert and do not use with other similar headache meds.
6. Practice reliable contraception; report if pregnancy suspected.
7. Store away from heat, light, and moisture; store in a safe place.
8. Avoid known triggers, i.e., chocolate, cheese, citrus fruit, caffeine, alcohol, missing sleep/meals, etc.
9. Report any unusual side effects, intolerance, or lack of response.

OUTCOMES/EVALUATE

Termination of migraine headaches

SKELETAL MUSCLE RELAXANTS, CENTRALLY ACTING

SEE ALSO THE FOLLOWING INDIVIDUAL ENTRIES:

Baclofen
Carisoprodol
Chlorzoxazone
Cyclobenzaprine hydrochloride
Dantrolene sodium
Diazepam
Methocarbamol
Tizanidine hydrochloride

ACTION/KINETICS

These drugs decrease muscle tone and involuntary movement. Many relieve anxiety and tension as well. Although the precise mechanism of action is unknown, most of these agents depress spinal polysynaptic reflexes. Their beneficial effects may also be attributable to their antianxiety activity. Several of the drugs in this group also manifest analgesic properties.

USES

Musculoskeletal and neurologic disorders associated with muscle spasms, hyperreflexia, and hypertonia, including parkinsonism, tetanus, tension headaches, acute muscle spasms caused by trauma, and inflammation (e.g., low back syndrome, sprains, arthritis, bursitis). They also may be useful in the management of cerebral palsy and multiple sclerosis.

SIDE EFFECTS

See individual drugs.

OD OVERDOSE MANAGEMENT

Symptoms: Often extensions of the side effects. Stupor, ***coma, shock-like syndrome, respiratory depression,*** loss of muscle tone, and impaired deep tendon reflexes may also occur. *Treatment:* Symptomatic. Emesis or gastric lavage (followed by activated charcoal). If necessary, artificial respiration, oxygen administration, pressor agents, and IV fluids may be used. It may be possible to increase the rate of excretion of selected drugs by diuretics (including mannitol), peritoneal dialysis, or hemodialysis.

DRUG INTERACTIONS

CNS depressants (e.g., alcohol, barbiturates, sedatives and hypnotics, and antianxiety agents) / ↑ Sedative and respiratory depressant effects

H *Kava Kava* / Additive effects

DOSAGE

See individual agents.

NURSING CONSIDERATIONS

ADMINISTRATION/STORAGE

1. If unable to swallow, crush tablets or empty capsules into a small amount of fruit juice.
2. If skeletal muscle relaxant is to be discontinued after long-term use, taper the dose to prevent rebound spasticity, hallucinations, or other withdrawal symptoms.
3. Determine the lowest dosage to treat symptoms.

ASSESSMENT

1. Document indications for therapy and characteristics of symptoms. List other agents prescribed and the outcome.
2. Note any prior seizures; may cause loss of seizure control.
3. Assess extent of musculoskeletal and neurologic disorders associated with muscle spasm. Note muscle stiffness, pain, and extent of ROM.
4. Document baseline mental status.

INTERVENTIONS

1. Monitor BP q 4 hr. Supervise ambulation/transfers and ensure safe environment. Sedentary or immobilized clients are more prone to hypotension upon ambulation.
2. Monitor urinary output; evaluate need for drugs to ↑ excretion rate.
3. Document level of mobility (ROM) and comfort (pain level) prior to and following drug administration.
4. Check muscle responses and DTRs for evidence of drug overdose.

CLIENT/FAMILY TEACHING

1. Take with meals to reduce GI upset.
2. If unable to swallow, crush tablets or empty capsules into a small amount of fruit juice.
3. These drugs may impair mental alertness; do not operate dangerous machinery or drive a car until drug effects realized.
4. Do not stop abruptly after prolonged use; may precipitate withdrawal symptoms, rebound spasticity, and hallucinations.
5. Review additional therapies that may be prescribed for muscle spasm (heat, rest, exercise, physical therapy) and importance of adhering to prescribed regimen.
6. Increase fluids and bulk in diet to prevent constipation.
7. Report if the urine becomes dark, the skin or sclera appears yellow, or itching develops.
8. Avoid alcohol and any other CNS depressants. Antihistamines may cause an additive depressant effect.
9. Report persistent nausea, anorexia, or changes in taste perception, as nutritional state may become impaired.
10. Report as scheduled for all lab and medical visits so therapy and symptoms can be evaluated and drug dosage/need assessed.

OUTCOMES/EVALUATE

- Improvement in extent/intensity of muscle spasm and pain
- ↑ ROM with measurable improvement in muscle tone, mobility, and involuntary movements
- Relief of tension headaches

SUCCINIMIDE ANTICONVULSANTS

SEE ALSO THE FOLLOWING INDIVIDUAL ENTRIES:

Ethosuximide
Methsuximide
Phensuximide

ACTION/KINETICS

Suppress the paroxysmal 3-cycle/sec spike and wave activity that is associated with lapses of consciousness seen in absence seizures. Act by depressing the motor cortex and by raising the threshold of the CNS to convulsive stimuli. Rapidly absorbed from the GI tract.

USES

Primarily absence seizures (petit mal). May be given concomitantly with other anticonvulsants if other types of epilepsy are manifested with absence seizures.

CONTRAINDICATIONS

Hypersensitivity to succinimides.

SPECIAL CONCERNS

Safe use during pregnancy has not been established. Use with caution in clients with abnormal liver and kidney function.

SIDE EFFECTS

CNS: Drowsiness, ataxia, dizziness, headaches, euphoria, lethargy, fatigue, insomnia, irritability, nervousness, dream-like state, hyperactivity. Psychiatric or psychologic aberrations such as mental slowing, hypochondriasis, sleep disturbances, inability to concentrate, depression, night terrors, instability, confusion, aggressiveness. Rarely, auditory hallucinations, paranoid psychosis, increased libido, suicidal behavior. **GI:** N&V, hiccoughs, anorexia, diarrhea, gastric distress, weight loss, abdominal and epigastric pain, cramps, constipation. **Hematologic:** Leukopenia, granulocytopenia, eosinophilia, ***agranulocytosis,*** pancytopenia with or without bone marrow suppression, monocytosis. **Dermatologic:** Pruritus, urticaria, erythema multiforme, lupus erythematosus, ***Stevens-Johnson syndrome,*** pruritic erythematous rashes, skin eruptions, alopecia, hirsutism, photophobia. **GU:** Urinary frequency, vaginal bleeding, renal damage, microscopic hematuria. **Miscellaneous:** Blurred vision, muscle weakness, hyperemia, hypertrophy of gums, swollen tongue, myopia, periorbital edema.

OD OVERDOSE MANAGEMENT

Symptoms (Acute Overdose): Confusion, sleepiness, slow shallow respiration, N&V, ***CNS depression with coma and respiratory depression,*** hypotension, cyanosis, hyper- or hypothermia, absence of reflexes, unsteadiness, flaccid muscles. *Symptoms (Chronic Overdose):* Ataxia, dizziness, drowsiness, confusion, depression, proteinuria, skin rashes, hangover, irritability, poor judgment, N&V, muscle weakness, periorbital edema, hepatic dysfunction, ***fatal bone marrow aplasia, delayed onset of coma,*** nephrosis, hematuria, casts. *Treatment:* General supportive measures. Charcoal hemoperfusion may be helpful.

DRUG INTERACTIONS

Succinimides may ↑ effects of hydantoins by ↓ breakdown by the liver.

DOSAGE

Individualized. See individual agents.

NURSING CONSIDERATIONS

SEE ALSO *NURSING CONSIDERATIONS* FOR *ANTICONVULSANTS*.

ASSESSMENT

Document onset and characteristics of seizures. List other therapies prescribed and the outcome.

CLIENT/FAMILY TEACHING

1. Take as directed and do not stop abruptly; may cause an increase in the severity and frequency of seizures.
2. Caution should be exercised while driving or performing other tasks requiring alertness and coordination; initially may cause, dizziness, blurred vision, headaches, N&V, and drowsiness.
3. Alert family to the possibility of transient personality changes, hypochondriacal behavior, and aggressiveness, which should be reported.
4. Report any increase in frequency of seizures or unusual side effects.
5. Any persistent fever, swollen glands, and bleeding gums may signal a blood dyscrasia and require reporting.
6. May discolor urine pinkish brown.
7. Report for CBC, liver and renal function studies as scheduled.

OUTCOMES/EVALUATE

↓ Frequency; ↑ control of seizures

SULFONAMIDES

SEE ALSO THE FOLLOWING INDIVIDUAL ENTRIES:

Mafenide acetate
Sulfacetamide sodium
Sulfadiazine
Sulfamethoxazole
Sulfasalazine
Sulfisoxazole
Sulfisoxazole diolamine
Trimethoprim and Sulfamethoxazole

ACTION/KINETICS

Structurally related to PABA and, as such, competitively inhibit the enzyme dihydropteroate synthetase, which is responsible for incorporating PABA into dihydrofolic acid. Thus, the synthesis of dihydrofolic acid is inhibited, resulting in a decrease in tetrahydrofolic acid, which is required for synthesis of DNA, purines, and thymidine. Are bacteriostatic. Readily absorbed from the GI tract. Distributed throughout all tissues, including the CSF, where concentrations attain 50%–80% of those found in the blood. Metabolized in the liver and primarily excreted by the kidneys. Small amounts are found in the feces, bile, breast milk, and other secretions.

USES

PO, Parenteral. See individual drugs. Uses include urinary tract infections, chancroid, meningitis caused by *Hemophilus influenzae,* meningogoccal meningitis, rheumatic fever, nocardiosis, trachoma, with pyrimethamine for toxoplasmosis, with quinine sulfate and pyrimethamine for chloroquine-resistant *Plasmodium falciparum,* and with penicillin for otitis media.

Ophthalmic. Conjunctivitis, corneal ulcer, and other superficial ocular infections due to susceptible organisms. Adjunct to systemic sulfonamides to treat trachoma.

Vaginal. Sulfanilamide is used to treat *Candida albicans* vulvovaginitis only.

CONTRAINDICATIONS

Hypersensitivity reactions to sulfonamides and chemically related drugs (e.g., thiazides, sulfonylureas, loop diuretics, carbonic anhydrase inhibitors, local anesthetics, PABA-containing sunscreens). Use in infants less than 2 years of age, except with pyrimethamine to treat congenital toxoplasmosis. Use at term during pregnancy. Use in premature infants who are nursing or those with hyperbilirubinemia or G6PD deficiency. Group A beta-hemolytic streptococcal infections.

SPECIAL CONCERNS

Use with caution, and in reduced dosage, in clients with impaired liver or renal function, intestinal or urinary tract obstructions, blood dyscrasias, allergies, asthma, and hereditary G6PD deficiency. Use with caution if exposed to sunlight or ultraviolet light as photosensitivity may occur. Superinfection is a possibility. Use ophthalmic products with caution in clients with dry eye. Safety and efficacy of ophthalmic use in children have not been determined.

SIDE EFFECTS

Systemic.

GI: N&V, diarrhea, abdominal pain, glossitis, stomatitis, anorexia, pseudomembranous enterocolitis, pancreatitis, hepatitis, ***hepatocellular necrosis.*** **Allergic:** Rash, pruritus, photosensitivity, erythema nodosum or multiforme, generalized skin eruptions, ***Stevens-Johnson syndrome,*** conjunctivitis, rhinitis, balanitis. Serum sickness, urticaria, pruritus, exfoliative dermatitis, ***anaphylaxis, toxic epidermal necrolysis*** with or without corneal damage, periorbital edema, conjunctival and scleral injection, allergic myocarditis, decreased pulmonary function with eosinophila, disseminated lupus erythematosus, periarteritis nodosa, arteritis. **CNS:** Headaches, mental depression, ***seizures,*** hallucinations, vertigo, insomnia, apathy, ataxia, drowsiness, restlessness. **Renal:** Crystalluria, toxic nephrosis with oliguria and anuria, elevated creatinine. **Hematologic:** ***Aplastic anemia,*** leukopenia, neutropenia, ***agranulocytosis,*** thrombocytopenia, hemolytic anemia, methemoglobinemia, purpura, hypoprothrombinemia. **Neurologic:** Peripheral neuropathy, polyneuritis, neuritis, optic neuritis. **Miscellaneous:** Jaundice, tinnitus, arthralgia, superinfection, hearing loss, drug fever, pyrexia, chills, lupus erythematosus phenomenon, transient myopia.

By killing the intestinal flora, the sulfonamides also reduce the bacterial synthesis of vitamin K. This may result in ***hemorrhage.*** Administration of vitamin K to clients on long-term sulfonamide therapy is recommended.

• **OPHTHALMIC USE.**

Headache, browache. Blurred vision, eye irritation, itching, transient epithelial keratitis, reactive hyperemia, conjunctival edema, burning and transient stinging. Rarely, ***Stevens-Johnson syndrome,*** exfoliative dermatitis, ***toxic epidermal necrolysis,*** photosensitivity, fever, skin rash, GI disturbances, and bone marrow depression.

OD OVERDOSE MANAGEMENT

Symptoms: N&V, anorexia, colic, dizziness, drowsiness, headache, unconsciousness, vertigo, toxic fever. More serious manifestations include ***acute hemolytic anemia, agranulocytosis,*** acidosis, maculopapular dermatitis, hepatic jaundice, sensitivity reactions, toxic neuritis, ***death*** (several days after the first dose). *Treatment:* Immediately discontinue the drug.

• Induce emesis or perform gastric lavage, especially if large doses were taken.

• To hasten excretion, alkalinize the urine and force fluids (if kidney function is normal). If there is renal blockage due to sulfonamide crystals, catheterization of the ureters may be needed.

• In the event of agranulocytosis, antibiotic therapy is needed to combat infection.

• To treat severe anemia or thrombocytopenia, blood or platelet transfusions are required.

DRUG INTERACTIONS

Anticoagulants, oral / ↑ Drug effects R/T ↓ plasma protein binding
Antidiabetics, oral / ↑ Hypoglycemic effect R/T ↓ plasma protein binding
Cyclosporine / ↓ Effect of cyclosporine and ↑ nephrotoxicity
Diuretics, thiazide / ↑ Risk of thrombocytopenia with purpura
Indomethacin / ↑ Effect of sulfonamides R/T ↓ plasma protein binding
Methenamine / ↑ Chance of sulfonamide crystalluria due to acid urine
Methotrexate / ↑ Risk of drug-induced bone marrow suppression
Phenytoin / ↑ Drug effect R/T ↓ liver breakdown
Probenecid / ↑ Effect of sulfonamides R/T ↓ plasma protein binding
Salicylates / ↑ Effect of sulfonamides R/T ↓ plasma protein binding
Silver products / Incompatible with ophthalmic products
Uricosuric agents / Potentiation of uricosuric action

LABORATORY TEST CONSIDERATIONS

False + or ↑ LFTs (amino acids, bilirubin, BSP), renal function (BUN, NPN, C_{CR}), blood counts, PT, Coombs' test. False + or ↑ urine glucose (copper reduction methods, such as Benedict's solution or Clinitest), protein, urobilinogen.

DOSAGE

See individual drugs.

NURSING CONSIDERATIONS

SEE ALSO *GENERAL NURSING CONSIDERATIONS FOR ALL ANTI-INFECTIVES.*

ADMINISTRATION/STORAGE

1. Do not use ophthalmic solutions if they have darkened or contain a precipitate.
2. Take care to avoid contamination of ophthalmic products.

ASSESSMENT

1. Obtain a thorough nursing and drug history. Note previous sulfonamide therapy and response.
2. Document indications for therapy, type, onset, and characteristics of symptoms. List other agents prescribed and the outcome.
3. Question concerning any condi-

tions that may preclude drug therapy, i.e., intestinal problems, urinary tract obstructions, G6PD deficiency (may precipitate hemolysis), or allergies.
4. Determine if pregnant; drug may be harmful to developing fetus.
5. Monitor CBC, BS, bleeding times, cultures, renal and LFTs.

INTERVENTIONS

1. During drug therapy, assess for any of the following reactions that may require drug withdrawal:
- Skin rashes, abdominal pain, anorexia, irritation of the mouth or tingling of the extremities
- Blood dyscrasias (characterized by sore throat, fever, pallor, purpura, jaundice, or weakness)
- Serum sickness (characterized by eruptions of purpuric spots and pain in limbs and joints); onset 7–10 days after initiation of therapy.
- Early S&S of Stevens-Johnson syndrome (characterized by high fever, severe headaches, stomatitis, conjunctivitis, rhinitis, urethritis, and balanitis [inflammation of the tip of the penis])
- Jaundice, indicating hepatic involvement; onset 3–5 days after initiation of therapy
- Renal involvement (characterized by renal colic, oliguria, anuria, hematuria, and proteinuria)
- Ecchymosis and hemorrhage (caused by decreased synthesis of vitamin K by intestinal bacteria)
- Hemolytic anemia especially in the elderly
- Behavioral changes or acute mental disturbances

2. Monitor I&O and record. Encourage adequate fluid intake to prevent crystalluria. Observe urinalysis for evidence of crystals. Minimum urine output should be 1.5 L/day. Test urine pH to determine excess acidity. Administration of a particularly insoluble sulfonamide may require urine alkalinization (i.e., $NaHCO_3$).
3. If administering long-acting sulfonamides, adequate fluid intake must be maintained for 24–48 hr after the drug has been discontinued.

CLIENT/FAMILY TEACHING

1. Take on time and as prescribed despite feeling better.
2. Do not perform activities that require mental alertness until drug effects realized.
3. May color urine orange-red or brown; not cause for alarm but report.
4. Take with 6–8 oz (180–240 mL) of water and maintain adequate fluid intake for 24–48 hr after therapy.
5. May cause N&V and loss of appetite. Monitor I&O and consume > 2.5 L/day of fluids.
6. Test urine pH and report changes in acidity as additional drug therapy may be necessary.
7. Avoid Vitamin C; may make the urine more acidic and contribute to crystal formation.
8. If also taking anticoagulants, report increased bleeding tendencies.
9. Avoid prolonged exposure to sunlight; may cause a photosensitivity reaction. Wear protective clothing, sunglasses, and sunscreen.
10. Report any changes in vision or hearing. With ophthalmic use, report if no improvement in 5–7 days, if condition worsens, or if pain, redness, itching, or eye swelling occurs.
11. Vaginal intercourse should be avoided when using vaginal products.
12. Report for labs as scheduled; notify provider if symptoms do not improve or worsen after 48–72 hr.

OUTCOMES/EVALUATE

- Negative C&S results (note any organism resistance to sulfonamide)
- Resolution of infection; symptomatic improvement

SYMPATHOMIMETIC DRUGS

SEE ALSO THE FOLLOWING INDIVIDUAL ENTRIES:

Albuterol
Bitolterol mesylate

Brimonidine tartrate
Dobutamine hydrochloride
Dopamine hydrochloride
Ephedrine sulfate
Epinephrine
Epinephrine bitartrate
Epinephrine borate
Epinephrine hydrochloride
Isoetharine hydrochloride
Isoproterenol hydrochloride
Isoproterenol sulfate
Levalbuterol hydrochloride
Levarterenol bitartrate
Mephentermine sulfate
Metaproterenol sulfate
Metaraminol bitartrate
Phenylephrine hydrochloride
Phenylpropanolamine hydrochloride
Pirbuterol acetate
Pseudoephedrine hydrochloride
Pseudoephedrine sulfate
Salmeterol xinafoate
Terbutaline sulfate

ACTION/KINETICS

Adrenergic drugs act: (1) by mimicking the action of norepinephrine or epinephrine by combining with alpha and/or beta receptors (directly acting sympathomimetics) or (2) by causing or regulating the release of the natural neurohormones from their storage sites at the nerve terminals (indirectly acting sympathomimetics). Some drugs exhibit a combination of both effects.

Adrenergic stimulation of receptors will manifest the following general effects:

Alpha-1-adrenergic: / Vasoconstriction, decongestion, constriction of the pupil of the eye, contraction of splenic capsule, contraction of the trigone-sphincter muscle of the urinary bladder.

Alpha-2-adrenergic: / Presynaptic to regulate amount of transmitter released; decrease tone, motility, and secretory activity of the GI tract (possibly involved in hypersecretory response also); decrease insulin secretion.

Beta-1-adrenergic: / Myocardial contraction (inotropic), regulation of heartbeat (chronotropic), improved impulse conduction, ↑ lipolysis.

Beta-2-adrenergic: / Peripheral vasodilation, bronchial dilation; ↓ tone, motility, and secretory activity of the GI tract; ↑ renin secretion.

Beta adrenergic drugs stimulate adenyl cyclase which catalyzes the formation of cyclic AMP from ATP. The formed cyclic AMP inhibits release of mediators from mast cells and basophils that cause hypersensitivity reactions. The increase in cyclic AMP leads to activation of protein kinase A, which inhibits phosphorylation of myosin and lowers intracellular ionic calcium levels causing relaxation.

USES

See individual drugs.

CONTRAINDICATIONS

Tachycardia due to arrhythmias; tachycardia or heart block caused by digitalis toxicity. See individual drugs.

SPECIAL CONCERNS

Use with caution in hyperthyroidism, diabetes, prostatic hypertrophy, seizures, degenerative heart disease, especially in geriatric clients or those with asthma, emphysema, or psychoneuroses. Also, use with caution in clients with coronary insufficiency, CAD, ischemic heart disease, CHF, cardiac arrhythmias, hypertension, or history of stroke. Asthma clients who rely heavily on inhaled beta-2-agonist bronchodilators may increase their chances of death. Thus, use to "rescue" clients but do not prescribe for regular long-term use. Beta-2 agonists may inhibit uterine contractions.

SIDE EFFECTS

See individual drugs; side effects common to most sympathomimetics are listed.

CV: Tachycardia, arrhythmias, palpitations, BP changes, anginal pain, precordial pain, pallor, skipped beats, chest tightness, hypertension. **GI:** N&V, heartburn, anorexia, altered taste or bad taste, GI distress, dry mouth, diarrhea. **CNS:** Restlessness, anxiety, tension, insomnia, hyperkinesis, drowsiness, weakness, vertigo, irritability, dizziness, headache, tremors, general CNS stimulation, nervousness, shakiness, hyperactivity. **Respiratory:** Cough, dyspnea, dry throat, pharyngitis, ***paradoxical bronchospasm,*** irritation. **Other:** Flushing, sweating, ***allergic reactions.***

OD OVERDOSE MANAGEMENT

Symptoms: Following inhalation: Exaggeration of side effects resulting in anginal pain, hypertension, hypokalemia, ***seizures.*** Following systemic use: CV symptoms include bradycardia, tachycardia, palpitations, extrasystoles, ***heart block,*** elevated BP, chest pain, hypokalemia. CNS symptoms include anxiety, insomnia, tremor, delirium, ***convulsions, collapse, and coma.*** Also, fever, chills, cold perspiration, N&V, mydriasis, and blanching of the skin.

Treatment:

- For overdosage due to inhalation: General supportive measures with sedatives given for restlessness. Use metoprolol or atenolol cautiously as they may induce an asthmatic attack in clients with asthma.
- For systemic overdosage: Discontinue or decrease dose. General supportive measures. For overdose due to PO agents, emesis, gastric lavage, or charcoal may be helpful. In severe cases, propranolol may be used but this may cause airway obstruction. Phentolamine may be given to block strong alpha-adrenergic effects.

DRUG INTERACTIONS

Ammonium chloride / ↓ Effect of sympathomimetics R/T ↑ kidney excretion

Anesthetics / Halogenated anesthetics sensitize heart to adrenergics—causes cardiac arrhythmias

Anticholinergics / Concomitant use aggravates glaucoma

Antidiabetics / Hyperglycemic effect of epinephrine may necessitate ↑ dosage of insulin or oral hypoglycemic agents

Beta-adrenergic blocking agents / Inhibit adrenergic stimulation of the heart and bronchial tree; cause bronchial constriction; hypertension, asthma, not relieved by adrenergic agents

Corticosteroids / Chronic use with sympathomimetics may result in or aggravate glaucoma; aerosols containing sympathomimetics and corticosteroids may be lethal in asthmatic children

Digitalis glycosides / Combination may cause cardiac arrhythmias

Furazolidone / ↑ Effects of mixed-acting sympathomimetics

Guanethidine / Direct-acting sympathomimetics ↑ drug effects, while indirect-acting sympathomimetics ↓ effects of guanethidine; also reversal of hypotensive drug effects

H *Indian snakeroot* / Initial significant ↑ BP

Lithium / ↓ Pressor effect of direct-acting sympathomimetics

MAO inhibitors / All effects of sympathomimetics are potentiated; symptoms include hypertensive crisis with possible intracranial hemorrhage, hyperthermia, convulsions, coma; death may occur

Methyldopa / ↑ Pressor response

Methylphenidate / Potentiates pressor effect of sympathomimetics; combination hazardous in glaucoma

Oxytocics / ↑ Chance of severe hypertension

Phenothiazines / ↑ Risk of cardiac arrhythmias

Reserpine / ↑ Risk of hypertension following use of direct-acting sympathomimetics and ↓ effect of indirect-acting sympathomimetics

Sodium bicarbonate / ↑ Effect of sympathomimetics R/T ↓ kidney excretion

Theophylline / Enhanced toxicity (especially cardiotoxicity); also ↓ drug levels

Thyroxine / Potentiation of pressor response of sympathomimetics

Tricyclic antidepressants / ↑ Effect of direct-acting sympathomimetics and ↓ effect of indirect-acting sympathomimetics

DOSAGE

See individual drugs.

NURSING CONSIDERATIONS

ADMINISTRATION/STORAGE

Discard colored solutions.

ASSESSMENT

1. Determine any sensitivity to adrenergic drugs.
2. Note previous experience with drugs in this class and the outcome.
3. Document any history of CAD, tachycardia, endocrine disturbances, or respiratory tract problems.
4. Obtain baseline data regarding general physical condition and hemodynamic status including ECG, VS, PFTs, and lab data and monitor.
5. Document indications for therapy, contributing factors, and anticipated response.

CLIENT/FAMILY TEACHING

1. Review prescribed drug therapy and potential drug side effects.
2. Take exactly as directed. Do not increase the dosage and do not take more frequently than prescribed. Consult provider if symptoms become more severe.
3. Take early in the day to prevent insomnia.
4. Feelings/symptoms of fear or anxiety may be evident; these drugs mimic body's stress response.
5. Avoid all OTC preparations.
6. Stop smoking to preserve current lung function. Attend formal smoking cessation classes.

SPECIAL NURSING CONSIDERATIONS FOR ADRENERGIC BRONCHODILATORS

ASSESSMENT

1. Obtain history and PE prior to starting drug therapy.
2. Note any experience with this class of drugs.
3. Monitor VS; assess CV response.
4. Document lung assessment, ABGs (or O_2 saturation), and PFTs. Note characteristics of cough and sputum production.
5. Evaluate cardiac function and note ejection fraction.

INTERVENTIONS

1. Observe effects on CNS; if pronounced, adjust dosage and frequency of administration.
2. With status asthmaticus and abnormal ABGs, continue to provide oxygen and ventilating assistance even though the symptoms appear to be relieved by the bronchodilator.
3. To prevent depression of respiratory effort, administer oxygen based on client's clinical symptoms and ABGs or O_2 saturations.
4. If three to five aerosol treatments of the same agent have been administered within the last 6–12 hr, with no relief, further evaluation is warranted.
5. If dyspnea worsens after repeated excessive use of the inhaler, paradoxical airway resistance may occur. Be prepared to assist with alternative therapy and respiratory support.

CLIENT/FAMILY TEACHING

1. Review technique for use and care of prescribed inhalers and respiratory equipment. Rinsing of equipment and of mouth after use is imperative in preventing oral fungal infections. Maintain record of peak flow readings and seek medical attention at identified levels.
2. If postural drainage prescribed, review how to cough productively and show family how to clap and vibrate the chest and position the client to promote good respiratory hygiene.
3. Regular, consistent use of the drug is essential for maximum benefit, but overuse can be life-threatening.
4. To improve lung ventilation and reduce fatigue during eating, start inhalation therapy upon arising in the morning and before meals.
5. A single aerosol treatment is usually enough to control an asthma attack. Overuse of adrenergic bronchodilators may result in reduced effectiveness, paradoxical reaction, and death from cardiac arrest.
6. Increased fluid intake will aid in liquefying secretions and removal.
7. Consult provider if dizziness or chest pain occurs, or if there is no relief when the usual dose is used.
8. Avoid OTC preparations and any other unprescribed adrenergic meds.
9. Consult provider if more than three (or prescribed #) aerosol treatments in a 24-hr period are required for relief.

10. If using inhalable meds and bronchodilators, use the bronchodilator first and wait 5 min before using the other medication.
11. **Stop smoking,** avoid crowds during "flu seasons," dress warmly in cold weather and cover mouth with scarf to filter cold air, receive the pneumonia vaccine and seasonal flu shot, and stay in air conditioning during hot, humid days to prevent exacerbations of illness. Identify triggers and practice avoidance.
12. Have family/significant other learn CPR.

TETRACYCLINES

SEE ALSO THE FOLLOWING INDIVIDUAL ENTRIES:

Doxycycline calcium
Doxycycline hyclate
Doxycycline monohydrate
Tetracycline hydrochloride

ACTION/KINETICS

Tetracyclines inhibit protein synthesis by microorganisms by binding to the ribosomal 50S subunit, thereby interfering with protein synthesis. They block the binding of aminoacyl transfer RNA to the messenger RNA complex. Cell wall synthesis is not inhibited. Are mostly bacteriostatic and are effective only against multiplying bacteria. Well absorbed from the stomach and upper small intestine. Well distributed throughout all tissues and fluids and diffuse through noninflamed meninges and the placental barrier. Are deposited in the fetal skeleton and calcifying teeth. **t½:** 7–18.6 hr (see individual agents); increased in the presence of renal impairment. They bind to serum protein (range: 20%–93%; see individual agents). Concentrated in the liver in the bile; excreted mostly unchanged in the urine and feces.

USES

See individual drugs. (1) Infections caused by *Rickettsiae* (Rocky Mountain spotted fever, typhus fever and the typhus group, Q fever, rickettsialpox, and tick fevers); *Mycoplasma pneumonia*; agents of psittacosis and ornithosis; agents of lymphogranuloma venerum and granuloma inguinale; *Borrelia recurrentis.* (2) Gram-negative infections caused by *Haemophilus ducreyi* (chancroid); *Yersinia pestis* and *Francisella tularensis; Bartonella bacilliformis, Bacteroides* species, *Campylobacter fetus, V. cholerae, Brucella* species (with streptomycin). (3) Infections caused by the following microorganisms when testing indicates appropriate susceptibility: *Escherichia coli, Enterobacter aerogenes, Shigella* species, *Acinetobacter calcoaceticus, H. influenzae* (respiratory infections), *Klebsiella* species (respiratory and urinary infections). *Streptococcus* species, including *S. pneumoniae. (Note:* Up to 44% of *S. pyogenes* strains and 74% of *S. faecalis* strains are resistant to tetracyclines. (4) Treatment of trachoma, although the infectious agent is not always eliminated. (5) When penicillin is contraindicated, including infections caused by *Nneisseria gonorrhoeae, Treponema pallidum,* and *T. pertenue* (syphilis and yaws). Also, *Listeria monocytogenes, Clostridium* species, *Bacillus anthracis, Fusobacterium fusiforme, Actinomycetes* species, *N. meningitidis* (IV only). (6) Acute intestinal ambebiasis. (7) PO in adults to treat uncomplicated urethral, endocervical, or rectal infections due to *Chlamydia trachomatis.* (8) PO as adjunctive therapy to treat severe acne. (9) PO with topical agents to treat inclusion conjunctivitis.

CONTRAINDICATIONS

Hypersensitivity. Use during tooth development stage (last trimester of pregnancy, neonatal period, during breast-feeding, and during childhood up to 8 years) because tetracyclines interfere with enamel formation and dental pigmentation. Never administer intrathecally.

SPECIAL CONCERNS

Use with caution and at reduced dosage in clients with impaired kidney function.

SIDE EFFECTS

GI (most common): N&V, thirst, diarrhea, anorexia, sore throat, flatulence, epigastric distress, bulky loose stools. Less commonly, stomatitis, dysphagia, black hairy tongue, glossitis, or inflammatory lesions of the anogenital area. Rarely, pseudomembranous colitis.

• **PO**

Dosage forms may cause esophageal ulcers, especially in clients with esophageal obstructive element or hiatal hernia. *Allergic* (rare): Urticaria, pericarditis, polyarthralgia, fever, rash, pulmonary infiltrates with eosinophilia, ***angioneurotic edema,*** worsening of SLE, ***anaphylaxis,*** purpura. **Skin:** photosensitivity, maculopapular and erythematous rashes,exfoliative dermatitis (rare), onycholysis, discoloration of nails. **CNS:** Dizziness, lightheadedness, unsteadiness, paresthesias. **Hematologic:** Eosinophilia, ***hemolytic anemia,*** neutropenia thrombocytopenia, thrombocytopenic purpura. **Hepatic:** Fatty liver, increases in liver enzymes; rarely, hepatotoxicity, hepatitis, hepatic cholestasis. **Miscellaneous:** Candidal superinfections including oral and vaginal candidiasis, discoloration of infants' and children's teeth, bone lesions, delayed bone growth, abnormal pigmentation of the conjunctiva, pseudotumor cerebri in adults and bulging fontanels in infants.

• **IV**

Administration may cause thrombophlebitis; IM injections are painful and may cause induration at the injection site.

Use of deteriorated tetracyclines may result in Fanconi-like syndrome characterized by N&V, acidosis, proteinuria, glycosuria, aminoaciduria, polydipsia, polyuria, hypokalemia.

DRUG INTERACTIONS

Aluminum salts / ↓ Effect of tetracyclines R/T ↓ GI tract absorption
Antacids, oral / ↓ Effect of tetracyclines R/T ↓ GI tract absorption
Anticoagulants, oral / IV tetracyclines ↑ hypoprothrombinemia
Bismuth salts / ↓ Effect of tetracyclines R/T ↓ GI tract absorption
H *Bromelain* / ↑ Plasma tetracycline levels
Bumetanide / ↑ Risk of kidney toxicity
Calcium salts / ↓ Effect of tetracyclines R/T ↓ GI tract absorption
Cimetidine / ↓ Effect of tetracyclines R/T ↓ GI tract absorption
Contraceptives, oral / ↓ Effect of oral contraceptives
Digoxin / ↑ Bioavailability of digoxin
Diuretics, thiazide / ↑ Risk of kidney toxicity
Ethacrynic acid / ↑ Risk of kidney toxicity
Furosemide / ↑ Risk of kidney toxicity
Insulin / May ↓ insulin requirements
Iron preparations / ↓ Effect of tetracyclines R/T ↓ GI tract absorption
Lithium / Either ↑ or ↓ drug levels
Magnesium salts / ↓ Effect of tetracyclines R/T ↓ GI tract absorption
Methoxyflurane / ↑ Risk of kidney toxicity
Penicillins / Tetracyclines may mask bactericidal effect of penicillins
Sodium bicarbonate / ↓ Effect of tetracyclines R/T ↓ GI tract absorption
Zinc salts / ↓ Effect of tetracyclines R/T ↓ GI tract absorption

LABORATORY TEST CONSIDERATIONS

False + or ↑ urinary catecholamines and urinary protein (degraded); ↑ coagulation time. False – or ↓ urinary urobilinogen, glucose tests (see *Nursing Considerations*). Prolonged use or high doses may change liver function tests and WBC counts.

DOSAGE

See individual drugs.

NURSING CONSIDERATIONS

SEE ALSO *GENERAL NURSING CONSIDERATIONS* FOR *ALL ANTI-INFECTIVES.*

ADMINISTRATION/STORAGE

1. Do not use outdated or deteriorated drugs as a Fanconi-like syndrome may occur (see *Side Effects*).
2. Administer IM into large muscle mass to avoid extravasation into subcutaneous or fatty tissue.

3. Continue treatment for 24–48 hr after symptoms and fever subside. Treat all infections due to group A β-hemolytic streptococci for 10 or more days.
IV 4. Avoid rapid IV administration.
5. Prolonged IV use may cause thrombophlebitis.

ASSESSMENT

1. Determine any drug allergens or sensitivity. IM form contains procaine HCl.
2. Document indications for therapy, onset, and characteristics of symptoms. List other agents trialed and the outcome.
3. Note any colitis or other bowel problems.
4. If pregnant, document trimester.
5. Monitor VS, weight, CBC, BUN, creatinine, electrolytes, and cultures. Assess for impaired kidney function.

INTERVENTIONS

1. Monitor VS and I&O. Maintain adequate I&O because renal dysfunction may result in drug accumulation, leading to toxicity. With impaired renal function assess for increased BUN, acidosis, anorexia, N&V, weight loss, and dehydration; latent symptoms may appear.
2. To prevent or treat pruritus ani, cleanse anal area with water several times a day and/or after each bowel movement. Observe for symptoms of enterocolitis, such as diarrhea, pyrexia, abdominal distention, and scanty urine; may need to discontinue drug and try another antibiotic.
3. If GI disturbances occur, avoid antacids that contain calcium, magnesium, or aluminum. May take with a light meal to reduce distress. An alternative would be to reduce the dose but increase the administration frequency.
4. Assess with IV therapy for N&V, chills, fever, and hypertension resulting from too rapid administration or an excessively high dose; slow rate and report. Observe infant for bulging fontanelle, which may also be caused by a too rapid infusion rate.
5. Side effects such as sore throat, dysphagia, fever, dizziness, hoarseness, and inflammation of mucous membranes or candidal superinfections may occur.
6. Assess for altered level of consciousness or other CNS disturbances with impaired hepatic or renal function; may cause toxicity.
7. May cause onycholysis (loosening or detachment of the nail from the nail bed) or discoloration.

CLIENT/FAMILY TEACHING

1. Take on an empty stomach at least 1 hr before or 2 hr after meals. Withhold antacids, iron salts, dairy foods, and other foods high in calcium for at least 2 hr after PO administration. Do not take with milk, cheese, ice cream or yogurt.
2. Zinc tablets or vitamin preparations containing zinc may interfere with drug absorption. Food sources high in zinc that should be avoided include oysters, fresh and raw; cooked lobster; dry oat flakes; steamed crabs; veal; and liver.
3. Avoid direct or artificial sunlight, which can cause a severe sunburn-like reaction; report if erythema occurs. Wear protective clothing, sunglasses, and a sunscreen for up to 3 weeks following therapy.
4. Tetracyclines interfere with formation of tooth enamel and dental pigmentation from the third trimester of pregnancy through age 8.
5. Prevent or treat pruritus ani by cleansing the anal area with water several times a day and/or after each bowel movement.
6. Use alternative method of birth control, as drug may interfere with oral contraceptives; may also cause a vaginal infection.
7. Take only as directed and complete full prescription. Discard any unused capsules to prevent reaction from deteriorated drugs.
8. Report loss of effectiveness or lack or response.

OUTCOMES/EVALUATE

- Resolution of infection (↓ temperature, ↓ WBCs, ↑ appetite)

- Symptomatic improvement
- Negative culture reports

THYROID DRUGS

SEE ALSO THE FOLLOWING INDIVIDUAL ENTRIES:

Levothyroxin sodium
Liothyronine sodium
Liotrix

ACTION/KINETICS

The thyroid manufactures two active hormones: thyroxine and triiodothyronine, both of which contain iodine. Thyroid hormones are released into the bloodstream where they are bound to protein. Synthetic derivatives include liothyronine (T_3), levothyronine (T_4), and liotrix (a 4:1 mixture of T_4 and T_3). Thyroid hormones regulate growth by controlling protein synthesis and regulating energy metabolism by increasing the resting or basal metabolic rate. This increases respiratory rate; body temperature; CO; oxygen consumption; HR; blood volume; enzyme system activity; rate of fat, carbohydrate, and protein metabolism; and growth and maturation. Excess thyroid hormone causes a decrease in TSH, and a lack of thyroid hormone causes an increase in the production and secretion of TSH. Normally, the ratio of T_4 to T_3 released from the thyroid gland is 20:1 with about 35% of T_4 being converted in the periphery (e.g., kidney, liver) to T_3.

USES

Replacement or supplemental therapy in hypothyroidism due to all causes except transient hypothyroidism during the recovery phase of subacute thyroiditis. To treat or prevent euthyroid goiters, including thyroid nodules, subacute or chronic lymphocytic thyroiditis, multinodular goiter, and to manage thyroid cancer. With antithyroid drugs for thyrotoxicosis (to prevent goiter or hypothyroidism). Diagnostically to differentiate suspected hyperthyroidism from euthyroidism. The treatment of choice for hypothyroidism is usually T_4 because of its consistent potency and its prolonged duration of action although it does have a slow onset and its effects are cumulative over several weeks.

CONTRAINDICATIONS

Uncorrected adrenal insufficiency, acute MI, hyperthyroidism, and thyrotoxicosis. When hypothyroidism and adrenal insufficiency coexist unless treatment with adrenocortical steroids is initiated first. To treat obesity or infertility

SPECIAL CONCERNS

Geriatric clients may be more sensitive to the usual adult dosage of these hormones. Use with extreme caution in the presence of angina pectoris, hypertension, and other CV diseases, renal insufficiency, and ischemic states. Use with caution during lactation.

SIDE EFFECTS

Thyroid preparations have cumulative effects, and overdosage (e.g., symptoms of hyperthyroidism) may occur.

CV: Arrhythmias, palpitations, angina, increased HR and pulse pressure, ***cardiac arrest,*** aggravation of CHF. **GI:** Cramps, diarrhea, N&V, appetite changes. **CNS:** Headache, nervousness, mental agitation, irritability, insomnia, tremors. **Miscellaneous:** Weight loss, hyperhidrosis, excessive warmth, irregular menses, heat intolerance, fever, dyspnea, allergic skin reactions (rare). Decreased bone density in pre- and postmenopausal women following long-term use of levothyroxine.

OD OVERDOSE MANAGEMENT

Symptoms: Signs and symptoms of hyperthyroidism including headache, irritability, sweating, tachycardia, nervousness, increased bowel motility, palpitations, vomiting, psychosis, menstrual irregularities, ***seizures,*** fever. Production or aggravation of angina or CHF, ***shock, arrhythmias, cardiac failure.***

DRUG INTERACTIONS

Anticoagulants / ↑ Effect of anticoagulants by ↑ hypoprothrombinemia

Antidepressants, tricyclic / ↑ Effect of antidepressants and ↑ effect of thyroid
Antidiabetic agents / Hyperglycemic effect of thyroid preparations may necessitate ↑ in dose of antidiabetic agent
Beta-adrenergic blockers / ↓ Effect of beta blockers when the hypothyroid state is converted to the euthyroid state
Calcium salts / ↓ Thyroid absorption from the GI tract
Cholestyramine / ↓ Effect of thyroid hormone R/T ↓ GI tract absorption
Colestipol / ↓ Effect of thyroid hormone R/T ↓ GI tract absorption
Corticosteroids / Thyroid preparations ↑ tissue demands for corticosteroids. Adrenal insufficiency must be corrected with corticosteroids before administering thyroid hormones. In clients already treated for adrenal insufficiency, dosage of corticosteroids must be increased when initiating therapy with thyroid drug
Digitalis compounds / ↓ Effect of digitalis, with worsening of arrhythmias or CHF
Epinephrine / CV effects ↑ by thyroid preparations
Estrogens / May ↑ requirements for thyroid hormone
Ketamine / Concomitant use may result in severe hypertension and tachycardia
Levarterenol / CV effects ↑ by thyroid preparations
Phenytoin / ↑ Effect of thyroid hormone by ↓ plasma protein binding
Salicylates / Salicylates compete for thyroid-binding sites on protein
H *Soy* / ↓ Absorption of supplemental thyroid hormones; space doses 2 hr apart
Theophylline / ↓ Theophylline clearance in hypothyroid client is returned to normal when euthyroid state is reached

LABORATORY TEST CONSIDERATIONS

Alter thyroid function tests. ↑ PT. ↓ Serum cholesterol. A large number of drugs alter thyroid function tests.

DOSAGE

See individual hormone products.

NURSING CONSIDERATIONS

ADMINISTRATION/STORAGE

1. Initiate treatment with small doses that are gradually increased.
2. A childs dosage may be the same as the dosage for an adult.
3. Due to differences from one brand of drug to another, brand interchange is not recommended without consulting with provider or pharmacist. Use caution to prevent overdosage or relapse.
4. Store in a cool, dark place away from moisture and light.

ASSESSMENT

1. Perform a thorough history, documenting onset and characteristics of symptoms and thyroid function tests (TFTs).
2. Review all meds currently receiving to be sure none interacts with antithyroid drug; especially antidiabetic or anticoagulant therapy.
3. Assess clinical presentation noting S&S consistent with hypothyroidism (i.e., fatigue, lethargy, weight gain, puffy face and eyelids, large tongue, thyroid nodules, cold intolerance, hair loss, and cardiomegaly).
4. Assess general physical condition (age, weight, disease severity/duration) and note angina, cardiac or other health problems.
5. Obtain/monitor ECG, labs, and TFTs.

INTERVENTIONS

1. Monitor thyroid function studies closely (for reduced T_3, T_4; ↑ radioimmunoassay of TSH).
2. Observe for drug side effects; report complaints of headache, insomnia, and tremors.
3. With anticoagulant therapy observe for purpura or ↑ bleeding. Monitor PT/PTT closely; anticoagulant potentiated by thyroid preparations.
4. Report any symptoms or history of CAD. Monitor VS and cardiac rhythms; report if HR > 100 bpm.
5. Note general response to therapy. Complaints of abdominal cramps,

weight gain, edema, dyspnea, palpitations, angina, fatigue, or ↑ pallor may indicate cardiac problems.
6. Monitor weights. Observe for heat intolerance and excessive weight loss.
7. Note agent prescribed; thyroid extracts from hog or sheep do not have as predictable a response as the synthetic agents, may see more reactions. Animal derivatives are less stable and will degrade with exposure to moisture.
8. Stop drug therapy 4 weeks before radioimmunoassay.

CLIENT/FAMILY TEACHING

1. Drug must be taken only under medical supervision and must be taken for life.
2. Side effects may not appear for 4–6 weeks after the start of therapy or when dosage is increased.
3. Take in a single morning dose, at the same time each day, to reduce the likelihood of insomnia.
4. Do not substitute or change brands without approval.
5. Record BP, pulse, and weight for review at each visit, to evaluate effectiveness of drug therapy.
6. Any excessive weight loss, palpitations, leg cramps, nervousness, or insomnia requires immediate reporting, as dosage may be too high.
7. Carefully monitor child's growth and chart.
8. With diabetes, thyroid preparations may require adjustment of insulin dosage. Monitor BS closely and report changes.
9. Certain foods, such as cabbage, turnips, pears, and peaches, are goitrogenic and may alter the requirements for thyroid hormone. Consult dietitian to discuss diet and assist with selecting foods according to increased energy demands resulting from the therapy.
10. Thyroid hormones increase client's toxicity to iodine. Therefore avoid foods high in iodine (dried kelp, iodized salt, saltwater fish/shellfish), multivitamins, dentifrices, and other nonprescription meds containing iodine.
11. Thyroid preparations potentiate the action of anticoagulants; if receiving anticoagulant therapy, report excessive bleeding.
12. Keep a record of menstrual cycles and report changes.
13. Children may experience temporary hair loss.
14. After several weeks of therapy, report if irritability, nervousness, and excitability occur; may indicate overdosage.
15. Report as scheduled for follow-up visits and lab tests.

OUTCOMES/EVALUATE

- Desired weight; normal sleep patterns
- TFTs within desired range
- Normal metabolism evidenced by ↑ mental alertness, improvement in hair and skin condition, ↓ fatigue, ↓ panic attacks, normal growth/development, normal HR and bowel function

TRANQUILIZERS/ ANTIMANIC DRUGS/ HYPNOTICS

SEE ALSO THE FOLLOWING INDIVIDUAL ENTRIES:

Alprazolam
Buspirone hydrochloride
Chlordiazepoxide
Clorazepate dipotassium
Diazepam
Estazolam
Flurazepam hydrochloride
Hydroxyzine hydrochloride
Hydroxyzine pamoate
Lithium carbonate
Lithium citrate
Lorazepam
Meprobamate
Midazolam hydrochloride
Oxazepam
Temazepam
Triazolam
Zaleplon
Zolpidem tartrate

ACTION/KINETICS

Benzodiazepines are the major antianxiety agents. They are thought to affect the limbic system and reticular formation to reduce anxiety by increasing or facilitating the inhibitory neurotransmitter activity of GABA. Two benzodiazepine receptor subtypes have been identified in the brain–BZ_1 and BZ_2. Receptor subtype BZ_1 is believed to be associated with sleep mechanisms, whereas receptor subtype BZ_2 is associated with memory, motor, sensory, and cognitive function. When used for 3–4 weeks for sleep, certain benzodiazepines may cause REM rebound when discontinued. Meprobamate and the benzodiazepines also possess varying degrees of anticonvulsant activity, skeletal muscle relaxation, and the ability to alleviate tension. The benzodiazepines generally have long half-lives (1–8 days); thus cumulative effects can occur. Several of the benzodiazepines are metabolized to active metabolites in the liver, which prolongs their duration of action. Benzodiazepines are widely distributed throughout the body. Approximately 70%–99% of an administered dose is bound to plasma protein. Metabolites of benzodiazepines are excreted through the kidneys. All tranquilizers have the ability to cause psychologic and physical dependence. Benzodiazepines have a wide margin of safety between therapeutic and toxic doses.

USES

See individual drugs. Depending on the drug, used as antianxiety agents, hypnotics, anticonvulsants, and muscle relaxants. Many drugs also have special uses (see individual drugs).

CONTRAINDICATIONS

Hypersensitivity, acute narrow-angle glaucoma, psychoses, primary depressive disorder, psychiatric disorders in which anxiety is not a signficiant symptom.

SPECIAL CONCERNS

Use with caution in impaired hepatic or renal function and in the geriatric or debilitated client. Use during lactation may cause sedation, weight loss, and possibly feeding difficulties in the infant. Geriatric clients may be more sensitive to the effects of benzodiazepines; symptoms may include oversedation, dizziness, confusion, or ataxia. When used for insomnia, rebound sleep disorders may occur following abrupt withdrawal of certain benzodiazepines.

SIDE EFFECTS

CNS: Drowsiness, fatigue, confusion, ataxia, sedation, dizziness, vertigo, depression, apathy, lightheadedness, delirium, headache, lethargy, disorientation, hypoactivity, crying, anterograde amnesia, slurred speech, stupor, ***coma,*** fainting, difficulty in concentration, euphoria, nervousness, irritability, akathisia, hypotonia, vivid dreams, "glassy-eyed," hysteria, ***suicide attempt,*** psychosis. Paradoxical excitement manifested by anxiety, acute hyperexcitability, increased muscle spasticity, insomnia, hallucinations, sleep disturbances, rage, and stimulation. **GI:** Increased appetite, constipation, diarrhea, anorexia, N&V, weight gain or loss, dry mouth, bitter or metallic taste, increased salivation, coated tongue, sore gums, difficulty in swallowing, gastritis, fecal incontinence. **Respiratory:** ***Respiratory depression and sleep apnea,*** especially in clients with compromised respiratory function. **Dermatologic:** Urticaria, rash, pruritus, alopecia, hirsutism, dermatitis, edema of ankles and face. **Endocrine:** Increased or decreased libido, gynecomastia, menstrual irregularities. **GU:** Difficulty in urination, urinary retention, incontinence, dysuria, enuresis. **CV:** Hypertension, hypotension, bradycardia, tachycardia, palpitations, edema, ***CV collapse.*** **Hematologic:** Anemia, ***agranulocytosis,*** leukopenia, eosinophilia, thrombocytopenia. **Ophthalmologic:** Diplopia, conjunctivitis, nystagmus, blurred vision. **Miscellaneous:** Joint pain, lymphadenopathy, muscle cramps, paresthesia, dehydration, lupus-like symptoms, sweating, SOB, flushing, hiccoughs, fever, hepatic dysfunction. **Following IM use:** Redness, pain, burning. **Following IV use:** Thrombosis and phlebitis at site.

OD OVERDOSE MANAGEMENT

Symptoms: Severe drowsiness, confusion with reduced or absent reflexes, tremors, slurred speech, staggering, hypotension, SOB, labored breathing, ***respiratory depression,*** impaired coordination, ***seizures,*** weakness, slow HR, ***coma.*** *NOTE:* Geriatric clients, debilitated clients, young children, and clients with liver disease are more sensitive to the CNS effects of benzodiazepines. *Treatment:* Supportive therapy. In the event of an overdose of a benzodizepine, have a benzodiazepine antagonist (flumazenil) readily available. Gastric lavage, provided that an ET tube with an inflated cuff is used to prevent aspiration of vomitus. Emesis only if drug ingestion was recent and client is fully conscious. Activated charcoal and saline cathartic may be given after emesis or lavage. Maintain adequate respiratory function. Reverse hypotension by IV fluids, norepinephrine, or metaraminol. **Do not** treat excitation with barbiturates.

DRUG INTERACTIONS

Alcohol / Potentiation or addition of CNS depressant effects. Concomitant use may lead to drowsiness, lethargy, stupor, respiratory collapse, coma, or death
Anesthetics, general / See *Alcohol*
Antacids / ↓ Rate of absorption of benzodiazepines
Antidepressants, tricyclic / Concomitant use with benzodiazepines may cause additive sedative effect and/or atropine-like side effects
Antihistamines / See *Alcohol*
Barbiturates / See *Alcohol*
Cimetidine / ↑ Effect of benzodiazepines R/T ↓ liver breakdown
CNS depressants / See *Alcohol*
Digoxin / Benzodiazepines ↑ serum digoxin levels
Disulfiram / ↑ Effect of benzodiazepines by ↓ liver breakdown
Erythromycin / ↑ Effect of benzodiazepines by ↓ liver breakdown
Fluoxetine / ↑ Effect of benzodiazepines R/T ↓ liver breakdown
Isoniazid / ↑ Effect of benzodiazepines R/T ↓ liver breakdown
H *Kava kava* / Additive CNS depressant effect
Ketoconazole / ↑ Effect of benzodiazepines R/T ↓ liver breakdown
Levodopa / Effect may be ↓ by benzodiazepines
Metoprolol / ↑ Effect of benzodiazepines R/T ↓ liver breakdown
Narcotics / See *Alcohol*
Neuromuscular blocking agents / Benzodiazepines may ↑, ↓, or have no effect on the action of neuromuscular blocking agents
Oral contraceptives / ↑ Effect of benzodiazepines R/T ↓ liver breakdown; or, ↑ rate of clearance of benzodiazepines that undergo glucuronidation (e.g., lorazepam, oxazepam)
Phenothiazines / See *Alcohol*
Phenytoin / Concomitant use with benzodiazepines may cause ↑ effect of phenytoin R/T ↓ liver breakdown
Probenecid / ↑ Effect of selected benzodiazepines R/T ↓ liver breakdown
Propoxyphene / ↑ Effect of benzodiazepines R/T ↓ liver breakdown
Propranolol / ↑ Effect of benzodiazepines R/T ↓ liver breakdown
Ranitidine / May ↓ absorption of benzodiazepines from the GI tract
Rifampin / ↓ Effect of benzodiazepines R/T ↑ liver breakdown
Sedative-hypnotics, nonbarbiturate / See *Alcohol*
Theophyllines / ↓ Sedative effect of benzodiazepines
H *Valerian* / Additive CNS depressant effect
Valproic acid / ↑ Effect of benzodiazepines R/T ↓ liver breakdown

LABORATORY TEST CONSIDERATIONS

↑ AST, ALT, LDH, alkaline phosphatase.

DOSAGE

See individual drugs.

NURSING CONSIDERATIONS

ADMINISTRATION/STORAGE

1. Persistent drowsiness, ataxia, or visual disturbances may require dosage adjustment.
2. Lower dosage is usually indicated for older clients. For example, diazepam, 3 mg or more equivalents/day, increases the risk of hip fracture in the elderly.
3. GI effects are decreased when drugs are given with meals or shortly afterward.
4. Withdraw drugs gradually.

ASSESSMENT

1. Document indications for therapy, onset of symptoms, and behavioral manifestations. Note any prior treatments, what was used, for how long, and the outcome.
2. List drugs currently prescribed to ensure none interact unfavorably. Note any adverse reactions to this class of drugs.
3. Assess life-style and general level of health; note any situations that may contribute to these symptoms.
4. Assess the manner in which client responds to questions/ problems.
5. Monitor CBC, liver and renal function studies; assess for blood dyscrasias or impaired function.
6. Review physical and history for any contraindications to therapy.

INTERVENTIONS

1. Document any symptoms consistent with overdosage.
2. Report any complaints of sore throat (other than those caused by NG or ET tubes), fever, or weakness and assess for blood dyscrasias; check CBC.
3. Monitor BP before and after IV dose of antianxiety medication. Keep recumbent for 2–3 hr after IV administration.
4. Administer the lowest possible effective dose, especially if elderly or debilitated.
5. When hospitalized and administered PO, remain until swallowed.
6. If client exhibits ataxia, or weakness or lack of coordination when ambulating, provide supervision/assistance. Use side rails once in bed and identify at risk for falls.
7. Note any S&S of cholestatic jaundice: nausea, diarrhea, upper abdominal pain, or the presence of high fever or rash; check LFTs.
8. Report if yellowing of sclera, skin, or mucous membranes evident (late sign of cholestatic jaundice and biliary tract obstruction); hold if overly sleepy/confused or becomes comatose.
9. With suicidal tendencies, anticipate drug will be prescribed in small doses. Report signs of increased depression immediately.
10. If history of alcoholism or if taking excessive quantities of drug, carefully supervise amount of drug prescribed and dispensed. Assess for manifestations of ataxia, slurred speech, and vertigo (symptoms of chronic intoxication and that client may be exceeding dose).
11. Note any evidence of physical or psychologic dependence. Assess frequency and quantity of refills.

CLIENT/FAMILY TEACHING

1. These drugs may reduce ability to handle potentially dangerous equipment, such as cars and machinery.
2. Take most of daily dose at bedtime, with smaller doses during the waking hours to minimize mental/motor impairment.
3. Avoid alcohol while taking antianxiety agents. Alcohol potentiates the depressant effects of both the alcohol and the medication.
4. Do not take any unprescribed or OTC medications without approval.
5. Arise slowly from a supine position and dangle legs over side of the bed before standing. If feeling faint sit/lie down immediately and lower the head.
6. Allow extra time to prepare for daily activities; take precautions before arising, to reduce one source of anxiety and stress.
7. Do not stop taking drug suddenly. Any sudden withdrawal after prolonged therapy or after excessive use

may cause a recurrence of the preexisting symptoms of anxiety. It may also cause a withdrawal syndrome, manifested by increased anxiety, anorexia, insomnia, vomiting, ataxia, muscle twitching, confusion, and hallucinations. May also develop seizures and convulsions.

8. Identify/practice relaxation techniques that may assist in lowering anxiety levels.

9. These drugs are generally for short-term therapy; follow-up is imperative to evaluate response and the need for continued therapy.

10. Attend appropriate counselling sessions as condition and length of therapy dictate.

OUTCOMES/EVALUATE

- Symptomatic improvement with ↓ anxiety/tension episodes
- Effective coping
- ↓ Frequency/intensity of muscle spasms/tremor
- Improved sleeping patterns; less frequent early morning awakenings
- Control of seizures
- Control of alcohol withdrawal symptoms

VACCINES

SEE TABLES 3, 4, AND 5.

GENERAL STATEMENT

Vaccines have played an important role in the health and life span of our population. They have been in use over 200 years, but since World War II, once the importance of disease prevention became evident, research into the area of vaccine development exploded.

Use of a vaccine (or actually contracting the disease) usually renders one temporary or permanent resistance to an infectious disease. Vaccines and toxoids promote the type of antibody production one would see if they had experienced the natural infection. This active immunization involves the direct administration of antigens to the host to cause them to produce the desired antibodies and cell-mediated immunity. These agents may consist of live attenuated agents or killed (inactivated) agents, or agents that alter the hosts genetic structure. Immunizations confer resistance without actually producing disease. Some vaccines (tetanus) are in short supply due to the push for immunization and are reserved for those individuals with wounds. Passive immunization occurs when immunologic agents are administered. Immunoglobulins and antivenins only offer passive short-term immunity and are usually administered for a specific exposure.

Aggressive pediatric immunization programs have helped reduce preventable infections and death in children worldwide. This focus should continue and be expanded to the adult population, many of whom have missed the natural infection and their past immunizations. A careful immunization history should be documented for every client, regardless of age. When in doubt or if unknown if had disease/infection or immunization, appropriate serologic evidence/titers may be drawn. Table 2 lists some of the more common diseases, the general recommended schedule to confer immunization, and the length of immunity conferred; Table 3 outlines the active childhood immunization schedule.

VITAMINS

SEE TABLES 6, 7, AND 8.

GENERAL STATEMENT

Vitamins are essential, carbon-containing, noncaloric substances that are required for normal metabolism. They are produced by living materials such as plants and animals and they are generally obtained from the diet. Vitamin D is synthesized in the diet to a limited extent and Vitamin B–12 is synthesized in the intestinal tract by bacterial flora.

Vitamins are essential for promoting growth, health, and life. They are necessary for the metabolic processes responsible for transforming foods into tissue or energy. Vitamins are also involved in the formation and maintenance of blood cells, chemicals supporting the nervous system, hormones, and genetic materials. Vitamins do not provide energy because they contain no calories. Yet, some do help convert the calories in fats, carbohydrates, and proteins into usable body energy.

Disease states caused by severe nutritional deficiencies prompted the discovery of vitamins because scientists were able to reverse the signs and symptoms of these disease states with vitamins. Severe deficiencies include scurvy, rickets, pellagra, pernicious anemia, xerophthalmia, beriberi, osteomalacia, infantile hemolytic anemia, and hemorrhagic diseases of the newborn. Moderate vitamin deficiencies may also produce symptoms of impaired health.

Environmental factors and genetic predisposition may influence individual requirements for specific vitamins. Disease processes, growth, hormone balance, and drugs may also alter the dietary requirements and function of vitamins.

Many deficiency states can be traced to special circumstances such as pernicious anemia after gastrectomy; pellagra in corn–eating populations, and scurvy in the elderly subsisting on soft foods (e.g., eggs, bread, milk) while neglecting citrus fruits. Generally, although not common in the United States, vitamin deficiency usually involves multiple rather than single deficiencies and usually can be attributed to poor lifestyle choices and poor dietary habits with an inadequate intake of many nutrients, including all vitamins.

There are two categories of vitamins: fat soluble and water soluble. Fat soluble vitamins A, D, E, and K are found in the fat or oil of foods and require digestible fat and bile salts for absorption in the small intestine. The water-soluble vitamins, C and B complex (B-1, B-2, niacin, B-6, folic acid, B-12, pantothenic acid, and biotin) are found in the watery portion of foods and are well absorbed by the GI tract. They are easily lost through overcooking and do not require fat for absorption. Water soluble vitamins mix easily in the blood, are excreted by the kidneys, and only small amounts are stored in the tissues, so regular daily intake is essential. Fat soluble vitamins are stored in the body after binding to specific plasma globulins in fat parts of the body.

Recommended Dietary Allow-ances (RDAs) are the recommended human vitamin and mineral intake requirements. These were developed by the Food and Nutrition Board, National Research Council of the National Academy of Sciences and have evolved over the past 50 years and are updated every 5 years. They are based on age, height, weight, and gender. These are only estimates of nutrient needs; each client and the surrounding factors warrant individualized evaluation when replacement is being considered. Clients with impaired liver function should not take large amounts of fat soluble vitamins (i.e.; A,D,E,K) unless specifically prescribed due to the toxicity potential from cumulative effects.

TABLE 3 Common Diseases, General Recommended Immunization Schedule, and Length of Immunity

DISEASE	IMMUNIZATION SCHEDULE	LENGTH OF IMMUNITY
Botulism	Pentavalent toxoid (types A,B,C,D,E) 0.5mL SQ available from USAMRIID)	post-exposure
Cholera	Two doses 1 week to 1 month apart	6 months
Diphtheria	Given as DPT; four doses at ages 2, 4, 6, and 15–18 months	10 years
Haemophilusinfluenzae (Hib)	Four doses at ages 2, 4, 6, and 15 months	Unknown
Hepatitis B	Three doses: at birth (or initial dose), 1 month later, and 6 months after second dose	Unknown
Influenza	One dose (or two doses of split virus if under 13 years)	1–3 years
Lyme Disease	Three doses at ages 15–70 years old; at 0, 1, and 12 months; plan 3rd dose just before tick season	1 yr; yearly booster
Measles	Given as MMR at ages 12–15 months and 4–6 years	Lifetime
Meningococcal meningitis	One dose (antibody response requires 5 days); antibiotic prophylaxis (Rifampin 600 mg or 10 mg/kg q 12 hr for four doses should be given to all contacts per exposure)	?Lifetime; not consistently effective in those <2 years of age
Mumps	Given as MMR at ages 12–15 months and 4–6 years	Lifetime
Pertussis	Given as DPT; four doses at ages 2, 4, 6, and 15–18 months	10 years
Pneumococcus	One dose (0.5 mL)	Approx. 5-10 years
Poliomyelitis	Four doses at ages 2, 4, and 6 months, then at age 4–6 years	Lifetime
Rabies	Postexposure: five doses on days 0, 3, 7, 14, and 28 with the rabies immune globulin; pre-exposure: two doses 1 week apart, third dose 2–3 weeks later	Approx. 2 years

Rubella	Given as MMR at ages 12–15 months and 4–6 years	Lifetime
Smallpox	One dose; this vaccine available at CDC (critical in less than 4 days of exposure) Vaccinia immune globulin in special cases-call USAMRIID	3 years
Tetanus	Given initially as DPT; four doses at ages 2, 4, 6, and 15–18 months	10 years; a tetanus booster is required q 10 years; 5 years if trauma
VZV (varicellazoster virus; chicken pox)	One dose (0.5 mL) age 12 months to 12 years; two injections of 0.5 mL 4–8 weeks apart in age 13 and older	?Lifetime
Yellow fever	One dose	10 years

TABLE 4 Active Childhood Immunization Schedule

	#1	#2	#3	#4
DPT	2 months	4 months	6 months	15–18 months
OPV	2 months	4 months	6 months	4–6 years
Hib	2 months	4 months	6 months	15–18 months
MMR	12 months	4 years		
Hep B	birth or initial dose	1 month after first dose	6 months or more after second dose	

TABLE 5 Active Adult Immunization Schedule

Tetanus	Tetanus booster every 10 years; with injury obtain one in 5 yrs
Pneumococcus	Every 5 years
Influenza	Every year
Lyme	Yearly booster in endemic areas after series completed

TABLE 6 Common Vitamin Requirements

Vitamin	RDA	Physiologic Effects Essential for:
A (retinol, retinaldehyde, retonic acid)	1400-6000 IU	Growth & development epithelial tissue maintenance; reproduction prevents night blindness
B complex:		
B-1 (thiamine)	0.3–1.5 mg	Energy metabolism: normal nerve function
B-2 (riboflavin)	0.4–1.8 mg	Reactions in energy cycle that produce ATP; oxidation of amino acids and hydroxy acids; oxidation of purines
B-3 Niacin (nicotinic acid, nicotinamide)	5–19 mg	Synthesis of fatty acids and cholesterol; blocks FFA; conversion of phenylalanine to tyrosine
B-6 (pyridoxine, pyridoxal, pyridoxamine)	0.3–2.5 mg	Amino acid metabolism; glycogenolysis, RBC/Hb synthesis; formation of neurotransmitters; formation of antibodies
Folacin (folic acid, pteroylglutamic acid)	50–800 mcg	DNA synthesis, formation of RBCs in bone marrow with cyanocobalamine
Pantothenic acid (calcium pantothenate, dexpanthenol)	10 mg	Synthesis of sterols, steroid hormones, porphyrins; synthesis and degradation of fatty acids; oxidative metabolism of carbohydrates, gluconeogenesis
B-12 (cyanocobalamin, hydroxocobalamin, extrinsic factor)	0.3–4.0 mcg	DNA synthesis in bone marrow; RBC production with folacin; nerve tissue maintenance
B-7 (Biotin)	No recommendation	Synthesis of fatty acids, generation of tricarboxylic acid cycle; formation of purines Coenzyme in CHO metabolism
C (ascorbic acid, ascorbate)	60 mg	Formation of collagen; conversion of cholesterol to bile acids; protects Aand E and polyunsaturated fats from excessive oxidation; absorption and utilization of iron; converts folacin to folinic acid; some role in clotting, adreno cortical hormones, and resistance to cancer and infections

TABLE 6 (continued)

Vitamin	RDA	Physiologic Effects Essential for:
D (calcitriol, cholecalciferol, dihydrotachysterol, ergocalciferol, viosterol)	400 IU	Intestinal absorption and metabolism of calcium and phosphorus as well as renal reabsorption; release of calcium from bone and resorption
E (tocopherol)	4–15 IU	May oppose destruction of Vit. A and fats by oxygen fragments called free radicals; antioxidant; may affect production of prostaglandins which regulate a variety of body processes
K (menadione, phytonadione)	No recommendation	Formation of prothrombin and other clotting proteins by the liver; blood coagulation

TABLE 7 Vitamins and Uses

Vitamin	Effect	Uses
A (retinoic acid)	Reduces formation of comedones; keratin production suppression	Acne, psoriasis, ichthyosis, Darier's disease xeropthalmia,intestinal infections, prevents night blindness
Niacin	Reduction of blood cholesterol and triglycerides blocks FFA release	Hypercholesterolemia, hyperbetalipoproteinemia
D (dihydrotachysterol)	Maintains calcium and phosphorus levels in bone and blood	Hypoparathyroidism increase intestinal absorption of calcium
C	Reduces urine pH; converts methemoglobin to hemoglobin clients	Idiopathic methemoglobin; recurrent UTIs in high risk aids in iron absorption
E	Reduces endogenous peroxidases	Hemolytic anemia in premature infants protects cell mebranes from oxidation
K	Increases liver production of thrombin	Warfarin toxicity essential for blood coagulation

TABLE 8 Vitamin Deficiency States

Vitamin	Deficiency	Signs & Symptoms
A	Xerophthalmia	Progressive eye changes: night blindness to xerosis of conjunctiva and cornea with scarring
	Keratomalacia	Degeneration of epithelial cells with hardening and shrinking
B-6	Beriberi	Fatigue, weight loss, weakness, irritability; headaches, insomnia, peripheral neuropathy, CHF, cardiomyopathy
Niacin	Pellagra	Depression, anorexia, beefy red glossitis, cheilosis, dermatitis
B-12	Pernicious anemia	Macrocytic, megaloblastic anemia; progressive neuropathy R/T demyelination
C	Scurvy	Joint pain, growth retardation, anemia, poor wound healing with increased susceptibility to infection; petechial hemorrhages
D	Rickets (child) Osteomalacia (adult)	Demineralization of bones and teeth with bone pain and skeletal muscle deformities
E	Hemolytic anemia in low birth weight infants	Macrocytic anemia; increased hemolysis of RBC's and increased capillarity fragility
K	Hemorrhagic disease in newborns	Increase tendency to hemorrhage

chapter 2

A–Z Listing of Drugs

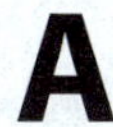

A

Abacavir sulfate

(uh-**BACK**-ah-veer)

PREGNANCY CATEGORY: C
CLASSIFICATION(S):
Antiviral, antiretroviral
Rx: Ziagen

SEE ALSO *ANTIVIRAL DRUGS.*

ACTION/KINETICS

Synthetic nucleoside analog. Converted intracellularly to the active carbovir triphosphate which inhibits the activity of HIV-1 reverse transcriptase by competing with the natural substrate deoxyguanosine-5′-triphosphate and by incorporation into viral DNA. The lack of a 3′-OH group in the incorporated nucleoside analog prevents the formation of the 5′ to 3′ phosphodiester linkage essential for DNA chain elongation. Thus, viral DNA growth is terminated. Cross resistance in vitro has been seen to lamivudine, didanosine, and zalcitabine. Rapidly absorbed after PO use. Metabolized in the liver and excreted in both the urine and feces.

USES

In combination with other antiretroviral drugs (e.g., lamivudine and zidovudine) to treat HIV-1 infection. Do not add as a single agent when antiretroviral regimens are changed due to loss of virologic response.

CONTRAINDICATIONS

Lactation.

SPECIAL CONCERNS

Fatal hypersensitivity reactions are possible (See *Side Effects*) even if no hypersensitivity seen previously. Efficacy for long-term suppression of HIV RNA or disease progression have not been determined. Not a cure for HIV infection; clients may continue to show illnesses associated with HIV infection, including opportunistic infections. Not shown to reduce the risk of transmission of HIV to others through sexual contact or blood. Use with caution with liver disease. May show cross resistance with other nucleoside reverse transcriptase inhibitors.

SIDE EFFECTS

Hypersensitivity.
Fever, skin rash, fatigue, N&V, diarrhea, abdominal pain, malaise, lethargy, myalgia, arthralgia, edema, SOB, pharyngitis, dyspnea, cough, paresthesia, lymphadenopathy, conjunctivitis, mouth ulcerations, maculopapular or urticarial rash, ***life-threatening hypotension, liver failure, renal failure, death; fatal hypersensitivity reactions***.
GI: N&V, diarrhea, loss of appetite, pancreatitis. **Miscellaneous:** Severe hepatomegaly with steatosis (may be fatal), lactic acidosis, pancreatitis, insomnia, other sleep disorders, headache, fever, skin rashes.

LABORATORY TEST CONSIDERATIONS

↑ LFTs, CPK, GGT, creatinine, glucose, triglycerides. Lymphopenia, anemia, neutropenia.

DRUG INTERACTIONS

Ethanol ↓ excretion of abacavir → ↑ exposure.

HOW SUPPLIED

Oral Solution: 20 mg/mL; *Tablets:* 300 mg

A

DOSAGE

• **ORAL SOLUTION, TABLETS**

Treat HIV-1 infection.

Adults: 300 mg b.i.d. with other antiretroviral drugs. **Pediatric, 3 months to 16 years:** 8 mg/kg b.i.d., not to exceed 300 mg b.i.d., in combination with other antiretroviral drugs.

NURSING CONSIDERATIONS

SEE ALSO *NURSING CONSIDERATIONS* FOR *ANTIVIRAL DRUGS*.

ADMINISTRATION/STORAGE

1. May give with/without food.
2. Do not restart abacavir therapy following a hypersensitivity reaction. More severe symptoms will occur within hours and may include life-threatening hypotension or death.
3. Store at 20–25°C (68–77°F). Do not freeze, although may be refrigerated.

ASSESSMENT

1. Note indications for therapy and other agents trialed.
2. Obtain lytes and LFTs; assess for liver enlargement and lactic acidosis.
3. Assess for any hypersensitivity reactions, including clients who present with acute respiratory disease, even if alternative diagnosis is possible. Once reactions experienced may never resume therapy with this drug.
4. If drug is discontinued and no hypersensitivity reactions were noted, it may be reintroduced with caution and only if medical care is readily accessible.
5. Providers must report hypersensitivity reactions to the registry @ 1-800-270-0425.

CLIENT/FAMILY TEACHING

1. Take drug orally as directed and with other antiretroviral agents. May take with or without food.
2. Review medication guide that accompanies this product.
3. Drug does not cure disease but works to lower viral count.
4. Immediately report any S&S of allergic reactions (fever, severe fatigue, skin rash, N &V, diarrhea or abdominal pain) and stop drug.
5. If allergic reaction is experienced with this drug, never restart therapy as it may be fatal.
6. Practice safe sex, drug does not prevent disease transmission.
7. Use reliable birth control; do not breast feed.

OUTCOMES/EVALUATE

Suppression of HIV RNA

Abciximab

(ab-**SIX**-ih-mab)

PREGNANCY CATEGORY: C
CLASSIFICATION(S):
Antiplatelet drug
Rx: ReoPro

ACTION/KINETICS

Abciximab is the Fab fragment of the chimeric human-murine monoclonal antibody 7E3. It binds to a glycoprotein receptor on human platelets, thus inhibiting platelet aggregation by preventing the binding of fibrinogen, von Willebrand factor, and other adhesive molecules to receptor sites on activated platelets. **t½, after IV bolus:** 30 min. Recovery of platelet function: About 48 hr, although the drug remains in the circulation bound to platelets for up to 10 days. Following IV infusion, free drug levels in the plasma decrease rapidly for about 6 hr and then decline at a slower rate.

USES

Inhibition of platelet aggregation. Adjunct to percutaneous coronary intervention (PCI) to prevent acute cardiac ischemic complications in clients at high risk for abrupt closure of the treated coronary vessel. Used with aspirin and heparin. *Investigational:* Early treatment of acute MI.

CONTRAINDICATIONS

Due to a potential for drug-induced bleeding, abciximab is contraindicated as follows: history of CVA (within 2 years) or CVA with a significant residual neurologic deficit; active internal bleeding; within 6 weeks of GI or GU bleeding of clinical significance; bleeding diathesis; within 7 days of administration of oral anticoagulants unless the PT is less than 1.2 times control; thrombocytopenia (less than 100,000 cells/μL); within 6 weeks of major surgery or trauma; intracranial neoplasm; arteriovenous malformation or aneurysm; severe uncontrolled hypertension; presumed or documented history of vasculitis; use of IV dextran before PCI or intent to use it during PCI; hypersensitivity to murine proteins.

SPECIAL CONCERNS

Assess benefits versus the risk of increased bleeding in clients who weigh less than 75 kg, are 65 years of age or older, have a history of GI disease, and are receiving thrombolytics and heparin. Conditions also associated with an increased risk of bleeding in the angioplasty setting and which may be additive to that of abciximab: PCI within 12 hr of onset of symptoms for acute MI, PCI lasting more than 70 min, and failed PCI. Use with caution during lactation and when abciximab is used with other drugs that affect hemostasis, including thrombolytics, oral anticoagulants, NSAIDs, dipyridamole, and ticlopidine. Safety and efficacy have not been determined in children.

SIDE EFFECTS

Bleeding tendencies.

Major bleeds, including intracranial hemorrhage. Minor bleeding, including spontaneous gross hematuria, spontaneous hematemesis. Loss of hemoglobin.

CV: Hypotension, bradycardia, atrial fibrillation or flutter, vascular disorder, pulmonary edema, incomplete or ***complete AV block,*** ventricular tachycardia, weak pulse, palpitations, nodal arrhythmia, limb embolism, thrombophlebitis, intermittent claudication, pericardial effusion, pseudoaneurysm, AV fistula, ventricular arrhythmia. **GI:** N&V, abdominal pain, diarrhea, dry mouth, dyspepsia, ileus, gastroesophageal reflux. **Hematologic:** Thrombocytopenia, anemia, leukocytosis, hemolytic anemia, petechiae. **CNS:** Hypesthesia, confusion, abnormal thinking, agitation, anxiety, dizziness, ***coma, brain ischemia,*** insomnia. **Respiratory:** Pleural effusion, pleurisy, pneumonia, rales, bronchitis, bronchospasm, ***pulmonary embolism,*** rhonchi. **Musculoskeletal:** Myopathy, cellulitis, myalgia, muscle contraction. **GU:** UTI, urinary retention, abnormal renal function, dysuria, frequent micturition, cystalgia, urinary incontinence, prostatitis. **Ophthalmic:** Diplopia, abnormal vision. **Miscellaneous:** Pain, peripheral edema, development of human antichimeric antibody, dysphonia, pruritus, increased sweating, asthenia, incisional pain, wound abscess, cellulitis, peripheral coldness, injection site pain, pallor, diabetes mellitus, hypertonia, enlarged abdomen, bullous eruption, inflammation..

DRUG INTERACTIONS

H *Bromelain* / Possible ↑ bleeding risk

H *Evening primrose oil* / Possible ↑ antiplatelet effect

H *Feverfew* / Possible ↑ antiplatelet effect

H *Garlic* / Possible ↑ antiplatelet effect

H *Ginger* / Possible ↑ antiplatelet effect

H *Ginkgo biloba* / Possible ↑ antiplatelet effect

H *Ginseng* / Possible ↑ antiplatelet effect

H *Grapeseed extract* / Possible ↑ antiplatelet effect

HOW SUPPLIED

Injection: 2 mg/mL

DOSAGE

• IV BOLUS FOLLOWED BY IV INFUSION

Clients undergoing percutaneous coronary intervention (PCI) with concomitant use of heparin and aspirin.

IV bolus: 0.25 mg/kg given 10–60 min before the start of the intervention. Followed by **continuous IV infusion:** 10 mcg/min for 12 hr. Those with unstable angina not responding to usual therapy and who require PCI within 24 hr may be given abciximab, 0.25 mg/kg IV bolus, followed by an 18–24 hr IV infusion of 10 mcg/min, ending 1 hr after the PCI.

NURSING CONSIDERATIONS

ADMINISTRATION/STORAGE

IV 1. Stop infusion after 12 hr to avoid prolonged platelet receptor blockade effects.

2. Stop continuous infusion with failed PCIs; no evidence effective in such situations.
3. Discontinue abciximab and heparin if serious bleeding occurs not controlled by compression.
4. Do not use if preparations contain visibly opaque particles.
5. If symptoms of an allergic reaction or anaphylaxis occur, stop infusion immediately and institute appropriate treatment. Have available epinephrine, dopamine, theophylline, antihistamines, and corticosteroids for immediate use.
6. Withdraw drug (2 mg/mL) through a sterile, nonpyrogenic, low-protein-binding 0.2- or 0.22-μm filter into a syringe; give bolus 10–60 min before procedure.
7. For continuous infusion, withdraw 4.5 mL of abciximab as #6 directs into a syringe. Inject into 250 mL of 0.9% NSS or D5% and infuse at a rate of 17 mL/hr (10 mcg/min) for 12 hr by infusion pump with an in-line sterile, nonpyrogenic, low-protein-binding 0.2- or 0.22-μm filter. Discard any unused drug after 12 hr.
8. Give drug through a separate IV line with no other medications added to infusion solution. No incompatibilities have been noted with glass bottles or PVC bags or IV sets.
9. Store vials at 2–8°C (36–46°F); do not freeze or shake vials.

ASSESSMENT

1. Obtain a thorough nursing history; note indications/goals of therapy.
2. Note any history of CVA, bleeding disorders, recent episodes of bleeding, trauma, or surgery.
3. List other agents prescribed/OTC and when last consumed to prevent any bleeding potential.
4. Monitor PT, INR, PTT, CBC, VS, and EKG. Check platelet count 2–4 hr after initial bolus and again in 24 hr.

INTERVENTIONS

1. Anticipate client undergoing PCI will be bolused with abciximab (0.25 mg/kg) 10–60 min before procedure followed by a continuous IV infusion (10 mcg/min) for 12 hr.
2. Insert separate IV lines with saline locks for blood draws.
3. Observe carefully during infusion; anaphylaxis may occur at any time.
4. Administer 325 mg aspirin orally 2 hr before procedure and prepare heparin bolus and infusion for administration as prescribed.
5. Observe for any potential bleeding sites: catheter insertion sites, needle punctures, GI, GU, and retroperitoneal sites. Remove tape/dressings gently.
6. If serious bleeding develops (not controlled with pressure), stop infusions of abciximab and heparin.
7. Keep on complete bedrest while vascular access sheath in place. Restrain limb straight and raise HOB no more than 30 degrees. Stop heparin infusion at least 4 hr before sheath removal. Palpate/monitor distal pulses of involved extremity.
8. Apply pressure for 30 min over femoral artery once sheath removed. When hemostasis evident, apply a pressure dressing (sandbag) and check frequently for evidence of bleeding. Monitor hematoma for enlargement. Enforce bedrest for 6–8 hr after infusion completed and sheath removed.

CLIENT/FAMILY TEACHING

1. Review indications for therapy, what to expect, clinical management, and anticipated results.
2. Review risks associated with this therapy, e.g., bleeding from intracranial hemorrhage, which may be lethal, or hematuria or hematemesis, may require blood/platelet transfusions.
3. Drug may cause formation of human antichimeric antibody, which may cause hypersensitivity reactions, thrombocytopenia, or diminished response on readministration.

OUTCOMES/EVALUATE

Prevention of abrupt coronary vessel closure with associated ischemic complications

Acarbose

(ah-**KAR**-bohs)

PREGNANCY CATEGORY: B
CLASSIFICATION(S):
Antidiabetic, oral; alpha-glucosidase inhibitor

A

Rx: Precose
★**Rx:** Prandase

ACTION/KINETICS
An oligosaccharide obtained from a fermentation process using the microorganism *Actinoplans utahensis.* Causes a competitive, reversible inhibition of pancreatic alpha-amylase and membrane-bound intestinal alpha-glucosidase hydrolase enzymes. This causes delayed glucose absorption resulting in a smaller increase in blood glucose following meals. Glycosylated hemoglobin levels are decreased in those with NIDDM. Additive effect with sulfonylureas due to different mechanism of action. Approximately 65% of an oral dose of acarbose remains in the GI tract, which is the site of action. Metabolized in the GI tract by both intestinal bacteria and intestinal enzymes. Acarbose and metabolites that are absorbed are excreted in the urine.

USES
Alone, with insulin or metformin, or with a sulfonylurea to treat type 2 diabetes mellitus. Diet control is essential.

CONTRAINDICATIONS
Diabetic ketoacidosis, cirrhosis, IBD, colonic ulceration, partial intestinal obstruction or predisposition to intestinal obstruction, chronic intestinal diseases associated with marked disorders of digestion or absorption, conditions that may deteriorate as a result of increased gas formation in the intestine. In significant renal dysfunction. Severe, persistent bradycardia. Lactation.

SPECIAL CONCERNS
Safety and efficacy have not been determined in children. Acarbose does not cause hypoglycemia; however, sulfonylureas and insulin can lower blood glucose sufficiently to cause symptoms or even life-threatening hypoglycemia.

SIDE EFFECTS
GI: Abdominal pain, diarrhea, flatulence. GI side effects may be severe and be confused with paralytic ileus.

LABORATORY TEST CONSIDERATIONS
↑ Serum transaminases (especially with doses greater than 50 mg t.i.d.). Small ↓ in hematocrit. Low plasma B_6 levels.

OD OVERDOSE MANAGEMENT
Symptoms: Flatulence, diarrhea, abdominal discomfort. *Treatment:* Reduce dose; symptoms will subside.

DRUG INTERACTIONS
Charcoal / ↓ Acarbose effect
Digestive enzymes / ↓ Acarbose effect
Digoxin / ↓ Serum digoxin levels
Insulin / ↑ Hypoglycemia; possible severe hypoglycemia
Sulfonylureas / ↑ Hypoglycemia; possible severe hypoglycemia

HOW SUPPLIED
Tablet: 25 mg, 50 mg, 100 mg

DOSAGE
• **TABLETS**

Type 2 diabetes mellitus.

Individualized, depending on effectiveness and tolerance. **Initial:** 25 mg 1–3 times/day with the first bite of each main meal. **Maintenance:** Increase dose to 50 mg t.i.d. Some may benefit from 100 mg t.i.d. The dosage can be adjusted at 4- to 8-week intervals. **Recommended maximum daily dose:** 50 mg t.i.d. for clients weighing less than 60 kg and 100 mg t.i.d. for those weighing more than 60 kg.

NURSING CONSIDERATIONS
ADMINISTRATION/STORAGE
1. Start with a low dose to reduce GI side effects and to help determine the minimum effective dose.
2. If dose missed, take usual dose at start of next main meal.

ASSESSMENT
1. Document indications for therapy, age at symptom onset, other agents trialed and the outcome.
2. Note any cirrhosis or chronic intestinal diseases with disorders of digestion or absorption.
3. Obtain baseline CBC, HbA1c, BS, electrolytes, U/A, liver and renal function tests; assess for B_6 deficiency. Monitor HbA1c and LFTs q 3 mo.
4. Initiate and titrate acarbose based on BS results. Ideally, a 1-hr postprandial

A

plasma glucose level should be measured to determine the effective dose.
5. Acarbose may enhance glycemic control with a sulfonylurea, but it may also be used alone.

CLIENT/FAMILY TEACHING

1. Take as prescribed, three times a day with the first bite of main meals. May be used with insulin or other oral agents.
2. Acarbose delays digestion of ingested carbohydrates (glucose) and is used in addition to diet and not instead of.
3. Caloric restrictions and weight loss, especially in the obese client, must be continued to control BS and prevent complications of diabetes; continue regular daily exercise.
4. The most common side effects are of GI origin (abdominal discomfort, diarrhea, gas); should subside in frequency and intensity.
5. Do frequent monitoring of glucose (finger sticks) and record to assess the therapeutic response.
6. Loss of glucose control may result when exposed to stress, such as fever, trauma, infection, or surgery. In these instances, temporary insulin therapy may be needed.
7. Candy bars should not be used to counteract hypoglycemia; use glucose tablets or gel or lactose.

OUTCOMES/EVALUATE

Control of BS in clients with NIDDM; HbA1C < 7

Acebutolol hydrochloride

(ays-**BYOU**-toe-lohl)

PREGNANCY CATEGORY: B
CLASSIFICATION(S):
Beta-adrenergic blocking agent
Rx: Sectral
✱**Rx:** Apo-Acebutolol, Gen-Acebutolol, Gen-Acebutolol (Type S), Monitan, Novo-Acebutolol, Nu-Acebutolol, Rhotral

SEE ALSO *BETA-ADRENERGIC BLOCKING AGENTS.*

ACTION/KINETICS

Predominantly beta-1 blocking activity; at higher doses, inhibits beta-2 receptors and decreases beta-1 selectivity. Some intrinsic sympathomimetic activity. Useful in arrhythmias due to prolongation of the effective refractory period of the AV node and slow AV conduction. **t½:** 3–4 hr. Low lipid solubility. **Duration:** 24–30 hr. Metabolized in liver and excreted in urine and bile. Fifteen to 20% excreted unchanged.

USES

Hypertension (either alone or with other antihypertensive agents such as thiazide diuretics). Premature ventricular beats.

ADDITIONAL CONTRAINDICATIONS

Severe, persistent bradycardia. Pheochromocytoma.

SPECIAL CONCERNS

Dosage not established in children. May be used with caution in bronchospastic disease in clients not responding to, or who cannot tolerate, other antihypertensive drugs.

ADDITIONAL DRUG INTERACTIONS

H *Aloe* / ↑ Acebutolol effect
H *Buckthorn* / ↑ Acebutolol effect
H *Cascara sagrada bark* / ↑ Acebutolol effect
H *Ephedra* / Possible dysrhythmia
H *Rhubarb root* / ↑ Acebutolol effect
H *Senna* / ↑ Acebutolol effect

HOW SUPPLIED

Capsule: 200 mg, 400 mg

DOSAGE

• **CAPSULES**

Hypertension.

Initial: 400 mg/day for uncomplicated mild–to–moderate hypertension (although 200 mg b.i.d. may be needed for optimum control); **then,** 400–800 mg/day (range: 200–1,200 mg/day).

PVCs.

Initial: 200 mg b.i.d.; **then,** increase dose gradually to 600–1,200 mg/day.

In those with impaired kidney or liver function, decrease dose by 50% when C_{CR} is <50 mL/min/1.73 m^2 and by 75% when it is <25 mL/min/1.73 m^2.

NURSING CONSIDERATIONS

SEE ALSO *NURSING CONSIDERATIONS* FOR *BETA-ADRENERGIC BLOCKING AGENTS* AND *ANTIHYPERTENSIVE AGENTS*.

ADMINISTRATION/STORAGE

1. When discontinued, gradually withdraw drug over a 2-week period.
2. Bioavailability increases in elderly clients; may require lower maintenance doses (no more than 800 mg/day).
3. May be combined with another antihypertensive agent.
4. Reduce dosage with impaired liver and renal function.

CLIENT/FAMILY TEACHING

1. Drug may cause drowsiness; do not perform tasks that require mental alertness until drug effects realized.
2. May cause an increased sensitivity to cold; dress appropriately.
3. Report any evidence of sudden weight gain, edema, SOB or lowered heart rate. Monitor BP and record.
4. Do not stop abruptly without provider approval.

OUTCOMES/EVALUATE

↓ BP; control of PVCs

Acetaminophen (APAP, Paracetamol)

(ah-**SEAT**-ah-**MIN**-oh-fen)

OTC: Caplets: Aspirin Free Anacid Maximum Strength, Aspirin Free Pain Relief, Genapap Extra Strength, Genebs Extra Strength Caplets, Panadol, Panadol Junior Strength, Tapanol Extra Strength, Tylenol Extended Relief, **Capsules:** Dapacin, **Drops:** Infants' Pain Reliever, Aspirin Free Anacin Maximum Strength, Children's Dynafed Jr., Children's Mapap, Dolono, Extra Strength Dynafed E.X., Liquiprin Drops for Children, **Elixir:** Aceta, Genapap Children's, Mapap Children's, Oraphen-PD, Ridenol, Silapap Children's, Tylenol Children's, **Gelcaps:** Aspirin Free Anacid Maximum Strength, Tapanol Extra Strength, Tylenol Extra Strength, **Oral Liquid/Syrup:** Halenol Children's, Panadol Children's, Tempra 2 Syrup, Tylenol Extra Strength, **Oral Solution:** Acetaminophen Drops, Apacet, Genapap Infants' Drops, Mapap Infant Drops, Panadol Infants' Drops, Silapap Infants, Tempra 1, Tylenol Infants' Drops, Uni-Ace, **Sprinkle Capsules:** Feverall Junior Strength, Feverall Children's, **Suppositories:** Acephen, Acetaminophen Uniserts, Children's Feverall, Infant's Feverall, Junior Strength Feverall, Neopap, **Tablet, Chewable:** Apacet, Children's Genapap, Children's Pain Reliever, Children's Pain Reliever Suspension, Children's Panadol, Children's Tylenol Soft Chews, Meda Cap, Tempra 3, Tylenol Caplets, Tylenol Children's, **Tablets:** Aceta, Aspirin Free Pain Relief, Genapap, Genapap Extra Strength, Genebs, Genebs Extra Strength, Mapap Extra Strength, Mapap Regular Strength, Maranox, Meda Tab, Panadol, Redutemp, Tapanol Extra Strength, Tapanol Regular Strength, Tempra, Tylenol Extra Strength, Tylenol Junior Strength, Tylenol Regular Strength

✱**OTC: Caplets:** Atasol, Atasol Forte, **Oral Liquid/Syrup:** Atasol, Children's Acetaminophen Elixir Drops, Pediatrix, Tempra, Tempra Children's Syrup, **Oral Solution:** Atasol, Children's Acetaminophen Oral Solution, Pediatrix, PMS-Acetaminophen, **Oral Suspension:** Tylenol Children's Suspension, Tylenol Infants' Suspension, **Suppositories:** Abenol 120, 325, 650 mg, **Tablet, Chewable:** Children's Chewable Acetaminophen, Tempra, Tylenol Junior Strength Chewable Tablets Fruit, **Tablets:** A.F. Anacin, A.F. Anacin Extra Strength, Apo-Acetaminophen, Atasol, Atasol Forte, Extra Strength Acetaminophen, Regular Strength Acetaminophen, Tylenol Tablets 325 mg, 500 mg

Acetaminophen, buffered

(ah-**SEAT**-ah-**MIN**-oh-fen)

OTC: Bromo Seltzer Effervescent Granules

CLASSIFICATION(S):

Non-narcotic analgesic

A

ACTION/KINETICS

Decreases fever by a hypothalamic effect leading to sweating and vasodilation. Also inhibits the effect of pyrogens on the hypothalamic heat-regulating centers. May cause analgesia by inhibiting CNS prostaglandin synthesis; however, due to minimal effects on peripheral prostaglandin synthesis, acetaminophen has no anti-inflammatory or uricosuric effects. Does not cause any anticoagulant effect or ulceration of the GI tract. Antipyretic and analgesic effects are comparable to those of aspirin.

Peak plasma levels: 30–120 min. **t½:** 45 min–3 hr. **Therapeutic serum levels** (analgesia): 5–20 mcg/mL. **Plasma protein binding:** Approximately 25%. Metabolized in the liver and excreted in the urine as glucuronide and sulfate conjugates. However, an intermediate hydroxylated metabolite is hepatotoxic following large doses of acetaminophen.

The extended-relief product uses a bilayer system that allows the outer layer to release acetaminophen rapidly while the inner layer is designed to release the remainder of the dose more slowly. This allows prolonged relief of symptoms.

The buffered product is a mixture of acetaminophen, sodium bicarbonate, and citric acid that effervesces when placed in water. This product has a high sodium content (0.76 g/¾ capful).

USES

Control of pain due to headache, earache, dysmenorrhea, arthralgia, myalgia, musculoskeletal pain, arthritis, immunizations, teething, tonsillectomy. To reduce fever in bacterial or viral infections. As a substitute for aspirin in upper GI disease, aspirin allergy, bleeding disorders, clients on anticoagulant therapy, and gouty arthritis. *Investigational:* In children receiving DPT vaccination to decrease incidence of fever and pain at injection site.

CONTRAINDICATIONS

Renal insufficiency, anemia. Clients with cardiac or pulmonary disease are more susceptible to acetaminophen toxicity.

SPECIAL CONCERNS

Toxicity, including serious liver damage, may occur with doses not far beyond labeled dosing. Use with caution in pregnancy. Consult a physician before use if more than three alcoholic drinks per day are consumed.

SIDE EFFECTS

Few when taken in usual therapeutic doses. Chronic and even acute toxicity can develop after long symptom-free usage.

Hematologic: Methemoglobinemia, ***hemolytic anemia,*** neutropenia, thrombocytopenia, pancytopenia, leukopenia. **Allergic:** Urticarial and erythematous skin reactions, skin eruptions, fever. **Miscellaneous:** CNS stimulation, hypoglycemic coma, jaundice, drowsiness, glossitis. Possible liver damage in those who consume three or more alcoholic drinks daily.

OD OVERDOSE MANAGEMENT

Symptoms: May be no early specific symptoms. Within first 24 hr: N&V, diaphoresis, anorexia, drowsiness, confusion, liver tenderness, cardiac arrhythmias, low BP, jaundice, acute hepatic and renal failure. Within 24–48 hr, increased AST, ALT, bilibrubin, PT levels. After 72–96 hr, peak hepatotoxicity with death possible due to liver necrosis. *Treatment:* Initially, induction of emesis, gastric lavage, activated charcoal. Oral *N*-acetylcysteine is said to reduce or prevent hepatic damage by inactivating acetaminophen metabolites, which cause liver toxicity.

DRUG INTERACTIONS

Alcohol, ethyl / Chronic use → ↑ toxicity of larger therapeutic doses of acetaminophen

Barbiturates / ↑ Potential of hepatotoxicity R/T ↑ liver breakdown of acetaminophen

Carbamazepine / ↑ Potential of hepatotoxicity R/T ↑ liver breakdown of acetaminophen

Charcoal, activated / ↓ Absorption of acetaminophen when given as soon as possible after overdose

Diuretics, loop / ↓ Effect R/T ↓ renal prostaglandin excretion and ↓ plasma renin activity

Hydantoins (including Phenytoin) / ↑ Potential of hepatotoxicity R/T ↑ liver breakdown of acetaminophen
Isoniazid / ↑ Potential of hepatotoxicity R/T ↑ liver breakdown of acetaminophen
Lamotrigene / ↓ Serum lamotrigene levels → ↓ effect
H *Milk thistle* / Helps prevent acetaminophen liver damage
Oral contraceptives / ↑ Liver breakdown of acetaminophen → ↓ t½
Propranolol / ↑ Effect R/T ↓ liver breakdown
Rifampin / ↑ Hepatotoxicity potential R/T ↑ liver breakdown of acetaminophen
Sulfinpyrazone / ↑ Hepatotoxicity potential R/T ↑ liver breakdown of acetaminophen
Zidovudine / ↓ Zidovudine effect R/T ↑ nonhepatic or renal clearance

HOW SUPPLIED

Acetaminophen: *Caplet:* 160 mg, 500 mg, 650 mg; *Capsule:* 325 mg, 500 mg; *Capsules, Sprinkle:* 80 mg, 160 mg; *Chew Tablet:* 80 mg, 160 mg; *Drops:* 80 mg/0.8 mL; *Gelcap:* 500 mg; *Elixir:* 80 mg/2.5 mL, 80 mg/5 mL, 120 mg/5 mL, 160 mg/5 mL; *Liquid:* 160 mg/5 mL, 500 mg/15 mL; *Solution:* 80 mg/1.66 mL, 100 mg/mL; *Suppository:* 80 mg, 120 mg, 125 mg, 300 mg, 325 mg, 650 mg; *Tablet:* 325 mg, 500 mg, 650 mg. Acetaminophen, buffered: *Granule, effervescent*

DOSAGE

• **CAPLETS, CAPSULES, CHEWABLE TABLETS, GELCAPS, ELIXIR, ORAL LIQUID, ORAL SOLUTION, ORAL SUSPENSION, SPRINKLE CAPSULES, SYRUP, TABLETS**

Analgesic, antipyretic.

Adults: 325–650 mg q 4 hr; doses up to a maximum of 1 g q.i.d. may be used. **Pediatric:** Doses given 4–5 times/day. **Up to 3 months:** 40 mg/dose; **4–11 months:** 80 mg/dose; **1–2 years:** 120 mg/dose; **2–3 years:** 160 mg/dose; **4–5 years:** 240 mg/dose; **6–8 years:** 320 mg/dose; **9–10 years:** 400 mg/dose; **11 years:** 480 mg/dose. **12–14 years:** 640 mg/dose. **Over 14 years:** 650 mg/dose. *Alternative pediatric dose:* 10–15 mg/kg q 4 hr.

• **EXTENDED RELIEF CAPLETS**

Analgesic, antipyretic.

Adults: 2 caplets (1,300 mg) q 8 hr.

• **SUPPOSITORIES**

Analgesic, antipyretic.

Adults: 650 mg q 4 hr, not to exceed 4 g/day for up to 10 days. Clients on long-term therapy should not exceed 2.6 g/day. **Pediatric, 3–11 months:** 80 mg q 6 hr. **1–3 years:** 80 mg q 4 hr; **3–6 years:** 120–125 mg q 4–6 hr, with no more than 720 mg in 24 hr. **6–12 years:** 325 mg q 4–6 hr with no more than 2.6 g in 24 hr. Given as needed while symptoms persist.

• **GRANULES, EFFERVESCENT**

Analgesic, antipyretic.

Adult, usual: 1 or 2 three-quarter capfuls are placed into an empty glass; add half a glass of cool water. May be taken while fizzing or after settling. Can be repeated q 4 hr as required or directed by provider.

NURSING CONSIDERATIONS

ADMINISTRATION/STORAGE

1. Do not exceed a dose of 4 g/24 hr in adults and 75 mg/kg/day in children.
2. Do not take for more than 5 days for pain in children, 10 days for pain in adults, or more than 3 days for fever in adults or children without consulting provider.
3. Store suppositories below 80°F (27°C).
4. Take extended-relief product with water; do not crush, chew, or dissolve before swallowing.
5. Bubble gum flavored OTC pediatric products (suspension liquid and chewable tablet) are available for children to treat fever and/or pain.

ASSESSMENT

1. Identify indications for therapy and expected outcomes.
2. If for long-term therapy, monitor CBC, liver and renal function studies.
3. Document presence of fever. Rate pain, noting type, onset, location, duration, and intensity.
4. Check urine for occult blood and albumin to assess for nephritis.

A

CLIENT/FAMILY TEACHING

1. Warn not to combine products containing acetaminophen, many of which are OTC. Read labels on all OTC products consumed.
2. Make sure parents know the difference between the concentrated dropper-dose formulation and the teaspoon dose formulation.
3. Take only as directed and with food or milk to minimize GI upset.
4. S&S of acute toxicity that require immediate reporting include N&V or abdominal pain. Any bluish coloration of the mucosa and nailbeds or complaints of dyspnea, weakness, headache, or vertigo are S&S of methemoglobinemia caused by anoxia and require immediate attention.
5. Report pallor, weakness, and palpitations; S&S of hemolytic anemia.
6. Dyspnea, rapid, weak pulse; cold extremities; unexplained bleeding, bruising, sore throat, malaise, feeling clammy or sweaty; or subnormal temperatures may also be symptoms of chronic poisoning; report.
7. Abdominal pain, yellow discoloration of skin and sclera, dark urine, itching, or clay-colored stools may indicate liver toxicity.
8. Phenacetin, the major active metabolite, may cause urine to become dark brown or wine-colored.
9. Headache and minor pain relievers containing combinations of salicylates, acetaminophen, and caffeine may be no more beneficial than aspirin alone.
10. Any unexplained pain or fever that persists for longer than 3–5 days requires medical evaluation.
11. Avoid alcohol as this may cause toxicity. Not for regular use in clients with any form of liver disease.

OUTCOMES/EVALUATE

- ↓ Fever
- Relief of pain

Acetazolamide

(ah-set-ah-**ZOE**-la-myd)

PREGNANCY CATEGORY: C

Rx: Dazamide, Diamox, Diamox Sequels
★**Rx:** Apo-Acetazolamide

Acetazolamide sodium

(ah-set-ah-**ZOE**-la-myd)

Rx: Diamox
CLASSIFICATION(S):
Anticonvulsant, carbonic anhydrase inhibitor

SEE ALSO *ANTICONVULSANTS.*

ACTION/KINETICS

Sulfonamide derivative possessing carbonic anhydrase inhibitor activity. As an anticonvulsant, beneficial effects may be due to inhibition of carbonic anhydrase in the CNS, which increases carbon dioxide tension resulting in a decrease in neuronal conduction. Systemic acidosis may also be involved. As a diuretic, the drug inhibits carbonic anhydrase in the kidney, which decreases formation of bicarbonate and hydrogen ions from carbon dioxide, thus reducing the availability of these ions for active transport. Use as a diuretic is limited because the drug promotes metabolic acidosis, which inhibits diuretic activity. This may be partially circumvented by giving acetazolamide on alternate days. Also reduces intraocular pressure.

Absorbed from the GI tract and widely distributed throughout the body, including the CNS. Excreted unchanged in the urine. **Tablets: Onset,** 60–90 min; **peak:** 1–4 hr; **duration:** 8–12 hr. **Sustained-release capsules: Onset,** 2 hr; **peak:** 3–6 hr; **duration:** 18–24 hr. **Injection (IV): Onset,** 2 min; **peak:** 15 min; **duration:** 4–5 hr. Eliminated mainly unchanged through the kidneys.

USES

Adjunct in the treatment of edema due to CHF or drug-induced edema. Absence (petit mal) and unlocalized seizures. Open-angle, secondary, or acute-angle closure glaucoma when delay of surgery is desired to lower

IOP. Prophylaxis or treatment of acute mountain sickness in climbers attempting a rapid ascent or in those who are susceptible to mountain sickness even with gradual ascent.

CONTRAINDICATIONS

Low serum sodium and potassium levels. Renal and hepatic dysfunction. Hyperchloremic acidosis, adrenal insufficiency, suprarenal gland failure, hypersensitivity to thiazide diuretics, cirrhosis. Chronic use in noncongestive angle-closure glaucoma.

SPECIAL CONCERNS

Use with caution in the presence of mild acidosis, advanced pulmonary disease, and during lactation. Increasing the dose does not increase effectiveness may but increase the risk of drowsiness or paresthesia. Safety and efficacy have not been established in children.

SIDE EFFECTS

GI: Anorexia, N&V, melena, constipation, alteration in taste, diarrhea. **GU:** Hematuria, glycosuria, urinary frequency, renal colic, renal calculi, crystalluria, polyuria, phosphaturia, decreased or absent libido, impotence. **CNS:** ***Seizures,*** weakness, malaise, fatigue, nervousness, drowsiness, depression, dizziness, disorientation, confusion, ataxia, tremor, headache, tinnitus, flaccid paralysis, lassitude, paresthesia of the extremities. **Hematologic:** ***Bone marrow depression,*** thrombocytopenic purpura, thrombocytopenia, ***hemolytic anemia,*** leukopenia, pancytopenia, agranulocytosis. **Dermatologic:** Pruritus, urticaria, skin rashes, erythema multiforme, ***Stevens-Johnson syndrome, toxic epidermal necrolysis,*** photosensitivity. **Other:** Weight loss, fever, acidosis, electrolyte imbalance, transient myopia, hepatic insufficiency. *NOTE:* Side effects similar to those produced by sulfonamides may also occur.

OD OVERDOSE MANAGEMENT

Symptoms: Drowsiness, anorexia, N&V, dizziness, ataxia, tremor, paresthesias, tinnitus. *Treatment:* Emesis or gastric lavage. Hyperchloremic acidosis may respond to bicarbonate. Administration of potassium may also be necessary. Observe carefully and give supportive treatment.

DRUG INTERACTIONS

ALSO SEE *DIURETICS*.

Amphetamine / ↑ Amphetamine effect by ↑ renal tubular reabsorption
Cyclosporine / ↑ Cyclosporine levels → possible nephrotoxicity and neurotoxicity
Diflunisal / Significant ↓ in IOP with ↑ side effects
Ephedrine / ↑ Ephedrine effect R/T ↑ renal tubular reabsorption
Lithium carbonate / ↓ Lithium effect R/T ↑ renal excretion
Methotrexate / ↓ Methotrexate effect R/T ↑ renal excretion
Primidone / ↓ Primidone effect R/T ↓ GI absorption
Pseudoephedrine / ↑ Pseudoephedrine effect by ↑ renal tubular reabsorption
Quinidine / ↑ Quinidine effect by ↑ renal tubular reabsorption
Salicylates / Accumulation and toxicity of acetazolamide (including CNS depression and metabolic acidosis). Also, acidosis due to ↑ CNS penetration of salicylates

HOW SUPPLIED

Acetazolamide: *Capsule, Extended Release:* 500 mg; *Tablet:* 125 mg, 250 mg. Acetazolamide sodium: *Powder for injection:* 500 mg

DOSAGE

• EXTENDED-RELEASE CAPSULES, TABLETS, IV

Epilepsy.

Adults/children: 8–30 mg/kg/day in divided doses. Optimum daily dosage: 375–1,000 mg (doses higher than 1,000 mg do not increase therapeutic effect).

Adjunct to other anticonvulsants.

Initial: 250 mg/day; dose can be increased up to 1,000 mg/day in divided doses if necessary.

Glaucoma, simple open-angle.

Adults: 250–1,000 mg/day in divided doses. Doses greater than 1 g/day do not increase the effect.

Glaucoma, closed-angle prior to surgery or secondary.

Adults, short-term therapy: 250 mg q 4 hr or 250 mg b.i.d. **Adults, acute therapy:** 500 mg followed by 125–250 mg q 4 hr using tablets. For extended-release capsules, give 500 mg b.i.d. in the morning and evening. IV therapy may be used for rapid decrease in intraocular pressure. **Pediatric:** 5–10 mg/kg/dose IM or IV q 6 hr or 10–15 mg/kg/day in divided doses q 6–8 hr using tablets.

Acute mountain sickness.

Adults: 250 mg b.i.d.–q.i.d. (500 mg 1–2 times/day of extended-release capsules). During rapid ascent, 1 g/day is recommended.

Diuresis in CHF.

Adults, initial: 250–375 mg (5 mg/kg) once daily in the morning. If the client stops losing edema fluid after an initial response, do not increase doses; rather, skip medication for a day to allow the kidney to recover. The best diuretic effect occurs when the drug is given on alternate days or for 2 days alternating with a day of rest.

Drug-induced edema.

Adults: 250–375 mg once daily for 1 or 2 days. Most effective if given every other day or for 2 days followed by a day of rest. **Children:** 5 mg/kg/dose PO or IV once daily in the morning.

NURSING CONSIDERATIONS

SEE ALSO *NURSING CONSIDERATIONS* FOR *ANTICONVULSANTS*.

ADMINISTRATION/STORAGE

1. Change over from other anticonvulsant therapy should be gradual.
2. Acetazolamide tablets may be crushed and suspended in a cherry, chocolate, raspberry, or other sweet syrup. Do not use vehicles containing glycerin or alcohol. As an alternative, 1 tablet may be submerged in 10 mL of hot water and added to 10 mL of honey or syrup.
3. Tolerance after prolonged use may necessitate dosage increase.
4. Do not administer the sustained-release dosage form as an anticonvulsant; it should be used only for glaucoma and acute mountain sickness.
5. With prophylaxis of mountain sickness, initiate dosage 1–2 days before ascent and continue for at least 2 days while at high altitudes.
6. Due to possible differences in bioavailability, do not interchange brands.

IV 7. IV administration is preferred; IM administration is painful due to alkalinity of solution.

8. For direct IV use, administer over at least 1 min. For intermittent IV use, further dilute in dextrose or saline solution and infuse over 4-8 hr. Reconstitute each 500-mg vial with at least 5 mL of sterile water for injection.
9. Use within 24 hr after reconstitution, although reconstituted solutions retain potency for 1 week if refrigerated.

ASSESSMENT

1. Note indications for therapy, type and onset of symptoms.
2. Review electrolytes, uric acid, and glucose. Note any liver and renal dysfunction prior to administering.
3. List drugs currently prescribed to ensure none interacts unfavorably.
4. With glaucoma, note baseline ophthalmic exam and intraocular pressures; assess for visual effects.
5. Perform CV/pulmonary assessment with CHF history.

CLIENT/FAMILY TEACHING

1. Taking drug with food may decrease gastric irritation and GI upset.
2. Determine drug effects before undertaking tasks that require mental alertness.
3. Drug increases voiding frequency; take early to avoid interrupting sleep.
4. Take only as directed. If prescribed every other day, record to enhance adherence.
5. Increase fluids (2–3 L/day) to prevent crystalluria/ stone formation.
6. Drug may increase blood glucose levels. Monitor FS and report increases; hypoglycemic agent may need adjustment.
7. Report if nausea, dizziness, rapid weight gain, muscle weakness, cramps, or any changes in the color/consistency of stools occur.
8. Report for labs to determine need for potassium replacement.

OUTCOMES/EVALUATE

- ↓ Seizure activity
- ↓ Intraocular pressure

A

- ↓ CHF-associated edema
- Prevention of mountain sickness

Acetylcysteine

(ah-see-till-**SIS**-tay-een)

PREGNANCY CATEGORY: B
CLASSIFICATION(S):
Mucolytic
Rx: Mucomyst, Mucosil-10 and -20
✱Rx: Parvolex

ACTION/KINETICS
Reduces the viscosity of purulent and nonpurulent pulmonary secretions and facilitates their removal by splitting disulfide bonds. Action increases with increasing pH (peak: pH 7–9). **Onset, inhalation:** Within 1 min; **by direct instillation:** immediate. **Time to peak effect:** 5–10 min. Also reduces liver injury due to acetaminophen overdosage by maintaining or restoring glutathione levels or by acting as an alternate substrate for the reactive metabolite of acetaminophen.

USES
Adjunct in the treatment of chronic emphysema, emphysema with bronchitis, chronic asthmastic bronchitis, tuberculosis, bronchiectasis, primary amyloidosis of lung, acute bronchopulmonary disease (bronchitis, pneumonia, tracheobronchitis). Routine care of clients with tracheostomy, pulmonary complications after thoracic or CV surgery, use during anesthesia, atelectasis due to mucus obstruction, and in posttraumatic chest conditions. Pulmonary complications of cystic fibrosis. Diagnostic bronchial studies. Antidote in acetaminophen poisoning to reduce or prevent hepatotoxicity. *Investigational:* As an ophthalmic solution for dry eye. As an enema to treat bowel obstruction due to meconium ileus or equivalent. Alzheimer's disease to increase reasoning skills.

CONTRAINDICATIONS
Sensitivity to drug.

SPECIAL CONCERNS
Use with caution during lactation, in the elderly, and in clients with asthma.

SIDE EFFECTS
Respiratory: Increased incidence of bronchospasm in clients with asthma. Increased amount of liquefied bronchial secretions, which must be removed by suction if cough is inadequate. Bronchial and tracheal irritation, tightness in chest, bronchoconstriction. **GI:** N&V, stomatitis. **Other:** Rashes, fever, drowsiness, rhinorrhea.

DRUG INTERACTIONS
Acetylcysteine is incompatible with antibiotics and should be administered separately.

HOW SUPPLIED
Solution (as sodium): 10%, 20%

DOSAGE

• 10% OR 20% SOLUTION: NEBULIZATION, DIRECT APPLICATION, OR DIRECT INTRATRACHEAL INSTILLATION

Nebulization into face mask, tracheostomy, mouth piece.
1–10 mL of 20% solution or 2–10 mL of 10% solution 3–4 times/day.

Closed tent or croupette.
Up to 300 mL of 10% or 20% solution/treatment.

Direct instillation into tracheostomy.
1–2 mL of 10% or 20% solution q 1–4 hr.

Percutaneous intratracheal catheter.
1–2 mL of 20% solution or 2–4 mL of 10% solution q 1–4 hr by syringe attached to catheter.

Instillation to particular portion of bronchopulmonary tree using small plastic catheter into the trachea.
2–5 mL of 20% solution instilled into the trachea by means of a syringe connected to a catheter.

Diagnostic procedures.
2–3 doses of 1–2 mL of 20% or 2–4 mL of 10% solution by nebulization or intratracheal instillation before the procedure.

Acetaminophen overdose.
Given PO, initial: 140 mg/kg; **then,** 70 mg/kg q 4 hr for a total of 17 doses.

NURSING CONSIDERATIONS

ADMINISTRATION/STORAGE

1. Use nonreactive plastic, glass, or stainless steel for administration.
2. May use 10% solution undiluted.
3. Use either water for injection or saline to dilute the 20% solution.
4. May administer via face mask, face tent, oxygen tent, head tent, or by positive-pressure apparatus.
5. Administer with compressed air for nebulization. Hand nebulizers are contraindicated.
6. After prolonged nebulization, dilute the last fourth of the medication with sterile water to prevent drug concentration.
7. Solution may develop a light purple color; does not affect action.
8. Closed bottles of solution remain stable for 2 years when stored at 20°C (68°F). Store open bottles at 2–8°C (35–46°F) and use within 96 hr. Once opened, record time/date to prevent use beyond 96 hr.
9. Incompatible with antibiotics; administer separately.
10. Have suction available for removal of increased secretions.

ASSESSMENT

1. Note pulmonary findings; determine when spasms occur.
2. Document conditions likely to cause congestion and wheezing.
3. Identify previous approaches (successful and unsuccessful) used to treat symptoms.
4. Determine smoking status. If currently taking antibiotics do not administer together.
5. With acetaminophen overdosage document time of ingestion. Administer drug within 8–10 hr following overdose to protect from hepatoxicity and death. Monitor LFTs and acetaminophen levels.

INTERVENTIONS

1. With bronchospasm, have bronchodilator, such as isoproterenol for aerosol inhalation, readily available.
2. Position to facilitate removal of secretions. If unable to cough up secretions, provide suction.
3. Monitor VS and I&O.
4. Wash face following nebulization treatments; medication may cause the face to become sticky.
5. Administration route for acetaminophen toxicity is oral and will consist of 17 doses.

CLIENT/FAMILY TEACHING

1. Use only as directed; do not exceed prescribed dosage.
2. Report unusual changes in sputum color, consistency, or characteristics.
3. The nauseous odor when the treatment begins will become less noticeable as therapy continues.
4. Avoid any triggers that may stimulate bronchospasm (i.e., cigarette smoke, dust, chemicals, cold air).
5. Attend smoking cessation classes and support groups to help stop smoking.

OUTCOMES/EVALUATE

- Improved airway exchange with ↓ viscosity; mobilization and expectoration of secretions
- ↓ Acetaminophen levels and associated liver toxicity

Acyclovir (Acycloguanosine)

(ay-**SYE**-kloh-veer, ay-**SYE**-kloh-**GWON**-oh-seen)

PREGNANCY CATEGORY: C
CLASSIFICATION(S):
Antiviral
Rx: Zovirax
✱Rx: Apo-Acyclovir, Avirax, Nu-Acyclovir

SEE ALSO *ANTIVIRAL DRUGS*.

ACTION/KINETICS

A synthetic acyclic purine nucleoside analog converted by HSV-infected cells to acyclovir triphosphate, which interferes with HSV DNA polymerase, thereby inhibiting DNA replication. Systemic absorption is slow from the GI tract (although therapeutic levels are reached) and following topical administration. It is preferentially taken up and converted to the active triphosphate form by herpes virus–infected cells. Food does not affect absorption. **Peak levels after PO:** 1.5–2 hr. Widely distributed in tissues and body fluids. The half-life and total body clearance depend on renal function. **$t^{1/2}$, PO, C_{CR}, greater than 80 mL/min/1.73 m^2:** 2.5 hr. Metabolites and unchanged drug (up to 85%) are excreted through the kidney. Reduce dosage in clients with impaired renal function. Clients who take acyclovir (600–800 mg/day) with Zidovudine had a significantly prolonged survival rate compared with clients taking only acyclovir.

USES

PO. Initial and recurrent genital herpes in immunocompromised and nonimmunocompromised clients. Prophylaxis of frequently recurrent genital herpes infections in nonimmunocompromised clients. Treatment of chickenpox in children ranging from 2 to 18 years of age. Acute treatment of herpes zoster (shingles).

Parenteral. Initial therapy for severe genital herpes in clients who are not immunocompromised; initial and recurrent mucosal and cutaneous HSV-1 and HSV-2 infections in immunocompromised individuals. Varicella zoster infections (shingles) in immunocompromised clients. HSE in clients over 6 months of age. Neonatal herpes simplex infections.

Topical. To decrease healing time and duration of viral shedding in initial herpes genitalis. Limited non-life-threatening mucocutaneous HSV infections in immunocompromised clients. No beneficial effect in recurrent herpes genitalis or in herpes labialis in nonimmunocompromised clients.

Investigational: Cytomegalovirus and HSV infection following bone marrow or renal transplantation; herpes simplex ocular infections; herpes simplex proctitis; herpes simplex labialis; herpes simplex whitlow; herpes zoster encephalitis; disseminated primary eczema herpeticum; herpes simplex–associated erythema multiforme; infectious mononucleosis; and varicella pneumonia.

CONTRAINDICATIONS

Hypersensitivity to formulation. Use in the eye. Use to prevent recurrent HSV infections.

SPECIAL CONCERNS

Use with caution during lactation or with concomitant intrathecal methotrexate or interferon. Safety and efficacy of PO form not established in children less than 2 years of age. Prolonged or repeated doses in immunocompromised clients may result in emergence of resistant viruses. Use of oral acyclovir does not eliminate latent HSV and is not a cure.

SIDE EFFECTS

• **PO**

Short-term treatment of herpes simplex.

GI: N&V, diarrhea, anorexia, sore throat, taste of drug. **CNS:** Headache, dizziness, fatigue. **Miscellaneous:** Edema, skin rashes, leg pain, inguinal adenopathy.

Long-term treatment of herpes simplex.

GI: Nausea, diarrhea. **CNS:** Headache. **Other:** Skin rash, asthenia, paresthesia.

Treatment of herpes zoster.

GI: N&V, diarrhea, constipation. **CNS:** Headache, malaise.

Treatment of chickenpox.

GI: Vomiting, diarrhea, abdominal pain, flatulence. **Dermatologic:** Rash.

• **PARENTERAL *(frequency greater than 1%).***

At injection site: Phlebitis, inflammation.

GI: N&V. **CNS:** Encephalopathic changes, including lethargy, obtundation, tremors, agitation, confusion, hallucination, ***seizures, coma*** , jitters, headache. **Miscellaneous:** Skin rashes, urticaria, itching, transient elevation of serum creatinine or BUN (most often following rapid IV infusion), elevation of transaminases, ***fatal renal failure, fatal thrombotic thrombocytopenic purpura or hemolytic uremic syndrome in immunocompromised clients.***

A

• **TOPICAL**

Transient burning, stinging, pain. Pruritus, rash, vulvitis, local edema. *NOTE:* All of these effects have also been reported with the use of a placebo preparation.

OD OVERDOSE MANAGEMENT

Symptoms: Increased BUN and serum creatinine, ***renal failure following parenteral overdose.*** *Treatment:* Hemodialysis (peritoneal dialysis is less effective).

DRUG INTERACTIONS

Probenecid / ↑ Bioavailability and half-life of acyclovir → ↑ effect
Zidovudine / Severe lethargy and drowsiness

HOW SUPPLIED

Capsule: 200 mg; *Injection:* 5 mg/mL; *Ointment:* 5%; *Powder for injection:* 500 mg/vial, 1000 mg/vial; *Suspension:* 200 mg/5 mL; *Tablet:* 400 mg, 800 mg

DOSAGE

• **CAPSULES, SUSPENSION, TABLETS**

Initial genital herpes.

200 mg q 4 hr 5 times/day for 10 days.

Chronic genital herpes.

400 mg b.i.d., 200 mg t.i.d., or 200 mg 5 times/day for up to 12 months.

Intermittent therapy for genital herpes.

200 mg q 4 hr 5 times/day for 5 days. Start therapy at the first symptom/sign of recurrence.

Herpes zoster, acute treatment.

800 mg q 4 hr 5 times/day for 7–10 days.

Chickenpox.

20 mg/kg (of the suspension) q.i.d. for 5 days. A single dose should not exceed 800 mg. Begin therapy at the earliest sign/symptom.

• **IV INFUSION**

Mucosal and cutaneous herpes simplex in immunocompromised clients.

Adults: 5 mg/kg infused at a constant rate over 1 hr, q 8 hr (15 mg/kg/day) for 7 days. **Children less than 12 years of age:** 250 mg/m^2 infused at a constant rate over 1 hr q 8 hr for 7 days.

Varicella-zoster infections (shingles) in immunocompromised clients.

Adults: 10 mg/kg infused at a constant rate over 1 hr q 8 hr for 7 days (not to exceed 500 mg/m^2 q 8 hr). **Children less than 12 years of age:** 500 mg/m^2 infused at a constant rate over at least 1 hr q 8 hr for 7 days.

Herpes simplex encephalitis.

Adults: 10 mg/kg infused at a constant rate over at least 1 hr q 8 hr for 10 days. **Children less than 12 years of age and greater than 6 months of age:** 500 mg/m^2 infused at a constant rate over at least 1 hr q 8 hr for 10 days.

• **TOPICAL (5% OINTMENT)**

Adults and children: Lesion should be covered with sufficient amount of ointment (0.5 in ribbon/4 in^2 of surface area) q 3 hr 6 times/day for 7 days. Initiate treatment as soon as possible after onset of symptoms.

NURSING CONSIDERATIONS

SEE ALSO *GENERAL NURSING CONSIDERATIONS FOR ALL ANTI-INFECTIVES* AND *ANTIVIRAL DRUGS.*

ADMINISTRATION/STORAGE

1. Store ointment in a dry place at room temperature.
2. Adjust both the PO and parenteral dose and/or dosing interval in acute or chronic renal impairment.
3. The suspension may be used to treat varicella zoster infections.
IV 4. Prepare IV solution by dissolving the contents of the 500- or 1000-mg vial in 10 or 20 mL sterile water for injection, respectively (final concentration of 50 mg/mL). Infusion concentrations of 7 mg/mL or lower are recommended; thus, the calculated dose must be added to an appropriate IV solution at the correct volume. Reconstituted solution should be used within 12 hr. Avoid bacteriostatic water containing benzyl alcohol or parabens; will cause a precipitate.
5. Administer infusion over 1 hr to prevent renal tubular damage; do not administer by rapid or bolus IV, IM, or SC injections.
6. Accompany IV infusion by hydration (3 L/day) to prevent precipitation in renal tubules (crystalluria).
7. If refrigerated, reconstituted solution may show a precipitate which dissolves at room temperature.

A

ASSESSMENT

1. Document indications for therapy and assess/analyze skin lesions.
2. Monitor CBC, electrolytes, renal and LFTs closely with IV therapy and if immunocompromised.
3. With chickenpox or herpes zoster, institute appropriate precautions for all susceptible individuals (i.e., pregnant women, immunocompromised clients, and those who have not had chickenpox [may check titer if unknown]).

CLIENT/FAMILY TEACHING

1. Drug is not a cure; use only to help manage symptoms. It will not prevent disease transmission to others or prevent reinfection.
2. Adequately cover all lesions with topical acyclovir as ordered; do not exceed dosage, frequency of application or treatment time.
3. Report any burning, stinging, itching, and rash when applying.
4. Complete all exams/tests to rule out presence of other STDs.
5. Acyclovir is ineffective for treatment of reinfection; return to provider if HSV recurs.
6. Apply ointment as directed with a finger cot or rubber glove to prevent transmission of infection to other body sites.
7. Use condoms for sexual intercourse to prevent reinfections while undergoing treatment. Abstain during acute outbreaks (lesions present) and use condoms at all other times.
8. The total dose and dosage schedule differ depending on whether the infection is initial or chronic and whether intermittent therapy regimen is being used. Therefore, follow prescribed dosage, dosage combinations (i.e., with Zidovudine) and duration of treatment.
9. Consume 2–3 L/day of fluids, especially during parenteral therapy, to prevent renal toxicity/crystalluria.
10. Females should have an annual Pap test; an increased risk of cervical cancer may be associated with genital herpes.
11. Do not exceed dosage and do not share meds.

OUTCOMES/EVALUATE

- Less severe and less frequent herpes outbreaks
- Crusting and healing of herpetic lesions
- ↓ Pain with shingles outbreak

Adenosine

(ah-**DEN**-oh-seen)

PREGNANCY CATEGORY: C
CLASSIFICATION(S):
Antiarrhythmic
Rx: Adenocard, Adenoscan

SEE ALSO *ANTIARRHYTHMIC AGENTS.*

ACTION/KINETICS

Found naturally in all cells of the body. It slows conduction time through the AV node, interrupts the reentry pathways through the AV node, and restores normal sinus rhythm in paroxysmal supraventricular tachycardia. May cause a transient slowing of ventricular response immediately after use. Competitively antagonized by caffeine and theophylline; potentiated by dipyridamole. **Onset, after IV:** 34 sec. **t¹/₂:** Less than 10 sec (taken up by erythrocytes and vascular endothelial cells). **Duration:** 1–2 min. Exogenous adenosine becomes part of the body pool and is metabolized mainly to inosine and AMP.

USES

Conversion to sinus rhythm of PSVT (including that associated with accessory bypass tracts). The phosphate salt is used for symptomatic relief of complications with stasis dermatitis in varicose veins. *Investigational:* With thallium-201 tomography in noninvasive assessment of clients with suspected CAD who cannot exercise adequately prior to being stress-tested. Adenosine is not effective in converting rhythms other than PSVT. The phosphate salt has been used to treat herpes infections and to increase blood flow to

brain tumors and in porphyria cutanea tarda.

CONTRAINDICATIONS

Second- or third-degree AV block or sick sinus syndrome (except in clients with a functioning artificial pacemaker), atrial flutter, atrial fibrillation, ventricular tachycardia. History of MI or cerebral hemorrhage.

SPECIAL CONCERNS

At time of conversion to normal sinus rhythm, new rhythms (PVC, atrial premature contractions, sinus bradycardia, skipped beats, varying degrees of AV block, sinus tachycardia) lasting a few seconds may occur. Use with caution in the elderly as severe bradycardia and AV block may occur and in clients with asthma due to possibility of bronchoconstriction. Safety and efficacy as a diagnostic agent have not been determined in clients less than 18 years of age.

SIDE EFFECTS

CV: Short lasting first-, second-, or ***third-degree heart block; cardiac arrest,*** sustained ventricular tachycardia, sinus bradycardia, ST-segment depression, sinus exit block, sinus pause, arrhythmias, T-wave changes, hypertension. prolonged asystole, Nonfatal MI, transient increase in BP, ***ventricular fibrillation***. Facial flushing (common), chest pain, sweating, palpitations, hypotension (may be significant). **CNS:** Lightheadedness, dizziness, numbness, headache, blurred vision, apprehension, paresthesia, drowsiness, emotional instability, tremors, nervousness. **GI:** Nausea, metallic taste, tightness in throat. **Respiratory:** SOB or dyspnea (common), urge to breathe deeply, chest pressure or discomfort, cough, hyperventilation, nasal congestion. **GU:** Urinary urgency, vaginal pressure. **Miscellaneous:** Pressure in head, burning sensation, neck and back pain, weakness, blurred vision, dry mouth, ear discomfort, pressure in groin, scotomas, tongue discomfort, discomfort (tingling, heaviness) in upper extremities, discomfort in throat, neck, or jaw.

DRUG INTERACTIONS

H *Aloe; Buckthorn bark/berry; Cascara sagrada bark; Rhubarb root; Senna pod and leaf* / Possible ↑ adenosine effect
Carbamazepine / ↑ AV block
Caffeine / Competitively antagonizes adenosine effect
Digoxin / Possibility of ventricular fibrillation (rare)
Dipyridamole / ↑ Adenosine effect
Theophylline / Competitively antagonizes adenosine effect
Verapamil / Possibility of ventricular fibrillation (rare)

HOW SUPPLIED

Injection: 3 mg/mL

DOSAGE

- **RAPID IV BOLUS ONLY**

Antiarrhythmic.

Initial: 6 mg over 1–2 sec. If the first dose does not reverse the SVT within 1–2 min, 12 mg should be given as a rapid IV bolus. The 12-mg dose may be repeated a second time, if necessary. Doses greater than 12 mg are not recommended.

- **IV INFUSION ONLY**

Diagnostic aid.

Adults: 140 mcg/kg/min infused over 6 min (total dose of 0.84 mg/kg).

- **IM ONLY**

Varicose veins.

Initial: 25–50 mg 1–2 times daily until symptoms subside. **Maintenance:** 25 mg 2 or 3 times weekly.

NURSING CONSIDERATIONS

SEE ALSO *NURSING CONSIDERATIONS* FOR *ANTIARRHYTHMIC AGENTS.*

ADMINISTRATION/STORAGE

IV 1. Drug can be stored at room temperature; crystallization may result if the drug is refrigerated. If crystals form, dissolve by warming to room temperature. The solution must be clear when administered.

2. Discard any unused portion; contains no preservatives.

3. Administer directly into a vein. If given into an IV line, introduce in the most proximal line and follow with a rapid saline flush.

4. When used as a diagnostic aid, the dose of thallium-201 should be given at the midpoint of the adenosine infusion (i.e., after 3 min).

A

ASSESSMENT

1. Document indications for therapy, onset of symptoms, and ECG confirmation of arrhythmia.
2. Monitor rhythm strips closely for evidence of varying degrees of AV block and increased arrhythmias during conversion to sinus rhythm. These are usually only transient.
3. Monitor BP and pulse. Report complaints of numbness, tingling in the arms, blurred vision, or apprehensiveness, as this may be an indication to discontinue drug therapy.
4. Document chest pressure, SOB, heaviness of the arms, palpitations, or dyspnea. Note any history of MI or CVA as drug is contraindicated; with asthma may cause bronchoconstriction.
5. In stasis dermatitis carefully assess extremities and note findings.

CLIENT/FAMILY TEACHING

1. Drug helps restore heart to a normal, slower rhythm.
2. Avoid caffeine and report if concurrently prescribed theophylline, digoxin, or dipyridamole.
3. Facial flushing is a common temporary side effect of therapy.

OUTCOMES/EVALUATE

- Conversion of PSVT to NSR
- Symptomatic relief with stasis dermatitis

Albuterol (Salbutamol)

(al-**BYOU**-ter-ohl)

PREGNANCY CATEGORY: C
CLASSIFICATION(S):
Sympathomimetic
Rx: AccuNeb, Airet, Proventil, Proventil HFA, Proventil Repetabs, Ventolin, Ventolin HFA, Ventolin Nebules, Ventolin Rotacaps, Volmax
✱**Rx:** Airomir, Alti-Salbutamol Sulfate, Asmavent, Gen-Salbutamol Respirator Solution, Gen-Salbutamol Sterinebs P.F., Novo-Salmol Tablets, Nu-Salbutamol, PMS-Salbutamol, Rhoxal-salbutamol, Salbutamol Nebuamp

SEE ALSO *SYMPATHOMIMETIC DRUGS.*

ACTION/KINETICS

Stimulates beta-2 receptors of the bronchi, leading to bronchodilation. Causes less tachycardia and is longer-acting than isoproterenol. Has minimal beta-1 activity. Available as an inhaler that contains no chlorofluorocarbons (Proventil HFA). **Onset, PO:** 15–30 min; **inhalation,** within 5 min. **Peak effect, PO:** 2–3 hr; **inhalation,** 60–90 min (after 2 inhalations). **Duration, PO:** 4–8 hr (up to 12 hr for extended-release); **inhalation,** 3–6 hr. Metabolites and unchanged drug excreted in urine and feces.

USES

Bronchial asthma; bronchospasm due to bronchitis or emphysema; bronchitis; children 4 years and older for treatment or prevention of bronchospasm with reversible obstructive pulmonary disease; exercise-induced bronchospasm, including those 4 years of age and older. Prophylaxis of bronchial asthma or bronchospasms. Proventil HFA may be used in clients 4 years of age and older. *Investigational:* Nebulized albuterol may be useful as an adjunct to treat serious acute hyperkalemia in hemodialysis clients.

CONTRAINDICATIONS

Aerosol for prevention of exercise-induced bronchospasm and tablets are not recommended for children less than 12 years of age. Use during lactation.

SPECIAL CONCERNS

Dosage not established for the syrup and solution for inhalation in children less than 2 years of age, for tablets and extended-release tablets in children less than 6 years of age, and the aerosol and inhalation powder in children less than 4 years of age. May delay preterm labor. Large IV doses may aggravate preexisting diabetes mellitus and ketoacidosis.

ADDITIONAL SIDE EFFECTS

GI: Diarrhea, dry mouth, appetite loss or stimulation, epigastric pain. **CNS:** Hyperkinesia, excitement, nervousness, tension, tremor, dizziness, vertigo, weakness, drowsiness, restlessness, headache, insomnia, malaise, emotional

A

lability, fatigue, lightheadedness, nightmares, disturbed sleep, aggressive behavior, irritability. **Respiratory:** Cough, wheezing, dyspnea, bronchospasm, dry throat, pharyngitis, throat irritation, bronchitis, epistaxis, hoarseness (especially in children), nasal congestion, increase in sputum. **CV:** Palpitations, tachycardia, BP changes, hypertension, tight chest, chest pain or discomfort, angina. **Hypersensitivity (may be immediate):** Urticaria, ***angioedema,*** rash, ***bronchospasm.*** **Miscellaneous:** Flushing, sweating, bad or unusual taste, change in smell, muscle cramps, pallor, teeth discoloration, conjunctivitis, dilated pupils, difficulty in urination, muscle spasm, voice changes, oropharyngeal edema.

OD OVERDOSE MANAGEMENT

Symptoms: Seizures, anginal pain, hypertension, hypokalemia, tachycardia (rate may increase to 200 beats/min).

SEE ALSO *SYMPATHOMIMETIC DRUGS.*

DRUG INTERACTIONS

H *Fir needle oil; Pine needle oil;* / ↑ Risk of bronchospasm

HOW SUPPLIED

Capsule for Inhalation: 200 mcg; *Inhalation Aerosol:* 90 mcg/inh; *Inhalation Solution:* 0.083%, 0.5%, 0.63 mg/3 mL, 1.25 mg/3 mL; *Syrup:* 2 mg/5 mL; *Tablet:* 2 mg, 4 mg; *Tablet, Extended Release:* 4 mg, 8 mg

DOSAGE

• **METERED DOSE INHALER (INHALATION AEROSOL)**

Bronchodilation.

Adults and children over 4 years of age: 180 mcg (2 inhalations) q 4–6 hr. In some clients 1 inhalation (90 mcg) q 4 hr may be sufficient.

Prophylaxis of exercise-induced bronchospasm.

Adults and children over 4 years of age: 180 mcg (2 inhalations) 15 min before exercise.

• **INHALATION SOLUTION**

Bronchodilation.

Adults and children over 12 years of age: 2.5 mg t.i.d.–q.i.d. by nebulization (dilute 0.5 mL of the 0.5% solution with 2.5 mL sterile NSS and deliver over 5–15 min). **Children, 2–12 years of age, initial:** 0.l–0.15 mg/kg/dose; titrate subsequent dosage based on desired clinical response, but not to exceed 2.5 mg t.i.d.–q.i.d. by nebulization.

• **INHALATION CAPSULES**

Bronchodilation.

Adults and children over 4 years of age: 200 mcg q 4–6 hr using a Rotahaler inhalation device. In some clients, 400 mcg q 4–6 hr may be required.

Prophylaxis of exercise-induced bronchospasm.

Adults and children over 4 years: 200 mcg (1 capsule) 15 min before exercise using a Rotahaler inhalation device.

• **SYRUP**

Bronchodilation.

Adults and children over 14 years of age: 2–4 mg (1–2 teaspoonfuls) t.i.d.–q.i.d., up to a maximum of 8 mg q.i.d. **Children, 6–14 years, initial:** 2 mg (1 teaspoonful) t.i.d.–q.i.d.; **then,** increase as necessary to a maximum of 24 mg/day in divided doses. **Children, 2–6 years, initial:** 0.1 mg/kg t.i.d.; **then,** increase as necessary up to 0.2 mg/kg, not to exceed 4 mg t.i.d.

• **TABLETS**

Bronchodilation.

Adults and children over 12 years of age, initial: 2–4 mg t.i.d.–q.i.d.; **then,** increase dose as needed up to a maximum of 8 mg t.i.d.–q.i.d. In geriatric clients or those sensitive to beta agonists, start with 2 mg t.i.d.–q.i.d. and then increase dose gradually, if needed, to a maximum of 8 mg t.i.d.–q.i.d. **Children, 6–12 years of age, usual, initial:** 2 mg t.i.d.–q.i.d.; **then,** if necessary, increase the dose in a stepwise fashion to a maximum of 24 mg/day in divided doses.

• **PROVENTIL REPETABS**

Bronchodilation.

Adults and children over 12 years of age: 4 or 8 mg q 12 hr up to a maximum of 32 mg/day. **Children 6–11 years of age, initial:** 4 mg q 12 hr. If necessary, increase the dosage stepwise to a maximum of 12 mg b.i.d. Clients on regular-release albuterol can be switched to the Repetabs (a 4-mg extended-release tablet q 12 hr is equivalent to a regular 2-mg tablet q 6 hr). Multiples of this regimen, up to the maximum recommended dose, also apply.

• **VOLMAX EXTENDED RELEASE TABLETS**

Bronchodilation.

Adults and children over 12 years of age: 8 mg q 12 hr; in some clients (e.g., low adult body weight), 4 mg q 12 hr may be sufficient initially and then increased to 8 mg q 12 hr, depending on the response. The dose can be increased stepwise and cautiously (under provider supervision) to a maximum of 32 mg/day in divided doses q 12 hr. **Children, 6–12 years of age:** 4 mg q 12 hr. The dose can be increased stepwise and cautiously (under provider supervision) to a maximum of 24 mg/day in divided doses q 12 hr.

NURSING CONSIDERATIONS

SEE ALSO *NURSING CONSIDERATIONS* FOR *SYMPATHOMIMETIC DRUGS.*

ADMINISTRATION/STORAGE

1. When given by nebulization, either a face mask or mouthpiece may be used. Use compressed air or oxygen with a gas flow of 6–10 L/min; a single treatment lasts from 5 to 15 min.
2. When given by IPPB, the inspiratory pressure should be from 10 to 20 cm water, with the duration of treatment ranging from 5 to 20 min depending on the client and instrument control.
3. The MDI may also be administered on a mechanical ventilator through an adapter.
4. Take extended-release tablets whole with the aid of liquids; do not chew or crush. The outer coating of Volmax Extended-Release Tablets is not absorbed and is excreted in the feces; empty outer coating may be seen in the stool.
5. The contents of the MDI container are under pressure. Do not store near heat or open flames and do not puncture the container.
6. Proventil HFA and Ventolin HFA contain hydrofluoroalkane as the propellant rather than chlorofluorocarbons.
7. AccuNeb, either 0.63 mg/3 mL or 1.25 mg/3 mL is intended for relief of bronchospasm in children 2–12 years of age with asthma.

ASSESSMENT

1. Obtain history and assess CNS status.
2. Document PFTs, CXR, and lung sounds. Note any anxiety; may contribute to air hunger.
3. Document symptom characteristics, onset, duration, frequency, and any precipitating factors.
4. Determine if able to self-administer medication. Assess environmental/home characteristics.
5. Monitor pulmonary status (i.e., breath sounds, VS, peak flow, or ABGs) for effects of the therapy.
6. Observe for evidence of allergic responses.

CLIENT/FAMILY TEACHING

1. Take only as directed; do not exceed prescribed dose.
2. Maintain a calm, reassuring approach. Do not leave client unattended if acutely short of breath.
3. Practice how to inhale through nose and exhale with pursed lip or diaphragmatic breathing in order to prolong expiration and keep the airways open longer, thus reducing the work of breathing.
4. Do not put lips around inhaler; go two fingerbreadths away before attempting to activate and inhale. May use a spacer to facilitate inhalation. Attend instruction on the correct method for administration.
5. A spacer used with the MDI may enhance drug dispersion. Always thoroughly rinse mouth and equipment with water following each use to prevent oral fungal infections.
6. When using albuterol inhalers, do not use other albuterol inhalation medication unless specifically prescribed.
7. Establish dosing regimens that fit life-style, i.e., 1–2 puffs q 6 hr or 4 puffs 4 times/day; the usual dosing is q 4–6 hr with an as-needed order, or before exercise. Check peak flows, call if requiring more puffs more frequently than prescribed or if dose of drug used previously does not provide relief.

8. To check inhaler content, may place in a glass of water: full inhalers sink, empty inhalers float and half-full are partially submerged.

OUTCOMES/EVALUATE

Improved breathing patterns/airway exchange

Aldesleukin (Interleukin-2; IL-2)

(al-des-**LOO**-kin)

PREGNANCY CATEGORY: C
CLASSIFICATION(S):
Antineoplastic, miscellaneous
Rx: Proleukin

SEE ALSO *ANTINEOPLASTIC AGENTS.*

ACTION/KINETICS

Is a human interleukin-2 (IL-2) product produced by recombinant DNA technology. The recombinant form differs from natural IL-2 in that aldesleukin is not glycosylated, the molecule has no N-terminal alanine, the molecule has serine substituted for cysteine at amino acid position 125, and the aggregation state of aldesleukin may be different from that of native IL-2. However, aldesleukin possesses the biologic activity of human native IL-2. Drug effects include activation of cellular immunity with profound lymphocytosis, eosinophilia, and thrombocytopenia; the production of cytokines, including tumor necrosis factor, IL-1, and gamma-interferon; and inhibition of tumor growth. The exact mechanism is not known but may induce the proliferation of natural killer and cytotoxic T cells, which recognize and fight tumor-specific antigens located on the surface of malignant cells. High plasma levels reached after a short IV infusion; rapidly distributed to the extravascular, extracellular space. Rapidly cleared from the circulation by both glomerular filtration and peritubular extraction; metabolized in the kidneys with little or no active form excreted through the urine. **t½, distribution:** 13 min; **t½, elimination:** 85 min.

USES

Metastatic renal cell carcinoma in adults 18 years of age and older. Metastatic melanona. *Investigational:* Kaposi's sarcoma in combination with zidovudine, metastatic melanoma in combination with low-dose cyclophosphamide, colorectal cancer and non-Hodgkin's lymphoma often in combination with lymphokine-activated killer cells.

CONTRAINDICATIONS

Hypersensitivity to IL-2 or any components of the product. Abnormal thallium stress test or pulmonary function tests. Organ allografts. Use in either men or women not practicing effective contraception. Lactation.

Retreatment is contraindicated in those who have experienced the following during a previous course of therapy: sustained ventricular tachycardia; uncontrolled or unresponsive cardiac rhythm disturbances; recurrent chest pain with ECG changes that are consistent with angina or MI; intubation required for more than 72 hr; pericardial tamponade; renal dysfunction requiring dialysis for more than 72 hr; coma or toxic psychosis lasting more than 48 hr; seizures that are repetitive or difficult to control; ischemia or perforation of the bowel; and GI bleeding requiring surgery.

SPECIAL CONCERNS

Symptoms may worsen in unrecognized or untreated CNS metastases. Use of medications known to be nephrotoxic or hepatotoxic may further increase toxicity to the kidney and liver caused by aldesleukin. May increase the risk of allograft rejection in transplant clients. Safety and efficacy have not been established in children less than 18 years of age.

SIDE EFFECTS

Side effects are frequent, often serious, and sometimes fatal. Most clients will experience fever, chills, rigors, pruritus, and GI side effects. The frequency and severity of side effects are usually dose-related and schedule-dependent. Incidence of side effects is greater in PS 1 clients than in PS 0 clients. The side effects listed have an incidence of 1% or greater.

Capillary leak syndrome (CLS): Results from extravasation of plasma proteins and fluid into the extracellular space with loss of vascular tone. This results in a drop in mean arterial BP within 2–12 hr after the start of treatment and reduced organ perfusion that may be severe and result in death. CLS causes hypotension, hypoperfusion, and extravasation that leads to edema and effusion. ***CLS may be associated with supraventricular and ventricular arrhythmias, MI,*** angina, respiratory insufficiency requiring intubation, GI bleeding or infarction, renal insufficiency, and changes in mental status.

CV: Hypotension (sometimes requiring vasopressor therapy), sinus tachycardia, ***arrhythmias (atrial, junctional, supraventricular, ventricular)***, bradycardia, PVCs, PACs, myocardial ischemia, ***MI, cardiac arrest, CHF,*** myocarditis, endocarditis, gangrene, ***stroke, pericardial effusion, thrombosis.*** **Respiratory:** Pulmonary congestion/edema, dyspnea, ***respiratory failure,*** tachypnea, pleural effusion, wheezing, apnea, pneumothorax, hemoptysis. **GI:** N&V, diarrhea, stomatitis, anorexia, ***GI bleeding*** (sometimes requiring surgery), dyspepsia, constipation, ***intestinal perforation,*** intestinal ileus, pancreatitis. **CNS:** Changes in mental status (may be an early indication of bacteremia or early bacterial sepsis), dizziness, sensory dysfunction, disorders of special senses (speech, taste, vision), syncope, motor dysfunction, ***coma, seizure***. **GU:** Oliguria or anuria, proteinuria, hematuria, dysuria, impaired renal function requiring dialysis, urinary retention/frequency. **Hepatic:** Jaundice, ascites, hepatomegaly. **Hematologic:** Anemia, thrombocytopenia, leukopenia, coagulation disorders, leukocytosis, eosinophilia. **Dermatologic:** Pruritus, erythema, rash, dry skin, exfoliative dermatitis, purpura, petechiae, urticaria, alopecia. **Musculoskeletal:** Arthralgia, myalgia, arthritis, muscle spasm. *Electrolyte and other disturbances:* Hypomagnesemia, acidosis, hypocalcemia/kalemia, hypophosphatemia, hyperuricemia, hypoalbuminemia/proteinemia, hyponatremia, hyperkalemia, alkalosis, hypo/hyperglycemia, hypocholesterolemia, hypercalcemia, hypernatremia/phosphatemia. **Miscellaneous:** Fever, chills, pain (abdominal, chest, back), fatigue, malaise, weakness, edema, infection (including the injection site, urinary tract, catheter tip, phlebitis, sepsis), weight gain/loss, headache, conjunctivitis, reactions at the injection site, allergic reactions, hypothyroidism.

LABORATORY TEST CONSIDERATIONS

↑ BUN, bilirubin, serum creatinine, transaminase, alkaline phosphatase. See also *Electrolyte and other disturbances* under Side Effects.

OD OVERDOSE MANAGEMENT

Symptoms: See *Side Effects*. *Treatment:* Side effects will usually reverse if the drug is stopped, especially because the serum half-life is short. Continuing toxicity is treated symptomatically. Life-threatening side effects have been treated by the IV administration of dexamethasone (which may result in loss of the therapeutic effectiveness of aldesleukin).

DRUG INTERACTIONS

Aminoglycosides / ↑ Risk of kidney toxicity
Antihypertensives / Potentiate hypotension R/T aldesleukin
Asparaginase / ↑ Risk of hepatic toxicity
Cardiotoxic agents / ↑ Risk of cardiac toxicity
Corticosteroids / Concomitant use may ↓ antitumor effectiveness of aldesleukin (although corticosteroids ↓ aldesleukin side effects)
Cytotoxic chemotherapy / ↑ Risk of myelotoxicity
Doxorubicin / ↑ Risk of cardiac toxicity
Hepatotoxic drugs / ↑ Risk of liver toxicity
Indinavir / ↑ Indinavir plasma levels R/T ↓ liver breakdown
Indomethacin / ↑ Risk of kidney toxicity
Methotrexate / ↑ Risk of hepatic toxicity

A

Myelotoxic agents / ↑ Risk of myelotoxicity
Nephrotoxic agents / ↑ Risk of kidney toxicity

HOW SUPPLIED

Powder for injection: 22 million IU/vial

DOSAGE

• **INTERMITTENT IV INFUSION**

Metastatic renal cell carcinoma in adults.

Each course of treatment consists of two 5-day treatment cycles separated by a rest period. **Adults:** 600,000 IU/kg (0.037 mg/kg) given q 8 hr by a 15-min IV infusion for a total of 14 doses. Following 9 days of rest, repeat schedule for another 14 doses, for a maximum of 28 doses per course. *NOTE:* Due to toxicity, clients may not be able to receive all 28 doses (median number of doses given is 20).

Retreatment for metastatic renal cell carcinoma.

Evaluate for a response about 4 weeks after completion of a course of therapy and again just prior to the start of the next treatment course. Give additional courses only if there is evidence of some tumor shrinkage following the last course and retreatment is not contraindicated (see preceding *Contraindications*). Separate each treatment course by at least 7 weeks from the date of hospital discharge.

NURSING CONSIDERATIONS

SEE ALSO *NURSING CONSIDERATIONS* FOR *ANTINEOPLASTIC AGENTS*.

ADMINISTRATION/STORAGE

IV 1. Undertake dose modification for toxicity by withholding or interrupting a dose rather than reducing the dose to be given.

2. *Permanently discontinue* therapy for the following toxicities:

• CV: Sustained VT, uncontrolled or unresponsive cardiac rhythm disturbances, recurrent chest pain with ECG changes indicating angina or MI, pericardial tamponade
• Pulmonary: Intubation > 72 hr
• Renal: Dialysis > 72 hr
• CNS: Coma or toxic psychosis > 48 hr, repetitive or difficult to control seizures
• GI: Bowel ischemia, bowel perforation, GI bleeding requiring surgery

3. Consult the product information carefully for held and subsequent doses of aldesleukin.

4. Reconstitute vials aseptically with 1.2 mL sterile water for injection; each mL will contain 18 million IU (1.1 mg) of aldesleukin. Such solutions should be clear and colorless to slightly yellow.

5. The vial is for a single use only; discard any unused portion. Not for use with transplant clients; risk of allograft rejection.

6. During reconstitution, direct the sterile water at the side of the vial. Swirl contents gently to avoid foaming. *Do not shake vial.*

7. The reconstituted drug may be diluted in 50 mL of D5/W and infused over 15 min.

8. Use plastic bags for more consistent drug delivery. Do *not* use in-line filters.

9. Due to increased aggregation, do not reconstitute using bacteriostatic water or 0.9% NaCl injection.

10. Dilution with albumin can alter the pharmacology of aldesleukin. Do not mix with other drugs.

11. After reconstitution, drug is stable for 48 hr if stored at room temperature or 2–8°C (36–46°F). Administer within 48 hr of reconstitution, bringing solution to room temperature before infusing. Do not freeze the product.

12. The undiluted drug is stable for 5 days if refrigerated in 1-mL B-D syringes.

13. The drug is compatible with glass, polyvinylchloride (preferred), or polypropylene syringes.

ASSESSMENT

1. Note any liver or renal dysfunction as well as cardiac, pulmonary, or CNS impairment.

2. The following baseline parameters should be determined prior to initiation of therapy and daily during drug use: CBC, blood chemistries, renal and LFTs, and CXRs. Obtain baseline PFTs with ABGs.

3. Screen with a thallium stress test to document normal ejection fraction and unimpaired wall motion. If minor abnormalities in wall motion are noted,

a stress echocardiogram may help to exclude significant CAD.
4. Assess for any S&S of infection. Obtain cultures to R/O any potential sources. Preexisting bacterial infections must be treated prior to initiation of therapy, as intensive treatment may cause impaired neutrophil function and an increased risk of disseminated infection leading to sepsis and bacterial endocarditis.
5. All clients with in-dwelling central lines should receive antibiotic prophylaxis against *Saccharomyces aureus*.

INTERVENTIONS

1. Initiate therapy in a closely monitored environment where VS and I&O are assessed often.
2. Cardiac function should be assessed daily by clinical examination and assessment of VS. Clients who have chest pain, murmurs, gallops, irregular rhythm, or palpitations should be further assessed with an ECG and CPK evaluation. If evidence of ischemia or CHF, get a repeat thallium or cardiolyte stress test.
3. Perform daily CV evaluations to identify any early S&S of drug toxicity. Monitor for symptoms of CLS characterized by hypotension and hypoperfusion, altered mental status, and decreased urine output. Mental status changes are usually transient but should be evaluated carefully. Alterations in urinary output may signal renal toxicity.Monitor for dehydration, liver or renal failure. Stop infusion and transport to ICU for intubation and dialysis if progressive toxicity is evident.

CLIENT/FAMILY TEACHING

1. Report any persistent abdominal pain/discomfort, unusual bruising or bleeding, fatigue, or ↑ SOB.
2. Review list of drug side effects and note those (dyspnea, palpitations, hemoptysis, confusion, chest pain, or impaired vision) requiring immediate intervention.
3. Practice reliable contraception.
4. Avoid any OTC drugs unless specifically ordered.

OUTCOMES/EVALUATE

Disease regression with evidence of ↓ tumor size and spread

Alemtuzumab

(**ah**-lem-**TOOZ**-uh-mab)

PREGNANCY CATEGORY: C
CLASSIFICATION(S):
Monoclonal antibody
Rx: Campath

ACTION/KINETICS

Recombinant DNA-derived humanized monoclonal antibody. Binds to CD52, a nonmodulating antigen, that is present on the surface of nearly all B and T lymphocytes, a majority of monocytes, macrophages, NK cells, and a subpopulation of granulocytes. Probably acts by lysis of leukemic cells following cell surface binding. **t½:** About 12 days.

USES

Treatment of B-cell chronic lymphocytic leukemia in clients previously treated with alkylating agents and who have failed fludarabine therapy.

CONTRAINDICATIONS

Active systemic infections, underlying immunodeficiency, or known Type I hypersensitivity or anaphylactic reaction to alemtuzumab or any of its components. Lactation.

SPECIAL CONCERNS

Due to immunosuppression by the drug, do not immunize with live viral vaccines those who have recently received alemtuzumab. Safety and efficacy have not been determined in children.

SIDE EFFECTS

Infusion-related: Hypotension, rigors, drug-related fever, N&V, SOB, bronchospasm, chills, rash, fatigue, urticaria, dyspnea, pruritus, headache, diarrhea. **GI:** N&V, diarrhea, stomatitis, ulcerative stomatitis, mucositis, abdominal pain, dyspepsia, constipation. **CNS:** Headache, dysesthesias, dizziness, insomnia, depression, trem-

A

or, somnolence. **CV:** Hypotension, tachycardia, SVT, hypertension. **Hematologic:** ***Myelosuppression,*** bone marrow aplasia, hypoplasia, ***severe/fatal autoimmune anemia,*** thrombocytopenia, neutropenia, purpura, pancytopenia. **Respiratory:** Dyspnea, cough, bronchitis, pneumonitis, pneumonia, pharyngitis, bronchospasm, rhinitis. **Musculoskeletal:** Skeletal pain, myalgias, back/chest pain. **Dermatologic:** Rash (including maculopapular, erythematous), urticaria, pruritus, increased sweating. **Miscellaneous:** Opportunistic infections (may be fatal), rigors, fever, fatigue, anorexia, ***sepsis,*** asthenia, edema, herpes simplex, malaise, moniliasis, temperature change sensation.

LABORATORY TEST CONSIDERATIONS

Interference with diagnostic serum tests that use antibodies.

HOW SUPPLIED

Solution for Injection: 30 mg/3 mL

DOSAGE

- **IV ONLY.**

B-cell chronic lymphocytic leukemia.

Initial: 3 mg given as a 2-hr infusion daily. When the 3 mg dose is tolerated (Grade 2 or less infusion-related toxicities), escalate the dose to 10 mg and continue as tolerated. When the 10 mg dose is tolerated, initiate maintenance dose of 30 mg/dose given 3 times/week on alternate days for 12 weeks or less. Escalation to 30 mg can usually be done in 3–7 days. Single doses greater than 30 mg or weekly doses greater than 90 mg are associated with an increased incidence of pancytopenia.

NURSING CONSIDERATIONS

ADMINISTRATION/STORAGE

IV 1. Do not give as an IV push or bolus.

2. Withdraw the correct amount of drug from the ampule into a syringe. Filter with a sterile, low protein-binding, non-fiber-releasing 5 micrometer filter prior to dilution. Do not use the vial if particulate matter is present or the solution is discolored. Do not shake ampule prior to use.

3. Inject amount withdrawn from vial into 100 mL sterile 0.9% NaCl or D5W. Gently invert the bag to mix the solution. Discard syringe and any unused drug product.

4. Do not add any other drug or simultaneously infuse any other drug through the same IV line.

5. Alemtuzumab contains no preservative. Thus, use within 8 hr after dilution. Store solutions at room temperature or refrigerate. Protect from light. Prior to dilution, store ampule at 2–8°C (36–46°F). Do not freeze. Discard if ampule has been frozen. Protect from direct sunlight.

6. To minimize infusion-related effects, give premedication prior to the first dose, at dose escalations, and as needed. Premedication consists of diphenhydramine, 50 mg, and acetaminophen, 650 mg, each given 30 min prior to alemtuzumab. If severe infusion-related symptoms occur, give hydrocortisone, 200 mg.

7. To minimize risk of serious opportunistic infections, anti-infectives may be given. One regimen is trimethoprim/sulfamethoxazole DS b.i.d. 3 times/week and famciclovir (or equivalent) 250 mg b.i.d. upon starting therapy. Continue prophylaxis for 2 months after completion of therapy or until CD_4^+ count is 200 or more cells/microliter (whichever occurs later).

8. Discontinue during serious infection, serious hematologic toxicity, or other serious toxicity, until resolution of problem. Permanently discontinue if autoimmune anemia or thrombocytopenia occurs. If severe neutropenia or thrombocytopenia occurs, use the following dose modification and reinitiation of therapy protocol:

- For first occurrence of ANC <250/mcL and/or platelet count 25,000/mcL or less, withhold therapy. When ANC is 500/mcL or more and platelet count is 50,000/mcL or more, resume therapy at the same dose. If delay between dosing is 7 days or more, start therapy at 3 mg and escalate to 10 mg and then 30 mg as tolerated.
- For second occurrence of ANC <250/mcL and/or platelet count 25,000/mcL or less, withhold therapy. When ANC is 500 /mcL or more and platelet count is

50,000/mcL or more, resume therapy at 10 mg. If delay between dosing is 7 days or more, initiate therapy at 3 mg and escalate to 10 mg only.

• For a third incidence of ANC <250/mcL and/or platelet count 25,000/mcL or less, discontinue therapy permanently.

• If there is a ↓ in ANC and/or platelet count of 50% or less of the baseline value in those who started therapy with a baseline ANC 500/mcL or less and/or a baseline platelet count of 25,000/mcL or less, withhold therapy. When ANC and platelet counts return to baseline value(s), resume therapy. If the delay between dosing is 7 days or more, start therapy at 3 mg and escalate to 10 mg and then to 30 mg as tolerated.

ASSESSMENT

1. Note indications for therapy, disease characteristics, and physical condition. Identify fludarabine failure and other alkylating agents used.
2. Premedicate with diphenhydramine 50 mg and acetaminophen 650 mg 30 min before infusion, at dose escalations, and as indicated. Hydrocortisone 200 mg may help decrease infusion-related events.
3. Administer over 2 hr. Monitor CBCs and platelets closely. Follow guidelines under IV #8 for resuming therapy if ANC depressed or CD_4 count<200 cells/mcL.
4. Assess clients carefully for evidence of infections; monitor VS and assess skin, urine, and lungs frequently. Infection prophylaxis may be followed under IV #7. Drug is extremely toxic and requires close client observation.

CLIENT/FAMILY TEACHING

1. Drug is used to treat CLL in those who have failed to respond to fludarabine and other alkylating agents.
2. Once the maintenance dose of 30 mg has been reached, the drug is given 3 x per week (over 2 hrs) on alternating days for up to 12 weeks. If the ANC or platelets drop, the dose may be modified.
3. Avoid live viral vaccines during therapy R/T drug-induced immunosuppression.
4. Report any unusual or adverse side effects immediately as the drug is highly toxic.
5. Women of child-bearing age and men of reproductive potential should practice reliable contraception during treatment and for a minimum of 6 months after therapy. Egg/sperm harvesting prior to therapy may be considered.

OUTCOMES/EVALUATE

Control of malignant cell proliferation in B-cell CLL

Alendronate sodium

(ay-**LEN**-droh-nayt)

PREGNANCY CATEGORY: C
CLASSIFICATION(S):
Bone growth regulator, bisphosphonate
Rx: Fosamax

ACTION/KINETICS

Binds to bone hydroxyapatite and inhibits osteoclast activity, thereby preventing bone resorption. Appears to reduce fracture risk and reverse the progression of osteoporosis. Does not inhibit bone mineralization. Well absorbed orally and initially distributed to soft tissues, but then quickly redistributed to bone. Not metabolized; excreted through the urine. **t½, terminal:** Believed to be more than 10 years, due to slow release from the skeleton.

USES

Daily dosing: Prevention and treatment of osteoporosis in postmenopausal women. Increase bone density in men with osteoporosis. Glucocorticoid-induced osteoporosis in men and women receiving daily dosage equivalent to 7.5 mg or greater of prednisone and who have low bone mineral density. Paget's disease of bone in those with alkaline phosphatase at least two times the upper limit of normal or for those who are sympto-

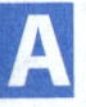

matic or at risk for future complications from the disease. **Weekly dosing:** Treatment or prevention of postmenopausal osteoporosis.

CONTRAINDICATIONS

In hypocalcemia. Severe renal insufficiency (C_{CR} less than 35 mL/min). Use of hormone replacement therapy with alendronate for osteoporosis in postmenopausal women. Lactation.

SPECIAL CONCERNS

Use with caution in those with upper GI problems, such as dysphagia, symptomatic esophageal diseases, gastritis, duodenitis, or ulcers. Safety and effectiveness have not been determined in children. Some elderly clients may be more sensitive to the drug effects.

SIDE EFFECTS

GI: Flatulence, acid regurgitation, esophageal ulcer, dysphagia, abdominal distention, gastritis, abdominal pain, constipation, diarrhea, dyspepsia, N&V. **Miscellaneous:** Musculoskeletal pain, pain, headache, taste perversion, rash and erythema (rare), back pain, glaucoma, accidental injury, edema, flu–like symptoms.

LABORATORY TEST CONSIDERATIONS

↓ Serum calcium and phosphate.

OD OVERDOSE MANAGEMENT

Symptoms: Hypocalcemia, hypophosphatemia, upset stomach, heartburn, esophagitis, gastritis, ulcer. *Treatment:* Consider giving milk or antacids to bind the drug.

DRUG INTERACTIONS

Antacids / ↓ Absorption of alendronate

Aspirin / ↑ Risk of upper GI side effects

Calcium supplements / ↓ Absorption of alendronate

Naproxen / ↑ Risk of drug-induced gastric ulcers

Ranitidine / ↑ Bioavailability of alendronate (significance not known)

HOW SUPPLIED

Tablet: 5 mg, 10 mg, 35 mg, 40 mg, 70 mg

DOSAGE

• **TABLETS**

Prevention of osteoporosis in postmenopausal women.

5 mg once a day in the morning ½ hr before the first food, beverage, or medication of the day with 6–8 oz of plain water. Or, 35 mg once a week.

Treatment of osteoporosis.

10 mg once a day in the morning ½ hr before the first food, beverage, or medication of the day with 6–8 oz of plain water. Or, 70 mg once a week.

Prevention of fractures in postmenopausal women with osteoporosis. Increase bone density in men with osteoporosis.

10 mg once a day in the morning ½ hr before the first food, beverage, or medication of the day with 6–8 oz of plain water. Or, 70 mg once a week. Safety of treatment for more than 4 years has not been determined.

Treatment of glucocorticoid-induced osteoporosis in men and women receiving daily dosage equivalent to 7.5 mg or greater of prednisone and who have low bone mineral density.

5 mg once daily for men or women with low bone mineral density and 10 mg once daily for treatment of low bone mineral density in postmenopausal women who are receiving glucocorticoid therapy but not estrogen.

Paget's disease of bone.

40 mg once a day for 6 months taken as for osteoporosis.

NOTE: The 35 mg dosage form is used for once weekly dosing to prevent postmenopausal osteoporosis; 70 mg dosage form is used for once weekly dosing to treat postmenopausal osteoporosis.

NURSING CONSIDERATIONS

ADMINISTRATION/STORAGE

1. To facilitate delivery to the stomach and reduce irritation of the esophagus, do not lie down for at least 30 min following administration.
2. Due to possible interference with absorption, at least 30 min should elapse before taking antacids or calcium supplements.
3. Retreatment for Paget's disease may be considered following a 6-month posttreatment evaluation in clients who have relapsed, based on increases in serum alkaline phospha-

tase. Retreatment may also be appropriate for those who failed to normalize their serum alkaline phosphatase.
4. Dosage adjustment is not needed for the elderly.

ASSESSMENT

1. Document indications for therapy: osteoporosis prevention or treatment in postmenopausal women or Paget's disease. Note symptoms, age at onset, and physical changes.
2. Obtain baseline calcium, liver and renal function studies and correct any calcium or vitamin D deficiencies.
3. Note any history of upper GI problems such as gastritis, dysphagia, duodenitis, or ulcers.
4. Document bone mineral density studies and/or skeletal X rays.
5. Assess for fractures and manage appropriately to prevent further injury and loss of function.
6. With Paget's disease, document baseline S&S and alkaline phosphatase; monitor.

CLIENT/FAMILY TEACHING

1. Osteoporosis occurs usually after age 40 and is a systemic skeletal disease characterized by low bone mass due to a higher amount of bone resorbed than formed.
2. Take only as prescribed. Benefit seen only when each tablet is taken with plain water the first thing in the morning at least 30 min before the first food, beverage, or medication of the day. Waiting > 30 min will improve absorption. Taking with juice or coffee will markedly reduce absorption. Once weekly therapy may enhance compliance.
3. Do not lie down after taking drug; wait at least 30 min.
4. Take calcium (500 mg) and vitamin D daily, especially if dietary intake or sun exposure is inadequate. Regular daily weight bearing exercise is enouraged.

OUTCOMES/EVALUATE

- Prevention of osteoporosis and bone resorption (↓ bone turnover)
- Inhibition of kyphosis and pain due to bone fracture or deformity
- ↓ Pain; ↓ Serum alkaline phosphatase levels with Paget's disease

Alfentanil hydrochloride

(al-**FEN**-tah-nil)

PREGNANCY CATEGORY: C
CLASSIFICATION(S):
Narcotic analgesic
Rx: Alfenta **C-II**

SEE ALSO *NARCOTIC ANALGESICS*.

ACTION/KINETICS
Onset: Immediate. **t½:** 1–2 hr (after IV use).

USES
Continuous infusion: As an analgesic with nitrous oxide/oxygen to maintain general anesthesia. *Incremental doses:* Adjunct with barbiturate/nitrous oxide/oxygen to maintain general anesthesia. *Anesthetic induction:* As primary agent when ET intubation and mechanical ventilation are necessary. Analgesic component for monitored anesthesia care.

CONTRAINDICATIONS
Use during labor and in children less than 12 years of age.

SPECIAL CONCERNS
Use with caution during lactation.

ADDITIONAL SIDE EFFECTS
Bradycardia, postoperative confusion, blurred vision, hypercapnia, shivering, and ***asystole***. Neonates with respiratory distress syndrome have manifested hypotension with doses of 20 mcg/kg.

ADDITIONAL DRUG INTERACTIONS
Fluconazole / ↑ Alfentanil plasma levels due to ↓ liver breakdown
H *Indian snakeroot* / Potentiation of alfentanil effects
H *Kava kava* / Potentiation of alfentanil effects

HOW SUPPLIED
Injection: 0.5 mg/mL

DOSAGE

Individualize dosage and titrate to desired effect according to body

weight, physical status, underlying disease states, use of other drugs, and type and duration of surgical procedure and anesthesia.

• **IV**

Continuous infusion, duration 45 min or more.

Initial for induction: 50–75 mcg/kg; **maintenance, with nitrous oxide/oxygen:** 0.5–3 mcg/kg/min (average infusion rate: 1–1.5 mcg/kg/min). Following the induction dose, reduce the infusion rate requirement by 30%–50% for the first hour of maintenance.

Induction of anesthesia, duration 45 min or more.

Initial for induction: 130–245 mcg/kg; **maintenance:** 0.5–1.5 mcg/kg/min. If a general anesthetic is used for maintenance, the concentration of inhalation agents should be reduced by 30%–50% for the first hour.

Anesthetic adjunct, 30–60 min duration, incremental injection to attenuate response to laryngoscopy and intubation.

Initial for induction: 20–50 mcg/kg; **maintenance:** 5–15 mcg/kg q 5–20 min, up to a total dose of 75 mcg/kg.

Anesthetic adjunct, less than 30 min duration, incremental injection, spontaneously breathing or assisted ventilation.

Initial for induction: 8–20 mcg/kg; **maintenance:** 3–5 mcg/kg q 5–20 min (or 0.5–1 mcg/kg/min, up to a total dose of 8–40 mcg/kg).

Monitored anesthesia care, less than 30 min duration, for sedated and responsive spontaneously breathing clients.

Initial for induction: 3–8 mcg/kg; **maintenance:** 3–5 mcg/kg every 5–20 min (or 0.25–1 mcg/kg/min, up to a total dose of 3–40 mg/kg).

NOTE: If there is a lightening of general anesthesia or the client manifests signs of surgical stress, the rate of administration of alfentanil may be increased to 4 mcg/kg/min or a bolus dose of 7 mcg/kg may be used. If the situation is not controlled following three bolus doses over 5 min, an inhalation anesthetic, a barbiturate, or a vasodilator should be used. If signs of lightening anesthesia are noted within the last 15 min of surgery, a bolus dose of 7 mcg/kg should be given rather than increasing the infusion rate. A potent inhalation anesthetic may be used as an alternative.

NURSING CONSIDERATIONS

SEE ALSO *NURSING CONSIDERATIONS* FOR *NARCOTIC ANALGESICS*.

ADMINISTRATION/STORAGE

IV 1. Individualize drug dosage for each client and for each use.

• Reduce dosage for elderly or debilitated clients.

• For those who are more than 20% above their ideal body weight, base dosage on lean body weight.

2. Use a tuberculin-type syringe to administer small volumes of drug.

3. The injectable form may be reconstituted with either NSS, D5/NSS, RL solution, or D5W. Direct IV administration over 1½–3 min. For continous IV administration dilute 20 cc of alfentanil in 230 mL diluent to provide a solution of 40 mcg/mL.

4. Discontinue infusion 10–15 min prior to the end of surgery.

ASSESSMENT

1. Note any history of drug hypersensitivity.

2. Obtain baseline weight and VS.

3. Report any muscular rigidity before giving the next dose.

4. Assess respiratory and CV status continuously during therapy.

CLIENT/FAMILY TEACHING

1. May experience dizziness, drowsiness, and orthostatic hypotension.

2. Avoid alcohol or any CNS depressants for at least 24 hr following drug administration.

OUTCOMES/EVALUATE

• Induction/maintenance of anesthesia

• Facilitation of intubation and mechanical ventilation

Alitretinoin

(**al**-eh-**TRET**-ih-**noh**-in)

PREGNANCY CATEGORY: D

CLASSIFICATION(S):
Retinoid
Rx: Panretin Gel

ACTION/KINETICS
Retinoid binds to and activates all known intracellular retinoid receptor subtypes. Upon activation, the receptors regulate the expression of genes that control cellular differentiation and proliferation in both healthy and cancerous cells. Inhibits growth of Kaposi's sarcoma cells in vitro. Little is absorbed through the skin.

USES
Treat cutaneous lesions in AIDS-related Kaposi's sarcoma.

CONTRAINDICATIONS
Hypersensitivity to retinoids. Use when systemic treatment of Kaposi's sarcoma is needed (i.e., 10 new sarcoma lesions in the prior month, symptomatic lymphedema, symptomatic pulmonary Kaposi's sarcoma, symptomatic visceral involvement). Lactation.

SPECIAL CONCERNS
Safety and efficacy have not been determined in children or in clients 65 years of age or older.

SIDE EFFECTS
Dermatologic: Rash (erythema, scaling, irritation, redness, dermatitis), pain, burning pain, pruritus, exfoliative dermatitis, paresthesia, edema, inflammation, vesiculation, skin disorder (excoriation, cracking, scabbing, crusting, drainage, eschar, fissure, oozing).

DRUG INTERACTIONS
Increased toxicity when combined with N,N-diethyl-m-toluamide (DEET), a common component of insect repellents.

HOW SUPPLIED
Gel: 0.1%

DOSAGE

• **GEL**

Kaposi's sarcoma cutaneous lesions.
Initial: Apply b.i.d. Can increase frequency of application to t.i.d. or q.i.d., according to individual lesion tolerance.

NURSING CONSIDERATIONS

ADMINISTRATION/STORAGE

1. A reponse may be seen within 2 weeks. However, most clients require 4–8 weeks of treatment; some require 14 or more weeks of treatment before beneficial effects are noted.
2. Continue application as long as the client is getting benefit.
3. Application frequency can be reduced if application site toxicity occurs. Discontinue for a few days if severe irritation occurs.

ASSESSMENT

1. Note size, location, and characteristics of cutaneous lesions.
2. Determine any sensitivity to retinoids.

CLIENT/FAMILY TEACHING

1. Use as directed, may take 4 to 8 weeks before improvement noted. May gradually increase application frequency from 2 to 3-4 times/day as tolerated. Reduce application frequency if site bcomes red and swollen. If reaction becomes intense with vesicles, stop for several days until symptoms subside and then may resume.
2. Apply sufficient gel to cover the lesion generously. Allow to dry for 3–5 min before covering with clothing.
3. Avoid application to healthy skin surrounding lesions or to mucosal surfaces as skin irritation may occur.
4. May cause photosensitivity, avoid direct exposures; cover treated sites.
5. Avoid insect repellents with DEET; may cause toxicity.
6. Practice reliable contraception; may cause fetal harm.

OUTCOMES/EVALUATE
Clearing of Kaposi's lesions

Allopurinol

(al-oh-**PYOUR**-ih-nohl)

PREGNANCY CATEGORY: C
CLASSIFICATION(S):
Antigout drug

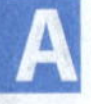

Rx: Zyloprim, Aloprim for Injection
✱**Rx:** Apo-Allopurinol

ACTION/KINETICS

Allopurinol and its major metabolite, oxipurinol, are potent inhibitors of xanthine oxidase, an enzyme involved in the synthesis of uric acid, without disrupting the biosynthesis of essential purine. Results in decreased uric acid levels. Also increases reutilization of xanthine and hypoxanthine for synthesis of nucleotide and nucleic acid by acting on the enzyme hypoxanthine-guanine phosphoribosyltransferase. The resultant increases in nucleotides cause a negative feedback to inhibit synthesis of purines and a decrease in uric acid levels. **Peak plasma levels, after PO:** 1.5 hr for allopurinol and 4.5 hr for oxipurinol. **Onset, after PO:** 2–3 days. **t½, after PO;** (allopurinol); 1–3 hr; **t½** (oxipurinol): 12–30 hr. **Peak serum levels after PO, allopurinol:** 2–3 mcg/mL; **oxipurinol:** 5–6.5 mcg/mL (up to 50 mcg/mL in clients with impaired renal function). **Maximum therapeutic effect, after PO:** 1–3 weeks. Well absorbed from GI tract, metabolized in liver, excreted in urine and feces (20%).

USES

IV: Clients with Leukemia, lymphoma, and solid tumor malignancies receiving cancer chemotherapy and which cause elevations of serum and urinary uric acid levels and who cannot tolerate PO therapy. **PO:** Primary or secondary gout (acute attacks, tophi, joint destruction, nephropathy, uric acid lithiasis). Clients with leukemia, lymphoma, or other malignancies in whom drug therapy causes elevations of serum and urinary uric acid. Recurrent calcium oxalate calculi where daily uric acid excretion exceeds 800 mg/day in males and 750 mg/day in females. *Investigational:* Mixed with methylcellulose as a mouthwash to prevent stomatitis following fluorouracil administration. Reduce the granulocyte suppressant effect of fluorouracil. Prevent ischemic reperfusion tissue damage. Reduce the incidence of perioperative mortality and postoperative arrhythmias in coronary artery bypass surgery. Reduce the rates of *Helicobacter pylori*-induced duodenal ulcers and treatment of hematemesis from NSAID-induced erosive esophagitis. Alleviate pain due to acute pancreatitis. Treatment of American cutaneous leishmaniasis and against *Trypanosoma cruzi.* Treat Chagas' disease. As an alternative in epileptic seizures refractory to standard therapy.

CONTRAINDICATIONS

Hypersensitivity to drug. Clients with idiopathic hemochromatosis or relatives of clients suffering from this condition. Children except as an adjunct in treatment of neoplastic disease. Severe skin reactions on previous exposure. To treat asymptomatic hyperuricemia.

SPECIAL CONCERNS

Use with caution during lactation and in clients with liver or renal disease. In children use has been limited to rare inborn errors of purine metabolism or hyperuricemia as a result of malignancy or cancer therapy.

SIDE EFFECTS

Dermatologic (most frequent): Pruritic maculopapular skin rash (may be accompanied by fever and malaise). Vesicular bullous dermatitis, eczematoid dermatitis, pruritus, urticaria, onycholysis, purpura, lichen planus, ***Stevens-Johnson syndrome, toxic epidermal necrolysis.*** Skin rash has been accompanied by hypertension and cataract development. **Allergy:** Fever, chills, leukopenia, eosinophilia, arthralgia, skin rash, pruritus, N&V, nephritis. **GI:** N&V, diarrhea, GI bleeding, splenomegaly, intestinal obstruction, flatulence, constipation, proctitis, gastritis, dyspepsia, abdominal pain (intermittent). **CNS:** Agitation, cerebral infarction, coma, dystonia, change in mental status, myoclonus, paralysis, seizures, ***status epilepticus,*** tremor, twitching. **Hematologic:** Leukopenia, eosinophilia, thrombocytopenia, anemia, bone marrow suppression, leukocytosis, ***DIC,*** marrow aplasia, neutropenia, pancytopenia. **Hepatic:** Hepatomegaly, cholestatic jaundice, ***hepatic necrosis, liver failure,*** hyperbilirubinemia, jaundice,

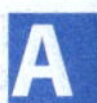

granulomatous hepatitis. **Neurologic:** Headache, peripheral neuropathy, paresthesia, somnolence, neuritis. **CV:** Bradycardia, ***cardiorespiratory arrest,*** CV disorder, decreased venous pressure, abnormal ECG, flushing, ***heart failure, hemorrhage,*** hypertension, hypotension, ***septic shock, stroke, ventricular fibrillation,*** thrombophlebitis, necrotizing angiitis, hypersensitivity vasculitis. **GU:** Renal failure/insufficiency, hematuria, abnormal kidney function, oliguria, UTI. **Respiratory:** Apnea, mucositis, pharyngitis, ***ARDS, respiratory failure,*** respiratory insufficiency, increased respiratory rate, ***pulmonary embolus.*** **Metabolic:** Abnormal electrolytes, glycosuria, hypercalcemia, hyperglycemia, hyperkalemia, hypernatremia, hyperphosphatemia, hyperuricemia, hypocalecmia, hypokalemia, hypomagnesemia, hyponatremia, lactic acidosis, metabolic acidosis, water intoxication. **Miscellaneous:** Ecchymosis, headache, blast crisis, edema, cellulitis, chills, diaphoresis, enlarged abdomen, hypervolemia, hypotonia, infection, pain, tumor lysis syndrome, arthralgia, epistaxis, taste loss, arthralgia, acute attacks of gout, fever, myopathy, renal failure, uremia, alopecia.

LABORATORY TEST CONSIDERATIONS

↑ ALT, AST, alkaline phosphatase, serum cholesterol. ↓ Serum glucose.

DRUG INTERACTIONS

ACE inhibitors / ↑ Risk of hypersensitivity reactions

Aluminum salts / ↓ Effect of allopurinol

Ampicillin / ↑ Risk of drug-induced skin rashes

Anticoagulants, oral / ↑ Anticoagulant effect R/T ↓ liver breakdown

Azathioprine / ↑ Azathioprine effect R/T ↓ liver breakdown

Chlorpropamide / ↑ t½ of chlorpropamide → hypoglycemia

Cyclophosphamide / ↑ Risk of bleeding or infection due to ↑ drug myelosuppressive effects

Cyclosporine / ↑ Cyclosporine levels

Iron preparations / Allopurinol ↑ hepatic iron concentrations

Mercaptopurine / ↑ Mercaptopurine effect R/T ↓ liver breakdown

Theophylline / Allopurinol ↑ plasma drug levels → possible toxicity

Thiazide diuretics / ↑ Risk of hypersensitivity reactions to allopurinol

Uricosuric agents / ↓ Effect of oxipurinol due to ↑ rate of excretion

HOW SUPPLIED

Injection: 500 mg/30 mL; *Tablet:* 100 mg, 300 mg

DOSAGE

- **IV INFUSION**

Lower serum uric acid in leukemia, lymphoma, or solid malignancies.

Adults: 200–400 mg/m²/day, to a maximum of 600 mg/day. **Children, initial:** 200 mg/m²/day. Reduce dose in those with impaired renal function as follows: C_{CR} 10–20 mL/min: 200 mg/day; C_{CR} 3–10 mL/min: 100 mg/day; C_{CR} less than 30 mL/min: 100 mg/day at extended intervals.

- **TABLETS**

Gout/hyperuricemia.

Adults: 200–600 mg/day, depending on severity (minimum effective dose: 100–200 mg/day), not to exceed 800 mg/day.

Prevention of uric acid nephropathy during treatment of neoplasms.

Adults: 600–800 mg/day for 2–3 days (with high fluid intake).

Prophylaxis of acute gout.

Initial: 100 mg/day; increase by 100 mg at weekly intervals to achieve serum uric acid level of 6 mg/100 mL or less.

Hyperuricemia associated with malignancy.

Pediatric, 6–10 years of age: 300 mg/day either as a single dose of 100 mg t.i.d.; **under 6 years of age:** 150 mg/day in three divided doses.

Recurrent calcium oxalate calculi.

200–300 mg/day in one or more doses (dose may be adjusted according to urinary levels of uric acid).

To ameliorate granulocyte suppressant effect of fluorouracil.

600 mg/day.

Reduce perioperative mortality and postoperative arrhythmias in coronary artery bypass surgery.

300 mg 12 hr and 1 hr before surgery.

Reduce relapse rates of H. pylori-*induced duodenal ulcers; treat hematemesis from NSAID-induced erosive gastritis.*

50 mg q.i.d.

Alleviate pain due to acute pancreatitis.

50 mg q.i.d.

Treat American cutaneous leishmaniasis and T. cruzi.

20 mg/kg for 15 days.

Treat Chagas' disease.

600–900 mg/day for 60 days.

Alternative to treat epileptic seizures refractory to standard therapy.

300 mg/day, except use 150 mg/day in those less than 20 kg.

• **MOUTHWASH**

Prevent fluorouracil-induced stomatitis.

20 mg in 3% methylcellulose (1 mg/mL compounded in the pharmacy).

NURSING CONSIDERATIONS

ADMINISTRATION/STORAGE

1. Keep urine slightly alkaline to prevent formation of uric acid stones.
2. Transfer from colchicine, uricosuric agents, and/or anti-inflammatory agents to allopurinol should be made gradually by decreasing the dosage of one and increasing the dosage of allopurinol until a normal serum uric acid level is achieved.
3. Reduce the PO dose as follows in impaired renal function: creatinine clearance (C_{CR}) less than 10 mL/min: 100 mg 3 times a week; C_{CR} 10 mL/min: 100 mg every other day; C_{CR} 20 mL/min: 100 mg/day; C_{CR} 40 mL/min: 150 mg/day; C_{CR} 60 mL/min: 200 mg/day.
4. **IV** For either adults or children, give daily dose as a single infusion or in equally divided infusions at 6–, 8–, or 12– hr intervals at a concentration not to exceed 6 mg/mL.
5. Whenever possible, administer 24–48 hr before the start of chemotherapy known to cause tumor cell lysis (including corticosteroids).
6. Do not mix allopurinol with or administer through the same IV port with agents which are incompatible (see package insert).
7. Dissolve the contents of each 30 mL vial with 25 mL of sterile water for injection. Then, dilute to the desired concentration with 0.9% NaCl or 5% dextrose injection (do not use sodium bicarbonate-containing solutions).
8. Store reconstituted solution at 20–25°C (68–77°F); begin administration within 10 hr after reconstitution.
9. Do not refrigerate either the reconstituted and/or diluted product.

ASSESSMENT

1. Take a complete drug history; note any drugs that may interact unfavorably.
2. Document indications for therapy, type and onset of symptoms, and any previous allopurinol use. Note location, severity, and frequency of attacks and joint deformity.
3. If female and of childbearing age, or if nursing, avoid allopurinol.
4. Determine any history of idiopathic hemochromatosis.
5. Monitor CBC, uric acid, liver and renal function studies. Reduce dose with renal dysfunction; xray joint.

CLIENT/FAMILY TEACHING

1. Take with food or immediately after meals to lessen gastric irritation. Consume at least 10–12 8-oz glasses of fluid/day to prevent stone formation.
2. When used IV, ensure sufficient fluid intake to yield a daily urinary output of at least 2 L in adults; maintain a neutral, or preferably, a slightly alkaline urine.
3. Monitor weight if experiencing N&V or other signs of gastric irritation. Report persistent weight loss.
4. Skin rashes may start after months of therapy. If drug related, must discontinue drug.
5. Do not take iron salts; high iron concentrations may occur in liver.
6. Avoid excessive intake of vitamin C; may cause kidney stones.
7. Avoid caffeine and alcoholic beverages; decreases allopurinol effect.
8. Avoid foods high in purine; these may include sardines, roe, salmon, scallops, anchovies, organ meats, and mincemeat.
9. Minimize exposure to UV light due to increased risk of cataracts. Report vision changes.

OUTCOMES/EVALUATE

- ↓ Uric acid levels (6 mg/dL)
- ↓ Joint pain and inflammation
- ↓ Frequency of gout attacks
- Inhibition of stomatitis following fluorouracil therapy

Almotriptan maleate

(**AL**-moh-**trip**-tin)

PREGNANCY CATEGORY: C
CLASSIFICATION(S):
Antimigraine drug
Rx: Axert

ACTION/KINETICS

As an agonist, binds to 5-HT_{1D}, 5-HT_{1B}, and 5-HT_{1F} receptors on the extracerebral, intracranial blood vessels that become dilated during a migraine headache, as well as on nerve terminals in the trigeminal system. Activation of these receptors causes cranial vessel vasoconstriction, inhibition of neuropeptide release, and reduced transmission in trigeminal nerve pathways. Well absorbed after PO use; **peak plasma levels:** 1–3 hr. **t½, mean:** 3–4 hr. Metabolized in the liver; metabolites and unchanged drug (40%) are excreted mainly in the urine.

USES

Acute treatment of migraine, with and without aura, in adults. Use only where there is a clear diagnosis of migraine.

CONTRAINDICATIONS

Use to prevent migraine or in management of hemiplegic or basilar migraine. Use in those with ischemic heart disease (angina pectoris, history of MI, documented silent ischemia) or who have symptoms or findings consistent with ischemic heart disease, coronary artery vasospasm (including Prinzmetal's variant angina), or other significant underlying CV disease. Use when unrecognized coronary artery disease is predicted by presence of risk factors such as hypertension, hypercholesterolemia, smoking, diabetes, strong family history of CAD, females with surgical or physiologic menopause, or males over 40 years of age unless a CV evaluation shows individual is reasonably free of CAD or ischemic myocardial disease. Use in uncontrolled hypertension, within 24 hr of treatment with another 5-HT_1 agonist or an ergotamine-containing or ergot-type medication (e.g., dihydroergotamine, methysergide). Use in children less than 18 years of age.

SPECIAL CONCERNS

Use with caution during lactation and in diseases that may alter the absorption, metabolism, or excretion of the drug, such as impaired hepatic or renal function. Safety and efficacy have not been determined in children less than 18 years of age or for cluster headaches (present in an older, predominately male population).

SIDE EFFECTS

CV: ***Acute MI, disturbances of cardiac rhythm, death, cerebral hemorrhage, subarachnoid hemorrhage, stroke, hypertensive crisis, ventricular fibrillation*** , peripheral vascular ischemia, transient myocardial ischemia, ventricular tachycardia, coronary artery vasospasm, vasodilation, palpitations, colonic ischemia (with abdominal pain and bloody diarrhea). **CNS:** Somnolence, dizziness, headache, parethesia, tremor, vertigo, anxiety, hypesthesia, restlessness, CNS stimulation, insomnia, shakiness. **GI:** N&V, dry mouth, abdominal cramps or pain, diarrhea, dyspepsia. **Body as a whole:** Asthenia, chills, back pain, chest pain, neck pain, fatigue, rigid neck. **Musculoskeletal:** Myalgia, muscular weakness. **Respiratory:** Pharyngitis, rhinitis, dyspnea, laryngismus, sinusitis, bronchitis, epistaxis. **Dermatologic:** Diaphoresis, dermatitis, erythema, pruritus, rash. **Ophthalmic:** Conjunctivitis, eye irritation. **Miscellaneous:** Ear pain, hyperacusis, taste alteration, dysmenorrhea. Sensations of tightness, pain, and heaviness in the precordium, throat, neck, and jaw.

LABORATORY TEST CONSIDERATIONS

↑ Serum creatine phosphokinase. Hyperglycemia.

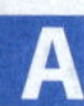

DRUG INTERACTIONS
Dihydroergotamine / Possible additive vasospastic effects; do not use within 24 hr of each other
Erythromycin / Possible ↑ almotriptan levels
Itraconazole / Possible ↑ almotriptan levels
Ketoconazole / Possible ↑ almotriptan levels
MAO inhibitors / ↓ Almotriptan clearance
Methysergide / Possible additive vasospastic effects; do not use within 24 hr of each other
Ritonavir / Possible ↑ almotriptan levels

HOW SUPPLIED
Tablet: 6.25 mg, 12.5 mg

DOSAGE

• **TABLETS**

Migraine headache.

Adults: Single dose of either 6.25 or 12.5 mg (more effective). Choice of dose is on an individual basis. If the headache returns, dose may be repeated after 2 hr, but give no more than 2 doses in a 24-hr period.

NURSING CONSIDERATIONS

ADMINISTRATION/STORAGE

1. If the first dose does not produce a response, reconsider the diagnosis of migraine before giving a second dose.
2. The safety of treating an average of more than 4 headaches in a 30-day period has not been studied.
3. For those with hepatic or renal impairment, do not exceed a maximum daily dose of 12.5 mg and a starting dose of 6.25 mg.

ASSESSMENT

1. Review symptom characteristics; ensure not hemiplegic or basilar migraine type of headaches.
2. Note drugs currently prescribed to ensure none interact.
3. Assess for CAD, uncontrolled HTN, and list cardiac risk factors.
4. Determine renal and LFTs; evaluate for dysfunction.

CLIENT/FAMILY TEACHING

1. Take only as directed for migraine headaches; do not share meds with another person regardless of symptoms; do not use for other types of headaches.
2. If headache returns may repeat dose in 2 hr; do not exceed 2 tablets in 24 hr.
3. Use caution if driving or performing activities that require mental alertness; may cause dizziness or drowsiness.
4. Store away from heat, light, and moisture; store in a safe place.
5. Drug acts to shrink swollen blood vessels surrounding the brain that cause migraine headaches. Keep a headache diary and identify factors/foods/events that surround migraine headaches.
6. Avoid known triggers, i.e., chocolate, cheese, citrus fruit, caffeine, alcohol, missing sleep/meals, etc.
7. Report any unusual side effects, intolerance, or lack of response.

OUTCOMES/EVALUATE
Resolution of migraine headaches

Alprazolam

(al-**PRAYZ**-oh-lam)

PREGNANCY CATEGORY: D
CLASSIFICATION(S):
Antianxiety drug, Benzodiazepine
Rx: Alprazolam Intensol, Xanax
✱Rx: Alti-Alprazolam, Apo-Alpraz,, Gen-Alprazolam, Novo-Alprazol, Nu-Alpraz, Xanax TS **C-IV**

SEE ALSO ***TRANQUILIZERS/ANTIMANIC DRUGS/HYPNOTICS.***

ACTION/KINETICS
Onset: Intermediate. **Peak plasma levels: PO,** 8–37 ng/mL after 1–2 hr. **t½:** 12–15 hr. 80% plasma protein bound. Metabolized to alpha-hydroxyalprazolam, an active metabolite. **t½:** 12–15 hr. Excreted in urine.

USES
Anxiety. Anxiety associated with depression with or without agoraphobia. *Investigational:* Agoraphobia with social phobia, depression, PMS.

CONTRAINDICATIONS
Use with itraconazole or ketoconazole.

A

ADDITIONAL DRUG INTERACTIONS

Azole antifungal drugs, clarithromycin, erythromycin, protease inhibitors or SSRIs decrease the metabolism of alprazolam. Decrease the dose of alprazolam by 50% to 75%.

H Possible lethargy and disorientation when combined with kava kava.

HOW SUPPLIED

Intensol: 1 mg/mL; *Oral Solution:* 0.5 mg/5 mL; *Tablet:* 0.25 mg, 0.5 mg, 1 mg, 2 mg

DOSAGE

- **INTENSOL, ORAL SOLUTION, TABLETS**

Anxiety disorder.

Adults, initial: 0.25–0.5 mg t.i.d.; **then,** titrate to needs of client, with total daily dosage not to exceed 4 mg. **In elderly or debilitated: initial;** 0.25 mg b.i.d.–t.i.d.; **then,** adjust dosage to needs of client.

Antipanic agent.

Adults: 0.5 mg t.i.d.; increase dose as needed up to a maximum of 10 mg/day.

Agoraphobia with social phobia.

Adults: 2–8 mg/day.

PMS.

0.25 mg t.i.d.

NURSING CONSIDERATIONS

SEE ALSO NURSING CONSIDERATIONS FOR TRANQUILIZERS/ANTIMANIC DRUGS/HYPNOTICS.

ADMINISTRATION/STORAGE

1. Do not decrease the daily dose more than 0.5 mg over 3 days if therapy is terminated or the dose decreased.
2. Reduce dosage in elderly and debilitated clients.

CLIENT/FAMILY TEACHING

1. May take with milk or food to decrease GI upset.
2. Include extra fluids and bulk in the diet to minimize constipation.
3. Seek appropriate psychological therapy as prolonged use may cause dependence.
4. Use support devices as needed, especially at night; elderly tend to become confused. Store drug away from bedside to prevent overdose.

OUTCOMES/EVALUATE

- Positive behaviors with phobias
- ↓ Anxiety/restlessness; Control of panic disorder
- Improvement in PMS symptoms

Alprostadil (PGE_1)

(al-**PROSS**-tah-dill)

CLASSIFICATION(S):

Prostaglandin

Rx: Caverject, Edex, Muse, Prostin VR Pediatric

✱**Rx:** Prostin VR

ACTION/KINETICS

Alprostadil is the naturally occurring acidic lipid prostaglandin E_1. It relaxes smooth muscle of the ductus arteriosus leading to increased pulmonary blood flow with increased blood oxygenation and lower body perfusion. Clients with low pO_2 values respond best. May also cause vasodilation, inhibit platelet aggregation, and stimulate both intestinal and uterine smooth muscle. When injected intracavernosally, alprostadil relaxes the trabecular cavernous smooth muscles and causes dilation of penile arteries. This results in increased arterial blood flow to the corpus cavernosa and thus swelling and elongation of the penis. **Onset, systemic:** 1.5–3 hr for acyanotic congenital heart disease and 15–30 min for cyanotic congenital heart disease. **Time to peak effect:** 3 hr for coarctation of the aorta and 1.5 hr for interruption of aortic arch. **Duration:** Closure of the ductus arteriosus usually begins 1–2 hr after infusion discontinued. Alprostadil is rapidly metabolized (80% in one pass) by oxidation in the lung, and metabolites are excreted by the kidney.

USES

Diagnosis and treatment of erectile dysfunction (male impotence) due to neurologic, vascular, psychologic, or mixed causes. Prostin VR Pediatric is

used in newborns with congenital heart defects to maintain patency of the ductus arteriosus. *Investigational:* Diagnostic peripheral arteriography. Treat atherosclerosis, gangrene, and pain due to peripheral vascular disease.

CONTRAINDICATIONS

Respiratory distress syndrome. Conditions that predispose to priapism: sickle cell anemia or trait, multiple myeloma, leukemia. In clients with anatomic deformation of the penis or in those with penile implants. Use in women, children, newborns, or men for whom sexual activity is not advisable or is contraindicated. Use for sexual intercourse with a pregnant woman unless a condom is used. Hyaline membrane disease.

SIDE EFFECTS

Respiratory: ***Apnea (in 10%–12% of neonates), especially in neonates less than 2 kg at birth;*** bronchial wheezing, bradypnea, hypercapnia, respiratory depression. Also, in adults, respiratory infection, flu syndrome, sinusitis, rhinitis, nasal congestion, cough. **CNS:** Fever, ***seizures,*** hypothermia, jitteriness, lethargy, ***cerebral bleeding,*** stiffness, hyperextension of the neck, irritability. **CV:** Flushing, especially after intra-arterial dosage, bradycardia, hypotension, tachycardia, edema, ***cardiac arrest, CHF, shock, arrhythmias.*** **GI:** Diarrhea, hyperbilirubinemia, gastric regurgitation. **Renal:** Hematuria, anuria. **Skeletal:** Cortical proliferation of long bones. **Hematologic:** ***Disseminated intravascular coagulation,*** thrombocytopenia, anemia, bleeding. **Miscellaneous:** ***Sepsis, peritonitis,*** hypoglycemia, hypokalemia or hyperkalemia.

Side effects when used for erectile dysfunction.

Penile pain, prolonged erection, penile fibrosis, hematoma at injection site, penile disorders, including numbness, yeast infection, irritation, sensitivity, phimosis, pruritus, erythema, venous leak, penile skin tear, strange feeling in penis, discoloration of penile head, itch at tip of penis. Painful erection, abnormal ejaculation, penile rash, penile edema, priapism, hematoma, ecchymosis, urethral pain, urethral burning, urethral bleeding or spotting, testicular pain.

LABORATORY TEST CONSIDERATIONS

↑ Bilirubin. ↓ Glucose, serum calcium. ↑ or ↓ Potassium.

OD OVERDOSE MANAGEMENT

Symptoms: ***Apnea,*** bradycardia, flushing, hypotension, pyrexia. *Treatment:* Reduce rate of infusion if symptoms of hypotension or pyrexia occur; discontinue infusion if symptoms of apnea or bradycardia occur.

DRUG INTERACTIONS

Cyclosporine / ↓ Cyclosporine blood levels

Heparin, Warfarin / ↑ Bleeding after intracavernosal injection

HOW SUPPLIED

Injection: 0.5 mg/mL; *Pellet:* 125 mcg, 250 mcg, 500 mcg, 1000 mcg; *Powder for Injection, lyophilized:* 5 mcg/mL, 10 mcg/mL, 20 mcg/mL, 40 mcg/mL.

DOSAGE

- **CONTINUOUS IV INFUSION OR UMBILICAL ARTERY**

Maintain patency of ductus arteriosus.

Initial: 0.05–0.1 mcg/kg/min; **then,** after response achieved, decrease infusion rate to lowest dose that will maintain response (e.g., 0.1–0.05 to 0.025–0.01 mcg/kg/min). *NOTE:* If 0.1 mcg/kg/min is insufficient, dosage can be increased up to 0.4 mcg/kg/min.

- **INTRACAVERNOSAL**

Erectile dysfunction due to vascular, psychogenic, or mixed etiology.

Individualize the dose for each client by careful titration. **Initial:** 2.5 mcg. If there is a partial response, increase the dose by 2.5 mcg to 5 mcg and then in increments of 5–10 mcg, depending on the erectile response, until a dose is reached that results in an erection suitable for intercourse but not exceeding 1 hr in duration. If there is no response to the initial 2.5-mcg dose, the second dose may be increased to 7.5 mcg, followed by increments of 5 to 10 mcg. **Maximum dose:** 60 mcg. Do not give the drug more than 3 times/week with at least 24 hr between each dose.

A

Erectile dysfunction due to pure neurogenic etiology (spinal cord injury).
Initial: 1.25 mcg. The dose may be increased by 1.25 mcg to 2.5 mcg, followed by an increment of 2.5 mcg to a dose of 5 mcg. The dose may be increased in 5-mcg increments until a dose is reached that produces an erection suitable for intercourse and not exceeding 1 hr in duration.

NURSING CONSIDERATIONS

ADMINISTRATION/STORAGE

1. For use in impotence, the diluent is mixed with alprostadil powder, and the solution is swirled gently. One mL of the reconstituted solution contains either 10 or 20 mcg of alprostadil. Use the solution immediately; do not store or freeze.
2. For treating impotence, alprostadil is injected into the corpus cavernosum using a small, thin needle (½ in., 27- to 30-gauge). Cleanse the injection site with an alcohol swab. The first injection should be administered in a physician's office.
3. Store ampules at 2–8°C (36–46°F).

IV 4. Administer infusions only in pediatric intensive care facilities. Use a Y set-up.
5. Dilute 500 mcg with either NaCl injection or dextrose injection in volumes appropriate for the infant's fluid intake and suitable for the type of infusion pump available.
6. Discard any unused solutions and prepare a fresh solution q 24 hr.
7. Infuse sterile solutions for the shortest time and at the lowest dose that will produce the desired effect.

ASSESSMENT

1. Document indications for therapy, onset of symptoms, and any associated predisposing factors.
2. Document VS and cardiac/respiratory function before administering.
3. Determine if the neonate has restricted pulmonary blood flow. Have a respirator readily available.
4. Note any evidence of bleeding tendencies or sickle cell anemia.
5. With sexual dysfunction, list all meds currently prescribed and those consumed. Note any altered psychosocial balance.

INTERVENTIONS

1. Monitor arterial pressure intermittently by umbilical artery catheter, auscultation, Dinemapp or with a Doppler transducer. Obtain written guidelines for arterial pressures; if pressure falls significantly, decrease flow rate and report.
2. Observe infant for apnea, bradycardia, pyrexia, flushing, and hypotension; symptoms of *overdose.* The following guidelines are appropriate.
   - With apnea or bradycardia, stop infusion, change to the unmedicated solution, and start resuscitation.
   - If infant develops pyrexia or hypotension, reduce flow rate until temperature and BP return to baseline.
   - Flushing may indicate an incorrect intra-arterial catheter placement and requires repositioning.
3. If infant has restricted pulmonary blood flow, monitor ABGs. A positive response to alprostadil is indicated by at least a 10 mm Hg increase in blood pO_2.
4. If systemic blood flow restricted, monitor BP and serum pH. If the infant has acidosis, a positive response to alprostadil would be indicated by an increased pH, an increase in BP, and a decreased PA to aortic pressure ratio.
5. Monitor neurological status and level of consciousness; stop drug and report seizures, hyperexcitability, or stiffness.
6. Treatment for impotence should be discontinued in clients who develop penile angulation, cavernosal fibrosis, or Peyronie's disease.

CLIENT/FAMILY TEACHING

1. Advise parents of infant's condition and why drug is indicated; review risks and benefits.
2. With erectile dysfunction, once initial injection response is evaluated, obtain instruction in the method for administration. Review written guidelines to ensure proper administration and dosing.
3. Do not exceed amount or frequency of use.

4. Report any foul discharge, pain, or local irritation and rash or problems voiding.
5. Report any unusual drug side effects. Seek immediate attention if an erection lasts longer than 6 hr and report for follow-up to detect signs of penile fibrosis.

OUTCOMES/EVALUATE

- Improved pulmonary blood flow with ↑ pO_2
- Closure of ductus arteriosus 1–2 hr following infusion
- Sustained penile erection

Alteplase, recombinant

(**AL**-teh-playz)

PREGNANCY CATEGORY: C
CLASSIFICATION(S):
Thrombolytic, tissue plasminogen activator
Rx: Cathflo Activase, Activase
✱Rx: Activase rt-PA

ACTION/KINETICS

Alteplase, a tissue plasminogen activator, is synthesized by a human melanoma cell line using recombinant DNA technology. This enzyme binds to fibrin in a thrombus, causing a conversion of plasminogen to plasmin. This conversion results in local fibrinolysis and a decrease in circulating fibrinogen. Within 10 min following termination of an infusion, 80% of the alteplase has been cleared from the plasma by the liver. The enzyme activity of alteplase is 580,000 IU/mg. **t½, initial:** 4 min; **final:** 35 min (elimination phase).

USES

Improvment of ventricular function following AMI, including reducing the incidence of CHF and decreasing mortality. Treat acute ischemic stroke, after intracranial hemorrhage has been excluded by CT scan or other diagnostic imaging. Acute pulmonary thromboembolism. Restoration of function to central venous access devices that have become occluded by a blood clot or thrombus (use Cathflo Activase). *Investigational:* Unstable angina pectoris.

CONTRAINDICATIONS

AMI or pulmonary embolism: Active internal bleeding, history of CVA, within 2 months of intracranial or intraspinal surgery or trauma, intracranial neoplasm, AV malformation or aneurysm, bleeding diathesis, severe uncontrolled hypertension.

Acute ischemic stroke: Symptoms of intracranial hemorrhage on pretreatment evaluation, suspected subarachnoid hemorrhage, recent intracranial surgery or serious head trauma, recent previous stroke, history of intracranial hemorrhage, uncontrolled hypertension (above 185 mm Hg systolic or above 110 Hg diastolic) at time of treatment, active internal bleeding, seizure at onset of stroke, intracranial neoplasm, AV malformation or aneurysm, bleeding diathesis.

SPECIAL CONCERNS

Use with caution in the presence of recent GI or GU bleeding (within 10 days), subacute bacterial endocarditis, acute pericarditis, significant liver dysfunction, concomitant use of oral anticoagulants, diabetic hemorrhagic retinopathy, septic thrombophlebitis or occluded arteriovenous cannula (at infected site), lactation, mitral stenosis with atrial fibrillation. Since fibrin will be lysed during therapy, careful attention should be given to potential bleeding sites such as sites of catheter insertion and needle puncture sites. Use with caution within 10 days of major surgery (e.g., obstetrics, coronary artery bypass) and in clients over 75 years of age. Safety and efficacy have not been established in children. *NOTE:* Doses greater than 150 mg have been associated with an increase in intracranial bleeding.

SIDE EFFECTS

Bleeding tendencies: *Internal bleeding* (including the GI and GU tracts and intracranial or retroperitoneal site). Superficial bleeding (e.g., gums, sites of recent surgery, venous cutdowns, arterial punctures). Ecchymosis, epistaxis. **CV:** Bradycardia, hypotension, cardiogenic shock, arrhythmias, ***heart failure, cardiac arrest, cardiac tamponade, myocardial rupture,*** recurrent ischemia, reinfarction, mitral regurgitation, pericardial effusion, pericarditis, venous thrombosis and embolism, electromechanical dissociation. **Allergic:** Rash, ***laryngeal edema, anaphylaxis.*** **GI:** N&V. **Miscellaneous:** Fever, urticaria, pulmonary edema, cerebral edema.

Due to accelerated infusion: ***Strokes, hemorrhagic stroke,*** nonfatal stroke. Incidence increases with age.

OD OVERDOSE MANAGEMENT

Symptoms: Bleeding disorders. *Treatment:* Discontinue therapy immediately as well as any concomitant heparin therapy.

DRUG INTERACTIONS

Abciximab / ↑ Risk of bleeding
Acetylsalicylic acid / ↑ Risk of bleeding
Dipyridamole / ↑ Risk of bleeding
Heparin / ↑ Risk of bleeding, especially at arterial puncture sites

HOW SUPPLIED

Powder for injection: 50 mg, 100 mg; *Single-patient vial (Cathflo Activase):* 2 mg

DOSAGE

• **IV INFUSION ONLY**

AMI, accelerated infusion.

Weight > 67 kg: 100 mg as a 15-mg IV bolus, followed by 50 mg infused over the next 30 min and then 35 mg infused over the next 60 min. **Weight < 67 kg:** 15 mg IV bolus, followed by 0.75 mg/kg infused over the next 30 min (not to exceed 50 mg) and then 0.50 mg/kg infused over the next 60 min (not to exceed 35 mg). The safety and efficacy of this regimen have only been evaluated using heparin and aspirin concomitantly.

AMI, 3-hr infusion.

100 mg total dose subdivided as follows: 60 mg (34.8 million IU) the first hour with 6–10 mg given in a bolus over the first 1–2 min and the remaining 50–54 mg given over the hour; 20 mg (11.6 million IU) over the second hour and 20 mg (11.6 million IU) given over the third hour. **Clients less than 65 kg:** 1.25 mg/kg given over 3 hr, with 60% given the first hour with 6%–10% given by direct IV injection within the first 1–2 min; 20% is given the second hour and 20% during the third hour. Doses of 150 mg have caused an increase in intracranial bleeding.

Pulmonary embolism.

100 mg over 2 hr; heparin therapy should be instituted near the end of or right after the alteplase infusion when the partial thromboplastin or thrombin time returns to twice that of normal or less.

Acute ischemic stroke.

0.9 mg/kg (maximum of 90 mg) infused over 60 min with 10% of the total dose given as an initial IV bolus over 1 min. Doses greater than 0.9 mg/kg may cause an increased incidence of intracranial hemorrhage. Use with aspirin and heparin during the first 24 hr after onset of symptoms has not been investigated.

Restoration of function to central venous access device.

2 mg in 2 mL of solution for clients weighing 30 kg or more; for those weighing between 10 and 30 kg, use a dose of 1 mg/mL solution equivalent to 110% of the volume of the catheter's internal lumen but not more than 2 mg. A second dose may be instilled if the catheter is not functioning 120 min after the first dose.

NURSING CONSIDERATIONS

ADMINISTRATION/STORAGE

IV 1. Initiate alteplase therapy as soon as possible after onset of symptoms and within 3 hr after the onset of stroke symptoms.

2. For acute MI, nearly 90% of clients also receive heparin concomitantly with alteplase and either aspirin or dipyridamole during or after heparin therapy.

3. Reconstitute with only sterile water for injection without preservatives immediately prior to use. The reconstituted preparation contains 1 mg/mL and is a colorless to pale yellow transparent solution.

4. Using an 18-gauge needle, direct the stream of sterile water into the lyophilized cake. Leave product undisturbed for several minutes to allow dissipation of any large bubbles.
5. If necessary, the reconstituted solution may be further diluted immediately prior to use in an equal volume of 0.9% NaCl injection or 5% dextrose injection to yield a concentration of 0.5 mg/mL. Dilute by gentle swirling or slow inversion.
6. Either glass bottles or polyvinylchloride bags may be used for administration.
7. Alteplase is stable for up to 8 hr following reconstitution or dilution. Stability will not be affected by light.
8. Do not use 50-mg vials if vacuum is not present (100-mg vials do not contain a vacuum). Reconstitute 50-mg vials with a large-bore needle (e.g., 18 gauge) directing stream of sterile water into lyophilized cake. For the 100-mg vial, use transfer device provided for reconstitution.
9. Use infusion device for administration. Do not add any other medications to the line. Anticipate 3 lines for access (1–alteplase; 1–heparin and other drugs such as lidocaine; 1–blood drawing and transfusions).
10. Store lyophilized alteplase at room temperatures not to exceed 30°C (86°F) or under refrigeration between 2–8°C (35–46°F).
11. Have available emergency drugs (especially aminocaproic acid) and resuscitative equipment.

ASSESSMENT

1. Note any history of hypertension, internal bleeding, PUD, or recent surgery.
2. Document onset and characteristics of chest pain and/or stroke symptoms; note deficits and monitor.
3. Assess and document overall physical condition; note CV and neurologic findings, weight, and ECG.
4. Obtain drug history. List what client is currently taking; note any anticoagulants/antiplatelets.
5. Obtain baseline hematologic parameters, type and cross, coagulation times, cardiac marker panel, and renal function studies.

INTERVENTIONS

1. Carefully review and follow instructions for drug reconstitution, review contraindications before initiating therapy, and document if accelerated or 3 hr infusion is prescribed.
2. Observe in a closely monitored environment; obtain VS and review and document monitor strips.
3. Anticipate and assess for reperfusion reactions such as:
   - Reperfusion arrhythmias usually of short duration. These may include accelerated idioventricular rhythm and sinus bradycardia.
   - Reduction of chest pain
   - Return of the elevated ST segment to near baseline levels
   - Smaller Q waves
4. Check all access sites for any evidence of bleeding.
5. During IV therapy, arterial sticks require 30 min of manual pressure followed by application of a pressure dressing.
6. In the event of any uncontrolled bleeding, terminate alteplase and heparin infusions and report.
7. Monitor neuro status; document q 15–30 min during infusion.
8. During treatment of stroke, note CT or MRI results.
9. During treatment for pulmonary embolism, ensure that the PTT or PT is no more than twice that of normal before heparin therapy is added.
10. Keep on bed rest and observe for S&S of abnormal bleeding (hematuria, hematemesis, melena, CVA, cardiac tamponade).
11. Obtain appropriate postinfusion labs (cardiac marker, platelets, H&H, PTT, ECG) as directed.

CLIENT/FAMILY TEACHING

1. Review the goals of therapy and inherent risks during acute coronary artery occlusion and/or stroke.
2. To be effective, the therapy should be instituted within 3 hr of stroke and 4–6 hr of MI symptoms.
3. Encourage family members to learn CPR.

OUTCOMES/EVALUATE

- Lysis of thrombi with reperfusion of ischemic cardiac and/or cerebral tissue

• ↓ Infarct size with restoration of coronary perfusion and improved ventricular function (↑ CO, ↓ incidence of CHF, ↓ mortality)

Altretamine (Hexylmethylmelamine)

(all-**TRET**-ah-meen)

PREGNANCY CATEGORY: D
CLASSIFICATION(S):
Antineoplastic, miscellaneous
Rx: Hexalen

SEE ALSO *ANTINEOPLASTIC AGENTS.*

ACTION/KINETICS
The mechanism of action is unknown, although metabolism of the drug is required for cytotoxicity. Well absorbed following PO ingestion; undergoes rapid demethylation in the liver, yielding the principal metabolites–pentamethylmelamine and tetramethylmelamine. **Peak plasma levels:** 0.5–3 hr. **t½:** 4.7–10.2 hr. Metabolites are excreted mainly through the kidney.

USES
Alone in the palliative treatment of persistent or recurrent ovarian cancer after first-line cisplatin- or alkylating agent-based combination therapy.

CONTRAINDICATIONS
Preexisting bone marrow depression or severe neurologic toxicity, although the drug has been used safely in clients with preexisting cisplatin neuropathies. Lactation.

SPECIAL CONCERNS
Safety and effectiveness have not been determined in children. High daily doses may result in gradual onset of N&V.

SIDE EFFECTS
GI: N&V (most common). **Neurologic:** Peripheral sensory neuropathy, fatigue, anorexia, seizures. **CNS:** Mood disorders, disorders of consciousness, ataxia, dizziness, vertigo. **Hematologic:** Leukopenia, thrombocytopenia, anemia. **Miscellaneous: *Hepatic toxicity,*** skin rash, pruritus, alopecia.

LABORATORY TEST CONSIDERATIONS
↑ Serum creatinine, BUN, alkaline phosphatase.

DRUG INTERACTIONS
Use with MAO inhibitors may cause severe orthostatic hypotension, especially in clients over the age of 60 years.

HOW SUPPLIED
Capsule: 50 mg

DOSAGE

• CAPSULES

Ovarian cancer.

260 mg/m²/day given either for 14 or 21 consecutive days in a 28-day cycle. The total daily dose is given as four divided doses PO after meals and at bedtime.

NURSING CONSIDERATIONS

SEE ALSO *NURSING CONSIDERATIONS* FOR *ANTINEOPLASTIC AGENTS.*

ADMINISTRATION/STORAGE
Discontinue temporarily (for 14 or more days) and restart at 200 mg/m²/day if any of the following occur: GI intolerance unresponsive to symptomatic treatment; WBCs less than 200/mm³ or granulocyte count less than 1000/mm³; platelet count less than 75,000/mm³; progressive neurotoxicity. Discontinue if neurologic symptoms fail to stabilize on a reduced dosage schedule.

ASSESSMENT
1. Document onset of symptoms and note all previous therapies.
2. Note neurologic findings.
3. Assess CBC and LFTs.

INTERVENTIONS
1. Anticipate neurotoxicity as a side effect of drug therapy. Assess neuro status prior to starting therapy and before each subsequent course.
2. Give pyridoxine to reduce severity of neurotoxic effects.
3. Monitor peripheral blood counts monthly, prior to the initiation of each course of therapy and as clinically indicated.

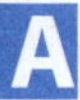

CLIENT/FAMILY TEACHING

1. Report any adverse symptoms, such as tingling, decreased sensation, dizziness, and N&V. Dose may need to be decreased or discontinued.
2. Practice barrier contraception; may cause fetal damage.
3. Report for monthly hematologic studies.

OUTCOMES/EVALUATE

Control of tumor growth and spread

Amantadine hydrochloride

(ah-**MAN**-tah-deen)

PREGNANCY CATEGORY: C
CLASSIFICATION(S):
Antiviral antiparkinson drug
Rx: Symmetrel
✱Rx: Endantadine, Gen-Amantadine

SEE ALSO *ANTIVIRAL DRUGS.*

ACTION/KINETICS

Believed to prevent penetration of the virus into cells, possibly by inhibiting uncoating of the RNA virus. May also prevent the release of infectious viral nucleic acid into the host cell. The reaction appears to be virus specific for influenza A but not host specific. The drug reduces symptoms (70% to 90% effective) of viral infections if given within 24–48 hr after onset of illness. For the treatment of parkinsonism, amantadine may increase the release of dopamine from dopaminergic nerve terminals in the substantia nigra of parkinson clients, resulting in an increase in dopamine levels in dopaminergic synapses. The drug decreases extrapyramidal symptoms, including akinesia, rigidity, tremors, excessive salivation, gait disturbances, and total functional disability. Well absorbed from GI tract. **Peak blood levels:** 4 hr. **Onset:** 48 hr. **Peak serum concentration:** 0.2 mcg/mL after 1–4 hr. **t½:** Approximately 15 hr; elimination half-life increases two- to threefold when C_{CR} is less than 40 mL/min/1.73 m^2. Renal clearance is reduced and plasma levels increased in otherwise healthy clients, aged 65 years and older. Ninety percent excreted unchanged in urine.

USES

Influenza A viral infections of the respiratory tract (prophylaxis and treatment of high-risk clients with immunodeficiency, CV, metabolic, neuromuscular, or pulmonary disease). Symptomatic treatment of idiopathic parkinsonism and parkinsonism syndrome resulting from encephalitis, carbon monoxide intoxication, drugs, or cerebral arteriosclerosis. Favorable results have been obtained in about 50% of the clients. Improvements can last for up to 30 months, although some clients report that the effect of the drug wears off in 1–3 months. A rest period or an increased dosage may reestablish effectiveness. For parkinsonism, amantadine hydrochloride is usually used concomitantly with other agents, such as levodopa and anticholinergic agents.

Amantadine is recommended for prophylaxis in the following situations:

- Short-term prophylaxis during the course of a presumed outbreak of influenza;
- Adjunct to late immunization in high-risk clients;
- To reduce disruption of medical care and to decrease spread of virus in high-risk clients when influenza A virus outbreaks occur;
- To supplement vaccination protection in clients with impaired immune responses;
- As chemoprophylaxis during flu season for those high-risk clients for whom influenza vaccine is contraindicated due to anaphylactic response to egg protein or prior severe reactions associated with flu vaccination

CONTRAINDICATIONS

Hypersensitivity to drug.

SPECIAL CONCERNS

Use with caution in clients with liver and renal disease, history of epilepsy, CHF, peripheral edema, orthostatic hypotension, recurrent eczematoid dermatitis, or severe psychosis, in clients taking CNS stimulant drugs, to those exposed to rubella, and to nursing mothers. Safe use in lactating moth-

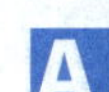

ers and in children less than 1 year has not been established.

SIDE EFFECTS

GI: N&V, constipation, anorexia, xerostomia. **CNS:** Depression, psychosis, ***convulsions,*** hallucinations, lightheadedness, confusion, ataxia, irritability, anxiety, headache, dizziness, fatigue, insomnia. **CV:** ***CHF,*** orthostatic hypotension, peripheral edema. **Miscellaneous:** Urinary retention, leukopenia, neutropenia, mottling of skin of the extremities due to poor peripheral circulation (livedo reticularis), skin rashes, visual problems, slurred speech, oculogyric episodes, dyspnea, weakness, eczematoid dermatitis.

OD OVERDOSE MANAGEMENT

Symptoms: Anorexia, N&V, CNS effects. *Treatment:* Gastric lavage or induction of emesis followed by supportive measures. Ensure that client is well hydrated; give IV fluids if necessary. To treat CNS toxicity: IV physostigmine, 1–2 mg given q 1–2 hr in adults or 0.5 mg at 5–10-min intervals (maximum of 2 mg/hr) in children. Sedatives and anticonvulsants may be given if needed; antiarrhythmics and vasopressors may also be required.

DRUG INTERACTIONS

Anticholinergics / Additive anticholinergic effects (including hallucinations, confusion), especially with trihexyphenidyl and benztropine

H *Belladonna leaf/root* / ↑ Anticholinergic effect

CNS stimulants / May ↑ CNS and psychic effects of amantadine; use cautiously together

H *Henbane leaf* / ↑ Anticholinergic effects

Hydrochlorothiazide/triamterene combination / ↓ Urinary excretion of amantadine → ↑ plasma levels

Levodopa / Potentiated by amantadine

H *Pheasant's eye herb* / ↑ Amantadine effect

H *Scopolia root* / ↑ Amantadine effect

HOW SUPPLIED

Capsule: 100 mg; *Syrup:* 50 mg/5 mL.

DOSAGE

• CAPSULES, SYRUP

Antiviral.

Adults: 200 mg/day as a single or divided dose. **Children, 1–9 years:** 4.4–8.8 mg/kg/day up to a maximum of 150 mg/day in one or two divided doses (use syrup); **9–12 years:** 100 mg b.i.d.

Prophylactic treatment.

Institute before or immediately after exposure and continue for 10–21 days if used concurrently with vaccine or for 90 days without vaccine.

Symptomatic management.

Initiate as soon as possible and continue for 24–48 hr after disappearance of symptoms. Decrease dose in renal impairment (see package insert). Reduce dose to 100 mg/day for persons with active seizure disorders due to the increased risk of seizure frequency using daily doses of 200 mg.

Parkinsonism.

Use as sole agent, usual: 100 mg b.i.d., up to 400 mg/day in divided doses, if necesssary. **Use with other antiparkinson drugs:** 100 mg 1–2 times/day.

Drug-induced extrapyramidal symptoms.

100 mg b.i.d. (up to 300 mg/day may be required in some). Reduce dose in impaired renal function.

NURSING CONSIDERATIONS

SEE ALSO *GENERAL NURSING CONSIDERATIONS FOR ALL ANTI-INFECTIVES* AND *ANTIVIRAL DRUGS*.

ADMINISTRATION/STORAGE

1. Protect capsules from moisture.
2. Initiate therapy for viral illness as soon as possible after symptoms begin and for 24–48 hr after symptoms disappear.

ASSESSMENT

1. Obtain history and note any evidence of seizures, CHF, and renal insufficiency.
2. With active seizure disorder reduce drug dosage to prevent breakthrough seizures. With an increase in seizure activity, take appropriate precautions and ensure that dosage is reduced to

A

100 mg/day to prevent loss of seizure control.
3. Monitor I&O; observe clients with renal impairment for crystalluria, oliguria, and increased BUN or creatinine levels.
4. With Parkinson's disease, following loss of drug effectiveness, benefits may be regained by increasing the dosage or discontinuing the drug for several weeks and then reinstituting it.

CLIENT/FAMILY TEACHING

1. Administer last dose several hours before bedtime to prevent insomnia.
2. Do not drive or work in a situation where alertness is important until drug effects realized; can affect vision, concentration, and coordination.
3. Rise slowly from a prone position because orthostatic hypotension may occur. Lie down if dizzy/weak to relieve symptoms.
4. Report diffuse patchy discoloration or skin mottling. Discoloration lessens when legs are elevated; usually fades completely within weeks after stopping drug.
5. Report any exposure to rubella; drug may increase disease susceptibility.
6. Susceptible individuals (elderly, immunocompromised) should avoid crowds during "flu" season, receive annual flu shot and the pneumonia vaccine.
7. Report any psychologic changes such as confusion, mental status changes, nervousness, or depression as well as any persistent, or new symptoms.
8. Avoid alcohol or any other unprescribed OTC products.
9. Clients with parkinsonism should not stop drug abruptly.
10. With seizure disorders, report any early S&S of seizure activity; dosage may require adjustment.

OUTCOMES/EVALUATE

- ↓ Drug-induced extrapyramidal S&S
- Improved motor control; ↓ tremor
- Influenza A prophylaxis; ↓ spread of infection to high-risk individuals during outbreaks

Amifostine

(**am**-ih-**FOS**-teen)

PREGNANCY CATEGORY: C
CLASSIFICATION(S):
Cytoprotective drug
Rx: Ethyol

ACTION/KINETICS

Amifostine, an organic thiophosphate prodrug, is dephosphorylated by alkaline phosphatase in tissue to the active free thiol metabolite. The thiol metabolite reduces the toxic effects of cisplatin. The ability to protect normal tissues differentially is due to the higher capillary alkaline phosphatase activity, higher pH, and better vascularity of normal tissues compared with tumor tissue. This results in a more rapid generation of the active thiol metabolite as well as greater uptake into tissues. The higher levels of the thiol metabolite in normal tissues binds to, and thus detoxifies, reactive metabolites of cisplatin; the thiol metabolite can also scavange free radicals that may be generated in tissues exposed to cisplatin. Rapidly cleared from the plasma. **t½, distribution:** less than 1 min; **t½, elimination:** about 8 min. The thiol metabolite is further broken down to a disulfide metabolite that is less active.

USES

To decrease cumulative renal toxicity due to repeated use of cisplatin in clients with advanced ovarian cancer and in those with non-small-cell lung cancer. Treat postoperative radiation-induced dry mouth in clients with head and neck cancer where the radiation port includes a significant part of the parotid glands. *Investigational:* Protect lung fibroblasts from damage by paclitaxel.

CONTRAINDICATIONS

Hypersensivity to aminothiol compounds or mannitol. Use in hypotensive or dehydrated clients, in those on antihypertensive therapy that cannot be terminated for 24 hr, and in clients receiving chemotherapy for malignancies that are potentially curable

(e.g., certain malignancies of germ cell origin). Use in clients receiving definitive radiotherapy, except during a clinical trial. Lactation.

SPECIAL CONCERNS

Safety has not been determined in clients over 70 years of age or in those with preexisting CV or cerebrovascular conditions, such as ischemic heart disease, arrhythmias, CHF, or history of stroke or transient ischemic attacks. Use with caution in those where N&V or hypotension may be more likely to have serious consequences. Safety and efficacy have not been determined in children.

SIDE EFFECTS

CV: Transient decrease in BP, hypotension. **GI:** Severe N&V. **CNS:** Dizziness, somnolence; rarely, reversible loss of consciousness or seizures. *Hypersensitivity:* Mild skin rash, fever, chills, dyspnea, urticaria, rigors, erythema multiforme; rarely, ***Stevens-Johnson syndrome, toxic epidermal necrolysis, anaphylaxis*** (hypoxia, laryngeal edema, chest tightness, cardiac arrest). **Miscellaneous:** Flushing or feeling of warmth, chills or feeling of coldness, hiccoughs, fever, sneezing, hypocalcemia.

DRUG INTERACTIONS

Amifostine may cause hypotension in clients receiving antihypertensive drugs or other drugs that may potentiate hypotension.

HOW SUPPLIED

Powder (lyophilized) for injection: 500 mg (anhydrous)

DOSAGE

• IV INFUSION

Cytoprotective agent used with cisplatin.

Initial: 910 mg/m² given once daily as a 15-min IV infusion, starting within 30 min prior to cisplatin chemotherapy.

Reduce dry mouth in postoperative radiation treatment for head and neck cancer.

200 mg/m² given once daily as a 3 min IV infusion, starting 15 to 30 min before standard fraction radiation therapy.

NURSING CONSIDERATIONS

ADMINISTRATION/STORAGE

IV 1. The 15-min infusion is better tolerated than infusions of longer duration.

2. Keep supine during administration; monitor BP every 5 min.

3. Give an antiemetic medication, including dexamethasone (20 mg IV) and a serotonin $5HT_3$ receptor antagonist, prior to and in conjunction with amifostine.

4. Stop infusion if the systolic BP decreases significantly from recommended baseline values. If BP returns to normal within 5 min and the client has no symptoms, the infusion may be restarted so the full dose of amifostine can be given. If the full dose of amifostine cannot be given, the dose for subsequent cycles should be 740 mg/m².

5. Reconstitute by adding 9.5 mL of 0.9% NaCl injection (use of other solutions is not recommended). The reconstituted solution contains 500 mg amifostine/10 mL and is stable for 5 hr at room temperature (25°C; 77°F) or up to 24 hr under refrigeration (2–8°C; 36–46°F).

ASSESSMENT

1. Note type of malignancy being managed, onset and duration of symptoms, other agents trialed, and the anticipated dose and length of cisplatin chemotherapy.

2. List drugs currently prescribed to ensure none interact unfavorably.

3. Obtain baseline VS, calcium, and renal function studies and monitor throughout therapy. Ensure that client is not dehydrated or hypotensive.

4. Monitor VS and I&O. Keep supine during 15 min infusion and check BP every 5 min.

5. Administer antiemetics prior to amifostine therapy; evaluate need for further antiemetic administration.

6. Review and follow manufacturer's guidelines for interrupting infusion due to decreased SBP and the suggested dose for readmission.

7. Monitor serum calcium in those at risk of hypocalcemia (e.g., nephrotic syndrome) or after multiple doses. If needed, give calcium supplements.

CLIENT/FAMILY TEACHING

1. Drug is given to protect the kidneys during repeated cisplastin therapy.
2. Stop BP medications 24 hr prior to therapy and ensure well hydrated.
3. Chills, flushing, dizziness, somnolence, hiccups, and sneezing may occur transiently.

OUTCOMES/EVALUATE

↓ Renal toxicity with cisplatin chemotherapy

Amikacin sulfate

(am-ih-**KAY**-sin)

PREGNANCY CATEGORY: D
CLASSIFICATION(S):
Antibiotic, aminoglycoside
Rx: Amikin

SEE ALSO *ANTI-INFECTIVES AND AMINOGLYCOSIDES.*

ACTION/KINETICS

Derived from kanamycin. Its spectrum is somewhat broader than that of other aminoglycosides, including *Serratia* and *Acinetobacter* species, as well as certain staphylococci and streptococci. Effective against both penicillinase- and non-penicillinase-producing organisms. **Peak therapeutic serum levels: IM,** 16–32 mcg/mL. **t½:** 2–3 hr. Toxic serum levels: >35 mcg/mL (peak measured after 1 hr) and >10 mcg/mL (trough measured before next dose).

USES

Short-term treatment of gram-negative bacterial infections including *Pseudomonas, Escherichia coli, Proteus, Providencia, Klebsiella, Enterobacter, Serratia,* and *Acinetobacter*. For infections due to gentamicin or tobramycin resistant strains of *Providencia rettgeri, P. stuartii, Serratia marcescens,* and *Pseudomonas aeruginosa.*

Infections include bacterial septicemia (including neonatal sepsis); serious infections of the respiratory tract, bones, joints, skin, soft tissue, and CNS (including meningitis); intra-abdominal infections (including peritonitis); burns; postoperative infections (including postvascular surgery). Also, serious complicated and recurrent infections of the urinary tract. May be used as initial therapy in certain situations in the treatment of known or suspected staphylococcal disease. *Investigational:* Intrathecal or intraventricular use. As part of multiple drug regimen for *Mycobacterium avium* complex (commonly seen in AIDS clients).

SPECIAL CONCERNS

Use with caution in premature infants and neonates.

HOW SUPPLIED

Injection: 250 mg/mL; *Pediatric Injection:* 50 mg/mL

DOSAGE

• **IM (PREFERRED) AND IV**

Adults, children, and older infants: 15 mg/kg/day in two to three equally divided doses q 8–12 hr for 7–10 days; **maximum daily dose:** 15 mg/kg.

Uncomplicated UTIs.

250 mg b.i.d.; **newborns:** loading dose of 10 mg/kg followed by 7.5 mg/kg q 12 hr.

Use in neonates.

Initial: Loading dose of 10 mg/kg; **then,** 7.5 mg/kg q 12 hr. Lower doses may be safer during the first 2 weeks of life.

Intrathecal or intraventricular use.

8 mg/24 hr.

As part of multiple drug regimen for M. avium complex.

15 mg/kg/day IV in divided doses q 8–12 hr.

In clients with impaired renal function.

Normal loading dose of 7.5 mg/kg; **then** monitor administration by serum level of amikacin (35 mcg/mL maximum) or creatinine clearance rates. Duration of treatment: **Usual:** 7–10 days.

NURSING CONSIDERATIONS

SEE ALSO *NURSING CONSIDERATIONS FOR AMINOGLYCOSIDES.*

ADMINISTRATION/STORAGE

IV 1. Add 500-mg vial to 200 mL of sterile diluent, such as NSS or D5W.

2. Administer over a 30- to 60-min period for adults.
3. Administer to infants in prescribed amount of fluid over 1–2 hr.
4. Store colorless liquid for no longer than 2 years at room temperature.
5. Potency is not affected if the solution turns a light yellow.

ASSESSMENT

1. Note indications for therapy and C&S results. Assess renal and LFTs.
2. Obtain audiometric assessment with high dosage or prolonged use.
3. Note any vestibular dysfunction and monitor for 8th CN impairment R/T elevated peak drug levels.

OUTCOMES/EVALUATE

- Resolution of infection
- Therapeutic drug levels (peak 30–35 mcg/mL; trough < 10 mcg/mL)

Amiloride hydrochloride

(ah-**MILL**-oh-ryd)

PREGNANCY CATEGORY: B
CLASSIFICATION(S):
Diuretic, potassium-sparing
Rx: Midamor

ACTION/KINETICS

Acts on the distal tubule to inhibit Na^+, K^+-ATPase, thereby inhibiting sodium exchange for potassium; this results in increased secretion of sodium and water and conservation of potassium. In the proximal tubule, amiloride inhibits the Na^+/H^+ exchange mechanism. Has weak diuretic and antihypertensive activity. **Onset:** 2 hr. **Peak effect:** 6–10 hr. **Peak plasma levels:** 3–4 hr. **Duration:** 24 hr. **t½:** 6–9 hr. Twenty-three percent is bound to plasma protein. Approximately 50% is excreted unchanged by kidney and 40% by the feces unchanged.

USES

Adjunct with thiazides or loop diuretics in the treatment of hypertension or edema due to CHF, hepatic cirrhosis, and nephrotic syndrome to help restore normal serum potassium or prevent hypokalemia. Prophylaxis of hypokalemia in clients who would be at risk if hypokalemia developed (e.g., digitalized clients or clients with significant cardiac arrhythmias). *Investigational:* To reduce lithium-induced polyuria. Aerosolized amiloride may slow the progression of pulmonary function reduction in adults with cystic fibrosis.

CONTRAINDICATIONS

Hyperkalemia (>5.5 mEq potassium/L). In clients receiving other potassium-sparing diuretics or potassium supplements. Impaired renal function. Diabetes mellitus. Use during lactation.

SPECIAL CONCERNS

Use with caution in metabolic or respiratory acidosis; during lactation. Geriatric clients may have a greater risk of developing hyperkalemia. Safety and efficacy have not been determined in children.

SIDE EFFECTS

Electrolyte: Hyperkalemia, hyponatremia, and hypochloremia if used with other diuretics. **CNS:** Headache, dizziness, encephalopathy, tremors, paresthesias, mental confusion, insomnia, decreased libido, depression, sleepiness, vertigo, nervousness. **GI:** Nausea, anorexia, vomiting, diarrhea, changes in appetite, gas and abdominal pain, dry mouth, flatulence, abdominal fullness, GI bleeding, GI disturbance, thirst, dyspepsia, heartburn, jaundice, constipation, activation of preexisting peptic ulcer. **Respiratory:** Dyspnea, cough, SOB. **Musculoskeletal:** Weakness; muscle cramps; fatigue; joint, chest and back pain; neck or shoulder ache; pain in extremities. **GU:** Impotence, polyuria, dysuria, bladder spasms, urinary frequency. **CV:** Angina, palpitations, ***arrhythmias,*** orthostatic hypotension. **Hematologic:** ***Aplastic anemia,*** neutropenia. **Dermatologic:** Skin rash, itching, pruritus, alopecia. **Miscellaneous:** Visual disturbances, nasal congestion, tinnitus, increased intraocular pressure, abnormal liver function.

OD OVERDOSE MANAGEMENT

Symptoms: Electrolyte imbalance, ***dehydration.*** *Treatment:* Induce emesis or gastric lavage. Treat hyperkalemia by IV sodium bicarbonate or oral or parenteral glucose with a rapid-acting insulin. Sodium polystyrene sulfonate, oral or by enema, may also be used.

DRUG INTERACTIONS

ACE inhibitors / ↑ Risk of significant hyperkalemia
Digoxin / Possible ↑ renal clearance and ↓ nonrenal clearance and possible ↑ inotropic effect of digoxin
Lithium / ↓ Renal excretion of lithium → ↑ chance of toxicity
NSAIDs / ↓ Therapeutic effect of amiloride
Potassium products / Hyperkalemia with possibility of cardiac arrhythmias or cardiac arrest
Spironolactone, Triamterene / Hyperkalemia, hyponatremia, hypochloremia

HOW SUPPLIED

Tablet: 5 mg

DOSAGE

• **TABLETS**

As single agent or with other diuretics.
Adults, initial: 5 mg/day; 10 mg/day may be necessary in some clients. Doses as high as 20 mg/day may be used, if needed, with careful monitoring of electrolytes.

Reduce lithium-induced polyuria.
10–20 mg/day.

Slow progression of pulmonary function reduction in cystic fibrosis.
Adults: Drug is dissolved in 0.3% saline and delivered by nebulizer.

NURSING CONSIDERATIONS

SEE ALSO ***NURSING CONSIDERATIONS*** FOR ***DIURETICS.***

ASSESSMENT

1. Monitor renal function studies, I&O, and weights.
2. Obtain serum electrolytes. Assess for hyperkalemia and indications for drug withdraw; may precipitate cardiac irregularities.

CLIENT/FAMILY TEACHING

1. Administer with food to reduce chance of GI upset.
2. Avoid potassium supplementation or foods rich in potassium because drug does not promote potassium excretion. Do not take with other potassium-sparing diuretics.

OUTCOMES/EVALUATE

- ↓ BP and enhanced diuresis
- Conservation of potassium
- ↓ Lithium-induced polyuria
- Maintenance of pulmonary function with cystic fibrosis

Amiodarone hydrochloride

(am-ee-**OH**-dah-rohn)

PREGNANCY CATEGORY: D
CLASSIFICATION(S):
Antiarrhythmic, class III
Rx: Pacerone, Cordarone
✱Rx: Alti-Amiodarone, Cordarone I.V., Gen-Amiodarone, Novo-Amiodarone

SEE ALSO ***ANTIARRHYTHMIC AGENTS.***

ACTION/KINETICS

Blocks sodium channels at rapid pacing frequencies, causing an increase in the duration of the myocardial cell action potential and refractory period, as well as alpha- and beta-adrenergic blockade. The drug decreases sinus rate, increases PR and QT intervals, results in development of U waves, and changes T-wave contour. After IV use, amiodarone relaxes vascular smooth muscle, reduces peripheral vascular resistance (afterload), and increases cardiac index slightly. No significant changes are seen in left ventricular ejection fraction after PO use. Absorption is slow and variable but food increases the rate and extent of absorption. **Maximum plasma levels:** 3–7 hr after a single dose. **Onset:** Several days up to 1–3 weeks. Drug may accumulate in the liver, lung, spleen, and adipose tissue. **Therapeutic serum levels:** 0.5–2.5 mcg/mL. **t½:** Biphasic: **initial t½:** 2.5–10 days; **final t½:** 26–107 days. Effects may persist for several weeks or months after therapy is terminated. Effective plasma concentrations are difficult to predict although concentrations below 1 mg/L are usually ineffective, whereas those above 2.5 mg/L are not necessary. Neither amiodarone nor its metabolite, desethylamiodarone, is dialyzable.

USES

Oral. Use should be reserved for life-threatening ventricular arrhythmias unresponsive to other therapy, such as recurrent ventricular fibrillation and recurrent, hemodynamically unstable ventricular tachycardia.

IV. Initial treatment and prophylaxis of frequently recurring ventricular fibrillation and hemodynamically unstable ventricular tachycardia in clients refractory to other therapy. Ventricular tachycardia/ventricular fibrillation clients unable to take PO medication. *Investigational:* Conversion of atrial fibrillation and maintenance of sinus rhythm, supraventricular tachycardia. IV to treat AV nodal reentry tachycardia.

CONTRAINDICATIONS

Parenteral use: Marked sinus bradycardia due to severe sinus node dysfunction, second- or third-degree AV block unless a functioning pacemaker is available, cardiogenic shock. **PO use:** Severe sinus-node dysfunction causing marked sinus bradycardia, second- and third-degree AV block, when bradycardia has caused syncope except when used with a pacemaker. **Parenteral and PO use:** Lactation.

SPECIAL CONCERNS

Safety and effectiveness in children have not been determined. Although not recommended for use in children, minimize the potential for the drug to leach out di-(2-ethylhexyl)phthalate (DEHP) from IV tubing during administration to children (DEHP may alter development of the male reproductive tract when given in high amounts). The drug may be more sensitive in geriatric clients, especially in thyroid dysfunction. Carefully monitor the IV product in geriatric clients and in those with severe left ventricular dysfunction.

SIDE EFFECTS

Adverse reactions, some potentially fatal, are common with doses greater than 400 mg/day. **Pulmonary:** Pulmonary infiltrates or fibrosis, interstitial/alveolar pneumonitis, hypersensitivity pneumonitis, alveolitis, pulmonary inflammation or fibrosis, ***ARDS (after parenteral use),*** lung edema, cough and progressive dyspnea. Oral use may cause a clinical syndrome of cough and progressive dyspnea accompanied by functional, radiographic, gallium scan, and pathologic data indicating pulmonary toxicity. **CV:** ***Worsening of arrhythmias, paroxysmal ventricular tachycardia,*** proarrhythmias, symptomatic bradycardia, sinus arrest, SA node dysfunction, ***CHF,*** edema, hypotension (especially with IV use), ***cardiac conduction abnormalities, coagulation abnormalities, cardiac arrest (after IV use).*** IV use may result in atrial fibrillation, nodal arrhythmia, prolonged QT interval, and sinus bradycardia. **Hepatic:** Abnormal LFTs, overt liver disease, nonspecific hepatic disorders, cholestatic hepatitis, cirrhosis, hepatitis. **CNS:** Malaise, tremor, lack of coordination, fatigue, ataxia, paresthesias, peripheral neuropathy, abnormal involuntary movements, sleep disturbances, dizziness, insomnia, headache, decreased libido, abnormal gait. **GI:** N&V, constipation, anorexia, abdominal pain, abnormal taste and smell, abnormal salivation. **Ophthalmologic:** Ophthalmic abnormalities, including optic neuropathy and/or optic neuritis (may progress to permanent blindness). Papilledema, corneal degeneration, photosensitivity, eye discomfort, scotoma, lens opacities, macular degeneration. Corneal microdeposits (asymptomatic) in clients on therapy for 6 months or more, photophobia, dry eyes, visual disturbances, blurred vision, halos. **Dermatologic:** Photosensitivity, solar dermatitis, blue discoloration of skin, rash, alopecia, spontaneous ecchymosis, flushing. **Miscellaneous:** Hypothyroidism or hyperthyroidism, vasculitis, flushing, pseudotumor cerebri, epididymitis, thrombocytopenia, angioedema. IV use may cause abnormal kidney function, Stevens-

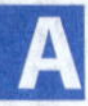

Johnson syndrome, respiratory syndrome, ***fatal "gasping syndrome" in neonates following IV use of benzyl alcohol-containing solutions,*** and ***shock.***

LABORATORY TEST CONSIDERATIONS

↑ AST, ALT, GGT. Alteration of thyroid function tests (↑ serum T_4, ↓ serum T_3).

OD OVERDOSE MANAGEMENT

Symptoms: Bradycardia, hypotension, ***disorders of cardiac rhythm, cardiogenic shock,*** AV block, hepatoxicity. *Treatment:* Use supportive treatment. Monitor cardiac rhythm and BP. Use a beta-adrenergic agonist or pacemaker to treat bradycardia; treat hypotension due to insufficient tissue perfusion with a vasopressor or positive inotropic agents. Cholestyramine may hasten the reversal of side effects by increasing elimination. Drug is not dialyzable.

DRUG INTERACTIONS

Anticoagulants / ↑ PT → bleeding disorders
Beta-adrenergic blocking agents / ↑ Bradycardia and hypotension
Calcium channel blockers / ↑ Risk of AV block with verapamil or diltiazem or hypotension with all calcium channel blockers
Cholestyramine / ↑ Elimination of amiodarone → ↓ serum levels and half-life
Cimetidine / ↑ Serum levels of amiodarone
Cyclosporine / ↑ Plasma drug levels → elevated creatinine levels (even with ↓ cyclosporine doses)
Dextromethorphan / Chronic use of PO amiodarone (> 2 weeks) impairs dextromethorphan metabolism
Digoxin / ↑ Serum digoxin levels → toxicity
Disopyramide / ↑ QT prolongation → possible arrhythmias
Fentanyl / Possibility of hypotension, bradycardia, ↓ CO
Flecainide / ↑ Plasma flecainide levels
Fluoroquinolones / ↑ Risk of life-threatening cardiac arrhythmias, including torsades de pointes
Indinavir / ↑ Plasma levels of amiodarone due to ↓ breakdown by liver
Methotrexate / Chronic use of PO amiodarone (> 2 weeks) ↓ methotrexate metabolism → toxicity
Phenytoin / ↑ Serum phenytoin levels → toxicity; also, ↓ amiodarone levels
Procainamide / ↑ Serum procainamide levels → toxicity
Quinidine / ↑ quinidine toxicity, including fatal cardiac arrhythmias
Pyridoxine / ↑ Amiodarone-induced photosensitivity
Rifampin / ↓ Serum levels of amiodarone due to ↑ breakdown by the liver
Ritonavir / ↑ Levels of amiodarone → ↑ risk of amiodarone toxicity
Theophylline / ↑ Serum theophylline levels → toxicity (effects may not be seen for 1 week and may last for a prolonged period after drug is discontinued)

HOW SUPPLIED

Injection: 50 mg/mL; *Tablet:* 200 mg, 400 mg

DOSAGE

Due to the drug's side effects, unusual pharmacokinetic properties, and difficult dosing schedule, administer amiodarone in a hospital only by physicians trained in treating life-threatening arrhythmias. Loading doses are required to ensure a reasonable onset of action.

- **IV INFUSION**

Life-threatening ventricular arrhythmias.

Loading dose, rapid: 150 mg over the first 10 minutes (15 mg/min). **Then, slow loading dose:** 360 mg over the next 6 hr (1 mg/min). **Maintenance dose:** 540 mg over the remaining 18 hr (0.5 mg/min). After the first 24 hr, continue maintenance infusion rate of 0.5 mg/min (720 mg/24 hr). This may be continued with monitoring for 2 to 3 weeks.

Once arrhythmias have been suppressed, the client may be switched to PO amiodarone. The following is intended only as a guideline for PO amiodarone dosage after IV infusion. **IV infusion less than 1 week:** Initial daily dose of PO amiodarone, 800–1,600 mg. **IV infusion from 1 to 3 weeks:** Initial daily dose of PO amiodarone, 600–800 mg. **IV infusion longer than**

A

3 weeks: Initial daily dose of PO amiodarone, 400 mg.

• **TABLETS**

Life-threatening ventricular arrhythmias.

Loading dose: 800–1,600 mg/day for 1–3 weeks (or until initial response occurs); **then,** reduce dose to 600–800 mg/day for 1 month. **Maintenance dose:** 400 mg/day (as low as 200 mg/day or as high as 600 mg/day may be needed in some clients). Give in divided doses with meals for total daily doses of 1,000 mg or higher or when GI intolerance occurs.

NURSING CONSIDERATIONS

SEE ALSO *NURSING CONSIDERATIONS* FOR *ANTIARRHYTHMIC AGENTS.*

ADMINISTRATION/STORAGE

1. Correct potassium or magnesium deficiencies before initiation of therapy since antiarrhythmics may be ineffective or arrhythmogenic in those with hypokalemia.
2. When initiating amiodarone therapy, gradually discontinue other antiarrhythmic drugs.
3. To minimize side effects, determine the lowest effective dose. If side effects occur, reduce the dose.
4. If dosage adjustments are required, monitor the client for an extended period of time due to the long and variable half-life of the drug and the difficulty in predicting the time needed to achieve a new steady-state plasma drug level.
5. Administer daily PO doses of 1,000 mg or more in divided doses with meals.
6. If additional antiarrhythmic therapy is required, the initial dose of such drugs should be about one-half the usual recommended dose.
7. IV For the first rapid loading dose, add 3 mL amiodarone IV (150 mg) to 100 mL D5W for a concentration of 1.5 mg/mL; infuse at a rate of 100 mL/10 min. For the slower loading dose, add 18 mL amiodarone IV (900 mg) to 500 mL of D5W for a concentration of 1.8 mg/mL.
8. IV concentrations of amiodarone greater than 3 mg/mL in D5W cause a high incidence of peripheral vein phlebitis; concentrations of 2.5 mg/mL or less are not as irritating. Thus, for infusions greater than 1 hr, the IV concentration should not exceed 2 mg/mL unless a central venous catheter is used.
9. Because amiodarone adsorbs to PVC, IV infusions exceeding 2 hr must be given in glass or polyolefin bottles containing D5W.
10. Cordarone I.V. has been found to leach out plasticizers, such as DEHP, which can adversely affect male reproductive tract development in fetuses, infants, and toddlers. Cordarone I.V. is not indicated to treat arrhythmias in pediatric clients.
11. Amiodarone IV in D5W is incompatible with aminophylline, cefamandole nafate, cefazolin sodium, mezlocillin sodium, heparin sodium, and sodium bicarbonate.
12. Store the injection at room temperature protected from light.

ASSESSMENT

1. Determine if client is taking any other antiarrhythmic medications.
2. Assess quality of respirations and breath sounds; note cardiac status and CV findings.
3. Note baseline VS and perfusion (skin temperature, color). Document ABGs and assess for circulatory impairment and hypotension.
4. Assess vision before therapy.
5. Monitor thyroid studies because drug inhibits conversion of T_4 to T_3.
6. Obtain baseline CBC, electrolytes, CXR, renal and LFTs.
7. Obtain ECG and document rhythm strips; note EPS findings. During administration, observe for increased PR and QRS intervals, increased arrhythmias, and HR < 60 bpm.
8. Anticipate reduced dosages of digoxin, warfarin, quinidine, procainamide, and phenytoin if administered concomitantly with amiodarone.

CLIENT/FAMILY TEACHING

1. Drug is used to control heart beat irregularities.

A

2. Report if crystals develop on the skin, producing a bluish color, so dosage can be adjusted.
3. Avoid direct exposure to sunlight. Wear protective clothing and a sunscreen when exposed.
4. Report all side effects, especially any abnormal swelling, bleeding, or bruising.
5. Complaints of painful breathing, wheezing, fever, coughing, or SOB are S&S of pulmonary problems and require prompt attention.
6. CNS symptoms such as tremor, lack of coordination, numbness, and dizziness require evaluation.
7. Complaints of headaches, depression, or insomnia as well as any change in behavior such as decreased interest in personal appearance or apparent hallucinations may require a change in therapy.
8. Schedule periodic eye exams because small yellow-brown granular corneal deposits may develop during prolonged therapy. Visual changes require prompt ophthalmic evaluation.
9. Therapy with this drug requires periodic lab studies and close medical evaluation.

OUTCOMES/EVALUATE

- Termination/control of arrhythmias
- Serum drug levels within therapeutic range (0.5–2.5 mcg/mL)

Amitriptyline hydrochloride

(ah-me-**TRIP**-tih-leen)

PREGNANCY CATEGORY: C
CLASSIFICATION(S):
Antidepressant, tricyclic
Rx: Elavil
✱Rx: Apo-Amitriptyline

SEE ALSO *ANTIDEPRESSANTS, TRICYCLIC.*

ACTION/KINETICS

Amitriptyline is metabolized to an active metabolite, nortriptyline. Has significant anticholinergic and sedative effects with moderate orthostatic hypotension. Very high ability to block serotonin uptake and moderate activity with respect to norepinephrine uptake. **Effective plasma levels of amitriptyline and nortriptyline:** Approximately 110–250 ng/mL. **Time to reach steady state:** 4–10 days. **t½:** 31–46 hr. Up to 1 month may be required for beneficial effects to be manifested.

USES

Relief of symptoms of depression, including depression accompanied by anxiety and insomnia. Chronic pain due to cancer or other pain syndromes. Prophylaxis of cluster and migraine headaches. *Investigational:* Pathologic laughing and crying secondary to forebrain disease, bulimia nervosa, antiulcer agent, enuresis. Adjunct analgesic for phantom limb pain, migraine, chronic tension headaches, diabetic neuropathy, tic douloureux, cancer pain, peripheral neuropathy with pain, postherpetic neuralgia, arthritic pain. Dermatologic disorders (chronic urticaria and angioedema, nocturnal pruritus in atopic eczema).

CONTRAINDICATIONS

Use in children less than 12 years of age.

ADDITIONAL DRUG INTERACTIONS

Guanethidine and similar drugs / Antihypertensive effect may be blocked
H *St. John's Wort* / ↓ Blood levels of amitriptyline and its metabolite

HOW SUPPLIED

Injection: 10 mg/mL; *Tablet:* 10 mg, 25 mg, 50 mg, 75 mg, 100 mg, 150 mg

DOSAGE

- **TABLETS**

Antidepressant.

Adults (outpatients): 75 mg/day in divided doses; may be increased to 150 mg/day. *Alternate dosage:* **Initial,** 50–100 mg at bedtime; **then,** increase by 25–50 mg, if necessary, up to 150 mg/day. **Hospitalized clients: initial,** 100 mg/day; may be increased to 200–300 mg/day. **Maintenance: usual,** 40–100 mg/day (may be given as a single dose at bedtime). **Adolescent and geriatric:** 10 mg t.i.d. and 20 mg at bedtime up to a maximum of 100 mg/day.

Chronic pain.
50–100 mg/day.
Enuresis.
Pediatric, over 6 years: 10 mg/day as a single dose at bedtime; dose may be increased up to a maximum of 25 mg. **Less than 6 years:** 10 mg/day as a single dose at bedtime.
Analgesic adjunct.
75–300 mg/day.
Dermatologic disorders.
10–50 mg/day.
- **IM ONLY**

Antidepressant.
Adults: 20–30 mg q.i.d.; switch to **PO** therapy as soon as possible.

NURSING CONSIDERATIONS

SEE ALSO *NURSING CONSIDERATIONS FOR ANTIDEPRESSANTS, TRICYCLIC.*

ADMINISTRATION/STORAGE

1. Initiate dosage increases late in the afternoon or at bedtime.
2. Sedative effects may be manifested prior to antidepressant effects.

CLIENT/FAMILY TEACHING

1. Take with food to minimize gastric upset.
2. Do not drive a car or operate hazardous machinery until drug effects realized; drug causes a high degree of sedation.
3. May take entire dose at bedtime if sedation is manifested during waking hours.
4. Rise slowly from a lying to a sitting position to reduce orthostatic drug effects.
5. Urine may appear blue-green in color; this is harmless.
6. Beneficial antidepressant effects may not be noted for 30 days.
7. Elderly clients may be at an increased risk for falls; start on low doses and observe closely.

OUTCOMES/EVALUATE

- ↓ Symptoms of depression
- Control of incontinence
- Enhanced pain control with chronic pain management
- Relief of insomnia

Amlodipine

(am-**LOH**-dih-peen)

PREGNANCY CATEGORY: C
CLASSIFICATION(S):
Calcium channel blocker
Rx: Norvasc

SEE ALSO *CALCIUM CHANNEL BLOCKING AGENTS.*

ACTION/KINETICS

Increases myocardial contractility; effect may be counteracted by reflex activity. CO is increased; pronounced decrease in peripheral vascular resistance. **Peak plasma levels:** 6–12 hr. **t½, elimination:** 30–50 hr. 90% metabolized in the liver to inactive metabolites; 10% excreted unchanged in the urine.

USES

Hypertension alone or in combination with other antihypertensives. Chronic stable or vasospastic (Prinzmetal's variant) angina alone or in combination with other antianginal drugs.

SPECIAL CONCERNS

Use with caution in clients with CHF and in those with impaired hepatic function or reduced hepatic blood flow. Safety and efficacy have not been determined in children.

SIDE EFFECTS

CNS: Headache, fatigue, lethargy, somnolence, dizziness, lightheadedness, sleep disturbances, depression, amnesia, psychosis, hallucinations, paresthesia, asthenia, insomnia, abnormal dreams, malaise, anxiety, tremor, hand tremor, hypoesthesia, vertigo, depersonalization, migraine, apathy, agitation, amnesia. **GI:** Nausea, abdominal discomfort, cramps, dyspepsia, diarrhea, constipation, vomiting, dry mouth, thirst, flatulence, dysphagia, loose stools. **CV:** Peripheral edema, palpitations, hypotension, syncope, bradycardia, unspecified arrhythmias, tachycardia, ventricular extrasystoles, peripheral ischemia, ***cardiac failure,*** pulse irregularity, increased risk of MI. **Dermatologic:** Dermatitis, rash, prurit-

A

us, urticaria, photosensitivity, petechiae, ecchymosis, purpura, bruising, hematoma, cold/clammy skin, skin discoloration, dry skin. **Musculoskeletal:** Muscle cramps, pain, or inflammation; joint stiffness or pain, arthritis, twitching, ataxia, hypertonia. **GU:** Polyuria, dysuria, urinary frequency, nocturia, sexual difficulties. **Respiratory:** Nasal or chest congestion, sinusitis, rhinitis, SOB, dyspnea, wheezing, cough, chest pain. **Ophthalmologic:** Diplopia, abnormal vision, conjunctivitis, eye pain, abnormal visual accommodation, xerophthalmia. **Miscellaneous:** Tinnitus, flushing, sweating, weight gain, epistaxis, anorexia, increased appetite, taste perversion, parosmia.

ADDITIONAL DRUG INTERACTIONS

Diltiazem ↑ plasma levels of amlodipine → further ↓ BP

HOW SUPPLIED

Tablet: 2.5 mg, 5 mg, 10 mg

DOSAGE

• **TABLETS**

Hypertension.

Adults, usual, individualized: 5 mg/day, up to a maximum of 10 mg/day. Titrate the dose over 7–14 days.

Chronic stable or vasospastic angina.

Adults: 5–10 mg, using the lower dose for elderly clients and those with hepatic insufficiency. Most clients require 10 mg.

NURSING CONSIDERATIONS

SEE ALSO *NURSING CONSIDERATIONS FOR CALCIUM CHANNEL BLOCKING AGENTS.*

ADMINISTRATION/STORAGE

1. Food does not affect the bioavailability of amlodipine.
2. Elderly clients, small/fragile clients, or those with hepatic insufficiency may be started on 2.5 mg/day. This dose may also be used when adding amlodipine to other antihypertensive therapy.

ASSESSMENT

1. Note any history of CAD or CHF.
2. Review list of drugs currently prescribed to prevent interactions.
3. Monitor VS, ECG, CBC, renal and LFTs. Reduce dose with cirrhosis.

CLIENT/FAMILY TEACHING

1. Take only as directed, once daily. May take with or without regard to meals.
2. Report any symptoms of chest pain, SOB, dizziness, swelling of extremities, irregular pulse, or altered vision immediately. Record BP.

OUTCOMES/EVALUATE

- Desired BP control
- ↓ Frequency/intensity of angina

Amoxapine

(ah-**MOX**-ah-peen)

PREGNANCY CATEGORY: C
CLASSIFICATION(S):
Antidepressant, tricyclic
Rx: Asendin

SEE ALSO *ANTIDEPRESSANTS, TRICYCLIC.*

ACTION/KINETICS

In addition to its effect on monoamines, this drug also blocks dopamine receptors. Significant anticholinergic effects, moderate sedation, and slight orthostatic hypotensive effect. Metabolized to the active metabolites 7-hydroxy- and 8-hydroxyamoxapine. **Peak blood levels:** 90 min. **Effective plasma levels:** 200–500 ng/mL. **Time to reach steady state:** 2–7 days. **$t^{1/2}$:** 8 hr; $t^{1/2}$ of major metabolite: 30 hr. Excreted in urine.

USES

Endogenous and psychotic, as well as neurotic or reactive depressions. Depression accompanied by anxiety or agitation.

CONTRAINDICATIONS

High dose levels in clients with a history of convulsive seizures. During acute recovery period after MI. Use in children less than 16 years of age.

SPECIAL CONCERNS

Safe use during lactation not established.

ADDITIONAL SIDE EFFECTS

Tardive dyskinesia. ***Overdosage may cause seizures (common), neuroleptic malignant syndrome,*** testicular swelling, impairment of sexual function, and breast enlargement in males and females. Also, renal failure may be seen 2–5 days after overdosage.

HOW SUPPLIED

Tablet: 25 mg, 50 mg, 100 mg, 150 mg

DOSAGE

• **TABLETS**

Antidepressant.

Adults, individualized, initial: 50 mg b.i.d.–t.i.d. Can be increased to 100 mg b.i.d.–t.i.d. during first week. Due to sedation, do not use doses greater than 300 mg/day unless this dose has been ineffective for at least 14 days. **Maintenance:** 300 mg as a single dose at bedtime. **Hospitalized clients:** Up to 150 mg q.i.d. **Geriatric, initial:** 25 mg b.i.d.–t.i.d. If necessary and tolerated, increase to 50 mg b.i.d.–t.i.d. after first week. **Maintenance:** Up to 300 mg/day at bedtime.

NURSING CONSIDERATIONS

SEE ALSO ***NURSING CONSIDERATIONS FOR ANTIDEPRESSANTS, TRICYCLIC.***

CLIENT/FAMILY TEACHING

1. Take with food to minimize gastric upset.
2. Take entire dose at bedtime if daytime sedation experienced.
3. Report early CNS manifestations of tardive dyskinesia, i.e., slow repetitive movements.
4. Report any side effects R/T overdosage, especially seizures, that require immediate medical care.

OUTCOMES/EVALUATE

- Improved coping mechanisms
- Control of depression; ↓ anxiety

Amoxicillin (Amoxycillin)

(ah-mox-ih-**SILL**-in)

CLASSIFICATION(S):

Antibiotic, penicillin

Rx: Amoxil, Amoxil Pediatric Drops, Trimox, Trimox Pediatric Drops, Wymox

✤Rx: Apo-Amoxi, Gen-Amoxicillin, Lin-Amox, Novamoxin, Nu-Amoxi, Scheinpharm Amoxicillin

SEE ALSO ***ANTI-INFECTIVES*** AND ***PENICILLINS.***

ACTION/KINETICS

Semisynthetic broad-spectrum penicillin closely related to ampicillin. Destroyed by penicillinase, acid stable, and better absorbed than ampicillin. From 50% to 80% of a PO dose is absorbed from the GI tract. **Peak serum levels: PO:** 4–11 mcg/mL after 1–2 hr. **t½:** 60 min. Mostly excreted unchanged in urine.

USES

1. Gram-positive streptococcal infections including *Streptococcus faecalis, S. pneumoniae,* and non-penicillinase-producing staphylococci.
2. Gram-negative infections due to *Hemophilus influenzae, Proteus mirabilis, Escherichia coli,* and *Neisseria gonorrhoeae.*
3. In combination with omeprazole or lansoprazole and clarithromycin to treat duodenal ulcers by eradicating *Helicobacter pylori.*

SPECIAL CONCERNS

Safe use during pregnancy has not been established.

HOW SUPPLIED

Capsule: 250 mg, 500 mg; *Chewable tablet:* 125 mg, 200 mg, 250 mg, 400 mg; *Powder for oral suspension:* 50 mg/mL, 125 mg/5 mL, 250 mg/5 mL; *Tablet:* 500 mg, 875 mg

DOSAGE

• **CAPSULES, ORAL SUSPENSION, CHEWABLE TABLETS, TABLETS**

Susceptible infections of ear, nose, throat, GU tract, skin and soft tissues.

Adults and children over 20 kg: 250–500 mg q 8 hr; alternatively, 500 mg or 875 mg q 12 hr. **Children under 20 kg:** 20–40 (or more) mg/kg/day in three equal doses. For children, give 200 mg q 12 as an alternative to 125 mg q 8 hr and give 400 mg q 12 hr in place of 250 mg q 8 hr. For children, do not exceed the maximum adult dose.

A

Infections of the lower respiratory tract.
Adults and children over 20 kg: 500 mg q 8 hr. **Children under 20 kg:** 40 mg/kg/day in divided doses q 8 hr.

Prophylaxis of bacterial endocarditis: dental, oral, or upper respiratory tract procedures in those at risk.
Adults: 2 g (50 mg/kg for children) PO 1 hr prior to procedure.

Prophylaxis of bacterial endocarditis: GU or GI procedures.
Adults, standard regimen: 2 g ampicillin plus 1.5 mg/kg gentamicin not to exceed 80 mg, either IM or IV, 30 min prior to procedure, followed by 1.5 g amoxicillin. **Children, standard regimen:** 50 mg/kg ampicillin plus 2 mg/kg gentamicin 30 min prior to procedure, followed by 25 mg/kg amoxcillin. **Adults, moderate risk:** 2 g PO 1 hr prior to procedure. **Children, moderate risk:** 50 mg/kg PO 1 hr pior to procedure. **Adults, alternate low-risk regimen:** 3 g 1 hr before procedure, followed by 1.5 g 6 hr after the initial dose.

Treat H. pylori *infections.*
Three regimens using amoxicillin may be used: (1) A ten day course of therapy consisting of amoxicillin, 1,000 mg b.i.d.; clarithromycin, 500 mg b.i.d.; and either omeprazole, 20 mg b.i.d. or lansoprazole, 30 mg b.i.d. A product, Prevpac, contains lansoprazole, clarithromycin, and amoxicillin. (2) A fourteen day course of therapy consisting of amoxicillin, 1,000 mg b.i.d., clarithromycin, 500 mg b.i.d., and omeprazole, 20 mg b.i.d.

Gonococcal infections, uncomplicated urethral, endocervical, or rectal infections.
Adults: 3 g as a single PO dose. **Children, over 2 years (prepubertal):** 50 mg/kg amoxicillin combined with 25 mg/kg probenecid as a single dose.

Chlamydia trachomatis *during pregnancy (as an alternative to erythromycin).*
0.5 g t.i.d. for 7 days.

NURSING CONSIDERATIONS

SEE ALSO *NURSING CONSIDERATIONS* FOR *PENICILLINS*.

ADMINISTRATION/STORAGE

1. The children's dose should not exceed the maximum adult dose.
2. Dry powder is stable at room temperature for 18–30 months. Reconstituted suspension is stable for 1 week at room temperature and for 2 weeks at 2–8°C (36–46°F).

CLIENT/FAMILY TEACHING

1. Take entire prescription; do not stop when feeling "better" as this creates antibiotic resistance.
2. With school-age child space medication evenly over the 24-hr period. Give suspension or tablet before school, upon arrival home, and at bedtime.
3. Chewable tablets are available for children; may be taken with food.
4. Pediatric drops are placed directly on the child's tongue for swallowing. Alternatively, the drops may be added to formula, milk, fruit juice, water, gingerale or cold drinks which must be taken immediately and consumed completely.
5. Report any unusual rash or lack of response.

OUTCOMES/EVALUATE

- Resolution of infection; symptomatic inprovement
- Therapeutic peak serum drug levels (4–11 mcg/mL)

—COMBINATION DRUG—

Amoxicillin and Potassium clavulanate

(ah-mox-ih-**SILL**-in, poh-**TASS**-ee-um klav-you-**LAN**-ayt)

PREGNANCY CATEGORY: B
CLASSIFICATION(S):
Antibiotic, penicillin
Rx: Augmentin, Augmentin ES-600
✱Rx: Clavulin

SEE ALSO *ANTI-INFECTIVES* AND *PENICILLINS*.

CONTENT

Tablets: '250' Tablet: 250 mg amoxicillin and 125 mg potassium clavulanate. '500' Tablet: 500 mg amoxicillin and 125 mg potassium clavulanate. '875' Tablet: 875 mg amoxicillin and 125 mg potassium clavulanate

Chewable Tablets: '125' Chewable Tablet: 125 mg amoxicillin and 31.25 mg potassium clavulanate. '200' Chewable Tablet: 200 mg amoxicillin and 28.5 mg potassium clavulanate. '250' Chewable Tablet: 250 mg amoxicillin and 62.5 mg potassium clavulanate. '400' Chewable Tablet: 400 mg amoxicillin and 57 mg potassium clavulanate.

Powder for Oral Suspension: '125' Powder for Oral Suspension: 125 mg amoxicillin and 31.25 mg potassium clavulanate/5 mL. '200' Powder for Oral Suspension: 200 mg amoxicillin and 28.5 mg potassium clavulanate/5 mL. '250' Powder for Oral Suspension: 250 mg amoxicillin and 62.5 mg potassium clavulanate/5 mL. '400' Powder for Oral Suspension : 400 mg amoxicillin and 57 mg potassium clavulanate/5 mL; Augmentin ES: 600 mg amoxicillin and 42.9 mg clavulanic acid/5 mL.

ACTION/KINETICS

For details, see Amoxicillin. Potassium clavulanate inactivates lactamase enzymes, which are responsible for resistance to penicillins. Effective against microorganisms that have manifested resistance to amoxicillin. For potassium clavulanate: **Peak serum levels:** 1–2 hr. **t½:** 1 hr.

USES

For beta-lactamase-producing strains of the following organisms: (1) Lower respiratory tract infections, otitis media, and sinusitis caused by *Hemophilus influenzae* and *Moraxella catarrhalis.* *(2)* Skin and skin structure infections caused by *Staphylococcus aureus, Escherichia coli,* and *Klebsiella.* (3) UTI caused by *E. coli, Klebsiella,* and *Enterobacter.* (4) Recurrent or persistent acute otitis media in children 3 months and older due to *Streptococcus pneumoniae, Haemophilus influenzae,* or *Moraxella catarrhalis.* *NOTE:* Mixed infections caused by organisms susceptible to ampicillin and organisms susceptible to amoxicillin/potassium clavulanate should not require an additional antibiotic.

HOW SUPPLIED

See Content.

DOSAGE

• ORAL SUSPENSION, CHEWABLE TABLETS, TABLETS

Susceptible infections.

Adults, usual: One 500-mg tablet q 12 hr or one 250-mg tablet q 8 hr. Adults unable to take tablets can be given the 125-mg/5 mL or the 250-mg/5 mL suspension in place of the 500-mg tablet or the 200-mg/5 mL or 400-mg/5 mL suspension can be given in place of the 875-mg tablet. **Children less than 3 months old:** 30 mg/kg/day amoxicillin in divided doses q 12 hr. Use of the 125-mg/5 mL suspension is recommended. **Children over 3 months old:** 25 mg/kg/day amoxicillin in divided doses q 12 hr or 20 mg/kg/day in divided doses q 8 hr.

Recurrent or persistent acute otitis media in children 3 months and older.

90 mg/kg/day in divided doses q 12 hr for 10 days.

Respiratory tract and severe infections.

Adults: One 875-mg tablet q 12 hr or one 500-mg tablet q 8 hr. **Children over 3 months old:** 45 mg/kg/day of amoxicillin in divided doses q 12 hr or 40 mg/kg/day amoxicillin in divided doses q 8 hr (these doses are used in children for otitis media, lower respiratory tract infections, or sinusitis). Treatment duration for otitis media is 10 days.

NURSING CONSIDERATIONS

SEE ALSO *NURSING CONSIDERATIONS* FOR *PENICILLINS*.

ADMINISTRATION/STORAGE

1. Both the "250" and "500" tablets contain 125 mg clavulanic acid; therefore, two "250" tablets are not the same as one "500" tablet. Also, the 250-mg tablet and the 250-mg chewable tablet do not contain the same amount of potassium clavulanate and are thus not interchangeable. The 250-mg tablet should not be used until children are over 40 kg.

2. Pediatric formulations are now available in fruit flavors for the oral suspension and chewable tablets. These formulations allow twice-daily dosing, which is more convenient than three-times daily dosing and, importantly, the incidence of diarrhea is significantly reduced.
3. The 200- and 400-mg suspensions and chewable tablets contain aspartame and should not be used by clients with (phenylketonuria.)

CLIENT/FAMILY TEACHING

1. Take exactly as directed and complete entire prescription.
2. May be taken without regard for meals; however, absorption is enhanced if taken just before a meal.
3. Report any rash, persistent diarrhea, lack of response or worsening of symptoms after 48–72 hr.
4. Refrigerate the reconstituted suspension and discard after 10 days.
5. Return as scheduled for follow-up evaluation.

OUTCOMES/EVALUATE

Resolution of infection; symptomatic improvement

Amphetamine sulfate

(am-**FET**-ah-meen)

PREGNANCY CATEGORY: C
CLASSIFICATION(S):
CNS stimulant
Rx: Adderall, Adderall XR
✱**Rx:** Dexedrine C-II

SEE ALSO *AMPHETAMINES AND DERIVATIVES.*

ACTION/KINETICS

Completely absorbed in 3 hr. **Peak effects:** 2–3 hr. **Duration:** 4–24 hr; **t½:** 10–30 hr, depending on urinary pH. Excreted in urine. Acidification increases excretion, whereas alkalinization decreases it. For every one unit increase in pH, the plasma half-life will increase by 7 hr.

USES

(ADHD) in children, narcolepsy: Adderall contains dextroamphetamine sulfate, dextroamphetamine saccharate, amphetamine sulfate, and amphetamine aspartate and is used in children aged three years and older who have ADHD or narcolepsy. Adderall provides similar relief as methylphenidate but with an extended duration of action, allowing for once or twice daily dosing.

CONTRAINDICATIONS

Use in children less than 3 years of age for attention deficit disorders and in children less than 6 years of age for narcolepsy. Use as an appetite suppressant.

HOW SUPPLIED

Tablet: 5 mg, 10 mg. *Adderall:* 5 mg, 7.5 mg, 10 mg, 12.5 mg, 15 mg, 20 mg, 30 mg. *Adderall XR Capsule:* 10 mg, 20 mg, 30 mg

DOSAGE

• **TABLETS**

Narcolepsy.

Adults: 5–20 mg 1–3 times/day. **Children over 12 years, initial:** 5 mg b.i.d.; increase in increments of 10 mg/day at weekly intervals until optimum dose is reached. **Children, 6–12 years, initial:** 2.5 mg b.i.d.; increase in increments of 5 mg at weekly intervals until optimum dose is reached (maximum is 60 mg/day).

Attention deficit disorders in children.

3–6 years, initial: 2.5 mg/day; increase by 2.5 mg/day at weekly intervals until optimum dose is achieved (usual range 0.1–0.5 mg/kg/dose each morning). **6 years and older, initial:** 5 mg 1–2 times/day; increase in increments of 5 mg/week until optimum dose is achieved (rarely over 40 mg/day). The dose of Adderall is 5–30 mg per day.

NURSING CONSIDERATIONS

SEE ALSO *NURSING CONSIDERATIONS* FOR *AMPHETAMINES AND DERIVATIVES.*

ASSESSMENT

1. Review CNS/neurologic status prior to initiating therapy.
2. Document symptom type and onset and pretreatment findings.
3. Determine if pregnant.
4. Monitor weight, CBC, chemistry profile, urinalysis, and ECG.

A

CLIENT/FAMILY TEACHING

1. When used for attention deficit disorders (ADD) or narcolepsy, give the first dose on awakening with an additional one or two doses given at intervals of 4–6 hr. Give the last dose 6 hr before bedtime.
2. Report any changes in mood or affect, including symptoms of impaired thinking.
3. Do not use caffeine or caffeine-containing products. Avoid any OTC preparations that contain caffeine, phenylpropanolamine, or other agents that affect CV system.
4. Avoid using heavy machinery or driving until drug effects realized.
5. Monitor weights and record.
6. Drink at least 2.5 L/day of fluids; increase intake of high-fiber foods/fruits to prevent constipation.
7. Chew sugarless gum/candies and rinse mouth frequently with nonalcoholic mouth rinses for dry mouth.
8. Children receiving amphetamines may have their growth retarded. Drug should periodically be discontinued by provider to allow growth to proceed normally and to evaluate the need for continued drug therapy.

OUTCOMES/EVALUATE

- Improved attention span
- ↓ Episodes of narcolepsy

Amphotericin B desoxycholate

(am-foe-**TER**-ih-sin)

PREGNANCY CATEGORY: B

CLASSIFICATION(S):

Antibiotic, antifungal

Rx: Amphocin, Fungizone Intravenous

SEE ALSO *ANTI-INFECTIVES*.

ACTION/KINETICS

Produced by *Streptomyces nodosus;* fungistatic or fungicidal depending on the level of drug in body fluids and susceptibility of the fungus. Binds to sterols in the cell membrane causing a change in membrane permeability leading to leakage of a variety of intracellular components. Can also bind to cholesterol in the mammalian cell leading to cytotoxicity. Highly protein bound (90%). **Peak plasma levels:** 0.5–2 mcg/mL. **t½, initial:** 24 hr; **second phase:** 15 days. Slowly excreted by the kidneys. Kinetics differ in adults and children.

USES

Drug is toxic; used mainly for clients with progressive and potentially fatal fungal infections. **Parenteral.** (1) Systemic, potentially fatal life-threatening invasive fungal infections, including aspergillosis; cryptococcosis; North American blastomycosis; systemic candidiasis; coccidiodomycosis; histoplasmosis; sporotrichosis; zygomycosis including mucormycosis caused by *Mucor, Rhizopus,* and *Absidia* species. (2) Infections due to susceptible species of *Conidiobolus* and *Basidiobolus.* (3) Secondary therapy to treat American mucocutaneous leishmaniasis. *Investigational:* Prophylaxis of fungal infection in bone marrow transplantation; treatment of primary amoebic meningoencephalitis due to *Naegleria fowleri*; subconjunctival or intravitreal injection in ocular aspergillosis; bladder irrigation for candidal cystitis; chemoprophylaxis for low dose IV, intranasal, or nebulized administration in immunocompromised clients at risk of aspergillosis; intrathecally in severe meningitis unresponsive to IV therapy; intra-articularly or IM for coccidioidal arthritis. **PO.** for treatment of oral candidiasis due to susceptible strains of *Candida albicans.* **Topical.** Cutaneous and mucocutaneous infections of *Candida (Monilia)*, especially in children, adults, and AIDS clients with thrush.

CONTRAINDICATIONS

Hypersensitivity to drug unless the condition is life-threatening and amenable only to amphotericin B therapy. Use to treat noninvasive forms of fungal disease such as oral thrush, vaginal candidiasis, and esophageal candidiasis in clients with normal neutrophil counts. Lactation.

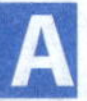

SPECIAL CONCERNS
The bone marrow depressant effects may result in increased incidence of microbial infection, delayed healing, and gingival bleeding. Although used in children, safety and efficacy have not been determined. Use with caution in clients receiving leukocyte transfusions.

SIDE EFFECTS
GI: Anorexia, N&V, diarrhea, dyspepsia, cramping, epigastric pain (common), acute liver failure, hepatitis, melena, jaundice, hemorrhagic gastroenteritis. **CNS:** Headache (most common), convulsions, tinnitus, vertigo (transient), peripheral neuropathy, encephalopathy, neurologic symptoms. **CV:** Hypotension (most common), ***cardiac arrest, cardiac failure, ventricular fibrillation,*** arrhythmias, hypertension. **Dermatologic:** Rash, especially maculopapular, pruritus. **Hematologic:** Normochromic anemia, normocytic anemia (most common), ***agranulocytosis,*** coagulation defects, thrombocytopenia, leukopenia, eosinophilia, leukocytosis. **GU:** Decreased renal function, azotemia, hyposthenuria, renal tubular acidosis, nephrocalcinosis. **Respiratory:** Tachypnea (most common), ***shock,*** pulmonary edema, hypersensitivity pneumonitis, dyspnea, bronchospasm, wheezing. **Ophthalmic:** Visual impairment, diplopia. **Miscellaneous:** Hearing loss, fever (with chills, shaking) occurring within 15 to 20 min after starting treatment, malaise, weight loss, pain at injection site (with or without phlebitis or thrombophlebitis), generalized pain (including muscle and joint pain), flushing, ***anaphylaxis*** and other allergic reactions.

LABORATORY TEST CONSIDERATIONS
↑ AST, ALT, GGT, LDH, alkaline phosphatase, serum creatinine, BUN, bilirubin. Hypomagnesemia, hyperkalemia, hypokalemia, hypercalcemia, hypercalemia, acidosis, hypoglycemia, hyperglycemia, hypermyalesmia, hyperuricemia, hypophosphatemia. Abnormal serum electrolytes, liver function, renal function.

OD OVERDOSE MANAGEMENT
Symptoms: Cardiopulmonary arrest. *Treatment:* Discontinue therapy, monitor clinical status, and provide supportive therapy.

DRUG INTERACTIONS
Aminoglycosides / Additive nephrotoxicity and/or ototoxicity
Antineoplastic drugs / ↑ Risk for renal toxicity, bronchospasm, and hypotension
Azole antifungals / ↑ Risk of fungal resistance to amphotericin B
Corticosteroids, Corticotropin / ↑ Risk of hypokalemia → cardiac dysfunction
Cyclosporine / ↑ Risk of renal toxicity
Digitalis glycosides / ↑ Risk of hypokalemia → ↑ incidence of digitalis toxicity
Flucytosine / ↑ Risk of flucytosine toxicity due to ↑ cellular uptake or ↓ renal excretion
Nephrotoxic drugs / ↑ Risk of nephrotoxicity
Skeletal muscle relaxants, surgical (e.g., succinylcholine, *d*-tubocurarine) / ↑ Muscle relaxation due to amphotericin B–induced hypokalemia
Tacrolimus / ↑ Serum creatinine levels
Thiazides / ↑ Electrolyte depletion, especially potassium
Zidovudine / ↑ Risk of myelotoxicity and nephrotoxicity

HOW SUPPLIED
Powder for Injection: 50 mg (as desoxycholate)

DOSAGE

- **IV.**

Test dose by slow IV infusion.

1 mg in 20 mL of 5% dextrose injection should be infused over 20 to 30 min to determine tolerance.

Severe and rapidly progressing fungal infection.

Initial: 0.25–0.3 mg/kg over 2 to 6 hr. *NOTE:* In impaired cardiorenal function or if a severe reaction to the test dose, initiate therapy with smaller daily doses (e.g., 5–10 mg). Depending on client status, the dose may be increased gradually by 5–10 mg/day to a final daily dose of 0.5–0.7 mg/kg, not exceed 1.5 mg/kg/day.

A

Aspergillosis.
1–1.5 mg/kg/day for a total dose of 3.6 g.
Blastomyces, Histoplasmosis.
0.5–0.6 mg/kg/day for 4 to 12 weeks.
Candidiasis, Coccidioidomycosis.
0.5–1 mg/kg/day for 4 to 12 weeks.
Cryptococcus.
0.5–0.7 mg/kg/day for 4 to 12 weeks.
Mucormycosis.
1–1.5 mg/kg/day for 4 to 12 weeks.
Rhinocerebral phycomyosis.
0.25–0.3 mg/kg/day, up to 1–1.5 mg/kg/day, for a total dose of 3 to 4 g.
Sporotrichosis.
0.5 mg/kg/day, up to 2.5 g total dose.
Leishmaniasis.
0.5 mg/kg/day given on alternate days for 14 doses (not recommended as primary therapy).
Prophylaxis of fungal infections in bone marrow transplants.
0.1 mg/kg/day.
Paracoccidioidomycosis.
0.4–0.5 mg/kg/day by slow IV infusion for 4 to 12 weeks.

• **BLADDER IRRIGATION**
Candidal cystitis.
Irrigate bladder with a 50 mcg/mL solution, instilled periodically or continuously for 5–10 days.

• **AMPHOTERICIN, INTRATHECAL**
Meningitis, coccidioidal or cryptococcal.
Initial: 0.25 mg intrathecally; gradually increase to the maximum tolerated dose (usually 0.25–1 mg q 2–5 days).

NURSING CONSIDERATIONS

SEE ALSO *GENERAL NURSING CONSIDERATIONS* FOR *ALL ANTI-INFECTIVES*.

ADMINISTRATION/STORAGE

IV 1. The following approaches may decrease severe side effects:

• Give aspirin, acetaminophen, antihistamines, and antiemetics before the infusion and maintain sodium balance.

• Give on alternate days to decrease anorexia and phlebitis.

• Small doses of IV corticosteroids before infusion may decrease febrile reactions.

• Adding a small amount of heparin (500–2000 units) to the infusion, removing the needle after infusion, rotating the infusion sites, giving through a large central vein, and using a pediatric scalp-vein may decrease the incidence of thrombophlebitis.

• Meperidine, 25–50 mg IV, may decrease the duration of shaking, chills, and fever that may occur.

2. *Preparation of amphotericin B desoxycholate:* To obtain an initial concentration of 5 mg/mL, rapidly inject 10 mL sterile water for injection (without a bacteriostatic agent) directly into the lyophilized cake, using a sterile 20-gauge needle. The vial should be shaken immediately until the colloidal solution is clear. To obtain the infusion solution of 0.1 mg/mL, further dilute 1:50 with 5% dextrose injection with a pH of 4.2 or above.

3. Determine the pH of each container of dextrose injection before use (pH is usually greater than 4.2). If the pH is less than 4.2, add 1 or 2 mL of buffer to the dextrose injection before it is infused to dilute the concentrated amphotericin B solution. The preferred buffer is dibasic sodium phosphate (anhydrous), 1.59 g; monobasic sodium phosphate (anhydrous), 0.96 g; and water for injection which is diluted to 100 mL. Sterilize the buffer before adding to the dextrose injection. Sterilize either by filtration through a bacterial retentive stone, mat, or membrane or by autoclaving for 30 min at 15 lb pressure and 121°C (249.8°F).

4. Strict aseptic technique must be used in preparation as there is no bacteriostatic agent in the medication.

5. **Do not** dilute or reconstitute with saline solution or mix with other drugs or electrolytes. If given through an existing IV line, flush with 5% dextrose for injection prior to and following infusion.

6. Do not use the initial concentrate if any precipitate is present.

7. Protect from light during administration. However, loss of drug activity during administration is likely negligible if the solution is exposed for 8 hr or less.

A

8. Initiate therapy in the most distal veins. When administered peripherally, changing sites with each dose may decrease phlebitis.
9. *Storage/stability of amphotericin B desoxycholate:* Vials should be refrigerated and protected from light. After reconstitution the concentrate may be stored in the dark at room temperature for 24 hr or under refrigeration for 1 week. Discard any unused solution. Use diluted solutions promptly after preparation. Protect from light during administration.

ASSESSMENT

1. Assess for any allergy to amphotericin B, adverse effects and hypersensitivity reactions.
2. Note mental status and age.
3. Describe characteristics of any severe systemic infections/lesions requiring therapy. Different organisms require different lengths of treatment i.e. sporotrichosis may require 9 mo of IV therapy, whereas topical lesions may require only 2-4 wks.
4. Review list of drugs prescribed to ensure none interact unfavorably.
5. Monitor CBC, liver and renal function, and cultures during therapy. Stop therapy and report any adverse effects. Monitor for bleeding, impaired kidney or liver function.

INTERVENTIONS

1. Ensure that correct prescribed form is prepared for administration; IV form in D5W only.
2. Determine that a 1-mg test dose has been administered (1 mg in 20 mL D5W over 20–30 min) and response.
3. Premedicate with antipyretics, antihistamines, corticosteroids, and/or antiemetic drugs to reduce side effects. See under administration/storage IV. Rashes, fevers, and chills may occur with this therapy.
4. Infuse slowly, monitoring VS every 15–30 min during first dose; interrupt infusion for adverse effects.
5. Monitor I&O; report change in output and cloudy urine.
6. Weigh twice weekly and assess for malnutrition or dehydration.
7. Anticipate hypokalemia with digoxin therapy. Observe for toxicity and muscle weakness and monitor K^+ and digoxin levels.
8. Intrathecal administration of amphotericin may cause inflammation of the spinal roots; report sensory loss or foot drop.

CLIENT/FAMILY TEACHING

1. GI effects may be reduced by an antihistamine or antiemetic before drug therapy and by administering the drug before mealtime. Try small frequent meals if diarrhea occurs.
2. Report any anorexia, N&V, headache, rashes, fever, or chills.
3. Report any decrease in I&O and extreme weight loss. Consume 2½ L/day of fluids to prevent nephrotoxic effects.
4. Amphotericin therapy usually requires long-term treatments (6–11 weeks) to ensure an adequate response and to prevent any relapse.
5. Neurologic symptoms such as tinnitus, blurred vision, or vertigo should be reported immediately.
6. Guidelines for therapy with creams and lotions:
• Does not stain skin when rubbed into lesion.
• Any discoloration of fabric caused by cream or lotion may be removed by washing with soap and water.
• Discoloration of clothing caused by ointment may be removed with a standard cleaning fluid.
• Report any worsening of condition, lack of response, itching, burning, or rash.
• Do not apply an occlusive dressing as this may promote yeast growth.

OUTCOMES/EVALUATE

• Resolution of fungal infection
• Reduction in number of skin lesions
• Symptomatic improvement

Amphotericin B Lipid-Based

(am-foe-**TER**-ih-sin)

PREGNANCY CATEGORY: B
CLASSIFICATION(S):
Antibiotic, antifungal
Rx: Abelcet, AmBisome, Amphotec

A

SEE ALSO *ANTI-INFECTIVES* AND *AMPHOTERICIN B DESOXYCHOLATE*

ACTION/KINETICS

See also *Amphotericin B desoxycholate*. Lipid-based products increase the circulation time and alter the biodistribution of amphotericin. Since lipid-based drugs stay in the circulation longer, they can localize and attain higher concentrations in areas with increased capillary permeability (e.g., inflammation, infection, solid tumors). Importantly, the three amphotericin lipid-based products have different physical and chemical properties that affect their use, pharmacokinetic properties, and side effects. Each of the products has a long terminal half-life and varies depending on the product (about 6.3–6.8 hr for AmBisome, 27.5–28.3 hr for Amphotec, and about 173.4 hr for Abelcet).

USES

Drug is toxic; use mainly for clients with progressive and potentially fatal fungal infections. Lipid products decrease the severe renal toxicity of amphotericin B and are indicated for use in those with renal impairment when amphotericin B can not or should not be used. (1) **Abelcet:** Systemic invasive fungal infections in those refractory to conventional amphotericin B desoxycholate therapy or when renal impairment or toxicity precludes use of the desoxycholate product. (2) **AmBisome:** Treatment of infections due to *Aspergillus, Candida,* or *Cryptococcus;* empirical treatment in febrile, neutropenic clients with presumed fungal infection; cryptococcal meningitis in HIV-infected clients; visceral leishmaniasis. (3) **Amphotec:**Treatment of invasive aspergillosis.

CONTRAINDICATIONS

See *Amphotericin B desoxycholate*.

SPECIAL CONCERNS

Use with caution in impaired renal function.

SIDE EFFECTS

• SIDE EFFECTS COMMON TO ALL PRODUCTS.

CV: Hypotension, hypertension, ***cardiac arrest,*** chest pain, tachycardia. **GI:** N&V, diarhea, abdominal pain, ***GI hemorrhage.*** **CNS:** Headache, anxiety, confusion, insomnia, leukoencephalopathy. **Respiratory:** ***Respiratory failure,*** dyspnea, respiratory disorder, hypoxia, increased cough, epistaxis, lung disorder, pleural effusion, rhinitis. **Hematologic:** Thrombocytopenia, anemia, leukopenia. **Dermatologic:** Rash, pruritus, sweating. **Infusion reactions:** Fever, shaking, chills, hypotension, anorexia, N&V, headache, tachypnea. **Miscellaneous:** Chills, fever, ***multiple organ failure, sepsis, anaphylactic reaction,*** infection, pain, kidney failure, asthenia, back pain, hematuria.

• SIDE EFFECTS REPORTED FOR ABELCET.

CV: ***Cardiac failure, MI, cardiomyopathy,*** arrhythmias, including ***ventricular fibrillation.*** **GI:** Melena, dyspepsia, cramping, epigastric pain. **CNS:** Convulsions, peripheral neuropathy, transient vertigo, encephalopathy, ***CVA,*** extrapyramidal syndrome and other neurologic symptoms. **Hematologic:** Coagulation defects, leukocytosis, eosinophilia. **GU:** Oliguria, decreased renal function, anuria, renal tubular acidosis, impotence, dysuria. **Respiratory:** Bronchospasm, wheezing, asthma, pulmonary edema, hemoptysis, ***pulmonary embolus,*** tachypnea, pleural effusion. **Hepatic:** Hepatitis, jaundice, ***acute liver failure,*** venoocclusive liver disease, hepatomegaly, cholangitis, cholecystitis. **Dermatologic:** Maculopapular rash, exfoliative dermatitis, erythema multiforme. **Musculoskeletal:** Myasthenia, bone pain, muscle pain, joint pain. **Ophthalmic:** Visual impairment, diplopia. **Otic:** Deafness, tinnitus, hearing loss. **Miscellaneous:** Malaise, weight loss, reaction at injection site (including inflammation, anaphylactoid and other allergic reactions), ***shock,*** thrombophlebitis, anorexia, acidosis.

• SIDE EFFECTS REPORTED FOR AMBISOME.

CV: Arrhythmia, atrial fibrillation, bradycardia, cardiomegaly, ***hemorrhage,*** postural hypotension, valvular heart disease, vascular disorder, flushing,

A

venoocclusive disease. **GI:** Anorexia, constipation, dry mouth/nose, dyspepsia, dysphagia, eructation, fecal incontinence, ***GI hemorrhage,*** hemorrhoids, gum/oral hemorrhage, hematemesis, hepatocellular damage, hepatomegaly, mucositis, rectal disorder, stomatitis, ulcerative stomatitis. **CNS:** Agitation, ***coma, convulsions,*** cough, depression, dysesthesia, dizziness, hallucinations, nervousness, paresthesia, somnolence, abnormal thinking, tremor. **Hematologic:** Coagulation disorder, ecchymosis, fluid overload, petechia, agranulocytosis. **GU:** Abnormal renal function, acute renal failure, dysuria, toxic nephropathy, urinary incontinence, vaginal hemorrhage, hemorrhagic cystitis. **Respiratory:** Asthma, atelectasis, hemoptysis, hiccough, hyperventilation, flu-like symptoms, lung edema, pharyngitis, pneumonia, sinusitis, cyanosis, hypoventilation, pulmonary edema. **Dermatologic:** Alopecia, dry skin, herpes simplex, inflammation at injection site, purpura, skin discoloration, skin disorder/ulcer, urticaria, vesiculobullous rash. **Musculoskeletal:** Arthralgia, bone pain, dystonia, myalgia, rigors. **Ophthalmic:** Conjunctivitis, dry eyes, eye hemorrhage. **Miscellaneous:** Enlarged abdomen, cellulitis, cell-mediated immunological reaction, face edema, graft-vs-host disease, malaise, neck pain, angioedema, erythema.

• **SIDE EFFECTS REPORTED FOR AMPHOTEC.**

CV: Postural hypotension, ***hemorrhage, shock,*** arrhythmia, atrial fibrillation, bradycardia, CHF, phlebitis, supraventricular tachycardia, syncope, vasodilation, venoocclusive liver disease, ventricular extrasystoles. **GI:** Dry mouth, hematemesis, jaundice, stomatitis, anorexia, bloody diarrhea, constipation, dyspepsia, fecal incontinence, GI disorder, gingivitis, glossitis, ***hepatic failure,*** melena, mouth ulceration, oral moniliasis, rectal disorder. **CNS:** Dizziness, somnolence, abnormal thinking, tremor, agitation, depression, ***convulsions,*** hallucinations, hypertonia, nervousness, neuropathy, paresthesia, psychosis, speech disorder, stupor. **Hematologic:** Coagulation disorder, ecchymosis, hypochromic anemia, leukocytosis, petechia. **GU:** Dysuria, oliguria, urinary incontinence/retention, urinary tract disorder. **Dermatologic:** Maculopapular rash, acne, alopecia, petechial rash, skin discoloration/disorder, skin nodule/ulcer, urticaria, vesiculobullous rash. **Respiratory:** Apnea, asthma, hyperventilation, hemoptysis, lung edema, pharyngitis, sinusitis. **Musculoskeletal:** Arthralgia, myalgia. **Ophthalmic:** Eye hemorrhage, amblyopia. **Otic:** Deafness, ear disorder, tinnitus. **Miscellaneous:** Peripheral edema, weight gain or loss, acidosis, dehydration, enlarged abdomen, facial edema, mucous membrane disorder, accidental injury, allergic reaction, ***death,*** hypothermia, immune system disorder, injection site inflammation/pain/reaction, neck pain.

LABORATORY TEST CONSIDERATIONS

Those common to all products. ↑ ALT, AST, creatine, BUN, alkaline phosphatase. Hyperbilirubinemia, hypokalemia, hypomagnesemia, hyperglycemia, hypernatremia, hypocalcemia, hypervolemia. Abnormal liver function tests. **Those for Abelcet.** Hyperkalemia, hypercalcemia, ↑ LDH, hyperamylasemia, hypoglycemia, hyperuricemia, hypophosphatemia. **Those for AmBisome.** ↑ Amylase, LDH, NPN. ↑ or ↓ Prothrombin. Hyperchloremia, hyperkalemia, hypermagnesemia, hyperphosphatemia, hyponatremia, hypophosphatemia, hypoproteinemia. **Those for Amphotec.** ↑ LDH, gamma glutamyl transpeptidase, fibrinogen. ↓ Prothrombin, thromboplastin. Hypophosphatemia, hyponatremia, hyperkalemia, hyperlipemia, hypoglycemia, hypoproteinemia, albuminuria, glycosuria.

OD OVERDOSE MANAGEMENT

See *Amphotericin B desoxycholate.*

DRUG INTERACTIONS

See *Amphotericin B desoxycholate.*

HOW SUPPLIED

Abelcet: *Suspenion for injection (as lipid complex):* 100 mg/20 mL. **AmBisome:** *Powder for injection (as liposomal):* 50 mg. **Amphotec:** *Powder for injection (as cholesteryl):* 50 mg, 100 mg

A

DOSAGE

• **Abelcet.**

Systemic fungal infections.

5 mg/kg/day prepared as a 1 mg/mL infusion and given at a rate of 2.5 mg/kg/hr. For children and those with CV disease, dilute the drug to a final concentration of 2 mg/mL. If the infusion exceeds 2 hr, mix the contents by shaking the infusion bag. Do not use an in-line filter.

• **AmBisome.**

Empircal fungal infections.

3 mg/kg/day using a controlled infusion device over about 2 hr. Can reduce infusion time to 60 min if well tolerated or increased if client is uncomfortable.

Infections due to Aspergillus, Candida, Cryptococcus.

3–5 mg/kg/day prepared as a 1–2 mg/mL infusion and given initially over 2 hr. Can reduce infusion time to 60 min if well tolerated or increased if client is uncomfortable. For infants and small children, infusion concentrations of 0.2–0.5 mg/mL may be better. A micron or more in-line filter may be used.

Cryptococcal meningitis in HIV.

6 mg/kg/day using a controlled infusion device over 2 hr. Can reduce infusion time to 60 min if well tolerated or increase if client is uncomfortable.

Leishmaniasis.

3 mg/kg/day on days 1 through 5, 14, and 21 to immunocompetent clients; repeat course may be given if parasite is not eradicated. Give 4 mg/kg/day on days 1 through 5, 10, 17, 24, 31, and 38 to immunosuppressed clients; if parasite is not eradicated, seek expert advice regarding further therapy.

• **AMPHOTEC.**

Systemic fungal infections.

Rec. Dosage: 3–4 mg/kg/day prepared as a 0.6 mg/mL (range: 0.16–0.83 mg/mL) infusion given at a rate of 1 mg/kg/hr. Give a test dose of 1.6–8.3 mg infused over 15–30 min. Do not filter or use and in-line filter.

NURSING CONSIDERATIONS

SEE ALSO *GENERAL NURSING CONSIDERATIONS* FOR *ALL ANTI-INFECTIVES.*

ADMINISTRATION/STORAGE

IV 1. The following approaches may decrease severe side effects:

• Give aspirin, acetaminophen, antihistamines, and antiemetics before the infusion and by maintain sodium balance.

• Give on alternate days to decrease anorexia and phlebitis.

• Small doses of IV corticosteroids before infusion may decrease febrile reactions.

• Adding a small amount of heparin (500–2000 units) to the infusion, removing the needle after infusion, rotating the infusion sites, giving through a large central vein, and using a pediatric scalp-vein may decrease the incidence of thrombophlebitis.

• Meperidine, 25–50 mg IV, may decrease the duration of shaking, chills, and fever that may occur.

2. *Preparation of amphotericin B lipid complex (Abelcet):* Shake vial gently until there is no yellow sediment at the bottom. Withdraw the appropriate dose from the required number of vials into one or more sterile 20-mL syringes using an 18-gauge needle. Remove the needle from each syringe filled with liposomal amphotericin B and replace with a 5-micron filter needle. Each filter needle is used for just one vial. Insert the filter needle on the syringe into an IV bag containing 5% dextrose injection and empty the syringe contents into the bag. The infusion concentration should be 1 mg/mL. For pediatric clients and those with CV disease, the drug may be diluted with 5% dextrose injection to a final infusion concentration of 2 mg/mL.

3. *Preparation of liposomal amphotericin B (AmBisome):* Add 12 mL of sterile water for injection to each vial to yield 4 mg/mL. Immediately shake the vial vigorously for 30 sec to completely disperse drug until a yellow, transluscent suspension is formed. After calculating the dose, withdraw the appropriate amount of reconstituted suspension into a sterile syringe. Attach the 5 micron filter provided and inject syringe contents through the fil-

ter needle into an appropriate volume of 5% dextrose for a final concentration of 1 to 2 mg/mL.
4. *Preparation of amphotericin B cholesteryl (Amphotec):* Reconstitute only with sterile water for injection. Using a sterile syringe and a 20-gauge needle, rapidly add the following volumes to the vial to provide a liquid containing 5 mg/mL. Shake gently by hand, rotating the vial until all solids have dissolved (fluid may be opalescent or clear). For 50 mg/vial add 10 mL sterile water; 100 mg/vial add 20 mL sterile water. For infusion, further dilute to a final concentration of about 0.6 mg/mL (range 0.16–0.83 mg/mL).
5. Strict aseptic technique must be used in preparation as there is no bacteriostatic agent in the medication.
6. Do not dilute or reconstitute with saline solution or mix with other drugs or electrolytes. If given through an existing IV line, flush with 5% dextrose for injection prior to and following infusion.
7. Do not use the initial concentrate if any precipitate is present.
8. Protect from light during administration. However, loss of drug activity during administration is likely negligible if the solution is exposed for 8 hr or less.
9. Initiate therapy in the most distal veins. When administered peripherally, changing sites with each dose may decrease phlebitis.
10. *Storage/stability of amphotericin B lipid complex (Abelcet):* Prior to admixture store at 2–8°C (36–46°F). Protect from exposure to light and do not freeze. Keep in the carton until used. Admixture may be stored for up to 48 hr at 2–8°C (36–46°F) and an additional 6 hr at room temperature.
11. *Storage/stability of liposomal amphotericin B (AmBisome):* Store unopened vials at 2–8°C (36–46°F), without freezing. Keep product in the carton until used. Store reconstituted product concentrate at 2–8°C (36–46°F) for up to 24 hr. Do not freeze. Use within 6 hr of dilution with 5% dextrose. Discard any unused drug.
12. *Storage/stability of amphotericin B cholesteryl (Amphotec):* Store unopened vials at 15–30°C (59–86°F). After reconstitution, refrigerate at 2–8°C (36–46°F) and use within 24 hr; do not freeze. After further dilution with 5% dextrose, store in refrigerator at 2–8°C (36–46°F); use within 24 hr.

ASSESSMENT

1. Assess for any allergy to amphotericin B, adverse effects and hypersensitivity reactions.
2. Note mental status and age.
3. Describe characteristics of any severe systemic infections requiring therapy. Different organisms require different lengths of treatment time.
4. Review list of drugs prescribed to ensure none interact unfavorably.
5. Monitor CBC, liver and renal function, and cultures during therapy. Stop therapy and report any adverse effects. Monitor for bleeding, progressive liver and kidney dysfunction. This form is generally used with kidney impairment.

INTERVENTIONS

1. Ensure that correct prescribed form is prepared for administration.
2. Premedicate with antipyretics, antihistamines, corticosteroids, and/or antiemetic drugs to reduce side effects. See under administration/storage IV. Rashes, fevers, and chills may occur with this therapy.
3. Infuse slowly until client response identified. May increase infusion time if well tolerated or decrease if not tolerated according to manufacturers guidelines and orders.
4. Monitor VS every 15–30 min during first dose; interrupt infusion for adverse effects.
5. Monitor I&O; report change in output and cloudy urine. Weigh twice weekly and assess for malnutrition or dehydration.
6. Assess for hypokalemia with digoxin therapy; and hyponatremia with this therapy. Observe for toxicity and muscle weakness and monitor K^+, Na, and digoxin levels.
7. Identify and protect those that are severely immunocompromised.

CLIENT/FAMILY TEACHING

1. GI effects may be reduced by an antihistamine or antiemetic before drug therapy and by administering

the drug before mealtime. Try small frequent meals if diarrhea occurs.
2. Report any anorexia, N&V, headache, rashes, fever, or chills.
3. Report any changes in I&O and extreme weight loss. Consume fluids as directed to prevent further nephrotoxic effects.
4. Amphotericin therapy usually requires long-term treatments to ensure an adequate response (eradication of organism) and to prevent any relapse.
5. Neurologic symptoms such as tinnitus, blurred vision, or vertigo should be reported immediately.
6. Fever reaction may diminish with prolonged therapy, muscle pain/aches may be r/t low potassium.
7. Report any bleeding, bruising, or soft tissue swelling as well as vertigo or hearing loss.

OUTCOMES/EVALUATE

- Resolution of fungal infection
- Eradication of parasites
- Symptomatic improvement

Ampicillin oral

(am-pih-**SILL**-in)

PREGNANCY CATEGORY: B
Rx: Marcillin, Omnipen, Principen, Totacillin
★Rx: Novo-Ampicillin

Ampicillin sodium, parenteral

(am-pih-**SILL**-in)

PREGNANCY CATEGORY: B
Rx: Omnipen-N
CLASSIFICATION(S):
Antibiotic, penicillin

SEE ALSO *ANTI-INFECTIVES* AND *PENICILLINS*.

ACTION/KINETICS
Synthetic, broad-spectrum antibiotic suitable for gram-negative bacteria. Acid resistant, destroyed by penicillinase. Absorbed more slowly than other penicillins. From 30% to 60% of PO dose absorbed from GI tract. **Peak serum levels: PO:** 1.8–2.9 mcg/mL after 2 hr; **IM,** 4.5–7 mcg/mL. **t½:** 80 min—range 50–110 min. Partially inactivated in liver; 25%–85% excreted unchanged in urine.

USES
Infections of respiratory, GI, and GU tracts caused by *Shigella, Salmonella, Escherichia coli, Hemophilus influenzae, Proteus mirabilis, Neisseria gonorrhoeae, N. meningitidis,* and *Enterococcus.* Also, otitis media in children, bronchitis, rat-bite fever, and whooping cough. Penicillin G-sensitive staphylococci, streptococci, pneumococci.

ADDITIONAL DRUG INTERACTIONS
Allopurinol / ↑ Skin rashes
Oral contraceptives/ ↓ Effect of ampicillin

HOW SUPPLIED
Ampicillin oral: *Capsule (either anhydrous or trihydrate):* 250 mg, 500 mg; *Powder for Oral Suspension (trihydrate):* 125 mg/5 mL, 250 mg/5 mL. **Ampicillin sodium, parenteral:** *Powder for injection:* 125 mg, 250 mg, 500 mg, 1 g, 2 g, 10 g

DOSAGE

• **AMPICILLIN ORAL: CAPSULES, ORAL SUSPENSION; AMPICILLIN SODIUM: IV, IM**

Respiratory tract and soft tissue infections.

PO, 20 kg or more: 250 mg q 6 hr; **less than 20 kg:** 50 mg/kg/day in equally divided doses q 6–8 hr. **IV, IM, 40 kg or more:** 250–500 mg q 6 hr; **less than 40 kg:** 25–50 mg/kg/day in equally divided doses q 6–8 hr.

Bacterial meningitis.

Adults and children: 150–200 mg/kg/day in divided doses q 3 to 4 hr. Initially give IV drip, followed by IM q 3 to 4 hr.

Bacterial endocarditis prophylaxis (dental, oral, or upper respiratory tract procedures).

Clients at moderate risk or those unable to take PO medications: **Adults, IM, IV:** 2 g 30 min prior to procedure; **children:** 50 mg/kg, 30 min prior to

A

procedure. Clients at high risk: **Adults, IM, IV:** 2 g ampicillin plus gentamicin, 1.5 mg/kg, given 30 min before procedure followed in 6 hr by ampicillin, 1 g IM or IV, or amoxicillin, 1 g PO. **Children, IM, IV:** Ampicillin, 50 mg/kg, plus gentamicin, 1.5 mg/kg, 30 min prior to procedure followed in 6 hr by ampicillin, 25 mg/kg IM or IV, or amoxicillin, 25 mg/kg PO.

Septicemia.

Adults/children: 150–200 mg/kg/day, IV for first 3 days, then IM q 3–4 hr.

GI and GU infections, other than N. gonorrhea.

Adults/children, more than 20 kg: 500 mg PO q 6 hr. Use larger doses, if needed, for severe or chronic infections. **Children, less than 20 kg:** 100 mg/kg/day q 6 hr.

N. gonorrhea *infections.*

PO: Single dose of 3.5 g given together with probenecid, 1 g. **Parenteral, Adults/children over 40 kg:** 500 mg IV or IM q 6 hr. **Children, less than 40 kg:** 50 mg/kg/day IV or IM in equally divided doses q 6 to 8 hr.

Urethritis in males caused by N. gonorrhea.

Parenteral, males over 40 kg: Two 500 mg doses IV or IM at an interval of 8 to 12 hr. Repeat treatment if necessary. In complicated gonorrheal urethritis, prolonged and intensive therapy is recommended.

NURSING CONSIDERATIONS

SEE ALSO *NURSING CONSIDERATIONS* FOR *PENICILLINS*.

ADMINISTRATION/STORAGE

1. Reconstituted PO solution is stable for 7 days at room temperature, not exceeding 25°C (77°F) or 14 days refrigerated.
2. For IM use, dilute only with sterile or bacteriostatic water for injection.
3. If the C_{CR} is less than 10 mL/min, the dosing interval should be increased to 12 hr.
4. IV After reconstitution for IM or direct IV administration, the solution **must be used within the hour**.
5. For IVPB, ampicillin may be reconstituted with NaCl injection.
6. Once reconstituted, give IV slowly over at least 10–15 min.
7. For administration by IV drip, check compatibility and length of time that drug retains potency in a particular solution. Use within one hr.

ASSESSMENT

1. Document type, onset, and characteristics of symptoms.
2. Note history of sensitivity/reactions to this drug or related drugs.
3. Monitor CBC, cultures, liver and renal function studies.
4. Advise that IM route may be painful; rotate and document sites.
5. Monitor urinary output and serum K^+ levels, especially elderly.

CLIENT/FAMILY TEACHING

1. Take 1 hr before or 2 hr after meals.
2. Review the appropriate method for administration and storage.
3. Take for the prescribed number of days even if the symptoms subside.
4. Ampicillin chewable tablets should not be swallowed whole.
5. Do not save for future use or share with family members/friends who have similar symptoms.
6. May decrease effectiveness of oral contraceptives; use additional contraception during therapy.
7. Report any "ampicillin rashes": a dull, red, itchy, flat or raised rash occurs more often with this drug than with other penicillins and is usually benign. If a late skin rash develops with symptoms of fever, fatigue, sore throat, generalized lymphadenopathy, and enlarged spleen, a heterophil antibody test may be ordered to rule out mononucleosis.

OUTCOMES/EVALUATE

- Resolution of S&S of infection; symptomatic improvement
- Negative culture reports

—COMBINATION DRUG—

Ampicillin sodium/Sulbactam sodium

(am-pih-**SILL**-in/sull-**BACK**-tam)

PREGNANCY CATEGORY: B
CLASSIFICATION(S):
Antibiotic, penicillin
Rx: Unasyn

SEE ALSO *ANTI-INFECTIVES* AND *PENICILLINS.*

CONTENT

Powder for Injection: 1 g ampicillin sodium/0.5 g sulbactam sodium, 2 g ampicillin sodium/1 g sulbactam sodium, or 10 g ampicillin/5 g sulbactam sodium.

ACTION/KINETICS

For details, see *Ampicillin oral.* Sulbactam is present in this product because it irreversibly inhibits beta-lactamases, thus ensuring activity of ampicillin against beta-lactamase-producing microorganisms. Thus, sulbactam broadens the antibiotic spectrum of ampicillin to those bacteria normally resistant to it. **Peak serum levels, after IV infusion:** 15 min. **t$^1/_2$, both drugs:** about 1 hr. From 75%–85% of both drugs is excreted unchanged in the urine within 8 hr after administration.

USES

Infections caused by beta-lactamase-producing strains of the following: (1) Skin and skin structure infections caused by *Staphylococcus aureus, Escherichia coli, Klebsiella* species (including *K. pneumoniae*), *Proteus mirabilis, Bacteroides fragilis, Enterobacter* species, and *Acinetobacter calcoaceticus;* (2) Intra-abdominal infections caused by *E. coli, Klebsiella* species (including *K. pneumoniae*), *Bacteroides* (including *B. fragilis* and *Enterobacter)* (3) Gynecologic infections caused by *E. coli* and *Bacteroides* (including *B. fragilis). NOTE:* Mixed infections caused by ampicillin-susceptible organisms and beta-lactamase-producing organisms are susceptible to this product; thus, additional antibiotics do not have to be used.

SPECIAL CONCERNS

Safety and efficacy in children 1 year of age and older have not been established for intra-abdominal infections or for IM administration.

SIDE EFFECTS

• **AT SITE OF INJECTION**
Pain and thrombophlebitis.
GI: Diarrhea, N&V, flatulence, abdominal distention, glossitis. **CNS:** Fatigue, malaise, headache. **GU:** Dysuria, urinary retention. **Miscellaneous:** Itching, chest pain, edema, facial swelling, erythema, chills, tightness in throat, epistaxis, substernal pain, mucosal bleeding, candidiasis.

LABORATORY TEST CONSIDERATIONS

↑ AST, ALT, alkaline phosphatase, LDH, creatinine, BUN; also, ↑ basophils, eosinophils, lymphocytes, monocytes, platelets. ↓ Serum albumin and total proteins, H&H, RBCs, WBCs, and platelets. Presence of RBCs and hyaline casts in urine.

OD OVERDOSE MANAGEMENT

Symptoms: ***Neurologic symptoms, including convulsions.*** *Treatment:* Both ampicillin and sulbactam may be removed by hemodialysis.

HOW SUPPLIED

See Content

DOSAGE

• **IV, IM**

Adults: 1 g ampicillin/0.5 g sulbactam to 2 g ampicillin/1 g sulbactam q 6 hr, not to exceed 4 g sulbactam daily. Doses must be decreased in renal impairment. **Children, over 40 kg:** Use adult doses; total sulbactam dose should not exceed 4 g/day. **Children, one year and older but less than 40 kg:** 200 mg ampicillin/kg/day and 100 mg sulbactam/kg/day in divided doses q 6 hr.

NURSING CONSIDERATIONS

SEE ALSO *NURSING CONSIDERATIONS* FOR *PENICILLINS* AND *AMPICILLIN.*

ADMINISTRATION/STORAGE

1. For IM use, may reconstitute with sterile water for injection or 0.5% or 2% lidocaine HCl injection.
2. Must use solutions for IM administration **within 1 hr** of preparation.
IV 3. After reconstitution, solutions should stand so that any foaming will dissipate; inspect the vial to ensure dissolution.

A

4. For IV use, mix reconstituted drug with any of the following: 5% dextrose injection, D5/0.45% NaCL, 10% invert sugar, RL injection, 0.9% NaCl, M/6 sodium lactate injection, or sterile water for injection.
5. May give by slow injection over 10–15 min or, if mixed with 50–100 mL of diluent, over 15–30 min.
6. If aminoglycosides are prescribed concomitantly, administer each separately (1 hr apart) because ampicillin will inactivate aminoglycosides.

CLIENT/FAMILY TEACHING

1. With impaired renal function, dose will be reduced.
2. IM injections are extremely painful; expect some discomfort.
3. Report any evidence of skin rash; if accompanied by fatigue, sore throat and enlarged spleen and lymph nodes, may be mononucleosis.

OUTCOMES/EVALUATE

- Resolution of infection
- Symptomatic improvement

Amprenavir

(am-**PREH**-nah-vir)

PREGNANCY CATEGORY: C
CLASSIFICATION(S):
Antiviral, protease inhibitor
Rx: Agenerase

ACTION/KINETICS
Inhibitor of HIV-1 protease. Binds to the active site of HIV-1 protease, thus preventing the processing of viral gag and gag-pol polyprotein precursors. Results in formation of immature noninfectious viral particles. Rapidly absorbed after PO. High fat meals decrease absorption. **Peak levels:** 1–2 hr after a single dose. The PO solution is 14% less bioavailable than the capsules necessitating a difference in dosing (see Dosage). Metabolized in the liver and excreted in both the urine and feces. **t½:** 7.1–10.6 hr.

USES
In combination with other antiretroviral drugs for the treatment of HIV-1 infections.

CONTRAINDICATIONS
Use with bepridil, dihydroergotamine, ergotamine, midazolam, rifampin, and triazolam. Lactation. Due to large amounts of propylene glycol ingestion and possible toxicity, do not use the solution in infants, children less than 4 years of age, pregnancy, in liver or kidney failure, and in those treated with disulfiram or metronidazole.

SPECIAL CONCERNS
Use with caution in those with impaired hepatic function and in the elderly. Safety and efficacy have not been determined in children less than 4 years of age. Use with caution in combination with sildenafil. Amprenavir is a sulfonamide; thus, there is potential for cross-sensitivity between drugs in the sulfonamide class. Possibility of resistance/cross-resistance among protease inhibitors.

SIDE EFFECTS
GI: N&V, diarrhea, abdominal pain, taste disorders. **CNS:** Depression, mood disorders. **Dermatologic:** Maculopapular rash, pruritus, oral/perioral paresthesia, peripheral paresthesia, ***Stevens-Johnson syndrome.*** **Metabolic:** New onset diabetes mellitus, exacerbation of preexisting diabetes mellitus, hyperglycemia, diabetic ketoacidosis. **Miscellaneous:** Spontaneous bleeding in clients with hemophilia A and B. Redistribution/accumulation of body fat, including central obesity, dorsocervical fat enlargement, peripheral wasting, breast enlargement, "cushinoid" appearance.

LABORATORY TEST CONSIDERATIONS
Hypercholesterolemia, hyperglycemia, hypertriglyceridemia.

DRUG INTERACTIONS
Amiodarone / Serious or life-threatening interactions; monitor levels
Antacids / ↓ Amprenavir absorption
Bepridil / Possible serious or life-threatening effects; do not use together
Carbamazepine / ↓ Amprenavir levels R/T ↑ liver metabolism; also, possible ↑ carbamazepine plasma levels
Cimetidine / ↑ Plasma amprenavir levels
Cisapride / Possible serious or life-threatening effects; do not use together

A

Clarithromycin / Possible ↑ plasma amprenavir levels and ↓ plasma clarithromycin levels
Clozapine / ↑ Plasma clozapine levels
Dapsone / ↑ Plasma dapsone levels
Delavirdine / ↑ Amprenavir serum levels
Efavirenz / ↓ Amprenavir serum levels
Ergot alkaloids / Possible serious or life-threatening effects; do not use together
Erythromycin / Possible ↑ plasma amprenavir levels and ↓ plasma erythromycin levels
HMG-CoA reductase inhibitors / ↑ Serum levels of HMG-CoA reductase inhibitors → ↑ activity or toxicity
Indinavir / ↑ Plasma amprenavir levels and ↓ plasma indinavir levels
Itraconazole / Possible ↑ plasma levels of both drugs
Ketoconazole / Possible ↑ plasma levels of both drugs
Lidocaine / Serious or life-threatening interactions; monitor levels
Loratidine / ↑ Plasma loratidine levels
Midazolam / Possible serious or life-threatening effects; do not use together
Nelfinavir / Possible ↓ plasma amprenavir levels and ↑ plasma nelfinavir levels
Nevirapine / ↓ Amprenavir serum levels
Oral contraceptives / ↓ Effectiveness of oral contraceptives; use alternate contraceptive measures
Phenobarbital / ↓ Amprenavir levels R/T ↑ liver metabolism
Phenytoin / ↓ Amprenavir levels R/T ↑ liver metabolism
Pimozide / ↑ Plasma pimozide levels
Quinidine / Serious or life-threatening interactions; monitor levels
Rifabutin / ↓ Amprenavir levels and significant ↑ rifabutin levels; reduce dose of rifabutin to at least one-half
Rifampin / ↓ (by 90%) Amprenavir plasma levels R/T ↑ liver metabolism
Ritonavir / ↑ Amprenavir plasma levels
Saquinavir / Possible ↑ saquinavir plasma levels and ↓ amprenavir plasma levels
Sildenafil / ↑ Risk of sildenafil side effects, including hypotension, visual changes, and priapism
Triazolam / Possible serious or life-threatening effects; do not use together
Tricyclic antidepressants / Serious or life-threatening interactions; monitor levels
Warfarin / Possible ↑ Plasma warfarin levels; monitor INR if used together
Zidovudine / ↑ Amprenavir and zidovudine plasma levels

HOW SUPPLIED

Capsules: 50 mg, 150 mg; *Oral Solution:* 15 mg/mL

DOSAGE

• **CAPSULES**

HIV-1 infection.

Adults and adolescents, aged 13–16 years old: 1200 mg (eight 150 mg capsules) b.i.d. in combination with other antiretroviral drugs. **Children, 4–12 years old or aged 13–16 years old with weight less than 50 kg:** 20 mg/kg b.i.d. or 15 mg/kg t.i.d., up to a maximum of 2400 mg daily in combination with other antiretroviral drugs.

Give capsules at a dose of 450 mg b.i.d. to clients with a Child-Pugh score from 5–8; give capsules at a dose of 300 mg b.i.d. to those with a Child-Pugh score from 9–12.

• **ORAL SOLUTION**

HIV-1 infection.

Children, 4–12 years old or aged 13–16 years old with weight less than 50 kg: 22.5 mg/kg (1.5 mL/kg) b.i.d. or 17 mg/kg (1.1 mL/kg) t.i.d., up to a maximum of 2800 mg daily in combination with other antiretroviral drugs.

NOTE: Capsules and Oral Solution are **not** interchangeable on a mg per mg basis.

NURSING CONSIDERATIONS

ADMINISTRATION/STORAGE

Store at 25° C (77° F).

ASSESSMENT

1. Document disease onset and previous agents used.
2. Note any evidence of sulfa allergy; potential cross-sensitivity.
3. Identify all drugs prescribed/consumed to ensure none interact.

4. Monitor CBC, chemistry, lipids, renal and LFTs; adjust dose with liver dysfunction.

CLIENT/FAMILY TEACHING

1. Take amprenavir at least 1 hr before or after antacids or didanosine.
2. May be taken with or without food; avoid high fat meals.
3. Take every day as prescribed in combination with other antiretroviral drugs.
4. Do not exchange capsule dose for solution dose as solution is less bioavailable.
5. Do not take supplemental Vitamin E; the Vitamin E content of amprenavir capsules and oral solution exceeds the Reference Daily Intake.
6. If using hormonal contraceptives, use alternate contraceptive measures.
7. Do not alter the dose or discontinue therapy without consulting provider. If a dose is missed, take as soon as possible and return to the normal schedule. If a dose is skipped, do not double the next dose.
8. If taking sildenafil and amprenavir, may be at an increased risk of experiencing hypotension, visual changes, and priapism.
9. May cause a redistribution of body fat with enlargement centrally and at the back of the neck; may also cause or aggravate DM. Report any unusual adverse effects.

OUTCOMES/EVALUATE

Treatment of HIV infections; ↓ viral load; ↑ CD_4 counts

Anagrelide hydrochloride

(an-**AG**-greh-lyd)

PREGNANCY CATEGORY: C
CLASSIFICATION(S):
Antiplatelet drug
Rx: Agrylin

ACTION/KINETICS

May act to reduce platelets by decreasing megakaryocyte hypermaturation. Does not cause significant changes in white cell counts or coagulation parameters. Inhibits platelet aggregation at higher doses than needed to reduce platelet count. **Peak plasma levels:** 5 ng/mL at 1 hr. **t½:** 1.3 hr; **terminal t½:** About 3 days. Metabolized in liver and excreted in urine and feces.

USES

Reduce platelet count in essential thrombocythemia. Treatment of polycythemia vera, chronic myelogenous leukemia, and other myeloproliferative diseases.

CONTRAINDICATIONS

Lactation.

SPECIAL CONCERNS

Use with caution in known or suspected heart disease and in impaired renal or hepatic function. Safety and efficacy have not been determined in those less than 16 years of age.

SIDE EFFECTS

CV: CHF, palpitations, chest pain, tachycardia, arrhythmias, angina, postural hypotension, hypertension, CVD, vasodilation, migraine, syncope, ***MI, cardiomyopathy, CHB, fibrillation, CVA, pericarditis, hemorrhage, heart failure,*** cardiomegaly, AF **GI:** Diarrhea, abdominal pain, pancreatitis, gastric/duodenal ulcers, N&V, flatulence, anorexia, constipation, GI distress, ***GI hemorrhage,*** gastritis, melena, aphthous stomatitis, eructations. **Respiratory:** Rhinitis, epistaxis, respiratory disease, sinusitis, pneumonia, bronchitis, asthma, pulmonary infiltrate, ***pulmonary fibrosis, pulmonary hypertension,*** dyspnea. **CNS:** Headache, ***seizures,*** dizziness, paresthesia, depression, somnolence, confusion, insomnia, nervousness, amnesia. **Musculoskeletal:** Arthralgia, myalgia, leg cramps. **Dermatologic:** Pruritus, skin disease, alopecia, rash, urticaria. **Hematologic:** Anemia, thrombocytopenia, ecchymosis, lymphadenoma. **Body as a whole:** Fever, flu symptoms, chills, photosensitivity, dehydration, malaise, asthenia, edema, pain. **Ophthalmic:** Amblyopia, abnormal vision, visual field abnormality, diplopia. **Miscellaneous:** Back pain, tinnitus.

LABORATORY TEST CONSIDERATIONS

↑ Liver enzymes.

OD OVERDOSE MANAGEMENT
Symptoms: Thrombocytopenia. *Treatment:* Close clinical monitoring. Decrease or stop dose until platelet count returns to within the normal range.

DRUG INTERACTIONS
H *Evening primrose oil* / Potential for ↑ antiplatelet effect
H *Feverfew* / Potential for ↑ antiplatelet effect
H *Garlic* / Potential for ↑ antiplatelet effect
H *Ginger* / Potential for ↑ antiplatelet effect
H *Ginkgo biloba* / Potential for ↑ antiplatelet effect
H *Ginseng* / Potential for ↑ antiplatelet effect
H *Grapeseed extract* / Potential for ↑ antiplatelet effect

HOW SUPPLIED
Capsules: 0.5 mg, 1 mg

DOSAGE

• **CAPSULES**

Essential thrombocythemia.

Initial: 0.5 mg q.i.d. or 1 mg b.i.d. Maintain for one week or more. **Then,** adjust to lowest effective dose to maintain platelet count less than 600,000/mcL. Can increase the dose by 0.5 mg or less/day in any 1 week. **Maximum dose:** 10 mg/day or 2.5 mg in single dose. Most respond at a dose of 1.5 to 3 mg/day.

NURSING CONSIDERATIONS

ASSESSMENT
1. Document etiology, onset, and duration of thrombocythemia.
2. Note any CAD, liver or renal dysfunction; document cardiovascular assessment and monitor closely.
3. Monitor VS, CBC, liver and renal function; check platelets every 2 days during first week and then weekly thereafter until stabilized.
4. Determine if pregnant.

CLIENT/FAMILY TEACHING
1. Take exactly as directed.
2. Drug is used to lower platelet counts. Increases usually occur within 4 days after therapy stopped.
3. Practice reliable contraception; may cause fetal harm.
4. Report any palpitations, SOB, dizziness, chest or abdominal pain, or unusual bleeding.

OUTCOMES/EVALUATE
Reduction in platelet counts; ↓ risk of thrombosis

Anakinra

(an-ah-KIN-rah)

PREGNANCY CATEGORY: B
CLASSIFICATION(S):
Antiarthritic drug
Rx: Kineret

ACTION/KINETICS
Interleukin-1 (IL-1) production is induced by inflammation. IL-1 degrades cartilage due to its induction of the rapid loss of proteoglycans, as well as stimulation of bone resorption. Anakinra acts by blocking activity of interleukin-1 by competitively inhibiting IL-1 binding to the interleukin-1 type I receptor found in many tissues and organs. Thus, symptoms of rheumatoid arthritis improve. **Maximum plasma levels:** 3–7 hr. **$t^{1/2}$, terminal:** 4–6 hr.

USES
Decrease signs and symptoms of moderate-to-severe active rheumatoid arthritis in clients 18 and older who have failed 1 or more disease modifying antirheumatic drugs (DMARD). Can be used alone or with DMARDs (except TNF blocking drugs).

CONTRAINDICATIONS
Known hypersensitivity to *E. coli*-derived proteins. Use of live vaccines concurrently with anakinra.

SPECIAL CONCERNS
Associated with an increased incidence of serious infections. Safety and efficacy has not been determined in immunosuppressed clients, in those with chronic infections, when used with tumor necrosis factor blocking agents, or with use for juvenile rheumatoid arthritis. Vaccination may not be effective in those receiving anakinra.

A

Use with caution during lactation, in treating geriatric clients, and in those with impaired renal function. Safety and efficacy for use in clients with juvenile rheumatoid arthritis have not been determined.

SIDE EFFECTS

Injection site reactions: Erythema, ecchymosis, inflammation, pain. **Body as a whole:** Serious infections, including cellulitis, pneumonia, bone and joint infections, bacterial pneumonia. Other infections, including URI, sinusitis, flu-like symptoms. Also, malignancies, headache. **Hematologic:** Neutropenia. **GI:** Nausea, diarrhea, abdominal pain.

LABORATORY TEST CONSIDERATIONS

↓ Total WBC, platelets, and absolute neutrophil blood counts. Small ↑ mean eosinophil differential percentage.

HOW SUPPLIED

Injection, single-use: 100 mg/0.67 mL

DOSAGE

• **SC.**

Rheumatoid arthritis.

100 mg/day given by SC injection.

NURSING CONSIDERATIONS

ADMINISTRATION/STORAGE

1. Give at about the same time every day.
2. Before administration, visually inspect for particulate matter or discoloration. If observed, do not use the prefilled syringe.
3. Give only one dose/day (i.e., entire contents of 1 prefilled glass syringe). Discard any unused portion as there is no preservative in the product.
4. Store in the refrigerator at 2–8°C (36–46°F). Do not freeze or shake. Protect from light.

ASSESSMENT

1. Document indications for therapy, extent and characteristics of disease, and other agents trialed/failed.
2. List other drugs taking to ensure none interact. Do not administer with TNF (tumor necrosis factor) blocking agents or to those with juvenile RA.
3. Monitor CBC, liver and renal function studies.

CLIENT/FAMILY TEACHING

1. Review drug insert and guidelines as needed.
2. Inject anakinra daily, at approximately the same time each day, into the sc tissues as instructed.
3. Drug comes in a single dose syringe and requires refrigeration. Check expiration date, protect from light, and do **not** shake or freeze.
4. Store drug safely out of reach; dispose of needles as instructed.
5. Injection site reactions may occur; rotate sites and report any pain, inflammation, or bruising at the sites.
6. Avoid immunizations with live vaccines while on drug therapy.
7. Stop drug and report if any infection is suspected. Drug is highly toxic and has been associated with an increased incidence of serious infections.
8. Anticipate frequent lab visits (q1mo x 3 mo then q 3 mo) for CBC and to be evaluated by rheumatologist.

OUTCOMES/EVALUATE

Control of RA progression; ↓ joint pain; ↓ bone erosion in those unresponsive to 1 or more DMARDs

Anastrozole

(an-**AS**-troh-zohl)

PREGNANCY CATEGORY: D
CLASSIFICATION(S):
Antineoplastic, hormone
Rx: Arimidex

SEE ALSO *ANTINEOPLASTIC AGENTS.*

ACTION/KINETICS

Growth of many breast cancers is due to stimulation of estrogen receptors by estrogens. In postmenopausal women the main source of circulating estrogen is conversion of androstenedione to estrone by aromatase in peripheral tissues with further conversion to estradiol. Anastrozole is a nonsteroidal aromatase inhibitor that significantly decreases serum estradiol levels. Has no effect on formation of adrenal corticosteroids or aldosterone. Well absorbed from the GI tract;

A

food does not affect the extent of absorption. **t½, terminal:** About 50 hr in postmenopausal women. Steady-state levels reached in about 7 days of once daily dosing. 40% plasma-protein bound. Metabolized by the liver and both unchanged drug (about 10%) and metabolites are excreted through the urine.

USES

First-line treatment in postmenopausal women with advanced or locally advanced breast cancer whose disease is hormone receptor positive or hormone receptor unknown. Advanced breast cancer in postmenopausal women with progression of the disease following tamoxifen therapy. *NOTE:* Clients with negative tumor estrogen receptors and those who do not respond to tamoxifen are rarely helped by anastrozole.

SPECIAL CONCERNS

Use with caution during lactation. Safety and efficacy have not been determined in children.

SIDE EFFECTS

GI: N&V, diarrhea, constipation, abdominal pain, anorexia, dry mouth, increased appetite, GI disturbances, anorexia. **CNS:** Headache, paresthesia, dizziness, depression, somnolence, confusion, insomnia, anxiety, nervousness, hypertonia, lethargy. **CV:** Hypertension, vasodilation, hypertension, thromboembolic disease, thrombophlebitis. **Musculoskeletal:** Asthenia, back pain, bone pain, myalgia, arthralgia, pathological fracture. **Respiratory:** Dyspnea, increased cough, pharyngitis, sinusitis, bronchitis, rhinitis. **Dermatologic:** Hot flushes, rash, sweating, hair thinning, pruritus. **GU:** Vaginal hemorrhage, UTI, breast pain, vaginal dryness, vaginal bleeding during first few weeks after changing from hormone therapy. **Hematologic:** Anemia, leukopenia, leukorrhea. **Miscellaneous:** Pain, peripheral edema, hot flushes, pelvic pain, chest pain, weight gain or loss, flu syndrome, fever, neck pain, malaise, accidental injury, infection, tumor flare.

LABORATORY TEST CONSIDERATIONS

↑ GGT, AST, ALT, alkaline phosphatase, total cholesterol, LDL cholesterol.

HOW SUPPLIED

Tablet: 1 mg

DOSAGE

• **TABLETS**

First-line treatment of advanced or locally advanced breast cancer. Advanced breast cancer following tamoxifen therapy.

1 mg daily.

NURSING CONSIDERATIONS

SEE ALSO *NURSING CONSIDERATIONS* FOR *ANTINEOPLASTIC AGENTS*.

ADMINISTRATION/STORAGE

1. Glucocorticoid or mineralocorticoid therapy is not required.
2. For first-line therapy, continue treatment until tumor regression is evident.
3. Dosage adjustment is not necessary in either hepatic or renal dysfunction.

ASSESSMENT

1. Document disease progression and last tamoxifen therapy.
2. Obtain baseline CBC, renal and LFT's and pregnancy test.

CLIENT/FAMILY TEACHING

1. Take as directed at the same time each day.
2. Use reliable birth control; may cause fetal harm and impair fertility.

OUTCOMES/EVALUATE

Control of malignant cell proliferation

Anistreplase

(an-ih-**STREP**-layz)

PREGNANCY CATEGORY: C

CLASSIFICATION(S):

Thrombolytic enzyme

Rx: Eminase

ACTION/KINETICS

Prepared by acylating human plasma derived from lys-plasminogen and purified streptokinase derived from

group C beta-hemolytic streptococci. When prepared, anistreplase is an inactive derivative of a fibrinolytic enzyme although the compound can still bind to fibrin. Anistreplase is activated by deacylation and subsequent release of the anisoyl group in the blood stream. The production of plasmin from plasminogen occurs in both the blood stream and the thrombus leading to thrombolysis. Lyses thrombi obstructing coronary arteries and reduces the size of infarcts. **t½:** 70–120 min.

USES

Management of AMI in adults, for lysis of thrombi obstructing coronary arteries, reduction of infarct size, improvement of ventricular function, and reduction of mortality. Initiate treatment as soon as possible after the onset of symptoms of AMI.

CONTRAINDICATIONS

Use in active internal bleeding; within 2 months of intracranial or intraspinal surgery; recent trauma, including cardiopulmonary resuscitation; history of CVA; intracranial neoplasm; arteriovenous malformation or aneurysm; known bleeding diathesis; severe, uncontrolled hypertension; severe allergic reactions to streptokinase.

SPECIAL CONCERNS

Use with caution in nursing mothers. Safety and effectiveness have not been determined in children.

NOTE: The risks of anistreplase therapy may be increased in the following conditions; thus, benefit versus risk must be assessed prior to use. Within 10 days of major surgery (e.g., CABG, obstetric delivery, organ biopsy, previous puncture of noncompressible vessels); cerebrovascular disease; within 10 days of GI or GU bleeding; within 10 days of trauma including cardiopulmonary resuscitation; SBP > 180 mm Hg or DBP > 110 mm Hg; likelihood of left heart thrombus (e.g., mitral stenosis with atrial fibrillation); SBE; acute pericarditis; hemostatic defects including those secondary to severe hepatic or renal disease; pregnancy; clients older than 75 years of age; diabetic hemorrhagic retinopathy or other hemorrhagic ophthalmic conditions; septic thrombophlebitis or occluded arteriovenous cannula at seriously infected site; clients on oral anticoagulant therapy; any condition in which bleeding constitutes a significant hazard or would be difficult to manage due to its location.

SIDE EFFECTS

Bleeding.

Including at the puncture site (most common), nonpuncture site hematoma, hematuria, hemoptysis, ***GI hemorrhage, intracranial bleeding,*** gum/mouth hemorrhage, epistaxis, anemia, eye hemorrhage.

CV: *Arrhythmias,* conduction disorders, hypotension; ***cardiac rupture,*** chest pain, emboli (causal relationship to use of anistreplase unknown). **Allergic: *Anaphylaxis, bronchospasm,*** angioedema, urticaria, itching, flushing, rashes, eosinophilia, delayed purpuric rash which may be associated with arthralgia, ankle edema, mild hematuria, GI symptoms, and proteinuria. **GI:** N&V. **Hematologic:** Thrombocytopenia. **CNS:** Agitation, dizziness, paresthesia, tremor, vertigo. **Respiratory:** Dyspnea, lung edema. **Miscellaneous:** Chills, fever, headache, shock.

LABORATORY TEST CONSIDERATIONS

↑ Transaminase levels, thrombin time, activated PTT, and PT. ↓ Plasminogen and fibrinogen.

DRUG INTERACTIONS

↑ Risk of bleeding or hemorrhage if used with heparin, oral anticoagulants, vitamin K antagonists, aspirin, or dipyridamole.

HOW SUPPLIED

Powder for injection, lyophilized: 30 U

DOSAGE

IV only: 30 units over 2–5 min into an IV line or vein as soon as possible after onset of symptoms.

NURSING CONSIDERATIONS

SEE ALSO *NURSING CONSIDERATIONS FOR ALTEPLASE, RECOMBINANT.*

ADMINISTRATION/STORAGE

IV 1. To reconstitute slowly add 5 mL of sterile water. To minimize foaming, gently roll vial after directing ster-

ile water stream against the side of the vial. Do not shake.
2. The reconstituted solution should be colorless to pale yellow without particulate matter or discoloration.
3. Do not further dilute the reconstituted solution before administration. Give IV over 2-5 min.
4. Do not add reconstituted solution to any infusion fluids; do not add any other medications to the vial or syringe.
5. Discard if not administered within 30 min of reconstitution.

ASSESSMENT

1. Note any history and/or evidence of excessive bleeding.
2. Take a full drug history, noting any aspirin, anticoagulant, or vitamin K antagonist use.
3. Note resistance to the effects of anistreplase, which may be observed if given between 5 days and 12 months after a previous dose, after streptokinase therapy, or after a streptococcal infection.
4. Increased antistreptokinase antibody levels between 5 days and 6 months after anistreplase or streptokinase administration may increase the risk of allergic reactions.
5. Obtain baseline hematologic parameters, type and cross, coagulation studies, cardiac marker panel, and renal function studies.

INTERVENTIONS

1. Avoid invasive procedures to minimize bleeding potential. Post bleeding precautions sign.
2. If an arterial puncture is necessary following use of anistreplase, use an upper extremity vessel accessible to compression. Apply 30 min of manual pressure followed by application of a pressure dressing. Puncture site should be checked frequently for bleeding.
3. Monitor ECG closely and document any reperfusion arrhythmias.

CLIENT/FAMILY TEACHING

1. Review goals of therapy and inherent risks during acute MI.
2. To be effective, therapy should be instituted as soon as possible after onset of S&S of MI.
3. Encourage family members to learn CPR.

OUTCOMES/EVALUATE

• Thrombilysis with restoration of blood flow to ischemic cardiac tissue
• ↓ Infarct size; ↓ mortality, and improved ventricular function

Antihemophilic factor (AHF, Factor VIII)

(an-tie-hee-moh-**FILL**-ick)

PREGNANCY CATEGORY: C
CLASSIFICATION(S):
Antihemophilic agent
Rx: Alphanate, Bioclate, Helixate FS, Hemofil M, Hyate:C (Porcine), Koate-DVI, Kogenate, Kogenate FS, Monoclate-P, Recombinate, ReFacto

ACTION/KINETICS

The potency and purity of preparations vary but each lot is standardized. Details on the package should be noted. Plasma protein (factor VIII) accelerates the conversion of Factor X to activated Factor X which converts prothrombin to thrombin. Thrombin then converts fibrinogen to fibrin resulting in clot formation. **t½:** 10–18 hr. One AHF unit is the activity found in 1 mL of normal pooled human plasma. *NOTE:* ReFacto is albumin free which reduces the risk of viral transmission.

USES

(1) Control of bleeding in clients suffering from hemophilia A (factor VIII deficiency and acquired factor VIII inhibitors). These products temporarily replace the missing clotting factor in order to correct or prevent bleeding episodes or to perform surgery. AHF is safe and effective for use in children of all ages, including neonates. (2) ReFacto only: Short-term prophylaxis to decrease frequency of spontaneous bleeding episodes. (3) Hyate C: Treatment and prevention of bleeding in congenital hemophilia A clients with antibodies to human Factor VIII. Also, for

previous nonhemophilic clients with spontaneously acquired inhibitors to human Factor VIII. *Note:* Not effective in controlling bleeding due to von Willebrand's disease.

CONTRAINDICATIONS

Use of monoclonal antibody-derived AHF in clients hypersensitive to bovine, hamster, or mouse protein or to murine or porcine factor.

SPECIAL CONCERNS

Since AHF is prepared from human plasma, there is a risk of transmitting hepatitis or AIDS. However, the products are carefully prepared and tested. Koate DVI has not been studied in children and limited studies have been conducted with Alphanate.

SIDE EFFECTS

CNS: Headache, somnolence, lethargy, fatigue, dizziness, jittery feeling, asthenia. **CV:** Increased bleeding tendency, flushing, angina pectoris, tachycardia, chest discomfort, slight hypotension, acute hemolytic anemia, hyperfibrinogenemia. **GI:** N&V, constipation, stomach ache, diarrhea, anorexia, taste changes, gastroenetritis, abdominal pain. **Dermatologic:** Rash, flushing of face, acne, increased perspiration. **Musculoskeletal:** Myalgia, muscle weakness. **Respiratory:** Nose bleeds, rhinitis, dyspnea, coughing. **Hematologic:** Forearm bleeding following venipuncture, anemia, infected hematoma, forehead bruises, permanent venous access catheter complications. Acute thrombocytopenia (rare) with Hyate:C. **Ophthalmic:** Blurred vision, eye disorder, abnormal vision. **Allergic:** Nausea, fever, hives, chills, urticaria, wheezing, hypotension, chest tightness, stinging at infusion site, hypotension, ***anaphylaxis.*** **Miscellaneous:** Sore throat, cold feet; tingling in arm, ear, and face; fever, chills, urticaria, depersonalization, adenopathy, cold sensation, finger pain. Antibodies may form to the mouse protein found in AHF derived from monoclonal antibodies. Approximately 10% of clients develop inhibitors to Factor VIII, which leads to a significantly decreased response. Antihemophilic factor contains traces of blood group A and B isohemagglutins. These may cause ***intravascular hemolysis*** in clients with types A, B, or AB blood. ***Both hepatitis and AIDS may be transmitted from AHF prepared from human plasma.***

HOW SUPPLIED

Powder for Injection: Wide range of concentrations, depending on product

DOSAGE

• IV ONLY

Individualized, depending on severity of bleeding, degree of deficiency, body weight, and presence of inhibitors of factor VIII. *NOTE:* AHF levels may rise 2% for every unit of AHF per kilogram administered. The following formula provides a guide for dosage calculation: Expected Factor VIII increase (in % of normal): AHF/IU administered × 2 ÷ body weight (in kg). Dosages given are only guidelines.

Prophylaxis of spontaneous hemorrhage.

Increase AHF levels to about 5% of normal; 30% of normal is the minimum required for hemostasis following surgery and trauma. A single dose of 10 IU/kg (increases of approximately 20%) may be sufficient for mild superficial bleeds or early hemorrhages. Smaller doses may be sufficient for early hemarthrosis.

Mild hemorrhage.

Single infusion to achieve AHF levels of at least 30%. Dosage should not be repeated.

Minor surgery, moderate hemorrhage.

AHF levels should be raised to 30%–50% of normal. **Initial:** 15–25 IU/kg; **maintenance, if necessary:** 10–15 IU/kg q 8–12 hr.

Severe hemorrhage.

Increase AHF levels to 80%–100% of normal. **Initial:** 40–50 IU/kg; **maintenance:** 20–25 IU/kg q 8–12 hr.

Major surgery.

Raise AHF levels to 80%–100% of normal. Administer 1 hr before surgery; one-half the priming dose may be given 5 hr after the first dose. AHF levels should be maintained at 30% of normal for at least 10–14 days.

Dental extraction.

Factor VIII level should be increased to 50% immediately before the procedure.

NURSING CONSIDERATIONS

ADMINISTRATION/STORAGE

IV 1. AHF is labile and is inactivated within 10 min at 56°C and within 3 hr at 49°C. Store vials at 2–8°C (35–46°F). Check expiration date. **Do not freeze.**

2. Do not store products stabilized with sucrose (e.g., Helixate FS, Helixate NexGen, Kogenate FS) at room temperature. Refrigerate at all times from 2–8°C (35–40°F).

3. Warm the concentrate and diluent to room temperature before reconstitution.

4. Place one needle in the concentrate to act as an airway and then aseptically with a syringe and needle add the diluent to the concentrate.

5. Gently agitate or roll the vial containing diluent and concentrate to dissolve the drug. **Do not shake vigorously.**

6. Administer drug within 3 hr of reconstitution, to avoid incubation if contamination occurrs with mixing.

7. Do not refrigerate after reconstitution, active ingredient may precipitate out.

8. Keep reconstituted drug at room temperature during infusion because, at a lower temperature, precipitation of active ingredients may occur.

9. Administer IV only using a plastic syringe (solutions stick to glass syringes). Administer at a rate of 2 mL/min, although rates up to 10 mL/min can be used if necessary. If the HR increases significantly, reduce rate or discontinue administration.

10. There are a large number of products available. It is important to note the actual AHF units, which are indicated on the vial.

ASSESSMENT

1. Note blood type. Clients with A, B, and AB are more prone to hemolytic reactions.

2. Determine any recent trauma or injury; assess joints carefully.

3. Document baseline hematologic parameters and factor VIII levels. Monitor H&H and factor levels and obtain Coombs' test during therapy.

INTERVENTIONS

1. Document baseline VS and monitor q 5–15 min during infusion. If tachycardia and hypotension occur, slow IV and report.

2. Premedicate (usually diphenhydramine) to reduce allergic S&S.

3. Should only be administered in a center with specially trained personnel familiar with drug therapy.

4. Document I&O. Assess urine for quantity, color, and occult blood.

5. To control spontaneous bleeding, 5% of normal Factor VIII must be present. For moderate bleeding or prior to surgery, 30-50% must be present and for severe bleeding associated with trauma or major surgery, 80-100% of the normal Factor VIII level must be present.

6. Give the first dose 1 hr before surgery, and the 2nd dose (1/2 of the first dose) 5-8 hr postop. Maintain Factor VIII levels at 30% of normal for 10-14 days postoperatively.

7. Slow infusion and report if client complains of headaches, flushing, numbness, back/joint pain, visual disturbances, or chest constriction.

CLIENT/FAMILY TEACHING

1. Review method for storing and administering AHF at home.

2. If product is prepared from human plasma identify the rare but associated potential risks, such as hepatitis and HIV. Heat treated or monoclonal antibody preparations may decrease risk.

3. Avoid any drugs/OTC agents that may alter clotting (i.e., ASA, NSAIDS).

4. Determine knowledge level concerning disease process and hereditary transmission. Identify areas necessary to ensure compliance.

5. Reinforce safety measures related to sports, work, risk taking, and sexual activity.

6. Identify local support groups that may assist to understand and cope with this disease.

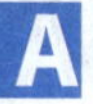

OUTCOMES/EVALUATE

- Prevention and control of bleeding with hemophilia A
- Promotion of normal clotting mechanisms
- Coagulation times and factor VIII levels within desired range

Antithrombin III (Human)

(an-tee-**THROM**-bin)

PREGNANCY CATEGORY: B
CLASSIFICATION(S):
Anticoagulant, antithrombin
Rx: Thrombate III

ACTION/KINETICS

Antithrombin III (AT-III) is the major plasma inhibitor of thrombin. For therapeutic use it is obtained from plasma of human volunteers. Inactivation of thrombin by AT-III results from formation of a covalent bond causing an inactive 1:1 stoichiometric complex between thrombin and AT-III. AT-III also inactivates other components of the coagulation cascade including factors IXa, Xa, XIa, and XIIa, and plasmin. **t½:** 2.5 days (based on immunologic assays).

USES

Hereditary AT-III deficiency in pregnant clients, in clients requiring surgery, and in individuals with thromboembolism.

SPECIAL CONCERNS

Safety and effectiveness have not been determined in children. Even though special precautions are taken to screen plasma donors, clients may develop S&S of viral infections, especially hepatitis C.

SIDE EFFECTS

GI: Nausea, foul taste in mouth, bowel fullness. **CNS:** Dizzness, lightheadedness. **Respiratory:** Chest tightness, shortness of breath, chest pain. **Miscellaneous:** Chills, cramps, film over eye, hives, fever, oozing, hematoma.

DRUG INTERACTIONS

↑ Heparin effect when used concomitantly with AT-III; ↓ heparin dose during AT-III therapy.

HOW SUPPLIED

Powder for injection, lyophilized: 500 IU, 1000 IU

DOSAGE

- **IV ONLY**

Individualize dose depending on the pretherapy plasma AT-III level. The dosage can be calculated from the following formula:

units required (IU) = [desired AT-III level (%) – baseline AT-III level (%)]/1.4 × body weight (kg)

The formula is based on an expected incremental recovery above baseline levels for AT-III of 1.4%/IU/kg given. Each bottle of AT-III has the functional activity, in international units (IU) stated on the label.

The following regimen may be used as a starting point for treatment; modification is based on actual plasma AT-III levels reached.

1. Calculate the initial loading dose to elevate plasma AT-III levels to 120%, assuming a rise over baseline plasma AT-III of 1.4% (functional activity)/IU/kg given.
2. Measure plasma AT-III levels preinfusion, 20 minutes postinfusion (peak), after 12 hr, and preceding the next infusion (trough level). Subsequently, measure AT-III levels preceding and 20 min after each infusion until predictable peak and trough levels have been reached (usually between 80% and 120%). Plasma levels between 80% and 120% may be maintained by giving maintenance doses of 60% of the initial loading dose q 24 hr. Adjust the maintenance dose or interval between doses based on actual plasma AT-III levels reached.

If AT-III therapy is indicated for a client with hereditary deficiency to control an acute thrombotic episode or to prevent thrombosis following surgical or obstetrical procedures, increase the AT-III plasma level to normal and maintain for 2–8 days. This will depend on the reason for treatment, type and extensiveness of surgery, medical condition and history of the client, and judgment of the physician.

NURSING CONSIDERATIONS

ADMINISTRATION/STORAGE

IV 1. Reconstitute with sterile water for injection. Filter through a sterile needle as supplied in the package. Do not shake product.
2. After reconstitution, bring to room temperature and administer within 3 hr.
3. Infuse over 10–20 min.
4. Once reconstituted, give the drug alone without mixing with other agents or diluting solutions.

ASSESSMENT

1. Perform a complete nursing history noting any positive family history of venous thrombosis.
2. Determine that AT-III levels have been obtained prior to drug therapy and as directed under dosage.
3. Document pretreatment weight.

INTERVENTIONS

1. Observe for dyspnea and elevated BP during IV administration; slow infusion rate and report if evident.
2. Monitor VS closely (q 5–15 min) during infusion.
3. Note early S&S of acute thrombosis. Perform routine vascular checks and monitor AT-III levels.
4. Observe for any evidence of bleeding. Anticipate a reduced dose of heparin when administered concomitantly with AT-III.
5. Anticipate that when AT-III is given for clients with hereditary deficiency to control an acute thrombosis or to prevent thrombosis due to surgery or in obstetrics, levels should be maintained for 2–8 days, depending on the status of the client.
6. For use only in facilities with personnel trained in drug use and selected patient management.

CLIENT/FAMILY TEACHING

1. Review the high risk of thrombosis during pregnancy and surgery in clients with hereditary deficiencies because AT-III levels are generally 50% of the level of normal.
2. The disease is inherited; obtain appropriate medical follow-up, counseling, and family planning.
3. Understand associated risks of drug therapy; product is derived from pooled human plasma.

OUTCOMES/EVALUATE

- Serum AT-III levels > 80% of normal during therapy for high-risk procedures
- Prevention of thrombus formation

Aprotinin

(ah-**PROH**-tih-nin)

PREGNANCY CATEGORY: B
CLASSIFICATION(S):
Hemostatic, systemic
Rx: Trasylol

ACTION/KINETICS

Aprotinin, a natural protease inhibitor derived from bovine lung, inhibits plasmin and kallikrein, thereby directly affecting fibrinolysis. It also inhibits the contact phase activation of coagulation which initiates coagulation and promotes fibrinolysis. Also preserves the adhesive glycoproteins in the platelet membrane, rendering them resistant to damage from the increased plasmin levels and mechanical injury that occur during cardiopulmonary bypass. The net effect is to inhibit both fibrinolysis and turnover of coagulation factors and to decrease bleeding. **t½, IV:** 150 min; **t½, terminal elimination:** 10 hr. Slowly broken down by lysosomal enzymes, although depending on the dose, up to 9% may be excreted through the urine unchanged.

USES

Prophylactically to reduce perioperative blood loss and the need for blood transfusions in clients undergoing cardiopulmonary bypass surgery in the course of repeat CABG surgery. In selected cases of primary CABG surgery where the risk of bleeding is high or where transfusion is unavailable or unacceptable. Use in CABG is based on the risk of renal dysfunction and

A

the risk of anaphylaxis (i.e., should a second procedure be required).

CONTRAINDICATIONS

Hypersensitivity to aprotinin.

SPECIAL CONCERNS

Give a test dose to assess for potential allergic reactions; due to the risk of anaphylaxis, use caution when administering aprotinin (including test doses) to clients who have received the drug previously. Safety and efficacy have not been determined in children.

SIDE EFFECTS

CV: AF, ***MI, heart failure, heart arrest***, atrial flutter, ***VT***, hypotension, CHF, SVT, pericarditis, phlebitis, heart block, hemolysis, ***CVA, VF***. Possibly an increased incidence of saphenous vein graft closure in clients undergoing primary or repeat CABG. **Respiratory:** Pneumonia, respiratory disorder, asthma, apnea, dyspnea, lung edema, pleural effusion, pneumothorax. **GU:** ***Acute kidney failure,*** kidney tubular necrosis. **CNS:** Confusion, ***convulsions, cerebral embolism.*** **Body as a whole:** Fever, sepsis, ***shock, allergic reactions, anaphylaxis.*** **Miscellaneous:** Liver damage.

LABORATORY TEST CONSIDERATIONS

↑ Creatinine, transaminases, creatine kinase, PTT, activated clotting time, serum glucose. ↑ Incidence of postoperative renal dysfunction.

DRUG INTERACTIONS

Captopril / Blockade of acute hypotensive effect

Fibrinolytic drugs / Inhibition of fibrinolytic effects

Heparin / Prolongation of activated clotting time

HOW SUPPLIED

Injection: 10,000 Kallikrein Inhibitor Units (KIU)/mL

DOSAGE

• **IV**

Coronary artery bypass graft surgery.

A 1-mL (1.4-mg or 10,000-KIU) test dose must be given 10 min prior to the loading dose. Follow the test dose by the loading dose using either regimen A or B; the loading dose is then followed by the constant infusion dose. In addition, the "pump prime" dose is added to the priming fluid of the cardiopulmonary bypass circuit by replacing an aliquot of the priming fluid prior to beginning cardiopulmonary bypass. **Regimen A, loading dose:** 280 mg (or 2 million KIU) with 280 mg (or 2 million KIU) into the pump prime volume; **constant infusion dose:** 70 mg/hr (500,000 KIU/hr). **Regimen B, loading dose:** 140 mg (or 1 million KIU) with 140 mg (or 1 million KIU) into the pump prime volume; **constant infusion dose:** 35 mg/hr (250,000 KIU/hr). Total doses greater than 7 million KIU have not been studied.

NURSING CONSIDERATIONS

ADMINISTRATION/STORAGE

IV 1. Experience with regimen B is limited. Regimen A seems more effective than regimen B in clients given aspirin preoperatively.

2. All IV doses are given through a central line. Do not administer any other drug through the same line.

3. Both regimens must include a 1-mL test dose, a loading dose, a dose to be added to the priming fluid of the cardiopulmonary bypass circuit, and a constant infusion dose.

4. The loading dose is given slowly over 20–30 min after induction of anesthesia (but prior to sternotomy) with the client in a supine position. This is followed by a constant infusion dose which is continued until client leaves the OR.

5. Aprotinin is incompatible in vitro with corticosteroids, heparin, tetracyclines, and nutrient solutions containing amino acids or fat emulsion. If these agents must be given, each should be given separately through different venous lines or catheters.

6. Store between 2–5°C (36–77°F); prevent from freezing.

ASSESSMENT

1. Determine if client has received this drug previously because there is an increased risk of anaphylaxis. Anticipate antihistamine administration before the loading dose if this is a re-exposure case.

2. Ensure that client has received a 1-mL test dose 10 min before the loading dose and note results.

A

INTERVENTIONS

1. Drug may cause increased serum glucose, CPK-MB fractions, transaminase levels, and postoperative renal dysfunction; monitor closely.
2. Drug prolongs whole blood clotting time of heparinized blood and lab results may not report true state of anticoagulation. Therefore, an activated clotting time greater than 400–450 sec may in fact lead to inadequate anticoagulation.
3. During cardiopulmonary bypass, administer standard loading doses of heparin. Additional heparin should be administered either in a fixed-dose regimen or based on client weight and duration of cardiopulmonary bypass, since the activated clotting time is not reliable.
4. Coordinate with the lab; a protamine titration test may be useful in determining heparin levels, as this is not altered by aprotinin.
5. Observe client closely for cardiac arrhythmias, hemorrhage, hypotension, and fever, as these are frequent drug-related side effects.

OUTCOMES/EVALUATE

↓ Perioperative blood loss in clients undergoing cardiopulmonary bypass surgery

Ardeparin sodium

(ar-dee-**PAH**-rin)

PREGNANCY CATEGORY: C
CLASSIFICATION(S):
Anticoagulant, low molecular weight heparin
Rx: Normiflo

SEE ALSO *HEPARINS, LOW MOLECULAR WEIGHT.*

ACTION/KINETICS

Plasma levels of ardeparin can not be measured directly; rather, serine protease activity is used. Well absorbed following SC administration. **t½, disposition:** 3.3 hr (for ardeparin anti-Xa) and 1.2 hr (for ardeparin anti-IIa).

USES

Prophylaxis of deep vein thrombosis (DVT) following total knee replacement (TKR) surgery. *Investigational:* Secondary prophylaxis for recurrent thromboembolic events.

ADDITIONAL CONTRAINDICATIONS

Hypersensitivity to propylparaben.

SPECIAL CONCERNS

SEE ALSO *HEPARINS, LOW MOLECULAR WEIGHT*. The product contains metabisulfite that may cause allergic reactions in susceptible persons.

SIDE EFFECTS

Bleeding events.

Intraoperative bleeding, postoperative surgical site or nonsurgical site hematoma or hemorrhage, bleeding requiring an invasive procedure; ecchymosis, ***GI hemorrhage,*** hematemesis, hematuria, melena, petechiae, ***rectal hemorrhage, retroperitoneal hemorrhage, CVA,*** abnormal stools. **GI:** N&V, constipation. *Allergic reaction:* Maculopapular rash, vesiculobullous rash, urticaria. **CNS:** Confusion, dizziness, headache, insomnia. **Miscellaneous:** Fever, pruritus, anemia, thrombocytopenia, arthralgia, chest pain, dyspnea, reactions at injection site (edema, hypersensitivity, inflammation, pain), peripheral edema.

HOW SUPPLIED

Injection: 5,000 U/0.5 mL; 10,000 U/0.5 mL

DOSAGE

• **SC ONLY**

Prophylaxis of DVT during TKR surgery.

Adults: 50 anti-Xa U/kg q 12 hr. Begin treatment evening of day of surgery or following morning and continue for up to 14 days or until client is fully ambulatory, whichever is shorter.

Prophylaxis of thromboembolic recurrence.

35–50 U/kg b.i.d.

NURSING CONSIDERATIONS

SEE ALSO *NURSING CONSIDERATIONS* FOR *HEPARINS, LOW MOLECULAR WEIGHT.*

A

ADMINISTRATION/STORAGE

1. Give by deep (intra-fat) SC injection in abdomen, avoiding navel, anterior aspect of thighs, or outer aspect of upper arms.
2. Before using, inspect visually for particulate matter and discoloration.
3. Do not mix with other injections or infusions.
4. Store at room temperature, 15–30°C (59–77°F).

ASSESSMENT

1. Take a complete history noting any conditions that may preclude drug therapy. Note any active major bleeding, bleeding disorders, or thrombocytopenia.
2. Drug dosage is based on weight; obtain reliable dry weight.
3. Note any sensitivity to heparin or pork products or metasulfites.
4. Monitor CBC, urinalysis, liver and renal function studies.

CLIENT/FAMILY TEACHING

1. Review indications for therapy and how to administer. Therapy consists of 2 injections deep SC q 12 hr while sitting or lying down. May be given in the abdomen; avoid navel, anterior aspect of thighs, or outer aspect of upper arms. Vary administration site with each injection.
2. To minimize bruising, do not rub site after giving injection.
3. Use Tubex® injector and follow printed guidelines for loading and removing Tubex®. Remove air and excess medication from unit before injection. Discard used needles safely.
4. Therapy is continued until fully ambulatory or for about 14 days.
5. Avoid aspirin and NSAIDs.
6. Report any unusual bruising, bleeding or dizziness.
7. CBC, FOB, and urinalysis will be ordered.

OUTCOMES/EVALUATE

DVT prophylaxis after TKR

Argatroban

(are-**GAT**-roh-ban)

PREGNANCY CATEGORY: B

CLASSIFICATION(S):

Anticoagulant, thrombin inhibitor

Rx: Acova

ACTION/KINETICS

A synthetic, direct thrombin inhibitor derived from L-arginine. Reversibly binds to the thrombin active site and does not require antithrombin III for antithrombotic activity. Acts by inhibiting thrombin-catalyzed or induced reactions, including fibrin formation; activation of coagulation factors V, VIII, and XIII; protein C; and platelet aggregation. Inhibits both free and clot-associated thrombin. The small molecule provides the needed anticoagulant effect without worsening hypercoagulable states. Has little or no effect on trypsin, factor Xa, plasmin, and kallikrein. Does not interact with heparin-induced antibodies. Distributes mainly in the extracellular fluid. Steady state reached, by IV infusion, in 1–3 hr and is continued until infusion is stopped. Metabolized in the liver by cytochrome P450 enzymes (CYP3A4/5). **t½, terminal:** 39–51 min. Excreted in the feces, primarily through biliary excretion.

USES

Prophylaxis or treatment of thrombosis in heparin-induced thrombocytopenia.

CONTRAINDICATIONS

Overt major bleeding, hypersensitivity to the product or any of its components. Lactation.

SPECIAL CONCERNS

Use with caution in hepatic disease and in disease states and circumstances with an increased danger of hemorrhage, including severe hypertension, immediately following lumbar puncture, spinal anesthesia, major surgery (especially the brain, spinal cord, or eye), congenital or acquired bleeding disorders, and GI lesions (e.g., ulcerations). Safety and efficacy have not been determined in children less than 18 years of age.

SIDE EFFECTS

Bleeding.

Major hemorrhagic events, including GI, GU/hematuria, decreased H&H,

multisystem hemorrhage and DIC, limb and BK amputation stump. Minor hemorrhagic events, including GI, GU/hematuria, groin, hemoptysis, brachial. Intracranial bleeding in clients with acute MI started on argatroban and streptokinase.
Allergic: Airway reactions (coughing, dyspnea), rash, bullous eruption, vasodilation. **GI:** Diarrhea, vomiting. **CV:** Hypotension, ***cardiac arrest, VT***, CV disorder, atrial fibrillation. **Respiratory:** Dyspnea, pneumonia, coughing. **GU:** UTI, abnormal renal function. **Miscellaneous:** Fever, pain, infection, abdominal pain, ***sepsis***.

LABORATORY TEST CONSIDERATIONS

Coadministration of argatroban and warfarin produces a combined effect on laboratory measurement of INR. However, concurrent therapy exerts no additional effect on vitamin K-dependent factor Xa activity, compared with warfarin monotherapy.

OD OVERDOSE MANAGEMENT

Symptoms: Major/minor bleeding events. *Treatment:* Discontinue argatroban or decrease infusion dose. Anticoagulation parameters usually return to baseline within 2–4 hr after discontinuing the drug. Reversal may take longer in hepatic impairment. No specific antidote is available. Provide symptomatic and supportive therapy.

DRUG INTERACTIONS

Concomitant use with antiplatelet drugs, thrombolytics, and other anticoagulants ↑ risk of bleeding.

HOW SUPPLIED

Injection: 100 mg/mL

DOSAGE

• IV INFUSION

Prevention and treatment of thrombosis.

Adults, initial, without hepatic impairment: 2 mcg/kg/min as a continuous IV infusion. The infusion rate depends on body weight. After the initial dose, adjust dose as clinically indicated, not to exceed 10 mcg/kg/min, until the steady state APTT is 1.5–3 times initial baseline value, not to exceed 100 seconds. **Adults, initial, moderate hepatic impairment:** 0.5 mcg/kg/min, based on about a 4-fold decrease in argatroban clearance compared with normal hepatic function.

NURSING CONSIDERATIONS

ADMINISTRATION/STORAGE

IV 1. To prepare for IV infusion, dilute argatroban in 0.9% NaCl, D5W, or LR injection to a final concentration of 1 mg/mL. Thus, dilute each 2.5 mL vial 100-fold by mixing with 250 mL of diluent.
2. Mix the reconstituted solution by repeated inversion of the diluent bag for 1 min. After preparation, the solution may be briefly hazy due to the formation of microprecipitates. These dissolve rapidly upon mixing.
3. If prepared correctly, the pH of the IV solution is 3.2–7.5.
4. Use of argatroban and warfarin results in prolongation of INR beyond that caused by warfarin alone. Measure INR daily if argatroban and warfarin are given together. Generally, with doses of argatroban of 2 mcg/kg/min or less, argatroban can be discontinued when the INR is greater than 4 on combined therapy. After argatroban is discontinued, repeat INR measurement in 4–6 hr. If the repeat INR is below the desired range, resume argatroban infusion and repeat the procedure daily until the desired therapeutic range on warfarin alone is reached.
5. For doses of argatroban greater than 2 mcg/kg/min, the relationship of INR on warfarin alone to the INR of both drugs given together is less predictable. Thus, temporarily reduce the dose of argatroban to 2 mcg/kg/min. Repeat the INR on argatroban and warfarin 4–6 hr after reducing the argatroban dose and follow the process outlined above for giving argatroban at doses of 2 mcg/kg/min or less.
6. Argatroban is a clear, colorless to pale yellow, slightly viscous solution. Discard vial if the solution is cloudy or an insoluble precipitate is observed.
7. Prepared solutions are stable at 15–30°C (59–85°F) for 24 hr at ambient indoor light. Prepared solutions

A

are stable for 48 hr or less when stored at 2–8°C (36–46°F) in the dark. Do not expose prepared solutions to direct sunlight.

ASSESSMENT

1. Note indications for therapy: thrombosis prophylaxis or treatment.
2. Review history noting any conditions that may preclude drug therapy. Note any active bleeding sites/disorders.
3. Stop heparin therapy. Obtain and monitor weight, INR, PT/PTT, CBC, and LFTs. Lower dosage with liver dysfunction.
4. Observe closely for evidence of abnormal bleeding or adverse effects. Perform routine vascular checks.

CLIENT/FAMILY TEACHING

1. Review goals of therapy and potential bleeding risks.
2. Report any unusual oozing or bleeding sites; wet bandages or bedding.
3. Encourage family members to learn CPR.

OUTCOMES/EVALUATE

Inhibition/treatment of thrombus formation with heparin-induced- thrombocytopenia

Asparaginase

(ah-**SPAIR**-ah-jin-ays)

PREGNANCY CATEGORY: C
CLASSIFICATION(S):
Antineoplastic, miscellaneous
Rx: Elspar
✱**Rx:** Kidrolase

SEE ALSO *ANTINEOPLASTIC AGENTS.*

ACTION/KINETICS

Asparaginase, derived from *Escherichia coli,* contains the enzyme L-asparagine amidohydrolase, type EC-2. Neoplastic cells are unable to synthesize sufficient asparagine, an amino acid, to meet their metabolic needs. The supply of asparagine is further decreased by the enzyme asparaginase, which breaks down asparagine to aspartic acid and ammonia. Asparaginase interferes with synthesis of DNA, RNA, and protein and is cell-cycle specific for the G_1 phase of cell division. **Time to peak plasma levels, after IM:** 14–24 hr. **t½, after IV:** 8–30 hr; **after IM:** 39–49 hr. Accumulates in plasma and tissue, and a small amount (1%) appears in CSF. Excretion is unknown. More toxic in adults than in children.

USES

Acute lymphocytic leukemia (ALL) in children; mostly used in combination with other drugs. Not to be used for maintenance therapy. *Investigational:* Acute myelocytic and myelomonocytic leukemia, chronic lymphocytic leukemia, Hodgkin's and non-Hodgkin's lymphomas, melanosarcoma.

CONTRAINDICATIONS

Anaphylactic reactions to asparaginase. Pancreatitis or a history of pancreatitis. Lactation.

SPECIAL CONCERNS

Use with caution in presence of liver dysfunction. Due to the possibility of an increased risk of hypersensitivity, institute retreatment with great care.

SIDE EFFECTS

GI: N&V, anorexia, abdominal cramps, ***pancreatitis (sometimes fulminant), acute hemorrhagic pancreatitis.*** **CNS:** Depression, somnolence, coma, confusion, fatigue, agitation, mild to severe hallucinations, headache, irritability, Parkinson-like syndrome with tremor and a progressive increase in muscle tone (rare). **Hematologic:** Marked leukopenia, bone marrow depression (rare). Depression of clotting factors; rarely, ***intracranial hemorrhage and fatal bleeding.*** **Hypersensitivity:** Skin rashes, urticaria, arthralgia, respiratory distress, ***acute anaphylaxis.*** **Renal:** Azotemia, proteinuria (rare), acute renal shutdown, ***fatal renal insufficiency.*** **Hepatic:** Hepatotoxicity, fatty changes in the liver. **Miscellaneous:** Hyperglycemia with glucosuria and polyuria. Marked hypoalbuminemia associated with peripheral edema, malabsorption syndrome, ***fatal hyperthermia,*** chills, fever, mild weight loss.

LABORATORY TEST CONSIDERATIONS

↑ Blood ammonia, BUN, glucose, uric acid, AST, ALT, alkaline phosphatase, bilirubin (direct and indirect). ↓ Serum

A

albumin, cholesterol (total and esters), plasma fibrinogen. ↑ or ↓ Total lipids. Interference with interpretation of thyroid function tests.

DRUG INTERACTIONS

Methotrexate / Asparaginase ↓ effect of methotrexate

Prednisone / Even though used with asparaginase, may cause ↑ toxicity

Vincristine / Even though used with asparaginase, may cause ↑ toxicity; ↑ hyperglycemic effect

HOW SUPPLIED

Powder for injection: 10,000 IU

DOSAGE

• **IV, IM**

When used as the sole agent for induction.

Adults and children: 200 IU/kg/day IV for 28 days.

Regimen I for ALL in children.

Prednisone: 40 mg/m²/day PO in three divided doses for 15 days, followed by tapering of dosage as follows: 20 mg/m²/day for 2 days, 10 mg/m²/day for 2 days, 5 mg/m²/day for 2 days, 2.5 mg/m²/day for 2 days, and then discontinue. Vincristine sulfate: 2 mg/m² IV once weekly on days 1, 8, and 15. The maximum single dose should not exceed 2 mg. Asparaginase: 1,000 IU/kg/day IV for 10 successive days beginning on day 22.

Regimen II for ALL in children.

Prednisone: 40 mg/m²/day PO in three divided doses for 28 days with the total daily dose to the nearest 2.5 mg; then, discontinue gradually over 14 days. Vincristine sulfate: 1.5 mg/m² IV weekly for four doses on days 1, 8, 15, and 22. The maximum single dose should not exceed 2 mg. Asparaginase: 6,000 IU/m² IM on days 4, 7, 10, 13, 16, 19, 22, 25, and 28. When remission is obtained with either regimen, appropriate maintenance therapy should be instituted. Do not use asparaginase for maintenance therapy.

NURSING CONSIDERATIONS

SEE ALSO *GENERAL NURSING CONSIDERATIONS* FOR *ANTINEOPLASTIC AGENTS.*

ADMINISTRATION/STORAGE

1. Give an intradermal skin test (0.1 mL of a 20-IU/mL solution) at least 1 hr before initial administration of drug and when 1 week or more has elapsed between treatments. Observe for at least 1 hr for wheal or erythema that indicates a positive reaction. A negative skin test reaction does not preclude the possibility of an allergic reaction.
2. A desensitization procedure, with increasing amounts of asparaginase may be carried out in those hypersensitive to the drug (1 IU, then double dose q 10 min until total dose for day or reaction occurs).
3. Due to the unpredictability of side effects, initiate treatment only in hospitalized clients.
4. Do not use asparaginase as sole induction agent unless a combined regimen is not possible due to toxicity or because client is refractory.
5. For IM use, reconstitute by adding 2 mL NaCl injection to the 10,000-unit vial. Use within 8 hr and only if clear. Give no more than 2 mL at a single injection site.
6. Handle the drug with care because it is a contact irritant.
7. Have emergency equipment readily available during each administration of asparaginase because a severe hypersensitivity reaction is more likely to occur with this drug.
8. Store both the lyophilized product and reconstituted solution at 2–8°C (36–46°F). Discard the reconstituted solution after 8 hr (sooner if cloudy).

IV 9. Follow administration guidelines.

10. For IV use, reconstitute the 10,000-unit vial with either 5 mL sterile water or NaCl injection. Give solution by direct IV administration within 8 hr following reconstitution. For infusion, dilute solutions with NaCl injection or 5% dextrose injection. Infuse over at least 30 min and within 8 hr only if solution is clear.

ASSESSMENT

1. Document indications for therapy and baseline labs. May cause mild

A

lymphocyte suppression. Nadir: 7–10 days; recovery 14 days.
2. Monitor LFTs, amylase, and lipase levels; check for S&S of pancreatitis.
3. Assess cardiopulmonary function and document ECG and CXR.

INTERVENTIONS

1. Anticipate antiemetic administration prior to drug therapy.
2. Administer vincristine and prednisone before asparaginase to reduce the toxic effects.
3. Asparaginase administration 9–10 days before or within 24 hr after methotrexate (MTX) may reduce the GI and hematologic effects of MTX.
4. Weigh weekly and monitor I&O; assess for any evidence of renal failure. Alkalinization of the urine and allopurinol therapy may help prevent urate stone formation.
5. Observe for peripheral edema due to hypoalbuminemia triggered by asparaginase.
6. Monitor for hyperglycemia, glycosuria, and polyuria, all of which may be precipitated by asparaginase. Have IV fluids and regular insulin available; stop therapy.

CLIENT/FAMILY TEACHING

1. Promptly report any stomach pain and N&V; S&S of pancreatitis.
2. Report any sudden increase in SOB, coughing, feet swelling, frequent urination, increased thirst, or fever.
3. Consume 2–3 L/day of fluids.
4. Drug may cause drowsiness, even several weeks after administration; therefore, do not drive a car or operate hazardous machinery.
5. Report shakiness or unusual body movements. A Parkinson-like condition may be precipitated by drug.
6. Avoid immunizations and contact with child who has recently taken poliovirus vaccine.
7. Avoid crowds, especially during flu season. Consider pneumoccal vaccine and annual flu shot.
8. Do not take any aspirin-containing compounds or drink alcohol.

OUTCOMES/EVALUATE

- Improved hematologic parameters
- Inhibition of malignant cell proliferation

Aspirin (Acetylsalicylic acid, ASA)

PREGNANCY CATEGORY: C

Rx: Easprin, ZORprin

OTC: ½ Halfprin, Arthritis Foundation Pain Reliever, Aspergum, Aspirin, Bayer Children's Aspirin, Bayer Low Adult Strength, Ecotrin Adult Low Strength, Ecotrin Caplets and Tablets, Ecotrin Maximum Strength Caplets and Tablets, Empirin, Extended Release Bayer 8-Hour Caplets, Extra Strength Bayer Enteric 500 Aspirin, Genprin, Genuine Bayer Aspirin Caplets and Tablets, Halfprin 81, Heartline, Maximum Bayer Aspirin Caplets and Tablets, Norwich Extra Strength, Regular Strength Bayer Enteric Coated Caplets, St. Joseph Adult Chewable Aspirin, Tri-Buffered Bufferin Caplets and Tablets, Adprin-B, Alka-Seltzer Extra Strength with Aspirin, Alka-Seltzer with Aspirin, Alka-Seltzer with Aspirin (flavored), Arthritis Pain Formula, Ascriptin A/D, Ascriptin Extra Strength, Ascriptin Regular Strength, Asprimox, Asprimox Extra Protection for Arthritis Pain, Asprimox Extra Protection for Arthritis Pain, Bayer Buffered Aspirin, Buffered Aspirin, Bufferin, Buffex, Cama Arthritis Pain Reliever, Extra-Strength Adprin-B, Extra-Strength Bayer Plus Caplets, Magnaprin, Magnaprin Arthritis Strength Captabs

✱OTC: Apo-Asa, Asaphen, Entrophen, MSD Enteric Coated ASA, Novasen

Aspirin, buffered

(ah-**SEE**-till-sal-ih-**SILL**-ick **AH**-sid)

PREGNANCY CATEGORY: C

CLASSIFICATION(S):

Nonsteroidal anti-inflammatory drug

Antipyretic

SEE ALSO NONSTEROIDAL ANTI-INFLAMMATORY DRUGS

ACTION/KINETICS

Exhibits antipyretic, anti-inflammatory, and analgesic effects. The antipyretic effect is due to an action on the hypothalamus, resulting in heat loss by vasodilation of peripheral blood vessels and promoting sweating. The anti-inflammatory effects are probably mediated through inhibition of cyclo-oxygenase, which results in a decrease in prostaglandin (implicated in the inflammatory response) synthesis and other mediators of the pain response. The mechanism of action for the analgesic effects of aspirin is not known fully but is partly attributable to improvement of the inflammatory condition. Aspirin also produces inhibition of platelet aggregation by decreasing the synthesis of endoperoxides and thromboxanes—substances that mediate platelet aggregation.

Large doses of aspirin (5 g/day or more) increase uric acid secretion, while low doses (2 g/day or less) decrease uric acid secretion. However, aspirin antagonizes drugs used to treat gout.

Rapidly absorbed after PO administration. Is hydrolyzed to the active salicylic acid, which is 70%–90% protein bound. **Blood levels for arthritis and rheumatic disease:** Maintain 150–300 mcg/mL. **Blood levels for analgesic and antipyretic:** 25–50 mcg/mL. **Blood levels for acute rheumatic fever:** 150–300 mcg/mL. Tinnitus occurs at serum levels above 200 mcg/mL and serious toxicity above 400 mcg/mL. **t½:** aspirin, 15–20 min; salicylic acid, 2–20 hr, depending on the dose. Salicylic acid and metabolites are excreted by the kidney. The bioavailability of enteric-coated salicylate products may be poor. The addition of antacids (buffered aspirin) may decrease GI irritation and increase the dissolution and absorption of such products.

USES

Analgesic: Pain from integumental structures, myalgias, neuralgias, arthralgias, headache, dysmenorrhea, and similar types of pain. Gout. May be effective in less severe postoperative and postpartum pain; pain secondary to trauma and cancer. **Antipyretic: Anti-Inflammatory:** Arthritis, ostgeoarthritis, SLE, acute rheumatic fever, gout, and many other conditions. Mucocutaneous lymph node syndrome (Kawasaki disease). **Cardiovascular:** Despite the increased risk of GI bleeding, low-dose aspirin should be used for the following CV events:

1. Reduce risk of death and nonfatal stroke in those who have had an ischemic stroke or TIA; also combined with dipyridamole for this purpose.
2. Reduce risk of vascular mortality with suspected acute MI.
3. Reduce the combined risk of recurrent MI and death after an MI or unstable angina.
4. Reduce risk of MI and sudden death in chronic stable angina.
5. Pre-existing need for aspirin following coronary artery bypass grafting, PTCA, or carotid endarterectomy.
6. Used with ticlopidine as adjunctuve therapy to reduce development of subacute stent thrombosis.

Investigational: Chronic use to prevent cataract formation; low doses to prevent toxemia of pregnancy; in pregnant women with inadequate uteroplacental blood flow. Reduce colon cancer mortality (low doses). Low doses of aspirin and warfarin to reduce risk of a second heart attack. In addition to treatment for CV risk factors, may reduce risk of dying from heart attack or stroke significantly.

CONTRAINDICATIONS

Hypersensitivity to salicylates. Clients with asthma, hay fever, or nasal polyps have a higher incidence of hypersensitivity reactions. Severe anemia, history of blood coagulation defects, in conjunction with anticoagulant therapy. Salicylates can cause congestive failure when taken in the large doses used for rheumatic diseases. Vitamin K deficiency; 1 week before and after surgery. In pregnancy, especially the last trimester as the drug may cause problems in the newborn child or complications during delivery. In children or teenagers with chicken-pox or flu due to possibility of development of Reye's syndrome.

Controlled-release aspirin is not recommended for use as an antipyretic or

short-term analgesic because adequate blood levels may not be reached. Also, controlled-release products are not recommended for children less than 12 years of age and in children with fever accompanied by dehydration.

SPECIAL CONCERNS

Use with caution during lactation and in the presence of gastric or peptic ulcers, in mild diabetes, erosive gastritis, bleeding tendencies, in cardiac disease, and in liver or kidney disease. Aspirin products now carry the following labeling: "It is especially important not to use aspirin during the last three months of pregnancy unless specifically directed to do so by a doctor because it may cause problems in the newborn child or complications during delivery."

SIDE EFFECTS

The toxic effects of the salicylates are dose-related.

GI: Dyspepsia, heartburn, anorexia, nausea, occult blood loss, epigastric discomfort, ***massive GI bleeding, potentiation of peptic ulcer***. Possible stomach bleeding in those who ingest three or more alcoholic drinks/day. **Allergic:** ***Bronchospasm, asthma-like symptoms, anaphylaxis,*** skin rashes, angioedema, urticaria, rhinitis, nasal polyps. **Hematologic:** Prolongation of bleeding time, thrombocytopenia, leukopenia, purpura, shortened erythrocyte survival time, decreased plasma iron levels. **Miscellaneous:** Thirst, fever, dimness of vision.

NOTE: Use of aspirin in children and teenagers with flu or chickenpox may result in the development of ***Reye's syndrome***. Also, dehydrated, febrile children are more prone to salicylate intoxication.

LABORATORY TEST CONSIDERATIONS

False + or ↑ : Amylase, AST, ALT, uric acid, PBI, urinary VMA (most tests), catecholamines, urinary glucose (Benedict's, Clinitest), and urinary uric acid (at high doses) values. False - or ↓ CO_2 content, glucose (fasting), potassium, urinary VMA (Pisano method), and thrombocyte values.

OD OVERDOSE MANAGEMENT

Symptoms of Mild Salicylate Toxicity (Salicylism): At serum levels between 150 and 200 mcg/mL. *GI:* N&V, diarrhea, thirst. *CNS:* Tinnitus (most common), dizziness, difficulty in hearing, mental confusion, lassitude. *Miscellaneous:* Flushing, sweating, tachycardia. Symptoms of salicylism may be observed with doses used for inflammatory disease or rheumatic fever. *Symptoms of Severe Salicylate Poisoning:* At serum levels over 400 mcg/mL. *CNS:* Excitement, confusion, disorientation, irritability, hallucinations, lethargy, stupor, ***coma, respiratory failure, seizures.*** *Metabolic:* Respiratory alkalosis (initially), respiratory acidosis and metabolic acidosis, dehydration. *GI:* N&V. *Hematologic:* Platelet dysfunction, hypoprothrombinemia, increased capillary fragility. *Miscellaneous:* ***Hyperthermia, hemorrhage, CV collapse, renal failure,*** hyperventilation, pulmonary edema, tetany, hypoglycemia (late).

Treatment (Toxicity):

1. If the client has had repeated administration of large doses of salicylates, document and report evidence of hyperventilation or complaints of auditory or visual disturbances (symptoms of salicylism).

2. Severe salicylate poisoning, whether due to overdose or accumulation, will have an exaggerated effect on the CNS and the metabolic system:

- Clients may develop a salicylate jag characterized by garrulous behavior. They may act as if they were inebriated.
- Convulsions and coma may follow.

3. When working with febrile children or the elderly who have been treated with aspirin, maintain adequate fluid intake. These clients are more susceptible to salicylate intoxication if they are dehydrated.

4. The following treatment approaches may be considered for treatment of *acute salicylate toxicity:*

- Initially induce vomiting or perform gastric lavage followed by activated charcoal (most effective if given within 2 hr of ingestion).
- Monitor salicylate levels and acid-base and fluid and electrolyte balance. If required, administer IV solutions of dextrose, saline, potassium, and sodium bicarbonate as well as vitamin K.

• Seizures may be treated with diazepam.
• Treat hyperthermia if present.
• Alkaline diuresis will enhance renal excretion. Hemodialysis is effective but should be reserved for severe poisonings.
• If necessary, administer oxygen and artificial ventilation

DRUG INTERACTIONS

Acetazolamide / ↑ CNS toxicity of salicylates; also, ↑ excretion of salicylic acid in alkaline urine
Alcohol, ethyl / ↑ Chance of GI bleeding caused by salicylates
Alteplase, recombinant / ↑ Risk of bleeding
Amino Salicylate / Possible ↑ effect of PAS due to ↓ excretion by kidney or ↓ plasma protein binding
Ammonium chloride / ↑ Effect of salicylates by ↑ renal tubular reabsorption
ACE inhibitors / ↓ Effect of ACE inhibitors possibly due to prostaglandin inhibition
Antacids / ↓ Salicylate levels in plasma due to ↑ rate of renal excretion
Anticoagulants, oral / ↑ Effect of anticoagulant by ↓ plasma protein binding and plasma prothrombin
Antirheumatics / Both are ulcerogenic and may cause ↑ GI bleeding
Ascorbic acid / ↑ Effect of salicylates by ↑ renal tubular reabsorption
Beta-adrenergic blocking agents / Salicylates ↓ action of beta-blockers, possibly due to prostaglandin inhibition
Charcoal, activated / ↓ Absorption of salicylates from GI tract
Corticosteroids / Both are ulcerogenic; also, corticosteroids may ↓ blood salicylate levels by ↑ breakdown by liver and ↑ excretion
Dipyridamole / Additive anticoagulant effects
H *Feverfew* / Possible ↑ antiplatelet effect
Furosemide / ↑ Risk of salicylate toxicity due to ↓ renal excretion; also, salicylates may ↓ effect of furosemide in clients with impaired renal function or cirrhosis with ascites
H *Garlic* / Possible ↑ antiplatelet effect
H *Ginkgo biloba* / Possible ↑ effect on platelet aggregation
H *Ginseng* / Possible ↓ effect on platelet aggregation
Griseofulvin / ↓ Salicylate levels
Heparin / Inhibition of platelet adhesiveness by aspirin may result in bleeding tendencies
Hypoglycemics, oral / ↑ Hypoglycemia R/T ↓ plasma protein binding and ↓ excretion
Indomethacin / Both are ulcerogenic → ↑ GI bleeding
Insulin / Salicylates ↑ hypoglycemic effect of insulin
Methionine / ↑ Effect of salicylates by ↑ renal tubular reabsorption
Methotrexate / ↑ Methotrexate effect by ↓ plasma protein binding; also, salicylates block drugs' renal excretion
Nitroglycerin / Combination may result in unexpected hypotension
Nizatidine / ↑ Serum levels of salicylates
NSAIDs / Additive ulcerogenic effects; also, aspirin may ↓ serum levels of NSAIDs
Phenytoin / ↑ Phenytoin effect by ↓ plasma protein binding
Probenecid / Salicylates inhibit uricosuric activity of probenecid
Sodium bicarbonate / ↓ Effect of salicylates by ↑ rate of excretion
Spironolactone / Aspirin ↓ diuretic drug effect
Sulfinpyrazone / Salicylates inhibit uricosuric drug activity
Sulfonamides / ↑ Sulfonamides effect by ↑ salicylate blood levels
Valproic acid / ↑ Valproic effect R/T ↓ plasma protein binding

HOW SUPPLIED

Acetylsalicylic Acid. *Chew tablet:* 81 mg; *Enteric coated tablet:* 81 mg, 165 mg, 325 mg, 500 mg, 650 mg, 975 mg; *Gum:* 227.5 mg; *Suppository:* 120 mg, 200 mg, 300 mg, 600 mg; *Tablet:* 325 mg, 500 mg; *Tablet, Delayed Release:* 81 mg; *Tablet, Extended Release:* 650 mg, 800 mg. **Acetylsalicylic Acid, Buffered. Caplets:** 325 mg; *Tablets:* 325 mg, 500 mg; *Tablets, Coated:* 325

mg, 500 mg; *Tablets, Effervescent:* 325 mg, 500 mg.

DOSAGE

• GUM, CHEWABLE TABLETS, COATED TABLETS, EFFERVESCENT TABLETS, ENTERIC-COATED TABLETS, SUPPOSITORIES, TABLETS DELAYED OR EXTENDED

Analgesic, antipyretic.

Adults: 325–500 mg q 3 hr, 325–600 mg q 4 hr, or 650–1,000 mg q 6 hr. As an alternative, the adult chewable tablet (81 mg each) may be used in doses of 4–8 tablets q 4 hr as needed. **Pediatric:** 65 mg/kg/day (alternate dose: 1.5 g/m^2/day) in divided doses q 4–6 hr, not to exceed 3.6 g/day. Alternatively, the following dosage regimen can be used: **Pediatric, 2–3 years:** 162 mg q 4 hr as needed; **4–5 years:** 243 mg q 4 hr as needed; **6–8 years:** 320–325 mg q 4 hr as needed; **9–10 years:** 405 mg q 4 hr as needed; **11 years:** 486 mg q 4 hr as needed; **12–14 years:** 648 mg q 4 hr.

Arthritis, rheumatic diseases.

Adults: 3.2–6 g/day in divided doses.

Juvenile rheumatoid arthritis.

60–110 mg/kg/day (alternate dose: 3 g/m^2) in divided doses q 6–8 hr. When initiating therapy at 60 mg/kg/day, dose may be increased by 20 mg/kg/day after 5–7 days and by 10 mg/kg/day after another 5–7 days.

Acute rheumatic fever.

Adults, initial: 5–8 g/day. **Pediatric, initial:** 100 mg/kg/day (3 g/m^2/day) for 2 weeks; **then,** decrease to 75 mg/kg/day for 4–6 weeks.

Reduce risk of death and nonfatal stroke following ischemic stroke or TIA

50–325 mg/day.

Reduce risk of vascular mortality in suspsected acute MI.

Initial: 160–162.5 mg, **then** daily for 30 days. Consider subsequent prophylactic therapy.

Reduce combined risk of recurrent MI and death in those with a previous MI or unstable angina or to reduce risk of MI and sudden death in those with chronic stable angina.

75–325 mg/day.

Pre-existing need for aspirin following coronary artery bypass grafting, PTCA, carotid endarterectomy.

Dosage varies by procedure.

Kawasaki disease.

Adults: 80–180 mg/kg/day during the febrile period. After the fever resolves, the dose may be adjusted to 10 mg/kg/day.

NOTE: Aspirin Regimen Bayer 81 mg with Calcium contains 250 mg calcium carbonate (10% of RDA) and 81 mg of acetylsalicylic acid for individuals who require aspirin to prevent recurrent heart attacks and strokes.

NURSING CONSIDERATIONS

SEE ALSO *NONSTEROIDAL ANTI-INFLAMMATORY DRUGS*

ADMINISTRATION/STORAGE

1. Enteric-coated tablets or buffered tablets are better tolerated by some.
2. Take with a full glass of water to prevent lodging of the drug in the esophagus.
3. Have epinephrine available to counteract hypersensitivity reactions should they occur. Asthma caused by hypersensitive reaction to salicylates may be refractory to epinephrine, so antihistamines should also be available for parenteral and PO use.

ASSESSMENT

1. Take a complete drug history and note any evidence of hypersensitivity. Individuals allergic to tartrazine should not take aspirin. Clients who have tolerated salicylates well in the past may suddenly have an allergic or anaphylactoid reaction.
2. If administered for pain, rate and determine the type and pattern of pain, if the pain is unusual, or if it is recurring. Note the effectiveness of aspirin if previously used for pain.
3. Note if client has asthma, hay fever, ulcer disease or nasal polyps.
4. Document age; drug is discouraged in those under 12. Assess for chickenpox or the flu.
5. Test stool and urine for blood; monitor CBC routinely during high-dose and chronic therapy.
6. Determine if diagnostic tests scheduled. Drug causes irreversible platelet effects. Anticipate 4–7 days for the body to replace these once drug discontinued; hence no salicylates one week prior to procedure.

A

7. Determine any history of peptic ulcers or bleeding tendencies. Obtain bleeding parameters with prolonged use.
8. Review drugs currently prescribed for drug interactions.
9. The therapeutic serum level of salicylate is 150–300 mcg/mL for adult and juvenile rheumatoid arthritis and acute rheumatic fever. Reassure that the higher dosage is necessary for anti-inflammatory effects.

CLIENT/FAMILY TEACHING

1. Take only as directed. To reduce gastric irritation or lodging in the esophagus, administer with meals, milk, a full glass of water, or crackers.
2. Do not take salicylates if product is off-color or has a strange odor. Note expiration date.
3. Report any toxic effects: ringing in the ears, difficulty hearing, dizziness or fainting spells, unusual increase in sweating, severe abdominal pain, or mental confusion.
4. Salicylates potentiate the effects of antidiabetic drugs. Monitor FS and report hypoglycemia.
5. When administering for antipyretic effect, follow temperature administration parameters.
• Obtain temperature 1 hr after administering to assess outcome.
• With marked diaphoresis, dry client, change linens, provide fluids, and prevent chilling.
6. Cardiac clients on large doses should report symptoms of CHF.
7. Tell dentist and other HCPs you are taking salicylates.
8. Before purchasing other OTC preparations, notify provider and note the quantity used per day.
9. Salicylates should be administered to children only upon specific medical recommendation due to increased risk of Reye's syndrome.
10. If child refuses medication or vomits it, consider aspirin suppositories or acetaminophen.
11. Children who are dehydrated and who have a fever are especially susceptible to aspirin intoxication from even small doses. Report any gastric irritation/pain; may be S&S of hypersensitivity or toxicity.
12. Sodium bicarbonate may decrease the serum level of aspirin, reducing its effectiveness.
13. Report any unusual bruising or bleeding. Large doses may increase PT and should be avoided. Aspirin and NSAIDs may interfere with blood-clotting mechanisms (antiplatelet effects) and are usually discontinued 1 week before surgery to prevent increased risk of bleeding.
14. Avoid indiscriminate use; store appropriately.

OUTCOMES/EVALUATE

• Relief of pain/discomfort; Improved joint mobility/function
• ↓ Fever; ↓ Vascular mortality
• Prophylaxis of MI/TIA

Atenolol

(ah-**TEN**-oh-lohl)

PREGNANCY CATEGORY: C
CLASSIFICATION(S):
Beta-adrenergic blocking agent
Rx: Tenormin
✱**Rx:** Apo-Atenol, Gen-Atenolol, Novo-Atenol, Nu-Atenol, PMS-Atenolol, Rhoxal-atenolol, Schein-pharm Atenolol, Tenolin

SEE ALSO *BETA-ADRENERGIC BLOCKING AGENTS.*

ACTION/KINETICS

Predominantly beta-1 blocking activity. Has no membrane stabilizing activity or intrinsic sympathomimetic activity. Low lipid solubility. **Peak blood levels:** 2–4 hr. **t½:** 6–9 hr. 50% eliminated unchanged in the feces.

USES

Hypertension (either alone or with other antihypertensives such as thiazide diuretics). Long-term treatment of angina pectoris due to coronary atherosclerosis. Acute MI. *Investigational:* Prophylaxis of migraine, alcohol withdrawal syndrome, situational anxiety, ventricular arrhythmias, prophylactically to reduce incidence of

A

supraventricular arrhythmias in coronary artery bypass graft surgery.

SPECIAL CONCERNS

Dosage not established in children.

HOW SUPPLIED

Injection: 0.5 mg/mL; *Tablet:* 25 mg, 50 mg, 100 mg

DOSAGE

• TABLETS

Hypertension.

Initial: 50 mg/day, either alone or with diuretics; if response is inadequate, 100 mg/day. Doses higher than 100 mg/day will not produce further beneficial effects. Maximum effects usually seen within 1–2 weeks.

Angina.

Initial: 50 mg/day; if maximum response is not seen in 1 week, increase dose to 100 mg/day (some clients require 200 mg/day).

Alcohol withdrawal syndrome.

50–100 mg/day.

Prophylaxis of migraine.

50–100 mg/day.

Ventricular arrhythmias.

50–100 mg/day.

Prior to coronary artery bypass graft surgery.

50 mg/day started 72 hr prior to surgery.

Adjust dosage in cases of renal failure to 50 mg/day if C_{CR} is 15–35 mL/min/1.73 m^2 and to 50 mg every other day if C_{CR} is less than 15 mL/min/1.73 m^2.

• IV

Acute myocardial infarction.

Initial: 5 mg over 5 min followed by a second 5-mg dose 10 min later. Begin treatment as soon as possible after client arrives at the hospital. In clients who tolerate the full 10-mg dose, give a 50-mg tablet 10 min after the last IV dose followed by another 50-mg dose 12 hr later. **Then,** 100 mg/day or 50 mg b.i.d. for 6–9 days (or until discharge from the hospital).

NURSING CONSIDERATIONS

SEE ALSO *NURSING CONSIDERATIONS FOR ANTIHYPERTENSIVE AGENTS AND BETA-ADRENERGIC BLOCKING AGENTS.*

ADMINISTRATION/STORAGE

1. For hemodialysis clients, give 25 or 50 mg in the hospital after each dialysis. Give under hospital supervision as significant decreases in BP may occur.

IV 2. For IV use, the drug may be diluted in NaCl injection, dextrose injection, or both.

3. If there is any question in using IV atenolol, eliminate IV administration and use tablets, 100 mg once daily or 50 mg b.i.d. for 7 or more days.

ASSESSMENT

1. Document indications for therapy, type, and onset of symptoms.

2. Note any history of diabetes, pulmonary disease, or cardiac failure.

CLIENT/FAMILY TEACHING

1. With angina, do not stop abruptly; may cause an anginal attack.

2. Report any changes in mood or affect, especially severe depression and/or fatigue.

3. May enhance sensitivity to cold.

4. With initiation of therapy or change in dosage stress importance of returning as scheduled for evaluation of drug response. Keep log of HR and BP.

OUTCOMES/EVALUATE

- ↓ BP; ↓ HR
- ↓ Frequency of anginal attacks
- Prevention of reinfarction

Atorvastatin calcium

(ah-**TORE**-vah-**stah**-tin)

PREGNANCY CATEGORY: X

CLASSIFICATION(S):

Antihyperlipidemic, HMG-CoA reductase inhibitor

Rx: Lipitor

SEE ALSO *ANTIHYPERLIPIDEMIC AGENTS—HMG-COA REDUCTASE INHIBITORS.*

ACTION/KINETICS

Undergoes first-pass metabolism to active metabolites. **t½:** 14 hr. Over 98% bound to plasma proteins. Plasma levels are not affected by renal disease but they are markedly increased with chronic alcoholic liver disease. Over 98% plasma-protein bound. Metabolized in the liver to active metabolites. Decreases in LDL cholesterol range from 35%–40% (10 mg/day) to 50%–60% (80 mg/day).

USES

(1) Adjunct to diet to decrease elevated total and LDL cholesterol, apo-B, and trigylceride levels and to increase HDL cholesterol in primary hypercholesterolemia (including heterozygous familial and nonfamilial) and mixed dyslipidemia (including Frederickson type IIa and IIb). (2) Adjunct to other lipid-lowering treatments to reduce total and LDL cholesterol in homozygous familial hypercholesterolemia. (3) Primary dysbetalipoproteinemia (Frederickson type III) in those not responding adequately to diet. (4) Adjunct to diet in elevated serum triglyceride levels (Frederickson type IV).

CONTRAINDICATIONS

Active liver disease or unexplained persistently high LFTs. Pregnancy, lactation.

SPECIAL CONCERNS

Safety and efficacy have not been determined in children less than 18 years of age.

SIDE EFFECTS

SEE ALSO *ANTIHYPERLIPIDEMIC AGENTS—HMG-CoA REDUCTASE INHIBITORS.*

GI: Altered LFTs (usually within the first 3 months of therapy), flatulence, dyspepsia. **CNS:** Headache, paresthesia, asthenia, insomnia. **Musculoskeletal:** Myalgia, leg pain, back pain, arthritis, arthralgia. **Respiratory:** Sinusitis, bronchitis, pharyngitis, rhinitis. **Miscellaneous:** Infection, rash, pruritus, allergy, influenza, accidental trauma, peripheral edema, chest pain, alopecia.

LABORATORY TEST CONSIDERATIONS

↑ CPK (due to myalgia).

ADDITIONAL DRUG INTERACTIONS

Antacids / ↓ Atorvastatin plasma levels

Colestipol / ↓ Atorvastatin plasma levels

Digoxin / ↑ Digoxin levels after 80 mg atorvastatin R/T ↑ digoxin absorption

Erythromycin / ↑ Atorvastatin plasma levels; possibility of severe myopathy or rhabdomyolysis

Oral contraceptives / ↑ Plasma levels of norethindrone and ethinyl estradiol

HOW SUPPLIED

Tablets: 10 mg, 20 mg, 40 mg, 80 mg

DOSAGE

• TABLETS

Hypercholesterolemias, homozygous familial hypercholesterolemia, dysbetalipoproteinemia, hypertriglyceridemia.

Initial: 10 mg/day; **then,** a dose range of 10–80 mg/day may be used.

NURSING CONSIDERATIONS

SEE ALSO *NURSING CONSIDERATIONS* FOR *ANTIHYPERLIPIDEMIC AGENTS—HMG-COA REDUCTASE INHIBITORS.*

ADMINISTRATION/STORAGE

1. Give as a single dose at any time of the day, with or without food.
2. Determine lipid levels within 2–4 weeks; adjust dosage accordingly.
3. For an additive effect, may be used in combination with a bile acid binding resin. Do not use atorvastatin with fibrates.

ASSESSMENT

1. Document indications for therapy, onset and duration of disease, and other agents and measures trialed.
2. Obtain baseline cholesterol profile and LFTs. Monitor LFTs at 6 and 12 weeks after starting therapy and with any dosage change then semiannually thereafter. If ALT or AST exceed 3 times the normal level, reduce dose or withdraw drug. Assess need for liver biopsy if elevations remain after stopping drug therapy.
3. Review dietary habits, weight, and exercise patterns; identify life-style changes needed.

CLIENT/FAMILY TEACHING

1. These drugs help to lower blood cholesterol and fat levels, which have been proven to promote CAD.
2. Drug may be taken with or without food.
3. Continue dietary restrictions of saturated fat and cholesterol, regular exercise and weight loss in the overall goal of lowering cholesterol levels.

A

See dietician for additional dietary recommendations.
4. Report immediately any unexplained muscle pain, weakness, or tenderness, especially if accompanied by fever or malaise.
5. Use UV protection (i.e., sunglasses, sunscreens, clothing/hat) to prevent photosensitivity.
6. Report for lab studies to evaluate effectiveness and need for dosage adjustments.

OUTCOMES/EVALUATE

Reduction in total and LDL cholesterol levels

Atovaquone

(ah-**TOV**-ah-kwohn)

PREGNANCY CATEGORY: C
CLASSIFICATION(S):
Antiprotozoal drug
Rx: Mepron

ACTION/KINETICS

The mechanism against *Pneumocystis carinii* is not known. However, in *Plasmodium,* appears to act by inhibiting electron transport resulting in inhibition of nucleic acid and ATP synthesis. The bioavailability is increased twofold when taken with food. Plasma levels in AIDS clients are about one-third to one-half the levels achieved in asymptomatic HIV-infected volunteers. **t ½:** 2.2 days in AIDS clients due to enterohepatic cycling and eventually fecal elimination. Not metabolized in the liver; over 94% is excreted unchanged in the feces.

USES

Acute oral treatment of mild to moderate *P. carinii* in clients who are intolerant to trimethoprim-sulfamethoxazole. Prophylaxis of *P. carinii* in clients intolerant to trimethoprim-sulfamethoxazole. Not effective for concurrent pulmonary diseases such as bacterial, viral, or fungal pneumonia or in mycobacterial diseases.

CONTRAINDICATIONS

Hypersensitivity to atovaquone or any components of the formulation; possible life-threatening allergic reactions.

SPECIAL CONCERNS

Use with caution during lactation, in elderly clients, and in severe hepatic impairment. Safety and efficacy have not been determined in children. GI disorders may limit absorption of atovaquone.

SIDE EFFECTS

Since many clients taking atovaquone have complications of HIV disease, it is often difficult to distinguish side effects caused by atovaquone from symptoms caused by the underlying medical condition.
GI: Nausea, diarrhea, vomiting, abdominal pain, constipation, dyspepsia, taste perversion. **CNS:** Headache, fever, insomnia, dizziness, anxiety, anorexia. **Dermatologic:** Rash (including maculopapular), pruritus. **Respiratory:** Cough, sinusitis, rhinitis. **Hematologic:** Anemia, neutropenia. **Miscellaneous:** Asthenia, oral monilia, pain, sweating, hypoglycemia, hyperglycemia, hypotension, hyponatremia, allergic reaction, infection.

LABORATORY TEST CONSIDERATIONS

↑ ALT, AST, alkaline phosphatase, amylase.

DRUG INTERACTIONS

Atovaquone is >99.9% bound to plasma proteins; use caution when given with other highly plasma protein-bound drugs with narrow therapeutic indices as competition for binding may occur.
Azithromycin / Possible ↓ peak serum levels of azithromycin in pediatric HIV-infected clients
Rifampin / Significant ↓ in average atovaquone steady-state plasma levels and ↑ in average rifampin steady-state plasma levels

HOW SUPPLIED

Suspension: 750 mg/5 mL

DOSAGE

• **SUSPENSION**

Treatment of mild to moderate Pneumocystis carinii *pneumonia.*
Adults and adolescents, 13–16 years of age: 750 mg (5 mL) given with food b.i.d. for 21 days (total daily dose: 1,500 mg).

Prevention of Pneumocystis carinii *pneumonia.*
Adults and adolescents, 13–16 years of age: 1,500 mg (10 mL) once daily with a meal.

NURSING CONSIDERATIONS

ADMINISTRATION/STORAGE

1. Failure to give with food may result in lower plasma levels and may limit the response to therapy.
2. Dispense drug in a well-closed container and store at 15–25°C (59–77°F). Do not freeze.

ASSESSMENT

1. Document previous therapy for *P. carinii,* drugs used, and results.
2. Assess baseline pulmonary status, CBC, and pulmonary culture results.
3. Clients with acute *P. carinii* must be carefully evaluated/screened for other related pulmonary diseases of viral, bacterial, or fungal origin and treated as indicated.

CLIENT/FAMILY TEACHING

1. This is not a cure but alleviates symptoms of *P. carinii.*
2. Take only as directed and with meals as food enhances absorption.
3. Review side effects noting those that require immediate reporting.
4. Do not exceed prescribed dose and do not share medication.
5. Continue precautions for safe sex; HIV transmission is not reduced.
6. Identify appropriate support groups and individuals to help understand and cope with disease.

OUTCOMES/EVALUATE

- Relief of symptoms R/T *P. carinii* three consecutive negative sputum cultures

Atracurium besylate

(ah-trah-**KYOUR**-ee-um)

PREGNANCY CATEGORY: C
CLASSIFICATION(S):
Skeletal muscle relaxant, nondepolarizing
Rx: Tracrium Injection

SEE ALSO *NEUROMUSCULAR BLOCKING AGENTS.*

ACTION/KINETICS
Prevents acetylcholine effects by competing for the cholinergic receptor at the motor end plate. May also release histamine, leading to hypotension. **Onset:** Within 2 min. **Peak effect:** 1–2 min. **Duration:** 20–40 min with balanced anesthesia. Recovery from blockade under balanced anesthesia begins about 20–35 min after injection; recovery is usually 95% complete within 60–70 min after injection. **t½:** 20 min. Recovery occurs more rapidly than recovery from *d*-tubocurarine, metocurine, and pancuronium. Metabolized in the plasma.

USES
Skeletal muscle relaxant during surgery; adjunct to general anesthesia; assist in ET intubation. *Investigational:* Treat seizures due to drugs or electrically induced.

CONTRAINDICATIONS
In clients with myasthenia gravis, Eaton-Lambert syndrome, electrolyte disorders, bronchial asthma.

SPECIAL CONCERNS
Use with caution during labor and delivery and when significant histamine release would be dangerous (e.g., CV disease, asthma). Safety and efficacy have not been determined during lactation. Children up to 1 month of age may be more sensitive to the effects of atracurium. No known effect on pain threshold or consciousness; use only with adequate anesthesia.

ADDITIONAL SIDE EFFECTS
CV: Flushing, tachycardia. *Dermatologic:* Rash, urticaria, reaction at injection site. *Musculoskeletal:* Prolonged block, inadequate block. *Respiratory:* Dyspnea, laryngospasm. *Hypersensitivity:* Allergic reactions. Other side effects may be due to histamine release and include flushing, erythema, wheezing, urticaria, bronchial secretions, BP and HR changes.

OD OVERDOSE MANAGEMENT
Symptoms: Hypotension, enhanced pharmacologic effects. *Treatment:* CV support. Ensure airway and ventila-

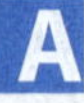

tion. An anticholinesterase reversing agent (e.g., neostigmine, edrophonium, pyridostigmine) with an anticholinergic agent (e.g., atropine, glycopyrrolate) may be used.

ADDITIONAL DRUG INTERACTIONS

Acetylcholinesterase inhibitors / Muscle relaxation is inhibited and neuromuscular block is reversed
Aminoglycosides / ↑ Muscle relaxation
Corticosteroids / Prolonged weakness
Enflurane / ↑ Muscle relaxation
Halothane / ↑ Muscle relaxation
Isoflurane / ↑ Muscle relaxation
Lithium / ↑ Muscle relaxation
Phenytoin / ↓ Effect of atracurium
Procainamide / ↑ Muscle relaxation
Quinidine / ↑ Muscle relaxation
Succinylcholine / ↑ Onset and depth of muscle relaxation
Theophylline / ↓ Effect of atracurium
Trimethaphan / ↑ Muscle relaxation
Verapamil / ↑ Muscle relaxation

HOW SUPPLIED

Injection: 10 mg/mL

DOSAGE

• **IV BOLUS ONLY**

Intubation and maintenance of neuromuscular blockade.

Adults and children over 2 years, initial: 0.4–0.5 mg/kg as IV bolus; **maintenance:** 0.08–0.1 mg/kg. The first maintenance dose is usually required 20–45 min after the initial dose. Give maintenance doses every 15–25 min under balanced anesthesia, slightly longer under isoflurane or enflurane anesthesia.

Following use of succinylcholine for intubation under balanced anesthesia.

Initial: 0.3–0.4 mg/kg; if using potent inhalation anesthetics, further reductions may be required.

Use in neuromuscular disease, severe electrolyte disorders, or carcinomatosis.

Consider dosage reductions where potentiation of neuromuscular blockade or difficulty with reversal have been noted.

Use after steady-state enflurane or isoflurane anesthesia established.

0.25–0.35 mg/kg (about ⅓ less than the usual initial dose).

Use in infants 1 month to 2 years of age under halothane anesthesia.

0.3–0.4 mg/kg. More frequent maintenance doses may be required.

• **IV INFUSION**

Balanced anesthesia.

IV infusion: 9–10 mcg/kg until the level of neuromuscular blockade is reestablished; **then,** rate of infusion is adjusted according to client needs (usually 5–9 mcg/kg/min although some clients may require as little as 2 mcg/kg/min and others as much as 15 mcg/kg/min).

For cardiopulmonary bypass surgery in which hypothermia is induced.

Reduce rate of infusion by 50%.

NURSING CONSIDERATIONS

SEE ALSO NURSING CONSIDERATIONS FOR NEUROMUSCULAR BLOCKING AGENTS.

ADMINISTRATION/STORAGE

IV 1. IM administration may cause tissue irritation.
2. Use only by those skilled in airway management and respiratory support. Equipment and personnel must be available immediately for intubation and support of ventilation. Have anticholinesterase reversal agents immediately available.
3. Reduce initial dose to 0.25–0.35 mg/kg if drug is being used with steady-state enflurane or isoflurane (smaller reductions with halothane).
4. Reduce dosage in clients with myasthenia gravis or other neuromuscular diseases, electrolyte disorders, or carcinomatosis.
5. Prepare infusion solutions by admixing atracurium with either D5W, 0.9% NaCL, or D5/0.9% NaCL. Do *not* mix with alkaline solutions, including LR injection.
6. Maintenance doses by continuous infusion of a diluted solution can be given to clients age 2 to adulthood.
7. Solutions containing 0.2 or 0.5 mg/mL can be stored either under refrigeration or at room temperature for 24 hr without significant loss of potency.
8. To preserve potency, refrigerate the drug at 2–8°C (36–46°F).

ASSESSMENT

1. Document indications for therapy, onset, duration, and characteristics of symptoms.

2. Utilize a peripheral nerve stimulator to assess neuromuscular response and recovery intraoperatively.
3. Obtain baseline ECG, VS, and lab studies and monitor. May cause vagal stimulation resulting in bradycardia, hypotension, and arrhythmias. IV atropine may be used to treat bradycardia.
4. Drug should only be used on a short-term basis and in a continuously monitored environment. Drug blocks the effect of acetylcholine at the myoneural junction thus preventing neuromuscular transmission.
5. Client may be fully conscious and aware of surroundings and conversations. Drug does not affect pain threshold or anxiety; administer analgesics and/or antianxiety agents regularly. Reassure that once drug wears off they may resume talking.

OUTCOMES/EVALUATE

- Skeletal muscle paralysis
- Facilitation of ET intubation; tolerance of mechanical ventilation
- Control of electrically/pharmacologically induced seizures

Atropine sulfate

(**AH**-troh-peen)

PREGNANCY CATEGORY: C
CLASSIFICATION(S):
Cholinergic blocking drug
Rx: Atropair, Atropine Sulfate Ophthalmic, Atropine-1 Ophthalmic, Atropine-Care Ophthalmic, Atropisol Ophthalmic, Isopto Atropine Ophthalmic
✽**Rx:** Minims Atropine

SEE ALSO *CHOLINERGIC BLOCKING AGENTS.*

ACTION/KINETICS

Blocks acetylcholine effects on postganglionic cholinergic receptors in smooth muscle, cardiac muscle, exocrine glands, urinary bladder, and the AV and SA nodes in the heart. Ophthalmologically, blocks acetylcholine effects on the sphincter muscle of the iris and the accommodative muscle of the ciliary body. This results in dilation of the pupil (mydriasis) and paralysis of the muscles required to accommodate for close vision (cycloplegia). **Peak effect:** *Mydriasis,* 30–40 min; *cycloplegia,* 1–3 hr. **Recovery:** Up to 12 days. **Duration, PO:** 4–6 hr. **t½:** 2.5 hr. Metabolized by the liver although 30%–50% is excreted through the kidneys unchanged.

USES

PO:
1. Adjunct in peptic ulcer treatment.
2. Relieve pylorospasm, small intestine hypertonicity, and colon hypermotility.
3. Relax biliary and ureteral colic spasm and bronchial spasms.
4. Decrease tone of the detrusor muscle of the urinary bladder in treating urinary tract disorders.
5. Preanesthetic to control salivation and bronchial secretions.
6. Control rhinorrhea of acute rhinitis or hay fever.
7. Has been used for parkinsonism but more effective drugs are available.

Parenteral:
1. Restore cardiac rate and arterial pressure during anesthesia when vagal stimulation, due to intra-abdominal surgical traction, causes a sudden decrease in pulse rate and cardiac action.
2. Decrease degree of AV heart block when increased vagal tone is a major factor in the conduction defect (e.g., due to digitalis).
3. Overcome severe bradycardia and syncope due to hyperactive carotid sinus reflex.
4. Relax upper GI tract and colon during hypertonic radiography.
5. Antidote (with external cardiac massage) for CV collapse from toxicity due to cholinergic drugs, pilocarpine, physostigmine, or isofluorophate.
6. Treat anticholinesterase poisoning from organophosphates; antidote for mushroom poisoning due to muscarine.
7. Control the crying and laughing episodes in clients with brain lesions.

A

8. To treat closed head injuries that cause acetylcholine to be released or be present in CSF, which causes abnormal EEG patterns, stupor, and neurological symptoms.
9. Relieve hypertonicity of uterine muscle.
10. As a preanesthetic or in dentistry to decrease secretions.

Ophthalmologic: Cycloplegic refraction or pupillary dilation in acute inflammatory conditions of the iris and uveal tract.

Investigational: Treatment and prophylaxis of posterior synechiae; pre- and postoperative mydriasis; treatment of malignant glaucoma.

ADDITIONAL CONTRAINDICATIONS

Ophthalmic use: Infants less than 3 months of age, primary glaucoma or a tendency toward glaucoma, adhesions between the iris and the lens, geriatric clients and others where undiagnosed glaucoma or excessive pressure in the eye may be present, in children who have had a previous severe systemic reaction to atropine.

SPECIAL CONCERNS

Use with caution in infants, small children, geriatric clients, diabetes, hypo- or hyperthyroidism, narrow anterior chamber angle, individuals with Down syndrome.

ADDITIONAL SIDE EFFECTS

Ophthalmologic: Blurred vision, stinging, increased intraocular pressure, contact dermatitis. Long-term use may cause irritation, photophobia, eczematoid dermatitis, conjunctivitis, hyperemia, or edema.

OD OVERDOSE MANAGEMENT

Treatment of Ocular Overdose: Eyes should be flushed with water or normal saline. A topical miotic may be necessary.

HOW SUPPLIED

Injection: 0.05 mg/mL, 0.1 mg/mL, 0.3 mg/mL, 0.4 mg/mL, 0.5 mg/mL, 0.8 mg/mL, 1 mg/mL; *Ophthalmic Ointment:* 1%; *Ophthalmic Solution:* 0.5%, 1%; *Tablet:* 0.4 mg

DOSAGE

- **TABLETS**

Anticholinergic or antispasmodic.

Adults: 0.3–1.2 mg q 4–6 hr. **Pediatric, over 41 kg:** same as adult; **29.5–41 kg:** 0.4 mg q 4–6 hr; **18.2–29.5 kg:** 0.3 mg q 4–6 hr; **10.9–18.2 kg:** 0.2 mg q 4–6 hr; **7.3–10.9 kg:** 0.15 mg q 4–6 hr; **3.2–7.3 kg:** 0.1 mg q 4–6 hr.

Prophylaxis of respiratory tract secretions and excess salivation during anesthesia.

Adults: 2 mg.

Parkinsonism.

Adults: 0.1–0.25 mg q.i.d.

- **IM, IV, SC**

Anticholinergic.

Adults, IM, IV, SC: 0.4–0.6 mg q 4–6 hr. **Pediatric, SC:** 0.01 mg/kg, not to exceed 0.4 mg (or 0.3 mg/m^2).

Treatment of toxicity from cholinesterase inhibitors.

Adults, IV, initial: 2–4 mg; **then,** 2 mg repeated q 5–10 min until muscarinic symptoms disappear and signs of atropine toxicity begin to appear. **Pediatric, IM, IV, initial:** 1 mg; **then,** 0.5–1 mg q 5–10 min until muscarinic symptoms disappear and signs of atropine toxicity appear.

Treatment of mushroom poisoning due to muscarine.

Adults, IM, IV: 1–2 mg q hr until respiratory effects decrease.

Treatment of organophosphate poisoning.

Adults, IM, IV, initial: 1–2 mg; **then,** repeat in 20–30 min (as soon as cyanosis has disappeared). Dosage may be continued for up to 2 days until symptoms improve.

Arrhythmias.

Pediatric, IV: 0.01–0.03 mg/kg.

Prophylaxis of respiratory tract secretions, excessive salivation, succinylcholine- or surgical procedure-induced arrhythmias.

Pediatric, up to 3 kg, SC: 0.1 mg; **7–9 kg:** 0.2 mg; **12–16 kg:** 0.3 mg; **20–27 kg:** 0.4 mg; **32 kg:** 0.5 mg; **41 kg:** 0.6 mg.

- **OPHTHALMIC SOLUTION**

Uveitis.

Adults: 1–2 gtt instilled into the eye(s) up to q.i.d. **Children:** 1–2 gtt of the 0.5% solution into the eye(s) up to t.i.d.

Refraction.
Adults: 1–2 gtt of the 1% solution into the eye(s) 1 hr before refracting. **Children:** 1–2 gtt of the 0.5% solution into the eye(s) b.i.d. for 1–3 days before refraction.
• **OPHTHALMIC OINTMENT**
Instill a small amount into the conjunctival sac up to t.i.d.

NURSING CONSIDERATIONS

SEE ALSO *NURSING CONSIDERATIONS* FOR *CHOLINERGIC BLOCKING AGENTS.*

ADMINISTRATION/STORAGE
1. After instillation of the ophthalmic ointment, compress the lacrimal sac by digital pressure for 1–3 min. to decrease systemic effects.
2. Have physostigmine available in the event of overdose.

ASSESSMENT
1. Document indications for therapy and any presenting symptoms.
2. Check for any history of glaucoma before ophthalmic administration; may precipitate an acute crisis.
3. Obtain VS and ECG; monitor CV status during IV therapy.

CLIENT/FAMILY TEACHING
1. When used in the eye, vision will be temporarily impaired. Close work, operating machinery, or driving a car should be avoided until drug effects have worn off.
2. Do not blink excessively; wait 5 min before instilling other drops.
3. Drug impairs heat regulation; avoid strenuous activity in hot environments; wear sunglasses.
4. Males with BPH may experience urinary retention and hesitancy.
5. Increase fluids and add bulk to diet to diminish constipating effects.
6. Use sugarless candies and gums to decrease dry mouth symptoms.

OUTCOMES/EVALUATE
• ↑ HR
• Desired pupillary dilatation
• ↓ GI activity; ↓ Salivation
• Reversal of muscarinic effects of anticholinesterase agents

Azathioprine

(ay-zah-**THIGH**-oh-preen)

PREGNANCY CATEGORY: D
CLASSIFICATION(S):
Immunosuppressant
Rx: Imuran
✱**Rx:** Alti-Azathioprine, Gen-Azathioprine

ACTION/KINETICS
Antimetabolite that is quickly split to form mercaptopurine. To be effective, must be given during the induction period of the antibody response. The precise mechanism in depressing the immune response is unknown, but it suppresses cell-mediated hypersensitivities and alters antibody production. Inhibits synthesis of DNA, RNA, and proteins and may interfere with meiosis and cellular metabolism. The mechanism for its effect on autoimmune diseases is not known. Is readily absorbed from the GI tract. The anuric client manifests increased effectiveness and toxicity (up to twofold). **Onset:** 6–8 weeks for rheumatoid arthritis. **t½:** 3 hr.

USES
As an adjunct to prevent rejection in renal homotransplantation. In adult clients meeting criteria for classic or definite rheumatoid arthritis as defined by the American Rheumatism Association. Restrict use to clients with severe, active, and erosive disease that is not responsive to conventional therapy. *Investigational:* Chronic ulcerative colitis, generalized myasthenia gravis, to control the progression of Behçet's syndrome (especially eye disease), Crohn's disease (low doses).

CONTRAINDICATIONS
Treatment of rheumatoid arthritis in pregnancy or in clients previously treated with alkylating agents. Pregnancy and lactation.

SPECIAL CONCERNS
Hematologic toxicity is dose-related and may occur late in the course of

A

therapy; may be more severe in renal transplant clients undergoing rejection. Although used in children, safety and efficacy have not been established.

SIDE EFFECTS

Hematologic: Leukopenia, thrombocytopenia, macrocytic anemia, ***severe bone marrow depression,*** selective erythrocyte aplasia. **GI:** N&V, diarrhea, abdominal pain, steatorrhea. **CNS:** Fever, malaise. **Other:** ***Increased risk of carcinoma,*** severe infections (fungal, viral, bacterial, and protozoal), and ***hepatotoxicity*** are major side effects. Also, skin rashes, alopecia, myalgias, increase in liver enzymes, hypotension, negative nitrogen balance.

OD OVERDOSE MANAGEMENT

Symptoms: Large doses may result in ***bone marrow hypoplasia,*** bleeding, infection, and death. *Treatment:* Approximately 45% can be removed from the body following 8 hr of hemodialysis.

DRUG INTERACTIONS

ACE inhibitors / ↑ Risk of severe leukopenia
Allopurinol / ↑ Azathioprine effects R/T ↓ liver breakdown
Anticoagulants / ↓ Anticoagulant effect
Corticosteroids / Possible muscle wasting after prolonged therapy
Cyclosporine / ↑ Plasma cyclosporine levels
H *Echinacea* / Do not give with azathioprine
Methotrexate / ↑ Plasma levels of the active metabolite, 6-mercaptopurine
Tubocurarine / ↓ Tubocurarine (and other nondepolarizing neuromuscular blocking agents) effects

HOW SUPPLIED

Powder For Injection: 100 mg (as sodium); *Tablet:* 50 mg

DOSAGE

• TABLETS, IV

Use in renal homotransplantation.

Adults and children, initial: 3–5 mg/kg (120 mg/m^2), 1–3 days before or on the day of transplantation; **maintenance:** 1–3 mg/kg (45 mg/m^2) daily.

Rheumatoid arthritis, SLE.

Adults and children, tablets, initial: 1 mg/kg (50–100 mg); **then,** increase dose by 0.5 mg/kg/day after 6–8 weeks and thereafter q 4 weeks, up to maximum of 2.5 mg/kg/day; **maintenance:** lowest effective dose. Dosage should be reduced in clients with renal dysfunction.

Myasthenia gravis.

2–3 mg/kg/day. However, side effects occur in more than 35% of clients.

To control progression of Behçet's syndrome.

2.5 mg/kg/day.

Crohn's disease.

75–100 mg/day.

NURSING CONSIDERATIONS

ADMINISTRATION/STORAGE

1. When used for rheumatoid arthritis, a therapeutic response may not be observed for 6–8 weeks.
2. May be discontinued abruptly, but delayed effects are possible.
3. When used with allopurinol, reduce dose of azathioprine by 25%–33% of the usual dose.
IV 4. Reconstitute drug (100 mg) with 10 mL of sterile water for injection and use within 24 hr. Further dilution with NSS or dextrose is usually made and infusion time ranges from 5 min to 8 hr.

ASSESSMENT

1. Document indications for therapy and include preassessment data.
2. Assess for drug interactions.
3. Monitor CBC, renal and LFTs. Observe for symptoms of bleeding abnormalities or hepatic dysfunction. Stop drug and report if jaundiced or abnormal LFTs.
4. Assess I&O and weigh daily. Report any decreases in urine volume, C_{CR} or oliguria; symptoms of kidney transplant rejection.

CLIENT/FAMILY TEACHING

1. If GI upset occurs, give in divided doses or take with food.
2. Take only as directed and do not skip or stop drug without approval; increase fluid intake.
3. Practice reliable contraception during and for 4 months following therapy.

4. Report any bruising, bleeding, S&S of infection, fever, rash, abdominal pain, yellow eyes or skin, itching, and/or clay-colored stools.
5. Must take this medication for life to prevent transplant rejection .
6. Avoid crowds or contact with any person who has taken oral poliovirus vaccine recently or persons with active infections.
7. When used for RA, improvement in joint pain, swelling, and stiffness may take 6–12 weeks. Client should be considered refractory if no beneficial effect is noted after 12 weeks.

OUTCOMES/EVALUATE

• Prevention of transplant rejection
• Suppression of cell-mediated immunity
• With RA ↓ joint pain and inflammation with improved mobility

Azelastine hydrochloride

PREGNANCY CATEGORY: C
CLASSIFICATION(S):
Antihistamine, second generation: phthalazinone
Rx: Astelin, Optivar

SEE ALSO *ANTIHISTAMINES.*

ACTION/KINETICS

Low to no sedation or anticholinergic activity.

USES

Nasal spray. Symptoms of seasonal allergic rhinitis, including rhinorrhea, sneezing, and nasal pruritis in adults and children 5 years and older. Symptoms of vasomotor rhinitis, including rhinorrhea, nasal congestion, and postnasal drip in adults and children 12 years and older. **Solution.** Itching of the eye associated with allergic conjunctivitis.

CONTRAINDICATIONS

Use to treat contact lens-related irritation.

SPECIAL CONCERNS

Use with caution during lactation. Safety and efficacy of the ophthalmic solution has not been determined in children less than 3 years of age.

SIDE EFFECTS

Nasal Spray.
CNS: Drowsiness, somnolence, headache, dizziness, fatigue, weight increase. **GI:** N&V. **Respiratory:** Dry mouth, nose, throat; pharyngitis, epistaxis. **Ophthalmic Solution. Ophthalmic:** Transient eye burning/stinging, conjunctivitis, eye pain, temporary blurring. **Respiratory:** Asthma, dyspnea, pharyngitis, rhinitis. **Miscellaneous:** Headache, bitter taste, fatigue, flu-like symptoms, pruritus.

HOW SUPPLIED

Nasal Spray: 137 mcg/spray; *Ophthalmic Solution:* 0.5 mg/mL

DOSAGE

• **NASAL SPRAY**
Seasonal allergic rhinitis.
Adults and children 12 years and older: 2 sprays per nostril b.i.d. **Children, 5–11 years:** 1 spray per nostril b.i.d.
Vasomotor rhinitis.
Adults and children 12 years and older: 2 sprays per nostril b.i.d.
• **OPHTHALMIC SOLUTION**
Allergic conjunctivitis.
Instill 1 gtt in each affected eye b.i.d.

NURSING CONSIDERATIONS

ADMINISTRATION/STORAGE

1. Before initial use, replace the screw cap with the pump unit. Prime the delivery system with 4 sprays or until a fine mist appears.
2. If 3 or more days elapse since last use, reprime the pump with 2 sprays or until a fine mist appears.
3. Do not spray in the eyes.
4. Advise those who wear soft contact lenses (and whose eyes are not red) to wait at least 10 min after instilling azelastine before inserting their lenses as the preservative, benzylkonium chloride, may be absorbed by the lenses.

CLIENT/FAMILY TEACHING

1. Before initial use, replace the screw cap with the pump unit. Prime the de-

A

livery system with 4 sprays or until a fine mist appears.
2. If 3 or more days elapse since last use, reprime the pump with 2 sprays or until a fine mist appears. Discard pump and delivery system after 3 mo.
3. Tilt head forward when instilling spray; do not spray in the eyes.
4. Advise those who wear soft contact lenses (and whose eyes are not red) to wait at least 10 min after instilling azelastine before inserting their lenses as the preservative, benzylkonium chloride, may be absorbed by the lenses.
5. Avoid driving or hazardous activities until drug effects realized.
6. Do not breast feed without medical clearance.

OUTCOMES/EVALUATE

Relief of seasonal allergic rhinitis/conjunctivitis

Azithromycin

(az-**zith**-roh-**MY**-sin)

PREGNANCY CATEGORY: B
CLASSIFICATION(S):
Antibiotic, macrolide
Rx: Zithromax
✱Rx: Z-Pak

ANTI-INFECTIVES

ACTION/KINETICS

A macrolide antibiotic derived from erythromycin. Acts by binding to the P site of the 50S ribosomal subunit and may inhibit RNA-dependent protein synthesis by stimulating the dissociation of peptidyl t-RNA from ribosomes. Rapidly absorbed and distributed widely throughout the body. Food increases the absorption of azithromycin. **Time to reach maximum concentration:** 2.2 hr. **t½, terminal:** 68 hr. A loading dose will achieve steady-state levels more quickly. Mainly excreted unchanged through the bile with a small amount being excreted through the kidneys.

USES

Adults: (1) Acute bacterial exacerbations of COPD due to *Hemophilus influenzae, Moraxella catarrhalis,* or *Streptococcus pneumoniae.* (2) Required initial IV therapy in community-acquired pneumonia (CAP) due to *S. pneumoniae, Chlamydia pneumoniae, Mycoplasma pneumoniae, H. influenzae, M. catarrhalis, Legionella pneumophila,* and *Staphylococcus aureus.* (3) Those who can take PO therapy in CAP due to *C. pneumoniae, M. pneumoniae, S. pneumoniae, or H. influenzae.* (4) PO for genital ulcer disease in men due to *Haemophilus ducreyi.* (5) Initial IV therapy in PID due to *Chlamydia trachomatis, Neisseria gonorrhoeae,* or *Mycoplasma hominis.* (6) As an alternative to first-line therapy to treat streptococcal pharyngitis or tonsillitis due to *Streptococcus pyogenes.* (7) PO for uncomplicated skin and skin structure infections due to *S. aureus, Staphyloccus pyogenes,* or *Streptococcus agalactiae.* Abscesses usually require surgical drainage. (8) PO for urethritis and cervicitis due to *C. trachomatis* or *N. gonorrhoeae.*

Children: (1) PO for acute otitis media due to *H. influenzae, M. catarrhalis,* or *S. pneumoniae* in children over 6 months of age. (2) PO for CAP due to *C. pneumoniae, H. influenzae, M. pneumoniae,* or *S. pneumoniae* in children over 6 months of age. (3) Pharyngitis/tonsillitis due to *S. pyogenes* in children over 2 years of age who cannot use first-line therapy.

Investigational: Uncomplicated gonococcal pharyngitis of the cervix, urethra, and rectum caused by *N. gonorrhoeae.* Gonococcal phayrngitis due to *N. gonorrhoeae.* Chlamydial infections due to *C. trachomatis.*

CONTRAINDICATIONS

Hypersensitivity to azithromycin, any macrolide antibiotic, or erythromycin. In clients who are not eligible for outpatient PO therapy (e.g., known or suspected bacteremia, immunodeficiency, functional asplenia, nosocomially acquired infections, geriatric or debilitated clients). Use with astemizole, cisapride, or pimozide.

SPECIAL CONCERNS

Use with caution in clients with impaired hepatic or renal function and during lactation. Safety and efficacy for acute otitis media have not been

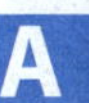

determined in children less than 6 months of age or for pharyngitis/tonsillitis in children less than 2 years of age.

SIDE EFFECTS

GI: N&V, diarrhea, loose stools, abdominal pain, dyspepsia, anorexia, gastritis, flatulence, melena, mucositis, oral moniliasis, taste perversion, cholestatic jaundice, pseudomembranous colitis. In children, gastritis, constipation, and anorexia have also been noted. **CNS:** Dizziness, headache, somnolence, fatigue, vertigo. In children, hyperkinesia, agitation, nervousness, insomnia, fever, and malaise have also been noted. **CV:** Chest pain, palpitations, ***ventricular arrhythmias (including ventricular tachycardia and torsades de pointes in clients with prolonged QT intervals observed with other macrolides).*** **GU:** Monilia, nephritis, vaginitis. **Allergic:** Angioedema, photosensitivity, rash, ***anaphylaxis.*** **Hematologic:** Leukopenia, neutropenia, decreased platelet count. **Miscellaneous:** Superinfection, bronchospasm, local IV site reactions. In children, pruritus, urticaria, conjunctivitis, and chest pain have been noted.

LABORATORY TEST CONSIDERATIONS

↑ Serum CPK, potassium, ALT, GGT, AST, serum alkaline phosphatase, bilirubin, BUN, creatinine, blood glucose, LDH, and phosphate.

DRUG INTERACTIONS

SEE ALSO *DRUG INTERACTIONS FOR ERYTHROMYCINS.*

Al– and Mg–containing antacids / ↓ Peak serum levels of azithromycin but not the total amount absorbed
Atovaquone / Possible ↓ peak serum levels of azithromycin in pediatric HIV-infected clients
Cyclosporine / ↑ Serum cyclosporine levels R/T ↓ metabolism → ↑ risk of nephrotoxicity and neurotoxicity
HMG-CoA reductase inhibitors / ↑ Risk of severe myopathy or rhabdomyolysis
Phenytoin / ↑ Serum phenytoin levels R/T ↓ metabolism
Pimozide / Possibility of sudden death

HOW SUPPLIED

Powder for Injection: 500 mg; *Powder for Oral Suspension:* 100 mg/5mL, 200 mg/5mL, 1 gm/packet; *Tablet:* 250 mg, 600 mg

DOSAGE

• SUSPENSION, TABLETS

Adults: Mild to moderate acute bacterial exacerbations of COPD, mild CAP, second-line therapy for pharyngitis/tonsillitis; uncomplicated skin and skin structure infections.

Adults and children over 16 years of age: 500 mg as a single dose on day 1 followed by 250 mg once daily on days 2–5 for a total dose of 1.5 g.

Nongonococcal urethritis and cervicitis due to C. trachomatis *or genital ulcer disease due to* H. ducreyi.

1 g given as a single dose.

Gonococcal urethritis/cervicitis due to N. gonorrhoeae.

2 g given as a single dose.

Uncomplicated gonococcal infections due to N. gonorrhoeae.

1 g given as a single dose plus a single dose of 400 mg PO cefixime, 125 mg IM ceftriaxone, 500 mg PO ciprofloxacin, or 400 mg PO ofloxacin.

Gonococcal pharyngitis.

1 g given as a single dose plus a single dose of 125 mg IM ceftriaxone, 500 mg ciprofloxacin, or 400 mg ofloxacin.

Chlamydial infections caused by C. trachomatis.

1 g given as a single dose.

• ORAL SUSPENSION

Pediatric: Otitis media or CAP.

10 mg/kg (not to exceed 500 mg) on day 1, followed by 5 mg/kg (not to exceed 250 mg/day) on days 2 through 5.

Pediatric: Pharyngitis/tonsillitis.

12 mg/kg once daily for 5 days, not to exceed 500 mg/day.

Chlamydial infections in children caused by C. trachomatis.

Children 45 kg or more and less than 8 years of age or over 8 years of age: 1 g given as a single dose.

• IV

CAP.

500 mg IV as a single daily dose for at least 2 days followed by a single daily

dose of 500 mg PO to complete a 7- to 10-day course of therapy.

PID.

500 mg IV as a single daily dose for 1 or 2 days followed by a single daily dose of 250 mg PO to complete a 7-day course of therapy.

NURSING CONSIDERATIONS

SEE ALSO *NURSING CONSIDERATIONS FOR ERYTHROMYCINS*.

ADMINISTRATION/STORAGE

1. Give suspension at least 1 hr prior to or at least 2 hr after a meal. Tablets may be taken with or without food, although increased tolerability increases with food. May be taken with milk.

IV 2. Infuse IV over 60 min or longer; do not give as a bolus or IM.

3. To obtain a concentration range of 1 to 2 mg/mL, transfer 5 mL of the 100-mg/mL solution into the appropriate amount of any of the following: 0.9% or 0.45% NaCl, D5W, RL solution, D5/0.45% NaCl with 20 mEq KCl, D5/RL solution, D5/0.3% NaCl, D5/0.45% NaCl, Normosol-M in D5%, or Normosol-R in D5%.

4. Infusion rate should be 1 mg/mL over 3 hr or 2 mg/mL over 1 hr.

5. The reconstituted solution for injection is stable for 24 hr if stored below 30°C (86°F) or for 7 days refrigerated at 5°C (41°F).

ASSESSMENT

1. Determine any history of sensitivity to erythromycins and note any previous therapy.

2. Determine other drugs prescribed; may cause an increase in serum concentrations of certain drugs (digoxin, carbamazepine, cyclosporine, dilantin).

3. Obtain documentation that clients with sexually transmitted cervicitis or urethritis are tested for gonorrhea and syphilis at the time of diagnosis. Ensure that appropriate drug therapy is instituted if necessary.

4. Obtain liver and renal function studies and cultures when warranted.

CLIENT/FAMILY TEACHING

1. Tablets may be taken with food or milk to improve tolerability. Food decreases absorption.

2. Avoid ingesting aluminum- or magnesium-containing antacids simultaneously with azithromycin.

3. Notify provider if N&V or diarrhea is excessive.

4. Avoid sun exposure and use protection when needed.

5. With STDs, encourage sexual partner to seek medical evaluation and treatment to prevent reinfections. Use condoms during intercourse throughout therapy.

OUTCOMES/EVALUATE

Resolution of S&S of infection; Negative cultures

Aztreonam for injection

(as-**TREE**-oh-nam)

PREGNANCY CATEGORY: B
CLASSIFICATION(S):
Antibiotic, monobactam
Rx: Azactam for Injection

SEE ALSO *ANTI-INFECTIVES*.

ACTION/KINETICS

Synthetic monobactam antibiotic. Bactericidal against gram-negative aerobic pathogens. Acts by inhibiting cell wall synthesis due to a high affinity of the drug for penicillin binding protein 3, resulting in cell lysis and death. Widely distributed to all body fluids. **Time to peak serum levels:** 0.6–1.3 hr. **t½:** 1.5–2 hr. (prolonged in clients with impaired renal function). Approximately 60%–75% excreted unchanged in the urine within 8 hr.

USES

(1) Complicated and uncomplicated UTIs (including pyelonephritis and cystitis) due to *Escherichia coli, Klebsiella pneumoniae, Proteus mirabilis, Pseudomonas aeruginosa, Enterobacter cloacae, Klebsiella oxytoca, Citrobacter* species, and *Serratia marcescens.* (2) Lower respiratory tract infections (including bronchitis and pneumonia) due to *E. coli, K. pneumoniae, P. aeruginosa, Hemophilus influenzae, P. mirabilis, Enterobacter* species, and *S. marcescens.* (3) Septicemia due to *E. coli, K. pneumoniae, P. aeruginosa, P. mirabilis,*

S. marcescens and *Enterobacter* species. (4) Skin and skin structure infections (including postoperative wounds, ulcers, and burns) caused by *E. coli, P. mirabilis, S. marcescens, Enterobacter* species, *P. aeruginosa, K. pneumoniae*, and *Citrobacter* species. (5) Intra-abdominal infections (including peritonitis) due to *E. coli, Klebsiella* species including *K. pneumoniae, Enterobacter* species including *E. cloacae, P. aeruginosa, Citrobacter* species including *C. freundii*, and *Serratia* species including *S. marcescens*. (6) Gynecologic infections (including endometritis and pelvic cellulitis) due to *E. coli, K. pneumoniae, P. mirabilis*, and *Enterobacter* species including *E. cloacae*.

As an adjunct to surgery to manage infections caused by susceptible organisms. As an alternative to spectinomycin in clients with acute uncomplicated gonorrhea who are resistant to penicillin. Concomitant initial therapy with other anti-infective drugs and aztreonam in seriously ill clients is recommended before the causative organism is known and who are at risk for an infection due to gram-positive aerobic pathogens.

CONTRAINDICATIONS

Allergy to aztreonam. Lactation.

SPECIAL CONCERNS

Safety and effectiveness have not been determined in infants less than 9 months of age or for use in children with septicemia or skin and skin-structure infections where the skin infection is due to *H. influenzae*, type b. Use with caution in clients allergic to penicillins or cephalosporins and in those with impaired hepatic or renal function.

SIDE EFFECTS

GI: N&V, diarrhea, abdominal cramps, mouth ulcers, numb tongue, halitosis, pseudomembranous colitis, *Clostridium difficile*-associated diarrhea or GI bleeding. **CNS:** Confusion, ***seizures,*** vertigo, headache, paresthesia, insomnia, dizziness. **Hematologic:** Anemia, neutropenia, thrombocytopenia, leukocytosis, thrombocytosis, pancytopenia, eosinophilia. **Dermatologic:** Rash, purpura, erythema multiforme, urticaria, petechiae, pruritus, diaphoresis, exfoliative dermatitis, ***toxic epidermal necrolysis.*** **CV:** Hypotension, transient ECG changes, flushing. *Following parenteral use:* Phlebitis and thrombophlebitis after IV use; discomfort and swelling at the injection site after IM use. **Allergic: *Anaphylaxis,*** angioedema, bronchospasm. **Miscellaneous:** Superinfection, weakness, fever, malaise, hepatitis, jaundice, muscle aches, tinnitus, diplopia, nasal congestion, altered taste, sneezing, vaginal candidiasis, vaginitis, breast tenderness, chest pain, dyspnea, wheezing.

LABORATORY TEST CONSIDERATIONS

↑ AST, ALT, alkaline phosphatase, serum creatinine, PT, PTT. Positive Coombs' test. Hepatobiliary dysfunction.

OD OVERDOSE MANAGEMENT

Treatment: Hemodialysis or peritoneal dialysis to reduce serum levels.

DRUG INTERACTIONS

Aminoglycosides / ↑ Risk of nephrotoxicity and ototoxicity
Cefoxitin / Inhibits aztreonam activity
Imipenem / Inhibits aztreonam activity

HOW SUPPLIED

Powder for injection (lyophilized cake): 500 mg, 1 g, 2 g

DOSAGE

- **IM, IV**

UTI's.

Adults: 0.5–1 g q 8–12 hr, not to exceed 8 g/day.

Mild to moderate infections in children.

Children: 30 mg/kg q 8 hr, not to exceed 120 mg/kg/day.

Moderate to severe systemic infections.

Adults: 1–2 g q 8–12 hr, not to exceed 8 g/day. **Children:** 30 mg/kg q 6– 8 hr, not to exceed 120 mg/kg/day.

Severe systemic or life-threatening infections.

2 g q 6–8 hr, not to exceed 8 g/day.

P. aeruginosa *infections in children.*

50 mg/kg q 4–6 hr.

NOTE: Reduce dose in impaired renal function.

NURSING CONSIDERATIONS

SEE ALSO *GENERAL NURSING CONSIDERATIONS FOR ANTI-INFECTIVES.*

ADMINISTRATION/STORAGE

1. Continue therapy for at least 48 hr after client becomes asymptomatic or until lab tests indicate infection eradicated.
2. For IM use, give drug in a large muscle mass.
3. Aztreonam is incompatible with cephradine, nafcillin sodium, and metronidazole.

IV 4. Use IV route for doses greater than 1 g or with septicemia.

5. For use as a bolus, dilute the 15-mL vial with 6–10 mL sterile water for injection. For IM use, dilute the 15-mL vial with at least 3 mL of either sterile water, NaCl injection, bacteriostatic water or bacteriostatic NaCl injection. Final dilution should not exceed 20 mg/mL.
6. An IV bolus injected slowly over 3–5 min may be used to initiate therapy. Give infusion over 20–60 min.
7. IV solutions prepared with 0.9% NaCl or D5% to which clindamycin, cefazolin, gentamicin, or tobramycin has been added are stable for 48 hr or less at room temperature or 7 days if refrigerated.

ASSESSMENT

1. Note any allergy to penicillins or cephalosporins.
2. Monitor CBC, liver and renal function studies; reduce dosage with impaired renal function.
3. Monitor renal and auditory function if used with an aminoglycoside (especially if high doses are used or if therapy is prolonged).

CLIENT/FAMILY TEACHING

1. During therapy an itchy, red rash and nasal congestion may occur.
2. A taste alteration may be experienced during IV therapy; report if eating is significantly impaired.

OUTCOMES/EVALUATE

Resolution of infecting organism; Symptomatic improvement

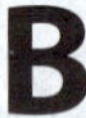

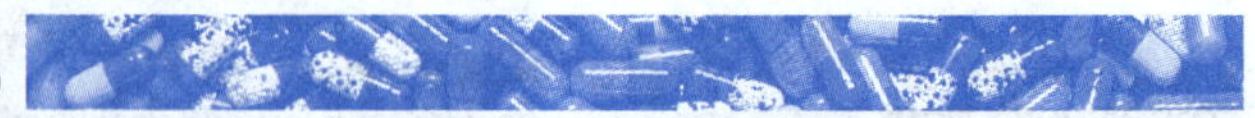

Bacampicillin hydrochloride

(bah-kam-pih-**SILL**-in)

PREGNANCY CATEGORY: B
CLASSIFICATION(S):
Antibiotic, penicillin
Rx: Spectrobid
✱Rx: Penglobe

SEE ALSO *ANTI-INFECTIVES AND PENICILLINS.*

ACTION/KINETICS

Semisynthetic, acid-resistant penicillin that is hydrolyzed to the active ampicillin in the GI tract. Food does not affect absorption. 98% absorbed from the GI tract and approximately 20% plasma protein bound. **Peak serum levels:** About 3 times equivalent doses of ampicillin after 0.9 hr. 75% excreted in the urine as active ampicillin within 8 hr.

USES

(1) Upper and lower respiratory tract infections (including acute exacerbations of chronic bronchitis) caused by beta-hemolytic streptococcus, *Staphylococcus pyogenes,* pneumococci, non-penicillinase-producing staphylococci, and *Haemophilus influenzae.* (2) UTIs caused by *Escherichia coli, Proteus mirabilis,* and *S. faecalis* (enterococci). (3) Skin and skin structure infections caused by streptococci and susceptible staphylococci. (4) Acute uncomplicated urogenital infections caused by *Neisseria gonorrhoeae.*

CONTRAINDICATIONS

History of penicillin allergy. Concomitant use with disulfiram (Antabuse).

LABORATORY TEST CONSIDERATIONS

False + reaction to Clinitest, Benedict's solution, and Fehling's solution. ↑ AST.

B

DRUG INTERACTIONS
Do not use concomitantly with disulfiram.
HOW SUPPLIED
Tablet: 400 mg; *Injection:* 0.3 mg/mL
DOSAGE
• **TABLETS**
Upper respiratory tract infections, otitis media, UTIs, skin and skin structure infections.
Adults: 400 mg q 12 hr; **pediatric, over 25 kg:** 25 mg/kg/day in equally divided doses q 12 hr. Dose may be doubled in cases of lower respiratory tract infections, severe infections, or in treating less susceptible organisms.
Gonorrhea.
Males and females: 1.6 g with 1 g probenecid as a single dose. No pediatric dosage has been established.

NURSING CONSIDERATIONS

SEE ALSO *GENERAL NURSING CONSIDERATIONS* FOR *ANTI-INFECTIVES*.
ADMINISTRATION/STORAGE
May be taken with meals.
CLIENT/FAMILY TEACHING
1. May take on an empty stomach or with meals.
2. Do not start disulfiram while taking bacampicillin.
3. Diabetics should monitor fingersticks to assess replacement needs.
4. With allopurinol therapy, report any skin rash.

OUTCOMES/EVALUATE
Resolution of infection; negative C&S results

Bacitracin intramuscular

(bass-ih-**TRAY**-sin)

PREGNANCY CATEGORY: C
Rx: Baci-IM

Bacitracin ointment

(bass-ih-**TRAY**-sin)

OTC: Baciguent

Bacitracin ophthalmic ointment

(bass-ih-**TRAY**-sin)

Rx: AK-Tracin
CLASSIFICATION(S):
Antibiotic, miscellaneous

SEE ALSO *ANTI-INFECTIVES*.
ACTION/KINETICS
Produced by *Bacillus subtilis*. Interferes with synthesis of cell wall, preventing incorporation of amino acids and nucleotides. Is bactericidal, bacteriostatic, and active against protoplasts. Not absorbed from the GI tract. When given parenterally, drug is well distributed in pleural and ascitic fluids. High nephrotoxicity. Systemic use is restricted to infants (see *Uses*). Carefully evaluate renal function prior to, and daily, during use. **Peak plasma levels: IM,** 0.2–2 mcg/mL after 2 hr. From 10% to 40% is excreted in the urine after IM administration.
USES
Parenteral: Limited to the treatment of staphylococcal-induced pneumonia or empyema in infants. **Topical:** Prophylaxis or treatment of infections in minor cuts, wounds, burns, and skin abrasions. As an aid to healing and for treating superficial infections of the skin due to susceptible organisms. **Ophthalmic:** Superficial ocular infections of the conjunctiva or cornea involving species of *Staphylococcus, S. aureus, Streptococcus, S. pneumoniae, S. pyogenes, Corynebacterium, Neisseria, N. gonorrhoeae,* and beta-hemolytic streptococci. Do not use topical antibiotics in deep-seated ocular infections or in those that are likely to become systemic.
CONTRAINDICATIONS
Hypersensitivity or toxic reaction to bacitracin. Pregnancy. Epithelial herpes simplex keratitis, vaccinia, varicella, mycobacterial eye infections, fungal diseases of the eye.

SPECIAL CONCERNS
Ophthalmic ointments may retard corneal epithelial healing. Prolonged or repeated use may result in bacterial or fungal overgrowth of nonsusceptible organisms leading to a secondary infection.

SIDE EFFECTS
• **PARENTERAL**
Nephrotoxicity due to tubular and glomerular necrosis, renal failure, toxic reactions, N&V.
• **TOPICAL**
Allergic contact dermatitis, superinfection.
• **OPHTHALMIC USE**
Transient burning, stinging, itching, irritation, inflammation, angioneurotic edema, urticaria, vesicular and maculopapular dermatitis.

DRUG INTERACTIONS
Aminoglycosides / Additive nephrotoxicity and neuromuscular blocking activity
Anesthetics / ↑ Neuromuscular blockade → possible muscle paralysis
Neuromuscular blocking agents / Additive neuromuscular blockade → possible muscle paralysis

HOW SUPPLIED
Bacitracin intramuscular: *Powder for Injection:* 50,000 U/vial; **Bacitracin ointment:** 500 U/g; **Bacitracin ophthalmic ointment:** 500 U/g

DOSAGE
• **IM ONLY**
Infants, 2.5 kg and below: 900 units/kg/day in two to three divided doses; **infants over 2.5 kg:** 1,000 units/kg/day in two to three divided doses.
• **OPHTHALMIC OINTMENT**
Acute infections.
½ in. in lower conjunctival sac q 3–4 hr until improvement occurs. Reduce treatment before the drug is discontinued.
Mild to moderate infections.
½ in. b.i.d.–t.i.d.
• **TOPICAL OINTMENT**
Apply a small amount equal to the surface area of a fingertip 1–3 times/day after cleaning the affected area. Do not use for more than 1 week.

NURSING CONSIDERATIONS

SEE ALSO *GENERAL NURSING CONSIDERATIONS FOR ANTI-INFECTIVES.*

ADMINISTRATION/STORAGE
1. When used IM, maintain adequate fluid intake either PO or parenterally.
2. Give IM in upper outer quadrant of buttocks; alternate sides and avoid multiple injections in the same region due to transient pain after injection.
3. To prepare for IM use, dissolve in NaCl injection containing 2% procaine HCl. Ensure the bacitracin concentration is not < 5,000 units/mL nor > 10,000 units/mL. Do not use diluents containing parabens. Reconstitution of the 50,000 unit vial with 9.8 mL of diluent results in a concentration of 5,000 units/ mL.
4. Refrigerate the unreconstituted drug at 2–8°C (36–46°F). Solutions are stable for 1 week if stored the same as the unreconstituted drug.
5. Do not mix bacitracin with glycerin or other polyalcohols that cause drug to deteriorate.
6. When used topically, the affected area may be covered with a sterile bandage.

ASSESSMENT
1. Document indications for therapy, type, onset, and duration of symptoms.
2. List any previous experiences with this type of infection (especially ocular), agents used, and results.
3. Recurrent ophthalmic infections should be cultured and carefully assessed by an ophthalmologist.

INTERVENTIONS
1. Monitor renal function studies and maintain adequate I&O with parenteral therapy.
2. Test urine pH daily; pH should be kept at 6 or greater to decrease renal irritation. Have $NaHCO_3$ or other alkali available if pH < 6.
3. Do not administer with a topical or systemic nephrotoxic drug.

CLIENT/FAMILY TEACHING
1. Apply as directed. Cleanse area thoroughly before applying bacitracin as a wet dressing or ointment.
2. Report any lack of response, rash, or unusual symptoms.

OUTCOMES/EVALUATE

- Resolution of S&S of infection
- Restoration of skin integrity

Baclofen

(**BAK**-low-fen)

PREGNANCY CATEGORY: C
CLASSIFICATION(S):
Skeletal muscle relaxant, centrally-acting
Rx: Lioresal
✱**Rx:** Apo-Baclofen, Gen-Baclofen, Lioresal Intrathecal, Liotec, Novo-Baclofen, Nu-Baclo, PMS-Baclofen

SEE ALSO *SKELETAL MUSCLE RELAXANTS, CENTRALLY ACTING.*

ACTION/KINETICS

Related chemically to GABA, an inhibitory neurotransmitter. May act by combining with the $GABA_B$ receptor subtype. It increases threshold for excitation of primary afferent nerves and decreases the release of excitatory amino acids from presynaptic sites. May also act at certain brain sites. Has CNS depressant effects. After PO use, baclofen is rapidly and extensively absorbed. **Peak serum levels, PO:** 2–3 hr. **Therapeutic serum levels:** 80–400 ng/mL. **t½, PO:** 3–4 hr. **Onset after intrathecal bolus:** 30–60 min; **peak effect after intrathecal bolus:** 4 hr; **duration after intrathecal bolus:** 4–8 hr. **t½ after bolus lumbar injection of 50 or 100 mcg:** 1.5 hr over the first 4 hr. **Onset after intrathecal continuous infusion:** 6–8 hr; **peak effect after intrathecal continuous infusion:** 24–48 hr. 70% to 80% is eliminated unchanged by the kidney.

USES

PO. Multiple sclerosis (flexor spasms, pain, clonus, and muscular rigidity) and diseases and injuries of the spinal cord associated with spasticity. Not effective for the treatment of cerebral palsy, stroke, parkinsonism, or rheumatic disorders. *Investigational:* Trigeminal neuralgia, tardive dyskinesia, intractable hiccoughs. **Intrathecal.** Severe spasticity of spinal cord of cerebral origin in clients unresponsive to PO baclofen therapy or who have intolerable CNS side effects. *Investigational:* Reduce spasticity in children with cerebral palsy.

CONTRAINDICATIONS

Hypersensitivity. PO to treat rheumatic disorders, spasm resulting from Parkinson's disease, stroke, cerebral palsy. Intrathecal product for IV, IM, SC, or epidural use.

SPECIAL CONCERNS

Use during lactation only if potential benefit outweighs the potential risk. Safe use of the oral product for children under 12 years of age and of the intrathecal product for children under 4 years of age not established. Use with caution in impaired renal function, in those with autonomic dysreflexia and where spasticity is used to sustain an upright posture and balance in locomotion; in those with psychotic disorders, schizophrenia, or confusional states as worsening of these conditions has occurred following PO use. Geriatric clients may be at higher risk for developing CNS toxicity, including mental depression, confusion, hallucinations, and significant sedation. Due to serious, life-threatening side effects after intrathecal use, physicians must be trained and educated in chronic intrathecal infusion therapy. Abrupt drug withdrawal may cause hallucinations and seizures.

SIDE EFFECTS

- **PO**

CNS: Drowsiness, dizziness, lightheadedness, weakness, lethargy, fatigue, confusion, headaches, insomnia, euphoria, excitement, depression, paresthesia, muscle pain, coordination disorder, tremor, ridigity, dystonia, ataxia, strabismus, dysarthria. Hallucinations following abrupt withdrawal. **CV:** Hypotension. Rarely, chest pain, syncope, palpitations. **GI:** N&V, constipation, dry mouth, anorexia, taste disorder, abdominal pain, diarrhea. **GU:** Urinary frequency, enuresis, urinary retention, dysuria, impotence, inability to ejaculate, nocturia.

B

Ophthalmic: Nystagmus, miosis, mydriasis, diplopia. **Miscellaneous:** Rash, pruritus, ankle edema, increased perspiration, weight gain, dyspnea, nasal congestion.

• **INTRATHECAL**

Spasticity of spinal origin.

CNS: Dizziness, somnolence, paresthesia, headache, ***convulsion,*** confusion, speech disorder, coma, ***death,*** insomnia, anxiety, depression, hallucinations. **GI:** N&V, constipation, dry mouth, diarrhea, anorexia. **GU:** Urinary retention, impotence, urinary incontinence, urinary frequency. **CV:** Hypotension, hypertension. **Miscellaneous:** Accidental injury, asthenia, amblyopia, pain, peripheral edema, dyspnea, hypoventilation, fever, urticaria, anorexia, diplopia, dysautonomia.

• **INTRATHECAL**

Spasticity of cerebral origin.

CNS: Somnolence, headache, ***convulsion,*** dizziness, paresthesia, abnormal thinking, agitation, coma, speech disorder, tremor. **GI:** N&V, increased salivation, constipation, dry mouth. **GU:** Urinary retention, urinary incontinence, impaired urination. **Miscellaneous:** Hypertonia, hypoventilation, hypotension, back pain, pain, pruritus, peripheral edema, asthenia, chills, pneumonia.

LABORATORY TEST CONSIDERATIONS

↑ AST, alkaline phosphatase, blood glucose.

OD OVERDOSE MANAGEMENT

Symptoms: Symptoms after PO use include vomiting, drowsiness, muscular hypotonia, muscle twitching, accommodation disorders, respiratory depression, seizures, coma. Symptoms after intrathecal use include drowsiness, dizziness, lightheadedness, somnolence, respiratory depression, rostral progression of hypotonia, ***seizures, loss of consciousness leading to coma (for up to 24 hr).***

Treatment:

1. After PO use:

• Induce vomiting (only if the client is alert and conscious) followed by gastric lavage.

• If the client is not alert and conscious, undertake only gastric lavage making sure the airway is secured with a cuffed ET tube.

• Maintain an adequate airway.

• Atropine may be used to improve HR, BP, ventilation, and core body temperature.

2. After intrathecal use:

• Remove residual solution from the pump as soon as possible.

• Intubate the client with respiratory depression until the drug is eliminated.

• IV physostigmine (total dose of 1–2 mg given over 5–10 min) may be tried, with caution.

• Can withdraw 30–60 mL of CSF to decrease baclofen levels (provided that lumbar puncture is not contraindicated).

DRUG INTERACTIONS

CNS depressants / Additive CNS depression

MAO Inhibitors / ↑ CNS depression and hypotension

Tricyclic antidepressants / Muscle hypotonia

HOW SUPPLIED

Kit: 0.05 mg/mL, 0.5 mg/mL, 2 mg/mL; *Tablet:* 10 mg, 20 mg

DOSAGE

• **TABLETS**

Muscle relaxant, spasticity.

Adults, initial: 5 mg t.i.d. for 3 days; **then,** 10 mg t.i.d. for 3 days, 15 mg t.i.d. for 3 days, and 20 mg t.i.d. for 3 days. Additional increases in dose may be required but do not exceed 20 mg q.i.d. **Children (treatment of spasticity), initial:** 10–15 mg/kg/day in 3 divided doses. Titrate to a maximum of 40 mg/day if less than 8 years of age and to a maximum of 80 mg/day if more than 8 years of age.

Trigeminal neuralgia.

50–60 mg/day.

Tardive dyskinesia.

40 mg/day used in combination with neuroleptics.

• **INTRATHECAL**

Initial screening bolus.

50 mcg/mL given into the intrathecal space by barbotage over a period of not less than 1 min. The client is observed for 4–8 hr for a positive response consisting of a decrease in muscle tone, frequency, and/or sever-

ity of muscle spasms. If the response is not adequate, a second bolus dose of 75 mcg/1.5 mL, 24 hr after the first bolus dose, can be given with the client observed for 4–8 hr. If the response is still inadequate, a final bolus screening dose of 100 mcg/2 mL can be given 24 hr later.

Postimplant dose titration.
To determine the initial daily dose of baclofen following the implant for intrathecal use, double the screening dose that gave a positive response and give over a 24-hr period. However, if the effectiveness of the bolus dose lasted for more than 12 hr, the daily dose should be the same as the screening dose but delivered over a period of 24 hr. After the first 24 hr, the dose can be increased slowly by 10%–30% increments only once each 24 hr until the desired effect is reached.

Maintenance therapy.
The maintenance dose may need to be adjusted during the first few months of intrathecal therapy. The daily dose may be increased by 10% to no more than 40% daily. If side effects occur, the daily dose may be decreased by 10%–20%. Daily doses for long-term continuous infusion have ranged from 12 to 1,500 mcg (usual maintenance is 300-800 mcg/day). Use the lowest dose producing optimal control.

Reduce spasticity of cerebral palsy in children.
25, 50, or 100 mcg.

NURSING CONSIDERATIONS

SEE ALSO *NURSING CONSIDERATIONS* FOR *SKELETAL MUSCLE RELAXANTS*, .

ADMINISTRATION/STORAGE

1. If beneficial effects are not noted, withdraw the drug slowly.
2. Check the manufacturer's manual for specific instructions and precautions for programming the implantable intrathecal infusion pump and refilling the reservoir.
3. Prior to intrathecal implantation of the pump, clients must show a positive response to a bolus dose of baclofen in a screening trial.
4. If there is not a significant clinical response to increases in the daily dose given intrathecally, check the pump for proper function and the catheter for patency.
5. During long-term intrathecal treatment, approximately 10% of clients become tolerant to increasing doses. If this occurs, a drug "holiday" consisting of a gradual decrease of intrathecal baclofen over a 2-week period can be considered. Alternate methods to treat spasticity must be undertaken. After a few days, sensitivity to baclofen may return. However, to avoid possible side effects or overdose, discontinue alternative medication slowly.
6. Filling of the reservoir for intrathecal use must be performed by fully trained/qualified personnel. Refill intervals must be carefully calculated to avoid reservoir depletion.
7. Use extreme caution when filling an FDA-approved implantable pump equipped with an injection port (i.e., that allows direct access to the intrathecal catheter). Direct injection into the catheter through the access port may result in a life-threatening overdose of baclofen.
8. For screening purposes, intrathecal baclofen, either 10 mg/20 mL or 10 mg/5 mL, must be diluted with sterile preservative-free NaCl for injection, to a concentration of 50 mcg/mL for bolus administration. For maintenance, baclofen must be diluted with sterile preservative-free NaCl for injection USP for clients who require concentrations other than 500 mcg/mL (i.e., the 10 mg/20 mL product) or 2,000 mcg/mL (i.e., the 10 mg/5 mL product).

ASSESSMENT

1. Document indications for therapy; note pretreatment findings.
2. With epilepsy assess for clinical S&S of disease. Obtain EEG at regular intervals to assess for reduced seizure control.
3. Obtain initial renal and LFTs.
4. Note if client has diabetes.

5. Clients must be closely monitored in a fully equipped and staffed facility during both the intrathecal screening phase and dose-titration period following the intrathecal implant. Resuscitative equipment should be readily available.
6. Ensure client is free from S&S of infection. Systemic infection may alter response to screening trials and (during pump implantation) may lead to surgical complications and interfere with the pump dosing rate.
7. Assess for level of useful spasticity (e.g., to aid in transfers or to maintain posture) as rigidity is important for gait in some clients.
8. In those who require hypertonicity to stand upright, to maintain balance when walking, or to increase functionality, baclofen may be contraindicated because it interferes with this coping mechanism.

INTERVENTIONS

1. Note any evidence of hypersensitivity reaction and report.
2. Monitor urine output; test for blood.
3. If improvement in condition does not occur within 6–8 weeks, the drug should be withdrawn gradually.
4. For clients with an intrathecal pump:
• Calculate pump refill interval to prevent an empty reservoir and return of severe spasticity.
• Access the pump reservoir percutaneously. Refill and program by one specifically trained in this procedure.
• When filling pumps with injection ports permitting direct access to the catheter, use care as an injection directly into the catheter can cause a lethal overdose. In this event, immediately remove any residual drug from the pump and follow guidelines for Treatment under Overdose Management.
• When the dose requirements suddenly escalate, assess for catheter kinks or dislodgement.
• When programming for increased dosage, e.g., at bedtime, the flow rate should be programmed to change 2 hr before desired effect.

CLIENT/FAMILY TEACHING

1. Take oral medication with meals or a snack to avoid gastric irritation. Report if GI S&S are severe/ persistent.
2. To prevent constipation, increase fluids and roughage in diet.
3. It may take several weeks of therapy before improvement occurs.
4. Monitor and record weight and I&O; note frequency and amount of each voiding; report any edema.
5. May alter insulin requirements.
6. Report impotence as a change of drug or dosage may be required. Do not stop abruptly.
7. With the intrathecal pump:
• Once screening trials completed, the "baclofen pump" will be surgically placed in the abdominal wall and attached to an implanted lumbar intrathecal catheter. Demonstrate proper postop site care and review S&S of infection that require immediate reporting.
• Maintain a log identifying when the spasms are greatest. This facilitates proper pump programming to ensure optimal control of spasticity and discomfort.
• Identify symptoms that require immediate medical intervention.
• Report as scheduled (usually monthly with maintenance) to ensure proper reservoir drug levels and to prevent loss of effect or air entering the reservoir.
• Drowsiness, dizziness, and lower extremity weakness may occur; report if persistent or progressive as dose may require adjustment.
• Those who become refractory to increasing doses may require hospitalization for a "drug holiday." This would consist of a *gradual reduction* of intrathecal baclofen over a 2-week period and alternative therapy with other agents. Sensitivity to baclofen usually returns after several days and may be resumed intrathecally at the initial continuous dose.

OUTCOMES/EVALUATE

• Improved muscle tone and involuntary movements; ↓ muscle spasticity and pain
• ↓ Painful/disabling symptoms permitting ↑ functioning level

B

Balsalazide disodium

(bal-**SAL**-ah-zide)

PREGNANCY CATEGORY: B
CLASSIFICATION(S):
Ulcerative colitis drug
Rx: Colazal

ACTION/KINETICS
Delivered intact to the colon where it is cleaved by bacteria to release equimolar amounts of mesalamine, which is the active portion of 4-aminobenzoyl-β-alanine. Exact mechanism unknown but the drug may act locally to diminish inflammation by blocking production of arachidonic acid metabolites in the colon. Absorption is low and variable. Metabolites and parent drug are mainly excreted in the feces.

USES
Treatment of mild to moderately active ulcerative colitis.

CONTRAINDICATIONS
Hypersensitivity to salicylates, components of balsalazide capsules, or balsalazide metabolites.

SPECIAL CONCERNS
Use with caution in those with known renal dysfunction, history of renal disease, and during lactation. Those with pyloric stenosis may have prolonged gastric retention of balsalazide capsules. Safety and efficacy have not been determined in children.

SIDE EFFECTS
GI: N&V, diarrhea, abdominal pain, rectal bleeding, flatulence, dyspepsia, frequent stools, dry mouth, constipation, cramps, bowel irregularity, aggravated ulcerative colitis, diarrhea with blood, diverticulosis, epigastric pain, eructation, fecal incontinence, abnormal feces, gastroenteritis, giardiasis, glossitis, hemorrhoids, melena, benign neoplasm, pancreatitis, ulcerative stomatitis, tenemus, tongue discoloration. **CNS:** Headache, insomnia, dizziness, aphasia, dysphonia, abnormal gait, hypertonia, hypoesthesia, paresis, generalized spasm, tremor, anxiety, depression, nervousness, somnolence. **CV:** Bradycardia, DVT, hypertension, leg ulcer, palpitations, pericarditis. **Respiratory:** Respiratory infection, rhinitis, pharyngitis, coughing, sinusitis, bronchospasm, dyspnea, hemoptysis. **Dermatologic:** Alopecia, angioedema, dermatitis, dry skin, erythema nodosum, erythematous rash, pruritus, pruritus ani, psoriasis, skin ulceration. **Hematologic:** Anemia, eosinophilia, granulocytopenia, leukocytosis, leukopenia, lymphadenopathy, lymphoma-like disorder, lymphopenia. ***hemorrhage***, thrombocytopenia. **GU:** Menstrual disorder, hematuria, interstitial nephritis, micturition frequency, polyuria, pyuria. **Musculoskeletal:** Myalgia, arthritis, arthropathy, leg stiffness. **Ophthalmic:** Conjunctivitis, iritis, abnormal vision. **Otic:** Earache/infection, tinnitus. **Body as a whole:** Fatigue, fever, pain, back pain, myalgia, flu-like disorder, viral infection, asthenia, chills, edema, hot flushes, malaise. **Miscellaneous:** Epistaxis, abnormal hepatic function, abscess, infection, moniliasis, weight increase/decrease, parosmia, taste perversion, enlarged abdomen, chest pain.

LABORATORY TEST CONSIDERATIONS
↑ Bilirubin, AST, ALT, creatine phosphokinase, LDH, plasma fibrinogen. Hypocalcemia, hypokalemia, hypoproteinemia. Increased/decreased prothrombin.

HOW SUPPLIED
Capsule: 750 mg

DOSAGE

• **CAPSULES**

Ulcerative colitis.

Three 750 mg capsules t.i.d. (total daily dose of 6.75 g) for 8 weeks. Some require treatment for 12 weeks or less. Safety and efficacy beyond 12 weeks have not been determined.

NURSING CONSIDERATIONS

ASSESSMENT

1. Note other agents used and the outcome.
2. Document character/frequency of stools. Assess abdomen for bowel sounds, distension, pain/tenderness.

3. Monitor CBC, LFTs, and renal function studies.

CLIENT/FAMILY TEACHING

1. Take exactly as directed (3 capsules 3x per day) to control bowel movements.
2. Practice reliable contraception and avoid therapy if nursing.
3. May experience headaches, N&V, diarrhea, abdominal pain and fatigue; report if persistent.
4. Report prolonged abdominal pain, yellowing of eyes or skin as drug may cause liver toxicity. Obtain blood tests and colon studies as scheduled and have regular F/U with provider.

OUTCOMES/EVALUATE

Control of abnormal/frequent liquid stools with ulcerative colitis

Basiliximab

(**bah**-zih-**LIX**-ih-mab)

PREGNANCY CATEGORY: B
CLASSIFICATION(S):
Immunosuppressant
Rx: Simulect

ACTION/KINETICS

An interleukin-2 (IL-2) receptor antagonist which is a monoclonal antibody produced by recombinant DNA technology. Acts as immunosuppressant by binding to and blocking the IL-2 receptor α-chain which is selectively expressed on the surface of activated T-lymphocytes. This competitively inhibits IL-2-mediated activation of lymphocytes which is a critical pathway in the cellular immune response involved in allograft rejection. To be effective, serum levels must exceed 0.2 mcg/mL. At the recommended dosing regimen, the mean duration of basiliximab saturation of IL-2Rα was 36 days. **t½, terminal, adults and adolescents:** 7.2 days; **t½, terminal, children:** 11.5 days.

USES

Prophylaxis of acute organ rejection in renal transplantation, including children. Used as part of an immunosuppresive regimen that includes cyclosporine and corticosteroids.

CONTRAINDICATIONS

Lactation.

SPECIAL CONCERNS

Increased risk for developing opportunistic infections and lymphoproliferative disorders. Possible severe acute hypersensitivity reactions within 24 hr of use with both first and subsequent doses.

SIDE EFFECTS

The incidence of side effects following basiliximab is no greater than placebo groups; however, 99% of clients in both groups reported side effects. Those with an incidence of 3% or greater are listed.

GI: Constipation, N&V, diarrhea, abdominal pain, dyspepsia, moniliasis, enlarged abdomen, flatulence, GI disorder, gastroenteritis, GI hemorrhage, gum hyperplasia, melena, esophagitis, ulcerative stomatitis. **CNS:** Headache, tremor, dizziness, insomnia, hypoesthesia, neuropathy, paresthesia, agitation, anxiety, depression. **CV:** Angina pectoris, cardiac failure, chest pain, abnormal heart sounds, aggravated hypertension, hypotension, arrhythmia, atrial fibrillation, tachycardia, vascular disorder. **GU:** Dysuria, UTI, impotence, genital edema, bladder disorder, hematuria, frequent micturition, oliguria, abnormal renal function, renal tubular necrosis, ureteral disorder, urinary retention. **Respiratory:** Dyspnea, URTI, coughing, rhinitis, pharyngitis, bronchitis, bronchospasm, abnormal chest sounds, pneumonia, pulmonary disorder, pulmonary edema, sinusitis. **Dermatologic:** Surgical wound complications, acne, cysts, herpes simplex, herpes zoster, hypertrichosis, pruritus, rash, skin disorder, skin ulceration. **Musculoskeletal:** Leg pain, back pain, arthralgia, arthropathy, bone fracture, cramps, hernia, myalgia. **Hematologic:** Hematoma, anemia, ***hemorrhage,*** purpura, thrombocytopenia, thrombosis, polycythemia. **Metabolic:** Acidosis, weight increase, dehydration, diabetes mellitus, fluid overload. **Ophthalmic:** Cataract, conjunctivitis, abnormal vision. **Miscellaneous:** Pain, peripheral edema, fever, viral infection, leg edema, asthenia, accidental trauma, chest pain, increased drug level, face edema, fatigue, infection, malaise, generalized edema, rigors, ***sepsis, hypersensitivity reactions (including anaphylaxis).***

LABORATORY TEST CONSIDERATIONS

↑ NPN, glucocorticoids. Albuminuria, hyper/hypokalemia, hyper/hypoglycemia, hyperuricemia, hypophosphatemia, hyper/hypocalcemia, hyperlipemia, hypercholesterolemia, hypoproteinemia, hypomagnesemia.

DRUG INTERACTIONS

H Do not give echinacea with basiliximab.

HOW SUPPLIED

Powder for injection: 20 mg

DOSAGE

• IV INFUSION, CENTRAL OR PERIPHERAL ONLY IV bolus

Prevent kidney transplant rejection.

Adults: Two 20-mg doses; give the first 20 mg within 2 hr prior to transplant surgery and the second 20 mg dose 4 days after transplantation. **Children, < 35 kg:** Two doses of 10 mg each. **Children, 35 kg and higher:** Two doses of 20 mg each. Space the doses as in adults. Withhold the second dose if complications occur (e.g., severe hypersensitivity).

NURSING CONSIDERATIONS

ADMINISTRATION/STORAGE

IV 1. To reconstitute, add 5 mL of sterile water for injection to the powder vial (20 mg/5 mL). Shake gently to dissolve.

2. After reconstitution, the solution should be colorless and clear to opalescent. If particulate matter is present or the solution is colored, do not use.

3. The reconstituted solution is isotonic. May be given as a bolus injection or diluted to a volume of 50 mL with NSS or D5W and infused over 20–30 min.

4. Do not add or infuse other drugs simultaneously through the same IV line.

5. Use the reconstituted solution immediately. If not used immediately, store at 2–8°C (36–46°F) for 24 hr or at room temperature for 4 hr. Discard if not used within 24 hr.

ASSESSMENT

1. Drug is used in conjunction with cyclosporine and corticosteroids.

2. Given as 2 doses: infuse the first dose 2 hr prior to transplant surgery and then give the 2nd dose 4 days after transplantation.

3. Assess carefully for any evidence of infection. Monitor labs and serum drug levels.

INTERVENTIONS

1. Have medications available for immediate use for treatment of hypersensitivity reactions.

2. Withhold the second dose if hypersensitivity reactions occur.

OUTCOMES/EVALUATE

• Prophylaxis of renal transplant rejection

• Serum drug levels of >0.2 mcg/mL

BCG, Intravesical

PREGNANCY CATEGORY: C

CLASSIFICATION(S):

Antineoplastic, miscellaneous

Rx: TheraCys, TICE BCG

ACTION/KINETICS

BCG promotes a local acute inflammatory and subacute granulomatous reaction with macrophage and lymphocyte infiltration in the urothelium and lamina propria of the urinary bladder. Precise mechanism is unknown but the anti-tumor effect seems to be T-lymphocyte dependent.

USES

Treatment and prophylaxis of carcinoma in situ (CIS) of the urinary bladder. Prophylaxis of primary or recurrent stage Ta and/or T1 papillary tumors after transurethral resection. Intravesical use to treat CIS in the absence of an associated invasive cancer of the bladder in the following situations: (1) primary treatment of CIS with or without papillary tumors after transurethral resection; (2) secondary treatment of CIS in those failing to respond or relapsing after intravesical therapy with other agents; (3) primary or secondary

B

treatment of CIS for those with medical contraindications to radical surgery.

CONTRAINDICATIONS

TheraCys, TICE BCG: Stage TaG1 papillary tumors unless there is a high risk of tumor recurrence. Positive Mantoux test, unless there is evidence of an active TB infection. Active tuberculosis. Use as an immunizing agent to prevent TB. Use in presence of a urinary tact infection or fever. Lactation. **TheraCys:** Immunosuppressed clients with congenital or acquired immune deficiencies, whether due to concurrent disease (e.g., AIDS, leukemia, lymphoma), cancer therapy (e.g., cytotoxic drugs, radiation), or immunosuppressive therapy (e.g., corticosteroids) due to the possibility of a systemic BCG infection. **TICE BCG:** Papillary tumors of stages higher than T1; concurrent infections.

SPECIAL CONCERNS

BCG contains live, attenuated mycobacteria; there is the potential risk for transmission; thus, prepare, handle, and dispose of as a biohazardous material. BCG infection of aneurysms and prosthetic devices is possible, although risk is small. Safety and efficacy have not been established in children.

SIDE EFFECTS

GU: Dysuria, cystitis, urinary urgency/frequency, hematuria, nocturia, urinary incontinence, UTI, foreign material in urine, renal toxicity, genital pain, contracted bladder, genital inflammation/abscess. **GI:** Diarrhea, N&V, anorexia, weight loss. **Hematologic:** Anemia, leukopenia, coagulopathy. **Musculoskeletal:** Arthralgia, myalgia, arthritis, rigors. **Respiratory:** Pulmonary infection. **Body as a whole:** Fever, flu-like symptoms, chills, malaise, fatigue, allergy, systemic infection, hypersensitivity reactions. **Miscellaneous:** Abdominal pain, cramps/pain, liver involvement, cardiac involvement, headache, dizziness, skin rash.

DRUG INTERACTIONS

Antimicrobial therapy / Possible interference with effectiveness of TICE BCG

Bone marrow depressants / Possible impaired response to BCG

Immunosuppressants / Possible impaired response to BCG

Radiation / Possible impaired response to BCG

HOW SUPPLIED

Powder for suspension, lyophilized: 1–8 x 10^8 CFU (TICE BCG), 10.5 +/- 8.7 x 10^8 CFU (TheraCys)

DOSAGE

• INTRAVESICALLY

Carcinoma in situ of the urinary bladder.

Allow 7–14 days to elapse if bladder catheterization has been traumatic or after bladder biopsy or transurethral resection before giving BCG. TheraCys: Instill 81 mg BCG (dry weight) into the bladder once a week for 6 weeks. Follow with maintenance therapy, consisting of 1 dose given at 3, 6, 12, 18, and 24 months after initial treatment. *TICE BCG:* One vial (about 50 mg) suspended in 50 mL preservative-free saline and instilled into the bladder once a week for 6 weeks. Schedule may be repeated if tumor remission has not been achieved. For both products, retain in bladder for 2 hr and then void in a seated position to avoid splashing of urine.

NURSING CONSIDERATIONS

ADMINISTRATION/STORAGE

1. Product contains viable attenuated mycobacteria. Handle as a biohazardous substance. Use aseptic technique. If the product can not be prepared in a biocontainment hood, the person preparing the product should wear gloves, mask, and gown to avoid inadvertant exposure to broken skin or inhalation of BCG organisms. Product should not be handled by individuals with an immunologic deficiency.

2. Reconstitute and dilute immediately before use. Any delay between reconstitution and administration must not exceed 2 hr.

3. For *TheraCys*, do not remove the rubber stopper from the vial. Reconstitute the contents of 1 vial with 3 mL of diluent provided. Shake gently until a fine, even suspension results. Further dilute in an additional 50 mL of sterile, preservative free saline provided to a final volume of 53 mL.

4. For *TICE BCG,* draw 1 mL of sterile preservative-free 0.9% NaCl into a small (e.g., 3 mL) syringe. Add to 1 vial of TICE BCG to resuspend. Gently swirl the vial until a homogenous suspension is obtained. Dispense the cloudy BCG suspension into the top end of a catheter-tip syringe containing 49 mL of sterile, preservative-free 0.9% NaCl. Gently rotate the syringe. Do not filter the contents.
5. Client should not drink fluids for 4 hr before treatment. Empty bladder prior to instillation.
6. Instill the suspension into the bladder slowly by gravity flow, via the catheter. Do not force the flow.
7. During the first hour following instillation, have the client lie for 15 min each in the prone and supine positions and on each side. Client can then be up but must retain the suspension for another hr (i.e., total of 2 hr).
8. Maintain adequate hydration.
9. After usage, place all equipment and materials used for product instillation into the bladder into plastic bags labeled "Infectious Waste" and dispose of properly as biohazardous waste.
10. Disinfect urine voided for 6 hr after instillation with an equal volume of 5% sodium hypochlorite solution (undiluted household bleach) and allow to stand for 15 min before flushing.

ASSESSMENT

1. Determine symptom onset, TUR, and staging results.
2. Avoid in immunocompromised individuals.
3. Handle and mix carefully away from other parental drugs, as drug contamination may occur.
4. Dispose of all equipment used to administer product according to institutional guidelines for hazardous waste.

CLIENT/FAMILY TEACHING

1. Drug is used to treat bladder cancer. It contains a viable mycobacteria and should be handled as a biohazard as it can make others ill.
2. Do not drink fluids for 4 hr before treatment. Empty bladder prior to instillation. Retain for 2 hr in the bladder before expelling.
3. Sit on toilet seat and void to prevent splashing. Disinfect urine for up to 6 hr after instillation with equal volumes of bleach; wait 15 min before flushing to ensure deactivation of bacteria.
4. Report any increase in symptoms associated with blood in the urine, rash, fever/chills, increased frequency/urgency, painful urination, or flu-like symptoms.
5. Any development of cough after BCG treatment requires immediate reporting as this may signal a toxic systemic infection.
6. Report as scheduled for F/U evaluations and cystogram to evaluate drug response.

OUTCOMES/EVALUATE

Control/resolution of bladder cancer

Becaplermin

(beh-**KAP**-ler-min)

PREGNANCY CATEGORY: C
CLASSIFICATION(S):
Topical drug, wound healing
Rx: Regranex

ACTION/KINETICS

Topical recombinant human platelet-derived growth factor. Promotes chemotactic recruitment and proliferation of cells involved in wound repair and enhances formation of granulation tissue.

USES

As adjunct to good ulcer care practices to treat lower extremity diabetic neuropathic ulcers that extend into SC tissue or beyond and have adequate blood supply. Use for diabetic neuropathic ulcers that do not extend through dermis into SC tissue or ischemic ulcers has not been studied.

CONTRAINDICATIONS

Known neoplasms at application site. Use in wounds that close by primary intention.

B

SPECIAL CONCERNS
Effect on exposed joints, tendons, ligaments, and bone has not been established. Use with other topical drugs has not been studied. Use with caution during lactation. Safety and efficacy have not been determined in children less than 16 years of age.
SIDE EFFECTS
General: Infection, cellulitis, osteomyelitis, erythematous rashes.
HOW SUPPLIED
Gel: 0.01%

DOSAGE
• **GEL, 0.01%**
Lower extremity diabetic neuropathic ulcers.
Dose depends on size of ulcer area. To determine length of gel to be applied, measure greatest length of ulcer by greatest width of ulcer in either inches or centimeters. To calculate length of gel in inches:
7.5 g or 15 g tube: length x width x 0.6
2 g tube: length x width x 1.3
Generally, each square inch of ulcer surface will require about ⅔ inch from 7.5 g or 15 g tube and about 1¼ inches from 2 g tube.
To calculate length of gel in centimeters:
7.5 g or 15 g tube: length x width divided by 4
2 g tube: length x width divided by 2
Generally, each square centimeter of ulcer surface will require about 0.25 cm of gel from 7.5 or 15 g tube or about 0.5 cm of gel from 2 g tube. Calculate amount to be applied at weekly or biweekly intervals depending on rate of change in ulcer area.

NURSING CONSIDERATIONS
ADMINISTRATION/STORAGE
1. Squeeze calculated length of gel onto a clean measuring surface (e.g., wax paper). Gel is transferred from clean measuring surface using an application aid and then spread over entire ulcer area. This should yield thin continuous layer of about 1/16 inch thickness.
2. Cover site with saline moistened dressing; leave in place for 12 hr.
3. Remove dressing after 12 hr and rinse ulcer with saline or water to remove residual gel. Cover again with second moist dressing without gel for remainder of day.
4. Apply once daily until complete ulcer healing has occurred.
5. If ulcer does not decrease in size by about 30% after 10 weeks of therapy or complete healing has not occurred in 20 weeks, reassess treatment.
6. Refrigerate gel but do not freeze. Do not use gel after expiration date at bottom of tube.

ASSESSMENT
1. Document onset, duration, size, and characteristics of area requiring treatment. May record initial wound assessment with photographs.
2. Assess area to ensure it is free from infection, cellulitis, rash, and osteomyelitis.
3. Ensure client is enrolled in active wound management program with ongoing debridement, relief of pressure (e.g., wheel chair, wedge shoe), systemic management of infections, and moist dressings changed b.i.d.

CLIENT/FAMILY TEACHING
1. Wash hands before application.
2. Apply gel with cotton swab or tongue depressor; do not let tube tip come in contact with wound or skin surfaces and cap tightly.
3. Squeeze calculated length of gel on firm, dry, surface. Spread gel over area requiring treatment and cover with saline moistened gauze dressing.
4. Gently rinse wound after 12 hr with saline or water to remove gel; cover wound with saline moistened dressing.
5. Report any changes in wound that resemble infection, such as purulent drainage, odor, swelling, redness, or increased pain.

OUTCOMES/EVALUATE
Regranulation with desired wound healing.

Beclomethasone dipropionate
(be-kloh-**METH**-ah-zohn)

PREGNANCY CATEGORY: C

CLASSIFICATION(S):
Glucocorticoid
Rx: Aerosol Inhaler: QVAR, Vanceril, Vanceril Double Strength. **Nasal Spray:** Beconase, Beconase AQ Nasal, Vancenase, Vancenase AQ 84 mcg, Vancenase Pockethaler
✱Rx: Apo-Beclomethasone, Nu-Beclomethasone, Rivanase AQ. **Aerosol Inhaler:** Alti-Beclomethasone Inhalation Aerosol. **Nasal Spray:** Alti-Beclomethasone Aqueous Suspension, Gen-Beclo Aq. **Topical:** Propaderm

SEE ALSO *CORTICOSTEROIDS*.

ACTION/KINETICS

t½, after intranasal: 0.5 hr. **t½, after inhalation:** 2.8 hr. Rapidly inactivated by the liver, resulting in few systemic effects. Excreted in the feces and urine.

USES

Relief of symptoms of seasonal or perennial rhinitis in clients not responsive to more conventional therapy and to prevent recurrence of nasal polyps following surgical removal. *Spray formulations:* to treat allergic or nonallergic (vasomotor) rhinitis.

Inhalation therapy for chronic asthma. *Vanceril Aerosol:* Only for those who require chronic steroid treatment for bronchial asthma. QVAR, *Vanceril Double Strength:* Prophylaxis of asthma for clients aged 12 and over who require systemic corticosteroids and where adding an inhaled corticosteroid may reduce or eliminate the need for systemic corticosteroids.

CONTRAINDICATIONS

Status asthmaticus, acute episodes of asthma, hypersensitivity to drug or aerosol ingredients.

SPECIAL CONCERNS

Safe use during lactation and in children under 6 years of age not established.

SIDE EFFECTS

Intranasal: Headache, pharyngitis, coughing, epistaxis, nasal burning, pain, conjunctivitis, myalgia, tinnitus. Rarely, ulceration of the nasal mucosa and nasal septum perforation.

HOW SUPPLIED

Aerosol Inhaler: 40 mcg/inh, 42 mcg/inh, 80 mcg/inh, 84 mcg/inh; *Nasal Spray:* 0.042%, 0.084%

DOSAGE

• AEROSOL INHALER (METERED DOSE)

Asthma, chronic.

QVAR: **Adults and children over 12 years of age:** If previous therapy was bronchodilators alone, start with 40–80 mcg b.i.d. The highest recommended dose is 320 mcg b.i.d. If previous therapy was inhaled corticosteroids, start with 40–160 mcg b.i.d. The highest recommended dose is 320 mcg b.i.d. *Vanceril:* **Adults:** Usually, 2 inhalations (84 mcg) t.id. or q.i.d. In some, 4 inhalations (168 mcg) b.i.d. has been effective. In those with severe asthma, start with 12–16 inhalations/day and adjust dose downward, depending on the response. Do not exceed 20 inhalations (840 mcg)/day in adults. **Children, 6–12 years of age:** Usually, 1–2 inhalations (42–84 mcg) t.i.d. or q.i.d. Alternative dose: 4 inhalations (168 mcg) b.i.d. Do not exceed 10 inhalations (420 mcg)/day in children. Insufficient information is available for use in children less than 6 years of age. *Vanceril Double Strength:* **Adults:** 2 inhalations (168 mcg) b.i.d. In those with severe asthma, start with 6–8 inhalations/day and adjust dose downward, depending on response. Do not exceed 10 inhalations/day (840 mcg) in adults. **Children, 6–12 years of age:** 2 inhalations (168 mcg) b.i.d. Do not exceed 5 inhalations/day (420 mcg) in children. Insufficient information is available for use in children less than 6 years of age. In clients also receiving systemic glucocorticosteroids, follow above dosage.

• NASAL AEROSOL OR SPRAY

Allergic or nonallergic rhinitis, prophylaxis of nasal polyps.

Adults and children over 12 years. *Beconase, Vancenase:* 1 inhalation (42 mcg) in each nostril b.i.d.–q.i.d. (i.e., total daily dose: 168–336 mcg). Clients can be maintained on a maxi-

B

mum dose of 1 inhalation in each nostril t.i.d. (252 mcg/day). *Beconase AQ:* 1 or 2 inhalations (42–84 mcg) in each nostril b.i.d. (168–336 mcg/day). *Vancenase Pockethaler:* 1 inhalation (42 mcg) in each nostril b.i.d.–q.i.d. (total dose of 168–336 mcg/day). **Maintenance:** 1 inhalation in each nostril t.i.d. (252 mcg/day).

Children 6–12 years: *Beconase, Vancenase:* 1 inhalation in each nostril t.i.d. (252 mcg/day). Do not use in children less than 6 years of age. *Beconase AQ:* Initially, 1 inhalation in each nostril b.i.d. Those not responding to 168 mcg or those with more severe symptoms may use 2 inhalations in each nostril b.i.d. (total of 336 mcg). Do not use in children less than 6 years of age. *Vancenase Pockethaler:* 1 inhalation in each nostril t.i.d. (252 mcg/day). Do not use in children less than 6 years of age.

Adults and children 6 years of age and older: *Vancenase AQ:* 1 or 2 inhalations in each nostril once daily (total dose of 168–336 mcg/day) at regular intervals. Not recommended for children less than 6 years of age.

NOTE: For nasal use, symptoms usually improve in a few days but relief may not be seen in some clients for up to 2 weeks. Do not continue therapy beyond 3 weeks if symptoms do not improve. For nasal polyps treatment may be required for several weeks or more before a beneficial result can be assessed. Recurrence of nasal polyps can occur after stopping treatment.

NURSING CONSIDERATIONS

SEE ALSO *NURSING CONSIDERATIONS* FOR *CORTICOSTEROIDS*.

ADMINISTRATION/STORAGE

1. To prevent explosion of contents under pressure, do not store or use near heat or open flame, or throw into a fire or incinerator. Keep secure from children.
2. If the canister is cold, the therapeutic effect may be decreased. Shake well before using.
3. Once canister is removed from the moisture-protected package, use within 6 months.
4. If a client is on systemic steroids, transfer to beclomethasone may be difficult because recovery from impaired renal function may be slow.

ASSESSMENT

1. Note any sensitivity to corticosteroids or fluorocarbon propellants.
2. Document indications for therapy, presenting symptoms, PFTs and pulmonary findings.

CLIENT/FAMILY TEACHING

1. Review use, care, and storage of inhaler. Rinse out mouth and wash mouth piece, spacer, sprayer; dry after each use.
2. A spacer may facilitate oral administration. With nasal administration aim toward the outer eye and not the inside nose to decrease nasal irritation. Review video/instruction to ensure proper use.
3. To administer with an inhaler:
   - Shake metal canister thoroughly immediately prior to use.
   - Exhale as completely as possible.
   - Place the mouthpiece of the inhaler/spacer into the mouth and tighten lips around it.
   - Inhale deeply through the mouth while pressing the metal canister down with forefinger.
   - Hold breath as long as possible.
   - Remove mouthpiece.
   - Exhale slowly.
   - A minimum of 60 sec must elapse between inhalations.
4. Inhaler is not to be used for acute asthma attacks but should be used regularly to prevent attacks.
5. Follow prescribed therapy; may take 1–4 weeks for any improvement to be realized.
6. To check inhaler content, may place in a glass of water: full inhalers sink, empty inhalers float, and half-full inhalers are partially submerged.
7. Report signs of adrenal insufficiency (i.e., muscular pain, lassitude, and depression) even if respiratory function has improved. Symptoms such as hypotension and weight loss are indications that the dosage of systemic steroid should be boosted temporarily, and then withdrawn more gradually.
8. More than 1 mg in adults or more than 500 mcg in children may precipi-

tate hypothalamic-pituitary axis depression, resulting in adrenal insufficiency. Do not overuse inhaler or exceed prescribed dosage.
9. Report immediately any symptoms of localized oral infections. Gargling and rinsing after treatments, rinsing of the spacer and/or administration port may help prevent infections. May require antifungal meds and possibly discontinuation of drug.
10. If also receiving bronchodilators by inhalation (i.e., Albuterol) use the bronchodilator first to open the airways and then use beclomethasone. This increases penetration of steroid and reduces toxicity from inhaled fluorocarbon propellants of both inhalers.
11. For those receiving systemic steroid therapy, initiate beclomethasone therapy *very* slowly, withdrawing the systemic steroids as ordered. The benefit of inhaled steroids is that a much lower dose, since it goes to the target organ and does not require weaning. Once systemic steroid is withdrawn, keep a supply of PO glucocorticoids and take immediately if subjected to unusual stress.
12. Carry ID with diagnosis, treatment, and possible need for systemic glucocorticoids, in the event of exposure to unusual stress.
13. Identify/practice relaxation techniques during stressful situations.

OUTCOMES/EVALUATE

- Control of asthma
- Relief of rhinitis
- Prophylaxis of nasal polyp recurrence

Benazepril hydrochloride

(beh-**NAYZ**-eh-prill)

PREGNANCY CATEGORY: D
CLASSIFICATION(S):
Antihypertensive, ACE inhibitor
Rx: Lotensin

SEE ALSO *ANGIOTENSIN-CONVERTING ENZYME INHIBITORS.*

ACTION/KINETICS
Both supine and standing BPs are reduced with mild-to-moderate hypertension and no compensatory tachycardia. Also an antihypertensive effect in clients with low-renin hypertension. Food does not affect the extent of absorption. Almost completely converted to the active benazeprilat, which has greater ACE inhibitor activity. **Onset:** 1 hr. **Duration:** 24 hr. **Peak plasma levels, benazepril:** 30–60 min. **Peak plasma levels, benazeprilat:** 1–2 hr if fasting and 2–4 hr if not fasting. **t½, benazeprilat:** 10–11 hr. **Peak reduction in BP:** 2–4 hr after dosing. **Peak effect with chronic therapy:** 1–2 weeks. Highly bound to plasma protein and excreted through the urine with about 20% of a dose excreted as benazeprilat.

USES
Alone or in combination with thiazide diuretics to treat hypertension.

CONTRAINDICATIONS
Hypersensitivity to benazepril or any other ACE inhibitor.

SPECIAL CONCERNS
Use with caution during lactation. Safety and effectiveness have not been determined in children.

SIDE EFFECTS
CNS: Headache, dizziness, fatigue, anxiety, insomnia, drowsiness, nervousness. **GI:** N&V, constipation, abdominal pain, gastritis, melena, pancreatitis. **CV:** Symptomatic hypotension, postural hypotension, syncope, angina pectoris, palpitations, peripheral edema, ECG changes. **Dermatologic:** Flushing, photosensitivity, pruritus, rash, diaphoresis. **GU:** Decreased libido, impotence, UTI. **Respiratory:** Cough, asthma, bronchitis, dyspnea, sinusitis, bronchospasm. **Neuromuscular:** Paresthesias, arthralgia, arthritis, asthenia, myalgia. **Hematologic:** Occasionally, eosinophilia, leukopenia, neutropenia, decreased hemoglobin. **Miscellaneous:** Angioedema, which may be associated with involvement of the tongue, glottis, or larynx, hypertonia, proteinuria, hyponatremia, infection.

LABORATORY TEST CONSIDERATIONS
↑ Serum creatinine, BUN, serum potassium. ↓ Hemoglobin. ECG changes.

DRUG INTERACTIONS
Diuretics / Excessive ↓ in BP
Lithium / ↑ Serum lithium levels with ↑ risk of lithium toxicity
Potassium-sparing diuretics, potassium supplements / ↑ Risk of hyperkalemia

HOW SUPPLIED
Tablet: 5 mg, 10 mg, 20 mg, 40 mg

DOSAGE

- **TABLETS**

Clients not receiving a diuretic.
Initial: 10 mg once daily; **maintenance:** 20–40 mg/day given as a single dose or in two equally divided doses. Total daily doses greater than 80 mg have not been evaluated.

Clients receiving a diuretic.
Initial: 5 mg/day.

C_{CR} < 30 mL/min/1.73 m². Starting with 5 mg/day; **maintenance:** titrate dose upward until BP is controlled or to a maximum total daily dose of 40 mg.

NURSING CONSIDERATIONS

SEE ALSO *NURSING CONSIDERATIONS* FOR *ANGIOTENSIN-CONVERTING ENZYME INHIBITORS* AND *ANTIHYPERTENSIVE AGENTS*.

ADMINISTRATION/STORAGE

1. Base dosage adjustment on measuring peak (2–6 hr after dosing) and trough responses. Consider increasing the dose or give divided doses if once-daily dosing does not provide an adequate trough response.
2. If BP not controlled by benazepril alone, add a diuretic.
3. If receiving a diuretic, discontinue the diuretic, if possible, 2–3 days before beginning benazepril therapy.

ASSESSMENT

1. Note any previous experience with this class of drugs.
2. Review diet, weight loss, exercise, and life-style changes necessary to control BP.
3. Monitor lytes, renal and LFTs.

CLIENT/FAMILY TEACHING

1. Take only as directed. May be taken with or without food.
2. Avoid concomitant administration of potassium-sparing diuretics/supplements; may lead to increased K+ levels.
3. Side effects such as headache, fatigue, dizziness, and cough have been associated with this drug therapy; report if persistent/bothersome.

OUTCOMES/EVALUATE
Control of hypertension

Benztropine mesylate

(**BENS**-troh-peen)

PREGNANCY CATEGORY: C
CLASSIFICATION(S):
Cholinergic blocking drug, antiparkinson drug
Rx: Cogentin
🍁**Rx:** Apo-Benztropine

SEE ALSO *CHOLINERGIC BLOCKING AGENTS*.

ACTION/KINETICS
Synthetic anticholinergic possessing antihistamine and local anesthetic properties. **Onset, PO:** 1–2 hr; **IM, IV:** Within a few minutes. Effects are cumulative; long-acting (24 hr). **Full effects:** 2–3 days. Low incidence of side effects.

USES
Adjunct in the treatment of parkinsonism (all types). To reduce severity of extrapyramidal effects in phenothiazine or other antipsychotic drug therapy (not effective in tardive dyskinesia).

CONTRAINDICATIONS
Use in children under 3 years of age.

SPECIAL CONCERNS
Geriatric and emaciated clients cannot tolerate large doses. Certain drug-induced extrapyramidal symptoms may not respond to benztropine.

HOW SUPPLIED
Injection: 1 mg/mL; *Tablet:* 0.5 mg, 1 mg, 2 mg

DOSAGE

- **TABLETS**

Parkinsonism.
Adults: 1–2 mg/day (range: 0.5–6.5 mg/day).

Idiopathic parkinsonism.
Adults, initial: 0.5–1 mg/day, in-

creased gradually to 4–6 mg/day, if necessary.

Postencephalitic parkinsonism.
Adults: 2 mg/day in one or more doses.

Drug-induced extrapyramidal effects.
Adults: 1–4 mg 1–2 times/day.

• IM, IV (RARELY)

Acute dystonic reactions.
Adults, initial: 1–2 mg; **then,** 1–2 mg PO b.i.d. usually prevents recurrence. Clients can rarely tolerate full dosage.

NURSING CONSIDERATIONS

SEE ALSO *NURSING CONSIDERATIONS* FOR *CHOLINERGIC BLOCKING AGENTS.*

ADMINISTRATION/STORAGE

1. When used as replacement for or supplement to other antiparkinsonism drugs, substitute or add gradually.
2. For difficulty swallowing tablets, may crush tablets and mix with a small amount of food or liquid.
3. Some may benefit by taking the entire dose at bedtime while others are best treated by taking divided doses, b.i.d.–q.i.d.
4. Initiate therapy with a low dose (e.g., 0.5 mg) and then increase in increments of 0.5 mg at 5–6-day intervals. Do not exceed 6 mg/day.

IV 5. If administered IV, may give undiluted at a rate of 1 mg over 1 min.

ASSESSMENT

1. Note if phenothiazines or TCAs are being used; may cause a paralytic ileus.
2. Note age; elderly clients require a lower dosage.

INTERVENTIONS

1. Monitor I&O. Assess for urinary retention and bowel sounds; especially important with limited mobility.
2. Inspect skin at regular intervals for evidence of skin changes.
3. Observe for extrapyramidal symptoms, i.e., drooling, muscle spasms, shuffling gait, muscle rigidity, and pill rolling.
4. If excitation or vomiting occurs, withdraw drug temporarily and resume at a lower dose.

CLIENT/FAMILY TEACHING

1. Review goals of therapy (control of parkinsonian symptoms, i.e., improved gait and balance and less rigidity and involuntary movements; control of extrapyramidal symptoms, i.e., less drooling, muscle spasms, shuffling gait, or pill rolling).
2. Use caution when performing tasks that require mental alertness; drug has a sedative effect and may also cause postural hypotension.
3. It usually takes 2–3 days for drug to exert a desired effect. Take as ordered unless side effects occur; these usually subside with continued drug use.
4. Avoid strenuous activity and increased heat exposure. Plan rest periods during the day as ability to tolerate heat will be reduced and heat stroke may occur.
5. Report any difficulty in voiding or inadequate emptying of the bladder.
6. Avoid alcohol and any other CNS depressants.

OUTCOMES/EVALUATE

- ↓ Involuntary movements and rigidity with improved gait and balance
- Control of extrapyramidal side effects of antipsychotic agents

Bepridil hydrochloride

(BEH-prih-dill)

PREGNANCY CATEGORY: C
CLASSIFICATION(S):
Calcium channel blocker
Rx: Vascor

SEE ALSO *CALCIUM CHANNEL BLOCKING AGENTS.*

ACTION/KINETICS

Inhibits the transmembrane influx of calcium ions into cardiac and vascular smooth muscle. Increases the effective refractory period of the atria, AV node, His-Purkinje fibers, and ventricles. Dilates peripheral arterioles and reduces total peripheral resistance; reduces HR and arterial pressure at rest and at a given level of exercise. Rapidly and completely absorbed following PO use. **Onset:** 60 min. **Time to peak plasma levels:** 2–3 hr. Greater than 99% bound to plasma protein. Food does not affect either the peak plasma levels or the extent of absorption. **Therapeutic serum levels:** 1–2 ng/mL. **t½, distribution:** 2 hr; **terminal elimination:** 24 hr. Steady-state blood levels do not occur for 8 days. Metabolized in the liver. Metabolites excreted through both the kidney (70%) and the feces (22%).

USES

Chronic stable angina (classic effort-associated angina) in clients who have failed to respond to other antianginal medications or who are intolerant to such medications. Used alone, with beta blockers, or wtih nitrates. Additive effect if used with propranolol.

CONTRAINDICATIONS

Clients with a history of serious ventricular arrhythmias, sick sinus syndrome, second- or third-degree heart block (except in the presence of a functioning ventricular pacemaker), hypotension (less than 90 mm Hg systolic), uncompensated cardiac insufficiency, congenital QT interval prolongation, and in those taking other drugs that prolong the QT interval (e.g., quinidine, procainamide, tricyclic antidepressants). Use in clients with MI during the previous 3 months. Lactation.

SPECIAL CONCERNS

Safety and effectiveness have not been determined in children. Use with caution in clients with CHF, left bundle block, sinus bradycardia (less than 50 beats/min), serious hepatic or renal disorders. New arrhythmias can be induced. Geriatric clients may require more frequent monitoring.

SIDE EFFECTS

CV: *Induction of new serious arrhythmias such as torsades de pointes/type ventricular tachycardia, prolongation of QTc and QT interval, increased PVC rates, new sustained VT and VT/VF,* sinus tachycardia, sinus bradycardia, hypertension vasodilation, palpitations. **GI:** Nausea (common), dyspepsia, GI distress, diarrhea, dry mouth, anorexia, abdominal pain, constipation, flatulence, gastritis, increased appetite. **CNS:** Nervousness, dizziness, drowsiness, insomnia, depression, vertigo, akathisia, anxiousness, tremor, hand tremor, syncope, paresthesia. **Respiratory:** Cough, pharyngitis, rhinitis, dyspnea, respiratory infection. **Body as a whole:** Asthenia, headache, flu syndrome, fever, pain, superinfection. **Dermatologic:** Rash, skin irritation, sweating. **Miscellaneous:** Tinnitus, arthritis, blurred vision, taste change, loss of libido, impotence, agranulocytosis.

LABORATORY TEST CONSIDERATIONS

↑ ALT, transaminase. Abnormal LFTs.

DRUG INTERACTIONS

Cardiac glycosides / Exaggerated depression of AV nodal conduction
Digoxin / Possible ↑ serum digoxin levels
Potassium-wasting diuretics / Hypokalemia → ↑ risk of serious ventricular arrhythmias
Procainamide / ↑ Risk of serious side effects due to exaggerated prolongation of the QT interval
Quinidine / ↑ Risk of serious side effects due to exaggerated prolongation of the QT interval
Tricyclic antidepressants / ↑ Risk of serious side effects due to exaggerated prolongation of the QT interval

HOW SUPPLIED

Tablet: 200 mg, 300 mg

DOSAGE

- **TABLETS**

Chronic stable angina.

Adults, initial: 200 mg once daily; after 10 days the dosage may be adjusted upward depending on the response of the client (e.g., ability to perform ADL, QT interval, HR, frequency and severity of angina). **Maintenance:** 300 mg/day, not to exceed 400 mg/day. The minimum effective dose is 200 mg.

NURSING CONSIDERATIONS

SEE ALSO *NURSING CONSIDERATIONS* FOR *CALCIUM CHANNEL BLOCKING AGENTS.*

ASSESSMENT

1. Note antianginal agents used previously and their effects.
2. Monitor VS, CBC, K+, and ECG.

3. List drugs currently prescribed; note any that may prolong QT interval (e.g., procainamide, quinidine, TCAs). Check QT intervals prior to initiating therapy, 1 to 3 weeks after beginning therapy, and periodically thereafter; especially after any dosage adjustment. Prolongation may lead to serious ventricular arrhythmias, especially torsades de pointes.
4. Note any evidence of AV block, new arrhythmias, or history of MI, and/or implanted ventricular pacemaker.
5. Geriatric clients require more frequent monitoring.
6. If diuretics required, use a potassium-sparing agent.

CLIENT/FAMILY TEACHING

1. Can be taken with meals or at bedtime if nausea occurs.
2. Take at about the same time each day. If a dose is missed, the next dose should *not* be doubled.
3. Continue nitroglycerin if prescribed.
4. Report dizziness, chest pain, altered mental status, ↑ SOB, or fainting.

OUTCOMES/EVALUATE

- Prophylaxis/control of angina
- Therapeutic levels (1–2 ng/mL)

Beractant

(beh-**RACK**-tant)

CLASSIFICATION(S):
Lung surfactant
Rx: Survanta

ACTION/KINETICS

Derived from natural bovine lung extract; contains phospholipids, fatty acids, neutral lipids, and surfactant-associated proteins (to which colfosceril palmitate, tripalmitin, and palmitic acid are added). The proteins in the product—SP-B and SP-C—are hydrophobic, low molecular weight, and surfactant associated. Beractant replenishes pulmonary surfactant and restores surface activity to the lungs of premature infants to reduce respiratory distress syndrome. Intended for intratracheal use only. Significant improvement is observed in the arterial-alveolar oxygen ratio and mean airway pressure. Significantly decreases the incidence of respiratory distress syndrome, mortality due to respiratory distress syndrome, and air leak complications.

USES

Prevention and treatment ("rescue") of respiratory distress syndrome (hyaline membrane disease) in premature infants.

SPECIAL CONCERNS

Can quickly affect oxygenation and lung compliance; thus, use only in a highly supervised setting with immediate availability of physicians experienced with intubation, ventilator management, and general care of premature infants.

SIDE EFFECTS

Commonly, side effects are associated with the dosing procedure and include transient bradycardia, oxygen desaturation, ET tube reflux, vasoconstriction, pallor, hypo/hypertension, ET tube blockage, hypo/hypercarbia, and ***apnea***. Other symptoms include ***intracranial hemorrhage,*** rales, moist breath sounds, and nosocomial sepsis.

OD OVERDOSE MANAGEMENT

Symptoms: ***Acute airway obstruction.***

HOW SUPPLIED

Intratracheal injection: 25 mg/mL

DOSAGE

- **INTRATRACHEAL ONLY**

4 mL/kg (100 mg phospholipids/kg birth weight).

NURSING CONSIDERATIONS

ADMINISTRATION/STORAGE

1. For prevention of respiratory distress syndrome in premature infants weighing less than 1,250 g at birth or with evidence of surfactant deficiency, give as soon as possible, preferably within 15 min of birth.
2. To treat infants with confirmed respiratory distress syndrome and who

require mechanical ventilation, give as soon as possible, preferably within 8 hr of birth.

B

3. Four doses can be given within the first 48 hr of life; doses should be given no sooner than q 6 hr.
4. Refrigerate at 2–8°C (36–46°F) and warm at room temperature for at least 20 min or in the hand for at least 8 min before administration. Does not have to be reconstituted or sonicated before use. If a prevention dose is required, preparation should begin before the infant is born. Do not warm and then return to the refrigerator for future use more than once.
5. Visually inspect vial before administration for discoloration (beractant is off-white to light brown). If settling occurs during storage, swirl the vial gently (do not shake) to redisperse although some foaming may occur at the surface during handling.
6. Each vial is for single use only; discard any residual drug.
7. Instill beractant through a 5 French end-hole catheter that has been inserted into the ET tube of the infant with the tip of the catheter protruding just beyond the end of the ET tube above the infant's carina. The length of the catheter should be shortened before inserting it through the ET tube. Do not give into a mainstem bronchus.
8. To ensure homogeneous distribution, divide each dose into four quarter-doses with each quarter-dose given with the infant in a different position—head and body inclined slightly *down*, with head turned to the right; then with head turned to the left; head and body inclined slightly *up*, with head turned to the right; then with head turned to the left.
9. For the first dose, determine the total dose based on the infant's birth weight and withdraw the entire contents of the vial into the plastic syringe using at least a 20-gauge needle. The premeasured 5 French end-hole catheter is attached to the syringe and the catheter filled with beractant. Discard any excess through the catheter so that only the total dose to be given remains in the syringe. Before giving the drug, proper placement and patency of the ET tube must be ensured (the tube may be suctioned before giving the drug). Allow infant to stabilize before proceeding with dosing.
10. If the first dose is to be used for prevention strategy, give to the stabilized infant as soon as possible after birth (preferably within 15 min). The infant is positioned appropriately and the first quarter-dose is gently injected through the catheter over 2–3 sec. After the first quarter-dose is given, the catheter is removed from the ET tube. To prevent cyanosis, manually ventilate with sufficient oxygen using a hand-bag (ambu type) at a rate of 60 breaths/min with sufficient positive pressure to provide adequate air exchange and chest wall excursion.
11. If rescue strategy is to be undertaken, give the first dose as soon as possible after the infant is placed on a ventilator for management of hyaline membrane disease. Studies have been undertaken in which the infant's ventilator settings were changed to a rate of 60/min (inspiratory time 0.5 sec and FiO_2 1) immediately before instilling the first quarter-dose. The infant is positioned appropriately and the first quarter-dose is gently injected through the catheter over 2–3 sec. The catheter is removed from the ET tube and the infant is returned to the mechanical ventilator.
12. When using both prevention and rescue strategies, the infant is ventilated for 20 sec or until stable. The infant is repositioned for instillation of the next quarter-dose. The remaining quarter-doses are given using the same procedures. After instillation of each quarter-dose, the catheter is removed and the infant is ventilated for 30 sec or until stabilized. After the final quarter-dose is instilled, the catheter is removed without flushing. The infant should not be suctioned for 1 hr after dosing unless signs of significant airway obstruction occur. After the dosing procedure is completed, resume usual ventilator management and care.
13. If repeat doses are necessary, the

dose is also 100 mg phospholipids/kg with the dose based on the infant's birth weight (the infant should not be reweighed). Additional doses are determined by evidence of continuing respiratory distress. Give repeat doses no sooner than 6 hr after the preceding dose if the infant remains intubated and requires a FiO_2 of at least 30 to maintain a pO_2 of less than or equal to 80 torr. X-ray confirmation of respiratory distress syndrome should be made before giving additional doses to infants who received a prevention dose.
14. Repeat doses are given by the same procedure as described for prevention strategy. However, studies have used different ventilator settings. For repeat doses, the FiO_2 was increased by 0.2 or an amount sufficient to prevent cyanosis. The ventilator delivered a rate of 30/min with an inspiratory time of less than 1 sec. If the infant's pretreatment rate was greater than or equal to 30, it was left unchanged during instillation. Manual hand-bag ventilation should *not* be used to give repeat doses.
15. Store unopened vials in the refrigerator at 2–8°C (36–46°F) and protect from light. Store vials in the carton until ready for use.
16. Ross Laboratories offers audiovisual instructional materials concerning administration procedures and dosing requirements.

ASSESSMENT

1. Note indications for therapy (prevention, rescue, or both).
2. The infant HR, color, chest expansion, facial expression, oximeter readings, and ET tube patency and position should be documented and monitored carefully.
3. Ascertain that the ET tube tip is in the trachea and not in the esophagus or right or left mainstem bronchus, before inserting the 5 French end-hole catheter, to ensure appropriate drug dispersion to all lung areas.
4. Document birth weight, ABGs, CXR, and physical assessments.

INTERVENTIONS

1. Follow administration guidelines carefully. Beractant is for intratracheal administration. It should only be administered by trained personnel in a highly supervised environment permitting continuous observation.
2. Auscultate lung fields frequently and avoid suctioning for 1 hr after dosing unless symptoms of significant airway obstruction are evident.
3. Monitor ECG, arterial BP, and transcutaneous oxygen saturation continuously. After beractant treatment, frequent ABGs should be measured to prevent postdosing hyperoxia and hypocarbia.
4. Monitor (during dosing) for any evidence of transient bradycardia and decreased oxygen saturation. If evident, the dosing procedure should be stopped and the infant treated symptomatically until stabilized; then the dosing procedure may be resumed.
5. Observe closely for air leaks and mucous plugs. If mucous plug is unrelieved by suctioning, the ET tube must be replaced immediately.

OUTCOMES/EVALUATE

- Improved airway exchange with ↓ pulmonary air leaks
- Oxygen saturation readings between 90% and 95%; improved pulmonary parameters more consistent with survival
- Prevention or successful treatment of respiratory distress syndrome in premature infants

Betamethasone

(bay-tah-**METH**-ah-zohn)

PREGNANCY CATEGORY: C
Rx: Celestone

Betamethasone dipropionate

(bay-tah-**METH**-ah-zohn)

Rx: Topical: Alphatrex, Diprolene, Diprolene AF, Diprosone, Maxivate, Teladar

✱Rx: Topical: Diprolene Glycol, Taro-Sone, Topilene, Topisone

Betamethasone sodium phosphate

(bay-tah-**METH**-ah-zohn)

Rx: Celestone Phosphate, Cel-U-Jec
✱Rx: Betnesol

Betamethasone sodium phosphate and Betamethasone acetate

(bay-tah-**METH**-ah-zohn)

Rx: Celestone Soluspan
✱Rx: Betaject

Betamethasone valerate

Rx: Topical: Betatrex, Beta-Val, Ectosone Regular, Luxiq, Psorion Cream, Valisone, Valisone Reduced Strength
✱Rx: Topical: Betaderm, Betnovate, Betnovate-1/2, Celestoderm-V, Celestoderm-V/2, Ectosone Mild, Ectosone Scalp Lotion, Prevex B

CLASSIFICATION(S):
Glucocorticoid

SEE ALSO ***CORTICOSTEROIDS.***

ACTION/KINETICS
Causes low degree of sodium and water retention, as well as potassium depletion. The injectable form contains both rapid-acting and repository forms of betamethasone (mixture of betamethasone sodium phosphate and betamethasone acetate). Long-acting. **t½:** over 300 min.

ADDITIONAL USES
Prevention of respiratory distress syndrome in premature infants.

CONTRAINDICATIONS
Replacement therapy in any acute or chronic adrenal cortical insufficiency due to weak sodium-retaining effects.

SPECIAL CONCERNS
Safe use during pregnancy and lactation not established.

HOW SUPPLIED
Betamethasone: *Syrup:* 0.6 mg/5 mL; *Tablet:* 0.6 mg. **Betamethasone dipropionate:** *Cream:* 0.05%; *Gel:* 0.05%; *Lotion:* 0.05%; *Ointment:* 0.05%; *Spray:* 0.1%. **Betamethasone sodium phosphate:** *Injection:* 4 mg/mL. **Betamethasone sodium phosphate and betamethasone acetate:** *Injection:* 3 mg/mL. **Betamethasone valerate:** *Cream:* 0.01%, 0.05%, 0.1%; *Foam:* 0.12%; *Lotion:* 0.1%; *Ointment:* 0.1%

DOSAGE

BETAMETHASONE

• SYRUP, TABLETS
0.6–7.2 mg/day.

BETAMETHASONE SODIUM PHOSPHATE

• IV, INTRA-ARTICULAR, INTRALESIONAL, SOFT TISSUE INJECTION
Initial: up to 9 mg/day; **then,** adjust dosage at minimal level to reduce symptoms.

BETAMETHASONE SODIUM PHOSPHATE AND BETAMETHASONE ACETATE

(contains 3 mg/mL each of the acetate and sodium phosphate)

• IM
Initial: 0.5–9 mg/day (dose ranges are ⅓–½ the PO dose given q 12 hr.)

• INTRA-ARTICULAR, INTRABURSAL, INTRADERMAL, INTRALESIONAL

Bursitis, peritendinitis, tenosynovitis.
1 mL.

Rheumatoid arthritis and osteoarthritis.
0.25–2 mL, depending on size of the joint.

Foot disorders, bursitis.
0.25–0.5 mL under heloma durum or heloma molle; 0.5 mL under calcaneal spur or over hallux rigidus or digiti quinti varus.

Tenosynovitis or periostitis of cuboid:
0.5 mL.

Acute gouty arthritis.
0.5–1 mL.

• INTRADERMAL
0.2 mL/cm² not to exceed 1 mL/week.

BETAMETHASONE DIPROPIONATE, BETAMETHASONE VALERATE

• TOPICAL SPRAY, CREAM, FOAM, GEL, LOTION, OINTMENT

Apply sparingly to affected areas and rub in lightly.

NURSING CONSIDERATIONS

SEE ALSO *NURSING CONSIDERATIONS* FOR *CORTICOSTEROIDS*.

ADMINISTRATION/STORAGE

Avoid injection into deltoid muscle because SC tissue atrophy may occur.

ASSESSMENT

Document indications for therapy, type, onset, and duration of symptoms; list agents trialed with the outcome.

CLIENT/FAMILY TEACHING

1. Review appropriate method/indication for therapy.
2. Report any S&S of infection, i.e., increased fever, any redness, odor, or purulent wound drainage. Avoid exposure to those with contagious diseases.
3. Cover lesions to avoid sun burn.
4. Do not overuse joint after injection; this may further injure joint.
5. Record weight; report any sudden weight gain or swelling in limbs, blood in stools, severe abdominal pain, bruising or lack of response.

OUTCOMES/EVALUATE

- ↓ Pain/inflammation; ↑ mobility
- Prevention of respiratory distress syndrome in premature infants
- Improved skin integrity; healing of lesions

Betaxolol hydrochloride

(beh-**TAX**-oh-lohl)

PREGNANCY CATEGORY: C
CLASSIFICATION(S):
Beta-adrenergic blocking agent
Rx: Betoptic, Betoptic S, Kerlone

SEE ALSO *BETA-ADRENERGIC BLOCKING AGENTS*.

ACTION/KINETICS

Inhibits beta-1-adrenergic receptors (beta-2 receptors inhibited at high doses). Has some membrane stabilizing activity but no intrinsic sympathomimetic activity. Low lipid solubility. Reduces the production of aqueous humor, thus, reducing IOP. No effect on pupil size or accommodation. **t½:** 14–22 hr. Metabolized in the liver with most excreted through the urine; about 15% is excreted unchanged.

USES

PO: Hypertension, alone or with other antihypertensive agents (especially thiazide diuretics). **Ophthalmic:** Ocular hypertension and chronic open-angle glaucoma (used alone or in combination with other antiglaucoma drugs).

SPECIAL CONCERNS

Use with caution during lactation. Safety and effectiveness have not been determined in children. Geriatric clients are at greater risk of developing bradycardia.

HOW SUPPLIED

Ophthalmic Solution: 0.5%; *Ophthalmic Suspension:* 0.25%; *Tablet:* 10 mg, 20 mg

DOSAGE

- **TABLETS**

Hypertension.

Initial: 10 mg once daily either alone or with a diuretic. If desired effect is not reached, may increase dose to 20 mg; doses higher than 20 mg will not increase the therapeutic effect. In geriatric clients the initial dose should be 5 mg/day.

- **OPHTHALMIC SOLUTION, SUSPENSION**

Ocular hypertension; chronic open-angle glaucoma.

Adults, usual: 1–2 gtt b.i.d. If used to replace another drug, continue the drug being used and add 1 gtt of betaxolol b.i.d. Discontinue the previous drug the following day. If transferring from several antiglaucoma drugs being used together, adjust one drug at a time at intervals of not less than 1 week. The agents being used can be continued and add 1 gtt betaxolol b.i.d. The next day another agent should be discontinued. The remaining antiglaucoma drug dosage can be decreased or discontinued depending on client response.

B

NURSING CONSIDERATIONS

SEE ALSO *NURSING CONSIDERATIONS* FOR *BETA-ADRENERGIC BLOCKING AGENTS* AND *ANTIHYPERTENSIVE AGENTS*.

ADMINISTRATION/STORAGE

1. Full antihypertensive effect usually observed within 7 to 14 days.
2. As PO dose is increased, the HR decreases.
3. Discontinue PO therapy gradually over a 2-week period.
4. Shake ophthalmic suspension well before use.
5. Store ophthalmic products at room temperature not to exceed 30°C (86°F).

CLIENT/FAMILY TEACHING

1. Review appropriate method/indications for therapy.
2. Drug may mask S&S of hypoglycemia, and cause increased cold sensitivity.
3. Avoid OTC products without approval.
4. With HTN, monitor BP and record; report any adverse drug effects.
5. With eye therapy, review instillation procedure. Wear sunglasses and avoid sun exposure; may cause photophobia.

OUTCOMES/EVALUATE

- ↓ BP (PO)
- ↓ Intraocular pressure (Ophthalmic)

Bexarotene

(bex-**AIR**-oh-teen)

PREGNANCY CATEGORY: X
CLASSIFICATION(S):
Antineoplastic, retinoid
Rx: Targretin

SEE ALSO *ANTINEOPLASTIC AGENTS*.

ACTION/KINETICS

Binds with and activates retinoid X receptor subtypes. Once activated, these receptors act as transcription factors that regulate the expression of genes that control cell differentiation and proliferation. Exact mechanism to treat cutaneous T-cell lymphoma is not known but the drug inhibits growth of some tumor cell lines, in vitro, of hematopoietic and squamous cell origin and induces tumor regression, in vitro, in some animal models. Maximum absorption within 2 hr. More than 99% bound to plasma proteins. Metabolized in the liver and excreted through the hepatobiliary system. **t½, terminal:** 7 hr. Absorption of the gel is insignificant.

USES

Capsules: Early and advanced stage cutaneous T-cell lymphoma in clients refractory to 1 or more prior systemic treatments. **Gel:** Early stage cutaneous T-cell lymphoma (Stage IA and IB) in those who have refractory or persistent disease after other therapies or who do not tolerate other therapies.

CONTRAINDICATIONS

Pregnancy, lactation.

SPECIAL CONCERNS

Use with caution in those with known hypersensitivity to other retinoids and in clients using insulin, sulfonylureas, or insulin-sensitizers due to possible enhanced hypoglycemic effect. Safety and efficacy have not been determined in children.

SIDE EFFECTS

- **SYSTEMIC USE**

Induces major lipid abnormalities (e.g., ↑ fasting triglycerides, total and LDL cholesterol; ↓ HDL).

GI: Acute pancreatitis, impaired hepatic function, abdominal pain, N&V, diarrhea, anorexia, constipation, dry mouth, flatulence, colitis, dyspepsia, cheilitis, gastroenteritis, gingivitis, **liver failure,** melena. **CNS:** Headache, insomnia, depression, agitation, ataxia, confusion, dizziness, hyperesthesia, hypesthesia, neuropathy. **CV:** ***CVA, hemorrhage,*** hypertension, angina pectoris, chest pain, syncope, tachycardia. **Hematologic:** Leukopenia, anemia, hypochromic anemia, eosinophilia, thrombocythemia, lymphocytosis, thrombocytopenia. **Dermatologic:** Dry skin, rash, exfoliative dermatitis, alopecia, skin ulcer, acne, skin nodule, maculopapular rash, pustular rash, serous drainage, vesicular bullous rash. **Respiratory:** Pharyngitis, rhinitis, dyspnea, pleural effusion, bronchitis, increased cough, lung edema, hemoptysis, hypoxia. **GU:** Urinary incontinence, UTI, urinary urgency, dysuria, abnormal kidney function, breast pain. **Musculoskeletal:** Arthralgia, myalgia, bone pain, myasthenia, arthrosis. **Ophthalmic:** Dry eyes, conjunctivitis, blepharitis, corneal lesion, keratitis, visual field defect. **Body as a whole:** Asthenia, bacterial infection, pneumonia, chills, fever, flu syndrome, peripheral edema, increase or decrease in weight, ***sepsis***. **Miscellaneous:** Clinical hypothyroidism, back pain, ear pain, otitis externa, cellulitis, monilia.

• **TOPICAL USE**

Dermatologic: Rash, pruritus, skin disorder, and pain at application site. Also, contact dermatitis, exfoliative dermatitis, maculopapular rash, sweating. **CV:** Edema, peripheral edema. **Hematologic:** Leukopenia, lymphadenopathy, abnormal WBCs. **Respiratory:** Increased cough, pharyngitis. **Body as a whole:** Infection, headache, asthenia, pain. **Miscellaneous:** Hyperlipemia, paresthesia.

LABORATORY TEST CONSIDERATIONS

↑ AST, ALT, alkaline phosphatase, LDH, creatinine, amylase. Bilirubinemia, hypercholesterolemia, hyperlipemia, hyperglycemia, hypocalcemia, hyponatremia, hypoproteinemia.

DRUG INTERACTIONS

Antidiabetic drugs (insulin, sulfonylureas) ↑ Risk of hypoglycemia
Erythromycin / ↑ Plasma bexarotene levels R/T ↓ liver metabolism
Gemfibrozil / Significant ↑ in plasma bexarotene levels
Grapefruit juice / ↑ Plasma bexarotene levels R/T ↓ liver metabolism
Itraconazole / ↑ Plasma bexarotene levels R/T ↓ liver metabolism
Ketoconazole / ↑ Plasma bexarotene levels R/T ↓ liver metabolism
Phenobarbital / ↓ Plasma bexarotene levels R/T ↑ liver metabolism
Phenytoin / ↓ Plasma bexarotene levels R/T ↑ liver metabolism
Rifampin / ↓ Plasma bexarotene levels R/T ↑ liver metabolism
Vitamin A / Additive toxic effects

HOW SUPPLIED

Capsules: 75 mg; *Gel:* 1%

DOSAGE

• **CAPSULES**

Cutaneous T-cell lymphoma.

Initial: 300 mg/m²/day; **then,** adjust for BSA as a single PO daily dose taken with a meal as follows: **0.88–1.12 m²:** 300 mg/day; **1.13–1.37 m²:** 375 mg/day; **1.38–1.62 m²:** 450 mg/day; **1.63–1.87 m²:** 525 mg/day; **1.88–2.12 m²:** 600 mg/day; **2.13–2.37 m²:** 675 mg/day; **2.38–2.62 m²:** 750 mg/day.

NOTE: If there is no response after 8 weeks of therapy and if the initial dose of 300 mg/m²/day is well tolerated, the dose can be increased to 400 mg/m²/day; monitor carefully. If toxic effects occur, the 300 mg/m²/day may be decreased to 200 mg/m²/day or 100 mg/m²/day. When toxicity is controlled, the dose can be readjusted upward.

• **GEL**

Cutaneous T-cell lymphoma.

Initial: Once every other day for the first week. **Then,** increase application frequency at weekly intervals to once daily, then twice daily, then three times daily, and finally four times daily, depending on individual lesion tolerance. If severe irritation occurs, temporarily discontinue for a few days until symptoms subside.

NURSING CONSIDERATIONS

SEE ALSO ***NURSING CONSIDERATIONS*** FOR ***ANTINEOPLASTIC AGENTS.***

ASSESSMENT

1. Note onset and characteristics of disease; list other agents/therapies trialed.
2. List drugs prescribed to ensure none interact (enhances hypoglycemic effects).
3. Monitor renal and LFTs. Use cautiously with impaired function; drug is liver metabolized.

CLIENT/FAMILY TEACHING

1. Take as directed; avoid grapefruit juice.

2. May experience flu-like symptoms. Report any unusual side effects including rashes, abnormal bruising/bleeding, UTI/URI, unsteady gait, confusion, dizziness/drowsiness, abdominal pain, yellow skin discoloration, depression or pain in extremities.
3. Practice reliable birth control.
4. Identify local support groups to assist with disease understanding/management.

OUTCOMES/EVALUATE

Inhibition of malignant cell proliferation

Bicalutamide

(**buy**-kah-**LOO**-tah-myd)

PREGNANCY CATEGORY: X
CLASSIFICATION(S):
Antineoplastic, antiandrogen
Rx: Casodex

SEE ALSO *ANTINEOPLASTIC AGENTS*.

ACTION/KINETICS

A nonsteroidal antiandrogen that competitively inhibits the action of androgens by binding to cytosolic androgen receptors in target tissues. Well absorbed after PO administration; food does not affect the rate or amount absorbed. Metabolized in the liver, and both parent drug and metabolites are eliminated in the urine and feces. **t½:** 5.8 days. **Mean steady-state concentration in prostatic cancer:** 8.9 mcg/mL.

USES

In combination therapy with a leutinizing hormone-releasing hormone analog for the treatment of advanced prostate cancer.

CONTRAINDICATIONS

Pregnancy. Use in women.

SPECIAL CONCERNS

Use with caution in clients with moderate to severe hepatic impairment and during lactation. Safety and efficacy have not been established in children.

SIDE EFFECTS

GI: Constipation, N&V, diarrhea, anorexia, dyspepsia, rectal hemorrhage, dry mouth, melena, flatulence, dysphagia, GI disorder, periodontal abscess, GI carcinoma, hepatotoxicity. **CNS:** Dizziness, paresthesia, insomnia, anxiety, depression, decreased libido, hypertonia, confusion, neuropathy, somnolence, nervousness. **GU:** Gynecomastia, breast pain, nocturia, hematuria, UTI, impotence, urinary incontinence/frequency, impaired urination, dysuria, urinary retention/urgency, hydronephrosis, urinary tract disorder. **CV:** Hot flashes (most common), hypertension, angina pectoris, CHF, ***MI, cardiac arrest,*** coronary artery disorder, syncope. **Metabolic:** Peripheral edema, hyperglycemia, weight loss or gain, dehydration, gout, edema. **Musculoskeletal:** Myasthenia, arthritis, myalgia, bone pain, leg cramps, pathologic fracture. **Respiratory:** Dyspnea, increased cough, pharyngitis, bronchitis, pneumonia, rhinitis, lung disorder, asthma, epistaxis, sinusitis, interstitial pneumonitis, pulmonary fibrosis. **Dermatologic:** Rash, sweating, dry skin, pruritus, alopecia, herpes zoster, skin carcinoma, skin disorder. **Hematologic:** Anemia, hypochromic and iron deficiency anemia. **Body as a whole:** General pain, back pain, asthenia, pelvic/abdominal/chest pain, flu syndrome, edema, neoplasm, fever, neck pain, chills, ***sepsis.*** **Miscellaneous:** Infection, bone pain, headache, hernia, cyst, specified cataract, diabetes mellitus.

LABORATORY TEST CONSIDERATIONS

↑ Alkaline phosphatase, creatinine, AST, ALT, bilirubin, BUN, liver enzyme tests. ↓ Hemoglobin, white cell count.

DRUG INTERACTIONS

Bicalutamide may displace coumarin anticoagulants from their protein-binding sites, resulting in an increased anticoagulant effect.

HOW SUPPLIED

Tablet: 50 mg

DOSAGE

• **TABLETS**

Prostatic carcinoma.

50 mg (1 tablet) once daily (morning or evening) in combination with an LHRH analog with or without food.

NURSING CONSIDERATIONS

SEE ALSO *NURSING CONSIDERATIONS* FOR *ANTINEOPLASTIC AGENTS*.

ADMINISTRATION/STORAGE

1. Take at the same time each day.
2. Start treatment at the same time as LHRH analog.

ASSESSMENT

1. Note indications for therapy, onset, duration of symptoms, and any other agents/therapies trialed.
2. Monitor liver and renal function studies, CBC, and PSA. (If transaminases increase 2 X normal, stop drug.)
3. If prescribed warfarin, monitor PT/INR closely; can displace from protein binding sites.

CLIENT/FAMILY TEACHING

1. Take at the same time each day, with prescribed LHRH analog (i.e., goserelin implant or leuprolide depot).
2. Side effects that require immediate attention include hemorrhage, urinary retention, yellow skin, fracture, and respiratory distress.
3. Periodic lab studies for PSA, CBC, liver and renal function will be required to assess response.

OUTCOMES/EVALUATE

- Symptomatic improvement
- Reduction of serum PSA and inhibition of tumor growth

Bimatoprost

(by-**MAH**-toh-prost)

PREGNANCY CATEGORY: C
CLASSIFICATION(S):
Antiglaucoma drug
Rx: Lumigan

ACTION/KINETICS

Bimatoprost selectively mimics the effects of the naturally occurring prostamides. Acts to lower IOP by increasing outflow of aqueous humor through the trabecular network and uveoscleral routes. **Onset:** About 4 hr after first administration. **Maxiumum effect:** About 8–12 hr.

USES

Reduce elevated intraocular pressure in open angle glaucoma or ocular hypertension.

SPECIAL CONCERNS

Has not been evaluated to treat angle closure, inflammatory, or neovascular glaucoma. May cause increased pigmentation and growth of eyelashes, may increase the amount of brown pigment in the iris and darken the eyelid skin, changes may be permanent. Bacterial keratitis, due to contamination of the product, is possible. Use with caution in active intraocular inflammation, in aphakic or pseudophakic clients with a torn posterior lens capsule, in those with known risk factors for macular edema, and during lactation. Safety and efficacy have not been determined in children.

SIDE EFFECTS

Ophthalmic: Conjunctival hyperemia, growth of eyelashes, ocular pruritus/burning/dryness, visual disturbances, foreign body sensation, eye pain/discharge, pigmenation of the periocular skin, blepharitis, cataract, superficial punctate keratitis, eyelid erythema, ocular irritation, eyelash darkening, tearing, photophobia, allergic conjunctivitis, asthenopia, increases in iris pigmentation, conjunctival edema, iritis. **Systemic:** Infections, headache, abnormal LFTs, asthenia, hirsutism.

HOW SUPPLIED

Solution, Ophthalmic: 0.03%

DOSAGE

- **OPHTHALMIC SOLUTION**

Elevated IOP.

1 gtt in the affected eye(s) once daily in the evening.

NURSING CONSIDERATIONS

ADMINISTRATION/STORAGE

Store in the original container at 15–25°C (59–77°F).

ASSESSMENT

1. Note indications for therapy, other agents trialed, and pressure readings. Used with open angle glaucoma or ocular hypertension.

B

2. Assess eye for inflammation, exudate, pain, and level of vision. Note iris color.
3. Note LFTs as drug may alter levels.

CLIENT/FAMILY TEACHING

1. Use once daily as directed, more frequent use may decrease the IOP-lowering effect.
2. Do not let tip of eye dropper come in contact with any eye or surrounding tissue. If contact suspected rinse well, do not share eye droppers.
3. May be used together with other topical ophthalmic drug products to lower IOP. If more than 1 eye drop is used, administer them at least 5 min apart.
4. Do not administer while wearing contact lenses. Remove contact lenses prior to instillation, lenses may be reinserted 15 min after drug administration. Bimatoprost contains benzalkonium chloride which may be absorbed by soft contact lenses.
5. May cause irreversible pigmentation changes to iris (brown color) and skin around the eye and lid. May also cause increased eyelash growth which may be of more concern if only one eye is being treated.
6. Report any unusual or intolerable side effects. Keep all F/U appointments to evaluate response to treatment. Do not drive or perform hazardous functions until vision clears.

OUTCOMES/EVALUATE

Reduction of IOP

Biperiden hydrochloride

(bye-**PER**-ih-den)

PREGNANCY CATEGORY: C
CLASSIFICATION(S):
Cholinergic blocking drug, antiparkinson drug
Rx: Akineton Hydrochloride

SEE ALSO *ANTIPARKINSON DRUGS* AND *CHOLINERGIC BLOCKING AGENTS*.

ACTION/KINETICS

Synthetic anticholinergic. Tremor may increase as spasticity is relieved. Slight respiratory and CV effects. **Time to peak levels:** 60–90 min. **Peak levels:** 4–5 mcg/L. **t½:** About 18–24 hr. Tolerance may develop.

USES

Parkinsonism, especially of the postencephalitic, arteriosclerotic, and idiopathic types. Drug-induced (e.g., phenothiazines) extrapyramidal manifestations.

ADDITIONAL CONTRAINDICATIONS

Children under the age of 3 years.

SPECIAL CONCERNS

Use with caution in older children.

ADDITIONAL SIDE EFFECTS

Muscle weakness, inability to move certain muscles.

HOW SUPPLIED

Injection: 5 mg/mL (as lactate); *Tablet:* 2 mg.

DOSAGE

• **TABLETS**

Parkinsonism.

Adults: 2 mg t.i.d.–q.i.d., to a maximum of 16 mg/day.

Drug-induced extrapyramidal effects.

Adults: 2 mg 1–3 times/day. Maximum daily dose: 16 mg.

• **IM, IV**

Drug-induced extrapyramidal effects.

2 mg. Repeat q 30 min until symptoms improve, but not more than 4 consecutive doses/24 hr.

NURSING CONSIDERATIONS

SEE ALSO *NURSING CONSIDERATIONS* FOR *ANTIPARKINSON DRUGS* AND *CHOLINERGIC BLOCKING AGENTS*.

ASSESSMENT

1. Note age; older clients should receive lower doses of biperiden.
2. Record drugs client taking to prevent any unfavorable interactions.

CLIENT/FAMILY TEACHING

1. Take after meals to avoid gastric irritation.
2. Do not use antacids or antidiarrheal for 1–2 hr after taking drug.
3. Record stools; increase intake of fluids, fruit juices, and fiber to avoid constipation.
4. Avoid overheating; drug decreases perspiration.

5. Record I&O; report urinary difficulty.
6. Use sugarless gum or candies and rinse mouth often to control dry mouth effects.

OUTCOMES/EVALUATE

Control of drug-induced (phenothiazine) extrapyramidal manifestations (i.e., ↓ muscle rigidity and drooling)

—COMBINATION DRUG—

Bismuth subsalicylate, Metronidazole, Tetracycline hydrochloride

(**BIS**-muth, meh-troh-**NYE**-dah-zohl, teh-trah-**SYE**-kleen)

PREGNANCY CATEGORY: B (METRONIDAZOLE), D (TETRACYCLINE)
CLASSIFICATION(S):
Treatment of *Helicobacter pylori*
Rx: Helidac

SEE ALSO *METRONIDAZOLE* AND *TETRACYCLINE HYDROCHLORIDE*.

ACTION/KINETICS

The information to follow was derived from each drug being given alone and not in the combination in this product. Bismuth subsalicylate is hydrolyzed in the GI tract to bismuth and salicylic acid. Less than 1% of bismuth from PO doses of bismuth subsalicylate is absorbed into the general circulation. However, more than 80% of salicylic acid is absorbed. Metronidazole is well absorbed from the GI tract. **Peak plasma levels, metronidazole:** 1–2 hr; **t½, elimination:** 8 hr. Metronidazole is metabolized by the liver and is excreted through both the urine (60% to 80%) and the feces (6% to 15%). Tetracyclines are readily absorbed from the GI tract. The relative contributions of systemic versus local antimicrobial activity against *H. pylori* for agents used in eradication therapy have not been determined.

USES

In combination with an H_2 antagonist to treat active duodenal ulcer associated with *H. pylori* infection.

CONTRAINDICATIONS

Use during pregnancy or lactation, in children, or in renal or hepatic impairment. Hypersensitivity to bismuth subsalicylate, metronidazole or other imidazole derivatives, and any tetracycline. Use in those allergic to aspirin or salicylates. Use of bismuth subsalicylate in children and teenagers who have or who are recovering from chicken pox or the flu due to the possibility of Reye's syndrome. Use of tetracyclines during tooth development in children (i.e., last half of pregnancy, infancy, and childhood to 8 years of age) due to the possibility of permanent tooth discoloration.

SPECIAL CONCERNS

Use with caution in elderly clients and in clients with evidence or history of blood dyscrasias. Safety and efficacy have not been determined in children.

SIDE EFFECTS

See also *Metronidazole* and *Tetracyclines* for specific side effects for these drugs. The following side effects were noted when the three drugs were given concomitantly.
GI: N&V, diarrhea, abdominal pain, melena, anal discomfort, anorexia, constipation. **CNS:** Dizziness, paresthesia, insomnia. **Miscellaneous:** Asthenia, pain, URI.

Excessive doses of bismuth subsalicylate may cause neurotoxicity, which is reversible if therapy is terminated. Large doses of metronidazole have been associated with seizures and peripheral neuropathy (characterized by numbness or paresthesia of an extremity). Metronidazole may exacerbate candidiasis. Tetracycline use may cause superinfection, benign intracranial hypertension (pseudotumor cerebri), and photosensitivity.

DRUG INTERACTIONS

See also *Metronidazole* and *Tetracyclines*. There may be a decrease in absorption of tetracycline due to the presence of bismuth or calcium carbonate (an excipient in bismuth subsalicylate tablets).

HOW SUPPLIED

Patient Pak. Capsule: Tetracycline hydrochloride, 500 mg; *Tablets:* Bismuth subsalicylate, 262.4 mg; Metronidzole, 250 mg.

DOSAGE

• TABLETS (BISMUTH SUBSALICYLATE, METRONIDAZOLE) AND CAPSULES (TETRACYCLINE HYDROCHLORIDE)

Treatment of H. pylori.

Each dose includes two pink, round chewable tablets (525 mg bismuth subsalicylate), one white tablet (250 mg metronidazole), and one pale orange and white capsule (500 mg tetracycline hydrochloride). Each dose is taken q.i.d. with meals and at bedtime for 14 days. *NOTE:* Concomitant therapy with an H_2 antagonist is also required.

NURSING CONSIDERATIONS

SEE ALSO *NURSING CONSIDERATIONS* FOR *METRONIDAZOLE* AND *TETRACYCLINE HYDROCHLORIDE*.

ADMINISTRATION/STORAGE

1. Bismuth subsalicylate may cause darkening of the tongue and black stools, do not confuse with melena.
2. The bismuth subsalicylate tablets should be chewed and swallowed. Take metronidazole and tetracycline whole with 8 oz of water.
3. Ingest adequate fluids, especially with the bedtime dose, in order to decrease the risk of esophageal irritation and ulceration.
4. If a dose is missed, it can be made up by continuing the normal dosage schedule until the medication is gone. Double doses are not to be taken. Report if more than four doses are missed.

ASSESSMENT

1. Note clinical presentation and characteristics of symptoms, including onset and duration.
2. Document any allergy to aspirin or salicylates.
3. Determine women of child-bearing age are not pregnant. Do not use in children under age 8.
4. Obtain CBC, liver and renal function studies; note dysfunction.
5. Document serum and/or endoscopic confirmation of organism.
6. Note agents prescribed; therapy requires an H_2 antagonist.

CLIENT/FAMILY TEACHING

1. Review the tablets: 2 pink round chewable (bismuth), 1 white tablet (metronidazole), and 1 pale orange and white capsule (tetracycline). All must be taken 4 times a day with meals and at bedtime for 14 days total. Chew and swallow the pink chewables (bismuth); swallow the others with a full glass of water. Consume plenty of fluids to prevent esophageal irritation. Avoid milk/dairy products; may alter tetracycline absorption. Also take H_2 antagonist as prescribed.
2. Do not double up on missed doses; take next dose and continue prescription as directed until completed. Frequent multiple missed doses should be reported.
3. Avoid alcohol during and for 24 hr following completion of therapy.
4. Use additional contraception with birth control pills; tetracycline may lower effectiveness.
5. Avoid prolonged sun exposure to prevent a photosensitivity reaction. Use sunglasses, sun screen, and protective clothing when exposed.
6. Tongue may darken and stools may appear black; this is only temporary. Report any unusual or persistent side effects.

OUTCOMES/EVALUATE

- Eradication of *H. pylori* infection
- ↓ Recurrence of duodenal ulcers

Bisoprolol fumarate

(**BUY**-soh-**proh**-lol)

PREGNANCY CATEGORY: C

CLASSIFICATION(S):

Beta-adrenergic blocking agent

Rx: Zebeta

🍁**Rx:** Monocor

SEE ALSO *BETA-ADRENERGIC BLOCKING AGENTS*.

B

ACTION/KINETICS
Inhibits beta-1-adrenergic receptors and, at higher doses, beta-2 receptors. No intrinsic sympathomimetic activity and no membrane-stabilizing activity. **t½:** 9–12 hr. Over 90% of PO dose is absorbed. Approximately 50% is excreted unchanged through the urine and the remainder as inactive metabolites; a small amount (less than 2%) is excreted through the feces.
USES
Hypertension alone or in combination with other antihypertensive agents. *Investigational:* Angina pectoris, SVTs, PVCs.
SPECIAL CONCERNS
Use with caution during lactation. Safety and efficacy have not been determined in children. Due to selectivity for beta-1 receptors, it may be used with caution in clients with bronchospastic disease who do not respond to, or who cannot tolerate, other antihypertensive therapy.
LABORATORY TEST CONSIDERATIONS
↑ AST, ALT, uric acid, creatinine, BUN, serum potassium, glucose, and phosphorus. ↓ WBCs and platelets.
HOW SUPPLIED
Tablet: 5 mg, 10 mg

DOSAGE
• **TABLETS**
Antihypertensive.
Dose must be individualized. **Adults, initial:** 5 mg once daily (in some, 2.5 mg/day may be appropriate). **Maintenance:** If the 5-mg dose is inadequate, the dose may be increased to 10 mg/day and then, if needed, to 20 mg once daily. In impaired renal (C_{CR} < 40 mL/min) or hepatic function (hepatitis or cirrhosis), initially give 2.5 mg with caution in titrating the dose upward.

NURSING CONSIDERATIONS

SEE ALSO *NURSING CONSIDERATIONS FOR BETA-ADRENERGIC BLOCKING AGENTS.*
ADMINISTRATION/STORAGE
1. Food does not affect bioavailability; may give without regard to meals.
2. Bisoprolol is not dialyzable so dose adjustments are not required in clients undergoing hemodialysis.
3. Dosage adjustment is not necessary in the elderly.
ASSESSMENT
1. Document indications for therapy, previous agents used, and outcome.
2. Monitor CBC, lytes, renal and LFTs; reduce dose with dysfunction.
3. Once baseline parameters determined, continue to monitor BP in both arms with client lying, sitting, and standing.
4. Document cardiac rhythm; note any arrhythmias.
OUTCOMES/EVALUATE
• ↓ BP; relief of angina
• Stable cardiac rhythm

Bitolterol mesylate

(bye-**TOHL**-ter-ohl)

PREGNANCY CATEGORY: C
CLASSIFICATION(S):
Bronchodilator
Rx: Tornalate

SEE ALSO *SYMPATHOMIMETIC DRUGS.*
ACTION/KINETICS
Prodrug converted by esterases to the active colterol. Colterol combines with beta-2-adrenergic receptors, producing dilation of bronchioles. Minimal beta-1-adrenergic activity. **Onset following inhalation:** 2–4 min. **Time to peak effect:** 30–60 min. **Duration:** 5–8 hr.
USES
Prophylaxis and treatment of bronchial asthma and reversible bronchospasms. May be used with theophylline and/or steroids.
SPECIAL CONCERNS
Safety has not been established for use during lactation and in children less than 12 years of age. Use with caution in ischemic heart disease, hypertension, hyperthyroidism, diabetes mellitus, cardiac arrhythmias, seizure disorders, or in those who respond unusually to beta-adrenergic agonists. There may be decreased effec-

tiveness in steroid-dependent asthmatic clients. Hypersensitivity reactions may occur.

ADDITIONAL SIDE EFFECTS

CNS: Hyperactivity, hyperkinesia, lightheadedness, tremor, dizziness, vertigo, nervousness, tension, headache, insomnia. **CV:** PVCs, palpitations, tachycardia, hypertension, chest tightness/pain/discomfort, angina. **Respiratory:** Dry throat, throat irritation, pharyngitis, cough, dyspnea, bronchospasm. **Other:** N&V, flushing.

LABORATORY TEST CONSIDERATIONS

↑ AST. ↓ Platelets, WBCs. Proteinuria.

DRUG INTERACTIONS

Additive effects with other beta-adrenergic bronchodilators.

HOW SUPPLIED

Aerosol 0.37 mg/inh; *Solution for Inhalation:* 0.2%

DOSAGE

• **AEROSOL**

Bronchospasm.

Adults and children over 12 years: 2 inhalations at an interval of 1–3 min (if necessary, a third inhalation may be taken). Do not exceed 3 inhalations q 6 hr or 2 inhalations q 4 hr.

Prophylaxis of bronchospasm.

Adults and children over 12 years: 2 inhalations q 8 hr.

• **SOLUTION FOR INHALATION**

Bronchospasm.

Continuous flow nebulization: **Usual:** 2.5 mg. (1.25 mL); **decreased dose:** 1.5 mg (0.75 mL); **increased dose:** 3.5 mg (1.75 mL). Intermittent flow nebulization: **Usual:** 1 mg (0.5 mL); **decreased dose:** 0.5 mg (0.25 mL); **increased dose:** 1.5 mg (0.75 mL)

Note: Usual frequency is t.i.d.; can increase to q.i.d. but interval between treatments should be 4 hr or more.

NURSING CONSIDERATIONS

SEE ALSO *NURSING CONSIDERATIONS* FOR *SYMPATHOMIMETIC DRUGS.*

ADMINISTRATION/STORAGE

1. Available as MDI; delivers 0.37 mg bitolterol per actuation.
2. Administer the solution for inhalation during a 10– to 15–minute period.
3. Up to 1 mL of the solution for inhalation (0.2%, 2 mg) can be given with the interimittent flow system to severely obstructed clients.
4. Do not store the medication above 120°F (49°C).

CLIENT/FAMILY TEACHING

1. With the inhaler in an upright position, breathe out completely in a normal fashion. Breathe in slowly and deeply, squeeze the canister and mouthpiece between the thumb and forefinger to activate the medication. Hold the breath for 10 sec and then slowly exhale. A spacer may facilitate drug dispersion. Review video/instruction for proper administration guidelines.
2. Do not exceed prescribed dosage; seek medical assistance if symptoms worsen.

OUTCOMES/EVALUATE

• Improved airway exchange with ↓ airway resistance

• Asthma/bronchospasm prophylaxis

Bivalirudin

(**by**-val-ih-**ROO**-din)

PREGNANCY CATEGORY: B

CLASSIFICATION(S):

Anticoagulant, thrombin inhibitor

Rx: Angiomax

SEE ALSO *ANTICOAGULANTS.*

ACTION/KINETICS

Direct-acting thrombin inhibitor by binding to both the catalytic site and to the anion-binding exosite of circulating and clot-bound thrombin. Binding to thrombin is reversible. When bound to thrombin, all effects of thrombin are inhibited, including activation of platelets, cleavage of fibrinogen, and activation of the positive amplification reactions of thrombin. Advantages over heparin include activity against clot-bound thrombin, more predictable anticoagulation, and no inhibition by components of the platelet release reaction. **t½, after IV:** 25 min. Metabolized in the liver with about 20% excreted unchanged in the urine.

USES

As an anticoagulant with aspirin in clients with unstable angina undergoing percutaneous transluminal coronary angioplasty (PTCA).

CONTRAINDICATIONS

Use in active major bleeding, cerebral aneurysm, intracranial hemorrhage. IM use.

SPECIAL CONCERNS

Reduce dose in moderate to severe impaired renal function. Increased risk of hemorrhage with GI ulceration or hepatic disease. Hypertension may increase risk of cerebral hemorrhage. Use with caution following recent surgery or trauma and during lactation. Safety and efficacy not established when used with glycoprotein IIb/IIIa inhibitors, in clients with unstable angina who are not undergoing PTCA, in those with other acute coronary syndromes, or in children.

SIDE EFFECTS

Major side effect is bleeding with possiblity (infrequent) of major hemorrhage, including ***intracranial hemorrhage*** and ***retroperitoneal hemorrhage***. **CV:** Hypotension, hypertension, bradycardia. **GI:** N&V, dyspepsia, abdominal pain. **CNS:** Headache, insomnia, anxiety, nervousness. **Dermatologic:** Hematoma, pain at injection site. **Miscellaneous:** Urinary retention, back pain, pain, pelvic pain, fever.

LABORATORY TEST CONSIDERATIONS

Prolongation of APTT, activated clotting time, thrombin time, and PT.

HOW SUPPLIED

Injection, lyophilized: 250 mg/vial

DOSAGE

• **IV**

Unstable angina undergoing PTCA

Adults: IV bolus dose of 1 mg/kg followed by a 4-hr IV infusion at a rate of 2.5 mg/kg/hr. After the initial 4-hr infusion, an additional IV infusion may be started at a rate of 0.2 mg/kg/hr for up to 20 hr, if needed. Use with aspirin (300–325 mg/day).

NURSING CONSIDERATIONS

ADMINISTRATION/STORAGE

IV 1. Initiate just prior to PTCA.

2. To reconstitute, add 5 mL sterile water to each 250 mg vial and gently swirl until material is dissolved. Each reconstituted vial is further diluted in 50 mL of D5%/W or 0.9% NaCL for a final concentration of 5 mg/mL.

3. Adjust dose according to client weight.

4. If the low-rate infusion (i.e., 0.2 mg/kg/hr) is needed, prepare as follows: reconstitute the 250 mg vial with 5 mL of sterile water and further dilute in 500 mL of D5%/W or 0.9% NaCL for a final concentration of 0.5 mg/mL.

5. Do not mix with any other medications before administration.

6. Do not use if the preparation contains particulate matter.

7. Do not freeze reconstituted or diluted drug.

8. Reconstituted drug may be stored at 2–8°C (36–46°F) for up to 24 hr. Diluted drug (0.5 mg/mL–5 mg/mL) is stable at room temperature for up to 24 hr.

ASSESSMENT

1. Document indications for and method of therapy.

2. Note any history of cerebral aneurysm or intracranial hemorrhage.

3. Monitor ECG, CBC, bleeding parameters, renal and LFTs; reduce dose with renal dysfunction.

4. Assess carefully for any evidence of bleeding abnormalities.

CLIENT/FAMILY TEACHING

1. Review procedure, dosage and frequency of administration. Rotate sites.

2. Report any adverse side effects or unusual bruising or bleeding. New onset SOB, chest pain or edema warrant evaluation.

3. Incorporate life style changes related to smoking, alcohol, diet and exercise into daily routine.

4. Encourage family member to learn CPR.

OUTCOMES/EVALUATE

• ↓ Ischemic complications during angioplasty
• DVT prophylaxis

B

Bleomycin sulfate

(blee-oh-**MY**-sin)

PREGNANCY CATEGORY: D
CLASSIFICATION(S):
Antineoplastic, antibiotic
Rx: Blenoxane (Abbreviation: BLM)

SEE ALSO *ANTINEOPLASTIC AGENTS.*

ACTION/KINETICS
Bleomycin is a mixture of cytotoxic glycopeptide antibiotics isolated from *Streptomyces verticillus.* Main effect is likely inhibition of DNA synthesis with less inhibition of RNA and protein synthesis. Most effective in the G_2 and M phases of cell division. Drug currently used is mostly a mixture of bleomycin A_2 and B_2. Relatively low bone marrow depressant activity; localizes in certain tissues.

Is an important component of some combination regimens. **Peak plasma levels** (after 4–5 days of therapy): 50 ng/mL. **t½, distribution, after IV:** 10–20 min. **Peak blood levels, after IM:** 30–60 min with levels that are about one-third that of IV. **t½, elimination, C_{CR} less than 35 mL/min:** About 2 hr; half-life increases exponentially as (C_{CR}) decreases below 35 mL/min. Two-thirds excreted in the urine as active bleomycin.

USES
Palliative treatment of cancers listed, either used alone or in combination.
1. Squamous cell carcinoma of the head and neck, including mouth, tongue, tonsil, nasopharynx, oropharynx, sinus, palate, lip, buccal mucosa, gingiva, epiglottis, skin, and larynx. Carcinoma of the skin, penis, cervix, and vulva.
2. Lymphomas, including Hodgkin's and non-Hodgkin's.
3. Testicular carcinoma, including embryonal cell, choriocarcinoma, and teratocarcinoma.
4. Sclerosing agent to prevent or treat malignant pleural effusions associated with cancer. *Investigational:* Soft tissue sarcomas, osteosarcoma, malignant effusions (peritoneal, pleural), ovarian tumors. Also for severe, recalcitrant common warts (verruca vulgaris).

CONTRAINDICATIONS
Lactation. Renal or pulmonary diseases. Pregnancy.

SPECIAL CONCERNS
Safety and efficacy have not been determined in children. When used in combination with other antineoplastic drugs, pulmonary toxicity may occur at lower doses.

SIDE EFFECTS
Pulmonary: Pneumonitis, ***pulmonary fibrosis, especially in older clients.*** **Hypersensitivity:** Hypotension, fever, chills, mental confusion, and wheezing in about 1% of lymphoma clients. **Integumentary and mucous membranes:** Erythema, rash, striae, vesiculation, hyperpigmentation, skin tenderness, hyperkeratosis, nail changes, alopecia, pruritus, stomatitis, skin toxicity. **GI:** Vomiting, anorexia, weight loss. **Miscellaneous:** Renal and hepatic toxicity.

DRUG INTERACTIONS
Digoxin / ↓ Serum digoxin levels
Filgrastim / ↑ Risk of pulmonary toxicity
Phenytoin / ↓ Serum phenytoin levels

HOW SUPPLIED
Powder for injection: 15 U, 30 U

DOSAGE

• **SC, IM, IV**

Hodgkin's disease.

Initial: 0.25–0.5 units/kg (10–20 units/m^2 once or twice weekly). **Maintenance:** After a 50% response, give 1 unit/day or 5 units/week IM or IV. Due to pulmonary toxicity, give doses greater than 400 units with great caution.

Squamous cell carcinoma, non-Hodgkin's lymphoma, testicular carcinoma.

0.25–0.5 units/kg (10–20 units/m^2) once or twice a week. Due to the possibility of anaphylaxis, give lymphoma clients 2 units or less for the first two doses; if no acute reaction occurs, follow the regular dosage schedule.

• **INTRAPLEURAL INJECTION**

Malignant pleural effusion.

60 units given as a single bolus dose by a thoracostomy tube following drain-

age of excess pleural fluid and confirmation of complete lung expansion.

- **INTRALESIONAL**

Warts.

0.2–0.8 unit (depending on the size) one or more times q 2–4 weeks (up to a maximum total dose of 2 units using a solution of 15 units of sterile bleomycin solution in 15 mL 0.9% saline or water for injection).

NURSING CONSIDERATIONS

SEE ALSO *NURSING CONSIDERATIONS* FOR *ANTINEOPLASTIC AGENTS*.

ADMINISTRATION/STORAGE

1. For IM or SC use, reconstitute drug with 1–5 mL (15-unit vial) or 2–10 mL (30-unit vial) 0.9% NaCl, sterile water, or bacteriostatic water for injection.
2. For intrapleural use, dissolve 60 units in 50–100 mL of 0.9% NaCl and give through a thoracostomy tube following drainage of excess pleural fluid and confirmation of complete lung expansion. The amount of drainage from the chest tube should be as minimal as possible before instillation of bleomycin. Clamp the thoracostomy tube after instillation. Move from supine to left and right lateral positions several times during the next 4 hr, followed by removal of the clamp to reestablish suction.
3. Do not reconstitute with D5W or other dextrose-containing dilutions due to loss of potency.
4. Hodgkin's disease and testicular tumors should respond within 2 weeks; squamous cell cancers require at least 3 weeks.
5. Bleomycin is stable for 24 hr at room temperature (14 days if refrigerated) in NaCl.

IV 6. For IV use, reconstitute the contents of the 15- or 30-unit vial with 5 or 10 mL, respectively, of 0.9% NaCl. Administer IV slowly over 10 min. Do not reconstitute with D5W or other dextrose-containing dilutions.

ASSESSMENT

1. Document reason for therapy, onset and symptom characteristics.
2. Obtain baseline CBC, LFTs, and PFTs. Assess for basilar rales, cough, dyspnea, and tachypnea, all of which are dose-related symptoms of pulmonary toxicity.
3. Document and avoid adhesive on the skin; drug accumulates in keratin and may discolor epithelium.
4. If receiving digoxin, monitor levels.
5. Clients with lymphoma may initially receive two test doses of 2 units each to assess for idiosyncratic response.
6. May cause mild granulocyte suppression. Nadir: 10 days; recovery: 14 days.

CLIENT/FAMILY TEACHING

1. Symptoms of idiosyncratic reaction (*hypoxia, fever, chills, confusion)* may occur with lymphoma.
2. Fever 3–6 hr after treatment is common; may use acetaminophen;.
3. Avoid vaccinations during therapy.
4. Practice safe contraception.
5. Report abnormal oral/skin rashes.
6. Smoking may aggravate pulmonary symptoms.

OUTCOMES/EVALUATE

- ↓ Tumor size/spread
- Resolution of recalcitrant common warts

Bosentan

(boh-**SEN**-tan)

PREGNANCY CATEGORY: X

CLASSIFICATION(S):

Vasodilator, endothelin receptor antagonist

Rx: Tracleer

ACTION/KINETICS

Bosentan is the first of a new class of drugs. Endothelin-1 (ET-1) is a neurohormone. Its effects are mediated by binding to ET_A and ET_B receptors in the endothelium and smooth muscle. ET-1 levels are increased in plasma and lung tissue of clients with pulmonary arterial hypertension. Bosentan is a specific and competitive antagonist at endothelin receptor types ET_A and ET_B. Bosentan is highly bound (> 98%) to plasma proteins. **Maximum**

plasma levels: 3–5 hr. Metabolized in the liver to three metabolites, one of which is active. Steady state reached in 3–5 days. Excreted in the bile. **t½, terminal:** About 5 hr.

USES

To improve exercise ability and decrease the rate of worsening in pulmonary arterial hypertension in those with WHO Class III or IV symptoms. *Note:* Because of potential liver injury and to decrease the chance as much as possible for fetal exposure, bosentan may be prescribed only through the Bosentan Access Program.

CONTRAINDICATIONS

Use in moderate or severe liver abnormalities or elevated aminotransferases >3 times ULN. Pregnancy, use with cyclosporine A or glyburide. Hypersensitivity to bosentan or any component of the medication. Lactation.

SPECIAL CONCERNS

Special attention must be paid to the possibility of serious liver damage and potential damage to a fetus. Use with caution in those with mildly impaired liver function. Safety and efficacy have not been determined in children.

SIDE EFFECTS

CV: Flushing, hypotension, palpitations, edema, lower limb edema. **Miscellaneous:** Headache, nasopharyngitis, abnormal liver function, dyspepsia, fatigue, pruritus.

LABORATORY TEST CONSIDERATIONS

↑ Liver transferases. Dose-related ↓ in H & H.

DRUG INTERACTIONS

Contraceptives, hormonal (oral, injectable, implantation) / Possible contraceptive failure due to ↑ liver metabolism of hormones

Cyclosporine A / ↑ Bosentan trough levels by about 30 fold and steady-state levels by 3–4 fold. ↓ Cyclosporine A levels by about 50%. **Do not give together**

Glyburide / ↓ Glyburide levels by about 40% and bosentan levels by about 30%. Also, ↑ risk of elevated liver aminotransferases. **Do not give together**

Ketoconazole / ↑ Bosentan plasma levels by about 2 fold

Simvastatin (and other statins) / ↓ Plasma statin levels by about 50%

Warfarin / ↓ Plasma warfarin levels

HOW SUPPLIED

Tablets: 62.5 mg, 125 mg

DOSAGE

• **TABLETS**

Pulmonary arterial hypertension.

Initial: 62.5 mg b.i.d. for 4 weeks. **Then,** increase to maintenance dose of 125 mg b.i.d. In those with a body weight less than 40 kg and who are over 12 years of age, the recommended inital and maintenance dose is 62.5 mg b.i.d.

NURSING CONSIDERATIONS

ADMINISTRATION/STORAGE

1. Use the following guidelines for dosage adjustment and monitoring in clients who develop aminotransferase abnormalities:

• If ALT/AST levels are >3 and 5 or less times ULN, confirm by another aminotransferase test. If confirmed, stop treatment and monitor aminotransferase levels at least every 2 weeks. If levels return to pretreatment values, continue or reintroduce the treatment as appropriate (see below).

• If ALT/AST levels are >5 and 8 or less times ULN, confirm by another aminotransferase test. If confirmed, stop treatment and monitor aminotransferase levels at least every 2 weeks. Once levels return to pretreatment values, consider reintroduction as described below.

• If ALT/AST levels are >8 times ULN, stop treatment and do not consider bosentan reintroduction.

2. If bosentan is reintroduced, begin again with the starting dose. Check aminotransferase levels within 3 days and thereafter.

3. If aminotransferase levels are accompanied by N&V, fever, abdominal pain, jaundice, unusual lethargy or fatigue (i.e., symptoms of liver injury) or increases in bilirubin 2 or more times ULN, stop treatment.

4. To avoid the potential for clinical deterioration after abrupt discontinuation, reduce dose gradually (i.e., 62.5 b.i.d. for 3–7 days).

ASSESSMENT

1. Note indications for therapy, other agents trialed, when diagnosed, and present class of pulmonary artery hypertension.
2. List drugs currently prescribed to ensure none interact adversely; drug is highly protein bound.
3. Ensure client is not pregnant; perform pregnancy test on all females of childbearing potential.
4. After initial labs, monitor LFTs and pregnancy tests monthly; H&H after 1 and 3 mo and then q 3 mo to assess for any deficiencies. CXR, ABGs, and PFTs as indicated.

CLIENT/FAMILY TEACHING

1. Review bosentan medication guide for safe drug administration. Take twice a day as directed and increase dosage after 4 weeks upon provider recommendation only.
2. Drug has two significant concerns: potential for serious liver damage and fetal damage. Thus, it is only administered through the Bosentan Access Program.
3. Drug is not a cure but may improve clinical symptoms of disease. Report all side effects and any changes in breathing or exercise tolerance.
4. Practice reliable contraception; use an additional form of contraception with the hormonal form as drug will cause major birth defects.
5. Continue all other therapies perscribed by pulmonologist. Keep all scheduled appointments with lab q mo and provider as scheduled.

OUTCOMES/EVALUATE

- Improved exercise tolerance
- ↓ Clinical worsening of pulmonary artery hypertension

Botulinum Toxin, Type A

(**bot**-you-**LIE**-num **TOX**-in)

PREGNANCY CATEGORY: C
CLASSIFICATION(S):
Botulinum toxin
Rx: Botox

ACTION/KINETICS

The product is a sterile, lyophilized form of purified botulinum toxin type A produced from *Clostridium botulinum* type A grown in a medium containing casein hydrolysate and yeast extract. The toxin blocks neuromuscular conduction by binding to receptor sites on motor nerve terminals, entering the nerve terminals, and inhibiting acetylcholine release. When given IM, the toxin produces a partial chemical denervation of the muscle, resulting in a localized reduction in muscle activity.

USES

Treatment of cervical dystonia in adults to decrease the severity of abnormal head position and neck pain. *Investigational:* Hemifacial spasms, spasmodic torticollis, oromandibular dystonia, spasmodic dysphonia, writer's cramp, and focal task-specific dystonia. Treatment of head and neck tremor unresponsive to other drug therapy. Is an orphan drug used to treat dynamic muscle contracture in pediatric cerebral palsy.

CONTRAINDICATIONS

Use if there is infection at the proposed injection site(s).

SPECIAL CONCERNS

Use with caution in those with peripheral motor neuropathic diseases (e.g., amyotropic lateral sclerosis, motor neuropathy) or neuromuscular junctional disorders (e.g., myasthenia gravis, Lambert-Eaton syndrome). Since the product contains albumin, there is an extremely remote risk for transmission of viral diseases or Creutzfeldt-Jakob disease. Use with caution in the presence of inflammation at the injection site(s), when excessive weakness or atrophy is present in target tissue(s), or in clients taking drugs that interfere with neuromuscular transmission. Formation of neutralizing antibodies may reduce the effectiveness by inactivating the biological activity. Use with caution during lactation. Safety and efficacy have not been determined in children less than 16 years of age.

B

SIDE EFFECTS

The most common side effects are dysphagia, URTI, neck pain, and headache. Other side effects include:

GI: Nausea, oral dryness. **CNS:** Dizziness, speech disorder, drowsiness. **CV:** Rarely, arrhythmia, ***MI*.** **Respiratory:** Increased cough, flu syndrome, rhinitis, dyspnea. **Dermatologic:** Skin rash, including erythema multiforme, urticaria, and psoriaform eruption, pruritus, allergic reaction. **Ophthalmic:** Ptosis, diplopia. **Local:** Soreness at injection site, localized pain, tenderness, bruising, weakness of adjacent muscles. **Miscellaneous:** Back pain, hypertonia, hypersensitivity (including ***anaphylaxis***).

DRUG INTERACTIONS

Effect of botulinum toxin may be potentiated by aminoglycosides or any other drug that interferes with neuromuscular transmission (e.g., curare-like drugs).

HOW SUPPLIED

Powder for Injection, Vacuum Dried: 100 units of *Clostridium botulinum* toxin type A neurotoxin complex

DOSAGE

- **INJECTION**

Cervical dystonia.

Clients with a known history of tolerance: The mean dose administered in the phase 3 study was 236 U and was divided among the affected muscles. Individualize both initial and subsequent doses based on the client's head and neck position, localization of pain, muscle hypertrophy, client response, and history of side effects. **Clients without prior use, initial:** Start with a lower dose and adjust based on individual response. Limiting the total dose injected into the sternocleidomastoid muscles to 100 units or less may decrease the occurrence of dysphagia.

NURSING CONSIDERATIONS

ADMINISTRATION/STORAGE

1. Safe and effective use depends on proper storage of the product, selection of the correct dose, and proper reconstitution and administration.

2. To reconstitute the vacuum dried powder for injection, use NSS without a preservative. Draw up the proper amount of diluent in the appropriate size syringe and slowly inject the diluent into the vial. Inject the diluent into the vial gently as bubbling or similar violent agitation denatures the toxin. Mix the toxin with the saline by gently rotating the vial. Record the date and time of reconstitution on the designated label space. Administer within 4 hr of reconstitution.

3. Discard the vial if a vacuum does not pull the diluent into the vial.

4. The usual injection volume is 0.1 mL. To obtain 10 U/0.1 mL, add 1 mL of diluent, for 5 U/0.1 mL, add 2 mL diluent, for 2.5 U/0.1 mL, add 4 mL diluent, and for 1.25 U/0.1 mL, add 8 mL of diluent. The diluent should be 0.9% NaCl injection.

5. Injection volume in excess of the intended dose is expelled through the needle into an appropriate waste container to assure patency of the needle and to confirm there is no syringe-needle leakage.

6. For superficial muscles use a 15-, 27-, or 30-gauge needle. Use a longer 22-gauge needle for deeper musculature. Use a new, sterile needle and syringe to enter the vial on each occasion for dilution or removal of the toxin.

7. Localization of the involved muscles with electromyographic guidance may be helpful.

8. Improvement usually begins within the first 2 weeks after injection with maximum benefit noted at about 6 weeks postinjection. Most clients will return to pretreatment status by 3 months posttreatment.

9. Do not exceed the recommended dose or frequency of administration since risks are not known. If accidental injection or PO ingestion occurs, monitor the client for several days (on an outpatient basis) for signs and symptoms of systemic weakness or muscle paralysis.

10. For the elderly, start at the low end of the dosing range.

11. Clients with smaller neck mass and those who require bilateral injections into the sternocleidomastoid muscle are at greater risk to develop dysphagia. Limiting the dose may decrease the occurrence.
12. Injections into the levator scapulae may increase the risk of URTIs and dysphagia.
13. Store the vacuum-dried product at or below -5°C (23°F). Give within 4 hr after the vial is removed from the freezer and reconstituted. During the 4-hr period, store the reconstituted toxin at 2–8°C (36–46°F).
14. The reconstituted toxin should be clear, colorless, and free of particulate matter.

ASSESSMENT

1. Note indications for therapy, extent of neck rigidity/jerking, positional dysfunction, pain level, associated characteristics, and other agents/therapies trialed.
2. Assess carefully for any evidence/history of neuropathic, neurologic, or neuromuscular disorders.
3. For use/administration only by those individuals trained to administer.
4. Review associated risk factors to ensure client understanding. Drug contains albumin which may present the remote risk of disease transmission of Creutzfeldt-Jakob disease (CJD).

CLIENT/FAMILY TEACHING

1. Drug is used to relieve abnormal muscle spasms/contractures of the head and neck, or spasticity of extremities permitting more controlled movement, improved posture, and increased activity.
2. Do not perform activities that require mental alertness until drug effects realized, may cause drowsiness. Resume activity slowly and carefully following administration.
3. The clostridium bacteria (A) that makes the toxin is not being injected directly; a sterilized byproduct of the bacteria is utilized. May experience a slight sting with injections.
4. Report any swallowing problems, SOB, respiratory disorders/infections, injection site abnormalities, drooping, or weakness.
5. Effects usually last up to 3 mo and repeat injections may be required.
6. Practice reliable contraception.
7. An antitoxin is available in the event of significant overdose or misinjection. Contact Allergan Pharmaceuticals at 1-800-433-8871 from 8a-4p or the CDC

OUTCOMES/EVALUATE

Relief of painful muscle spasms/contractures permitting improved posture, movement, and activity

Botulinum Toxin, Type B

(**bot**-you-**LIE**-NUM **TOX**-in)

PREGNANCY CATEGORY: C
CLASSIFICATION(S):
Botulinum toxin
Rx: Myobloc

ACTION/KINETICS

The product is a sterile liquid formulation of a purified neurotoxin derived from fermentation of *Clostridium botulinum* type B. It acts at the neuromuscular junction to produce flaccid paralysis by inhibiting acetylcholine release at the neuromuscular junction.

USES

Treatment of cervical dystonia to reduce the severity of abnormal head position and neck pain.

SPECIAL CONCERNS

Use with caution in those with peripheral motor neuropathic diseases (e.g., amyotropic lateral sclerosis, motor neuropathy) or neuromuscular junctional disorders (e.g., myasthenia gravis, Lambert-Eaton syndrome). Since the product contains albumin, there is an extremely remote risk for transmission of viral diseases or Creutzfeldt-Jakob disease. The effect of giving different botulinum neurotoxin serotypes at the same time or within less than 4 months of each other is unknown; neuromuscular paralysis may be potentiated by coadministration or overlapping administration of different botulinum toxin serotypes. Use with caution during lactation. Safety and efficacy have not been determined in children.

SIDE EFFECTS

The most common side effects are dry mouth, dysphagia, dyspepsia, and pain at the injection site. Other side effects include:

GI: N&V, GI disorder, glossitis, stomatitis, tooth disorder. **CNS:** Dizziness, neck pain related to cervical dystonia, headache, torticollis, pain related to cervical dystonia or torticollis, migraine, anxiety, tremor, hyperesthesia, somnolence, confusion. **Respiratory:** Increased cough, rhinitis, dyspnea, lung disorder, pneumonia. **Musculoskeletal:** Arthralgia, back pain, myasthenia, arthritis, joint disorder. **GU:** UTI, cystitis, vaginal moniliasis. **Dermatologic:** Pruritus, ecchymosis. **Ophthalmic:** Amblyopia, abnormal vision. **Otic:** Otitis media, tinnitus. **Body as a whole:** Infection, pain, flu syndrome, accidental injury, fever, chills, malaise, viral infection. **Miscellaneous:** Injection site pain, peripheral edema, hypercholesterolemia, taste perversion, allergic reaction, chest pain, hernia, abscess, cyst, neoplasm, vasodilation.

DRUG INTERACTIONS

Effect of botulinum toxin may be potentiated by aminoglycosides or any other drug that interferes with neuromuscular transmission (e.g., curare-like drugs).

HOW SUPPLIED

Injectable Solution: 5,000 U/mL

DOSAGE

- **INJECTION**

Cervical dystonia.

Clients with a history of tolerating botulinum toxin, initial: 2,500–5,000 U divided among the affected muscles. **Clients without a history of tolerating botulinum toxin:** Use a lower initial dose. Individualize subsequent dosing based on individual client response.

NURSING CONSIDERATIONS

ADMINISTRATION/STORAGE

1. The duration of effect in those responding to the toxin is between 12 and 16 weeks at doses of 5,000 U or 10,000 U.
2. Administration of the toxin should only be by physicians familiar and experienced in assessing and managing clients with cervical dystonia.
3. Units of biological activity of botulinum toxin, type B can not be compared or converted into units of any other botulinum toxin.
4. If a client ingests the drug or is accidentally overdosed, monitor for up to several weeks for signs and symptoms of systemic weakness or paralysis.
5. There is an increased incidence of dysphagia with an increased dose in the sternocleidomastoid muscle.
6. The incidence of dry mouth may increase when the toxin is used in the splenius capitis, trapezius, and sternocleidomastoid muscles.
7. Store under refrigeration at 2–8°C (36–46°F) for up to 21 months. Do not freeze or shake.
8. After dilution with normal saline, use within 4 hr as the product does not contain a preservative.

ASSESSMENT

1. Note indications for therapy, level of pain, extent of abnormal head/neck positioning, and other agents/therapies trialed.
2. Assess carefully for any evidence/history of neuropathic, neurologic, or neuromuscular disorders.
3. For use/administration only by those individuals trained to administer.
4. Do not use within 4 mo of any other botulinum toxin serotype.
5. Review associated risk factors to ensure client understanding. Drug contains albumin which may present the remote risk of disease transmission of Creutzfeldt-Jakob disease (CJD).

CLIENT/FAMILY TEACHING

1. Drug is used to release abnormal muscle spasms/contractures permitting more controlled movements, mobility, and freedom.

2. The clostridium bacteria (B) that makes the toxin is not being injected directly; a sterilized byproduct of the bacteria is utilized. May experience a slight sting with injections and dryness of mouth.
3. Do not perform activities that require mental alertness until drug effects realized, may experience dizziness, anxiety, confusion. Resume activity slowly and carefully following administration.
4. Report any swallowing problems, SOB, respiratory disorders/infections, injection site abnormalities, drooping, or weakness.
5. Effects usually last from 12-16 weeks when reinjection may be necessary to reattain desired results.
6. Practice reliable contraception.
7. An antitoxin is available in the event of significant overdose or misinjection. Contact Elan Pharmaceuticals at 1-888-638-7605, or the CDC

OUTCOMES/EVALUATE

Relief of painful neck spasms/contractures with cervical dystonia

Bretylium tosylate

(breh-**TILL**-ee-um **TOZ**-ill-ayt)

PREGNANCY CATEGORY: C
CLASSIFICATION(S):
Antiarrhythmic, class III

ACTION/KINETICS

Inhibits catecholamine release at nerve endings by decreasing excitability of the nerve terminal. Initially there is a release of norepinephrine, which may cause tachycardia and a rise in BP; this is followed by a blockade of release of catecholamines. Also increases the duration of the action potential and the effective refractory period, which may assist in reversing arrhythmias. **Peak plasma concentration and effect:** 1 hr after IM. Antifibrillatory effect within a few minutes after IV use. Suppression of ventricular tachycardia and ventricular arrhythmias takes 20–120 min, whereas suppression of PVCs does not occur for 6–9 hr. **Therapeutic serum levels:** 0.5–1.5 mcg/mL. **t½:** Approximately 5–10 hr. **Duration:** 6–8 hr. From 0% to 8% is protein bound. Up to 90% of drug is excreted unchanged in the urine after 24 hr.

USES

Life-threatening ventricular arrhythmias that have failed to respond to other antiarrhythmics. Prophylaxis and treatment of ventricular fibrillation. For short-term use only. *Investigational:* Second-line drug (after lidocaine) for advanced cardiac life support during CPR.

CONTRAINDICATIONS

Severe aortic stenosis, severe pulmonary hypertension.

SPECIAL CONCERNS

Safety and efficacy in children have not been established. Dosage adjustment required in impaired renal function.

SIDE EFFECTS

CV: Hypotension (including postural hypotension), transient hypertension, increased frequency of PVCs, bradycardia, precipitation of anginal attacks, initial increase in arrhythmias, sensation of substernal pressure. **GI:** N&V (especially after rapid IV administration), diarrhea, abdominal pain, hiccoughs. **CNS:** Vertigo, dizziness, lightheadedness, syncope, anxiety, paranoid psychosis, confusion, mood swings. **Miscellaneous:** Renal dysfunction, flushing, hyperthermia, SOB, nasal stuffiness, diaphoresis, conjunctivitis, erythematous macular rash, lethargy, generalized tenderness.

OD OVERDOSE MANAGEMENT

Symptoms: Marked hypertension followed by hypotension. *Treatment:* Treat hypertension with nitroprusside or another short-acting IV antihypertensive. Treat hypotension with appropriate fluid therapy and pressor agents such as norepinephrine or dopamine.

DRUG INTERACTIONS

Digoxin / Bretylium may aggravate toxicity due to initial release of norepinephrine

B

Procainamide, Quinidine / Concomitant use ↓ inotropic effect of bretylium and ↑ hypotension

HOW SUPPLIED

Injection: 50 mg/mL

DOSAGE

• **IV INFUSION**

Ventricular fibrillation, hemodynamically unstable VT.

Adults: 5 mg/kg of undiluted solution given rapidly. Can increase to 10 mg/kg if ventricular fibrillation persists, repeat as needed. **Maintenance, IV infusion:** 1–2 mg/min, or, 5–10 mg/kg q 6 hr of diluted drug infused over more than 8 min. **Children:** 5 mg/kg/dose IV followed by 10 mg/kg at 15–30-min intervals for a maximum total dose of 30 mg/kg, **maintenance:** 5–10 mg/kg q 6 hr.

Other ventricular arrhythmias.

• **IV INFUSION**

5–10 mg/kg of diluted solution over more than 8 min. **Maintenance:** 5–10 mg/kg q 6 hr over a period of 8 min or more or 1–2 mg/min by continuous IV infusion. **Children:** 5–10 mg/kg/dose q 6 hr.

• **IM**

Other ventricular arrhythmias.

Adults: 5–10 mg/kg of undiluted solution followed, if necessary, by the same dose at 1–2-hr intervals, **then,** give same dosage q 6–8 hr.

NURSING CONSIDERATIONS

SEE ALSO *NURSING CONSIDERATIONS FOR ANTIARRHYTHMIC AGENTS.*

ADMINISTRATION/STORAGE

1. For IM, use drug undiluted.
2. Rotate injection sites so that no more than 5 mL of drug is given at any site to avoid atrophy, necrosis, fibrosis, vascular degeneration, or inflammation.
3. Keep supine during therapy, observe for postural hypotension.
4. Start on an oral antiarrhythmic medication as soon as possible.

IV 5. For IV infusion, bretylium is compatible with D5W, 0.9% NaCl, D5/0.45% NaCl, D5/0.9% NaCl, D5/RL, 5% $NaHCO_3$, 20% mannitol, 1/6 molar sodium lactate, RL, $CaCl_2$ (54.5 mEq/L) in 5% dextrose, and KCl (40 mEq/L) in 5% dextrose.

6. For direct IV, administer undiluted over 15–30 sec, may repeat in 15–30 min if symptoms persist. May further dilute 500 mg in 50 cc and infuse over 10–30 min.

ASSESSMENT

1. Document indications for therapy, pretreatment ECG, and VS.
2. If taking digitalis, may aggravate digitalis toxicity.

INTERVENTIONS

1. Monitor VS and rhythm strips as dose is titrated on client response.
2. To reduce N&V, administer IV slowly over 10 min while supine. Once infusion complete remain supine until the BP has stabilized.
3. Supervise once ambulation is permitted, may experience lightheadedness and vertigo.
4. Bretylium often causes a fall in supine BP within 1 hr of IV administration. If SBP < 75 mm Hg, anticipate need for pressor agents.
5. If clients develop side effects, stay to reassure and reorient as needed.

OUTCOMES/EVALUATE

• Termination of life-threatening ventricular arrhythmia, stable cardiac rhythm
• Serum drug levels (0.5–1.5 mcg/mL)

Brimonidine tartrate

(brih-**MOH**-nih-deen)

PREGNANCY CATEGORY: B
CLASSIFICATION(S):
Sympathomimetic
Rx: Alphagan, Alphagan P

SEE ALSO *SYMPATHOMIMETIC DRUGS.*

ACTION/KINETICS

An alpha-2 adrenergic receptor agonist that reduces aqueous humor production and increases uveoscleral outflow. **Peak plasma levels after intraocular administration:** 1–4 hr. **t½, systemic:** About 3 hr. Metabolized by the liver and excreted through the urine as unchanged drug and metabolites.

B

USES
Lower intraocular pressure in open-angle glaucoma or ocular hypertension.
CONTRAINDICATIONS
Use with MAO inhibitor therapy. Lactation.
SPECIAL CONCERNS
Use with caution in those with renal or hepatic impairment; in severe CV disease, depression, cerebral or coronary insufficiency, Raynaud's phenomenon, orthostatic hypotension, or thromboangiitis obliterans. Safety and efficacy have not been determined in children. Benzylkonium chloride, a preservative in the product, may be absorbed by soft contact lenses.
SIDE EFFECTS
Ophthalmic: Ocular hyperemia, burning and stinging, blurring, foreign body sensation, conjunctival follicles, ocular allergic reactions, ocular pruritus, corneal staining or erosion, photophobia, eyelid erythema, ocular ache or pain, ocular dryness, tearing, eyelid edema, conjunctival edema, blepharitis, ocular irritation, conjunctival blanching, abnormal vision, lid crusting, conjunctival hemorrhage, conjunctival discharge. **CNS:** Headache, fatigue, drowsiness, dizziness, insomnia, depression, anxiety. **Miscellaneous:** Upper respiratory symptoms, GI symptoms, asthenia, muscle pain, abnormal taste, hypertension, palpitations, nasal dryness, syncope.
HOW SUPPLIED
Solution: 0.15%, 0.2%

DOSAGE
- **SOLUTION, 0.15%, 0.2%**

Open-angle glaucoma or ocular hypertension.
Adults: 1 gtt in the affected eye(s) t.i.d., with doses about 8 hr apart.

NURSING CONSIDERATIONS

SEE ALSO *NURSING CONSIDERATIONS* FOR *SYMPATHOMIMETIC DRUGS*.

ADMINISTRATION/STORAGE
1. Alphagan P (0.15%) contains less preservative than Alphagan (0.2%) causing less conjunctival hyperemia and fewer other side effects.
2. Store at or below 25°C (77°F).
ASSESSMENT
1. Document ophthalmic findings and ensure routine screenings.
2. Note if MAO inhibitor ordered as this precludes drug therapy.
CLIENT/FAMILY TEACHING
1. Wash hands before and after instillation. Use as directed: 1 gtt every 8 hr to affected eye(s).
2. Remove and do not reinsert soft contact lenses for at least 15 min following instillation of drops.
3. Use caution when performing activities that require mental alertness as drug may cause fatigue and drowsiness. Report any unusual or intolerable side effects.
4. Avoid alcohol and any other CNS depressants.
5. Report for follow-up ophthalmic evaluations.
OUTCOMES/EVALUATE
↓ IOP

Brinzolamide ophthalmic suspension

(brin-**ZOH**-lah-myd)

PREGNANCY CATEGORY: C
CLASSIFICATION(S):
Antiglaucoma drug
Rx: Azopt

ACTION/KINETICS
Inhibits carbonic hydrase in the ciliary processes of the eye, thus decreasing aqueous humor production and reducing intraocular pressure (IOP). Is absorbed into the systemic circulation following ocular use. It can then distribute to RBCs. Eliminated unchanged mainly through the urine.
USES
Treatment of elevated IOP in ocular hypertension or open-angle glaucoma.

B

CONTRAINDICATIONS
Use in severe renal impairment (C_{CR} less than 30 mL/min). Concomitant use with oral carbonic anhydrase inhibitors. Lactation.
SPECIAL CONCERNS
Is a sulfonamide; thus, similar side effects can occur. Use with caution in hepatic impairment. Safety and efficacy have not been determined in children.
SIDE EFFECTS
Ophthalmic: Blurred vision following dosing, blepharitis, dry eye, foreign body sensation, hyperemia, ocular discharge, ocular discomfort, ocular keratitis, ocular pain, ocular pruritus, rhinitis, conjunctivitis, diplopia, eye fatigue, keratoconjunctivitis, keratopathy, lid margin crusting or sticky sensation, tearing, hypertonia. **GI:** Bitter, sour, or unusual taste; nausea, diarrhea, dry mouth, dyspepsia. **CNS:** Headache, dizziness. **Miscellaneous:** Dermatitis, allergic reactions, alopecia, chest pain, dyspnea, kidney pain, pharyngitis, urticaria.
DRUG INTERACTIONS
Possible additive effects with oral carbonic anhydrase inhibitors.
HOW SUPPLIED
Ophthalmic Suspension: 1%

DOSAGE
- **OPHTHALMIC SUSPENSION**
  Increased IOP.
1 gtt in the affected eye(s) t.i.d.

NURSING CONSIDERATIONS

ADMINISTRATION/STORAGE
Shake well before use. Benzalkonium chloride, the preservative in the product, may be absorbed by soft contact lenses. Remove lenses during administration; reinsert 15 min after administration.
ASSESSMENT
1. Note any sulfonamide sensitivity.
2. Obtain renal and LFTs; do not use with severe impairment.
CLIENT/FAMILY TEACHING
1. Shake well, wash hands, and administer as directed.
2. Do not permit the tip of the container to touch the eye or surrounding structures; contamination may occur.
3. Use care operating machinery/car; may temporarily blur vision after dosing.
4. If more than one topical ophthalmic drug is being used, administer at least 10 min apart.
5. Report any S&S of infection, eye trauma or surgery.
6. Benzalkonium chloride, the preservative in the product, may be absorbed by soft contact lenses. Remove lenses during administration; wait 15 min to reinsert.
OUTCOMES/EVALUATE
↓ IOP

Brompheniramine maleate

(brohm-fen-**EAR**-ah-meen)

PREGNANCY CATEGORY: B
CLASSIFICATION(S):
Antihistamine, first generation, alkylamine
Rx: Brompheniramine Maleate Injection
OTC: Dimetapp Allergy

SEE ALSO *ANTIHISTAMINES*.

ACTION/KINETICS
Fewer sedative effects. **t½:** 25 hr. **Time to peak effect:** 3–9 hr. **Duration:** 4–25 hr.
USES
PO. Allergic rhinitis. **Parenteral.** To treat allergic reactions to blood or plasma; adjunct to treat anaphylaxis; uncomplicated allergic conditions when PO therapy is not possible or is contraindicated.
CONTRAINDICATIONS
Use in neonates.
SPECIAL CONCERNS
Geriatric clients may be more sensitive to the usual adult dose.
HOW SUPPLIED
Injection: 10 mg/mL; *Liqui-Gels:* 4 mg

DOSAGE
- **LIQUI-GELS**
  Allergic rhinitis.
Adults and children over 12 years: 4

mg q 4–6 hr, not to exceed 24 mg/ day.

• **IM, IV, SC**

Adults: usual, 10 mg (range: 5–20 mg) b.i.d. (maximum daily dose: 40 mg); **pediatric, under 12 years:** 0.5 mg/kg/day (15 mg/m² /day) divided into three or four doses.

NURSING CONSIDERATIONS

SEE ALSO *NURSING CONSIDERATIONS* FOR *ANTIHISTAMINES*.

ADMINISTRATION/STORAGE

1. For IM or SC, use undiluted or diluted 1:10 with NSS.

IV 2. Do not use solutions containing preservatives for IV injection.

3. For IV, the 10-mg/mL preparation may be used undiluted or diluted 1:10 with sterile saline for injection. Administer over 1 min. slowly, preferably to a recumbent client.

4. May add to NSS, 5% dextrose, or whole blood for IV use.

CLIENT/FAMILY TEACHING

1. Drug may cause drowsiness.
2. Consume 1.5–2 L of fluids/day to decrease secretion viscosity.
3. Avoid alcohol.
4. Report any persistent or bothersome side effects and loss of drug responsiveness.

OUTCOMES/EVALUATE

Relief of allergic manifestations; ↓ congestion

Budesonide

(byou-**DES**-oh-nyd)

PREGNANCY CATEGORY: C
CLASSIFICATION(S):
Glucocorticoid
Rx: Entocort EC, Pulmicort Respules, Pulmicort Turbuhaler, Rhinocort, Rhinocort Aqua
✱**Rx:** Entocort, Gen-Budesonide Aq., Pulmicort Nebuamp, Rhinocort Turbuhaler

SEE ALSO *CORTICOSTEROIDS*.

ACTION/KINETICS

Exerts a direct local anti-inflammatory effect with minimal systemic effects when used intranasally. Entocort EC Capsules contain micronized budesonide which has been coated to prevent release in the stomach. Bbudesonide is released in the intestine resulting in decreased inflammation by a local action. When taken PO, not absorbed into the body. Exceeding the recommended dose may result in suppression of hypothalamic-pituitary-adrenal function. **Onset, nasal spray:** 10 hr. **t½:** 2–3 hr. Liver metabolism of absorbed drug is rapid. Excreted through both urine and feces.

USES

1. Treat symptoms of seasonal or perennial allergic rhinitis in adults and children over 6 years of age.
2. Nonallergic perennial rhinitis in adults.
3. The Turbuhaler is used for maintenance treatment of asthma as prophylaxis in adults and children 6 years of age and older; also for those requiring oral corticosteroid therapy for asthma.
4. Respules are used for prophylaxis of and maintenance treatment of asthma in children and infants 12 months to 8 years.
5. Mild-to-moderate active Crohn's disease involving the ileum and/or ascending colon (Entocort EC).

CONTRAINDICATIONS

Hypersensitivity to the drug. Untreated localized nasal mucosa infections. Lactation. Use in children less than 6 years of age or for acute or life-threatening asthma attacks, including status asthmaticus.

SPECIAL CONCERNS

Use with caution in clients already on alternate day corticosteroids (e.g., prednisone); in clients with active or quiescent tuberculosis infections of the respiratory tract, or in untreated fungal, bacterial; systemic viral infections; or ocular herpes simplex. Use with caution in clients with recent nasal septal ulcers, recurrent epistaxis, nasal surgery, or trauma. Avoid exposure to chicken pox or measles.

SIDE EFFECTS

Respiratory: Nasopharyngeal irritation, nasal irritation, pharyngitis, increased cough, hoarseness, nasal pain, burning, stinging, dryness, epistaxis, bloody mucus, rebound congestion, ***bronchial asthma,*** occasional sneezing attacks (especially in children), rhinorrhea, reduced sense of smell, throat discomfort, ulceration of the nasal mucosa, sore throat, dyspnea, localized infections of nose and pharynx with *Candida albicans*, wheezing (rare). **CNS:** Lightheadedness, headache, nervousness. **GI:** Nausea, loss of sense of taste, bad taste in mouth, dry mouth, dyspepsia. **Miscellaneous:** Watery eyes, ***immediate and delayed hypersensitivity reactions,*** moniliasis, facial edema, rash, pruritus, herpes simplex, alopecia, arthralgia, myalgia, contact dermatitis (rare).

OD OVERDOSE MANAGEMENT

Symptoms: Symptoms of hypercorticism, including menstrual irregularities, acneiform lesions, and cushingoid features (all are rarely seen, however). *Treatment:* Discontinue the drug slowly using procedures that are acceptable for discontinuing oral corticosteroids.

ADDITIONAL DRUG INTERACTIONS

Grapefruit juice and ketoconazole increase systemic levels of budesonide twofold and eightfold, respectively.

HOW SUPPLIED

Capsules: 3mg; *Inhalation Powder:* 200 mcg/inh; *Aerosol Aqua Nasal Spray:* 32 mcg/inh; *Aerosol Nasal Spray:* 32 mcg/inh; *Aerosol Liquid:* 0.25 mg/inh, 0.5 mg/inh

DOSAGE

• INHALATION AEROSOL POWDER

Seasonal or perennial rhinitis.

Adults and children 6 years of age and older, initial: 256 mcg/day given as either 2 sprays in each nostril in the morning and evening or 4 sprays in each nostril in the morning. Doses greater than 256 mcg/day are not recommended. **Maintenance:** Reduce initial dose to the smallest amount necessary to control symptoms; decrease dose q 2–4 weeks as long as desired effect is maintained. If symptoms return,. the dose may be increased briefly to the initial dose.

• AEROSOL AQUA NASAL SPRAY

Seasonal and perennial allergic rhinitis.

Adults and children over 6 years, initial: 1 spray/nostril once daily. **Maximum:** 2 sprays/nostril for children and 4 sprays/nostril for adults. Maximum benefit seen in 2 weeks.

• PULMICORT TURBUHALER

Prevention or treatment of asthma.

Adults: 200–400 mcg b.i.d., not to exceed 400 mcg b.i.d. For mild to moderate asthmatics well controlled on inhaled corticosteroids, initial dose is 200–400 mcg (1–2 inhalations) once daily either in the morning or evening. **Children, over 6 years of age:** 200 mcg b.i.d., not to exceed 400 mcg b.i.d. Each actuation actually delivers about 160 mcg of budesonide to the client however.

• PULMICORT RESPULES

Prophalaxis or maintenance treatment of asthma.

If previous therapy was bronchodilators alone: 0.5 mg total daily dose given either once daily or b.i.d. in divided doses (maximum daily dose: 0.5 mg). If previous therapy was inhaled corticosteroids: 0.5 mg total daily dose given either once daily or b.i.d. in divided doses (maximum daily dose: 1 mg). If previous therapy was oral corticosteroids: 1 mg total daily dose given either as 0.5 mg b.i.d. or 1 mg daily (maximum daily dose: 1 mg).

• CAPSULES

Crohn's disease.

9 mg once daily in the a.m. for up to 8 weeks. If the disease recurs, another 8-week course may be given.

NURSING CONSIDERATIONS

SEE ALSO *NURSING CONSIDERATIONS FOR CORTICOSTEROIDS.*

ADMINISTRATION/STORAGE

1. The Turbuhaler contains no chlorofluorocarbon propellants; drug delivered by client's inhalation.

2. Turbuhaler does not require a spacer; it delivers about twice the

amount of drug per inhalation to the airway as metered dose inhalers.
3. Pulmicort Respules may be used in children as young as 12 months.

ASSESSMENT

1. Note indications for therapy, onset and frequency of symptoms.
2. List drugs prescribed to ensure that none interact unfavorably.

CLIENT/FAMILY TEACHING

1. Review the appropriate method and frequency for administration. Review video/instruction for proper administration guidelines.
2. Rinse mouth (especially children) and equipment thoroughly after each use to prevent oral fungal infections.
3. Prior to using, clear nasal passages of secretions. If nasal passages are blocked, use decongestant first.
4. Maximum benefit is usually not seen for 3–7 days, although a decrease in symptoms can be seen within 24 hr. Report if no improvement noted within 3 weeks.
5. Shake canister well before administering. Store valve down and away from areas of high humidity. Once aluminum pouch is opened, use or discard within 6 months.
6. Avoid persons with chicken pox or communicable diseases.
7. Symptoms of hoarseness may be evident but should subside upon completion of therapy.
8. Drug is a steroid; chronic use in excessive amounts may lead to adverse systemic reactions.
9. Identify triggers and avoid irritants to control symptoms.

OUTCOMES/EVALUATE

Relief of nasal congestion/allergic manifestations

Bumetanide

(byou-**MET**-ah-nyd)

PREGNANCY CATEGORY: C
CLASSIFICATION(S):
Diuretic, loop
Rx: Bumex
✱**Rx:** Burinex

SEE ALSO *DIURETICS, LOOP.*

ACTION/KINETICS

Inhibits reabsorption of both sodium and chloride in the proximal tubule and the ascending loop of Henle. Possible activity in the proximal tubule to promote phosphate excretion. **Onset, PO:** 30–60 min. **Peak effect, PO:** 1–2 hr. **Duration, PO:** 4–6 hr (dose-dependent). **Onset, IV:** Several minutes. **Peak effect, IV:** 15–30 min. **Duration, IV:** 3.5–4 hr. **t½:** 1–1.5 hr. Metabolized in the liver although 45% excreted unchanged in the urine.

USES

Edema associated with CHF, nephrotic syndrome, hepatic disease. Adjunct to treat acute pulmonary edema. Especially useful in clients refractory to other diuretics. *Investigational:* Treatment of adult nocturia. Not effective in males with prostatic hypertrophy.

CONTRAINDICATIONS

Anuria. Hepatic coma or severe electrolyte depletion until condition improved/corrected. Hypersensitivity to drug. Lactation.

SPECIAL CONCERNS

Safety and efficacy in children under 18 have not been established. Geriatric clients may be more sensitive to the hypotensive and electrolyte effects and are at greater risk for developing thromboembolic problems and circulatory collapse. SLE may be activated or made worse. Clients allergic to sulfonamides may show cross sensitivity to bumetanide. Sudden changes in electrolyte balance may cause hepatic encephalopathy and coma in clients with hepatic cirrhosis and ascites.

SIDE EFFECTS

Electrolyte and fluid changes: Excess water loss, ***dehydration,*** electrolyte depletion including hypokalemia, hypochloremia, hyponatremia, hypovolemia, thromboembolism, ***circulatory collapse.*** **Otic:** Tinnitus, reversible and irreversible hearing impairment, deafness, vertigo (with a sense of fullness in the ears). **CV:** ***Reduction in blood volume may cause circulatory collapse and vascular thrombosis and embolism, especially in geriatric***

B

clients. Hypotension, ECG changes, chest pain. **CNS:** Asterixis, encephalopathy with preexisting liver disease, vertigo, headache, dizziness. **GI:** Upset stomach, dry mouth, N&V, diarrhea, GI pain. **GU:** Premature ejaculation, difficulty maintaining erection, renal failure. **Musculoskeletal:** Arthritic pain, weakness, muscle cramps, fatigue. **Hematologic:** Agranulocytosis, thrombocytopenia. **Allergic:** Pruritus, urticaria, rashes. **Miscellaneous:** Sweating, hyperventilation, rash, nipple tenderness, photosensitivity, pain following parenteral use.

LABORATORY TEST CONSIDERATIONS

Alterations in LDH, AST, ALT, alkaline phosphatase, creatinine clearance, total serum bilirubin, serum proteins, cholesterol. Changes in hemoglobin, PT, hematocrit, WBCs, platelet and differential counts, phosphorus, carbon dioxide content, bicarbonate, and calcium. ↑ Urinary glucose and protein, serum creatinine. Also, hyperuricemia, hypochloremia, hypokalemia, azotemia, hyponatremia, hyperglycemia.

OD OVERDOSE MANAGEMENT

Symptoms: Profound loss of water, electrolyte depletion, dehydration, decreased blood volume, ***circulatory collapse (possibility of vascular thrombosis and embolism).*** Symptoms of electrolyte depletion include: anorexia, cramps, weakness, dizziness, vomiting, and mental confusion. *Treatment:* Replace electrolyte and fluid losses and monitor urinary and serum electrolyte levels. Emesis or gastric lavage. Oxygen or artificial respiration may be necessary. General supportive measures.

HOW SUPPLIED

Injection: 0.25 mg /mL; *Tablet:* 0.5 mg, 1 mg, 2 mg

DOSAGE

• **TABLETS**

Adults: 0.5–2 mg once daily; if response is inadequate, a second or third dose may be given at 4–5-hr intervals up to a maximum of 10 mg/day.

• **IV, IM**

Adults: 0.5–1 mg; if response is inadequate, a second or third dose may be given at 2–3-hr intervals up to a maximum of 10 mg/day. Initiate PO dosing as soon as possible.

NURSING CONSIDERATIONS

SEE ALSO *NURSING CONSIDERATIONS* FOR *DIURETICS, LOOP*.

ADMINISTRATION/STORAGE

1. The recommended PO medication schedule is on alternate days or for 3–4 days with a 1–2-day rest period in between.
2. Bumetanide, at a 1:40 ratio of bumetanide:furosemide, may be ordered if allergic to furosemide.
3. Reserve IV or IM administration for clients in whom PO use is not practical or absorption from the GI tract is impaired.
4. IV In severe chronic renal insufficiency, a continuous infusion (12 mg over 12 hr) may be more effective and cause fewer side effects than intermittent bolus therapy.
5. Prepare solutions fresh for IM or IV; use within 24 hr.
6. Ampules may be reconstituted with D5W, NSS, or RL solution.
7. Administer IV solutions slowly over 1–2 min.

ASSESSMENT

1. Document indications for therapy and pretreatment findings.
2. Note any sulfonamide allergy; may be cross sensitivity.
3. Monitor electrolytes, liver and renal function studies; assess for ↓ K^+.
4. Review history; note any hearing impairment, lupus, or thromboembolic events.
5. *NOTE:* 1 mg of bumetanide is equivalent to 40 mg of furosemide.
6. Monitor VS. Rapid diuresis may cause dehydration and circulatory collapse (especially in the elderly). Hypotension may occur when administered with antihypertensives.
7. Assess hearing and for ototoxicity, especially if receiving other ototoxic drugs

CLIENT/FAMILY TEACHING

1. Take early in the day to prevent nighttime voidings.

2. Do not perform activities that require mental alertness until drug effects realized.
3. Review dietary requirements such as reduced sodium and high potassium; may see dietitian.
4. Record weights; report any sudden weight gain or evidence of swelling in the hands or feet.
5. Report any unusual side effects.

OUTCOMES/EVALUATE

↓ Peripheral and sacral edema; Enhanced diuresis

Buprenorphine hydrochloride

(byou-pren-**OR**-feen)

PREGNANCY CATEGORY: C
CLASSIFICATION(S):
Narcotic agonist/antagonist
Rx: Buprenex **C-V**

SEE ALSO *NARCOTIC ANALGESICS*.

ACTION/KINETICS

Semisynthetic opiate possessing both narcotic agonist and antagonist activity. Limited activity at the mu receptor. **IM, onset:** 15 min; **Peak effect:** 1 hr; **Duration:** 6 hr. **t½:** 2–3 hr. May also be given IV with shorter onset and peak effect. Is about equipotent with naloxone as a narcotic antagonist.

USES

Moderate to severe pain.

SPECIAL CONCERNS

Use during lactation only if benefits outweigh risks. Use in children less than 2 years of age has not been established. Use with caution in clients with compromised respiratory function, in head injuries, in impairment of liver or renal function, Addison's disease, prostatic hypertrophy, biliary tract dysfunction, urethral stricture, myxedema, and hypothyroidism. Administration to individuals physically dependent on narcotics may result in precipitation of a withdrawal syndrome.

SIDE EFFECTS

CNS: Sedation, dizziness, confusion, headache, euphoria, slurred speech, depression, paresthesia, psychosis, malaise, hallucinations, coma, dysphoria, agitation, seizures. **GI:** N&V, constipation, dyspepsia, loss of appetite, dry mouth. **Ophthalmologic:** Miosis, blurred/double vision, conjunctivitis. **CV:** Hypotension, bradycardia, tachycardia, Wenckebach block. **Respiratory:** Decreased respiratory rate, cyanosis, dyspepsia. **Dermatologic:** Sweating, rash, pruritus, flushing. **Other:** Urinary retention, chills, tinnitus.

DRUG INTERACTIONS

Additive CNS depression with alcohol, general anesthetics, antianxiety agents, sedative-hypnotics, phenothiazines, and other narcotic analgesics.

HOW SUPPLIED

Injection: Equivalent to 0.3 mg/mL buprenorphine

DOSAGE

- **IM, SLOW IV**

Analgesia.

Over 13 years of age: 0.3 mg q 6 hr; repeat once (up to 0.3 mg) if needed, 30-60 min. after initial dose. **Children, 2–12 years of age:** 2–6 mcg/kg q 4–6 hr. Do not give single doses greater than 6 mcg/kg.

NURSING CONSIDERATIONS

SEE ALSO *NURSING CONSIDERATIONS* FOR *NARCOTIC ANALGESICS*.

ADMINISTRATION/STORAGE

1. Not all children may clear buprenorphine faster than adults. Thus, fixed interval or "round the clock" dosing should not be undertaken until the proper interdose interval has been established.
2. Some pediatric clients may not need to be remedicated for 6–8 hr.
3. Have naloxone to reverse drug-induced respiratory depression.
4. Avoid storage in excessive heat and light
IV 5. Do not mix with solutions containing diazepam or lorazepam.

6. May be mixed with solutions containing haloperidol, glycopyrrolate, scopolamine hydrobromide, hydroxyzine chloride, or droperidol.
7. May be mixed with isotonic saline, RL solution, and D5/0.9% NaCl.
8. May be administered undiluted IV, slowly.

ASSESSMENT

1. Document indications for therapy, onset, location, and intensity/pain level.
2. Determine any respiratory depression; drug is contraindicated.
3. Report head injuries immediately.
4. If receiving narcotics, observe for withdrawal symptoms.
5. Assess for liver or renal dysfunction, diseases of the biliary tract, or BPH.

CLIENT/FAMILY TEACHING

1. Drug may cause drowsiness, dizziness, and orthostatic effects.
2. Cough and deep breathe every 2 hr to prevent atelectasis.
3. Avoid alcohol.

OUTCOMES/EVALUATE

Relief of pain

Bupropion hydrochloride

(byou-**PROH**-pee-on)

PREGNANCY CATEGORY: B
CLASSIFICATION(S):
Antidepressant, miscellaneous smoking deterrent
Rx: Wellbutrin, Wellbutrin SR, Zyban

ACTION/KINETICS

Mechanism of action is not known; the drug does not inhibit MAO and it only weakly blocks neuronal uptake of epinephrine, serotonin, and dopamine. Exerts moderate anticholinergic and sedative effects, but only slight orthostatic hypotension. **Peak plasma levels:** 2–3 hr. **t½:** 8–24 hr. **Time to steady state:** Within 8 days. Significantly metabolized by a first-pass effect through the liver to both active and inactive metabolites. Can induce drug-metabolizing enzymes. During chronic use the plasma levels of two active metabolites may be higher than bupropion. Excreted through both the urine (87%) and the feces (10%). Zyban is a sustained-release formulation.

USES

Short-term (6 weeks or less) treatment of depression. Aid to stop smoking (Zyban); may be combined with a nicotine transdermal system.

CONTRAINDICATIONS

Seizure disorders; presence or history of bulimia or anorexia nervosa due to the higher incidence of seizures in such clients. Concomitant use of an MAO inhibitor. Wellbutrin, Wellbutrin SR, and Zyban all contain bupropion; do not use together. Lactation.

SPECIAL CONCERNS

Use with caution in clients with cranial trauma, with drugs that lower the seizure threshold (e.g., alcohol use; addiction to opiates, cocaine, or stimulants; use of OTC stimulants and anorectics, antipsychotics, other antidepressants, theophylline, systemic steroids; diabetes treated with oral hypoglycemics or insulin); and, situations that might cause seizures (e.g., abrupt cessation of a benzodiazepine). Use with extreme caution in severe hepatic cirrhosis (do not exceed 150 mg every other day). Use with caution and in lower doses in clients with liver or kidney disease and in those with a recent history of MI or unstable heart disease. Safety and efficacy have not been established in clients less than 18 years of age.

SIDE EFFECTS

Listed are side effects with an incidence of 0.1% or greater.
CNS: Agitation, restlessness, anxiety, insomnia, headache, migraine, dizziness, seizures, excessive sweating, tremor, sedation, akinesia, bradykinesia, nervousness, sensory disturbances, impaired sleep quality, somnolence, irritability, decreased memory, pseudoparkinsonism, akathisia, hyperkinesia, paresthesia, CNS stimulation, confusion, hostility, disturbed concentration, increased/ decreased libido, delusions, euphoria, ataxia, dyskinesia, dystonia, hypertonia, hypesthesia, vertigo, depersonalization, dysphoria,

suicidal ideation, mania/hypomania, incoordination, myoclonus, hallucinations, depression, psychosis, unstable moods, paranoia, formal thought disorder, frigiditiy. **GI:** Constipation, weight loss/gain, N&V, anorexia, dry mouth, diarrhea, increased appetite, dyspepsia, dysphagia, increased salivary flow, stomatitis, bruxism, glossitis, thirst disturbance, jaundice, liver damage, toothache, gum irritation, oral edema, gastric reflux, gingivitis, mouth ulcers, thirst, taste perversion. **CV:** Tachycardia, cardiac arrhythmias, hyper/hypotension, palpitations, syncope, ECG abnormalities, chest pain. **Respiratory:** Pharyngitis, sinusitis, increased cough, upper respiratory complaints, SOB, dyspnea, bronchitis. **Musculoskeletal:** Arthritis, myalgia, arthralgia, twitch/muscle spasms, musculoskeletal chest pain. **GU:** Menstrual complaints, impotence, urinary frequency/retention/urgency, vaginal hemorrhage, UTI, vaginal irritation, testicular swelling, painful erection, retarded ejaculation, polyuria, prostate disorder. **Dermatologic:** Rash, pruritus, urticaria, flushing, hot flushes, rashes, angioedema, exfoliative dermatitis, alopecia, dry skin, ecchymosis. **Ophthalmic:** Blurred vision, amblyopia, visual disturbances, abnormal accommodation, dry eye. **Otic:** Auditory disturbance, tinnitus. **Miscellaneous:** Infection, fatigue, pain, fever, chills, cutaneous temperature disturbance, flu-like symptoms, nonspecific pain.

OD OVERDOSE MANAGEMENT

Symptoms: Seizures, hallucinations, loss of consciousness, tachycardia, multiple uncontrolled seizures, bradycardia, fever, muscle rigidity, hypotension, rhabdomyolsis, stupor, ***coma, respiratory failure, cardiac failure*** and ***cardiac arrest prior to death***. *Treatment:* Client should be hospitalized. If conscious, give syrup of ipecac to induce vomiting followed by activated charcoal q 6 hr during the first 12 hr after ingestion. Monitor both ECG and EEG for 48 hr; fluid intake must be adequate. If the client is in a stupor, is comatose, or is convulsing, gastric lavage may be undertaken provided intubation of the airway has been performed. Seizures may be treated with IV benzodiazepines and other supportive procedures.

DRUG INTERACTIONS

Alcohol / ↓ Seizure threshold; may precipitate seizures
Amantadine / Psychotic reactions
Antiarrhythymics, type 1C / ↑ Antiarrhythmic side effects R/T ↓ liver metabolism
Antipsychotics (haloperidol, risperidone, thioridazine) / ↑ Antipsychotic side effects R/T ↓ liver metabolism
Carbamazepine / ↑ Bupropion metabolism → ↓ plasma levels
Cimetidine / Inhibits metabolism of bupropion
Fluoxetine / Panic symptoms and psychotic reactions
Levodopa / ↑ Risk of side effects
MAO inhibitors / ↑ Acute toxicity to bupropion, especially phenelzine
Metoprolol / ↑ Metoprolol side effects R/T ↓ liver metabolism
Phenobarbital / ↑ Bupropion metabolism → ↓ plasma levels
Phenytoin / ↑ Bupropion metabolism → ↓ plasma levels
Retonavir / ↑ Risk of bupropion toxicity
Tricyclic antidepressants (TCAs) / ↑ TCA side effects R/T ↓ liver metabolism

HOW SUPPLIED

Tablet: 75 mg, 100 mg; *Tablet Extended Release:* 100 mg, 150 mg

DOSAGE

- **TABLETS, IMMEDIATE RELEASE**
  Antidepressant.

Adults, initial: 100 mg in the morning and evening for the first 3 days; **then,** 100 mg t.i.d., given in the morning, midday, and in the evening (6 hr should elapse between doses). If no response is observed after 4 weeks or longer, the dose may be increased to a maximum of 450 mg/day with individual doses not to exceed 150 mg. **Maintenance:** Lowest dose to control depression. Several months of treatment may be necessary.

B

• **TABLETS, SUSTAINED RELEASE**

Antidepressant.

Adults, initial: 150 mg once daily in the a.m. If 150 mg is tolerated, increase to 300 mg/day given as 150 mg b.i.d., allowing 8 or more hr between successive doses. Do not exceed a daily dose of 400 mg given as 200 mg b.i.d. in clients where no clinical improvement was noted after several weeks of 300 mg/day.

Smoking deterrent. (Zyban)

Initial: 150 mg/day for the first 3 days; **then,** 150 mg b.i.d. for 7–12 weeks (up to 6 months). Eight hours or more should elapse between successive doses.

NURSING CONSIDERATIONS

ADMINISTRATION/STORAGE

1. Administer in a way to minimize risk of seizures; the total daily dose should not exceed 450 mg to treat depression or 300 mg as a smoking deterrent. Each single dose should not exceed 150 mg; increase doses gradually.
2. Several months of treatment may be necessary to control acute depression.
3. Intitiate treatment while the client is still smoking since about 1 week of treatment is needed to reach steady-state blood levels. A "target quit date," usually in the second week, should be set. Continue treatment for 7 to 12 weeks. If significant progress has not been made by week 7 of treatment, it is not likely the client will stop smoking during this attempt. Thus, discontinue treatment.

ASSESSMENT

1. Document indications for therapy, presenting behaviors, and duration of symptoms.
2. Note any history of seizures, recent MI, bulimia or anorexia nervosa.
3. Determine if client of childbearing age and lactating.
4. Monitor weight, ECG, liver and renal function studies; reduce dose with renal/liver dysfunction.
5. Assess mental stability and potential for compliance. Fewer side effects (no CV effects, drug interactions, sedation, and weight gain) with bupropion than other antidepressants.
6. With tobacco abuse, ensure client is ready to quit; note numbers of cigarettes smoked per day, nicotine content, other failures, and date desired to quit so that treatment can be started 1 week prior.

CLIENT/FAMILY TEACHING

1. May experience changes in taste perception; may result in appetite/weight loss. Record weights and report changes.
2. May cause menstrual irregularities and impotence. Report changes in urinary output.
3. Beneficial drug effects may not be evident for 5–21 days. Continue and do not be discouraged by the delayed response.
4. Dizziness may occur. Do not arise from a supine position suddenly. If dizziness occurs during the day, sit until it subsides.
5. Report for follow-up so that drug therapy and dosage may be evaluated and adjusted as needed.
6. Report any mood swings or suicidal ideations immediately.
7. May cause drowsiness, hyperactivity, GI upset, diarrhea, constipation, and dry mouth.
8. With the sustained-released formulation, for smoking cessation, drug will be started at a low dose for b.i.d. consumption. Take last dose 4 to 6 hr before bedtime to prevent insomnia. GlaxoWellcome operates a toll- free number (1-800-u can quit, 822-6784) for assistance and support during withdrawal of nicotine; they can also be reached on the Internet at www.glaxowellcome.com.

OUTCOMES/EVALUATE

- Improvement in S&S of depression such as ↓ fatigue, improved eating and sleeping patterns, and ↑ socialization
- Successful nicotine withdrawal

Buspirone hydrochloride

(byou-**SPYE**-rohn)

PREGNANCY CATEGORY: B

CLASSIFICATION(S):
Antianxiety drug, nonbenzodiazepine
Rx: BuSpar
✱Rx: Apo-Buspirone, Buspirex, Bustab, Gen-Buspirone, Lin-Buspirone, Novo-Buspirone, Nu-Buspirone, PMS-Buspirone

ACTION/KINETICS

The mechanism of action is unknown. Not chemically related to the benzodiazepines; no anticonvulsant, muscle relaxant properties, or significant sedation seen. Binds to serotonin ($5\text{-}HT_{1A}$) and dopamine (D_2) receptors in the CNS; is possible that dopamine-mediated neurologic disorders may occur. These include dystonia, Parkinson-like symptoms, akathisia, and tardive dyskinesla. **Peak plasma levels:** 1–6 ng/mL 40–90 min after a single PO dose of 20 mg. **t½:** 2–3 hr. Extensive first-pass metabolism; active and inactive metabolites excreted in the urine and through the feces.

USES

Short-term use to relieve symptoms of anxiety due to motor tension, apprehension, autonomic hyperactivity, or hyperattentiveness.

CONTRAINDICATIONS

Psychoses, severe liver or kidney impairment, lactation. Not usually indicated for treatment of anxiety and tension due to stress of everyday living.

SPECIAL CONCERNS

Safety and efficacy in children less than 18 years of age not established. A decrease in dose may be necessary in geriatric clients due to age-related impairment of renal function.

SIDE EFFECTS

CNS: Dizziness, drowsiness, insomnia, fatigue, nervousness, excitement, dream disturbances, dysphoria, noise intolerance, euphoria, depersonalization, akathisia, hallucinations, suicidal ideation, seizures, decreased concentration, confusion, anger or hostility, depression. **CV:** Nonspecific chest pain, hypotension, palpitations, tachycardia, syncope, hypertension. **GI:** N&V, diarrhea, constipation, abdominal distress, dry mouth, altered taste, increased appetite, irritable colon. **Ophthalmologic:** Redness and itching of eyes, conjunctivitis, photophobia, eye pain. **Dermatologic:** Skin rash, pruritus, dry skin, edema of face, acne, easy bruising, flushing. **Neurologic:** Paresthesia, tremor, numbness, incoordination. **GU:** Urinary hesitancy/frequency, enuresis, amenorrhea, PID. **Miscellaneous:** Tinnitus, sore throat, nasal congestion, altered smell, muscle aches/pains, skin rash, headache, sweating, hyperventilation, SOB, hair loss, galactorrhea, decreased/increased libido, delayed ejaculation.

OD OVERDOSE MANAGEMENT

Symptoms: Dizziness, drowsiness, N&V, gastric distress, miosis. *Treatment:* Immediate gastric lavage; general symptomatic and supportive measures.

DRUG INTERACTIONS

Grapefruit juice / ↑ Plasma levels of buspirone → excess sedation
Itraconazole / ↑ Plasma itraconazole levels → ↑ effects and toxicity
MAO inhibitors / ↑ BP

HOW SUPPLIED

Tablet: 5 mg, 7.5 mg, 10 mg, 15 mg, 30 mg

DOSAGE

• **TABLETS**

Adults: 5 mg t.i.d. May increase dose in increments of 5 mg/day q 2–3 days to achieve optimum effects; do not exceed a total daily dose of 60 mg. BuSpar is available in a 15-mg tablet that is scored in 5-mg increments and notched in 7.5-mg increments so clients can take the drug b.i.d. rather than t.i.d.

NURSING CONSIDERATIONS

ADMINISTRATION/STORAGE

1. No cross-tolerance with other sedative-hypnotic drugs, including benzodiazepines.
2. Buspirone will not block the withdrawal syndrome, which may occur following cessation of sedative-hypnotics. Thus, withdraw clients on chronic sedative-hypnotic therapy gradually prior to beginning buspirone therapy.

3. To date, no potential for abuse, tolerance, or either physical or psychologic dependence.
4. Up to 2 weeks may be required before beneficial antianxiety effects are manifested.

ASSESSMENT

1. Document indications for therapy and note pretreatment findings.
2. Determine support systems and encourage active family involvement in treatment plan.
3. Assess for recent benzodiazepine therapy; drug may be less effective.
4. Document mental status and note age; good agent to use in elderly because of less CNS suppression.
5. Determine causative factor/event that precipitated disorder.

CLIENT/FAMILY TEACHING

1. Take with food or snack to decrease nausea, a common side effect; report if persistant/severe.
2. May cause drowsiness or dizziness. Use caution when operating a motor vehicle or performing tasks that require mental alertness.
3. Avoid the use of alcohol.
4. Do not stop suddenly as withdrawal symptoms such as N&V, dry mouth, nasal congestion, or sore throat may occur.
5. Report any weakness, restlessness, nervousness, headaches, or feelings of depression.
6. Report any involuntary, repetitive movements of the face or neck muscles, Parkinson-like symptoms or suicide ideations immediately.
7. Avoid all OTC agents.
8. Separate buspirone dosage by 6–8 hr from ingestion of grapefruit juice.

OUTCOMES/EVALUATE

Relief of agitated depressive S&S; ↓ anxiety

Busulfan

(byou-**SUL**-fan)

PREGNANCY CATEGORY: D
CLASSIFICATION(S):
Antineoplastic, alkylating
Rx: Myleran , Busulfex

SEE ALSO *ANTINEOPLASTIC AGENTS* AND *ALKYLATING AGENTS.*

ACTION/KINETICS

Is cell cycle-phase nonspecific; acts predominately against cells of the granulocytic type by alkylating cellular thiol groups. Cross-linking of nucleoproteins occurs. May cause severe bone marrow depression. Leukocyte count drops during the second or third week; thus, weekly laboratory tests are mandatory. Resistance may develop; thought to be due to the altered transport into the cell and/or increased intracellular inactivation. Rapidly absorbed from the GI tract; appears in serum 0.5–2 hr after PO administration. **t½:** 2.5 hr. Extensively metabolized and excreted in the urine. Clearance is more rapid in children than in adults.

Increased appetite and sense of well-being may occur a few days after therapy is started. Sometimes administered with allopurinol to prevent symptoms of clinical gout.

USES

Injection: With cyclophosphamide as a conditioning treatment prior to allogeneic hematopoietic progenitor cell transplantation for chronic myelogenous leukemia (CML). **Tablets:** Palliative treatment of CML (granulocytic, myelocytic, myeloid). Less effective in individuals with CML who lack the Philadelphia (Ph[1]) chromosome. Not effective in individuals where the disease is in the "blastic" phase.

CONTRAINDICATIONS

Use of tablets unless a diagnosis of CML has been adequately established. Lactation.

SPECIAL CONCERNS

Safety and efficacy have not been established in children. Take caution not to confuse Alkeran (melphalan), Leukeran (chlorambucil), and Myleran (busulfan).

SIDE EFFECTS

Hematologic: ***Pancytopenia, severe bone marrow hypoplasia,*** anemia, leukopenia, thrombocytopenia. **GI:** N&V, stomatitis, anorexia, diarrhea, abdominal pain/enlargement, dyspepsia, constipation, dry mouth, rectal disorder/discomfort, jaundice, hepatomegaly, ***hepatotoxicity,*** hematemesis, pancreatitis. **CNS:** Insomnia, anxiety, dizziness, depression, confusion, lethargy, hallucinations, delirium, encephalopathy, agitation, seizures, somnolence, ***cerebral hemorrhage/coma.*** **Respiratory: *Bronchopulmonary dysplasia with interstitial pulmonary fibrosis.*** Rhinitis, lung disorder, cough, epistaxis, dyspnea, pharyngitis, hiccup, asthma, avelolar hemorrhage, hemoptysis, pleural effusion, sinusitis, atelectasis, hypoxia. **CV:** Tachycardia, hypertension, thrombosis, vasodilation, hypotension, arrhythmia, cardiomegaly, atrial fibrillation, abnormal ECG, heart block, left-sided heart failure, pericardial effusion, ventricular extrasystoles, ***endocardial fibrosis. Cardiac tamponade in children with thalessemia. Ophthalmologic:*** Cataracts after prolonged use. **Dermatologic:** Hyperpigmentation, especially in clients with a dark complexion. Rash, pruritus, alopecia, vesicular rash, vesiculo-bullous rash, maculopapular rash, acne, exfoliative dermatitis, erythema nodosum. **Metabolic:** Syndrome resembling adrenal insufficiency, including symptoms of weakness, severe fatigue, weight loss, anorexia, N&V, and melanoderma (especially after prolonged use). Also, hyperuricemia/uricosuria in clients with CML. **GU:** Oliguria, hematuria, dysuria, hemorrhagic cystitis. **Miscellaneous:** Cellular dysplasia in various organs, including lymph nodes, pancreas, thyroid, adrenal glands, bone marrow, and liver. Also, cataracts after prolonged use, fever, edema, headache, asthenia, infection, chills, pain, allergic reaction, chest/back pain, myalgia, inflammation at injection site, arthralgia, pneumonia, ear disorder.

LABORATORY TEST CONSIDERATIONS

↑ Uric acid in blood and urine.

OD OVERDOSE MANAGEMENT

Symptoms: ***Bone marrow toxicity, CNS stimulation with convulsions and death on the first day.*** *Treatment:* If ingestion is recent, gastric lavage or induction of vomiting followed by activated charcoal. Hematologic status must be monitored.

DRUG INTERACTIONS

Acetaminophen / ↓ Busulfan clearance
Cyclophosphamide / Cardiac tamponade in clients with thalessemia (rare), but possibly fatal
Itraconazole / ↓ Busulfan clearance
Phenytoin / ↑ Busulfan clearance
Thioguanine / ↑ Risk of esophageal varices with abnormal LFTs

HOW SUPPLIED

Injection: 6 mg/mL; *Tablet:* 2 mg

DOSAGE

• **TABLETS**

CML.

Adults or children, remission, induction, usual dose: 4–8 mg/day (about 60 mcg/kg or 1.8 mg/m² per day) until leukocyte count falls below 15,000/mm³; then, withdraw drug. **Maintenance, when leukocyte reaches about 50,000/mcL:** Resume treatment with induction dosage. When remission is less than 3 mo, consider 1–3 mg/day that may keep client under control and prevent rapid relapse.

• **INJECTION**

With cyclophosphamide prior to allogeneic hematopoietic progenitor cell transplantation.

Adults: 0.8 mg/kg of IBW or actual body weight (whichever is lower) of busulfan q 6 hr for 4 days (i.e., total of 16 doses). For obese or severely obese clients, calculate the dose of busulfan based on adjusted IBW. For cyclophosphamide, 60 mg/kg given on each of 2 days as a 1-hr infusion beginning on BMT day minus 3, 6 hr following the 16th busulfan dose.

NURSING CONSIDERATIONS

SEE ALSO *NURSING CONSIDERATIONS* FOR *ANTINEOPLASTIC AGENTS*.

ADMINISTRATION/STORAGE

1. Do not administer without supervision and facilities for weekly CBCs.

IV 2. Busulfan is given IV via a central catheter as a 2-hr infusion (using an infusion pump) q 6 hr for 4 consecutive days. Cyclophosphamide is given IV as a 1-hr infusion each day for 2 days beginning 6 hr following the 16th busulfan dose.

B

3. Dilute busulfan prior to use with either 0.9% NaCl injection or D5W. The diluent quantity should be 10 times the volume of busulfan, ensuring the final concentration is about 0.5 mg/mL or more. To prepare the final solution for infusion, add 9.3 mL of busulfan to 93 ml of diluent. Always add the busulfan to the diluent, not the diluent to the busulfan. Mix thoroughly by inverting several times.
4. Diluted busulfan is stable at room temperature for up to 8 hr; infusion must be completed by that time. Busulfan diluted in 0.9% NaCl is stable for up to 12 hr if refrigerated; infusion must be completed by that time.
5. Exercise caution in handling and preparing busulfan solutions as skin reactions may occur with accidental exposure. Use a vertical laminar flow safety hood; wear gloves and protective clothing.
6. Do not infuse rapidly or at the same time with any other IV solution of unknown compatibility.

ASSESSMENT

1. Note previous experience with drug therapy and any resistance.
2. Monitor CBC, renal and LFTs.
3. In clients with CML note presence of Philadelphia (Ph^1) chromosome.
4. Document when disease in "blastic" phase as drug is not effective.
5. Drug may cause moderate to severe granulocyte suppression. Monitor appropriate weekly hematologic profiles. Nadir: 21 days; recovery: 42–56 days.

CLIENT/FAMILY TEACHING

1. Take at the same time each day.
2. May take on an empty stomach if N&V occur. Extra fluid intake may be required during therapy.
3. Report any early symptoms of sore throat or infection; expect weekly CBC studies .
4. Avoid vaccinations and all OTC agents without approval.
5. Any skin rash should be reported immediately; drug may cause increased pigmentation.
6. Allopurinol may be prescribed to decrease urate crystal formation.
7. Increased cough and visual difficulties may be symptoms of toxicity; Report increased weight loss, fatigue, loss of appetite, or weakness.

OUTCOMES/EVALUATE

• Maintenance of leukocytes at 20,000/mm^3
• Absence of blasts on peripheral blood smear; ↓ spleen size

Butenafine hydrochloride

(byou-**TEN**-ah-feen)

PREGNANCY CATEGORY: B
CLASSIFICATION(S):
Antifungal
Rx: Mentax

SEE ALSO ANTI-INFECTIVES.

ACTION/KINETICS

Acts by inhibiting epoxidation of squalene, thus blocking the synthesis of ergosterol, an essential component of fungal cell membranes. Depending on the concentration and the fungal species, the drug may be fungicidal. Although applied topically, some of the drug is absorbed into the general circulation.

USES

Treatment of interdigital tinea pedia (athlete's foot), tinea corporis (ringworm), and tinea cruris (jock itch) due to *Epidermophyton floccosum, Trichophyton mentagrophytes, T. rubrum,* or *T. tonsurans*. Treatment of tinea (pityriasis) versicolor due to *Malassezia fufur*.

SPECIAL CONCERNS

Use with caution during lactation and in clients sensitive to allylamine antifungal drugs as the drugs may be cross-reactive. Safety and efficacy have not been determined in children less than 12 years of age.

SIDE EFFECTS

Dermatologic: Contact dermatitis, burning or stinging, worsening of the condition, erythema, irritation, itching.

HOW SUPPLIED

Cream: 1%

DOSAGE

- **CREAM, 1%**

Tinea versicolor, tinea corporis, tinea cruris.

Apply the cream to cover the affected area and immediate surrounding skin once daily for 2 weeks.

Interdigital tinea pedis.

Apply b.i.d. for 7 days or once daily for 4 weeks.

NURSING CONSIDERATIONS

SEE ALSO *GENERAL NURSING CONSIDERATIONS FOR ALL ANTI-INFECTIVES.*

ADMINISTRATION/STORAGE

1. For external use only; not for ophthalmic, PO, or intravaginal use.
2. Store the drug between 5 – 30°C (41–86°F).

ASSESSMENT

1. Document indications for therapy, onset, duration, and characteristics of symptoms.
2. Describe clinical presentation.

CLIENT/FAMILY TEACHING

1. Review method for site preparation and application of cream; wash hands before and after applying.
2. After bathing, dry feet thoroughly and carefully between each toe before applying. Avoid occlusive dressings.
3. Avoid contact with the eyes, nose, mouth, and other mucous membranes.
4. Do not stop therapy when condition shows improvement; continue for full prescribed time.
5. Report any increased swelling, itching, burning, blistering, drainage, irritation, or lack of improvement.

OUTCOMES/EVALUATE

Resolution of fungal infection

Butoconazole nitrate

(byou-toe-**KON**-ah-zohl)

PREGNANCY CATEGORY: C

CLASSIFICATION(S):

Antifungal

Rx: Gynazole-1

OTC: Femstat 3, Mycelex-3

ACTION/KINETICS

By permeating chitin in the fungal cell wall, butoconazole increases membrane permeability to intracellular substances, leading to reduced osmotic resistance and viability of the fungus. Approximately 5.5% of drug is absorbed following vaginal administration; plasma. **t½:** 21–24 hr.

USES

Vulvovaginal fungal infections caused by *Candida* species.

CONTRAINDICATIONS

Use during first trimester of pregnancy.

SPECIAL CONCERNS

Pediatric dosage has not been established. Use with caution during lactation.

SIDE EFFECTS

GU: Vaginal burning, vulvar burning or itching, discharge; soreness, swelling, and itching of the fingers.

HOW SUPPLIED

Vaginal cream: 2%

DOSAGE

Vulvovaginal infections.

One applicatorful of Gynazole-1 intravaginally once (remains in vaginal vault for approximately four days). Or, one applicatorful a day of either Femstat 3 or Mycelex-3, preferably at bedtime, for three consecutive days.

NURSING CONSIDERATIONS

ADMINISTRATION/STORAGE

1. During pregnancy, use of a vaginal applicator may be contraindicated.
2. If there is no response, repeat studies to confirm the diagnosis before reinstituting antifungal therapy.
3. Not to be stored above 40°C (104°F).

ASSESSMENT

1. Document onset and characteristics of symptoms.
2. Determine if pregnant.
3. Obtain appropriate cultures and lab studies as needed.

CLIENT/FAMILY TEACHING

1. Review administration technique; insert cream high into the vagina.
2. Use as prescribed and continue during menstrual cycle.

3. Report any irritation or burning.
4. Use sanitary napkins to prevent soiling and staining of undergarments and clothing.
5. To prevent reinfection, partner should use a condom during intercourse and receive treatment if symptomatic.
6. If having recurrent vaginal infections and exposed to HIV, consult provider to determine the cause of symptoms. If the symptoms return within 2 months, R/O pregnancy or a serious underlying medical cause (e.g., diabetes, HIV infection).

OUTCOMES/EVALUATE

Eradication of fungal infection; symptomatic improvement.

Butorphanol tartrate

(byou-**TOR**-fah-nohl)

PREGNANCY CATEGORY: C
CLASSIFICATION(S):
Narcotic agonist/antagonist
Rx: Stadol NS , Stadol **C-IV**

SEE ALSO *NARCOTIC ANALGESICS.*

ACTION/KINETICS

Has both narcotic agonist and antagonist properties. Analgesic potency may be up to 7 times that of morphine and 30–40 times that of meperidine. Overdosage responds to naloxone. After IV use, CV effects include increased PA pressure, PCWP, LVED pressure, system arterial pressure, PVR, and increased cardiac work load. **Onset, IM:** 10–15 min; **IV:** rapid; **nasal:** within 15 min. **Duration, IM, IV:** 3–4 hr; **nasal:** 4–5 hr. **Peak analgesia, IM, IV:** 30–60 min; **nasal:** 1–2 hr. **t½, IM:** 2.1–8.8 hr; **nasal:** 2.9–9.2 hr. The t½ is increased up to 25% in clients over 65 years of age. Metabolized in the liver and excreted by the kidney. The drug has about 1/40 the narcotic antagonist activity as naloxone. ***Note:*** 1 mg of tartrate salt is equal to 0.68 mg base.

USES

Parenteral and nasal: Moderate to severe pain, especially after surgery. **Parenteral:** Preoperative medication (as part of balanced anesthesia). Pain during labor. **Nasal:** Treatment of migraine headaches.

CONTRAINDICATIONS

Use of the nasal form during labor or delivery.

SPECIAL CONCERNS

Safe use during pregnancy, during labor for premature infants, or in children under 18 years not established. Use with extreme caution in clients with AMI, ventricular dysfunction, and coronary insufficiency (morphine or meperidine are preferred). Use in clients physically dependent on narcotics will result in precipitation of a withdrawal syndrome. Geriatric clients may be more sensitive to side effects, especially dizziness.

ADDITIONAL SIDE EFFECTS

Most common: Somnolence, dizziness, N&V. The nasal product commonly causes nasal congestion and insomnia.

ADDITIONAL DRUG INTERACTIONS

Barbiturate anesthetics may increase respiratory and CNS depression of butorphanol.

HOW SUPPLIED

Injection: 1 mg/mL, 2 mg/mL; *Spray:* 10 mg/mL

DOSAGE

- **IM**

Analgesia.

Adults, usual: 2 mg q 3–4 hr, as necessary; **range:** 1–4 mg q 3–4 hr. Single doses should not exceed 4 mg.

Preoperative/preanesthetic.

Adults: 2 mg 60–90 min before surgery. Individualize dosage.

Labor.

Adults: 1–2 mg if at full term and during early labor. May be repeated after 4 hr.

- **IV**

Analgesia.

Adults, usual: 1 mg q 3–4 hr; **range:** 0.5–2 mg q 3–4 hr. **Not recommended for use in children.**

Balanced anesthesia.

Adults: 2 mg just before induction or 0.5–1 mg in increments during anesthesia. The increment may be up to

0.06 mg/kg, depending on drugs previously given. Total dose range: less than 4 mg to less than 12.5 mg.

Labor.

Adults: 1–2 mg if at full term and during early labor. May be repeated after 4 hr.

• **NASAL SPRAY**

Analgesia.

Adults: 1 spray (1 mg) in one nostril. If pain relief is not reached within 60–90 min, an additional 1 mg may be given. The two-dose sequence may be repeated in 3–4 hr if necessary. In severe pain, 2 mg (1 spray in each nostril) may be given initially followed in 3–4 hr by additional 2-mg doses if needed. **Geriatric clients, initial:** 1 mg; wait 90–120 min before determining if a second 1-mg dose is required.

NURSING CONSIDERATIONS

SEE ALSO *NURSING CONSIDERATIONS* FOR *NARCOTIC ANALGESICS*.

ADMINISTRATION/STORAGE

1. Have naloxone available for treatment of overdose.
2. Store the nasal product below 86°F (30°C).

IV 3. If administered by direct IV infusion, may give undiluted at a rate of 2 mg or less over 3–5-min.

ASSESSMENT

1. Determine if narcotic dependent; antagonist property of drug may precipitate withdrawal symptoms.
2. Monitor VS and CNS status during therapy.
3. With CV problems, morphine may be a preferred drug to use.
4. Give geriatric clients one-half the usual dose at twice the usual interval.
5. With renal/hepatic impairment, increase the initial dosage interval to 6–8 hr with subsequent intervals determined by client response.

OUTCOMES/EVALUATE

Relief of pain; termination of migraine headache

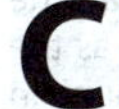

Calcipotriene (Calcipotriol)

(kal-**SIH**-poh-tren)

PREGNANCY CATEGORY: C
CLASSIFICATION(S):
Antipsoriasis drug
Rx: Dovonex

ACTION/KINETICS

Synthetic vitamin D_3 analog. Vitamin D_3 receptors are located in skin cells known as keratinocytes. Abnormal growth and production of keratinocytes cause the scaly red patches of psoriasis. Calcipotriene regulates production and development of these skin cells. About 6% of a topically applied dose is absorbed into the systemic circulation where it is converted to inactive metabolites.

USES

Cream, Ointment: Treatment of moderate plaque psoriasis in adults. **Solution**: Control moderately severe scalp psoriasis.

CONTRAINDICATIONS

Demonstrated hypercalcemia or evidence of vitamin D toxicity. Use on the face; oral, ophthalmic, intravaginal use.

SPECIAL CONCERNS

Side effects are more common in geriatric clients. Use with caution during lactation. Safety and efficacy for use of topical calcipotriene in dermatoses other than psoriasis have not been studied. Safety and efficacy have not been determined in children. Children have a higher ratio of skin surface to body mass; thus, children are at a greater risk than adults of systemic side effects following use of topical medication.

C

SIDE EFFECTS

• **TOPICAL**
Most commonly burning, itching, skin irritation. Also, erythema, dry skin, peeling, rash, worsening of psoriasis, dermatitis, skin atrophy, hyperpigmentation, hypercalcemia, folliculitis. Irritation of lesions and surrounding uninvolved skin.

• **SYSTEMIC**
Transient, rapidly reversible hypercalcemia.

OD OVERDOSE MANAGEMENT

Symptoms: Hypercalcemia and other systemic effects. *Treatment:* Discontinue use until normal calcium levels are restored.

HOW SUPPLIED

Cream: 0.005%; *Ointment:* 0.005%; *Scalp Solution:* 0.005%

DOSAGE

• **OINTMENT, CREAM, SOLUTION (EACH 0.005%)**
Treatment of psoriasis.
Apply a thin layer to the affected skin b.i.d. (ointment can be used once daily); rub in gently and completely.

NURSING CONSIDERATIONS

ADMINISTRATION/STORAGE

1. For external use only. Avoid contact with the face and eyes.
2. Safety and efficacy have been shown for use up to 8 weeks.

ASSESSMENT

1. Describe psoriatic lesions requiring therapy; assess extent, location/characteristics.
2. Monitor calcium levels with extended use.

CLIENT/FAMILY TEACHING

1. Apply a thin layer directly to psoriatic lesions; wash hands before and after application.
2. Use only as directed and do not exceed prescribed dosage; avoid contact with face and eyes.
3. Do not mix or apply at the same time as other topical products.
4. Transient burning and stinging may occur. Avoid use on the face if possible; report if erythema and facial dermatitis occur.

OUTCOMES/EVALUATE

Clearing and healing of psoriatic lesions

Calcitonin-human

(kal-sih-**TOH**-nin)

PREGNANCY CATEGORY: C

Calcitonin-salmon

(kal-sih-**TOH**-nin)

PREGNANCY CATEGORY: C
Rx: Calcimar, Miacalcin, Osteocalcin, Salmonine
Rx: Caltine, Miacalcin NS
CLASSIFICATION(S):
Calcium regulator

ACTION/KINETICS

Calcitonins are polypeptide hormones produced in mammals by the parafollicular cells of the thyroid gland. Calcitonin isolated from salmon has the same therapeutic effect as the human hormone, except for a greater potency per milligram and a somewhat longer duration of action. Calcitonin-human is a synthetic product that has the same sequence of amino acids as the naturally occurring calcitonin found in human beings. Ineffective when administered PO. Beneficial in Paget's disease of bone by reducing the rate of turnover of bone; the drug acts to both block initial bone resorption, decreasing alkaline phosphatase levels in the serum, and urinary hydroxyproline excretion. Its effectiveness in treating osteoporosis or hypercalcemia is due to decreased serum calcium levels from direct inhibition of bone resorption. Use of the nasal spray for osteoporosis results in significant increases in bone mass density within 6 months. **Time to peak plasma levels, calcitonin-salmon: 16–25 min for the injection and 31–39 min for the spray. Duration, calcitonin-salmon: 6–8 hr for hypercalcemia. t$^1/_2$:** 60 min for calcitonin-human and 43 min for calcitonin-salmon. The onset of calcitonin-human in reducing serum alkaline phosphatase levels and urinary hydroxyproline excretion in Paget's disease may take 6–24 months. Metabolized to inactive compounds in the kidneys, blood, and peripheral tissues. *NOTE:* Calcitonin human is now an orphan drug.

USES

Injection: (1) Prevention of progressive loss of bone mass in postmenopausal osteoporosis in women who are more than 5 years past menopause and who have low bone mass compared with women before menopause. Also, for women who cannot or will not take estrogens. (2) Moderate to severe Paget's disease characterized by polyostotic involvement with elevated serum alkaline phosphatase and urinary hydroxyproline excretion. (3) With other therapies for early treatment of hypercalcemic emergencies. **Nasal:** Postmenopausal osteoporosis (see above for injection).

CONTRAINDICATIONS

Allergy to calcitonin-salmon or its gelatin diluent.

SPECIAL CONCERNS

Use with caution during lactation. Safe use in children not established.

SIDE EFFECTS

Side effects listed are for calcitonin-salmon.

GI: N&V, anorexia, epigastric discomfort, salty taste, flatulence, increased appetite, gastritis, diarrhea, dry mouth, abdominal pain, dyspepsia, constipation. **CNS:** Dizziness, paresthesia, insomnia, anxiety, vertigo, migraine, neuralgia, agitation, depression (rare). **CV:** Hypertension, tachycardia, palpitation, bundle branch block, ***MI, CVA, thrombophlebitis,*** angina pectoris (rare). **Respiratory:** Sinusitis, URTI, pharyngitis, bronchitis, pneumonia, coughing, dyspnea, taste perversion, parosmia, ***bronchospasm.*** **Musculoskeletal:** Arthrosis, arthritis, polymyalgia rheumatica, stiffness, myalgia. **Dermatologic:** Inflammatory reactions at the injection site, flushing of face or hands, pruritus of ear lobes, edema of feet, skin rash/ulceration, eczema, alopecia, increased sweating. **Endocrine:** Goiter, hyperthyroidism. **Ophthalmic:** Abnormal lacrimation, conjunctivitis, eye pain, blurred vision, vitreous floater. **Otic:** Tinnitus, hearing loss, earache. **Hematologic:** Lymphadenopathy, anemia, infection. **Metabolic:** Mild tetanic symptoms, asymptomatic mild hypercalcemia, cholelithiasis, thirst, hepatitis, weight increase. **Miscellaneous:** Flu-like symptoms, fatigue, nocturia, feverish sensation. Use of the nasal spray may cause rhinitis, nasal irritation/redness/sores, back pain, arthralgia, epistaxis, and headache.

LABORATORY TEST CONSIDERATIONS

↓ Alkaline phosphatase and 24-hr urinary excretion of hydroxyproline are indicative of successful therapy. Monitor urine for casts (indicative of kidney damage).

OD OVERDOSE MANAGEMENT

Symptoms: N&V.

HOW SUPPLIED

Calcitonin-salmon: *Injection:* 200 IU/mL; *Nasal Spray:* 200 IU/activation

DOSAGE

CALCITONIN-HUMAN

• SC

Paget's disease.

Adults, initial: 0.5 mg/day; **then,** depending on severity of disease, dosage may range from 0.5 mg 2–3 times/week to 0.25 mg/day.

CALCITONIN-SALMON

• IM, SC

Paget's disease.

Adults, initial: 100 IU/day; **maintenance, usual:** 50 IU/day, every other day, or 3 times/week.

Hypercalcemia.

Adults, initial: 4 IU/kg q 12 hr; **then,** increase the dose, if necessary after 1 or 2 days (i.e., if unsatisfactory response), to 8 IU/kg q 12 hr up to a maximum of 8 IU/kg q 6 hr. If the volume to be injected exceeds 2 mL by the SC route, give the dose IM with multiple sites used.

Postmenopausal osteoporosis.

Adults: 100 IU/day given with calcium carbonate (1.5 g/day) and vitamin D (400 units/day).

• NASAL SPRAY

Adults: 200 IU/day, alternating nostrils daily, given with calcium carbonate (1.5 g/day) and vitamin D (400 units/day).

C

NURSING CONSIDERATIONS

ADMINISTRATION/STORAGE

1. Activate the pump for the nasal spray before use. To do this, hold the bottle upright and depress the two white side arms toward the bottle six times, until a faint spray is emitted. The pump has been activated once the first faint spray is emitted. Place the nozzle firmly into the nostril with the head in the upright position and depress the pump toward the bottle. It is not necessary to reactivate the pump before each dose.
2. Store calcitonin-salmon injection at a temperature between 2–6°C (36–43°F).
3. Store the unopened calcitonin nasal spray between 2–8°C (36– 46°F). Once pump is activated, may be stored at room temperature.
4. With Paget's disease, more than 1 year of therapy may be required to treat neurologic lesions.
5. Check for hypersensitivity reactions before administering either medication. Administer 1 IU intracutaneously in the inner forearm and observe for 15 min.

ASSESSMENT

1. Note any hypersensitivity to drug or its gelatin diluent.
2. Document indications for therapy, noting baseline assessments.
3. Review diet and intake of calcium and vitamin D; obtain levels as needed.
4. Before initiating therapy, determine serum alkaline phosphatase level and urinary hydroxyproline excretion. Repeat at the end of 3 months and q 3–6 months thereafter.

INTERVENTIONS

1. Perform test dose; note local inflammatory reactions at site; assess for systemic allergic reactions.
2. Observe for hypocalcemic tetany, i.e., muscular fibrillation, twitching, tetanic spasms, and convulsions. Check at least q 10 min for the next 30 min following injection; have IV calcium available.
3. Check for evidence of hypercalcemia and report, i.e., increased thirst, anorexia, polyuria, and N&V.
4. Assess for facial flushing, abdominal/epigastric distress, anorexia, diarrhea, or changes in taste perception. Record weights, I&O, and report if S&S persist.
5. If good clinical response initially, then client has a relapse, check for antibody formation to drug.

CLIENT/FAMILY TEACHING

1. Identify what to observe for with Paget's disease and how to assess the response to therapy.
2. Review aseptic methods of reconstituting solution, proper injection technique, and importance of alternating injection sites.
3. With the spray: take with vitamin D (400 IU) and calcium (1,500 mg) daily, alternate nostrils, and do not exceed prescribed dosage.
4. N&V may occur at the onset of therapy, but should subside as treatment continues; report if persists.
5. Report increased urine sediment; have periodic urine tests to assess for kidney damage.
6. Continue regular exercise/activity to minimize bone loss.
7. May take in the evening to minimize flushing.
8. See dietitian for dietary adjustments.

OUTCOMES/EVALUATE

- ↓ Serum calcium, ↓ alkaline phosphatase, and ↓ 24-hr urinary excretion of hydroxyproline
- Promotion of bone formation with ↑ bone mass density
- ↓ Bone pain
- Halt in postmenopausal osteoporosis

Calcium carbonate

(**KAL**-see-um **KAR**-bon-ayt)

CLASSIFICATION(S):
Calcium salt

OTC: Alka-Mints, Amitone, Antacid Tablets, Cal Carb-HD, Calci-Chew, Calciday-667, Calci-Mix, Calcium 600, Cal-Guard Softgels, Cal-Plus, Caltrate 600, Caltrate Jr., Chooz, Dicarbosil, Equilet, Extra Strength Alkets Antacid, Extra Strength Antacid, Extra Strength Tums E-X, Fem-Cal, Gencalc 600, Maalox Antacid Caplets, Malla-

mint, Mylanta Lozenges, Nephro-Calci, Os-Cal 500, Os-Cal 500 Chewable, Oysco 500 Chewable, Oyst-Cal 500, Oyster Shell Calcium-500, Oystercal 500, Tums, Tums 500, Tums Ultra
✱OTC: Apo-Cal,, Calcite 500, Calcium 500, Calcium Oyster Shell

SEE ALSO *CALCIUM SALTS.*

USES
Mild hypocalcemia, antacid, antihyperphosphatemic.

SPECIAL CONCERNS
Dosage not established in children.

HOW SUPPLIED
Capsule: 125 mg, 1250 mg; *Chew Tablet:* 350 mg, 420 mg, 500 mg, 750 mg, 850 mg, 1000 mg, 1250 mg; *Gum Tablets:* 500 mg; *Lozenge:* 600 mg; *Powder:* 6500 mg/packet; *Suspension:* 1250 mg/5 mL; *Tablet:* 250 mg, 500 mg, 600 mg, 650 mg, 667 mg, 1000 mg, 1250 mg, 1500 mg

DOSAGE

• CHEWABLE TABLETS, TABLETS, SUSPENSION, GUM, LOZENGES
Adults: 0.5–1.5 g, as needed.

• CAPSULES, SUSPENSION, TABLETS, CHEWABLE TABLETS
Hypocalcemia, nutritional supplement.
Adults: 1.25–1.5 g 1–3 times/day with or after meals.
Antihyperphosphatemic.
Adults: 5–13 g/day in divided doses with meals.
NOTE: The preparation contains 40% elemental calcium and 400 mg elemental calcium/g (20 mEq/g).

NURSING CONSIDERATIONS

SEE ALSO *NURSING CONSIDERATIONS* FOR *CALCIUM SALTS.*

OUTCOMES/EVALUATE
• Desired serum calcium levels
• ↓ Gastric acidity

Calcium chloride

(**KAL**-see-um **KLOH**-ryd)

PREGNANCY CATEGORY: C

CLASSIFICATION(S):
Calcium salt

SEE ALSO *CALCIUM SALTS.*

USES
(1) Mild hypocalcemia due to neonatal tetany, tetany due to parathyroid deficiency or vitamin D deficiency, and alkalosis. (2) Prophylaxis of hypocalcemia during exchange transfusions. (3) Intestinal malabsorption. (4) Treat effects of serious hyperkalemia as measured by ECG. (5) Cardiac resuscitation after open heart surgery when epinephrine fails to improve weak or ineffective myocardial contractions. (6) Adjunct to treat insect bites or stings to relieve muscle cramping. (7) Depression due to magnesium overdosage. (8) Acute symptoms of lead colic. (9) Rickets, osteomalacia. (10) Reverse symptoms of verapamil overdosage.

CONTRAINDICATIONS
Use to treat hypocalcemia of renal insufficiency.

SPECIAL CONCERNS
Use usually restricted in children due to significant irritation and possible tissue necrosis and sloughing caused by IV calcium chloride.

ADDITIONAL SIDE EFFECTS
Peripheral vasodilation with moderate decreases in BP. Extravasation can cause severe necrosis, sloughing, or abscess formation following IM or SC use.

HOW SUPPLIED
Injection: 100 mg /mL

DOSAGE

• IV ONLY
Hypocalcemia, replenish electrolytes.
Adults: 0.5–1 g q 1–3 days (given at a rate not to exceed 13.6–27.3 mg/min). **Pediatric:** 25 mg/kg (0.2 mL/kg up to 1–10 mL/kg) given slowly.
Magnesium intoxication.
0.5 g promptly; observe for recovery before other doses given.
Cardiac resuscitation.
0.5–1 g IV or 0.2–0.8 g injected into the ventricular cavity as a single dose. **Pediatric:** 0.2 mL/kg.
Hyperkalemia.
Sufficient amount to return ECG to normal.

NOTE: The preparation contains 27.2% calcium and 272 mg calcium/g (13.6 mEq/g).

NURSING CONSIDERATIONS

C

SEE ALSO *NURSING CONSIDERATIONS FOR CALCIUM SALTS.*

ADMINISTRATION/STORAGE

1. Never administer IM.

IV 2. May give undiluted by IV push.

OUTCOMES/EVALUATE

- Desired serum calcium levels
- ↓ Magnesium and potassium levels

Calcium gluconate

(**KAL**-see-um **GLUE**-koh-nayt)

CLASSIFICATION(S):
Calcium salt
Rx: injection
OTC: tablets

SEE ALSO *CALCIUM SALTS.*

USES

(1) Mild hypocalcemia due to neonatal tetany, tetany due to parathyroid deficiency or vitamin D deficiency, and alkalosis. (2) Prophylaxis of hypocalcemia during exchange transfusions. (3) Intestinal malabsorption. (4) Adjunct to treat insect bites or stings to relieve muscle cramping. (5) Depression due to magnesium overdosage. (6) Acute symptoms of lead colic. (7) Rickets, osteomalacia. (8) Reverse symptoms of verapamil overdosage. (9) Decrease capillary permeability in allergic conditions, nonthrombocytopenic purpura, and exudative dermatoses (e.g., dermatitis herpetiformis). (10) Pruritus due to certain drugs. (11) Hyperkalemia to antagonize cardiac toxicity (as long as client is not receiving digitalis).

CONTRAINDICATIONS

IM, intramyocardial, or SC use due to severe tissue necrosis, sloughing, and abscess formation.

HOW SUPPLIED

Injection: 100 mg /mL; *Tablet:* 500 mg, 650 mg, 975 mg, 1000 mg

DOSAGE

- **CHEWABLE TABLETS, TABLETS**

Treatment of hypocalcemia.

Adults: 8.8–16.5 g/day in divided doses; **pediatric:** 0.5–0.72 g/kg/day in divided doses.

Nutritional supplement.

Adults: 8.8–16.5 g/day in divided doses.

- **IV ONLY**

Treatment of hypocalcemia.

Adults: 2.3–9.3 mEq (5–20 mL of the 10% solution) as needed (range: 4.65–70 mEq/day). **Children:** 2.3 mEq/kg/day (or 56 mEq/m^2/day) given well diluted and slowly in divided doses. **Infants:** No more than 0.93 mEq (2 mL of the 10% solution).

Emergency elevation of serum calcium.

Adults: 7–14 mEq (15–30.1 mL). **Children:** 1–7 mEq (2.2–15 mL). **Infants:** Less than 1 mEq (2.2 mL). Depending on client response, the dose may be repeated q 1–3 days.

Hypocalcemic tetany.

Children: 0.5–0.7 mEq/kg (1.1–1.5 mL/kg) t.i.d.–q.i.d. until tetany is controlled. **Infants:** 2.4 mEq/kg/day (5.2 mL/kg/day) in divided doses.

Hyperkalemia with cardiac toxicity.

2.25–14 mEq (4.8–30.1 mL) while monitoring the ECG. If needed, the dose can be repeated after 1–2 min.

Magnesium intoxication.

Initial: 4.5–9 mEq (9.7–19.4 mL). Subsequent dosage based on client response.

Exchange transfusion.

Adults: 1.35 mEq (2.9 mL) concurrent with each 100 mL citrated blood. **Neonates:** 0.45 mEq (1 mL)/100 mL citrated blood.

- **IM**

Hypocalcemic tetany.

Adults: 4.5–16 mEq (9.7–34.4 mL) until a therapeutic response is noted.

Magnesium intoxication.

If IV administration is not possible: 2–5 mEq (4.3–10.8 mL) in divided doses as needed.

NOTE: The preparation contains 9% calcium and 90 mg calcium/g (4.5 mEq/g).

NURSING CONSIDERATIONS

SEE ALSO *NURSING CONSIDERATIONS* FOR *CALCIUM SALTS*.

ADMINISTRATION/STORAGE

1. If a precipitate is noted in the syringe, do not use.
2. If a precipitate is noted in the vials or ampules, heat to 80°C (146°F) in a dry heat oven for 1 hr to dissolve. Shake vigorously and allow to cool to room temperature. Do not use if precipitate remains.
IV 3. IV rate should not exceed 0.5–2 mL/min.
4. Give by intermittent IV infusion at a rate not exceeding 200 mg (19.5 mg calcium ion)/min. Can also be given by continuous IV infusion.

OUTCOMES/EVALUATE

- Restoration of serum calcium levels
- ↓ Magnesium/potassium levels

Calfactant

(kal-**FAK**-tant)

CLASSIFICATION(S):
Lung surfactant
Rx: Infasurf

ACTION/KINETICS
Lung surfactant which contains phospholipids, neutral lipids, and hydrophobic surfactant-associated proteins B and C from calf lungs. Calfactant modifies alveolar surface tension thus stabilizing alveoli. Adsorbs rapidly to the surface of the air:liquid interface and modifies surface tension similarly to natural lung surfactant. Treatment often rapidly improves oxygenation and lung compliance.

USES
Prevention and treatment of respiratory distress syndrome in premature infants.

SPECIAL CONCERNS
For endotracheal use only. Possible increased proportion of clients with both intraventricular hemorrhage and periventricular leukomalacia. These conditions were not associated with increased mortality.

SIDE EFFECTS
Cyanosis, airway obstruction, bradycardia, reflux of surfactant into the endotracheal tube, requirement for manual ventilation, reintubation, intraventricular hemorrhage, periventricular leukomalacia.

HOW SUPPLIED
Suspension, intratracheal: 35 mg phospholipids/mL and 0.65 mg proteins

DOSAGE

- **INTRATRACHEAL SUSPENSION**

Prophylaxis of respiratory distress syndrome at birth.

Instill 3 mL/kg of birth weight as soon as possible after birth. Give as 2 doses of 1.5 mL/kg each. Care and stabilization of the premature infant born with hypoxemia or bradycardia should precede calfactant therapy.

Treatment of respiratory distress syndrome within 72 hr of birth.

Instill 3 mL/kg of birth weight, given as 2 doses of 1.5 mL/kg. Repeat doses of 3 mL/kg of birth weight may be given, up to a total of 3 doses 12 hr apart.

NURSING CONSIDERATIONS

ADMINISTRATION/STORAGE

1. Begin calfactant prophylaxis as soon as possible, preferably within 30 minutes after birth.
2. Give only through an endotracheal tube. Draw dose into a syringe from the single–dose vial using a 20–gauge or larger needle. Avoid excessive foaming. Give only under the supervision of a clinician experienced in the acute care of newborns with respiratory failure who require intubation.
3. Does not require reconstitution. Do not dilute, sonicate, or shake. Gently swirl or agitate the vial for redispersion. Visible flecks in the suspension and foaming at the surface are normal. Drug does not have to be warmed before administration.
4. Unopened, unused vials warmed to room temperature may be returned to the refrigerator within 24 hr for future use. Avoid repeated warming to room temperature.
5. Refrigerate at 2–8°C (36–46°F) and protect from light.

6. Vials are for single use only; discard any unused drug after opening.

ASSESSMENT

1. If side effects occur, stop administration and take appropriate measures to alleviate. Dosing can resume once stabilized.
2. Monitor infant carefully so that oxygen therapy and ventilatory support can be adjusted in response to changes in respiratory status.

OUTCOMES/EVALUATE

Prophylaxis/management of respiratory distress syndrome

Candesartan cilexetil

(**kan**-deh-**SAR**-tan)

PREGNANCY CATEGORY: C (FIRST TRIMESTER), D (SECOND AND THIRD TRIMESTERS)
CLASSIFICATION(S):
Antihypertensive, angiotensin II receptor blocker
Rx: Atacand

SEE ALSO *ANGIOTENSIN II RECEPTOR ANTAGONISTS* AND *ANTIHYPERTENSIVE DRUGS*.

ACTION/KINETICS

Is rapidly and completely bioactivated to candesartan by ester hydrolysis during absorption from the GI tract. Food does not affect bioavailability. Effect somewhat less in blacks. **t½, elimination:** 9 hr. Excreted mainly unchanged in the urine and feces.

SIDE EFFECTS

GI: N&V, abdominal pain, diarrhea, dyspepsia, gastroenteritis. **CNS:** Headache, dizziness, paresthesia, vertigo, anxiety, depression, somnolence. **CV:** Tachycardia, palpitation; rarely, angina pectoris, MI. **Body as a whole:** Fatigue, asthenia, fever, peripheral edema. **Respiratory:** URTI, pharyngitis, rhinitis, bronchitis, coughing, dyspnea, sinusitis, epistaxis. **GU:** Impaired renal function, hematuria. **Dermatologic:** Rash, increased sweating. **Miscellaneous:** Backpain, chest pain, arthralgia, myalgia, angioedema.

LABORATORY TEST CONSIDERATIONS

↑ Creatine phosphatase. Albuminuria, hyperglycemia/triglyceridemia/uricemia.

HOW SUPPLIED

Tablets: 4 mg, 8 mg, 16 mg, 32 mg

DOSAGE

• **TABLETS**

Hypertension, monotherapy.

Adults, usual initial: 16 mg once daily for monotherapy in those not volume depleted. Can be given once or twice daily in doses from 8 to 32 mg. If BP is not controlled, a diuretic can be added.

NURSING CONSIDERATIONS

ADMINISTRATION/STORAGE

1. Maximum BP reduction is reached within 4 to 6 weeks.
2. Initiate dosage under close supervision in those with possible depletion of intravascular volume (e.g., after a diuretic). Consider giving a lower dose.
3. May give with or without food.
4. If BP is not controlled by candesartan alone, a diuretic may be added.

ASSESSMENT

1. Note onset and duration, other agents trialed and outcome.
2. Assess lytes, renal and LFTs.
3. Ensure adequate hydration, especially with diuretic therapy in renal dysfunction.

CLIENT/FAMILY TEACHING

1. Take as directed with or without food.
2. Practice reliable birth control; report if pregnancy suspected.
3. Continue life style modifications, i.e. diet, regular exercise, stress reduction, no smoking, and moderate alcohol intake to ensure BP control.

OUTCOMES/EVALUATE

↓ BP

Capecitabine

(cap-**SITE**-ah-bean)

PREGNANCY CATEGORY: D
CLASSIFICATION(S):
Antineoplastic, antimetabolite
Rx: Xeloda

SEE ALSO *ANTINEOPLASTIC AGENTS*.

ACTION/KINETICS

An oral prodrug of 5′-deoxy-5-fluorouridine (5′DFUR) that is converted to 5-fluorouracil (5-FU). 5-FU is metabolized to 5-fluoro-2-deoxyuridine monophosphate (FdUMP) and 5-fluorouridine triphosphate (FUTP) which cause cell injury in two ways. First, FdUMP and the folate cofactor, N^{5-10}-methylenetetrahydrofolate, bind to thymidylate synthase to form a ternary complex which inhibits the formation of thymidylate from uracil. Thymidylate is essential for the synthesis of DNA so a deficiency inhibits cell division. Secondly, nuclear transcriptional enzymes can mistakenly incorporate FUTP in place of uridine triphosphate during RNA synthesis; this interferes with RNA processing and protein synthesis. Readily absorbed from the GI tract. **Peak blood levels, capecitabine:** 1.5 hr; **peak blood levels, 5-FU:** 2 hr. Food reduces the rate and extent of absorption. **t½, capecitabine and 5-FU:** 45 min. Metabolites excreted in the urine.

USES

(1) First-line therapy for metastatic colorectal cancer when treatment with fluoropyrimidine therapy alone is preferred. (2) In combination with docetaxel to treat metastatic breast cancer in those for whom anthracycline therapy has failed. (3) Metastatic breast cancer in those resistant to both paclitaxel and an anthracycline-containing chemotherapy regimen or resistant to paclitaxel and for whom further anthracycline therapy is not indicated (e.g., those who have received cumulative doses of 400 mg/m² of doxorubicin or doxorubicin equivalents).

CONTRAINDICATIONS

Use in cancer clients with severe renal impairment (C_{CR} less than 30 mL/min). Hypersensitivity to 5-fluorouracil.

SPECIAL CONCERNS

Use with caution in impaired renal function and in the elderly. Patients 80 years of age or older may experience a greater incidence of side effects. Patients with severe diarrhea should be carefully monitored. Discontinue drug if nursing. Safety and efficacy in children less than 18 years of age have not been determined. When combined with docetaxel, more frequent side effects occur, including N&V and fatigue. Use caution not to confuse Xeloda (capecitabine) with Xenical (orlistat).

SIDE EFFECTS

GI: Diarrhea (may be severe), N&V, stomatitis, abdominal pain, constipation, dyspepsia, intestinal obstruction, rectal bleeding, ***GI hemorrhage,*** esophagitis, gastritis, colitis, duodenitis, hematemesis, ***necrotizing enterocolitis,*** oral/GI/esophageal candidiasis, gastroenteritis. **CV:** Cardiotoxicity (***MI,*** angina, dysrhythmias, ECG changes, ***cardiogenic shock, sudden death***), angina pectoris, ***cardiomyopathy,*** hypo/hypertension, venous phlebitis, thrombophlebitis, DVT, lymphedema, ***pulmonary embolism, CVA***. **Hematologic:** Neutropenia (grade 3 or 4), thrombocytopenia, decreased hemoglobin, anemia, lymphopenia, coagulation disorder, IT, pancytopenia, ***sepsis***. **Dermatologic:** Hand-and-foot syndrome, dermatitis, nail disorder, increased sweating, photosensitivity, radiation recall syndrome. **Neurological:** Paresthesia, fatigue, headache, dizziness, insomnia. **CNS:** Ataxia, encephalopathy, decreased level/loss of consciousness, confusion. **Metabolic:** Anorexia, dehydration, cachexia, hypertriglyceridemia. **Respiratory:** Dyspnea, epistaxis, bronchospasm, respiratory distress, URTI, bronchitis, pneumonia, bronchopneumonia, laryngitis. **Musculoskeletal:** Myalgia, pain in limb, bone pain, joint stiffness. **GU:** Nocturia, UTI. **Hepatic:** Hepatic fibrosis, cholestatic hepatitis, hepatitis. **Miscellaneous:** Hyperbilirubinemia (grade 3 or 4), eye irritation, pyrexia, edema, chest pain, drug hypersensitivity.

OD OVERDOSE MANAGEMENT

Symptoms: N&V, diarrhea, GI irritation and bleeding, bone marrow suppression. *Treatment:* Supportive medical interventions, dose interruption, adjust dose.

DRUG INTERACTIONS

Antacids / ↑ Capecitabine plasma levels

Coumarin derivatives (warfarin) / ↑ Risk of bleeding and altered coagulation test results
Leucovorin / ↑ 5-FU levels → ↑ toxicity; deaths from severe enterocolitis, diarrhea, and dehydration seen in elderly clients receiving both drugs
Phenytoin / ↑ Phenytoin levels; phenytoin dose may need to be ↓
Warfarin ↑ Anticoagulant effect; caution with other CYP2C9 substrates

HOW SUPPLIED

Tablets: 150 mg, 500 mg

DOSAGE

• **TABLETS**

Metastatic breast cancer.

For all indications: 1250 mg/m² twice daily (for a total of 2500 mg/m²/day). Each dose should be taken about 12 hours apart at the end of a meal for 2 weeks. Follow by a 1-week rest period (i.e., give as 3-week cycles). Reduce the dose to 75% of the starting dose in clients with moderate renal impairment (C_{CR}, 30–50 mL/min). Interrupt and/or reduce dose if toxicity occurs; readjust according to adverse effects.

NURSING CONSIDERATIONS

SEE ALSO *NURSING CONSIDERATIONS* FOR *ANTINEOPLASTIC AGENTS*.

ADMINISTRATION/STORAGE

If the dose has to be reduced due to toxicity, do not increase at a later time.

ASSESSMENT

1. Assess for CAD, any sensitivitiy to 5-FU, and other therapies/agents trialed/failed.
2. Monitor weights, CBC, INR or PT, renal and LFTs.
3. Administer cautiously with impaired liver/renal function and in the elderly.

CLIENT/FAMILY TEACHING

1. Take within 30 min after meals and twice/day with water. Will take for 14 days and rest for 7 days in a three week cycle.
2. Review package insert for administration guidelines; expect dose adjustments during therapy.
3. May experience nausea/ vomiting, diarrhea, mouth ulcers, and painful, swollen joints. Stop therapy immediately and report:
• grade 2 diarrhea (>4-6 stools per day or at nighttime)
• grade 2 nausea (loss of appetite with decreased food intake)
• grade 2 vomiting (2-5 times/day)
• grade 2 stomatitis (painful, red ulcers in mouth/tongue)
• grade 2 hand-and-foot syndrome (red swollen hands/feet)
• temperature over 100.5 °F or evidence of infection.
4. Practice reliable birth control, may harm fetus; do not nurse.

OUTCOMES/EVALUATE

↓ Tumor size

Capsaicin

(kap-**SAY**-ih-sin)

CLASSIFICATION(S):

Analgesic, topical

Rx: Capsin, Capzasin-P, Dolorac, No Pain-HP, Pain Doctor, Pain-X, R-Gel, Zostrix, Zostrix-HP

✱**Rx:** Antiphlogistine Rub A-535 Capsaicin, Capsaicin HP

ACTION/KINETICS

Derived from natural sources from plants of the Solanaceae family. May act to deplete and prevent the reaccumulation of substance P, thought to be the main mediator of pain impulses from the periphery to the CNS.

USES

Temporary relief of pain due to rheumatoid arthritis and osteoarthritis. Pain following herpes zoster (shingles), painful diabetic neuropathy. *Investigational:* Possible use in psoriasis, vitiligo, intractable pruritus, reflex sympathetic dystrophy, postmastectomy, vulvar vestibulitis, apocrine chromhidrosis, and postamputation and postmastectomy neuroma.

SPECIAL CONCERNS

For external use only.

SIDE EFFECTS

Skin: Transient burning following application, stinging, erythema.
Respiratory: Cough, respiratory irritation.

HOW SUPPLIED
Cream: 0.025%, 0.075%, 0.25%; *Gel:* 0.025%, 0.05%; *Lotion:* 0.025%, 0.075%; *Roll-On:* 0.075%

DOSAGE

• **CREAM, GEL LOTION, ROLL-ON, 0.025% OR 0.075%**

Adults and children over 2 years of age: Apply to affected area no more than 3–4 times/day.

NURSING CONSIDERATIONS

CLIENT/FAMILY TEACHING

1. Drug is for external use only. Avoid eyes and broken/irritated skin. Expect transient burning/stinging.
2. Wash hands before and immediately after application. May use a tongue blade to apply or wear glove to prevent contamination of eyes, mouth etc.
3. Do not bandage area tightly.
4. Regular use (3–4 times/day) is required for desired response; drug interferes with substance P (pain neurotransmitter).
5. Report if condition worsens, if symptoms persist > 3 weeks, or if clear then recur within a few days.

OUTCOMES/EVALUATE

Relief of pain

Captopril

(**KAP**-toe-prill)

PREGNANCY CATEGORY: C (FIRST TRIMESTER); D (SECOND AND THIRD TRIMESTERS)
CLASSIFICATION(S):
Antihypertensive, angiotensin synthesis inhibitor
Rx: Capoten
★**Rx:** Alti-Captopril, Apo-Capto, Gen-Captopril, Novo-Captoril, Nu-Capto, PMS-Captopril

SEE ALSO ***ANGIOTENSIN-CONVERTING ENZYME INHIBITORS.***

ACTION/KINETICS
Onset: 60–90 min. **Peak serum levels:** 30–90 min; presence of food decreases absorption by 30%–40%. **Plasma protein binding:** 25%–30%. **Time to peak effect:** 60–90 min. **Duration:** 6–12 hr. **t½, normal renal function:** 2 hr; **t½, impaired renal function:** 3.5–32 hr. More than 95% of absorbed dose excreted in urine (40%–50% unchanged). Food decreases bioavailability of captopril by 30%–40%.

USES
(1) Antihypertensive, alone or in combination with other antihypertensive drugs, especially thiazide diuretics. May be used as initial therapy for those with normal renal function. (2) In combination with diuretics and digitalis in treatment of CHF. (3) To improve survival following MI in clinically stable clients with LV dysfunction manifested as an ejection fraction of 40% or less; to reduce the incidence of overt heart failure and subsequent hospitilization for CHF in these clients. (4) Treatment of diabetic nephropathy (proteinuria > 500 mg/day) in those with type I insulin-dependent diabetes and retinopathy. *Investigational:* Rheumatoid arthritis, hypertensive crisis, neonatal and childhood hypertension, hypertension related to scleroderma renal crisis, diagnosis of anatomic renal artery stenosis, diagnosis of primary aldosteronism, Raynaud's syndrome, diagnosis of renovascular hypertension, enhance sensitivity and specificity of renal scintigraphy, idiopathic edema, and Bartter's syndrome.

CONTRAINDICATIONS
Use with a history of angioedema related to previous ACE inhibitor use.

SPECIAL CONCERNS
Use with caution in cases of impaired renal function and during lactation. Use in children only if other antihypertensive therapy has proven ineffective in controlling BP. May cause a profound drop in BP following the first dose or if used with diuretics.

SIDE EFFECTS
Dermatologic: Rash (usually maculopapular) with pruritus and occasionally fever, eosinophilia, and arthralgia. Alopecia, erythema multiforme, photosensitivity, exfoliative dermatitis,

C

Stevens-Johnson syndrome, reversible pemphigoid-like lesions, bullous pemphigus, onycholysis, flushing, pallor, scalded mouth sensation. **GI:** N&V, anorexia, constipation or diarrhea, gastric irritation, abdominal pain, dysgeusia, peptic/aphthous ulcers, dyspepsia, dry mouth, glossitis, pancreatitis. **Hepatic:** Jaundice, cholestasis, hepatitis. **CNS:** Headache, dizziness, insomnia, malaise, fatigue, paresthesias, confusion, depression, nervousness, ataxia, somnolence. **CV:** Hypotension, angina, ***MI,*** Raynaud's phenomenon, chest pain, palpitations, tachycardia, ***CVA, CHF, cardiac arrest,*** orthostatic hypotension, rhythm disturbances, cerebrovascular insufficiency. **Renal:** Renal insufficiency/failure, proteinuria, urinary frequency, oliguria, polyuria, nephrotic syndrome, interstitial nephritis. **Respiratory: *Bronchospasm,*** cough, dyspnea, asthma, ***pulmonary embolism/infarction.*** **Hematologic:** Agranulocytosis, neutropenia, thrombocytopenia, pancytopenia, ***aplastic/hemolytic anemia.*** **Other:** Decrease/loss of taste perception with weight loss (reversible), angioedema, asthenia, syncope, fever, myalgia, arthralgia, vasculitis, blurred vision, impotence, hyperkalemia, hyponatremia, myasthenia, gynecomastia, rhinitis, eosinophilic pneumonitis.

LABORATORY TEST CONSIDERATIONS

False + test for urine acetone.

OD OVERDOSE MANAGEMENT

Symptoms: Hypotension with SBP of < 80 mm Hg a possibility. *Treatment:* Volume expansion with NSS (IV) is the treatment of choice to restore BP.

ADDITIONAL DRUG INTERACTIONS

Indomethacin / ↓ 24-hr antihypertensive effects of Captopril

Probenecid / ↑ Captopril blood levels R/T ↓ renal excretion

HOW SUPPLIED

Tablet: 12.5 mg, 25 mg, 50 mg, 100 mg

DOSAGE

• **TABLETS**

Hypertension.

Adults, initial: 25 mg b.i.d.–t.i.d. If unsatisfactory response after 1–2 weeks, increase to 50 mg b.i.d.–t.i.d.; if still unsatisfactory after another 1–2 weeks, add a thiazide diuretic (e.g., hydrochlorothiazide, 25 mg/day). May increase dose 100–150 mg b.i.d.–t.i.d., not to exceed 450 mg/day.

Accelerated or malignant hypertension.

Stop current medication (except for the diuretic) and initiate captopril at 25 mg b.i.d.–t.i.d. May increase dose q 24 hr until a satisfactory response is obtained or the maximum dose reached. Furosemide may be indicated.

Heart failure.

Initial: 25 mg t.i.d.; **then,** if necessary, increase dose to 50 mg t.i.d. and evaluate response; **maintenance:** 50–100 mg t.i.d., not to exceed 450 mg/day.

NOTE: For adults, give an initial dose of 6.25–12.5 mg (0.15 mg/kg t.i.d. in children) b.i.d.–t.i.d. to clients who are sodium- and water-depleted due to diuretics, who will continue to be on diuretic therapy, and who have renal impairment.

Left ventricular dysfunction after MI.

Therapy may be started as early as 3 days after the MI. **Initial dose:** 6.25 mg; **then,** begin 12.5 mg t.i.d. and increase to 25 mg t.i.d. over the next several days. The target dose is 50 mg t.i.d. over the next several weeks. Other treatments for MI may be used concomitantly (e.g., aspirin, beta blockers, thrombolytic drugs).

Diabetic nephropathy.

25 mg t.i.d. for chronic use. Other antihypertensive drugs (e.g., beta blockers, centrally-acting drugs, diuretics, vasodilators) may be used with captopril if additional drug therapy is needed to reduce BP.

Hypertensive crisis.

Initial: 25 mg; **then,** 100 mg 90–120 min later, 200–300 mg/day for 2–5 days (then adjust dose). Sublingual captopril, 25 mg, has also been used successfully.

Rheumatoid arthritis.

75–150 mg/day in divided doses.

Severe childhood hypertension.

Initial: 0.3 mg/kg titrated to 6 mg or less given in 2 to 3 divided doses.

NOTE: For all uses, reduce dose in clients with renal impairment.

NURSING CONSIDERATIONS

SEE ALSO *NURSING CONSIDERATIONS FOR ACE INHIBITORS* AND *ANTIHYPERTENSIVE AGENTS*.

ADMINISTRATION/STORAGE

1. Do not discontinue without the provider's consent.
2. Give 1 hr before meals.
3. Discontinue previous antihypertensive medication 1 week before starting captopril, if possible.
4. The tablets can be used to prepare a solution of captopril if desired.

ASSESSMENT

1. Monitor hematologic, renal, and LFTs.
2. Determine if diuretics, or nitrates prescribed; may act synergistically and cause a more pronounced response.
3. Document any ACE intolerance.
4. Determine ability to understand/ comply with therapy.
5. Note ejection fraction (at or below 40%) in stable, post-MI clients.
6. Usually very effective with heart failure, diabetes, and arthritis.

INTERVENTIONS

1. Observe for precipitous drop in BP within 3 hr after initial dose if on diuretic therapy and a low-salt diet.
2. If BP falls rapidly, place supine; have saline infusion available.
3. Check for proteinuria monthly and for 9 mo during therapy.
4. Withhold potassium-sparing diuretics; hyperkalemia may result. Hyperkalemia may occur several months after administration of spironolactone and captopril.

CLIENT/FAMILY TEACHING

1. Take 1 hr before meals, on an empty stomach; food interferes with drug absorption.
2. Report any fever, skin rash, sore throat, mouth sores, fast or irregular heartbeat, chest pain, or cough.
3. May develop dizziness, fainting, or lightheadedness; usually disappear once body adjusts to drug. Avoid sudden changes in posture to prevent dizziness/fainting.
4. Loss of taste may be experienced for the first 2–3 months; report if persists/interferes with nutrition.
5. Carry ID and a list of medications currently prescribed.
6. Call with any questions concerning symptoms or effects of drug therapy; do not stop taking abruptly. Report for regular F/U of BP, electrolytes and urine protein.
7. Insulin-dependent clients may experience hypoglycemia; monitor FS closely.
8. Avoid OTC agents without approval.

OUTCOMES/EVALUATE

- ↓ BP
- Improvement in symptoms of CHF (↓ preload, ↓ afterload)
- Improved mortality post-MI

Carbamazepine

(kar-bah-**MAYZ**-eh-peen)

PREGNANCY CATEGORY: C
CLASSIFICATION(S):
Anticonvulsant, miscellaneous
Rx: Atretol, Carbitrol, Epitol, Tegretol, Tegretol XR
★**Rx:** Apo-Carbamazepine, Gen-Carbamazepine CR, Novo–Carbamaz, Nu–Carbamazepine, PMS-Carbamazepine, Taro-Carbamazepine, Tegretol Chewtabs, Tegretol CR

SEE ALSO *ANTICONVULSANTS*.

ACTION/KINETICS

Chemically similar to the cyclic antidepressants. It also manifests antimanic, antineuralgic, antidiuretic, anticholinergic, antiarrhythmic, and antipsychotic effects. The anticonvulsant action is not known but may involve depressing activity in the nucleus ventralis anterior of the thalamus, resulting in a reduction of polysynaptic responses and blocking posttetanic potentiation. Due to the potentially serious blood dyscrasias, a benefit-to-risk evaluation should be undertaken before the drug is instituted. **Peak ser-**

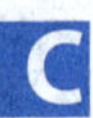

um levels: 4–5 hr. **t½** (serum): 12–17 hr with repeated doses. **Therapeutic serum levels:** 4–12 mcg/mL. Metabolized in the liver to the active epoxide derivative with a half-life of 5–8 hr. Metabolites are excreted through the feces and urine.

USES

(1) Partial seizures with complex symptoms (psychomotor, temporal lobe). (2) Tonic-clonic seizures, diseases with mixed seizure patterns or other partial or generalized seizures. Carbamazepine is often a drug of choice. (3) For children with epilepsy who are less than 6 years of age for the treatment of partial seizures, generalized tonic-clonic seizures, and mixed seizure patterns and for treating trigeminal neuralgia. (4) To treat pain associated with tic douloureux (trigeminal neuralgia) and glossopharyngeal neuralgia. *Investigational:* Bipolar disorders, unipolar depression, schizoaffective illness, resistant schizophrenia, dyscontrol syndrome associated with limbic system dysfunction, intermittent explosive disorder, PTSD, atypical psychosis. Management of alcohol, cocaine, and benzodiazepine withdrawal symptoms. Restless leg syndrome, nonneuritic pain syndromes, neurogenic or central diabetes insipidus, hereditary and nonhereditary chorea in children.

CONTRAINDICATIONS

History of bone marrow depression. Hypersensitivity to drug or tricyclic antidepressants. Lactation. Use for relief of general aches and pains.

SPECIAL CONCERNS

Safety and effectiveness have not been established in children less than 6 years of age. Use with caution in glaucoma and in hepatic, renal, CV disease, and a history of hematologic reaction. Use with caution in clients with mixed seizure disorder that includes atypical absence seizures (carbamazepine is not effective and may be associated with an increased frequency of generalized convulsions). Use in geriatric clients may cause an increased incidence of confusion, agitation, AV heart block, syndrome of inappropriate antidiuretic hormone, and bradycardia. In clients taking MAO inhibitors, discontinue for 14 days before taking carbamazepine.

SIDE EFFECTS

GI: N&V (common), diarrhea, constipation, gastric distress, abdominal pain, anorexia, glossitis, stomatitis, dry mouth and pharynx. **Hematologic:** ***Aplastic anemia,*** leukopenia, eosinophilia, thrombocytopenia, ***agranulocytosis,*** leukocytosis, pancytopenia, ***bone marrow depression.*** **CNS:** Dizziness, drowsiness, disturbances of coordination, headache, fatigue, confusion, speech disturbances, visual hallucinations, depression with agitation, talkativeness, hyperacusis, abnormal involuntary movements, behavioral changes in children. **CV:** CHF, aggravation of hypertension, hypotension, syncope and collapse, edema, recurrence of or primary thrombophlebitis, aggravation of CAD, paralysis and other symptoms of cerebral arterial insufficiency, thromboembolism, ***arrhythmias (including AV block).*** **GU:** Urinary frequency, acute urinary retention, oliguria with hypertension, impotence, renal failure, azotemia, albuminuria, glycosuria, increased BUN, microscopic deposits in urine. **Pulmonary:** Pulmonary hypersensitivity characterized by fever, dyspnea, pneumonitis, or pneumonia. **Dermatologic:** Pruritus, urticaria, photosensitivity, exfoliative dermatitis, erythematous rashes, alterations in pigmentation, alopecia, sweating, purpura, ***toxic epidermal necrolysis*** (Lyell's syndrome), ***Stevens-Johnson syndrome,*** aggravation of disseminated lupus erythematosus, alopecia, erythema nodosum/multiforme. **Ophthalmologic:** Nystagmus, double/blurred vision, oculomotor disturbances, conjunctivitis; scattered, punctate cortical lens opacities. **Hepatic:** Abnormal LFTs, cholestatic/hepatocellular jaundice, hepatitis, acute intermittent porphyria. **Other:** Peripheral neuritis, paresthesias, tinnitus, fever, chills, joint/muscle aches and leg cramps, adenopathy/lymphadenopathy, SIADH, frank water intoxication with hyponatremia and confusion.

LABORATORY TEST CONSIDERATIONS

↓ Calcium, thyroid function tests. Interference with some pregnancy tests.

OD OVERDOSE MANAGEMENT

Symptoms: First appear after 1 to 3 hours. Neuromuscular disturbances are the most common. *Pulmonary:* Irregular breathing, ***respiratory depression.*** *CV:* Tachycardia, hypo- or hypertension, conduction disorders, ***shock.*** *CNS:* Seizures (especially in small children), impaired consciousness (deep coma possible), motor restlessness, muscle twitching or tremors, athetoid movements, ataxia, drowsiness, dizziness, nystagmus, mydriasis, psychomotor disturbances, hyperreflexia followed by hyporeflexia, opisthotonos, dysmetria, dizziness, EEG may show dysrhythmias. *GI:* N&V. *GU:* Anuria, oliguria, urinary retention. *Treatment:* Stomach should be irrigated completely even if more than 4 hr has elapsed following drug ingestion, especially if alcohol has been ingested. Activated charcoal, 50–100 g initially, using a NGT (dose of 12.5 or more g/hr until client is symptom free). Diazepam or phenobarbital may be used to treat seizures (although they may aggravate respiratory depression, hypotension, and coma). Respiration, ECG, BP, body temperature, pupillary reflexes, and kidney and bladder function should be monitored for several days.

If significant bone marrow depression occurs, discontinue and determine daily CBC, platelet and reticulocyte counts. Perform bone marrow aspiration and trephine biopsy immediately and repeat often enough to monitor recovery.

DRUG INTERACTIONS

Acetaminophen / ↑ Acetaminophen breakdown → ↓ effect and ↑ risk of hepatotoxicity
Bupropion / ↓ Bupropion effect R/T ↑ liver breakdown
Charcoal / ↓ Carbamazepine effect R/T ↓ GI tract absorption
Cimetidine / ↑ Carbamazepine effect R/T ↓ liver breakdown
Contraceptives, oral / ↓ OC effect R/T ↑ liver breakdown
Cyclosporine / ↓ Cyclosporine effect R/T ↑ liver breakdown
Danazol / ↑ Carbamazepine effect R/T ↓ liver breakdown
Diltiazem / ↑ Carbamazepine effect R/T ↓ liver breakdown
Doxycycline / ↓ Doxycycline effect R/T ↑ liver breakdown
Erythromycin / ↑ Carbamazepine effect R/T ↓ liver breakdown
Felbamate / Possible ↓ serum levels of either drug
Felodipine / ↓ Felodipine effect
Fluoxetine / ↑ Carbamazepine levels → possible toxicity
Fluvoxamine / ↑ Carbamazepine levels → possible toxicity
Grapefruit juice / ↑ Peak levels of carbamazepine
Haloperidol / ↓ Haloperidol effect R/T ↑ liver breakdown
Isoniazid / ↑ Carbamazepine effect R/T ↓ liver breakdown; also, carbamazepine may ↑ risk of drug-induced hepatotoxicity
Lamotrigene / ↓ Lamotrigene effect; also, ↑ levels of active metabolite of carbamazepine
Lithium / ↑ CNS toxicity
Macrolide antibiotics (e.g., Clarithromycin, Troleandomycin) / ↑ Carbamazepine effect R/T ↓ liver breakdown
Melatonin / ↑ Melatonin bioavailability
Methylphenidate / ↓ Blood levels of methylphenidate
Muscle relaxants, nondepolarizing / Resistance to or reversal of the neuromuscular blocking effects
Oral Contraceptives / ↓ Oral contraceptive effect R/T ↑ liver breakdown
Phenobarbital / ↓ Carbamazepine effect R/T ↑ liver breakdown
Phenytoin / ↓ Carbamazepine effect R/T ↑ liver breakdown; also, phenytoin levels may ↑ or ↓
Primidone / ↓ Carbamazepine effect R/T ↑ liver breakdown
Propoxyphene / ↑ Carbamazepine effect R/T ↓ liver breakdown
Sertraline / ↓ Sertraline effect R/T ↑ liver breakdown

Thyroxine/Triiodothyronine / ↑ Elimination of thyroid hormone R/T ↑ liver breakdown
Ticlopidine / ↑ Carbamazepine effect R/T ↓ liver breakdown
Tricyclic antidepressants (TCA) / ↓ TCA effects R/T ↑ liver breakdown; also, ↓ levels of TCAs
Valproic acid / ↓ Valproic acid effect R/T ↑ liver breakdown; half-life of carbamazepine may be ↑
Vasopressin / ↑ Vasopressin effect
Verapamil / ↑ Carbamazepine effect R/T ↓ liver breakdown
Warfarin sodium / ↓ Anticoagulant effect R/T ↑ liver breakdown

HOW SUPPLIED

Capsule, Extended Release: 200 mg, 300 mg; *Chew Tablet:* 100 mg; *Suspension:* 100 mg/5 mL; *Tablet:* 200 mg; *Tablet, Extended Release:* 100 mg, 200 mg, 400 mg

DOSAGE

• ORAL SUSPENSION, EXTENDED RELEASE CAPSULES, TABLETS, CHEWABLE TABLETS, EXTENDED-RELEASE TABLETS

Anticonvulsant.

Adults and children over 12 years, initial: 200 mg b.i.d. on day 1 (100 mg q.i.d. of suspension). Increase by 200 mg/day or less at weekly intervals until best response is attained. Divide total dose and administer q 6–8 hr; the extended-release tablets may be used for twice-daily dosing instead of dosing 3 or 4 times a day. **Maximum dose, children 12–15 years:** 1,000 mg/day; **adults and children over 15 years:** 1,200 mg/day. **Maintenance:** decrease dose gradually to minimum effective level, usually 800–1,200 mg/day. **Children, 6–12 years: initial,** 100 mg b.i.d. on day 1 (50 mg q.i.d. of suspension); **then,** increase slowly, at weekly intervals, by 100 mg/day or less; dose is divided and given q 6–8 hr. Do not exceed 1,000 mg/day. **Maintenance:** 400–800 mg/day. **Children, less than 6 years:** 10–20 mg/kg/day in two to three divided doses (4 times/day with suspension); dose can be increased slowly in weekly increments to maintenance levels of 35 mg/kg/day (not to exceed 400 mg/day).

Trigeminal neuralgia.

Initial: 100 mg b.i.d. on day 1 (50 mg q.i.d. of suspension); increase by no more than 200 mg/day, using increments of 100 mg q 12 hr as needed, up to maximum of 1,200 mg/day. **Maintenance: Usual:** 400–800 mg/day (range: 200–1,200 mg/day). Attempt discontinuation of drug at least 1 time q 3 months.

Manage alcohol withdrawal.

200 mg q.i.d., up to 1,000 mg/day.

Manage cocaine or benzodiazepine withdrawal.

200 mg b.i.d., up to 800 mg/day.

Restless legs syndrome.

100–300 mg at bedtime.

Hereditary or nonhereditary chorea in children.

15–25 mg/kg/day.

Neurogenic or central diabetes.

200 mg b.i.d.–t.i.d.

NURSING CONSIDERATIONS

SEE ALSO *NURSING CONSIDERATIONS* FOR *ANTICONVULSANTS*.

ADMINISTRATION/STORAGE

1. Do not administer for a minimum of 2 weeks after client has received MAO inhibitor drugs.
2. Protect tablets from moisture.
3. Start therapy gradually using lowest dose to minimize adverse reactions.
4. Add gradually to other anticonvulsant therapy which may be maintained or decreased except for phenytoin, which may need to be increased.
5. If carbamazepine therapy must be discontinued due to side effects, abrupt withdrawal may lead to seizures or status epilepticus.

ASSESSMENT

1. Document indications for therapy. With seizures, describe type, frequency, and characteristics.
2. Assess for a history of psychosis; drug may activate symptoms.
3. Obtain baseline hematologic, renal, and LFTs; assess for dysfunction. With high doses, perform weekly CBC for the first 3 mo, then monthly to assess extent of bone marrow depression. At first sign of blood dyscrasia, slowly discontinue drug
4. Obtain eye exams; assess for opacities and intraocular pressures.

5. Obtain EEG periodically during therapy. Use seizure precautions with quick withdrawal; may precipitate status epilepticus.
6. During dosage adjustment, monitor I&O and VS for evidence of fluid retention, renal failure, or CV complications.

CLIENT/FAMILY TEACHING

1. Take with meals to minimize GI upset. The coating for extended release capsules is not absorbed and may be noticeable in the stool.
2. Withhold drug and report if any of the following symptoms occur:
• Fever, sore throat, mouth ulcers, easy bruising/bleeding; early signs of bone marrow depression.
• Urinary frequency, retention, reduced output, sexual impotence.
• Symptoms that require immediate attention: CHF, fainting, collapse, swelling, blood clot, or cyanosis.
• Loss of symptom control.
3. Use caution in operating a car or other dangerous machinery; may interfere with vision/coordination.
4. Report any skin eruptions or pigmentation changes.
5. Avoid excessive sunlight; wear protective clothing and sunscreen.
6. Use nonhormonal birth control.
7. Obtain labs to assess for early blood/organ dysfunction.

OUTCOMES/EVALUATE

• Control of refractory seizures
• Control of alcohol/drug withdrawal S&S
• ↓ Pain with trigeminal neuralgia
• Therapeutic serum drug levels (4–12 mcg/mL)

Carbenicillin indanyl sodium

(kar-ben-ih-**SILL**-in)

PREGNANCY CATEGORY: B
CLASSIFICATION(S):
Antibiotic, penicillin
Rx: Geocillin

SEE ALSO *ANTI-INFECTIVES* AND *PENICILLINS.*

ACTION/KINETICS

Acid stable drug. **Peak serum levels: PO:** 6.5 mcg/mL after 1 hr. **t½:** 60 min. Rapidly excreted unchanged in urine.

USES

(1) Upper and lower UTIs or bacteriuria due to *Escherichia coli, Proteus vulgaris* and *P. mirabilis, Morganella morganii, Providencia rettgeri, Enterobacter, Pseudomonas,* and enterococci. (2) Prostatitis due to *E. coli, Streptococcus faecalis* (enterococci), *P. mirabilis,* and *Enterobacter* species.

SPECIAL CONCERNS

Safe use in children not established. Use with caution in clients with impaired renal function.

ADDITIONAL SIDE EFFECTS

Neurotoxicity in clients with impaired renal function.

ADDITIONAL DRUG INTERACTIONS

Gentamicin / Enhanced effect of carbenicillin when used for *Pseudomonas* infection
Probenecid / ↑ Carbenicillin blood levels
Tobramycin / Enhanced effect of carbenicillin when used for *Pseudomonas* infection

HOW SUPPLIED

Tablet: 382 mg

DOSAGE

• **TABLETS**

UTIs due to E. coli, Proteus, Enterobacter.
382–764 mg carbenicillin q.i.d.

Prostatitis due to E. coli, P. mirabilis, Enterobacter, and enterococci. UTIs due to *Pseudomonas and enterococci.*
764 mg carbenicillin q.i.d.

NURSING CONSIDERATIONS

SEE ALSO *GENERAL NURSING CONSIDERATIONS* FOR *ALL ANTI-INFECTIVES* AND *PENICILLINS.*

ADMINISTRATION/STORAGE

1. Protect from moisture.
2. Store at temperature of 30°C (86°F) or less.

CLIENT/FAMILY TEACHING

1. Perform frequent mouth care to minimize nausea and unpleasant aftertaste.

2. Report any neurotoxicity, manifested by hallucinations, impaired sensorium, muscular irritability, and seizures or lack of improvement.
3. Hemorrhagic manifestations, such as bruising, discolored skin, and frank bleeding of gums and/or rectum should be reported.

OUTCOMES/EVALUATE

- Negative C&S results
- Resolution of infection; symptomatic improvement

Carbidopa

(**KAR**-bih-doh-pah)

PREGNANCY CATEGORY: C
Rx: Lodosyn

Carbidopa/Levodopa

(**KAR**-bih-doh-pah/**LEE**-voh-doh-pah)

Rx: Sinemet CR, Sinemet-10/100, -25/100, or -25/250
✱Rx: Apo-Levocarb, Endo Levodopa Carbidopa, Nu-Levocarb
CLASSIFICATION(S):
Antiparkinson drug

SEE ALSO *LEVODOPA*.

CONTENT

Carbidopa/Levodopa: Each 10/100 tablet contains: carbidopa, 10 mg, and levodopa, 100 mg. Each 25/100 tablet contains: carbidopa, 25 mg, and levodopa, 100 mg. Each 25/250 tablet contains: carbidopa, 25 mg, and levodopa, 250 mg. Each sustained-release tablet contains: carbidopa, 50 mg, and levodopa, 200 mg.

ACTION/KINETICS

Carbidopa inhibits peripheral, but not central, decarboxylation of levodopa because it does not cross the blood-brain barrier. Since peripheral decarboxylation is inhibited, more levodopa is available for transport to the brain, where it will be converted to dopamine, thus relieving the symptoms of parkinsonism. Carbidopa and levodopa are given together (e.g., Sinemet). However, *the dosage of levodopa must be reduced by up to 80% when combined with carbidopa.* This decreases the incidence of levodopa-induced side effects. *NOTE:* Pyridoxine will not reverse the action of carbidopa/levodopa. **t½, carbidopa:** 1–2 hr; when given with levodopa, the t½ of levodopa increases from 1 hr to 2 hr (may be as high as 15 hr in some clients). About 30% carbidopa is excreted unchanged in the urine.

USES

Parkinsonism (idiopathic, postencephalitic, following injury to the nervous system due to carbon monoxide and manganese intoxication). Not effective in drug-induced extrapyramidal symptoms. Carbidopa alone is used in clients who require individual titration of carbidopa and levodopa. *Investigational:* Postanoxic intention myoclonus. **Warning:** Discontinue levodopa at least 8 hr before carbidopa/levodopa therapy is initiated.

CONTRAINDICATIONS

History of melanoma. Lactation.

SPECIAL CONCERNS

Use during pregnancy only if benefits outweigh risks. Safety and efficacy in children less than 18 years of age have not been determined. Lower doses may be necessary in geriatric clients due to aged-related decreases in peripheral dopa decarboxylase. Stop MAO inhibitors 2 weeks before therapy.

SIDE EFFECTS

See *Levodopa.* Because more levodopa reaches the brain, dyskinesias may occur at lower doses with carbidopa/levodopa than with levodopa alone. Clients abruptly withdrawn from levodopa may experience neuroleptic malignant-like syndrome including symptoms of muscular rigidity, hyperthermia, increased serum phosphokinase, and changes in mental status.

LABORATORY TEST CONSIDERATIONS

↓ Creatinine, BUN, and uric acid.

DRUG INTERACTIONS

Use with tricyclic antidepressants → hypertension and dyskinesia.

HOW SUPPLIED

Carbidopa: *Tablet:* 25 mg. **Carbidopa/Levodopa:** See Content

DOSAGE

• **TABLETS**

Parkinsonism, clients not receiving levodopa.

Initial: 1 tablet of 10 mg carbidopa/100 mg levodopa t.i.d.–q.i.d. or 25 mg carbidopa/100 mg levodopa t.i.d.; **then,** increase by 1 tablet q 1–2 days until a total of 8 tablets/day is taken. If additional levodopa is required, substitute 1 tablet of 25 mg carbidopa/250 mg levodopa t.i.d.–q.i.d.

Parkinsonism, clients receiving levodopa.

Initial: Carbidopa/levodopa dosage should be about 25% of prior levodopa dosage (levodopa dosage is discontinued 8 hr before carbidopa/levodopa is initiated); **then,** adjust dosage as required. Suggested starting dose is 1 tablet of 25 mg carbidopa/250 mg levodopa t.i.d.–q.i.d. for clients taking more than 1500 mg levodopa or 25 mg carbidopa/100 mg levodopa for clients taking less than 1500 mg levodopa.

• **SUSTAINED-RELEASE TABLETS**

Parkinsonism, clients not receiving levodopa.

1 tablet b.i.d. at intervals of not less than 6 hr. Depending on the response, dosage may be increased or decreased. Usual dose is 2–8 tablets/day in divided doses at intervals of 4–8 hr during waking hours (if divided doses are not equal, the smaller dose should be given at the end of the day).

Parkinsonism, clients receiving levodopa.

1 tablet b.i.d. Carbidopa is available alone for clients requiring additional carbidopa (i.e., inadequate reduction in N&V); in such clients, carbidopa may be given at a dose of 25 mg with the first daily dose of carbidopa/levodopa. If necessary, additional carbidopa, at doses of 12.5 or 25 mg, may be given with each dose of carbidopa/levodopa.

Clients receiving carbidopa/levodopa who require additional carbidopa.

In clients taking 10 mg carbidopa/100 mg levodopa, 25 mg carbidopa may be given with the first dose each day. Additional doses of 12.5 or 25 mg may be given during the day with each dose. If the client is taking 25 mg carbidopa/250 mg levodopa, a dose of 25 mg carbidopa may be given with any dose, as needed. The maximum daily dose of carbidopa is 200 mg.

NURSING CONSIDERATIONS

SEE ALSO *NURSING CONSIDERATIONS* FOR *LEVODOPA*.

ADMINISTRATION/STORAGE

1. Dosage must be individualized.
2. Assess for drug interactions.
3. Do not administer carbidopa/levodopa with levodopa.
4. Administration of sustained-release form of carbidopa/levodopa with food results in increased levodopa availability by 50% and increased peak levodopa levels by 25%.
5. Do not crush or chew the sustained-release form of Sinemet; may administer as whole or half tablets.
6. Allow a minimum of 3 days to elapse between dosage adjustments of the sustained-release product.
7. When carbidopa is used as a supplement to carbidopa/levodopa, 1 tablet of carbidopa may be added or omitted per day.
8. If general anesthesia is necessary, continue therapy as long as PO fluids and other medication are allowed. Resume therapy when able to take PO medication.

ASSESSMENT

1. Note indications for therapy. Assess and document motor function, reflexes, gait, strength of grip, and amount of tremor.
2. Observe extent of tremors, noting muscle weakness, muscle rigidity, difficulty walking, or changing directions. During dosage adjustment, any involuntary movement may require dosage reduction.
3. Determine usual sleep patterns; assess mental status.
4. Note any history of CV disease, cardiac arrhythmias, or COPD.

5. List drugs currently prescribed. Elderly clients may require a reduced dosage.
6. Obtain baseline ECG, VS, and respiratory assessment and determine level of bladder function. Monitor BP while supine and standing to detect postural hypotension.
7. Assess need for a drug "holiday" periodically based on decreased drug response. Ensure regular neurologic F/U.

CLIENT/FAMILY TEACHING

1. Food may alter availability; do not crush or chew sustained-release form of Sinemet. May take as whole or half tablets.
2. Report side effects as dose of drug may need to be reduced or temporarily discontinued. May be asked to tolerate certain side effects because of the overall benefits gained with therapy.
3. With improvement, may resume normal activity gradually; with increased activity, other medical conditions must be considered.
4. Do not withdraw abruptly. When changing medication, one drug should be withdrawn slowly and the other started in small doses under supervision. To facilitate adjustment, take the last dose of levodopa at bedtime and start carbidopa/levodopa upon arising.
5. Drug may discolor or darken urine and/or sweat.
6. Muscle/eyelid twitching may indicate toxicity; report immediately.

OUTCOMES/EVALUATE

Control of parkinsonian symptoms (e.g., improvement in motor function, reflexes, gait, strength of grip, and amount of tremor)

Carboplatin for Injection

(**KAR**-boh-plah-tin)

PREGNANCY CATEGORY: D
CLASSIFICATION(S):
Antineoplastic, alkylating
Rx: Paraplatin
✱Rx: Paraplatin-AQ

SEE ALSO *ANTINEOPLASTIC* AND *ALKYLATING AGENTS*.

ACTION/KINETICS

Related to cisplatin. Acts by producing interstrand DNA cross-links; thought to be cell-cycle nonspecific. **t½, initial:** 1.1–2 hr; **postdistribution:** 2.6–5.9 hr. Not bound to plasma proteins, although platinum from carboplatin is irreversibly bound to plasma protein with a slow half-life (5 days). Eliminated unchanged in the urine at a rate related to C_{CR}.

USES

(1) Initial treatment of advanced ovarian cancer in combination with other chemotherapeutic agents. (2) Palliative treatment of recurrent ovarian cancer either initially or previously treated with chemotherapy, including cisplatin. *Investigational:* Small cell lung carcinoma (in combination with etoposide); advanced or recurrent squamous cell tumors of the head and neck (in combination with fluorouracil); seminoma of testicular cancer; advanced endometrial cancer; relapsed or refractory acute leukemia.

ADDITIONAL CONTRAINDICATIONS

History of severe allergy to mannitol or platinum compounds (including cisplatin). Severe bone marrow depression, significant bleeding, lactation.

ADDITIONAL SIDE EFFECTS

Bone marrow suppression may be severe. Vomiting (common). **Neurologic:** Central neurotoxicity, peripheral neuropathies (more common in ages 65 and over), ototoxicity. **GU:** Nephrotoxicity (including increased BUN and serum creatinine). **Electrolytes:** Loss of calcium, magnesium, potassium, sodium. **Allergic:** Rash, urticaria, pruritus, erythema; ***bronchospasm*** and hypotension (rare). **Miscellaneous:** Pain, alopecia, asthenia. CV, respiratory, mucosal side effects, ***anaphylaxis.***

LABORATORY TEST CONSIDERATIONS

↑ Alkaline phosphatase, AST, total bilirubin.

OD OVERDOSE MANAGEMENT

Symptoms: ***Bone marrow suppression, hepatic toxicity.*** *Treatment:* Monitor bone marrow and LFTs. Treat symptomatically.

C

DRUG INTERACTIONS
Aluminum / Precipitate formation and loss of potency R/T reaction with Al (e.g., needles, IV adminstration sets)
Phenytoin / ↓ Serum phenytoin levels → loss of therapeutic effect
HOW SUPPLIED
Powder for injection: 50 mg, 150 mg, 450 mg

DOSAGE

• **IV**

Ovarian cancer, as a single agent.
360 mg/m² q 4 weeks on day 1. Lower doses are recommended in clients with low C_{CR}.

In combination with cyclophosphamide.
Carboplatin, 300 mg/m² plus cyclophosphamide, 600 mg/m², both on day 1 q 4 weeks for 6 cycles.

NURSING CONSIDERATIONS

SEE ALSO *NURSING CONSIDERATIONS* FOR *ANTINEOPLASTIC AGENTS.*

ADMINISTRATION/STORAGE

IV 1. Do not repeat single intermittent doses of carboplatin until neutrophil count is at least 2,000/mm³ and platelet count 100,000/mm³.
2. May escalate dose by no more than 125% of the starting dose if platelet count greater than 100,000/mm³ and neutrophil counts greater than 2,000/mm³. If platelet count is less than 50,000/mm³ and neutrophil count is less than 500/mm³, subsequent doses should be 75% of the prior dose.
3. With impaired kidney function, adjust dose: C_{CR} of 41–59 mL/min, 250 mg/m² on day 1; C_{CR} of 16–40 mL/min, 200 mg/m². There is no recommended dose if the C_{CR} is less than 15 mL/min.
4. Cisplatin easily confused with carboplatin. Post signs in storage areas warning of the name mix-ups. Do not refer to as "platinum."
5. Do not use with needles or IV sets containing aluminum.
6. Immediately before use, reconstitute with either sterile water, D5W, or NaCl to a final concentration of 10 mg/mL. May be further diluted to concentrations as low as 0.5 mg/mL with D5W or NaCl injection. The dose is administered by infusion lasting 15 min or longer.
7. Reconstituted solutions are stable for 8 hr at room temperature. Discard after 8 hr; (no antibacterial preservative in the formulation).
8. Store unopened vials at room temperature, protected from light.

ASSESSMENT

1. Determine any allergic reactions to mannitol or platinum compounds.
2. Note any evidence of kidney impairment.
3. Document and assess for any neurologic disorders to determine if those occuring at a later date are drug related or exacerbations of a prior condition.
4. Assess CBC for drug-induced anemia, a frequent drug side effect.
5. Monitor alkaline phosphatase, AST, and total bilirubin.

INTERVENTIONS

1. Premedicate with antiemetics; vomiting is a frequent side effect.
2. Drug dose is based on CBC and C_{CR}; reduce dose with impaired liver/renal function.
3. With kidney impairment, initially give 1–2 L of fluids slowly. Use diuretics if overhydrated.

CLIENT/FAMILY TEACHING

1. N&V may be experienced.
2. Report if a skin rash, itching, or redness develops.
3. Maintain adequate fluid intake using fluids with electrolytes (K, Ca), since these may be lost in excess with therapy.
4. Report any sore throat, fever, fatigue, breathing problems, or mouth sores; may indicate bone marrow depression, which can be severe with this drug therapy.

OUTCOMES/EVALUATE

↓ Size and spread of tumor; stabilization of malignant process

Carisoprodol

(kar-eye-so-**PROH**-dohl)

C

PREGNANCY CATEGORY: C
CLASSIFICATION(S):
Skeletal muscle relaxant, centrally-acting
Rx: Soma

SEE ALSO ***SKELETAL MUSCLE RELAXANTS, CENTRALLY ACTING.***

ACTION/KINETICS
Does not directly relax skeletal muscles. Sedative effects may be responsible for muscle relaxation. **Onset:** 30 min. **Duration:** 4–6 hr. **Peak serum levels:** 4–7 mcg/mL. **t½:** 8 hr. Metabolized in the liver and excreted in urine.

USES
As an adjunct to rest, PT, and other measures to treat skeletal muscle disorders including bursitis, low back disorders, contusions, fibrositis, spondylitis, sprains, muscle strains, and cerebral palsy.

CONTRAINDICATIONS
Acute intermittent porphyria. Hypersensitivity to carisoprodol or meprobamate. Children under 12 years of age.

SPECIAL CONCERNS
Use with caution during lactation and in impaired liver or kidney function. May cause GI upset and sedation in infants.

SIDE EFFECTS
CNS: Ataxia, dizziness, drowsiness, excitement, tremor, syncope, vertigo, insomnia, irritability, headache, depressive reactions. **GI:** N&V, gastric upset, hiccoughs. **CV:** Flushing of face, postural hypotension, tachycardia. **Allergic reactions:** Pruritus, skin rashes, erythema multiforme, eosinophilia, fever, dizziness, angioneurotic edema, asthmatic symptoms, "smarting" of the eyes, weakness, hypotension, ***anaphylaxis.***

OD OVERDOSE MANAGEMENT
Symptoms: Stupor, coma, shock, respiratory depression, and rarely, death. *Treatment:* Supportive measures. Diuresis, osmotic diuresis, peritoneal dialysis, hemodialysis. Monitor urinary output to avoid overhydration. Observe client for possible relapse due to incomplete gastric emptying and delayed absorption.

DRUG INTERACTIONS
Alcohol / Additive CNS depressant effects
Antidepressants, tricyclic / ↑ Carisoprodol effect
Barbiturates / Possible ↑ Carisoprodol effect, followed by inhibition of carisoprodol
Chlorcyclizine / ↓ Carisoprodol effect
CNS depressants / Additive CNS depression
MAO inhibitors / ↑ Carisoprodol effect R/T ↓ liver breakdown
Phenobarbital / ↓ Carisoprodol effect R/T ↑ liver breakdown
Phenothiazines / Additive depressant effects

HOW SUPPLIED
Tablet: 350 mg

DOSAGE

• **TABLETS**
Skeletal muscle disorders.
Adults: 350 mg q.i.d. (take last dose at bedtime).

NURSING CONSIDERATIONS

SEE ALSO ***NURSING CONSIDERATIONS FOR SKELETAL MUSCLE RELAXANTS, CENTRALLY ACTING.***

ASSESSMENT
1. Note any hypersensitivity to meprobamate or carisoprodol.
2. Record extent of skeletal muscular disorders noting baseline ROM, stiffness, and level of discomfort.
3. Review drugs prescribed to ensure no interactions.

CLIENT/FAMILY TEACHING
1. If unable to swallow tablets, mix with syrup, chocolate, or a jelly mixture.
2. Administer with food if gastric upset occurs.
3. Report side effects of ataxia, or tremors should they occur.
4. Establish a schedule so the last dose is taken at bedtime.
5. Due to the possibility of drug-induced dizziness, drowsiness, and palpitations, use caution when driving or

undertaking tasks requiring mental alertness. Report if severe; may necessitate drug withdrawal.
6. Avoid OTC agents and alcohol.
7. Psychologic dependence may occur.

OUTCOMES/EVALUATE

Improvement in skeletal muscle pain and spasticity; ↑ ROM

Carmustine (BCNU)

(kar-**MUS**-teen)

PREGNANCY CATEGORY: D
CLASSIFICATION(S):
Antineoplastic, alkylating
Rx: Gliadel, BiCNU

SEE ALSO *ANTINEOPLASTIC AND ALKYLATING AGENTS.*

ACTION/KINETICS

Alkylates DNA and RNA, as well as inhibits several enzymes by carbamoylation of amino acids in proteins. Cell-cycle nonspecific. Not cross-resistant with other alkylating agents. Rapidly cleared from plasma and metabolized. Crosses blood-brain barrier (concentration in CSF at least 50% greater than in plasma). **t½:** 15–30 min. Thirty percent excreted in urine after 24 hr, 60%–70% after 96 hr. Wafers are biodegradable in the brain when implanted into the cavity after tumor resection. Released carmustine diffuses into the surrounding brain tissue.

USES

Injection: (1) Alone or in combination with other antineoplastic agents for palliative treatment of primary (e.g., brain stem glioma, astrocytoma, glioblastoma, ependymoma, medulloblastoma) and metastatic brain tumors. (2) Multiple myeloma (in combination with prednisone). (3) Advanced Hodgkin's disease and non-Hodgkin's lymphomas (not the drug of choice) in those who relapse or who fail to respond to primary therapy. *Investigational:* GI cancer, malignant melanoma, mycosis fungoides. **Wafer:** Adjunct to surgery to prolong survival in recurrent glioblastoma multiforme when surgical resection is indicated.

CONTRAINDICATIONS

Lactation.

SPECIAL CONCERNS

Delayed bone marrow toxicity. Safety and effectiveness not established in children.

ADDITIONAL SIDE EFFECTS

GI: N&V within 2 hr after administration, lasting 4–6 hr. **GU:** Renal failure, azotemia, decrease in kidney size. **Hepatic:** Reversible increases in alkaline phosphatase, bilirubin, and transaminase. **Other:** Rapid IV administration may produce transitory intense flushing of skin and conjunctiva (onset: after 2 hr; duration: 4 hr). ***Pulmonary fibrosis,*** ocular toxicity including retinal hemorrhage.

DRUG INTERACTIONS

Cimetidine / Additive bone marrow suppression
Digoxin / ↓ Serum digoxin levels → ↓ effect
Mitomycin / Corneal and conjunctival epithelial damage
Phenytoin / ↓ Serum phenytoin levels → ↓ effect

HOW SUPPLIED

Powder for injection: 100 mg; *Wafer Implant:* 7.7 mg

DOSAGE

• **IV**

In previously untreated clients.

150–200 mg/m² q 6 weeks as a single dose. Alternate dosing schedule: 75–100 mg/m² on 2 successive days q 6 weeks. Reduce subsequent dosage if platelet levels are less than 100,000/mm³ and leukocyte levels are less than 4,000/mm³.

• **WAFER IMPLANT**

Recurrent glioblastoma multiforme.

Eight wafers placed in the resection cavity if size and shape of the cavity allow. If this is not possible, use the maximum number of wafers allowed.

NURSING CONSIDERATIONS

SEE ALSO *NURSING CONSIDERATIONS* FOR *ANTINEOPLASTIC AGENTS.*

C

ADMINISTRATION/STORAGE

1. Slight overlap of the wafer in the cavity is acceptable. A wafer broken in half may be used; discard wafers broken into more than two pieces.
2. To secure wafers against the cavity surface, oxidized regenerated cellulose may be placed over the wafers.
3. Irrigate resection cavity after wafer placement; dura should be closed in a watertight fashion.
4. Unopened foil pouches of wafers may be kept at ambient room temperature for a maximum of 6 hr. Store at or below –20°C (–4°F).

IV 5. Discard vials in which powder has become an oily liquid.
6. Reconstitute powder with absolute ethyl alcohol (provided); then add sterile water. For injection, dilutions stable for 24 hr when stored as noted in #13.
7. Stock solutions diluted to 500 mL with 0.9% NaCl or D5% are stable for 48 hr when stored as noted in #13.
8. Administer IV over 1–2-hr; faster injection may produce intense pain and burning at injection site.
9. Check for extravasation if burning/pain at injection site; discomfort may be from alcohol diluent. If no extravasation but burning experienced, reduce rate of flow.
10. Slow rate of infusion and report intense flushing of skin and/or redness of conjunctiva.
11. Skin contact with reconstituted carmustine may result in hyperpigmentation (transient). If occurs, wash the skin/mucosa thoroughly with soap and water.
12. *Do not use vial for multiple doses;* no preservatives.
13. Store unopened vials at 2–8°C (36–46°F) and protect from light. Store diluted solutions at 4°C (39°F) and protect from light.

ASSESSMENT

1. Obtain baseline renal and LFTs. Monitor CBC up to 6 weeks after drug dose; delayed bone marrow toxicity may develop. Drug causes granulocyte and bone marrow suppression. Nadir: 21 days; recovery: 35–42 days.
2. Document/monitor baseline oral and ophthalmic exams.

CLIENT/FAMILY TEACHING

1. Report any S&S of fever/infection; increased SOB, abnormal bruising/bleeding.
2. Avoid vaccinations during therapy.
3. Avoid smoking as this enhances pulmonary toxicity.
4. May experience hair loss.
5. Severe flushing after IV dose should subside in 2–4 hr; may also experience N&V 2 hr after infusion.
6. Report if mouth sores develop; a special mouthwash or anesthetic can be prescribed.

OUTCOMES/EVALUATE

↓ Size/spread of metastatic process

Carteolol hydrochloride

(kar-**TEE**-oh-lohl)

PREGNANCY CATEGORY: C
CLASSIFICATION(S):
Beta-adrenergic blocking agent
Rx: Cartrol, Ocupress

SEE ALSO *BETA-ADRENERGIC BLOCKING AGENTS.*

ACTION/KINETICS

Has both beta-1 and beta-2 receptor blocking activity. Has no membrane-stabilizing activity but does have moderate intrinsic sympathomimetic effects. Low lipid solubility. **t½:** 6 hr. **Duration, ophthalmic use:** 12 hr. Approximately 50%–70% excreted unchanged in the urine.

USES

PO. Hypertension alone or with other antihypertensive drugs. *Investigational:* Reduce frequency of anginal attacks. **Ophthalmic.** Alone or with other drugs to lower IOP in chronic open-angle glaucoma and intraocular hypertension.

CONTRAINDICATIONS

Severe, persistent bradycardia. Bronchial asthma or bronchospasm, including severe COPD.

SPECIAL CONCERNS

Dosage not established in children.

ADDITIONAL SIDE EFFECTS
Ophthalmic: Transient irritation, burning, tearing, conjunctival hyperemia, edema, blurred/cloudy vision, photophobia, decreased night vision, ptosis, blepharoconjunctivitis, abnormal corneal staining, corneal sensitivity.
HOW SUPPLIED
Ophthalmic solution: 1%; *Tablet:* 2.5 mg, 5 mg

DOSAGE
• TABLETS
Hypertension.
Initial: 2.5 mg once daily either alone or with a diuretic. If response inadequate, may increase dose gradually to 5 mg, then 10 mg/day as a single dose. **Maintenance:** 2.5–5 mg once daily. Doses greater than 10 mg/day not likely to increase beneficial effect and may decrease response. Increase dosage interval in clients with renal impairment as follows: C_{CR} 20–60 mL/min: Dosage interval q 48 hr; C_{CR} <20 mL/min: Dosage interval q 72 hr.
Reduce frequency of anginal attacks.
10 mg/day.
• OPHTHALMIC SOLUTION
Usual: 1 gtt in affected eye b.i.d. If response unsatisfactory, concomitant therapy may be initiated.

NURSING CONSIDERATIONS

SEE ALSO *NURSING CONSIDERATIONS FOR BETA-ADRENERGIC BLOCKING AGENTS* AND *ANTIHYPERTENSIVE AGENTS.*

ASSESSMENT
1. Document indications for therapy and note baseline findings.
2. Assess renal function; reduce dose with impairment.

CLIENT/FAMILY TEACHING
1. Do not exceed prescribed dose; may alter desired response.
2. May cause increased sensitivity to cold; dress appropriately.
3. Report symptoms of bleeding, infection, dizziness, confusion, depression, SOB, weight gain, or rash.
4. Reinforce diet, exercise, and weight reduction.
5. With ophthalmic solution, report any persistent burning, pain, or visual impairment.

OUTCOMES/EVALUATE
• ↓ BP; ↓ anginal attacks
• ↓ Intraocular pressure

Carvedilol

(kar-**VAY**-dih-lol)

PREGNANCY CATEGORY: C
CLASSIFICATION(S):
Alpha-beta adrenergic blocking agent
Rx: Coreg

SEE ALSO *ALPHA-1 AND BETA-ADRENERGIC BLOCKING AGENTS.*

ACTION/KINETICS
Has both alpha- and beta-adrenergic blocking activity. Decreases cardiac output, reduces exercise- or isoproterenol-induced tachycardia, reduces reflex orthostatic hypotension, causes vasodilation, and reduces peripheral vascular resistance. Significant beta-blocking activity occurs within 60 min while alpha-blocking action is observed within 30 min. BP is lowered more in the standing than in the supine position. Significantly lowers plasma renin activity when given for at least 4 weeks. Rapidly absorbed after PO administration; significant first-pass effect. **Terminal t½:** 7–10 hr. Food delays absorption rate. Over 98% is bound to plasma protein. Plasma levels average 50% higher in geriatric compared with younger clients. Extensively metabolized in the liver; metabolites excreted primarily via the bile into the feces.

USES
(1) Essential hypertension used either alone or in combination with other antihypertensive drugs, especially thiazide diuretics. (2) Used with digitalis, diuretics, and ACE inhibitors to reduce the progression of mild to moderate CHF of ischemic or cardiomyopathic origin. (3) Treat severe heart failure. *Investigational:* Angina pectoris, idiopathic cardiomyopathy.

C

CONTRAINDICATIONS

Clients with NYHA Class IV decompensated cardiac failure, bronchial asthma, or related bronchospastic conditions, second- or third-degree AV block, SSS (unless a permanent pacemaker is in place), cardiogenic shock, severe bradycardia, drug hypersensitivity. Hepatic impairment. Lactation.

SPECIAL CONCERNS

Use with caution in hypertensive clients with CHF controlled with digitalis, diuretics, or an ACE inhibitor. Use with caution in PVD, in surgical procedures using anesthetic agents that depress myocardial function, in diabetics receiving insulin or oral hypoglycemic drugs, in those subject to spontaneous hypoglycemia, or in thyrotoxicosis. Clients with a history of severe anaphylactic reaction to a variety of allergens may be more reactive to repeated challenge while taking beta blockers. Safety and efficacy have not been established in children less than 18 years of age.

SIDE EFFECTS

CV: Bradycardia, postural hypotension, dependent/peripheral edema, AV block, extrasystoles, hyper/hypotension, palpitations, peripheral ischemia, syncope, angina, ***cardiac failure,*** myocardial ischemia, tachycardia, CV disorder. **CNS:** Dizziness, headache, somnolence, insomnia, ataxia, hypesthesia, paresthesia, vertigo, depression, nervousness, migraine, neuralgia, paresis, amnesia, confusion, sleep disorder, impaired concentration, abnormal thinking, paranoia, emotional lability. **Body as a whole:** Fatigue, viral infection, rash, allergy, asthenia, malaise, pain, injury, fever, infection, somnolence, sweating, ***sudden death.*** **GI:** Diarrhea, abdominal pain, bilirubinemia, N&V, flatulence, dry mouth, anorexia, dyspepsia, melena, periodontitis, increased hepatic enzymes, ***GI hemorrhage***. **Respiratory:** Rhinitis, pharyngitis, sinusitis, bronchitis, dyspnea, ***asthma, bronchospasm,*** pulmonary edema, respiratory alkalosis, dyspnea, respiratory disorder, URTI, coughing. **GU:** UTI, albuminuria, hematuria, frequency of micturition, abnormal renal function, impotence. **Dermatologic:** Pruritus; erythematous, maculopapular, and psoriaform rashes, photosensitivity reaction, exfoliative dermatitis. **Metabolic:** Hypertriglyceridemia, hypercholesterolemia, hyperglycemia, hypo/hypervolemia, hyperuricemia, increased weight, gout, dehydration, glycosuria, hyponatremia, hypo/hyperkalemia, diabetes mellitus. **Hematologic:** Thrombocytopenia, anemia, leukopenia, pancytopenia, purpura, atypical lymphocytes. **Musculoskeletal:** Back pain, arthralgia, myalgia, arthritis. **Otic:** Decreased hearing, tinnitus. **Miscellaneous:** Hot flushes, leg cramps, abnormal vision, ***anaphylactoid reaction.***

LABORATORY TEST CONSIDERATIONS

↑ ALT, AST, BUN, NPN, alkaline phosphatase. ↓ HDL.

OD OVERDOSE MANAGEMENT

Symptoms: Severe hypotension, bradycardia, cardiac insufficiency, ***cardiogenic shock, cardiac arrest, generalized seizures,*** respiratory problems, bronchospasms, vomiting, lapse of consciousness. *Treatment:* Place client in a supine position, monitor carefully, and treat under intensive care conditions. Continue treatment for a sufficient period consistent with the 7- to 10-hr drug half-life.

- Gastric lavage or induced emesis shortly after ingestion.
- For excessive bradycardia, atropine, 2 mg IV. If bradycardia is resistant to therapy; use pacemaker therapy.
- To support cardiovascular function, give glucagon, 5–10 mg IV rapidly over 30 sec, followed by a continuous infusion of 5 mg/hr. Sympathomimetics (dobutamine, isoproterenol, epinephrine) may be given.
- For peripheral vasodilation, give epinephrine or norepinephrine with continuous monitoring of circulatory conditions.
- For bronchospasm, give beta sympathomimetics as aerosol or IV or use aminophylline IVPB.
- With seizures, give diazepam or clonazepam slowly IV.

C

DRUG INTERACTIONS

Antidiabetic agents / ↑ Hypoglycemic effects due to beta blockade
Calcium channel blocking agents / ↑ Risk of conduction disturbances
Clonidine / Potentiation of BP and heart rate lowering effects
Cyclosporine / ↑ Cyclosporine blood levels R/T ↓ liver breakdown
Digoxin / ↑ Digoxin levels
Rifampin / ↓ Plasma carvedilol levels

HOW SUPPLIED

Tablet: 3.125 mg, 6.25 mg, 12.5 mg, 25 mg

DOSAGE

• **TABLETS**

Essential hypertension.

Initial: 6.25 mg b.i.d. If tolerated, using standing systolic pressure measured about 1 hr after dosing, maintain dose for 7–14 days. **Then,** increase to 12.5 mg b.i.d., if necessary, based on trough BP, using standing systolic pressure 2 hr after dosing. Maintain this dose for 7–14 days; adjust upward to 25 mg b.i.d. if necessary and tolerated. Do not exceed 50 mg/day.

Congestive heart failure.

Initial: 3.125 mg b.i.d. for 2 weeks. If tolerated, increase to 6.25 mg b.i.d. Double dose every 2 weeks to the highest tolerated level, up to a maximum of 25 mg b.i.d. in those weighing less than 85 kg and 50 mg b.i.d. in those weighing over 85 kg.

Angina pectoris.

25–50 mg b.i.d.

Idiopathic cardiomyopathy.

6.25–25 mg b.i.d.

NURSING CONSIDERATIONS

SEE ALSO *NURSING CONSIDERATIONS* FOR *ANTIHYPERTENSIVE AGENTS* AND *ALPHA-1 AND BETA-ADRENERGIC BLOCKING AGENTS.*

ADMINISTRATION/STORAGE

1. The full antihypertensive effect is seen within 7–14 days.
2. Addition of a diuretic can produce additive effects and exaggerate the orthostatic effect.

ASSESSMENT

1. Document indications for therapy, type/onset of symptoms, other agents trialed, and outcome.
2. Note any history/evidence of bronchospastic conditions, asthma, advanced AV block, or severe bradycardia; drug contraindicated.
3. Obtain baseline CBC, and renal and LFTs.

CLIENT/FAMILY TEACHING

1. Take as prescribed with food to slow absorption and decrease incidence of orthostatic effects.
2. Avoid activities that require mental acuity until drug effects realized.
3. Do not stop abruptly due to beta-blocking activity (especially with ischemic heart disease); call provider.
4. To prevent orthostatic hypotension, sit or lie until symptoms subside; rise slowly from a sitting or lying position. Concomitant therapy with a diuretic may aggravate orthostatic drug effects.
5. Decreased lacrimation may be noted by contact lens wearers.
6. Dosing adjustments will be made every 7–14 days based on standing SBP measured 1 hr after dosing.

OUTCOMES/EVALUATE

• Desired reduction of BP
• ↓ Progression of CHF

Caspofungin acetate

(**kas**-poh-**FUN**-jin)

PREGNANCY CATEGORY: C
CLASSIFICATION(S):
Antifungal
Rx: Cancidas

ACTION/KINETICS

Inhibits the synthesis of β (1,3)–D–glucan, an essential component of the cell wall of susceptible filamentous fungi. The glucan is not present in human cells. The drug is active on active cell growth of the hyphae of *Aspergillus fumigatus.* About 97% plasma protein bound. Plasma levels decline in a polyphasic manner after a 1-hr IV infusion—a short α-phase immediately postinfusion followed by a β-phase (t½: 9–11 hr). An additional longer half-life phase of 40–50 hr also occurs. Slowly metabolized. Excreted through both the urine and feces.

USES

Treatment of invasive aspergillosis in those who are refractory to or intolerant of other therapies, including amphotericin B, lipid formulations of amphotericin B, and/or itraconazole.

CONTRAINDICATIONS

Hypersensitivity to any component of the product. Concomitant use with cyclosporine unless potential benefit outweighs potential risk to the client.

SPECIAL CONCERNS

Safety and efficacy have not been determined in children under 18 years of age. Use with caution during lactation.

SIDE EFFECTS

Histamine-mediated symptoms: Rash, facial swelling, pruritus, sensation of warmth, ***anaphylaxis.*** **GI:** N&V, anorexia, diarrhea. **CNS:** Headache, paresthesia. **CV:** Infused vein complications, phlebitis, thrombophlebitis, tachycardia. **Respiratory:** Pulmonary edema, ***ARDS*** , tachypnea. **Dermatologic:** Flushing, induration, sweating. **Musculoskeletal:** Myalgia, musculoskeletal pain. **Body as a whole:** Fever, chills, flu-like illness, pain, anemia. **Miscellaneous:** Radiographic infiltrates, abdominal pain.

LABORATORY TEST CONSIDERATIONS

↑ Serum alkaline phosphatase, eosinophils, AST, ALT, urine protein/RBCs, PT. ↓ Serum albumin/potassium, H&H, neutrophils, platelets, WBC.

DRUG INTERACTIONS

Cyclosporine / ↑ Area under the curve of caspofungin and ↑ ALT and AST

Tacrolimus / ↓ Tacrolimus area under the curve, peak blood levels, and 12-hr blood level

HOW SUPPLIED

Powder/cake for injection, lyophilized: 50 mg, 70 mg

DOSAGE

• **IV INFUSION**

Aspergillosis.

Initial: A single 70-mg dose on Day 1; **then,** 50 mg daily thereafter. For clients with moderate hepatic insufficiency (Chile-Pugh score 7–9), give 35 mg/day *after* the initial 70-mg loading dose. Base duration of treatment on severity of underlying disease, recovery from immunosuppression, and clinical response.

NURSING CONSIDERATIONS

ADMINISTRATION/STORAGE

IV 1. Administer by slow IV infusion over about 1 hr.

2. Do not mix or co-infuse with other drugs.

3. **Do not use diluents containing dextrose.**

4. To prepare either the 70-mg Day 1 loading dose infusion or the daily 50-mg infusion:

• Equilibrate the refrigerated vial to room temperature.

• Aseptically add 10.5 mL of 0.9% NaCl injection to the vial. This reconstituted solution may be stored for up to 1 hr at 25°C or less (77°F or less).

• Aseptically transfer 10 mL of reconstituted drug to an IV bag or bottle containing 250 mL 0.9% NaCl.

5. To prepare a 35-mg daily dose for those with moderate hepatic insufficiency, reconstitute one 50-mg vial (as outlined above). Aseptically transfer 7 mL of the reconstituted drug from the vial to 250 mL of 0.9% NaCl or, if medically necessary, to 100 mL of 0.9% NaCl injection.

6. Store lyophilized vials in the refrigerator at 2–8°C (36–46°F).

7. The final infusion solution in the IV bag or bottle can be stored at 25°C or less (77°F or less) for 24 hr.

ASSESSMENT

1. Note onset of invasive aspergillosis and other therapies trialed as failed or intolerant.

2. Reduce dose with liver dysfunction.

3. Monitor labs, xrays and respiratory status.

CLIENT/FAMILY TEACHING

1. Respiratory aspergillosis is a fungus of the respiratory tract that will only respond to certain drugs. It impairs the ability of one to breathe normally and requires drug treatment to resolve.

2. Some of the drugs used to treat this fungal infection can be toxic to the client, thus others may be trialed.
3. Report any increased SOB, stridor, itching, facial swelling, or rash immediately.

OUTCOMES/EVALUATE

Improved radiographic findings and resolution of respiratory fungus.

Cefaclor

(**SEF**-ah-klor)

PREGNANCY CATEGORY: B
CLASSIFICATION(S):
Cephalosporin, second generation
Rx: Ceclor, Ceclor CD
★Rx: Apo-Cefaclor, Novo-Cefaclor, Nu-Cefaclor, PMS-Cefaclor, Scheinpharm Cefaclor

SEE ALSO *ANTI-INFECTIVES* AND *CEPHALOSPORINS*.

ACTION/KINETICS

Peak serum levels: 5–15 mcg/mL after 1 hr. **t½: PO,** 36–54 min. Well absorbed from GI tract. From 60% to 85% excreted in urine within 8 hr.

USES

(1) Otitis media due to *Streptococcus pneumoniae, Hemophilus influenzae, Streptococcus pyogenes*, and staphylococci. (2) Upper respiratory tract infections (including pharyngitis and tonsillitis) caused by *S. pyogenes*. (3) Lower respiratory tract infections (including pneumonia) due to *S. pneumoniae, H. influenzae*, and *S. pyogenes*. (4) Skin and skin structure infections due to *Staphylococcus aureus* and *S. pyogenes*. (5) UTIs (including pyelonephritis and cystitis) caused by *Escherichia coli, Proteus mirabilis, Klebsiella*, and coagulase-negative staphylococci.

Extended-release tablets: (1) Acute bacterial exacerbations of chronic bronchitis due to non-β-lactamase-producing strains of *H. influenzae, Moraxella catarrhalis* (including β-lactamase-producing strains), or *S. pneumoniae*. (2) Secondary bacterial infections of acute bronchitis due to *H. influenzae* (non-β-lactamase-producing strains only), *M. catarrhalis* (including β-lactamase-producing strains), or *S. pneumoniae*. (3) Pharyngitis or tonsillitis due to *S. pyogenes*. (4) Uncomplicated skin and skin structure infections due to *S. aureus* (methicillin-susceptible). *Investigational:* Acute uncomplicated UTIs in select populations using a single dose of 2 g.

SPECIAL CONCERNS

Safety in infants less than 1 month of age not established.

ADDITIONAL SIDE EFFECTS

Cholestatic jaundice, lymphocytosis.

HOW SUPPLIED

Capsule: 250 mg, 500 mg; *Powder for Oral Suspension:* 125 mg/5 mL, 187 mg/5 mL, 250 mg/5 mL, 375 mg/5 mL; *Tablet, Extended Release:* 375 mg, 500 mg

DOSAGE

- **CAPSULES, ORAL SUSPENSION**

All uses.

Adults: 250 mg q 8 hr. May double dose in more severe infections or those caused by less susceptible organisms. Do not exceed 4 g/day. **Children:** 20 mg/kg/day in divided doses q 8 hr. May double dose in more serious infections, otitis media, or for infections caused by less susceptible organisms. For otitis media and pharyngitis, the total daily dose may be divided and given q 12 hr. Do not exceed a total dose of 2 g/day.

- **TABLETS, EXTENDED RELEASE**

Acute bacterial exacerbations, chronic bronchitis, secondary bacterial infections of acute bronchitis.

500 mg q 12 hr for 7 days.

Pharyngitis, tonsillitis.

375 mg q 12 hr for 10 days.

Uncomplicated skin and skin structure infections.

375 mg q 12 hr for 7–10 days.

NURSING CONSIDERATIONS

SEE ALSO *NURSING CONSIDERATIONS FOR ANTI-INFECTIVES* AND *CEPHALOSPORINS*.

ADMINISTRATION/STORAGE

1. Refrigerate suspension after reconstitution; discard after 2 weeks.
2. The extended-release tablet can not be assumed to be equivalent to the capsule or suspension.
3. The total daily dose for otitis media and pharyngitis can be divided and given q 12 hr.

ASSESSMENT

1. Document type, onset, duration of symptoms, and agents trialed.
2. Note allergic reactions to penicillin; cross-sensitivity reaction may occur.

CLIENT/FAMILY TEACHING

1. Take entire prescription as directed; do not stop when feeling better.
2. Take extended-release tablets with food to enhance absorption. Food does not affect capsule absorption.
3. Report any adverse response or lack of improvement after 48–72 hr.

OUTCOMES/EVALUATE

Resolution of infection; symptomatic improvement

Cefadroxil monohydrate

(sef-ah-**DROX**-ill)

PREGNANCY CATEGORY: B
CLASSIFICATION(S):
Cephalosporin, first generation
Rx: Duricef
✱**Rx:** Novo-Cefadroxil

SEE ALSO *ANTI-INFECTIVES* AND *CEPHALOSPORINS*.

ACTION/KINETICS

Peak serum levels: PO, 15–33 mcg/mL after 90 min. **t½: PO,** 78–96 min. 90% excreted unchanged in urine within 24 hr.

USES

(1) UTIs caused by *Escherichia coli, Proteus mirabilis,* and *Klebsiella.* (2) Skin and skin structure infections due to staphylococci or streptococci. (3) Pharyngitis and tonsillitis due to group A beta-hemolytic streptococci.

SPECIAL CONCERNS

Safe use in children not established. Determine C_{CR} in clients with renal impairment.

HOW SUPPLIED

Capsule: 500 mg; *Powder for Oral Suspension:* 125 mg/5 mL, 250 mg/5 mL, 500 mg/5 mL; *Tablet:* 1 g

DOSAGE

• CAPSULES, ORAL SUSPENSION, TABLETS

Pharyngitis, tonsillitis.

Adults: 1 g/day in single or two divided doses for 10 days. **Children:** 30 mg/kg/day in single or two divided doses (for beta-hemolytic streptococcal infection; give dose for 10 or more days).

Skin and skin structure infections.

Adults: 1 g/day in single or two divided doses. **Children:** 30 mg/kg/day in divided doses q 12 hr.

UTIs.

Adults: 1–2 g/day in single or two divided doses for uncomplicated lower UTI (e.g., cystitis). For all other UTIs, the usual dose is 2 g/day in two divided doses. **Children:** 30 mg/kg/day in divided doses q 12 hr.

For clients with C_{CR} rates below 50 mL/min.

Initial: 1 g; **maintenance,** 500 mg at following dosage intervals: q 36 hr for C_{CR} rates of 0–10 mL/min; q 24 hr for C_{CR} rates of 10–25 mL/min; q 12 hr for C_{CR} rates of 25–50 mL/min.

NURSING CONSIDERATIONS

SEE ALSO *GENERAL NURSING CONSIDERATIONS* FOR *ANTI-INFECTIVES* AND *CEPHALOSPORINS*.

ADMINISTRATION/STORAGE

1. Give without regard to meals.
2. Shake the suspension well before using.
3. For beta-hemolytic streptococcal infections, continue treatment for 10 days.
4. Refrigerate the reconstituted suspension; discard after 14 days.

ASSESSMENT

1. Document indications for therapy, type/onset of symptoms, and pretreatment culture results.
2. Note any penicillin allergy.

CLIENT/FAMILY TEACHING

1. Take as directed with or without food.

2. Report adverse side effects or lack of response.

OUTCOMES/EVALUATE

- Symptomatic improvement
- Negative culture reports

Cefazolin sodium

(sef-**AYZ**-oh-lin)

PREGNANCY CATEGORY: B
CLASSIFICATION(S):
Cephalosporin, first generation
Rx: Ancef, Kefzol, Zolicef

SEE ALSO *ANTI-INFECTIVES* AND *CEPHALOSPORINS*.

ACTION/KINETICS

Peak serum concentration: IM 17–76 mcg/mL after 1 hr. **t½: IM, IV:** 90–120 min. From 60% to 80% excreted unchanged in urine.

USES

(1) Respiratory tract infections due to *Streptococcus pneumoniae, Klebsiella, Haemophilus influenzae, Staphylococcus aureus,* and group A β-hemolytic streptococci. (2) GU infections (prostatitis, epididymitis) due to *Escherichia coli, Proteus mirabilis, Klebsiella,* and some strains of *Enterobacter* and *enterococci.* (3) Skin and skin structure infections due to *S. aureus,* group A β-hemolytic streptococci, and other strains of streptococci. (4) Biliary tract infections due to *E. coli,* various strains of streptococci, *P. mirabilis, Klebsiella,* and *S. aureus.* (5) Bone and joint infections due to *S. aureus.* (6) Septicemia due to *S. pneumoniae, S. aureus, P. mirabilis, E. coli,* and *Klebsiella.* (7) Endocarditis due to *S. aureus* and group A β-hemolytic streptococci. (8) Perioperative prophylaxis may reduce the incidence of certain postoperative infections in those having contaminated or potentially contaminated surgical procedures (e.g., vaginal hysterectomy or cholescystectomy).

SPECIAL CONCERNS

Safety in infants under 1 month of age not determined.

ADDITIONAL SIDE EFFECTS

When high doses are used in renal failure clients: extreme confusion, ***tonic-clonic seizures,*** mild hemiparesis.

HOW SUPPLIED

Injection: 500 mg, 1 g; *Powder for injection:* 250 mg, 500 mg, 1 g, 5 g, 10 g, 20 g

DOSAGE

- **IM, IV ONLY**

Mild infections due to gram-positive cocci.

Adults: 250–500 mg q 8 hr.

Mild to moderate infections.

Children over 1 month: 25–50 mg/kg/day in three to four doses.

Moderate to severe infections.

Adults: 0.5–1 g q 6–8 hr.

Acute, uncomplicated UTIs.

Adults: 1 g q 12 hr. *For severe infections,* up to 100 mg/kg/day may be used.

Endocarditis, septicemia.

Adults: 1–1.5 g q 6 hr (rarely, up to 12 g/day).

Pneumococcal pneumonia.

Adults: 0.5 g q 12 hr.

Preoperative prophylaxis.

Adults: 1 g 30–60 min prior to surgery.

During surgery of 2 or more hours.

Adults: 0.5–1 g.

Postoperative prophylaxis.

Adults: 0.5–1 g q 6–8 hr for 24 hr (may be given for 3–5 days, especially in open heart surgery or prosthetic arthroplasty).

Impaired renal function.

Initial: 0.5 g; **then,** give maintenance doses, depending on C_{CR}, according to schedule provided by manufacturer.

NURSING CONSIDERATIONS

SEE ALSO *GENERAL NURSING CONSIDERATIONS* FOR *ANTI-INFECTIVES* AND *CEPHALOSPORINS*.

ADMINISTRATION/STORAGE

1. For IM, inject into a large muscle mass. Pain on injection is infrequent.
2. For IM use, reconstitute with sterile water, bacteriostatic water, or 0.9% NaCL injection. Shake well until dissolved.

IV 3. Follow manufacturer guidelines for dosage with renal dysfunction.
4. For direct IV administration, reconstituted 0.5 or 1 g may be diluted in 5 mL of sterile water and infused over 3–5 min.
5. For intermittent IV use, further dilute 0.5 or 1 g in 50–100 mL NSS; 5% or 10% dextrose injection; D5/RL; D5% and 0.2%, 0.45%, or 0.9% NaCl; RL injection; 5% or 10% invert sugar in sterile water for injection; 5% $NaHCO_3$; Ringer's injection; Normosol-Ionosol B w/ dextrose 5%; or Plasma-Lyte with 5% dextrose. Assess carefully for phlebitis.
6. Discard reconstituted solution after 24 hr at room temperature and after 96 hr when refrigerated.

ASSESSMENT

Document indications for therapy, type and onset of symptoms, and culture results.

OUTCOMES/EVALUATE

- Resolution of infection
- Negative culture reports

Cefdinir

(**SEF**-dih-near)

PREGNANCY CATEGORY: B
CLASSIFICATION(S):
Cephalosporin, third generation
Rx: Omnicef

SEE ALSO *CEPHALOSPORINS.*

ACTION/KINETICS

Maximum plasma levels: 2–4 hr. **t½, elimination:** 1.7 hr. Excreted through the urine.

USES

Adults: (1) Community-acquired pneumonia or acute exacerbations of chronic bronchitis due to *Haemophilus influenzae* (including β-lactamase producing strains), *Haemophilus parainfluenzae* (including β-lactamase producing strains), *Streptococcus pneumoniae* (penicillin-susceptible strains only), and *Moraxella catarrhalis* (including β-lactamase producing strains). (2) Acute maxillary sinusitis due to *Haemophilus influenzae* (including β-lactamase producing strains), *Streptococcus pneumoniae* (penicillin-susceptible strains only), and *Moraxella catarrhalis* (including β-lactamase producing strains). (3) Uncomplicated skin and skin structure infections due to *Staphylococcus aureus* (including β-lactamase producing strains) and *Streptococcus pyogenes.*

Children (6 months through 12 years): (1) Acute bacterial otitis media due to *H. influenzae* (including β-lactamase producing strains), *S. pneumoniae* (penicillin-susceptible strains only), and *M. catarrhalis* (including β-lactamase producing strains). (2) Pharyngitis/tonsillitis due to *S. pyogenes.* Acute maxillary sinusitis. (3) Uncomplicated skin and skin structure infections due to *S. aureus* (including β-lactamase producing strains) and *S. pyogenes.*

NOTE: The suspension is approved for use for all infections in children indicated above.

CONTRAINDICATIONS

Allergy to cephalosporins.

SPECIAL CONCERNS

Reduce dose in compromised renal function. Safety and efficacy have not been determined in infants less than 6 months of age.

SIDE EFFECTS

See *Cephalosporins.*

DRUG INTERACTIONS

Antacids, aluminum– or magnesium–containing / ↓ Cefdinir absorption
Probenecid / ↑ Plasma cefdinir levels → ↑ effect

HOW SUPPLIED

Capsules: 300 mg; *Oral Suspension:* 125 mg/5mL

DOSAGE

- **CAPSULES**

Community-acquired pneumonia, uncomplicated skin and skin structure infections.

Adults and adolescents age 13 and older: 300 mg q 12 hr for 10 days.

Acute exacerbations of chronic bronchitis, acute maxillary sinusitis, or pharyngitis/tonsillitis.

Adults and adolescents age 13 and older: 300 mg q 12 hr or 600 mg q 24 hr for 10 days (5–10 days for pharyngitis/tonsillitis). Alternatively, 300 mg b.i.d. for 5 days for acute exacerbations of chronic bronchitis.

• **ORAL SUSPENSION**

Acute bacterial otitis media, acute maxillary sinusitis, pharyngitis/tonsillitis.

Children, 6 months through 12 years: 7 mg/kg q 12 hr or 14 mg/kg q 24 hr for 10 days (5 days for acute otitis media and 5–10 days for pharyngitis/tonsillitis).

Uncomplicated skin and skin structure infections.

Children, 6 months through 12 years: 7 mg/kg q 12 hr for 10 days.

NURSING CONSIDERATIONS

SEE ALSO *NURSING CONSIDERATIONS* FOR *CEPHALOSPORINS*.

ASSESSMENT

1. Determine any cephalosporin or PCN allergy.
2. Note indications for therapy, onset, duration, and characteristics of symptoms.
3. Assess liver and renal function; if C_{CR} < 30 mL/min, reduce dose.

CLIENT/FAMILY TEACHING

1. May be taken without regard to food.
2. Iron supplements, multivitamins containing iron, interfere with drug absorption and antacids with aluminum or magnesium; if needed, take either 2 hr before or 2 hr after cefdinir.
3. Oral suspension contains 2.86 grams of sucrose per teaspoon; use capsules for clients with diabetes.
4. May administer suspension in iron fortified infant formula without losing potency.
5. Report if diarrhea is persistent or exceeds 4 episodes/day.
6. Stools may be discolored red; this should subside.

OUTCOMES/EVALUATE

Resolution of infection

Cefditoren pivoxil

(sef-**DIH**-tor-en)

PREGNANCY CATEGORY: B

CLASSIFICATION(S):
Cephalosporin, third generation
Rx: Spectracef

SEE ALSO *ANTI-INFECTIVES* AND *CEPHALOSPORINS*.

ACTION/KINETICS

Absorbed from the GI tract and hydrolyzed to cefditoren by esterases. **Maximum plasma levels:** 1.5–3 hr. High fat meals increase plasma levels. Primarily bound (88%) to serum albumin. **t½, terminal:** 1.6 hr. Not appreciably metabolized; mainly excreted through the urine. Clearance is decreased in renal insufficiency.

USES

(1) Acute bacterial exacerbation of chronic bronchitis due to *Haemophilus influenzae* (including β–lactamase–producing strains), *Haemophilus parainfluenzae* (including β–lactamase–producing strains), *Streptococcus pneumoniae* (penicillin-susceptible strains only), and *Moraxella catarrhalis* (including β–lactamase–producing strains). (2) Pharyngitis/tonsillitis due to *Streptococcus pyogenes*. Eradicates *S. pyogenes* from the oropharynx. (3) Uncomplicated skin and skin-structure infections due to *Staphylococcus aureus* (including β–lactamase–producing strains) and *Streptococcus pyogenes*.

CONTRAINDICATIONS

Use with known allergy to cephalosporin antibiotics, in those with carnitine deficiency or inborn errors of metabolism that may result in clinically significant carnitine deficiency, and in those with milk protein hypersensitivity (not lactose intolerance).

SPECIAL CONCERNS

Use with caution in clients hypersensitive to other cephalosporins, pencillins, or other drugs. Long-term use may cause carnitine deficiency or emergence and overgrowth of resistant organisms. Use with caution during lactation. Safety and efficacy have not been determined in children less than 12 years of age.

SIDE EFFECTS

GI: Diarrhea, N&V, abdominal pain, dyspepsia, pseudomembranous colitis, constipation, dry mouth, eructation, flatulence, gastritis, GI disorder, mouth ulceration, abnormal LFT, oral moniliasis, stomatitis, taste perversion. **CNS:** Headache, abnormal dreams, dizziness, insomnia, nervousness, somnolence. **Body as a whole:** Asthenia, fever, fungal infection, pain, sweating, urticaria, weight loss. **Respiratory:** Pharyngitis, rhinitis, sinusitis. **GU:** Vaginal moniliasis, urinary frequency, vaginitis, hematuria. **Miscellaneous:** Allergic reaction, increased coagulation time, hyperglycemia, increased appetite, leukopenia, leukorrhea, myalgia, peripheral edema, pruritus, rash, thrombocytopenia.

LABORATORY TEST CONSIDERATIONS

Possible positive direct Coomb's test. ↑ Urine WBCs, glucose. ↓ Hematocrit.

OD OVERDOSE MANAGEMENT

Symptoms: N&V, epigastric distress, diarrhea, convulsions. *Treatment:* Hemodialysis, especially if renal function is compromised. Treat symptomatically. Institute supportive measures.

DRUG INTERACTIONS

Antacids / ↓ Cefditoren absorption
H-2 receptor antagonists / ↓ Cefditoren absorption
Probenecid / ↑ Plasma cefditoren levels

HOW SUPPLIED

Tablets: 200 mg

DOSAGE

• TABLETS

Acute bacterial exacerbation of chronic bronchitis.

Adults: 400 mg b.i.d. for 10 days.

Pharyngitis, tonsillitis, uncomplicated skin and skin structure infections.

Adults: 200 mg b.i.d. for 10 days.

NURSING CONSIDERATIONS

SEE ALSO NURSING CONSIDERATIONS FOR ANTI-INFECTIVES AND CEPHALOSPORINS.

ADMINISTRATION/STORAGE

1. No dose adjustment is needed with mild renal impairment (C_{CR} of 50–80 mL/min/1.73 m^2). Do not give more than 200 mg b.i.d. to those with moderate renal impairment (C_{CR} of 30–49 mL/min/1.73 m^2) and 200 mg per day to those with severe renal impairment (C_{CR} of <30 mL/min/1.73 m^2).
2. Store between 15–30°C (59–86°F). Protect from light and moisture.
3. Dispense in tight, light resistant containers.

ASSESSMENT

1. Note indications for therapy, symptom onset, and characteristics.
2. Obtain C&S, CBC, liver and renal function studies; note any dysfunction as dosage may require adjustment.
3. Assess carefully for any sensitivity to this drug, cephalosporins, or penicillins; cross sensitivity may occur.
4. Drug is not for use in those with carnitine deficiency or those with milk protein hypersensitivity.

CLIENT/FAMILY TEACHING

1. Take twice a day as directed. To enhance absorption, take with meals. Complete entire prescription and do not share medications.
2. Do not take at the same time as antacids or other drugs that decrease stomach acid.
3. Those with milk protein hypersensitivity (not lactose intolerance) should not consume this drug.
4. Report lack of response, worsening of symptoms, or severe diarrhea and mouth pain.

OUTCOMES/EVALUATE

Resolution of infection; symptomatic improvement

Cefepime hydrochloride

(**SEF**-eh-pim)

PREGNANCY CATEGORY: B
CLASSIFICATION(S):
Cephalosporin, third generation
Rx: Maxipime

SEE ALSO CEPHALOSPORINS AND ANTI-INFECTIVES.

ACTION/KINETICS

Antibacterial activity against both gram-negative and gram-positive pathogens, including those resistant to other β-lactam antibiotics. High affinity for the multiple penicillin-binding proteins that are essential for cell wall synthesis. **Peak serum levels, after IV:** 78 mcg/mL. **t½, terminal:** 2 hr. About 85% of the drug is excreted unchanged in the urine.

USES

Adults: (1) Uncomplicated and complicated UTIs (including pyelonephritis) caused by *Escherichia coli* or *Klebsiella pneumoniae;* when the infection is severe or caused by *E. coli, K. pneumoniae,* or *Proteus mirabilis;* when the infection is mild to moderate, including infections associated with concurrent bacteremia with these microorganisms. (2) Uncomplicated skin and skin structure infections caused by *Staphylococcus aureus* (methicillin-susceptible strains only) or *Streptococcus pyogenes.* (3) Moderate to severe pneumonia due to *Streptococcus pneumoniae,* including cases associated with concurrent bacteremia, *Pseudomonas aeruginosa, K. pneumoniae,* or *Enterobacter* species. (4) Monotherapy for empiric treatment of febrile neutropenia. (5) Complicated intra-abdominal infections due to *E. coli,* viridans group streptococci, *P. aeruginosa, K. pneumoniae, Enterobacter* species, or *Bacteroides fragilis.*

Children, 2 months to 16 years: Treatment of complicated and uncomplicated UTIs including pyelonephritis, uncomplicated skin and skin structure infections, pneumonia, and as empiric therapy for febrile neutropenic clients.

CONTRAINDICATIONS

Use after a hypersensitivity reaction to cefepime, cephalosporins, pencillins, or any other β-lactam antibiotics.

SPECIAL CONCERNS

Use with caution during lactation. Safety and efficacy have not been determined in children less than 12 years of age.

SIDE EFFECTS

See *Cephalosporins.* The most common side effects include rash, phlebitis, pain, and/or inflammation.

LABORATORY TEST CONSIDERATIONS

↑ ALT, AST, alkaline phosphatase, BUN, creatinine, potassium, total bilirubin. ↓ Hematocrit, neutrophils, platelets, WBCs. ↑ or ↓ Calcium, phosphorus. Positive Coombs' test. Abnormal PTT, PT.

DRUG INTERACTIONS

Aminoglycosides / ↑ Risk of nephrotoxicity and ototoxicity
Furosemide / ↑ Risk of nephrotoxicity

HOW SUPPLIED

Powder for injection: 500 mg, 1 g, 2 g

DOSAGE

- **IM, IV**

Mild to moderate uncomplicated or complicated UTIs, including pyelonephritis, due to E. coli, K. pneumoniae, *or* P. mirabilis.

Adults: 0.5–1 g IV or IM (for *E. coli* infections) q 12 hr for 7–10 days.

Severe uncomplicated or complicated UTIs, including pyelonephritis, due to E. coli *or* K. pneumoniae.

Adults: 2 g IV q 12 hr for 10 days.

Moderate to severe pneumonia due to S. pneumoniae, P. aeruginosa, K. pneumoniae, *or* Enterobacter *species.*

Adults: 1–2 g IV q 12 hr for 10 days.

Moderate to severe uncomplicated skin and skin structure infections due to S. aureus *or* S. pyogenes.

Adults: 2 g IV q 12 hr for 10 days.

Febrile neutropenia.

2 g IV q 8 hr for 7 days, or until resolution of neutropenia.

Complicated intra-abdominal infections due to E. coli, P. aeruginosa, K. pneumoniae, B. fragilis, Enterobacter *species, or viridans group streptococci.*

Adults: 2 g IV q 12 hr for 7–10 days.

Infections in children 2 months to 16 years.

Up to 40 kg: 50 mg/kg b.i.d. (q 8 hr for febrile neutropenia) for 7–10 days, depending on the type and severity of infection. Do not exceed the adult dose.

NURSING CONSIDERATIONS

SEE ALSO *NURSING CONSIDERATIONS FOR ANTI-INFECTIVES* AND *CEPHALOSPORINS*.

ADMINISTRATION/STORAGE

1. To reconstitute for IM use, dilute with 0.9% NaCl, D5%, 0.5% or 1% lidocaine HCl, sterile water, or bacteriostatic water for injection with parabens or benzyl alcohol.

IV 2. Adjust the dose (see package insert) for impaired renal function (C_{CR} 60 mL/min).

3. To reconstitute for IV use, dilute with 50–100 mL of 0.9% NaCl injection, 5% and 10% dextrose injection, M/6 sodium lactate injection, D5/0.9% NaCl injection, D5/RL, or Normosol-R or Normosol-M in D5% injection and administer over 30 min. Cefepime is compatible at concentrations of 1–40 mg/mL with the above solutions.

4. Solutions of cefepime should not be added to ampicillin at a concentration of 40 mg/mL and should not be added to aminophylline, gentamicin, metronidazole, netilmicin sulfate, tobramycin, or vancomycin. If necessary, each of these antibiotics can be given separately.

5. Protect reconstituted drug from light and store at room temperature 20–25°C (68–77°F) for 24 hr or refrigerate at 2–8°C (36–46°F) for 7 days.

ASSESSMENT

1. Document indications for therapy, onset, location, duration, and characteristics of symptoms. List agents prescribed and outcome.

2. Note any previous sensitivity to penicillin, cephalosporins, or other antibiotics.

3. Obtain baseline cultures, CBC, renal and LFTs. Reduce dose with renal dysfunction.

4. List other agents prescribed; aminoglycosides and furosemide may increase the risk of nephrotoxicity or ototoxicity.

CLIENT/FAMILY TEACHING

1. Must perform regular dosing to maintain therapeutic serum levels.

2. Drug may cause a positive Coombs' test.

3. Pain and inflammation may occur at infusion site; may see a rash.

4. Report any prolonged or persistent diarrhea; an overgrowth of colon flora may have occurred and requires additional therapy.

OUTCOMES/EVALUATE

Symptomatic improvement with resolution of infective organism

Cefixime oral

(seh-**FIX**-eem)

PREGNANCY CATEGORY: B
CLASSIFICATION(S):
Cephalosporin, third generation
Rx: Suprax

SEE ALSO *ANTI-INFECTIVES* AND *CEPHALOSPORINS*.

ACTION/KINETICS

Stable in the presence of beta-lactamase enzymes. **Peak serum levels:** 2–6 hr. **t½:** Averages 3–4 hr. About 50% excreted unchanged in the urine and approximately 10% in the bile.

USES

(1) Uncomplicated UTIs caused by *E. coli* and *P. mirabilis.* (2) Otitis media due to *H. influenzae* (beta-lactamase positive and negative strains), *Moraxella catarrhalis,* and *S. pyogenes.* (3) Pharyngitis and tonsillitis caused by *S. pyogenes.* (4) Acute bronchitis and acute exacerbations of chronic bronchitis caused by *S. pneumoniae* and *H. influenzae* (beta-lactamase positive and negative strains). (5) Uncomplicated cervical or urethral gonorrhea due to *N. gonorrhoeae* (both penicillinase- and non-penicillinase-producing strains).

SPECIAL CONCERNS

Safe use in infants less than 6 months old not established.

ADDITIONAL SIDE EFFECTS

GI: Flatulence. **Hepatic:** Elevated alkaline phosphatase levels. **Renal:** Transient increases in BUN or creatinine.

ADDITIONAL LABORATORY TEST CONSIDERATIONS

False + test for ketones using nitroprusside test.

HOW SUPPLIED

Powder for Oral Suspension: 100 mg/5 mL; *Tablet:* 200 mg, 400 mg

DOSAGE

• **ORAL SUSPENSION, TABLETS**

Adults: Either 400 mg once daily or 200 mg q 12 hr. **Children:** Either 8 mg/kg once daily or 4 mg/kg q 12 hr. Clients on renal dialysis or in whom C_{CR} is 21–60 mL/min, the dose should be 75% of the standard dose (i.e., 300 mg/day). If the C_{CR} is less than 20 mL/min, the dose should be 50% of the standard dose (i.e., 200 mg/day).

Uncomplicated gonorrhea.

One 400-mg tablet daily.

NURSING CONSIDERATIONS

SEE ALSO *NURSING CONSIDERATIONS* FOR *ANTI-INFECTIVES* AND *CEPHALOSPORINS*.

ADMINISTRATION/STORAGE

1. Continue therapy for at least 10 days when treating *S. pyogenes*.
2. Give adult dose if over age 12 or weight over 50 kg.
3. Treat otitis media using the suspension as higher blood levels are achieved compared with the tablet given at the same dose.
4. Once reconstituted, keep the suspension at room temperature where it maintains potency for 14 days.

ASSESSMENT

1. Note any prior sensitivity to cephalosporins or penicillins.
2. Anticipate reduced dose with impaired renal function.
3. Use suspension in children and when treating otitis media.

CLIENT/FAMILY TEACHING

1. May cause GI upset; report persistent side effects, especially diarrhea.
2. Once-a-day dosing should be taken at the same time each day; cost may be prohibitive.
3. May alter results of urine glucose and ketone testing; do finger sticks for more accurate results.
4. Consult provider if child's condition does not improve or deteriorates after 48–72 hr. Return as scheduled.

OUTCOMES/EVALUATE

Resolution of infection; symptomatic improvement

Cefoperazone sodium

(sef-oh-**PER**-ah-zohn)

PREGNANCY CATEGORY: B
CLASSIFICATION(S):
Cephalosporin, third generation
Rx: Cefobid

SEE ALSO *ANTI-INFECTIVES* AND *CEPHALOSPORINS*.

ACTION/KINETICS

Peak serum levels: 73–153 mcg/mL. **t½:** 102–156 min. Approximately 30% excreted unchanged in the urine.

USES

(1) Respiratory tract infections due to *Streptococcus pneumoniae, Haemophilus influenzae, Staphylococcus aureus* (penicillinase/non-penicillinase producing), *S. pyogenes* (group A β–hemolytic streptococci), *Pseudomonas aeruginosa, Klebsiella pneumoniae, Escherichia coli, Proteus mirabilis,* and *Enterococcus* species. (2) Peritonitis and other intra–abdominal infections due to *E. coli, P. aeruginosa,* enterococci, anaerobic gram–negative bacilli (including *Bacteroides fragilis).* (3) Bacterial septicemia due to *S. pneumoniae, S. agalactiae, S. aureus,* enterococci, *P. aeruginosa, E. coli, Klebsiella* species, *Proteus* species, *Clostridium* species, and anaerobic gram–positive cocci. (4) Skin and skin structure infections due to *S. aureus, S. pyogenes, P. aeruginosa,* and enterococci. (5) PID, endometritis, and other female genital tract infections due to *N. gonorrhoeae, S. epidermidis, S. agalactiae, E. coli, Clostridium* species, enterococci, *Bacteroides* species, anaerobic gram–positive cocci. (6) UTIs due to enterococci, *E. coli,* and *P. aeruginosa*.

SPECIAL CONCERNS

Use with caution in hepatic disease or biliary obstruction. Safety and effectiveness not determined in children.

ADDITIONAL SIDE EFFECTS
Hypoprothrombinemia resulting in bleeding and/or bruising.

ADDITIONAL DRUG INTERACTIONS
Possible Antabuse-like reaction if used with ethanol.

HOW SUPPLIED
Injection: 1 g, 2, g, 10 g; *Powder for injection:* 1 g, 2 g

DOSAGE

• **IM, IV**

Adults, usual: 2–4 g/day in equally divided doses q 12 hr (up to 12–16 g/day has been used in severe infections or for less sensitive organisms).

NOTE: Significantly excreted in the bile; do not exceed 4 g/day in hepatic disease or biliary obstruction.

NURSING CONSIDERATIONS

SEE ALSO *NURSING CONSIDERATIONS* FOR *CEPHALOSPORINS*.

ADMINISTRATION/STORAGE

1. For IM use, reconstitute with 0.5% lidocaine HCl, bacteriostatic or sterile water for injection. Do not use preparations containing benzyl alcohol in infants.
2. For IM, any of the following diluents may be used following reconstitution: D5%, D5/RL, D5/0.2% or 0.9% NaCl, D10%, LR, 0.5% lidocaine HCl injection, 0.9% NaCl, D5/Normosol M, Normosol R, bacteriostatic or sterile water for injection. If concentrations of 250 mg/mL or more needed, prepare solutions using 0.5% lidocaine HCl injection.
3. After reconstituition for IM or IV use, allow any foaming to dissipate; visually inspect for complete solubilization. Vigorous prolonged agitation may be necessary to solubilize concentrations of 333 mg/mL or higher.
4. IV For IV use, reconstitute with any of the solutions listed for IM, except 0.5% lidocaine HCL, bacteriostatic or sterile water for injection.
5. When used for intermittent infusion, further dilute reconstituted product in 20–40 mL of diluent/g and give over 15–30 min.
6. When used IVPB for continuous infusion, dilute to a final concentration between 2 and 25 mg/mL.
7. Reconstituted drug may be frozen; however, after thawing, discard any unused portion.
8. Protect unreconstituted powder from light and store in refrigerator.
9. Do not mix cefoperazone directly with an aminoglycoside. If concomitant therapy is needed, use sequential intermittent IV infusion provided that separate secondary IV tubing is used and the primary IV tubing is irrigated between doses. Give prior to the aminoglycoside.

ASSESSMENT

1. Note any penicillin sensitivity. Assess for bruising, hematuria, black stools, or S&S of bleeding.
2. Obtain baseline coagulation studies and monitor; drug may cause hypoprothrombinemia. Assess need for prophylactic vitamin K administration (usually 10 mg/week).
3. With skin lesions, inspect lesions closely, noting size, location, and extent of involvement.
4. Assess for excessive alcohol use. Reduce dose with liver or biliary tract disease.

CLIENT/FAMILY TEACHING

1. Avoid alcohol and any alcohol-containing products during and for 72 hr after last dose; an Antabuse-like reaction may occur.
2. Report any unusual bruising/bleeding or lack of response.

OUTCOMES/EVALUATE

• ↓ Size and number of skin lesions; wound healing
• Resolution of infection

Cefotaxime sodium

(sef-oh-**TAX**-eem)

PREGNANCY CATEGORY: B
CLASSIFICATION(S):
Cephalosporin, third generation
Rx: Claforan

SEE ALSO *ANTI-INFECTIVES* AND *CEPHALOSPORINS*.

ACTION/KINETICS
t½: 1 hr. **Peak serum levels after 1 g IV:** 42–102 mcg/mL. 60% excreted unchanged in the urine.

C

USES

(1) Infections of the GU tract, lower respiratory tract (including pneumonia), skin, skin structures, bones, joints, and CNS (including ventriculitis and meningitis). (2) Intra-abdominal infections (including peritonitis), gynecologic infections (including endometritis, pelvic cellulitis, PID), septicemia, bacteremia, and prophylaxis in surgery. Used with aminoglycosides for gram-positive or gram-negative sepsis where the causative agent has not been identified.

The IV route is preferable for clients with severe or life-threatening infections; for clients after surgery; or for those manifesting malnutrition, trauma, malignancy, heart failure, or diabetes, especially if shock is present or possible.

HOW SUPPLIED

Injection: 1 g, 2 g; *Powder for Injection:* 500 mg, 1 g, 2 g, 10 g

DOSAGE

• **IV, IM**

Uncomplicated infections.

Adults: 1 g q 12 hr.

Moderate to severe infections.

Adults: 1–2 g q 8 hr.

Septicemia.

Adults, IV: 2 g q 6–8 hr, not to exceed 12 g/day.

Life-threatening infections.

Adults, IV: 2 g q 4 hr, not to exceed 12 g/day.

Gonorrhea.

Adults, IM: Single dose of 1 g for rectal gonorrhea in males. **IM:** Single dose of 0.5 g for rectal gonorrhea in females or gonococcoal urethritis/cervicitis in males and females.

Preoperative prophylaxis.

Adults: 1 g 30–90 min prior to surgery.

Cesarean section.

IV: 1 g when the umbilical cord is clamped; **then,** give 1 g 6 and 12 hr after the first dose.

Use in children.

Pediatric, 1 month to 12 years, IM, IV: 50–180 mg/kg/day in four to six divided doses; **1–4 weeks, IV:** 50 mg/kg q 8 hr; **0–1 week, IV:** 50 mg/kg q 12 hr. *NOTE:* Use adult dose in children 50 kg or over.

Use in impaired renal function.

If C_{CR} is less than 20 mL/min/1.73m^2, reduce the dose by 50%. If only serum creatinine is available, use the following formulas to calculate C_{CR}:

Males: Weight (kg) x (140 - age) / 72 x serum creatinine (mg/dL).

Females: 0.85 x male value.

NURSING CONSIDERATIONS

SEE ALSO *NURSING CONSIDERATIONS* FOR *CEPHALOSPORINS*.

ADMINISTRATION/STORAGE

1. Continue therapy for a minimum of 10 days for group A beta-hemolytic streptococcal infections to minimize risk of glomerulonephritis/rheumatic fever.

2. For IM use, reconstitute with sterile/bacteriostatic water for injection. Inject deeply into large muscle. Divide doses of 2 g and administer into different sites.

IV 3. Discontinue other IV solutions during therapy. Do not mix cefotaxime with aminoglycosides for continuous IV infusion; give each separately.

4. Cefotaxime is maximally stable at a pH of 5–7; do not prepare with diluents having a pH greater than 7.5 (e.g., $NaHCO_3$ injection).

5. Add recommended amount of diluent, shake to dissolve. Do not administer if particles are present or solution discolored. The normal solution color ranges from light yellow to amber.

6. For direct IV administration, mix 1 or 2 g cefotaxime with 10 mL sterile water for injection and administer over 3–5 min. For intermittent administration, dilute in 50–100 mL of solution and infuse over 30 min.

7. After reconstitution, the drug remains stable for 24 hr at room temperature, 5 days refrigerated, and 13 weeks frozen. Thaw frozen samples at room temperature before use. Do not refreeze; discard unused portions.

8. Store dry cefotaxime below 30°C (86°F) and protect from excess heat/light to prevent darkening.

C

ASSESSMENT

1. With joint infections, assess ROM and freedom of movement.
2. With gynecologic infections, determine extent of infection, duration, and characteristics of symptoms.
3. Monitor labs and review culture results for organism resistance; reduce dose with renal dysfunction.

CLIENT/FAMILY TEACHING

1. Review drugs prescribed, side effects, and expected outcomes.
2. Complete course of therapy as prescribed despite feeling better.
3. Review appropriate technique/frequency for administration and proper storage. Inspect site for pain and redness; IM may cause thrombophlebitis.
4. Record I&O; report any reduction in urinary output or persistent diarrhea.
5. Avoid alcohol in any form; an antabuse-type reaction may occur.

OUTCOMES/EVALUATE

- Resolution of infection; symptomatic improvement
- Negative culture reports

Cefotetan disodium

(sef-oh-**TEE**-tan)

PREGNANCY CATEGORY: B
CLASSIFICATION(S):
Cephalosporin, second generation
Rx: Cefotan

SEE ALSO *ANTI-INFECTIVES* AND *CEPHALOSPORINS*.

ACTION/KINETICS

t½: 3–4.6 hr. **Peak serum levels after 1 g IV:** 158 mcg/mL. From 50% to 80% is excreted unchanged in the urine.

USES

(1) UTIs due to *Escherichia coli*, *Klebsiella* species, *Proteus vulgaris*, *Providencia rettgeri*, and *Morganella morganii*. (2) Lower respiratory tract infections due to *Streptococcus pneumoniae*, *Staphylococcus aureus*, *H. influenzae* (including ampicillin–resistant strains), *Klebsiella* species, *Proteus mirabilis*, *Serratia marcescens*, and *E. coli*. (3) Skin/skin structure infections due to *S. aureus*, *S. epidermidis*, *S. pyogenes*, *Streptococcus* species (excluding enterococci), *Klebsiella* pneumoniae, *Peptococcus niger*, *Peptostreptococcus* species, and *E. coli*. (4) Gynecologic infections due to *S. aureus*, *S. epidermidis*, *Streptococcus* species (excluding enterococcus), *S. agalactiae*, *E. coli*, *P. mirabilis*, *N. gonorrhoeae*, *Bacteroides* species (excluding *B. distasonis*, *B. ovatus*, *B. thetaiotaomicron*), *Fusobacterium* species and gram–positive anaerobic cocci (including *Peptococcus* and *Peptostreptococcus* species). (5) Intra–abdominal infections due to *E. coli*, *Klebsiella* species (including *K. pneumoniae*), *Streptococcus* species (excluding enterococci), *Bacteroides* species (excluding *B. distasonis*, *B. ovatus*, *B. thetaiotaomicron*), and *Clostridium* species. (6) Bone/joint infections due to *S. aureus*. (7) Perioperatively to prevent infections in those underoing C-section, abdominal or vaginal hysterectomy, transurethral surgery, or GI and biliary tract surgery.

The IV route is preferred with bacterial septicemia, bacteremia, or other severe or life-threatening infections. It's also preferred for poor-risk clients as the result of malnutrition, surgery, diabetes, trauma, heart failure, malignancy, or if shock is present or impending.

SPECIAL CONCERNS

Safety and effectiveness have not been determined in children.

ADDITIONAL SIDE EFFECTS

Concomitant use with ethanol produces a disulfiram-type reaction and hypotension.

ADDITIONAL LABORATORY TEST CONSIDERATIONS

May affect measurement of creatinine levels by the Jaffe reaction.

HOW SUPPLIED

Injection: 1 g/50 mL, 2 g/50 mL; *Powder for Injection:* 1 g, 2 g, 10 g

DOSAGE

- **IV OR IM**

Mild to moderate skin/skin structure infections.

Adults: 2 g q 24 hr IV or 1 g q 12 hr IV or IM.

Klebsiella pneumoniae skin/skin structure infections.

1 or 2 g q 12 hr IV or IM.

Severe skin/skin structure infections.
Adults, IV: 2 g q 12 hr.
UTIs.
Adults: Either 0.5 g q 12 hr IV or IM, 1 or 2 g q 24 hr IV or IM, or 1 or 2 g q 12 hr IV or IM.
Infections of other sites.
Adults: 1 or 2 g q 12 hr IV or IM.
Severe infections.
Adults, IV: 2 g q 12 hr.
Life-threatening infections.
Adults, IV: 3 g q 12 hr.
Prophylaxis of postoperative infection.
Adults, IV: 1–2 g 30–60 min prior to surgery.
Use in impaired renal function.
May maintain q 12 hr dosing but reduce dose by ½ if the C_{CR} is 10–30 mL/min and reduce the dose by ¼ if the C_{CR} is less than 10 mL/min. If only serum creatinine is available, use the following formulas to calculate the C_{CR}:
Males: Weight (kg) x (140 - age) / 72 x serum creatinine (mg/dL).
Females: 0.85 x male value.

NURSING CONSIDERATIONS

SEE ALSO *NURSING CONSIDERATIONS* FOR *CEPHALOSPORINS*.

ADMINISTRATION/STORAGE

1. For IM use, reconstitute with sterile water, NSS, bacteriostatic water for injection, or 0.5% or 1% lidocaine HCl.
2. Give IM well within a large muscle (e.g., gluteus maximus).
IV 3. Direct IV administration may be completed over 3–5 min following reconstitution (1 g in 10 mL of sterile water for injection). May further dilute in 50–100 mL D5W or NSS and infuse over 30–60 min.
4. Reconstituted solutions maintain potency for 24 hr at room temperature, for 96 hr if refrigerated, and for 1 week if frozen. Discard any unused portion after these times; do not refreeze.
5. Do not mix cefotetan with solutions containing aminoglycosides. If both drugs are to be given, administer separately.

ASSESSMENT

1. Note any penicillin sensitivity or excessive alcohol use.
2. Monitor renal function and coagulation studies as drug may cause hypoprothrombinemia; assess for bruising, hematuria, black stools, or other evidence of bleeding.
3. Evaluate need for prophylactic vitamin K administration (usually 10 mg/week).
4. Reduce dose with impaired renal function; according to C_{CR}.

CLIENT/FAMILY TEACHING

1. Avoid alcohol ingestion during and for 72 hr after therapy; an Antabuse-like reaction may occur.
2. Report any unusual diarrhea, bruising/bleeding, decreased urine output, or lack of response.

OUTCOMES/EVALUATE

• Resolution of infection with symptomatic improvement
• Surgical infection prophylaxis

Cefoxitin sodium

(seh-**FOX**-ih-tin)

PREGNANCY CATEGORY: B
CLASSIFICATION(S):
Cephalosporin, second generation
Rx: Mefoxin

SEE ALSO *ANTI-INFECTIVES* AND *CEPHALOSPORINS*.

ACTION/KINETICS

Broad-spectrum cephalosporin that is penicillinase- and cephalosporinase-resistant and is stable in the presence of beta-lactamases. **Peak serum level after 1 g IV:** 110 mcg/mL. **t½:** 40–60 min; 85% of drug excreted unchanged in urine after 6 hr.

USES

(1) Lower respiratory tract infections (pneumonia and abcess) due to *Streptococcus pneumoniae,* other streptococci (excluding enterococci such as *S. faecalis*), *Staphylococcus aureus, Escherichia coli, Klebsiella* species, *Haemophilus influenzae,* and *Bacteroides* species. (2) UTIs due to *E. coli, Klebsiel-*

C

la species, *Proteus mirabilis, Morganella morganii, Proteus vulgaris,* and *Providencia* species (including *P. rettgeri).* (3) Uncomplicated gonorrhea due to *Neisseria gonorrhoeae* (penicillinase/non–penicillinase producing). Intra–abdominal infections (peritonitis and intra–abdominal abscess) due to *E. coli, Klebsiella* species, *Bacteroides* species (including *B. fragilis),* and *Clostridium* species. (4) Gynecological infections (endometritis, pelvic cellulitis, PID) due to *E. coli, N. gonorrhoeae, Bacteroides* species (including *B. fragilis* group), *Clostridium* species, *Peptococcus* species, *Peptostreptococcus* species, and group B streptococci. (5) Septicemia due to *S. pneumoniae, S. aureus, E. coli, Klebsiella* species, and *Bacteroides* species (including *B. fragilis).* (6) Bone/joint infections due to *S. aureus.* (7) Skin/skin structure infections due to *S. aureus, S. epidermidis,* streptococci (excluding enterococci, especially *S. faecalis), E. coli, P. mirabilis, Klebsiella* species, *Bacteroides* species (including the *B. fragilis* group), *Clostridium* species, *Peptococcus* species, and *Peptostreptococcus* species. (8) Perioperative prophylaxis, including vaginal hysterectomy, GI surgery, TURP, prosthetic arthroplasty, and C-section.

NOTE: Many gram-negative infections resistant to certain cephalosporins and penicillins respond to cefoxitin.

ADDITIONAL SIDE EFFECTS

Higher doses have caused increased incidence of eosinophilia and increased AST levels in children over 3 months of age.

ADDITIONAL LABORATORY TEST CONSIDERATIONS

High concentrations may interfere with the measurement of creatinine by the Jaffe method.

HOW SUPPLIED

Injection: 1 g/50 mL, 2 g/50 mL; *Powder for Injection:* 1 g, 2 g, 10 g

DOSAGE

• **IM, IV**

Uncomplicated infections (cutaneous, pneumonia, urinary tract).

Adults, IV: 1 g q 6–8 hr.

Moderately severe or severe infections.

Adults, IV: 1 g q 4 hr or 2 g q 6–8 hr.

Infections requiring higher dosage (e.g., gas gangrene).

Adults, IV: 2 g q 4 hr or 3 g q 6 hr.

Gonorrhea.

Adults, IV: 2 g IM with 1 g probenecid PO.

Prophylaxis in surgery.

Adults, IV: 2 g IV 30–60 min before surgery followed by 2 g q 6 hr after first dose for 24 hr only (72 hr for prosthetic arthroplasty).

Cesarean section, prophylaxis.

2 g

IV: when cord is clamped; **then,** give two additional doses 4 and 8 hr later.

TURP, prophylaxis.

1 g before surgery; **then,** 1 g q 8 hr for up to 5 days.

Impaired renal function.

Initial: 1–2 g; **then,** follow maintenance schedule provided by manufacturer. When only creatinine level is available, use the following formulas to obtain C_{CR}:

Males: Weight (kg) x (140 - age) / 72 x serum creatinine (mg/dL).

Females: 0.85 x male value.

Use in children for infections.

Children over 3 months: 80–160 mg/kg/day in four to six divided doses. Total daily dosage not to exceed 12 g.

Use in children for prophylaxis.

Children over 3 months: 30–40 mg/kg q 6 hr.

NURSING CONSIDERATIONS

SEE ALSO NURSING CONSIDERATIONS FOR CEPHALOSPORINS.

ADMINISTRATION/STORAGE

1. For IM injections, reconstitute each g with 2 mL sterile water or 2 mL 0.5% lidocaine HCl (without epinephrine) to reduce pain at injection site.

IV 2. For IV administration reconstitute 1 g with 10 or more mL of sterile water and 2 g with 10–20 mL. The 10 g vial may be reconstituted with 43 or 93 mL sterile water or other compatible solutions (see package insert). Do not use solutions containing benzyl alcohol in infants.

3. For intermittent IV administration, give 1 or 2 g in 10 mL sterile water over 3 to 5 min. For continuous IV ad-

ministration (e.g., for higher doses), add solution to 50-100 mL of D5, NSS, D5/0.9% NaCl, or D5%/ 0.02% $NaHCO_3$ solution and give over 15-30 min.
4. Do not mix with aminoglycosides. If both must be used, administer separately.
5. Store premixed products (for IV use only) at less than -20°C (-5°F). Will maintain potency after thawing for 24 hr at room temperature and 21 days if refrigerated. Discard any unused thawed solutions; do not refreeze.
6. Store dry powder below 30°C (86°F). The dry powder, solutions darken depending on storage conditions. Potency is unaffected.

ASSESSMENT

1. Document indications for therapy, onset and characteristics of symptoms.
2. Monitor I&O; report any significant reduction in urinary output.
3. Assess infusion site for pain and redness; may cause thrombophlebitis.

OUTCOMES/EVALUATE

- Resolution of infection
- Surgical infection prophylaxis

Cefpodoxime proxetil

(sef-poh-**DOX**-eem)

PREGNANCY CATEGORY: B
CLASSIFICATION(S):
Cephalosporin, third generation
Rx: Vantin

SEE ALSO *ANTI-INFECTIVES* AND *CEPHALOSPORINS*.

ACTION/KINETICS

t½, after PO: 2–3 hr. From 29% to 33% is excreted unchanged in the urine.

USES

(1) Acute, community-acquired pneumonia due to *Streptococcus pneumoniae* or *Hemophilus influenzae* (non-β-lactamase-producing strains only). (2) Acute bacterial exacerbation of chronic bronchitis caused by *S. pneumoniae,* non-beta-lactamase-producing *H. influenzae,* or *M. catarrhalis.* (3) Acute otitis media caused by *S. pneumoniae, H. influenzae* (including beta-lactamase-producing strains), and *Moraxella catarrhalis.* (4) Pharyngitis or tonsillitis due to *Streptococcus pyogenes.* (5) Acute, uncomplicated urethral and cervical gonorrhea caused by *Neisseria gonorrhoeae* (including penicillinase-producing strains). (6) Acute, uncomplicated anorectal infections in women due to *N. gonorrhoeae* (including penicillinase-producing strains). (7) Uncomplicated skin and skin structure infections due to *Staphylococcus aureus* (including penicillinase-producing strains) or *S. pyogenes.* (8) Uncomplicated UTIs (cystitis) due to *Escherichia coli, Klebsiella pneumoniae, Proteus mirabilis,* or *Staphylococcus saprophyticus.* (9) Mild to-moderate acute maxillary sinusitis.

HOW SUPPLIED

Granule for Oral Suspension: 50 mg/5 mL, 100 mg/5 mL; *Tablet:* 100 mg, 200 mg

DOSAGE

- **TABLETS, ORAL SUSPENSION**

Acute community-acquired pneumonia.

Adults and children over 13 years: 200 mg q 12 hr for 14 days.

Acute bacterial exacerbations of chronic bronchitis.

Adults and children over 13 years: 200 mg q 12 hr for 10 days. Use the tablets.

Uncomplicated gonorrhea (men and women) and rectal gonococcal infections (women).

Adults and children over 13 years: Single dose of 200 mg.

Skin and skin structure infections.

Adults and children over 13 years: 400 mg q 12 hr for 7–14 days.

Pharyngitis, tonsillitis.

Adults and children over 13 years: 100 mg q 12 hr for 5–10 days. **Children, 5 months–12 years:** 5 mg/kg (maximum of 100 mg/dose) q 12 hr (maximum daily dose: 200 mg) for 5–10 days.

C

Uncomplicated UTIs.
Adults and children over 13 years: 100 mg q 12 hr for 7 days.
Acute otitis media.
Children, 2 months–12 years: 5 mg/kg q 12 hr for 5 days.

NURSING CONSIDERATIONS

SEE ALSO *GENERAL NURSING CONSIDERATIONS* FOR *ANTI-INFECTIVES* AND *CEPHALOSPORINS*.

ADMINISTRATION/STORAGE

1. In severe renal impairment (C_{CR} < 30 mL/min), increase dosing interval to q 24 hr. If on hemodialysis, use a dosage frequency of 3 times/week after hemodialysis. Adjustment not required with cirrhosis.
2. May use the following formula to estimate C_{CR} (mL/min): **males: weight (kg) × (140 - age)/72 × serum creatinine (mg/100 mL); females: 0.85 × male value.**
3. Prepare suspension by adding a total of 58 mL of distilled water to the 50 mg/mL product or 57 mL of distilled water to the 100 mg/5 mL product. Tap bottle gently to loosen the powder, then add 25 mL of water and shake vigorously for 15 sec to wet the powder. Add the remainder of the water and shake the bottle vigorously for 3 min or until all particles are suspended. Shake well before using.
4. After reconstitution, store in the refrigerator; discard after 14 days.

ASSESSMENT

1. Note any reactions to cephalosporins/penicillins; cross-sensitivity can occur.
2. Document source of infection; obtain baseline cultures.
3. Note any renal dysfunction; alter dosage if evident.
4. Obtain serologic test for syphilis with gonorrhea treatment.
5. Monitor VS and I&O; evaluate persistent diarrhea for other causes, such as *C. difficile*.
6. Discontinue therapy/report if seizures occur.

CLIENT/FAMILY TEACHING

1. Take tablets with food to enhance absorption. The oral suspension may be given with/without food.
2. Report any persistent N&V or diarrhea as drug or dosage may require adjustment.
3. If receiving treatment for gonorrhea, have partner tested and treated and use barrier contraception to prevent reinfections. Drug is not effective against syphilis; all partners should be tested so that appropriate treatment may be provided.

OUTCOMES/EVALUATE

- Resolution of infection
- Symptomatic improvement

Cefprozil

(**SEF**-proh-zill)

PREGNANCY CATEGORY: B
CLASSIFICATION(S):
Cephalosporin, second generation
Rx: Cefzil

SEE ALSO *ANTI-INFECTIVES* AND *CEPHALOSPORINS*.

ACTION/KINETICS

t½, after PO: 78 min. Sixty percent is recovered in the urine unchanged.

USES

(1) Pharyngitis and tonsillitis due to *Streptococcus pyogenes.* (2) Acute bacterial sinusitis due to *Streptococcus pneumoniae, Staphylococcus aureus, Haemophilus influenzae* (including β-lactamase producing strains), and *Morazella catarrhalis* (including β-lactamase producing strains). (3) Otitis media caused by *S. pneumoniae, H. influenzae,* and *M. catarrhalis.* (4) Uncomplicated skin and skin structure infections due to *S. aureus* (including penicillinase-producing strains) and *S. pyogenes.* (5) Secondary bacterial infection of acute bronchitis and acute bacterial exacerbation of chronic bronchitis due to *S. pneumoniae, H. influenzae* (beta-lactamase positive and negative strains), and *M. catarrhalis.*

HOW SUPPLIED

Powder for Oral Suspension: 125 mg/5 mL, 250 mg/5 mL; *Tablet:* 250 mg, 500 mg

DOSAGE

• **SUSPENSION, TABLETS, ORAL SUSPENSION**

Pharyngitis, tonsillitis.

Adults and children over 13 years: 500 mg q 24 hr for at least 10 days (for *S. pyogenes* infections, give 10 or more days). **Children, 2–12 years:** 7.5 mg/kg q 12 hr for at least 10 days (for *S. pyogenes* infections, give 10 or more days).

Acute sinusitis.

Adults and children over 13 years: 250 mg q 12 hr or 500 mg q 12 hr for 10 days. Use the higher dose for moderate to severe infections. **Children, 6 months–12 years:** 7.5 mg/kg q 12 hr or 15 mg/kg q 12 hr for 10 days. Use the higher dose for moderate to severe infections.

Secondary bacterial infections of acute bronchitis and acute bacterial exacerbation of chronic bronchitis.

Adults and children over 13 years: 500 mg q 12 hr for 10 days.

Uncomplicated skin and skin structure infections.

Adults and children over 13 years: Either 250 mg q 12 hr, 500 mg q 24 hr, or 500 mg q 12 hr (all for a duration of 10 days). **Children, 2–12 years:** 20 mg/kg q 24 hr for 10 days.

Otitis media.

Infants and children 6 months–12 years: 15 mg/kg q 12 hr for 10 days.

NURSING CONSIDERATIONS

SEE ALSO *GENERAL NURSING CONSIDERATIONS* FOR *ANTI-INFECTIVES* AND *CEPHALOSPORINS*.

ADMINISTRATION/STORAGE

1. With impaired renal function (C_{CR} of 0–30 mL/min), give 50% of the usual dose at standard intervals.
2. After reconstitution, refrigerate suspension; discard any unused portion after 14 days.

ASSESSMENT

Reduce dose with impaired renal function; monitor I&O and VS.

CLIENT/FAMILY TEACHING

1. Take exactly as directed. Report lack of response.
2. Refrigerate suspension; discard any unused portion after 14 days.

OUTCOMES/EVALUATE

- Symptomatic improvement
- Resolution of infection

C

Ceftazidime

(sef-**TAY**-zih-deem)

PREGNANCY CATEGORY: B
CLASSIFICATION(S):
Cephalosporin, third generation
Rx: Ceptaz, Fortaz, Tazicef, Tazidime

SEE ALSO *ANTI-INFECTIVES* AND *CEPHALOSPORINS*.

ACTION/KINETICS

Only for IM or IV use. **t½:** 114–120 min. From 80% to 90% is excreted unchanged in the urine.

USES

(1) Lower respiratory tract infections (including pneumonia) due to *Pseudomonas aeruginosa* and other *Pseudomonas* species, *Haemophilus influenzae* (including ampicillin-resistant strains), *Klebsiella* species, *Enterobacter* species, *Proteus mirabilis, Escherichia coli, Serratia* species, *Citrobacter* species, *Streptococcus pneumoniae, Staphylococcus aureus* (methicillin-susceptible strains). (2) Skin and skin structure infections due to *P. aeruginosa, Klebsiella* species, *E. coli, Proteus* species (including *P. mirabilis* and indole-positive *Proteus*), *Enterobacter* species, *Serratia* species, *S. aureus* (methicillin-susceptible strains), *S. pyogenes* (group A β-hemolytic streptococci). (3) UTIs, both complicated and uncomplicated, due to *P. aeruginosa, Enterobacter* species, *Proteus* species (including *P. mirabilis* and indole-positive *Proteus*), *Klebsiella* species, and *E. coli.* (4) Bacterial septicemia due to *P. aeruginosa, Klebsiella* species, *H. influenzae, E. coli, Serratia* species, *S. pneumoniae, S. aureus* (methicillin-susceptible strains). (5) Bone and joint infections due to *P. aeruginosa, Klebsiella* species, *Enterobacter* species, *S. aureus* (methicillin-susceptible strains). (6) Gynecologic infec-

C

tions, including endometritis, pelvic cellulitis, and other infections of the female genital tract, due to *E. coli.* (7) Intra-abdominal infections, including peritonitis, due to *E. coli, Klebsiella* species, *S. aureus* (methicillin-susceptible strains); polymicrobial infections due to aerobic and anaaerobic organisms and *Bacteroides* species (many strains of *B. fragilis* are resistant). (8) CNS infections, including meningitis, due to *H. influenzae* and *Neisseria meningitidis* (limited effect against *P. aeruginosa* and *S. pneumoniae*). *NOTE:* May be used with aminoglycosides, vancomycin, and clindamycin in severe and life-threatening infections and in the immunocompromised client.

SPECIAL CONCERNS

A sodium carbonate formulation should be used if the drug is indicated for children less than 12 years of age. Possible resistance when used to treat *Pseudomonas aeruginosa* infections.

HOW SUPPLIED

Injection: 1 g, 2 g; *Powder for Injection:* 500 mg, 1 g, 2 g, 6 g, 10 g

DOSAGE

• **IM, IV**

Usual infections.

Adults, IM, IV: 1 g q 8–12 hr.

UTIs, uncomplicated.

Adults, IM, IV: 0.25 g q 12 hr.

UTIs, complicated.

Adults, IM, IV: 0.5 g q 8–12 hr.

Uncomplicated pneumonia, mild skin and skin structure infections.

Adults, IM, IV: 0.5–1 g q 8 hr.

Bone and joint infections.

Adults, IV: 2 g q 12 hr.

Serious gynecologic or intra-abdominal infections, meningitis, severe or life-threatening infections (especially in immunocompromised clients).

Adults, IV: 2 g q 8 hr.

Pseudomonal lung infections in cystic fibrosis clients with normal renal function.

IV: 30–50 mg/kg q 8 hr, not to exceed 6 g/day.

Use in neonates, infants, and children.

Neonates, 0–4 weeks, IV: 30 mg/kg q 12 hr, not to exceed the adult dose.

Infants and children, 1 month–12 years, IV: 30–50 mg/kg q 8 hr not to exceed 6 g/day.

NURSING CONSIDERATIONS

SEE ALSO *GENERAL NURSING CONSIDERATIONS* FOR *ANTI-INFECTIVES* AND *CEPHALOSPORINS.*

ADMINISTRATION/STORAGE

1. For IM administration, reconstitute in sterile water or bacteriostatic water for injection, or 0.5% or 1% lidocaine HCl injection.
2. If administering IM, use large muscle mass and inject deeply.
3. IV The IV route is preferred with bacterial septicemia, peritonitis, bacterial meningitis, or other severe/ life-threatening infections. Also, use IV route if poor risks due to malnutrition, surgery, diabetes, trauma, heart failure, malignancy, or if shock present/imminent.
4. For direct IV administration, reconstitute 1 g in 10 mL sterile water for injection; give over 3–5 min.
5. For intermittent administration, further dilute in 50–100 mL of solution and administer over 30–60 min. It is compatible with 0.9% NaCl, Ringer's/RL injection, D5% or D10%, M/6 sodium lactate injection, D5% and 0.225%, 0.45%, or 0.9% NaCl, 10% invert sugar in water. $NaHCO_3$ injection should not be used for reconstitution; however, a sodium carbonate formulation should be used for children less than 12 years.
6. For use as an IV infusion, the 1- or 2-g infusion pack is reconstituted with 100 mL sterile water for injection (or a compatible IV solution).
7. Do not add ceftazidime to solutions containing aminoglycosides. Give separately.

ASSESSMENT

1. Note indications for therapy; assess for any penicillin allergy.
2. Obtain renal function studies; reduce dose with impaired function (see package insert).

OUTCOMES/EVALUATE

- Resolution of infection
- Negative culture reports

Ceftibuten

PREGNANCY CATEGORY: B
CLASSIFICATION(S):
Cephalosporin, third generation
Rx: Cedax

SEE ALSO *CEPHALOSPORINS*.

ACTION/KINETICS
Resistant to beta-lactamase. Is well absorbed from the GI tract. Food delays the time to peak serum concentration, lowers the peak concentration, and decreases the total amount of drug absorbed. **Peak serum levels:** 2 to 3 hours. **t½:** 144 min. 56% excreted in the urine unchanged.

USES
(1) Acute bacterial exacerbations of chronic bronchitis due to *Haemophilus influenzae* (including β-lactamase-producing strains), *Moraxella catarrhalis* (including β-lactamase-producing strains), and penicillin-susceptible strains of *Streptococcus pneumoniae*. (2) Acute bacterial otitis media due to *H. influenzae* (including β-lactamase-producing strains), *M. catarrhalis* (including β-lactamase-producing strains), and *Staphylococcus pyogenes*. (3) Pharyngitis and tonsillitis due to *S. pyogenes*.

SPECIAL CONCERNS
Although ceftibuten has been approved for pharyngitis or tonsillitis, only penicillin has been shown to be effective in preventing rheumatic fever.

SIDE EFFECTS
See *Cephalosporins*. Ceftibuten is usually well tolerated. The most common side effect is diarrhea.

HOW SUPPLIED
Capsules: 400 mg; *Powder for Oral Suspension*: 90 mg/5mL, 180 mg/5 mL.

DOSAGE

• **CAPSULES, ORAL SUSPENSION**

All uses.

Adults and children over 12 years: 400 mg once daily for 10 days. The maximum daily dose is 400 mg. Adjust the dose in clients with a creatinine clearance (C_{CR}) less than 50 mL/min as follows. If the C_{CR} is between 30 and 49 mL/min, the recommended dose is 4.5 mg/kg or 200 mg once daily. If the C_{CR} is between 5 and 29 mL/min, the recommended dose is 2.25 mg/kg or 100 mg once daily. In clients undergoing hemodialysis 2 or 3 times/week, a single 400-mg dose of ceftibuten capsules or a single dose of 9 mg/kg (maximum of 400 mg) of PO suspension can be given at the end of each hemodialysis session.

Pharyngitis, tonsillitis, acute bacterial otitis media.

Children: 9 mg/kg, up to a maximum of 400 mg daily, for a total of 10 days. Give children over 45 kg the maximum daily dose of 400 mg.

NURSING CONSIDERATIONS

SEE ALSO *NURSING CONSIDERATIONS* FOR *CEPHALOSPORINS*.

ADMINISTRATION/STORAGE
1. Follow directions for mixing ceftibuten suspension carefully, depending on the final concentration and the bottle size. First, tap bottle to loosen powder; then add the appropriate amount of water in two portions. Shake well after each portion.
2. After mixing, the suspension may be kept for 14 days under refrigeration. Keep the container tightly closed and shake well before each use. Discard any unused drug after 14 days.

ASSESSMENT
1. Document type, onset, duration, and characteristics of symptoms.
2. Obtain cultures and renal function studies; reduce dose with dysfunction.
3. Review conditions requiring treatment as drug is only approved for chronic bronchitis, bacterial otitis media, and pharyngitis or tonsillitis, based on the infective organisms.

CLIENT/FAMILY TEACHING
1. Suspension must be consumed on an empty stomach, at least 2 hr before or 1 hr after a meal.
2. Complete entire prescription; do not stop despite feeling better.
3. Report persistent diarrhea.

4. Return for F/U (e.g., ear check, throat culture, X-ray).

OUTCOMES/EVALUATE

- Resolution of underlying infection
- Symptomatic improvement

C

Ceftizoxime sodium

(sef-tih-**ZOX**-eem)

PREGNANCY CATEGORY: B
CLASSIFICATION(S):
Cephalosporin, third generation
Rx: Cefizox

SEE ALSO *ANTI-INFECTIVES* AND *CEPHALOSPORINS*.

ACTION/KINETICS

t½: Approximately 1–2 hr. **Peak serum levels after 1 g IV:** 60–87 mcg/mL. Approximately 80% excreted unchanged in the urine.

USES

(1) Lower respiratory tract infections due to *Streptococcus* species (including *S. pneumoniae,* but excluding enterococci), *Klebsiella* species, *Proteus mirabilis, Escherichia coli, Haemophilus influenzae* (including ampicillin-resistant strains), *Staphylococcus aureus* (penicillinase/nonpenicillinase-producing), *Serratia* species, *Enterobacter* species, and *Bacteroides* species. (2) UTIs due to *S. aureus, E. coli, Pseudomonas* species (including *P. aeruginosa*), *P. mirabilis, P. vulgaris, Providencia rettgeri, Morganella morganii, Klebsiella* species, *Serratia* species (including *S. marcescens*), and *Enterobacter* species. (3) Uncomplicated cervical and urethral gonorrhea due to *N. gonorrhoeae.* (4) PID due to *N. gonorrhoeae, E. coli,* or *S. agalactiae.* (5) Intra-abdominal infections due to *E. coli, S. epidermidis, Streptococcus* species (excluding enterococci), *Enterobacter* species, *Klebsiella* species, *Bacteroides* species (including *B. fragilis*), and anaerobic cocci (including *Peptococcus* and *Peptostreptococcus* species). (6) Septicemia due to *Streptococcus* species (including *S. pneumoniae,* but excluding enterococci), *S. aureus, E. coli, Bacteroides* species (including *B. fragilis*), *Klebsiella* species, and *Serratia* species. (7) Skin and skin structure infections due to *S. aureus, S. epidermidis, E. coli, Klebsiella* species, *Streptococcus* species (including *S. pyogenes,* but excluding enterococci), *P. mirabilis, Serratia* species, *Enterobacter* species, *Bacteroides* species (including *B. fragilis*), and anaerobic cocci (including *Peptococcus* and *Peptostreptococcus* species). (8) Bone and joint infections due to *S. aureus, Streptococcus* species (excluding enterococci), *P. mirabilis, Bacteroides* species (including B. fragilis), and anaerobic cocci (including *Peptococcus* and *Peptostreptococcus* species). (9) Meningitis due to *H. influenzae* and limited use for *S. pyogenes.*

ADDITIONAL SIDE EFFECTS

Transient increased levels of eosinophils, AST, ALT, and CPK have been seen in children over 6 months of age.

HOW SUPPLIED

Injection: 1 g/50 mL, 2 g/50 mL; *Powder for Injection:* 500 mg, 1 g, 2 g, 10 g

DOSAGE

- **IM, IV**

Uncomplicated UTIs.

Adults: 0.5 g q 12 hr IM or IV.

Severe or resistant infections.

Adults: 1 g q 8 hr or 2 g q 8–12 hr IM or IV.

Life-threatening infections.

Adults: Up to 3–4 g q 8 hr IV.

PID.

2 g q 8 hr IV (doses up to 2 g q 4 hr have been used).

Infections at other sites.

Adults: 1 g q 8–12 hr IM or IV.

- **IV**

Uncomplicated gonorrhea.

Adults: 1 g as a single dose **IM.**

Use in children.

Pediatric, over 6 months: 50 mg/kg q 6–8 hr up to 200 mg/kg/day (not to exceed the maximum adult dose).

Impaired renal function.

Initial, IM, IV: 0.5–1 g; **then,** use maintenance schedule in package insert.

NURSING CONSIDERATIONS

SEE ALSO *GENERAL NURSING CONSIDERATIONS FOR CEPHALOSPORINS*.

ADMINISTRATION/STORAGE

1. For IM doses of 2 g, divide the dose equally and give in different large muscle masses.

IV 2. For direct IV administration, reconstitute 1 g in 10 mL sterile water and give slowly over 3–5 min.

3. For intermittent administration or continuous infusion, dilute reconstituted solution in 50–100 mL in one of the compatible solutions (see package insert).

4. For piggyback vials, reconstitute with 50–100 mL of any of the recommended IV solutions (see package insert). Shake well and administer as a single dose with primary IV fluids over 30 min.

5. A solution of 1 g ceftizoxime in 13 mL sterile water for injection is isotonic.

6. Reconstituted solutions are stable at room temperature for 8 hr and for 48 hr if refrigerated.

7. For frozen solutions, thaw container at room temperature. After thawing, the solution is stable for 24 hr at room temperature or for 10 days if refrigerated. Do not refreeze or introduce additives into the solution.

OUTCOMES/EVALUATE

- Negative culture reports
- Resolution of S&S of infection

Ceftriaxone sodium

(sef-try-**AX**-ohn)

PREGNANCY CATEGORY: B
CLASSIFICATION(S):
Cephalosporin, third generation
Rx: Rocephin

SEE ALSO *ANTI-INFECTIVES* AND *CEPHALOSPORINS*.

ACTION/KINETICS

t½: Approximately 6–8 hr. Significantly protein bound. **Serum levels after 1 g IV:** 151 mcg/mL. One-third to two-thirds excreted unchanged in the urine.

USES

(1) Lower respiratory tract infections due to *Streptococcus pneumoniae, Staphylococcus aureus, Haemophilus influenzae, H. parainfluenzae, Klebsiella pneumonia, Serratia marcescens, Escherichia coli, E. aerogenes,* and *Proteus mirabilis.* (2) Skin and skin structure infections due to *S. aureus, S. epidermidis, S. pyogenes,* Viridins group streptococci, *E. coli, Enterobacter cloacae, K. oxytoca, K. pneumoniae, P. mirabilis, Pseudomonas aeruginosa, Morganella morganii, S. marcescens. Acinetobacter calcoaceticus, Bactgeroides fragilis, Peptostreptococcus* species. UTIs (complicated and uncomplicated) due to *E. coli, P. mirabilis, P. vulgaris, M. morganii,* and *K. pneumoniae.* (3) Uncomplicated cervical/urethral and rectal gonorrhea due to *Neisseria gonorrhoeae,* including penicillinase/nonpenicillinase producing strains. (4) Pharyngeal gonorrhea due to nonpenicillinase producing strains of *N. gonorrhoeae.* PID due to *N. gonorrhoeae.* (5) Bacterial septicemia due to *S. aureus, S. pneumoniae, E. coli, H. influenzae,* and *K. pneumoniae.* (6) Bone and joint infections due to *S. aureus, S. pneumoniae, E. coli, P. mirabilis, K. pneumoniae,* and *Enterobacter* species. (7) Intra-abdominal infections due to *E. coli, K. pneumoniae, B. fragilis, Clostridium* species (most strains of *C. difficle* are resistant) and *Peptostreptococcus* species. (8) Meningitis due to *H. influenzae, N. meningitidis,* and *S. pneumoniae.* (9) Single preoperative doses may decrease the incidence of postoperative infections following vaginal or abdominal hysterectomy or in coronary artery bypass surgery. (10) Pediatric otitis media. *Investigational:* Neurologic complications, arthritis, and carditis associated with Lyme disease in clients refractory to penicillin G.

ADDITIONAL SIDE EFFECTS

Increase in serum creatinine, presence of casts in the urine, alteration of PTs (rare).

HOW SUPPLIED

Injection: 1 g/50 mL, 2 g/50 mL; *Powder for Injection:* 250 mg, 500 mg, 1 g, 2 g, 10 g

C

DOSAGE

- **IV, IM**

General infections.

Adults, usual: 1–2 g/day in single or divided doses q 12 hr, not to exceed 4 g/day. Maintain therapy for 4–14 days, depending on the infection. **Pediatric:** *Other than meningitis:* 50–75 mg/kg/day not to exceed total daily dose of 2 g given in divided doses q 12 hr.

Meningitis.

Pediatric: 100 mg/kg/day, not to exceed total daily dose of 4 g given once daily or in equally divided doses q 12 hr for 7–14 days.

Skin and skin structure infections.

Pediatric: 50–75 mg/kg once daily or in equally divided doses q 12 hr. Do not exceed a daily dose of 2 g.

Preoperative for prophylaxis of infection in surgery.

1 g 30–120 min prior to surgery.

Uncomplicated gonorrhea.

Adults, IM: 125 mg as a single dose plus doxycycline, 100 mg b.i.d. for 7 days or azithromycin, 1 g, as a single PO dose. Or, a single dose of cefpriaxone 250 mg IM.

Disseminated gonococcal infection.

Adults: 1 g IM or IV q 24 hr.

Gonococcal meningitis or endocarditis.

Adults: 1–2 g IV q 12 hr for 10–14 days (meningitis) or 4 weeks (endocarditis).

Gonococcal conjunctivitis.

Adults and children over 20 kg: 1 g given as a single IM dose.

Haemophilus ducreyi infection.

250 mg IM as a single dose.

Acute PID.

250 mg IM plus doxycycline or tetracycline.

Lyme disease in those refractory to Pencillin G.

IV: 2 g/day for 14–28 days.

NOTE: Dosage adjustment is not required for renal or hepatic impairment; however, monitor blood levels.

Acute bacterial otitis media.

IM: Single dose of 50 mg/kg, not to exceed 1 g.

NURSING CONSIDERATIONS

SEE ALSO *GENERAL NURSING CONSIDERATIONS* FOR *ANTI-INFECTIVES* AND *CEPHALOSPORINS*.

ADMINISTRATION/STORAGE

1. IM injections should be deep into the body of a large muscle.

IV 2. IV infusions should contain concentrations of 10–40 mg/mL. Reconstitute 500 mg in 4.8 mL of sterile water, NSS, or D5W. Then further dilute in 50–100 mL D5W or NSS and infuse over 30–60 min.

3. Do not mix drug with other antibiotics.

4. Stability of solutions for IM or IV use varies depending on the diluent used; check package insert carefully.

5. Maintain dosage for at least 2 days after symptoms have disappeared (usual course is 4–14 days, although complicated infections may require longer therapy).

6. Continue dosage for at least 10 days when treating *Streptococcus pyogenes* infections.

ASSESSMENT

1. Document indications for therapy and include pretreatment findings.

2. Note any history of GI disease, especially colitis; use drug cautiously.

3. Note any penicillin reactions.

4. Monitor coagulation studies; drug may alter PTs. Use vitamin K (10 mg/week) prophylactically if bleeding occurs.

OUTCOMES/EVALUATE

- Resolution of S&S of infection
- Negative culture reports

Cefuroxime axetil

(sef-your-**OX**-eem)

PREGNANCY CATEGORY: B
Rx: Ceftin

Cefuroxime sodium

(sef-your-**OX**-eem)

PREGNANCY CATEGORY: B
Rx: Kefurox, Zinacef
CLASSIFICATION(S):
Cephalosporin, second generation

SEE ALSO *ANTI-INFECTIVES* AND *CEPHALOSPORINS*.

ACTION/KINETICS

Cefuroxime axetil is used PO, whereas cefuroxime sodium is used either IM or IV. **IM, IV: t½, 80 min. Peak serum levels after 1.5 g IV:** 100 mcg/mL. 66%–100% is excreted unchanged in the urine. t½ will be prolonged in clients with renal failure.

USES

PO (axetil). Pharyngitis, tonsillitis, otitis media, acute bacterial maxillary sinusitis, acute bacterial exacerbations of chronic bronchitis and secondary bacterial infections of acute bronchitis, uncomplicated UTIs, uncomplicated skin and skin structure infections, uncomplicated gonorrhea (urethral and endocervical) caused by non-penicillinase-producing strains of *Neisseria gonorrhoeae.* Early Lyme disease due to *Borrelia burgdorferi.* The suspension is indicated for children from 3 months to 12 years to treat pharyngitis, tonsillitis, acute bacterial otitis media, bacterial maxillary sinusitis, and impetigo.

IM, IV (sodium). Infections of the urinary tract, lower respiratory tract (including pneumonia), skin and skin structures, bones, and joints. Septicemia, meningitis, uncomplicated and disseminated gonococcal infections due to penicillinase- or non-penicillinase-producing strains of *N. gonorrhoeae* in men and women. Mixed infections in which several organisms have been identified. Prophylaxis of postoperative infections in surgical procedures such as vaginal hysterectomy.

ADDITIONAL SIDE EFFECTS

Decrease in H&H.

ADDITIONAL LABORATORY TEST CONSIDERATIONS

False – reaction in the ferricyanide test for blood glucose.

HOW SUPPLIED

Cefuroxime axetil: *Powder for Oral Suspension:* 125 mg/5 mL, 250 mg/5 mL; *Tablet:* 125 mg, 250 mg, 500 mg **Cefuroxime sodium:** *Injection:* 750 mg/50 mL, 1.5 g/50 mL; *Powder for Injection:* 750 mg, 1.5 g, 7.5 g

DOSAGE

CEFUROXIME AXETIL

• **TABLETS**

Pharyngitis, tonsillitis.

Adults and children over 13 years: 250 mg q 12 hr for 10 days. **Children:** 125 mg q 12 hr for 10 days.

Acute bacterial exacerbations of chronic bronchitis and secondary bacterial infections of acute bronchitis, uncomplicated skin and skin structure infections.

Adults and children over 13 years: 250 or 500 mg q 12 hr for 10 days (5 days for secondary bacterial infections of acute bronchitis).

Uncomplicated UTIs.

Adults and children over 13 years: 125 or 250 mg q 12 hr for 7–10 days. **Infants and children less than 12 years:** 125 mg b.i.d.

Acute otitis media.

Children: 250 mg b.i.d. for 10 days.

Uncomplicated gonorrhea.

Adults and children over 13 years: 1,000 mg as a single dose.

Early Lyme disease.

500 mg/day for 20 days.

• **SUSPENSION**

Pharyngitis, tonsillitis.

Children, 3 months to 12 years: 20 mg/kg/day in 2 divided doses, not to exceed 500 mg total dose/day, for 10 days.

Acute otitis media, impetigo.

Children, 3 months to 12 years: 30 mg/kg/day in 2 divided doses, not to exceed 1,000 mg total dose/day, for 10 days.

CEFUROXIME SODIUM

• **IM, IV**

Uncomplicated infections, including urinary tract, uncomplicated pneumonia, disseminated gonococcal, skin and skin structure.

Adults: 750 mg q 8 hr. **Pediatric, over 3 months:** 50–100 mg/kg/day in divided doses q 6–8 hr (not to exceed adult dose for severe infections).

Severe or complicated infections; bone and joint infections.

Adults: 1.5 g q 8 hr. **Pediatric, over 3 months:** *bone and joint infections,* **IV:**

150 mg/kg/day in divided doses q 8 hr (not to exceed adult dose).

Life-threatening infections or those due to less susceptible organisms.
Adults: 1.5 g q 6 hr.

Bacterial meningitis.
Adults: Up to 3 g q 8 hr. **Pediatric, over 3 months, initial, IV:** 200–240 mg/kg/day in divided doses q 6–8 hr; **then,** after clinical improvement, 100 mg/kg/day.

Gonorrhea (uncomplicated).
1.5 g as a single IM dose given at two different sites together with 1 g PO probenecid.

Prophylaxis in surgery.
Adults, IV: 1.5 g 30–60 min before surgery; if procedure is of long duration, **IM, IV:** 0.75 g q 8 hr.

Open heart surgery, prophylaxis.
IV: 1.5 g when anesthesia is initiated; **then,** 1.5 g q 12 hr for a total of 6 g.
NOTE: Reduce the dose in impaired renal function as follows: C_{CR} over 20 mL/min: 0.75–1.5 g q 8 hr; C_{CR}, 10–20 mL/min: 0.75 g q 12 hr; C_{CR}, less than 10 mL/min: 0.75 g q 24 hr.

NURSING CONSIDERATIONS

SEE ALSO *NURSING CONSIDERATIONS* FOR *CEPHALOSPORINS*.

ADMINISTRATION/STORAGE

1. Cefuroxime axetil for PO use is available in tablet and suspension forms. Swallow tablets whole and do not crush; crushed tablet has a strong, bitter, persistent taste. The tablets may be taken without regard for food; however, the suspension must be taken with food. Protect tablets from excessive moisture.
2. To reconstitute suspension, loosen powder by shaking the bottle. Add appropriate amount of water (depending on bottle size). Invert bottle and shake vigorously. Shake before each use. Store reconstituted suspension either at room temperature or refrigerate. Discard any unused portion after 10 days.
3. Tablet and suspension are not bioequivalent and not substitutable on a mg-per-mg basis.
4. For IM use, inject deep into a large muscle mass.

IV 5. Use IV route for severe or life-threatening infections such as septicemia or in poor-risk clients, especially in presence of shock.
6. For direct IV, reconstitute 750 mg in 8 mL sterile water; give over 3–5 min. For intermittent IV, further dilute in 100 mL of dextrose or saline solution; infuse over 30 min.
7. For direct intermittent IV administration, slowly inject drug over 3 to 5 min, or give in tubing of other IV solutions. For intermittent IV infusion with a Y-type setup, may give dose in the tubing through which client is receiving other medications; however, during drug infusion, discontinue administration of other solutions. For continuous IV infusion, the drug may be added to 0.9% NaCl, D5% or D10%, D5/0.45% or 0.9% NaCl, and M/6 sodium lactate injection.
8. Do not add cefuroxime sodium to solutions of aminoglycosides; if both required, give separately.
9. Prior to reconstitution, protect drug from light. The powder and reconstituted drug may darken without affecting potency.
10. Continue therapy for at least 10 days in infections due to *Streptococcus pyogenes*.

ASSESSMENT

1. Document indications for therapy and note baseline assessments.
2. Assess for any evidence of anemia or renal dysfunction. Reduce dose with impaired renal function.

CLIENT/FAMILY TEACHING

1. Take tablets and/or suspension with food to enhance absorption.
2. Report S&S of anemia (SOB, dizziness, pale skin, etc.) immediately.
3. Crushed tablets have a distinctive bitter taste even when hidden in foods. If intolerable, report so alternative drug therapy may be instituted.

OUTCOMES/EVALUATE

- Resolution of S&S of infection
- Surgical infection prophylaxis

Celecoxib

(**sell**-ah-**KOX**-ihb)

PREGNANCY CATEGORY: C

C

CLASSIFICATION(S):
Nonsteroidal anti-inflammatory drug, COX-2 inhibitor
Rx: Celebrex

SEE ALSO ***NONSTEROIDAL ANTI-INFLAMMATORY DRUGS.***

ACTION/KINETICS
Inhibits prostaglandin synthesis, primarily by inhibiting cyclooxygenase-2 (COX-2); it does not inhibit the cyclooxygenase-1 (COX-1) isoenzyme. Does not affect platelet aggregation; renal effects similar to other NSAIDs. Causes fewer GI complications, such as bleeding and perforation, compared with other NSAIDs. **Peak plasma levels:** 3 hr. About 97% protein bound. **t½, terminal:** 11 hr when fasting; low solubility prolongs absorption. Metabolized in the liver to inactive compounds; excreted in the urine and feces. Blacks show a 40% increase in the total amount absorbed compared with Caucasians.

USES
(1) Relief of signs and symptoms of rheumatoid arthritis in adults and of osteoarthritis. (2) Treat acute pain and menstrual pain in adults. (3) To reduce the number of adenomatous colorectal polyps in familial adenomatous polyposis.

CONTRAINDICATIONS
Use in severe hepatic impairment, in those who have shown an allergic reaction to sulfonamides, or in those who have experienced asthma, urticaria, or allergic-type reactions after taking aspirin or other NSAIDs. Use in late pregnancy (may cause premature closure of ductus arteriosus). Lactation.

SPECIAL CONCERNS
Use with caution in pre-existing asthma, with drugs that are known to inhibit P450 2C9 in the liver, or when initiating the drug in significant dehydration. Use with extreme caution in those with a prior history of ulcer disease or GI bleeding. Possible serious cardiovascular side effects. Safety and efficacy have not been determined in clients less than 18 years of age. Use caution not to confuse Celebrex with Celexa (an antidepressant) or Cerebyx (injectable fosphenytoin to treat seizures).

SIDE EFFECTS
Listed are side effects with a frequency of 0.1% or greater.
GI: Dyspepsia, diarrhea, abdominal pain, N&V, dry mouth, flatulence, constipation, GI bleeding/ulceration, ***GI hemorrhage,*** diverticulitis, dysphagia, eructation, esophagitis, gastritis, gastroenteritis, GERD, hemorrhoids, hiatal hernia, melena, stomatitis, tooth disorder, abnormal hepatic function. **CNS:** Headache, dizziness, insomnia, anorexia, anxiety, depression, nervousness, somnolence, hypertonia, hypoesthesia, migraine, neuropathy, paresthesia, vertigo, increased appetite. **CV:** Aggravated hypertension, angina pectoris, CAD, ***MI,*** palpitation, tachycardia, thrombocythemia, thrombotic events, CHF-related adverse effects. **Respiratory:** URI, sinusitis, pharyngitis, rhinitis, bronchitis, bronchospasm, coughing, dyspnea, laryngitis, pneumonia. **Dermatologic:** Rash, ecchymosis, alopecia, dermatitis, nail disorder, photosensitivity, pruritus, erythematous/ maculopapular rash, skin disorder, dry skin, increased sweating, urticara. **Body as a whole:** Accidental injury, back/chest pain, peripheral edema, aggravated allergy, allergic reaction, asthenia, fluid retention, generalized edema, fatigue, fever, hot flushes, flu-like symptoms, pain/peripheral pain, weight increase. **Musculoskeletal:** Arthralgia, arthrosis, bone disorder, accidental fracture, myalgia, stiff neck, synovitis, tendinitis. **Infections:** Bacterial/fungal, or viral infection; herpes simplex/ zoster, soft tissue infection, moniliasis, genital moniliasis, otitis media. **GU:** Cystitis, dysuria, frequent urination, renal calculus, urinary incontinence, UTI, breast fibroadenosis/neoplasm/pain, dysmenorrhea, menstrual disorder, vaginal hemorrhage, vaginitis, prostatic disorder. **Ophthalmic:** Glaucoma, blurred vision, cataract, conjunctivitis, eye pain. **Otic:** Deafness, ear abnormality, ear-

ache, tinnitus. **Miscellaneous:** Tenesmus, facial edema, leg cramps, diabetes mellitus, epistaxis, anemia, taste perversion.

LABORATORY TEST CONSIDERATIONS

↑ ALT, AST, BUN, CPK, NPN, creatinine, alkaline phosphatase. Hypercholesterolemia, hyperglycemia, hypokalemia, albuminuria, hematuria.

DRUG INTERACTIONS

ACE Inhibitors / ↓ Antihypertensive effect
Antacids, aluminum- and magnesium-containing / ↓ Celecoxib absorption
Aspirin / ↑ Risk of GI ulceration
Fluconazole / ↑ Plasma celecoxib levels
Furosemide / ↓ Natriuretic drug effect
Lithium / ↑ Plasma lithium levels
Thiazide diuretics / ↓ Natriuretic drug effects
Warfarin / Possible ↑ PT with bleeding, especially in the elderly

HOW SUPPLIED

Capsules: 100 mg, 200 mg

DOSAGE

• **CAPSULES**

Osteoarthritis.

Adults: 100 mg b.i.d. or 200 mg as a single dose.

Rheumatoid arthritis.

Adults: 100–200 mg b.i.d.

Familial adenomatous polyposis.

400 mg (2–200 mg capsules) b.i.d. with food. Continue usual medical care (e.g., endoscopic surveillance, surgery). Reduce the dose by about 50% in moderate hepatic impairment (Child-Pugh Class II).

NURSING CONSIDERATIONS

SEE ALSO *NURSING CONSIDERATIONS FOR NONSTEROIDAL ANTI-INFLAMMATORY DRUGS.*

ASSESSMENT

1. Document indications for therapy, onset and characteristics of disease, ROM, deformity/loss of function, level of pain, other agents trialed and the outcome.
2. Determine any GI bleed or ulcer history, sulfonamide allergy or aspirin or other NSAID-induced asthma, urticaria, or allergic-type reactions.
3. List drugs prescribed to ensure none interact.
4. Assess for liver/renal dysfunction; monitor lytes, renal and LFTs.

CLIENT/FAMILY TEACHING

1. Seek the lowest dose for each client. Take exactly as directed and generally at the same time each day.
2. Report any unusual or persistent side effects including dyspepsia, abdominal pain, dizziness, and changes in stool or skin color.
3. Avoid therapy during pregnancy.
4. Report weight gain, swelling of ankles, chest pain, or SOB.

OUTCOMES/EVALUATE

• Relief of joint pain and inflammation with improved mobility

Cephalexin hydrochloride monohydrate

(sef-ah-**LEX**-in)

PREGNANCY CATEGORY: B
Rx: Keftab

Cephalexin monohydrate

(sef-ah-**LEX**-in)

PREGNANCY CATEGORY: B
Rx: Biocef, Keflex
✱**Rx:** Apo-Cephalex, Novo-Lexin, Nu-Cephalex, PMS-Cephalexin
CLASSIFICATION(S):
Cephalosporin, first generation

SEE ALSO *ANTI-INFECTIVES* AND *CEPHALOSPORINS.*

ACTION/KINETICS

Peak serum levels: PO, 9–39 mcg/mL after 1 hr. **t½, PO:** 50–80 min. Absorption delayed in children. The HCl monohydrate does not require conversion in the stomach before absorption. Ninety percent of drug excreted unchanged in urine within 8 hr.

USES

(1) Respiratory tract infections caused by *Streptococcus pneumoniae* and group A β-hemolytic streptococci. (2)

Otitis media due to *S. pneumoniae, Hemophilus influenzae, Moraxella catarrhalis* (use monohydrate only), staphylococci, streptococci, and *N. catarrhalis*. (3) GU infections (including acute prostatitis) due to *Escherichia coli, Proteus mirabilis,* or *Klebsiella* species. (4) Bone infections caused by *P. mirabilis* or staphylococci. (5) Skin and skin structure infections due to staphylococci and streptococci.

SPECIAL CONCERNS

Safety and effectiveness of the HCl monohydrate have not been determined in children.

ADDITIONAL SIDE EFFECTS

Nephrotoxicity, cholestatic jaundice.

HOW SUPPLIED

Cephalexin hydrochloride monohydrate: *Tablet:* 500 mg. **Cephalexin monohydrate:** *Capsule:* 250 mg, 500 mg; *Powder for Oral Suspension:* 125 mg/5 mL, 250 mg/5 mL; *Tablet:* 250 mg, 500 mg

DOSAGE

• CAPSULES, ORAL SUSPENSION, TABLETS

General infections.

Adults, usual: 250 mg q 6 hr up to 4 g/day. **Pediatric:** *Monohydrate,* 25–50 mg/kg/day in four equally divided doses.

Infections of skin and skin structures, streptococcal pharyngitis, uncomplicated cystitis, over 15 years.

Adults: 500 mg q 12 hr. Large doses may be needed for severe infections or for less susceptible organisms. For streptococcal pharyngitis in children over 1 year and for skin and skin structure infections, the total daily dose should be divided and given q 12 hr. In severe infections, the dose should be doubled.

Otitis media.

Pediatric: 75–100 mg/kg/day in four divided doses.

NURSING CONSIDERATIONS

SEE ALSO *NURSING CONSIDERATIONS* FOR *CEPHALOSPORINS.*

ADMINISTRATION/STORAGE

1. After reconstitution, refrigerate; discard after 14 days.
2. If the total daily dose is more than 4 g, use parenteral therapy.
3. Continue for at least 10 days for beta-hemolytic streptococcal infections.
4. Dosage may have to be reduced with impaired renal function or increased for severe infections. Drug action can be prolonged by concurrent use of probenecid.

CLIENT/FAMILY TEACHING

1. Use full prescription; may take with meals for GI upset.
2. Consume 2–3 L/day of fluids to prevent dehydration.
3. Report changes in elimination patterns, yellow discoloration of the skin/eyes, or lack of response.

OUTCOMES/EVALUATE

- Resolution of infection
- Symptomatic improvement

Cephapirin sodium

(sef-ah-**PIE**-rin)

PREGNANCY CATEGORY: B
CLASSIFICATION(S):
Cephalosporin, first generation
Rx: Cefadyl

SEE ALSO *ANTI-INFECTIVES* AND *CEPHALOSPORINS.*

ACTION/KINETICS

Peak serum levels after 1 g IV: 73 mcg/mL. **t½, IM, IV:** 21–47 min. 70% excreted unchanged in the urine.

USES

(1) Respiratory tract infections due to *Streptococcus pneumoniae, Staphylococcus aureus* (penicillinase/nonpenicillinase producing), *Klebsiella* species, *Haemophilus influenzae,* and group A β-hemolytic streptococci. (2) Skin and skin structure infections due to *S. aureus, S. epidermidis* (methicillin-susceptible strains), *Escherichia coli, Proteus mirabilis, Klebsiella* species, and group A β-hemolytic streptococci. (3) UTIs due to *S. aureus, E. coli, P. mirabilis,* and *Klebsiella* species. (4) Septicemia due

to *S. aureus, S. viridans, E. coli, Klebsiella* species, and group A β-hemolytic streptococci. (4) Endocarditis due to *S. aureus* and *S. viridans.* (5) Osteomyelitis due to *S. aureus, Klebsiella* species, *P. mirabilis,* and group A β-hemolytic streptococci. (6) Preoperatively and postoperatively to reduce chance of infection during vaginal hysterectomy, open heart surgery, and prosthetic arthroplasty.

SPECIAL CONCERNS

Assess benefits versus risks before use in children less than 3 months.

LABORATORY TEST CONSIDERATIONS

Increase in serum bilirubin.

HOW SUPPLIED

Powder for Injection: 1 g

DOSAGE

- **IM, IV ONLY**

General infections.

Adults: 0.5–1 g q 4–6 hr up to 12 g/day for serious or life-threatening infections. **Pediatric, over 3 months:** 40–80 mg/kg/day in four equally divided doses, not to exceed adult doses.

Preoperatively.

Adults: 1–2 g 30–60 min before surgery.

During surgery.

Adults: 1–2 g.

Postoperatively.

Adults: 1–2 g q 6 hr for 24 hr.

In clients with impaired renal function, a dose of 7.5–15 mg/kg q 12 hr may be adequate.

NURSING CONSIDERATIONS

SEE ALSO *NURSING CONSIDERATIONS* FOR *CEPHALOSPORINS*.

ADMINISTRATION/STORAGE

1. For IM use, reconstitute the 1 g vial with sterile or bacteriostatic water for injection. Each 1.2 mL contains 500 mg cephapirin.
2. Inject IM deep into the muscle mass.
IV 3. For intermittent IV administration reconstitute 1 g in 10 mL or more of solution and infuse over 3–5 min or give with IV infusions.
4. Solutions can be frozen immediately after reconstitution and stored at –15°C (5°F) for 60 days. After thawing at room temperature, solutions are stable for 12 or more hours at room temperature or 10 days when refrigerated.
5. Stable and compatible for 24 hr at room temperature at concentrations between 2 and 30 mg/mL in a variety of solutions (check package insert).

ASSESSMENT

Note any previous antibiotic reactions; reduce dose with impaired renal function.

OUTCOMES/EVALUATE

- Resolution of infection
- Surgical infection prophylaxis

Cephradine

(**SEF**-rah-deen)

PREGNANCY CATEGORY: B
CLASSIFICATION(S):
Cephalosporin, first generation
Rx: Velosef

SEE ALSO *ANTI-INFECTIVES* AND *CEPHALOSPORINS*.

ACTION/KINETICS

Similar to cephalexin. Rapidly absorbed PO or IM (30 min–2 hr); 60%–90% excreted after 6 hr. **Peak serum levels: PO,** 8–24 mcg/mL after 30–60 min; **IM,** 5.6–13.6 mcg/mL after 1–2 hr. **t½:** 42–80 min; 80%–95% excreted in urine unchanged.

USES

Oral. (1) Respiratory tract infections (tonsillitis, pharyngitis, lobar pneumonia) due to *Streptococcus pneumoniae* and group A β–hemolytic streptococci. (2) Otitis media due to group A β–hemolytic streptococci, *S. pneumoniae, Haemophilus influenzae,* and staphylococci. (3) Skin and skin structure infections due to staphylococci (penicillinase/nonpenicillinase–producing) and β–streptococci. (4) UTIs (including prostatitis) due to *Escherichia coli, Proteus mirabilis,* and *Klebsiella* species.

Parenteral. (1) Respiratory tract infections due to *S. pneumoniae, Klebsiella* species, *H. influenzae, S. aureus* (penicillinase/nonpenicillinase–producing), and group A β–hemolytic streptococci. (2) UTIs due to *E. coli, P. mirabilis,* and *Klebsiella* species. (3) Skin and skin structure infections due to *S. aureus* and group A β–hemolytic streptococci. (4) Bone infections due to *S. aureus.* (5) Septicemia due to *S. pneumoniae, S. aureus, P. mirabilis,* and *E. coli.* (6) To prevent infections before, during, and after surgery for vaginal hysterectomy and other surgical procedures.

SPECIAL CONCERNS

Safe use during pregnancy, of the parenteral form in infants under 1 month of age, and of the PO form in children less than 9 months of age have not been established.

ADDITIONAL LABORATORY TEST CONSIDERATIONS

False + reactions using sulfosalicylic acid for urinary protein tests. High concentrations may interfere with measurement of creatinine by the Jaffe method.

HOW SUPPLIED

Capsule: 250 mg, 500 mg; *Powder for Injection:* 250 mg, 500 mg, 1 g, 2 g; *Powder for Oral Suspension:* 125 mg/5 mL, 250 mg/5 mL

DOSAGE

• **CAPSULES, ORAL SUSPENSION**

Skin and skin structures, respiratory tract infections (other than lobar pneumonia).

Adults, usual: 250 mg q 6 hr or 500 mg q 12 hr.

Lobar pneumonia.

Adults: 500 mg q 6 hr or 1 g q 12 hr.

Uncomplicated UTIs.

Adults, usual: 500 mg q 12 hr.

More serious UTIs and prostatitis.

500 mg q 6 hr or 1 g q 12 hr (severe, chronic infections may require up to 1 g q 6 hr).

Use in children.

Pediatric, over 9 months: 25–50 mg/kg/day in equally divided doses q 6–12 hr (75–100 mg/kg/day for otitis media). Do not exceed 4 g/day.

• **DEEP IM, IV**

General infections.

Adults: 2–4 g/day in equally divided doses q.i.d.

Surgical prophylaxis.

Adults: 1 g 30–90 min before surgery; **then,** 1 g q 4–6 hr for one to two doses (or up to 24 hr postoperatively).

Cesarean section, prophylaxis.

IV: 1 g when the umbilical cord is clamped; **then,** give two additional 1-g doses **IV or IM** 6 and 12 hr after the initial dose.

Use in children.

Pediatric, over 1 year: 50–100 mg/kg/day in equally divided doses q.i.d. Do not exceed adult dose.

NOTE: For clients not on dialysis, use the following dosage in renal impairment: C_{CR}, over 20 mL/min: 500 mg q 6 hr; C_{CR}, 5–20 mL/min: 250 mg q 6 hr; C_{CR}, less than 5 mL/min: 250 mg q 12 hr. For those on chronic, intermittent hemodialysis, give 250 mg initially; repeat at 12 hr and after 36–48 hr.

NURSING CONSIDERATIONS

SEE ALSO *NURSING CONSIDERATIONS FOR CEPHALOSPORINS.*

ADMINISTRATION/STORAGE

1. Administer oral medication without regard to meals.
2. Do not store oral suspension above 30°C (86°F) before reconstitution. After reconstitution, suspension retains potency for 7 days at room temperature and 14 days if refrigerated.
3. For IM, reconstitute with sterile or bacteriostatic water for injection.
4. Inject IM into large muscle; rotate injection sites. Sterile abscesses from accidental SC injection may occur.
IV 5. For direct IV administration, add 5 mL of diluent to the 250 or 500 mg vials, 10 mL to the 1 g vial, or 20 mL to the 2 g vial. Inject slowly over 3–5 min or give through tubing. Diluents include sterile water, D5%, and NaCl injection.
6. For continuous or intermittent IV infusion, add 10 or 20 mL sterile water (or other diluent—see package insert) to the 1 g vial or 2 g bottle, respectively. Withdraw contents and transfer to an IV infusion container; give over 30-60 min.
7. Do not mix cephradine with other antibiotics or with LR solution.

8. Use IM or direct IV solutions within 2 hr at room temperature. Solutions refrigerated at 5°C (41°F) retain potency for 24 hr. The IV infusion retains potency for 10 hr at room temperature or 48 hr at 5°C (42°F). Infusion solutions in sterile water, frozen immediately after reconstitution are stable for 6 weeks at -20°C (-4°F).
9. To ensure stability, replace medication infusion solution during prolonged IV administration q 10 hr.

ASSESSMENT

Note any previous penicillin reaction; reduce dose with renal dysfunction.

OUTCOMES/EVALUATE

- Resolution of S&S of infection
- Infection prophylaxis in surgery
- Negative culture reports

Cetirizine hydrochloride

(seh-**TIH**-rah-zeen)

PREGNANCY CATEGORY: B
CLASSIFICATION(S):
Antihistamine, second generation, piperazine
Rx: Zyrtec
✱Rx: Apo-Cetirizine, Reactine

SEE ALSO *ANTIHISTAMINES.*

ACTION/KINETICS

Potent H_1-receptor antagonist. Mild bronchodilator that protects against histamine-induced bronchospasm; negligible anticholinergic and sedative activity. Rapidly absorbed after PO administration; Food delays the time to peak serum levels but does not decrease the total amount of drug absorbed. Poorly penetrates the CNS, but high levels are distributed to the skin. **t½:** 8.3 hr (longer in elderly clients and in those with impaired liver or renal function). Excreted mostly unchanged (95%) in the urine; 10% is excreted in the feces.

USES

Relief of symptoms associated with seasonal allergic rhinitis due to ragweed, grass, and tree pollens. Perennial allergic rhinitis due to allergens such as dust mites, animal dander, and molds. Chronic idiopathic urticaria.

CONTRAINDICATIONS

Lactation. In those hypersensitive to hydroxyzine. In children less than 6 years of age with impaired renal or hepatic function.

SPECIAL CONCERNS

Due to the possibility of sedation, use with caution in situations requiring mental alertness. Safety and efficacy have not been determined in children less than 12 years of age.

SIDE EFFECTS

See *Antihistamines*. The most common side effects are somnolence, dry mouth, fatigue, pharyngitis, and dizziness.

OD OVERDOSE MANAGEMENT

Symptoms: Somnolence. *Treatment*: Symptomatic and supportive. Dialysis is not effective in removing the drug from the body.

HOW SUPPLIED

Syrup: 1 mg/mL; *Tablets:* 5 mg, 10 mg.

DOSAGE

- **SYRUP, TABLETS**

Seasonal or perennial allergic rhinitis, chronic urticaria.

Adults and children 12 years and older, initial: Depending on the severity of the symptoms, 5 or 10 mg (most common initial dose) once daily. **Children, 2–5 years:** 2.5 mg once daily, up to a maximum of 5 mg daily given as 2.5 mg q 12 hr. In clients 12 years and older with decreased renal function (C_{CR} 11–31 mL/min), in hemodialysis clients (C_{CR} less than 7 mL/min), and in those with impaired hepatic function, use 5 mg once daily.

NURSING CONSIDERATIONS

SEE ALSO *NURSING CONSIDERATIONS* FOR *ANTIHISTAMINES.*

ASSESSMENT

1. Document type, onset, and characteristics of symptoms; note triggers.
2. Note any hypersensitivity to hydroxyzine.

CLIENT/FAMILY TEACHING

1. May take with or without food; time of administration may be varied depending on client needs.

2. Use caution when performing activities that require mental alertness until drug effects realized; may cause drowsiness.
3. Drug may cause dry mouth and fatigue; report adverse effects that inhibit compliance with therapy.
4. Avoid alcohol/CNS depressants.
5. Review allergens that trigger symptoms, e.g., ragweed, dust mites, molds, animal dander, etc., and instruct in how to control and avoid contact.

OUTCOMES/EVALUATE

• Symptom relief with seasonal and perennial allergic rhinitis
• ↓ Occurrence, duration, and severity of hives; ↓ pruritus

Cetrorelix acetate

PREGNANCY CATEGORY: X
CLASSIFICATION(S):
Gonadotropin-releasing hormone antagonist
Rx: Cetrotide

ACTION/KINETICS
Synthetic decapeptide that competes with natural gonadotropin releasing hormone (GnRH) for binding to membrane receptors on pituitary cells, thus controlling the release of LH and FSH in a dose-dependent manner. **Onset:** About 1 hr with the 3 mg dose and 2 hr with the 0.25 mg dose. Suppression of release of LH and FSH is maintained by continuous treatment; there is a more pronounced effect on LH than on FSH. Effects are reversible if treatment is discontinued. Readily absorbed. About 86% plasma-protein bound. **t½:** 62.8 hr following a single 3-mg dose, 5 hr following a single 0.25-mg dose, and 20.6 hr following multiple 0.25-mg doses.

USES
Inhibition of premature LH surges in women undergoing controlled ovarian stimulation.

CONTRAINDICATIONS
Hypersensitivity to cetrorelix acetate, extrinsic peptide hormones, mannitol, GnRH, other GnRH analogs. Clients 65 years of age and over. Known or suspected pregnancy. Lactation.

SPECIAL CONCERNS
Use caution in monitoring clients hypersensitive to cetrorelix as severe reactions are possible.

SIDE EFFECTS
GI: Nausea. **CNS:** Headache. **GU:** Ovarian hyperstimulation syndrome. **Hypersensitivity:** ***Anaphylaxis,*** cough, rash, hypotension. **At reaction site:** Redness, erythema, bruising, itching, swelling, pruritus.

LABORATORY TEST CONSIDERATIONS
↑ ALT, AST, GGT, alkaline phosphatase.

HOW SUPPLIED
Injection: 0.25 mg, 3 mg

DOSAGE

• **SC**
Inhibition of premature LH surges.
Single dose regimen: 3 mg when the serum estradiol level indicates an appropriate stimulation response (usually on stimulation day 7 — range 5–9 days). If HCG has not been given within 4 days after injection of 3 mg cetrorelix, give cetrorelix, 0.25 mg once daily until the day of HCG administration. **Multiple dose regimen:** 0.25 mg cetrorelix given on either stimulation day 5 (a.m. or p.m.) or day 6 (a.m.) and continued daily until the day of HCG administration.

NURSING CONSIDERATIONS

ADMINISTRATION/STORAGE
Directions for Use of Cetrorelix
1. Wash hands thoroughly with soap and water.
2. Flip off the plastic cover of the vial and wipe the aluminum ring and the rubber stopper with an alcohol swab.
3. Put the injection needle with the yellow mark (20 gauge) on the prefilled syringe.
4. Push the needle through the rubber stopper of the vial and slowly inject the solvent into the vial.
5. Leave the syringe on the vial and gently agitate the vial until the solu-

tion is clear and without residue. Avoid forming bubbles.
6. Draw the total contents of the vial into the syringe. If necessary, invert the vial and pull back the needle as far as needed to withdraw the entire contents of the vial.
7. Remove the needle and replace with the injection needle (27 gauge) with the grey mark.

ASSESSMENT

1. Note indications for therapy, other agents/therapies trialed for infertility and outcome.
2. Monitor VS and LFTs.
3. Obtain ultrasound to assess for follicle number and size and to R/O pregnancy.

CLIENT/FAMILY TEACHING

1. If self-administering have client demonstrate technique in office. Review patient leaflet for administration guidelines.
2. Review time committment that therapy requires for desired outcome. Frequent monitoring, lab tests and ultrasounds are required to prevent adverse effects and for desired results.
3. Drug may cause birth defects.
4. Stop drug and report if pregnancy suspected.
5. Report any abdominal pain, cough, injection site rash, or yellowing of eyes or skin.

OUTCOMES/EVALUATE

Desired pregnancy

Cevimeline hydrochloride

(sih-**VIH**-meh-lan)

PREGNANCY CATEGORY: C
CLASSIFICATION(S):
Cholinergic agonist
Rx: Evoxac

ACTION/KINETICS

Cholinergic agonist that binds to muscarinic receptors, resulting in increased secretion of saliva and sweat and increased tone of GI and urinary tract smooth muscle. Rapidly absorbed; **peak levels:** 1.5–2 hr. Metabolized in the liver and excreted in the urine. **t½:** About 5 hr.

USES

Treat dry mouth in those with Sjogren's syndrome.

CONTRAINDICATIONS

Uncontrolled asthma, when miosis is not desired (acute iritis, narrow-angle glaucoma). Lactation.

SPECIAL CONCERNS

Use with caution, and with close medical supervision, in clients with a history of CVD (e.g., angina pectoris, MI) cholelithiasis, or nephrolithiasis and in those with asthma, chronic bronchitis, COPD, or a deficiency of CYP2D6 activity. Safety and efficacy have not been determined in children.

SIDE EFFECTS

Listed are those side effects with an incidence of 1% or greater.
GI: N&V, diarrhea, dyspepsia, abdominal pain, excessive salivation, constipation, salivary gland pain/enlargement, GERD, tooth disorder, flatulence, toothache, ulcerative stomatitis, dry mouth, hiccough, sialadenitis, eructation. **CNS:** Headache, dizziness, insomnia, anxiety, vertigo, anorexia, depression, migraine. **Respiratory:** Sinusitis, URTI, rhinitis, coughing, pharyngitis, bronchitis, pneumonia, epistaxis. **Dermatologic:** Excessive sweating, rash, flushing. **GU:** UTI, urinary frequency, polyuria, vaginitis, cystitis. **Dermatologic:** Pruritus, erythematous rash, skin disorder. **Ophthalmic:** Conjunctivitis, abnormal vision, eye pain/infection, eye abnormality, xerophthalmia. **Body as a whole:** Fatigue, pain, hot flushes, rigors, asthenia, tremor, peripheral edema, fever, flu-like symptoms, hyporeflexia, infection, fungal infection, edema, allergy, abscess, allergic reaction. **Miscellaneous:** Injury, chest/back/skeletal pain, arthralgia, hypertonia, myalgia, earache, postoperative pain, otitis media, anemia, hypoesthesia, leg cramps, moniliasis, palpitations.

OD OVERDOSE MANAGEMENT

Symptoms: Headache, visual disturbance, lacrimation, sweating, respiratory distress, GI spasm, N&V, diarrhea, AV block, tachy/bradycardia, hypo/hypertension, shock, mental confusion, cardiac arrhythmias. *Treatment:* Institute general supportive measures. Atropine may be used. Epinephrine in presence of severe CV depression or bronchoconstriction.

DRUG INTERACTIONS

Antimuscarinics / Blockade of effects of cevimeline
Beta blockers / Possibility of conduction disturbances
Parasympathomimetics / Additive cholinergic effects

HOW SUPPLIED

Capsules: 30 mg

DOSAGE

• **CAPSULES**

Dry mouth in Sjogren's syndrome.

Adults: 30 mg t.i.d.

NURSING CONSIDERATIONS

ASSESSMENT

1. Note type and frequency of symptoms, other agents trialed and when diagnosed with Sjogren's syndrome.
2. Avoid use with asthma, acute iritis, or narrow angle glaucoma.
3. Use cautiously with any history of CAD, COPD, kidney and/or gallbladder stones.
4. Monitor electrolytes, renal and LFTs.

CLIENT/FAMILY TEACHING

1. Take as directed; three times/day to control symptoms.
2. May experience flu-like symptoms. Report any unusual/prolonged side effects; dose may require adjustment.
3. Disease is seen mostly in postmenopausal women and includes rheumatoid arthritis, dryness of mouth, and dryness and redness of the conjunctiva; thought to be an immune disorder.

OUTCOMES/EVALUATE

↑ Saliva/sweat production with relief of dry mouth in Sjogren's syndrome

Chloral hydrate

(**KLOH**-ral **HY**-drayt)

PREGNANCY CATEGORY: C

CLASSIFICATION(S):

Sedative-hypnotic, nonbenzodiazepine

Rx: Aquachloral Supprettes, Somnote **C-IV**

✱Rx: PMS-Chloral Hydrate

ACTION/KINETICS

Metabolized to trichloroethanol, which is the active metabolite causing CNS depression. Produces only slight hangover effects and is said not to affect REM sleep. High doses lead to severe CNS depression, as well as depression of respiratory and vasomotor centers (hypotension). Both psychologic and physical dependence develop. **Onset:** Within 30 min. **Duration:** 4–8 hr. **t½, trichloroethanol:** 7–10 hr. Readily absorbed from the GI tract and distributed to all tissues; passes the placental barrier and appears in breast milk. Metabolites excreted by kidneys.

USES

Short-term hypnotic. Daytime sedative and sedation prior to EEG procedures. Preoperative sedative and postoperative as adjunct to analgesics. Prevent or reduce symptoms of alcohol withdrawal.

CONTRAINDICATIONS

Marked hepatic or renal impairment, severe cardiac disease, lactation. PO use in clients with esophagitis, gastritis, or gastric or duodenal ulcer.

SPECIAL CONCERNS

Use by nursing mothers may cause sedation in the infant. Dose decrease may be necessary in geriatric clients due to age-related decrease in both hepatic and renal function.

SIDE EFFECTS

CNS: Paradoxical paranoid reactions. Sudden withdrawal in dependent clients may result in "chloral delirium." ***Sudden intolerance to the drug following prolonged use may result in respiratory depression, hypotension, cardiac effects, and possibly death.*** **GI:** N&V, diarrhea, bad taste in mouth, gastritis, increased peristalsis. **GU:** Renal damage, decreased urine flow and uric acid excretion. **Miscella-**

neous: Skin reactions, hepatic damage, allergic reactions, leukopenia, eosinophilia. Chronic toxicity is treated by gradual withdrawal and rehabilitative measures such as those used in treatment of the chronic alcoholic. Poisoning by chloral hydrate resembles acute barbiturate intoxication; the same supportive treatment is indicated (see *Phenobarbital.*)

LABORATORY TEST CONSIDERATIONS

↑ 17-Hydroxycorticosteroids. Interference with fluorescence tests for catecholamines and copper sulfate test for glucose.

DRUG INTERACTIONS

Anticoagulants, oral / ↑ Anticoagulant effect by ↓ plasma protein binding
CNS depressants / Additive CNS depression; concomitant use may lead to drowsiness, lethargy, stupor, respiratory collapse, coma, or death
Furosemide (IV) / Concomitant use results in diaphoresis, tachycardia, hypertension, flushing

HOW SUPPLIED

Capsule: 500 mg; *Suppository:* 324 mg, 500 mg, 648 mg; *Syrup:* 250 mg/5 mL; 500 mg/5 mL

DOSAGE

• **CAPSULES, SYRUP**

Daytime sedative.

Adults: 250 mg t.i.d. after meals.

Preoperative sedative.

Adults: 0.5–1.0 g 30 min before surgery.

Hypnotic.

Adults: 0.5–1 g 15–30 min before bedtime. **Pediatric:** 50 mg/kg (1.5 g/m^2) at bedtime (up to 1 g may be given as a single dose).

Daytime sedative.

Pediatric: 8.3 mg/kg (250 mg/m^2) up to a maximum of 500 mg t.i.d. after meals.

Premedication prior to EEG procedures.

Pediatric: 20–25 mg/kg.

• **SUPPOSITORIES, RECTAL**

Daytime sedative.

Adults: 325 mg t.i.d. **Pediatric:** 8.3 mg/kg (250 mg/m^2) t.i.d.

Hypnotic.

Adults: 0.5–1 g at bedtime. **Pediatric:** 50 mg/kg (1.5 g/m^2) at bedtime (up to 1 g as a single dose).

NURSING CONSIDERATIONS

SEE ALSO *NURSING CONSIDERATIONS* FOR *PHENOBARBITAL SODIUM*.

ADMINISTRATION/STORAGE

1. **PO:** Give capsules after meals with a full glass of water. Give the syrup with half a glass of juice, water, or ginger ale.
2. PO syrups have an unpleasant taste, which can be reduced by chilling the syrup before administration.
3. Have emergency drugs and equipment available should the client require supportive, physiologic treatment of acute poisoning.

ASSESSMENT

1. Document indications for therapy; evaluate sleep habits/patterns and life-style.
2. Assess mental status and response to stimuli. Monitor level/pattern of alertness and compare with the premedication history.
3. Observe respiratory and cardiac responses; document evidence of vasomotor depression and dilatation of cutaneous blood vessels.
4. Note any history of cardiac disease, liver or renal dysfunction. Monitor labs for evidence of impairment; drug is metabolized to an alcohol component.
5. Report any psychologic/physical dependence; symptoms resemble those of acute alcoholism, but with more severe gastritis.

CLIENT/FAMILY TEACHING

1. Take only as directed.
2. Store away from the bedside.
3. Avoid activities that require mental alertness. Use measures that promote comfort and relaxation. To protect from injury, ambulate with assistance, use side rails, call for help, and use a night light.
4. Drug is for short-term use only; may cause psychologic and physical dependence.
5. Review methods to enhance sleep, i.e., no caffeine, increased exercise, muscle relaxation exercises, no daytime napping.
6. Review drug side effects, note those that require immediate attention.

OUTCOMES/EVALUATE
- Desired level of sedation
- ↓ Alcohol withdrawal symptoms
- Improved sleep patterns

Chlorambucil (CHL)

(klor-**AM**-byou-sill)

PREGNANCY CATEGORY: D
CLASSIFICATION(S):
Antineoplastic, alkylating
Rx: Leukeran

SEE ALSO *ANTINEOPLASTIC AGENTS* AND *ALKYLATING AGENTS*.

ACTION/KINETICS
Cell-cycle nonspecific; cytotoxic to nonproliferating cells and has immunosuppressant activity. Forms an unstable ethylenimmonium ion which binds (alkylates) with intracellular substances such as nucleic acids. The cytotoxic effect is due to cross-linking of strands of DNA and RNA and inhibition of protein synthesis. Rapidly absorbed from the GI tract. **Peak plasma levels:** 1 hr. **$t^{1}/_{2}$, plasma:** 1.5 hr. 99% bound to plasma proteins, especially albumin. Extensively metabolized by the liver; at least one metabolite is active. Fifteen to 60% is excreted through the urine 24 hr after drug administration; 40% is bound to tissues, including fat.

USES
Palliation in chronic lymphocytic leukemia, malignant lymphomas (including lymphosarcoma), giant follicular lymphomas, and Hodgkin's disease. *Investigational:* Uveitis and meningoencephalitis associated with Behçet's syndrome. With a corticosteroid for idiopathic membranous nephropathy. Rheumatoid arthritis. Possible alternative to MOPP in combination with oncovin (vinblastine), procarbazine, and prednisone.

SPECIAL CONCERNS
Use during lactation only if benefits outweigh risks. Safety and efficacy have not been established in children. The drug is carcinogenic in humans and may be both mutagenic and teratogenic in humans. It also affects fertility. May be cross-hypersensitivity with other alklyating agents. Use care not to confuse chlorambucil (Leukeran) with busulfan (Myleran).

ADDITIONAL SIDE EFFECTS
Hepatic: Hepatotoxicity with jaundice. *Pulmonary:* ***Pulmonary fibrosis,*** bronchopulmonary dysplasia. **CNS:** Children with nephrotic syndrome have an increased risk of seizures. **Miscellaneous:** Keratitis, drug fever, sterile cystitis, interstitial pneumonia, peripheral neuropathy. Cross-sensitivity (skin rashes) may occur with other alkylating agents.

LABORATORY TEST CONSIDERATIONS
↑ Uric acid levels in serum and urine.

OD OVERDOSE MANAGEMENT
Symptoms: Pancytopenia (reversible), ataxia, agitated behavior, ***clonic-tonic seizures.*** *Treatment:* General supportive measures. Monitor blood profiles carefully; blood transfusions may be required.

HOW SUPPLIED
Tablet: 2 mg

DOSAGE
- **TABLETS**

Leukemia, lymphomas.
Individualized according to response of client. **Adults, children, initial dose:** 0.1–0.2 mg/kg (or 4–10 mg) daily in single or divided doses for 3–6 weeks; **maintenance:** 0.03–0.1 mg/kg/day depending on blood counts.

Alternative for chronic lymphocytic leukemia.
Initial: 0.4 mg/kg; **then,** repeat this dose every 2 weeks increasing by 0.1 mg/kg until either toxicity or control of condition is observed.

Nephrotic syndrome, immunosuppressant.
Adults, children: 0.1–0.2 mg/kg body weight daily for 8–12 weeks.

Uveitis and meningoencephalitis associated with Behçet's syndrome.
0.1 mg/kg/day.

Idiopathic membranous nephropathy. 0.1–0.2 mg/kg/day every other month, alternating with a corticosteroid for 6 months duration.
Rheumatoid arthritis.
0.1–0.3 mg/kg/day.

C

NURSING CONSIDERATIONS

SEE ALSO *NURSING CONSIDERATIONS* FOR *ANTINEOPLASTIC AGENTS*.

ADMINISTRATION/STORAGE

Store at 15–25°C (59–77°F) in a dry place.

ASSESSMENT

1. Document indications for therapy, noting pretreatment lab and physical assessment findings.
2. Drug may cause severe granulocyte and lymphocyte suppression. Nadir: 21 days; recovery: 42–56 days.

CLIENT/FAMILY TEACHING

1. Take 1 hr before breakfast or 2 hr after the evening meal.
2. Consume 2–3 L/day of fluids to decrease urate crystals.
3. Report side effects; skin rash may result from cross-sensitivity with other alkylating agents.
4. Drug is carcinogenic and may also be mutagenic and teratogenic; practice reliable birth control.

OUTCOMES/EVALUATE

- Positive tumor response evidenced by ↓ tumor size/spread; suppression of malignant cell proliferation
- Immunosuppressant activity

Chloramphenicol

(klor-am-**FEN**-ih-kohl)

PREGNANCY CATEGORY: D
Rx: Chloromycetin (Cream and Otic)
✱Rx: Pentamycetin

Chloramphenicol ophthalmic

(klor-am-**FEN**-ih-kohl)

PREGNANCY CATEGORY: C
Rx: AK Chlor, Chloromycetin Ophthalmic, Chloroptic Ophthalmic, Chloroptic S.O.P. Ophthalmic
✱Rx: Diochloram, Ophtho-Chloram

Chloramphenicol sodium succinate

(klor-am-**FEN**-ih-kohl)

Rx: Chloromycetin Sodium Succinate, Mychel-S
✱Rx: Chloromycetin Injection
CLASSIFICATION(S):
Antibiotic, chloramphenicol

SEE ALSO *ANTI-INFECTIVES*.

ACTION/KINETICS

Interferes with or inhibits protein synthesis in bacteria by binding to 50S ribosomal subunits. Therapeutic serum concentrations: **peak,** 10–20 mcg/mL; **trough**: 5–10 mcg/mL (less for neonates). **Peak serum concentration: IM,** 2 hr. **t½:** 4 hr. Metabolized in the liver; 75%–90% excreted in urine within 24 hr, as parent drug (8%–12%) and inactive metabolites. Mostly bacteriostatic. Well absorbed from the GI tract and distributed to all parts of the body, including CSF, pleural, and ascitic fluids; saliva; milk; and aqueous and vitreous humors.

USES

Not to be used for trivial infections, prophylaxis of bacterial infections, or to treat colds, flu, or throat infections. **Systemic:** (1) Treatment of choice for typhoid fever but not for typhoid carrier state. (2) Serious infections caused by *Salmonella, Rickettsia, Chlamydia,* and lymphogranuloma-psittacosis group. (3) Meningitis due to *Haemophilus influenzae.* (4) Brain abscesses due to *Bacteroides fragilis.* (5) Cystic fibrosis anti-infective. (6) Meningococcal or pneumococcal meningitis. **Topical:** (1) Otitis externa. (2) Prophylaxis of infection in minor cuts, wounds, skin abrasions, burns; promote healing in superficial infections of the skin. **Ophthalmic:** Superficial ocular infections due to *Staphylococcus aureus; Streptococcus* species, including *S. pneumoniae; Escherichia coli, H. influenzae, H. aegyptius, H. ducreyi, Klebsiella* species, *Neisseria* species, *Enterobacter* species, *Moraxella* species, and *Vibrio* species. Use only for serious ocular infections for which less dangerous drugs are either contraindicated or ineffective.

CONTRAINDICATIONS

Hypersensitivity to chloramphenicol; pregnancy, especially near term and during labor; lactation. Avoid simultaneous administration of other drugs that may depress bone marrow. Ophthalmically in the presence of dendritic keratitis, vaccinia, varicella, mycobacterial or fungal eye infections, or following removal of a corneal foreign body. Topical products should not be used near or in the eye.

SPECIAL CONCERNS

Use with caution in clients with intermittent porphyria or G6PD deficiency. To avoid gray syndrome, use with caution and in reduced doses in premature and full-term infants. Ophthalmic ointments may retard corneal epithelial healing.

SIDE EFFECTS

Hematologic (most serious): ***Aplastic anemia, hypoplastic anemia,*** thrombocytopenia, granulocytopenia, ***hemolytic anemia,*** pancytopenia, hemoglobinuria (paroxysmal nocturnal). *Hematologic studies should be undertaken before and every 2 days during therapy.* **GI:** N&V, diarrhea, glossitis, stomatitis, unpleasant taste, enterocolitis, pruritus ani. **Allergic:** Fever, angioedema, macular and vesicular rashes, urticaria, hemorrhages of the skin, intestine, bladder, mouth, ***anaphylaxis.*** **CNS:** Headache, delirium, confusion, mental depression. **Neurologic:** Optic neuritis, peripheral neuritis.

Following topical use: Burning, itching, irritation, redness of skin. Hypersensitive clients may exhibit ***angioneurotic edema,*** urticaria, vesicular and maculopapular dermatoses. **Miscellaneous:** Superinfection. Jaundice (rare). Herxheimer-like reactions when used for typhoid fever (may be due to release of bacterial endotoxins). ***Gray syndrome in infants:*** Rapid respiration, ashen gray color, failure to feed, abdominal distention with or without vomiting, progressive pallid cyanosis, vasomotor collapse, death. Can be reversed when drug is discontinued. *NOTE: Neonates should be observed closely, since the drug accumulates in the bloodstream and the infant is thus subject to greater hazards of toxicity.*

After ophthalmic use: Temporary blurring of vision, stinging, itching, burning, redness, irritation, swelling, decreased vision, persistent or worse pain.

DRUG INTERACTIONS

Acetaminophen / ↑ Chloramphenicol effect R/T ↑ serum levels
Anticoagulants, oral / ↑ Anticoagulant effect R/T ↓ liver breakdown
Antidiabetics, oral / ↑ Hypoglycemic effect R/T ↓ liver breakdown
Barbiturates / ↑ Barbiturate effect R/T ↓ liver breakdown; also, ↓ serum chloramphenicol levels
Chymotrypsin / Chloramphenicol will inhibit chymotrypsin
Cyclophosphamide / Delayed ↓ activation of cyclophosphamide
Iron preparations / ↑ Serum levels
Penicillins / Either ↑ or ↓ effect when combined to treat certain microorganisms
Phenytoin / ↑ Phenytoin effect R/T ↓ liver breakdown; also, chloramphenicol levels may be ↑ or ↓
Rifampin / ↓ Chloramphenicol effect R/T ↑ liver breakdown
Tacrolimus / ↑ Tacrolimus blood levels R/T ↓ liver breakdown
Vitamin B_{12} / ↓ Vitamin B_{12} response when treating pernicious anemia

HOW SUPPLIED

Chloramphenicol: *Capsules:* 250 mg; *Otic Solution.* 0.5% **Chloramphenicol ophthalmic:** *Ointment:* 1%; *Powder for reconstitution:* 25 mg; *Solution:* 0.5% **Chloramphenicol sodium succinate:** *Powder for injection:* 1 g

DOSAGE

CHLORAMPHENICOL

• **PO**

Adults: 50 mg/kg/day in four equally divided doses q 6 hr. Can be increased to 100 mg/kg/day in severe infections, but dosage should be reduced as soon as possible. **Neonates and children with immature metabolic function:** 25 mg/kg once daily in divided doses q 12 hr. **Neonates, less than 2 kg:** 25 mg/kg once daily. **Neonates, over 2 kg, over 7 days of age:** 50 mg/kg/day q 12 hr in divided doses. **Neonates, over 2 kg, from birth to 7 days of age:** 50 mg/kg once daily. **Children:** 50–75 mg/kg/day in divided doses q 6 hr (50–100 mg/kg/day in divided doses q 6 hr for meningitis). *NOTE:* Carefully follow dosage for premature and newborn infants less than 2 weeks of age because blood levels differ significantly from those of other age groups.

CHLORAMPHENICOL SODIUM SUCCINATE

• **IV ONLY**

Same dosage as chloramphenicol (see the preceding). Switch to **PO** as soon as possible.

CHLORAMPHENICOL

• **OPHTHALMIC OINTMENT 1%**

0.5-in. ribbon placed in lower conjunctival sac q 3–4 hr for acute infections and b.i.d.–t.i.d. for mild to moderate infections.

• **OPHTHALMIC SOLUTION 0.5%**

1–2 gtt in lower conjunctival sac 2–6 times/day (or more for acute infections).

• **OTIC SOLUTION 0.5%**

2–3 gtt in ear t.i.d.

• **TOPICAL CREAM 1%**

Apply 1–4 times/day.

NURSING CONSIDERATIONS

SEE ALSO *GENERAL NURSING CONSIDERATIONS* FOR *ANTI-INFECTIVES*.

ADMINISTRATION/STORAGE

IV Administer IV as a 10% solution over at least a 60-sec interval. Reconstitute 1 g in 10 mL of water for injection or 5% dextrose injection. May further dilute in 50–100 mL of dextrose or saline solution and infuse over 30–60 min.

ASSESSMENT

1. Note any hypersensitivity, or previous reaction to other agents.
2. Document type, onset, and duration of symptoms; list other agents prescribed. If receiving drugs that cause bone marrow depression, use of chloramphenicol is contraindicated.
3. If nursing, transmission of the drug to breast milk can result in the infant also receiving the drug; infants have underdeveloped capacity to metabolize chloramphenicol.
4. If taking oral hypoglycemic agents, may need insulin during therapy.
5. Arrange for frequent hematologic studies to detect early signs of bone marrow depression; may develop weeks to months after therapy.
6. Reduce dose with impaired renal function and in newborn infants.

INTERVENTIONS

1. Note drugs that enhance chloramphenicol; monitor closely for evidence of severe toxicity.
2. Avoid repeated courses of therapy; drug is highly toxic.
3. Monitor for the development of any of the following and report:
• *Bone marrow depression* characterized by weakness, fatigue, sore throat, and bleeding.
• *Optic neuritis* characterized by bilaterally reduced visual acuity.
• *Peripheral neuritis* characterized by pain and sensation disturbance.
• Development of *gray syndrome* in premature and newborn infants, characterized by rapid respiration, failure to feed, abdominal distention with or without vomiting, loose green stools, progressive cyanosis, and vasomotor collapse.
4. Assess for toxic and irritative effects, such as N&V, unpleasant taste, diarrhea, and perineal irritation following PO administration. Differentiation of drug-induced diarrhea from that caused by a superinfection is critical and may be accomplished by assessment and analysis of all presenting symptoms.

CLIENT/FAMILY TEACHING

1. Take 1 hr before or 2 hr after meals; if GI upset occurs, may be taken with food.
2. Take at regularly spaced intervals *around the clock*.
3. Avoid alcohol during therapy.
4. Do not take salicylates/NSAIDs.
5. When used topically for skin infections, may use sterile bandage. Report any signs of hypersensitivity; e.g., itching and rash.

6. Report any sore throat or any unusual fatigue, bruising, or bleeding.
7. To instill in the eye, place head back and instill in the conjunctival sac; close eyes. Apply light finger pressure on the lacrimal sac for 1 min. Ophthalmic solutions may cause blurred vision immediately after instillation; this should clear.
8. To avoid contamination, do not touch the tip of the ophthalmic products with any surface.
9. Do not wear contact lenses if treating bacterial conjunctivitis. If contact lenses are required, do not insert the lenses for at least 15 min after using any solutions that contain benzalkonium chloride (may be absorbed by the lens).
10. During IV administration a bitter taste may be experienced; should subside after several minutes.

OUTCOMES/EVALUATE

- Resolution of infection
- Therapeutic levels (peak 10–20 mcg/mL; trough 5–10 mcg/mL)

Chlordiazepoxide

(klor-dye-**AYZ**-eh-**POX**-eyed)

PREGNANCY CATEGORY: D
CLASSIFICATION(S):
Antianxiety drug, benzodiazepine
Rx: Libritabs, Mitran, Reposans-10 , Librium **C-IV**
✱**Rx:** Apo-Chlordiazepoxide, Novo–Poxide

SEE ALSO *TRANQUILIZERS/ANTIMANIC DRUGS/HYPNOTICS*.

ACTION/KINETICS
Onset: PO, 30–60 min; **IM,** 15–30 min (absorption may be slow and erratic); **IV,** 3–30 min. **Peak plasma levels (PO):** 0.5–4 hr. **Duration: t½:** 5–30 hr. About 96% protein bound. Is metabolized to four active metabolites: desmethylchlordiazepoxide, desmethyldiazepam, oxazepam, and demoxepam. Has less anticonvulsant activity and is less potent than diazepam.

USES
Anxiety, acute withdrawal symptoms in chronic alcoholics. Sedative-hypnotic. Preoperatively to reduce anxiety and tension. Tension headache. Antitremor agent (PO). Antipanic (parenteral).

ADDITIONAL SIDE EFFECTS
Jaundice, acute hepatic necrosis, hepatic dysfunction.

LABORATORY TEST CONSIDERATIONS
↑ 17-Hydroxycorticosteroids, 17-ketosteroids, alkaline phosphatase, bilirubin, serum transaminase, porphobilinogen. ↓ PT (clients on Coumarin).

HOW SUPPLIED
Capsule: 5 mg, 10 mg, 25 mg; *Powder for Injection:* 100 mg; *Tablet:* 10 mg, 25 mg

DOSAGE

- **CAPSULES, TABLETS**

Anxiety and tension.
Adults: 5–10 mg t.i.d.–q.i.d. (up to 20–25 mg t.i.d.–q.i.d. in severe cases). Reduce dose to 5 mg b.i.d.–q.i.d. in geriatric or debilitated clients. **Pediatric, over 6 years, initial,** 5 mg b.i.d.–q.i.d. May be increased to 10 mg b.i.d.–q.i.d.

Preoperatively.
Adults: 5–10 mg t.i.d.–q.i.d. on day before surgery.

Alcohol withdrawal/sedative-hypnotic.
Adults: 50–100 mg; may be increased to 300 mg/day; **then,** reduce to maintenance levels.

- **IM, IV (NOT RECOMMENDED FOR CHILDREN UNDER 12 YEARS)**

Acute/severe agitation, anxiety.
Initial: 50–100 mg; **then,** 25–50 mg t.i.d.–q.i.d.

Preoperatively.
Adults: 50–100 mg IM 1 hr before surgery.

Alcohol withdrawal.
Adults: 50–100 mg IM or IV; repeat in 2–4 hr if necessary. Dosage should not exceed 300 mg/day.

Antipanic.
Adults, initial: 50–100 mg; dose may be repeated in 4–6 hr if needed.

NURSING CONSIDERATIONS

SEE ALSO NURSING CONSIDERATIONS FOR TRANQUILIZERS/ANTIMANIC DRUGS/HYPNOTICS.

C

ADMINISTRATION/STORAGE

1. **IM:** Prepare solution immediately before administration by adding provided diluent to ampule. Shake until dissolved. Discard any unused solution. Inject slowly into upper, outer quadrant of gluteal muscle.

IV 2. Prepare immediately before administration by diluting with 5 mL of sterile water for injection or sterile 0.9% NaCl solution. Inject directly into vein over 1-min period. Do not add to IV infusion because of instability of drug. Do not use IV solution for IM administration.

ASSESSMENT

1. Document indications for therapy and pretreatment symptoms.
2. Maintain a quiet, supervised environment; keep recumbent for 3 hr following parenteral administration.
3. Obtain LFTs to R/O impairment.

CLIENT/FAMILY TEACHING

1. Take with food and as directed.
2. Consume extra fluids and bulk to minimize constipating effects.
3. Use caution, may cause dizziness and drowsiness.
4. Avoid all OTC agents, alcohol, and any other CNS depressants.

OUTCOMES/EVALUATE

- ↓ Tremors; ↓ anxiety; sedation
- Termination of panic attacks
- ↓ Alcohol withdrawal symptoms

Chloroquine hydrochloride

(**KLOR**-oh-kwin)

PREGNANCY CATEGORY: C
Rx: Aralen HCl

Chloroquine phosphate

(**KLOR**-oh-kwin)

Rx: Aralen Phosphate

CLASSIFICATION(S):
4-aminoquinoline, antimalarial amebicide

ACTION/KINETICS

Several mechanisms have been proposed for the action of 4-aminoquinolines. These include (1) an active chloroquine-concentrating mechanism in the acid vesicles of the parasite causing inhibition of growth, (2) release of aggregates of ferriprotoporphyrin IX from erythrocytes in the parasite causing membrane damage and erythrocyte or parasite lysis, (3) interference with hemoglobin digestion by the parasite, and (4) interference with synthesis of nucleoprotein by the parasite. 4-Aminoquinolines are active against the erythrocytic forms of *Plasmodium vivax* and *P. malariae* as well as most strains of *P. falciparum.* They are rapidly and almost completely absorbed from the GI tract and are widely distributed throughout the body. **Peak serum levels:** 1–6 hr. Very slowly excreted; presence of drug has been demonstrated in the bloodstream weeks and even months after the drug has been discontinued. Up to 70% may be excreted unchanged. Urinary excretion is increased by acidifying the urine; excretion is slowed by alkalinization.

USES

(1) Treatment or prophylaxis of acute attacks of malaria caused by *P. vivax, P. ovale, P. malariae,* and susceptible strains of *P. falciparum*. Will cause a radical cure of vivax and malariae malaria if combined with primaquine. Effective only against the erythrocytic stages and therefore will not prevent infections. However, complete cure of infections due to sensitive strains of falciparum malaria is possible. (2) As an alternative to mefloquine for travelers to areas where chloroquine-resistant *P. falciparum* is endemic and for whom mefloquine is contraindicated (e.g., pregnant women, children less than 15 kg). (3) Extraintestinal amebiasis caused by *Entamoeba histolytica. Investigational:* Discoid or lupus erythematosus, scleroderma, pemphi-

gus, lichen planus, polymyositis, sarcoidosis, porphyria cutanea tarda.

CONTRAINDICATIONS

Hypersensitivity. Changes in retinal or visual field. Lactation. Use in psoriasis or porphyria only if benefits clearly outweigh risks. Concomitantly with gold or in clients receiving drugs that depress blood-forming elements of bone marrow.

SPECIAL CONCERNS

Use during pregnancy only if benefits outweigh risks. Use with extreme caution in the presence of hepatic, severe GI, neurologic, and blood disorders. Infants and children are sensitive to the effects of 4-aminoquinolines. Certain strains of *P. falciparum* are resistant to 4-aminoquinolines. Infants and children are extremely susceptible to overdosage with severe reactions and possible death.

SIDE EFFECTS

GI: N&V, diarrhea, cramps, anorexia, epigastric distress, stomatitis, dry mouth. **CNS:** Headache, fatigue, nervousness, anxiety, irritability, agitation, apathy, confusion, personality changes, depression, psychoses, ***seizures.*** **CV:** Hypotension, ECG changes (inversion or depression of T wave, widening of QRS complex). **Dermatologic:** Pruritus, changes in pigment of skin and mucous membranes, dermatoses, bleaching of hair. **Hematologic:** Neutropenia, ***aplastic anemia,*** thrombocytopenia, ***agranulocytosis.*** **Ocular:** Retinopathy that may be permanent and may lead to blindness. Blurred vision, difficulty in focusing or in accommodation; chronic use may lead to corneal deposits or keratopathy. **Miscellaneous:** Peripheral neuritis, ototoxicity, neuromyopathy manifested by muscle weakness, worsening of psoriasis (may precipitate an acute attack).

LABORATORY TEST CONSIDERATIONS

Colors urine brown.

OD OVERDOSE MANAGEMENT

Symptoms: Headache, drowsiness, visual disturbances, ***CV collapse, seizures followed by sudden and early respiratory and cardiac arrest.*** Infants and children have manifested respiratory depression, ***CV collapse, shock, seizures, and death following overdoses of parenteral chloroquine.*** ECG changes include nodal rhythm, atrial standstill, prolonged intraventricular conduction, and bradycardia, which lead to ***ventricular fibrillation or arrest.*** *Treatment:* Undertake gastric lavage or emesis followed by activated charcoal. Seizures should be controlled prior to gastric lavage. Seizures due to anoxia can be treated by oxygen, mechanical ventilation, or vasopressors (in shock with hypotension). Tracheostomy or tracheal intubation may be required. Forced fluids and acidification of the urine may hasten excretion. Peritoneal dialysis and exchange transfusions may also help.

DRUG INTERACTIONS

Acidifying agents, urinary (ammonium chloride, etc.) / ↑ Urinary excretion of chloroquine → ↓ effect
Alkalinizing agents, urinary (bicarbonate, etc.) / ↓ Excretion of chloroquine → ↑ effect
Antipsoriatics / 4-Aminoquinolines inhibit antipsoriatic drugs
Cimetidine / ↓ Oral clearance rate and metabolism of chloroquine
Kaolin / ↓ Effect of chloroquine due to ↓ GI absorption
Magnesium trisilicate / ↓ Effect of chloroquine due to ↓ GI absorption
MAO inhibitors / ↑ Toxicity of 4-aminoquinolines due to ↓ liver breakdown

HOW SUPPLIED

Chloroquine hydrochloride: *Injection:* 50 mg/mL **Chloroquine phosphate:** *Tablet:* 250 mg, 500 mg

DOSAGE

CHLOROQUINE HYDROCHLORIDE

- **IM**

Acute malarial attack.

Adults, initial: 200–250 mg (160–200 mg base); repeat dosage in 6 hr if necessary. Total daily dose in first 24 hr should not exceed 1 g (800 mg base). Begin PO therapy as soon as possible and continue for 3 days until about

1.5 g has been given. **Children and infants:** 6.25 mg/kg (5 mg base/kg) repeated in 6 hr; do not exceed 12.5 mg/kg/day (10 mg base/kg/day).

Extraintestinal amebiasis.

200–250 mg/day (160–200 mg of the base) for 10–12 days. Begin PO therapy as soon as possible.

CHLOROQUINE PHOSPHATE

• **TABLETS**

Malarial suppression.

Adults: 300 mg (base) per week, on the same day each week. Begin 1–2 weeks prior to exposure and continue for 4 weeks after leaving the endemic area. **Children:** 5 mg base/kg weekly, up to a maximum adult dose of 300 mg base. If suppressive therapy is not started before exposure, double the initial loading dose (i.e., adults, 600 mg base and children, 10 mg base/kg) and give in 2 divided doses, 6 hr apart.

Acute malarial attack.

Adults, Day 1: 1 g (600 mg base); **then,** 500 mg (300 mg base) 6 hr later. **Days 2 and 3:** 500 mg/day (300 mg base/day). **Children, Day 1:** 10 mg base/kg; **then,** 5 mg base/kg 6 hr later. **Days 2 and 3:** 5 mg base/kg/day.

Extraintestinal amebiasis.

Adults: 1 g (600 mg base) given as 250 mg q.i.d. for 2 days; **then,** 500 mg (300 mg base) given as 250 mg b.i.d. for 2–3 weeks (combine with an intestinal amebicide). **Children:** 10 mg/kg (not to exceed 500 mg) daily for 3 weeks.

NURSING CONSIDERATIONS

SEE ALSO *GENERAL NURSING CONSIDERATIONS* FOR *ANTI-INFECTIVES*.

ADMINISTRATION/STORAGE

1. Store in amber–colored containers.
2. Chloroquine HCl, 50 mg, is equivalent to 40 mg chloroquine base.
3. Chloroquine phosphate, 500 mg, is equivalent to 300 mg chloroquine base.

ASSESSMENT

1. Document indications for therapy and onset of symptoms. Note if prophylaxis or acute drug therapy; identify source and exposure dates.
2. Determine any history of psoriasis; drug may exacerbate condition and precipitate an acute attack.
3. Note drugs currently prescribed to prevent adverse interactions.
4. Obtain cultures. Note any hepatic, neurologic, or blood disorders; monitor lab parameters.
5. Assess for retinopathy manifested by visual disturbances. Retinal changes are not reversible. Mandate regular eye exams during prolonged therapy.

INTERVENTIONS

1. Observe for overdosage and symptoms of acute toxicity (headache, drowsiness, visual disturbances, CV collapse, convulsions, and cardiac arrest) which develop within 30 min of ingestion. Death may occur within 2 hr; see *Overdose Management*.
2. Monitor VS, I&O, and state of consciousness.
3. With some therapies, fluids will have to be forced and ammonium chloride administered for weeks to months to acidify urine and promote renal excretion of the drug.
4. Check toxic effects of other drugs being used because the combination with chloroquine may intensify toxic effects.

CLIENT/FAMILY TEACHING

1. Take only as directed; complete prescribed course of therapy. Take with the evening meal with discoid lupus erythematosus.
2. May take with food to ↓ GI upset.
3. Avoid activities that require mental alertness until drug effects realized; drug may cause dizziness.
4. When used for suppressive therapy, take on the same day each week, immediately before or after meals to minimize gastric irritation (e.g., hydroxychloroquine).
5. Ensure that adequate fluid intake as well as the meds to acidify urine are taken as prescribed. Some drugs may discolor urine dark yellow or reddish brown.
6. Report any persistent, new, or bothersome side effects.
7. Report as scheduled for F/U and labs to prevent relapse.
8. Avoid direct sun exposure; wear protective clothing, sunscreens and sunglasses to prevent photophobia.
9. Review appropriate methods for protection against mosquitoes, i.e., long pants and long-sleeved shirts, repellents, and netting or screens.

10. Avoid ingestion of alcohol in any form.
11. Keep in child-proof containers and out of child's reach.

OUTCOMES/EVALUATE

- Understanding of disease/adherence with prescribed therapy
- Malaria prophylaxis
- Elimination of causative organism
- Symptomatic improvement

Chlorothiazide

(klor-oh-**THIGH**-ah-zyd)

PREGNANCY CATEGORY: C
Rx: Diurigen, Diuril

Chlorothiazide sodium

(klor-oh-**THIGH**-ah-zyd)

PREGNANCY CATEGORY: C
Rx: Sodium Diuril
CLASSIFICATION(S):
Diuretic, thiazide

SEE ALSO *DIURETICS, THIAZIDES.*

ACTION/KINETICS

Onset: 2 hr for PO, 15 min for IV; **Peak effect:** 4 hr for PO, 30 min for IV; **Duration:** 6–12 hr. **t½:** 45–120 min. Incompletely absorbed from the GI tract. Produces a greater diuretic effect if given in divided doses.

SPECIAL CONCERNS

Geriatric clients may be more sensitive to the usual adult dose.

ADDITIONAL SIDE EFFECTS

Hypotension, renal failure/dysfunction, interstitial nephritis. Following IV use: Alopecia, hematuria, exfoliative dermatitis, toxic epidermal necrolysis, erythema multiforme, ***Stevens-Johnson syndrome.***

HOW SUPPLIED

Chlorothiazide: *Oral Suspension:* 250 mg/5 mL; *Tablet:* 250 mg, 500 mg. **Chlorothiazide sodium:** *Powder for Injection, Lyophilized:* 0.5 g

DOSAGE

- **ORAL SUSPENSION, TABLETS, IV**

Diuretic.

Adults: 0.5–2 g 1–2 times/day either PO or IV (reserved for clients unable to take PO medication or in emergencies). Some clients may respond to the drug given 3–5 days each week.

Antihypertensive.

Adults, IV, PO: 0.5–1 g/day in one or more divided doses. **Pediatric, 6 months and older, PO:** 22 mg/kg/day (10 mg/lb/day) in two divided doses; **6 months and younger, PO:** 33 mg/kg/day (15 mg/lb/day) in two divided doses. Thus, children up to 2 years of age may be given 125–375 mg/day in two doses while children 2–12 years of age may be given 375 mg–1 g/day in two doses. IV use in children is not recommended.

NURSING CONSIDERATIONS

SEE ALSO *NURSING CONSIDERATIONS* FOR *DIURETICS, (THIAZIDES)* AND *ANTIHYPERTENSIVE AGENTS.*

ADMINISTRATION/STORAGE

1. Do not give SC or IM.
IV 2. Reserve IV use for adults in emergency situations or those unable to take medication PO.
3. To obtain an isotonic solution for injection, add 18 mL sterile water for injection to 500 mg powder and administer over 5 min.
4. Avoid simultaneous administration of whole blood or derivatives.
5. IV solution is compatible with NaCl or dextrose solutions.
6. Discard unused reconstituted solutions after 24 hr.

ASSESSMENT

List drugs currently prescribed; note any sulfa allergy.

CLIENT/FAMILY TEACHING

1. May cause orthostatic hypotension; use caution when rising or changing positions.
2. Follow high-potassium diet.
3. Use sun screens (avoid ones with PABA), sunglasses, and protective clothing to ↓ photosensitivity.
4. Avoid alcohol and OTC agents.

OUTCOMES/EVALUATE

- ↓ BP
- Enhanced diuresis with ↓ edema

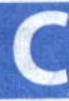

Chlorpheniramine maleate

(klor-fen-**EAR**-ah-meen)

PREGNANCY CATEGORY: B
CLASSIFICATION(S):
Antihistamine, first generation, alkylamine
Rx: Capsules, Sustained Release: Chlorpheniramine maleate .
OTC: Chewable Tablets: Aller-Chlor, Allergy, Chlo-Amine, Chlor-Trimeton Allergy 4 Hour, **Timed release Tablets:** Chlor-Trimeton 8 Hour and 12 Hour
✱OTC: Chlor-Tripolon

SEE ALSO *ANTIHISTAMINES.*

ACTION/KINETICS
Moderate anticholinergic and low sedative activity. **Onset:** 15–30 min **t½:** 21–27 hr. **Time to peak effect:** 6 hr. **Duration:** 3–6 hr.

USES
Allergic rhinitis, including sneezing; itchy, watery eyes; itchy throat, and runny nose due to hay fever and other upper respiratory allergies.

CONTRAINDICATIONS
IV or intradermal use. Parenteral route for neonates. Use for children under 6 years of age.

SPECIAL CONCERNS
Geriatric clients may be more sensitive to the adult dose.

HOW SUPPLIED
Capsules, Sustained-Release: 8 mg, 12 mg; *Syrup:* 2 mg/5 mL; *Tablet:* 4 mg; *Tablet, Chewable:* 2 mg; *Tablet, Timed Release:* 8 mg, 12 mg

DOSAGE

Allergic rhinitis.

• **SYRUP, TABLETS, CHEWABLE TABLETS**
Adults and children over 12 years: 4 mg q 6 hr, not to exceed 24 mg in 24 hr. **Pediatric, 6–12 years:** 2 mg (break 4-mg tablets in half) q 4–6 hr, not to exceed 12 mg in 24 hr. **2–6 years:** 1 mg (¼ of a 4-mg tablet) q 4–6 hr.

• **TIMED-RELEASE TABLETS**
Adults and children over 12 years: 8 mg q 8–12 hr or 12 mg q 12 hr, not to exceed 24 mg in 24 hr.

• **SUSTAINED-RELEASE CAPSULES**
Adults and children over 12 years: 8 or 12 mg q 12 hr, up to 16 or 24 mg/day. **Children, 6–12 hr:** 8 mg at bedtime or during the day as indicated.

NURSING CONSIDERATIONS

SEE ALSO *NURSING CONSIDERATIONS FOR ANTIHISTAMINES.*

CLIENT/FAMILY TEACHING

1. Food delays absorption.
2. May cause drowsiness; use caution.
3. Avoid alcohol in any form.
4. Anticipate dry mouth and use appropriate remedies.

OUTCOMES/EVALUATE
↓ Nasal congestion and allergic manifestations

Chlorpromazine hydrochloride

(klor-**PROH**-mah-zeen)

PREGNANCY CATEGORY: C
CLASSIFICATION(S):
Antipsychotic, phenothiazine
Rx: Thorazine Spansules , Thorazine
✱Rx: Chlorpromanyl, Largactil

SEE ALSO *ANTIPSYCHOTIC AGENTS, PHENOTHIAZINES.*

ACTION/KINETICS
Has significant antiemetic, hypotensive, and sedative effects; moderate anticholinergic and extrapyramidal effects. **Peak plasma levels:** 2–3 hr after both PO and IM administration. **t½** (after IV, IM): **Initial,** 4–5 hr; **final,** 3–40 hr. Extensively metabolized in the intestinal wall and liver; certain of the metabolites are active. **Steady-state plasma levels** (in psychotics): 10–1,300 ng/mL. After 2–3 weeks of therapy, plasma levels decline, possibly because of reduction in drug absorption and/or increase in drug metabolism.

C

USES
Acute and chronic psychoses, including schizophrenia; manic phase of manic-depressive illness. Acute intermittent porphyria. Preanesthetic, adjunct to treat tetanus, intractable hiccoughs, severe behavioral problems in children, and N&V. *Investigational:* Treatment of phencyclidine psychosis. IM or IV to treat migraine headaches.

SPECIAL CONCERNS
Use during pregnancy only if benefits outweigh risks. Safety for use during lactation has not been established. PO dosage for psychoses and N&V has not been established in children less than 6 months of age. Take care not to confuse chlorpropamide with chlorpromazine.

LABORATORY TEST CONSIDERATIONS
Possible ↑ plasma cholesterol.

ADDITIONAL DRUG INTERACTIONS
Epinephrine / Chlorpromazine ↓ peripheral vasoconstriction and may reverse action of epinephrine
Norepinephrine / Chlorpromazine ↓ pressor effect and eliminates bradycardia R/T norepinephrine
Valproic acid / ↑ Valproic acid effect R/T ↓ clearance

HOW SUPPLIED
Capsule, Sustained Release: 30 mg, 75 mg, 150 mg; *Concentrate:* 30 mg/mL, 100 mg/mL; *Injection:* 25 mg/mL; *Rectal Suppository:* 25 mg, 100 mg; *Syrup:* 10 mg/5 mL; *Tablet:* 10 mg, 25 mg, 50 mg, 100 mg, 200 mg

DOSAGE

• TABLETS, SUSTAINED-RELEASE CAPSULES, ORAL CONCENTRATE, SYRUP

Outpatients, general uses.

Adults: 10 mg t.i.d.–q.i.d. or 25 mg b.i.d.–t.i.d. For more serious cases, 25 mg t.i.d. After 1 or 2 days, increase daily dose by 20 to 50 mg semiweekly, until client becomes calm and cooperative. Maximum improvement may not be seen for weeks or months. Continue optimum dosage for 2 weeks; then, reduce gradually to maintenance levels (200 mg/day is usual). Up to 800 mg/day may be needed in discharged mental clients.

Psychotic disorders, less acutely disturbed.

Adults and adolescents: 25 mg t.i.d.; dosage may be increased by 20–50 mg/day q 3–4 days as needed, up to 400 mg/day.

Behavioral disorders in children.

Outpatients: 0.5 mg/kg (0.25 mg/lb) q 4–6 hr, as needed. **Hospitalized:** Start with low doses and increase gradually. For severe conditions: 50–100 mg/day. In older children, 200 mg or more/day may be needed.

N&V.

Adults and adolescents: 10–25 mg (of the base) q 4 hr; dosage may be increased as needed. **Pediatric:** 0.55 mg/kg (15 mg/m^2) q 4–6 hr.

Preoperative sedation.

Adults and adolescents: 25–50 mg 2–3 hr before surgery. **Pediatric:** 0.5 mg/kg (15 mg/m^2) 2–3 hr before surgery.

Hiccoughs or porphyria.

Adults and adolescents: 25–50 mg t.i.d.–q.i.d.

• IM

Psychotic disorders, acutely manic or disturbed.

Adults, initial: 25 mg. If necessary, give an additional 25–50 mg in 1 hr. Increase gradually over several days; up to 400 mg q 4–6 hr may be needed in severe cases. Client usually becomes quiet and cooperative within 24–48 hr. Substitute PO dosage and increase until client is calm (usually 500 mg/day). **Pediatric, over 6 months:** 0.5 mg/kg (0.25 mg/lb) q 6–8 hr as needed. Do not exceed 75 mg/day in children 5 to 12 years of age or 40 mg/day in children up to 5 years of age.

Intraoperative to control N&V.

Adults: 12.5 mg; repeat in 30 min if necessary and if no hypotension occurs. **Pediatric:** 0.25 mg/kg (0.125 mg/lb); repeat in 30 min if necessary and if no hypotension occurs.

Preoperative sedative.

Adults: 12.5–25 mg 1–2 hr before surgery. **Pediatric:** 0.5 mg/kg (0.25 mg/lb) 1–2 hr before surgery.

Hiccoughs.

Adults: 25–50 mg (base) t.i.d.–q.i.d.

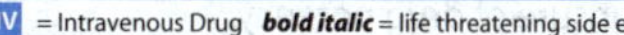

C

Acute intermittent porphyria.
Adults: 25 mg q 6–8 hr until client can take PO therapy.
Tetanus.
Adults: 25–50 mg t.i.d.–q.i.d., usually with barbiturates.
• **IV**
Intraoperative to control N&V.
Adults: 2 mg/fractional injection at 2–min intervals, not to exceed 25 mg (dilute with 1 mg/mL saline). **Pediatric:** 1 mg/fractional injection at 2–min intervals, not to exceed IM dosage (always dilute to 1 mg/mL saline).
Tetanus.
Adults: 25–50 mg diluted to 1 mg/mL with 0.9% NaCl injection and given at a rate of 1 mg/min. **Pediatric:** 0.5 mg/kg diluted to 1 mg/mL with 0.9% NaCl injection and given at a rate of 1 mg/2 min. Do not exceed 40 mg/day in children who weigh up to 23 kg (50 lb) or 75 mg/day in children who weigh 23–45 kg (50–100 lb).
• **SUPPOSITORIES**
Behavioral disorders in children.
1 mg/kg (0.5 mg/lb) q 6–8 hr, as needed.

NURSING CONSIDERATIONS

SEE ALSO *NURSING CONSIDERATIONS* FOR *ANTIPSYCHOTIC AGENTS, PHENOTHIAZINES.*

ADMINISTRATION/STORAGE

1. The maximum daily PO and parenteral dose for adults and adolescents should be 1 g of the base.
2. Swallow sustained-release capsules whole.
3. The concentrate (to be used in hospitals only) can be mixed with 60 mL or more of fruit or tomato juice, orange or simple syrup, milk, carbonated drinks, coffee, tea, water, or semisolid foods (e.g., soup, pudding).
4. When administering the drug IM, select a large, well-developed muscle mass. Use the dorsogluteal site or rectus femoris in adults and the vastus lateralis in children; rotate sites.
5. Solutions may cause contact dermatitis; avoid contact with hands or clothing.
6. Slight discoloration of IM/IV or PO solutions will not affect drug action.
IV 7. Discard solutions with marked discoloration. Consult with pharmacist if unsure of drug potency.
8. A precipitate or discoloration may occur when chlorpromazine is mixed with morphine, meperidine, or other drugs preserved with creosols.

ASSESSMENT

1. Document indications for therapy and behavioral manifestations.
2. Note any seizure disorders; drug may be contraindicated.
3. Obtain baseline CBC, liver and renal function studies.
4. Assess male clients for S&S of prostatic hypertrophy.

CLIENT/FAMILY TEACHING

1. Review side effects; report any extrapyramidal symptoms, especially uncontrolled twitching.
2. Urine may become discolored pinkish to brown.
3. Protect from sun exposure; skin may develop pigmentation changes.
4. Use caution when performing activities that require mental acuity.
5. Avoid alcohol and any other CNS depressants; may potentiate orthostatic hypotension.
6. Perform frequent toothbrushing and flossing to discourage oral fungal infections.
7. Report unusual bruising/bleeding, fever, sore throat, or malaise.
8. Avoid temperature extremes; drug may impair body's ability to regulate temperature.
9. Therapeutic psychologic effects may require 7–8 weeks of therapy.

OUTCOMES/EVALUATE

- ↓ Psychotic/manic manifestations
- Control of N&V
- Cessation of hiccoughs
- Sedation; ↓ muscular twitching

Chlorthalidone

(klor-**THAL**-ih-dohn)

PREGNANCY CATEGORY: B
CLASSIFICATION(S):
Diuretic, thiazide
Rx: Hygroton, Thalitone
✱Rx: Apo-Chlorthalidone

SEE ALSO *DIURETICS, THIAZIDES.*

ACTION/KINETICS
Onset: 2–3 hr. **Peak effect:** 2–6 hr. **Duration:** 24–72 hr. **t½:** 40 hr. Bioavailability may be dose-dependent.
ADDITIONAL USES
To potentiate and reduce dosage of other antihypertensive agents.
SPECIAL CONCERNS
Geriatric clients may be more sensitive to the usual adult dose.
ADDITIONAL SIDE EFFECTS
Exfoliative dermatitis, toxic epidermal necrolysis.
HOW SUPPLIED
Tablet: 15 mg, 25 mg, 50 mg, 100 mg

DOSAGE

• **TABLETS**

Edema.

Adults, initial: 50–100 mg/day (30–60 mg Thalitone) or 100 mg (60 mg Thalitone) on alternate days. Some clients require 150 or 200 mg (90–120 mg Thalitone). **Maximum daily dose:** 200 mg (120 mg Thalitone). **Pediatric:** All uses, 2 mg/kg (60 mg/m^2) 3 times/week.

Hypertension.

Adults, initial: Single dose of 25 mg (15 mg Thalitone); if response is not sufficient, dose may be increased to 50 mg (30 mg Thalitone). For additional control, increase the dose to 100 mg/day (except Thalitone) or a second antihypertensive drug may be added to the regimen. **Maintenance:** Determined by client response. *NOTE:* Doses greater than 25 mg/day are likely to increase potassium excretion but not cause further benefit in sodium excretion or BP reduction.

NURSING CONSIDERATIONS

SEE *NURSING CONSIDERATIONS* FOR *DIURETICS (THIAZIDES)* AND *ANTIHYPERTENSIVE AGENTS*.

ADMINISTRATION/STORAGE
1. Initiate with the lowest possible dose. Maintenance doses may be lower than initial doses.
2. Doses higher than 25 mg/day will increase potassium excretion but will not cause further benefit in sodium excretion or reduction of BP.

ASSESSMENT
1. Note indications for therapy, other agents trialed, and the outcome.
2. Monitor CBC, electrolytes, glucose, BUN, and creatinine.

CLIENT/FAMILY TEACHING
Take in the morning with food.

OUTCOMES/EVALUATE
- Enhanced diuresis; ↓ edema
- ↓ BP

Chlorzoxazone
(klor-**ZOX**-ah-zohn)

PREGNANCY CATEGORY: C
CLASSIFICATION(S):
Skeletal muscle relaxant, centrally-acting
Rx: Paraflex, Parafon Forte DSC, Remular-S

SEE ALSO *SKELETAL MUSCLE RELAXANTS, CENTRALLY ACTING.*

ACTION/KINETICS
Inhibits polysynaptic reflexes at both the spinal cord and subcortical areas of the brain. Effects may also be due to sedation. **Onset:** 1 hr. **Time to peak blood levels:** 1–2 hr. **Peak serum levels:** 10–30 mcg/mL (after 750-mg dose). **Duration:** 3–4 hr. **t½:** 1 hr. Metabolized in the liver and inactive metabolites excreted in the urine.
USES
As adjunct to rest, physical therapy, and other approaches for treatment of acute, painful musculoskeletal conditions (e.g., muscle spasms, sprains, muscle strain).
SPECIAL CONCERNS
Use during pregnancy only if benefits clearly outweigh risks. Use with caution in clients with known allergies or a history of allergic reactions to drugs.
SIDE EFFECTS
CNS: Dizziness, drowsiness, lightheadedness, overstimulation, malaise. **Dermatologic:** Allergic-type skin rashes, petechiae, ecchymoses (rare). **GI:** GI upset, GI bleeding (rare). **Allergic Reactions:** ***Angioneurotic edema, anaphylaxis*** (rare). **Miscellaneous:** Discoloration of urine, liver damage.

OD OVERDOSE MANAGEMENT

Symptoms: N&V, diarrhea, drowsiness, dizziness, lightheadedness, headache, malaise, sluggishness. May be followed by marked loss of muscle tone (voluntary movement may be impossible), decreased or absent deep tendon reflexes, respiratory depression, decreased BP. *Treatment:* Supportive.

ADDITIONAL DRUG INTERACTIONS

Isoniazid ↑ plasma levels of chlorzoxazone due to ↓ liver breakdown.

HOW SUPPLIED

Caplet: 250 mg, 500 mg; *Tablet:* 250 mg, 500 mg

DOSAGE

- **TABLETS, CAPLETS**

Skeletal muscle disorders.

Adults: 250–750 mg t.i.d.–q.i.d. with meals and at bedtime; **pediatric:** 125–500 mg t.i.d.–q.i.d. (or 20 mg/kg in three to four divided doses daily).

NURSING CONSIDERATIONS

SEE ALSO *NURSING CONSIDERATIONS* FOR *SKELETAL MUSCLE RELAXANTS, CENTRALLY ACTING.*

ASSESSMENT

1. Document indications for therapy; note pain level and pretreatment findings.
2. During physical exam test for weakness, stiffness, ROM, reflexes; with low-back pain, perform rectal exam and note sphincter tone.
3. Obtain baseline renal and LFTs; assess for dysfunction.

CLIENT/FAMILY TEACHING

1. May take with food if GI upset occurs. May be mixed with food or beverages for children.
2. Do not operate dangerous machinery or drive a car until drug effects evident; causes drowsiness.
3. Drug may cause urine to have an orange or purple-red color when exposed to the air.
4. Review importance of RICE (rest, ice, compression, and elevation) in the setting of an acute injury.
5. Do not overuse extremity during therapy; drug may mask pathology.
6. Return to provider in 3 weeks if no improvement in symptoms.

OUTCOMES/EVALUATE

Relief of musculoskeletal spasm and pain

Cholestyramine resin

(koh-less-**TEER**-ah-meen)

PREGNANCY CATEGORY: B

CLASSIFICATION(S):

antihyperlipdemic, bile acid sequestrant

Rx: LoCHOLEST, LoCHOLEST Light, Prevalite, Questran, Questran Light

✱Rx: Novo-Cholaine Light, Novo-Cholamine, PMS-Cholestyramine, Questran Light Sugar Free

ACTION/KINETICS

Binds sodium cholate (bile salts) in the intestine; thus, the principal precursor of cholesterol is not absorbed due to formation of an insoluble complex, which is excreted in the feces. Decreases cholesterol and LDL and either has no effect or increases triglycerides, VLDL, and HDL. Also, itching is relieved as a result of removing irritating bile salts. The antidiarrheal effect results from the binding and removal of bile acids. **Onset, to reduce plasma cholesterol:** Within 24–48 hr, but levels may continue to fall for 1 yr; **to relieve pruritus:** 1–3 weeks; **relief of diarrhea associated with bile acids:** 24 hr. Cholesterol levels return to pretreatment levels 2–4 weeks after discontinuance. Fat-soluble vitamins (A, D, K) and possibly folic acid may have to be administered IM during long-term therapy because cholestyramine binds these vitamins in the intestine.

USES

(1) Adjunct to reduce elevated serum cholesterol in primary hypercholesterolemia in those who do not respond adequately to diet. (2) Pruritus associated with partial biliary obstruction. (3) Diarrhea due to bile acids. *Investigational:* Antibiotic-induced pseudomembranous colitis (i.e., due to toxin produced by *Clostridium difficile*), digitalis toxicity, treatment of chlordecone (Kepone) poisoning,

treatment of thyroid hormone overdose.

CONTRAINDICATIONS

Complete obstruction or atresia of bile duct.

SPECIAL CONCERNS

Use during pregnancy only if benefits outweigh risks. Use with caution during lactation and in children. Long-term effects and efficacy in decreasing cholesterol levels in pediatric clients are not known. Geriatric clients may be more likely to manifest GI side effects as well as adverse nutritional effects. Exercise caution in clients with phenylketonia as Prevalite contains 14.1 mg phenylalanine per 5.5-g dose.

SIDE EFFECTS

GI: Constipation (may be severe), N&V, diarrhea, heartburn, GI bleeding, anorexia, flatulence, belching, abdominal distention/pain or cramping, loose stools, indigestion, aggravation of hemorrhoids, rectal bleeding or pain, black stools, bleeding duodenal ulcer, peptic ulceration, GI irritation, dysphagia, dental bleeding, hiccoughs, sour taste, pancreatitis, diverticulitis, cholescystitis, cholelithiasis. Fecal impaction in elderly clients. Large doses may cause steatorrhea. **CNS:** Migraine/sinus headaches, dizziness, anxiety, vertigo, insomnia, fatigue, lightheadedness, syncope, drowsiness, femoral nerve pain, paresthesia. **Hypersensitivity:** Urticaria, dermatitis, asthma, wheezing, rash. **Hematologic:** Increased PT, ecchymosis, anemia. **Musculoskeletal:** Muscle or joint pain, backache, arthritis, osteoporosis. **GU:** Hematuria, dysuria, burnt odor to urine, diuresis. **Other:** Bleeding tendencies (due to hypoprothrombinemia). Deficiencies of vitamins A and D. Uveitis, weight loss or gain, osteoporosis, swollen glands, increased libido, weakness, SOB, edema, swelling of hands/feet; hyperchloremic acidosis in children, rash/irritation of the skin, tongue, and perianal area.

LABORATORY TEST CONSIDERATIONS

Liver function abnormalities.

OD OVERDOSE MANAGEMENT

Symptoms: GI tract obstruction.

DRUG INTERACTIONS

Anticoagulants, PO / ↓ Anticoagulant effect R/T ↓ GI tract absorption
Aspirin / ↓ Aspirin absorption from GI tract
Clindamycin / ↓ Clindamycin absorption from GI tract
Clofibrate / ↓ Clofibrate absorption from GI tract
Digoxin / ↓ Digitalis effect R/T ↓ GI tract absorption
Furosemide / ↓ Furosemide absorption from GI tract
Gemfibrozil / ↓ Gemfibrozil bioavailability
Glipizide / ↓ Serum glipizide levels
Hydrocortisone / ↓ Hydrocortisone effect R/T ↓ GI tract absorption
Imipramine / ↓ Imipramine absorption from GI tract
Iopanoic acid / Results in abnormal cholecystography
Lovastatin / Effects may be additive
Methyldopa / ↓ Methyldopa absorption from GI tract
Nicotinic acid / ↓ Nicotinic acid absorption from GI tract
Penicillin G / ↓ Penicillin G effect R/T ↓ GI tract absorption
Phenytoin / ↓ Phenytoin absorption from GI tract
Phosphate supplements / ↓ Phosphate absorption from GI tract
Piroxicam / ↑ Piroxicam elimination
Propranolol / ↓ Propranolol effect R/T ↓ GI tract absorption
Tetracyclines / ↓ Tetracycline effects R/T ↓ GI tract absorption
Thiazide diuretics / ↓ Thiazide effects R/T ↓ GI tract absorption
Thyroid hormones, Thyroxine / ↓ Thyroid effects R/T ↓ GI tract absorption
Tolbutamide / ↓ Tolbutamide absorption from GI tract
Troglitazone / ↓ Troglitazone absorption from the GI tract
Ursodiol / ↓ Ursodiol effects R/T ↓ GI tract absorption
Vitamins A, D, E, K / Malabsorption of fat-soluble vitamins
Vitamin C / ↑ Vitamin C absorption

NOTE: These drug interactions may also be observed with colestipol.

HOW SUPPLIED

Powder for Suspension: 4 g/dose, 4 g/5.5 g powder, 4 g/5.7 g powder, 4 g/6.4 g powder, 4 g/9 g powder

C

DOSAGE

• **POWDER**

Adults, initial: 4 g 1–2 times/day. Dose is individualized. For Prevalite, give 1 packet or 1 level scoopful (5.5 g Prevalite: 4 g anhydrous cholestyramine). **Maintenance:** 2–4 packets or scoopfuls/day (8–16 g anhydrous cholestyramine resin) mixed with 60–180 mL water or noncarbonated beverage. The recommended dosing schedule is b.i.d. but it can be given in one to six doses/day. Maximum daily dose: 6 packets or scoopsful (equivalent to 24 g cholestyramine).

NURSING CONSIDERATIONS

ADMINISTRATION/STORAGE

1. Always mix powder with 60–180 mL water or noncarbonated beverage before administering; resin may cause esophageal irritation or blockage. Highly liquid soups or pulpy fruits such as applesauce or crushed pineapple may be used.
2. After placing contents of 1 packet of resin on the surface of 4–6 oz of fluid, allow it to stand without stirring for 2 min, occasionally twirling the glass, and then stir slowly (to prevent foaming) to form a suspension.
3. Avoid inhaling powder; may be irritating to mucous membranes.
4. Cholestyramine may interfere with the absorption of other drugs taken orally; thus, take other drug(s) 1 hr before or 4–6 hr after dosing.

ASSESSMENT

1. Document type and onset of symptoms, and other agents trialed.
2. Determine onset of pruritus and note bile acid level.
3. Monitor CBC, cholesterol profile, and liver and renal function studies.
4. Vitamins A, D, E, K, and folic acid will need to be administered in a water-miscible form during long-term therapy.
5. Assess skin and eyes for evidence of jaundice or bile deposits.

CLIENT/FAMILY TEACHING

1. Other prescribed medications should be taken at least 1 hr before or 4 hr after taking drug. These drugs interfere with the absorption and desired effects of other medications.
2. Review constipating effects of drug and ways to control: daily exercise, fluid intake of 2.5–3 L/day, increased intake of citrus fruits, fruit juices, and high-fiber foods; also, a stool softener may help. If constipation persists, a change in dosage or drug may be indicated.
3. If diarrhea develops, stop constipation measures, record I&O, and weight and report.
4. Clients with high cholesterol levels should follow dietary restrictions of fat and cholesterol as well as smoking cessation, alcohol reduction, and regular exercise.
5. Report tarry stools or abnormal bleeding as supplemental vitamin K (10 mg/week) may be necessary. CBC, PT, and renal function tests should be done routinely.
6. Pruritus may subside 1–3 weeks after taking the drug but may return after the medication is discontinued. Corn starch or oatmeal baths may also assist to alleviate symptoms.

OUTCOMES/EVALUATE

- Control of pruritus
- ↓ Serum cholesterol levels
- ↓ Diarrheal stools
- ↓ Bile acid levels

Choriogonadotropin alfa

(**KOR**-ee-oh-goh-**nah**-dah-**troh**-pin **AL**-fah)

PREGNANCY CATEGORY: X

CLASSIFICATION(S):

Ovarian stimulant

Rx: Ovidrel

ACTION/KINETICS

The physicochemical, biologic, and immunologic effects of recombinant choriogonadotropin (HCG) are comparable to those of HCG derived from placental and human pregnancy urine. HCG stimulates late follicular maturation and resumption of ooctye meiosis and initiates rupture of the preovulatory ovarian follicle. Choriogonadotropin alfa binds to the LH/hCG receptor of the granulosa and theca cells of the ovary and initiates its effects in the absence of an endogenous LH surge. Choriogonadotropin alfa is given when sufficient follicular development has occured following FSH treatment for ovulation induction. **Maximum serum levels:** 12–24 hr. **t$^1/_2$, distribution, initial:** About 4.5 hr; **t$^1/_2$ terminal:** About 29 hr.

USES

(1) Induction of final follicular maturation and early luteinization in infertile women who have undergone pituitary desensitization and who have been pretreated appropriately with FSH as part of an assisted reproductive technology program (e.g., in vitro fertilization and embryo transfer). (2) For the induction of ovulation and pregnancy in anovulatory infertile clients where the cause of infertility is functional and not due to primary ovarian failure.

CONTRAINDICATIONS

Hypersensitivity to HCG products and their components; primary ovarian failure; uncontrolled thyroid or adrenal dysfunction; uncontrolled organic intracranial lesions (e.g., pituitary tumor); abnormal uterine bleeding of undetermined origin; ovarian cyst or enlargement of undetermined origin; sex hormone-dependent tumors of the reproductive tract and accessory organs; pregnancy.

SPECIAL CONCERNS

Ovarian enlargement, ovarian hyperstimulation syndrome, or multiple births may occur. Use with caution during lactation.

SIDE EFFECTS

Ovarian enlargement: Abdominal distention/pain. **Ovarian hyperstimulation syndrome:** Increase in vascular permeability resulting in rapid accumulation of fluid in the peritoneal cavity, thorax, and potentially the pericardium. Early warning signs include severe pelvic pain, N&V, weight gain. Symptoms include abdominal pain/distention, N&V, diarrhea, severe ovarian enlargement, weight gain, dsypnea, oliguria. Also, hypovolemia, hemoconcentration, electrolyte imbalances, ascites, hemoperitoneum, pleural effusions, hydrothorax, ***acute pulmonary distress, thromboembolism.***

Side effects when used for assisted reproductive technology. GI: GI system disorder, abdominal pain, N&V, flatulence, diarrhea, hiccough. **GU:** Ectopic pregnancy, intermenstrual bleeding, breast pain, vaginal hemorrhage, cervical lesion, ovarian hyperstimulation, leukorrhea, uterine disorders, vaginitis, vaginal discomfort, UTI, urinary incontinence, dysuria, albuminuria, genital moniliasis, genital herpes, cervical carcinoma. **CNS:** Dizziness, headache, paresthesias, emotional lability, insomnia. **Respiratory:** URI, cough. **CV:** Cardiac arrhythmias, heart murmur. **At injection site:** Pain/bruising. **Miscellaneous:** Body/back pain, fever, hot flashes, malaise, leukocytosis.

Side effects when used for induction of ovulation. At injection site: Pain, bruising, inflammation. **GU:** Ovarian cyst, ovarian hyperstimulation, breast pain. **GI:** Abdominal pain, GI system disorders, flatulence, abdominal enlargement. **Respiratory:** URTI, pharyngitis. **Miscellaneous:** Hyperglycemia, pruritus.

Effects in pregnancies resulting from HCG therapy. Spontaneous abortion, ectopic pregnancy, premature labor, postpartum fever, congenital abnormalities.

HOW SUPPLIED

Powder for injection, lyophilized: 285 mcg r-HCG (to deliver 250 mcg r-HCG after reconstitution)

DOSAGE

- **SC**

Infertile women undergoing assisted reproductive technology; Induction of ovulation in infertile women.

250 mcg 1 day following the last dose of FSH. Do not give until adequate fol-

licular development is confirmed by serum estradiol and vaginal ultrasonography. Withhold when there is an excessive ovarian response as indicated by clinically significant ovarian enlargment or excessive estradiol production.

NURSING CONSIDERATIONS

ADMINISTRATION/STORAGE

1. Give as a single SC injection following reconstitution with 1 mL sterile water for injection. Use immediately after reconstitution.
2. Discard any unused reconstituted drug.
3. Vials may be stored refrigerated or at room temperature. Protect from light.

ASSESSMENT

1. Document indications for therapy: induction of ovulation or for in vitro fertilization program, symptom onset, and clinical presentation.
2. Note any drug sensitivity. Ensure FSH treatment for ovulation induction.
3. Assess for any pituitary or sex hormone dependent tumors; uncontrolled thyroid or adrenal dysfunction or abnormal uterine bleeding as these preclude therapy.
4. Obtain estradiol levels and vaginal ultrasound to assess follicular development. If levels too high or follicles significantly enlarged hold therapy.

CLIENT/FAMILY TEACHING

1. Review indications for therapy and the anticipated results.
2. Follow self administration guidelines pamphlet once initial injection done in office. May cause pain at injection site.
3. Record daily weights and report extent of edema which is common.
4. Delayed menses, excessive menstrual bleeding, pain in the pelvic region, weakness, and fatigue are S&S of ectopic pregnancy; report now.
5. May experience multiple births .
6. Therapy requires a long term commitment.
7. Report headache, easy fatigue, and restlessness; if increasingly irritable, depressed, and changes in attention to physical appearance occur, may have to stop drug.
8. Report for scheduled lab tests and ultrasound studies as scheduled.
9. Some pregnancies may result in abortion or birth defects.

OUTCOMES/EVALUATE

Ovulation with desired pregnancy

Chorionic gonadotropin (HCG)

(kor-ee-**ON**-ik go-**NAD**-oh-troh-pin)

PREGNANCY CATEGORY: X
CLASSIFICATION(S):
Ovarian stimulant
Rx: A.P.L., Chorex-5 and -10, Choron 10, Gonic, Pregnyl, Profasi

ACTION/KINETICS

The actions of HCG, produced by the trophoblasts of the fertilized ovum and then by the placenta, resemble those of LH. In males, HCG stimulates androgen production by the testes, the development of secondary sex characteristics, and testicular descent when no anatomic impediment is present. In women, HCG stimulates progesterone production by the corpus luteum and completes expulsion of the ovum from a mature follicle. No significant evidence that HCG causes a more attractive or "normal" distribution of fat or that it decreases hunger and discomfort due to calorie-restricted diets.

USES

Males: Prepubertal cryptorchidism, hypogonadism due to pituitary insufficiency. **Females:** Infertility not due to primary ovarian failure (used with menotropins).

CONTRAINDICATIONS

Precocious puberty, prostatic cancer or other androgen-dependent neoplasm, hypersensitivity to drug. Development of precocious puberty is cause for discontinuance of therapy. Pregnancy.

SPECIAL CONCERNS
Since HCG increases androgen production, drug should be used with caution in clients in whom androgen-induced edema may be harmful (epilepsy, migraines, asthma, cardiac or renal diseases). Use with caution during lactation. Safety and efficacy have not been shown in children less than 4 years of age.

SIDE EFFECTS
CNS: Headache, irritability, restlessness, depression, fatigue, aggressive behavior. **GU:** Precocious puberty, ovarian hyperstimulation syndrome, ovarian malignancy (rare), ***enlargement of preexisting ovarian cysts with possible rupture.*** **Miscellaneous:** Edema, gynecomastia, pain at injection site, fluid retention, arterial thromboembolism.

HOW SUPPLIED
Powder for Injection: 5,000 units, 10,000 units, 20,000 units

DOSAGE
- **IM ONLY**

Prepubertal cryptorchidism, not due to anatomic obstruction.
Various regimens including (1) 4,000 USP units 3 times/week for 3 weeks; (2) 5,000 USP units every other day for 4 injections; (3) 15 injections over a period of 6 weeks of 500–1,000 USP units/injection; (4) 500 USP units 3 times/week for 4–6 weeks; may be repeated after 1 month using 1,000 USP units.

Hypogonadotropic hypogonadism in males.
The following regimens may be used: (1) 500–1,000 USP units 3 times/week for 3 weeks; **then,** same dose twice weekly for 3 weeks; (2) 4,000 USP units 3 times/week for 6–9 months; use induction of ovulation and pregnancy 5000–10,000 USP units 3 days following the last dose of menotropins then, 2,000 USP units 3 times/week for 3 more months; (3) 1,000–2,000 USP units 3 times/week.

NURSING CONSIDERATIONS

ADMINISTRATION/STORAGE
1. Reconstituted solutions are stable for 1–3 months, depending on manufacturer, when stored at 2–8°C (35–46°F).
2. Have emergency drugs and equipment available in the event of an acute allergic response.

ASSESSMENT
1. Document indications for therapy, symptom onset, and clinical presentation.
2. Note any drug sensitivity.
3. Assess prepubescent male for appearance of secondary sex characteristics; drug is contraindicated.

CLIENT/FAMILY TEACHING
1. Review indications for therapy and the anticipated results.
2. May cause pain at injection site.
3. Record daily weights and report extent of edema which is common.
4. Delayed menses, excessive menstrual bleeding, pain in the pelvic region, weakness, and fatigue are S&S of ectopic pregnancy; report now.
5. When used with menotropins may experience multiple births .
6. With corpus luteum deficiency, if bleeding occurs after day 15 of therapy, hold drug and report.
7. Report headache, easy fatigue, and restlessness; if increasingly irritable, depressed, and changes in attention to physical appearance occur, may have to stop drug.
8. Gynecomastia may develop in young males. Report the beginning of secondary sex characteristics, as this is an indication of sexual precocity and drug should be withdrawn
9. With cryptorchidism, examine weekly for testicular descent.
10. Return for follow-up visits to monitor drug effectiveness.

OUTCOMES/EVALUATE
- Testicular descent
- Functional spermatozoa
- ↑ Progesterone → ovum release
- Sexual maturation

Ciclopirox olamine

(sye-kloh-**PEER**-ox)

PREGNANCY CATEGORY: B
CLASSIFICATION(S):
Antifungal
Rx: Loprox, Penlac Nail Lacquer

ACTION/KINETICS
At lower concentrations the drug blocks the transport of amino acids into the cell, whereas at higher concentrations the cell membrane of the fungus is altered so that intracellular material leaks out. May also inhibit synthesis of RNA, DNA, and protein in growing fungal cells. A small amount of drug is absorbed through the skin; it also penetrates to the sebaceous glands and dermis as well as into the hair.

USES
Loprox: Effective against dermatophytes, yeast, *Malassezia furfur, Trichophyton rubrum, T. mentagrophytes, Epidermophyton floccosum, Microsporum canis,* and *Candida albicans* that cause tinea pedis, tinea corporis, tinea cruris, tinea versicolor, candidiasis. The gel is also used to treat seborrheic dermatitis. **Penlac Nail Lacquer:** As part of total program for the topical treatment in immunocompetent clients with mild to moderate onychomycosis, due to *T. rubrum,* of the fingernails and toenails without lunula involvement

CONTRAINDICATIONS
Use in or around the eyes.

SPECIAL CONCERNS
Safety and efficacy in lactation and in children under 10 years of age not established.

SIDE EFFECTS
Dermatologic: Irritation, redness, burning, pain, skin sensitivity, pruritus at application site, periungual erythema, erythema of proximal nail fold, nail disorders. Loprox may worsen signs and symptoms.

HOW SUPPLIED
Cream: 1%; Gel: 0.77%; *Lotion:* 1%; *Topical Solution*: 8%

DOSAGE

• CREAM, GEL, LOTION
Massage gently into the affected area and surrounding skin morning and evening. If there is no improvement after 4 weeks, reevaluate diagnosis.

• SOLUTION
Apply once daily preferably at bedtime or 8 hr before washing to all affected nails using the applicator brush provided. Apply evenly over the entire nail plate and 5 mm of surrounding skin.

NURSING CONSIDERATIONS

ASSESSMENT
1. Document indications for therapy, onset and duration of symptoms.
2. Describe lesion presentation and obtain scrapings.
3. Weigh the risk of removing the unattached, infected nail before prescribing in clients with insulin-dependent diabetes or with diabetic neuropathy.

CLIENT/FAMILY TEACHING
1. Cleanse skin with soap and water and dry thoroughly. Apply cream with a glove; wash hands before and after therapy.
2. Avoid occlusive dressings or wrappings; adult incontinence pads/diapers are occlusive.
3. Even if symptoms have improved, use for the full time.
4. Change shoes and socks at least once daily. Shoes should be well-fitted and ventilated.
5. Report any evidence of blistering, burning, itching, oozing, redness, or swelling.
6. When using the solution, apply to the nail bed, hyponychium, and under the surface of the nail plate when it is free of the nail bed. Do not remove on a daily basis; rather, apply daily over the previous coat and remove with alcohol every 7 days. Up to 48 weeks may be needed, along with weekly nail trimmings and monthly professional removal of the unattached, infected nail.
7. For Penlac, avoid skin contact other than skin immediately surrounding the treated nail(s).

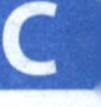

OUTCOMES/EVALUATE

- Resolution of infection; wound healing
- Symptomatic improvement

Cidofovir

(sih-**DOF**-oh-veer)

PREGNANCY CATEGORY: C
CLASSIFICATION(S):
Antiviral
Rx: Vistide

SEE ALSO *ANTIVIRAL DRUGS*.

ACTION/KINETICS
A nucleotide analog that suppresses CMV replication by selective inhibition of viral DNA synthesis. The drug inhibits CMV DNA polymease. Must be administered with probenecid.

USES
Treatment of CMV retinitis in clients with AIDS.

CONTRAINDICATIONS
History of severe hypersensitivity to probenecid or other sulfa-containing drugs. Use by direct intraocular injection. In clients with a serum creatinine greater than 1. 5 mg/dL, a calculated C_{CR} of 55 mL/min or less, or a urine protein of 100 mg/dL or more (equivalent to 2+ proteinuria or more). Lactation.

SPECIAL CONCERNS
Safety and efficacy have not been determined for children or for treatment of other CMV infections, including pneumonitis, gastroenteritis, congenital or neonatal CMV disease, or CMV disease in non-HIV-infected clients. Increased risk of ocular hypotony in those with preexisting diabetes. Use caution in clients with risk factors for nephrotoxicity.

SIDE EFFECTS
GU: Nephrotoxicity, Fanconi's syndrome and decreases in serum bicarbonate associated with renal tubular damage, proteinuria, elevated serum creatinine, glycosuria, hematuria, urinary incontinence, UTI, ***acute renal failure***. **GI:** N&V, diarrhea, anorexia, abdominal pain, colitis, constipation, tongue discoloration, dyspepsia, dysphagia, flatulence, gastritis, hepatomegaly, abnormal LFTs, melena, oral candidiasis, rectal disorder, stomatitis, aphthous stomatitis, mouth ulceration, dry mouth. **CNS:** Headache, asthenia, amnesia, anxiety, confusion, ***convulsions,*** depression, dizziness, abnormal gait, hallucinations, insomnia, neuropathy, paresthesia, somnolence. **CV:** Hypotension, postural hypotension, pallor, syncope, tachycardia, vasodilation. **Hematologic:** Neutropenia, granulocytopenia, thrombocytopenia, anemia. **Respiratory:** Asthma, bronchitis, coughing, dyspnea, hiccup, increased sputum, lung disorder, pharyngitis, pneumonia, rhinitis, sinusitis. **Dermatologic:** Alopecia, rash, acne, skin discoloration, dry skin, herpes simplex, pruritus, rash, sweating, urticaria. **Musculoskeletal:** Arthralgia, myasthenia, myalgia. **Metabolic:** Edema, dehydration, weight loss. **Ophthalmic:** Ocular hypotony, amblyopia, conjunctivitis, eye disorder, iritis, retinal detachment, uveitis, abnormal vision. **Miscellaneous:** Allergic reactions, facial edema, malaise, back/chest/neck pain, ***sarcoma, sepsis,*** fever, infections, chills, taste perversion.

LABORATORY TEST CONSIDERATIONS
↑ AST, ALT, alkaline phosphatase. Hyperglycemia, hyperlipemia, hypocalcemia, hypokalemia.

DRUG INTERACTIONS
Amphotericin B / ↑ Risk of nephrotoxicity
Aminoglycosides / ↑ Risk of nephrotoxicity
Foscarnet / ↑ Risk of nephrotoxicity
Pentamidine, IV / ↑ Risk of nephrotoxicity
Zidovudine / ↓ Zidovudine clearance

HOW SUPPLIED
Injection: 75 mg/mL

DOSAGE

- **IV INFUSION**

CMV retinitis.

Induction: 5 mg/kg given once weekly for 2 consecutive weeks as an IV infusion at a constant rate over 1 hr.

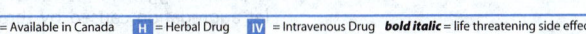

Maintenance: 5 mg/kg given once q 2 weeks as an IV infusion at a constant rate over 1 hr. With each dose of cidofovir, probenecid, 2 g PO, must be given 3 hr prior to the cidofovir dose and 1 g PO given at 2 hr and again at 8 hr after completion of the 1-hr cidofovir infusion. Also, with each dose of cidofovir, the client should receive a total of 1 L of 0.9% NaCl solution IV over a 1- to 2-hr period just before the cidofovir infusion. If the client can tolerate it, give a second liter of 0.9% NaCl solution either at the start of the cidofovir infusion or immediately afterward and infuse over a 1- to 3-hr period. If serum creatinine increases by 0.3 to 0.4 mg/dL, reduce the dose of cidofovir from 5 to 3 mg/kg. Discontinue cidofovir if the serum creatinine increases by 0.5 mg/dL or more or if there is development of 3+ or more proteinuria.

NURSING CONSIDERATIONS

SEE ALSO *NURSING CONSIDERATIONS* FOR *ANTIVIRAL DRUGS*.

ADMINISTRATION/STORAGE

IV 1. A full course of probenecid and IV saline prehydration must be taken with each dose of cidofovir.
2. Use probenecid after a meal or with an antiemetic to decrease nausea.
3. Prior to administration, dilute cidofovir in 100 mL of 0.9% NaCl solution; administer over 1 hr.
4. If taking a nephrotoxic agent, discontinue 7 days or more before starting cidofovir.
5. Admixtures may be stored at 2–8°C (36–46°F) for no more than 24 hr. Bring to room temperature prior to use.

ASSESSMENT

1. Document indications, onset, duration, and symptom characteristics.
2. Note sensitivity to probenecid or sulfa drugs; note ophthalmic exam.
3. Monitor CBC, renal function studies, and urinalysis.
4. To minimize potential for nephrotoxicity:
• Initiate therapy only if serum creatinine is less than or equal to 1.5 mg/dL, a C_{CR} greater than 55 mL/min, and urine protein less than 100 mg/mL.
• Monitor renal function before each dose; modify/discontinue drug as indicated.
• Prehydrate with at least 1L IV of NSS and ensure adequate fluid volume status.
• Coadminster PO probenecid, 4 g total, with each cidofovir dose.
• Avoid concomitant nephrotoxic drugs at least 7 days before initiating cidofovir.

CLIENT/FAMILY TEACHING

1. This is not a cure but controls symptoms. Retinitis may progress as well as other CMV symptoms; must have regular medical/eye exams.
2. Stop Zidovudine or decrease dose by 50% on cidofovir days; probenecid inhibits Zidovudine clearance.
3. Report any change or decrease in urinary output.
4. Complete full probenecid course with each cidofovir dose; take after meals or use antiemetics to decrease nausea.
5. Women should use reliable contraception during and for 1 month following therapy. Men should practice barrier contraception during and for 3 months following therapy. Infertility may result; identify if candidates for sperm/egg harvesting.

OUTCOMES/EVALUATE

Control of symptoms of CMV retinitis

Cilostazol

(sih-**LESS**-tah-zohl)

PREGNANCY CATEGORY: C
CLASSIFICATION(S):
Antiplatelet drug
Rx: Pletal

ACTION/KINETICS

Inhibits cellular phosphodiesterase (PDE), especially PDE III. Cilostazol and several metabolites inhibit cyclic AMP PDE III. Suppression of this isoenzyme causes increased levels of cyclic AMP resulting in vasodilation and inhibition of platelet aggregation. Inhibits platelet aggregation caused by thrombin,

ADP, collagen, arachidonic acid, epinephrine, and shear stress. High fat meals significantly increase absorption. Significantly plasma protein bound. Extensively metabolized by the liver with two of the metabolites being active. Primarily excreted through the urine (74%) with the rest in the feces.

USES

Reduce symptoms of intermittent claudication.

CONTRAINDICATIONS

CHF of any severity (may cause a decreased survival rate in clients with class III-IV CHF). Concurrent use of grapefruit juice. Lactation.

SPECIAL CONCERNS

Safety and efficacy have not been determined in children.

SIDE EFFECTS

GI: Abnormal stool, diarrhea, dyspepsia, flatulence, N&V, abdominal pain, anorexia, cholelithiasis, colitis, duodenal ulcer, duodenitis, esophageal hemorrhage, esophagitis, gastritis, gastroenteritis, gum hemorrhage, hematemesis, melena, gastric ulcer, periodontal abscess, rectal hemorrhage, stomach ulcer, tongue edema. **CNS:** Headache, dizziness, vertigo, anxiety, insomnia, neuralgia. **CV:** Palpitation, tachycardia, hypertension, angina pectoris, atrial fibrillation/flutter, cerebral infarct, cerebral ischemia, CHF, ***heart arrest, hemorrhage,*** hypotension, MI, myocardial ischemia, nodal arrhythmia, postural hypotension, supraventricular tachycardia, syncope, varicose veins, vasodilation, ventricular extrasystole or ***ventricular tachycardia.*** **Respiratory:** Rhinitis, pharyngitis, increased cough, dyspnea, bronchitis, asthma, epistaxis, hemoptysis, pneumonia, sinusitis. **Musculoskeletal:** Back pain, myalgia, asthenia, leg cramps, arthritis, arthralgia, bone pain, bursitis. **Dermatologic:** Rash, dry skin, furunculosis, skin hypertrophy, urticaria. **GU:** Hematuria, UTI, cystitis, urinary frequency, vaginal hemorrhage, vaginitis. **Hematologic:** Anemia, ecchymosis, iron deficiency anemia, polycythemia, purpura. **Ophthalmic:** Amblyopia, blindness, conjunctivitis, diplopia, eye hemorrhage, retinal hemorrhage. **Miscellaneous:** Infection, peripheral edema, hyperesthesia, paresthesia, flu syndrome, ear pain, tinnitus, chills, facial edema, fever, generalized edema, malaise, neck rigidity, pelvic pain, ***retroperitoneal hemorrhage,*** diabetes mellitus.

LABORATORY TEST CONSIDERATIONS

↑ GGT, creatinine. Albuminuria, hyperlipemia, hyperuricemia.

OD OVERDOSE MANAGEMENT

Symptoms: Severe headache, diarrhea, hypotension, tachycardia, possible cardiac arrhythmias. *Treatment:* Observe client carefully and provide symptomatic treatment.

DRUG INTERACTIONS

Diltiazem, erythromycin, grapefruit juice, itraconazole, ketoconazole, macrolide antibiotics, and omeprazole inhibit liver enzymes that breakdown cilostazol, resulting in ↑ plasma levels. Reduce dose of these drugs if used concomitantly.

HOW SUPPLIED

Tablets: 50 mg, 100 mg

DOSAGE

• TABLETS

Intermittent claudication.

100 mg b.i.d. taken 30 min or more before or 2 hr after breakfast and dinner. Consider a dose of 50 mg b.i.d. during coadministration of diltiazem, erythromycin, itraconazole, or ketoconazole.

NURSING CONSIDERATIONS

ADMINISTRATION/STORAGE

The dosage of cilostazol may be reduced or discontinued without platelet hyperaggregability.

ASSESSMENT

1. Determine onset and characteristics of symptoms. Measure distance walked before pain elicited.
2. Determine any history or evidence of CHF.
3. Monitor labs for liver or renal dysfunction.
4. Assess extent/amount/duration of nicotine use.

CLIENT/FAMILY TEACHING

1. Take 30 minutes before or 2 hr after meals. Avoid consuming grapefruit juice.
2. Read the patient package insert carefully before starting therapy and each time therapy is renewed.
3. May experience headaches, GI upset, dizziness, or runny nose; report if bothersome.
4. Do not smoke; enroll in formal smoking cessation program.
5. Walk past the point of severe pain, until resting; then resume walking, to improve symptoms.
6. Beneficial effects may be seen in 2 to 4 weeks, but up to 12 weeks may be needed before evident.

OUTCOMES/EVALUATE

- Increased walking distance without pain
- ↓ S&S intermittent claudication

Cimetidine

(sye-**MET**-ih-deen)

PREGNANCY CATEGORY: B
CLASSIFICATION(S):
Histamine H-2 receptor blocking drug
Rx: Cimetidine Oral Solution, Tagamet
OTC: Tagamet HB
✱**OTC:** Apo-Cimetidine, Gen-Cimetidine, Novo-Cimetine, Nu-Cimet, PMS-Cimetidine

SEE ALSO *HISTAMINE H_2 ANTAGONISTS.*

ACTION/KINETICS

Reduces postprandial daytime and nighttime gastric acid secretion by about 50%–80%. May increase gastromucosal defense and healing in acid-related disorders (e.g., stress-induced ulcers) by increasing production of gastric mucus, increasing mucosal secretion of bicarbonate and gastric mucosal blood flow as well as increasing endogenous mucosal synthesis of prostaglandins. It also inhibits cytochrome P-450 and P-448, which will affect metabolism of drugs. Also possesses antiandrogenic activity and will increase prolactin levels following an IV bolus injection. Well absorbed from GI tract. **Peak plasma level, PO:** 45–90 min. **Time to peak effect, after PO:** 1–2 hr. **Peak plasma levels, after PO use:** 0.7–3.2 mcg/mL (after a 300 mg dose; **after IV:** 3.5–7.5 mcg/mL. **Protein binding:** 13%–25%. **Duration, nocturnal:** 6–8 hr; **basal:** 4–5 hr. **t½:** 2 hr, longer in presence of renal impairment. After PO use, most metabolized in liver; after parenteral use, about 75% of drug excreted unchanged in the urine.

USES

Rx. (1) Treatment and maintenance of active duodenal ulcers. (2) Short-term (6 weeks) treatment of benign gastric ulcers (in rare cases, healing has occurred). (3) As part of multidrug regimen to eradicate *Helicobacter pylori.* (4) Management of gastric acid hypersecretory states (Zollinger-Ellison syndrome, systemic mastocytosis). (5) GERD, including erosive esophagitis. (6) Prophylaxis of UGI bleeding in critically ill hospitalized clients. *Investigational:* Prior to surgery to prevent aspiration pneumonitis, secondary hyperparathyroidism in chronic hemodialysis clients, prophylaxis of stress-induced ulcers, hyperparathyroidism, dyspepsia, herpes virus infections, tinea capitis, hirsute women, chronic idiopathic urticaria, dermatologic anaphylaxis, acetaminophen overdosage, warts, colorectal cancer.

OTC. Relief of symptoms of heartburn, acid indigestion, and sour stomach.

CONTRAINDICATIONS

Children under 16, lactation. Cirrhosis, impaired liver and renal function.

SPECIAL CONCERNS

In geriatric clients with impaired renal or hepatic function, confusion is more likely to occur. Not recommended for children less than 16 years of age.

SIDE EFFECTS

GI: Diarrhea, pancreatitis (rare), hepatitis, hepatic fibrosis. **CNS:** Dizziness, sleepiness, headache, confusion, delirium, hallucinations, double vision, dysarthria, ataxia. Severely ill clients may manifest agitation, anxiety, depression, disorientation, hallucinations, mental confusion, and psychosis. **CV:** Hypotension and arrhythmias following rapid IV administration. **Hematologic:** Agranulocytosis, thrombocytopenia, ***hemolytic or aplastic anemia,*** granulocytopenia. **GU:** Impotence (high doses for prolonged periods of time), gynecomastia (long-term treatment). **Dermatologic:** Exfoliative dermatitis, erythroderma, erythema multiforme. **Musculoskeletal:** Arthralgia, reversible worsening of joint symptoms with preexisting arthritis (including gouty arthritis). **Other:** Hypersensitivity reactions, pain at injection site, myalgia, rash, cutaneous vasculitis, peripheral neuropathy, galactorrhea, alopecia, bronchoconstriction.

DRUG INTERACTIONS

Antacids / ↓ Effect of cimetidine R/T ↓ GI tract absorption
Anticholinergics / ↓ Effect of cimetidine R/T ↓ GI tract absorption
Benzodiazepines / ↑ Benzodiazepine effects R/T ↓ liver breakdown
Beta-adrenergic blocking drugs / ↑ Beta-adrenergic effects R/T ↓ liver breakdown
Caffeine / ↑ Caffeine effect R/T ↓ liver breakdown
Calcium channel blockers / ↑ Calcium channel blocker effects R/T ↓ liver breakdown
Carbamazepine / ↑ Carbamazepine effect R/T ↓ liver breakdown
Carmustine / Additive bone marrow depression
Chloroquine / ↑ Chloroquine effects R/T ↓ liver breakdown
Chlorpromazine / ↓ Chlorpromazine effect R/T ↓ GI tract absorption
Cyanocobalamin / ↓ Cyanocobalamin absorption
Digoxin / ↓ Serum digoxin levels
Flecainide / ↑ Flecainide effect
Fluconazole / ↓ Fluconazole effect R/T ↓ GI tract absorption
Fluorouracil / ↑ Serum fluorouracil levels following chronic cimetidine use
Indomethacin / ↓ Indomethacin effect R/T ↓ GI tract absorption
Iron salts / ↓ Iron salt effects R/T ↓ GI tract absorption
Ketoconazole / ↓ Ketoconazole effect R/T ↓ GI tract absorption
Labetalol / ↑ Labetalol effect R/T ↓ liver breakdown
Lidocaine / ↑ Lidocaine effect R/T ↓ liver breakdown
Metoclopramide / ↓ Cimetidine effect R/T ↓ GI tract absorption
Metoprolol / ↑ Metoprolol effect R/T ↓ liver breakdown
Metronidazole / ↑ Metronidazole effect R/T ↓ liver breakdown
Moricizine / ↑ Moricizine effect R/T ↓ liver breakdown
Narcotics / Possible ↑ toxic effects (respiratory depression) of narcotics
Pentoxifylline / ↑ Pentoxifylline effect R/T ↓ liver breakdown
Phenytoin / ↑ Phenytoin effect R/T ↓ liver breakdown
Procainamide / ↑ Procainamide effect R/T ↓ kidney excretion
Propafenone / ↑ Propafenone effect R/T ↓ liver breakdown
Propranolol / ↑ Propranolol effect R/T ↓ liver breakdown
Quinidine / ↑ Quinidine effect R/T ↓ liver breakdown
Quinine / ↑ Quinine effect R/T ↓ liver breakdown
Sildenafil / ↑ Sildenafil effect R/T ↓ liver breakdown
Succinylcholine / ↑ Neuromuscular blockade → respiratory depression and extended apnea
Sulfonylureas / ↑ Sulfonylurea effects R/T ↓ liver breakdown
Tacrine / ↑ Tacrine effect R/T ↓ liver breakdown
Tetracyclines / ↓ Tetracycline effects R/T ↓ GI tract absorption
Theophyllines / ↑ Theophylline effects R/T ↓ liver breakdown
Tocainide / ↓ Tocainide effect
Triamterene / ↑ Triamterene effect R/T ↓ liver breakdown
Tricyclic antidepressants / ↑ TCA effects R/T ↓ liver breakdown
Valproic acid / ↑ Valproic acid effect R/T ↓ liver breakdown
Warfarin / ↑ Anticoagulant effects R/T ↓ liver breakdown

HOW SUPPLIED

Injection: 150 mg/mL, 300 mg/2 mL; 300 mg/50 mL; *Liquid:* 300 mg/5 mL; *Tablet:* 100 mg (OTC), 200 mg, 300 mg, 400 mg, 800 mg

C

DOSAGE

• **TABLETS, ORAL SOLUTION**

Duodenal ulcers, short-term.

Adults: 800 mg at bedtime. Alternate dosage: 300 mg q.i.d. with meals and at bedtime for 4–6 weeks (administer with antacids, staggering the dose of antacids) or 400 mg b.i.d. (in the morning and evening). **Maintenance:** 400 mg at bedtime.

Active benign gastric ulcers.

Adults: 800 mg at bedtime (preferred regimen) or 300 mg q.i.d. with meals and at bedtime for no more than 8 weeks.

Pathologic hypersecretory conditions.

Adults: 300 mg q.i.d. with meals and at bedtime up to a maximum of 2,400 mg/day for as long as needed.

Erosive gastroesophageal reflux disease.

Adults: 800 mg b.i.d. or 400 mg q.i.d. for 12 weeks. Use beyond 12 weeks has not been determined.

Dyspepsia.

Adults: 400 mg b.i.d.

Prophylaxis of aspiration pneumonitis.

Adults: 400–600 mg 60–90 min before anesthesia.

Primary hyperparathyroidism, secondary hyperparathyroidism in chronic hemodialysis clients.

Up to 1 g/day.

• **SUSPENSION, TABLETS**

Heartburn, acid indigestion, sour stomach (OTC only).

200 mg, as symptoms present, up to b.i.d. Take tablets with water.

• **IM, IV, IV INFUSION**

Hospitalized clients with pathologic hypersecretory conditions or intractable ulcers or those unable to take PO medication.

Adults: 300 mg IM or IV q 6–8 hr. If an increased dose is necessary, administer 300 mg more frequently than q 6–8 hr, not to exceed 2,400 mg/day.

Prophylaxis of upper GI bleeding.

Adults: 50 mg/hr by continuous IV infusion. If C_{CR} is less than 30 mL/min, use one-half the recommended dose. Treatment beyond 7 days has not been studied.

Prophylaxis of aspiration pneumonitis.

Adults: 300 mg IV 60–90 min before induction of anesthetic.

NURSING CONSIDERATIONS

SEE ALSO *NURSING CONSIDERATIONS* FOR *HISTAMINE H_2 ANTAGONISTS.*

ADMINISTRATION/STORAGE

1. Do not use the OTC product continuously for more than 2 weeks except under medical supervision.
2. If antacids are used, stagger dose with that of cimetidine; antacids (but not food) decrease absorption.
3. Administer PO medication with meals and with a snack at bedtime.
4. In renal dysfunction, a dose of 300 mg PO or IV q 12 hr may be necessary. The dose may be given, with caution, q 8 hr if needed.
5. For IM use, give undiluted.
6. IV For IV injections, dilute 300 mg in 0.9% NaCl (or other compatible solution) to a total volume of 20 mL. Inject over at least 2 min.
7. For intermittent IV infusion, dilute 300 mg in at least 50 mL of dextrose or saline solution and infuse over 15–20 min.
8. For continuous IV infusion, give a loading dose of 150 mg (by intermittent IV infusion); then, administer 37.5 mg/hr (900 mg/day) in 0.9% NaCl, D5% or 10%, 5% $NaHCO_3$ injection, RL solution, or as part of TPN. Stable for 24 hr at room temperature if mixed with these diluents.
9. May be diluted in 100–1,000 mL; if the volume for a 24-hr infusion is less than 250 mL, use a pump.
10. Do *not* introduce drugs/additives to solutions in plastic containers.
11. Cimetidine is incompatible with aminophylline and barbiturates in IV solutions and in the same syringe with pentobarbital sodium and a pentobarbital sodium/atropine sulfate combination.

12. Do not expose premixed single-dose product to excessive heat; store at 15–30°C (59–86°F).

ASSESSMENT

1. Note general client condition. Those receiving radiation therapy or myelosuppressive drugs may have additional side effects.
2. List drugs prescribed to ensure none interact unfavorably.
3. Document indications for therapy, type/onset of symptoms, and anticipated length of therapy.
4. Assess location, characteristics, extent of abdominal pain; note blood in emesis, stool, or gastric aspirate. Maintain gastric pH above 5 to enhance mucosal healing.
5. Document radiologic/endoscopic findings; check for *H. Pylori*.
6. Monitor CBC, I&O, electrolytes, renal and LFTs, especially in the elderly, severely ill, or with renal impairment.

CLIENT/FAMILY TEACHING

1. Take with meals/snack at bedtime. Avoid antacids 1 hr before or after dose; establish regular schedule.
2. Take entire prescription even if symptoms disappear.
3. Review dietary modifications, especially if being treated for GI problems; consult dietitian as needed.
4. Do not perform tasks that require mental alertness until effects realized.
5. Report any breast swelling/discharge/pain.
6. Report if abdominal pain, bloody stools, or other S&S of reactivated ulcer are evident.
7. Avoid alcohol, caffeine, spicy foods, and aspirin-containing products; may enhance GI irritation.
8. Do not smoke after the last dose of cimetidine to ensure optimal suppression of nocturnal gastric acid secretion. Attend smoking cessation program if unable to quit.
9. Report any new symptoms of confusion/mood swings; more common with elderly.
10. Note any increased susceptibility to infections; may develop agranulocytosis, thrombocytopenia, or anemia; obtain periodic CBC.
11. If diarrhea develops, maintain adequate hydration, monitor frequency and severity, and report.
12. Report skin rashes/changes.
13. May alter response to skin tests with allergenic extracts; stop drug 48–72 hr prior to testing.

OUTCOMES/EVALUATE

- ↓ Abdominal pain; ulcer healing
- Control of acid hypersecretion
- Prophylaxis of GI bleeding

Ciprofloxacin hydrochloride

(sip-row-**FLOX**-ah-sin)

PREGNANCY CATEGORY: C
CLASSIFICATION(S):
Antibiotic, fluoroquinolone
Rx: Ciloxan Ophthalmic, Cipro, Cipro Cystitis Pack, Cipro I.V.
✱**Rx:** Cipro Oral Suspension

SEE ALSO *FLUOROQUINOLONES*.

ACTION/KINETICS

Effective against both gram-positive and gram-negative organisms. Rapidly and well absorbed following PO administration. Food delays absorption of the drug. **Maximum serum levels:** 2–4 mcg/mL 1–2 hr after dosing. **t½:** 4 hr for PO use and 5–6 hr for IV use. Avoid peak serum levels above 5 mcg/mL. About 40%–50% of a PO dose and 50%–70% of an IV dose is excreted unchanged in the urine.

USES

Systemic. (1) UTIs caused by *Escherichia coli, Enterobacter cloacae, Citrobacter diversus, Citrobacter freundii, Klebsiella pneumoniae, Proteus mirabilis, Providencia rettgeri, Pseudomonas aeruginosa, Morganella morganii, Serratia marcescens, Serratia epidermidis, Enterococcus faecalis, Staphylococcus saprophyticus,* and *Streptococcus faecalis.* (2) Uncomplicated cervical, rectal, and urethral gonorrhea due to *Neisseria gonorrhoeae.* (3) Chancroid due to *Haemophilus ducreyi*; uncomplicated or disseminated gonococcal infections. (4) Mild to moderate chron-

C

ic bacterial prostatitis due to *E. coli* or *P. mirabilis*. (5) Acute sinusitis due to *S. pneumoniae, H. influenzae*, or *M. catarrhalis*. (6) Lower respiratory tract infections caused by *E. coli, E. cloacae, K. pneumoniae, P. mirabilis, P. aeruginosa, Haemophilus influenzae, H. parainfluenzae*, and *Streptococcus pneumoniae*. PO to treat acute exacerbations of chronic bronchitis due to *M. catarrhalis*. (7) Bone and joint infections due to *E. cloacae, P. aeruginosa*, and *S. marcescens*. (8) Skin and skin structure infections caused by *E. coli, E. cloacae, Citrobacter freundii, M. morganii, K. pneumoniae, P. aeruginosa, P. mirabilis, Proteus vulgaris, Providencia stuartii, Staphylococcus pyogenes, Staphylococcus epidermidis*, and penicillinase- and nonpenicillinase-producing strains of *staphylococcus aureus*. (9) PO for Infectious diarrhea caused by enterotoxigenic strains of *E. coli*. Also, *Campylobacter jejuni, Shigella boydii, Shigella dysenteriae, Shigella flexneri*, and *Shigella sonnei*. (10) PO for typhoid fever (enteric fever) due to *Salmonella typhi*. Efficacy in eradicating the chronic typhoid carrier state has not been shown. (11) IV with piperacillin sodium as empirical therapy in febrile neutropenia. (12) IV for nosocomial pneumonia due to *H. influenzae* or *K. pneumoniae*. (13) PO for acute uncomplicated cystitis in females due to *E. coli* or *S. saprophyticus*. (14) With metronidazole for complicated intra-abdominal infections due to *E. coli, P.aeruginosa, P. mirabilis, K. pneumoniae*, or *B. fragilis*. (15) Postexposure prophylaxis of inhalational *Bacillus anthracis*, the bacterium that causes anthrax (i.e., in the event of biological warfare or terrorism).

Investigational: Clients, over 14 years of age, with cystic fibrosis who have pulmonary exacerbations due to susceptible microorganisms. Malignant external otitis. In combination with rifampin and other tuberculostatics for tuberculosis.

Ophthalmic. Superficial ocular infections due to *Staphylococcus* species (including *S. aureus*), *Streptococcus* species (including *S. pneumoniae, S. pyogenes*), *E. coli, H. ducreyi, H. influenzae, H. parainfluenzae, K. pneumoniae, N. gonorrhoeae, Proteus* species, *Klebsiella* species, *Acinetobacter calcoaceticus, Enterobacter aerogenes, P. aeruginosa, S. marcescens, Chlamydia trachomatis, Vibrio* species, and *Providencia* species.

CONTRAINDICATIONS

Hypersensitivity to quinolones. Use in children. Lactation. Ophthalmic use in the presence of dendritic keratitis, varicella, vaccinia, and mycobacterial and fungal eye infections and after removal of foreign bodies from the cornea.

SPECIAL CONCERNS

Safety and effectiveness of ophthalmic, PO, or IV use have not been determined in children. Possible antibiotic resistence when used to treat *Pseudomonas aeruginosa* infections.

ADDITIONAL SIDE EFFECTS

SEE ALSO *SIDE EFFECTS* FOR *FLUOROQUINOLONES*.

GI: N&V, abdominal pain/discomfort, diarrhea, dry/painful mouth, dyspepsia, heartburn, constipation, flatulence, pseudomembranous colitis, oral candidiasis, ***intestinal perforation,*** anorexia, GI bleeding, bad taste in mouth. **CNS:** Headache, dizziness, fatigue, lethargy, malaise, drowsiness, restlessness, insomnia, nightmares, hallucinations, tremor, lightheadedness, irritability, confusion, ataxia, mania, weakness, psychotic reactions, depression, depersonalization, seizures. **GU:** Nephritis, hematuria, cylindruria, renal failure, urinary retention, polyuria, vaginitis, urethral bleeding, acidosis, renal calculi, interstitial nephritis, vaginal candidiasis. **Skin:** Urticaria, photosensitivity, hypersensitivity, flushing, erythema nodosum, cutaneous candidiasis, hyperpigmentation, rash, paresthesia, edema (of lips, neck, face, conjunctivae, hands), angioedema, ***toxic epidermal necrolysis***, exfoliative dermatitis, ***Stevens-Johnson syndrome.*** **Ophthalmic:** Blurred or disturbed vision, double vision, eye pain, nystagmus. **CV:** Hypertension, syncope, angina pectoris, palpitations, atrial flutter, ***MI, cerebral thrombosis,*** ventricular ectopy, ***cardiopulmonary arrest,*** postural hypotension. **Respiratory:** Dyspnea, ***bronchospasm, pulmonary embolism, edema of larynx or lungs,*** hemoptysis, hiccoughs, epistaxis. **Hematologic:** Eosinophilia, pancytopenia, leukopenia, anemia, leukocytosis, ***agranulocytosis,*** bleeding diathesis. **Miscellaneous:** Superinfections; fever; chills; tinnitus; joint pain or stiffness; back, neck, or chest pain; flare-up of gout; flushing; worsening of myasthenia gravis; ***hepatic necrosis;*** cholestatic jaundice; hearing loss, dysphasia.

After ophthalmic use: Irritation, burning, itching, angioneurotic edema, urticaria, maculopapular and vesicular dermatitis, crusting of lid margins, conjunctival hyperemia, bad taste in mouth, corneal staining, keratitis, keratopathy, allergic reactions, photophobia, decreased vision, tearing, lid edema. Also, a white, crystalline precipitate in the superficial part of corneal defect (onset within 1–7 days after initiating therapy; lasts about 2 weeks and does not affect continued use of the medication).

LABORATORY TEST CONSIDERATIONS

↑ ALT, AST, alkaline phosphatase, serum bilirubin, LDH, serum creatinine, BUN, GGT, amylase, uric acid, blood monocytes, potassium, PT, triglycerides, cholesterol. ↓ H&H. Either ↑ or ↓ blood glucose, platelets.

ADDITIONAL DRUG INTERACTIONS

Azlocillin / ↓ Excretion of ciprofloxacin → possible ↑ effect
Caffeine / ↓ Excretion of caffeine → ↑ pharmacologic effects
Cyclosporine / ↑ Nephrotoxic effects
Hydantoins / ↓ Phenytoin serum levels
Theophylline / Do not take with ciprofloxacin

HOW SUPPLIED

Injection: 200 mg, 400 mg; *Ophthalmic solution:* 3.5 mg/mL; *Ophthalmic ointment:* 0.3%; *Powder for Oral Suspension:* 250 mg/5 mL, 500 mg/5 mL; *Tablet:* 100 mg, 250 mg, 500 mg, 750 mg

DOSAGE

• **SUSPENSION, TABLETS**

UTIs.

100 or 250 mg q 12 hr for 3 days for acute, uncomplicated infections. 250 mg (mild to moderate) to 500 mg (severe/complicated) q 12 hr for 7–14 days.

Mild to moderate chronic bacterial prostatitis.

Adults: 500 mg q 12 hr for 28 days.

Mild to moderate acute sinusitis.

Adults: 500 mg q 12 hr for 10 days.

Urethral or cervical gonococcal infections, uncomplicated.

250 mg in a single dose.

Infectious diarrhea, mild to severe.

500 mg q 12 hr for 5–7 days.

Skin, skin structures, lower respiratory tract, bone and joint infections.

500 mg (mild to moderate) to 750 mg (severe or complicated) q 12 hr for 7–14 days. Treatment may be required for 4–6 weeks in bone and joint infections.

Intra-abdominal infections, complicated.

500 mg q 12 hr for 7–14 days.

Typhoid fever, mild to moderate.

500 mg q 12 hr for 10 days.

*Chancroid (*H. ducreyi *infection).*

500 mg b.i.d. for 3 days.

Uncomplicated gonococcal infections.

500 mg in a single dose plus doxycycline, 100 mg b.i.d. for 7 days or azithromycin, 1 g in a single dose.

Postexposure prophylaxis of inhalational anthrax.

500 mg b.i.d. started as soon as possible after exposure; continue for 60 days.

NOTE: Dose must be reduced with a C_{CR} less than 50 mL/min. The PO dose should be 250–500 mg q 12 hr if the C_{CR} is 30–50 mL/min and 250–500 mg q 18 hr (IV: 200–400 mg q 18–24 hr) if the C_{CR} is 5–29 mL/min. If the client is on hemodialysis or peritoneal dialysis, the PO dose should be 250–500 mg q 24 hr after dialysis.

• **CIPRO CYSTITIS PACK**

Uncomplicated UTI infections.

100 mg b.i.d. for 3 days. The pack contains six 100-mg tablets of ciprofloxacin and is intended to increase compliance.

• **IV INFUSION**

UTIs.

200 mg (mild to moderate) to 400 mg (severe or complicated) q 12 hr for 7–14 days.

C

Skin, skin structures, respiratory tract, bone and joint infections.
400 mg (for mild to moderate infections) q 12 hr for 7–14 days. Up to 4–6 weeks may be needed for bone and joint infections.
Nosocomial pneumonia.
400 mg q 8 hr.
Febrile neutropenic clients, empirical therapy.
400 mg q 8 hr. If severe, 400 mg q 8 hr with piperacillin, 50 mg/kg q 4 hr, not to exceed 24 g/day.
Acute sinusitis.
400 mg q 12 hr for 10 days.
Chronic bacterial prostatitis.
400 mg q 12 hr for 28 days.
Intra-abdominal infections.
500 mg q 12hr for 7–14 days.
Disseminated gonococcal infections.
500 mg **IV** for 24–48 hr after improvement begins; then, 500 mg PO b.i.d. for 7 days.

• **OPHTHALMIC SOLUTION**
Acute infections.
Initial, 1–2 gtt q 15–30 min; **then,** reduce dosage as infection improves.
Moderate infections.
1–2 gtt 4–6 (or more) times/day.

• **OPHTHALMIC OINTMENT**
Acute infections.
Initial: Apply ½ in. ribbon to conjunctival sac t.i.d. for the first 3 days; **then,** ½ in. ribbon b.id. for the next 5 days.

NURSING CONSIDERATIONS

SEE ALSO *NURSING CONSIDERATIONS* FOR *ANTI-INFECTIVES* AND *FLUOROQUINOLONES*.

ADMINISTRATION/STORAGE

1. Although food delays absorption of the drug, it may be taken with or without meals; recommended dosing time is 2 hr after a meal.
2. Clients on theophylline or probenecid require close observation and potential medication adjustments.
3. Do not administer to children.
4. Following instillation of ophthalmic solution, apply light finger pressure to lacrimal sac for 1 min.

IV 5. Reconstitute the IV solution dose to 0.5–2 mg/mL and give over 60 min. To minimize discomfort and irritation, slowly infuse a dilute solution into a large vein.
6. Product can be diluted with 0.9% NaCl or 5% dextrose injection. Such dilutions are stable up to 14 days at refrigerated or room temperatures; do not freeze.
7. Ciprofloxin in admixture is incompatible with aminophylline, amoxicillin sodium, amoxicillin sodium/potassium clavulanate, clindamycin, and mezlocillin.

ASSESSMENT

1. Note indications for therapy; obtain cultures prior to use.
2. Determine age. Not for use in children under 18 as irreversible collagen destruction has occurred.
3. Note meds currently prescribed. Fatal reactions have been reported with concurrent administration of IV ciprofloxacin and theophylline.

CLIENT/FAMILY TEACHING

1. Take 2 hr after meals; food may delay absorption, as will antacids containing magnesium or aluminum.
2. Drink 2–3 L/day of fluids to keep the urine acidic and to minimize the risk of crystalluria.
3. May cause dizziness; use caution in any activity that requires mental alertness or coordination.
4. Report any persistent joint pain (esp. knee) or GI symptoms such as diarrhea, vomiting, or abdominal pain.
5. Review side effects; note those that should be reported immediately.

OUTCOMES/EVALUATE

• Symptomatic improvement; ↓ fever, ↓ WBCs, ↑ appetite
• Negative culture reports

Cisatracurium besylate

(sis-ah-trah-**KYOU**-ree-um)

PREGNANCY CATEGORY: B
CLASSIFICATION(S):
Neuromuscular blocking drug
Rx: Nimbex

SEE ALSO *NEUROMUSCULAR BLOCKING AGENTS*.

ACTION/KINETICS

Nondepolarizing neuromuscular blocking agent that binds competitively to cholinergic receptors on the motor end-plate, resulting in antagonism of the action of acetylcholine and therefore neuromuscular blockade. The neuromuscular blocking potency of cisatracurium is about three times greater than that for atracurium. Intermediate onset and duration. **Time to maximum blockade**: 2 min. **Time to recovery**: Approximately 55 min. Continuous infusion for up to 3 hr may be undertaken without tachyphylaxis or cumulative neuromuscular blockade. The time required for recovery following successive maintenance doses does not change with the number of doses given, provided that partial recovery is allowed to occur between doses. Onset, duration, and recovery are faster in children. About 95% of a dose is excreted as metabolites and unchanged drug (10%) in the urine and 4% is eliminated through the feces. Laudanosine, a major biologically active metabolite with no neuromuscular activity, may cause transient hypotension and cerebral excitatory effects (in high doses).

USES

Neuromuscular blocking agent for in- and out-patients as an adjunct to general anesthesia, to facilitate tracheal intubation, and to cause skeletal muscle relaxation during surgery or mechanical ventilation in the intensive care unit.

CONTRAINDICATIONS

Hypersensitivity to cisatracurium or other bis-benzylisoquinolinium agents or hypersensitivity to benzyl alcohol. Use for rapid-sequence ET intubation due to its intermediate onset of action.

SPECIAL CONCERNS

Since the drug has no effect on consciousness, pain threshold, or cerebration, administration should not be undertaken before unconsciousness. May cause a profound effect in those with myasthenia gravis or the myasthenic syndrome. Burn clients may require higher doses. Onset time is faster (about 1 min) and recovery is slower (by about 1 min) in clients with impaired hepatic function. The time to maximum blockage is about 1 min slower in geriatric clients and in those with impaired renal function. Use with caution during lactation. Safety and efficacy have not been determined in children less than 2 years of age.

SIDE EFFECTS

Bradycardia, hypotension, flushing, bronchospasm, rash.

OD OVERDOSE MANAGEMENT

Symptoms: Neuromuscular blockade beyond the time needed for surgery and anesthesia. *Treatment*: Maintain a patent airway and control ventilation until recovery of normal function is assured. Once recovery begins, facilitate the process by using neostigmine or edrophonium with an anticholinergic drug. Do not give these antidotes when complete blockade is evident.

DRUG INTERACTIONS

Aminoglycosides / ↑ Cisatracurium effect
Bacitracin / ↑ Cisatracurium effect
Carbamazepine / Resistance to neuromuscular blockage → slightly shorter duration.
Clindamycin / ↑ Cisatracurium effect
Colistin, sodium colistimethate / ↑ Cisatracurium effect
Enflurane/nitrous oxide/oxygen / ↑ Cisatracurium duration
Isoflurane/nitrous oxide/oxygen / ↑ Cisatracurium duration
Lincomycin / ↑ Cisatracurium effect
Lithium / ↑ Cisatracurium effect
Local anesthetics / ↑ Cisatracurium effect
Magnesium salts / ↑ Cisatracurium effect
Phenobarbital / Resistance to neuromuscular blockade → slightly shorter duration
Polymyxins / ↑ Cisatracurium effect
Procainamide / ↑ Cisatracurium effect
Quinidine / ↑ Cisatracurium effect
Succinylcholine / Time to onset of maximum block of cisatracurium is about 2 min faster
Tetracyclines / ↑ Cisatracurium effect

HOW SUPPLIED

Injection: 2 mg/mL, 10 mg/mL.

DOSAGE

• **IV BOLUS**

Neuromuscular blockade.

Adults, initial: Depending on the desired time to intubation and the anticipated length of surgery, either 0.15 or 0.2 mg/kg is used. These doses are components of a propofol/nitrous oxide/oxygen induction-intubation technique. **Maintenance during prolonged surgery:** 0.03 mg/kg given 40–50 min following an initial dose of 0.15 mg/kg and 50–60 min following an initial dose of 0.2 mg/kg.

Children, 2–12 years of age: 0.1 mg/kg over 5–10 sec during either halothane or opioid anesthesia. When given during stable opioid/nitrous oxide/oxygen anesthesia, 0.1 mg/kg produces maximum effects in about 2.8 min and a clinically effective blockade for 28 min.

• **IV INFUSION**

Neuromuscular blockade during extended surgery or in the ICU.

In the OR or ICU, following an initial bolus dose, a diluted solution can be given by continuous infusion to both adults and children over 2 years of age. The rate is dependent on the response of the client determined by peripheral nerve stimulation. An infusion rate of 3 mcg/kg/min can be used to counteract rapid spontaneous recovery of neuromuscular blockade. Thereafter, an infusion rate of 1–2 mcg/kg/min is usually adequate to maintain blockade. Reduce infusion rate by 30%–40% when given during stable isoflurane or enflurane anesthesia.

NURSING CONSIDERATIONS

SEE ALSO *NURSING CONSIDERATIONS* FOR *NEUROMUSCULAR BLOCKING AGENTS.*

ADMINISTRATION/STORAGE

IV 1. Due to slower times of onset in geriatric clients and those with impaired renal function, extend interval between drug administration and intubation.

2. Spontaneous recovery following infusion will proceed at a rate comparable to that following administration of a bolus dose.

3. Cisatracurium is acidic; thus, it may not be compatible with alkaline solutions with a pH greater than 8.5 (e.g., barbiturate solutions).

4. Drug is compatible with D5%, 0.9% NaCl, D5/0.9% NaCl, sufentanil, alfentanil HCl, fentanyl, midazolam HCl, and droperidol. Not compatible with propofol or ketorolac for Y-site administration.

5. Refrigerate vials at 2–8°C (36–46°F) and protect from light. Once removed from the refrigerator, use vials within 21 days, even if rerefrigerated.

6. Cisatracurium diluted in D5%, 0.9% NaCl, or D5/0.9% NaCl may be refrigerated or stored at room temperature for 24 hr without significant loss of potency. Dilutions to 0.1 or 0.2 mg/mL in D5%/RL may be refrigerated for 24 hr. Due to chemical instability, do not dilute in RL.

ASSESSMENT

1. Document indications for therapy, other agents trialed, and anticipated duration of therapy.

2. Note any hypersensitivity to benzyl alcohol.

3. Document baseline neurologic assessment and labs.

INTERVENTIONS

1. To be administered only by those trained in administration of neuromuscular blocking agents.

2. Client requires constant monitoring and respiratory support.

3. Medicate with analgesics for pain and agents for anxiety based on assessed need.

4. Utilize a peripheral nerve stimulator to evaluate response to therapy and to ensure partial recovery between doses.

OUTCOMES/EVALUATE

- Facilitation of ET intubation
- Skeletal muscle relaxation

Cisplatin

(sis-**PLAH**-tin)

PREGNANCY CATEGORY: D

CLASSIFICATION(S):
Antineoplastic, alkylating
Rx: Platinol-AQ (Abbreviation: CDDP)

SEE ALSO *ANTINEOPLASTIC AGENTS*.

ACTION/KINETICS
Binds to DNA and causes production of intrastrand cross-links and formation of DNA adducts. The drug is cell-cycle nonspecific. **t½, plasma:** 20–30 min. **Terminal t½, blood cells:** 36–47 days. Incomplete urinary excretion (only 35%–51% after 5 days). Concentrates in liver, kidneys, and large and small intestines, with low penetration of CNS. Over 90% bound to plasma protein.

USES
Palliative therapy. (1) Combination therapy in metastatic testicular tumors and for metastatic ovarian tumors (e.g., with cyclophosphamide) in those who have received appropriate surgical or radiotherapeutic procedures. (2) Single agent in metastatic ovarian tumors as secondary therapy in those refractive to standard therapy who have not previously received cisplatin. (3) Single agent in transitional cell bladder cancer that is no longer amenable to surgery or radiotherapy.

ADDITIONAL CONTRAINDICATIONS
Lactation. Preexisting renal impairment, myelosuppression, impaired hearing, history of allergic reactions to platinum compounds.

ADDITIONAL SIDE EFFECTS
Renal: Severe cumulative renal toxicity, including renal tubular damage and renal insufficiency. **Electrolytes:** Low levels of calcium, magnesium, potassium, phosphate, and sodium. **Neurologic:** Seizures, taste loss, peripheral neuropathies. Neurotoxicity may occur 4–7 months after prolonged therapy. **Otic:** Ototoxicity characterized by tinnitus, especially in children. **Ophthalmologic:** Papilledema, cerebral blindness, optic neuritis. High doses have resulted in blurred vision and altered color perception. **Body as a whole:** Asthenia, alopecia. **Miscellaneous:** ***Anaphylactic reactions,*** hyperuricemia, hepatotoxicity, vascular toxicities (rare).

LABORATORY TEST CONSIDERATIONS
↑ Plasma iron levels. Nephrotoxicity results in ↑ serum uric acid, BUN, and creatinine and ↓ C_{CR}.

OD OVERDOSE MANAGEMENT
Symptoms: Liver and kidney failure, deafness, ocular toxicity (including retinal detachment), significant myelosuppression, intractable N&V, neuritis, death. *Treatment:* General supportive measures.

ADDITIONAL DRUG INTERACTIONS
Aminoglycosides / Cumulative nephrotoxity
Anticonvulsants / Anticonvulsant plasma levels may become subtherapeutic
Loop diuretics / Additive ototoxicity
Phenytoin / ↓ Phenytoin effect R/T ↓ plasma levels

HOW SUPPLIED
Injection: 1 mg/mL

DOSAGE
- **IV ONLY**

Metastatic testicular tumors.
20 mg/m²/day for 5 days/cycle.

Metastatic ovarian tumors.
Cisplatin: 75–100 mg/m² once every 4 weeks/cycle. Cyclophosphamide: 600 mg/m² once every 4 weeks on day 1. Administer cisplatin and cyclophosphamide sequentially.

Advanced bladder cancer.
50–70 mg/m² per cycle once q 3–4 weeks, depending on prior radiation or chemotherapy. For those heavily pretreated, give an initial dose of 50 mg/m²/cycle repeated q 4 weeks.

NOTE: Repeat courses should not be administered until (1) serum creatinine is below 1.5 mg/dL and/or the BUN is below 25 mg/dL; (2) platelets are equal to or greater than 100,000/mm³ and leukocyte count is equal to or greater than 4,000/mm³; and (3) auditory activity is within the normal range.

NURSING CONSIDERATIONS

SEE ALSO *NURSING CONSIDERATIONS FOR ANTINEOPLASTIC AGENTS*.

C

ADMINISTRATION/STORAGE

IV 1. Add dosage recommended from vial to 2 L of 5% dextrose in one-half or one-third NSS containing 37.5 g mannitol. Infuse over a period of 6–8 hr. Furosemide may be used instead of mannitol. Maintain adequate hydration and urinary output for 24 hr following infusion.
2. Before administration of cisplatin, hydrate client with 1–2 L of IV fluid over a period of 8–12 hr.
3. Do *not* use any equipment with aluminum for preparing or administering because a black precipitate will form and loss of potency will occur.
4. Platinol-AQ is a sterile, multidose vial without preservatives. Unopened containers should be stored at 15–25°C (59–77°F), protected from light. Once opened, solution is stable for 28 days protected from light, or 7 days under fluorescent lights.
5. Cisplatin has been confused with carboplatin. Place signs/label warnings of the name mix-ups. Do not refer to as "platinum."
6. Have emergency equipment available for anaphylactic reaction.

ASSESSMENT

1. Document indications for therapy and anticipated results. Identify previous treatments (XRT, chemotherapy).
2. Obtain audiometry testing before and after therapy to ensure hearing has not been affected.
3. *During therapy monitor for:*
• Facial edema, bronchoconstriction, tachycardia, and shock.
• Tremors that may progress to seizures due to hypomagnesemia.
• Tetany, confusion, or signs of hypocalcemia associated with hypomagnesemia; monitor Ca/Mg levels.
4. Hydrate well to prevent urate deposits; monitor I&O for 24 hr after treatment.
5. Obtain baseline CBC, uric acid, renal and LFTs. May cause severe cumulative renal toxicity; additional doses of cisplatin should not be administered until renal function has returned to baseline and usually not more frequently than every 3–4 weeks. Assess for mild granulocyte suppression. Nadir: 14 days; recovery: 21 days.

CLIENT/FAMILY TEACHING

1. Report any numbness, tingling, swelling, or joint pain.
2. Avoid vaccinations.
3. Report any ringing in ears, difficulty hearing, edema of lower extremities, or decreased urination.
4. Avoid alcohol and salicylates as these may increase gastric bleeding.
5. Use reliable birth control; may cause infertility. Identify candidates for egg/sperm harvesting.

OUTCOMES/EVALUATE

↓ Tumor size; suppression of malignant cell proliferation

Citalopram hydrobromide

(sigh-**TAL**-oh-pram)

PREGNANCY CATEGORY: C
CLASSIFICATION(S):
Antidepressant, selective serotonin reuptake inhibitor
Rx: Celexa

SEE ALSO *ANTIDEPRESSANTS*.

ACTION/KINETICS

Acts to inhibit reuptake of serotonin into CNS neurons resulting in increased levels of serotonin in synapses. Has minimal effects on reuptake of norepinephrine and dopamine. **Peak plasma levels:** 120–150 nmol/L after 2–4 hr. **t½, terminal:** 35 hr. Half-life is increased in geriatric clients. **Steady state plasma levels:** About 1 week. Metabolized in the liver and excreted in the urine (35%) and feces (65%).

USES

Treatment of depression in those with DSM-IV category of major depressive disorder. *Investigational:* Treatment of alcoholism, panic disorder, premenstrual dysphoria, social phobia, trichotillomania.

CONTRAINDICATIONS

Use with MAO inhibitors or with alcohol. Lactation.

SPECIAL CONCERNS
Use with caution in severe renal impairment (dosage adjustment not necessary), a history of seizure disorders, or in diseases or conditions that produce altered metabolism or hemodynamic responses. Safety and efficacy have not been determined in children. Do not confuse citalopram with Celebrex (celecoxib used as a NSAID) or Cerebyx (fosphenytoin sodium injection used to treat seizures).

SIDE EFFECTS
CNS: Activation of mania/hypomania, dizziness, insomnia, agitation, somnolence, anorexia, paresthesia, migraine, hyperkinesia, vertigo, hypertonia, extrapyramidal disorder, neuralgia, dystonia, abnormal gait, hypesthesia, ataxia, aggravated depression, suicide attempt, confusion, aggressive reaction, drug dependence, depersonalization, hallucinations, euphoria, psychotic depression, delusions, paranoid reaction, emotional lability, panic reaction, psychosis. **GI:** N&V, dry mouth, diarrhea, dyspepsia, abdominal pain, increased salivation, flatulence, gastritis, gastroenteritis, stomatitis, eructation, hemorrhoids, dysphagia, teeth grinding, gingivitis, esophagitis. **CV:** Tachycardia, postural hypotension, hypertension, bradycardia, edema of extremities, angina pectoris, extrasystoles, ***cardiac failure, MI, CVA,*** flushing, myocardial ischemia. **Musculoskeletal:** Arthralgia, myalgia, arthritis, muscle weakness, skeletal pain, leg cramps, involuntary muscle contraction. **Hematologic:** Purpura, anemia, leukocytosis, lymphadenopathy. **Metabolic/nutritional:** Decreased/increased weight, thirst. **GU:** Ejaculation disorder, impotence, dysmenorrhea, decreased/increased libido, amenorrhea, galactorrhea, breast pain, breast enlargement, vaginal hemorrhage, polyuria, frequent micturition, urinary incontinence/retention, dysuria. **Respiratory:** Coughing, epistaxis, bronchitis, dyspnea, pneumonia. **Dermatologic:** Rash, pruritus, photosensitivity reaction, urticaria, acne, skin discoloration, eczema, dermatitis, dry skin, psoriasis. **Ophthalmic:** Abnormal accommodation, conjunctivitis, eye pain. **Body as a whole:** Asthenia, fatigue, fever. **Miscellaneous:** Hyponatremia, increased sweating, yawning, hot flushes, rigors, alcohol intolerance, syncope, flu-like symptoms, taste perversion, tinnitus.

LABORATORY TEST CONSIDERATIONS
↑ Hepatic enzymes, alkaline phosphatase. Abnormal glucose tolerance.

OD OVERDOSE MANAGEMENT
Symptoms: Dizziness, sweating, N&V, tremor, somnolence, sinus tachycardia. Rarely, amnesia, confusion, coma, convulsions, hyperventilation, cyanosis, rhabdomyolysis, ECG changes (including QTc prolongation, nodal rhythm, ventricular arrhythmias). *Treatment:* Establish and maintain an airway. Gastric lavage with use of activated charcoal. Monitor cardiac and vital signs. General symptomatic and supportive care.

DRUG INTERACTIONS
See also *Drug Interactions* for *Selective Serotonin Reuptake Inhibitors.*
Azole antifungals / ↑ Citalopram plasma levels
Beta blockers / ↑ Effect of beta blocker; reduce initial beta blocker dose
Carbamazepine / ↓ Citalopram plasma levels; ↑ serum carbamazepine levels
Imipramine / ↑ Drug metabolite (desimpramine) by 50%
Lithium / Possible ↑ serotonergic effects of citalopram
Macrolide antibiotics (e.g., erythromycin)/ ↑ Citalopram plasma levels
MAO inhibitors / Possible serious and sometimes fatal reactions, including hyperthermia, rigidity, myoclonus, autonomic instability, mental status changes (extreme agitation, delirium, coma)

HOW SUPPLIED
Oral Solution: 10 mg/5 mL; *Tablets:* 20 mg, 40 mg

DOSAGE
- **ORAL SOLUTION, TABLETS**

Depression.
Adults, initial: 20 mg once daily in the a.m. or p.m. with or without food. Increase the dose in increments of 20 mg at intervals of no less than 1 week. Dos-

C

es greater than 40 mg/day are not recommended. For the elderly or those with hepatic impairment, 20 mg/day is recommended; titrate to 40 mg/day only for nonresponders. Initial treatment is continued for 6 or 8 weeks. **Maintenance:** Up to 24 weeks following 6 or 8 weeks of initial treatment.

Panic disorder.

20–30 mg/day.

NURSING CONSIDERATIONS

SEE ALSO *NURSING CONSIDERATIONS* FOR *ANTIDEPRESSANTS*.

ADMINISTRATION/STORAGE

Allow at least 14 days to elapse between discontinuation of a monoamine oxidase inhibitor and initiation of citalopram or vice versa.

ASSESSMENT

1. Note indications for therapy, onset and characteristics of symptoms. List other agents trialed and outcome.
2. Note other drugs prescribed to ensure none interact. Avoid use with MAOs or within 14 days before or after MAO use.
3. Determine any liver or renal dysfunction or seizure disorder.
4. Assess for altered metabolic/hemodynamics; reduce dose with liver or renal dysfunction.

CLIENT/FAMILY TEACHING

1. Take as directed, once daily, with or without food.
2. Use caution operating machines or cars until drug effects known.
3. Avoid alcohol or other CNS depressants.
4. Use reliable birth control.
5. May see improvement in 1 to 4 weeks; continue therapy as prescribed.

OUTCOMES/EVALUATE

Relief/control of depression

Cladribine injection

(**KLAD**-rih-bean)

PREGNANCY CATEGORY: D
CLASSIFICATION(S):
Antineoplastic, antimetabolite
Rx: Leustatin

SEE ALSO *ANTINEOPLASTIC AGENTS*.

ACTION/KINETICS

By inhibiting both DNA synthesis and repair, toxicity occurs to both actively dividing and quiescent lymphocytes and monocytes. Results in accumulation of 2-chloro-2′-deoxy-beta-D-adenosine monophosphate (2-CdAMP), which is subsequently converted to the active triphosphate deoxynucleotide (2-CdATP). Cells with high deoxycytidine kinase and low deoxynucleotidase activities (as in lymphocytes and monocytes) will be selectively killed as toxic deoxynucleotides accumulate intracellularly. **t½:** 5.4 hr. Excreted mainly through the urine.

USES

Hairy cell leukemia as defined by clinically significant anemia, neutropenia, thrombocytopenia, or disease-related symptoms. *Investigational:* Advanced cutaneous T-cell lymphomas; chronic lymphocytic leukemia; non-Hodgkin's lymphomas; acute myeloid leukemia; autoimmune hemolytic anemia; mycosis fungoides or the Sezary syndrome.

CONTRAINDICATIONS

Lactation.

SPECIAL CONCERNS

Use with caution in clients with known or suspected renal or hepatic insufficiency. Benzyl alcohol, a constituent of the 7-day infusion solution, has been associated with a fatal "gasping syndrome" in premature infants. Although used in children, safety and efficacy have not been established.

SIDE EFFECTS

Hematologic: Neutropenia, anemia, thrombocytopenia, prolonged depression of CD_4 counts, prolonged bone marrow hypocellularity. **Body as a whole:** Fever, infections (including septicemia, pneumonia), fatigue, chills, asthenia, diaphoresis, malaise, trunk pain. **GI:** Nausea, decreased appetite, vomiting, diarrhea, constipation, abdominal pain. **CV:** Edema, tachycardia, purpura, petechiae, epistaxis. **CNS:** Headache, dizziness, insomnia. **Dermatologic:** Rashes, reactions at injection site, pruritus, pain, erythema. **Respiratory:** Abnormal breath sounds, cough, abnormal chest sounds, SOB.

Musculoskeletal: Myalgia, arthralgia. **Following IV injection:** Redness, swelling pain, thrombosis, phlebitis.

OD OVERDOSE MANAGEMENT

Symptoms: Irreversible neurologic toxicity (paraparesis/quadriparesis), ***acute nephrotoxicity, severe bone marrow suppression.*** *Treatment:* Discontinue infusion of the drug. Institute appropriate supportive measures as there is no antidote for cladribine.

HOW SUPPLIED

Injection: 1 mg/mL

DOSAGE

- **IV INFUSION**

  Hairy cell leukemia.

A single course given by continuous infusion for 7 consecutive days at a dose of 0.09 mg/kg/day.

NURSING CONSIDERATIONS

SEE ALSO *NURSING CONSIDERATIONS* FOR *ANTINEOPLASTIC AGENTS*.

ADMINISTRATION/STORAGE

IV 1. If neuro/renal toxicity occur, delay or discontinue drug therapy.

2. Aseptic technique and proper environmental precautions must be observed; contains no antimicrobial preservative.

3. To prepare a single daily dose, 0.09 mg/kg or 0.09 mL/kg of cladribine is added to an infusion bag containing 500 mL of 0.9% NaCl. The use of 5% dextrose is not recommended due to increased drug degradation. Admixtures of cladribine are stable for 24 hr at room temperature under normal room fluorescent light in Baxter Viaflex PVC infusion containers.

4. To prepare the 7-day infusion, mix the drug only with bacteriostatic 0.9% NaCl (benzyl alcohol preserved). To minimize the risk of microbial contamination, pass both the cladribine and diluent through a sterile 0.22-μm disposable hydrophilic syringe filter as each solution is being introduced into the infusion reservoir. The calculated dose of cladribine (0.09 mg/kg or mL/kg for 7 days) is first added to the infusion reservoir through the sterile filter; then, a calculated amount of bacteriostatic 0.9% NaCl injection is run through the filter to bring the total volume of the solution to 100 mL. After preparation of the solution, clamp the line, disconnect and discard the filter. Aseptically aspirate air bubbles from the reservoir as necessary using the syringe and a dry second sterile filter assembly. Admixtures for the 7-day infusion are stable in Pharmacia Deltic medication cassettes.

5. Adherence to recommended diluents/infusion systems is advised due to limited compatibility data.

6. Do not mix solutions containing cladribine with other IV drugs or additives or infuse simultaneously in a common IV line.

7. Refrigerate unopened vial at 2–8°C (36–46°F); protect from light. Although freezing does not affect solution, a precipitate may form at low temperatures. The drug may be resolubilized by allowing the solution to warm naturally to room temperature and by shaking vigorously. The solution is not to be heated or microwaved. Once thawed, do not refreeze solution.

8. Once diluted, promptly inject or store in the refrigerator for no more than 8 hr prior to administration.

9. Vials of cladribine are for single use only; discard any unused portion.

ASSESSMENT

1. Document type/onset of symptoms; note therapies trialed.

2. Reconstituted infusion solution contains benzyl alcohol.

3. Client should be infection free prior to administration. Fevers during the first 1–2 months following therapy should be evaluated (e.g., labs, cultures, X rays) to determine need for antibiotics.

4. High dose therapy may precipitate acute nephrotoxity and delayed neurotoxity (from demyelination).

5. With large tumor burdens; use allopurinol for hyperuricemia and tumor lysis syndrome.

6. Obtain baseline CBC, liver and renal function studies. Monitor hemato-

logic profile closely for 4–8 weeks after therapy; blood transfusions and to a lesser extent platelet transfusions may be required due to severe myelosuppressive effects.

C

CLIENT/FAMILY TEACHING

1. The recommended dosing requires a continuous infusion for 7 consecutive days.
2. Report any evidence of abnormal bleeding, pain, or fever.
3. Nausea may be relieved with chlorpromazine; report if evident.
4. Fever and fatigue are common side effects; report if prolonged or debilitating. Schedule activities to include frequent rest periods.
5. Drug is teratogenic; practice safe form of contraception.
6. Bone marrow aspiration and biopsy will be repeated to confirm pharmacologic response.

OUTCOMES/EVALUATE

- Normalization of hematologic profile
- Absence of hairy cells in peripheral blood and bone marrow
- Inhibition of pathologic and clinical disease progression

Clarithromycin

(klah-**rith**-roh-**MY**-sin)

PREGNANCY CATEGORY: C
CLASSIFICATION(S):
Antibiotic, macrolide
Rx: Biaxin, Biaxin XL

SEE ALSO *ANTI-INFECTIVES*.

ACTION/KINETICS

Macrolide antibiotic that acts by binding to the 50S ribosomal subunit of susceptible organisms, thus interfering with or inhibiting microbial protein synthesis. Rapidly absorbed from the GI tract although food slightly delays the onset of absorption and the formation of the active metabolite but does not affect the extent of the bioavailability. **Peak serum levels:** When fasting, 2 hr for the tablet and 3 hr for the suspension. **Steady-state peak serum levels:** 1 mcg/mL within 2–3 days after 250 mg q 12 hr and 2–3 mcg/mL after 500 mg q 12 hr. Clarithromycin and 14-OH clarithromycin (active metabolite) are readily distributed to body tissues and fluids. **t½, elimination:** 3–7 hr (depending on the dose) for clarithromycin and 5–6 hr for 14-OH clarithromycin. Up to 30% of a dose is excreted unchanged in the urine.

USES

Mild to moderate infections caused by susceptible strains of the following. **Adults.** (1) Pharyngitis/tonsillitis due to *Streptococcus pyogenes.* (2) Acute maxillary sinusitis or acute bacterial exacerbaton of chronic bronchitis due to *Streptococcus pneumoniae, Haemophilus influenzae,* and *Moraxella catarrhalis.* The active metabolite, 14-OH clarithromycin, has significant activity (twice the parent compound) against *H. influenzae.* (3) Pneumonia due to *Mycoplasma pneumoniae, S. pneumoniae,* or *Chlamydia pneumoniae.* Community-acquired pneumonia due to *Haeomophilus influenzae.* (4) Uncomplicated skin and skin structure infections due to *Staphylococcus aureus* or *S. pyogenes.* (5) Treatment of disseminated mycobacterial infections due to *Mycobacterium avium* (commonly seen in AIDS clients) and *M. intracellulare.* Prevention of disseminated *M. avium* complex in individuals with advanced HIV. (6) Used with omeprazole and ranitidine bismuth citrate (Tritec) or with amoxicillin and lansoprazole (Prevpac) for the eradication of *Helicobacter pylori* infection in clients with active duodenal ulcers associated with *H. pylori* infection. (7) Community-acquired pneumonia due to *H. influenzae.*

The extended release tablet is used to treat (1) Acute bacterial exacerbation of chronic bronchitis due to *H. influenzae, H. parainfluenzae, M. catarrhalis,* and *Streptococcus pneumoniae.* (2) Acute maxillary sinusitis due to *Haemophilus influenzae, Streptococcus pneumoniae,* and *Moraxella catarrhalis.* (3) Mild-to-moderate community-acquired pneumonia in adults due to *H. influenzae, H. parainfluenzae, Moraxella catarrhalis, Streptococcus pneumoniae, Chlamydia pneumoniae,* and *Mycoplasma pneunoniae.*

C

Children. (1) Pharyngitis or tonsillitis due to *S. pyogenes.* (2) Acute maxillary sinusitis or acute otitis media due to *S. pneumoniae, H. influenzae,* and *M. catarrhalis.* (3) Uncomplicated skin and skin structure infections due to *S. aureus* or *S. pyogenes.* (4) Disseminated mycobacterial infections due to *M. avium* or *M. intracellulare.* Prevention of disseminated *M. avium* complex disease in clients with advanced HIV infection. (5) Community-acquired pneumonia caused by *M. pneumoniae, Chlamydia pneumoniae,* and *S. pneumoniae.*

CONTRAINDICATIONS

Hypersensitivity to clarithromycin, other macrolide antibiotics, or erythromycin. Clients taking pimozide. Use with ranitidine bismuth citrate in those with a history of acute porphyria.

SPECIAL CONCERNS

Use with caution in severe renal impairment with or without concomitant hepatic impairment and during lactation. Safety and effectiveness in children less than 6 months of age have not been determined. Safety has not been determined in MAC clients less than 20 months of age.

SIDE EFFECTS

GI: Diarrhea, nausea, abnormal taste, dyspepsia, abdominal discomfort or pain, pseudomembranous colitis, glossitis, stomatitis, oral moniliasis, vomiting. **CNS:** Headache, dizziness, behavioral changes, confusion, depersonalization, disorientation, hallucinations, insomnia, nightmares, vertigo. **Allergic:** Urticaria, mild skin eruptions and, rarely, ***anaphylaxis and Stevens-Johnson syndrome.*** **Hepatic:** Hepatocellular cholestatic hepatitis with or without jaundice, increased liver enzymes, ***hepatic failure.*** **Miscellaneous:** Hearing loss (usually reversible), alteration of sense of smell (usually with taste perversion).

In children, the most common side effects are diarrhea, vomiting, abdominal pain, rash, and headache.

LABORATORY TEST CONSIDERATIONS

↑ ALT, AST, GGT, alkaline phosphatase, LDH, total bilirubin, BUN, serum creatinine, PT. ↓ WBC count.

DRUG INTERACTIONS

See also *Drug Interactions* for *Erythromycins.*

Anticoagulants / ↑ Anticoagulant effects

Benzodiazepines / ↑ Plasma levels of certain benzodizepines → ↑ and prolonged CNS effects

Buspirone / ↑ Buspirone plasma levels → ↑ risk of side effects

Carbamazepine / ↑ Carbamazepine blood levels

Cyclosporine ↑ Cyclosporine levels → ↑ risk of nephrotoxicity and neurotoxicity

Digoxin / ↑ Digoxin plasma levels R/T ↓ digoxin metabolism by the gut flora

Disopyramide / ↑ Plasma levels → arrhythmias and ↑ QT intervals

Ergot alkaloids / Acute drug toxicity, including severe peripheral vasospasm and dysesthesia

Fluconazole / ↑ Clarithromycin blood levels

HMG–CoA Reductase Inhibitors / ↑ Risk of severe myopathy or rhabdomyolysis

Omeprazole / ↑ Plasma levels of omeprazole, clarithromycin, and 14-OH-clarithromycin

Pimozide / ↑ Risk of sudden death due to cardiac effects; do not use together

Ranitidine bismuth citrate / ↑ Levels of ranitidine, bismuth citrate, and 14–OH clarithromycin

Repaglinide / ↑ Repaglinide plasma levels likely R/T ↓ liver metabolism

Rifabutin, Rifampin / ↓ Effect of clarithromycin and ↑ GI side effects

Tacrolimus / ↑ Tacrolimus plasma levels → ↑ risk of toxicity (e.g., nephrotoxicity)

Theophylline / ↑ Theophylline serum levels

Triazolam / ↑ Risk of somnolence and confusion

Verapamil / Possible severe hypotension and bradycardia

Zidovudine/ ↓ Steady-state AZT levels in HIV-infected clients; however, peak serum AZT levels may be ↑ or ↓

HOW SUPPLIED

Granules for Oral Suspension after Reconstitution: 125 mg/5 mL, 187.5 mg/

mL, 250 mg/5 mL; *Tablet:* 250 mg, 500 mg; *Extended Release Tablet:* 500 mg.

DOSAGE

• **TABLETS, ORAL SUSPENSION**

Pharyngitis, tonsillitis.

Adults: 250 mg q 12 hr for 10 days.

Acute exacerbation of chronic bronchitis due to S. pneumoniae *or M. catarrhalis; pneumonia due to* S. pneumoniae *or M. pneumoniae; uncomplicated skin and skin structure infections.*

Adults: 250 mg q 12 hr for 7–14 days.

Acute maxillary sinusitis, acute exacerbation of chronic bronchitis due to H. influenzae.

Adults: 500 mg q 12 hr for 7–14 days. Or, 1-500 mg Extended Release Tablet daily.

Disseminated M. avium complex or prophylaxis of *M. avium complex.*

Adults: 500 mg b.i.d.; **children:** 7.5 mg/kg b.i.d. up to 500 mg b.i.d.

NOTE: The usual daily dose for children is 15 mg/kg q 12 hr for 10 days.

Community-acquired pneumonia.

Adults: 1 g once daily for 7 days. **Children:** 15 mg/kg/day of the suspension, divided and given q 12 hr for 10 days.

Active duodenal ulcers associated with H. pylori *infection.*

The following drug regimens are used: (a) Clarithromycin, 500 mg b.i.d., amoxicillin, 1,000 mg b.i.d., and lansoprazole, 30 mg b.i.d. each for 10–14 days. (b) Clarithromycin, 500 mg b.i.d., amoxicillin, 1,000 mg b.i.d., and omeprazole, 20 mg b.i.d. each for 10 or 14 days. (c) Clarithromycin, 500 mg b.i.d., metronidazole, 500 mg b.i.d., and *either* lansoprazole, 30 mg b.i.d., *or* omeprazole, 20 mg b.i.d., each for 14 days.

• **TABLETS, EXTENDED-RELEASE**

Maxillary sinusitis.

Adults: 1000 mg once daily for 14 days.

Acute exacerbation of chronic bronchitis, acquired pneumonia.

Adults: 1000 mg once daily for 7 days.

NURSING CONSIDERATIONS

SEE ALSO *NURSING CONSIDERATIONS* FOR *ERYTHROMYCINS*.

ADMINISTRATION/STORAGE

1. May be given with or without food, and both tablets and suspension can be given with milk. Food delays both the onset of absorption and the formation of 14-OH clarithromycin (the active metabolite).
2. Consider decreased doses or prolonging the dosing interval with severe renal impairment with or without hepatic impairment.
3. Shake the reconstituted suspension well before each use; use within 14 days and do not refrigerate.

ASSESSMENT

1. Note any sensitivity to erythromycin or any of the macrolide antibiotics.
2. Document type, severity, onset, and duration of symptoms.
3. List drugs currently prescribed to prevent any interactions.
4. Obtain baseline cultures, CBC, liver and renal function studies.

CLIENT/FAMILY TEACHING

1. May take with or without meals; food delays onset of absorption. Drug may cause a bitter taste.
2. Report any persistent diarrhea; an antibiotic-associated colitis may be precipitated by *C. difficile* and require alternative management.
3. Report if no symptom improvement after 48–72 hr.

OUTCOMES/EVALUATE

- Symptomatic improvement
- Negative follow-up cultures

Clemastine fumarate

(kleh-**MAS**-teen)

PREGNANCY CATEGORY: B

CLASSIFICATION(S):

Antihistamine, first generation, ethanolamine

Rx: Tavist

OTC: Antihist-1, Dayhist-1, Tavist Allergy

SEE ALSO *ANTIHISTAMINES*.

ACTION/KINETICS

Moderate sedative effects, high anticholinergic activity, and moderate to high antiemetic effects. **Peak blood levels:** 2–4 hr. **Peak effects:** 5–7 hr.

Duration: 10–12 hr (up to 24 hr in some clients). Metabolized in the liver and excreted through the urine.

USES

Allergic rhinitis. Urticaria and angioedema.

CONTRAINDICATIONS

Use in newborns or premature infants. Lactation. Treatment of lower respiratory tract symptoms, including asthma. Use with monoamine oxidase (MAO) inhibitors.

SPECIAL CONCERNS

Use with caution in clients with narrow angle glaucoma, stenosing peptic ulcer, pyloroduodenal obstruction, symptomatic prostatic hypertrophy, and bladder neck obstruction. Use with caution in clients 60 years of age and older and in those with a history of bronchial asthma, increased intraocular pressure, hyperthyroidism, CV disease, and hypertension. Safety and efficacy have not been determined in children less than 12 years of age.

SIDE EFFECTS

CNS: Drowsiness (common), sedation, sleepiness, dizziness, incoordination, fatigue, confusion, restlessness, excitation, nervousness, tremor, irritability, insomnia, euphoria, paresthesia, blurred vision, diplopia, vertigo, tinnitus, acute labyrinthitis, hysteria, neuritis, ***convulsions.*** **GI:** Epigastric distress, anorexia, N&V, diarrhea, constipation. **CV:** Hypotension, headache, palpitations, tachycardia, extrasystoles. **Respiratory:** Thickening of bronchial secretions, tightness of chest, wheezing, nasal stuffiness. **Hematologic:** Hemolytic anemia, thrombocytopenia, agranulocytosis. **GU:** Urinary frequency/difficulty/retention, early menses.

HOW SUPPLIED

Syrup: 0.5 mg base/5 mL; *Tablets:* 1.34 mg (OTC), 2.68 mg.

DOSAGE

• **SYRUP, TABLETS**

Allergic rhinitis.

Adults and children over 12 years of age, initial: 1.34 mg (1 mg clemastine) b.i.d., up to a maximum dose of 8.04 mg (60 mL of syrup or 6 tablets) daily. **Children, aged 6 to 12 years of age, initial:** 0.67 mg (0.5 mg clemastine) b.i.d., up to a maximum of 4.02 mg (3 mg base) daily. Use only the syrup in children.

Urticaria and angioedema.

Adults and children over 12 years of age, initial: 2.68 mg (use tablet) 1–3 times/day, not to exceed 8.04 mg daily. **Children, aged 6 to 12 years, initial:** 1.34 mg (use syrup only) b.i.d., not to exceed 4.02 mg daily.

NURSING CONSIDERATIONS

SEE ALSO *NURSING CONSIDERATIONS* FOR *ANTIHISTAMINES*.

ADMINISTRATION/STORAGE

Store the syrup below 77°F (25°C) in a tight, amber glass bottle. Store tablets at room temperatures between 15–30°C (59–86°F) in a tight, light-resistant container.

ASSESSMENT

1. Document onset and characteristics of symptoms; identify triggers.
2. Assess for evidence/history of asthma, BPH, HTN, PUD, or glaucoma.
3. Obtain baseline CBC, VS, ECG, ENT, and CP assessments.

CLIENT/FAMILY TEACHING

1. Take as directed; do not exceed prescribed dose.
2. Do not perform activities that require mental alertness until drug effects realized; dizziness and drowsiness may occur.
3. Avoid alcohol and any other CNS depressants.
4. Use sugarless gum and candy or sips of water for dry mouth symptoms. Report any intolerable side effects or loss of symptom control.

OUTCOMES/EVALUATE

Relief of allergic manifestations.

Clindamycin hydrochloride

(klin-dah-**MY**-sin)

PREGNANCY CATEGORY: B (VAGINAL CREAM, TOPICAL GEL, LOTION, SOLUTION)

PREGNANCY CATEGORY: B
Rx: Cleocin
✤Rx: Alti-Clindamycin, Dalacin C

Clindamycin palmitate hydrochloride

(klin-dah-**MY**-sin)

PREGNANCY CATEGORY: B
Rx: Cleocin Pediatric
✤Rx: Dalacin C Flavored Granules

Clindamycin phosphate

(klin-dah-**MY**-sin)

PREGNANCY CATEGORY: B (VAGINAL CREAM, TOPICAL GEL, LOTION, SOLUTION)
Rx: C/T/S, Cleocin T, Cleocin Vaginal Cream, Clinda-Derm, Clindets , Cleocin Phosphate
✤Rx: Dalacin C Phosphate Sterile Solution, Dalacin T Topical Solution, Dalacin Vaginal Cream

CLASSIFICATION(S):
Antibiotic, lincosamide

SEE ALSO *ANTI-INFECTIVES.*

ACTION/KINETICS
A semisynthetic antibiotic that suppresses protein synthesis by microorganisms by binding to ribosomes (50S subunit) and preventing peptide bond formation. Is both bacteriostatic and bactericidal. **Peak serum concentration: PO,** 4 mcg/mL after 300 mg; **IM,** 4.9 mcg/mL after 300 mg; **IV,** 14.7 mcg/mL after 300 mg. **t½:** 2.4–3 hr. In serious infections the rate of IV administration is adjusted to maintain appropriate serum drug concentrations: 4–6 mcg/mL.

USES
Should not be used for trivial infections. **Systemic.** (1) *Anareobes:* Serious respiratory tract infections (e.g., empyema, lung abscess, anaerobic pneumonitis). (2) Serious skin and soft tissue infections, septicemia, intra-abdominal infections (e.g., peritonitis, intra–abdominal abscess), infections of the female pelvis and genital tract (e.g., PID, endometritis, nongonococcal tubo–ovarian abscess, pelvic cellulitis, postsurgical vaginal cuff infection). (3) *Streptococci/staphylococci:* Serious respiratory tract infections, serious skin and soft tissue infections, septicemia (parenteral use), acute staphylococcal hematogenous osteomyelitis (parenteral use). (4) *Pneumonococcus:* Serious respiratory tract infections. (5) Adjunct to surgery for chronic bone/joint infections. *Investigational:* Alternative to sulfonamides in combination with pyrimethamine in the acute treatment of CNS toxoplasmosis in AIDS clients. In combination with primaquine to treat *Pneumocystis carinii* pneumonia. Chlamydial infections in women. Bacterial vaginosis due to *Gardnerella vaginalis.* **Topical.** (1) Used topically for inflammatory acne vulgaris. (2) Vaginally to treat bacterial vaginosis. *Investigational:* Treatment of rosacea (lotion used).

CONTRAINDICATIONS
Hypersensitivity to either clindamycin or lincomycin. Use in treating viral and minor bacterial infections or in clients with a history of regional enteritis, nonbacterial infections (e.g., most URIs), ulcerative colitis, meningitis, or antibiotic-associated colitis. Lactation.

SPECIAL CONCERNS
Use with caution in infants up to 1 month of age, in clients with GI disease, liver or renal disease, or a history of allergy or asthma. Safety and efficacy of topical products have not been established in children less than 12 years of age.

SIDE EFFECTS
GI: N&V, diarrhea, ***pseudomembranous colitis*** (more frequent after **PO Use:** abdominal pain, esophagitis, unpleasant or metallic taste (after high IV doses), glossitis, stomatitis. **CV:** Hypotension, ***rarely, cardiopulmonary arrest after too rapid IV use.*** **Allergic:** Morbilliform rash (most common), skin rashes, urticaria, erythema multiforme, ***anaphylaxis, Stevens-Johnson-like syndrome,*** maculopapular rash, angioneurotic edema. **Hemato-**

logic: Leukopenia, neutropenia, thrombocytopenia, transient eosinophilia, ***agranulocytosis, aplastic anemia.*** **Hepatic:** Jaundice, abnormal LFTs. **GU:** Renal dysfunction (azotemia, oliguria, proteinuria), vaginitis. **Miscellaneous:** Superinfection, tinnitus, polyarthritis. Also sore throat, fatigue, urinary frequency, headache. **Following IV use:** Thrombophlebitis, erythema, pain, swelling. *Following IM use:* Pain, induration, sterile abscesses. **Following topical use:** Erythema, irritation, dryness, peeling, itching, burning, oiliness of skin. **Following vaginal use:** Cervicitis, vaginitis, vulvar irritation, urticaria, rash.

NOTE: The injection contains benzyl alcohol, which has been associated with ***a fatal "gasping syndrome"*** in infants.

LABORATORY TEST CONSIDERATIONS

↓ Levels of AST, ALT, NPN, alkaline phosphatase, bilirubin, BSP retention, and ↓ platelet count.

DRUG INTERACTIONS

Antiperistaltic antidiarrheals (opiates, Lomotil) / ↑ Diarrhea R/T ↓ toxin removal from colon

Ciprofloxacin HCl / Additive antibacterial activity

Cyclosporine / ↓ Cyclosporine serum levels

Erythromycin / Cross-interference → ↓ effect of both drugs

Kaolin/Pectin (e.g., Kaopectate) / ↓ Effect R/T ↓ GI tract absorption

Neuromuscular blocking agents / ↑ Effect of blocking agents

HOW SUPPLIED

Clindamycin hydrochloride: *Capsule:* 75 mg, 150 mg, 300 mg. **Clindamycin palmitate hydrochloride:** *Granule for oral solution: 75 mg/5 mL.* **Clindamycin phosphate:** *Gel:* 1%; *Injection:* 150 mg/mL; *Lotion:* 1%; *Topical Solution:* 1%; *Vaginal cream:* 2%

DOSAGE

• **CAPSULES, ORAL SOLUTION**

Serious infections.

Adults: 150–300 mg q 6 hr. **Pediatric, Clindamycin hydrochloride:** 8–16 mg/kg/day divided into three or four equal doses. **Pediatric, clindamycin palmitate hydrochloride:** 8–12 mg/kg/day divided into three or four equal doses.

More severe infections.

Adults: 300–450 mg q 6 hr. **Pediatric, Clindamycin hydrochloride:** 16–20 mg/kg/day divided into three or four equal doses. **Pediatric, clindamycin palmitate hydrochloride:** 13–25 mg/kg/day divided into three or four equal doses. **Children less than 10 kg:** Minimum recommended dose is 37.5 mg t.i.d.

• **IM, IV**

Serious infections due to aerobic gram–positive cocci.

Adults: 600–1,200 mg/day in two to four equal doses. **Pediatric, over 1 month to 16 years:** 350 mg/m²/day.

More severe infections due to B. fragilis, Peptococcus, or *Clostridium (other than* C. perfringens).

Adults: 1,200–2,700 mg/day in two to four equal doses. May have to be increased in more serious infections. **Pediatric, over 1 month to 16 years:** 450 mg/m²/day.

Life-threatening infections.

Adults: 4.8 g IV. **Pediatric, 1 month to 16 years:** 20–40 mg/kg/day in three to four equal doses depending on severity of infections. **Pediatric, less than 1 month of age:** 15–20 mg/kg/day in three or four equal doses.

Acute pelvic inflammatory disease.

IV: 900 mg q 8 hr plus gentamicin loading dose of 2 mg/kg IV or IM; **then,** gentamicin, 1.5 mg/kg q 8 hr IV or IM. Therapy may be discontinued 24 hr after client improves. After discharge from the hospital, continue with doxycycline PO, 100 mg b.i.d. for 10–14 days. Alternatively, give clindamycin, PO, 450 mg q.i.d. for 14 days.

• **TOPICAL GEL, LOTION, OR SOLUTION**

Apply thin film b.i.d. to affected areas. One or more pledgets may also be used.

• **VAGINAL CREAM (2%)**

Bacterial vaginosis.

One applicatorful (containing about 100 mg clindamycin phosphate), preferably at bedtime, for 3 (nonpregnant women) or 7 (pregnant and nonpregnant women) consecutive days.

NURSING CONSIDERATIONS

SEE ALSO *GENERAL NURSING CONSIDERATIONS* FOR *ANTI-INFECTIVES*.

ADMINISTRATION/STORAGE

1. For anaerobic infections, use the parenteral form initially; may be followed by PO therapy.
2. For β–hemolytic streptococci infections, continue treatment for at least 10 days.
3. Reduce dosage in severe renal impairment.
4. Single IM injections greater than 600 mg are not advisable. Inject deeply into muscle to prevent induration, pain, and sterile abscesses.
5. Do not refrigerate the reconstituted solution as it may become thickened and difficult to pour.
6. Shake lotion well just before using.

IV 7. Give parenteral clindamycin only to hospitalized clients.

8. Dilute IV injections to maximum concentration of 18 mg/mL, with no more than 1,200 mg administered in 1 hr.
9. Administer IV over a period of 20–60 min, depending on dose and desired therapeutic serum concentration.
10. The phosphate is stable in NSS, D5/W, and RL solution in both glass or PVC containers at concentrations of 6, 9, and 12 mg/mL for 8 weeks frozen, 32 days refrigerated, or 16 days at room temperature.

ASSESSMENT

1. Document indications for therapy, type and onset of symptoms.
2. Auscultate lungs and note extent of respiratory tract infections.
3. Describe skin and soft tissue infections; note complaints indicative of PID or intra-abdominal infections.
4. Obtain baseline cultures, liver and renal function studies. Note any history of liver or renal disease, allergies, or GI problems.
5. With IV therapy, observe for hypotension; keep in bed for 30 min following infusion. Advise that a bitter taste may be evident.
6. Observe for drug interactions caused by concurrent administration of neuromuscular blocking agents. Be alert to hypotension, bronchospasms, cardiac disturbances, hyperthermia, and respiratory depression.
7. Observe closely for:
   - Skin rash; frequently reported
   - Renal and/or hepatic impairment and newborns for organ dysfunction
   - GI disturbances, such as abdominal pain, diarrhea, anorexia, N&V, bloody/tarry stools, and excessive flatulence.

CLIENT/FAMILY TEACHING

1. Take oral medication with a full glass of water to prevent esophageal ulceration. May be taken with or without food.
2. Report any side effects such as persistent vomiting, diarrhea, fever, or abdominal pain and cramping.
3. Pseudomembranous colitis may occur 2–9 days or several weeks after initiation of therapy. Fluids, electrolytes, protein supplements, systemic corticosteroids, and oral antibiotics may be needed. Do not use antiperistaltic agents if diarrhea occurs because these can prolong or aggravate condition. Kaolin will reduce absorption of antibiotic; if prescribed, take 3 hr before drug.
4. The vaginal cream contains mineral oil, which may weaken latex or rubber products, such as condoms or vaginal contraceptive diaphragms; avoid for 72 hr following treatment.
5. Do not engage in intercourse when using the vaginal cream as this may enhance irritation.
6. Do not use any acne or topical mercury preparations containing a peeling agent in affected area; severe irritation may occur.

OUTCOMES/EVALUATE

- Resolution of infection
- Symptomatic improvement
- Therapeutic drug levels with IV therapy (4–6 mcg/mL)

Clobetasol propionate

(kloh-**BAY**-tah-sohl)

PREGNANCY CATEGORY: C

CLASSIFICATION(S):
Glucocorticoid
Rx: Clobevate Gel, Cormax, Embeline E 0.05%, Olux, Temovate, Temovate Emollient
✱Rx: Alti-Clobetasol, Dermovate, Gen-Clobetasol Cream/Ointment, Gen-Clobetasol Scalp Application, Novo-Clobetasol

SEE ALSO ***CORTICOSTEROIDS.***

ACTION/KINETICS
Has anti-inflammatory, antipruritic, and vasoconstrictive effects.

USES
Relief of inflammatory and pruritic dermatoses of the skin and scalp, including eczema, atopic dermatitis, contact dermatitis, seborrhea.

CONTRAINDICATIONS
Use in children less than 12 years old, use for more than 2 weeks, to treat rosacea or perioral dermatitis, and use on face, groin, axillae.

SPECIAL CONCERNS
May suppress hypothalamic-pituitary-adrenal (HPA) axis at doses as low as 2 g/day. Use with caution during lactation.

SIDE EFFECTS
Dermatologic: Burning sensation, itching, stinging, irritation, dryness, pruritus, erythema, folliculitis, hypertrichosis, acneform eruptions, hypopigmentation, perioral dermatitis, allergic contact dermatitis, skin maceration, secondary infection, striae, millaria, cracking and fissuring of the skin, skin atrophy, numbness of fingers, telangiectasia. **Miscellaneous:** Cushing's syndrome.

HOW SUPPLIED
Cream: 0.05%; *Foam*: 0.05%; *Gel:* 0.05%; *Ointment:* 0.05%; *Scalp Application:* 0.05%

DOSAGE

• TOPICAL CREAM, FOAM, GEL, OINTMENT

Dermatoses.

Apply thin layer to affected skin or scalp b.i.d. once in the morning and once in the evening. Rub in gently and completely. Use no more than 50 g/week.

NURSING CONSIDERATIONS

ADMINISTRATION/STORAGE
1. Do not use occlusive dressings.
2. Do not refrigerate.
3. Do not use the gel on the face, groin, or axillae.

ASSESSMENT
1. Document onset, location, and characteristics of symptoms (photograph); note agents trialed/outcome.
2. Drug is a potent corticosteroid for short term use; assess for S&S of HPA axis suppression-may use ACTH stimulation test, a.m. cortisol, and urinary free cortisol test.

CLIENT/FAMILY TEACHING
1. Apply thin layer to affected area and gently rub in. Use only as directed, externally, avoid eye contact.
2. Wash hands before and after application. Do not cover, wrap, or bandage treatment area.
3. Report any failure to heal as this may indicate an allergic contact dermatitis from agent.
4. If skin infections develop, may also need antifungal or antibacterial agent; report if evident.
5. Report any severe burning, stinging, swelling, numbness, or lack of response.

OUTCOMES/EVALUATE
Relief/healing of inflamed/pruritic skin manifestations

Clofazimine

(kloh-**FAYZ**-ih-meen)

PREGNANCY CATEGORY: C
CLASSIFICATION(S):
Leprostatic
Rx: Lamprene

ACTION/KINETICS
Inhibits mycobacterial growth (is bactericidal) and binding to mycobacterial DNA in *Mycobacterium leprae.* Is also anti-inflammatory by controlling erythema nodosum leprosum reactions. Cross-resistance with rifampin or dapsone is not observed. Concentrated in fatty tissues and the reticuloendothe-

lial system. **Average serum levels:** 0.7 mcg/mL after 100 mg/day and 1 mcg/mL after 300 mg/day. **t½:** 70 days. Excreted in the feces via the bile, as well as in sputum, sweat, and sebum.

USES

Lepromatous leprosy (including dapsone-resistant leprosy and leprosy complicated by erythema nodosum leprosum). In combination with other drugs to prevent resistance in multibacillary leprosy.

SPECIAL CONCERNS

Use with caution in clients with abdominal pain or diarrhea. Use during lactation only if benefits outweigh risks. Safety and efficacy have not been determined in children.

SIDE EFFECTS

GI: N&V, diarrhea, abdominal or epigastric pain, GI intolerance/ bleeding, intestinal obstruction, anorexia, constipation, enlarged liver, eosinophilic enteritis, taste disorder. **Dermatologic:** Pink to brownish black skin pigmentation in nearly all clients, ichthyosis, skin dryness, pruritus, rash, erythroderma, acneiform eruptions, monilial cheilosis. **Ophthalmologic:** Pigmentation of conjunctiva/cornea (due to clofazimine crystals), phototoxicity, decreased vision, eye irritation/burning/itching/dryness. **CNS:** Headache, dizziness, drowsiness, neuralgia, fatigue, depression, giddiness. Depression due to skin discoloration. **Miscellaneous:** Jaundice, weight loss, hepatitis, anemia, ***thromboembolism,*** bone pain, edema, cystitis, fever, vascular pain, lymphadenopathy, eosinophilia, hypokalemia. Discoloration of urine, feces, sweat, or sputum.

LABORATORY TEST CONSIDERATIONS

↑ AST, serum bilirubin, albumin, blood sugar, ESR.

OD OVERDOSE MANAGEMENT

Treatment: Gastric lavage or induction of vomiting. General supportive measures.

HOW SUPPLIED

Capsule: 50 mg

DOSAGE

• **CAPSULES**

Leprosy resistant to dapsone.

100 mg/day together with one or more other leprostatic drugs for a period of 3 years; **maintenance:** clofazimine alone, 100 mg/day.

Erythema nodosum leprosum.

Dosage depends on severity of symptoms, but doses greater than 200 mg/day are not recommended. Goal is 100 mg/day.

NURSING CONSIDERATIONS

ADMINISTRATION/STORAGE

1. Give with one or more other leprostatic agents to prevent the development of resistance to each drug.
2. Clinical improvement can usually be seen after 1–3 months and is clearly evident within 6 months.
3. When treating dapsone-sensitive multibacillary leprosy, give clofazimine with at least two other antileprosy drugs for at least 2 years or until negative skin smears are obtained. Monotherapy can then be instituted.
4. Store capsules below 30°C (86°F) and protect from moisture.

CLIENT/FAMILY TEACHING

1. Take as directed and with food to minimize GI irritation. Should be taken with one or more leprostatic agent to prevent drug resistance.
2. Report any increased GI distress, depression, and/or unusual side effects immediately.
3. Although reversible, clofazimine will cause pink to brownish black skin discoloration, which may persist after therapy.
4. Do not be alarmed; all body fluids become discolored during therapy.
5. Oil baths and frequent lotion application may minimize itchy, dry skin formation.

OUTCOMES/EVALUATE

- Symptomatic improvement
- ↓ Size and number of skin lesions

Clofibrate

(kloh-**FYE**-brayt)

PREGNANCY CATEGORY: C
CLASSIFICATION(S):
Antihyperlipidemic, fibric acid derivative
Rx: Atromid-S

ACTION/KINETICS

Decreases triglycerides and VLDL; cholesterol and LDL are decreased less predictably and less effectively. Mechanism may be due to inhibition of hepatic release of VLDL, potentiation of the action of lipoprotein lipase, and increased fecal excretion of neutral sterols. Cholesterol formation is inhibited early in the biosynthetic chain. **Peak plasma levels:** 3–6 hr. **t½, plasma:** 15 hr. **Therapeutic effect: Onset,** 2–5 days; **maximum effect:** 3 weeks. Triglycerides return to pretreatment levels 2–3 weeks after therapy is terminated. Hydrolyzed to the active *p*-chlorophenoxyisobutyric acid which is further metabolized and excreted in the urine. Drug may concentrate in fetal blood. LFTs should be performed during therapy.

USES

Dysbetalipoproteinemia (type III hyperlipidemia) not responding to diet. Hyperlipidemia (types IV and V) with a risk of abdominal pain and pancreatitis not responding to diet.

CONTRAINDICATIONS

Clinically significant impaired hepatic or renal function, primary biliary cirrhosis, lactation, pregnancy, children.

SPECIAL CONCERNS

Use with caution in clients with gout, peptic ulcer, or with a history of jaundice or hepatic disease. Reduced dosage may be required in geriatric clients due to age-related decreases in renal function. Safety and efficacy have not been determined in children.

SIDE EFFECTS

GI: Nausea, dyspepsia, weight gain, gastritis, vomiting, bloating, flatulence, abdominal distress, stomatitis, loose stools, diarrhea, hepatomegaly, cholelithiasis, gallstones, hepatic abnormalities. **CNS:** Headaches, dizziness, fatigue, weakness, drowsiness. **CV:** Changes in blood-clotting time, arrhythmias, increased or decreased angina, intermittent claudication, thromboembolic events, thrombophlebitis, swelling and phlebitis at xanthoma site, pulmonary embolism. **Skeletal muscle:** Asthenia, arthralgia, myalgia, weakness, muscle cramps, aches, myositis, myopathy, rhabdomyolysis (with or without CPK elevation). **GU:** Impotence, dysuria, hematuria, decreased urine output, decreased libido, proteinuria. **Hematologic:** Anemia, leukopenia, eosinophilia. **Dermatologic:** Allergic reactions, including urticaria, skin rash, dry skin, pruritus, dry brittle hair, alopecia. **Other:** Dyspnea, polyphagia, flu-like symptoms, ***noncardiovascular death.***

LABORATORY TEST CONSIDERATIONS

↑ AST, ALT, thymol turbidity, CPK, BSP retention. Proteinuria.

DRUG INTERACTIONS

Anticoagulants / ↑ Anticoagulant effect by ↓ plasma protein binding
Antidiabetics (sulfonylureas) / ↑ Hypoglycemic effects
Furosemide / Exaggerated diuretic response
Insulin / ↑ Insulin effect
Probenecid / ↑ Therapeutic and toxic effects of clofibrate R/T ↓ liver breakdown and ↓ kidney excretion
Ursodiol / ↑ Risk of gallstone formation

HOW SUPPLIED

Capsule: 500 mg

DOSAGE

• **CAPSULES**

Antihyperlipidemic.

Adults: 500 mg q.i.d. Therapeutic response may take several weeks to become apparent. Drug must be administered on a continuous basis because lowered levels of cholesterol and other lipids will return to elevated state within several weeks after administration is stopped. Discontinue after 3 months if response is poor.

NURSING CONSIDERATIONS

ASSESSMENT

Obtain baseline CBC, liver and renal function studies; document cholesterol profile and pregnancy test if appropriate.

CLIENT/FAMILY TEACHING

1. If GI upset occurs, take with food. Nausea usually decreases with continued therapy or reduced dose.

2. With anticoagulant therapy, report any abnormal bruising/bleeding; may require dose reduction.
3. Report symptoms of hypoglycemia because of possible drug interactions with oral antidiabetic agents.
4. Use contraception during and for several months after drug therapy if pregnancy is planned; drug may be teratogenic.
5. Review potential risks of drug therapy (e.g., gallstones, tumors); report any unusual side effects.
6. Stress importance of adhering to dietary restrictions, daily exercise, weight loss, and regular labs in the overall management of high cholesterol.

OUTCOMES/EVALUATE

Desired ↓ in serum triglyceride levels

Clomiphene citrate

(**KLOH**-mih-feen)

PREGNANCY CATEGORY: X
CLASSIFICATION(S):
Ovarian stimulant
Rx: Clomid, Milophene, Serophene

ACTION/KINETICS

Combines with estrogen receptors, thus decreasing the number of available receptor sites. Through negative feedback, the hypothalamus and pituitary are thus stimulated to increase secretion of LH and FSH. Under the influence of increased levels of these hormones, an ovarian follicle develops, followed by ovulation and corpus luteum development. Most women ovulate after the first course of therapy. Further treatment may be inadvisable if pregnancy fails to occur after ovulatory responses. Readily absorbed from the GI tract and excreted in the feces. **t½:** 5–7 days. **Time to peak effect:** 4–10 days after the last day of treatment for ovulation.

USES

To treat ovulatory failure in women desiring pregnancy and whose partners are fertile and potent. Normal liver function and normal levels of endogenous estrogen are necessary criteria to clomiphene use. Therapy is ineffective in clients with ovarian or pituitary failure. *Investigational:* Male infertility (controversial).

CONTRAINDICATIONS

Pregnancy, liver disease or history thereof, abnormal bleeding of undetermined origin. Ovarian cysts or enlargement not due to polycystic ovarian syndrome. Uncontrolled thyroid or adrenal dysfunction, organic intracranial lesion (e.g., pituitary tumor). The absence of neoplastic disease should be established before treatment is initiated.

SPECIAL CONCERNS

Multiple births are possible.

SIDE EFFECTS

Ovarian: Ovarian overstimulation/enlargement and subsequent symptoms resembling those of PMS. **Ophthalmologic:** Blurred vision, spots, or flashes, may be due to intensification of after images. Although cause and effect have not been established, the following have been noted in users of clomiphene: posterior capsular cataract, detachment of the posterior vitreous, spasm of retinal arteriole, and thrombosis of temporal arteries of retina. **GI:** Abdominal distention/pain/bloating/soreness; N&V. **GU:** Abnormal uterine bleeding, breast tenderness, increased urination. **CNS:** Insomnia, nervousness, headache, depression, fatigue, lightheadedness, dizziness. **Other:** Hot flashes, allergic dermatitis, urticaria, weight gain, alopecia (reversible).

LABORATORY TEST CONSIDERATIONS

↑ Serum thyroxine, thyroxine-binding globulin, BSP retention.

HOW SUPPLIED

Tablet: 50 mg

DOSAGE

- **TABLETS**

First course.

50 mg/day for 5 days. Therapy may be initiated at any time in clients who have had no recent uterine bleeding.

Second course.

Same dosage if ovulation has occurred. In absence of ovulation, dose may be increased to 100 mg/day for 5 days. This course may be started as early as 30 days after the previous one.

Third course.
Most clients who are going to respond will do so during the first course of therapy. Three courses are an adequate therapeutic trial. If ovulatory menses has not occurred, reevaluate diagnosis.

NURSING CONSIDERATIONS

ADMINISTRATION/STORAGE

If client has had recent uterine bleeding, start therapy on the fifth day of the cycle.

ASSESSMENT

1. Obtain menstrual history and any history of abnormal bleeding of undetermined origin.
2. Note history of hepatic dysfunction; document LFTs and abdominal US.
3. Determine if pregnant.

CLIENT/FAMILY TEACHING

1. Take basal temperature and chart on graph to determine if ovulation has occurred; usually 4–10 days after treatment.
2. Take at the same time each day.
3. Discontinue drug and report if pain in the pelvic area or abdominal distention occurs; may indicate ovarian enlargement, presence of an ovarian cyst or rupture.
4. Stop drug if blurred vision or spots or flashes in the eyes occur and report for eye exam.
5. Avoid performing hazardous tasks involving body coordination or mental alertness; drug may cause lightheadedness, dizziness, or visual disturbances.
6. Stop drug and report if pregnancy is suspected; drug may have teratogenic effects.
7. Potential for multiple pregnancy exists.

OUTCOMES/EVALUATE

- ↑ Levels of FSH and LH
- Ovulation → pregnancy

Clonazepam

(kloh-**NAY**-zeh-pam)

CLASSIFICATION(S):
Anticonvulsant, miscellaneous

Rx: Klonopin **C-IV**
✱**Rx:** Alti-Clonazepam, Apo-Clonazepam, Clonapam, Gen-Clonazepam, Novo-Clonazepam, Nu-Clonazepam, PMS–Clonazepam, Rho-Clonazepam, Rivotril

SEE ALSO *ANTICONVULSANTS.*

ACTION/KINETICS

Benzodiazepine derivative which increases presynaptic inhibition and suppresses the spread of seizure activity. **Peak plasma levels:** 1–2 hr. **t½:** 18–50 hr. **Therapeutic serum levels:** 20–80 ng/mL. About 97% bound to plasma protein; metabolized almost completely in the liver to inactive metabolites, which are excreted in the urine.

Even though a benzodiazepine, clonazepam is used only as an anticonvulsant. However, contraindications, side effects, and so forth are similar to those for diazepam.

USES

Absence seizures (petit mal) including Lennox-Gastaut syndrome, akinetic and myoclonic seizures. Some effectiveness in clients resistant to succinimide therapy. *Investigational:* Parkinsonian dysarthria, acute manic episodes of bipolar affective disorder, leg movements (periodic) during sleep, adjunct in treating schizophrenia, neuralgias, multifocal tic disorders.

CONTRAINDICATIONS

Sensitivity to benzodiazepines. Severe liver disease, acute narrow-angle glaucoma. Pregnancy.

SPECIAL CONCERNS

Effects on lactation not known.

ADDITIONAL SIDE EFFECTS

In clients in whom different types of seizure disorders exist, clonazepam may elicit or precipitate ***grand mal seizures.***

DRUG INTERACTIONS

CNS depressants / Potentiation of clonazepam CNS depressant effect
Phenobarbital / ↓ Clonazepam effect R/T ↑ liver breakdown
Phenytoin / ↓ Clonazepam effect R/T ↑ liver breakdown

Valproic acid / ↑ Chance of absence seizures

HOW SUPPLIED

Tablet: 0.5 mg, 1 mg, 2 mg

DOSAGE

• TABLETS

Seizure disorders.

Adults, initial: 0.5 mg t.i.d. Increase by 0.5–1 mg/day q 3 days until seizures are under control or side effects become excessive; **maximum:** 20 mg/day. **Pediatric up to 10 years or 30 kg:** 0.01–0.03 mg/kg/day in two to three divided doses up to a maximum of 0.05 mg/kg/day. Increase by increments of 0.25–0.5 mg q 3 days until seizures are under control or maintenance of 0.1–0.2 mg/kg is attained.

Parkinsonian dysarthria.

Adults: 0.25–0.5 mg/day.

Acute manic episodes of bipolar affective disorder.

Adults: 0.75–16 mg/day.

Periodic leg movements during sleep.

Adults: 0.5–2 mg nightly.

Adjunct to treat schizophrenia.

Adults: 0.5–2 mg/day.

Neuralgias.

Adults: 2–4 mg/day.

Multifocal tic disorders.

Adults: 1.5–12 mg/day.

NURSING CONSIDERATIONS

SEE ALSO *NURSING CONSIDERATIONS* FOR *HYPNOTICS*, AND *ANTICONVULSANTS*.

ADMINISTRATION/STORAGE

1. About one-third of clients show some loss of anticonvulsant activity within 3 mo; dosage adjustment may reestablish effectiveness.
2. Adding clonazepam to existing anticonvulsant therapy may increase the depressant effects.
3. Divide the daily dose in three equal doses; if doses cannot be divided equally, give the largest dose at bedtime.

ASSESSMENT

1. Document indications for therapy, onset/cause of symptoms, other agents prescribed, and the outcome.
2. Obtain baseline CBC, renal and LFTs.

CLIENT/FAMILY TEACHING

1. Take as directed; report any loss of seizure control or adverse side effects.
2. Assess drug effects before performing activities that require mental alertness.

OUTCOMES/EVALUATE

↓ Number and frequency of recurrent seizures

Clonidine hydrochloride

(**KLOH**-nih-deen)

PREGNANCY CATEGORY: C

CLASSIFICATION(S):

Antihypertensive, centrally-acting

Rx: Catapres, Catapres-TTS-1, -2, and -3, Duraclon

✱Rx: Apo-Clonidine, Dixarit, Novo–Clonidine, Nu-Clonidine

SEE ALSO *ANTIHYPERTENSIVE AGENTS*.

ACTION/KINETICS

Stimulates alpha-adrenergic receptors of the CNS, which results in inhibition of the sympathetic vasomotor centers and decreased nerve impulses. Thus, bradycardia and a fall in both SBP and DBP occur. Plasma renin levels are decreased, while peripheral venous pressure remains unchanged. Few orthostatic effects. Although NaCl excretion is markedly decreased, potassium excretion remains unchanged. To relieve spasticity, it decreases excitatory amino acids by central presynaptic α–receptor agonism. Tolerance to the drug may develop. **Onset, PO:** 30–60 min; **transdermal:** 2–3 days. **Peak plasma levels, PO:** 3–5 hr; **transdermal:** 2–3 days. **Maximum effect, PO:** 2–4 hr. **Duration, PO:** 12–24 hr; **transdermal:** 7 days (with system in place). **t½:** 12–16 hr. Approximately 50% excreted unchanged in the urine; 20% excreted through the feces.

The transdermal dosage form contains the following levels of drug: Catapres-TTS-1 contains 2.5 mg clonidine (surface area 3.5 cm^2), with 0.1 mg released daily; Catapres-TTS-2 contains 5 mg clonidine (surface area 7 cm^2), with 0.2 mg released daily; and Catapres-TTS-3 contains 7.5 mg clonidine (surface area 10.5 cm^2), with 0.3 mg released daily.

Epidural use causes analgesia at presynaptic and postjunctional alpha-2-adrenergic receptors in the spinal cord due to prevention of pain signal transmission to the brain. **t½, distribution, epidural:** 19 min; **elimination:** 22 hr.

USES

Oral, Transdermal: Mild to moderate hypertension. A diuretic or other antihypertensive drugs, or both, are often used concomitantly. Treat spasticity. *Investigational:* Alcohol withdrawal, atrial fibrillation, attention deficit hyperactivity disorder, constitutional growth delay in children, cyclosporine-associated nephrotoxicity, diabetic diarrhea, Gilles de la Tourette's syndrome, hyperhidrosis, hypertensive emergencies, mania, menopausal flushing, opiate detoxification, diagnosis of pheochromocytoma, postherpetic neuralgia, psychosis in schizophrenia, reduce allergen-induced inflammatory reactions in extrinsic asthma, restless leg syndrome, facilitate smoking cessation, ulcerative colitis.

Epidural: With opiates for severe pain in cancer clients not relieved by opiate analgesics alone. Most effective for neuropathic pain.

CONTRAINDICATIONS

Epidurally: Presence of an injection site infection, clients on anticoagulant therapy, in bleeding diathesis, administration above the C4 dermatome. For obstetric, postpartum, or perioperative pain.

SPECIAL CONCERNS

Use with caution during lactation and in the presence of severe coronary insufficiency, recent MI, cerebrovascular disease, or chronic renal failure. Safe use in children not established; when used for attention deficit disorder, even one extra dose can be harmful. Geriatric clients may be more sensitive to the hypotensive effects; a decreased dosage may also be necessary in these clients due to age-related decreases in renal function. For children, restrict epidural use to severe intractable pain from malignancy that is not responsive to epidural or spinal opiates or other analgesic approaches.

SIDE EFFECTS

CNS: Drowsiness (common), sedation, confusion, dizziness, headache, fatigue, malaise, nightmares, nervousness, restlessness, anxiety, mental depression, increased dreaming, insomnia, hallucinations, delirium, agitation. **GI:** Dry mouth (common), constipation, anorexia, N&V, parotid pain, weight gain, hepatitis, parotitis, ileus, pseudo-obstruction, abdominal pain. **CV:** CHF, severe hypotension, Raynaud's phenomenon, abnormalities in ECG, palpitations, tachycardia/bradycardia, postural hypotension, conduction disturbances, sinus bradycardia, ***CVA***. **Dermatologic:** Urticaria, skin rashes, sweating, ***angioneurotic edema,*** pruritus, thinning of hair, alopecia, skin ulcer. **GU:** Impotence, urinary retention, decreased sexual activity, loss of libido, nocturia, difficulty in urination, UTI. **Respiratory:** Hypoventilation, dyspnea. **Musculoskeletal:** Muscle or joint pain, leg cramps, weakness. **Other:** Gynecomastia, increase in blood glucose (transient), increased sensitivity to alcohol, chest pain, tinnitus, hyperaesthesia, pain, infection, thrombocytopenia, syncope, blurred vision, withdrawal syndrome, dryness of mucous membranes of nose; itching, burning, dryness of eyes; skin pallor, fever.

NOTE: When used for ADHD in children, can cause serious side effects, including bradycardia, hypotension, and respiratory depression.

Transdermal products: Localized skin reactions, pruritus, erythema, allergic contact sensitization and contact dermatitis, localized vesiculation, hyperpigmentation, edema, excoriation, burning, papules, throbbing, blanching, generalized macular rash.

NOTE: Rebound hypertension may be manifested if clonidine is withdrawn abruptly.

LABORATORY TEST CONSIDERATIONS
Transient ↑ blood glucose, serum phosphatase, and serum CPK. Weakly + Coombs' test. Alteration of electrolyte balance.

OD OVERDOSE MANAGEMENT
Symptoms: Hypotension, bradycardia, respiratory and CNS depression, hypoventilation, hypothermia, apnea, miosis, agitation, irritability, lethargy, ***seizures, cardiac conduction defects, arrhythmias,*** transient hypertension, diarrhea, vomiting. *Treatment:* Maintain respiration; perform gastric lavage followed by activated charcoal. Magnesium sulfate may be used to hasten the rate of transport through the GI tract. IV atropine sulfate (0.6 mg for adults; 0.01 mg/kg for children). Epinephrine, tolazoline, or dopamine to treat persistent bradycardia. IV fluids and elevation of the legs are used to reverse hypotension; if unresponsive to these measures, dopamine (2–20 mcg/kg/min) or tolazoline (1 mg/kg IV, up to a maximum of 10 mg/dose) may be used. To treat hypertension, diazoxide, IV furosemide, or an alpha-adrenergic blocking drug may be used.

DRUG INTERACTIONS
Alcohol / ↑ Depressant effects
Beta-adrenergic blocking agents / Paradoxical hypertension; also, ↑ severity of rebound hypertension following clonidine withdrawal
CNS depressants / ↑ CNS depressant effect
Levodopa / ↓ Levodopa effect
Local anesthetics / Epidural clonidine → prolonged duration of epidural local anesthetics
Mirtazapine / Loss of BP control due to antagonism of α–2 adrenergic receptors
Prazosin / ↓ Clonidine antihypertensive effect
Narcotic analgesics / Potentiation of clonidine hypotensive effect
Tolazoline / Blocks antihypertensive effect
Tricyclic antidepressants / Blocks antihypertensive effect
Verapamil / ↑ Risk of AV block and severe hypotension

HOW SUPPLIED
Film, Extended Release, Transdermal: 0.1 mg/24 hr, 0.2 mg/24 hr, 0.3 mg/24 hr; *Injection:* 0.1/mL, 0.5 mg/mL; *Tablet:* 0.1 mg, 0.2 mg, 0.3 mg

DOSAGE

• TABLETS

Hypertension.
Initial: 100 mcg b.i.d.; **then,** increase by 100–200 mcg/day until desired response is attained; **maintenance:** 200–600 mcg/day in divided doses (maximum: 2400 mcg/day). Tolerance necessitates increased dosage or concomitant administration of a diuretic. Gradual increase of dosage after initiation minimizes side effects. **Pediatric:** 50–400 mcg b.i.d.
NOTE: In hypertensive clients unable to take PO medication, clonidine may be administered sublingually at doses of 200–400 mcg/day.

Treat spasticity.
Adults and children: 0.1–0.3 mg/day, given in divided doses.

Alcohol withdrawal.
300–600 mcg q 6 hr.

Atrial fibrillation.
75 mcg 1–2 times/day with or without digoxin.

Attention deficit hyperactivity disorder.
5 mcg/kg/day for 8 weeks.

Constitutional growth delay in children.
37.5–150 mcg/m²/day.

Diabetic diarrhea.
100–600 mcg q 12 hr.

Gilles de la Tourette syndrome.
150–200 mcg/day.

Hyperhidrosis.
250 mcg 3–5 times/day.

Hypertensive urgency (diastolic > 120 mm Hg).
Initial: 100–200 mcg; **then,** 50– 100 mcg q hr to a maximum of 800 mcg.

Menopausal flushing.
100–400 mcg/day.

Withdrawal from opiate dependence.
15–16 mcg/kg/day.

Diagnosis of pheochromocytoma.
300 mcg/day.

Postherpetic neuralgia.
200 mcg/day.

Psychosis in schizophrenia.
Less than 900 mcg/day.

Reduce allergen-induced inflammation in extrinsic asthma.
150 mcg for 3 days or 75 mcg/1.5 mL saline by inhalation.

Restless leg syndrome.
100–300 mcg/day, up to 900 mcg/day.

Facilitate cessation of smoking.
150–750 mcg/day for 3–10 weeks.

Ulcerative colitis.
300 mcg t.i.d.

• **TRANSDERMAL**

Hypertension.
Initial: Use 0.1-mg system; **then,** if after 1–2 weeks adequate control has not been achieved, can use another 0.1-mg system or a larger system. The antihypertensive effect may not be seen for 2–3 days. The system should be changed q 7 days.

Treat spasticity.
Adults and children: 0.1–0.3 mg; apply patch q 7 days.

Cyclosporine-associated nephrotoxicity.
100–200 mcg/day.

Diabetic diarrhea.
0.3 mg/24 hr patch (1 or 2 patches/week).

Menopausal flushing.
100 mcg/24-hr patch.

Facilitate cessation of smoking.
200 mcg/24-hr patch.

• **EPIDURAL INFUSION**

Analgesia.
Initial: 30 mcg/hr. Dose may then be titrated up or down, depending on pain relief and side effects.

NURSING CONSIDERATIONS

SEE ALSO *NURSING CONSIDERATIONS* FOR *ANTIHYPERTENSIVE AGENTS.*

ADMINISTRATION/STORAGE

1. It may take 2–3 days to achieve effective blood levels using the transdermal system. Therefore, reduce any prior drug dosage gradually.
2. Clients with severe hypertension may require other antihypertensive drug therapy in addition to transdermal clonidine.
3. If the drug is to be discontinued, do gradually over a period of 2–4 days.
4. Do not use a preservative when given epidurally.
5. Store injection at controlled room temperature. Discard any unused portion.

ASSESSMENT

1. Document indications for therapy, onset, type of symptoms, and previous treatments.
2. Obtain baseline CBC, liver and renal function studies.
3. Note occupation; drug may interfere with the ability to work.
4. List drugs currently prescribed to prevent any interactions. With propranolol, observe for a paradoxical hypertensive response. With tolazoline or TCA, be aware that these may block the antihypertensive action of clonidine; clonidine dosage may need to be increased
5. Note evidence of alcohol, drug, or nicotine addiction. These agents usually work well for BP control in this group of clients (especially the once-a-week patch).
6. Initially, monitor BP closely. BP decreases occur within 30–60 min after administration and may persist for 8 hr. Note any fluctuations to determine whether to use clonidine alone or concomitantly with a diuretic. A stable BP reduces orthostatic effects with postural changes.

CLIENT/FAMILY TEACHING

1. With the transdermal system, apply to a hairless area of skin, such as upper arm or torso. Change the system q 7 days and use a different site with each application.
2. If taken PO, take last dose of the day at bedtime to ensure overnight control of BP.
3. Do not engage in activities that require mental alertness, such as operating machinery or driving a car; may cause drowsiness.
4. Do not change regimen or discontinue drug abruptly. Withdrawal should be gradual to prevent rebound hypertension.

5. Record weight daily, in the morning, in clothing of the same weight, to determine if there is edema caused by sodium retention. Any fluid retention should disappear after 3–4 days.
6. Clonidine may reduce the effect of levodopa; report any increase in the S&S of Parkinson's disease previously controlled with levodopa.
7. Report any depression (may be precipitated by drug), especially with history of mental depression.

OUTCOMES/EVALUATE

- ↓ BP; ↓ menopausal S&S
- Control of withdrawal symptoms
- Control of neuropathic pain

Clopidogrel bisulfate

(kloh-**PID**-oh-grel)

PREGNANCY CATEGORY: B
CLASSIFICATION(S):
Antiplatelet drug
Rx: Plavix

ACTION/KINETICS

Inhibits platelet aggregation by inhibiting binding of adenosine diphosphate (ADP) to its platelet receptor and subsequent ADP-mediative activation of glycoprotein GPIIb/IIIa complex. Modifies receptor irreversibly; thus, platelets are affected for remainder of their lifespan. Also inhibits platelet aggregation caused by agonists other than ADP by blocking amplification of platelet activation by released ADP. Rapidly absorbed from GI tract; food does not affect bioavailability. **Peak plasma levels:** About 1 hr. Extensively metabolized in liver; about 50% excreted in urine and 46% in feces. **t½, elimination:** 8 hr.

USES

Reduction of MI, stroke, and vascular death in clients with atherosclerosis documented by recent stroke, MI, or established peripheral arterial disease. *Investigational:* With aspirin to pretreat clients with acute coronary syndrome undergoing percutaneous coronary intervention (improves outcome). With aspirin to treat clients with non-ST-segment elevation acute coronary syndromes whether or not they undergo percutaneous coronary intervention.

CONTRAINDICATIONS

Lactation. Active pathological bleeding such as peptic ulcer or intracranial hemorrhage.

SPECIAL CONCERNS

Use with caution in those at risk of increased bleeding from trauma, surgery, or other pathological conditions. Safety and efficacy have not been determined in children.

SIDE EFFECTS

CV: Edema, hypertension, ***intracranial hemorrhage***. **GI:** Abdominal pain, dyspepsia, diarrhea, nausea, hemorrhage, ulcers (peptic, gastric, duodenal). **CNS:** Headache, dizziness, depression. **Body as a whole:** Chest pain, accidental injury, flu-like symptoms, pain, fatigue. **Respiratory:** URTI, dyspnea, rhinitis, bronchitis, coughing. **Hematologic:** Purpura, thrombotic thrombocytopenic purpura, epistaxis. **Musculoskeletal:** Arthralgia, back pain. **Dermatologic:** Disorders of skin/appendages, rash, pruritus. **Miscellaneous:** UTI.

LABORATORY TEST CONSIDERATIONS

Hypercholesterolemia.

DRUG INTERACTIONS

H *Evening primrose oil* / Potential for ↑ antiplatelet effect
H *Feverfew* / Potential for ↑ antiplatelet effect
H *Garlic* / Potential for ↑ antiplatelet effect
H *Ginger* / Potential for ↑ antiplatelet effect
H *Ginkgo biloba* / Potential for ↑ antiplatelet effect
H *Grapeseed extract* / Potential for ↑ antiplatelet effect
NSAIDs / ↑ Risk of occult blood loss
Warfarin / Clopidogrel prolongs bleeding time; safety of use with warfarin not established

HOW SUPPLIED

Tablets: 75 mg

DOSAGE

- **TABLETS**

Reduction of atherosclerotic events.

Adults: 75 mg once daily with or without food.

NURSING CONSIDERATIONS

ADMINISTRATION/STORAGE

Dosage adjustment not necessary for geriatric clients or with renal disease.

ASSESSMENT

1. Document atherosclerotic event (MI, stroke) or established peripheral arterial disease requiring therapy.
2. Assess for any active bleeding as with ulcers or intracranial bleeding.

CLIENT/FAMILY TEACHING

1. Take exactly as directed; may take without regard to food.
2. Avoid OTC agents especially aspirin and NSAIDs unless prescribed.
3. Report any unusual bruising or bleeding; advise all providers of prescribed therapy.
4. Drug should be discontinued 7 days prior to elective surgery.

OUTCOMES/EVALUATE

- Inhibition of platelet aggregation
- Reduction of atherosclerotic events

Clorazepate dipotassium

(klor-**AYZ**-eh-payt)

PREGNANCY CATEGORY: D
CLASSIFICATION(S):
Antianxiety drug, benzodiazepine; anticonvulsant, miscellaneous
Rx: Gen-Xene, Tranxene, Tranxene-SD, Tranxene-SD Half Strength, Tranxene-T **C-IV**
✱Rx: Apo-Clorazepate, Novo-Clopate

SEE ALSO *TRANQUILIZERS*.

ACTION/KINETICS

Peak plasma levels: 1–2 hr. **t½:** 40–50 hr. Hydrolyzed in the stomach to desmethyldiazepam, the active metabolite. Oxazepam is also an active metabolite. **t½, desmethyldiazepam:** 30–100 hr; **t½, oxazepam:** 5–15 hr. **Time to peak plasma levels:** 0.5–2 hr. Bound 97%–98% to plasma protein and slowly excreted by the kidneys.

USES

Anxiety, tension. Acute alcohol withdrawal, as adjunct in treatment of seizures. Adjunct for treating partial seizures.

ADDITIONAL CONTRAINDICATIONS

Depressed clients, nursing mothers.

SPECIAL CONCERNS

Use with caution with impaired renal or hepatic function.

HOW SUPPLIED

Capsule: 3.75 mg, 7.5 mg, 15 mg; *Tablet:* 3.75 mg, 7.5 mg, 15 mg; *Tablet, Extended Release:* 11.25 mg, 22.5 mg

DOSAGE

• EXTENDED-RELEASE TABLETS, TABLETS, CAPSULES

Anxiety.

Initial: 7.5–15 mg b.i.d.–q.i.d.; **maintenance:** 15–60 mg/day in divided doses. **Elderly or debilitated clients, initial:** 7.5–15 mg/day. **Alternative.** Single daily dosage: **Adult, initial,** 15 mg; **then,** 11.25–22.5 mg once daily.

Acute alcohol withdrawal.

Day 1, initial: 30 mg; **then,** 15 mg b.i.d.–q.i.d. the first day; **day 2:** 45–90 mg in divided doses; **day 3:** 22.5–45 mg in divided doses; **day 4:** 15–30 mg in divided doses. Thereafter, reduce to 7.5/day and discontinue as soon as possible. Maximum daily dose: 90 mg.

Partial seizures.

Adults and children over 12 years, initial: 7.5 mg t.i.d.; increase no more than 7.5 mg/week to maximum of 90 mg/day. **Children (9–12 years), initial:** 7.5 mg b.i.d.; increase by no more than 7.5 mg/week to maximum of 60 mg/day. Not recommended for children under 9 years of age.

NURSING CONSIDERATIONS

SEE ALSO *NURSING CONSIDERATIONS FOR TRANQUILIZERS/ANTIMANIC DRUGS/HYPNOTICS*.

ASSESSMENT

1. Note indications for therapy and characteristics; assess for evidence of depression.
2. With excessive alcohol intake, determine time of last drink.

CLIENT/FAMILY TEACHING

1. Avoid activities requiring mental alertness until drug effects realized.
2. Avoid alcohol and any other CNS depressants.

OUTCOMES/EVALUATE

- ↓ Anxiety and tension
- ↓ S&S of alcohol withdrawal
- Control of seizures

Clotrimazole

(kloh-**TRY**-mah-zohl)

PREGNANCY CATEGORY: C (SYSTEMIC USE); B (TOPICAL/VAGINAL USE)
CLASSIFICATION(S):
Antifungal
Rx: Fungoid, Lotrimin, Mycelex Twin Pack, Mycelex-G
OTC: FemCare, Gyne-Lotrimin 3, Gyne-Lotrimin 3 Combination Pack, Gyne-Lotrimin 7, Gyne-Lotrimin Combination Pack, Lotrimin AF, Mycelex OTC, Mycelex-7, Neo-Zol, Prescription Strength Desenex, Sweet'n Fresh Clotrimazole-7, Mycelex-7 Combination Pack
✱OTC: Canesten Topical/Vaginal, Clotrimaderm, Scheinpharm Clotrimazole

SEE ALSO *ANTI-INFECTIVES*.

ACTION/KINETICS

Depending on concentration, may be fungistatic or fungicidal. Acts by inhibiting the biosynthesis of sterols, resulting in damage to the cell wall and subsequent loss of essential intracellular elements due to altered permeability. May also inhibit oxidative and peroxidative enzyme activity and inhibit the biosynthesis of triglycerides and phospholipids by fungi. When used for *Candida albicans,* the drug inhibits transformation of blastophores into the invasive mycelial form. Poorly absorbed from the GI tract and metabolized in the liver to inactive compounds that are excreted through the feces. **Duration:** up to 3 hr.

USES

Broad-spectrum antifungal. **Oral troche:** Oropharyngeal candidiasis. Reduce incidence of oropharyngeal candidiasis in clients who are immunocompromised due to chemotherapy, radiotherapy, or steroid therapy used for leukemia, solid tumors, or kidney transplant. **Topical OTC products:** Treat tinea pedis, tinea cruris, and tinea corporis due to *T. rubrum, T. mentagrophytes, E. floccosum,* and *M. canis.* **Topical Rx products:** Treat candidiasis due to *C. albicans* and tinea versicolor due to *M. furfur.* **Vaginal products:** Vulvovaginal candidiasis.

CONTRAINDICATIONS

Hypersensitivity. First trimester of pregnancy. Topically in children less than 2 years of age. Use around the eyes.

SPECIAL CONCERNS

Use with caution during lactation. Safety and effectiveness for PO use in children age 3 or under has not been determined. For topical use, supervise children under age12.

SIDE EFFECTS

Skin: Irritation including rash, stinging, pruritus, urticaria, erythema, burning, peeling, blistering, edema. **Vaginal:** Lower abdominal cramps; urinary frequency; bloating; vaginal irritation, itching or burning; dyspareunia. **Hepatic:** Abnormal liver function tests. **GI:** N&V following use of troche.

HOW SUPPLIED

Topical: *Cream:* 1%; *Lotion:* 1%; *Solution:* 1%. **Oral: Troche:** 10 mg. **Vaginal:** *Cream:* 1%, 2%; **Combination/Twin Packs:** Suppositories/Cream: 100 mg/1%, 200 mg/1%; **Suppositories:** 200 mg

DOSAGE

• TROCHE

Treatment of oropharyngeal candidiasis.

One troche (10 mg) 5 times/day for 14 consecutive days.

Prophylaxis of oropharyngeal candidiasis.

One troche t.i.d. for duration of chemotherapy or until maintenance doses of steroids are instituted.

• TOPICAL CREAM, LOTION, SOLUTION (EACH 1%)

OTC for Tinea pedis/corporis.

Use daily for 4 weeks. If no improvement, consult provider.

OTC for Tinea cruris.
Use daily for 2 weeks. If no improvement, consult provider.
OTC cream for vaginal yeast infections.
Apply to affected areas morning and evening for 7 consecutive days or as needed.
Rx for candidiasis and tinea versicolor.
Massage into affected skin and surrounding areas b.i.d. in morning and evening. Diagnosis should be reevaluated if no improvement occurs in 4 weeks.

- **VAGINAL SUPPOSITORIES**

Insert 1 suppository (200 mg) at bedtime for 3 consecutive days.

- **VAGINAL CREAM**

Insert one full applicator at bedtime for 3–7 consecutive days.

NURSING CONSIDERATIONS

SEE ALSO *GENERAL NURSING CONSIDERATIONS* FOR *ANTI-INFECTIVES.*

ADMINISTRATION/STORAGE

1. Store Mycelex-G vaginal cream at 2–30°C (36–86°F). Do not store Mycelex-G 100-mg vaginal troche above 35°C (95°F); store the 500-mg vaginal troche below 30°C (86°F).
2. Slowly dissolve the troche in the mouth.
3. Do not allow topical products to come in contact with the eyes.

CLIENT/FAMILY TEACHING

1. Review goals of therapy; appropriate method for administration. Wash hands before and after treatments. Unless otherwise directed, apply only after cleaning the affected area.
2. With vaginal infections, do not engage in intercourse; or, to prevent reinfection, have partner wear a condom.
3. To prevent staining of clothes, use a sanitary napkin with vaginal tablets or cream.
4. If exposed to HIV and recurrent vaginal yeast infections occur, seek prompt medical intervention to determine cause of the symptoms.

OUTCOMES/EVALUATE

- Eradication of fungal infection
- Symptomatic improvement

Cloxacillin sodium

(klox-ah-**SILL**-in)

PREGNANCY CATEGORY: B
CLASSIFICATION(S):
Antibiotic, penicillin
Rx: Cloxapen
✱Rx: Apo-Cloxi, Novo-Cloxin, Nu-Cloxi

SEE ALSO *ANTI-INFECTIVES* AND *PENICILLINS.*

ACTION/KINETICS

Penicillinase resistant and acid stable. **Peak plasma levels:** 7–15 mcg/mL after 30–60 min. **t½:** 30 min. Protein binding: 95%. Well absorbed from GI tract. Mostly excreted in urine, but some excreted in bile.

USES

Infections caused by penicillinase-producing staphylococci, including pneumococci, group A beta-hemolytic streptococci, and penicillin G-sensitive and penicillin G-resistant staphylococci.

HOW SUPPLIED

Capsule: 250 mg, 500 mg; *Powder for Oral Suspension:* 125 mg/5 mL when reconstituted

DOSAGE

- **CAPSULES, ORAL SOLUTION**

Skin and soft tissue infections, mild to moderate URTIs.
Adults and children over 20 kg: 250 mg q 6 hr; **pediatric, less than 20 kg:** 50 mg/kg/day in divided doses q 6 hr.
Lower respiratory tract infections or disseminated infections.
Adults and children over 20 kg: 500 mg q 6 hr; **pediatric, less than 20 kg:** 100 mg/kg/day in divided doses q 6 hr. Alternatively, a dose of 50–100 mg/kg/day (up to a maximum of 4 g/day) divided q 6 hr may be used for infants and children.

NURSING CONSIDERATIONS

SEE ALSO *NURSING CONSIDERATIONS* FOR *PENICILLINS.*

ADMINISTRATION/STORAGE

1. To reconstitute the oral solution, add amount of water stated on label in

two portions; shake well after each addition.
2. Shake well before pouring each dose.
3. Refrigerate reconstituted solution and discard unused portion after 14 days.

ASSESSMENT

Note any sensitivity to penicillin; obtain baseline CBC, LFTs, and cultures.

CLIENT/FAMILY TEACHING

1. Review appropriate guidelines for administration; include frequency and amount. Shake well before using; refrigerate and discard after 14 days.
2. Take as directed, 1 hr before or 2 hr after meals; food interferes with drug absorption.
3. Complete prescription despite feeling better. Report lack of improvement or worsening of S&S.

OUTCOMES/EVALUATE

- Eradication of infection
- ↓ Fever, ↓ WBCs, improved symptoms

Clozapine

(**KLOH**-zah-peen)

PREGNANCY CATEGORY: B
CLASSIFICATION(S):
Antipsychotic
Rx: Clozaril

ACTION/KINETICS

Interferes with the binding of dopamine to both D-1 and D-2 receptors; more active at limbic than at striatal dopamine receptors. Thus, is relatively free from extrapyramidal side effects and does not induce catalepsy. Also acts as an antagonist at adrenergic, cholinergic, histaminergic, and serotonergic receptors. Increases the amount of time spent in REM sleep. Food does not affect the bioavailability of clozapine. **Peak plasma levels:** 2.5 hr. **Average maximum concentration at steady state:** 122 ng/mL plasma after 100 mg b.i.d. Highly bound to plasma proteins. **t½:** 12 hr. Metabolized in the liver to inactive compounds and excreted through the urine (50%) and feces (30%).

USES

Severely ill schizophrenic clients who do not respond adequately to conventional antipsychotic therapy, either because of ineffectiveness or intolerable side effects from other drugs. May be effective in chronic refractory schizophrenia. Due to the possibility of development of agranulocytosis and seizures, avoid continued use in clients failing to respond.

CONTRAINDICATIONS

Myeloproliferative disorders. Use in those with a history of clozapine–induced agranulocytosis or severe granulocytopenia; use with other agents known to suppress bone marrow function. Severe CNS depression or coma due to any cause. Lactation.

SPECIAL CONCERNS

Use with caution in clients with known CV disease, prostatic hypertrophy, narrow angle glaucoma, hepatic or renal disease.

SIDE EFFECTS

Hematologic: *Agranulocytosis,* leukopenia, neutropenia, eosinophilia. **CNS: *Seizures*** (appear to be dose dependent), drowsiness/sedation, dizziness, vertigo, headache, tremor, restlessness, nightmares, hypokinesia, akinesia, agitation, akathisia, confusion, rigidity, fatigue, insomnia, hyperkinesia, weakness, lethargy, slurred speech, ataxia, depression, anxiety, epileptiform movements. **CV:** Orthostatic hypotension (especially initially), tachycardia, syncope, hypertension, angina, chest pain, ***cardiac abnormalities,*** changes in ECG. **Neuroleptic malignant syndrome: *Hyperpyrexia,*** muscle rigidity, altered mental status, irregular pulse or BP, tachycardia, diaphoresis, cardiac dysrhythmias. **GI:** Constipation, nausea, heartburn, abdominal discomfort, vomiting, diarrhea, anorexia. **GU:** Urinary abnormalities, incontinence, abnormal ejaculation, urinary frequency/urgency/retention. **Musculoskeletal:** Muscle weakness, pain (back, legs, neck), muscle spasm/ache. **Respiratory:** Dyspnea, SOB, throat discomfort, nasal congestion. **Miscellaneous:** Salivation, sweating, visual disturbances, fever (transient), dry mouth, rash, weight gain, numb or sore tongue.

LABORATORY TEST CONSIDERATIONS
Hyperprolactinemia.

OD OVERDOSE MANAGEMENT
Symptoms: Drowsiness, delirium, tachycardia, ***respiratory depression,*** hypotension, hypersalivation, ***seizures, coma.*** *Treatment:* Establish airway; maintain with adequate oxygenation and ventilation. Give activated charcoal and sorbitol. Monitor cardiac status and VS. General supportive measures.

DRUG INTERACTIONS
Anticholinergic drugs / Additive anticholinergic effects
Antihypertensive drugs / Additive hypotensive effects
Benzodiazepines / Possible respiratory depression/collapse
Digoxin / ↑ Digoxin effect R/T ↓ plasma protein binding
Epinephrine / Clozapine may reverse effects when given for hypotension
Phenobarbital / ↓ Clozapine plasma levels R/T ↑ liver breakdown
H *St. John's wort* / Possible ↓ clozapine plasma levels R/T ↑ metabolism
Warfarin / ↑ Warfarin effect R/T ↓ plasma protein binding

HOW SUPPLIED
Tablet: 25 mg, 100 mg

DOSAGE

• **TABLETS**

Schizophrenia.

Adults, initial: 25 mg 1–2 times/day; **then,** if drug is tolerated, the dose can be increased by 25–50 mg/day to a dose of 300–450 mg/day at the end of 2 weeks. Subsequent dosage increments should occur no more often than once or twice a week in increments not to exceed 100 mg. **Usual maintenance dose:** 300–600 mg/day (although doses up to 900 mg/day may be required in some clients). Total daily dose should not exceed 900 mg.

NURSING CONSIDERATIONS

ADMINISTRATION/STORAGE

1. Clozapine is available through independent "Clozaril treatment systems" based on a plan developed by physicians and pharmacists to ensure safe use of the drug with respect to weekly CBC monitoring, data reporting, and drug dispensing. Prescriptions are limited to 1-week supplies, and the drug may only be dispensed following receipt, by the pharmacist, of weekly WBC test results that fall within the established limits. All weekly blood test results must be reported by participating pharmacists to the Clozaril National Registry.
2. If drug is effective, seek the lowest maintenance doses possible to maintain remission.
3. If termination of therapy is planned, gradually reduce the dose over a 1–2-week period. If cessation of therapy is abrupt due to toxicity, observe client carefully for recurrence of psychotic symptoms.
4. Clozapine therapy may be initiated immediately upon discontinuation of other antipsychotic medication; however, a 24-hr "washout period" is desirable.

ASSESSMENT

1. Document indications for therapy; assess behavioral manifestations. List other therapies trialed and the outcome.
2. Note history of seizure disorder.
3. Document baseline VS and ECG; report any irregular pulse, tachycardia, hyperpyrexia, or hypotension.
4. Obtain CBC and LFTs prior to initiating therapy. If WBCs fall below 2,000/mm^3 or granulocyte counts fall below 1,000/mm^3, the drug should be discontinued. Such clients should *not* be restarted on clozapine therapy.
5. Monitor and report WBCs once weekly for the first six months of therapy, then every 2 weeks if stable.
6. Assess risks versus benefits of therapy with family/client. Periodically reassess to determine continued need for therapy.

CLIENT/FAMILY TEACHING

1. Take only as directed; do not stop abruptly.
2. Report immediately symptoms of lethargy, weakness, fever, sore throat, malaise, mucous membrane ulceration, or signs of infection.

3. Rinse mouth frequently and perform regular oral care to minimize potential for candidiasis.
4. Avoid driving or other hazardous activity due to possibility of seizures.
5. Because of orthostatic hypotension, use care when rising from a supine or sitting position.
6. Avoid hot showers or baths and hot weather exposure.
7. Report if pregnancy occurs or desires to become pregnant.
8. Do not breast-feed.
9. Do not take any prescription drugs, OTC drugs, or alcohol.
10. Stress importance of weekly WBC to assess for agranulocytosis. These are reported to a national registry and must be completed before prescriptions will be issued and filled.

OUTCOMES/EVALUATE

- Improved behavior patterns with ↓ agitation, ↓ hyperactivity, ↓ delusions, paranoia, and hallucinations
- Improved coping behaviors and thought patterns

Coagulation Factor VIIa (Recombinant)

PREGNANCY CATEGORY: C
CLASSIFICATION(S):
Antihemophilic agent
Rx: NovoSeven

ACTION/KINETICS

Structurally similar to human plasma-derived Factor VIIa. The purification process removes exogenous viruses. To eliminate the risk of human viral contamination, no human serum or other proteins are used to produce the product. Promotes hemostasis by activating the intrinsic pathway of the coagulation cascade. When complexed with tissue factor, the drug can activate coagulation Factor X to Factor Xa, as well as coagulation Factor IX to Factor IXa. Factor Xa, in complex with other factors, converts prothrombin to thrombin leading to formation of a hemostatic plug by converting fibrinogen to fibrin. **t½:** 2.3 hr. **Median in vivo plasma recovery:** 44%.

USES

Treatment of bleeding episodes in hemophilia A or B clients with inhibitors to Factor VIII or Factor IX.

CONTRAINDICATIONS

Hypersensitivity to the product or to mouse, hamster, or bovine proteins. Lactation.

SPECIAL CONCERNS

Clients with DIC, advanced artherosclerotic disease, crush injury, or septicemia may have an increased risk of developing thrombotic events.

SIDE EFFECTS

CV: Hemorrhage NOS, decreased plasma fibrinogen, hypertension, bradycardia, coagulation disorder, DIC, increased fibrinolysis, hypotension, decreased prothrombin, thrombosis. **Dermatologic:** Injection site reaction, pruritus, purpura, rash. **Hypersensitivity:** Hives, urticaria, tightness of chest, wheezing, hypotension, **anaphylaxis. Miscellaneous:** Fever, allergic reaction, arthrosis, hemarthrosis, edema, headache, pain, pneumonia, abnormal renal function, vomiting.

DRUG INTERACTIONS

Potential interaction with activated prothrombin complex concentrates or prothrombin complex concentrates; avoid simultaneous use.

HOW SUPPLIED

Powder for injection, lyophilized: 1.2 mg/vial, 4.8 mg/vial

DOSAGE

• IV BOLUS ONLY

Hemophilia A or B with inhibitors

90 mcg/kg q 2 hr until hemostasis is achieved or until treatment is deemed to be inadequate. Dosage (35–120 mcg/kg) and administration interval may be adjusted based on severity of bleeding and degree of hemostasis achieved. Clients treated for joint or muscle bleeds showed beneficial effects within 8 doses, although more doses are required for severe bleeds. The appropriate duration of post-hemostatic dosing has not been determined. For severe bleeds, continue dosing at 3–6 hr intervals after hemostasis is achieved. The biological and clinical effects of prolonged elevated levels of Factor VIIa have not been

studied; thus, minimize duration of post-hemostatic dosing. Monitor clients during this time.

NURSING CONSIDERATIONS

ADMINISTRATION/STORAGE

IV 1. Use the following procedure to reconstitute:

- Bring the lyophilized powder and the diluent (sterile water for injection) to room temperature, but no higher than 37°C (98.6°F).
- Remove cap from the vial to expose the central portion of the rubber stopper. Cleanse the stopper with an alcohol swab and allow to dry.
- Draw back the plunger of a sterile syringe/needle and admit air into the syringe.
- Insert the needle of the syringe into the diluent vial. Inject air into the vial and withdraw the quanity required for reconstitution. For the 1.2 mg vial, add 2.2 mL of diluent and for the 4.8 mg vial add 8.5 mL of diluent.
- Insert the syringe/needle containing the diluent into the vial with the powder through the center of the rubber stopper. Aim the needle against the side so that the stream of liquid runs down the vial wall. Do not inject the diluent directly on the powder.
- Gently swirl the vial until all powder is dissolved. After reconstitution, each vial contains about 0.6 mg/mL rFVIIa. The reconstituted solution is clear and colorless (do not use if particulate matter or discoloration is observed). Use within 3 hr after reconstitution.

2. Administer the reconstituted solution as follows:

- Draw back the plunger of a sterile syringe/needle and admit air into the syringe.
- Insert needle into the vial of reconstituted rFVIIa and inject air into the vial. Withdraw the appropriate amount of reconstituted drug into the syringe.
- Remove and discard the needle from the syringe and attach a suitable IV needle. Administer as a slow bolus injection over 2–5 min, depending on the dose.
- Discard any unused reconstituted solution after 3 hr.

3. Do not mix rFVIIa with infusion solutions (data are not available).
4. Prior to reconstitution refrigerate at 2–8°C (36–46° F). Avoid exposure to direct sunlight.
5. After reconstitution, store either at room temperature or refrigerate for 3 hr or less. Do not freeze reconstituted drug or store it in syringes.

ASSESSMENT

1. Document indications for therapy i.e.; uncontrolled bleeding in hemophilia A/B clients with inhibitors to Factor VIII or IX.
2. Assess renal function, PT, PTT, and plasma FVII clotting activity. Evaluate any swelling or pain for hidden bleed.
3. Clients with DIC, advanced ASHD, crush injuries, or septicemia have increased risk of developing a thrombotic event; monitor closely.

CLIENT/FAMILY TEACHING

1. Review indications for therapy and risks/benefits associated with therapy.
2. Report S&S of hypersensitivity i.e.; wheezing, chest tightness, itching, hives, ↓ BP, and shock.
3. Avoid activities that may cause injury such as contact sports and jolting/falling activities. Report any unusual swelling or joint pains.

OUTCOMES/EVALUATE

Control of bleeding episodes in hemophilia A/B clients

Codeine phosphate

(**KOH**-deen)

PREGNANCY CATEGORY: C

Codeine sulfate

(**KOH**-deen)

PREGNANCY CATEGORY: C
CLASSIFICATION(S):
Narcotic analgesic
C-II

SEE ALSO *NARCOTIC ANALGESICS*.

C

ACTION/KINETICS
Produces less respiratory depression and N&V than morphine. Moderately habit-forming and constipating. Dosages over 60 mg often cause restlessness and excitement and irritate the cough center. In lower doses it is a potent antitussive and is an ingredient in many cough syrups. **Onset:** 10–30 min. **Peak effect:** 30–60 min. **Duration:** 4–6 hr. **t½:** 3–4 hr. Codeine is two-thirds as effective PO as parenterally.

USES
Relief of mild to moderate pain. Antitussive to relieve chemical or mechanical respiratory tract irritation. In combination with aspirin or acetaminophen to enhance analgesia.

CONTRAINDICATIONS
Premature infants or during labor when delivery of a premature infant is expected.

SPECIAL CONCERNS
May increase the duration of labor. Use with caution and reduce the initial dose in clients with seizure disorders, acute abdominal conditions, renal or hepatic disease, fever, Addison's disease, hypothyroidism, prostatic hypertrophy, ulcerative colitis, urethral stricture, following recent GI or GU tract surgery, and in the young, geriatric, or debilitated clients.

ADDITIONAL DRUG INTERACTIONS
Combination with chlordiazepoxide may induce coma.

HOW SUPPLIED
Codeine Phosphate: *Injection:* 30 mg/mL, 60 mg/mL; *Oral Solution:* 15 mg/5 mL. **Codeine Sulfate:** *Tablet:* 15 mg, 30 mg, 60 mg

DOSAGE

• **ORAL SOLUTION, TABLETS, IM, IV, SC**

Analgesia.

Adults: 15–60 mg q 4–6 hr, not to exceed 360 mg/day. **Pediatric, over 1 year:** 0.5 mg/kg or 15 mg/m² q 4–6 hr. Do not give IV in children.

Antitussive.

Adults: 10–20 mg PO q 4–6 hr, not to exceed 120 mg/day. **Pediatric, 2–6 years:** 2.5–5 mg PO q 4–6 hr, not to exceed 30 mg/day; **6–12 years:** 5–10 mg PO q 4–6 hr, not to exceed 60 mg/day.

NURSING CONSIDERATIONS

SEE ALSO *NURSING CONSIDERATIONS* FOR *NARCOTIC ANALGESICS*.

CLIENT/FAMILY TEACHING

1. Take only as directed. Tylenol or aspirin act synergistically with codeine and are usually given together.
2. Increase intake of fluids, fruits, and fiber to diminish constipation.
3. May cause dizziness/drowsiness.
4. Avoid alcohol/CNS depressants.
5. Report altered mental patterns.
6. If taking codeine syrups to suppress coughs, do not overuse. If productive coughing is suppressed, may cause additional congestion.

OUTCOMES/EVALUATE

- Relief of pain
- Control of coughing with improved sleeping patterns

Colchicine

(**KOHL**-chih-seen)

PREGNANCY CATEGORY: C (ORAL USE); D (PARENTERAL USE)
CLASSIFICATION(S):
Antigout drug

ACTION/KINETICS
Colchicine is not uricosuric. It may reduce the crystal-induced inflammation by reducing lactic acid production by leukocytes (resulting in a decreased deposition of sodium urate), by inhibiting leukocyte migration, and by reducing phagocytosis. May also inhibit the synthesis of kinins and leukotrienes. **t½, plasma:** 10–60 min. **Onset, IV:** 6–12 hr; **PO:** 12 hr. **Time to peak levels, PO:** 0.5–2 hr. It concentrates in leukocytes (t½, about 46 hr). Metabolized in the liver and mainly excreted in the feces with 10%–20% excreted unchanged through the urine.

USES
Prophylaxis and treatment of acute attacks of gout. *Investigational:* To slow progression of chronic progressive multiple sclerosis, to decrease fre-

quency and severity of fever and to prevent amyloidosis in familiar Mediterranean fever, primary biliary cirrhosis, hepatic cirrhosis, adjunct in the treatment of primary amyloidosis, Behçet's disease, pseudogout due to chondrocalcinosis, refractory idiopathic thrombocytopenic purpura, progressive systemic sclerosis, dermatologic disorders including dermatitis herpetiformis, psoriasis, palmoplantar pustulosis, and pyoderma associated with Crohn's disease.

CONTRAINDICATIONS

Blood dyscrasias. Serious GI, hepatic, cardiac, or renal disorders.

SPECIAL CONCERNS

Use with caution during lactation. Dosage has not been established for children. Geriatric clients may be at greater risk of developing cumulative toxicity. Use with extreme caution for elderly, debilitated clients, especially in the presence of chronic renal, hepatic, GI, or CV disease. May impair fertility.

SIDE EFFECTS

The drug is toxic; thus clients must be carefully monitored. **GI:** N&V, diarrhea, abdominal cramping. **Hematologic:** ***Aplastic anemia, agranulocytosis,*** or thrombocytopenia following long-term therapy. **Miscellaneous:** Peripheral neuritis, purpura, myopathy, neuropathy, alopecia, reversible azoospermia, dermatoses, hypersensitivity, thrombophlebitis at injection site (rare), liver dysfunction. If such symptoms appear, discontinue drug at once and wait at least 48 hr before reinstating drug therapy.

LABORATORY TEST CONSIDERATIONS

Alters liver function tests. ↑ Alkaline phosphatase, AST. False + for hemoglobin or RBCs in urine.

OD OVERDOSE MANAGEMENT

Symptoms (Acute Intoxication): Characterized at first by violent GI tract symptoms such as N&V, abdominal pain, and diarrhea. The latter may be profuse, watery, bloody, and associated with severe fluid and electrolyte loss. Also, burning of throat and skin, hematuria and oliguria, rapid and weak pulse, general exhaustion, muscular depression, and CNS involvement. ***Death is usually caused by respiratory paralysis.*** *Treatment (Acute Poisoning):* Gastric lavage, symptomatic support, including atropine and morphine, artificial respiration, hemodialysis, peritoneal dialysis, and treatment of shock.

DRUG INTERACTIONS

Acidifying agents / Inhibit colchicine action

Alkalinizing agents / Potentiate colchicine action

CNS depressants / Clients may be more sensitive to CNS depressant effects

Sympathomimetic agents / Enhanced by colchicine

Vitamin B_{12} / Colchicine may interfere with gut absorption

HOW SUPPLIED

Injection: 0.5 mg/mL; *Tablet:* 0.5 mg, 0.6 mg

DOSAGE

• **TABLETS**

Acute attack of gout.

Adults, initial: 1–1.2 mg followed by 0.5–1.2 mg q 1–2 hr until pain is relieved or nausea, vomiting, or diarrhea occurs. **Total amount required:** 4–8 mg.

Prophylaxis for gout.

Adults: 0.5–0.6 mg/day for 3–4 days a week if the client has less than one attack per year or 0.5–0.6 mg/day if the client has more than one attack per year.

Prophylaxis for surgical clients.

Adults: 0.5–0.6 mg t.i.d. for 3 days before and 3 days after surgery.

• **IV ONLY**

Acute attack of gout.

Adults, initial: 2 mg; **then,** 0.5 mg q 6 hr until pain is relieved; give no more than 4 mg in a 24-hr period. Some physicians recommend a single IV dose of 3 mg while others recommend no more than 1 mg for the initial dose, followed by 0.5 mg once or twice daily, if needed. If pain recurs, 1–2 mg/day may be given for several days; however, colchicine should not be given by any route for at least 7 days after a full course of IV therapy (i.e., 4 mg).

Prophylaxis or maintenance of recurrent or chronic gouty arthritis.
0.5–1 mg 1–2 times/day. However, PO colchicine is preferred (usually with a uricosuric drug).

C

NURSING CONSIDERATIONS

ADMINISTRATION/STORAGE

1. Store in tight, light-resistant containers.
IV 2. Parenterally, give only IV; SC or IM causes severe local irritation.
3. For parenteral administration, give undiluted or may dilute in 10–20 mL of NSS without a bacteriostatic agent or with sterile water. Administer over 2–5 min.
4. Do not use turbid solutions.
5. Not compatible with dextrose-containing solutions.

ASSESSMENT

1. Determine symptom onset; any other attacks, frequency, and any preventative therapy prescribed.
2. Note age and general physical condition.
3. Document joint involvement, noting pain, swelling, and degree of mobility; may need to aspirate joint for definitive diagnosis.
4. Monitor CBC, joint X ray, uric acid levels, and renal and LFTs.

CLIENT/FAMILY TEACHING

1. If prescribed for use in acute attacks take at the first S&S of attack to diminish severity. Stop uricosuric agent (if prescribed) during acute attack.
2. Start or increase dosage of colchicine as prescribed; at the first sign of joint pain or other symptom of impending gout attack. The maximum dose is 10 tablets or 10 mg in 24 hr; do not exceed. It usually takes 12–48 hr for relief of symptoms.
3. Acute episodes may be precipitated by aspirin, alcohol, or foods high in purine.
4. Stop drug and report if N&V, or diarrhea develops; signs of toxicity. With severe diarrhea, medication (paregoric) may be needed.
5. Report any evidence of liver dysfunction (yellow discoloration of eyes, skin, or stool). LFTs may be scheduled during long-term use.
6. Females should avoid pregnancy.
7. Consume 3–3.5 L/day of fluids to enhance excretion.
8. NSAIDs may help with pain and inflammation; use as prescribed.

OUTCOMES/EVALUATE

- ↓ Joint pain/swelling/destruction
- Termination of acute gout attacks

Colesevelam hydrochloride

(**koh**-leh-**SEV**-eh-lam)

PREGNANCY CATEGORY: B
CLASSIFICATION(S):
Antihyperlipidemic, bile acid sequestrant
Rx: WelChol

ACTION/KINETICS

Binds bile acids, including glycocholic acid (the major bile acid in humans), in the intestine, impeding their reabsorption. As the bile acid pool becomes depleted, the hepatic enzyme, cholesterol 7-α-hydroxylase, is upregulated which increases the conversion of cholesterol to bile acids. This causes an increased demand for cholesterol in liver cells, resulting in the effects of both increasing transcription and activity of the cholesterol biosynthetic enzyme (HMG-CoA) reductase and increasing the number of hepatic LDL receptors. The result is an increased clearance of LDL cholesterol from the blood, thus lowering serum LDL cholesterol levels. Is not absorbed from the GI tract. Maximum response achieved within 2 weeks.

USES

Given alone or with an HMG-CoA reductase inhibitor, in addition to diet and exercise, to reduce elevated LDL cholesterol in those with primary hypercholesterolemia (Fredrickson Type IIa).

CONTRAINDICATIONS

Use in bowel obstruction.

SPECIAL CONCERNS

Use with caution in clients with triglyceride levels greater than 300 mg/dL and in those with a susceptibility to vitamin K or fat soluble vitamin deficiencies. Safety and efficacy have not been established in children or for use in clients with dysphagia, swallowing disorders, severe GI motility disorders, or major GI tract surgery.

SIDE EFFECTS

GI: Flatulence, constipation, diarrhea, nausea, dyspepsia. **Respiratory:** Sinusitis, rhinitis, increased cough, pharyngitis. **Body as a whole:** Infection, headache, pain, back pain, abdominal pain, flu syndrome, accidental injury, asthenia, myalgia.

DRUG INTERACTIONS

Give consideration to monitoring drug levels or effects when giving other drugs for which alterations in blood levels could have clinical significance on safety or efficacy.

HOW SUPPLIED

Tablet: 625 mg

DOSAGE

• **TABLETS**

Primary hypercholesterolemia.

Monotherapy, initial: Three tablets b.i.d. with meals or 6 tablets once per day with a meal. Can be increased to 7 tablets, depending on desired effect. **Combination therapy:** Three tablets b.i.d. with meals or 6 tablets once per day with a meal. Doses of 4–6 tablets/day can be taken safely with a HMG-CoA reductase inhibitor or when the 2 drugs are dosed apart.

NURSING CONSIDERATIONS

ADMINISTRATION/STORAGE

Store at room temperature and protect from moisture.

ASSESSMENT

1. Note indications for therapy, other agents trialed and the outcome.
2. Prior to starting therapy, secondary causes of hypercholesterolemia (e.g., poorly controlled diabetes, hypothyroidism, nephrotic syndrome, dysproteinemias, obstructive liver disease, other drug therapy, alcholism) should be ruled out.
3. Obtain a 12 hr fasting lipid profile prior to therapy; assess total-C, HDL/LDL-C, and Triglycerides. Avoid/monitor carefully if Triglycerides > 300. Periodically assess serum cholesterol as outlined in the National Cholesterol Education Program guidelines to confirm a favorable initial and chronic response.
4. Determine if client suffers from vitamin K or fat soluble vitamin deficiency, bowel, GI motility or swallowing dysfunction, or major GI tract surgery as these may preclude therapy.

CLIENT/FAMILY TEACHING

1. Take as directed with a liquid and a low fat/low cholesterol meal.
2. Continue to make lifestyle changes that lower coronary risk factors such as smoking cessation, reduction in alcohol intake, low fat/low cholesterol diet, regular daily exercise, weight loss, and reduction in stress.
3. Practice reliable birth control; stop drug and report if pregnancy suspected.

OUTCOMES/EVALUATE

Reduced LDL cholesterol levels

Colestipol hydrochloride

(koh-**LESS**-tih-poll)

PREGNANCY CATEGORY: B
CLASSIFICATION(S):
Antihyperlipidemic, bile acid sequestrant
Rx: Colestid

ACTION/KINETICS

An anion exchange resin that binds bile acids in the intestine, forming an insoluble complex excreted in the feces. The loss of bile acids results in increased oxidation of cholesterol to bile acids and a decrease in LDL and serum cholesterol. Does not affect (or may increase) triglycerides or HDL and may increase VLDL. Not absorbed from the GI tract. **Onset:** 1–2 days; **maximum effect:** 1 month. Return to pretreatment cholesterol levels after discontinuance of therapy: 1 month.

USES

As adjunctive therapy in hyperlipoproteinemia (types IIA and IIB) to reduce serum cholesterol in clients who do not respond adequately to diet. *Investigational:* Digitalis toxicity.

CONTRAINDICATIONS

Complete obstruction or atresia of bile duct.

SPECIAL CONCERNS

Use during pregnancy only if benefits outweigh risks. Use with caution during lactation and in children. Children may be more likely to develop hyperchloremic acidosis although dosage has not been established. Clients over 60 years of age may be at greater risk of GI side effects and adverse nutritional effects.

SIDE EFFECTS

GI: Constipation (may be severe and accompanied by fecal impaction), N&V, diarrhea, heartburn, GI bleeding, anorexia, flatulence, steatorrhea, abdominal distention/cramping, bloating, loose stools, indigestion, rectal bleeding/pain, black stools, hemorrhoidal bleeding, ***bleeding duodenal ulcer, peptic ulceration,*** ulcer attack, GI irritation, dysphagia, dental bleeding/caries, hiccoughs, sour taste, pancreatitis, diverticulitis, cholecystitis, cholelithiasis. **CV:** Chest pain, angina, tachycardia (rare). **CNS:** Migraine or sinus headache, anxiety, vertigo, dizziness, lightheadedness, insomnia, fatigue, tinnitus, syncope, drowsiness, femoral nerve pain, paresthesia. **Hematologic:** Ecchymosis, anemia, beeding tendencies due to hypoprothrombinemia. **Allergic:** Urticaria, dermatitis, asthma, wheezing, rash. **Musculoskeletal:** Backache, muscle/joint pain, arthritis. **Renal:** Hematuria, burnt odor to urine, dysuria, diuresis. **Miscellaneous:** Uveitis, fatigue, weight loss or gain, increased libido, swollen glands, SOB, edema, weakness, swelling of hands/feet, osteoporosis, calcified material in biliary tree and gall bladder, hyperchloremic acidosis in children.

DRUG INTERACTIONS

See *Cholestyramine.*

HOW SUPPLIED

Granules: 5 g/dose, 5 g/7.5 g powder; *Tablet:* 1 g

DOSAGE

• **GRANULES**

Antihyperlipidemic.

Adults, initial: 5 g 1–2 times/day; **then,** can increase 5 g/day at 1–2-month intervals. **Total dose:** 5–30 g/day given once or in two to three divided doses.

• **TABLETS**

Adults, initial: 2 g 1–2 times/day. Dose can be increased by 2 g, once or twice daily, at 1–2-month intervals. **Total dose:** 2–16 g/day given once or in divided doses.

NURSING CONSIDERATIONS

SEE ALSO *NURSING CONSIDERATIONS* FOR *CHOLESTYRAMINE.*

ADMINISTRATION/STORAGE

1. If compliance is good and side effects acceptable but the desired effect is not obtained with 2–16 g/day using tablets, consider combined therapy or alternative treatment.
2. Granules are available in an orange-flavored product.

CLIENT/FAMILY TEACHING

1. Take 30 min before meals, preferably with the evening meal, since cholesterol synthesis is increased during the evening hours. Take other drugs 1 hr before or 4 hr after colestipol to reduce interference with their absorption.
2. Never take dose in dry form. Always mix granules with 90 mL or more of fruit juice, milk, water, carbonated beverages, applesauce, soup, cereal, or pulpy fruit before administering to disguise unpalatable taste and to prevent resin from causing esophageal irritation or blockage.
3. Rinse glass with a small amount of additional beverage and swallow ensure the total amount of the drug is taken.
4. Tablets should be swallowed whole (i.e., they should not be cut, crushed, or chewed); may be taken with water or other fluids.
5. Consume adequate amounts of fluids, fruits, and fiber to diminish constipating drug effects.
6. Continue to follow dietary restrictions of fat and cholesterol, regular

exercise program, smoking cessation, and weight reduction in the overall goal of cholesterol reduction.
7. Serum cholesterol level will return to pretreatment levels within 1 month if drug is discontinued.

OUTCOMES/EVALUATE

↓ LDL—C levels

Colfosceril palmitate (Dipalmitoylphosphatidylcholine, DPPC)

(kohl-**FOSS**-sir-ill)

CLASSIFICATION(S):
Lung surfactant
Rx: Exosurf Neonatal

ACTION/KINETICS

Contains dipalmitoylphosphatidylcholine (DPPC), which reduces surface tension in the lungs, as well as cetyl alcohol, which acts as a spreading agent for DPPC on the air–fluid surface. Also contains tyloxapol, which is a nonionic surfactant that assists in dispersion of DPPC and cetyl alcohol, and NaCl to adjust osmolality. The drug can rapidly affect oxygenation and lung compliance. DPPC is reabsorbed from the alveoli into lung tissue where it is broken down and reutilized for further phospholipid synthesis and secretion.

USES

Prophylaxis of respiratory distress syndrome in infants with birth weights of less than 1,350 g and in infants with birth weights greater than 1,350 g who manifest pulmonary immaturity. Treatment of infants who have developed respiratory distress syndrome. Such infants should be on mechanical ventilation and should have been diagnosed as having respiratory distress syndrome.

SPECIAL CONCERNS

Use of colfosceril should be undertaken only by medical personnel trained and experienced in airway and clinical management of unstable premature infants. Although colfosceril is effective in reducing mortality due to premature birth, infants may still develop severe complications resulting in either death or survival but with permanent handicaps. Benefits versus risks should be carefully assessed before using colfosceril in infants weighing 500–700 g.

SIDE EFFECTS

Respiratory: ***Pulmonary hemorrhage/air leak (pneumothorax, pneumomediastinum, pneumopericardium, pulmonary interstitial emphysema), ET tube mucous plugs, apnea,*** congenital/nosocomial pneumonia. **CV:** ***Intraventricular hemorrhage,*** patent ductus arteriosus, hypotension, bradycardia, tachycardia, exchange transfusion, persistent fetal circulation. **Changes in blood gases:** Fall/rise in oxygen saturation, fall/ rise in transcutaneous pO_2/pCO_2. **Miscellaneous:** ***Necrotizing enterocolitis, seizures*** major anomalies, hyperbilirubinemia, gagging, thrombocytopenia.

HOW SUPPLIED

Lyophilized Powder for Endotracheal Use: 108 mg.

DOSAGE

• ENDOTRACHEAL

Prophylaxis.

5 mL/kg (as two 2.5-mL/kg half-doses) ASAP after birth. A second and third dose should be given 12 and 24 hr later to infants who are still on mechanical ventilation.

Rescue treatment.

5 mL/kg (as two 2.5-mL/kg half-doses) ASAP after the diagnosis of respiratory distress syndrome is confirmed. A second 5-mL/kg dose is given after 12 hr to infants who are still on mechanical ventilation. The safety and effectiveness of additional doses are not known.

NURSING CONSIDERATIONS

ADMINISTRATION/STORAGE

1. Reconstitute according to manufacturer's directions immediately pri-

or to use with the diluent provided (preservative-free sterile water). Reconstituted product is a milky white suspension.
2. Ensure that the reconstituted suspension is uniformly dispersed before administration. Do not use if the vial contains large flakes or particulate matter.
3. Five different-sized ET tube adapters are provided with each vial of colfosceril. The adapters are clean but not sterile. Use adapters according to manufacturer instructions.
4. Administered directly into the trachea through the sideport on the special ET tube adapter without interruption of mechanical ventilation.
5. Each half-dose is given slowly over 1–2 min in small bursts timed with inspiration.
6. The first 2.5-mL/kg dose is given with the infant in the midline position; after the first half-dose is given, the infant's head and torso are first turned 45° to the right for 30 sec and then 45° to the left for 30 sec while continuing mechanical ventilation. This allows for gravity to help with lung distribution of the drug.
7. Refluxing of colfosceril into the ET tube may occur if the drug is given rapidly. If reflux is noted, stop drug administration and increase the peak inspiratory pressure on the ventilator by 4–5 cm water until the ET tube clears.
8. Undertake colfosceril administration only by experienced neonatologists and other individuals experienced at neonatal intubation and ventilatory management.

ASSESSMENT

1. Review indications for drug therapy to ensure that infant meets criteria and document as rescue or prophylactic treatment.
2. The infant's color, chest expansion, facial expression, oximeter readings, HR, and ET tube patency and position should be documented and monitored carefully before and during colfosceril dosing.
3. Ascertain that the ET tube tip is in the trachea and not in the esophagus or right or left mainstem bronchus to ensure drug dispersion to all lung areas.
4. Document baseline weight, ABGs, VS, CXR, and physical assessment findings.

INTERVENTIONS

1. Confirm brisk and symmetrical chest movement and equal breath sounds in the two axillae with each mechanical inspiration prior to and at the conclusion of each dosing.
2. Infant should be suctioned before drug administration but not for 2 hr after colfosceril administration (unless clinically necessary).
3. Continuous monitoring of ECG, arterial BP, and transcutaneous oxygen saturation must be undertaken during dosing. After either prophylactic or rescue treatment, frequent ABGs should be measured to prevent post-dosing hyperoxia and hypocarbia.
4. The volume of the 5-mL/kg dose may cause a transient impairment of gas exchange due to physical blockage of the airway. Infants may show a decrease in oxygen saturation during dosing, especially if they are on low ventilator settings. If evident, increase the FiO_2 and peak inspiratory pressure on the ventilator by 4–5 cm water for 1–2 min.
5. If chest expansion improves significantly after dosing, reduce the peak ventilator inspiratory pressure immediately. Failure to do this may cause lung overdistention and fatal pulmonary air leak.
6. If the infant becomes pink and transcutaneous oxygen saturation is more than 95%, reduce the FiO_2 in small but repeated steps until saturation is 90%–95%. Failure to do this may cause hyperoxia.
7. If arterial or transcutaneous CO_2 levels are less than 30 mm Hg, reduce the ventilator rate immediately; may cause significant hypocarbia, which reduces cerebral blood flow.
8. After dosing, confirm the position of the ET tube by listening for equal breath sounds in both axillae. Pay particular attention to chest expansion, skin color, transcutaneous O_2 saturation, and ABGs; remain at bedside for at least 30 min after dosing.
9. Observe for air leaks and mucous plugs. If mucous plug is unrelieved by

suctioning, replace the ET tube immediately.

OUTCOMES/EVALUATE

- Oxygen saturation between 90% and 95%; pulmonary parameters more consistent with survival
- ↓ Pulmonary air leaks and prevention of alveolar collapse

Conjugated estrogens and Medroxyprogesterone acetate

(**KON**-jyou-**gay**-ted **ES**- troh-jens, meh-**drox**-see-proh-**JESS**-ter- ohn)

PREGNANCY CATEGORY: X
CLASSIFICATION(S):
Sex homones
Rx: Premphase, PremPro

SEE ALSO *CONJUGATED ESTROGENS AND MEDROXYPROGESTERONE ACETATE.*

CONTENT

PremPro: Each tablet contains: conjugated estrogens, 0.625 mg, and medroxyprogesterone acetate, 2.5 mg or 5 mg. *Premphase:* Tablets contain either conjugated estrogens, 0.625 mg or conjugated estrogens, 0.625 mg, and medroxyprogesterone acetate, 5 mg.

USES

(1)Moderate to severe vasomotor symptoms associated with menopause in women with an intact uterus. (2) Vulvular and vaginal atrophy. (3) Prevention of osteoporosis.

CONTRAINDICATIONS

Known or suspected pregnancy, including use for missed abortion or as a diagnostic test for pregnancy. Known or suspected cancer of the breast or estrogen-dependent neoplasia. Undiagnosed abnormal genital bleeding. Active or past history of thrombophlebitis, thromboembolic disease, or stroke. Liver dysfunction or disease. Lactation.

SPECIAL CONCERNS

Estrogens reportedly increase the risk of endometrial carcinoma in postmenopausal women. Use with caution in conditions aggravated by fluid retention, including asthma, epilepsy, migraine, and cardiac or renal dysfunction. Estrogens may cause significant increases in plasma triglycerides that may cause pancreatitis and other complications in clients with familial defects of lipoprotein metabolism.

SIDE EFFECTS

See individual drug entries.

DRUG INTERACTIONS

See individual drug entries.

HOW SUPPLIED

See Content

DOSAGE

- **TABLETS**

Vasomotor symptoms due to menopause, vulvar and vaginal atrophy, prevention of osteoporosis.

PremPro: One 0.625/2.5 mg tablet once daily. *Premphase:* One 0.625 mg conjugated estrogen tablet once daily on days 1 to 14 and one 0.625/2.5 mg tablet once daily on days 15 to 28.

NURSING CONSIDERATIONS

SEE ALSO *NURSING CONSIDERATIONS* FOR *CONJUGATED ESTROGENS AND MEDROXYPROGESTERONE ACETATE.*

ASSESSMENT

1. Document indications for therapy (hormone replacement for menopausal symptoms or osteoporosis prevention), onset and duration of symptoms, and length of therapy.
2. Note any history or experience with replacement therapy. Do not give for cardiac protection; give for postmenopausal symptom control only.
3. Evaluate for any active or past conditions that may preclude drug therapy: liver dysfunction, thrombophlebitis, thromboembolic disorders, cancer of the breast or estrogen-dependent neoplasia, or any undiagnosed abnormal vaginal bleeding.

CLIENT/FAMILY TEACHING

1. Take only as directed; two cards are provided, marked cards 1 and 2.
2. Stress importance of follow-up exams to assess need for continued therapy. When used for treating vasomotor symptoms or vulval and vaginal atrophy, reevaluate every 3–6-mo to assess treatment results.
3. When used to prevent osteoporosis, monitor closely for signs of endometrial cancer. Consider other available therapies if for fracture prevention. Diagnostic procedures should be undertaken to rule out malignancy in the event of persistent or recurring AVB.

OUTCOMES/EVALUATE

- Osteoporosis prophylaxis
- ↓ Menopausal symptoms

C

Corticotropin injection (ACTH, Adrenocorticotropic hormone)

(kor-tih-koh-**TROH**-pin)

PREGNANCY CATEGORY: C
Rx: ACTH, Acthar

Corticotropin repository injection (ACTH gel, Corticotropin gel)

(kor-tih-koh-**TROH**-pin)

PREGNANCY CATEGORY: C
Rx: ACTH-80, H.P. Acthar Gel
CLASSIFICATION(S):
Anterior pituitary hormone

SEE ALSO *CORTICOSTEROIDS*.

ACTION/KINETICS

The hormone stimulates the functional adrenal cortex to secrete its entire spectrum of hormones, including the corticosteroids. Thus, the overall physiologic effects of corticotropin are similar to those of cortisone. Since the latter is more easily obtainable, is more predictable, and has more prolonged activity, it is usually used for therapeutic purposes. Is useful for the diagnosis of Addison's disease and other conditions in which the functionality of the adrenal cortex is to be determined. *Corticotropin cannot elicit a hormonal response from a nonfunctioning adrenal gland.* **Peak plasma levels (corticotropin injection):** 1 hr. **t½:** 15 min. The repository injection contains ACTH in a gelatin base to delay the rate of absorption and increase the duration. **Duration** (repository form): Up to 3 days.

USES

Diagnosis of adrenal insufficiency syndromes, nonsuppurative thyroiditis, hypercalcemia associated with cancer, tuberculous meningitis with subarachnoid block or impending block (with tuberculostatic drugs). *Investigational:* Infant spasm, multiple sclerosis. For same diseases as glucocorticosteroids.

ADDITIONAL CONTRAINDICATIONS

Cushing's syndrome, psychotic or psychopathic clients, active tuberculosis, active peptic ulcers. Lactation.

SPECIAL CONCERNS

Use with caution in clients who have diabetes and hypotension.

ADDITIONAL SIDE EFFECTS

In the treatment of myasthenia gravis, corticotropin may cause severe muscle weakness 2–3 days after initiation of therapy. Equipment for respiratory assistance must be on hand for such emergencies. Muscle strength returns and increases 2–7 days after cessation of treatment, and improvement lasts for about 3 months.

LABORATORY TEST CONSIDERATIONS

↓ I^{131} uptake and suppress skin test reactions. False ↓ levels of estradiol and estriol using the Brown method. False – estrogens using colorimetric or fluorometric tests.

HOW SUPPLIED

Corticotropin injection: *Powder for injection:* 25 U/vial, 40 U/vial. **Corticotropin repository injection:** *Injection:* 40 U/mL, 80 U/mL.

DOSAGE

• INJECTION: SC, IM, OR SLOW IV DRIP

Most uses.

Highly individualized. Usual, using aqueous solution IM or SC: 20 units q.i.d. **IV:** 10–25 units of aqueous solution in 500 mL 5% dextrose injection over period of 8 hr. Infants and young children require larger dose per body weight than do older children or adults.

Acute exacerbation of multiple sclerosis.

IM: 80–120 units/day for 2–3 weeks.

Infantile spasms.

IM: 20–40 units/day or 80 units every other day for 3 months (or 1 month after cessations of seizures).

• REPOSITORY GEL: IM, SC

40–80 units q 24–72 hr. A dose of 12.5 units q.i.d. causes little metabolic disturbance; 25 units q.i.d. causes definite metabolic alterations.

As a general rule, clients are started on 10–12.5 units q.i.d. If no clinical effect is noted in 72–96 hr, dosage is increased by 5 units every few days to a final maximum of 25 units q.i.d.

NURSING CONSIDERATIONS

SEE ALSO *NURSING CONSIDERATIONS FOR CORTICOSTEROIDS*.

ADMINISTRATION/STORAGE

Check label carefully for IV administration. *The label must say product is for IV use.* Administer IV slowly, over 8 hr. *The label must say product is for IV use.* Administer IV slowly, over 8 hr.

ASSESSMENT

1. Document indications for therapy, type and onset of symptoms.
2. Before administering IV, ensure client allergic to porcine proteins has been tested for any sensitivity to brand of corticotropin to be used.
3. Potassium requirements will be increased during IV administration of ACTH; monitor electrolytes.
4. Report mental status changes such as exaggerated euphoria and nervousness or complaints of insomnia and depression. Administer sedatives as needed.
5. Monitor BP, I&O, and weight; report any marked changes.
6. Plot and record growth and height in children regularly; drug may inhibit growth.

CLIENT/FAMILY TEACHING

1. Drug may mask S&S of infection.
2. Increased stress may require an increased dosage.
3. Avoid vaccinations during therapy.
4. Avoid alcohol, salicylates, and NSAIDs.
5. Report any unusual bruising or bleeding.
6. Do not discontinue abruptly; drug should be tapered.

OUTCOMES/EVALUATE

- Adrenal cortex function
- ↓ Serum calcium levels
- ↑ Muscle strength with MS

Cortisone acetate (Compound E)

(**KOR**-tih-zohn)

PREGNANCY CATEGORY: D
CLASSIFICATION(S):
Glucocorticoid
Rx: Cortone Acetate, Cortone Acetate Sterile Suspension
✱Rx: Cortone

SEE ALSO *CORTICOSTEROIDS*.

ACTION/KINETICS

Possesses both glucocorticoid and mineralocorticoid activity. Short-acting. **t½, plasma:** 30 min; **t½, biologic:** 8–12 hr.

USES

Replacement therapy in chronic cortical insufficiency. Short-term (due to strong mineralocorticoid effect) for inflammatory or allergic disorders. **Sterile suspension:** Congenital adrenal hyperplasia in children.

SPECIAL CONCERNS

Use during pregnancy only if benefits outweigh risks.

HOW SUPPLIED

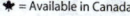

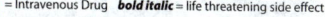

Injection: 50 mg/mL; *Tablet:* 5 mg, 10 mg, 25 mg

C

DOSAGE

• **TABLETS, INJECTION**

Initial or during crisis.

25–300 mg/day. Decrease gradually to lowest effective dose.

Anti-inflammatory.

25–150 mg/day, depending on severity of the disease.

Acute rheumatic fever.

200 mg b.i.d. day 1, thereafter, 200 mg/day.

Addison's disease.

Maintenance: 0.5–0.75 mg/kg/day.

NURSING CONSIDERATIONS

SEE ALSO *NURSING CONSIDERATIONS* FOR *CORTICOSTEROIDS*.

ADMINISTRATION/STORAGE

Single course of therapy should not exceed 6 weeks. Rest periods of 2–3 weeks are indicated between treatments.

OUTCOMES/EVALUATE

- Replacement with insufficiency
- Relief of allergic manifestations
- Normal plasma cortisol levels (138–635 nmol/L at 8 a.m.)

Cosyntropin

(koh-**SIN**-troh-pin)

PREGNANCY CATEGORY: C
CLASSIFICATION(S):
ACTH derivative, synthetic
Rx: Cortrosyn

SEE ALSO *CORTICOSTEROIDS*.

ACTION/KINETICS

Synthetic ACTH derivative that causes effects similar to those of ACTH, although fewer hypersensitivity reactions have been noted. The activity of 0.25 mg cosyntropin is equal to 25 units of ACTH.

USES

Diagnosis of adrenocortical insufficiency.

HOW SUPPLIED

Powder for injection: 0.25 mg

DOSAGE

• **IM, SC**

Adults, usual: 0.25 mg dissolved in sterile saline. Range: 0.25–0.75 mg. **Pediatric, under 2 years:** 0.125 mg IM.

• **IV**

Adults: 0.25 mg given over a 2-min period.

• **IV INFUSION**

Adults: 0.25 mg given at a rate of 0.04 mg/hr over a 6-hr period.

NURSING CONSIDERATIONS

SEE ALSO *NURSING CONSIDERATIONS* FOR *CORTICOSTEROIDS*.

ADMINISTRATION/STORAGE

1. For IM use, dissolve drug (usually 0.25 mg) in sterile saline.

IV 2. When given by IV infusion, 0.25 mg cosyntropin is added to dextrose or NSS and given at a rate of 0.04 mg/hr over 6 hr.

OUTCOMES/EVALUATE

Diagnosis of adrenal gland insufficiency (i.e., primary or secondary)

Cromolyn sodium (Sodium cromoglycate)

(**CROH**-moh-lin)

PREGNANCY CATEGORY: B
CLASSIFICATION(S):
Antiasthmatic drug, antiallergic drug
Rx: Children's Nasalcrom, Gastrocrom, Intal
★**Rx:** Apo-Cromolyn, Nalcrom, Nu-Cromolyn, Opticrom
OTC: Nasalcrom

ACTION/KINETICS

Acts locally to inhibit the degranulation of sensitized mast cells that occurs after exposure to certain antigens. Prevents the release of histamine, slow-reacting substance of anaphylaxis, and other endogenous substances causing hypersensitivity reactions. When effective, reduces the number and intensity of asthmatic attacks as well as decreasing allergic reactions in the eye. No antihistaminic, anti-inflammatory, or bronchodilator effects and has no role in terminating an acute attack of asthma. After inhalation, some drug is absorbed systemically. **t½:** 81 min; from lungs: 60 min. About 50% excreted unchanged through the urine and 50% through the bile. When used in the eye, approximately 0.03% is absorbed. **Onset, ophthalmic:** Several days. **Onset, nasal:** Less than 1 week. **Time to peak effect, nasal:** Up to 4 weeks.

USES

Inhalation: Prophylactic and adjunct in the management of bronchial asthma in clients who have a significant bronchodilator-reversible component to their airway obstruction. Prophylaxis of exercise-induced bronchospasms and bronchospasms due to allergens, cold dry air, or environmental pollutants. **Nasal, OTC:** Prophylaxis and treatment of allergic rhinitis, including children 2 years and older. **PO:** Mastocytosis (improves symptoms including diarrhea, flushing, headaches, vomiting, urticaria, nausea, abdominal pain, and itching). **Ophthalmic:** Treat vernal keratoconjunctivitis, vernal conjunctivitis, and vernal keratitis. *Investigational:* PO to treat food allergies. Ulcerative colitis, proctitis, urticaria, post-exercise bronchospasm.

CONTRAINDICATIONS

Hypersensitivity. Acute attacks and status asthmaticus. For mastocytosis in premature infants. Use of nasal product in children less than 6 years of age.

SPECIAL CONCERNS

Safety and efficacy have not been established for the aerosol in children less than 5 years of age, for the nebulizer in children less than 2 years of age, and for the ophthalmic solution in children less than 4 years of age. Reserve use in children less than 2 years of age to severe disease in which potential benefits clearly outweigh potential risks. Due to the propellants in the aerosol, use with caution in coronary artery disease or cardiac arrhythmias. Use with caution for long periods of time, in the presence of renal or hepatic disease, and during lactation.

SIDE EFFECTS

Respiratory: ***Bronchospasm (may be severe and associated with a precipitous fall in pulmonary function), laryngeal edema (rare),*** cough, eosinophilic pneumonia, pharyngeal irritation, nasal congestion, wheezing, nasal stinging or sneezing. **CNS:** Dizziness, drowsiness, headache. **Allergic:** Urticaria, rash, angioedema, serum sickness, ***anaphylaxis.*** **Other:** Nausea, urinary frequency, dysuria, joint swelling and pain, lacrimation, swollen parotid gland.

Following nebulization: Sneezing, wheezing, nasal itching, cough, nose bleeds, burning, nasal congestion, nausea, drowsiness, serum sickness, stomach ache. **Following aerosol:** Lacrimation, swollen parotid gland, dysuria, urinary frequency, dizziness, headache, rash, urticaria, angioedema, joint swelling and pain, nausea, dry or irritated throat, bad taste, cough, wheezing, substernal burning, myopathy (rare). **Following nasal solution:** Burning, stinging, irritation of nose; sneezing, nose bleeds, headache, bad taste in mouth, postnasal drip, rash.

Following PO use: GI: Diarrhea, taste perversion, spasm of esophagus, flatulence, dysphagia, burning of mouth and throat. **CNS:** Headache, dizziness, fatigue, migraine, paresthesia, anxiety, depression, psychosis, behavior changes, insomnia, hallucinations, lethargy, lightheadedness after eating. **Dermatologic:** Flushing, angioedema, urticaria, skin burning, skin erythema. **Musculoskeletal:** Arthralgia, stiffness and weakness in legs. **Miscellaneous:** Altered liver function test, dyspnea, dysuria, polycythemia, neutropenia.

HOW SUPPLIED

Oral Concentrate: 100 mg/5 mL; *Metered dose inhaler:* 0.8 mg/inh; *Solution for Nebulization:* 10 mg/mL; *Nasal spray:* 5.2 mg/inh; *Ophthalmic Solution:* 4%

DOSAGE

- **NEBULIZER SOLUTION**

Prophylaxis of bronchial asthma.

Adults and children over 2 years of age, initial: 20 mg inhaled q.i.d. at regular intervals.

Prophylaxis of exercise-induced bronchospasm.
Inhale 20 mg of the nebulizer solution no more than 1 hr (the shorter the interval between the dose and exercise, the better the effect) before anticipated exercise. Repeat as required for protection during prolonged exercise.

• **METERED DOSE INHALER**

Management of bronchial asthma.
Adults and children 5 years and older, initial: 2 metered sprays inhaled q.i.d. at regular intervals. Do not exceed this dose.

Prophylaxis of exercise-induced bronchospasm.
Inhalation of 2 metered dose sprays 10–15 min (but not more than 60 min) before exposure to precipitating factor.

• **NASAL SPRAY**

Allergic rhinitis.
Adults and children 6 years and older: 1 spray in each nostril 3–6 times/day at regular intervals q 4–6 hr. Maximum effect may not be seen for 1–2 weeks.

• **ORAL CONCENTRATE**

Mastocytosis.
Adults and children 13 years and older: 200 mg (i.e., 2 ampules) q.i.d. 30 min before meals and at bedtime. **Pediatric, 2–12 years:** 100 mg (i.e., 1 ampule) q.i.d. 30 min before meals and at bedtime. If relief is not seen within 2–3 weeks, dose may be increased, but should not exceed 40 mg/kg/day. **Maintenance:** Reduce dose to minimum amount to maintain client with minimum symptoms.

• **OPHTHALMIC SOLUTION**

Vernal keratoconjunctivitis, conjunctivitis, keratitis.
1–2 gtt in each eye 4–6 times/day at regular intervals. 1 gtt contains 1.6 mg cromolyn sodium.

NURSING CONSIDERATIONS

ADMINISTRATION/STORAGE

Continue corticosteroid dosage when initiating cromolyn therapy. If improvement occurs, taper the steroid dosage slowly. May have to reinstitute steroids if cromolyn inhalation is impaired, in times of stress, or in adrenocortical insufficiency.

CLIENT/FAMILY TEACHING

1. Institute only after acute episode is over, when airway is clear and able to inhale adequately.
2. Directions for using Aerosol:
• Remove cap from mouthpiece and shake the inhaler with canister in place for 5–10 seconds.
• Breathe out to the end of a normal breath. Place mouthpiece into mouth or position mouthpiece 2–3 finger widths from open mouth.
• Slightly tilt head back. Breathe in through mouth slowly for 3–5 sec and press the top of the canister at the same time.
• Remove inhaler from mouth and hold breath for about 10 sec; allow at least 1 min between inhalations.
3. Directions for using nebulizer solution:
• Assemble the face mask or mouthpiece and connect the tubing from the port to the compressor unit.
• Sit in an upright and comfortable position. Put the mask over your nose and mouth, making sure it fits properly to prevent mist from going into the eyes. If a mouthpiece is used, place it into your mouth.
• Turn on compressor and take slow, deep breaths. If possible, hold breath for 10 sec before slowly exhaling. Continue until medication chamber is empty.
4. Do not swallow nebulizer solution as it is poorly absorbed.
5. When using nebulizer solution, do not mix different types of medications without provider permission.
6. Directions for using nasal solution:
• Blow nose before using spray.
• Hold pump with thumb at bottom and nozzle between fingers. When using for the first time, prime the pump by initially spraying 5 times into the air until a fine mist appears.
• Insert nozzle into nostril, spray upward while breathing through the nose. Repeat in other nostril.
• Wipe nozzle to remove debris; cleanse.
• If the pump has not been used for 2 weeks, spray 2 times into the air before using again.
• Consult provider if used continously for more than 12 weeks.

7. Directions for PO use:
• Take at least 30 min before meals.
• Break open ampule and squeeze contents into a glass of water. Do not mix with fruit juice, milk, or foods.
• Stir solution and drink all of the liquid.
8. Continue prescribed medications; may take up to 4 weeks for frequency of asthmatic attacks to decrease.
9. With exposure induced bronchoconstriction, use inhaler within 10–15 min prior to precipitating agent (i.e., exercise, antigen, environmental pollutants) for best results.
10. Use a peak expiratory flow meter to monitor asthma control; establish level to seek medical assistance.
11. Do not discontinue inhalation or nasal medication abruptly. Rapid withdrawal of the drug may precipitate an asthmatic attack, and concomitant corticosteroid therapy may require adjustment.

OUTCOMES/EVALUATE
• ↓ Frequency of asthmatic attacks
• Prevention of exposure-induced bronchoconstriction
• Control of symptoms of mastocytosis (↓ diarrhea, N&V, headache, flushing, and abdominal pain)
• Relief of nasal allergic manifestations

Cyanocobalamin (Vitamin B_{12})

(sye-**an**-oh-koh-**BAL**-ah-min)

PREGNANCY CATEGORY: A (C IN DOSES THAT EXCEED THE RDA)
Rx: Nasal Gel: Nascobal
★**Rx:** Bedoz, Schweinpharm B12
OTC: Tablets: Big Shot B-12

Cyanocobalamin crystalline

(sye-**an**-oh-koh-**BAL**-ah-min)

PREGNANCY CATEGORY: C
Rx: Crystamine, Crysti 1000, Cyanoject, Cyomin, Rubesol-1000

CLASSIFICATION(S):
Vitamin B 12

ACTION/KINETICS
Required for hematopoiesis, cell reproduction, nucleoprotein and myelin synthesis. Plasma vitamin B_{12} levels: 150–750 pg/mL. Rapidly absorbed following IM or SC administration. Following absorption, vitamin B_{12} is carried by plasma proteins to the liver where it is stored until required for various metabolic functions. **t½:** 6 days (400 days in the liver). **Time to peak levels, after PO:** 8–12 hr; **after intranasal:** 1–2 hr.

USES
Cyanocobalamin Lozenges/Tablets: Nutritional vitamin B_{12} deficiency; not to be used for treatment of pernicious anemia. **Cyanocobalamin Gel/Parenteral:** Vitamin B_{12} deficiency due to malabsorption syndrome as seen in pernicious anemia. GI pathology, dysfunction, or surgery. Fish tapeworm infestation, maligancy of pancreas or bowel, gluten enteropathy, small bowel overgrowth of bacteria, sprue, accompanying folic acid deficiency, or total or partial gastrectomy.

CONTRAINDICATIONS
Hypersensitivity to cobalt, Leber's disease.

SPECIAL CONCERNS
Use with caution in clients with gout.

SIDE EFFECTS
Following parenteral use.
Allergic: Urticaria, itching, transitory exanthema, ***anaphylaxis, shock, death.*** **CV: *Peripheral vascular thrombosis,*** CHF, ***pulmonary edema.*** **Other:** Polycythemia vera, optic nerve atrophy in clients with hereditary optic nerve atrophy, diarrhea, hypokalemia, body feels swollen.

Following intranasal use. **GI:** Glossitis, N&V. **Miscellaneous:** Asthenia, headache, infection (sore throat, common cold), paresthesia, rhinitis.

NOTE: Benzyl alcohol, which is present in certain products, may cause ***fatal "gasping syndrome"*** in premature infants.

C

LABORATORY TEST CONSIDERATIONS

Antibiotics, methotrexate, or pyrimethamine invalidate folic acid and vitamin B_{12} diagnostic blood assays.

DRUG INTERACTIONS

Alcohol / ↓ Vitamin B_{12} absorption
Aminosalicylic acid / ↓ Vitamin B_{12} effect. Also, abnormal Schilling test and symptoms of vitamin B_{12} deficiency
Chloramphenicol / ↓ Response to vitamin B_{12} in pernicious anemia
Cholestyramine / ↓ Vitamin B_{12} absorption
Cimetidine / ↓ Digestion and release of vitamin B_{12}; ↓ absorption of cyanocobalamin
Colchicine / ↓ Vitamin B_{12} absorption
Neomycin / ↓ Vitamin B_{12} absorption
Amino salicylate / ↓ Vitamin B_{12} absorption
Potassium, timed-release / ↓ Vitamin B_{12} absorption

HOW SUPPLIED

Cyanocobalamin: *Gel, Intranasal:* 500 mcg/0.1 mL; *Lozenge:* 100 mcg, 250 mcg, 500 mcg; Tablet: 100 mcg, 500 mcg, 1000 mcg, 5000 mcg; **Cyanocobalamin crystalline:** *Injection:* 100 mcg/mL, 1,000 mcg/mL; *Tablets;* 500 mcg, 1000 mcg

DOSAGE

CYANOCOBALAMIN

• **TABLETS**

Nutritional supplement.

Adults: 1 mcg/day (up to 25 mcg for increased requirements). The RDA is 2 mcg/day. **Pediatric, up to 1 year:** 0.3 mcg/day; **over 1 year:** 1 mcg/day.

Nutritional deficiency.

25–250 mcg/day.

• **NASAL GEL**

Malabsorption in remission following parenteral therapy.

500 mcg/0.1 mL weekly given intranasally.

CYANOCOBALAMIN CRYSTALLINE

• **IM, DEEP SC**

Addisonian pernicious anemia.

Adults: 100 mcg/day for 6–7 days; **then,** if improvement is noted along with a reticulocyte response, give 100 mcg every other day for seven doses and then 100 mcg q 3–4 days for 2–3 weeks. **Maintenance, IM:** 100 mcg once a month for life. Give folic acid if necessary.

Vitamin B_{12} deficiency.

Adults: 30 mcg daily for 5–10 days; **then,** 100–200 mcg/month. Doses up to 1,000 mcg have been recommended. **Pediatric, for hematologic signs:** 10–50 mcg/day for 5–10 days followed by 100–250 mcg/dose q 2–4 weeks. **Pediatric, for neurologic signs:** 100 mcg/day for 10–15 days; **then,** 1–2 times/week for several months (can possibly be tapered to 250–1,000 mcg/month by 1 year).

Diagnosis of vitamin B_{12} deficiency.

Adults: 1 mcg/day IM for 10 days plus low dietary folic acid and vitamin B_{12}. Loading dose for the Schilling test is 1,000 mcg given IM.

NURSING CONSIDERATIONS

ADMINISTRATION/STORAGE

1. Protect cyanocobalamin crystalline injection from light. Do not freeze.
2. With pernicious anemia, the drug cannot be administered PO.
3. Clients should be in hematologic remission before use of the nasal gel.

ASSESSMENT

1. Document indications for therapy, type and onset of symptoms.
2. Determine if allergic to cobalt.
3. Note if prescribed chloramphenicol; this drug antagonizes the hematopoietic response to vitamin B_{12}.
4. Perform a baseline assessment of peripheral pulses and assess for neuropathy.
5. Monitor CBC, potassium, and B_{12} levels if being treated for megaloblastic anemia.
6. With pernicious anemia and malabsorption syndromes, administer intrinsic factor simultaneously.

CLIENT/FAMILY TEACHING

1. With pernicious anemia, *must take* vitamin B_{12} replacement for life.
2. When repository vitamin B_{12} used, it provides drug for 4 weeks.
3. The stinging, burning sensation after injection is transitory.
4. If vitamin B_{12} therapy is the result of dietary deficiency, identify foods (such as meats, especially liver, fermented cheeses, egg yolks, and seafood) high in B_{12} and review diet.
5. Avoid alcohol; interferes with drug absorption.

6. Report any symptoms of urticaria, itching, and evidence of anaphylaxis immediately.
7. If diarrhea occurs, record the frequency, quantity, and consistency of stools; may require a drug change.

OUTCOMES/EVALUATE

- Cause of B_{12} deficiency state
- Symptomatic improvement
- Plasma vitamin B_{12} levels of 350–750 pg/mL

Cyclobenzaprine hydrochloride

(sye-kloh-**BENZ**-ah-preen)

PREGNANCY CATEGORY: B
CLASSIFICATION(S):
Skeletal muscle relaxant, centrally-acting
Rx: Flexeril
✱**Rx:** Apo-Cyclobenzaprine, Flexitec, Gen-Cyclobenzaprine, Novo-Cycloprine, Nu-Cyclobenzaprine

SEE ALSO *SKELETAL MUSCLE RELAXANTS, CENTRALLY ACTING.*

ACTION/KINETICS

Related to the tricyclic antidepressants; possesses both sedative and anticholinergic properties. Thought to inhibit reflexes by reducing tonic somatic motor activity. **Onset:** 1 hr. **Time to peak plasma levels:** 4–6 hr. **Therapeutic plasma levels:** 20–30 ng/mL. **Duration:** 12–24 hr. **t½:** 1–3 days. Highly bound to plasma protein. Inactive metabolites are excreted in the urine.

USES

Adjunct to rest and physical therapy for relief of muscle spasms associated with acute and/or painful musculoskeletal conditions. Not indicated for the treatment of spastic diseases or for cerebral palsy. *Investigational:* Adjunct in the treatment of fibrositis syndrome.

CONTRAINDICATIONS

Hypersensitivity. Arrhythmias, heart block or conduction disturbances, CHF, or during acute recovery phase of MI. Hyperthyroidism. Concomitant use of MAO inhibitors or within 14 days of their discontinuation.

SPECIAL CONCERNS

Safe use during lactation and in children under age 15 has not been established. Due to atropine-like effects, use with caution in situations where cholinergic blockade is not desired (e.g., history of urinary retention, angle-closure glaucoma, increased intraocular pressure). Geriatric clients may be more sensitive to cholinergic blockade.

SIDE EFFECTS

Since cyclobenzaprine resembles tricyclic antidepressants, side effects to these drugs should also be noted.

GI: Dry mouth, N&V, constipation, dyspepsia, unpleasant taste, anorexia, diarrhea, GI pain, gastritis, thirst, flatulence, ageusia, paralytic ileus, discoloration of tongue, stomatitis, parotid swelling. **CNS:** Drowsiness, dizziness, fatigue, asthenia, blurred vision, nervousness, headache, ***convulsions,*** ataxia, vertigo, dysarthria, paresthesia, hypertonia, tremors, malaise, abnormal gait, delusions, Bell's palsy, alteration in EEG patterns, extrapyramidal symptoms. Psychiatric symptoms include: confusion, insomnia, disorientation, depressed mood, abnormal sensations, anxiety, agitation, abnormal thinking or dreaming, excitement, hallucinations. **CV:** Tachycardia, syncope, ***arrhythmias,*** vasodilation, palpitations, hypotension, edema, chest pain, hypertension, MI, heart block, stroke. **GU:** Urinary frequency or retention, impaired urination, dilation of urinary tract, impotence, decreased or increased libido, testicular swelling, gynecomastia, breast enlargement, galactorrhea. **Dermatologic:** Sweating, skin rashes, urticaria, pruritus, photosensitivity, alopecia. **Musculoskeletal:** Muscle twitching, weakness, myalgia. **Hematologic:** Purpura, bone marrow depression, leukopenia, eosinophilia, thrombocytopenia. **Hepatic:** Abnormal liver function, hepatitis, jaundice, cholestasis. **Miscellaneous:**

Tinnitus, diplopia, peripheral neuropathy, increase and decrease of blood sugar, weight gain or loss, ***edema of the face and tongue,*** inappropriate ADH syndrome, dyspnea.

OD OVERDOSE MANAGEMENT

Symptoms: Temporary confusion, disturbed concentration, transient visual hallucinations, agitation, hyperactive reflexes, muscle rigidity, vomiting, ***hyperpyrexia.*** Also, drowsiness, hypothermia, tachycardia, ***cardiac arrhythmias such as bundle branch block, ECG evidence of impaired conduction,*** CHF, dilated pupils, ***seizures, severe hypotension,*** stupor, ***coma,*** paradoxical diaphoresis. *Treatment:* In addition to the treatment outlined for Physostigmine salicylate, 1–3 mg IV may be used to reverse symptoms of severe cholinergic blockade, however, profound bradycardia and asystole may occur.

DRUG INTERACTIONS

NOTE: Because of the similarity of cyclobenzaprine to tricyclic antidepressants, the drug interactions for tricyclics should also be consulted.

Anticholinergics / Additive anticholinergic side effects

CNS depressants / Additive depressant effects

Guanethidine / Cyclobenzaprine may block effect

MAO inhibitors / Hypertensive crisis, severe convulsions

Tricyclic antidepressants / Additive side effects

HOW SUPPLIED

Tablet: 10 mg

DOSAGE

- **TABLETS**

Skeletal muscle disorders.

Adults: 20–40 mg/day in three to four divided doses (usual: 10 mg t.i.d.), up to a maximum of 60 mg/day in divided doses.

NURSING CONSIDERATIONS

SEE ALSO *NURSING CONSIDERATIONS* FOR *SKELETAL MUSCLE RELAXANTS, CENTRALLY ACTING.*

ADMINISTRATION/STORAGE

1. Use only for 2–3 weeks.
2. If taking an MAO inhibitor, do not administer cyclobenzaprine for at least 2 weeks after discontinuing.

ASSESSMENT

1. Document indications for therapy, extent of acute or painful musculoskeletal condition, DTRs, ROM, and evidence of weakness. Review RICE (rest, ice, compression, and elevation) with acute injury to reduce swelling and recovery time.
2. Note any hypersensitivity or spastic diseases.
3. Check for evidence of cardiac arrhythmias; note history of MI. Obtain ECG, CBC, and LFTs.
4. With injury/fall assess need for xrays.

CLIENT/FAMILY TEACHING

1. Report any unusual fatigue, sore throat, fever, easy bruising/bleeding; S&S of blood dyscrasia.
2. Report nausea or abdominal pain, itchy skin, or evidence of yellow sclera or skin; S&S of hepatic toxicity.
3. Symptoms of dry mouth, blurred vision, dizziness, tachycardia, or urinary retention should be reported.
4. Due to drug-induced drowsiness, dizziness, and/or blurred vision, observe caution if performing activities that require mental alertness.
5. Notify provider if S&S do not improve within 2–3 weeks of therapy.

OUTCOMES/EVALUATE

Relief of musculoskeletal spasms/pain; ↑ ROM

Cyclophosphamide (CYC)

(sye-kloh-**FOS**-fah-myd)

PREGNANCY CATEGORY: D

CLASSIFICATION(S):

Antineoplastic, alkylating

Rx: Cytoxan , Cytoxan Lyophilized, Neosar

✱Rx: Procytox

SEE ALSO *ANTINEOPLASTIC AGENTS* AND *ALKYLATING AGENTS.*

ACTION/KINETICS

Metabolized in the liver to both active antineoplastic alkylating agents and inactive metabolites. The active metabolites alkylate nucleic acids, thus interfering with the growth of neoplastic and normal tissues. The cytotoxic action is due to cross-linking of strands of DNA and RNA and inhibition of protein synthesis. Also possesses immunosuppressive activity. **t½:** 3–12 hr, but remnants of drug and/or metabolites detectable in serum after 72 hr; in children, the **t½** averages 4.1 hr. Metabolites are excreted through the urine with up to 25% of cyclophosphamide excreted unchanged. Cyclophosphamide is also excreted in milk.

USES

Often used in combination with other antineoplastic drugs. (1) *Malignancies:* Malignant lymphomas (Stages III and IV, Ann Arbor Staging System), Hodgkin's disease, lymphocytic lymphoma (nodular or diffuse), mixed-cell-type lymphoma, histiocytic lymphoma, Burkitt's lymphoma, multiple myeloma, neuroblastoma (disseminated), adenocarcinoma of the ovary, retinoblastoma, carcinoma of the breast. (2) *Leukemias:* Chronic lymphocytic and granulocytic leukemia, acute myelogenous and monocytic leukemia, acute lymphoblastic leukemia in children. (3) *Other:* Mycosis fungoides, nephrotic syndrome in children. *Investigational:* Rheumatic diseases including rheumatoid arthritis and lupus erythematosus, Wegemer's granulomatosis, multiple sclerosis, polyarteritis nodosa, polymyositis (use with corticosteroids), severe neuropsychiatric lupus erythematosus.

CONTRAINDICATIONS

Lactation. Severe bone marrow depression.

SPECIAL CONCERNS

Use with caution in clients with thrombocytopenia, leukopenia, previous radiation therapy, bone marrow infiltration of tumor cells, previous therapy causing cytotoxicity, and impaired liver and kidney function. May interfere with wound healing.

ADDITIONAL SIDE EFFECTS

Acute hemorrhagic cystitis. ***Bone marrow depression*** appears frequently during days 9–14 of therapy. Alopecia occurs more frequently than with other drugs. ***Secondary neoplasia (especially of urinary bladder), pulmonary fibrosis, cardiotoxicity,*** darkening of skin or fingernails. Interference with oogenesis and spermatogenesis.

LABORATORY TEST CONSIDERATIONS

↑ Uric acid in blood and urine; false + Pap test; ↓ serum pseudocholinesterase. Suppression of certain skin tests.

OD OVERDOSE MANAGEMENT

Treatment: General supportive measures. Dialysis.

DRUG INTERACTIONS

Allopurinol / ↑ Chance of bone marrow toxicity
Anticoagulants / ↑ Anticoagulant effects
Chloramphenicol / ↓ Metabolism of cyclophosphamide to active metabolites → ↓ pharmacologic effect
Digoxin / ↓ Serum digoxin levels
Doxorubicin / ↑ Cardiotoxicity
Insulin / ↑ Hypoglycemia
Phenobarbital / ↑ Rate of metabolism of cyclophosphamide in liver
Quinolone antibiotics / ↓ Antimicrobial effect of quinolones
Succinylcholine / ↑ Neuromuscular blockade R/T ↓ cholinesterase activity
Thiazide diuretics / ↑ Chance of leukopenia

HOW SUPPLIED

Powder for injection: 100 mg cyclophosphamide/75 mg mannitol, 100 mg cyclophosphamide/82 mg sodium bicarbonate; *Tablet:* 25 mg, 50 mg

DOSAGE

- **IV**

  Malignancies.

Initial, with no hematologic deficiency: 40–50 mg/kg in divided doses over 2–5 days. **Alternative therapy:** 10–15 mg/kg q 7–10 days or 3–5 mg/kg twice weekly.

- **TABLETS**

  Malignancies.

Initial and maintenance: 1–5 mg/kg depending on client tolerance. Attempt to maintain leukocyte count at 3,000–4,000/mm³. Adjust dosage for kidney or liver disease.

Nephrotic syndrome in children. 2.5–3 mg/kg/day for 60–90 days.

NURSING CONSIDERATIONS

SEE ALSO *NURSING CONSIDERATIONS* FOR *ANTINEOPLASTIC AGENTS*.

ADMINISTRATION/STORAGE

1. Prepare PO solution by dissolving injectable cyclophosphamide in aromatic elixir.
2. The initial loading dose may need to be reduced by one-third to one-half if previously received cytotoxic drugs or XRT.
IV 3. IV/IM: Dissolve 100 mg cyclophosphamide in appropriate amount (depending on vial strength) of sterile water for injection.
4. Solutions may be given IV, IM, intraperitoneally, or intrapleurally. May be infused IV with D5W, D5/0.9% NaCl, D5%/Ringer's injection, RL, 0.45% NaCl, or 1/6M sodium lactate injection.
5. Store reconstituted solution at room temperature for 24 hr or for 6 days if refrigerated at 2–8°C (36–46°F).

ASSESSMENT

1. Note any prior radiation or chemotherapy; dose requires reduction.
2. Assess skin condition and integrity noting evidence of breakdown; may interfere with wound healing.
3. Monitor for cardiotoxicity: increased SOB, rales, increased coughing, or tachycardia. Obtain periodic CXR and PFTs.
4. Check for dysuria and hematuria; monitor urinalysis with specific gravity to assess for SIADH.
5. Monitor CBC; may cause granulocyte suppression. Nadir: 14 days; recovery: 17–21 days.

CLIENT/FAMILY TEACHING

1. Take PO meds on an empty stomach; may take with meals if GI upset occurs.
2. Increase fluid intake before, during, and for 24 hr after therapy.
3. Take in the morning so kidneys can eliminate drug before bedtime; void frequently. Stay well hydrated to prevent hemorrhagic cystitis R/T excessive urinary concentrations.
4. May discolor skin and nails.
5. Report any unusual bruising, bleeding, or fever.
6. Avoid vaccinations during therapy.
7. With alopecia, hair should grow back when drug is stopped or when a maintenance dosage is given.
8. Drug may cause a false positive Pap test. May also cause sterility and menstrual irregularities; identify candidates for egg/sperm harvesting.
9. Practice reliable contraception (both sexes) during therapy.
10. S&S of hypoglycemia may be precipitated by drug interactions with insulin; monitor sugars closely and consult with provider for insulin dosage adjustment.
11. Report any evidence of injury or delayed wound healing.
12. May suppress skin test response for *Candida*, mumps, trichophyton, and PPD.

OUTCOMES/EVALUATE

- Improved hematologic profile
- ↓ Tumor size and spread

Cycloserine

(sye-kloh-**SEE**-reen)

PREGNANCY CATEGORY: C
CLASSIFICATION(S):
Antitubercular drug
Rx: Seromycin

ACTION/KINETICS

Produced by a strain of *Streptomyces orchidaceus* or *Garyphalus lavendulae.* Acts by inhibiting cell wall synthesis by interfering with the incorporation of the amino acid alanine. Well absorbed from the GI tract and widely distributed in body tissues. **Time to peak plasma levels:** 4–8 hr. CSF, pleural fluid, fetal blood, and breast milk levels are similar to those in plasma. **t½:** 10 hr. From 60% to 70% is excreted unchanged in urine.

USES

(1) With other drugs to treat active pulmonary and extrapulmonary tuberculosis only when primary therapy cannot be used. (2) To treat acute UTIs due to *Enterobacter* species and *Escherichia coli.* Usually less effective than other drugs. Use only when more conventional therapy has failed

and when sensitivity to organism has been shown.

CONTRAINDICATIONS

Hypersensitivity to cycloserine, epilepsy, depression, severe anxiety, psychosis, severe renal insufficiency, and alcoholism. Lactation.

SPECIAL CONCERNS

Safe use in children has not been established, although there is a recommended pediatric dose.

SIDE EFFECTS

CNS: Drowsiness, headache, somnolence, dysarthria, mental confusion, tremors, vertigo, disorientation with loss of memory, psychoses (possibly with ***suicidal tendencies),*** character changes, hyperirritability, aggression, increased reflexes, ***seizures*** (major and minor clonic), paresthesias, paresis, coma. Neurotoxic effects depend on blood levels of cycloserine. Hence, frequent determinations of cycloserine blood levels are indicated, especially during the initial period of therapy. **Other:** Sudden development of CHF, skin rashes (e.g., allergic dermatitis), allergy, anemia, increased transaminase.

OD OVERDOSE MANAGEMENT

Symptoms: CNS depression, including drowsiness, mental confusion, headache, vertigo, paresthesias, dysarthrias, hyperirritability, psychosis, paresis, ***seizures,*** and ***coma.*** *Treatment:* Supportive therapy. Charcoal may be more effective than emesis or gastric lavage. Hemodialysis may be used for life-threatening toxicity. Pyridoxine, 200–300 mg/day may treat neurotoxic effects.

DRUG INTERACTIONS

Ethanol / ↑ Risk of epileptic episodes
Ethionamide / Potentiation of neurotoxic side effects
Isoniazid / ↑ Risk of cycloserine CNS side effects (especially dizziness)
Phenytoin / Phenytoin metabolism inhibited

HOW SUPPLIED

Capsule: 250 mg

DOSAGE

• CAPSULES

Adults, initially: 250 mg q 12 hr for first 2 weeks; **then,** 0.5–1 g/day in divided doses based on blood levels. Dosage should not exceed 1 g/day. **Pediatric:** 10–20 mg/kg/day, not to exceed 0.75–1 g/day. *NOTE:* Pyridoxine, 200–300 mg/day may prevent neurotoxic effects. Also, increased dosing interval in renal impairment: q 24 hr if C_{CR} is 10–50 mL/min and q 36–48 hr if C_{CR} is less than 10 mL/min.

NURSING CONSIDERATIONS

SEE ALSO *GENERAL NURSING CONSIDERATIONS FOR ALL ANTI-INFECTIVES.*

ADMINISTRATION/STORAGE

Anticonvulsant or sedative drugs may help to control CNS toxicity, including seizures, anxiety, and tremor.

ASSESSMENT

1. Note any evidence of depression, anxiety, seizures, or excessive alcohol use. Report any psychotic or neurologic reactions that may necessitate temporary drug withdrawal.
2. Monitor I&O; observe for any S&S of CHF with high-dose therapy.
3. Monitor renal and LFTs and cycloserine levels (<25–30 mcg/mL) with therapy.

CLIENT/FAMILY TEACHING

1. May cause drowsiness and dizziness; do not perform tasks that require mental alertness; report if symptoms persist.
2. Consume 2–3 L/day of fluids.
3. Avoid alcohol.
4. Immediately report any SOB, skin rashes, or overt behavioral changes, especially suicide ideations.

OUTCOMES/EVALUATE

• Negative sputum cultures for acid-fast bacilli
• Improved CXR and PFTs

Cyclosporine

(sye-kloh-**SPOR**-een)

PREGNANCY CATEGORY: C
CLASSIFICATION(S):
Immunosuppressant
Rx: Cyclosporine Softgel Capsules, Gengraf, Neoral, Sandimmune
★**Rx:** Sandimmune I.V.

C

ACTION/KINETICS

Thought to act by inhibiting the immunocompetent lymphocytes in the G_0 or G_1 phase of the cell cycle. T-lymphocytes are specifically inhibited; both the T-helper cell and the T-suppressor cell may be affected. Also inhibits interleukin 2 or T-cell growth factor production and release. Absorption from the GI tract is incomplete and variable. Children often require larger PO doses than adults, which may be due to the smaller absorptive surface area of their intestines. **Peak plasma levels:** 3.5 hr. Food may both delay and impair drug absorption. **t½:** Approximately 19 hr for adults and 7 hr in children. Metabolized by the liver; inactive metabolites are excreted mainly through the bile.

Neoral immediately forms a microemulsion in an aqueous environment. This product has better bioequivalency; thus, Sandimmune and Neoral are not bioequivalent and cannot be used interchangeably without medical supervision. **Time to peak blood levels:** 1.5–2 hr. Food decreases the amount of drug absorbed.

USES

(1) Prophylaxis of rejection in kidney, liver, and heart allogeneic transplants. Sandimmune is always to be taken with adrenal corticosteroids while Neoral has been used in combination with azathioprine and corticosteroids. (2) NEORAL MICROEMULSION: Alone or in combination with methotrexate for severe, active rheumatoid arthritis which has not responded to methotrexate alone. (3) NEORAL MICROEMULSION: Severe recalcitrant plaque psoriasis. (4) SANDIMMUNE: Treatment of chronic rejection in clients previously treated with other immunosuppressants. Sandimmune has been used in children as young as 6 months with no unusual side effects. *Investigational:* Aplastic anemia, myasthenia gravis, atopic dermatitis, Crohn's disease, Graves ophthalmology, severe psoriasis, multiple sclerosis, polymyositis, Behçet's disease, biliary cirrhosis, corneal transplantation (or other diseases of the eye which have an autoimmune component), dermatomyositis, IDDM, lichen planus, lupus nephritis, nephrotic syndrome, pemphigus and pemphigoid, psoriatic arthritis, pulmonary sarcoidosis, pyoderma gangrenosum, alopecia areata, ulcerative colitis, uveitis.

CONTRAINDICATIONS

Hypersensitivity to cyclosporine or polyoxyethylated castor oil. Lactation. Use of potassium-sparing diuretics. Neoral in psoriasis or rheumatoid arthritis with abnormal renal function, uncontrolled hypertension, or malignancies. Neoral together with PUVA or UVB in psoriasis.

SPECIAL CONCERNS

Use with caution in clients with impaired renal or hepatic function. Safety and efficacy have not been established in children. Clients with malabsorption may not achieve therapeutic levels following PO use.

SIDE EFFECTS

GI: N&V, diarrhea, gum hyperplasia, anorexia, gastritis, hiccoughs, peptic ulcer, abdominal discomfort, UGI bleeding, pancreatitis, constipation, mouth sores, swallowing difficulty. **Hematologic:** Leukopenia, lymphoma, thrombocytopenia, anemia, microangiopathic hemolytic anemia syndrome. **Allergic:** ***Anaphylaxis (rare).*** **CV:** Hypertension, edema, chest pain, cramps, ***MI*** (rare). **CNS:** Headache, tremor, confusion, fever, ***seizures,*** anxiety, depression, weakness, lethargy, ataxia. **GU:** Renal dysfunction, glomerular capillary thrombosis, nephrotoxicity. **Dermatologic:** Acne, hirsutism, brittle finger nails, hair breaking, pruritus. **Miscellaneous:** Hepatotoxicity, flushing, paresthesia, sinusitis, gynecomastia, conjunctivitis, hearing loss, tinnitus, muscle pain, infections (including fungal, viral), *Pneumocystis carinii* pneumonia, hematuria, blurred vision, weight loss, joint pain, night sweats, tingling, hypomagnesemia in some clients with seizures, infectious complications, increased risk of cancer.

LABORATORY TEST CONSIDERATIONS

↑ Serum creatinine, potassium, BUN, total bilirubin, alkaline phosphatase. Possibly ↑ cholesterol, LDL, and apolipoprotein B. Hyperglycemia/kalemia/uricemia.

OD OVERDOSE MANAGEMENT

Symptoms: Transient hepatotoxicity and nephrotoxicity. *Treatment:* Induction of vomiting (up to 2 hr after ingestion). General supportive measures.

DRUG INTERACTIONS

Aminoglycosides / ↑ Risk of nephrotoxicity
Amiodarone / ↑ Cyclosporine blood levels → ↑ risk of nephrotoxicity
Amphotericin B / ↑ Risk of nephrotoxicity
Azathioprine / ↑ Immunosuppression R/T suppression of lymphocytes → possible infection and malignancy
Bromocriptine / ↑ Cyclosporine plasma level R/T ↓ liver breakdown
Calcium channel blockers / ↑ Cyclosporine plasma levels R/T ↓ liver breakdown; ↑ risk of toxicity
Carbamazepine / ↓ Cyclosporine plasma level R/T ↑ liver breakdown
Carvedilol / ↑ Carvedilol blood levels R/T ↓ liver breakdown
Chloramphencil / ↑ Cyclosporine blood levels in renal transplant clients
Cimetidine / ↑ Risk of nephrotoxicity
Clarithromycin / ↑ Cyclosporine plasma levels R/T ↓ liver breakdown; ↑ risk of nephro-/neurotoxicity
Clindamycin / ↓ Cyclosporine serum levels
Colchicine / Severe side effects, including GI, hepatic, renal, and neuromuscular toxicity
Corticosteroids / ↑ Immunosuppression R/T suppression of lymphocytes → possible infection and malignancy
Cyclophosphamide / ↑ Immunosuppression R/T suppression of lymphocytes → possible infection and malignancy
Danazol / ↑ Cyclosporine plasma level R/T ↓ liver breakdown
Diclofenac / ↑ Risk of nephrotoxicity
Digoxin / ↑ Digoxin levels R/T ↓ clearance; also, ↓ volume of distribution of digoxin → toxicity
Diltiazem / ↑ Cyclosporine plasma level R/T ↓ liver breakdown → possible nephrotoxicity
H *Echinacea* / Do not give with cyclosporine
Erythromycin / ↑ Cyclosporine plasma level R/T ↓ liver breakdown and ↓ biliary excretion → possible nephrotoxicity
Etoposide / ↓ Etoposide renal clearance → increased toxicity
Fluconazole / ↑ Cyclosporine plasma level R/T ↓ gut and liver metabolism → possible nephrotoxicity
Foscarnet ↑ Risk of renal failure
Grapefruit juice / ↑ Cyclosporine blood levels due to ↓ liver breakdown
Griseofulvin / ↓ Cyclosporine levels → ↓ effect
HIV protease inhibitors / ↑ Cyclosporine plasma levels R/T ↓ liver breakdown → toxicity
Imipenem-cilastatin / ↑ Cyclosporine blood levels → CNS toxicity
Isoniazid / ↓ Cyclosporine plasma level R/T ↑ liver breakdown
Itraconazole / ↑ Plasma level of cyclosporine R/T ↓ liver breakdown
Ketoconazole / ↑ Cyclosporine plasma level R/T ↓ breakdown by gut and liver metabolism → possible nephrotoxicity
Lovastatin / ↑ Risk of myopathy and rhabdomyolysis R/T ↓ cyclosporine breakdown
Melphalan / ↑ Risk of nephrotoxicity
Methylprednisolone / ↑ Cyclosporine blood levels R/T ↓ liver breakdown → toxicity
Metoclopramide / ↑ Cyclosporine plasma level R/T ↓ liver breakdown → toxicity
Mycophenolate / Possible ↑ Mycophenolate side effects if cyclosporine discontinued
Naproxen / ↑ Risk of nephrotoxicity
Nephrotoxic drugs / Additive nephrotoxicity
Nicardipine / ↑ Cyclosporine plasma level R/T ↓ liver breakdown → possible nephrotoxicity
Nifedipine / ↑ Risk of gingival hyperplasia
Octreotide / ↓ Cyclosporine plasma level R/T ↑ liver breakdown
Oral contraceptives / ↑ Cyclosporine plasma level R/T ↓ liver breakdown; possible severe hepatotoxicity

Orlistat / Possible ↓ cyclosporine blood levels R/T ↓ absorption
Phenobarbital / ↓ Cyclosporine plasma level R/T ↑ liver breakdown
Phenytoin / ↓ Cyclosporine plasma levels R/T ↑ liver breakdown
Probucol / ↓ Cyclosporine bioavailability → ↓ clinical effect
Ranitidine / ↑ Risk of nephrotoxicity
Rifabutin/Rifampin / ↓ Cyclosporine plasma level R/T ↑ liver breakdown
Saquinavir / ↑ Cyclosporine blood levels
Simvastatin / ↑ Risk of myopathy and rhabdomyolysis R/T ↓ cyclosporine breakdown
H *St. John's Wort* / Possible induction of liver enzymes → ↓ cyclosporine effect
Sulfamethoxazole and/or trimethoprim / ↑ Risk of nephrotoxicity; also, ↓ cyclosporine serum levels → possible organ rejection
Sulindac / ↑ Risk of nephrotoxicity
Tacrolimus / ↑ Risk of nephrotoxicity
Vancomycin / ↑ Risk of nephrotoxicity
Verapamil / ↑ Immunosuppression

HOW SUPPLIED

Capsule, Soft Gelatin: 25 mg, 50 mg, 100 mg; *Capsule, Soft Gelatin for Microemulsion:* 25 mg 100 mg; *Injection:* 50 mg/mL; *Oral Solution:* 100 mg/mL; *Oral Solution for Microemulsion:* 100 mg/mL

DOSAGE

• **CAPSULES, ORAL SOLUTION**

Allogenic transplants.

Adults and children, initial: A single 15 mg/kg dose given 4–12 hr before transplantation; there is a trend to use lower initial doses of 10–14 mg/kg/day. The dose should be continued postoperatively for 1–2 weeks followed by 5% decrease in dose per week to maintenance dose of 5–10 mg/kg/day (some have used a dose of 3 mg/kg/day successfully). Compared with Sandimmune, lower maintenance doses of Neoral may be sufficient.

If converting from Sandimmune to Neoral, start with a 1:1 conversion. Then, adjust the Neoral dose to reach the pre-conversion cyclosporine blood trough levels. Until this level is reached, monitor the cyclosporine trough level q 4–7 days.

Rheumatoid arthritis (Neoral only).

Initial: 1.25 mg/kg b.i.d. PO. Salicylates, NSAIDs, and PO corticosteroids may be continued. If sufficient beneficial effect is not seen and the client is tolerating the medication, the dose may be increased by 0.5–0.75 mg/kg/day after 8 weeks and again after 12 weeks to a maximum dose of 4 mg/kg/day. If no benefit is seen after 16 weeks, discontinue therapy. If Neoral is combined with methotrexate, the same initial dose and dose range of Neoral can be used.

Psoriasis (Neoral only).

Initial: 1.25 mg/kg b.i.d. PO. Maintain this dose for 4 weeks if tolerated. If significant improvement is not seen, increase the dose at 2-week intervals. Based on client response, make dose increases of about 0.5 mg/kg/day to a maximum of 4 mg/kg/day. Discontinue treatment if beneficial effects can not be achieved after 6 weeks at 4 mg/kg/day. Once beneficial effects are seen, decrease the dose (doses less than 2.5 mg/kg/day may be effective). To control side effects, make dose decreases by 25% to 50% at any time.

• **IV (ONLY IN CLIENTS UNABLE TO TAKE PO MEDICATION)**

Allogenic transplants.

Adults: 5–6 mg/kg/day 4–12 hr prior to transplantation and postoperatively until client can be switched to PO dosage. *NOTE:* Steroid therapy must be used concomitantly.

Investigational uses.

Oral doses ranging from 1 to 10 mg/kg/day.

NURSING CONSIDERATIONS

ADMINISTRATION/STORAGE

1. Sandimmune and Neoral are not bioequivalent and should not be used interchangeably without the supervision of someone experienced in immunosuppressive therapy. Conversion from Neoral to Sandimmune using a 1:1 ratio (mg/kg/day) may result in lower cyclosporine blood levels.

2. Sandimmune capsules and oral solution are bioequivalent. Neoral capsules and oral solution are bioequivalent.

3. May dilute the PO solution with milk, chocolate milk, orange or apple juice immediately before administering. Dilute Neoral, preferably, with orange or apple juice; grapefruit juice affects metabolism of cyclosporine and is not to be used. After removal of the protective cover, transfer the solution, using the dosing syringe supplied, and transfer the solution to a glass of diluent. Stir well and drink at once. Do not allow diluted solution to stand before drinking. Use a glass container (not plastic). Rinse the glass with more diluent and swallow to ensure the total dose is taken. Do not store PO solutions in the refrigerator; contents should be used within 2 months after being opened.

4. At temperatures less than 20°C (68°F), Neoral solution may gel; light flocculation or the formation of a light sediment may also occur. This will not affect product peformance or dosing using the syringe provided. Allow to warm to room temperature to reverse such changes.

5. Due to variable absorption of the PO solution, monitor blood levels.

6. Clients with malabsorption from the GI tract may not achieve appropriate blood levels.

IV 7. Dilute IV concentrate 1 mL (50 mg) in 20–100 mL 0.9% NaCl or D5% injection; give infusion slowly over 2–6 hr. Do not refrigerate once cyclosporine has been added to an IV solution.

8. Following addition to an IV solution, shake vigorously to disperse the drug.

9. Protect IV solution from light.

10. The polyoxyethylated castor oil found in the concentrate for IV infusion may cause phthalate stripping from PVC.

11. Due to possibility of anaphylaxis, monitor clients receiving IV cyclosporine closely for 30 min at the start of therapy. Have epinephrine (1:1,000) for anaphylaxis.

ASSESSMENT

1. Document indications for therapy; note any previous treatments. List drugs prescribed and note any potential interactions. Anticipate concomitant administration of adrenal corticosteroids.

2. Monitor VS, CBC, cyclosporine levels, liver and renal function studies. Drug may increase BP, serum K, lipid, and uric acid levels.

3. Differentiate nephrotoxicity from rejection using criteria provided by the manufacturer.

CLIENT/FAMILY TEACHING

1. Review importance of following the written guidelines for medication therapy explicitly. Drug must be taken throughout one's lifetime to prevent transplant rejection.

2. Because this drug is so important in preventing rejection, a written list of all possible drug side effects and those which need to be reported will be provided.

3. Taking the drug with food may reduce nausea and GI upset. If PO form unpalatable, mix with milk or orange juice in a glass container to minimize container adherence. Measure dose accurately and take immediately after mixing.

4. Do not take with grapefruit juice due to biometabolic concerns.

5. Do not stop abruptly; must be discontinued gradually.

6. Record BP, I&O, and daily weights. Report any persistent diarrhea and N&V.

7. Avoid crowds and persons with infectious illnesses.

8. Practice reliable birth control.

9. Use nystatin swish and swallow to prevent development of thrush; perform oral care and routine dental exams.

10. May develop acne and hirsutism; report as dermatology referral may be needed.

11. Yellow discoloration of eyes, skin, or stools; fever; other signs of hepatotoxicity require reporting.

12. Report increased fatigue, malaise, unexplained bleeding or bruising, or hematuria.

OUTCOMES/EVALUATE
• Prevention of transplant rejection; improved organ function
• Cyclosporine trough levels (100–200 ng/mL)

C

Cysteamine bitartrate

(**SIS**-tee-**ah**-meen)

PREGNANCY CATEGORY: C
CLASSIFICATION(S):
Urinary tract drug
Rx: Cystagon

ACTION/KINETICS
Lowers cystine levels of cells in cystinosis, which is an inherited defect of lysosomal transport. In those with cystinosis, cystine transport out of lysosomes is abnormal, resulting in the formation of crystals which damage the kidney. Other tissues are damaged as well, including the retina, muscles, and CNS. Acts within the cell to convert cystine into both cysteine and cysteine-cysteamine mixed disulfide, which can leave the lysosome in those with cystinosis.
USES
Management of nephropathic cystinosis in adults and children.
CONTRAINDICATIONS
Hypersensitivity to cysteamine or penicillamine. Use during lactation.
SIDE EFFECTS
CNS: Lethargy, somnolence, depression, encephalopathy, ***seizures,*** headache, ataxia, confusion, tremor, hyperkinesia, dizziness, jitteriness, nervousness, abnormal thinking, emotional lability, hallucinations, nightmares. **GI:** N&V, anorexia, abdominal pain (may be severe), diarrhea, bad breath, dyspepsia, constipation, gastroenteritis, duodenitis, duodenal ulceration. **Hematologic:** Reversible leukopenia, anemia. **Miscellaneous;** Decreased hearing, fever, rash, dehydration, hypertension, urticaria.
LABORATORY TEST CONSIDERATIONS
Abnormal LFTs.
OD OVERDOSE MANAGEMENT
Symptoms: Extension of side effects, respiratory symptoms. *Treatment:* Support the cardiovascular and respiratory systems. Hemodialysis may be effective in removing the drug from the body.
HOW SUPPLIED
Capsule: 50 mg, 150 mg
DOSAGE
• CAPSULES
Nephropathic cystinosis.
Initial: New clients should be started on one-fourth to one-sixth of the maintenance dose. The dose is then raised gradually over 4–6 weeks to avoid intolerance. **Maintenance, children up to age 12 years:** 1.3 g/m^2/day (of the free base) given in four divided doses. **Maintenance, children over 12 years and over 110 lb:** 2 g/day in four divided doses.

NURSING CONSIDERATIONS
ADMINISTRATION/STORAGE
1. Initiate therapy in children and adults promptly after the diagnosis has been confirmed by increased white cell cystine levels.
2. Do not give intact cysteamine capsules to children less than 6 years of age due to the possibility of aspiration. Sprinkle contents of the capsule over food.
3. The goal is to keep leukocyte cystine levels less than 1 nmol/½ cystine/mg protein 5–6 hr following administration of cysteamine. Those with intolerance to cysteamine can still get a beneficial effect if cystine levels are less than 2 nmol/½ cystine/mg protein. To achieve this level, the dose of cysteamine may be increased to a maximum of 1.95 g/m^2/day.
4. Cystinotic clients taking cysteamine HCl or phosphocysteamine solutions may be transferred to equimolar doses of cysteamine bitartrate capsules. Clients being transferred should have their white cell cystine levels measured in 2 weeks and every 3 months thereafter.
ASSESSMENT
Obtain baseline CBC, renal and LFTs, C_{CR} and white cell cystine levels; repeat levels 5–6 hr after therapy.

CLIENT/FAMILY TEACHING

1. Take only as directed. May be given with electrolyte and mineral replacements, vitamin D, and thyroid hormone to manage adverse renal effects.
2. Report rash; provider will withhold drug until cleared and then reinstitute at a lower dose with gradual increases to therapeutic dose. This may also have to be done if CNS or GI side effects occur.
3. Obtain labs to assess for leukocyte cystine levels, abnormal liver function, or reversible leukopenia.

OUTCOMES/EVALUATE

- Prevention of organ damage R/T cystine accumulation
- White cell cystine levels of <1 nmol/½ cystine/mg protein

Cytarabine (ARA-C, Cytosine arabinoside)

(sye-**TAIR**-ah-bean)

PREGNANCY CATEGORY: D
Rx: Cytosar-U, Tarabine PFS
★**Rx:** Cytosar

Cytarabine, Liposomal

(sye-**TAIR**-ah-bean)

PREGNANCY CATEGORY: D
Rx: DepoCyt
CLASSIFICATION(S):
Antineoplastic, antimetabolite

SEE ALSO *ANTINEOPLASTIC AGENTS.*

ACTION/KINETICS

Available as conventional and liposomal products. Converted intracellularly to the active cytarabine-5′-triphosphate, which inhibits DNA polymerase. Is cell-phase specific, acting in the S phase to kill cells undergoing DNA synthesis and also blocking the progression of cells from the G_1 phase to the S phase. May also decrease the immune response. Conventional cytarabine is not effective PO. **Conventional: Peak plasma levels, after IM or SC:** 20–60 min. **t½, after IV:** About 10 min for distributive phase and 1–3 hr for elimination phase. **Liposomal:** Given intrathecally. **Peak levels in ventricle and lumbar sac:** Within 5 hr. **t½, terminal:** 100–263 hr. Metabolized in the liver to uracil arabinoside, which is excreted in the urine. Crosses blood-brain barrier. Eighty percent eliminated in urine in 24 hr.

USES

Conventional: Induction and maintenance of remission in acute non-lymphocytic leukemia in adults and children, acute myelocytic leukemia in adults and children, acute lymphocytic leukemia in adults and children, chronic myelocytic leukemia, and meningeal leukemia. **Liposomal:** Intrathecal treatment of lymphomatous meningitis.

CONTRAINDICATIONS

Lactation. Use of liposomal product in active meningeal infection or benzyl alcohol-containing products intrathecally.

SPECIAL CONCERNS

Anaphylaxis has occurred, causing acute cardiopulmonary arrest. Use with caution in clients with impaired renal or hepatic function. Safety and efficacy of the liposomal product have not been determined in children (use the conventional product for children). The liposomal product may cause serious toxicity.

SIDE EFFECTS

Conventional and liposomal cytarabine.

CNS: Confusion, somnolence, abnormal gait. **GI:** N&V, constipation. **Hematologic:** Thrombocytopenia, neutropenia, anemia. **Miscellaneous:** Headache, fever, asthenia, back pain, pain, peripheral edema, urinary incontinence.

Conventional cytarabine.

"Cytarabine syndrome" (6–12 hr following drug administration) manifested by bone pain, fever, myalgia, maculopapular rash, conjunctivitis, chest pain, or malaise. **GI:** Anorexia, diarrhea, oral and anal inflammation/ulceration, hepatic dysfunction, esophageal ulceration, esophagitis, bowel necrosis, abdominal pain, pancreatitis, jaundice. **Respiratory:** Pneumonia, shortness of breath. **Dermatologic:** Rash, cellulitis at injection site, skin ulceration, freckling, alopecia, pruritus, urticaria. **Miscellaneous:** Thrombophlebitis, bleeding (all sites), sepsis, urinary retention, renal dysfunction, neuritis or neural toxicity, peripheral motor and sensory neuropathies, sore throat, chest pain, pericarditis, conjunctivitis (with rash), dizziness, acute pancreatitis, ***anaphylaxis,*** allergic edema, headache. Intrathecal administration may result in systemic side effects including N&V, fever, and rarely neurotoxicity and paraplegia.

Liposomal cytarabine.

Arachnoiditis which includes symptoms of neck rigidity, neck pain, meningism, N&V, headache, fever, back pain, or CSF pleocytosis.

LABORATORY TEST CONSIDERATIONS

Hyperuricemia. *Liposomal product:* Transient ↑ CSF protein and WBCs. The liposomal particles are similar in size and appearance to WBCs; take care in interpreting CSF exams after giving the liposomal product.

OD OVERDOSE MANAGEMENT

Symptoms: CNS toxicity. *Treatment:* General supportive measures.

DRUG INTERACTIONS

Absorption of digoxin may be impaired when cytarabine is used with other antineoplastics.

HOW SUPPLIED

Cytarabine Conventional. *Injection:* 20 mg/mL, 100 mg/mL; *Powder for injection:* 100 mg, 500 mg, 1 g, 2 g. **Cytarabine Liposomal.** *Injection:* 10 mg/mL

DOSAGE

NOTE: Cytarabine is frequently used in combination with other drugs; thus, dosage varies and must be carefully checked.

CYTARABINE, CONVENTIONAL

• **IV INFUSION**

Acute lymphocytic leukemia.

Consult current literature.

Acute nonlymphocytic leukemia (in combination with other drugs).

100 mg/m²/day by continuous IV infusion (days 1–7) or 100 mg/m² q 12 hr (days 1–7).

Refractory acute leukemia.

High dose cytarabine: 3 g/m² given over 2 hr, q 12 hr for 4–12 doses; repeat at 2–3-wk intervals.

• **INTRATHECAL**

Meningeal leukemia.

Usual: 30 mg/m² (range: 5–75 mg/m²) once daily for 4 days to once q 4 days with hydrocortisone, sodium succinate and methotrexate, each at a dose of 15 mg/m², until CSF findings are normal, followed by one additional dose.

NOTE: The drug should be discontinued if platelet level falls to 50,000/mm³ or less or polymorphonuclear granulocyte level falls to 1,000/mm³ or less.

CYTARABINE LIPOSOMAL

• **INTRATHECAL**

Lymphomatous meningitis

Induction: 50 mg q 14 days for 2 doses (weeks 1 and 3). **Consolidation therapy:** 50 mg q 14 days for 3 doses (weeks 5, 7, and 9). **Maintenance:** 50 mg q 28 days for 4 doses (weeks 17, 21, 25, and 29). Give either intraventricularly or by lumbar puncture. If drug-related neurotoxicity occurs, reduce the dose to 25 mg followed by 1 additional dose at week13 dexamethasone, 4 mg b.i.d., either PO or IV for 5 days starting on the day of liposomal cytarabine.

NURSING CONSIDERATIONS

SEE ALSO *NURSING CONSIDERATIONS* FOR *ANTINEOPLASTIC AGENTS*.

ADMINISTRATION/STORAGE

1. Conventional cytarabine may be given SC, IV infusion, or IV injection. It is ineffective PO.
2. Do not use benzyl alcohol for reconstitution if the drug is to be used intrathecally; use 0.9% saline or Elliott's B solution.
3. With liposomal product use dexamethasone to prevent chemical arachnoiditis.

4. For administration of cytarabine liposomal:
• Withdraw from the vial just before use. The liposomal product is a single-use vial and does not contain any preservative. Use within 4 hr after withdrawal.
• Allow vials to warm to room temperature and gently agitate or invert the vials just prior to withdrawal to resuspend the particles. Do not agitate aggressively.
• No reconstitution or dilution is required.
• Do not mix with any other medications.
• Do not use in-line filters. Give directly into the CSF via an intraventricular reservoir or by direct injection into the lumbar sac.
• Inject slowly over a period of 1–5 min. If lumbar puncture is used, have the client lie flat for 1 hr.
• Refrigerate at 2–8°C (36–46°F). Protect from freezing.

IV 5. Reconstitute the 100-mg vial of conventional cytarabine with 5 mL bacteriostatic water for injection with benzyl alcohol (0.9%) to yield a solution containing 20 mg/mL. Reconstitute the 500-mg vial with 10 mL of bacteriostatic water for injection with benzyl alcohol (0.9%) to yield a solution containing 50 mg/mL cytarabine.
6. To administer direct IV, reconstitute the 100-mg vial and administer over 1–3 min. May be further diluted into 100 mL of D5W or NSS and infused over 30 min.
7. Store reconstituted solution at room temperature and use within 48 hr. Discard if hazy.
8. Have appropriate resuscitative drugs and equipment readily available in the event of anaphylaxis.

ASSESSMENT

1. Obtain CBC, uric acid, liver and renal function; note impaired hepatic function.
2. Document any previous therapy for leukemia and outcome.
3. Systemic toxicity may result from use of liposomal cytarabine or intrathecal use. To prevent chemical arachnoiditis, treat all clients receiving the liposomal product with dexamethasone.
4. Some clients with neoplastic meningitis receiving liposomal cytarabine may require concurrent radiation or systemic treatment with other chemotherapy; this increases the incidence of side effects and may alter dosage.
5. Obtain hematologic parameters to interrupt therapy; drug causes severe granulocyte and platelet toxicity. Nadir: 10 days; recovery: 21 days.

CLIENT/FAMILY TEACHING

1. Report any unusual bruising, bleeding, fever, or S&S of anemia (fatigue, SOB, dizziness).
2. Consume 2–3 L/day of fluids to prevent renal damage from hyperuricemia related to cell lysis. Alkalinization of the urine may enhance uric acid excretion.
3. Report any inflammation of the eye, which may require treatment with steroid eye drops.
4. Avoid crowds, persons with known infections, and vaccinations during therapy.
5. Use birth control during and for at least 4 months following therapy.

OUTCOMES/EVALUATE

• ↓Tumor size and spread
• Improved hematologic parameters; evidence of disease remission

Cytomegalovirus Immune Globulin Intravenous, Human (CMV-IGIV)

(**sigh**-toh-**meg**-ah-lo-**VIGH**-rus im-**MYOUN GLOB**-you-lin)

PREGNANCY CATEGORY: C
CLASSIFICATION(S):
Immune globulin
Rx: CytoGam

ACTION/KINETICS

Obtained from pooled adult human plasma that has been selected for

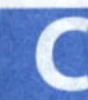

high titers of antibody for CMV. Is purified. When reconstituted, each mL contains 50 mg of immunoglobulin that is primarily IgG with trace amounts of IgA and IgM; albumin is also present. In individuals exposed to CMV, the immune globulin can increase the relevant antibodies to levels that prevent or reduce the incidence of serious CMV disease.

USES

Attenuation of primary CMV disease for kidney transplant recipients who are seronegative for CMV and who receive a kidney from a CMV seropositive donor. With ganciclovir to prevent CMV in clients undergoing liver, lung, pancreas, and heart transplants from CMV-seropositive donors to CMS-seronegaitve recipients. (*NOTE:* There is a 50% decrease in primary CMV disease in renal transplant clients given this product.)

CONTRAINDICATIONS

Use in clients with a history of a prior severe reaction to this product or other human immunoglobulin preparations.

SPECIAL CONCERNS

Individuals with selective immunoglobulin (Ig) A deficiency may develop antibodies to IgA and could develop anaphylactic reactions to subsequent administration of blood products that contain IgA.

SIDE EFFECTS

Usually minor and often due to the rate of infusion; the infusion schedule should be adhered to closely.

GI: N&V. **Body as a whole:** Flushing, chills, fever. **Musculoskeletal:** Muscle cramps, back pain. **Respiratory:** Wheezing. Hypotension and allergic reactions such as ***angioneurotic edema*** and ***anaphylactic shock*** are possible but have not been observed.

OD OVERDOSE MANAGEMENT

Symptoms: Major effects would be those related to volume overload. Also possible are anaphylaxis and a drop in BP. *Treatment:* Discontinue the infusion immediately and have epinephrine and diphenhydramine available for treatment of acute allergic symptoms.

DRUG INTERACTIONS

The antibodies present in this product may interfere with the immune response to live virus vaccines, including measles, mumps, and rubella. Thus, such vaccinations should be deferred until at least 3 months after administration of CMV immune globulin or revaccination may be required.

HOW SUPPLIED

Injection: 50± 10 mg/mL

DOSAGE

• **IV**

Prevention of rejection of kidney transplants.

The maximum total dose/infusion is 150 mg/kg given according to the following schedule:

Within:

72 hr of transplant: 150 mg/kg
2–8 weeks of transplant: 100 mg/kg
12–16 weeks of transplant: 50 mg/kg

The rate of infusion for the initial dose is 15 mg/kg/hr. If no side effects occur after 30 min, the rate may be increased to 30 mg/kg/hr. If no side effects occur after a subsequent 30-min period, the dose may be increased to 60 mg/kg/hr at a volume not to exceed 7.5 mL/hr. **This rate of infusion must not be exceeded.** For subsequent doses, the rate of infusion is 15 mg/kg/hr for 15 min. If no side effects occur, increase the rate to 30 mg/kg/hr for 15 min and then increase to a maximum rate of 60 mg/kg/hr at a volume not to exceed 7.5 mL/hr. **This rate of infusion must not be exceeded.**

NURSING CONSIDERATIONS

ADMINISTRATION/STORAGE

IV 1. The reconstituted solution should be colorless and translucent. Do not use solution if turbid.

2. After removing tab portion of the vial cap, the rubber stopper is cleaned with 70% alcohol or equivalent. Reconstitute the lyophilized powder with 50 mL of sterile water for injection using a double-ended transfer needle or large syringe. When using a double-ended transfer needle, insert one end first into the vial of water. The lyophilized powder is supplied in an

evacuated vial; thus, the water should transfer by suction. To avoid foaming, do not shake vial. After water is transferred into the evacuated vial, release the residual vacuum to hasten dissolution. Rotate container gently to wet all the undissolved powder. Allow 30 min for complete dissolution of the powder.
3. This product does not contain a preservative. After reconstitution, enter the vial only once and begin the infusion within 6 hr and complete within 12 hr.
4. Administer drug through a separate IV line using a constant infusion pump. If not possible, the drug may be "piggybacked" into a preexisting line that contains either NaCl or one of the following dextrose solutions (with or without NaCl added): 2.5%, 5%, 10%, or 20% dextrose in water. If used with a preexisting line, do not dilute drug more than 1:2 with any solutions. See *Dosage* for administration guidelines.
5. If minor side effects occur, slow or temporarily interrupt the infusion.

ASSESSMENT

1. Determine any previous experience with human immunoglobulin preparations.
2. Document any IgA deficiency as these clients may experience anaphylactic reactions with subsequent exposures to IgA products.
3. Follow infusion dosing schedules carefully and assess closely during each rate change. Monitor VS continuously; if side effects develop, slow/stop infusion and report.

CLIENT/FAMILY TEACHING

1. If client is seronegative for CMV and receives a seropositive donor kidney, CMV disease may develop.
2. Identify side effects that would indicate an acute allergic reaction and warrant immediate attention.
3. Avoid vaccinations for at least 3 mo following therapy; may require revaccination. Antibodies in suspension may interfere with immune response to live virus vaccines.
4. In order to prevent transmission of infectious agents/hepatitis virus from one client to another, sterile disposable syringes and needles should be used; do not reuse.
5. Identify support groups that may assist to cope with chronic disease condition.

OUTCOMES/EVALUATE

CMV prophylaxis in renal transplant recipients

D

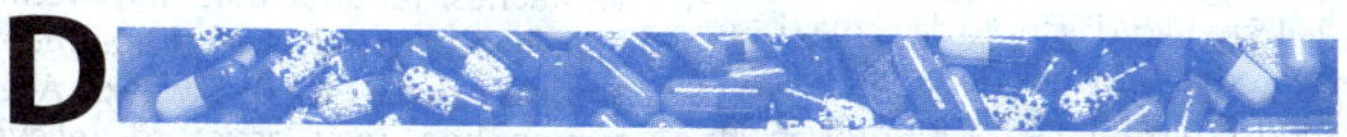

Dacarbazine

(dah-**KAR**-bah-zeen)

PREGNANCY CATEGORY: C
CLASSIFICATION(S):
Antineoplastic, alkylating
Rx: Imidazole Carboxamide, (Abbreviation: DTIC) , DTIC-Dome
✱**Rx:** DTIC

SEE ALSO *ANTINEOPLASTIC AGENTS* AND *ALKYLATING AGENTS*.

ACTION/KINETICS

Mechanisms of action: alkylation by an activated carbonium ion, antimetabolite to inhibit DNA and RNA synthesis, and alkylation by combining with protein sulfhydryl groups. Is cell-cycle nonspecific. **t½, biphasic, initial:** 19 min; **terminal:** 5 hr. The t½ is increased to 55 min and 7.2 hr in those with renal and hepatic dysfunction. Probably localizes in liver. Limited amounts (14% of plasma level) enter CSF. Approximately 40% of drug excreted in urine unchanged within 6 hr. Secreted through the kidney tubules rather than filtered through the glomeruli.

USES

Metastatic malignant melanoma. Hodgkin's disease (with other agents).

Investigational: In combination with cyclophosphamide and vincristine for malignant pheochromocytoma; in combination with tamoxifen for metastatic malignant melanoma.

CONTRAINDICATIONS

Lactation.

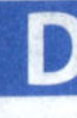

SPECIAL CONCERNS

Dosage not established in children.

ADDITIONAL SIDE EFFECTS

Hematologic: Hemopoietic depression, especially ***leukopenia and thrombocytopenia which may cause death*.** **GI:** N&V (more than 90% of clients within 1 hr after initial administration, which persists for 12–48 hr), anorexia, diarrhea. **Dermatologic:** Erythematous and urticarial rashes, photosensitivity reactions, alopecia, facial flushing, paresthesia. **Miscellaneous:** Flu-like syndrome, including fever, myalgia, and malaise. Hepatotoxicity, hypersensitivity, ***anaphylaxis*.**

LABORATORY TEST CONSIDERATIONS

↑ AST, ALT, and other enzymes.

OD OVERDOSE MANAGEMENT

Treatment: Monitor blood cell counts; supportive treatment.

HOW SUPPLIED

Injection: 10 mg/mL.

DOSAGE

- **IV ONLY**

Malignant melanoma.

2–4.5 mg/kg/day for 10 days; may be repeated at 4-week intervals; or 250 mg/m²/day for 5 days; may be repeated at 3-week intervals.

Hodgkin's disease.

150 mg/m²/day for 5 days in combination with other drugs, and repeated q 4 weeks; or, 375 mg/m² on day 1, with other drugs and repeated q 15 days.

NURSING CONSIDERATIONS

SEE ALSO *NURSING CONSIDERATIONS* FOR *ANTINEOPLASTIC AGENTS*.

ADMINISTRATION/STORAGE

IV 1. Avoid extravasation.

2. Reconstitute with sterile water for injection—9.9 mL for the 100-mg vials and 19.7 mL for the 200-mg vials for a final concentration of 10 mg/mL. Drug can be given by IV push over 1-min period. May further dilute with 5% dextrose or NaCl injection and given (preferred) over 15–30 min.

3. Protect dry vials from light and store at 2–8°C (36–46°F).

4. Reconstituted solutions are stable for up to 72 hr at 4°C (39°F) or for 8 hr at 20°C (68°F). More dilute solutions for IV infusions are stable for 24 hr when stored at 2–8°C (36–46°F).

ASSESSMENT

1. Ascertain how fluid status is to be handled (fast for 4–6 hr before treatment to reduce emesis or have fluids up to 1 hr before administration to minimize).

2. Administer antiemetic before and throughout therapy. Have phenobarbital and/or prochlorperazine available for palliation of vomiting.

3. Monitor client and labs closely for evidence of bone marrow depression, liver or renal toxicity, or hypersensitivity reaction. Anticipitate mild granulocyte toxicity. Nadir: 10 days; recovery: 21 days.

CLIENT/FAMILY TEACHING

1. To minimize adverse GI effects, antiemetics, fasting, and limited fluid intake (4–6 hr preceding treatment) have been suggested. After the first 1–2 days of therapy, vomiting should cease as tolerance develops.

2. Report any flu-like symptoms (fever, aches, fatigue) that may occur. Usually occurs 1 week after treatment and may persist for 1–3 weeks. Acetaminophen may assist to relieve symptoms.

3. Avoid prolonged exposure to sun or UV light and wear protective clothing; photosensitivity reaction may occur.

4. Prepare for hair loss; report any blurred vision or paresthesia.

5. Practice contraception during and for several months following therapy.

OUTCOMES/EVALUATE

↓ Tumor size/spread with suppression of malignant cell proliferation

Daclizumab

(dah-**KLIZ**-you-mab)

PREGNANCY CATEGORY: C

CLASSIFICATION(S):
Immunosuppressant
Rx: Zenapax

ACTION/KINETICS
Humanized IgG1 monoclonal antibody produced by recombinant DNA technology. As an antagonist, it binds to the alpha subunit (Tac subunit) of the human high affinity interleukin-2 (IL-2) receptor found on the surface of activated lymphocytes. This results in inhibition of IL-2 mediated activation of lymphocytes, a critical pathway in the cellular immune response involved in allograft rejection. **t½, terminal:** Estimated to be 20 days.

USES
Prophylaxis of acute organ rejection in renal transplants. Used with cyclosporine and corticosteroids.

CONTRAINDICATIONS
Lactation.

SPECIAL CONCERNS
Increased risk for developing lymphoproliferative disorders and opportunistic infections. Use with caution in geriatric clients. Adequate studies have not been performed in children.

SIDE EFFECTS
Incidence of 2% or more is reported. **GI:** Constipation, N&V, abdominal pain, pyrosis, dyspepsia, abdominal distention, epigastric pain, flatulence, gastritis, hemorrhoids. **CNS:** Tremor, headache, dizziness, prickly sensation, depression, anxiety. **CV:** Hypertension, hypotension, aggravated hypertension, tachycardia, thrombosis, bleeding. **Respiratory:** Dyspnea, pulmonary edema, coughing atelectasis, congestion, pharyngitis, rhinitis, hypoxia, rales, abnormal breathing sounds, pleural effusion. **GU:** Oliguria, dysuria, renal tubular necrosis, renal damage, hydronephrosis, urinary tract bleeding, urinary tract disorder, renal insufficiency, urinary retention. **Dermatologic:** Impaired wound healing without infection, acne, pruritus, hirsutism, rash, night sweats, increased sweating. **Musculoskeletal:** Musculoskeletal pain, back pain, arthralgia, leg cramps, myalgia. **Body as a whole:** Post-traumatic pain, chest pain, fever, pain, fatigue, insomnia, lymphocele, shivering, general weakness, injection site reaction, infections. **Metabolic:** Peripheral edema, edema, fluid overload, diabetes mellitus, hyperglycemia. **Miscellaneous:** Blurred vision.

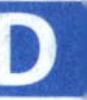

DRUG INTERACTIONS
H Do not give echinacea with daclizumab.

HOW SUPPLIED
Injection concentrate: 25 mg/5mL

DOSAGE
- **IV**

Prevent kidney transplant rejection.
1 mg/kg q 14 days for total of five doses. Regimen also includes cyclosporine and corticosteroids.

NURSING CONSIDERATIONS

ADMINISTRATION/STORAGE

IV 1. Give the first dose 24 hr or less before transplantation.
2. Mix the calculated volume of daclizumab with 50 mL of NSS solution. Give by peripheral or central vein over 15-min period.
3. When mixing, gently invert bag to avoid foaming; do not shake.
4. Contains no preservatives or bacteriostatic agents; once prepared, give within 4 hr. If solution must be held longer, refrigerate between 2–8°C (36–46°F); discard after 24 hr. Discard any unused solution.
5. Do not add or infuse other drugs simultaneously through same IV line.

ASSESSMENT

1. Document indications/date of kidney transplant.
2. Therapy includes cyclosporine and corticosteroids. Initiate therapy within 24 hr pretransplant and subsequent doses every 14 days for total of 5 doses.
3. Monitor VS, I&O, suture line, CBC, electrolytes, liver and renal function studies.

CLIENT/FAMILY TEACHING

1. Review importance of following written guidelines for medication therapy explicitly. Must take meds ex-

actly as prescribed to prevent transplant rejection.
2. Review written list of all possible drug side effects and those which must be reported.
3. Record BP, I&O, and daily weights and report sudden changes.
4. Practice reliable birth control.
5. May develop acne and excessive hair growth or impaired wound healing; may need dermatologic referral.
6. Report increased fatigue, malaise, breathing problems, unexplained bleeding/bruising or hematuria.

OUTCOMES/EVALUATE
Prophylaxis of acute organ rejection

Dactinomycin (Actinomycin D)

(dack-tin-oh-**MY**-sin)

PREGNANCY CATEGORY: C
CLASSIFICATION(S):
Antineoplastic, antibiotic
Rx: Cosmegen

SEE ALSO *ANTINEOPLASTIC AGENTS.*

ACTION/KINETICS
Chromopeptide antibiotic produced by *Streptomyces parvullus.* Acts by intercalating into the purine-pyrimidine base pair, thereby inhibiting synthesis of messenger RNA. Is cell-cycle nonspecific, although the maximum number of cells are destroyed in the G_1 phase. Cleared from the blood within 2 min and concentrated in nucleated cells. **t½:** 36 hr. Does not cross the blood-brain barrier and is excreted mainly unchanged.

USES
(1) In combination with vincristine, surgery, and/or irradiation for treatment of Wilms' tumor (nephroblastoma) and its metastases. In combination with methotrexate to treat metastatic and nonmetastatic choriocarcinoma. (2) In combination with cyclophosphamide, doxorubicin, and vincristine to treat rhabdomyosarcoma. (3) Nonseminomatous testicular carcinoma. (4) With cyclophosphamide and radiotherapy to treat Ewing's sarcoma. (5) In combination with radiotherapy to treat sarcoma botryoides. (6) Endometrial carcinoma. *Investigational:* Ovarian cancer, Kaposi's sarcoma, osteosarcoma, malignant melanoma.

CONTRAINDICATIONS
Concurrent infection with chickenpox or herpes zoster (death may result). Lactation. Infants less than 6–12 months of age.

SPECIAL CONCERNS
When used with Xray therapy, erythema is seen in normal skin and the buccal and pharyngeal mucosa.

ADDITIONAL SIDE EFFECTS
Appearance of toxic manifestations may be delayed by several weeks. ***Anaphylaxis.*** Due to corrosiveness, extravasation causes severe damage to soft tissues. Hypocalcemia. When combined with radiation, increased severity of skin reactions, GI toxicity, and ***bone marrow depression (irreversible in clients with preexisting renal, hepatic, or bone marrow impairment).***

LABORATORY TEST CONSIDERATIONS
Interferes with bioassay tests used to determine antibacterial drug levels.

HOW SUPPLIED
Powder for injection, lyophilized: 0.5 mg

DOSAGE

• IV

Carcinomas.

Adults, usual: 0.5 mg/m²/week for 3 weeks; or, 0.01–0.015 mg/kg/day for a maximum of 5 days q 4–6 weeks. Dose is individualized. **Pediatric:** 10–15 mcg/kg (0.45 mg/m²) daily for 5 days; **alternatively,** a total dose of 2.4 mg/m² over 1 week. Total daily dosage for both adults and children should not exceed 15 mcg/kg over a 5-day period. Course of treatment may be repeated after 3 weeks unless contraindicated due to toxicity. If no toxicity, second course can be given after 3 weeks.

• ISOLATION PERFUSION

Ewing's sarcoma/sarcoma botryoides.

0.05 mg/kg for pelvis and lower extremities and 0.035 mg/kg for upper extremities.

NURSING CONSIDERATIONS

SEE ALSO *NURSING CONSIDERATIONS FOR ANTINEOPLASTIC AGENTS*.

ADMINISTRATION/STORAGE

IV 1. For IV use, available in a lyophilized dactinomycin-mannitol mixture that turns a gold color upon reconstitution with sterile water. Use only sterile water without a preservative to reconstitute drug for IV use, as it will precipitate. Do not expose solutions to direct sunlight.
2. Exercise extreme care in reconstituting and administering dactinomycin so that the dust or vapors are not inhaled or come in contact with skin or mucous membranes. Take special care to prevent contact with the eyes. Prepare under a laminar hood.
3. *Drug is extremely corrosive;* most safely administered through the tubing of a running IV (e.g., 5% dextrose or NaCl). May be given directly into the vein. The needle used to draw up the solution should be discarded and another sterile needle attached, before injection, to prevent SC reaction and thrombophlebitis.
4. Discard any unused solution.
5. For direct IV administration, reconstitute 0.5-mg vial with 1.1 mL of sterile water for injection and infuse at a rate of 500 mcg/min. May be further diluted in 50 mL of D5W or NSS and infused over 10–15 min.

ASSESSMENT

1. Determine if pregnant, lactating, or infected with herpes, all of which contraindicate therapy.
2. Interferes with bioassay test used to measure antibacterial drug levels; monitor response to antibiotic therapy carefully. Inhibits action of penicillin; do not use for infection.
3. Monitor CBC, uric acid, liver and renal function studies. Drug may cause severe granulocyte and platelet toxicity. Nadir: 10 days; recovery 21–28 days.
4. During therapy, leukocyte counts should be performed daily, and platelet counts q 3 days. Frequent liver and kidney function tests are recommended.

CLIENT/FAMILY TEACHING

1. Report erythema of the skin, which can lead to desquamation and sloughing, particularly in areas previously affected by radiation. Erythema may be noted in normal skin and buccal and pharyngeal mucosa; use topical viscous xylocaine as needed.
2. Consume 2–3 L/day of fluids to prevent dehydration and urate crystal formation; may need allopurinol therapy if inadequate fluid intake.
3. May be administered intermittently if N&V persist even when an antiemetic is given.
4. Report unusual bruising, bleeding, fever, stomatitis, or persistent diarrhea.
5. Avoid vaccinations.
6. Practice contraception during and for 4 weeks following therapy. Evaluate for egg/sperm harvesting.
7. May experience hair loss 7–10 days after therapy.

OUTCOMES/EVALUATE

↓ Tumor size/spread and suppression of malignant cell proliferation

Dalteparin sodium

(**DAL**-tih-**pair**-in)

PREGNANCY CATEGORY: B
CLASSIFICATION(S):
Anticoagulant, low molecular weight heparin
Rx: Fragmin

SEE ALSO *HEPARINS, LOW MOLECULAR WEIGHT*.

ACTION/KINETICS

Peak plasma levels: 4 hr. **t½, SC:** 3–5 hr. t½ increased in those with chronic renal insufficiency requiring hemodialysis.

USES

(1) To prevent deep vein thrombosis (DVT) in clients undergoing hip replacement or abdominal surgery who are at risk for thromboembolic complications (i.e., pulmonary embolism). High risk includes obesity, general anesthesia more than 30 min, malignan-

cy, history of DVT or pulmonary embolism, age 40 and over. (2) To prevent ischemic complications due to blood clot formation in life-threatening unstable angina and non-Q-wave MI in clients on concurrent aspirin therapy. *Investigational:* Systemic anticoagulation in venous and arterial thromboembolic complications.

D

SPECIAL CONCERNS

See also *Heparins, Low Molecular Weight.* Also, the multiple dose vial contains benzyl alcohol that has been associated with a fatal "gasping syndrome" in premature infants.

SIDE EFFECTS

CV: ***Hemorrhage,*** hematoma at injection site, wound hematoma, reoperation due to bleeding, postoperational transfusions. **Hematologic:** Thrombocytopenia. **Hypersensitivity:** Allergic reactions, including pruritus, rash, fever, injection site reaction, bullous eruption, skin necrosis (rare), ***anaphylaxis.*** **Miscellaneous:** Pain at injection site.

HOW SUPPLIED

Injection: 2,500 IU/0.2 mL, 5,000 IU/0.2 mL, 10,000 IU/mL

DOSAGE

- **SC ONLY**

Prevention of DVT in abdominal surgery.

Adults: 2,500 IU each day starting 1–2 hr prior to surgery and repeated once daily for 5–10 days postoperatively. High-risk clients: 5,000 IU the night before surgery and repeated once daily for 5–10 days. In malignancy: 2,500 IU 1–2 hr before surgery followed by 2,500 IU 12 hr later and 5,000 IU once daily for 5–10 days.

Prevention of DVT following hip replacement surgery.

Adults: 2,500 IU within 2 hr before surgery with a second dose of 2,500 IU in the evening on the day of surgery (six or more hr after the first dose). If surgery occurs in the evening, omit the second dose on the day of surgery. On the first postoperative day, give 5,000 IU once daily for 5–10 days. Alternatively, can give 5,000 IU the evening before surgery, followed by 5,000 IU once daily for 5–10 days, starting the evening of the day of surgery.

Prevent ischemic complications in unstable angina/non-Q-wave MI.

Adults: 120 IU/kg, not to exceed 10,000 IU q 12 hr with concurrent PO aspirin (75–165 mg/day). Continue treatment until client is clinically stabilized (usually 5–8 days).

Systemic anticoagulation.

200 IU/kg SC daily or 100 IU b.i.d.

NURSING CONSIDERATIONS

ADMINISTRATION/STORAGE

1. Available in single-dose prefilled syringes affixed with a 27-gauge × ½-inch needle.
2. Before withdrawing the drug, inspect the vial visually for particulate matter or discoloration.
3. Do not mix with other infusions or injections unless compatibility data are known.
4. Store the drug at controlled room temperature of 20–25°C (68–77°F).

ASSESSMENT

1. Determine any sensitivity to heparin or pork products.
2. Note any evidence of active major bleeding, any bleeding disorders, or thrombocytopenia.
3. Monitor CBC with platelets, urinalysis, and FOB during therapy.
4. List criteria for inclusion (i.e., over 40, obese, prolonged general anesthesia, additional risk factors).

CLIENT/FAMILY TEACHING

1. Review indications for therapy, self-administration technique, and site rotation.
2. Give by deep SC injection while sitting or lying down. May give in a U-shape area around the navel, the upper outer side of the thigh, or the upper outer quadrangle of the buttock. Change injection site daily.
3. If the area around the navel or thigh is used, a fold of skin must be lifted, using the thumb and forefinger, while giving the injection.
4. Insert the entire length of the needle at a 45–90-degree angle.
5. Report any unusual bleeding or hemorrhage. Therapy may last for 5–10 days.

OUTCOMES/EVALUATE

DVT prophylaxis

Danaparoid sodium

(dah-**NAP**-ah-royd)

PREGNANCY CATEGORY: B
CLASSIFICATION(S):
Anticoagulant, glycosaminoglycan
Rx: Orgaran

ACTION/KINETICS
A low molecular weight sulfated glycosaminoglycan obtained from porcine mucosa. Prevents fibrin formation in the coagulation pathway via thrombin generation inhibition by anti-Xa and anti-IIa effects. Minimal effect on clotting assays, fibrinolytic activity, or bleeding time. 100% bioavailable with SC use. **t½:** About 24 hr. Excreted primarily through the kidneys.

USES
Prophylaxis of postoperative deep vein thrombosis (DVT) in clients undergoing elective hip replacement surgery. *Investigational:* Disseminated intravascular coagulation, diabetic nephropathy, ischemic stroke or thromboembolic complications of hemorrhagic stroke, treatment measure for DVT, routine anticoagulant therapy in those requiring hemodialysis. Also, to treat thromboembolism, hemofiltration during CV operations, in pregnant clients at increased risk for thrombosis.

CONTRAINDICATIONS
Use in hemophilia, idiopathic thrombocytopenic purpura, active major bleeding state (including hemorrhagic stroke in the acute phase), and type II thrombocytopenia associated with a positive in vitro test for antiplatelet antibody in the presence of danaparoid. Hypersensitivity to pork products. IM use.

SPECIAL CONCERNS
Cannot be dosed interchangeably (unit for unit) with either heparin or low molecular weight heparins. Use with extreme caution in disease states where there is an increased risk of hemorrhage, including severe uncontrolled hypertension, acute bacterial endocarditis, congenital or acquired bleeding disorders, active ulcerative and angiodysplastic GI disease, nonhemorrhagic stroke, postoperative indwelling epidural catheter use, and shortly after brain, spinal, or ophthalmologic surgery. In those in whom epidural/spinal anesthesia or spinal puncture is used, there is an increased risk of epidural or spinal hematoma that may cause long-term or permanent paralysis. Use with caution during lactation and in those with severely impaired renal function. Use with caution in clients receiving oral anticoagulants or platelet inhibitors. Safety and efficacy have not been determined in children.

SIDE EFFECTS
CV: Intraoperative blood loss, postoperative blood loss. **GI:** N&V, constipation. **CNS:** Insomnia, headache, dizziness. **Dermatologic:** Rash, pruritus. **GU:** UTI, urinary retention. **Miscellaneous:** Fever, pain at injection site, peripheral edema, joint disorder, edema, asthenia, anemia, pain, infection.

OD OVERDOSE MANAGEMENT
Symptoms: Bleeding disorders, including hemorrhage. *Treatment:* Protamine sulfate partially neutralizes the anti-Xa activity of the drug; however, there is no evidence that protamine sulfate will reduce severe non-surgical bleeding. For serious bleeding, discontinue danaparoid and give blood or blood product transfusions as needed.

HOW SUPPLIED
Injection: 750 anti-Xa units/0.6 mL.

DOSAGE

- **SC ONLY**

Prophylaxis of DVT in hip replacement surgery.

Adults: 750 anti-Xa units b.i.d. SC, beginning 1 to 4 hr preoperatively and then not sooner than 2 hr postoperatively. Continue treatment throughout the postoperative period until the risk of deep vein thrombosis has decreased. Average duration of treatment is 7 to 10 days, up to 14 days.

NURSING CONSIDERATIONS

ADMINISTRATION/STORAGE

Protect from light; store at 2–30°C (36–86°F).

ASSESSMENT

1. Note any pork or sulfite sensitivity.
2. Assess for any medical conditions that may preclude drug use (i.e., active hemorrhagic disease, bleeding dyscrasias, ITTP, etc.).
3. Monitor VS, I&O, CBC, U/A, and renal function studies; note any urinary retention or altered VS.

CLIENT/FAMILY TEACHING

1. Drug is used to prevent the formation of blood clots, especially in the legs. Usually given 1-4 hr before surgery and then 2 hr after surgery for 7 to 10 days.
2. To administer, lie down and grasp a fold of skin on the abdomen between the thumb and forefinger. Insert the entire length of the needle straight in; use a 25- to 26-gauge needle to minimize tissue trauma. Hold the skin fold throughout the injection; do not rub or massage area after administration; rotate sites with each injection.
3. Alternate administration between the left and right anterolateral and posterolateral abdominal walls.
4. Report any unusual bruising or bleeding, acute SOB, itching, rash, chest pain, and swelling.

OUTCOMES/EVALUATE

DVT prophylaxis

Danazol

(**DAN**-ah-zohl)

PREGNANCY CATEGORY: X
CLASSIFICATION(S):
Androgen, synthetic
Rx: Danocrine
★Rx: Cyclomen

ACTION/KINETICS

Inhibits the release of gonadotropins (FSH and LH) by the anterior pituitary; thus, inhibits synthesis of sex steroids and competitively inhibits binding of steroids to their cytoplasmic receptors in target tissues. In women this action arrests ovarian function, induces amenorrhea, and causes atrophy of normal and ectopic endometrial tissue. Has weak androgenic effects. **Onset, fibrocystic disease:** 4 weeks. **Time to peak effect, amenorrhea and anovulation:** 6–8 weeks; **fibrocystic disease:** 2–3 months to eliminate breast pain and tenderness and 4–6 months for elimination of nodules. **t½:** 4.5 hr. **Duration:** Ovulation and cyclic bleeding usually resume 60–90 days after cessation of therapy.

USES

Endometriosis amenable to hormonal management in clients who cannot tolerate or who have not responded to other drug therapy. Fibrocystic breast disease. Hereditary angioedema in males and females. *Investigational:* Gynecomastia, menorrhagia, precocious puberty, idiopathic immune thrombocytopenia, lupus-associated thrombocytopenia, and autoimmune hemolytic anemia.

CONTRAINDICATIONS

Undiagnosed genital bleeding; markedly impaired hepatic, renal, and cardiac function; porphyria; pregnancy and lactation.

SPECIAL CONCERNS

Use with caution in children treated for hereditary angioedema due to the possibility of virilization in females and precocious sexual development in males. Use with caution in conditions aggravated by fluid retention (e.g., epilepsy, migraine, cardiac, or renal dysfunction). Geriatric clients may have an increased risk of prostatic hypertrophy or prostatic carcinoma.

SIDE EFFECTS

Androgenic: Acne, edema, mild hirsutism, seborrhea, decrease in breast size, oily hair and skin, weight gain, deepening of voice and hair growth, clitoral hypertrophy, testicular atrophy. **Estrogen deficiency:** Flushing, sweating, vaginitis, vaginal dryness/irritation, decreased breast size, nervousness, changes in emotions. **GU:** Menstrual disturbances (e.g., spotting), alteration of the timing cycle, amenorrhea (may be persistent), abnormalities in semen volume, viscosity, sperm count, and motility with long-term use. **GI:** N&V, constipation, gastroenteritis. **Hepatic:** Jaundice, dysfunction, peliosis hepatitis and benign hepatic adenoma (***intra-abdominal hemorrhage possible***) with long term use. **CV:*Thromboembolism,*** thrombotic and thrombophlebitic events including sagittal sinus thrombosis and ***life-threatening or fatal strokes.*** **CNS:** Fatigue, tremor, headache, dizziness, sleep problems, paresthesia of extremities, anxiety, depression, appetite changes, pseudotumor cerebri. **Musculoskeletal:** Muscle cramps or spasms, joint swelling or lock-up, pain in back, legs, or neck. **Miscellaneous:** Allergic reactions (skin rashes and rarely nasal congestion), hematuria, increased BP, chills, pelvic pain, carpal tunnel syndrome, hair loss, change in libido.

LABORATORY TEST CONSIDERATIONS

↓ HDL and ↑ LDL (temporary but may be severe). Interference with lab determinations of testosterone, androstenedione, and dehydroepiandrosterone.

DRUG INTERACTIONS

Carbamazepine / ↑ Carbamazepine levels

Cyclosporine / ↑ Cyclosporine blood levels → possible nephrotoxicity

Insulin / ↑ Insulin requirements

Warfarin / ↑ PT in warfarin-stabilized clients

HOW SUPPLIED

Capsule: 50 mg, 100 mg, 200 mg

DOSAGE

• **CAPSULES**

Endometriosis.

400 mg b.i.d. (moderate to severe) or 100–200 mg b.i.d. (mild) for 3–6 months (up to 9 months may be required in some clients). Begin therapy during menses, if possible, to be sure that client is not pregnant.

Fibrocystic breast disease.

50–200 mg b.i.d. beginning on day 2 of menses. Begin therapy during menses to assure client is not pregnant.

Hereditary angioedema.

Initial: 200 mg b.i.d.–t.i.d.; after desired response, decrease dosage by 50% (or less) at 1–3-month intervals. Treat subsequent attacks by giving up to 200 mg/day. No more than 800 mg/day should be given to adults.

NURSING CONSIDERATIONS

ADMINISTRATION/STORAGE

Breast pain and tenderness in fibrocystic disease are usually relieved within 30 days and eliminated in 2–3 mo; elimination of nodularity requires 4–6 mo of uninterrupted therapy. Treatment may be reinstituted if symptoms recur (50% have recurring symptoms within 6 mo).

ASSESSMENT

1. Note reports of endometrial pain, breast pain, tenderness, and the presence of any nodules. Perform regular breast exams. Exclude breast carcinoma before initiating therapy for fibrocystic disease.
2. Determine any undiagnosed vaginal bleeding; note onset, frequency, extent, and precipitating factors.
3. CTS may develop due to drug-induced edema with compression of median nerve.
4. Obtain baseline CBC, renal and LFTs; determine if pregnant.
5. Identify factors that trigger angioedema (e.g.; C-1 inhibitor deficiency).

CLIENT/FAMILY TEACHING

1. Take with meals to ↓ GI upset.
2. Virilization may occur with drug therapy (e.g., abnormal hair growth, acne, reduced breast size, increased skin oiliness, enlarged clitoris, voice deepening); report so dosage can be adjusted to prevent voice damage. Hypoestrogenic side effects usually disappear once discontinued; ovulation will resume in 60–90 days.
3. Wear cotton underwear and pay careful attention to hygiene to diminish danazol-induced vaginitis.
4. Practice birth control as ovulation may not be suppressed until 6-8 weeks of therapy; continue breast self-exams and report changes
5. Clients with a history of epilepsy, migraines, and cardiac or renal dysfunction may develop fluid retention; stop drug and report.

6. With cystic breast disease, pain and discomfort usually resolve in 2-3 mo while nodules take 4-6 mo.

OUTCOMES/EVALUATE

- ↓ Endometrial pain (3–6 mo)
- ↓ Breast pain (2–3 mo)

Dantrolene sodium

(**DAN**-troh-leen)

PREGNANCY CATEGORY: C (PARENTERAL USE)
CLASSIFICATION(S):
Skeletal muscle relaxant, centrally-acting
Rx: Dantrium , Dantrium IV

SEE ALSO ***SKELETAL MUSCLE RELAXANTS, CENTRALLY ACTING.***

ACTION/KINETICS

Not related to other skeletal muscle relaxants. Acts directly on skeletal muscle, probably by dissociating the excitation-contraction coupling mechanism as a result of interference of release of calcium from the sarcoplasmic reticulum. This results in a decreased force of reflex muscle contraction and a reduction of hyperreflexia, spasticity, involuntary movements, and clonus. Effectiveness in malignant hyperthermia is due to an inhibition of release of calcium from the sarcoplasmic reticulum. This results in prevention or reduction of the increased myoplasmic calcium ion concentration that activates the acute catabolic processes associated with malignant hyperthermia. Absorption is slow and incomplete, but consistent. **Peak plasma levels:** 4–6 hr. **t½: PO,** 9 hr after a dose of 100 mg; **t½: IV,** 4–8 hr. Significant plasma protein binding.

USES

PO: (1) Muscle spasticity associated with severe chronic disorders, such as multiple sclerosis, cerebral palsy, spinal cord injury, and stroke. (2) Preoperatively to prevent or reduce the development of signs of malignant hyperthermia. (3) To prevent recurrence following a malignant hyperthermia crisis. **IV:** (1) Malignant hyperthermia due to hypermetabolism of skeletal muscle. (2) Preoperatively or postoperatively to prevent or reduce the development of signs of malignant hyperthermia in susceptible clients. *Investigational:* Exercise-induced muscle pain, heat stroke, and neuroleptic malignant syndrome.

CONTRAINDICATIONS

Orally in active hepatitis or cirrhosis, where spasticity is used to sustain upright posture and balance in locomotion or to obtain or maintain increased function, and to treat skeletal muscle spasm due to rheumatic disease. Pregnancy, lactation, or children under 5 years of age.

SPECIAL CONCERNS

Use with caution in clients with impaired pulmonary function, especially those with obstructive pulmonary disease; severely impaired cardiac function due to myocardial disease; and a history of previous liver disease or dysfunction.

SIDE EFFECTS

Following PO use: Side effects are dose-related and decrease with usage. ***Fatal*** and nonfatal ***hepatotoxicity.*** **CNS:** Drowsiness, dizziness, weakness, malaise, lightheadedness, headaches, insomnia, seizures, speech disturbances, fatigue, confusion, depression, nervousness. **GI:** Diarrhea (common), anorexia, constipation, GI bleeding, dysphagia, gastric irritation, abdominal cramps. **Musculoskeletal:** Backache, myalgia. **Dermatologic:** Rash (acne-like), photosensitivity, pruritus, urticaria, hair growth, sweating, eczematoid eruption. **CV:** BP changes, phlebitis, tachycardia. **GU:** Urinary retention, increased urinary frequency, urinary incontinence, hematuria, crystalluria, nocturia, impotence. **Ophthalmic:** Visual disturbances, diplopia. **Miscellaneous:** Chills, fever, tearing, feeling of suffocation, alteration of taste, ***pleural effusion with pericarditis.*** **Following IV use:** Pulmonary edema, ***thrombophlebitis,*** urticaria, erythema.

OD OVERDOSE MANAGEMENT

Symptoms: Extension of side effects. *Treatment:* Immediate gastric lavage. Maintain airway and have artificial resuscitation equipment available. Large quantities of IV fluids to prevent crystalluria. Monitor ECG.

DRUG INTERACTIONS
Clofibrate / ↓ Plasma protein binding of dantrolene
CNS depressants / ↑ CNS depression
Estrogens / ↑ Risk of hepatotoxicity
Warfarin / ↓ Plasma protein binding of dantrolene

HOW SUPPLIED
Capsule: 25 mg, 50 mg, 100 mg; *Powder for injection:* 20 mg/vial

DOSAGE

- **CAPSULES**

Spastic conditions.

Adults, initial: 25 mg once daily; **then,** increase to 25 mg b.i.d.–q.i.d.; dose may then be increased by 25-mg increments up to 100 mg b.i.d.–q.i.d. (doses in excess of 400 mg/day not recommended). **Pediatric: initial,** 0.5 mg/kg b.i.d.; **then,** increase to 0.5 mg/kg t.i.d.–q.i.d.; dose may then be increased by increments of 0.5 mg/kg to 3 mg/kg b.i.d.–q.i.d. (doses should not exceed 400 mg/day).

Malignant hyperthermia, preoperatively.

Adults and children: 4–8 mg/kg/day in three to four divided doses 1–2 days before surgery with the last dose given 3 to 4 hr before surgery.

Postmalignant hyperthermic crisis.

Adults and children: 4–8 mg/kg/day in four divided doses for 1–3 days.

- **IV INFUSION**

Malignant hyperthermia, crisis treatment.

Adults and children, initial: 2.5 mg/kg 60 min prior to surgery and infused over 1 hr. Additional IV dantrolene may be given during anesthesia and surgery, depending on symptoms.

- **IV PUSH**

Malignant hyperthermia, crisis treatment.

Initial: At least 1 mg/kg; continue administration until symptoms decrease or a cumulative dose of 10 mg/kg has been administered.

NURSING CONSIDERATIONS

SEE ALSO *NURSING CONSIDERATIONS* FOR *SKELETAL MUSCLE RELAXANTS, CENTRALLY ACTING.*

ADMINISTRATION/STORAGE

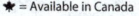

1. When administered PO, may be mixed with fruit juice or other liquids.
2. With spasticity, beneficial effects may take up to a week; discontinue after 6 weeks if none are evident.
3. Due to potential hepatotoxicity, long-term benefits must be evaluated for each client.
4. IV For IV use, reconstitute powder by adding 60 mL of sterile water for injection to each 20-mg vial.
5. Protect reconstituted solutions from light; use within 6 hr. Store reconstituted solutions at controlled room temperatures of 15–30°C (59–86°F).

ASSESSMENT

1. Note mental status and general appearance.
2. Monitor CBC, liver and renal function studies; hepatic dysfunction more likely in women over age 35.
3. Assess lung and heart sounds regularly during therapy. Note any evidence of impaired pulmonary function, cardiac disorders, active hepatitis or cirrhosis, or history of any benign or malignant breast tumors.
4. Note extent of muscle spasticity, involuntary movements, and clonus. Determine if spasticity is necessary to sustain an upright posture or for mobility as drug should be avoided.
5. Obtain and monitor VS, I&O, electrolytes, and ECG during acute therapy.

CLIENT/FAMILY TEACHING

1. Do not operate dangerous machinery or drive a car; drug causes drowsiness.
2. If double vision occurs, reassure that this and many of the other bothersome side effects may lessen with continued use.
3. Report any insomnia or depression, increased muscle weakness or impaired physical ability. Several weeks may be required before improvements will be noted.
4. Report any marked changes in BP and diarrhea or blood in the urine or stool. If slurred speech, drooling, inability to perform usual physical functions, or enuresis develops, drug may require withdrawal.

5. Avoid alcohol and any other CNS depressants.
6. Avoid sun exposure and use protection to prevent photosensitivity reactions.
7. Females should have mammograms and perform BSE to detect any drug-induced mammary tumors. Most important in women with a family history of malignant or benign breast tumors.
8. Males may develop impotence.
9. With malignant hyperthermia, carry ID and notify providers.

OUTCOMES/EVALUATE

- ↓ Muscle spasticity and/or pain
- ↓ Exercise-induced muscle pain
- ↓ Temperature (R/T hypermetabolism of skeletal muscle)

Dapiprazole hydrochloride

(dah-**PIP**-rah-zol)

PREGNANCY CATEGORY: B
CLASSIFICATION(S):
Alpha-adrenergic blocking drug, ophthalmic
Rx: Rev-Eyes

ACTION/KINETICS

Produces miosis by blocking the alpha-adrenergic receptors on the dilator muscle of the iris. No significant action on ciliary muscle contraction; thus, there are no changes in the depth of the anterior chamber of the thickness of the lens. Does not alter the IOP either in normal eyes or in eyes with elevated IOP. The rate of pupillary constriction may be slightly slower in clients with brown irides than in clients with blue or green irides.

USES

To reverse diagnostic mydriasis induced by adrenergic (e.g., Phenylephrine) or parasympatholytic (e.g., tropicamide) agents.

CONTRAINDICATIONS

Acute iritis or other conditions where miosis is not desirable. To reduce intraocular pressure or to treat open-angle glaucoma.

SPECIAL CONCERNS

Use with caution during lactation. Safety and effectiveness have not been determined in children. The drug may cause difficulty in adaptation to dark and may reduce the field of vision.

SIDE EFFECTS

Ophthalmic: Conjunctival injection lasting 20 min, burning on instillation, ptosis, lid erythema, itching, lid edema, chemosis, corneal edema, punctate keratitis, photophobia, tearing and blurring of vision, dryness of eyes. **Miscellaneous:** Headaches, browache.

HOW SUPPLIED

Ophthalmic Powder, Lyophilized, for Reconstitution: 20 mg (0.5% solution when reconstituted)

DOSAGE

- **OPHTHALMIC SOLUTION**

Reverse mydriasis.

2 gtt followed in 5 min by 2 more gtt applied to the conjunctiva of the eye after ophthalmic examination.

NURSING CONSIDERATIONS

ADMINISTRATION/STORAGE

1. Do not use more frequently than once a week.
2. To prepare solution, remove and discard aluminum seals and rubber plugs from drug and diluent vials. Pour diluent into drug vial; remove dropper assembly from its sterile wrapping and attach to drug vial. Shake container for several minutes to ensure adequate mixing.
3. Store reconstituted eye drops at room temperature for 21 days. Discard solution if not clear and colorless.

ASSESSMENT

1. Determine any hypersensitivity to alpha-adrenergic blocking agents.
2. Note eye color. Pupillary constriction may be slightly slower in clients with brown irides as opposed to those with blue or green irides.

CLIENT/FAMILY TEACHING

May cause burning on instillation. Use care; may impair adaptation to dark and reduce field of vision.

OUTCOMES/EVALUATE
Reversal of drug-induced mydriasis (constriction of pupils)

Darbepoetin alfa

(**DAR**-beh-**poh**-eh-tin **AL**-fah)

PREGNANCY CATEGORY: C
CLASSIFICATION(S):
Erythropoietin, human recombinant
Rx: Aranesp

ACTION/KINETICS
Darbepoetin alfa stimulates erythropoiesis-stimulating protein and is produced in Chinese hamster ovary cells by recombinant DNA technology. Production of endogenous erythropoietin is decreased in those with chronic renal failure and a deficiency in erythropoietin is the causative factor. Darbepoetin interacts with progenitor stem cells to increase RBC production. Usually takes 2–6 weeks to see increased hemoglobin levels. Darbepoetin has about a 3-fold longer terminal t½ when given IV or SC than does epoetin alfa. **t½, after IV:** About 1.4 hr (distribution) and about 21 hr (terminal). **t½, after SC:** 49 hr (terminal). **Peak levels after SC:** 34 hr. With once weekly dosing, steady-state serum levels are reached in 4 weeks.

USES
Anemia associated with chronic renal failure, whether or not on dialysis.

CONTRAINDICATIONS
Uncontrolled hypertension.

SPECIAL CONCERNS
Increased risk of CV events, including death. Product is formulated with two different excipients (one containing polysorbate 80 and the other containing albumin); there is a remote risk for transmission of viral diseases with the albumin product. There is the potential for immunogenicity to develop. Use with caution during lactation. Safety and efficacy have not been determined in children.

SIDE EFFECTS
CV: Vascular access thrombosis, ***access hemorrhage,*** CHF, cardiac arrhythmia, ***cardiac arrest, acute MI, stroke,*** TIA, angina pectoris, cardiac chest pain, hypertension, hypotension. **CNS:** Seizures, headache, dizziness. **GI:** Diarrhea, N&V, abdominal pain, constipation. **Body as a whole:** ***Sepsis,*** infection, fever, fatigue, flu-like symptoms, asthenia, ***death.*** **Musculoskeletal:** Myalgia, arthralgia, limb/back pain. **Respiratory:** URTI, dyspnea, cough, bronchitis. **Hypersensitivity reaction:** Skin rash, urticaria, ***anaphylaxis.*** **Miscellaneous:** Chest pain, pruritus, peripheral edema, injection site pain, fluid overload, access infection.

HOW SUPPLIED
Solution for Injection: 25 mcg/mL, 40 mcg/mL, 60 mcg/mL, 100 mcg/mL, 200 mcg/mL.

DOSAGE
- **IV, SC**

Anemia associated with chronic renal failure.

0.45 mcg/kg once weekly. Titrate doses so as not to exceed a target hemoglobin concentration of 12 g/dL.

NURSING CONSIDERATIONS

ADMINISTRATION/STORAGE

IV 1. For those who respond to darbepoetin with a rapid increase in hemoglobin (e.g., > 1 g/dL in any 2 week period), reduce the dose by 25%.
2. For many clients (especially predialysis clients), the maintenance dose will be lower than the starting dose.
3. Some clients have been successfully treated with SC doses given every 2 weeks.
4. Check the package insert carefully to determine the conversion process from epoetin alfa to darbepoetin alfa.
5. Do not increase the darbepoetin dose more often than once a month. If the hemoglobin is increasing and approaching 12 g/dL, reduce the dose by 25%. If hemoglobin continues to increase, withhold darbepoetin dose temporarily until the hemoglobin be-

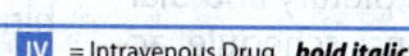
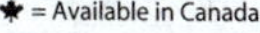
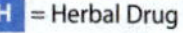

gins to decrease. Therapy can then be restarted at a dose of about 25% below the previous dose.
6. If hemoglobin increases by < 1 g/dL over 4 weeks and iron stores are adequate, the darbepoetin dose may be increased by about 25% of the previous dose. Make further dose increases at 4-week intervals.
7. When preparing the injection, do not shake as vigorous shaking may denature the drug.
8. Visually inspect vials; do not use if there is particulate matter and/or discoloration.
9. Do not dilute the product and do not give with any other drug solutions.
10. Discard any unused portion as the drug is packaged in single-use vials and contains no preservative. Do not pool unused portions.
11. Store at 2–8°C (36–46°F). Do not freeze; protect from light.

ASSESSMENT

1. Note indications for therapy , other agents trialed, the outcome, and if epoetin alfa conversion.
2. Assess for seizure history, uncontrolled HTN, and other medical conditions that may preclude therapy.
3. Obtain baseline iron panel, H&H, and BP. Monitor weekly until stabilized or until dosage change. Add supplemental iron therapy if serum ferritin <100 mcg/L or saturation < 20 %.
4. Review product literature for administration guidelines carefully.

CLIENT/FAMILY TEACHING

1. Review appropriate method for administration. Store safely out of reach and discard syringes as directed.
2. Administer exactly as directed. Do not increase or skip dose.
3. Do not shake vial; inactivates drug. Keep refrigerated.
4. Supplemental iron and vitamins may be prescribed to enhance drug effects.
5. Report as scheduled for F/U labs so drug dose can be adjusted.
6. Review list of drug side effects; report any persistent and/or bothersome ones, practice reliable contraception during therapy.
7. Follow prescribed dietary and dialysis recommendations; schedule activities to permit rest periods. Monitor BP and record.
8. Do not perform any tasks that require mental alertness until drug effects realized.

OUTCOMES/EVALUATE

↑ RBC production in anemia from CRF

Daunorubicin hydrochloride (DNR)

(daw-noh-**ROO**-bih-sin)

PREGNANCY CATEGORY: D
Rx: Cerubidine

Daunorubicin Citrate Liposomal

(daw-noh-**ROO**-bih-sin)

PREGNANCY CATEGORY: D
Rx: DaunoXome
CLASSIFICATION(S):
Antineoplastic, antibiotic

SEE ALSO *ANTINEOPLASTIC AGENTS*.

ACTION/KINETICS

Anthracycline antibiotic produced by *Streptomyces coeruleorubidus* or *S. peucetius*. The liposomal product contains an aqueous solution of the citrate salt of daunorubicin encapsulated within lipid vesicles which are composed of a lipid bilayer of distearoylphosphatidylcholine and cholesterol. Most active in the S phase of cell division but is not cell-cycle specific. Inhibits synthesis of nucleic acid by inserting into the double helix of DNA. Also possesses immunosuppressive, cytotoxic, and antimitotic activity. Rapidly cleared from the plasma. The liposomal preparation helps protect daunorubicin from chemical and enzymatic breakdown; also, it minimizes protein binding and decreases uptake by normal tissues. Is released from the liposomal preparation over time and improves selectivity for solid tumors. Metabolized to the active daunorubicinol. **t½:** daunorubicin (nonliposomal product), 18.5 hr; daunorubinicol, 27 hr. **t½, elimination:** 4.4 hr for liposomal form. Drug rapidly taken up by heart, kidneys, lung, liver, and spleen. Chiefly excreted in bile (40%) and unchanged in urine (25%). Does not pass blood-brain barrier.

USES

Daunorubicin HCl: (1) In combination with other drugs (e.g., cytarabine) for remission induction in acute nonlymphocytic leukemia (erythroid, monocytic, myelogenous) in adults. (2) Remission induction in acute lymphocytic leukemia in children and adults (increased effectiveness when combined with prednisone and vincristine). **Daunorubicin liposomal:** First-line cytotoxic therapy for advanced HIV-associated Kaposi's sarcoma. *Investigational:* Ewing's sarcoma, chronic myelocytic leukemia, neuroblastoma, non-Hodgkin's lymphomas, Wilms' tumor.

CONTRAINDICATIONS

Lactation. Hypersensitivity to previous doses. IM or SC use.

SPECIAL CONCERNS

Use with caution in preexisting heart disease or bone marrow depression, renal or hepatic failure (reduce dose). Cardiotoxicity may be more frequent in children and in the elderly.

SIDE EFFECTS

Myocardial toxicity: *Potentially fatal CHF,* *(especially if total dosage exceeds 550 mg/m² for adults, 300 mg/m² for children more than 2 years of age, and 10 mg/kg for children less than 2 years of age.)* Mucositis (3–7 days after administration), red-colored urine, hyperuricemia. Severe tissue necrosis if extravasation occurs. Cross-resistance with doxorubicin (produced by similar microorganism) and vinca alkaloids. Hyperuricemia may occur due to lysis of leukemic cells; give allopurinol as a precaution, before starting antileukemic therapy.

For the liposomal product.

CNS: Fatigue, headache, neuropathy, malaise, dizziness, depression, insomnia, amnesia, anxiety, ataxia, confusion, seizures, emotional lability, abnormal gait, hallucinations, hyperkinesia, hypertonia, meningitis, somnolence, abnormal thinking, tremors. **Hematologic:** Myelosuppression, especially of the granulocytic series. Neutropenia. **CV:** Cardiomyopathy associated with a decrease in left ventricular ejection fraction (especially in clients who have received prior anthracyclines or who have preexisting cardiac disease). Also, hot flushes, hypertension, palpitation, syncope, tachycardia. **GI:** Nausea, diarrhea, anorexia, abdominal pain, vomiting, stomatitis, constipation, increased appetite, dysphagia, ***GI hemorrhage,*** gastritis, gingival bleeding, hemorrhoids, hepatomegaly, melena, dry mouth, tooth caries. **Respiratory:** Cough, dyspnea, rhinitis, sinusitis, hemoptysis, hiccoughs, pulmonary infiltration, increased sputum. **Musculoskeletal:** Rigors, back pain, myalgia, arthralgia. **Dermatologic:** Alopecia, pruritus, foliculitis, seborrhea, dry skin. **GU:** Dysuria, nocturia, polyuria. **Ophthalmic:** Abnormal vision, conjunctivitis, eye pain. **Otic:** Deafness, ear pain, tinnitus. **Miscellaneous:** Fever, allergic reactions, sweating, chest pain, edema, taste perversion, tenesmus, flu-like symptoms, opportunistic infections, inflammation at injection site, lymphadenopathy, splenomegaly, dehydration, thirst. Back pain, flushing, and chest tightness have been reported within the first 5 min of the infusion.

LABORATORY TEST CONSIDERATIONS

Hyperuricemia secondary to rapid lysis of leukemic cells.

OD OVERDOSE MANAGEMENT

Symptoms: Granulocytopenia, fatigue, N&V. Also, extension of side effects.

DRUG INTERACTIONS

Cyclophosphamide / ↑ Risk of cardiotoxicity

Methotrexate / Impaired liver function → ↑ risk of toxicity

Myelosuppressive drugs / Reduce dose of daunorubicin

HOW SUPPLIED

Daunorubicin HCl. *Powder for Injection, lyophilized:* 5 mg/mL. **Daunorubicin Citrate Liposomal.** *Injection:* 2 mg/mL, 5 mg/mL

DOSAGE

• IV INFUSION OF DAUNORUBICIN HCL

Acute nonlymphocytic leukemia. **Adults, less than 60 years old:** Daunorubicin, 45 mg/m^2/day on days 1, 2, and 3 of the first course and days 1 and 2 of additional courses; cytosine arabinoside (Ara-C), 100 mg/m^2/day, by IV infusion, for 7 days during first course and for 5 days during any additional courses of treatment. **Adults, over 60 years old:** Daunorubicin, 30 mg/m^2/day on days 1, 2, and 3 of the first course and days 1 and 2 of additional courses. Use the same dose of cytosine arabinoside as for adults less than 60 years old. Up to three courses may be required.

Acute lymphocytic leukemia. **Adults:** Daunorubicin, 45 mg/m^2, IV, on days 1, 2, and 3; vincristine, 2 mg IV, on days 1, 8, and 15; prednisone, PO, 40 mg/m^2/day for days 1–22 and then taper between days 22 and 29; and, L-asparaginase, IV, 500 IU/kg/day on days 22–32.

Acute lymphocytic leukemia. **Children:** Daunorubicin, 25 mg/m^2, and vincristine, 1.5 mg/m^2, each IV, on day 1 every week with prednisone, 40 mg/m^2, PO, daily. Usually four courses will induce remission. *NOTE:* Calculate the dose on the basis of milligrams per kilogram if the child is less than 2 years of age or if the body surface is less than 0.5 m^2.

• IV INFUSION OF DAUNORUBICIN CITRATE LIPOSOMAL

Advanced HIV-associated Kaposi's sarcoma. 40 mg/m^2 given over 1 hr. Dose is repeated q 2 weeks. This regimen is continued until there is progression of the disease or other complications of HIV disease preclude continued therapy.

Reduce dosage for renal or hepatic disease. Recommended dose for liposomal product: three-fourths of normal dose if serum bilirubin is 1.2 to 3 mg/dL; one-half of normal dose if serum bilirubin is less than 3 mg/dL and serum creatinine is greater than 3 mg/dL.

NURSING CONSIDERATIONS

SEE ALSO *NURSING CONSIDERATIONS* FOR *ANTINEOPLASTIC AGENTS*.

ADMINISTRATION/STORAGE

IV 1. Dilute in vial with 4 mL sterile water for injection USP. Agitate gently until dissolved (solution contains 5 mg daunorubicin/mL). Withdraw desired dose into syringe containing 10–15 mL isotonic saline.

2. Inject into tubing of rapidly flowing D5W or NSS IV and administer over 3–5 min. May further dilute in 50 mL of D5W or NSS and infuse over 10–15 min (or in 100 mL of solution and infuse over 30–45 min).

3. Give into a rapidly flowing IV infusion. *Never administer IM or SC as severe local tissue necrosis will result.*

4. Reconstituted solution stable for 24 hr at room temperature; 48 hr refrigerated. Protect from sunlight.

5. Do not mix with other drugs.

6. Extravasation may cause severe local tissue necrosis.

7. Dilute the liposomal product 1:1 with 5% dextrose injection before use. Do not use an in-line filter.

8. Refrigerate the liposomal product at 2–8°C (36–46°F). Do not store the reconstituted solution for longer than 6 hr; do not freeze; protect from light.

ASSESSMENT

1. Assess during and following therapy for myocardial toxicity, manifested by changes in baseline ECG, edema, dyspnea, and cyanosis. A 30% decrease in QRS voltage and a reduction in the systolic ejection fraction may be early signals of cardiomyopathy. Clients with a cardiac history who receive doses above 550 mg/m^2 are more susceptible to CHF.

2. Follow appropriate guidelines for dose adjustment in liver dysfunction (e.g., bilirubin 1.2–3.0 mg%, give 75% of dose; bilirubin greater than 3.0 mg%, give 50% of dose).

3. Drug may precipitate hyperuricemia; administer allopurinol.

4. Monitor liver and renal function studies and hematologic profile as drug may cause severe granulocyte and platelet toxicity; allow bone marrow recovery before subsequent treat-

ments. Nadir: 10 days; recovery: 21–28 days.

CLIENT/FAMILY TEACHING

1. Report any S&S of cardiac toxicity (i.e., increased SOB, increased fatigue, and edema).
2. Report S&S of infection, or if mouth ulcers or pain interferes with eating. N&V usually controlled with antiemetics.
3. Urine may appear red for several days following therapy; not blood.
4. Consume 1.5–2 L/day of fluids. Record I&O and report alterations.
5. Avoid alcohol and foods high in purines.
6. Practice contraception during and for at least 1 mo after therapy.
7. Avoid crowds and those with active infections, vaccinations.
8. Anticipate hair loss; should grow back about 5 weeks later.

OUTCOMES/EVALUATE

Suppression of malignant cell proliferation

Deferoxamine mesylate

(deh-fer-**OX**-ah-meen)

PREGNANCY CATEGORY: C
CLASSIFICATION(S):
Antidote, heavy metal antagonist
Rx: Desferal

ACTION/KINETICS

Binds to free iron, iron from ferritin, and hemosiderin to form ferrioxamine, which is a water-soluble chelate excreted by the kidneys (urine is a reddish color) as well as in the feces via the bile. Iron is not removed from hemoglobin, myoglobin, or cytochromes. Must be given parenterally for systemic activity. Adequate renal function is necessary for effectiveness. **t½, IV:** 60 min. Rapidly metabolized by plasma enzymes and excreted in the urine.

USES

Adjunct in treatment of acute iron intoxication. Chronic iron overload including thalassemia. *Investigational:* Accumulation of aluminum in bone in renal failure and in encephalopathy due to aluminum. May be helpful in Alzheimer's disease and some cancers.

CONTRAINDICATIONS

Severe renal disease, anuria. Treatment of primary hemochromatosis.

SPECIAL CONCERNS

Use in pregnancy only if clearly necessary. Use with caution for clients with pyelonephritis. Should not be used in children under the age of 3 years unless mobilization of 1 mg iron/day or more can be shown. Use deferoxamine and ascorbic acid with caution in geriatric clients due to a greater risk of cardiac decompensation.

SIDE EFFECTS

Following long-term therapy. **Allergic:** Rash, itching, wheal formation, ***anaphylaxis.*** **GI:** Abdominal discomfort, diarrhea. **Ophthalmologic:** Blurred vision. Rarely, impaired peripheral, night, or color vision; cataracts, decreased visual acuity, retinal pigmentation abnormalities. **Other:** Dysuria, leg cramps, fever, tachycardia, high-frequency hearing loss.

Following rapid IV use. Hypotension, urticaria, erythema.

Following SC use. Local pain, erythema, swelling, pruritus, skin irritation.

HOW SUPPLIED

Powder for injection: 0.5 g, 2 g

DOSAGE

• **IM, IV, SC**

Acute iron intoxication.

Adults and children over 3 years of age, IM (preferred), initial: 1 g; **then,** 0.5 g q 4 hr for two doses; if necessary, then give 0.5 g q 4–12 hr, not to exceed 6 g/day. **IV infusion** (*only in emergencies such as CV collapse:*) Same as IM at a rate not to exceed 15 mg/kg/hr. Begin IM therapy as soon as possible.

Chronic iron overload.

IM: 0.5–1.0 g/day; **SC:** 1–2 g (20–40 mg/kg/day) given by mini-infusion pump over an 8–24-hr period; **IV:** 2 g (given separately but at same time as each unit of blood and in addition to IM administration); IV rate not to exceed 15 mg/kg/hr.

NURSING CONSIDERATIONS

ADMINISTRATION/STORAGE

1. Dissolve by adding 2 mL of sterile water to each ampule.
2. Pain and induration may occur at IM injection site.
3. Have epinephrine available to treat allergic reactions. With iron intoxication or acidosis, have emergency equipment available.
IV 4. For IV administration use NSS, D5W, or RL solution and administer *slowly* at a rate not exceeding 15 mg/kg/hr.
5. Discard dissolved drug if not used within 1 week. Protect from light and store above 25°C (77°F).

ASSESSMENT

1. Document indications for therapy, onset of symptoms, and any evidence of pyelonephritis.
2. In poisoning, note time and amount ingested and type of preparation. Document early S&S of iron toxicity: abdominal pain, emesis, and bloody diarrhea; and late S&S: decreased level of consciousness, metabolic acidosis, and shock.
3. Monitor serum iron, TIBC, ferritin, and urinary iron levels. Report if anuric as chelated iron is excreted by the kidneys. Conduct renal function studies; determine if pregnant.
4. Drug is oto and ocular toxic; obtain baseline exams.

CLIENT/FAMILY TEACHING

1. Pain and induration may occur at administration site.
2. Drug may give the urine a reddish color due to the chelated iron.
3. With a history of pyelonephritis, report hematuria or pain; may be caused by a deferoxamine-induced disease exacerbation.
4. Report any sudden hearing loss or complaints of visual disturbances such as changes in color vision or altered visual acuity; may be drug induced. Report for periodic ophthalmologic and audiometric exams.
5. Practice reliable birth control.

OUTCOMES/EVALUATE

- Relief of symptoms of iron toxicity
- ↓ Serum iron levels

Delavirdine mesylate

(deh-lah-**VIR**-deen)

PREGNANCY CATEGORY: C
CLASSIFICATION(S):
Antiviral, non-nucleoside reverse transcriptase inhibitor
Rx: Rescriptor

SEE ALSO *ANTIVIRAL DRUGS.*

ACTION/KINETICS

Non-nucleoside reverse transcriptase inhibitor that binds directly to reverse transcriptase and blocks RNA-dependent and DNA-dependent DNA polymerase activities. Effect is additive if used with other antiviral drugs. Delavirdine may confer cross-resistance to other non-nucleoside reverse transcriptase inhibitors when used alone or in combination. Rapidly absorbed. **Peak plasma levels:** About 1 hr. Median area under the curve is about 30% higher in females than males. Extensively bound (about 98%) to plasma albumin. Converted to inactive metabolites which are excreted in urine and feces. It inhibits its own metabolism. **t½, plasma:** 2–11 hr.

USES

Treatment of HIV-1 infections in combination with appropriate antiretroviral agents.

CONTRAINDICATIONS

Lactation.

SPECIAL CONCERNS

Use with caution in impaired hepatic function. Safety and efficacy in combination with other antiretroviral drugs have not been determined in HIV-1-infected clients less than 16 years of age.

SIDE EFFECTS

Body as a whole: Headache, fatigue, asthenia, allergic reaction, chest pain, chills, general or local edema, fever, flu syndrome, lethargy, malaise, neck rigidity, general or local pain, trauma. **CV:** Bradycardia, migraine, pallor, palpitation, postural hypotension, syncope, tachycardia, vasodilation. **CNS:** Abnormal coordination, agitation, amnesia, anxiety, change in dreams, cognitive impairment, confusion, decreased libido, depression, disorientation, dizziness, emotional lability, hallucinations, hyperesthesia, hyperreflexia, hypesthesia, impaired coordination, insomnia, mania, nervousness, neuropathy, nightmares, paralysis, paranoia, paresthesia, restlessness, somnolence, tingling, tremor, vertigo, weakness. **GI:** N&V, diarrhea, anorexia, aphthous stomatitis, bloody stool, colitis, constipation, appetite decreased or increased, diarrhea, duodenitis, dry mouth, diverticulitis, dyspepsia, dysphagia, fecal incontinence, flatulence, enteritis, esophagitis, gastritis, gagging, gastroesophageal reflux, GI bleeding or disorder, gingivitis, gum hemorrhage, increased saliva, increased thirst, mouth ulcer, abdominal cramps/distention/pain, lip edema, hepatitis (nonspecified), pancreatitis, rectal disorder, sialadenitis, stomatitis, tongue edema, ulceration. **Dermatologic:** Skin rashes, maculopapular rash, pruritus, angioedema, dermal leukocytoblastic vasculitis, dermatitis, desquamation, diaphoresis, dry skin, erythema, erythema multiforme, folliculitis, fungal dermatitis, alopecia, nail disorder, petechial rash, seborrhea, skin disorder, skin nodule, ***Stevens-Johnson syndrome,*** vesiculobullous rash, sebaceous cyst. **GU:** Breast enlargement, kidney calculi, epididymitis, hematuria, hemospermia, impotence, kidney pain, metrorrhagia, nocturia, polyuria, proteinuria, vaginal moniliasis. **Musculoskeletal:** Back pain, neck rigidity, arthritis or arthralgia of single or multiple joints, bone disorder or pain, leg cramps, muscle weakness, myalgia, tendon disorder, tenosynovitis, tetany, muscle cramps. **Respiratory:** Upper respiratory infection, bronchitis, chest congestion, cough, dyspnea, epistaxis, laryngismus, pharyngitis, rhinitis, sinusitis. **Hematologic:** Anemia, bruises, ecchymosis, eosinophilia, granulocytosis, neutropenia, pancytopenia, petechiae, purpura, spleen disorder, thrombocytopenia. **Ophthalmic:** Nystagmus, blepharitis, conjunctivitis, diplopia, dry eyes, photophobia. **Miscellaneous:** Alcohol intolerance, peripheral edema, weight increase or decrease, taste perversion, tinnitus, ear pain.

D

LABORATORY TEST CONSIDERATIONS

↑ ALT, AST, bilirubin, GGT, lipase, serum alkaline phosphatase, serum amylase, serum creatinine phosphatase, serum creatinine. Bilirubinemia, hyperkalemia, hyperuricemia, hypocalcemia, hyponatremia, hypophosphatemia

DRUG INTERACTIONS

Antacids / ↓ Delavirdine absorption; separate doses by 1 hr
Amprenavir / ↑ Amprenavir plasma levels
Anticonvulsants (Carbamazepine, Phenobarbital, Phenytoin) / ↓ Delavirdine plasma levels R/T ↑ hepatic metabolism
Benzodiazpines / Possible serious or life-threatening drug side effects R/T ↓ metabolism
Calcium channel blockers, dihydropyridine-type / Possible serious or life-threatening drug side effects R/T ↓ metabolism
Clarithromycin / Significant ↑ in amount absorbed of both drugs; possible serious side effects
Dapsone / Possible serious or life-threatening drug side effects of dapsone R/T ↓ metabolism
Didanosine / ↓ Absorption of both drugs; separate administration by at least 1 hr
Ergot derivatives / Possible serious or life-threatening ergot side effects R/T ↓ metabolism
Fluoxetine / ↑ Trough levels of delavirdine by 50%
Indinavir / ↑ Indinavir levels R/T ↓ metabolism; possible serious side effects (reduce indinavir dose to 600 mg t.i.d.)
Quinidine / Possible serious or life-threatening drug side effects R/T ↓ metabolism
Rifabutin, Rifampin / ↓ Delavirdine plasma levels R/T ↑ hepatic metab-

olism; also, possible ↑ rifabutin plasma levels
Saquinavir / ↑ Saquinavir levels R/T ↓ metabolism; possible serious side effects. Also, possible ↓ delavirdine area under the curve
Sildenafil / ↑ Sildenafil plasma levels (do not exceed a single 25 mg dose of sildenafil in a 48-hr period)
Warfarin / ↑ Warfarin plasma levels → possible serious or life-threatening warfarin side effects R/T ↓ metabolism

HOW SUPPLIED
Tablets: 100 mg, 200 mg

DOSAGE

• **TABLETS**
HIV-1 infection.
400 mg t.i.d. in combination with other antiretroviral therapy.

NURSING CONSIDERATIONS

ADMINISTRATION/STORAGE

1. Give with or without food.
2. In achlorhydria, take with an acidic beverage (e.g., cranberry or orange juice).

ASSESSMENT

1. Document disease onset/exposure times, likelihood of transmission, and disease characteristics such as stage of infection, viral load.
2. List drugs prescribed.
3. Monitor CBC, LFTs, viral load, CD_4 counts.
4. Assesss lifestyle and potential to resume risky behaviors.

CLIENT/FAMILY TEACHING

1. Take as directed, with or without food. Take antacids 1 hr before or 1 hr after drug ingestion.
2. Tablets may be dispersed with water prior to consumption. To prepare, add 4 tablets to at least 3 ounces of water and allow to stand for a few minutes. Stir until a uniform dispersion occurs and consume promptly. Rinse glass and swallow to ensure entire dose is taken.
3. Always administer with other antiretroviral therapy. Drug is not a cure for HIV; may continue to acquire opportunistic infections.
4. Rash on upper body and arms may necessitate interruption of therapy. Report especially if accompanied by fever, blistering, myalgia, eye or mouth lesions.
5. Avoid OTC agents without approval.
6. Continue barrier contraception; does not reduce risk of transmission.

OUTCOMES/EVALUATE

Post-exposure prophylaxis; ↓ viral load

Denileukin diftitox

(den-ih-**LOO**-kin **DIF**-tih-tox)

PREGNANCY CATEGORY: C
CLASSIFICATION(S):
Antineoplastic, miscellaneous
Rx: Ontak

ACTION/KINETICS
A recombinant DNA-derived cytotoxic protein produced in an *Escherichia coli* expression system. It is designed to direct the cytocidal action of diphtheria toxin to cells that express the IL-2 receptor. The human IL-2 receptor consists of three forms — a low (CD25), intermediate (CD122/CD132), and high affinity (CD25/CD122/CD132). The high affinity form is usually found only on activated T-lymphocytes, activated B-lymphocytes, and activated macrophages. Malignant cells expressing 1 or more of the subunits of the IL-2 receptor are found in certain leukemias and lymphomas, including cutaneous T-cell lymphoma. It is believed denileukin interacts with the high affinity IL-2 receptor on the cell surface leading to inhibition of cellular protein synthesis and cell death within hours. **t½, distribution:** About 2–5 min; **t½, terminal:** About 70–80 min. Metabolized by proteolytic degradation. Development of antibodies significantly impacts clearance rates.

USES
Treatment of persistent or recurrent cutaneous T- cell lymphoma whose malignant cells express the CD25 component of the IL-2 receptor.

D

CONTRAINDICATIONS

Hypersensitivity to denileukin, diphtheria toxin, interleukin-2, or excipients in the product. Lactation.

SPECIAL CONCERNS

Use only by those experienced with antineoplastic therapy and management of cancer clients; give in a facility equipped and staffed for CPR and where the client can be closely monitored. Safety and efficacy have not been determined in pediatric clients or in cutaneous T-cell lymphoma whose malignant cells do *not* express the CD25 component of the IL-2 receptor. Preexisting low serum albumin levels may predict and predispose clients to the vascular leak syndrome.

SIDE EFFECTS

Up to 5% of side effects are severe or life-threatening. **Hypersensitivity:** Hypotension, back pain, dyspnea, vasodilation, rash, chest pain or tightness, tachycardia, dysphagia or laryngismus, syncope, allergic reaction, ***anaphylaxis. Vascular leak syndrome:*** Hypotension, edema, hypoalbuminemia. **GI:** N&V, anorexia, diarrhea, constipation, dyspepsia, dysphagia, pancreatitis. **CNS:** Dizziness, paresthesia, nervousness, confusion, insomnia. **CV:** Hypotension, vasodilation, tachycardia, thrombotic events, hypertension, arrhythmia. **Dermatologic:** Acute or delayed onset rash (generalized maculopapular, petechial, vesicular bullous, urticarial, or eczematous), pruritus, sweating. **GU:** Hematuria, albuminuria, pyuria, acute renal insufficiency, microscopic hematuria. **Hematologic:** Anemia, thrombocytopenia, leukopenia. **Metabolic:** Edema, weight decrease, dehydration (due to GI events). **Respiratory:** Dyspnea, increased cough, pharyngitis, rhinitis, lung disorder. **Musculoskeletal:** Myalgia, arthralgia. **Body as a whole:** Chills, fever, asthenia, infection, pain, headache, flu-like syndrome. **Miscellaneous:** Chest pain, injection site reaction, infectious complications (decreased lymphocyte counts), hyperthyroidism, hypothyroidism.

LABORATORY TEST CONSIDERATIONS

↑ Creatinine, transaminase. Hypoalbuminemia, hypocalcemia, hypokalemia.

HOW SUPPLIED

Solution for injection, frozen: 150 mcg/mL

DOSAGE

• **IV ONLY**

Cutaneous T-cell lymphoma.

For each treatment cycle, give 9 or 18 mcg/kg/day for 5 consecutive days q 21 days. Infuse over 15 or more min.

NURSING CONSIDERATIONS

ADMINISTRATION/STORAGE

IV 1. If side effects occur during IV infusion, discontinue or reduce the rate, depending on the severity of the reaction.

2. The optimal duration of therapy has not been determined.

3. Prepare and hold diluted denileukin in plastic syringes or soft plastic IV bags (adsorption will occur if glass containers are used).

4. The concentration of denileukin must be 15 or more mcg/mL during all steps in the preparation of the solution for IV infusion. Ensure this by withdrawing the calculated dose from the vial(s) and injecting it into an empty IV infusion bag. For each 1 mL of denileukin removed from the vial(s), no more than 9 mL of sterile saline without preservative should be added to the IV bag.

5. Store frozen at −10°C (14°F) or lower. Bring to room temperature before preparing the dose. Vials may be thawed in the refrigerator for 24 hr or less or at room temperature for 1–2 hr. Do not heat. Administer prepared solutions within 6 hr. Do not refreeze.

6. Mix the solution in the vial by gently swirling (do not shake vigorously). After thawing a haze may be visible which should clear when the solution reaches room temperature. Do not use unless clear, colorless, and without visible particulate matter.

7. Infuse over 15 or more min. Do not administer as a bolus injection.

8. Do not physically mix with other drugs or administer through an in-line filter.
9. Administer prepared solution within 6 hr, using a syringe pump or IV infusion bag.
10. Discard any unused portion immediately.

ASSESSMENT

1. Note onset of disease, other agents trialed and the outcome.
2. Assess albumin levels and delay administration until levels are >3 g/dL. Low albumin levels may predispose client to vascular leak syndrome.
3. Manage hypersensitivity reactions as follows:
• Interrupt or decrease rate of infusion, depending on severity of reaction.
• IV antihistamines, corticosteroids, and epinephrine may be required.
• Have resuscitative equipment readily available during administration.
4. Observe for S&S of infection.
5. Obtain CBC, chemistry, renal and LFTs and monitor weekly during therapy.

OUTCOMES/EVALUATE

Inhibition of malignant cell proliferation; ↓ tumor burden

Desipramine hydrochloride

(dess-**IP**-rah-meen)

PREGNANCY CATEGORY: C
CLASSIFICATION(S):
Antidepressant, tricyclic
Rx: Norpramin
🍁Rx: Alti-Desipramine, Apo-Desipramine, Novo-Desipramine, Nu-Desipramine, PMS-Desipramine,

---

SEE ALSO *ANTIDEPRESSANTS, TRICYCLIC*.

ACTION/KINETICS

Slight anticholinergic, sedative, and orthostatic hypotensive effects. **Effective plasma levels:** 125–300 ng/mL. **t½:** 12–24 hr. **Time to reach steady state:** 2–11 days. Response usually seen within the first week.

USES

Symptoms of depression. Bulimia nervosa. To decrease craving and depression during cocaine withdrawal. To treat severe neurogenic pain. Cataplexy associated with narcolepsy. Attention deficit disorders with or without hyperactivity in children over 6 years of age.

CONTRAINDICATIONS

Use in children less than 12 years of age.

SPECIAL CONCERNS

Safe use during pregnancy has not been established. Safety and efficacy have not been established in children.

ADDITIONAL SIDE EFFECTS

Bad taste in mouth, hypertension during surgery.

HOW SUPPLIED

Tablet: 10 mg, 25 mg, 50 mg, 75 mg, 100 mg, 150 mg

DOSAGE

• **TABLETS**
Antidepressant.
Initial: 100–200 mg/day in single or divided doses. **Maximum daily dose:** 300 mg in severely ill clients. **Maintenance:** 50–100 mg/day. **Geriatric and adolescent clients:** 25–100 mg/day in single or divided doses up to a maximum of 150 mg/day.
Cocaine withdrawal.
50–200 mg/day.

NURSING CONSIDERATIONS

SEE ALSO *NURSING CONSIDERATIONS FOR ANTIDEPRESSANTS, TRICYCLIC*.

ADMINISTRATION/STORAGE

1. Initiate in a hospital setting for those requiring 300 mg/day.
2. Give maintenance doses for at least 2 months following a satisfactory response.

CLIENT/FAMILY TEACHING

1. Take as directed; may take 4—6 weeks to note desired effects.
2. Take single daily dose or any dosage increases at bedtime to reduce daytime sedation.
3. Drowsiness, dizziness, or postural hypotension may occur; may require dosage reduction.

OUTCOMES/EVALUATE

- ↓ Perceived depression; ↑ self-worth
- Relief of neurogenic pain
- Therapeutic levels (125–300 ng/mL)

Desloratadine

(**des**-lor-**AT**-ah-deen)

PREGNANCY CATEGORY: C
CLASSIFICATION(S):
Antihistamine, second generation, piperidine
Rx: Clarinex

SEE ALSO *ANTIHISTAMINES (H_1 BLOCKERS).*

ACTION/KINETICS

Desloratadine, a major metabolite of loratadine, is a long-acting selective histamine-H_1 receptor antagonist. **Maximum plasma levels:** About 3 hr. Neither food nor grapefruit juice affect bioavailability. Metabolized to 3-hydroxydesloratadine which is also active. There are both slow and normal metabolizers of desloratadine; Blacks have a higher frequency of slow metabolism. **t½, elimination:** 27 hr. Reduce dose in clients with renal or hepatic impairment.

USES

(1) Relief of the nasal and nonnasal symptoms of allergic rhinitis (seasonal or perennial) in clients 12 years and older. (2) Symptomatic relief of pruritus, reduction in the number of hives and size of hives, in chronic idiopathic urticaria in clients 12 years and older.

CONTRAINDICATIONS

Lactation.

SPECIAL CONCERNS

Use with caution in elderly clients.

SIDE EFFECTS

See also *Antihistamines*. Common side effects are listed. **CNS:** Fatigue, somnolence, headache, fatigue, dizziness. **GI:** Dry mouth, nausea, dyspepsia. **Miscellaneous:** Pharyngitis, myalgia, dysmenorrhea, tachycardia, rarely hypersensivity reactions (e.g., rash, pruritus, urticaria, edema, dyspnea, ***anaphylaxis***).

LABORATORY TEST CONSIDERATIONS

↑ Liver enzymes, bilirubin.

HOW SUPPLIED

Tablet: 5 mg

DOSAGE

- **TABLETS**

Allergic rhinitis, chronic idiopathic urticaria.

Adults and children over 12 years: 5 mg once daily. In those with liver or renal impairment, start with 5 mg every other day.

NURSING CONSIDERATIONS

SEE ALSO *NURSING CONSIDERATIONS* FOR *ANTIHISTAMINES (H_1 BLOCKERS).*

ADMINISTRATION/STORAGE

The drug is heat sensitive. Avoid temperatures above 30°C (86°F). Protect from excessive moisture.

ASSESSMENT

1. Note indications for therapy, onset, and characteristics of symptoms. List other agents trialed and outcome.
2. Assess liver and renal function, reduce dose/frequency of administration with dysfunction.

CLIENT/FAMILY TEACHING

1. May be taken without regard to meals.
2. Do not increase dose or dosing frequency as effectiveness is not increased and sleepiness may occur.
3. Avoid activities that require mental alertness until drug effects realized.
4. Keep a diary and attempt to identify triggers.
5. Report any unusual side effects, lack of response, or worsening of symptoms.

OUTCOMES/EVALUATE

- Control of S&S of seasonal/allergic rhinitis
- Relief from idiopathic urticaria

Desmopressin acetate

(des-moh-**PRESS**-in)

PREGNANCY CATEGORY: B
CLASSIFICATION(S):
Antidiuretic hormone, synthetic

Rx: DDAVP, Stimate
✱Rx: DDAVP Injection/Spray/Tablets, DDAVP Rhinyle Nasal Solution, Octostim

D

ACTION/KINETICS

A synthetic analog of arginine vasopressin which possesses antidiuretic activity but is devoid of vasopressor and oxytocic effects. Acts to increase absorption of water in the kidney by increasing permeability of cells in the collecting ducts. **Onset:** 1 hr. **Peak, intranasal:** 1–5 hr.; **peak, PO:** 4–7 hr. **Duration:** 8–20 hr. **t½:** initial, 8 min; final: 75 min. Effect ceases abruptly. It also increases factor VIII levels (**onset:** 30 min; **peak:** 1.5–2 hr) and von Willebrand's factor activity. **Time to reach maximum plasma levels, after PO or intranasal:** 0.9–1.5 hr.

USES

DDAVP: Primary noctural enuresis (intranasal), central cranial diabetes insipides (DI) (intranasal, oral, parenteral), hemophilia A with factor VIII levels greater than 5% (intranasal, parenteral), von Willebrand's disease (type I) with factor VIII levels greater than 5% (intranasal, parenteral). **Stimate:** Hemophilia A with factor VIII levels greater than 5%, von Willebrand's disease with factor VIII levels greater than 5%.

Investigational: Chronic autonomic failure (nocturnal polyuria, overnight weight loss, morning postural hypotension).

CONTRAINDICATIONS

Hypersensitivity to drug. Use for treatment of hemophilia A with factor VIII levels less than or equal to 5%, treatment of hemophilia B or in clients who have factor VIII antibodies. Treatment of severe classic von Willebrand's disease (type I) and when an abnormal molecular form of factor VIII antigen is present. Use for type IIB von Willebrand's disease. Parenteral administration for DI in infants under 3 months and intranasal administration in infants less than 11 months. Nephrogenic DI, polyuria due to psychogenic DI, renal disease, hypercalcemia, hyperkalemia, or administration of demeclocycline or lithium.

SPECIAL CONCERNS

Safety for use during lactation not established. Use with caution and with restricted fluid intake in infants due to an increased risk of hyponatremia and water intoxication. Geriatric clients may have a greater risk of developing hyponatremia and water intoxication. Use with caution in clients with coronary artery insufficiency and/or hypertensive CV disease. Use cautiously with other pressor agents. Safety and efficacy have not been determined in children less than 12 years of age (parenteral) or less than 2 months of age (intranasal) with DI.

SIDE EFFECTS

- **INTRANASAL DDAVP**

Transient headaches, nausea, nasal congestion, rhinitis, facial flushing, asthenia, chills, conjunctivitis, cough, dizziness, epistaxis, eye edema, GI disorder, lacrimation, nosebleed, nostril pain, sore throat, URIs.

- **STIMATE DDAVP**

Agitation, balanitis, chest pain, chills, dizziness, dyspepsia, edema, insomnia, itch or light-sensitive eyes, pain, palpitations, somnolence, tachycardia, vomiting, warm feeling.

- **PARENTERAL DDAVP**

Mild abdominal pain, facial flushing, transient headache, nausea, vulval pain, BP changes, burning pain, edema, local erythema, ***anaphylaxis (rare).***

OD OVERDOSE MANAGEMENT

Symptoms: Headache, abdominal cramps, facial flushing, dyspnea, fluid retention, mucous membrane irritation. *Treatment:* Reduce dose, decrease frequency of administration, or withdraw the drug depending on the severity of the condition.

DRUG INTERACTIONS

Chlorpropamide, clofibrate, and carbamazepine may potentiate desmopressin effects.

HOW SUPPLIED

Injection: 4 mcg/mL; *Nasal Solution:* 0.1 mg/mL, 1.5 mg/mL; *Tablet:* 0.1 mg, 0.2 mg

DOSAGE

- **SC, DIRECT IV**

Neurogenic DI.

Adults: 0.5–1 mL/day in two divided

doses, adjusted separately for an adequate diurnal rhythm of water turnover. If switching from intranasal to IV, the comparable IV antidiuretic dose is about 1/10 the intranasal dose.

Hemophilia A, von Willebrand's disease (type I).

Adults: 0.3 mcg/kg diluted in 50 mL 0.9% NaCl injection infused IV over 15–30 min; dose may be repeated, if necessary. **Pediatric, 3 months or older, weighing 10 kg or less, IV:** 0.3 mcg/kg diluted in 10 mL of 0.9% NaCl injection and given over 15–30 min; repeat if necessary. **Pediatric, 3 months or older, weighing 10 kg or more, IV:** 0.3 mcg/kg diluted in 50 mL of 0.9% NaCl injection and given over 15–30 min; repeat if necessary.

• **INTRANASAL**

Neurogenic DI.

Adults: 0.1–0.4 mL/day, either as a single dose or divided into two to three doses (usual: 0.2 mL/day in two divided doses). Adjust morning and evening doses separately for an adequate diurnal rhythm of water turnover. **Children, 3 months to 12 years:** 0.05–0.3 mL/day, either as a single dose or two divided doses.

Nocturnal enuresis.

Age 6 years and older, initial: 20 mcg (0.2 mL) at bedtime with one-half the dose in each nostril; if no response, the dose may be increased to 40 mcg.

Hemophilia A and type I von Willenbrand's disease.

In clients weighing 50 kg or more: One spray per nostril (total dose of 300 mcg). **In clients weighing less than 50 kg:** Given as a single spray of 150 mcg. The drug may be given 2 hr prior to minor surgery in the same doses as described above.

Renal concentration capacity test.

Adults: 40 mcg (20 mcg in each nostril) given any time during the day. **Children, 3–12 years:** 20 mcg given in the morning.

• **TABLETS**

Central cranial DI.

Adults, initial: 0.05 mg b.i.d.; adjust individually to optimum therapeutic dose and adjust each dose for an adequate diurnal rhythm of water turnover. Total daily dose should be increased or decreased (range 0.1–1.2 mg divided b.i.d.–t.i.d.) as needed to obtain adequate antidiuresis. **Children, initial:** 0.05 mg. Careful restriction of fluid intake in children is required to prevent hyponatremia and water intoxication.

Primary nocturnal enuresis.

Age 6 years and older, initial: 0.2 mg at bedtime. May be increased to 0.6 mg, depending on client response.

D

NURSING CONSIDERATIONS

ADMINISTRATION/STORAGE

1. Measure the dosage exactly because the drug is potent.
2. Note the three graduation marks on the soft flexible plastic nasal tube: 0.2, 0.1, and 0.05 mL. The 0.05-level is not designated by number. Cleanse and dry tube appropriately.
3. Stimate nasal spray pump can only deliver 0.1 mL (150 mcg). The pump must be primed prior to the first use by pressing down four times. Discard the bottle after 25 (150 mcg) doses since the amount delivered thereafter may be significantly less than 150 mcg.
4. Refrigerate nasal solution at 2–8°C (36–46° F) although the product will be stable for up to 3 weeks when stored at room temperature. Refrigerate the injection at the same temperature as the nasal spray.
5. If used for hemophilia A or von Willebrand's disease, do not use it more often than q 2 days as tachyphylaxis may occur.
6. To determine the renal concentration capacity in adults, the urine voided within 1 hr after drug administration is discarded; the two subsequent urines collected within 8 hr are saved and tested for osmolality. In children, osmolality is measured on urine voided during 3–5 hr after drug administration. Advise to drink only small amounts of fluid during the test day.

IV 7. For direct IV administration (with neurogenic DI) give each dose

over 1 min. With hemophilia, may dilute drug in 50 mL of NSS and infuse over 15–30 min.
8. Refrigerate the solution and injection at 4°C (39.2°F).

ASSESSMENT

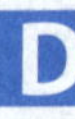

1. Monitor CBC, calcium, blood sugar, electrolytes, and factor levels.
2. Observe for early S&S of water intoxication (drowsiness, headache, and vomiting, excessive fluid consumption, weight gain, and/or seizures). Adjust fluid intake to avoid water intoxication and hyponatremia; if excessive retention, may treat with a diuretic.
3. With hemophilia, monitor BP and HR closely during IV therapy.
4. With neurogenic DI, monitor urine osmolarity and volume; weigh daily; assess for edema/dehydration.
5. Monitor duration of sleep. The amount of sleep, together with the client's daily I&O, provide parameters to estimate the clinical response to drug therapy with enuresis.

CLIENT/FAMILY TEACHING

1. If spray is prescribed, review administration technique using the special catheter provided. Insert tip of catheter into nose and blow on the other end of the catheter to deliver the medication deep into the nasal cavity. (A syringe filled with air may be used in children and comatose persons; rinse after use).
2. Review recommendations concerning fluid intake. Measure I&O and keep an accurate record of fluid status. Report any symptoms of water intoxication and hyponatremia.
3. Notify provider at the earliest signs of trouble, such as ↓ urinary output; headaches or severe nasal congestion which may be mistaken for an URI.
4. Avoid alcohol in any form.
5. Tolerance may develop over time and response may be diminished.

OUTCOMES/EVALUATE

- Prevention of hemorrhage
- Control of nocturnal enuresis
- Desired antidiuretic effects (↓ urine volume, ↑ urine osmolarity, and relief of polydipsia) with DI

Dexamethasone

(dex-ah-**METH**-ah-zohn)

PREGNANCY CATEGORY: C
CLASSIFICATION(S):
Glucocorticoid
Rx: Ophthalmic: Maxidex Ophthalmic **Oral:** Decadron, Dexameth, Dexamethasone Intensol, Dexone, Hexadrol **Topical:** Aeroseb-Dex, Decaspray
✱**Rx:** Alti-Dexamethasone, Dexasone, PMS-Dexamethasone.

SEE ALSO *CORTICOSTEROIDS*.

ACTION/KINETICS

Long-acting. Low degree of sodium and water retention. Diuresis may ensue when transferred from other corticosteroids to dexamethasone. **t½:** 110–210 min.

ADDITIONAL USES

(1) In acute allergic disorders, PO dexamethasone may be combined with dexamethasone sodium phosphate injection and used for 6 days. (2) To test for adrenal cortical hyperfunction. (3) Cerebral edema due to brain tumor, craniotomy, or head injury. *Investigational:* Diagnosis of depression. Antiemetic in cisplatin-induced vomiting. Prophylaxis or treatment of acute mountain sickness. Decrease hearing loss in bacterial meningitis. Hirsutism.

CONTRAINDICATIONS

Use for replacement therapy in adrenal cortical insufficiency.

SPECIAL CONCERNS

Use during pregnancy only if benefits outweigh risks.

ADDITIONAL DRUG INTERACTIONS

Ephedrine / ↓ Dexamethasone effect R/T ↑ liver breakdown
Oral Contraceptives / ↓ Effect of oral contraceptives R/T ↑ liver breakdown

HOW SUPPLIED

Aerosol, Topical: 0.01%, 0.04%; *Elixir:* 0.5 mg/5 mL; *Oral Solution:* 0.5 mg/0.5 mL, 0.5 mg/5 mL; *Ophthalmic Suspension:* 0.1%; *Tablet:* 0.25 mg, 0.5 mg, 0.75 mg, 1 mg, 1.5 mg, 2 mg, 4 mg, 6 mg; Therapeutic Pack

DOSAGE

- **ORAL SOLUTION, TABLETS, ELIXIR**

Most uses.

Initial: 0.75–9 mg/day; **maintenance:** gradually reduce to minimum effective dose (0.5–3 mg/day).

Suppression test for Cushing's syndrome.

0.5 mg q 6 hr for 2 days for 24-hr urine collection (or 1 mg at 11 p.m. with blood withdrawn at 8 a.m. for blood cortisol determination).

Suppression test to determine cause of pituitary ACTH excess.

2 mg q 6 hr for 2 days (for 24-hr urine collection).

Acute allergic disorders or acute worsening of chronic allergic disorders.

Day 1: Dexamethasone sodium phosphate injection, 4–8 mg IM. **Days 2 and 3:** Two 0.75-mg dexamethasone tablets b.i.d. **Day 4:** One 0.75-mg dexamethasone tablet b.i.d. **Days 5 and 6:** One 0.75-mg dexamethasone tablet. **Day 7:** No treatment. **Day 8:** Follow-up visit to physician.

- **TOPICAL AEROSOL, CREAM**

Apply sparingly as a light film to affected area b.i.d.–t.i.d.

- **OPHTHALMIC SUSPENSION**

1–2 gtt in the conjunctival sac q hr during day and q 2 hr during night until a satisfactory response obtained; **then,** 1 gtt q 4 hr and finally 1 gtt q 6–8 hr.

NURSING CONSIDERATIONS

SEE ALSO *NURSING CONSIDERATIONS FOR CORTICOSTEROIDS.*

CLIENT/FAMILY TEACHING

1. Use exactly as directed; do not exceed dose and do not stop abruptly unless ordered.
2. May take with food to decrease GI upset.
3. Report loss of response, worsening of symptoms, excessive thirst and urinary frequency.

OUTCOMES/EVALUATE

- Status of adrenal cortical function
- ↓ Symptoms of allergic response
- ↓ Cerebral edema

Dexamethasone acetate

(dex-ah-**METH**-ah-zohn)

CLASSIFICATION(S):
Glucocorticoid
Rx: Cortastat LA, Dalalone D.P., Dalalone L.A., Decadron-LA, Decaject-L.A., Dexasone L.A., Dexone LA, Solurex LA

SEE ALSO *CORTICOSTEROIDS.*

ACTION/KINETICS

Practically insoluble; provides the prolonged activity suitable for repository injections, although it has a prompt onset of action. Not for IV use.

SPECIAL CONCERNS

Use during pregnancy only if benefits outweigh risks.

HOW SUPPLIED

Injection: 8 mg/mL, 16 mg/mL

DOSAGE

- **REPOSITORY INJECTION, IM**

8–16 mg q 1–3 weeks, if necessary.

- **INTRALESIONAL**

0.8–1.6 mg.

- **SOFT TISSUE AND INTRA-ARTICULAR**

4–16 mg repeated at 1–3-week intervals.

NURSING CONSIDERATIONS

SEE ALSO *NURSING CONSIDERATIONS FOR CORTICOSTEROIDS.*

CLIENT/FAMILY TEACHING

Do not overuse joint/limb as futher injury may occur.

OUTCOMES/EVALUATE

- ↓ Inflammation
- Symptomatic improvement

Dexamethasone sodium phosphate •

(dex-ah-**METH**-ah-zohn)

PREGNANCY CATEGORY: C

D

CLASSIFICATION(S):
Glucocorticoid
Rx: Inhaler: Decadron Phosphate Respihaler, **Nasal:** Decadron Phosphate Turbinaire, **Ophthalmic:** AK-Dex, Decadron Phosphate Ophthalmic **Otic:** AK-Dex, Decadron, I-Methasone, **Systemic:** Cortastat, Dalalone, Decadron Phosphate, Decaject, Dexasone, Dexone, Hexadrol Phosphate, Solurex, **Topical:** Decadron Phosphate
✱**Rx:** Diodex, PMS-Dexamethasone Injection

SEE ALSO *CORTICOSTEROIDS*.

ACTION/KINETICS
Rapid onset and short duration of action.

ADDITIONAL USES
For IV or IM use in emergency situations when dexamethasone cannot be given PO. Intranasally for nasal polyps, allergic or inflammatory nasal conditions.

CONTRAINDICATIONS
Acute infections, persistent positive sputum cultures of *Candida albicans*. Lactation.

SPECIAL CONCERNS
Use during pregnancy only if benefits outweigh risks.

SIDE EFFECTS
Following inhalation: Nasal and nasopharyngeal irritation, burning, dryness, stinging, headache.

HOW SUPPLIED
Cream: 0.1%; *Injection:* 4 mg/mL, 10 mg/mL, 20 mg/mL, 24 mg/mL; *Ophthalmic ointment:* 0.05%; *Ophthalmic solution:* 0.1%

DOSAGE

• **IM, IV**

Most uses.

Range: 0.5–9 mg/day (⅓–½ the PO dose q 12 hr).

Cerebral edema.

Adults, initial: 10 mg IV; **then,** 4 mg IM q 6 hr until maximum effect obtained (usually within 12–24 hr). Switch to PO therapy (1–3 mg t.i.d.) as soon as feasible and then slowly withdraw over 5–7 days.

Shock, unresponsive.

Initial: either 1–6 mg/kg IV or 40 mg IV; **then,** repeat IV dose q 2–6 hr as long as necessary.

• **INTRALESIONAL, INTRA-ARTICULAR, SOFT TISSUE INJECTIONS**

0.4–6 mg, depending on the site (e.g., small joints: 0.8–1 mg; large joints: 2–4 mg; soft tissue infiltration: 2–6 mg; ganglia: 1–2 mg; bursae: 2–3 mg; tendon sheaths: 0.4–1 mg.

• **OPHTHALMIC OINTMENT**

Instill a small amount of the ointment into the conjunctival sac t.i.d.–q.i.d. As response is obtained, reduce the number of applications.

• **OPHTHALMIC SOLUTION**

Initial: Instill 1–2 gtt into the conjunctival sac q hr during the day and q 2 hr at night until response obtained. After a favorable response, reduce to 1 gtt q 4 hr and later 1 gtt t.i.d.–q.i.d.

• **TOPICAL CREAM**

Apply sparingly to affected areas and rub in.

NURSING CONSIDERATIONS

SEE ALSO *NURSING CONSIDERATIONS* FOR *CORTICOSTEROIDS*.

ADMINISTRATION/STORAGE

1. For intranasal use, some are controlled using 1 spray in each nostril b.i.d.
2. The ophthalmic ointment is useful when an eye pad is used and for situations when prolonged contact of dexamethasone with ocular tissues is required.
3. **IV** For IV administration may give undiluted over 1 min. Do not use preparation containing lidocaine IV.

CLIENT/FAMILY TEACHING

Review appropriate method/frequency for administration and use as directed; report loss of response or worsening of symptoms.

OUTCOMES/EVALUATE

• Improved airway exchange
• Relief of allergic manifestations
• Suppression of inflammatory response; enhanced tissue perfusion

---

Dexmedetomidine hydrochloride

(dex-**med**-ih-**TOM**-ih-deen)

PREGNANCY CATEGORY: C

CLASSIFICATION(S):
Sedative-hypnotic, nonbenzodiazepine
Rx: Precedex

ACTION/KINETICS
An alpha$_2$–adrenoceptor agonist with sedative effects. No evidence of respiratory depression when given at recommended doses. Rapidly distributed; **t½:** About 6 min. Almost completely metabolized in the liver; excreted in the urine and feces. **t½, terminal:** About 2 hr.

USES
For sedation in initially intubated and mechanically ventilated clients for treatment in an intensive care setting. *Investigational:* Single-dose premedication 15 min before thiopental-induced anesthesia in minor gynecologic surgery. Relieve pain and reduce opioid use following laparoscopic tubal ligation. Adjunct anesthetic in ophthalmic surgery. Treat shivering. As a premedication to attenuate the cardiostimulatory and postanesthetic delirium of ketamine.

CONTRAINDICATIONS
Use for infusions lasting over 24 hr, during labor and delivery, or in pediatric patients under 18 years of age.

SPECIAL CONCERNS
A higher incidence of hypotension and bradycardia is seen in geriatric clients; consider a dose reduction. Use with caution in advanced heart block. If chronically given and then abruptly discontinued, withdrawal symptoms (e.g., nervousness, agitation, headaches, increase in BP) may occur.

SIDE EFFECTS
CV: Bradycardia, sinus arrest, hypotension, atrial fibrillation, BP fluctuation, heart disorder, aggravated hypertension, arrhythmia, ventricular arrhythmia, AV block, ***cardiac arrest, ventricular tachycardia,*** extrasystoles, atrial fibrillation, heart block, T-wave inversion, tachycardia, supraventricular tachycardia. **GI:** N&V, abdominal pain, diarrhea. **CNS:** Dizziness, headache, neuralgia, neuritis, speech disorder, agitation, confusion, delirium, hallucinations, illusions, somnolence. **Respiratory:** Hypoxia, pleural effusion, pulmonary edema, apnea, bronchospasm, dyspnea, hypercapnia, hypoventilation, hypoxia, pulmonary congestion. **Body as a whole:** Thirst, anemia, pain, infection, leukocytosis, fever, hyperpyrexia, rigors, increased sweating. **Miscellaneous:** Oliguria, hypovolemia, photopsia, abnormal vision.

LABORATORY TEST CONSIDERATIONS
↑ AST, ALT, SGGT, alkaline phosphatase. Acidosis, respiratory acidosis, hyperkalemia.

DRUG INTERACTIONS
Possible enhanced CNS depression when given with anesthetics, hypnotics, narcotics, or sedatives. Consider dosage reduction.

HOW SUPPLIED
Injection: 100 mcg/mL

DOSAGE

• **IV INFUSION**

Sedation in intensive care setting.

Adults: Loading infusion of 1 mcg/kg over 10 min, followed by a maintenance infusion of 0.2–0.7 mcg/kg/hr. Adjust rate to achieve desired level of sedation. Reduce dosage in impaired hepatic function.

NURSING CONSIDERATIONS

ADMINISTRATION/STORAGE

IV 1. Administer using a controlled infusion device.

2. To prepare the infusion, withdraw 2 mL and add to 48 mL of 0.9% NaCl injection (i.e., total of 50 mL). Shake gently to mix. Ampules and vials are intended for single use only.

3. Dexmedetomidine is compatible with lactated Ringer's, D5W, 0.9% NaCl in water, 20% mannitol, thiopental sodium, etomidate, vecuronium bromide, pancuronium bromide, succinylcholine, atracurium besylate, mivacurium chloride, glycopyrrolate bromine, phenylephedrine HCl, atropine sulfate, midazolam, morphine sulfate, fentanyl citrate, and plasma substitute.

4. May adsorb to some types of natural rubber; use administration compo-

nents made with synthetic or coated natural rubber gaskets.
5. Store at controlled room temperature of 25°C (77°F).

ASSESSMENT

1. Note indications for use, goals of therapy and intended length of use.
2. Administer in a continously monitored environment. Client may develop cardiac arrhythmias, heart block, GI upset, and respiratory distress.
3. With chronic use, taper dosage to prevent withdrawal symptoms.
4. Monitor renal and LFTs, reduce dose with hepatic dysfunction and in older clients.

CLIENT/FAMILY TEACHING

Drug is used to sedate before surgery and during procedures. Do not attempt to get up or walk without assistance. May cause atrial fibrillation, burning at injection site, change in mental status, and respiratory suppression. Therefore is only administered in a carefully monitored environment by trained personnel.

OUTCOMES/EVALUATE

Desired sedation; control of intubated clients being mechanically ventilated

Dexmethylphenidate hydrochloride

(dex-**meth**-il-**FEN**-ah-dayt)

PREGNANCY CATEGORY: C
CLASSIFICATION(S):
CNS stimulant
Rx: Focalin **C-II**

ACTION/KINETICS

Precise mechanism to treat attention deficit disorder is not known. Drug is thought to block reuptake of norepinephrine and dopamine into the presynaptic neuron and increase the release of these neurotransmitters into the extraneuronal space. Rapidly absorbed; **maximum levels:** 1–1.5 hr. Food delays the time to maximum levels. Metabolized in the liver; 90% excreted through the urine. **t½, elimination:** About 2.2 hr.

USES

As part of a total program to treat attention deficit hyperactivity disorder. Effectiveness for use for more than 6 weeks has not been studied.

CONTRAINDICATIONS

Clients with marked anxiety, tension, and agitation. Those with glaucoma, motor tics, or with a family history of Tourette's syndrome, during treatment with MAO inhibitors or within a minimum of 14 days following discontinuation of a MAO inhibitor (hypertensive crisis may result). Use to treat severe depression or to prevent or treat normal fatigue states.

SPECIAL CONCERNS

Use with caution in those with a history of drug dependence or alcoholism. Chronic, abusive use may lead to marked tolerance and psychological dependence with abnormal behavior. Parenteral abuse may result in frank psychotic episodes. In psychotic children, worsening of symptoms of behavior disturbance and thought disorder may occur. Use with caution during lactation and in medical conditions that might be compromised by increases in BP or HR (e.g., preexisting hypertension, heart failure, recent MI, hyperthyroidism). Safety and efficacy have not been determined in children less than 6 years of age.

SIDE EFFECTS

CNS: Nervousness, insomnia, dizziness, drowsiness, dyskinesia, headache, Tourette's syndrome (rare), toxic psychosis (rare), transient depressed mood, lowering of seizure threshold in those with a history of seizures or with prior EEG abnormalities. **GI:** Abdominal pain, anorexia, nausea. **CV:** Tachycardia, angina, arrhythmia, palpitations, increased or decreased pulse/BP, cerebral arteritis or occlusion. **Dermatologic:** Skin rash, urticaria, exfoliative dermatitis, erythema multiforme with findings of necrotizing vasculitis, thrombocytopenia purpura. **Hematologic:** Leukopenia, anemia. **Ophthalmic:** Difficulties with accommodation and blurring of vision. **Miscellaneous:** Fever, arthralgia, scalp hair loss, neuroleptic malignant syndrome (rare).

LABORATORY TEST CONSIDERATIONS

Abnormal liver function (ranging from ↑ transaminase levels to hepatic coma).

OD OVERDOSE MANAGEMENT

Symptoms: Vomiting, agitation, tremors, hyperreflexia, muscle twitching, convulsions (may be followed by coma), euphoria, confusion, hallucinations, delirium, sweating, flushing, headache, hyperpyrexia, tachycardia, palpitations, cardiac arrhythmias, hypertension, mydriasis, dryness of mucous membranes. *Treatment:* Appropriate supportive measures. Protect against self-injury and external stimuli. Gastric lavage, control agitation and seizures before gastric lavage. Administration of activated charcoal and a cathartic. Maintain adequate circulation and respiratory exchange. External cooling procedures to treat hyperpyrexia.

DRUG INTERACTIONS

Antihypertensives / ↓ Effect of antihypertensives

Clonidine / Possible serious side effects

MAO inhibitors / Possible hypertensive crisis, hyperthermia, convulsions, coma

Phenobarbital / ↑ Effect of phenobarbital R/T ↓ metabolism

Phenytoin / ↑ Effect of phenytoin R/T ↓ metabolism

Primidone / ↑ Effect of primidone R/T ↓ metabolism

Selective serotonin reuptake inhibitors / ↑ Effect of SSRIs R/T ↓ metabolism

Tricyclic antidepressants / ↑ TCA effect R/T ↓ metabolism

Warfarin / ↓ Metabolism of warfarin; monitor coagulation times when starting or stopping therapy

HOW SUPPLIED

Tablet: 2.5 mg, 5 mg, 10 mg

DOSAGE

- **TABLETS**

Attention deficit hyperactivity disorder.

Children aged 6 and older new to methylphenidate: Initially, 2.5 mg b.i.d. of dexmethylphenidate. May adjust dose in 2.5–5 mg increments up to a maximum of 20 mg/day (10 mg b.i.d.). Dosage adjustments may be made at weekly intervals. **Children aged 6 and older currently taking methylphenidate:** Start dexmethylphenidate at one-half the dose of racemic methylphenidate being used. Maximum recommended dose is 20 mg/day (10 mg b.i.d.).

NURSING CONSIDERATIONS

ADMINISTRATION/STORAGE

1. Give b.i.d. at least 4 hr apart, with or without food.
2. If extended treatment is deemed necessary, periodically evaluate long-term usefulness with periods off the drug to determine client ability to function without the medication.
3. If paradoxical aggravation of symptoms or other side effects occur, decrease or discontinue the drug.
4. Discontinue the drug if improvement is not seen after appropriate dosage adjustment over a 1-month period.
5. Withdrawal from abuse use may cause severe depression.
6. Withdrawal from chronic therapeutic use may unmask symptoms of the underlying disorder.
7. Protect from light and moisture.

ASSESSMENT

1. Document indications for therapy, symptom characteristics, other agents trialed and outcome. Note other drugs prescribed that may interact unfavorably.
2. Assess for family history of Tourette's syndrome, evidence of glaucoma, tics, or depression as these preclude therapy.
3. Ensure psychologic evaluations show no evidence of psychotic disorder or severe stress/anxiety reaction.
4. Obtain baseline VS, LFTs, CBC, CNS evaluation, and ECG and monitor.
5. Assess for possible growth suppression. Monitor height and weight especially with long-term therapy and provide periodic "drug holiday" to determine need for continued therapy.

D

CLIENT/FAMILY TEACHING

1. Take before/with breakfast and lunch to avoid interference with sleep.
2. Store safely out of reach, may cause tolerance and psychological dependence.
3. Do NOT stop suddenly with long-term therapy, consult provider and do so with supervised direction.
3. Use caution when driving or operating hazardous machinery as drug may mask fatigue and/or cause physical incoordination, dizziness, or drowsiness.
4. Record weight 2 times/week and report any significant loss, weight loss may occur.
5. Report any overt changes in client mood or attention span.
6. Any adverse S&S as well as skin rashes, fever, or joint pains should be reported immediately.
7. Therapy may be interrupted periodically ("drug holiday") to determine if it is still necessary in those responsive to therapy and in some to permit normal growth.

OUTCOMES/EVALUATE

Ability to sit quietly and concentrate

Dexrazoxane

(dex-rah-**ZOX**-ayn)

PREGNANCY CATEGORY: C
CLASSIFICATION(S):
Antidote for doxorubicin toxicity
Rx: Zinecard

ACTION/KINETICS

A derivative of EDTA that is a potent chelating agent. It readily penetrates cell membranes, although its mechanism of action as a cardioprotective agent when using anthracyclines (e.g., doxorubicin) is not known. May act by interfering with iron-mediated free-radical generation that may be responsible, in part, for anthracycline-induced cardiomyopathy. **t½, elimination:** Approximately 2.5 hr. Metabolized in the liver and both unchanged drug and metabolites excreted through the urine. Not bound to plasma proteins.

USES

To reduce the incidence and severity of cardiomyopathy associated with doxorubicin administration in women with metastatic breast cancer and who have received a cumulated doxorubicin dose of 300 mg/m^2 and who need additional doxorubicin therapy.

CONTRAINDICATIONS

Use with the initiation of doxorubicin therapy, as there is evidence it may interfere with the antitumor efficacy of the regimen (i.e., fluorouracil, doxorubicin, cyclophosphamide). Use with chemotherapy regimens that do not contain an anthracycline. Lactation.

SPECIAL CONCERNS

Safety and efficacy have not been determined in children.

SIDE EFFECTS

NOTE: The side effects listed may be due to the fluorouracil, doxorubicin, cyclophosphamide regimen.
GI: N&V, anorexia, stomatitis, diarrhea, esophagitis, dysphagia. **CNS:** Fatigue, malaise, fever, neurotoxicity. **Dermatologic:** Alopecia, streaking/erythema, extravasation, urticaria, recall skin reaction. **CV:** ***Hemorrhage,*** phlebitis. **Hematologic:** Leukopenia, thrombocytopenia, granulocytopenia. **Miscellaneous:** Pain on injection, infection, ***sepsis.***

LABORATORY TEST CONSIDERATIONS

Marked interference with hepatic or renal function tests.

OD OVERDOSE MANAGEMENT

Symptoms: Extensions of the side effects, including myelosuppression. *Treatment:* Supportive care, including treatment of infections, fluid regulation, maintenance of nutrition, treatment of myelosuppression. Peritoneal dialysis or hemodialysis may be helpful in removing the drug.

DRUG INTERACTIONS

Dexrazoxane may increase the myelosuppression caused by chemotherapeutic drugs.

HOW SUPPLIED

Powder for injection: 250 mg, 500 mg

DOSAGE

- **SLOW IV PUSH OR RAPID IV INFUSION FROM A BAG**

Prevent doxorubicin cardiomyopathy. The recommended dosage ratio of dexrazoxane-doxorubicin is 10:1 (i.e., 500 mg/m² dexrazoxane to 50 mg/m² doxorubicin).

NURSING CONSIDERATIONS

ADMINISTRATION/STORAGE

IV 1. Reconstitute with 0.167 M (M/6) sodium lactate injection, to give a concentration of 10 mg/mL.
2. The reconstituted solution may be diluted with either 0.9% NaCl or D5W to a concentration range of 1.3–5 mg/mL.
3. Do not mix with other drugs.
4. Do not give doxorubicin prior to the IV injection of dexrazoxane; give doxorubicin within 30 min after beginning dexrazoxane infusion.
5. Use gloves and caution in the handling and preparation of reconstituted dexrazoxane. If drug or solution comes in contact with the skin or mucous membranes, wash immediately with soap and water.
6. Store the powder for injection at controlled room temperatures of 15–30°C (59–86°F). Reconstituted and diluted solutions are stable for 6 hr at controlled room temperature or under refrigeration of 2–8°C (36–46°F). Discard unused solutions.

ASSESSMENT

1. Note dose of prescribed doxorubicin therapy.
2. Monitor CBC and observe for increased myelosuppression.
3. Perform baseline cardiac assessment, noting any evidence of rales, S_3 gallop, PND, increased DOE, or cardiomegaly on X ray/ECG or echo. Assess for altered cardiac function; cardiomyopathy may still occur.

OUTCOMES/EVALUATE

↓ Incidence/severity of doxorubicin-induced cardiomyopathy

Dextroamphetamine sulfate

(dex-troh-am-**FET**-ah-meen)

PREGNANCY CATEGORY: C

CLASSIFICATION(S):
CNS stimulant
Rx: Dexedrine, Dextrostat **C-II**

SEE ALSO AMPHETAMINES AND DERIVATIVES.

ACTION/KINETICS

Stronger CNS effects and weaker peripheral action than amphetamine; thus, dextroamphetamine manifests fewer undesirable CV effects. After PO, completely absorbed in 3 hr. **Duration: PO,** 4–24 hr; **t½, adults:** 10–12 hr; **children:** 6–8 hr. Excreted in urine. Acidification will increase excretion, while alkalinization will decrease it.

USES

Attention deficit disorders in children, narcolepsy.

ADDITIONAL CONTRAINDICATIONS

Lactation. Use for obesity.

SPECIAL CONCERNS

Use of extended-release capsules for attention deficit disorders in children less than 6 years of age and the elixir or tablets for attention deficit disorders in children less than 3 years of age is not recommended. Dosage for narcolepsy has not been determined in children less than 6 years of age.

HOW SUPPLIED

Capsule, Extended Release: 5 mg, 10 mg, 15 mg; *Tablet:* 5 mg, 10 mg

DOSAGE

• **TABLETS**

Attention deficit disorders in children.

3–5 years, initial: 2.5 mg/day; increase by 2.5 mg/day at weekly intervals until optimum dose is achieved (usual range 0.1–0.5 mg/kg/dose each morning). **6 years and older, initial:** 5 mg 1–2 times/day; increase in increments of 5 mg/week until optimum dose is achieved (rarely over 40 mg/day).

Narcolepsy.

Adults: 5–60 mg in divided doses daily. **Children over 12 years, initial:** 10 mg/day; increase in increments of 10 mg/day at weekly intervals until optimum dose is reached. **Children, 6–12 years, initial:** 5 mg/day; increase in increments of 5 mg/week until optimum dose is reached (maximum is 60 mg/day).

• **EXTENDED-RELEASE CAPSULE**

Attention deficit disorders.

Children, 6 years and older: 5–15 mg/day.

Narcolepsy.

Adults: 5–30 mg/day. **Children, 6–12 years:** 5–15 mg/day; **12 years and older:** 10–15 mg/day.

D

NURSING CONSIDERATIONS

SEE ALSO *NURSING CONSIDERATIONS* FOR *AMPHETAMINES AND DERIVATIVES.*

ADMINISTRATION/STORAGE

1. Long-acting products may be used for once-a-day dosing in attention deficit disorders and narcolepsy.
2. When tablets or elixir are used for ADD or narcolepsy, give first dose upon awakening with one or two additional doses given at intervals of 4–6 hr. Give the last dose 6 hr before bedtime.
3. If receiving an MAO inhibitor, wait 14 days after stopping before initiating dextroamphetamine.

CLIENT/FAMILY TEACHING

1. Take last dose at least 6 hr before bedtime to ensure adequate rest.
2. Avoid activities that require alertness until drug effects realized.
3. Check weight weekly to ensure no significant loss. Eat regular meals with snacks to prevent wt loss.

OUTCOMES/EVALUATE

• Improved attention span and concentration levels
• ↓ Daytime sleeping

Dextromethorphan hydrobromide

(dex-troh-meth-**OR**-fan)

PREGNANCY CATEGORY: C
CLASSIFICATION(S):
Antitussive, nonnarcotic
Rx: Balminil DM
OTC: Benylin Adult, Benylin DM, Benylin DM Pediatric, Children's Hold, Creo-Terpin, Delsym, DexAlone, Diabetes CF, Drixoral Cough Liquid Caps, Hold DM, Pediatric Vicks 44D Dry Hacking Cough and Head Congestion, Pertussin CS, Pertussin ES, Robitussin Cough Calmers, Robitussin Pediatric, Scot-Tussin DM Cough Chasers, Silphen DM, St. Joseph Cough Suppressant, Sucrets 4-Hour Cough, Sucrets Cough Control, Suppress, Trocal, Vick's Dry Hacking Cough
✱OTC: Balminil DM Children, Koffex DM Children, Koffex DM Syrup, Novahistex DM, Novahistine DM, Robitussin Honey Cough DM

ACTION/KINETICS

Selectively depresses the cough center in the medulla. Dextromethorphan 15–30 mg is equal to 8–15 mg codeine as an antitussive. Does not produce physical dependence or respiratory depression. Well absorbed from GI tract. **Onset:** 15–30 min. **Duration:** 3–6 hr. The sustained liquid contains dextromethorphan plistirex equivalent to 30 mg dextromethorphan hydrobromide per 5 mL.

USES

Symptomatic relief of nonproductive cough due to colds or inhaled irritants.

CONTRAINDICATIONS

Persistent or chronic cough or when cough is accompanied by excessive secretions. Use during first trimester of pregnancy unless directed otherwise by physician. Use in children less than 2 years of age.

SPECIAL CONCERNS

Use with caution in clients with nausea, vomiting, high fever, rash, or persistent headache.

SIDE EFFECTS

CNS: Dizziness, drowsiness. **GI:** N&V, stomach pain.

OD OVERDOSE MANAGEMENT

Symptoms: ***Adults:*** Dysphoria, slurred speech, ataxia, altered sensory perception. ***Children:*** Ataxia, ***convulsions, respiratory depression.*** *Treatment:* Treat symptoms and provide support.

DRUG INTERACTIONS

MAO inhibitors / May cause nausea, hypotension, hyperpyrexia, myoclonic leg jerks, and coma.

Silbutramine / Accumulation of brain serotonin → serotonin syndrome (myoclonus, hyperreflexia, confusion, disorientation, agitation, hypomania, rigidity, tremor, sweating, shivering, seizures, coma, hypertension)

HOW SUPPLIED

Capsule: 30 mg; *Gelcap:* 30 mg; *Liquid:* 3.5 mg/5 mL, 7.5 mg/5 mL, 15 mg/5 mL, 10 mg/15 mL; *Lozenge/Troche:* 2.5 mg, 5 mg, 7.5 mg, 15 mg; *Suspension, Extended Release:* 30 mg/5 mL; *Syrup:* 1 mg/mL, 10 mg/5 mL

DOSAGE

- **CAPSULES, LIQUID, LOZENGES, SYRUP, CONCENTRATE, TABLETS**

Antitussive.

Adults and children over 12 years: 10–30 mg q 4–8 hr, not to exceed 120 mg/day; **pediatric, 6–12 years:** either 5–10 mg q 4 hr or 15 mg q 6–8 hr, not to exceed 60 mg/day; **pediatric, 2–6 years:** either 2.5–7.5 mg q 4 hr or 7.5 mg q 6–8 hr of the syrup, not to exceed 30 mg/day.

- **GELCAPS**

Antitussive

Adults and children over 12 years: 30 mg q 6–8 hr.

- **SUSTAINED-RELEASE SUSPENSION**

Antitussive.

Adults: 60 mg q 12 hr. **Pediatric, 6–12 years:** 30 mg q 12 hr, not to exceed 60 mg/day; **pediatric, 2–6 years:** 15 mg q 12 hr, not to exceed 30 mg/day.

NURSING CONSIDERATIONS

ADMINISTRATION/STORAGE

1. Increasing the dose of dextromethorphan will not increase its effectiveness but will increase the duration of action.
2. Do not give lozenges to children under 6 years of age.

ASSESSMENT

1. Document sputum production and characteristics. Note duration of cough, if persists beyond several weeks, stop drug and reassess cause.
2. Determine presence of nausea, vomiting, persistent headaches, or a high fever.
3. If pregnant, determine trimester; contraindicated in first trimester.
4. Assess lung sounds and determine need for CXR.

CLIENT/FAMILY TEACHING

1. Avoid tasks that require mental alertness until drug effects realized.
2. Avoid alcohol in any form.
3. Add humidity to environment.
4. Increase fluids to decrease viscosity of secretions.
5. Cigarette smoke, dust, and chemical fumes are irritants that may aggravate condition.
6. Symptoms that persist for more than a week require medical intervention; record onset, triggers, characteristics of secretions, medications, and response to therapy.

OUTCOMES/EVALUATE

Control of cough with improved sleep patterns

Dextrose and electrolytes

(**DEX**-trohs)

CLASSIFICATION(S):

Dextrose and electrolytes

Rx: Naturalyte, Pedialyte, Pediatric Electrolyte Solution, Rehydralyte, Resol

ACTION/KINETICS

PO products that contain varying amounts of sodium, potassium, chloride, citrate, and dextrose (Resol contains 20 g/L whereas Pedialyte and Rehydralyte contain 25 g/L). In addition, Resol contains magnesium, calcium, and phosphate. **Time to peak effect:** 8–12 hr.

USES

Diarrhea. Prophylaxis and treatment of electrolyte depletion in diarrhea or in continuing fluid loss. Maintenance of hydration.

CONTRAINDICATIONS

Anuria, oliguria. Severe dehydration including severe diarrhea (IV therapy is necessary for prompt replacement of fluids and electrolytes). Malabsorption of glucose. Severe and sustained vomiting when the client is unable to drink. Intestinal obstruction, perforated bowel, paralytic ileus.

SPECIAL CONCERNS

Use with caution in premature infants.

D

SIDE EFFECTS

Overhydration indicated by puffy eyelids. Hypernatremia, vomiting (usually shortly after treatment has started).

HOW SUPPLIED

Oral Solution

DOSAGE

- **ORAL SOLUTION**

Mild dehydration.

Adults and children over 10 years, initial: 50 mL/kg over 4–6 hr; **maintenance:** 100–200 mL/kg over 24 hr until diarrhea stops.

Moderate dehydration.

Adults and children over 10 years, initial: 100 mL/kg over 6 hr; **maintenance:** 15 mL/kg q hr until diarrhea stops.

Moderate to severe dehydration.

Pediatric, 2–10 years, initial: 50 mL/kg over the first 4–6 hr followed by 100 mL/kg over the next 18–24 hr; **less than 2 years, initial:** 75 mL/kg during the first 8 hr and 75 mL/kg during the next 16 hr.

NURSING CONSIDERATIONS

ADMINISTRATION/STORAGE

1. Give no more than 1,000 mL/hr to adults and no more than 100 mL/20 min to children.
2. Adjust the amount and rate of solution depending on need, thirst, and response.
3. Assist infants and small children in drinking the solution slowly and frequently in small quantities and, if necessary, feed by a spoon.
4. Do not dilute rehydration solutions with water.

CLIENT/FAMILY TEACHING

1. Soft foods such as bananas, cereal, cooked peas, beans, and potatoes should be given to maintain nutrition.
2. Report if fluid output exceeds intake, if there is no weight gain, or if S&S of dehydration persist.
3. If vomiting occurs after PO therapy initiated, continue but give small amounts, frequently and slowly.
4. If dehydration is severe, seek medical attention immediately. IV fluids and electrolytes should be started since the onset of action of PO solution is too slow. Oral solution can be used later for maintenance.

OUTCOMES/EVALUATE

- Adequate hydration
- Prevention of electrolyte depletion

Dezocine

(**DEZ**-oh-seen)

PREGNANCY CATEGORY: C
CLASSIFICATION(S):
Narcotic agonist/antagonist
Rx: Dalgan

SEE ALSO *NARCOTIC ANALGESICS*.

ACTION/KINETICS

Parenteral narcotic analgesic possessing both agonist and antagonist activity. Similar to morphine with respect to analgesic potency and onset and duration of action. Less risk of abuse due to the mixed agonist-antagonist properties of the drug. The narcotic antagonist activity is greater than that of pentazocine. **Onset:** Approximately 30 min after IM and approximately 15 min after IV. **Peak effect:** 30–150 min. **Peak plasma levels:** 10–38 ng/mL after a 10-mg dose. **Duration:** 2–4 hr. **t½, after IV:** 2.4 hr. Approximately two-thirds of a dose is excreted in the urine mostly as the glucuronide conjugate.

USES

Analgesic when use of a narcotic is desirable.

CONTRAINDICATIONS

Lactation. Individuals dependent on narcotics. SC administration.

SPECIAL CONCERNS

Elderly clients are at an increased risk for altered respiratory patterns and mental changes.

SIDE EFFECTS

CNS: Sedation (common), dizziness, vertigo, confusion, anxiety, crying, sleep disturbances, delusions, headache, depression, delirium. **Respira-**

tory: Respiratory depression, atelectasis. **CV:** Hypotension, irregular heart/pulse, hypertension, chest pain, pallor, thrombophlebitis. **GI:** N&V, dry mouth, constipation, abdominal pain, diarrhea. **Dermatologic:** Reactions at the injection site, pruritus, rash, erythema. **EENT:** Diplopia, blurred vision, congestion in ears, tinnitus. **GU:** Urinary frequency, retention, or hesitancy. **Miscellaneous:** Sweating, chills, edema, flushing, low hemoglobin, muscle cramps or aches, muscle pain, slurred speech.

OD OVERDOSE MANAGEMENT

Treatment: Naloxone IV with appropriate supportive measures including oxygen, IV fluids, vasopressors, and artificial respiration.

DRUG INTERACTIONS

Additive depressant effect when used with general anesthetics, sedatives, antianxiety drugs, hypnotics, alcohol, and other opiate analgesics.

HOW SUPPLIED

Injection: 5 mg/mL, 10 mg/mL, 15 mg/mL

DOSAGE

• **IM**

Analgesia.

Adults: 5–20 mg (usual is 10 mg) as a single dose; dose may be repeated q 3–6 hr with dosage adjusted, if necessary, depending on the status of the client.

• **IV**

Analgesia.

Adults: 2.5–10 mg (usual initial dose is 5 mg) repeated q 2–4 hr.

NURSING CONSIDERATIONS

SEE ALSO *NURSING CONSIDERATIONS* FOR *NARCOTIC ANALGESICS*.

ADMINISTRATION/STORAGE

1. Do not exceed a maximum single dose of 20 mg or a maximum daily dose of 120 mg.
2. Store at room temperature protected from light. Do not use if a precipitate is present.

ASSESSMENT

1. Note any sulfite sensitivity; drug contains sodium metabisulfite. Monitor for evidence of allergic reaction.
2. Determine any history or current use of opiate drugs; may precipitate an acute withdrawal syndrome.
3. Document location, onset, duration, and intensity of pain; rate pain and note alleviating factors.
4. Note any evidence of impaired renal or liver function; anticipate reduced dose with dysfunction.
5. Assess for any evidence of head injury or increased ICP. If administered with CNS depressants, reduce the dose of one or both agents.
6. Geriatric clients should receive reduced doses and be evaluated for subsequent dose levels.

CLIENT/FAMILY TEACHING

1. Do not drive or operate dangerous machinery until drug effects have worn off.
2. Avoid alcohol and the use of any unprescribed sedatives, hypnotics, or antianxiety agents.

OUTCOMES/EVALUATE

Effective pain control, as evidenced by ↑ activity, improved appetite, and reports of relief

Diazepam

(dye-**AYZ**-eh-pam)

PREGNANCY CATEGORY: D

CLASSIFICATION(S):

Antianxiety drug, benzodiazepine

Rx: Diastat, Diazepam Intensol , Valium **C-IV**

✱**Rx:** Apo-Diazepam, Diazemuls, Valium Roche, Vivol

SEE ALSO *TRANQUILIZERS/ANTIMANIC DRUGS/HYPNOTICS*.

ACTION/KINETICS

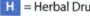

The skeletal muscle relaxant effect of diazepam may be due to enhancement of GABA-mediated presynaptic inhibition at the spinal level as well as in the brain stem reticular formation. **Onset: PO,** 30–60 min; **IM,** 15–30 min; **IV,** more rapid. **Peak plasma levels: PO,** 0.5–2 hr; **IM,** 0.5–1.5; **IV,** 0.25 hr. **Duration:** 3 hr. **t½:** 20–50 hr. Metabolized in the liver to the active metabolites desmethyldiazepam, oxazepam, and temazepam. Diazepam and metabolites are excreted through the urine. Diazepam is 97%–99% bound to plasma protein.

USES

(1) Anxiety, tension (more effective than chlordiazepoxide), alcohol withdrawal, muscle relaxant, adjunct to treat seizure disorders, antipanic drug. (2) Used prior to gastroscopy and esophagoscopy, preoperatively and prior to cardioversion. (3) In dentistry to induce sedation. (4) Treatment of status epilepticus. (5) Relief of skeletal muscle spasm due to inflammation of muscles or joints or trauma; spasticity caused by upper motor neuron disorders such as cerebral palsy and paraplegia; athetosis; and stiff-man syndrome. (6) Relieve spasms of facial muscles in occlusion and temporomandibular joint disorders. **IV:** Status epilepticus, severe recurrent seizures, and tetanus. **Rectal gel:** (1) Treat epilepsy in those with stable regimens of anticonvulsant drugs who require intermittent diazepam to control increased seizure activity. (2) To interrupt clusters of repetitive seizures in epilepsy clients.

ADDITIONAL CONTRAINDICATIONS

Narrow-angle glaucoma, children under 6 months, lactation, and parenterally in children under 12 years.

SPECIAL CONCERNS

When used as an adjunct for seizure disorders, diazepam may increase the frequency or severity of clonic-tonic seizures, for which an increase in the dose of anticonvulsant medication is necessary. Safety and efficacy of parenteral diazepam have not been determined in neonates less than 30 days of age. Prolonged CNS depression has been observed in neonates, probably due to inability to biotransform diazepam into inactive metabolites.

ADDITIONAL DRUG INTERACTIONS

(1) Diazepam potentiates antihypertensive effects of thiazides and other diuretics.
(2) Diazepam potentiates muscle relaxant effects of *d*-tubocurarine and gallamine.
Fluoxetine / ↑ Half-life of diazepam.
Isoniazid / ↑ Half-life of diazepam.
Ranitidine / ↓ GI absorption of diazepam.

HOW SUPPLIED

Injection: 5 mg/mL; *Rectal Gel:* 2.5 mg, 5 mg, 10 mg, 15 mg, 20 mg; *Oral Solution:* 5 mg/mL, 5 mg/5 mL; *Solution Intensol:* 5 mg/mL; *Tablet* 2 mg, 5 mg, 10 mg

DOSAGE

• TABLETS, ORAL SOLUTION, SOLUTION INTENSOL

Antianxiety, anticonvulsant, adjunct to skeletal muscle relaxants.

Adults: 2–10 mg b.i.d.–q.i.d. **Elderly, debilitated clients:** 2–2.5 mg 1–2 times/day. May be gradually increased to adult level. **Pediatric, over 6 months, initial:** 1–2.5 mg (0.04–0.2 mg/kg or 1.17–6 mg/m^2) b.i.d.–t.i.d.

Alcohol withdrawal.

Adults: 10 mg t.i.d.–q.i.d. during the first 24 hr; **then,** decrease to 5 mg t.i.d.–q.i.d. as required.

Anticonvulsant.

Adults: 15–30 mg once daily.

• RECTAL GEL

Anticonvulsant.

Over 12 years: 0.2 mg/kg. **Children, 6–11 years:** 0.3 mg/kg; **2–5 years:** 0.5 mg/kg. If required, a second dose can be given 4 to 12 hr after the first dose. Do not treat more than five episodes per month or more than one episode every 5 days. Adjust dose downward in elderly or debilitated clients to reduce ataxia or oversedation.

• IM, IV

Preoperative or diagnostic use.

Adults: 10 mg IM 5–30 min before procedure.

Adjunct to treat skeletal muscle spasm.

Adults, initial: 5–10 mg IM or IV; **then,** repeat in 3–4 hr if needed (larger doses may be required for tetanus).

Moderate anxiety.

Adults: 2–5 mg IM or IV q 3–4 hr if necessary.

Severe anxiety, muscle spasm.

Adults: 5–10 mg IM or IV q 3–4 hr, if necessary.

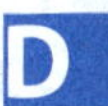

Acute alcohol withdrawal.
Initial: 10 mg IM or IV; **then,** 5–10 mg q 3–4 hr.
Preoperatively.
Adults: 10 mg IM prior to surgery.
Endoscopy.
IV: 10 mg or less although doses up to 20 mg can be used; **IM:** 5–10 mg 30 min prior to procedure.
Cardioversion.
IV: 5–15 mg 5–10 min prior to procedure.
Tetanus in children.
IM, IV, over 1 month: 1–2 mg, repeated q 3–4 hr as necessary; **5 years and over:** 5–10 mg q 3–4 hr.
• **IV**
Status epilepticus.
Adults, initial: 5–10 mg; **then,** dose may be repeated at 10–15-min intervals up to a maximum dose of 30 mg. Dosage may be repeated after 2–4 hr. **Children, 1 month–5 years:** 0.2–0.5 mg q 2–5 min, up to maximum of 5 mg. Can be repeated in 2–4 hr. **5 years and older:** 1 mg q 2–5 min up to a maximum of 10 mg; dose can be repeated in 2–4 hr, if needed.

NOTE: Elderly or debilitated clients should not receive more than 5 mg parenterally at any one time.

NURSING CONSIDERATIONS

SEE ALSO *NURSING CONSIDERATIONS FOR TRANQUILIZERS/ANTIMANIC DRUGS/HYPNOTICS.*

ADMINISTRATION/STORAGE

1. Mix Intensol solution with beverages such as water, soda, and juices or soft foods such as applesauce or puddings. Use only the calibrated dropper provided to withdraw drug. Once the medication is withdrawn and mixed, use immediately.
2. Except for the deltoid muscle, absorption from IM sites is slow and erratic.
IV 3. The IV route is preferred in the convulsing client.
4. Dizac, which is an emulsified injection, should only be given IV; it is not to be given IM or SC.
5. Parenteral administration may cause bradycardia, respiratory or cardiac arrest; have emergency equipment and drugs available.
6. Diazepam interacts with plastic; therefore, introducing diazepam into plastic containers or administration sets will decrease drug availability.
7. To reduce reactions at the IV site, give diazepam slowly (5 mg/min); avoid small veins or intra-arterial administration. For pediatric use, give the IV solution slowly over a 3-min period at a dose not exceeding 0.25 mg/kg. The initial dose can be repeated after 15–30 min.
8. Due to the possibility of precipitation and instability, do not infuse diazepam. Do not mix or dilute with other solutions or drugs in the syringe or infusion container.

ASSESSMENT

1. Document indications for therapy and time for anticipated results.
2. Determine any depression or drug abuse. Avoid simultaneous use of CNS depressants.
3. Reduce drug gradually to avoid withdrawal symptoms such as anxiety, tremors, anorexia, insomnia, weakness, headache, and N&V.
4. Monitor CBC, renal, and LFTs.
5. Review anxiety level and identify any contributing factors.
6. Elderly clients may experience adverse reactions more quickly than younger clients; use a lower dose in this group.

CLIENT/FAMILY TEACHING

1. Drug may cause dizziness and drowsiness. Avoid activities that require mental alertness until drug effects realized.
2. Avoid alcohol and any other CNS depressants.
3. Notify provider if pregnancy suspected.

OUTCOMES/EVALUATE

- ↓ Anxiety/tension episodes
- Control alcohol withdrawal
- Control of status epilepticus
- Relief of muscle spasms
- Effective sedation

Diazoxide IV

(dye-az-**OX**-eyed)

PREGNANCY CATEGORY: C
CLASSIFICATION(S):
Antihypertensive, direct-acting
Rx: Hyperstat IV

D

SEE ALSO *ANTIHYPERTENSIVE AGENTS* AND *DIAZOXIDE ORAL*.

ACTION/KINETICS
Exerts a direct action on vascular smooth muscle to cause arteriolar vasodilation and decreased peripheral resistance. **Onset:** 1–5 min. **Time to peak effect:** 2–5 min. **Duration** (variable): usual, 3–12 hr. Excreted through the kidney (50% unchanged).

USES
May be the drug of choice for hypertensive crisis (malignant and nonmalignant hypertension) in hospitalized adults and children. Often given concomitantly with a diuretic. Especially suitable for clients with impaired renal function, hypertensive encephalopathy, hypertension complicated by LV failure, and eclampsia. Ineffective for hypertension due to pheochromocytoma.

CONTRAINDICATIONS
Hypersensitivity to drug or thiazide diuretics. Treatment of compensatory hypertension due to aortic coarctation or AV shunt. Dissecting aortic aneurysm.

SPECIAL CONCERNS
A decrease in dose may be necessary in geriatric clients due to age-related decreases in renal function. If given prior to delivery, fetal or neonatal hyperbilirubinemia, thrombocytopenia, or altered carbohydrate metabolism may result. Use with caution during lactation and in clients with impaired cerebral or cardiac circulation.

SIDE EFFECTS
CV: Hypotension (may be severe enough to cause shock), sodium and water retention, especially in clients with impaired cardiac reserve, ***atrial or ventricular arrhythmias, cerebral or myocardial ischemia,*** marked ECG changes with possibility of ***MI,*** palpitations, bradycardia, SVT, chest discomfort or nonanginal chest tightness. **CNS:** Cerebral ischemia manifested by unconsciousness, ***seizures,*** paralysis, confusion, numbness of the hands. Headache, dizziness, weakness, drowsiness, lightheadedness, somnolence, lethargy, euphoria, weakness of short duration, apprehension, anxiety, malaise, blurred vision. **Respiratory:** Tightness in chest, cough, dyspnea, sensation of choking. **GI:** N&V, diarrhea, anorexia, parotid swelling, change in sense of taste, salivation, dry mouth, ileus, constipation, acute pancreatitis (rare). **Other:** Hyperglycemia (may be serious enough to require treatment), sweating, flushing, sensation of warmth, transient neurologic findings due to alteration in regional blood flow to the brain, hyperosmolar coma in infants, tinnitus, hearing loss, retention of nitrogenous wastes, acute pancreatitis, back pain, increased nocturia, lacrimation, hypersensitivity reactions, papilledema, hirsutism, decreased libido. Pain, cellulitis without sloughing, warmth or pain along injected vein, phlebitis at injection site, extravasation.

LABORATORY TEST CONSIDERATIONS
False + or ↑ uric acid.

OD OVERDOSE MANAGEMENT
Symptoms: Hypotension, excessive hyperglycemia. *Treatment:* Use the Trendelenburg position to reverse hypotension.

DRUG INTERACTIONS
Anticoagulants, oral / ↑ Anticoagulant effect R/T ↓ plasma protein binding
Nitrites / ↑ Hypotensive effect
Phenytoin / ↓ Anticonvulsant effect of phenytoin
Sulfonylureas / Destablization of the client → hyperglycemia
Thiazide diuretics / ↑ Hyperglycemic, hyperuricemic, and antihypertensive diazoxide effect
Vasodilators, peripheral / ↑ Hypotensive effect

HOW SUPPLIED
Injection: 15 mg/mL

DOSAGE

- **IV PUSH (30 SEC OR LESS)**

Hypertensive crisis.

Adults: 1–3 mg/kg up to a maximum of 150 mg; may be repeated at 5–15-min intervals until adequate BP response obtained. Drug may then be repeated at 4–24-hr intervals for 4–5 days or until oral antihypertensive therapy can be initiated. **Pediatric:** 1–3 mg/kg (30–90 mg/m²) using the same dosing intervals as adults.

Repeated use can result in sodium and water retention; therefore, a diuretic may be needed to avoid CHF and for maximum reduction of BP.

NURSING CONSIDERATIONS

SEE ALSO *NURSING CONSIDERATIONS* FOR *ANTIHYPERTENSIVE AGENTS* AND *DIAZOXIDE ORAL.*

ADMINISTRATION/STORAGE

IV 1. Do not administer IM or SC. Medication is highly alkaline.
2. Ensure patency and inject rapidly (30 sec) undiluted into a peripheral vein to maximize response.
3. Assess site for signs of irritation or extravasation. If extravasation occurs, apply ice packs.
4. Protect from light, heat, and freezing.
5. Have a sympathomimetic drug, such as norepinephrine, to treat severe hypotension should it occur.
6. Protect ampules from light and store between 2– 30°C (36–86°F).

ASSESSMENT

1. Assess for sensitivity to thiazide diuretics, sulfa drugs, or diazoxide.
2. With diabetics, can cause serious elevations in blood sugar levels. Note complaints of sweating, flushing, or evidence of hyperglycemia.
3. Obtain uric acid level and assess for evidence of hyperuricemia.
4. Monitor BP frequently until stabilized, then hourly until crisis resolved. Obtain final BP upon arising, prior to ambulation. Keep recumbent during and for 30 min after injection to avoid orthostatic hypotension; for 8–10 hr if furosemide is also administered.

OUTCOMES/EVALUATE

Reduction in BP during hypertensive crisis

Diazoxide oral

(dye-az-**OX**-eyed)

PREGNANCY CATEGORY: C
CLASSIFICATION(S):
Insulin antagonist
Rx: Proglycem

ACTION/KINETICS

Related to the thiazide diuretics. It inhibits the release of insulin from beta islet cells of the pancreas, leading to an increase in blood glucose levels. Effect is dose related. Causes sodium, potassium, uric acid, and water retention. Other effects include increased pulse rate, increased serum uric acid levels, increased serum free fatty acids, decreased para-aminohippuric acid clearance from the kidneys (little effect on GFR). **Onset:** 1 hr. **t½:** 24–36 hr (up to 53 hr in clients with anuria). **Duration:** 8 hr. Over 90% bound to plasma proteins. Metabolized in the liver although 50% is excreted through the kidneys unchanged.

USES

(1) Management of hypoglycemia due to hyperinsulinism, including inoperable islet cell adenoma or carcinoma or extrapancreatic malignancies in adults. (2) In children, for treatment of hyperinsulinemia due to leucine sensitivity, islet cell hyperplasia, nesidioblastosis, extrapancreatic malignancy, islet cell adenoma or adenomatosis. (3) Preoperatively as a temporary measure and postoperatively if hypoglycemia persists. The drug is used parenterally as an antihypertensive agent (see *Diazoxide IV*).

CONTRAINDICATIONS

Functional hypoglycemia, hypersensitivity to diazoxide or thiazides.

SPECIAL CONCERNS

Infants are particularly prone to development of edema. Use with extreme caution in clients with history of gout and in those in whom edema presents a risk (cardiac disease).

SIDE EFFECTS

CV: Sodium/fluid retention (common); precipitation of CHF in clients with compromised cardiac reserve, palpitations, increased HR, hypotension, transient hypertension, chest pain (rare). **Metabolic:** Hyperglycemia, glycosuria, ***diabetic ketoacidosis, hyperosmolar nonketotic coma.*** **GI:** N&V, diarrhea, transient taste loss, anorexia, ileus, abdominal pain. **CNS:** Weakness, headache, insomnia, extrapyramidal symptoms, dizziness, paresthesia, fever, malaise, anxiety, polyneuritis. **Hematologic:** Thrombocytopenia with or without purpura, eosinophilia, neutropenia, decreased hemoglobin/hematocrit/IgG, excessive bleeding. **Dermatologic:** Skin rashes, hirsutism, herpes, loss of hair from scalp, monilial dermatitis, pruritus. **GU:** Hematuria, decrease in urine production, nephrotic syndrome (reversible), azotemia, albuminuria. **Ophthalmologic:** Blurred/double vision, lacrimation, transient cataracts, ring scotoma, subconjunctival hemorrhage. **Other:** Pancreatitis, ***pancreatic necrosis,*** galactorrhea, gout, premature aging of bone, polyneuritis, enlargement of lump in breast.

LABORATORY TEST CONSIDERATIONS

↑ Serum uric acid, AST, alkaline phosphatase; ↓ C_{CR}

OD OVERDOSE MANAGEMENT

Symptoms: Hypotension, excessive hyperglycemia. *Treatment:* Insulin to treat hyperglycemia; use Trendelenburg position to reverse hypotension.

DRUG INTERACTIONS

Alpha-adrenergic blocking agents / ↓ Diazoxide effect

Anticoagulants, oral / ↑ Anticoagulant effect R/T ↓ plasma protein binding

Antihypertensives / Excessive ↓ BP due to additive effects

Phenothiazines / ↑ Diazoxide effects, including hyperglycemia

Phenytoin / ↓ Phenytoin effect R/T ↑ liver breakdown

Sulfonylureas / ↓ Effect of both drugs

Thiazide diuretics / ↑ Hyperglycemic and hyperuricemic effects; hypotension may occur.

HOW SUPPLIED

Capsule: 50 mg; *Oral Suspension:* 50 mg/mL

DOSAGE

- **CAPSULES, ORAL SUSPENSION**

  Diabetes.

Dosage is individualized on the basis of blood glucose level and response of client. **Adults and children, usual, initial:** 1 mg/kg q 8 hr (adjust according to response); **maintenance:** 3–8 mg/kg/day divided into two or three equal doses q 8–12 hr. **Infants and newborns, initial:** 3.3 mg/kg q 8 hr (adjust according to response); **maintenance:** 8–15 mg/kg/day divided into two or three equal doses q 8–12 hr.

NURSING CONSIDERATIONS

ADMINISTRATION/STORAGE

1. Blood glucose levels and urinary glucose and ketones must be monitored carefully until stabilized, which usually takes 1 week. Have insulin and IV fluids to counteract possible ketoacidosis. Discontinue if effect has not been established within 2–3 weeks.
2. Take on a regular basis with no skipped and no extra doses taken.
3. Protect the suspension from light.

ASSESSMENT

1. Document indications for therapy and time for expected results. Note sensitivity to thiazides.
2. Determine any gout or CAD.
3. Monitor BP for potentiation of antihypertensive effect if currently taking an antihypertensive agent.
4. With overdosage, observe closely for the first 7 days until blood sugar level is again within normal limits (80–110 mg/100 mL).
5. Review list of drug side effects to determine if clinical presentations may be drug related.

CLIENT/FAMILY TEACHING

1. Report unusual bruising or bleeding; may require discontinuation.
2. With history of CHF, observe carefully for fluid retention; could precipitate heart failure.
3. Excessive hair growth should subside once drug discontinued.

OUTCOMES/EVALUATE

Control of hypoglycemia with restoration of BS

Diclofenac potassium

(dye-**KLOH**-fen-ack)

PREGNANCY CATEGORY: B
Rx: Cataflam
✱Rx: Novo-Difenac-K, Riva-Diclofenac K, Voltaren Rapide

Diclofenac sodium

(dye-**KLOH**-fen-ack)

PREGNANCY CATEGORY: B
Rx: Diclotec, Solaraze, Voltaren, Voltaren Ophthalmic, Voltaren-XR
✱Rx: Apo-Diclo, Apo-Diclo SR, Novo–Difenac, Novo–Difenac SR, Nu-Diclo, Nu-Diclo-SR, PMS-Diclofenac SR, Riva-Diclofenac, Voltaren Ophtha, PMS-Diclofenac
CLASSIFICATION(S):
Nonsteroidal anti-inflammatory drug

SEE ALSO ***NONSTEROIDAL ANTI-INFLAMMATORY DRUGS.***

ACTION/KINETICS
Available as both the potassium (immediate-release) and sodium (delayed-release) salts. *Immediate-release product.* **Onset:** 30 min. **Peak plasma levels:** 1 hr. **Duration:** 8 hr. *Delayed-release product.* **Peak plasma levels:** 2–3 hr. **t½:** 1–2 hr. For all dosage forms, food will affect the rate, but not the amount, absorbed from the GI tract. Metabolized in the liver and excreted by the kidneys.

USES
PO, Immediate-release: Analgesic, primary dysmenorrhea. **PO, Immediate- or Delayed-release:** Rheumatoid arthritis, osteoarthritis, ankylosing spondylitis. **PO, Delayed-release:** Osteoarthritis, rheumatoid arthritis. *Investigational:* Mild to moderate pain, juvenile rheumatoid arthritis, acute painful shoulder, sunburn. **Ophthalmic:** Postoperative inflammation following cataract or corneal refractive surgery. **Topical Gel:** Actinic keratoses.

CONTRAINDICATIONS
Wearers of soft contact lenses. Use of the gel in those with hypersensitivity to benzyl alcohol, polyethylene glycol monomethyl ether 350, or hyaluronate sodium. Use of the gel during lactation or in children.

SPECIAL CONCERNS
Use with caution during lactation. Safety and effectiveness have not been determined in children. When used ophthalmically, may cause increased bleeding of ocular tissues in conjunction with ocular surgery. Healing may be slowed or delayed.

SIDE EFFECTS
Following ophthalmic use: Keratitis, increased IOP, ocular allergy, N&V, anterior chamber reaction, viral infections, transient burning/stinging on administration. When used with soft contact lenses, may cause ocular irritation, including redness/burning.

HOW SUPPLIED
Diclofenac potassium. *Tablet:* 50 mg. **Diclofenac sodium.** *Enteric Coated Tablet:* 25 mg, 50 mg, 75 mg; *Gel:* 3%; *Ophthalmic solution:* 0.1%; *Tablet, Extended Release:* 100 mg

DOSAGE

• IMMEDIATE-RELEASE TABLETS, EXTENDED-RELEASE TABLETS

Analgesia, primary dysmenorrhea.

Adults: 50 mg t.i.d. of immediate-release tablets. In some, an initial dose of 100 mg followed by 50-mg doses may achieve better results. After the first day, the total daily dose should not exceed 150 mg.

Rheumatoid arthritis.

Adults: 150–200 mg/day in divided doses (e.g., 50 mg t.i.d. or q.i.d.; 75 mg b.i.d. of the sodium salt). For chronic therapy, use extended-release tablets, 100 mg once or twice daily, not to exceed 225 mg/day.

Osteoarthritis.

Adults: 100–150 mg/day in divided doses (e.g., 50 mg b.i.d. or t.i.d.; 75 mg b.i.d. of the sodium salt). For chronic therapy, use extended-release tablets, 100 mg/day. Doses greater than 200 mg/day have not been evaluated.

Ankylosing spondylitis.

Adults: 25 mg q.i.d. with an extra 25-mg dose at bedtime, if necessary. Doses greater than 125 mg/day have not been evaluated.

• **OPHTHALMIC SOLUTION, 0.1%**

Following cataract surgery.

1 gtt in the affected eye q.i.d. beginning 24 hr after cataract surgery and for 2 weeks thereafter.

Corneal refractive surgery.

1–2 gtt within 1 hr prior to surgery; then, apply 1–2 gtt within 15 min of surgery and continue q.i.d. for three days or less.

• **TOPICAL GEL, 3%**

Actinic keratoses.

Apply gel b.i.d. to lesion areas for 60–90 days.

NURSING CONSIDERATIONS

SEE ALSO *NURSING CONSIDERATIONS* FOR *NONSTEROIDAL ANTI-INFLAMMATORY DRUGS.*

ADMINISTRATION/STORAGE

Up to 3 weeks may be required for beneficial effects to be realized when used for rheumatoid arthritis or osteoarthritis.

ASSESSMENT

1. Assess for redness, infection, pain, or vision changes with ophthalmic therapy.
2. With arthritis, assess joints for inflammation, ROM, and loss of function. Rate pain level.
3. Monitor CBC, liver and renal function studies; perform FOB with long-term therapy.
4. Ensure that drug is administered in high enough doses for anti-inflammatory effect when needed and in low doses for an analgesic effect.

CLIENT/FAMILY TEACHING

1. May take with meals, a full glass of water or milk if GI upset occurs.
2. Do not crush or chew delayed-release tablets.
3. Limit intake of sodium, monitor weights, and report any evidence of edema or unusual weight gain.
4. Clients with diabetes should monitor BS levels closely; may alter response to antidiabetic agents.
5. Avoid alcohol and OTC products.
6. Do not wear contacts when taking drug.
7. Maintain fluid intake of 2 L/day.
8. Report any changes in stools.

OUTCOMES/EVALUATE

• Relief of joint pain/inflammation with improved mobility

• ↓ Eye inflammation

Dicloxacillin sodium

(dye-klox-ah-**SILL**-in)

PREGNANCY CATEGORY: B

CLASSIFICATION(S):

Antibiotic, penicillin

Rx: Dycill, Dynapen, Pathocil

SEE ALSO *ANTI-INFECTIVES* AND *PENICILLINS.*

ACTION/KINETICS

Penicillinase-resistant and acid-stable. **Peak serum levels: IM, PO,** 4–20 mcg/mL after 1 hr. **t½:** 40 min. 98% bound to plasma proteins. Chiefly excreted in urine.

USES

Infections due to penicillinase-producing staphylococci. To initiate therapy in any suspected staphylococcal infection. Infections due to *Streptococcus pneumoniae.*

CONTRAINDICATIONS

Treatment of meningitis. Use in newborns.

HOW SUPPLIED

Capsule: 125 mg, 250 mg, 500 mg; *Powder for reconstitution:* 62.5 mg/5 mL

DOSAGE

• **CAPSULES, ORAL SUSPENSION**

Skin and soft tissue infections, mild to moderate URTIs.

Adults and children over 40 kg: 125 mg q 6 hr; **pediatric, less than 40 kg:** 12.5 mg/kg/day in four equal doses given q 6 hr.

More severe lower respiratory tract infections or disseminated infections.

Adults and children over 40 kg: 250 mg q 6 hr, up to a maximum of 4 g/day; **pediatric, less than 40 kg:** 25 mg/kg/day in four equal doses given q 6 hr.

NURSING CONSIDERATIONS

SEE ALSO *GENERAL NURSING CONSIDERATIONS* FOR *ANTI-INFECTIVES* AND *PENICILLINS.*

ADMINISTRATION/STORAGE

1. To prepare PO suspension, shake container to loosen powder, measure water for reconstitution as indicated on label, add half of the water, and immediately shake vigorously because usual handling may cause lumps. Add the remainder of the water and again shake vigorously.
2. Shake well before pouring each dose.
3. The reconstituted PO solution is stable for 7 days at room temperature, 10 days if refrigerated, and 21 days if frozen.

ASSESSMENT

Note indications for therapy, onset and duration of symptoms. Obtain cultures when indicated.

CLIENT/FAMILY TEACHING

Preferable to take on an empty stomach 1–2 hr before meals. Report any unusual side effects or lack of response.

OUTCOMES/EVALUATE

Symptomatic relief; negative cultures with resolution of infection

Dicyclomine hydrochloride

(dye-**SYE**-kloh-meen)

PREGNANCY CATEGORY: C
CLASSIFICATION(S):
Cholinergic blocking drug
Rx: Antispas, Bentyl, Byclomine, Dibent, Dilomine, Di-Spaz, Or-Tyl
✱Rx: Bentylol, Formulex, Lomine

SEE ALSO *CHOLINERGIC BLOCKING AGENTS.*

ACTION/KINETICS

t½, initial: 1.8 hr; **secondary:** 9–10 hr.

USES

Hypermotility and spasms of GI tract associated with irritable colon and spastic colitis, mucous colitis.

ADDITIONAL CONTRAINDICATIONS

Use for peptic ulcer.

SPECIAL CONCERNS

Lower doses may be needed in elderly clients due to confusion, agitation, excitement, or drowsiness.

ADDITIONAL SIDE EFFECTS

Brief euphoria, slight dizziness, feeling of abdominal distention. **Use of the syrup in infants less than 3 months of age: *Seizures,*** syncope, respiratory symptoms, fluctuations in pulse rate, ***asphyxia,*** muscular hypotonia, ***coma.***

HOW SUPPLIED

Capsules: 10 mg; *Injection:* 10 mg/mL; *Syrup:* 10 mg/5 mL; *Tablets:* 20 mg

DOSAGE

- **CAPSULES, SYRUP, TABLETS**

Hypermotility and spasms of GI tract.

Adults: 10–20 mg t.i.d.–q.i.d.; **then,** may increase to total daily dose of 160 mg if side effects do not limit this dosage. **Pediatric, 6 years and older, capsules or tablets:** 10 mg t.i.d.–q.i.d.; adjust dosage to need and incidence of side effects. **Pediatric, 6 months–2 years, syrup:** 5–10 mg t.i.d.–q.i.d.; **2 years and older:** 10 mg t.i.d.–q.i.d. The dose should be adjusted to need and incidence of side effects.

- **IM**

Hypermotility and spasms of GI tract.

Adults: 20 mg q 4–6 hr. **Not for IV use.**

NURSING CONSIDERATIONS

SEE ALSO *NURSING CONSIDERATIONS* FOR *CHOLINERGIC BLOCKING AGENTS.*

ADMINISTRATION/STORAGE

Can be administered to clients with glaucoma.

ASSESSMENT

1. Document indications for therapy, onset and characteristics of symptoms.
2. List other agents trialed and the outcome.
3. Determine presence/history of PUD.

CLIENT/FAMILY TEACHING

Take as directed and report any loss of response or adverse side effects.

OUTCOMES/EVALUATE

Restoration of normal bowel function/GI motility

Didanosine (ddI, dideoxyinosine)

(die-**DAN**-oh-seen)

PREGNANCY CATEGORY: B
CLASSIFICATION(S):
Antiviral, nucleoside reverse transcriptase inhibitor
Rx: Videx, Videx EC

SEE ALSO *ANTIVIRAL AGENTS*.

ACTION/KINETICS
A nucleoside analog of deoxyadenosine. After entering the cell, it is converted to the active dideoxyadenosine triphosphate (ddATP) by cellular enzymes. Due to the chemical structure of ddATP, its incorporation into viral DNA leads to chain termination and therefore inhibition of viral replication. ddATP also inhibits viral replication by interfering with the HIV–RNA-dependent DNA polymerase by competing with the natural nucleoside triphosphate for binding to the active site of the enzyme. Didanosine has shown in vitro antiviral activity in a variety of HIV-infected T cell and monocyte/macrophage cell cultures. Is broken down quickly at acidic pH; therefore, PO products contain buffering agents to increase the pH of the stomach. Food decreases the rate of absorption. Oral availability differs between adults (aboust 42%) and children (about 25%). **t½, elimination:** 1.5 hr for adults and 0.8 hr for children. Metabolized in the liver and excreted mainly through the urine.

USES
Videx: In combination with other antiretroviral drugs to treat HIV-1 infections. **Videx EC:** In combination with other antiretriviral drugs to treat HIV-1 infection in adults where treatment requires once-daily treatment of didanosine or an alternative didanosine formulation.

CONTRAINDICATIONS
Lactation.

SPECIAL CONCERNS
Use with caution in renal and hepatic impairment and in those on sodium-restricted diets. Opportunistic infections and other complications of HIV infection may continue to develop; thus, keep clients under close observation. Fatal and nonfatal pancreatitis in both treatment naive or treatment experienced clients, regardless of the degree of immunosuppression; especially seen in those receiving stavudine with or without hydroxyurea.

SIDE EFFECTS
Commonly pancreatitis (fatal or nonfatal) and peripheral neuropathy (manifested by distal numbness, tingling, or pain in the feet or hands). Lactic acidosis. Neuropathy occurs more frequently in clients with a history of neuropathy or neurotoxic drug therapy.

In adults. GI: Diarrhea, abdominal pain, N&V, anorexia, dry mouth, ileus, colitis, constipation, eructation, flatulence, gastroenteritis, ***GI hemorrhage,*** severe hepatomegaly with steatosis, oral moniliasis, stomatitis, mouth sores, sialadenitis, ***stomach ulcer hemorrhage,*** melena, oral thrush, liver abnormalities, ***pancreatitis***. **CNS:** Headache, ***tonic-clonic seizures,*** abnormal thinking, anxiety, nervousness, twitching, confusion, depression, acute brain syndrome, amnesia, aphasia, ataxia, dizziness, hyperesthesia, hypertonia, incoordination, ***intracranial hemorrhage,*** paralysis, paranoid reaction, psychosis, insomnia, sleep disorders, speech disorders, tremor. **Hematologic:** Leukopenia, granulocytopenia, thrombocytopenia, microcytic anemia, ***hemorrhage,*** ecchymosis, petechiae. **Dermatologic:** Rash, pruritus, herpes simplex, skin disorder, sweating, eczema, impetigo, excoriation, erythema. **Musculoskeletal:** Asthenia, myopathy, arthralgia, arthritis, myalgia, muscle atrophy, decreased strength, hemiparesis, neck rigidity, joint disorder, leg cramps. **CV:** Chest pain, hypertension, hypotension, migraine, palpitation, peripheral vascular disorder, syncope, vasodilation, arrhythmias. **Body as a whole:** Chills, fever, infection, allergic reaction, pain, abscess, cellulitis, cyst, dehydration, malaise, flu syndrome, numbness of hands and feet, weight loss, alopecia, ***lactic acidosis***. **Respiratory:** Pneumonia, dyspnea, asthma, bronchitis, increased cough, rhinitis, rhinorrhea, epistaxis, laryngitis, decreased lung function, pharyngitis, hypoventilation, sinusitis, rhonchi, rales, congestion, interstitial pneumonia, respiratory disorders. **Ophthalmic:** Blurred vision, conjunctivitis, diplopia, dry eye, glaucoma, retinitis, photophobia, strabismus, optic neuritis, retinal changes. **Otic:** Ear disorder, otitis (externa and media), ear pain. **GU:** Impotency, kidney calculus, kidney failure, abnormal kidney function, nocturia, urinary frequency, vaginal hemorrhage. **Miscellaneous:** Peripheral edema, sarcoma, hernia, hypokalemia, lymphoma-like reaction.

In children. GI: Diarrhea, N&V, liver abnormalities, abdominal pain, stomatitis, mouth sores, pancreatitis, anorexia, increase in appetite, constipation, oral thrush, melena, dry mouth. **CNS:** Headache, nervousness, insomnia, dizziness, poor coordination, lethargy, neurologic symptoms, ***seizures.*** **Hematologic:** Ecchymosis, ***hemorrhage,*** petechie, leukopenia, granulocytopenia, thrombocytopenia, anemia. **Dermatologic:** Rash, pruritus, skin disorder, eczema, sweating, impetigo, excoriation, erythema. **Musculoskeletal:** Arthritis, myalgia, muscle atrophy, decreased strength. **Body as a whole:** Chills, fever, asthenia, pain, malaise, failure to thrive, weight loss, flu syndrome, alopecia, dehydration, lactic acidosis. **CV:** Vasodilation, arrhythmia. **Respiratory:** Cough, rhinitis, dyspnea, asthma, rhinorrhea, epistaxis, pharyngitis, hypoventilation, sinusitis, rhonchi, rales, congestion, pneumonia. **Ophthalmic:** Photophobia, strabismus, visual impairment, optic neuritis. **Otic:** Ear pain, otitis. **Miscellaneous:** Urinary frequency, diabetes mellitus, diabetes insipidus, liver abnormalities.

LABORATORY TEST CONSIDERATIONS

↑ AST, ALT, alkaline phosphatase, bilirubin, uric acid, amylase, lipase.

OD OVERDOSE MANAGEMENT

Symptoms: Pancreatitis, peripheral neuropathy, diarrhea, hyperuricemia, hepatic dysfunction. *Treatment:* There are no antidotes; treatment should be symptomatic.

DRUG INTERACTIONS

Allopurinol / ↑ Didanosine plasma levels
Antacids, Mg- or Al-containing / ↑ Risk of side effects due to antacid components
Antifungal drugs (azoles) / ↓ Absorption of azole antifungals
Antiretroviral drugs (Delavirdine, Indinavir) / Significant ↓ plasma levels of antiretroviral drugs
Ganciclovir / ↑ Didanosine plasma levels; ↓ ganciclovir plasma levels
Itraconazole / ↓ Itraconazole effect; give 2 or more hr before didanosine
Ketoconazole / ↓ Ketoconazole absorption R/T gastric pH change caused by buffering agents in didanosine
Methadone / ↓ Didanosine levels
Pentamidine (IV) / ↑ Risk of pancreatitis
Quinolone antibiotics / ↓ Plasma quinolone levels R/T ↓ absorption
Ranitidine / ↓ Ranitidine absorption R/T gastric pH change caused by buffering agents in didanosine
Stavudine / ↑ Risk of fatal lactic acidosis in pregnant women, especially when combined with other drugs
Tetracyclines / ↓ Tetracycline absorption gastric pH changes caused by R/T buffering agents in didanosine

HOW SUPPLIED

Videx: *Chew Tablet, Buffered:* 25 mg, 50 mg, 100 mg, 150 mg, 200 mg; *Powder for Oral Solution, Buffered:* 100 mg, 167 mg, 250 mg; *Powder for Oral Solution, Pediatric:* 2 g, 4 g. **Videx EC:** *Delayed Release Capsule:* 125 mg, 200 mg, 250 mg, 400 mg

DOSAGE

• CHEWABLE/DISPERSIBLE BUFFERED TABLETS, BUFFERED POWDER FOR ORAL SOLUTION, ENTERIC-COATED CAPSULE, POWDER FOR PEDIATRIC ORAL SOLUTION

Adults, initial, over 60 kg: 200 mg q 12

hr (or 400 mg/day) for tablets; 250 mg b.i.d. for buffered oral solution; or, 400 mg/day for enteric-coated capsules. **Adults, less than 60 kg:** 125 mg q 12 hr (or 250 mg/day) for tablets; 167 mg b.i.d. for buffered oral solution; or, 250 mg/day for enteric-coated capsules. **Pediatric:** 120 mg/m² b.i.d. Once daily dosing may lower the virologic response; twice-daily dosing is preferred.

For adults with impaired renal function, the following dosage regimens are used: (1) **C_{CR} 60 mL or more/min:** See above. (2) **C_{CR} 30–59 mL/min, 60 kg or more:** 200 mg daily or 100 mg b.i.d. for tablets; or, 100 mg daily for buffered oral solution; or, 200 mg/day for enteric-coated capsules. **C_{CR} 30–59 mL/min, less than 60 kg:** 150 mg daily or 75 mg b.i.d. for tablets; or, 100 mg b.i.d. for buffered oral solution; or, 125 mg daily for enteric-coated capsules. (3) **C_{CR} 10–29 mL/min, 60 kg or more:** 150 mg daily for tablets; or,167 mg/day for buffered oral solution; or, 125 mg/day for enteric-coated capsules. **C_{CR} 10–29 mL/min, less than 60 kg:** 100 mg daily for tablets; or, 100 mg daily for buffered oral solution; or, 125 mg daily for enteric-coated capsules. (4) **C_{CR} less than 10 mL/min, 60 kg or more:** 100 mg daily for tablets; or,100 mg buffered oral solution; or, 125 mg daily for enteric coated capsules. **C_{CR} less than 10 mL/min, less than 60 kg:** 75 mg daily for tablets or 100 mg daily for buffered oral solution (do not use enteric-coated capsules in these clients).

NOTE: For clients requiring continuous ambulatory peritoneal dialysis or hemodialysis, give ¼ of the total daily dose once daily. For clients with a C_{CR} less than 10 mL/min, do not give a supplemental dose of didanosine following hemodialysis.

NURSING CONSIDERATIONS

SEE ALSO *NURSING CONSIDERATIONS* FOR *ANTIVIRAL AGENTS*.

ADMINISTRATION/STORAGE

1. Twice daily dosing may be more effective than once daily dosing.
2. Administer all formulations 30 min before or 1 hr after meals. Didanosine EC should be given on an empty stomach and be swallowed intact. Didanosine EC has not been studied in children.
3. For either once- or twice-daily dosing, clients must take at least 2 of the appropriate strength tablets at each dose to provide adequate buffering and to prevent gastric acid degradation of didanosine.
4. To reduce GI side effects, do not give clients more than 4 tablets at each dose.
5. To disperse tablets, add 2 tablets (for adults) to about 1 oz of water. Stir until a uniform dispersion forms and drink entire dispersion immediately. The dispersion may be diluted with 1 oz of clear apple juice. Pediatric dispersion is prepared similarly.
6. To prepare the buffered powder for PO solution for adults, mix with 4 oz of drinking water; do not mix the powder with fruit juice or other acid-containing beverages. Stir the mixture until the powder dissolves completely (about 2–3 min). Consume the entire solution immediately.
6. To prepare the powder for pediatric oral solution, mix the dry powder with purified water to an initial concentration of 20 mg/mL. The resulting solution is then mixed with antacid (e.g., Mylanta Double Strength Liquid, Extra Strength Maaolox Plus Suspension, or Maalox TC Suspension) to a final concentration of 10 mg/mL. Shake this admixture thoroughly prior to use. May be stored in a tightly closed container in the refrigerator for up to 30 days.

ASSESSMENT

1. Document all previous experience with zidovudine therapy; list reasons for transfer to didanosine.
2. Monitor CBC, CD_4 counts/viral load, liver and renal function studies.
3. Anticipate reduced dose with liver and renal impairment. Note baseline VS and weight.

CLIENT/FAMILY TEACHING

1. Food decreases the rate of drug absorption; take 30 min before or 1 hr after meals.

2. Do not swallow tablets whole. Tablets may be chewed or crushed thoroughly before taking or dispersed in at least 1 oz of drinking water (stir thoroughly and drink immediately).
3. Report any symptoms of neuropathy (numbness, burning, or tingling in the hands or feet); drug should be discontinued until symptoms subside. May tolerate a reduced dose once these symptoms resolved.
4. Report any abdominal pain and N&V immediately; may be clinical signs of pancreatitis. Stop drug and report; resume only after pancreatitis has been ruled out.
5. With Na-restricted diets, sodium content is more in the single-dose packet than the two-tablet dose. Each single-dose packet of buffered powder for oral solution contains 1,380 mg sodium.
6. Chewable/dispersible buffered tablets contain 73 mg phenylalanine per 2-tablet dose).
7. Increase fluid intake; report S&S of diarrhea or hyperuricemia.
8. Any changes in vision should be evaluated by an ophthalmologist. Get retinal exams every 6 mo to rule out depigmentation with children.
9. Avoid alcohol and any other drugs that may exacerbate toxicity of didanosine.
10. Drug is not a cure, but alleviates the symptoms of HIV infections; may continue to acquire opportunistic infections.
11. *Does not* reduce the risk of transmission of HIV to others through sexual contact or blood contamination; use appropriate precautions.
12. Identify local support groups that may assist client/family to understand and cope with disease.

OUTCOMES/EVALUATE

Control of symptoms of AIDS, ARC, and opportunistic infections in clients with HIV who are intolerant or have clinically deteriorated during zidovudine therapy

—COMBINATION DRUG—

Difenoxin hydrochloride with Atropine sulfate

(dye-fen-**OX**-in, **AH**-troh-peen)

PREGNANCY CATEGORY: C
CLASSIFICATION(S):
Antidiarrheal
Rx: Motofen

SEE ALSO CHOLINERGIC BLOCKING AGENTS.

CONTENT

Each tablet contains: *Antidiarrheal:* Difenoxin HCl, 1 mg. *Anticholinergic:* Atropine sulfate, 0.025 mg.

ACTION/KINETICS

Related chemically to meperidine; thus, atropine sulfate is incorporated to prevent deliberate overdosage. Difenoxin is the active metabolite of diphenoxylate and is effective at one-fifth the dosage of diphenoxylate. Slows intestinal motility by a local effect on the GI wall. **Peak plasma levels:** 40–60 min. The drug and its inactive metabolites are excreted through both the urine and feces.

USES

Management of acute nonspecific diarrhea and acute worsening of episodes of chronic functional diarrhea.

CONTRAINDICATIONS

Diarrhea caused by *Escherichia coli, Salmonella,* or *Shigella;* pseudomembranous colitis caused by broad-spectrum antibiotics; jaundice; children less than 2 years of age. Hypersensitivity to difenoxin or atropine. Lactation.

SPECIAL CONCERNS

Use with caution in ulcerative colitis, liver and kidney disease, lactation, and in clients receiving dependence-producing drugs or in those who are addiction prone. Safety and effectiveness in children less than 12 years of age have not been determined.

D

SIDE EFFECTS

GI: N&V, dry mouth, epigastric distress, constipation. **CNS:** Lightheadedness, dizziness, drowsiness, headache, tiredness, nervousness, confusion, insomnia. **Ophthalmic:** Blurred vision, burning eyes. Due to the small amount of atropine, significant anticholinergic side effects are not likely, except perhaps in children.

OD OVERDOSE MANAGEMENT

Symptoms: Initially include dry skin and mucous membranes, hyperthermia, flushing, and tachycardia. These are followed by hypotonic reflexes, nystagmus, miosis, lethargy, coma, and ***respiratory depression*** (may occur up to 30 hr after overdose taken). *Treatment:* Naloxone may be used to treat respiratory depression (duration of difenoxin may be longer than naloxone; supplemental naloxone may be necessary). Gastric lavage, establish a patent airway, mechanically assisted respiration.

DRUG INTERACTIONS

Antianxiety agents / Potentiation or addition of CNS depressant effects
Barbiturates / Potentiation or addition of CNS depressant effects
Ethanol / Potentiation or addition of CNS depressant effects
MAO inhibitors / Precipitation of hypertensive crisis
Narcotics / Potentiation or addition of CNS depressant effects

HOW SUPPLIED

See Content

DOSAGE

• **TABLETS**

Adults, initial: 2 tablets (2 mg difenoxin); **then,** 1 tablet (1 mg difenoxin) after each loose stool or 1 tablet q 3–4 hr as needed, not to exceed 8 mg (i.e., 8 tablets)/24 hr.

NURSING CONSIDERATIONS

ADMINISTRATION/STORAGE

Treatment beyond 48 hr is usually not necessary for acute diarrhea or acute exacerbation of functional diarrhea and generally not recommended if clinical improvement is not noted.

ASSESSMENT

1. Note the onset, characteristics, and frequency of diarrhea; identify precipitating factors, e.g., travel, stress, food, medication regimens.
2. Assess for evidence of dehydration (weakness, weight loss, poor skin turgor, higher temperature, rapid weak pulse, or decreased urinary output) or electrolyte imbalance (weakness, irritability, anorexia, nausea, and dysrhythmias).
3. Send stool for analysis; C&S.
4. Monitor LFTs; may precipitate hepatic coma with dysfunction.
5. Contains atropine sulfate.
6. May precipitate hypertensive crisis with MAO inhibitors.
7. With overdose, hospitalize, since latent (12–30 hr later) respiratory depression may occur.

CLIENT/FAMILY TEACHING

1. Do not perform tasks that require mental alertness until drug effects are realized.
2. Take only as directed; do not share.
3. Chew sugarless gum; use sugarless candy or ice chips for dry mouth. Report any swelling of gums or extremity numbness.
4. Keep out of child's reach; may be fatal if ingested.
5. Do *not* take if breast feeding.
6. Avoid alcohol or any other unprescribed CNS depressants.
7. May take 24–36 hr before effects are evident. Record the number, frequency, and characteristics of the stools; report if S&S persist more than 5 days.

OUTCOMES/EVALUATE

↓ Frequency/number of diarrheal stools

Diflunisal

(dye-**FLEW**-nih-sal)

PREGNANCY CATEGORY: C
CLASSIFICATION(S):
Nonsteroidal anti-inflammatory drug
Rx: Dolobid
✱Rx: Apo-Diflunisal, Novo-Diflunisal, Nu-Diflunisal

ACTION/KINETICS

Salicylic acid derivative, although not metabolized to salicylic acid. Mechanism not known; may be an inhibitor of prostaglandin synthetase. **Onset:** 20 min (analgesic, antipyretic). **Peak plasma levels:** 2–3 hr. **Peak effect:** 2–3 hr. **Duration:** 4–6 hr **t½:** 8–12 hr. Ninety-nine percent protein bound. Metabolites excreted in urine.

USES

(1) Analgesic (2) rheumatoid arthritis, osteoarthritis, ankylosing spondylitis, psoriatic arthritis, musculoskeletal pain. (3) Prophylaxis and treatment of vascular headaches.

CONTRAINDICATIONS

Hypersensitivity to diflunisal, aspirin, or other anti-inflammatory drugs. Acute asthmatic attacks, urticaria, or rhinitis precipitated by aspirin. During lactation and in children less than 12 years of age.

SPECIAL CONCERNS

Use with caution in presence of ulcers or in clients with a history thereof, in clients with hypertension, compromised cardiac function, or in conditions leading to fluid retention. Use with caution in only first two trimesters of pregnancy. Geriatric clients may be at greater risk of GI toxicity.

SIDE EFFECTS

GI: Nausea, dyspepsia, GI pain and bleeding, diarrhea, vomiting, constipation, flatulence, peptic ulcer, eructation, anorexia. **CNS:** Headache, fatigue, fever, malaise, dizziness, somnolence, insomnia, nervousness, vertigo, depression, paresthesias. **Dermatologic:** Rashes, pruritus, sweating, ***Stevens-Johnson syndrome,*** dry mucous membranes, erythema multiforme. **CV:** Palpitations, syncope, edema. **Other:** Tinnitus, asthenia, chest pain, hypersensitivity reactions, ***anaphylaxis,*** dyspnea, dysuria, muscle cramps, thrombocytopenia.

OD OVERDOSE MANAGEMENT

Symptoms: Drowsiness, N&V, diarrhea, tachycardia, hyperventilation, stupor, disorientation, diminished urine output, ***coma, cardiorespiratory arrest.*** *Treatment:* Supportive measures. To empty the stomach, induce vomiting, or perform gastric lavage. Hemodialysis may not be effective since the drug is significantly bound to plasma protein.

DRUG INTERACTIONS

Acetaminophen / ↑ Acetaminophen plasma levels
Antacids / ↓ Diflunisal plasma levels
Anticoagulants / ↑ PT
Furosemide / ↓ Furosemide hyperuricemic effect
Hydrochlorothiazide / ↑ Hydrochlorothiazide plasma drug levels and ↓ hyperuricemic effect
Indomethacin / ↓ Indomethacin renal clearance → ↑ plasma levels
Naproxen / ↓ Urinary naproxen and metabolite excretion

HOW SUPPLIED

Tablet: 250 mg, 500 mg

DOSAGE

• **TABLETS**

Mild to moderate pain.

Adults, initial: 1,000 mg; **then,** 250–500 mg q 8–12 hr.

Rheumatoid arthritis, osteoarthritis.

Adults: 250–500 mg b.i.d. Doses in excess of 1,500 mg/day are not recommended. For some, an initial dose of 500 mg followed by 250 mg q 8–12 hr may be effective. Reduce dosage with impaired renal function.

NURSING CONSIDERATIONS

ADMINISTRATION/STORAGE

Maximum relief occurs in 2–3 weeks when used for the pain and swelling of arthritis. Serum salicylate levels are not used as a guide to dosage or toxicity because the drug is not hydrolyzed to salicylic acid.

ASSESSMENT

1. Note any hypersensitivity to salicylates or other NSAIDs.
2. Determine any history of PUD, HTN, or cardiac dysfunction.
3. Check for pregnancy; avoid drug or use with extreme caution during the first two trimesters.
4. Give in high enough doses for anti-inflammatory effects when needed and use the lower dose for analgesic effects.
5. With long-term therapy, monitor CBC, liver and renal function studies.

CLIENT/FAMILY TEACHING

1. May be given with water, milk, or meals to reduce gastric irritation. Do not crush or chew tablets.

2. Report unusual bruising or bleeding; may inhibit platelet aggregation which is reversible with drug discontinuation. Do not give with acetaminophen or aspirin.
3. May cause dizziness or drowsiness; use care when operating machinery or driving.
4. Report stool color changes or diarrhea; can cause an electrolyte imbalance or GI bleed.
5. Must take on a regular basis to sustain the anti-inflammatory effect.
6. Report for medical follow-up; drug needs to be adjusted according to age, condition, and changes in disease activity.

OUTCOMES/EVALUATE

- ↓ Pain and inflammation; ↑ joint mobility
- Prevention of vascular headaches

D

Digoxin

(dih-**JOX**-in)

PREGNANCY CATEGORY: A
CLASSIFICATION(S):
Cardiac glycoside
Rx: Digitek, Digoxin Injection, Pediatric, Lanoxicaps, Lanoxin

ACTION/KINETICS

Digoxin increases the force and velocity of myocardial contraction (positive inotropic effect) by increasing the refractory period of the AV node and increasing total peripheral resistance. This effect is due to inhibition of sodium/potassium–ATPase in the sarcolemmal membrane, which alters excitation–contraction coupling. Inhibiting sodium, potassium–ATPase results in increased calcium influx and increased release of free calcium ions within the myocardial cells, which then potentiate the contractility of cardiac muscle fibers. Digoxin also decreases the rate of conduction and increases the refractory period of the AV node due to an increase in parasympathetic tone and a decrease in sympathetic tone. Clinical effects are not seen until steady-state plasma levels are reached. The initial dose of digoxin is larger (loading dose) and is traditionally referred to as the *digitalizing dose;* subsequent doses are referred to as *maintenance doses.* **Onset: PO,** 0.5–2 hr; **time to peak effect:** 2–6 hr. **Duration:** Over 24 hr. **Onset, IV:** 5–30 min; **time to peak effect:** 1–4 hr. **Duration:** 6 days. **t½:** 30–40 hr. **Therapeutic serum level:** 0.5–2.0 ng/mL. From 20% to 25% is protein bound. Serum levels above 2.5 ng/mL indicate toxicity. Fifty percent to 70% is excreted unchanged by the kidneys. Bioavailability depends on the dosage form: tablets (60%–80%), capsules (90%–100%), and elixir (70%–85%). Thus, changing dosage forms may require dosage adjustments.

USES

CHF, including that due to venous congestion, edema, dyspnea, orthopnea, and cardiac arrhythmia. May be drug of choice for CHF because of rapid onset, relatively short duration, and ability to be administered PO or IV.

Control of rapid ventricular contraction rate in clients with atrial fibrillation or flutter. Slow HR in sinus tachycardia due to CHF. SVT. Prophylaxis and treatment of recurrent paroxysmal atrial tachycardia with paroxysmal AV junctional rhythm. Cardiogenic shock (value not established).

CONTRAINDICATIONS

Ventricular fibrillation or tachycardia (unless congestive failure supervenes after protracted episode not due to digitalis), in presence of digoxin toxicity, hypersensitivity to cardiac glycosides, beriberi heart disease, certain cases of hypersensitive carotid sinus syndrome.

SPECIAL CONCERNS

Use with caution in clients with ischemic heart disease, acute myocarditis, hypertrophic subaortic stenosis, hypoxic or myxedemic states, Adams-Stokes or carotid sinus syndromes, cardiac amyloidosis, or cyanotic heart and lung disease, including emphysema and partial heart block. Those with carditis associated with rheumatic fever or viral myocarditis are especially sensitive to digoxin-induced disturbances in rhythm. Electric pacemakers may sensitize the myocardium to cardiac glycosides. Also use with caution and at reduced dosage in elderly, debilitated clients, pregnant women and nursing mothers, and newborn, term, or premature infants who have immature renal and hepatic function and in reduced renal and/or hepatic function.

The half-life of digoxin is prolonged in the elderly; anticipate smaller drug doses. Be especially alert to cardiac arrhythmias in children. This sign of toxicity occurs more frequently in children than in adults.

SIDE EFFECTS

Digoxin is extremely toxic and has caused death even in clients who have received the drugs for long periods of time. There is a narrow margin of safety between an effective therapeutic dose and a toxic dose. Overdosage caused by the cumulative effects of the drug is a constant danger in therapy. Digoxin toxicity is characterized by a wide variety of symptoms, which are hard to differentiate from those of the cardiac disease itself.

One of the most serious side effects of digoxin is hypokalemia. This may lead to cardiac arrhythmias, muscle weakness, hypotension, and respiratory distress. Other agents causing hypokalemia reinforce this effect and increase the chance of digitalis toxicity. Such reactions may occur in clients who have been on digoxin maintenance for a long time. **CV:** Changes in the rate, rhythm, and irritability of the heart and the mechanism of the heartbeat. Extrasystoles, bigeminal pulse, coupled rhythm, ectopic beat, and other forms of arrhythmias have been noted. ***Death most often results from ventricular fibrillation.*** Discontinue digoxin in adults when pulse rate falls below 60 beats/min. All cardiac changes are best detected by the ECG, which is also most useful in clients suffering from intoxication. ***Acute hemorrhage.*** **GI:** Anorexia, N&V, excessive salivation, epigastric distress, abdominal pain, diarrhea, bowel necrosis. Clients on digoxin therapy may experience two vomiting stages. The first is an early sign of toxicity and is a direct effect of digoxin on the GI tract. Late vomiting indicates stimulation of the vomiting center of the brain, which occurs after the heart muscle has been saturated with digoxin. **CNS:** Headaches, fatigue, lassitude, irritability, malaise, muscle weakness, insomnia, stupor. Psychotomimetic effects (especially in elderly or arteriosclerotic clients or neonates) including disorientation, confusion, depression, aphasia, delirium, hallucinations, and, rarely, ***convulsions.*** **Neuromuscular:** Neurologic pain involving the lower third of the face and lumbar areas, paresthesia. **Visual disturbances:** Blurred vision, flickering dots, white halos, borders around dark objects, diplopia, amblyopia, color perception changes. **Hypersensitivity (5–7 days after starting therapy):** Skin reactions (urticaria, fever, pruritus, facial and ***angioneurotic edema***). **Other:** Chest pain, coldness of extremities.

LABORATORY TEST CONSIDERATIONS

May ↓ PT. Alters tests for 17-ketosteroids and 17-hydroxycorticosteroids.

OD OVERDOSE MANAGEMENT

The relationship of digoxin levels to symptoms of toxicity varies significantly from client to client; thus, it is not possible to identify digoxin levels that would define toxicity accurately. *Symptoms (Toxicity): GI:* Anorexia, N&V, diarrhea, abdominal discomfort, or pain. *CNS:* Blurred, yellow, or green vision and halo effect; headache, weakness, drowsiness, mental depression, apathy, restlessness, disorientation, confusion, ***seizures,*** EEG abnormalities, delirium, hallucinations, neuralgia, psychosis. *CV:* VT, unifocal or multiform PVCs (especially in bigeminal or trigeminal patterns), paroxysmal/nonparoxysmal nodal rhythms, AV dissociation, accelerated junctional rhythm, excessive slowing of the pulse, ***AV block (may proceed to complete block),*** atrial fibrillation, ***ventricular fibrillation (most common cause of death).*** *Children:* Visual disturbances, headache, weakness, apathy, and psychosis occur but may be difficult to recognize. *CV:* Conduction disturbances, supraventricular tachyarrhythmias (e.g., ***AV block***), atrial tachycardia with or without block, nodal tachycardia, unifocal or multiform ventricular premature contractions, ventricular tachycardia, sinus bradycardia (especially in infants). *Treatment in Adults:*

- Discontinue drug, admit to ICU for continuous ECG monitoring.
- If serum potassium is below normal, KCl should be administered in divided PO doses totaling 3–6 g (40–80 mEq). Potassium should not be used when severe or complete heart block is due to digitalis and not related to tachycardia.
- *Atropine:* A dose of 0.01 mg/kg IV to treat severe sinus bradycardia or slow ventricular rate due to secondary AV block.
- *Cholestyramine, colestipol, activated charcoal:* To bind digitalis in the intestine, thus preventing enterohepatic recirculation.
- *Digoxin immune FAB:* See drug entry. Given in approximate equimolar quantities as digoxin, it reverses S&S of toxicity, often with improvement within 30 min.
- *Lidocaine:* A dose of 1 mg/kg given over 5 min followed by an infusion of 15–50 mcg/kg/min to maintain normal cardiac rhythm.
- *Phenytoin:* For atrial or ventricular arrhythmias unresponsive to potassium, can give a dose of 0.5 mg/kg at a rate not exceeding 50 mg/min (given at 1–2 hr intervals). The maximum dose should not exceed 10 mg/kg/day.
- *Countershock:* A direct-current countershock can be used *only as a last resort.* If required, initiate at low voltage levels.

Treatment in Children: Give potassium in divided doses totaling 1–1.5 mEq/kg (if correction of arrhythmia is urgent, a dose of 0.5 mEq/kg/hr can be used) with careful monitoring of the ECG. The potassium IV solution should be dilute to avoid local irritation although IV fluid overload must be avoided. Digoxin immune FAB may also be used.

Digoxin is not removed effectively by dialysis, by exchange transfusion, or during cardiopulmonary bypass as most of the drug is found in tissues rather than the circulating blood.

DRUG INTERACTIONS

The following drugs increase serum digoxin levels, leading to possible toxicity: Aminoglycosides, amiodarone, anticholinergics, atorvastatin, benzodiazepines, captopril, diltiazem, erythromycin, esmolol, flecainide, hydroxychloroquine, ibuprofen, indomethacin, itraconazole, nifedipine, quinidine, quinine, telmisartan, tetracyclines, tolbutamide, verapamil.

Albuterol / ↑ Digoxin binding to skeletal muscle

H *Aloe* / Potential for ↑ digoxin effect R/T aloe-induced hypokalemia

Amiloride / ↓ Digoxin inotropic effects

Aminoglycosides / ↓ Digoxin effect R/T ↓ GI tract absorption

Aminosalicylic acid / ↓ Digoxin effect R/T ↓ GI tract absorption

Amphotericin B / ↑ K depletion caused by digoxin; ↑ risk of digitalis toxicity

Antacids / ↓ Digoxin effect of R/T ↓ GI tract absorption

Beta blockers / Complete heart block possible

H *Buckthorn bark/berry* / Potential for ↑ digoxin effect R/T to buckthorn-induced hypokalemia

Calcium preparations / Cardiac arrhythmias following parenteral calcium

H *Cascara sagrada bark* / Potential for ↑ digoxin effect R/T to cascara-induced hypokalemia

Chlorthalidone / ↑ K and Mg loss with ↑ chance of digitalis toxicity

Cholestyramine / Binds digoxin in the intestine and ↓ its absorption

Colestipol / Binds digoxin in the intestine and ↓ its absorption

Disopyramide / May alter effect of digoxin

H *Ephedra* / ↑ Chance of cardiac arrhythmias

Ephedrine / ↑ Chance of cardiac arrhythmias

Epinephrine / ↑ Chance of cardiac arrhythmias

Ethacrynic acid / ↑ K and Mg loss with ↑ chance of digitalis toxicity

Fluoxetine / Possible ↑ serum digoxin levels

Furosemide / ↑ K and Mg loss with ↑ chance of digoxin toxicity
H *German chamomile flower* / Potential for ↑ digoxin effect R/T to chamomile-induced hypokalemia
H *Ginseng* / ↑ Digoxin levels
Glucose infusions / Large infusions of glucose may cause ↓ in serum potassium and ↑ chance of digoxin toxicity
H *Hawthorn* / Potentiation of digoxin effect
Hypoglycemic drugs / ↓ Effect of digitalis glycosides due to ↑ breakdown by liver
H *Iceland moss* / Potential for ↑ digoxin effect R/T to iceland moss-induced hypokalemia
H *Indian snakeroot* / ↑ Risk of bradycardia
H *Ivy leaf* / Potential for ↑ digoxin effect R/T to ivy leaf-induced hypokalemia
Levothyroxine / ↓ Serum levels and therapeutic digoxin effect
H *Licorice* / Potential for ↑ digoxin effect R/T to licorice-induced hypokalemia
H *Marshmallow root* / Potential for ↑ digoxin effect R/T to marshmallow root-induced hypokalemia
Methimazole / ↑ Chance of toxic effects of digitalis
Metoclopramide / ↓ Digoxin effect R/T ↓ GI tract absorption
Muscle relaxants, nondepolarizing / ↑ Risk of cardiac arrhythmias
Penicillamine / ↓ Serum digoxin levels.
Propranolol / Potentiates digitalis-induced bradycardia
H *Rhubarb root* / Potential for ↑ digoxin effect R/T to rhubarb root-induced hypokalemia
H *St. John's wort* / ↓ Digoxin plasma levels R/T ↑ renal excretion
H *Sarsaparilla root* / Potential for ↑ absorption of digoxin
H *Senna pod/leaf* / Potential for ↑ digoxin effect R/T to senna-induced hypokalemia
Spironolactone / Either ↑ or ↓ toxic effects of digoxin
Succinylcholine / ↑ Chance of cardiac arrhythmias
Sulfasalazine / ↓ Digoxin effect of R/T ↓ GI tract absorption
Sympathomimetics / ↑ Chance of cardiac arrhythmias
Thiazides / ↑ K and Mg loss with ↑ chance of digoxin toxicity
Thioamines / ↑ Effect and toxicity of digoxin
Thyroid / ↓ Digoxin effect
Triamterene / ↑ Digoxin effects

HOW SUPPLIED

Capsule: 0.05 mg, 0.1 mg, 0.2 mg; *Elixir, Pediatric:* 0.05 mg/mL; *Injection:* 0.1 mg/mL, 0.25 mg/mL; *Tablet:* 0.125 mg, 0.25 mg

DOSAGE

• **CAPSULES**

Digitalization: Rapid.

Adults: 0.4–0.6 mg initially followed by 0.1–0.3 mg q 6–8 hr until desired effect achieved.

Digitalization: Slow.

Adults: A total of 0.05–0.35 mg/day divided in two doses for a period of 7–22 days to reach steady-state serum levels. **Pediatric.** Digitalizing dosage is divided into three or more doses with the initial dose being about one-half the total dose; doses are given q 4–8 hr. **Children, 10 years and older:** 0.008–0.012 mg/kg. **5–10 years:** 0.015–0.03 mg/kg. **2–5 years:** 0.025–0.035 mg/kg. **1 month–2 years:** 0.03–0.05 mg/kg. **Neonates, full-term:** 0.02–0.03 mg/kg. **Neonates, premature:** 0.015–0.025 mg/kg.

Maintenance.

Adults: 0.05–0.35 mg once or twice daily. **Premature neonates:** 20%–30% of total digitalizing dose divided and given in two to three daily doses. **Neonates to 10 years:** 25%–35% of the total digitalizing dose divided and given in two to three daily doses.

• **ELIXIR, TABLETS**

Digitalization: Rapid.

Adults: A total of 0.75–1.25 mg divided into two or more doses each given at 6–8-hr intervals.

Digitalization: Slow.

Adults: 0.125–0.5 mg/day for 7 days. **Pediatric.** (Digitalizing dose is divided into two or more doses and given at

6–8-hr intervals.) **Children, 10 years and older, rapid or slow:** Same as adult dose. **5–10 years:** 0.02–0.035 mg/kg. **2–5 years:** 0.03–0.05 mg/kg. **1 month–2 years:** 0.035–0.06 mg/kg. **Premature and newborn infants to 1 month:** 0.02–0.035 mg/kg.

Maintenance.

Adults: 0.125–0.5 mg/day. **Pediatric:** One-fifth to one-third the total digitalizing dose daily. *NOTE:* An alternate regimen (referred to as the "small-dose" method) is 0.017 mg/kg/day. This dose causes less toxicity.

• **IV**

Digitalization.

Adults: Same as tablets. **Maintenance:** 0.125–0.5 mg/day in divided doses or as a single dose. **Pediatric:** Same as tablets.

NURSING CONSIDERATIONS

ADMINISTRATION/STORAGE

1. Measure liquids precisely, using a calibrated dropper or syringe.
2. Obtain written parameters indicating the pulse rates, both high and low, at which cardiac glycosides are to be held; changes in rate or rhythm may indicate toxicity.
3. Lanoxicaps gelatin capsules are more bioavailable than tablets. Thus, the 0.05-mg capsule is equivalent to the 0.0625-mg tablet; the 0.1- mg capsule is equivalent to the 0.125-mg tablet, and the 0.2-mg capsule is equivalent to the 0.25-mg tablet.
4. Differences in bioavailability have been noted between products; monitor clients when changing from one product to another.
5. Protect from light.

IV 6. Give IV injections over 5 min (or longer) either undiluted or diluted fourfold or greater with sterile water for injection, 0.9% NaCl, RL injection, or D5W.

ASSESSMENT

For clients starting on a digitalizing dose

1. Document type, onset, and characteristics of symptoms. If administered for heart failure, note causes; ensure that failure not solely related to diastolic dysfunction as drug's positive inotropic effect may increase cardiac outflow obstruction with hypertrophic cardiomyopathy.
2. Note any drugs prescribed that would adversely interact with digoxin and monitor; diuretics may increase toxicity.
3. Monitor CBC, serum electrolytes, calcium, magnesium, liver and renal function tests.
4. Obtain ECG; note rhythm/rate.
5. Document cardiopulmonary findings; note presence of S3, JVD, HJR, displaced PMI, HR above 100 bpm, rales, peripheral edema, DOE, PND, and echo, MUGA, and/or cardiac catheterization findings. Note New York Heart Association Classification based on client symptoms.
6. Elderly clients must be observed for early S&S of toxicity (N&V, anorexia, confusion, and visual disturbances) because their rate of drug elimination is slower.

INTERVENTIONS

For clients being digitalized and for clients on a maintenance dose of digoxin

1. During digitalization, monitor closely.
2. Observe monitor for bradycardia and/or arrhythmias, or count apical rate for at least 1 min before administering the drug. Obtain written parameters (e.g., HR > 50 or 60) for drug administration.
   - Document adult HR below 50 bpm or if an arrhythmia (irregular pulse) occurs.
   - If child's HR is 90–110 bpm or if an arrhythmia is present, withhold drug and report.
3. Anticipate more than once daily dosing in most children (up to age 10) due to higher metabolic activity.
4. With co-worker simultaneously take the apical and radial pulse for 1 min, and report pulse deficit (e.g., the wrist rate is less than the apical rate); may indicate an adverse drug reaction.
5. Monitor weights and I&O. Weight gain may indicate edema. Adequate intake will help prevent cumulative toxic drug effects.
6. If taking non-potassium-sparing

diuretics as well as digoxin, will need potassium supplements. Provide the most palatable preparation available. (Liquid potassium preparations are usually bitter.)
7. If gastric distress experienced, use an antacid. Antacids containing aluminum or magnesium and kaolin/pectin mixtures should be given 6 hr before or 6 hr after dose of cardiac glycoside to prevent decreased therapeutic effects.
8. When given to newborns, use a cardiac monitor to identify early evidence of toxicity: excessive slowing of sinus rate, sinoatrial arrest, or prolonged PR interval.
9. Monitor digoxin levels periodically and assess for symptoms of toxicity; draw specimen more than 6 hr after last dose. Have digoxin antidote available (digoxin immune FAB) for severe toxicity.
10. Use caution; digoxin withdrawal may worsen heart failure.

CLIENT/FAMILY TEACHING

1. Take after meals to lessen gastric irritation.
2. Maintain a written record of pulse rates and weights; review guidelines for withholding medication and reporting abnormal pulse rates.
3. Do not change brands; different preparations have variations in bioavailability and could cause toxicity or loss of effect.
4. Follow directions carefully for taking the medication. If one dose of drug is accidentally missed, do not double up on the next dose.
5. Report toxic drug symptoms: anorexia, N&V, abdominal pain and diarrhea are often early symptoms and are due to the toxic effects on the GI tract and CTZ stimulation. Disorientation, agitation, visual disturbances, changes in color perception, irregular heart beat and hallucinations may also occur.
6. Maintain a sodium-restricted diet. Read labels and review foods low in sodium; consult dietitian for assistance in food selection, meal planning, and preparation.
7. Consult provider before taking any other medications, whether prescribed or OTC, because drug interactions occur frequently with cardiac glycosides.
8. Report any persistent cough, difficulty breathing, or edema (S&S of CHF).
9. Identify community health agencies available to assist in maintaining health.
10. Return for scheduled follow-up visits and lab tests.

OUTCOMES/EVALUATE

- Stable cardiac rate and rhythm, improved breathing patterns, ↓ severity of S&S of CHF, improved CO, improved activity tolerance, ↓ weight, and improved diuresis
- Serum drug levels within therapeutic range (e.g., digoxin 0.5–2.0 ng/mL)

Digoxin Immune Fab (Ovine)

(dih-**JOX**-in)

PREGNANCY CATEGORY: C
CLASSIFICATION(S):
Antidote for digoxin poisoning
Rx: Digibind

ACTION/KINETICS

Digoxin immune Fab are antibodies that bind to digoxin making them unavailable to bind at their site of action. In cases of digoxin toxicity, the antibodies bind to digoxin and the complex is excreted through the kidneys. As serum levels of digoxin decrease, digoxin bound to tissue is released into the serum to maintain equilibrium and this is then bound and excreted. The net result is a decrease in both tissue and serum digoxin. **Onset:** Less than 1 min. Improvement in signs of toxicity occurs within 30 min. **t½:** 15–20 hr (after IV administration). Each vial contains 38 mg of pure digoxin immune Fab, which will bind approximately 0.5 mg digoxin.

USES

Life-threatening digoxin toxicity or overdosage. Symptoms of toxicity include severe sinus bradycardia, second- or third-degree heart block which does not respond to atropine, ventricular tachycardia, ventricular fibrillation.

NOTE: Cardiac arrest can be expected if a healthy adult ingests more than 10 mg digoxin or a healthy child ingests more than 4 mg. Also, steady-state serum concentrations of digoxin greater than 10 ng/mL or potassium concentrations greater than 5 mEq/L as a result of digoxin therapy require use of digoxin immune Fab.

SPECIAL CONCERNS

Use with caution during lactation. Use in infants only if benefits outweigh risks. Clients sensitive to products of sheep origin may also be sensitive to digoxin immune Fab. Skin testing may be appropriate for high-risk clients.

SIDE EFFECTS

CV: Worsening of CHF or low CO, atrial fibrillation (all due to withdrawal of the effects of digoxin). **Other:** Hypokalemia. Rarely, hypersensitivity reactions occur, including fever and ***anaphylaxis.***

HOW SUPPLIED

Injection: 38 mg/vial

DOSAGE

• **IV**

Dosage depends on the serum digoxin concentration. A large dose has a faster onset but there is an increased risk of allergic or febrile reactions. The package insert should be carefully consulted. **Adults, usual:** Six vials (228 mg) is usually enough to reverse most cases of toxicity. **Children, less than 20 kg:** A single vial (38 mg) should be sufficient. However 20 vials (760 mg) are sufficient to treat most life-threatening cases in both adults and children.

NURSING CONSIDERATIONS

ADMINISTRATION/STORAGE

IV 1. To calculate the dose (in # of vials) of Digibind, divide the total digitalis body load (in mg) by 0.5 (i.e., amount of digitalis bound/vial).

2. Reconstitute lyophilized material with 4 mL of sterile water for injection to give a concentration of 10 mg/mL. If small doses required (e.g., in infants), can be further diluted with 36 mL sterile isotonic saline for a concentration of 1 mg/mL.

3. Administer over a 30-min period through a 0.22-µm membrane filter; may use bolus injection if immediate danger of cardiac arrest.

4. Use reconstituted antibody immediately. May store up to 4 hr at 2–8°C (36–46°F).

5. If acute digoxin ingestion results in severe symptoms and serum concentration is not known, 800 mg (20 vials) of digoxin immune Fab may be given. Monitor for volume overload in small children.

6. Administer to infants with a tuberculin syringe.

ASSESSMENT

1. Determine amount, time of drug ingestion, and serum digoxin level.

2. If previous reaction suspected or high-risk client, perform skin testing: Prepare a 10-mL solution (0.1 mL of drug in 9.9 mL NSS). Administer 0.1 mL intradermally or perform a scratch test by placing 1 drop of solution on the skin and making a scratch through the drop with a sterile needle; assess site in 20 min. *Do not* use if reaction is positive: urticarial wheal with erythematous surrounding skin.

3. Do not administer to those with known allergy to sheep proteins.

4. Monitor VS and cardiac rhythm. Assess for electrolyte imbalance; note hypokalemia or evidence of increased CHF.

5. Wait several days for redigitalization to ensure complete elimination of digibind. Levels will take 5–7 days to stabilize following treatment, although improvement in S&S of toxicity should be evident in 30 min.

OUTCOMES/EVALUATE

• Resolution of digoxin toxicity
• Controlled cardiac rhythm

Dihydroergotamine mesylate

(dye-hy-droh-er-**GOT**-ah-meen)

PREGNANCY CATEGORY: X

CLASSIFICATION(S):
Antimigraine drug
Rx: Migranal Nasal Spray , D.H.E. 45
✱**Rx:** Dihydroergotamine (DHE) Sandoz

ACTION/KINETICS
Manifests alpha-adrenergic receptor blocking activity as well as a direct stimulatory action on vascular smooth muscle of peripheral and cranial blood vessels, resulting in vasoconstriction, thus preventing the onset of a migraine attack. Manifests greater adrenergic blocking activity, less pronounced vasoconstriction, less N&V, and less oxytocic properties than does ergotamine. More effective when given early in the course of a migraine attack. **Onset: IM,** 15–30 min; **IV,** < 5 min. **Duration: IM,** 3–4 hr. **t½: initial,** 1.4 hr; **final,** 18–22 hr. Metabolized in liver and excreted in feces with less than 10% excreted through the urine.
USES
IM, IV. To prevent or abort migraine, migraine variant, histaminic cephalalgia (cluster headaches). Especially useful when rapid effect is desired or when other routes of administration are not possible. **Nasal Spray.** Acute treatment of migraine headaches with or without aura.
CONTRAINDICATIONS
Lactation. Pregnancy. Peripheral vascular disease, coronary heart disease, hypertension, impaired hepatic or renal function, sepsis, hypersensitivity, malnutrition, severe pruritus, presence of infection.
SPECIAL CONCERNS
Safety and efficacy have not been determined in children. Geriatric clients may be more affected by peripheral vasoconstriction that results in hypothermia. Prolonged administration may cause ergotism and gangrene.
SIDE EFFECTS
CV: Precordial pain, transient tachycardia or bradycardia. Large doses may cause increased BP, vasoconstriction of coronary arteries, and bradycardia. **GI:** N&V, diarrhea. **Other:** Numbness and tingling of fingers and toes, muscle pain in extremities, weakness in legs, localized edema, and itching. **Prolonged use:** Gangrene, ergotism.
OD OVERDOSE MANAGEMENT
Symptoms: N&V, pain in limb muscles, tachycardia or bradycardia, precordial pain, numbness and tingling of fingers and toes, weakness of the legs, hypertension or hypotension, localized edema, S&S of ischemia due to vasoconstriction of peripheral arteries and arterioles. Symptoms of ischemia include the feet and hands becoming cold, pale, and numb; muscle pain, gangrene. Occasionally confusion, depression, drowsiness, and ***seizures.*** *Treatment:* Maintain adequate circulation. IV nitroglycerin and nitroprusside to treat vasospasm. IV heparin and low molecular weight dextran to minimize thrombosis.
DRUG INTERACTIONS
Beta-adrenergic blockers / ↑ Peripheral ischemia resulting in cold extremities and possibly peripheral gangrene
Macrolide antibiotics / Acute ergotism resulting in peripheral ischemia
Nitrates / ↑ Bioavailability of hydroergotamine and ↓ anginal effects of nitrates
HOW SUPPLIED
Injection: 1 mg/mL; *Nasal Spray:* 4 mg/mL

DOSAGE
- **IM**

Suppress vascular headache.

Adults, initial: 1 mg at first sign of headache; repeat q hr for a total of 3 mg (not to exceed 6 mg/week).
- **IV**

Suppress vascular headache.

Similar to IM but to a maximum of 2 mg/attack or 6 mg/week.
- **NASAL SPRAY**

Acute migraine headaches.

Single treatment of 0.5 mg spray in each nostril followed in 15 min by a second 0.5 mg spray in each nostril (i.e., total of 2 mg).

NURSING CONSIDERATIONS
ADMINISTRATION/STORAGE
Adjust dosage if client complains of severe headaches; use this dose when subsequent headaches begin.

ASSESSMENT

1. Obtain a thorough nursing, diet, and drug history; note any contributing factors (i.e., smoking, alcohol ingestion, OTC agents, stress).
2. Do not take with nitrates or if any sensitivity to ergotamine.
3. Determine severity and characteristics of headaches and what relieved them.
4. Assess for pregnancy; has an oxytocic effect.
5. Note any liver or renal dysfunction, HTN, PVD, or CAD.

CLIENT/FAMILY TEACHING

1. Take at the onset of migraine; most effective when administered early in an attack.
2. Seek bed rest in a darkened room for 1–2 hr after drug ingestion.
3. Practice alternative methods for dealing with stress, such as relaxation.
4. Report evidence of cold extremities and numbness or tingling (to avoid gangrene.)
5. Take only as directed and do not stop abruptly.
6. Keep a headache diary; list foods, events, activities surrounding onset.

OUTCOMES/EVALUATE

Relief of migraine headaches

Diltiazem hydrochloride

(dill-**TIE**-ah-zem)

PREGNANCY CATEGORY: C

CLASSIFICATION(S):

Calcium channel blocker

Rx: Cardizem, Cardizem CD, Cardizem-SR, Dilacor XR, Diltiazem HCl Extended Release, Nu-Diltiaz-CD, Taztia XT, Tiamate, Tiazac , Cardizem Injectable

✱**Rx:** Alti-Diltiazem, Alti-Diltiazem CD, Apo-Diltiaz, Apo-Diltiaz CD, Gen-Diltiazem, Gen-Diltiazem SR, Novo-Diltazem, Novo-Diltazem SR, Nu-Diltiaz

SEE ALSO *CALCIUM CHANNEL BLOCKING AGENTS.*

ACTION/KINETICS

Decreases SA and AV conduction and prolongs AV node effective and functional refractory periods. Also decreases myocardial contractility and peripheral vascular resistance. **Tablets: Onset,** 30–60 min; **time to peak plasma levels:** 2–3 hr; **t1/2, first phase:** 20–30 min; **second phase:** about 3–4.5 hr (5–8 hr with high and repetitive doses); **duration:** 4–8 hr. **Extended-Release Capsules: Onset,** 2–3 hr; **time to peak plasma levels:** 6–11 hr; **t1/2:** 5–7 hr; **duration:** 12 hr. **Therapeutic serum levels:** 0.05–0.2 mcg/mL. Metabolized to desacetyldiltiazem, which manifests 25%–50% of the activity of diltiazem. Excreted through both the bile and urine.

USES

Tablets: Chronic stable angina (classic effort-associated angina), especially in clients who cannot use beta-adrenergic blockers or nitrates or who remain symptomatic after clinical doses of these agents. **Capsules:** Essential hypertension. Vasospastic angina (Prinzmetal's variant), chronic stable angina. **Parenteral:** Atrial fibrillation or flutter. Paroxysmal SVT. Cardizem Lyo-Ject is used on an emergency basis for atrial fibrillation or atrial flutter. Cardizem Monovial is used to maintain control of HR for up to 24 hr in atrial fibrillation or flutter. *Investigational:* Prophylaxis of reinfarction of nonQ wave MI; tardive dyskinesia, Raynaud's syndrome.

CONTRAINDICATIONS

Hypotension. Second- or third-degree AV block and sick sinus syndrome except in presence of a functioning ventricular pacemaker. Acute MI, pulmonary congestion. Lactation.

SPECIAL CONCERNS

Safety and effectiveness in children have not been determined. The half-life may be increased in geriatric clients. Use with caution in hepatic disease and in CHF. Abrupt withdrawal may cause an increase in the frequency and duration of chest pain. Use with beta blockers or digitalis is usually well tolerated, although the effects of coadministration cannot be predicted (especially in clients with left ventricular dysfunction or cardiac conduction abnormalities).

SIDE EFFECTS

CV: AV block, bradycardia, CHF, hypotension, syncope, palpitations, peripheral edema, ***arrhythmias,*** angina, tachycardia, ***abnormal ECG, ventricular extrasystoles.*** **GI:** N&V, diarrhea, constipation, anorexia, abdominal discomfort, cramps, dry mouth, dysgeusia. **CNS:** Weakness, nervousness, dizziness, lightheadedness, headache, depression, psychoses, hallucinations, disturbances in sleep, somnolence, insomnia, amnesia, abnormal dreams. **Dermatologic:** Rashes, dermatitis, pruritus, urticaria, erythema multiforme, ***Stevens-Johnson syndrome.*** **Other:** Photosensitivity, joint pain or stiffness, flushing, nasal or chest congestion, dyspnea, SOB, nocturia/polyuria, sexual difficulties, weight gain, paresthesia, tinnitus, tremor, asthenia, gynecomastia, gingival hyperplasia, petechiae, ecchymosis, purpura, bruising, hematoma, leukopenia, double vision, epistaxis, eye irritation, thirst, alopecia, ***bundle branch block,*** abnormal gait, hyperglycemia.

LABORATORY TEST CONSIDERATIONS

↑ Alkaline phosphatase, CPK, LDH, AST, ALT.

ADDITIONAL DRUG INTERACTIONS

Amlodipine / ↑ Plasma amlodipine levels possibly R/T ↓ liver metabolism
Anesthetics / ↑ Risk of depression of cardiac contractility, conductivity, and automaticity as well as vascular dilation
Carbamazepine / ↑ Diltiazem effect R/T ↓ liver breakdown
Cimetidine / ↑ Diltiazem bioavailability
Cyclosporine / ↑ Cyclosporine effect → possible renal toxicity
Digoxin / Possible ↑ serum digoxin levels
Lithium / ↑ Risk of neurotoxicity
Ranitidine / ↑ Diltiazem bioavailability
Theophyllines / ↑ Risk of pharmacologic and toxicologic theophylline effects

HOW SUPPLIED

Capsule, Extended Release: 60 mg, 90 mg, 120 mg, 180 mg, 240 mg, 300 mg, 360 mg; *Injection:* 5 mg/mL; *Tablet:* 30 mg, 60 mg, 90 mg, 120 mg; *Tablet, Extended Release:* 120 mg, 180 mg, 240 mg

DOSAGE

• **TABLETS**

Angina.

Adults, initial: 30 mg q.i.d. before meals and at bedtime; **then,** increase gradually to total daily dose of 180–360 mg (given in three to four divided doses). Increments may be made q 1–2 days until the optimum response is attained.

• **CAPSULES, EXTENDED-RELEASE**

Angina.

Cardizem CD: Adults, initial: 120 or 180 mg once daily. Up to 480 mg/day may be required. One-360 mg capsule of microgranules may be given once daily. Dosage adjustments should be carried out over a 7–14-day period.

Dilacor XR: Adults, initial: 120 mg once daily; **then,** dose may be titrated, depending on the needs of the client, up to 480 mg once daily. Titration may be carried out over a 7–14-day period.

Hypertension.

Cardizem CD: Adults, initial: 180–240 mg once daily. Maximum antihypertensive effect usually reached within 14 days. Usual range is 240–360 mg once daily.

Cardizem SR: Adults, initial: 60–120 mg b.i.d.; **then,** when maximum antihypertensive effect is reached (approximately 14 days), adjust dosage to a range of 240–360 mg/day.

Dilacor XR: Adults, initial: 180–240 mg once daily. Usual range is 180–480 mg once daily. The dose may be increased to 540 mg/day with little or no increased risk of side effects.

Tiazac: Adults, initial: 120–240 mg once daily. Usual range is 120–360 mg once daily, although doses up to 540 mg once daily have been used.

• **IV BOLUS**

Atrial fibrillation/flutter; paroxysmal SVT.

Adults, initial: 0.25 mg/kg (average 20 mg) given over 2 min; **then,** if re-

D

sponse is inadequate, a second dose may be given after 15 min. The second bolus dose is 0.35 mg/kg (average 25 mg) given over 2 min. Subsequent doses should be individualized. Some clients may respond to an initial dose of 0.15 mg/kg (duration of action may be shorter).

D

• **IV INFUSION**

Atrial fibrillation/flutter.

Adults: 10 mg/hr following IV bolus dose(s) of 0.25 mg/kg or 0.35 mg/kg. Some clients may require 5 mg/hr while others may require 15 mg/hr. Infusion may be maintained for 24 hr.

NURSING CONSIDERATIONS

SEE ALSO *NURSING CONSIDERATIONS FOR CALCIUM CHANNEL BLOCKING AGENTS*.

ADMINISTRATION/STORAGE

1. Sublingual nitroglycerin may be taken concomitantly for acute angina. Diltiazem may also be taken together with long-acting nitrates.
2. Clients taking other forms of diltiazem can be safely switched to Dilacor XR at the nearest equivalent total daily dose. Titration to larger or smaller doses may be necessary.
3. Use with beta blockers or digitalis is usually well tolerated, but the combined effects cannot be predicted, especially with cardiac conduction abnormalities or LV dysfunction.

IV 4. May be administered by direct IV over 2 min or as an infusion (see *Dosage*). For IV infusion, drug may be mixed with NSS, D5W, or D5/0.45% NaCl.

5. The infusion may be maintained for up to 24 hr; beyond 24 hr is not recommended.
6. The injection should be refrigerated at 2–8°C (36–46°F). May be stored at room temperature for 1 mo; then, discard remaining solution.

ASSESSMENT

1. Document indications for therapy, symptom onset, and any previous treatments.
2. Note any edema or CHF; review ECG for evidence of AV block.
3. Monitor renal and LFTs; reduce dose with impaired function.
4. Drug half-life may be prolonged in elderly; monitor closely.

CLIENT/FAMILY TEACHING

1. Take the extended-release capsules on an empty stomach. Do not open, chew, or crush; should be swallowed whole.
2. May cause drowsiness/dizziness.
3. Rise slowly from a lying to a sitting and standing position; may cause postural hypotension.
4. Report persistent and bothersome side effects including constipation, unusual tiredness, or weakness.
5. Continue carrying short-acting nitrites (nitroglycerin) at all times and use as directed.
6. Continue diet (low fat and low Na), regular exercise, and decreased intake of caffeine, tobacco, and alcohol.

OUTCOMES/EVALUATE

- ↓ Frequency and intensity of vasospastic anginal attacks
- ↓ BP; stable cardiac rhythm

Dimenhydrinate

(dye-men-**HY**-drih-nayt)

PREGNANCY CATEGORY: B
CLASSIFICATION(S):
Cholinergic blocking drug, Antiemetic
Rx: Chewable Tablets: Dramamine, Dimetabs , **Injection:** Dinate, Dramanate, Dymenate, Hydrate
✱**Rx: Chewable Tablets:** Apo-Dimenhydrinate, Gravol, **Injection:** Dimenhydrinate Injection, Gravol
OTC: Chewable Tablets: Calm-X, Dramamine, Travamine, Triptone

SEE ALSO *ANTIHISTAMINES AND ANTIEMETICS*.

ACTION/KINETICS

Contains both diphenhydramine and chlorotheophylline. Antiemetic mechanism not known, but it does depress labyrinthine and vestibular function. May mask ototoxicity due to aminoglycosides. Possesses anticholinergic activity. **Duration:** 3–6 hr.

USES

Motion sickness, especially to relieve nausea, vomiting, or dizziness. Treat vertigo.

SPECIAL CONCERNS
Use of the injectable form is not recommended in neonates. Geriatric clients may be more sensitive to the usual adult dose.
HOW SUPPLIED
OTC. *Chew Tablet:* 50 mg; *Liquid:* 12.5 mg/4 mL, 12.5 mg/5 mL. **Rx.** *Injection:* 50 mg/mL; *Liquid:* 15.62 mg/5 mL

DOSAGE

• **ELIXIR, SYRUP, TABLETS, CHEWABLE TABLETS, INJECTION**
Motion sickness.
Adults: 50–100 mg q 4 hr, not to exceed 400 mg/day. **Pediatric, 6–12 years:** 25–50 mg q 6–8 hr, not to exceed 150 mg/day; **2–6 years:** 12.5–25 mg q 6–8 hr, not to exceed 75 mg/day.
• **IM, IV**
Adults: 50 mg as required. **Pediatric, over 2 years:** 1.25 mg/kg (37.5 mg/m^2) q.i.d., not to exceed 300 mg/day.
• **IV**
Adults: 50 mg in 10 mL sodium chloride injection given over 2 min; may be repeated q 4 hr as needed. **Pediatric:** 1.25 mg/kg (37.5 mg/m^2) in 10 mL of 0.9% sodium chloride injection given slowly over 2 min; may be repeated q 6 hr, not to exceed 300 mg/day.

NURSING CONSIDERATIONS

SEE ALSO *NURSING CONSIDERATIONS* FOR *ANTIHISTAMINES* AND *ANTIEMETICS*.

ASSESSMENT
Document indications for therapy and symptom onset; assess for vestibular damage when administered with antihistamines.

CLIENT/FAMILY TEACHING
1. Take at least 30 min before departure and may repeat before meals and upon retiring for motion sickness prophylaxis.
2. Avoid activities that require mental alertness until effects realized.
3. May alter skin testing results; wait 72 h after use.

OUTCOMES/EVALUATE
Prevention of N&V; control of vertigo

Dinoprostone (PGE_2)
(die-noh-PROS-tohn)

PREGNANCY CATEGORY: C
CLASSIFICATION(S):
Abortifacient
Rx: Cervidil, Prepidil Gel, Prostin E_2
✱**Rx:** Prostin E_2 Vaginal Gel

ACTION/KINETICS
Interacts with prostaglandin receptor to produce changes in the consistency, dilatation, and effacement of the cervix. May also stimulate the smooth muscle of the GI tract, causing vomiting and diarrhea. Extensively metabolized in the lungs on first pass through the pulmonary circulation. Metabolites are excreted through the kidneys. **t½:** 2.5–5 min.
USES
Ripening of an unfavorable cervix in pregnant women at or near term with a medical or obstetric need for induction of labor.
CONTRAINDICATIONS
Use when oxytocic drugs are contraindicated or when prolonged uterine contractions are inappropriate (e.g., history of cesarean section or major uterine surgery), presence of cephalopelvic disproportion, history of difficult labor and/or traumatic delivery, grand multiparae with six or more previous term pregnancies, non-vertex presentation, hyperactive or hypertonic uterine patterns, fetal distress where delivery is not imminent, obstetric emergencies when surgical intervention may be favored. Also, use is contraindicated in ruptured membranes, hypersensitivity to prostaglandins or constituents of the gel, placenta previa or unexplained vaginal bleeding during current pregnancy, or when vaginal delivery is contraindicated (e.g., vasa previa or active herpes genitalis). Use in conjunction with oxytocic agents.
SPECIAL CONCERNS
Uterine rupture is possible when high-tone uterine contractions are

sustained. Use with caution in clients with asthma or a history thereof, glaucoma, increased intraocular pressure, or impaired hepatic or renal function.

SIDE EFFECTS

• **GEL**

Maternal: Uterine contractile abnormality, GI effects, back pain, warm feeling in vagina, fever, premature rupture of membranes, uterine rupture. **Fetal:** Abnormality in fetal HR, bradycardia, deceleration, ***fetal depression.*** Extra-amniotic administration has resulted in amnionitis and ***intrauterine fetal sepsis.***

• **VAGINAL INSERT**

Uterine hyperstimulation with or without fetal distress, fetal distress without hyperstimulation, fever, N&V, diarrhea, abdominal pain.

OD OVERDOSE MANAGEMENT

Symptoms: Uterine hypercontractility, uterine hypertonus. *Treatment:* Symptoms may be relieved by changing maternal position, giving oxygen to the mother, or the use of beta-adrenergic drugs to treat hyperstimulation.

DRUG INTERACTIONS

Dinoprostone may ↑ action of other oxytocics.

HOW SUPPLIED

Vaginal Gel/Jelly: 0.5 mg/3 g; *Vaginal suppository:* 20 mg; *Vaginal insert, controlled release:* 0.3 mg/hr

DOSAGE

• **GEL**

Initial: 0.5 mg. If there is no cervical/uterine response, repeat doses of 0.5 mg may given q 6 hr. The maximum cumulative dose for 24 hr is 1.5 mg dinoprostone.

• **VAGINAL INSERT**

One insert (10 mg), designed to release approximately 0.3 mg dinoprostone/hr over a 12-hr period. The insert should be removed upon onset of active labor or 12 hr after insertion.

• **VAGINAL SUPPOSITORIES**

20 mg repeated every 3–5 hr; dose adjusted according to client response.

NURSING CONSIDERATIONS

ADMINISTRATION/STORAGE

1. Bring gel to room temperature just prior to administration.
2. Avoid contact with the skin; wash hands thoroughly with soap and water after administration.
3. The gel is intended for endocervical placement; do not administer above the level of the internal os. The degree of cervical effacement will regulate shielded catheter size to be used (20-mm catheter for no effacement and 10-mm catheter for 50% effacement).
4. Administer gel by sterile technique and introduce just below the level of the internal os.
5. Keep supine for at least 15–30 min after administration.
6. If desired response is obtained from the initial dose, the recommended interval before giving oxytocin is 6–12 hr. A dosing interval of at least 30 min is recommended following removal of vaginal insert.
7. The insert is placed transversely in the posterior fornix of the vagina immediately after removal from the foil package. Insertion does not require sterile conditions. Do not use insert without its retrieval system.
8. Insert may be placed in the vagina with a minimal amount of water-miscible lubricant. Prevent excess contact or coating with the lubricant, thus preventing optimal swelling and release of the drug.
9. The gel has a shelf life of 24 months when stored under refrigeration of 2–8°C (36–46°F). Store the insert in a freezer between –20 to –10°C (–4 to –14°F). When stored in a freezer, the insert is stable for up to 3 years.

ASSESSMENT

1. Document calculated and ultrasound-derived due date; note fetopelvic relationships.
2. Examine cervix for degree of effacement (shortening of cervical canal); to determine size of shielded endocervical catheter needed.
3. Document system used, time of insertion, and dosing intervals. Insert must be removed with retrieval system after 12 hr or onset of labor.
4. Monitor uterine contractions, fetal heart tones, cervical dilation and effacement by visual assessment, auscultation and electronic fetal monitor.

5. Continuous monitoring of uterine activity and fetal status should be undertaken with history of hypertonic uterine contractility or tetanic uterine contractions. Monitor for uterine rupture with sustained high-tone myometrial contractions.

CLIENT/FAMILY TEACHING

1. Explain purpose of therapy and anticipated outcome.
2. Gel may produce increased vaginal warmth.
3. Must remain supine for 30 min after gel insertion.
4. Avoid douches, tampons, intercourse and tub baths for at least 2 weeks. Monitor temperature (late afternoon) for a few days after discharge and report any new onset fever, bleeding, cramps/pain or foul smelling discharge.

OUTCOMES/EVALUATE

Desired cervical presentation to facilitate induction of labor. Evacuation of uterus

Diphenhydramine hydrochloride

(dye-fen-**HY**-drah-meen)

PREGNANCY CATEGORY: B
CLASSIFICATION(S):
Anhistamine, second generation, ethandamine

Rx: Banophen Allergy, Diphen AF, Scot-Tussin Allergy Relief Formula Clear, Benadryl, Hyrexin-50

OTC: Allergy Medication, AllerMax, AllerMax Allergy & Cough Formula, Banophen Caplets & Capsules, Benadryl Allergy, Benadryl Allergy Ultratabs, Benadryl Dye-Free Allergy, Benadryl Dye-Free Allergy Liqui Gels, Bydramine, Diphen Cough, Diphenhist, Diphenhydramine 50, Genahist, Midol PM, Scot-Tussin Allergy DM, Siladryl, Silphen Cough, Tusstat, Twilite, Uni-Bent Cough, **Sleep Aids:** Compoz Nighttime Sleep Aid, 40 Winks, Dormin, Maximum Strength Nytol, Miles Nervine, Nighttime Sleep Aid, Nytol, Sleep-eze 3, Sleepwell 2-nite, Snooze Fast, Sominex

✤OTC: Allerdryl, Nytol Extra Strength, PMS-Diphenhydramine

SEE ALSO *ANTIHISTAMINES, ANTIEMETICS, AND ANTIPARKINSON DRUGS.*

ACTION/KINETICS

High sedative, anticholinergic, and antiemetic effects.

USES

Hypersensitivity reactions, motion sickness (PO only), parkinsonism (postencephalitic, arteriosclerotic, idiopathic, drug/chemical induced), nighttime sleep aid (PO only), antitussive (syrup only).

CONTRAINDICATIONS

Topically to treat chickenpox, poison ivy, or sunburn. Topically on large areas of the body or on blistered or oozing skin.

ADDITIONAL DRUG INTERACTIONS

Diphenhydramine ↑ effects of metoprolol.

HOW SUPPLIED

Capsule: 25 mg, 50 mg; *Capsule, Soft Gels:* 25 mg; *Chew Tablet:* 12.5 mg; *Elixir::* 12.5 mg/5 mL; *Injection:* 50 mg/mL; *Liquid:* 6.25 mg/5 mL, 12.5 mg/5 mL; *Solution:* 12.5 mg/5 mL; *Syrup:* 12.5 mg/5 mL; *Tablet:* 25 mg, 50 mg

DOSAGE

• CAPSULES, SOFT GEL CAPSULES, CHEWABLE TABLETS, ELIXIR, LIQUID, SOLUTION, SYRUP, TABLETS

Antihistamine, antiemetic, antimotion sickness, parkinsonism.

Adults: 25–50 mg t.i.d.–q.i.d.; **pediatric, over 10 kg:** 12.5–25 mg t.i.d.–q.i.d. (or 5 mg/kg/day not to exceed 300 mg/day or 150 mg/m²/day).

Sleep aid.

Adults and children over 12 years: 50 mg at bedtime.

Antitussive (Syrup only).

Adults: 25 mg q 4 hr, not to exceed 100 mg/day; **pediatric, 6–12 years:** 12.5–25 mg q 4 hr, not to exceed 50 mg/day; **pediatric, 2–6 years:** 6.25 mg q 4 hr, not to exceed 25 mg/day.

• IV, DEEP IM

Parkinsonism.

Adults: 10–50 mg up to 100 mg if needed (not to exceed 400 mg/day);

pediatric: 1.25 mg/kg (or 37.5 mg/m²) q.i.d., not to exceed a total of 300 mg/day.

NURSING CONSIDERATIONS

SEE ALSO *NURSING CONSIDERATIONS* FOR *ANTIHISTAMINES, ANTIEMETICS,* AND *ANTIPARKINSON DRUGS.*

D

ADMINISTRATION/STORAGE

1. With motion sickness, give the full prophylactic dose 30 min prior to travel and 1–2 hr before exposures that precipitate sickness.
2. Take similar doses with meals and at bedtime.
3. Do not use more than 2 weeks to treat insomnia.

IV 4. For IV, may give undiluted; each 25 mg over at least 1 min.

CLIENT/FAMILY TEACHING

1. May cause drowsiness; use caution until drug effects realized.
2. Use sun protection; may cause photosensitivity reaction.
3. Use sugarless gum/candy to diminish dry mouth effects.
4. Avoid alcohol and any other CNS depressants unless prescribed.

OUTCOMES/EVALUATE

- ↓ Allergic manifestations
- Relief of nausea
- Promotion of sleep
- Relief of dyskinesias/extrapyramidal symptoms with parkinsonism

—COMBINATION DRUG—

Diphenoxylate hydrochloride with Atropine sulfate

(dye-fen-**OX**-ih-layt, **AH**-troh-peen)

PREGNANCY CATEGORY: C
CLASSIFICATION(S):
Antidiarrheal
Rx: Logen, Lomanate, Lomotil, Lonox
C-V

SEE ALSO *CHOLINERGIC BLOCKING AGENTS.*

CONTENT

Each tablet or 5 mL of liquid contains: *Antidiarrheal:* Diphenoxylate HCl, 2.5 mg. *Anticholinergic:* Atropine sulfate, 0.025 mg.

ACTION/KINETICS

Chemically related to the narcotic analgesic drug meperidine but without the analgesic properties. Inhibits GI motility and has a constipating effect. May aggravate diarrhea due to organisms that penetrate the intestinal mucosa (e.g., *Escherichia coli, Salmonella, Shigella)* or in antibiotic-induced pseudomembranous colitis. High doses over prolonged periods may cause euphoria and physical dependence. The product also contains small amounts of atropine sulfate which will prevent abuse by deliberate overdosage. **Onset:** 45–60 min. **$t^{1/2}$, diphenoxylate:** 2.5 hr; **diphenoxylic acid:** 12–24 hr. **Duration:** 2–4 hr. Metabolized in the liver to the active diphenoxylic acid and excreted through the urine.

USES

(1) Symptomatic treatment of chronic and functional diarrhea. Also, diarrhea associated with gastroenteritis, irritable bowel, regional enteritis, malabsorption syndrome, ulcerative colitis, acute infections, food poisoning, postgastrectomy, and drug-induced diarrhea. Therapeutic results for control of acute diarrhea are inconsistent. (2) Control of intestinal passage time in clients with ileostomies and colostomies.

CONTRAINDICATIONS

Obstructive jaundice, liver disease, diarrhea associated with pseudomembranous enterocolitis after antibiotic therapy or enterotoxin-producing bacteria, children under the age of 2.

SPECIAL CONCERNS

Use with caution during lactation, when anticholinergics may be contraindicated, and in advanced hepatic-renal disease or abnormal renal functions. Children (especially those with Down syndrome) are susceptible to atropine toxicity. Children and geriatric clients may be more sensitive to the respiratory depressant effects of diphenoxylate. Dehydration, especially in young children, may cause a delayed diphenoxylate toxicity.

SIDE EFFECTS

GI: N&V, anorexia, abdominal discomfort, paralytic ileus, megacolon.

Allergic: Pruritus, ***angioneurotic edema,*** swelling of gums. **CNS:** Dizziness, drowsiness, malaise, restlessness, headache, depression, numbness of extremities, ***respiratory depression, coma.***

• **DERMATOLOGIC**

Dry skin and mucous membranes, flushing.

Other: Tachycardia, urinary retention, hyperthermia.

OD OVERDOSE MANAGEMENT

Symptoms: Dry skin and mucous membranes, flushing, ***hyperthermia,*** mydriasis, restlessness, tachycardia followed by miosis, lethargy, hypotonic reflexes, nystagmus, ***coma, severe (and possibly fatal) respiratory depression.*** *Treatment:* Gastric lavage, induce vomiting, establish a patent airway, and assist respiration. Activated charcoal (100 g) given as a slurry. IV administration of a narcotic antagonist. Administration may be repeated after 10–15 min. Observe client and readminister antagonist if respiratory depression returns.

DRUG INTERACTIONS

Alcohol / Additive CNS depression
Antianxiety agents / Additive CNS depression
Barbiturates / Additive CNS depression
MAO inhibitors / ↑ Chance of hypertensive crisis
Narcotics / ↑ Effect of narcotics

HOW SUPPLIED

(See Content)

PEDIATRIC/DOSE

2–3 years / 0.75–1.5 mg q.i.d.*3–4 years* / 1–1.5 mg q.i.d.*4–5 years* / 1–2 mg q.i.d.*5–6 years* / 1.25–2.25 mg q.i.d.*6–9 years* / 1.25–2.5 mg q.i.d.*9–12 years* / 1.75–2.5 mg q.i.d.

Based on 4 mL/tsp or 2 mg of diphenoxylate. Each tablet or 5 mL of liquid preparation contains 2.5 mg diphenoxylate hydrochloride and 25 mcg of atropine sulfate. Dosage should be maintained at initial levels until symptoms are under control; then reduce to maintenance levels.

See Content

DOSAGE

• **ORAL SOLUTION, TABLETS**

Adults, initial: 2.5–5 mg (of diphenoxylate) t.i.d.–q.i.d.; **maintenance:** 2.5 mg b.i.d.–t.i.d. **Pediatric, 2–12 years:** 0.3–0.4 mg/kg/day (of diphenoxylate) in divided doses.

NURSING CONSIDERATIONS

SEE ALSO *NURSING CONSIDERATIONS* FOR *CHOLINERGIC BLOCKING AGENTS.*

ADMINISTRATION/STORAGE

1. For liquid preparations, use only the plastic dropper supplied by the manufacturer to measure dosage.
2. If clinical improvement is not evident after 10 days with a maximum dose of 20 mg/day, further use will not likely control symptoms.

ASSESSMENT

1. Document indications for therapy, onset, and frequency of stools, and other agents trialed.
2. Determine fluid and electrolyte status. Dehydration occurs rapidly in young children: may cause delayed toxicity. Correct before therapy.
3. Review culture reports to determine if drug is appropriate if not effective after 24–36 hr.
4. Note any hepatic or renal dysfunction.
5. Assess GI function and for abdominal distension and toxic megacolon.

CLIENT/FAMILY TEACHING

Take only as prescribed; do not exceed dosage, report lack of response. May cause drowsiness; use caution.

OUTCOMES/EVALUATE

Relief of diarrhea

Dipyridamole

(dye-peer-**ID**-ah-mohl)

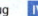

PREGNANCY CATEGORY: B
CLASSIFICATION(S):
Anticoagulant, platelet adhesion inhibitor
Rx: Persantine, Persantine IV
✱Rx: Apo-Dipyridamole FC, Novo-Dipiradol

D

ACTION/KINETICS

In higher doses may act by several mechanisms, including inhibition of red blood cell uptake of adenosine, itself an inhibitor of platelet reactivity; inhibition of platelet phosphodiesterase, which leads to accumulation of cAMP within platelets; direct stimulation of release of prostacyclin or prostaglandin D_2; and/or inhibition of thromboxane A_2 formation. Dipyridamole prolongs platelet survival time in clients with valvular heart disease and has maintained platelet count in open heart surgery. Also causes coronary vasodilation which may be due to inhibition of adenosine deaminase in the blood, thus allowing accumulation of adenosine which is a potent vasodilator. Vasodilation may also be caused by delaying the hydrolysis of cyclic 3′,5′-adenosine monophosphate as a result of inhibition of the enzyme phosphodiesterase. Incompletely absorbed from the GI tract. **Peak plasma levels, after PO:** 45–150 min. **t½, after PO: initial,** 40–80 min; **terminal,** 10–12 hr. Metabolized in the liver and mainly excreted in the bile.

USES

PO. (1) As an adjunct to coumarin anticoagulants in preventing post-operative thromboembolic complications of cardiac valve replacement. (2) With aspirin to reduce the risk of stroke in clients who have had a stroke or a TIA previously. **IV.** As an alternative to exercise in thallium myocardial perfusion imaging for the evaluation of CAD in those who cannot exercise adequately. *Investigational:* Alone or as an adjunct to treat angina, to prevent graft occlusion in those undergoing arterial reconstructive bypass surgery, intralingual bypass grafts, and to prevent deterioration of coronary vessel patency after percutaneous transluminal angioplasty. Use with aspirin for preventing migraine headaches, MI, to reduce platelet aggregation at the carotid endarterectomy, to slow progression of peripheral occlusive arterial disease, to reduce incidence of DVT, to reduce the number of platelets deposited on dacron aortofemoral artery grafts, and TIAs.

NOTE: Not effective for the treatment of acute episodes of angina and is not a substitute for the treatment of angina pectoris.

SPECIAL CONCERNS

Use with caution in hypotension and during lactation. Safety and efficacy have not been determined in children less than 12 years of age.

SIDE EFFECTS

• **AFTER PO USE**

GI: GI intolerance, N&V, diarrhea. **CNS:** Dizziness, headache, syncope. **CV:** Peripheral vasodilation, flushing. Rarely, angina pectoris or aggravation of angina pectoris (usually at the beginning of therapy). **Miscellaneous:** Weakness, rash, pruritus.

• **AFTER IV USE**

Most common side effects (1% or greater) are listed.

GI: Nausea, dyspepsia. **CNS:** Headache, dizziness, paresthesia, fatigue. **CV:** Chest pain, angina pectoris, ECG abnormalities (ST-T changes, extrasystoles, tachycardia), precipitation of acute myocardial ischemia in clients with CAD, hypotension, flushing, blood pressure lability, hypertension. **Miscellaneous:** Dyspnea, unspecified pain.

OD OVERDOSE MANAGEMENT

Symptoms: Hypotension of short duration. *Treatment:* Use of a vasopressor may be beneficial. Due to the high percentage of protein binding of dipyridamole, dialysis is not likely to be beneficial.

DRUG INTERACTIONS

H *Evening primrose oil* / Potential for ↑ antiplatelet effect

H *Feverfew* / Potential for ↑ antiplatelet effect

H *Garlic* / Potential for ↑ antiplatelet effect

H *Ginger* / Potential for ↑ antiplatelet effect

H *Ginkgo biloba* / Potential for ↑ antiplatelet effect

H *Ginseng* / Potential for ↑ antiplatelet effect

H *Grapeseed extract* / Potential for ↑ antiplatelet effect

HOW SUPPLIED
Injection: 5 mg/mL; *Tablets:* 25 mg, 50 mg, 75 mg.

DOSAGE

• **TABLETS**

Adjunct in prophylaxis of thromboembolism after cardiac valve replacement.

Adults: 75–100 mg q.i.d. as an adjunct to warfarin therapy.

Prevention of thromboembolic complications in other thromboembolic disorders.

Adults: 150–400 mg/day in combination with another platelet-aggregation inhibitor (e.g., aspirin) or an anticoagulant.

• **IV**

Adjunct to thallium myocardial perfusion imaging.

Adjust the dose according to body weight. Recommended dose is 0.142 mg/kg/min infused over 4 min. Total dose should not exceed 60 mg.

NURSING CONSIDERATIONS

ADMINISTRATION/STORAGE

IV 1. When used IV, to prevent irritation, dilute the injection in at least a 1:2 ratio with D5W, 0.45% NaCl, or 0.9% NaCl injection. The total volume should be 20 to 50 mL.
2. With imaging, give thallium-201 within 5 min after the IV injection.
3. Do not mix with other drugs in the same syringe or infusion container.

ASSESSMENT

1. Document indications for therapy, type, onset, duration, and characteristics of symptoms.
2. List all drugs currently prescribed to ensure none interact unfavorably.
3. Document mental status, skin color, and cardiopulmonary findings.
4. Monitor VS, ECG, CBC, PT, PTT, and INR.

CLIENT/FAMILY TEACHING

1. Drug helps prevent clots by inhibiting platelet stickiness; may also decrease frequency of chest pain and increase exercise tolerance. May take several months of therapy before effects evident.
2. Avoid alcohol and tobacco due to hypotensive vasoconstrictive effects; and any other unprescribed drugs including aspirin without approval.
3. Drug may cause dizziness and lightheadedness; change positions slowly.
4. Try small frequent meals if nausea or gastric distress is experienced.
5. Report any increased chest pain, skin rash, fainting or severe headaches.

OUTCOMES/EVALUATE

• CAD evaluation with imaging
• Prevention of thromboembolism

Dirithromycin

(die-**rih**-throw-**MY**-sin)

PREGNANCY CATEGORY: C
CLASSIFICATION(S):
Antibiotic, macrolide
Rx: Dynabac, Dynabac D5-Pak

ACTION/KINETICS
Rapidly absorbed and converted during intestinal absorption to the active erythromycylamine. Distributed throughout the body, including the lungs, GI tract, skin, soft tissues, and GU tract. Erythromycylamine acts by binding to the 50S ribosomal subunits of microorganisms, resulting in inhibition of protein synthesis. **$t^1/_2$:** 2–36 hr. From 81% to 97% of erythromycylamine is excreted in the feces via the bile.

USES
(1) Acute bacterial exacerbations of chronic bronchitis due to *Haemophilus influenzae, Moraxella catarrhalis* or *Streptococcus pneumoniae.* (2) Secondary bacterial infections of acute bronchitis due to *M. catarrhalis* or *S. pneumoniae.* (3) Community-acquired pneumonia due to *Legionella pneumophila, Mycoplasma pneumoniae,* or *S. pneumoniae.* (4) Pharyngitis or tonsillitis due to *Streptococcus pyogenes.* (5) Uncomplicated infections of the skin and skin structures due to *Staphylococcus aureus* or *S. pyogenes.*

CONTRAINDICATIONS
Hypersensitivity to erythromycin or any other macrolide antibiotic. Use in children less than 12 years of age. Use in clients with known, suspected, or potential bacteremias since serum levels of the drug are not high enough in the serum to be effective. Use for the empiric treatment of acute bacterial exacerbations of chronic or secondary bacterial infections of acute bronchitis or for empiric treatment of uncomplicated skin and skin structure infections.

SPECIAL CONCERNS
Although dirithromycin eradicates *S. pyogenes* from the nasopharynx, data are lacking as to its effectiveness in preventing rheumatic fever. Use with caution during lactation. Safety and efficacy have not been determined in children less than 12 years of age.

SIDE EFFECTS
GI: ***Pseudomembranous colitis,*** abdominal pain, nausea, diarrhea, vomiting, dyspepsia, GI disorder, flatulence, abnormal stools, constipation, dry mouth, gastritis, gastroenteritis, mouth ulceration, taste perversion, thirst, dysphagia. **CNS:** Headache, dizziness, vertigo, insomnia, anxiety, depression, nervousness, paresthesia, somnolence. **CV:** Palpitation, vasodilation, syncope. **GU:** Dysmenorrhea, urinary frequency, vaginal moniliasis, vaginitis. **Dermatologic:** Rash, pruritus, urticaria, sweating. **Respiratory:** Increased cough, dyspnea, hyperventilation. **Miscellaneous:** Nonspecific pain, asthenia, anorexia, dehydration, edema, epistaxis, eye disorder, fever, flu syndrome, hemoptysis, malaise, peripheral edema, ***allergic reaction,*** amblyopia, myalgia, neck pain, tinnitus, tremor, thirst.

LABORATORY TEST CONSIDERATIONS
↑ ALT, AST, alkaline phosphatase, potassium, serum CPK, bands, segs, basophils, eosinophils, platelet count, total bilirubin, creatinine, GGT, leukocyte count, lymphocytes, monocytes, phosphorus, uric acid, Ca, hematocrit, hemoglobin. ↓ Platelet count, albumin, chloride, hematocrit, hemoblobin, lymphocytes, segmented neutrophils, phosphorus, serum alkaline phosphatase, serum uric acid, total protein.

OD OVERDOSE MANAGEMENT
Symptoms: N&V, epigastric distress, diarrhea. *Treatment:* Treat symptoms.

DRUG INTERACTIONS
Antacids / Slightly ↑ absorption of dirithromycin
H_2-Antagonists / Slightly ↑ absorption of dirithromycin
Pimozide / Not to be used together due to possible sudden death

HOW SUPPLIED
Enteric-coated tablet: 250 mg

DOSAGE

• TABLETS, ENTERIC-COATED

Acute bacterial exacerbations of chronic bronchitis. Secondary bacterial infection of acute bronchitis.
Adults and children over 12 years of age: 500 mg once a day for 7 days.

Community-acquired pneumonia.
Adults and children over 12 years of age: 500 mg once a day for 14 days.

Pharyngitis or tonsillitis.
Adults and children over 12 years of age: 500 mg once a day for 10 days.

Uncomplicated skin and skin structure infections.
Adults and children over 12 years of age: 500 mg once a day for 5–7 days.

NURSING CONSIDERATIONS

SEE ALSO *GENERAL NURSING CONSIDERATIONS* FOR *ANTI-INFECTIVES*.

ASSESSMENT
1. Document indications for therapy, type, and symptom duration.
2. Obtain renal and LFTs and cultures for C&S initially; assess for any superinfections.
3. Does not appear to cause CV problems. Note other drugs prescribed, may increase theophylline blood levels.

CLIENT/FAMILY TEACHING
1. Take as prescribed with food or within 1 hr of eating.
2. Do not crush, cut, or chew enteric-coated tablets.
3. Report new diarrhea; drug alters normal colon flora, permitting clostridia overgrowth; requires drug withdrawal and symptom management.

OUTCOMES/EVALUATE
- Resolution of infection
- Negative culture reports

Disopyramide phosphate

(dye-so-**PEER**-ah-myd)

PREGNANCY CATEGORY: C
CLASSIFICATION(S):
Antiarrhythmic Class IA
Rx: Norpace, Norpace CR
🍁**Rx:** Rythmodan-LA

ACTION/KINETICS
Decreases the rate of diastolic depolarization (phase 4), decreases the upstroke velocity (phase 0), increases the action potential duration (of normal cardiac cells), and prolongs the refractory period (phases 2 and 3). Weak anticholinergic effects; fewer side effects than quinidine. Does not affect BP significantly; can be used in digitalized and nondigitalized clients. **Onset:** 30 min. **Peak plasma levels:** 2 hr. **Duration:** average of 6 hr (range 1.5–8 hr). **t½:** 4–10 hr. **Therapeutic serum levels:** 2–4 mcg/mL. Do not use serum levels to adjust the dose because of variance in protein binding and potential toxicity of unbound drug. **Protein binding:** 40%–60%. Bioavailability of the controlled-release capsules appears to be similar to that of the immediate-release capsules. Both unchanged drug (50%) and metabolites (30%) are excreted through the urine. Approximately 15% is excreted through the bile.

USES
Life-threatening ventricular arrhythmias (e.g., sustained ventricular tachycardia). Not been shown to improve survival in clients with ventricular arrhythmias. *Investigational:* Paroxysmal SVT.

CONTRAINDICATIONS
Hypersensitivity to drug. Cardiogenic shock, heart failure, heart block (especially preexisting second- and third-degree AV block if no pacemaker is present), congenital QT prolongation, asymptomatic ventricular premature contractions, sick sinus syndrome, glaucoma, urinary retention, myasthenia gravis. Use of controlled-release capsules in clients with severe renal insufficiency. Lactation.

SPECIAL CONCERNS
Safe use during childhood, labor, and delivery has not been established. Use with caution in Wolff-Parkinson-White syndrome or bundle branch block. Decrease dosage in impaired hepatic function. Geriatric clients may be more sensitive to the anticholinergic effects of this drug. The drug may be ineffective in hypokalemia and toxic in hyperkalemia.

SIDE EFFECTS
Increased risk of death when used in clients with non-life-threatening cardiac arrhythmias.
CV: Hypotension, CHF, ***worsening of arrhythmias,*** edema, weight gain, cardiac conduction disturbances, SOB, syncope, chest pain, AV block, ***severe myocardial depression (with hypotension and increased venous pressure).*** **Anticholinergic:** Dry mouth, urinary retention, constipation, blurred vision, dry nose, eyes, and throat. **GU:** Urinary frequency and urgency, urinary retention, impotence, dysuria. **GI:** Nausea, pain, flatulence, anorexia, diarrhea, vomiting, severe epigastric pain. **CNS:** Headache, nervousness, dizziness, fatigue, depression, insomnia, psychoses. **Dermatologic:** Rash, dermatoses, itching. **Other:** Fever, respiratory problems, gynecomastia, ***anaphylaxis,*** malaise, muscle weakness, numbness, tingling, angle-closure glaucoma, hypoglycemia, reversible cholestatic jaundice, symptoms of lupus erythematosus (usually in clients switched to disopyramide from procainamide).

LABORATORY TEST CONSIDERATIONS
↑ Creatinine, BUN, cholesterol, triglycerides, and liver enzymes.

OD OVERDOSE MANAGEMENT
Symptoms: Apnea, loss of consciousness, ***cardiac arrhythmias*** (widening of QRS complex and QT interval, conduction disturbances), hypotension, bradycardia, anticholinergic symptoms, ***loss of spontaneous respiration, death.*** *Treatment:* Induction of vomiting, gastric lavage, or a cathartic

followed by activated charcoal. Monitor ECG. IV isoproterenol, IV dopamine, cardiac glycosides, diuretics, intra-aortic balloon counterpulsation, artificial respiration, hemodialysis. Use endocardial pacing to treat AV block and neostigmine to treat anticholinergic symptoms.

DRUG INTERACTIONS

Anticoagulants / ↓ PT after discontinuing disopyramide
Beta-adrenergic blockers / Possible ↓ clearance of disopyramide; sinus bradycardia, hypotension
Digoxin / ↑ Serum digoxin levels (may be beneficial)
Erythromycin / ↑ Disopyramide levels → arrhythmias and ↑ QTc intervals
Phenytoin / ↓ Effect R/T ↑ liver breakdown; ↑ anticholinergic effects
Quinidine / ↑ Disopyramide serum levels or ↓ quinidine levels
Rifampin / ↓ Effect R/T ↑ liver breakdown

HOW SUPPLIED

Capsule: 100 mg, 150 mg; *Capsule, Extended Release:* 100 mg, 150 mg

DOSAGE

• **IMMEDIATE-RELEASE CAPSULES**

Antiarrhythmic.

Adults, initial loading dose: 300 mg of immediate-release capsule (200 mg if client weighs less than 50 kg); **maintenance:** 400–800 mg/day in four divided doses (usual: 150 mg q 6 hr). **For clients less than 50 kg, maintenance:** 100 mg q 6 hr. **Children, less than 1 year:** 10–30 mg/kg/day in divided doses q 6 hr; **1–4 years of age:** 10–20 mg/kg/day in divided doses q 6 hr; **4–12 years of age:** 10–15 mg/kg/day in divided doses q 6 hr; **12–18 years of age:** 6–15 mg/kg/day in divided doses q 6 hr.

Severe refractory tachycardia.

Up to 400 mg q 6 hr may be required.

Cardiomyopathy.

Do not administer a loading dose; give 100 mg q 6 hr of immediate-release or 200 mg q 12 hr for controlled-release.

• **EXTENDED-RELEASE CAPSULES**

Antiarrhythmic, maintenance only.

Adults: 300 mg q 12 hr (200 mg q 12 hr for body weight less than 50 kg).

NOTE: For all uses, decrease dosage in clients with renal or hepatic insufficiency.

Moderate renal failure or hepatic failure.

100 mg q 6 hr (or 200 mg/12 hr of sustained-release form).

Severe renal failure.

100 mg q 8–24 hr depending on severity (with or without an initial loading dose of 150 mg).

NURSING CONSIDERATIONS

SEE ALSO *NURSING CONSIDERATIONS* FOR *ANTIARRHYTHMIC AGENTS*.

ADMINISTRATION/STORAGE

1. Administer drug only after ECG assessment has been done.
2. Reserve use with other antiarrhythmics (e.g., class IA or propranolol) for life-threatening arrhythmias unresponsive to a single agent.
3. Do not use the controlled-release capsule for initial dosage. These are intended for maintenance therapy.
4. When being transferred from the regular PO capsule, give the first controlled-release capsule 6 hr after the last regular dose.
5. For children, a 1–10-mg/mL suspension may be made; add contents of the immediate-release capsule (do NOT use the controlled-release capsule) to cherry syrup. Syrup is stable for 1 month if refrigerated; shake thoroughly before use and dispense in an amber bottle.

ASSESSMENT

1. Document indications for therapy, and characteristics of symptoms.
2. If taking other antiarrhythmic agents, note response.
3. Assess for drug hypersensitivity.
4. Note any urine dribbling, frequency, or sensation of bladder fullness; drug may worsen. Important with BPH and in elderly clients who have had prior urinary tract problems; palpate bladder if hesitancy is severe.
5. Obtain ECG, liver and renal function studies; check serum potassium levels and correct if low.
6. Monitor for hypotensive effect; clients with poor LV function are more likely to develop hypotension.

7. If receiving drug in the hospital, monitor ECG for QRS widening, QT prolongation, or first-degree heart block. Hold drug and report if evident.

CLIENT/FAMILY TEACHING

1. Take at the same time each day.
2. Increase intake of fruit juices and bulk foods to prevent constipation.
3. For dry mouth, use mouth rinses, sugarless gum/hard candy.
4. Avoid alcohol in any form.
5. Report symptoms of CHF (edema, cough, weight gain, ↑ SOB).
6. Change positions slowly; avoid hot showers, temperature extremes, sun exposure, or prolonged standing.
7. Report any mental status changes or confusion.

OUTCOMES/EVALUATE

Control of ventricular arrhythmias; stable cardiac rhythm

Disulfiram

(dye-**SUL**-fih-ram)

CLASSIFICATION(S):
Treatment of alcoholism
Rx: Antabuse

ACTION/KINETICS

Produces severe hypersensitivity to alcohol. Inhibits liver enzymes that participate in the normal degradation of alcohol. This results in accumulation of acetaldehyde in the blood. High levels of acetaldehyde produce a series of symptoms referred to as the disulfiram-alcohol reaction or syndrome. The specific symptoms are listed under *Side Effects*. The symptoms vary individually, are dose-dependent with respect to both alcohol and disulfiram, and persist for periods ranging from 30 min to several hours. A single dose of disulfiram may be effective for 1–2 weeks. **Onset:** May be delayed up to 12 hr because disulfiram is initially localized in fat stores.

USES

To prevent further ingestion of alcohol in chronic alcoholics. Should be given only to cooperating clients fully aware of the consequences of alcohol ingestion.

CONTRAINDICATIONS

Alcohol intoxication. Severe myocardial or occlusive coronary disease. Use of paraldehyde or alcohol-containing products such as cough syrups. If client is exposed to ethylene dibromide.

SPECIAL CONCERNS

Use in pregnancy only if benefits outweigh risks. Use with caution in narcotic addicts or clients with diabetes, goiter, epilepsy, psychosis, hypothyroidism, hepatic cirrhosis, or nephritis.

SIDE EFFECTS

In the absence of alcohol, the following symptoms have been reported: Drowsiness (most common), headache, restlessness, fatigue, psychoses, peripheral neuropathy, dermatoses, hepatotoxicity, metallic or garlic taste, arthropathy, impotence. **In the presence of alcohol,** the following symptoms may be manifested. **CV:** Flushing, chest pain, palpitations, tachy-cardia, hypotension, syncope, arrhyth-mias, ***CV collapse, MI, acute CHF.*** **CNS:** Throbbing headaches, vertigo, weakness, uneasiness, confusion, unconsciousness, ***seizures, death.*** **GI:** Nausea, severe vomiting, thirst. **Respiratory:** Respiratory difficulties, dyspnea, hyperventilation, ***respiratory depression.*** **Other:** Throbbing in head and neck, sweating. In the event of an Antabuse-alcohol interaction, measures should be undertaken to maintain BP and treat shock. Oxygen, antihistamines, ephedrine, and/or vitamin C may also be used.

DRUG INTERACTIONS

Anticoagulants, oral / ↑ Anticoagulant effects by ↑ hypoprothrombinemia
Barbiturates / ↑ Barbiturate effects R/T ↓ liver breakdown
Chlordiazepoxide, diazepam / ↑ Chlordiazepoxide/diazepam effects R/T ↓ plasma clearance
Isoniazid / ↑ Isoniazid side effects (especially CNS)
Metronidazole / Acute toxic psychosis or confusional state
Paraldehyde / Antabuse-like effects

Phenytoin / ↑ Phenytoin effects R/T ↓ liver breakdown
Tricyclic antidepressants / Acute organic brain syndrome

HOW SUPPLIED

Tablet: 250 mg, 500 mg

D

DOSAGE

- **TABLETS**

Alcoholism.

Adults, initial (after alcohol-free interval of 12–48 hr): 500 mg/day for 1–2 weeks; **maintenance: usual,** 250 mg/day (range: 120–500 mg/day). Do not exceed 500 mg/day.

NURSING CONSIDERATIONS

CLIENT/FAMILY TEACHING

1. Tablets can be crushed or mixed with liquid.
2. Never give without client's knowledge. Ingesting 30 mL of 100-proof alcohol (e.g., one shot) may cause severe symptoms (within 15 min; lasting several hours) and possibly death. Avoid alcohol in any form, in foods, sauces, or other meds, such as cough syrups or tonics; avoid vinegar, paregoric, skin products, linaments, or lotions containing alcohol. Read all labels before consuming.
3. CNS side effects should lessen with continued therapy.
4. May feel tired, experience drowsiness and headaches, and develop a metallic or garlic-like taste; should subside after 2 weeks of therapy.
5. May have occasional impotence, usually transient; report.
6. Report if skin eruptions occur; an antihistamine may be prescribed.
7. Carry card stating "taking disulfiram" and describing symptoms and treatment if a disulfiram reaction occurs. Include provider and phone number. (Cards may be obtained from the Wyeth-Ayerst Laboratories, P.O. Box 8299, Philadelphia, PA 19101-1245; attention: Professional Services.)
8. Attend local support group meetings, e.g., Alcoholics Anonymous and Al-Anon, to gain the support, structure, referral, and encouragement to obtain an alcohol-free life.

OUTCOMES/EVALUATE

Freedom from alcohol and its effects; sobriety

Divalproex sodium

(dye-**VAL**-proh-ex)

PREGNANCY CATEGORY: D
Rx: Depakote
🍁Rx: Apo-Divalproex, Epival, Novo-Divalproex, Nu-Divalproex

SEE *VALPROIC ACID.*

HOW SUPPLIED

Enteric Coated Capsule: 125 mg; *Enteric Coated Tablet:* 125 mg, 250 mg, 500 mg; *Tablet, Extended-Release:* 500 mg

Dobutamine hydrochloride

(doh-**BYOU**-tah-meen)

PREGNANCY CATEGORY: B
CLASSIFICATION(S):
Sympathomimetic direct-acting
Rx: Dobutrex

SEE ALSO *SYMPATHOMIMETIC DRUGS.*

ACTION/KINETICS

Stimulates beta-1 receptors (in the heart), increasing cardiac function, CO, and SV, with minor effects on HR. Decreases afterload reduction although SBP and pulse pressure may remain unchanged or increase (due to increased CO). Also decreases elevated ventricular filling pressure and helps AV node conduction. **Onset:** 1–2 min. **Peak effect:** 10 min. **t½:** 2 min. **Therapeutic plasma levels:** 40–190 ng/mL. Metabolized by the liver and excreted in urine.

USES

Short-term treatment of cardiac decompensation in adults secondary to depressed contractility due to organic heart disease or cardiac surgical procedures. *Investigational:* Congenital heart disease in children undergoing diagnostic cardiac catheterization.

CONTRAINDICATIONS
Idiopathic hypertrophic subaortic stenosis.
SPECIAL CONCERNS
Safe use during childhood or after AMI not established.
SIDE EFFECTS
CV: Marked increase in HR, BP, and ***ventricular ectopic activity,*** precipitous drop in BP, premature ventricular beats, anginal and nonspecific chest pain, palpitations. **Hypersensitivity:** Skin rash, pruritus of the scalp, fever, eosinophilia, ***bronchospasm.*** **Other:** Nausea, headache, SOB, fever, phlebitis, and local inflammatory changes at the injection site.
OD OVERDOSE MANAGEMENT
Symptoms: Excessive alteration of BP, anorexia N&V, tremor, anxiety, palpitations, headache, SOB, anginal and nonspecific chest pain, ***myocardial ischemia, ventricular fibrillation or tachycardia.*** *Treatment:* Reduce the rate of administration or discontinue temporarily until the condition stabilizes. Establish an airway, ensuring oxygenation and ventilation. Initiate resuscitative measures immediately. Treat severe ventricular tachyarrhythmias with propranolol or lidocaine.
ADDITIONAL DRUG INTERACTIONS
Concomitant use with nitroprusside causes ↑ CO and ↓ PAWP.
HOW SUPPLIED
Injection: 12.5 mg/mL

DOSAGE
• **IV INFUSION**
Adults, individualized, usual: 2.5–15 mcg/kg/min (up to 40 mcg/kg/min). Rate of administration and duration of therapy depend on response of client, as determined by HR, presence of ectopic activity, BP, and urine flow.

NURSING CONSIDERATIONS

SEE ALSO *NURSING CONSIDERATIONS* FOR *SYMPATHOMIMETIC DRUGS.*
ADMINISTRATION/STORAGE
IV 1. Reconstitute solution according to manufacturer directions; takes place in two stages.
2. Before administration, the solution is diluted further according to the fluid needs of the client. This more dilute solution should be used within 24 hr. Solutions that can be used for further dilution include D5W, D5/0.45% NaCl injection, D5/0.9% NaCl injection, D10%/W, Isolyte M with 5% dextrose injection, RL injection, D5/RL, Normosol-M in D5W, 20% Osmitrol in water for injection, 0.9% NaCl injection, and sodium lactate injection.
3. The more concentrated solution may be refrigerated for 48 hr or stored at room temperature for 6 hr. After dilution (in glass or Viaflex containers), the solution is stable for 24 hr at room temperature. Dilute solutions may darken; does not affect potency when used within designated time spans.
4. Drug is incompatible with alkaline solutions. Do not give with agents or diluents containing both sodium bisulfite and ethanol. Is physically incompatible with hydrocortisone sodium succinate, cefazolin, cefamandole, neutral cephalothin, penicillin, sodium ethacrynate, and heparin sodium.
5. Drug is compatible when given through same tubing with dopamine, lidocaine, tobramycin, verapamil, nitroprusside, KCl, and protamine sulfate.
6. Give using an electronic infusion device. Carefully reconstitute and calculate dosage according to weight and desired response.
ASSESSMENT
Ensure adequately hydrated prior to infusion.
INTERVENTIONS
1. Monitor CVP to assess vascular volume and cardiac pumping efficiency. Normal range 5–10 cm water (1–7 mm Hg). Elevated CVP may indicate disruption of CO, as in pump failure or pulmonary edema; low CVP may indicate hypovolemia.
2. Monitor PAWP to assess the pressures in the left atrium and ventricle and to measure the efficiency of CO; usual range is 6–12 mm Hg.
3. Monitor ECG and BP continuously during drug administration; review written parameters for SBP and titrate infusion.

D

4. Record I&O.
5. Monitor glucose in diabetics; increased insulin may be needed.

OUTCOMES/EVALUATE

- ↑ CO; ↑ urine output
- SBP > 90 mm Hg

Docetaxel

(doh-seh-**TAX**-ell)

PREGNANCY CATEGORY: D
CLASSIFICATION(S):
Antineoplastic, miscellaneous
Rx: Taxotere

SEE ALSO *ANTINEOPLASTIC AGENTS.*

ACTION/KINETICS

Prepared with a precursor extracted from the yew plant. Effect is due to disruption of the microtubular network in cells that is required for mitotic and interphase cellular functions. **t½, 3 phases:** 4 min, 36 min, and 11.1 hr. Metabolized in the liver, and metabolites and small amounts of unchanged drug are excreted through both the feces (75%) and urine (6%).

USES

(1) Locally advanced or metastatic breast cancer after failure of prior chemotherapy. (2) In combination with capecitabine to treat metastatic breast cancer whose anthracycline treatment has failed. (3) Locally advanced or metastatic non-small cell lung cancer after failure of prior platinum-based chemotherapy. *Investigational:* Cancer of the stomach, head and neck, ovary, pancreas, prostate, urothelia. Melanoma, non-Hodgkin's lymphoma, soft-tissue sarcoma.

CONTRAINDICATIONS

Severe hypersensitivity to docetaxel or to other drugs formulated with polysorbate 80. Use in those with neutrophil counts less than 1,500 cells/mm^3, in those with bilirubin greater than the upper limit of normal (ULN), or in those with AST or ALT greater than 1.5 times the ULN. Lactation.

SPECIAL CONCERNS

The incidence of treatment-related mortality is increased in clients with abnormal liver function and in those receiving higher doses. Safety and efficacy have not been determined in children less than 16 years of age.

SIDE EFFECTS

Hematologic: Neutropenia (virtually in 100% of clients given 100 mg/m^2). Leukopenia, thrombocytopenia, anemia, febrile neutropenia. **GI:** N&V, diarrhea, stomatitis, abdominal pain, constipation, ulcer, esophagitis, ***GI hemorrhage,*** intestinal obstruction, ileus. **CV:** Fluid retention (even with premedication), hypotension, atrial fibrillation, ***DVT,*** ECG abnormalities, thrombophlebitis, ***pulmonary embolism, heart failure,*** syncope, tachycardia, sinus tachycardia, atrial flutter, dysrhythmia, unstable angina, pulmonary edema, hypertension (rare). **Respiratory:** Dyspnea, ***acute pulmonary edema, ARDS.*** **Dermatologic:** Reversible cutaneous reactions characterized by a rash, including localized eruptions on the hands, feet, arms, face, or thorax, and usually associated with pruritus. Nail changes, alopecia. **Hypersensitivity:** Flushing, localized skin reactions. Severe hypersensitivity reactions characterized by hypotension, bronchospasm, or generalized rash/erythema. **Musculoskeletal:** Myalgia, arthralgia. **Neurologic:** Paresthesia, dysesthesia, pain in those with anthracycline-resistant breast cancer. Distal extremity weakness. **Reactions at infusion site:** Hyperpigmentation, inflammation, redness or dryness of the skin, phlebitis, extravasation, mild swelling of the vein. **Miscellaneous:** ***Septic death, nonseptic death,*** infections, fever in absence of infections, asthenia, diffuse pain, chest pain, renal insufficiency, confusion.

LABORATORY TEST CONSIDERATIONS

↑ ALT, AST, alkaline phosphatase.

OD OVERDOSE MANAGEMENT

Symptoms: Bone marrow suppression, peripheral neurotoxicity, mucositis. *Treatment:* No known antidote. Keep client in a specialized unit to monitor vital functions. Give therapeutic G-CSF as soon as possible after overdose discovered. Treat symptomatically.

DRUG INTERACTIONS

The metabolism of docetaxel may be modified by drugs that inhibit, induce, or are metabolized by the cytochrome P4503A4 system, including cyclosporine, erythromycin, ketoconazole, and troleandomycin.

HOW SUPPLIED

Injection: 20 mg/0.5 mL, 80 mg/2 mL

DOSAGE

- **IV**

Breast cancer.

60–100 mg/m² given IV over 1 hr q 3 weeks. Reduce the dose to 75 mg/m² or discontinue therapy in those who are dosed initially at 100 mg/m² and who experience febrile neutropenia, neutrophils less than 500/mm³ for more than 1 week, severe or cumulative cutaneous reactions, or severe peripheral neuropathy. Those who are dosed at 60 mg/m² and do not experience these symptoms may tolerate higher doses.

Non-small cell lung cancer.

75 mg/m² IV over 1 hr q 3 weeks. Withhold treatment until toxicity is resolved for those who experience either febrile neutropenia, neutrophils less than 500/mm³ for more than 1 week, severe or cumulative cutaneous reactions, or severe peripheral neuropathy. Resume at 55 mg/m². Discontinue entirely if clients develop grade 3 or greater of peripheral neuropathy.

NURSING CONSIDERATIONS

SEE ALSO *NURSING CONSIDERATIONS* FOR *ANTINEOPLASTIC AGENTS*.

ADMINISTRATION/STORAGE

IV 1. To reduce severity of fluid retention and hypersensitivity reactions, premedicate with PO corticosteroids (e.g., dexamethasone, 16 mg/day) for 5 days starting 1 day prior to therapy.

2. Allow vials to stand at room temperature for about 5 min before using. Both the injection concentrate and the diluent vials contain an overfill. The 20-mg vial contains 23.6 mg and the 80-mg vial contains 94.4 mg of the drug. Only the final concentration of 10 mg/mL, prepared with the supplied diluent, should be used for preparing doses. Using the entire vial content for each 20- or 80-mg dose may result in a significant overdose when using multiple vials.

3. The diluted concentrate of 10 mg/mL is then used to prepare the solution for infusion. Withdraw the required amount of docetaxel using a calibrated syringe. Inject into a 250-mL infusion bag or bottle of either 0.9% NaCl injection or D5W to produce a final concentration of 0.3–0.9 mg/mL; administer as a 1-hr infusion. If doses greater than 240 mg are required, use more solution so that the concentration to be infused does not exceed 0.9 mg/mL.

4. Protect the drug from light and refrigerate at 2–8°C (36–46°F). The premixed solution is stable for 8 hr. Do not store in PVC bags.

ASSESSMENT

1. Document indications for therapy, disease onset, previous agents used, and the outcome.

2. Note any previous experience with this drug. If previous hypersensitivity, do not rechallenge.

3. List other drugs prescribed to ensure none interact unfavorably.

4. Monitor CBC and LFTs. Drug causes bone marrow suppression. Nadir: 8 days.

CLIENT/FAMILY TEACHING

1. May experience a rash 1 week after treatment; this should subside.

2. Prepare for hair loss.

3. Report any evidence of infection, fever, or illness. Avoid crowds and people with contagious diseases.

OUTCOMES/EVALUATE

Control of metastatic process

Docusate calcium (Dioctyl calcium sulfosuccinate)

(**DEW**-kyou-sayt)

PREGNANCY CATEGORY: C

OTC: DC Softgels, Pro-Cal-Sof, Sulfalax Calcium, Surfak Liquigels

★**OTC:** PMS-Docusate Calcium

Docusate sodium (Dioctyl sodium sulfosuccinate)

(**DEW**-kyou-sayt)

D

PREGNANCY CATEGORY: C
OTC: Colace, Dioto, Docu, D.O.S., D-S-S, Ex-Lax Stool Softener, Gena Soft, Modane Soft, Non-Habit Forming Stool Softener, Phillips Liqui-Gels, Regulex SS, Silace Stool Softener
✱OTC: PMS-Docusate Sodium, Selax, Soflax
CLASSIFICATION(S):
Laxative, emollient

SEE ALSO *LAXATIVES.*

ACTION/KINETICS
Acts by lowering the surface tension of the feces and promoting penetration by water and fat, thus increasing the softness of the fecal mass. Not absorbed systemically and does not seem to interfere with the absorption of nutrients. A microenema formulation is available for clients aged 3 and older. **Onset:** 24–72 hr.

USES
To lessen strain of defecation in persons with hernia or CV diseases or other diseases in which straining at stool should be avoided. Megacolon or bedridden clients. Constipation associated with dry, hard stools. The microemulsion formulation is indicated for relief of occasional constipation in children over the age of 3 years.

CONTRAINDICATIONS
Nausea, vomiting, abdominal pain, and intestinal obstruction.

DRUG INTERACTIONS
Docusate may ↑ absorption of mineral oil from the GI tract.

HOW SUPPLIED
Docusate calcium: *Capsule:* 50 mg, 240 mg. **Docusate sodium:** *Capsule:* 50 mg, 100 mg, 250 mg; *Capsule, Soft-Gel:* 50 mg, 100 mg, 250 mg; *Oral Liquid:* 150 mg/15 mL; *Syrup:* 20 mg/5 mL, 50 mg/15 mL, 60 mg/15 mL, 100 mg/30 mL; *Tablet:* 100 mg

DOSAGE

DOCUSATE CALCIUM
• **CAPSULES**
Adults: 240 mg/day until bowel movements are normal; **pediatric, over 6 years:** 50–150 mg/day.

DOCUSATE SODIUM
• **CAPSULES, SOFT-GEL CAPSULES, ORAL LIQUID, SYRUP, TABLETS**
Adults and children over 12 years: 50–500 mg; **pediatric, under 3 years:** 10–40 mg; **3–6 years:** 20–60 mg; **6–12 years:** 40–120 mg.
• **RECTAL SOLUTION**
Flushing or retention enema.
Adults: 50–100 mg.

NURSING CONSIDERATIONS

SEE ALSO *NURSING CONSIDERATIONS* FOR *LAXATIVES.*

CLIENT/FAMILY TEACHING
1. May give PO solutions with milk or juices to help mask bitter taste.
2. Drink a glass of water with each PO dose.
3. When used in enemas, add 50–100 mg (5–10 mL) to a retention or flushing enema.
4. Because docusate salts are minimally absorbed, it may require 1–3 days to soften fecal matter.

OUTCOMES/EVALUATE
Elimination of a soft, formed stool; ↓ straining

Dofetilide

(doh-**FET**-ih-lyd)

PREGNANCY CATEGORY: C
CLASSIFICATION(S):
Antiarrhythmic
Rx: Tikosyn

SEE ALSO *ANTIARRHYTHMIC DRUGS.*

ACTION/KINETICS
Acts by blocking the cardiac ion channel carrying the rapid component of the delayed rectifier potassium currents. Blocks only I_{Kr} with no significant block of other repolarizing potassium currents (e.g., I_{Ks}, I_{K1}). No effect on sodium channels or adrenergic re-

ceptors. Dofetilide increases the monophasic action potential duration due to delayed repolarization. **Maximum plasma levels:** 2–3 hr during fasting. Steady state plasma levels reached in 2–3 days. Metabolized in the liver and excreted in the urine. **t½, terminal:** About 10 hr. Women have lower oral clearances than men.

USES

(1) Conversion of atrial fibrillation or atrial flutter to normal sinus rhythm. (2) Maintenance of normal sinus rhythm in clients witih atrial fibrillation/atrial flutter of more than 1 week duration and who have been converted to normal sinus rhythm. Reserve for those in whom atrial fibrillation/atrial flutter is highly symptomatic due to life-threatening ventricular arrhythmias. *NOTE:* Available only to hospitals and prescribers who receive dosing and treatment initiation education through the *Tikosyn* education program.

CONTRAINDICATIONS

Congenital or acquired long QT syndromes, in those with a baseline QT interval greater than 440 msec (500 msec in clients with ventricular conduction abnormalities), severe renal impairment (C_{CR} less than 20 mL/min). Concomitant use of verapamil, cimetidine, trimethoprim (alone or with sulfamethoxazole), ketoconazole, prochlorperazine, megestrol. Lactation.

SPECIAL CONCERNS

There is a greater risk of dofetilide-induced TdP (type of ventricular tachycardia) in female clients than in male clients. Use with caution in severe hepatic impairment. Use with drugs that prolong the QT interval has not been studied with dofetilide use; therefore, do not use bepridil, certain macrolide antibiotics, phenothiazines, or TCAs with dofetilide. Safety and efficacy have not been determined in children less than 18 years of age.

SIDE EFFECTS

CV: Ventricular arrhythmias (especially TdP type ventricular tachycardia), ***torsades de pointes,*** angina pectoris, atrial fibrillation, hypertension, palpitation, supraventricular tachycardia, ventricular tachycardia, bradycardia, cerebral ischemia, ***CVA, MI, heart arrest, ventricular fibrillation,*** AV block, bundle branch block, heart block. **CNS:** Headache, dizziness, insomnia, anxiety, paresthesia. **GI:** Nausea, diarrhea, abdominal pain. **Respiratory:** Respiratory tract infection, dyspnea, increased cough. **Miscellaneous:** Chest pain, flu syndrome, accidental injury, back pain, rash, arthralgia, asthenia, pain, peripheral edema, sweating, UTI, angioedema, edema, facial paralysis, flaccid paralysis, liver damage, paralysis, **sudden death,** syncope.

OD OVERDOSE MANAGEMENT

Symptoms: Excessive prolongation of QT interval. *Treatment:* Symptomatic and supportive. Initiate cardiac monitoring. Can use charcoal slur but is effective only when given within 15 min of dofetilide. To treat TdP or overdose, may give isoproterenol infusion, with or without cardiac pacing. IV magnesium sulfate may be useful to manage TdP. Monitor until QT interval returns to normal.

DRUG INTERACTIONS

Amiloride / Possible ↑ dofetilide levels
Amiodarone / Possible ↑ dofetilide levels
Cannabinoids / Possible ↑ dofetilide levels
Cimetidine / ↑ Risk of arrhythmia (TdP) R/T ↓ liver metabolism of dofetilide
Digoxin / ↑ Risk of torsades de pointes
Diltiazem / Possible ↑ dofetilide levels
Grapefruit juice / Possible ↑ dofetilide levels
Ketoconazole / ↑ Risk of arrhythmia (TdP) R/T ↓ liver metabolism of dofetilide
Macrolide antibiotics / Possible ↑ dofetilide levels
Metformin / Possible ↑ dofetilide levels
Megestrol / Possible ↑ dofetilide levels → arrhythmias
Nefazadone / Possible ↑ dofetilide levels

Norfloxacin / Possible ↑ dofetilide levels
Potassium-depleting diuretics / Hypokalemia or hypomagnesemia may occur, → ↑ potential for torsades de pointes
Prochlorperazine / Possible ↑ dofetilide levels → arrhythmias
Quinine / Possible ↑ dofetilide levels
Triamterene / Possible ↑ dofetilide levels
Trimethoprim or Trimethoprim/Sulfamethoxazole / ↑ Risk of arrhythmia (TdP) R/T ↓ liver metabolism of dofetilide
Verapamil / Possible ↑ dofetilide levels → arrhythmias
Zafirlukast / Possible ↑ dofetilide levels

HOW SUPPLIED

Capsules: 125 mcg, 250 mcg, 500 mcg

DOSAGE

• CAPSULES

Conversion of atrial fibrillation/flutter; maintenance of normal sinus rhythm.

The dosing for dofetilide must be undertaken using the following steps:
1. Before giving the first dose, determine the QTc using an average of 5–10 beats. If the QTc is greater than 440 msec (500 msec in those with ventricular conduction abnormalities), dofetilide is contraindicated. Also, do not use if the heart rate is less than 60 bpm.
2. Before giving the first dose, calculate the C_{CR} using the following formulas: *Males:* Weight (kg) x (140 - age)/ 72 x serum creatinine (mg/dL) *Females:* 0.84 x male value
3. Determine the starting dose of dofetilide as follows: **C_{CR} greater than 60 mL/min:** 500 mcg b.i.d.; **C_{CR} 40–60 mL/min:** 250 mcg b.i.d.; **C_{CR} 20–less than 40 mL/min:** 125 mcg b.i.d.; **C_{CR} less than 20 mL/min:** DO NOT USE DOFETILIDE; CONTRAINDICATED IN THESE CLIENTS. The maximum daily dose is 500 mcg b.i.d.
4. Give the adjusted dose based on C_{CR} and begin continuous ECG monitoring.
5. At 2–3 hr after giving the first dofetilide dose, determine the QTc. If the QTc has increased by more than 15% compared with the baseline established in Step 1 or if the QTc is 500 msec (550 msec in those with ventriciular conduction abnormalities), adjust subsequent dosing as follows: If the starting dose based on C_{CR} is 500 mcg b.i.d., the adjusted dose (for QTc prolongation) is 250 mcg b.i.d. If the starting dose is 250 mcg b.i.d., the adjusted dose (for QTc prolongation) is 125 mcg b.i.d. If the starting dose is 125 mcg b.i.d., the adjusted dose (for QTc prolongation) is 125 mcg once daily.
6. At 2–3 hr after each subsequent dose of dofetilide, determine QTc for in-hospital doses 2 through 5. No further down titration of dofetilide based on QTc is recommended. Discontinue if at any time after the second dose of dofetilide, the QTc is greater than 500 msec (550 msec in those with ventricular conduction abnormalities).
7. Continuously monitor by ECG for a minimum of 3 days or for a minimum of 12 hr after electrical or pharmacologic conversion to normal sinus rhythm, whichever time is greater.

NURSING CONSIDERATIONS

SEE ALSO *NURSING CONSIDERATIONS* FOR *ANTIARRHYTHMIC DRUGS*.

ADMINISTRATION/STORAGE

1. Therapy must be started (and, if necessary, reinitiated) in a setting where continuous ECG monitoring and personnel trained in the management of serious ventricular arrhthymias are available for a minimum of 3 days.
2. Do not discharge clients within 12 hr of electrical or pharmacologic conversion to normal sinus rhythm.
3. Prior to electrical or pharmacologic cardioversion, anticoagulate clients with atrial fibrillation according to usual medical practices. Anticoagulants may be continued after cardioversion. Correct hypokalemia before starting dofetilide therapy.
4. Re-evaluate renal function q 3 months or as warranted. Discontinue dofetilide if the QTc is greater than 500 msec (550 msec in those with ventricular conduction abnormalities)

and monitor carefully until QTc returns to baseline levels. If renal function decreases, adjust the dose as described under Dosage.

5. The highest dose of 500 mcg b.i.d. is the most effective. However, the risk of torsades de pointes is increased. Thus, a lower dose may be used. If at any time the lower dose is increased, the client must be hospitalized for 3 days. Previous tolerance of higher doses does not eliminate the need for hospitalization.

6. Do not consider electrical conversion if the client does not convert to normal sinus rhythm within 24 hr after starting dofetilide.

7. Withdraw previous antiarrhythmic drug therapy before starting dofetilide therapy; during withdrawal, carefully monitor for a minimum of 3 plasma half-lives. Do not initiate dofetilide following amiodarone therapy until amiodarone plasma levels are less than 0.3 mcg/mL or until amiodarone has been withdrawn for 3 or more months.

8. Protect from moisture and humidity. Dispense in tight containers.

ASSESSMENT

1. Identify arrhythmia and duration. Note any S&S associated with arrhythmia.

2. Note drugs prescribed to ensure none interact. Avoid use of drugs that prolong the QT interval.

3. Monitor renal and LFTs; avoid use with dysfunction.

4. Drug is available only through the Tikosyn Dosing Program with provider education.

CLIENT/FAMILY TEACHING

1. Take exactly as prescribed; avoid grapefruit juice.

2. Do not double the next dose if a dose is missed. Take next dose at usual time.

3. Report any change in prescriptions or OTC/supplement use. Inform all providers especially if hospitalized or prescribed a new medication for any condition.

4. Read the package insert prior to use. Drug adherance is imperative with this therapy. Must report as scheduled for ECG evaluation and report any side effects to ensure no serious drug related complications.

OUTCOMES/EVALUATE

Conversion of atrial fibrillation/flutter to NSR; maintenance of NSR once converted

D

Dolasetron mesylate

(dohl-**AH**-seh-tron)

PREGNANCY CATEGORY: B

CLASSIFICATION(S):

Antinauseant, serotonin 5-HT_3 antagonist

Rx: Anzemet

ACTION/KINETICS

Selective serotonin 5-HT_3 antagonist that prevents N&V by inhibiting released serotonin from combining with receptors on vagal efferents that initiate vomiting reflex. May also cause acute, usually reversible, PR and QT_c prolongation and QRS widening, perhaps due to blockade of sodium channels by active metabolite of dolasetron. Well absorbed from GI tract. Metabolized to active hydrodolasetron: **peak plasma levels:** 1 hr; **t½:** 8.1 hr. Food does not affect bioavailability. Hydrodolasetron is excreted through urine and feces. Is eliminated more quickly in children than in adults.

USES

(1) Prevention of N&V associated with emetogenic (including high-dose cisplatin) cancer chemotherapy (initially and repeat courses). (2) Prevention of postoperative N&V. *Investigational:* Radiotherapy-induced N&V.

SPECIAL CONCERNS

Use with caution during lactation and in those who have or may develop prolongation of cardiac conduction intervals, including QT_c. These include clients with hypokalemia or hypomagnesemia, those taking diuretics with potential for electrolyte abnormalities, in congenital QT syndrome, those taking anti-arrhythmic drugs or other drugs which lead to QT prolongation, and cumulative high dose anthracycline therapy. Safety and efficacy in children less than 2 years of age have not been determined.

SIDE EFFECTS

Chemotherapy clients. Headache, fatigue, diarrhea, bradycardia, dizziness, pain, tachycardia, dyspepsia, chills, shivering. ***Postoperative clients.*** Headache, hypotension, dizziness, fever, pruritus, oliguria, hypertension, tachycardia. ***Chemotherapy or postoperative clients.*** **CV:** Hypotension, edema, peripheral edema, peripheral ischemia, thrombophlebitis, phlebitis. **GI:** Constipation, dyspepsia, abdominal pain, anorexia, pancreatitis, taste perversion. **CNS:** Flushing, vertigo, paresthesia, tremor, ataxia, twitching, agitation, sleep disorder, depersonalization, confusion, anxiety, abnormal dreaming. **Dermatologic:** Rash, increased sweating. **Hematologic:** Hematuria, epistaxis, anemia, purpura, hematoma, thrombocytopenia. **Hypersensitivity:** Rarely, ***anaphylaxis,*** facial edema, urticaria. **Musculoskeletal:** Myalgia, arthralgia. **Respiratory:** Dyspnea, bronchospasm. **GU:** Dysuria, polyuria, acute renal failure. **Ophthalmic:** Abnormal vision, photophobia. **Miscellaneous:** Tinnitus.

LABORATORY TEST CONSIDERATIONS

↑ PTT, AST, ALT, alkaline phosphatase. Prolonged prothrombin time.

DRUG INTERACTIONS

Possible interaction with drugs that the prolong QT_c interval.

HOW SUPPLIED

Injection: 20 mg/mL; *Tablet:* 50 mg, 100 mg

DOSAGE

• TABLETS

Prevention of N&V during chemotherapy.

Adults: 100 mg within 1 hr before chemotherapy. **Children, 2 to 16 years:** 1.8 mg/kg within 1 hr before chemotherapy, up to a maximum of 100 mg.

Prevention of postoperative N&V.

Adults: 100 mg within 2 hr before surgery. **Children, 2 to 16 years:** 1.2 mg/kg within 2 hr before surgery, up to a maximum of 100 mg.

• IV

Prevention of N&V during chemotherapy.

Adults: 1.8 mg/kg as a single dose about 30 min before chemotherapy. Alternatively, a fixed dose of 100 mg can be given over 30 seconds. **Children, 2 to 16 years:** 1.8 mg/kg as a single dose about 30 min before chemotherapy, up to a maximum of 100 mg.

Prevention of postoperative N&V.

Adults: 12.5 mg given as a single dose. **Children, 2 to 16 years:** 0.35 mg/kg, up to a maximum of 12.5 mg. For adults and children, give about 15 min before cessation of anesthesia or as soon as nausea and vomiting presents.

NOTE: For children, injection may be mixed with apple or apple-grape juice and used for oral dosing. When injection is used PO, recommended dose for prevention of cancer chemotherapy N&V is 1.8 mg/kg (up to a maximum of 100 mg) and dose for prevention of postoperative N&V is 1.2 mg/kg (up to a maximum of 100 mg). Diluted injection may be kept up to 2 hr at room temperature before use.

NURSING CONSIDERATIONS

ADMINISTRATION/STORAGE

IV 1. Injection can be safely infused as rapidly as 100 mg/30 seconds. May also be diluted to 50 mL with 0.9% NaCl, D5W, D5/0.45% NaCl, D5/RL, RL, and 10% mannitol injection. Dilutions are given over 15 min. Diluted product is stable for 24 hr (48 hr if refrigerated).

2. Do not mix with any other drugs.

3. Flush infusion line before and after administration of dolasetron.

4. Inspect visually for particulate matter and discoloration before using.

5. Store injection at controlled room temperature protected from light.

ASSESSMENT

1. Note indications for therapy.

2. List drugs prescribed to ensure none interact unfavorably.

3. Monitor CBC, electrolytes, Mg and ECG.
4. Give 1 hr before chemotherapy or 2 hrs before surgery to gain desired effect. May experience headache.
5. With children, calculate appropriate dose (cancer chemotherapy or postop N&V); may administer orally with apple or apple-grape juice.

OUTCOMES/EVALUATE

Inhibition of chemotherapy induced/postop N&V

Donepezil hydrochloride

(dohn-**EP**-eh-zil)

PREGNANCY CATEGORY: C
CLASSIFICATION(S):
Treatment of Alzheimer's disease
Rx: Aricept

ACTION/KINETICS

A decrease in cholinergic function may be the cause of Alzheimer's disease. Donepezil is a cholinesterase inhibitor and exerts its effect by enhancing cholinergic function by increasing levels of acetylcholine. No evidence that the drug alters the course of the underlying dementing process. Well absorbed from the GI tract. **Peak plasma levels:** 3–4 hr. Food does not affect the rate or extent of absorption. Metabolized in the liver, and both unchanged drug and metabolites are excreted in the urine and feces.

USES

Treatment of mild to moderate dementia of the Alzheimer's type.

CONTRAINDICATIONS

Hypersensitivity to piperidine derivatives.

SPECIAL CONCERNS

Use with caution in clients with a history of asthma or obstructive pulmonary disease. Safety and efficacy have not been determined for use in children.

SIDE EFFECTS

NOTE: Side effects with an incidence of 1% or greater are listed.
GI: N&V, diarrhea, anorexia, fecal incontinence, GI bleeding, bloating, epigastric pain. **CNS:** Insomnia, dizziness, depression, abnormal dreams, somnolence. **CV:** Hypertension, vasodilation, atrial fibrillation, hot flashes, hypotension, bradycardia. **Body as a whole:** Headache, pain (in various locations), accident, fatigue, influenza, chest pain, toothache. **Musculoskeletal:** Muscle cramps, arthritis, bone fracture. **Dermatologic:** Diaphoresis, urticaria, pruritus. **GU:** Urinary incontinence, nocturia, frequent urination. **Respiratory:** Dyspnea, sore throat, bronchitis. **Ophthalmic:** Cataract, eye irritation, blurred vision. **Miscellaneous:** Dehydration, syncope, ecchymosis, weight loss.

OD OVERDOSE MANAGEMENT

Symptoms: Cholinergic crisis characterized by severe N&V, salivation, sweating, bradycardia, hypotension, respiratory depression, collapse, convulsions, increased muscle weakness (may cause death if respiratory muscles are involved). *Treatment:* Atropine sulfate at an initial dose of 1–2 mg IV with subsequent doses based on the response. General supportive measures.

DRUG INTERACTIONS

Anticholinergic drugs / The cholinesterase inhibitor activitiy of donepezil interferes with the activity of anticholinergics
Bethanechol / Synergistic effect
Ketoconazole / ↑ Peak plasma levels of donepezil R/T ↓ breakdown by liver
NSAIDs / ↑ Gastric acid secretion → ↑ risk of active or occult GI bleeding
Succinylcholine / ↑ Muscle relaxant effect

HOW SUPPLIED

Tablet: 5 mg, 10 mg

DOSAGE

• **TABLETS**

Alzheimer's disease.

Initial: 5 mg. Use of a 10-mg dose did not provide a clinical effect greater than the 5-mg dose; however, in some clients, 10 mg daily may be superior. Do not increase the dose to 10 mg until clients have been on a daily dose of 5 mg for 4 to 6 weeks.

NURSING CONSIDERATIONS

ADMINISTRATION/STORAGE

Store at controlled room temperatures from 15–30°C (59–86°F).

ASSESSMENT

1. Document onset/duration, other agents trialed, and the outcome.
2. Describe clinical presentation.
3. Note any history of asthma or COPD.
4. Obtain ECG and labs.

CLIENT/FAMILY TEACHING

1. Take in the evening, just prior to bedtime.
2. May take with or without food.
3. Report any irregular pulse or dizzy spells, lack of response or worsening of symptoms.

OUTCOMES/EVALUATE

Improved cognitive functioning with Alzheimer's.

Dopamine hydrochloride

(**DOH**-pah-meen)

PREGNANCY CATEGORY: C
CLASSIFICATION(S):
Sympathomimetic, direct- and indirect-acting
Rx: Intropin

SEE ALSO *SYMPATHOMIMETIC DRUGS*.

ACTION/KINETICS
Dopamine is the immediate precursor of epinephrine in the body. Exogenously administered, it produces direct stimulation of beta-1 receptors and variable (dose-dependent) stimulation of alpha receptors (peripheral vasoconstriction). Will cause a release of norepinephrine from its storage sites. These actions result in increased myocardial contraction, CO, and SV, as well as increased renal blood flow and sodium excretion. Exerts little effect on DBP and induces fewer arrhythmias than are seen with isoproterenol. **Onset:** 5 min. **Duration:** 10 min. **t½:** 2 min. Does not cross the blood-brain barrier. Metabolized in liver and excreted in urine.

USES
Cardiogenic shock due to MI, trauma, endotoxic septicemia, open heart surgery, renal failure, and chronic cardiac decompensation (as in CHF). Clients most likely to respond include those in whom urine flow, myocardial function, and BP have not deteriorated significantly. Best responses are observed when the time is short between onset of symptoms of shock and initiation of dopamine and volume correction. *Investigational:* COPD, CHF, respiratory distress syndrome in infants.

ADDITIONAL CONTRAINDICATIONS
Pheochromocytoma, uncorrected tachycardia or arrhythmias. Pediatric clients.

SPECIAL CONCERNS
Use with caution during lactation. Safety and efficacy have not been established in children. Dosage may have to be adjusted in geriatric clients with occlusive vascular disease.

ADDITIONAL SIDE EFFECTS
CV: Ectopic heartbeats, tachycardia, anginal pain, palpitations, vasoconstriction, hypotension, hypertension. Infrequently: aberrant conduction, bradycardia, widened QRS complex. **Other:** Dyspnea, headache, mydriasis. Infrequently: piloerection, azotemia, polyuria. High doses may cause mydriasis and ventricular arrhythmia. Extravasation may result in necrosis and sloughing of surrounding tissue.

OD OVERDOSE MANAGEMENT
Symptoms: Extravasation. *Treatment:* To prevent sloughing and necrosis, infiltrate as soon as possible with 10–15 mL of 0.9% NaCl solution containing 5–10 mg phentolamine using a syringe with a fine needle. Infiltrate liberally throughout the ischemic area.

ADDITIONAL DRUG INTERACTIONS
Diuretics / Additive or potentiating effect
Phenytoin / Hypotension and bradycardia
Propranolol / ↓ Effect of dopamine

HOW SUPPLIED
Injection: 40 mg/mL, 80 mg/mL, 160 mg/mL

DOSAGE

• **IV INFUSION**

Shock.

Initial: 2–5 mcg/kg/min; **then,** increase in increments of 1–4 mcg/kg/min at 10–30-min intervals until desired response is obtained.

Severely ill clients.

Initial: 5 mcg/kg/min; **then,** increase rate in increments of 5–10 mcg/kg/min up to 20–50 mcg/kg/min as needed.

NOTE: Dopamine is a potent drug. Be sure to dilute the drug before administration. The drug should not be given as a bolus dose.

NURSING CONSIDERATIONS

SEE ALSO *NURSING CONSIDERATIONS* FOR *SYMPATHOMIMETIC DRUGS*.

ADMINISTRATION/STORAGE

IV 1. Must be diluted before use—see package insert.

2. For reconstitution use dextrose or saline solutions: 200 mg/250 mL for a concentration of 0.8 mg/mL or 800 mcg/mL; 400 mg/250 mL for a concentration of 1.6 mg/mL or 1,600 mcg/mL. Alkaline solutions such as 5% $NaHCO_3$, oxidizing agents, or iron salts will inactivate drug.

3. Dilute just prior to administration, solution stable for 24 hr at room temperature; protect from light.

4. To prevent fluid overload, may use more concentrated solutions with higher doses.

5. Administer using an electronic infusion device. Carefully reconstitute and calculate dosage.

6. When discontinuing, gradually decrease dose; sudden cessation may cause marked hypotension.

ASSESSMENT

Ensure adequate hydration prior to infusion.

INTERVENTIONS

1. Monitor VS, I&O, and ECG; titrate infusion to maintain SBP as ordered.

2. Be prepared to monitor CVP and PAWP.

3. Report any ectopy, palpitations, anginal pain, or vasoconstriction.

OUTCOMES/EVALUATE

• SBP > 90; ↑ urine output

• Improved organ perfusion

Dornase alfa recombinant

(**DOR**-nace **AL**-fah)

PREGNANCY CATEGORY: B

CLASSIFICATION(S):

Treatment of cystic fibrosis

Rx: Pulmozyme

ACTION/KINETICS

This drug is a highly purified solution of recombinant human deoxyribonuclease I (rhDNase), an enzyme that selectively cleaves DNA. It is produced by genetically engineered Chinese hamster ovary cells that contain DNA encoded for the native human protein, deoxyribonuclease (DNase). The amino acid sequence is identical to that of the native human enzyme. Cystic fibrosis (CF) clients have viscous purulent secretions in the airways that contribute to reduced pulmonary function and worsening of infection. These secretions contain high concentrations of extracellular DNA released by degenerating leukocytes that accumulate as a result of infection. Dornase alfa hydrolyzes the DNA in sputum of CF clients, thereby reducing sputum viscoelasticity and reducing infections.

USES

In CF clients in conjunction with standard therapy to decrease the frequency of respiratory infections that require parenteral antibiotics and to improve pulmonary function.

CONTRAINDICATIONS

Known sensitivity to dornase alfa or products from Chinese hamster ovary cells.

SPECIAL CONCERNS

Safety and effectiveness of daily use have not been demonstrated in clients with forced vital capacity (FVC) of less than 40% of predicted, or for

longer than 12 months. Use with caution during lactation.

SIDE EFFECTS

Respiratory: Pharyngitis, voice alteration, and laryngitis are the most common. Also, ***apnea,*** bronchiectasis, bronchitis, change in sputum, cough increase, dyspnea, hemoptysis, lung function decrease, nasal polyps, pneumonia, pneumothorax, rhinitis, sinusitis, sputum increase, wheezing. **Body as a whole:** Abdominal pain, asthenia, fever, flu syndrome, malaise, sepsis, weight loss. **GI:** Intestinal obstruction, gall bladder disease, liver disease, pancreatic disease. **Miscellaneous:** Rash, urticaria, chest pain, conjunctivitis, diabetes mellitus, hypoxia.

HOW SUPPLIED

Solution for Inhalation: 1 mg/mL

DOSAGE

• **INHALATION SOLUTION**

Cystic fibrosis.

One 2.5-mg single-dose ampule inhaled once daily using a recommended nebulizer (see Administration/Storage). Older clients and clients with baseline FVC above 85% may benefit from twice daily dosing.

NURSING CONSIDERATIONS

ADMINISTRATION/STORAGE

1. Approved nebulizers include the disposable jet nebulizer Hudson T Udraft II, disposable jet nebulizer Marquest Acorn II in conjunction with a Pulmo-Aide compressor, and the reusable PARI LC Jet+ nebulizer in conjunction with the PARI PRONEB compressor. Safety and efficacy have been demonstrated with these only.
2. Do not dilute or mix with other drugs in nebulizer. Mixing could lead to adverse physicochemical or functional changes in dornase alfa.
3. Must be stored in the refrigerator at 2–8°C (36–46°F) in the protective foil pouch and protected from strong light.
4. Refrigerate when transported and do not expose to room temperature for a total time of 24 hr.
5. Discard if cloudy or discolored.
6. Product does not contain a preservative; thus, once opened, entire ampule must be used or discarded.

ASSESSMENT

1. Document age of CF symptom onset, other therapies trialed, and outcome.
2. Drug is produced by genetically engineered Chinese hamster ovary cells; assess for sensitivity.
3. Monitor PFTs.

CLIENT/FAMILY TEACHING

1. Drug is administered by inhalation of an aerosol mist generated by a compressed air-driven nebulizer system; review dose, frequency, and method for inhalation. Ensure familiarity with use, care, and storage of equipment and drug. Rinse equipment and mouth after each use.
2. Must be performed on a daily schedule to obtain full benefits. Must continue standard therapies for CF, e.g., chest PT, antibiotics, bronchodilators, oral and inhaled corticosteroids, enzyme supplements, vitamins, and analgesics during therapy.
3. Report symptoms that require immediate medical intervention: severe rashes, itching, respiratory distress, fever. Learn CPR.
4. Identify support groups that may assist to cope with this disease.

OUTCOMES/EVALUATE

• ↓ Respiratory tract infectious exacerbations; ↓ sputum viscosity

• Improved PFTs

Dorzolamide hydrochloride ophthalmic solution

(dor-**ZOH**-lah-myd)

PREGNANCY CATEGORY: C

CLASSIFICATION(S):

Antiglaucoma drug

Rx: Trusopt

ACTION/KINETICS

Decreases aqueous humor secretion in the ciliary processes of the eye by inhibiting carbonic anhydrase. Occurs by decreasing the formation of bicarbonate ions with a reduction in sodium and fluid transport and a subsequent decrease in intraocular pressure. The drug may reach the systemic circulation, where it and the metabolite are excreted through the urine. The drug and metabolite also accumulate in RBCs.

USES

Elevated intraocular pressure (IOP) in those with ocular hypertension or open-angle glaucoma.

CONTRAINDICATIONS

Use with severe renal impairment (C_{CR} < 30 mL/min) or in soft contact lens wearers as the preservative (benzalkonium chloride) may be absorbed by the lenses. Lactation.

SPECIAL CONCERNS

Dorzolamide is a sulfonamide and, as such, may cause similar systemic reactions, including side effects and allergic reactions, as sulfonamides. Use with caution in hepatic impairment. Due to additive effects, concurrent use of dorzolamide with systemic carbonic anhydrase inhibitors is not recommended. Safety and efficacy have not been determined in children. It is possible geriatric clients may show greater sensitivity to the drug.

SIDE EFFECTS

Ophthalmic: Conjunctivitis, lid reactions, bacterial keratitis (due to contamination by concurrent corneal disease). Ocular burning, stinging, or discomfort immediately following administration. Also, superficial punctate keratitis, ocular allergic reaction, blurred vision, tearing, dryness, photophobia, iridocyclitis (rare). **Miscellaneous:** Acid-base and electrolyte disturbances (i.e., similar to systemic use of carbonic anhydrase inhibitors). Also, bitter taste following instillation, headache, nausea, asthenia, fatigue. Rarely, skin rashes, urolithiasis.

HOW SUPPLIED

Solution: 2%

DOSAGE

- **OPHTHALMIC SOLUTION**

Increased intraocular pressure.

Adults: 1 gtt in the affected eye(s) t.i.d.

NURSING CONSIDERATIONS

ADMINISTRATION/STORAGE

Protect from light and store at 15–30°C (59–86°F).

ASSESSMENT

Document visual symptoms and baseline IOP. Note any sensitivity to sulfonamides or impaired renal function.

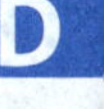

CLIENT/FAMILY TEACHING

1. Do not let dispenser tip come in contact with eye or surrounding structures; contamination may result.
2. Use only as prescribed. Report any evidence of conjunctivitis or eye or lid reaction. Burning or stinging may accompany administration; a bitter taste may also be noted.
3. May be used with other topical ophthalmic drugs. If more than one is being used, give them at least 10 min apart.
4. Do not administer drops while wearing contact lenses as they may absorb solution preservative.

OUTCOMES/EVALUATE

↓ IOP

Doxacurium chloride

(dox-ah-**KYOUR**-ee-um **KLOR**-ide)

PREGNANCY CATEGORY: C
CLASSIFICATION(S):
Skeletal muscle relaxant, nondepolarizing
Rx: Nuromax

SEE ALSO *NEUROMUSCULAR BLOCKING AGENTS.*

ACTION/KINETICS

Binds to cholinergic receptors on the motor end-plate to block the action of acetylcholine, resulting in a blockade of neuromuscular transmission. Up to 3 times more potent than pancuronium and up to 12 times more potent than metocurine. The time to maximum neuromuscular blockade during balanced anesthesia is dose-dependent and ranges from 9.3 min (following doses of 0.025 mg/kg) to 3.5 min (following doses of 0.08 mg/kg). The time to 25% recovery from blockade following balanced anesthesia ranges from 55 min for doses of 0.025 mg/kg to 160 min for doses of 0.08 mg/kg. **t½, elimination:** Dose-dependent, ranging from 86 to 123 min. The half-life is prolonged in kidney transplant clients. Children require higher doses on a mg/kg basis than adults to achieve the same level of blockade. Also, the onset, time, and duration of block are shorter in children than adults. The blockade may be reversed by anticholinesterase agents. Excreted unchanged through the urine and bile.

USES

Adjunct to general anesthesia to provide skeletal muscle relaxation during surgery. Skeletal muscle relaxation for ET intubation or to facilitate mechanical ventilation.

SPECIAL CONCERNS

Use with caution during lactation. Safety and effectiveness have not been determined in children less than 2 years of age. The duration of action may be up to twice as long for clients over 60 years of age and those who are obese (more than 30% more than ideal body weight for height). Malignant hyperthermia may occur in any client receiving a general anesthetic. A profound effect may be noted in clients with neuromuscular diseases such as myasthenia gravis and the myasthenic syndrome.

SIDE EFFECTS

Neuromuscular: Skeletal muscle weakness, ***profound and prolonged skeletal muscle paralysis causing respiratory insufficiency and apnea;*** difficulty in reversing the neuromuscular blockade. **CV:** Hypotension, flushing, ***ventricular fibrillation, MI.*** **Respiratory:** Wheezing, ***bronchospasm.*** **Dermatologic:** Urticaria, reaction at injection site. **Miscellaneous:** Fever, diplopia.

OD OVERDOSE MANAGEMENT

Symptoms: Prolonged neuromuscular block. *Treatment:* Maintain a patent airway and use controlled ventilation if necessary until recovery of normal neuromuscular function. Once recovery begins, it can be facilitated by giving neostigmine, 0.06 mg/kg.

DRUG INTERACTIONS

Aminoglycosides / ↑ Doxacurium effect
Bacitracin / ↑ Doxacurium effect
Carbamazepine / ↑ Doxacurium onset of effects and ↓ duration of action
Clindamycin / ↑ Doxacurium effect
Colistin / ↑ Doxacurium effect
Enflurane / ↓ Amount of doxacurium necessary to cause blockade and ↑ duration of action
Halothane / ↓ Amount of doxacurium necessary to cause blockade and ↑ duration of action
Isoflurane / ↓ Amount of doxacurium necessary to cause blockade and ↑ duration of action
Lincomycin / ↑ Doxacurium effect
Lithium / ↑ Doxacurium effect
Local anesthetics / ↑ Doxacurium effect
Magnesium salts / ↑ Doxacurium effect
Phenytoin / ↑ Doxacurium onset of effects and ↓ duration of action
Polymyxins / ↑ Doxacurium effect
Procainamide / ↑ Doxacurium effect
Quinidine / ↑ Doxacurium effect
Sodium colistimethate / ↑ Doxacurium effect
Tetracyclines / ↑ Doxacurium effect

HOW SUPPLIED

Injection: 1 mg/mL

DOSAGE

• IV ONLY

As a component of thiopental/narcotic induction-intubation, to produce neuromuscular blockade of long duration.

Adults, initial: 0.05 mg/kg.

If administered during steady-state enflurane, halothane, or isoflurane anesthesia.

Reduce dose by one-third. **Children:** 0.03 mg/kg for blockade lasting about 30 min or 0.05 mg/kg for blockade lasting about 45 min when used during halothane anesthesia. Maintenance doses are required more frequently in children.

Used with succinylcholine to facilitate ET intubation.

Initial: 0.025 mg/kg will provide approximately 60 min of effective blockade. **Maintenance doses:** Required about 60 min after an initial dose of 0.025 mg/kg or 100 min after an initial dose of 0.05 mg/kg during balanced anesthesia. Maintenance doses between 0.005–0.01 mg/kg provide an average of 30 min and 45 min, respectively, of additional neuromuscular blockade.

NURSING CONSIDERATIONS

SEE ALSO *NURSING CONSIDERATIONS* FOR *NEUROMUSCULAR BLOCKING AGENTS.*

ADMINISTRATION/STORAGE

IV 1. Individualize dose.
2. Reduce dose in those with neuromuscular disease, severe electrolyte abnormalities, debilitation, and carcinomatosis.
3. May need to increase dose in burn clients.
4. The dose for obese clients is determined using the ideal body weight (IBW), calculated as follows:
• For men: IBW (kg) = (106 + [6 × inches in height above 5 feet])/2.2
• For women: IBW (kg) = (106 + [5 × inches in height above 5 feet])/2.2
5. May not be compatible with alkaline solutions with a pH more than 8 (e.g., barbiturates).
6. May be mixed with D5W, D5/0.9% NaCl, 0.9% NaCl, RL injection, and D5/RL. Drug also compatible with alfentanil, fentanyl, and sufentanil.
7. Doxacurium diluted 1:10 with D5% or 0.9% NaCl is stable for 24 hr if stored in polypropylene syringes at 5–25°C (41–77°F). However, when diluted, immediate use is preferable. Discard any unused diluted portion after 8 hr at room temperature.

ASSESSMENT

1. Determine any neuromuscular disease (e.g., myasthenia gravis).
2. List drugs prescribed.
3. Obtain baseline weight, VS, and serum electrolyte levels.

INTERVENTIONS

1. To be administered only by those experienced with skeletal muscle relaxants, in a monitored setting.
2. Use a peripheral nerve stimulator to monitor drug response and recovery; have antagonist available.
3. Do not administer before unconsciousness (to avoid client stress); doxacurium has no effect on consciousness, pain threshold, or cerebration. Determine need and medicate for anxiety, pain, and sedation.
4. Explain all procedures and provide emotional support. Reassure client will be able to talk and move once the drug effects are reversed.
5. Position for comfort and proper body alignment. Turn and perform mouth/eye care frequently.
6. Provide continuous ventilatory support. Ventilator alarms should be set and on at all times.
7. Explain direction of recovery, i.e., facial muscles, diaphragm, legs, arms, and torso. Residual weakness and respiratory difficulty may slow recovery.

OUTCOMES/EVALUATE

• Skeletal muscle relaxation
• Facilitation of ET intubation; tolerance of mechanical ventilation
• Suppression of twitch response

Doxazosin mesylate

(dox-**AYZ**-oh-sin)

PREGNANCY CATEGORY: B
CLASSIFICATION(S):
Antihypertensive, peripherally-acting
Rx: Cardura
✱**Rx:** Apo-Doxazosin, Cardura-1, -2, -4, Gen-Doxazosin

ACTION/KINETICS

Blocks the alpha-1 (postjunctional) adrenergic receptors resulting in a decrease in systemic vascular resistance and a corresponding decrease in BP. **Peak plasma levels:** 2–3 hr. **Peak effect:** 2–6 hr. Significantly bound (98%) to plasma proteins. Metabolized in the liver to active and inactive metabolites, which are excreted through the feces and urine. **t½:** 22 hr.

USES

Alone or in combination with diuretics, calcium channel blockers, or beta blockers to treat hypertension. Treatment of BPH.

CONTRAINDICATIONS

Clients allergic to prazosin or terazosin.

SPECIAL CONCERNS

Use with caution during lactation, in impaired hepatic function, or in those taking drugs known to influence hepatic metabolism. Safety and effectiveness have not been demonstrated in children. Due to the possibility of severe hypotension, do not use the 2-, 4-, and 8-mg tablets for initial therapy.

SIDE EFFECTS

CV: Dizziness (most frequent), syncope, vertigo, lightheadedness, edema, palpitation, arrhythmia, postural hypotension, tachycardia, peripheral ischemia. **CNS:** Fatigue, headache, paresthesia, kinetic disorders, ataxia, somnolence, nervousness, depression, insomnia. **Musculoskeletal:** Arthralgia, arthritis, muscle weakness, muscle cramps, myalgia, hypertonia. **GU:** Polyuria, sexual dysfunction, urinary incontinence, urinary frequency. **GI:** Nausea, diarrhea, dry mouth, constipation, dyspepsia, flatulence, abdominal pain, vomiting. **Respiratory:** Fatigue or malaise, rhinitis, epistaxis, dyspnea. **Miscellaneous:** Rash, pruritus, flushing, abnormal vision, conjunctivitis, eye pain, tinnitus, chest pain, asthenia, facial edema, generalized pain, slight weight gain.

OD OVERDOSE MANAGEMENT

Symptoms: Hypotension. *Treatment:* IV fluids.

HOW SUPPLIED

Tablet: 1 mg, 2 mg, 4 mg, 8 mg

DOSAGE

• **TABLETS**

Hypertension.

Adults: initial, 1 mg once daily at bedtime; **then,** depending on the response (client's standing BP both 2–6 hr and 24 hr after a dose), the dose may be increased to 2 mg/day. A maximum of 16 mg/day may be required to control BP.

Benign prostatic hyperplasia.

Initial: 1 mg once daily. **Maintenance:** Depending on the urodynamics and symptoms, dose may be increased to 2 mg daily and then 4–8 mg once daily (maximum recommended dose). The recommended titration interval is 1–2 weeks.

NURSING CONSIDERATIONS

ADMINISTRATION/STORAGE

1. To minimize the possibility of severe hypotension, limit initial dosage to 1 mg/day.
2. Increasing the dose higher than 4 mg/day increases the possibility of severe syncope, postural dizziness, vertigo, and postural hypotension.

ASSESSMENT

1. Note any allergy to prazosin or terazosin; a quinazoline derivative.
2. Assess liver function and standing BP.
3. With BPH, numerically score severity.

CLIENT/FAMILY TEACHING

1. Take once daily; do not stop abruptly.
2. Record BP/weight; note edema.
3. Rise slowly to a sitting position before attempting to stand to prevent postural hypotension. Postural effects may occur 2–6 hr after a dose.
4. Driving and hazardous tasks should be avoided for 24 hr after first dose until effects are evident.
5. Report if S&S do not improve after several weeks of therapy as drug dosage may need adjustment.

OUTCOMES/EVALUATE

- ↓ BP
- ↓ S&S BPH/Nocturia

Doxepin hydrochloride

(**DOX**-eh-pin)

PREGNANCY CATEGORY: C

CLASSIFICATION(S):

Antidepressant, tricyclic

Rx: Prudoxin Cream 5%, Sinequan, Sinequan Concentrate, Zonalon

✱**Rx:** Alti-Doxepin, Apo-Doxepin, Novo-Doxepin

SEE ALSO *ANTIDEPRESSANTS, TRICYCLIC.*

ACTION/KINETICS

Metabolized to the active metabolite, desmethyldoxepin. Moderate anticholinergic effects and orthostatic hypotension; high sedative effects. **Therapeutic plasma levels of both doxepin and desmethyldoxepin:** 100–200 ng/mL. **Time to reach steady state:** 2–8 days. **t½:** 8–24 hr.

USES

Systemic. Psychoneurotic clients with depression or anxiety. Depression or anxiety due to organic disease or alcoholism. Psychotic depressive disorders with associated anxiety, including involutional depression and manic-depressive disorders. Depression or anxiety associated with organic disease. PUD. **Topical.** Dermatologic disorders including chronic urticaria, angioedema, atopic dermatitis, lichen simplex chronicus in adults, and nocturnal pruritus due to atopic eczema.

CONTRAINDICATIONS

Use in children less than 12 years of age. Glaucoma or a tendency for urinary retention.

SPECIAL CONCERNS

Safety has not been determined in pregnancy.

ADDITIONAL SIDE EFFECTS

Doxepin has a high incidence of side effects, including a high degree of sedation, decreased libido, extrapyramidal symptoms, dermatitis, pruritus, fatigue, weight gain, edema, paresthesia, breast engorgement, insomnia, tremor, chills, tinnitus, and photophobia. **After topical use:** Burning, stinging, drowsiness, dry mouth.

HOW SUPPLIED

Capsule: 10 mg, 25 mg, 50 mg, 75 mg, 100 mg, 150 mg; Oral *Concentrate:* 10 mg/mL; *Cream:* 5%

DOSAGE

• **CAPSULES, ORAL CONCENTRATE**

Antidepressant, mild to moderate anxiety or depression.

Adults, initial: 25 mg t.i.d. (or up to 150 mg can be given at bedtime); **then,** adjust dosage to individual response (usual optimum dosage: 75–150 mg/day). **Geriatric clients, initially:** 25–50 mg/day; dose can be increased as needed and tolerated.

Severe symptoms.

Initial: 50 mg t.i.d.; **then,** gradually increase to 300 mg/day.

Emotional symptoms with organic disease.

25–50 mg/day.

Antipruritic.

10–30 mg at bedtime.

• **CREAM (5%)**

Apply a thin film q.i.d. with at least a 3–4 hr interval between applications.

NURSING CONSIDERATIONS

SEE ALSO NURSING CONSIDERATIONS FOR ANTIDEPRESSANTS, TRICYCLIC.

ADMINISTRATION/STORAGE

1. Oral concentrate is to be diluted with 4 oz water, milk, or orange, grapefruit, tomato, prune, or pineapple juice just before ingestion. Do not mix the concentrate with carbonated beverages or grape juice.
2. Do not prepare or store bulk dilutions.
3. The antianxiety effect is manifested rapidly; however, it may take 2 to 3 weeks to observe the optimum antidepressant effect.

ASSESSMENT

1. Document type, onset and characteristics of symptoms. List any other prescribed therapy and the outcome.
2. Document clinical presentation and identify any contributing factors.

CLIENT/FAMILY TEACHING

1. Beneficial antidepressant effects may take up to 3 weeks, whereas antianxiety effects occur rapidly.
2. Do not perform activities that require mental alertness until drug effects realized.
3. Avoid alcohol and any other CNS depressants.

OUTCOMES/EVALUATE

- ↓ S&S of anxiety/depression
- Improved sleeping patterns
- Control of neurogenic pain
- Relief of nocturnal pruritus

Doxorubicin hydrochloride, conventional (ADR)

(dox-oh-**ROO**-bih-sin)

D

PREGNANCY CATEGORY: D
Rx: Adriamycin PFS, Adriamycin RDF, Rubex

Doxorubicin hydrochloride liposomal

PREGNANCY CATEGORY: D
Rx: Doxil
🍁Rx: Caelyx
CLASSIFICATION(S):
Antineoplastic, antibiotic

SEE ALSO *ANTINEOPLASTIC AGENTS.*

ACTION/KINETICS
Produced by *Streptomyces peucetius*. Cell-cycle specific for the S phase of cell division. Antineoplastic activity may be due to binding to DNA by intercalating between base pairs resulting in inhibition of synthesis of DNA and RNA by template disordering and steric obstruction. The liposomal product is produced with surface-bound methoxypolyethylene in order to protect liposomes from detection by mononuclear phagocytes and to increase blood circulation time. It is believed the liposomes are able to penetrate altered and often compromised vasculature of tumors. Conventional doxorubicin is significantly bound to tissue and plasma proteins whereas the liposomal product is confined mostly to the vascular fluid and does not bind to plasma proteins. Metabolized in the liver to the active doxorubicinol as well as inactive metabolites, which are excreted through the bile. **t½, doxorubicin, conventional: triphasic:** 12 min, 3.3 hr, and 29.6 hr. **t½, liposomes:** About 55 hr.

USES
Conventional doxorubicin: Acute lymphoblastic leukemia, acute myeloblastic leukemia, Wilms' tumor, soft tissue and osteogenic sarcomas, neuroblastoma, cancer of the breast, ovaries, lungs, bladder, and thyroid, lymphomas (Hodgkin's and non-Hodgkin's), bronchogenic carcinoma (especially small cell histologic type) and gastric carcinoma. *Investigational:* Cancer of the head and neck, cervix, liver, pancreas, prostate, testes, and endometrium.

Liposomal doxorubicin: AIDS-related Kaposi's sarcoma in clients where the disease has progressed on prior combination therapy or in those who are intolerant of such therapy. Third-line treatment of metastatic ovarian cancer in women who have failed or relapsed after cisplatin- or paclitaxel-based chemotherapy.

CONTRAINDICATIONS
Malignant melanoma, cancer of the kidney, large bowel carcinoma, brain tumors and metastases to the CNS (not responsive to doxorubicin therapy). Initiation of therapy in those with marked myelosuppression induced by previous treatment with other drugs or with radiotherapy. Use in preexisting heart disease. Previous treatment with complete cumulative doses of doxorubicin or daunorubicin. Lactation. Depressed bone marrow or cardiac disease. IM or SC use.

SPECIAL CONCERNS
Use with caution in impaired hepatic function and necrotizing colitis. Cardiotoxicity may be more frequent in children.

ADDITIONAL SIDE EFFECTS
Myocardial toxicity: Potentially fatal ***CHF***. **Infusion reactions liposomal product:** Flushing, SOB, facial swelling, headache, chills, back pain, tightness in chest and throat, hypotension. *GI:* N&V, mucositis (stomatitis, esophagitis), anorexia, diarrhea. ***Ulceration and necrosis of the colon.*** **Dermatologic:** Reversible complete alopecia, hyperpigmentation of nail beds and dermal creases (especially in children), onycholysis, recall of skin reaction to prior radiotherapy, palmar-plantar erythrodysesthesia (swelling, pain, erythema, and desquamation of the skin on the hands and feet). **Local:** Severe cellulitis, vesication, and tissue necrosis if the drug is extravasated. Er-

ythematous streaking along the vein next to injection site. **Hypersensitivity:** Fever, chills, urticaria, cross-sensitivity with lincomycin, ***anaphylaxis.*** **Hematologic:** Myelosuppression. **Ophthalmic:** Conjunctivitis, lacrimation.

OD OVERDOSE MANAGEMENT

Symptoms: Mucositis, leukopenia, thrombocytopenia, pancytopenia. Increased risk of ***cardiomyopathy*** and subsequent ***CHF*** with chronic overdosage. *Treatment:* If the client is myelosuppressed, antibiotics and platelet and granulocyte transfusions may be necessary. Treat symptoms of mucositis. Treat CHF with digitalis preparations and diuretics as well as peripheral vasodilators.

DRUG INTERACTIONS

Actinomycin-D / Acute "recall" pneumonitis in pediatric clients
Cyclophosphamide / ↑ Risk of hemorrhagic cystitis
Cyclosporine / ↑ Doxorubicin levels → more profound and prolonged hematologic toxicity
Digoxin / ↓ Digoxin plasma levels
6-Mercaptopurine / ↑ Risk of hemorrhagic cystitis
Paclitaxel / ↓ Doxorubicin clearance → more profound neutropenic and stomatitis episodes
Phenobarbital / ↑ Plasma clearance of doxorubicin
Phenytoin / Possible ↓ phenytoin levels
Progesterone / More pronounced doxorubicin-induced neutropenia and thrombocytopenia
Radiation / ↑ Radiation-induced toxicity to the myocardium, mucosa, skin, and liver
Streptozocin / Possible inhibition of doxorubicin hepatic metabolism

HOW SUPPLIED

Conventional. *Aqueous Injection:* 2 mg/mL; *Powder for injection, lyophilized:* 10 mg, 20 mg, 50mg, 100 mg, 150 mg. **Liposomal.** *Injection:* 20 mg

DOSAGE

• **IV ONLY**

CONVENTIONAL DOXORUBICIN

Adults, highly individualized: 60–75 mg/m² as a single injection q 21 days. Use the lower dose for clients with inadequate marrow reserves due to old age, prior therapy, or neoplastic marrow infiltration. Use reduced dosage in clients with hepatic dysfunction, depending on serum bilirubin level. If bilirubin is 1.2–3 mg/100 mL, give 50% of usual dose; if it is greater than 3 mg/100 mL, give 25% of usual dose.

LIPOSOMAL DOXORUBICIN

AIDS-related Kaposi's sarcoma.

Adults: 20 mg/m² over 30 min once q 3 weeks, as long as the client responds satisfactorily and tolerates the drug. For clients with hepatic dysfunction, use the same dosing schedule as conventional doxorubicin.

Metastatic ovarian carcinoma.

50 mg/m² at an initial rate of 1 mg/min. If no adverse effects occur, increase the rate of infusion to complete administration in 1 hr.

NURSING CONSIDERATIONS

SEE ALSO *NURSING CONSIDERATIONS* FOR *ANTINEOPLASTIC AGENTS*.

ADMINISTRATION/STORAGE

IV 1. Initiate while hospitalized. Give by slow IV into the tubing of a running NaCl or D5W infusion attached to a butterfly needle inserted into a large vein. Avoid veins over joints or in extremities with compromised venous or lymphatic drainage. Although infusion rate depends on vein size, do not administer in less than 3 to 5 min.

2. Reconstitute conventional drug with saline to give a final concentration of 2 mg/mL (e.g., dilute 10-mg vial with 5 mL, 20-mg vial with 10 mL, the 50-mg vial with 25 mL, and the 150-mg vial with 75 mL of 0.9% NaCl) and administer over 3–5 min. The reconstituted solution is stable for 24 hr at room temperature and 48 hr if stored at 2–8°C (36–46°F). The liposomal product is diluted, up to 90 mg, in 250 mL of D5W prior to administration. Do not use in-line filters. Refrigerate diluted liposomal doxorubicin at 2–8°C (36–46°F). Short-term freezing (less than 1 mo) should not affect liposomal product.

3. If the powder or solution comes in contact with the skin or mucous membranes, wash with soap and water thoroughly.
4. *Do not administer SC or IM because severe necrosis of tissue may result.* To minimize danger of extravasation, inject as directed. Monitor carefully; stinging, burning, or edema may indicate extravasation. Stop infusion and change sites to avoid tissue necrosis.
5. Be prepared with an injectable corticosteroid for local infiltration and flood site with NSS. Examine area frequently for ulceration which may necessitate early wide excision followed by plastic surgery.
6. Do not give liposomal product as a bolus injection or as undiluted solution. Rapid infusion may increase risk of infusion-related events.
7. Do not mix conventional doxorubicin with heparin, dexamethasone sodium phosphate, or cephalothin; a precipitate may form. Mixing with aminophylline or 5-FU will result in a change from red to blue-purple indicating decomposition. Do not mix liposomal doxorubicin with other drugs and do not use with any diluent other than D5W. Liposomal doxorubicin is a translucent, red liposomal dispersion.
8. Check package insert carefully for alternate dosing regimens for liposomal doxorubicin in clients with palmar-plantar erythrodysesthesia, hematologic toxicity, or stomatitis.

ASSESSMENT

1. Observe for cardiac arrhythmias, ST segment depression, sinus tachycardia, and/or respiratory difficulties indicative of cardiac toxicity. Have dexrazoxane available to prevent drug-induced cardiomyopathy. Monitor for late-onset (up to 6 mo) CHF.
2. Administer antiemetics 30–45 min before therapy and ATC as needed.
3. Monitor VS and I&O; encourage fluid intake of 2–3 L/day. Anticipate allopurinol administration and alkalinization of urine to decrease urate stone formation.
4. Monitor CBC, uric acid, liver and renal function studies; drug may cause granulocyte toxicity. Nadir: 10-14 days; recovery: 21 days.

CLIENT/FAMILY TEACHING

1. If medication reactivates previous radiotherapy damage, such as erythema, edema, and desquamation; should disappear after 7 days.
2. Consume 2–3 L/day of fluids. May experience increased tearing; avoid rubbing eyes.
3. Urine will turn red-brown for 1–2 days; this is not blood.
4. Nail beds may become discolored.
5. Any hair loss should grow back 2–3 months after therapy.
6. Report any flu-like symptoms; causes severe myelosuppression.
7. Avoid vaccinations.
8. Practice contraception during and for 4 months after therapy.
9. Report mouth ulcers; stomatitis may occur 5–10 days after dose and last for 3–7 days. A special mouth rinse may help decrease symptoms.

OUTCOMES/EVALUATE

Inhibition of malignant cell proliferation

Doxycycline calcium

(dox-ih-**SYE**-kleen)

PREGNANCY CATEGORY: D
Rx: Vibramycin

Doxycycline hyclate

(dox-ih-**SYE**-kleen)

PREGNANCY CATEGORY: D
Rx: Atridox, Bio-Tab, Doryx, Doxy-Caps, Periostat, Vibramycin, Vibra-Tabs, Vivox, Doxy 100 and 200, Doxy-chel Hyclate, Vibramycin IV
✱**Rx:** Apo-Doxy, Apo-Doxy-Tabs, Doxycin, Doxytec, Novo-Doxylin, Nu-Doxycycline, Vibra-Tabs C-Pak

Doxycycline monohydrate

(dox-ih-**SYE**-kleen)

PREGNANCY CATEGORY: D
Rx: Adoxa, Monodox, Vibramycin
CLASSIFICATION(S):
Antibiotic, tetracycline

SEE ALSO *ANTI-INFECTIVES* AND *TETRACYCLINES*.

ACTION/KINETICS
More slowly absorbed, and thus more persistent, than other tetracyclines. Preferred for clients with impaired renal function for treating infections outside the urinary tract. From 80% to 95% is bound to serum proteins. **t½:** 15–25 hr; 30%–42% excreted unchanged in urine. High lipid solubility.
ADDITIONAL USES
PO: (1) Uncomplicated gonococcal infections in adults (except anorectal infections in males); acute epididymo-orchitis caused by *Neisseria gonorrhoeae* and *Chlamydia trachomatis;* gonococcal arthritis-dermatitis syndrome; nongonococcal urethritis caused by *C. trachomatis* and *Ureaplasma urealyticum.* (2) Prophylaxis of malaria due to *Plasmodium falciparum* in short-term travelers (< 4 months) to areas with chloroquine- or pyrimethamine-sulfadoxine-resistant strains. (3) Treatment of anthrax, including cutaneous and inhalation anthrax (post-exposure). **Dental:** Atridox to reduce bacteria associated with periodontal disease. Periostat as an adjunct to scaling and root planing to promote attachment level gain and reduce pocket depth in adult periodontitis.
CONTRAINDICATIONS
Prophylaxis of malaria in pregnant individuals and in children less than 8 years old. Use during pregnancy (may stunt fetal growth) and in children up to 8 years of age (tetracycline may cause permanent discoloration of the teeth). Lactation.
SPECIAL CONCERNS
Safety for IV use in children less than 8 years of age has not been established.
ADDITIONAL DRUG INTERACTIONS
Barbiturates, Carbamazepine, Phenytoin / ↓ Effect of doxycycline by ↑ liver breakdown
Methotrexate / Possible GI and hematologic toxicity after high doses of methotrexate
HOW SUPPLIED
Doxycycline calcium: *Syrup:* 50 mg/5 mL. **Doxycyline hyclate:** *Capsule:* 20 mg, 50 mg, 100 mg; *Enteric Coated Capsule:* 100 mg; *Gel:* 10%; *Powder for injection:* 100 mg, 200 mg; *Tablet:* 20 mg, 100 mg. **Doxycycline monohydrate:** *Capsule:* 50 mg, 100 mg; *Powder for Oral Suspension:* 25 mg/5 mL

DOSAGE
• CAPSULES, DELAYED-RELEASE CAPSULES, ORAL SUSPENSION, SYRUP, TABLETS, IV
Infections.
Adult: First day, 100 mg q 12 hr; **maintenance:** 100–200 mg/day, depending on severity of infection. **Children, over 8 years (45 kg or less): First day,** 4.4 mg/kg in 1–2 doses; **then,** 2.2–4.4 mg/kg/day in divided doses depending on severity of infection. Children over 45 kg should receive the adult dose.
Lyme disease.
Single PO dose of 200 mg within 72 hr after removing the tick.
Acute gonorrhea.
200 mg at once given PO; **then,** 100 mg at bedtime on first day, followed by 100 mg b.i.d. for 3 days. Alternatively, 300 mg immediately followed in 1 hr with 300 mg.
Syphilis (primary/secondary).
300 mg/day in divided PO doses for 10 days.
C. trachomatis *infections.*
100 mg b.i.d. PO for minimum of 7 days.
Prophylaxis of "traveler's diarrhea."
100 mg/day given PO.
Prophylaxis of malaria.
Adults: 100 mg PO once daily; **children, over 8 years of age:** 2 mg/kg/day up to 100 mg/day.
Anthrax, all forms.
Adults: 100 mg q 12 hr for severe disease. **Children:** 2.2 mg/kg q 12 hr for children less than 45 kg.
Adjunct to promote attachment and level gain and to reduce pocket depth in adult periodontitis.
20 mg (either capsule or tablet) b.i.d. following scaling and planing. May be used for up to 9 months. Do not exceed recommended dose.
• IV
Endometritis, parametritis, peritonitis, salpingitis.
100 mg b.i.d. with 2 g cefoxitin, IV, q.i.d. continued for at least 4 days or 2

days after improvement observed. This is followed by doxycycline, PO, 100 mg b.i.d. for 10–14 days of total therapy.

NOTE: The Centers for Disease Control and Prevention have established treatment schedules for STDs.

D

• **GEL, 10%**

Reduce bacteria due to periodontal disease.

Apply to affected area; gel conforms to shape of the periodontal pocket and solidfies. It releases doxycycline for about 7 days.

NURSING CONSIDERATIONS

SEE ALSO *GENERAL NURSING CONSIDERATIONS FOR ANTI-INFECTIVES* AND *TETRACYCLINES*.

ADMINISTRATION/STORAGE

1. Prophylaxis for malaria can begin 1–2 days before travel begins, during travel, and for 4 weeks after leaving the malarious area.
2. The powder for suspension expires 12 months from date of issue.
3. Solution is stable for 2 weeks when stored in refrigerator.
4. IV Follow directions on vial for dilution. Concentrations should be no lower than 0.1 mg/mL and no higher than 1.0 mg/mL. Administer at a rate of 100 mg over 1-4 hr; complete infusion within 12 hr of dilution.
5. During infusion protect solution from light.
6. Administer solutions diluted with NaCl, D5W, Ringer's injection, and 10% invert sugar within 12 hr.
7. Administer solutions diluted with RL or D5/RL within 6 hr.

CLIENT/FAMILY TEACHING

1. May take with food; take with a full glass of water to prevent esophageal ulceration.
2. Avoid direct exposure to sunlight and wear protective clothing and sunscreens when exposed .
3. With STDs advise that partner be tested and treated. Use condoms until medically cleared.
4. Take entire prescription; do not stop if symptoms subside.

OUTCOMES/EVALUATE

• Resolution of infection
• Symptomatic improvement

Dronabinol (Delta-9-tetrahydro-cannabinol)

(droh-**NAB**-ih-nohl)

PREGNANCY CATEGORY: B
CLASSIFICATION(S):
Antinauseant, miscellaneous
Rx: Marinol, **C-III, C-II**

ACTION/KINETICS

As the active component in marijuana, significant psychoactive effects may occur. (See *Side Effects.*) In therapeutic doses, the drug also causes conjunctival injection and an increased HR. Antiemetic effect may be due to inhibition of the vomiting center in the medulla. **Onset:** 0.5–1 hr. **Peak plasma levels:** 2–4 hr. **Duration:** 4–6 hr. Significant first-pass effect. The 11-hydroxytetrahydrocannabinol metabolite is active. **t½, biphasic:** 4 hr and 25–36 hr. **t½, 11-hydroxy-THC:** 15–18 hr. Metabolized in the liver and mainly excreted in the feces. Cumulative toxicity using clinical doses may occur. Highly bound to plasma proteins and may thus displace other protein-bound drugs.

USES

Nausea and vomiting associated with cancer chemotherapy, especially in clients who have not responded to other antiemetic treatment. To stimulate appetite and prevent weight loss in AIDS clients.

CONTRAINDICATIONS

Nausea and vomiting from any cause other than cancer chemotherapy. Lactation. Hypersensitivity to sesame oil. Use for AIDS-related anorexia in children.

SPECIAL CONCERNS

Monitor pediatric and geriatric clients carefully due to an increased risk of psychoactive effects. Use with caution in clients with hypertension, occasional hypotension, syncope, tachycardia; those with a history of substance abuse, including alcohol abuse or dependence; clients with mania, depression, or schizophrenia (the drug may exacerbate these illnesses); clients receiving sedatives, hypnotics, or other psychoactive drugs (due to the potential for additive or synergistic CNS effects).

SIDE EFFECTS

CNS: Side effects are due mainly to the psychoactive effects of the drug and, in addition to those listed in the preceding, include dizziness, muddled thinking, coordination difficulties, irritability, weakness, headache, ataxia, cannabinoid "high," paresthesia, hallucinations, visual distortions, depersonalization, confusion, nightmares, disorientation, and confusion. **CV:** Palpitations, tachycardia, vasodilation, facial flush, hypotension. **GI:** Abdominal pain, N&V, diarrhea, dry mouth, fecal incontinence, anorexia. **Respiratory:** Cough, rhinitis, sinusitis. **Other:** Asthenia, conjunctivitis, myalgias, tinnitus, speech difficulty, vision difficulties, chills, headache, malaise, sweating, elevated hepatic enzymes.

Symptoms of Abstinence Syndrome: An abstinence syndrome has been reported following discontinuation of doses greater than 210 mg/day for 12–16 days. Symptoms include irritability, insomnia, and restlessness within 12 hr; within 24 hr, symptoms include "hot flashes," sweating, rhinorrhea, loose stools, hiccoughs, and anorexia. Disturbed sleep may occur for several weeks.

OD OVERDOSE MANAGEMENT

Symptoms: Extension of the pharmacologic effects. Symptoms of mild overdose include: drowsiness, euphoria, heightened sensory awareness, altered time perception, reddened conjunctiva, dry mouth, and tachycardia. Symptoms of moderate toxicity include impaired memory, depersonalization, mood alteration, urinary retention, and reduced bowel motility. Severe intoxication symptoms include decreased motor coordination, lethargy, slurred speech, and postural hypotension. Seizures may occur in clients with existing seizure disorders. Hallucinations, psychotic episodes, ***respiratory depression,*** and ***coma*** have been reported. *Treatment:* Clients with depressive, hallucinatory, or psychotic reactions should be placed in a quiet environment and provided supportive treatment, including reassurance. Diazepam (5–10 mg PO) may be used for extreme agitation. Hypotension usually responds to IV fluids and Trendelenburg position. In unconscious clients with a secure airway, administer activated charcoal (30–100 g in adults and 1–2 g/kg in children); this may be followed by a saline cathartic.

DRUG INTERACTIONS

Amphetamine / Additive hypertension, tachycardia, possibly cardiotoxicity
Anticholinergics / Additive/super additive tachycardia; drowsiness
CNS depressants / Additive depression
Cocaine / See *Amphetamine*
Antidepressants, tricyclic / Additive tachycardia, hypertension, drowsiness
Ethanol / During subchronic dronabinol use, lower and delayed peak alcohol blood levels
Sympathomimetics / See *Amphetamine*
Theophylline / Possible increased drug metabolism

HOW SUPPLIED

Capsule: 2.5 mg, 5 mg, 10 mg

DOSAGE

• **CAPSULES**

Antiemetic.

Adults and children, initial: 5 mg/m² 1–3 hr before chemotherapy; **then,** 5 mg/m² q 2–4 hr for a total of four to six doses/day. If ineffective, this dose may be increased by 2.5 mg/m² to a maximum of 15 mg/m²/dose. However, the incidence of serious psychoactive side effects increases dramatically at these higher dose levels.

Appetite stimulation.

Initial: 2.5 mg b.i.d. before lunch and dinner. If unable to tolerate 5 mg/day, reduce the dose to 2.5 mg/day as a single evening or bedtime dose. If side effects are absent or minimal and an increased effect is desired, the dose may be increased to 2.5 mg before lunch and 5 mg before dinner (or 5 mg at lunch and 5 mg after dinner). The dose may be increased to 20 mg/day in divided doses. The incidence of side effects increases at higher doses.

D

NURSING CONSIDERATIONS

ADMINISTRATION/STORAGE

1. Due to its CNS effects, use only when client closely supervised.
2. Due to abuse potential, limit prescriptions to one course of chemotherapy (i.e., several days) and reorder PRN.

ASSESSMENT

1. Note any allergy to sesame oil or seeds.
2. Document onset of symptoms; assess if N&V may be caused by anything other than chemotherapy.
3. List other agents trialed.
4. Assess for symptoms of abstinence syndrome which may be seen following withdrawal of doses greater than 210 mg/day for 12–16 days.

CLIENT/FAMILY TEACHING

1. Take 1–3 hr before chemotherapy.
2. Avoid sudden position changes; dizziness may occur.
3. Do not drive or perform hazardous tasks requiring mental acuity.
4. Potential for psychoactive symptoms, visual distortions, and mental confusion; these may be minimized by a quiet, supportive environment.
5. Keep out of child's reach; do not share regardless of symptoms.

OUTCOMES/EVALUATE

- Relief of chemotherapy-induced N&V
- ↑ Appetite; ↓ weight loss

Drotrecogin alfa (Activated)

(droh-treh-**KOH**-jin **AL**-fah)

PREGNANCY CATEGORY: C
CLASSIFICATION(S):
Sepsis drug
Rx: Xigris

ACTION/KINETICS
Drotrecogin alfa is a recombinant human activated Protein C. Activated Protein C exerts an antithrombotic effect by inhibiting Factors Va and VIIIa. Activated Protein C has indirect profibrolytic activity by inhibiting plasminogen activator inhibitor-1 and limiting generation of activated thrombin-activatable-fibrinolysis-inhibitor. Activated Protein C may also exert an anti-inflammatory effect by inhibiting tumor necrosis factor production by monocytes, by blocking leukocyte adhesion to selectins, and by limiting the thrombin-induced inflammatory responses within the microvascular endothelium. Activated Protein C levels in those with severe sepsis are below detectable levels. Infusion of drotrecogin alfa rapidly produces steady-state levels that are proportional to infusion rates. In most clients, plasma levels of drotrecogin alfa fall below detectable levels within 2 hr after stopping infusion.

USES
Reduce mortality in adults with sepsis associated with acute organ dysfunction who have a high risk of death.

CONTRAINDICATIONS
Due to increased risk of bleeding, use in active internal bleeding, within 3 months of hemorrhagic stroke, within 2 months of intracranial or intraspinal surgery or severe head trauma, trauma with an increased risk of life-threatening bleeding, presence of an epidural catheter, and intracranial neoplasm or mass lesion with evidence of cerebral herniation. Hypersensitivity to the drug or any component of the product. Lactation.

SPECIAL CONCERNS
Efficacy has not been determined in adults with severe sepsis and a lower risk of death. Safety and efficacy have not been determined in children with severe sepsis. Use with caution with other drugs that affect hemostasis; however concomitant use of low dose heparin does not affect safety.

SIDE EFFECTS
Hematologic: Bleeding (most common side effect), including the follow-

ing sites of hemorrhage: ***intracranial, GI, intra-abdominal, intrathoracic, retroperitoneal, GU, skin/soft tissue.***

LABORATORY TEST CONSIDERATIONS

Prolongation of APTT. Interference with factor VIII, IX, and XI assays (values obtained that are lower than the true concentrations).

HOW SUPPLIED

Powder for infusion, lyophilized: 5 mg, 20 mg

DOSAGE

• **IV**

Sepsis.

IV, at an infusion rate of 24 mcg/kg/hr for a total duration of 96 hr. Do **not** adjust dose based on clinical or lab parameters. If infusion is interrupted, restart at the 24 mcg/kg/hr infusion rate.

NURSING CONSIDERATIONS

ADMINISTRATION/STORAGE

IV 1. Do not escalate dose or give by bolus injection.

2. Stop infusion immediately if clinically important bleeding occurs.

3. Discontinue 2 hr before undergoing an invasive surgical procedure or procedures with an inherent risk of bleeding. Once adequate hemostasis has been achieved, drotrecognin alfa may be reconsidered 12 hr after any major invasive procedure or surgery and may be restarted immediately after uncomplicated less invasive procedures.

ASSESSMENT

1. Note indications for therapy, characteristics of symptoms, other agents trialed, and organ failure status.

2. Evaluate client carefully and weigh anticipated benefits versus potential risks of therapy. Certain conditions are likely to increase the risk of bleeding. In clients with 1 or more of the following conditions, consider using drotrecogin alfa therapy:

- Concurrent therapeutic heparin (15 or more units/kg/hr)
- Platelet count <30,000 x 10^6/L, even if platelet count is elevated after transfusions
- Prothrombin time-(INR) > 3
- Within 6 weeks of GI bleeding
- Within 3 days of thrombolytic therapy
- Within 7 days of oral anticoagulants or glycoprotein IIb/IIIa inhibitors
- Within 7 days of aspirin, > 650 mg/day or other platelet inhibitors
- Within 3 months of ischemic stroke
- Intracranial arteriovenous malformation or aneurysm
- Known bleeding diathesis
- Chronic severe hepatic disease
- Any other condition in which bleeding constitutes a significant hazard or would be difficult to manage because of its location

3. Place in a carefully monitored environment which permits continous assessment for any evidence of significant active bleeding. If evident, stop infusion and report.

4. Monitor VS, cultures, CBC, PT/INR, renal and LFTs. Sepsis predisposes one to a coagulopathy associated with prolongation of PTT/PT. Drotrecogin alfa may alter the PTT thus making it an unreliable test to assess the clients' coagulopathy status.

CLIENT/FAMILY TEACHING

Those with severe sepsis and organ failure may experience many adverse events that are life threatening; predisposes this population to a high risk of death. The benefits must far outweigh the risks when this therapy is selected.

OUTCOMES/EVALUATE

Improved mortality with severe sepsis

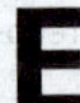

Edetate disodium (EDTA)

(**ED**-eh-tayt)

PREGNANCY CATEGORY: C
CLASSIFICATION(S):
Antidote, heavy metal antagonist
Rx: Endrate

ACTION/KINETICS
Forms a soluble calcium chelate in the blood which is excreted through the urine. This leads to a lowering of serum calcium and a mobilization of calcium stores, especially from bone. When used to treat digitalis toxicity, edetate disodium exerts a negative inotropic effect on the heart and thus the chronotropic and inotropic effects of digitalis on the heart are antagonized. Also forms chelates with magnesium, zinc, and other trace elements. Does not chelate with potassium but may increase potassium excretion.

USES
Hypercalcemia. Ventricular arrhythmias associated with digitalis toxicity.

CONTRAINDICATIONS
Anuria. Ventricular arrhythmias. To treat arteriosclerosis, atherosclerotic vascular disease, lead poisoning, or renal calculi by retrograde irrigation.

SPECIAL CONCERNS
Use during pregnancy only if the benefits clearly outweigh the risks. Use with extreme caution in digitalized clients as EDTA and calcium may reverse the desired effect of digitalis. Use with caution in clients with heart disease (e.g., CHF) or hypokalemia. Rapid IV infusion or a high serum EDTA level may result in a precipitous drop in serum calcium leading to death.

SIDE EFFECTS
Metabolic: Electrolyte imbalance including hypocalcemia, hypokalemia, hypomagnesemia, hyperuricemia may occur during treatment. **CV:** Decrease in both systolic and diastolic pressure, thrombophlebitis, anemia. **GI:** N&V, diarrhea. **CNS:** Headache, numbness, circumoral paresthesia, fever. **Other:** Exfoliative dermatitis, nephrotoxicity, ***reticuloendothelial system damage with hemorrhagic tendencies. Rapid injection may produce hypocalcemic tetany and convulsions, respiratory arrest, and severe arrhythmias.***

LABORATORY TEST CONSIDERATIONS
↓ Alkaline phosphatase levels.

OD OVERDOSE MANAGEMENT
Symptoms: Precipitous drop in calcium. *Treatment:* IV calcium gluconate which should be available at all times.

HOW SUPPLIED
Injection: 150 mg/mL

DOSAGE

• **IV**

Hypercalcemia, digitalis toxicity.
Individualized and depending on degree of hypercalcemia. **Adults, usual:** 50 mg/kg over 24 hr (up to 3 g/day may be prescribed); dose may be repeated for 5 consecutive days followed by a 2-day rest period with repeated courses, if needed, up to 15 doses. **Pediatric:** 40 mg/kg over 24 hr up to a maximum of 70 mg/kg/day. An alternative dosing regimen is 15–50 mg/kg/day, to a maximum of 3 g/day followed by a 5-day rest period between courses.

• **OPHTHALMIC**

Calcium deposits, calcium hydroxide burns.
Adults and children: 0.35%–1.85% solution as an irrigation for 15–20 min.

Zinc chloride injury.
Adults and children: 1.7% solution as an irrigation for 15 min.
NOTE: No ophthalmic product available in the U.S. However, the injection can be used to prepare the ophthalmic dosage form.

NURSING CONSIDERATIONS

ADMINISTRATION/STORAGE
IV 1. Check label on vial carefully to ensure drug is disodium edetate, not calcium disodium edetate.

2. For use in adults, dilute in 500 mL of D5W or NSS solution. For pediatric use, dissolve in either D5W or 0.9% NaCl; the final concentration should not exceed 3%.
3. Repeated use of the same vein may result in thrombophlebitis. Greater solution dilution and slower infusion reduce this incidence if the same vein must be used.
4. Infuse slowly over 3–4 hr, while in a Fowler's position. Do not exceed recommended dose, concentration, rate of administration, or cardiac reserve of the client.

ASSESSMENT

1. Document indications for therapy, symptom onset, and anticipated results.
2. Use cautiously with heart disease, seizures, and/or tuberculosis. Assess I&O.
3. Monitor calcium, zinc, magnesium, phosphorous, electrolytes, urinalysis, and renal function studies.
4. Transitory hypotension may occur; place supine until BP stabilized.
5. Be alert to a generalized systemic reaction that may occur from 4 to 8 hr after drug infusion (usually subsides within 12 hr). Provide supportive care if fever, chills, back pain, vomiting, muscle cramps, or urinary urgency occur.
6. With lead toxicity, notify local health department; identify source and need for further investigation.

CLIENT/FAMILY TEACHING

1. Review goals of therapy and frequency of administration.
2. May cause hypoglycemia; consult provider concerning management of diabetes (i.e., reduce insulin dosage or increase food intake).
3. Report unusual bruising/bleeding.

OUTCOMES/EVALUATE

- ↓ Calcium; ↓ digoxin levels
- Lead levels < 50 mcg/dL
- Dissolution of corneal deposits

Edrophonium chloride

(ed-roh-**FOH**-nee-um)

PREGNANCY CATEGORY: C
Rx: Enlon, Reversol, Tensilon

—COMBINATION DRUG—

Edrophonium chloride and Atropine sulfate

(ed-roh-**FOH**-nee-um)

PREGNANCY CATEGORY: C
Rx: Enlon-Plus
CLASSIFICATION(S):
Cholinesterase inhibitor, indirectly-acting

SEE ALSO *NEOSTIGMINE* AND *ATROPINE SULFATE*.

ACTION/KINETICS

By increasing the duration of action at the motor end plate, edrophonium causes a transient increase in muscle strength in myasthenia gravis clients and either no change or a slight weakness in muscle strength in clients with other disorders. Atropine counteracts the muscarinic side effects that will occur due to edrophonium (e.g., increased secretions, bradycardia, bronchoconstriction). **Onset: IM,** 2–10 min; **IV,** <1 min. **Duration: IM,** 5–30 min; **IV,** 10 min. Eliminated through the kidneys.

USES

Edrophonium: Differential diagnosis of myasthenia gravis. Adjunct to evaluate requirements for treating myasthenia gravis. Adjunct to treat respiratory depression due to curare and similar nondepolarizing agents such as gallamine, pancuronium, and tubocurarine.

Edrophonium and Atropine: To antagonize or reverse nondepolarizing neuromuscular blocking agents. Adjunct to treat respiratory depression caused by overdosage of curare.

CONTRAINDICATIONS

Edrophonium combined with atropine in the differential diagnosis of myasthenia gravis.

SPECIAL CONCERNS

Edrophonium combined with atropine is not effective against depolarizing neuromuscular blocking agents.

HOW SUPPLIED

Edrophonium chloride: *Injection:* 10 mg/mL. **Edrophonium chloride and Atropine sulfate:** *Injection:* 10 mg-0.14 mg/mL

DOSAGE

• **EDROPHONIUM, IV**

Differential diagnosis of myasthenia gravis.

IV, Adults: 2 mg initially over 15–30 sec; with needle in place, wait 45 sec; if no response occurs after 45 sec inject an additional 8 mg. If a cholinergic reaction is obtained following 2 mg (muscarinic side effects, skeletal muscle fasciculations, increased muscle weakness), test is discontinued and atropine, 0.4–0.5 mg, is given IV. The test may be repeated in 30 min. **Pediatric, up to 34 kg, IV:** 1 mg; if no response after 45 sec, can give up to 5 mg. **Pediatric, over 34 kg, IV:** 2 mg; if no response after 45 sec, can give up to 10 mg in 1-mg increments q 30–45 sec. **Infants:** 0.5 mg. If IV injection is not feasible, IM can be used.

To evaluate treatment needs in myasthenic clients.

1 hr after PO administration of drug used to treat myasthenia, give edrophonium IV, 1–2 mg. (*NOTE:* Response will be myasthenic in undertreated clients, adequate in controlled clients, and cholinergic in overtreated clients.)

Curare antagonist.

Slow IV: 10 mg over 30–45 sec to detect onset of cholinergic reaction; repeat if necessary to maximum of 40 mg. Should not be given before use of curare, gallamine, or tubocurarine.

• **EDROPHONIUM, IM**

Differential diagnosis of myasthenia gravis.

Adults: 10 mg; if hyperreactivity occurs, retest after 30 min with 2 mg IM to rule out false negative. **Pediatric, up to 34 kg:** 2 mg; **more than 34 kg:** 5 mg. (There is a 2–10-min delay in reaction with IM route.)

• **EDROPHONIUM AND ATROPINE, IV**

Adults: 0.5–1 mg/kg edrophonium and 0.007–0.014 mg/kg atropine.

NURSING CONSIDERATIONS

SEE ALSO NURSING CONSIDERATIONS FOR NEOSTIGMINE AND ATROPINE SULFATE.

ADMINISTRATION/STORAGE

IV 1. Do not give edrophonium before curare or curare-like drugs.
2. Have IV atropine sulfate available to use as an antagonist.
3. When atropine is combined with edrophonium, monitor carefully; assisted or controlled ventilation should be undertaken.
4. Recurarization has not been noted following satisfactory reversal with edrophonium and atropine.

ASSESSMENT

1. Document therapy indications.
2. List drugs currently prescribed.
3. Note any history of asthma, seizures, CAD, or hyperthyroidism.
4. Assess client closely during administration; effects last up to 30 min. Monitor VS and I&O at least q 4 hr.
5. Document any increased salivation, bronchial spasm, bradycardia, and cardiac arrhythmia; especially important with the elderly.
6. When administered as an antidote for curare, assess for each dose effect; do not administer the next dose unless prior effects have been observed. Larger doses may potentiate effects.
7. Evaluate respiratory effort and provide assisted ventilation prn.
8. With the edrophonium test for myasthenia gravis all cholinesterase inhibitors (anticholinesterases) should be discontinued for a least 8 hr before test. A brief improvement in muscle strength unaccompanied by lingual or skeletal muscle fasciculations is considered a positive response to the edrophonium test.
9. In evaluation of myasthenic treatment: with myasthenic response see immediate subjective improvement with increased muscle strength, absence of muscle fasciculations indicates that client requires larger dose of anticholinesterase agent or longer acting drug.
10. During cholinergic crisis, monitor state of consciousness closely; see abdominal cramps, diarrhea, N&V, tear-

ing, sweating and decrease in muscle strength. Usually indicates over treatment with cholinesterase inhibitor.

11. With an adequate response to treatment there is no change in muscle strength, muscle fasciculations may be present or absent, and minimal cholinergic side effects will be observed in those at or near optimal treatment levels.

OUTCOMES/EVALUATE

- With myasthenia gravis (transient ↑ muscle strength, improved gait)
- Curare antagonist
- Reversal of respiratory depression
- Differentiation of myasthenic from cholinergic crisis

Efavirenz

(eh-**FAH**-vih-rehnz)

PREGNANCY CATEGORY: C
CLASSIFICATION(S):
Antiviral, non-nucleoside reverse transcriptase inhibitor
Rx: Sustiva

SEE ALSO *ANTIVIRAL AGENTS.*

ACTION/KINETICS

A non-nucleoside reverse transcriptase inhibitor of HIV-1 that acts mainly by non-competitive inhibition of HIV-1. **Peak plasma levels:** 3–5 hr. **Steady-state plasma levels:** 6–10 days. Highly protein bound (99.5–99.75%). Metabolized by the cytochrome P450 system to inactive metabolites which are excreted in the urine and feces. Will induce its own metabolism. **t½, terminal:** 52–76 hr after a single dose and 40–55 hr after multiple doses.

USES

In combination with other antiretroviral drugs to treat HIV-1 infection.

CONTRAINDICATIONS

Use as a single agent to treat HIV (resistant virus emerges rapidly) or added on as a sole agent to a failing regimen. High fat meals (increase absorption). Use with cisapride, ergot derivatives, midazolam, or triazolam. Lactation (to prevent postnatal transmission of HIV infection).

SPECIAL CONCERNS

Use with caution in impaired hepatic function.

SIDE EFFECTS

CNS: Delusions, inappropriate behavior (especially in those with a history of mental illness or substance abuse), severe acute depression with suicidal ideation/attempts, psychosis, dizziness, impaired concentration, somnolence, abnormal dreams, insomnia, fatigue, headache, hypoesthesia, depression, anorexia, nervousness, ataxia, confusion, convulsions, impaired coordination, migraine headaches, neuralgia, paresthesia, peripheral neuropathy, speech disorder, tremor, vertigo, aggravated depression, agitation, amnesia, anxiety, apathy, emotional lability, euphoria, hallucinations, psychosis. **Dermatologic:** Skin rash, including moist or dry desquamation, ulceration, erythema, pruritus, diffuse maculopapular rash, vesiculation, erythema multiforme. Increased sweating, alopecia, eczema, folliculitis, urticaria, nail disorders, skin discoloration. Rarely, ***Stevens-Johnson syndrome, toxic epidermal necrolysis,*** necrosis requiring surgery, exfoliative dermatitis. **GI:** N&V, diarrhea, dyspepsia, abdominal pain, flatulence, dry mouth, pancreatitis. **GU:** Hematuria, renal calculus. **CV:** Flushing, palpitations, tachycardia, thrombophlebitis. **Musculoskeletal:** Arthralgia, myalgia, myopathy. **Ophthalmic:** Abnormal vision, diplopia. **Miscellaneous:** Parosmia, taste perversion, alcohol intolerance, allergic reaction, asthenia, fever, hot flushes, malasie, pain, peripheral edema, syncope, tinnitus, hepatitis, asthma.

LABORATORY TEST CONSIDERATIONS

↑ AST, ALT, total cholesterol, serum amylase, serum triglycerides. False+ urine cannabinoid tests using the CEDIA DAU Multi-Level THC assay.

OD OVERDOSE MANAGEMENT

Symptoms: Increased nervous system symptoms. *Treatment:* General supportive measures, including monitoring of vital signs. Activated charcoal may be used to aid removal of unabsorbed drug.

DRUG INTERACTIONS
Amprenavir / ↓ Serum amprenavir levels
Clarithromycin / ↓ Clarithromycin plasma levels and ↑ levels of metabolite; use alternative therapy such as azithromycin
CNS depressants / Additive CNS depression
Ergot derivatives / Inhibition of ergot metabolism → possible cardiac arrhythmias, prolonged sedation, or respiratory depression
Indinavir / ↑ Indinavir levels R/T enzyme induction
Methadone / ↑ Risk of methadone withdrawal symptoms R/T ↑ liver breakdown
Midazolam / Inhibition of midazolam metabolism → possible cardiac arrhythmias, prolonged sedation, or respiratory depression
Rifampin / ↓ Efavirenz plasma levels
Ritonavir / Higher frequency of dizziness, nausea, paresthesia, and elevated liver enzymes
Saquinavir / ↓ Saquinavir AUC and C_{max}
Triazolam / Inhibition of triazolam metabolism → possible cardiac arrhythmias, prolonged sedation, or respiratory depression

HOW SUPPLIED
Capsules: 50 mg, 100 mg, 200 mg

DOSAGE

• **CAPSULES**
HIV-1 infections.
Adults: 600 mg once daily in combination with a protease inhibitor or nucleoside analog reverse transcriptase inhibitors. **Children, 3 years and older. 10– < 15 kg:** 200 mg once daily; **15– < 20 kg:** 250 mg once daily; **20– < 25 kg:** 300 mg once daily; **25– < 32.5 kg:** 350 mg once daily; **32.5– < 40 kg:** 400 mg once daily; **40 kg or more:** 600 mg once daily.

NURSING CONSIDERATIONS

SEE ALSO *NURSING CONSIDERATIONS FOR ANTIVIRAL AGENTS.*

ADMINISTRATION/STORAGE
1. Always initiate therapy with 1 or more other new antiretroviral drugs to which the client has not been previously exposed.
2. May be taken with or without food; however, high-fat meals may increase the absorption and are to be avoided.
3. Use bedtime dosing during the first 2 to 4 weeks to improve tolerability of nervous system side effects.

ASSESSMENT
1. Note indications for therapy and other agents trialed.
2. May cause false-positive cannabinoid urine test.

CLIENT/FAMILY TEACHING
1. Take as directed and with other anti-retroviral agents.
2. May take with food but avoid high fat meals as these may increase drug absorption.
3. Drug does not cure disease but works to reduce viral load.
4. Practice reliable barrier contraception with additional form of birth control; do not breast feed.
5. May cause dizziness, drowsiness, delusions, and impaired concentration. Take at bedtime to increase tolerability; avoid tasks requiring concentration and dexterity until effects realized.
6. Most clients will experience a rash. This should resolve after several weeks; report if persistent or extensive.
7. Avoid alcohol and any OTC agents.

OUTCOMES/EVALUATE
↓ HIV-RNA levels; ↑ CD_4 cell counts

Emedastine difumarate

(em-eh-**DAS**-teen)

PREGNANCY CATEGORY: B
CLASSIFICATION(S):
Antihistamine, ophthalmic
Rx: Emadine

SEE ALSO *ANTIHISTAMINES.*

ACTION/KINETICS
Selective H_1 antagonist which inhibits histamine–stimulated vascular permeability in the conjunctiva. Very little reaches the systemic circulation.

USES

Relieve signs and symptoms of allergic conjunctivitis.

CONTRAINDICATIONS

Parenteral or oral use. Use to treat contact lens-related irritation.

SPECIAL CONCERNS

Use with caution during lactation. Safety and efficacy have not been established in children less than 3 years of age.

SIDE EFFECTS

Ophthalmic: Blurred vision, burning or stinging, corneal infiltrates, corneal staining, dry eyes, foreign body sensation, hyperemia, keratitis, tearing. **CNS:** Headache, abnormal dreams. **Respiratory:** Pruritus, rhinitis, sinusitis. **Miscellaneous:** Asthenia, bad taste, dermatitis, discomfort.

HOW SUPPLIED

Solution: 0.05%

DOSAGE

- **SOLUTION**

  Allergic conjunctivitis.

One drop in the affected eye(s) up to q.i.d.

NURSING CONSIDERATIONS

SEE ALSO *NURSING CONSIDERATIONS* FOR *ANTIHISTAMINES.*

ADMINISTRATION/STORAGE

Store at 4–30°C (39–86°F).

ASSESSMENT

Note time of year and events/triggers that surround symptoms.

CLIENT/FAMILY TEACHING

1. Use as directed; avoid triggers that precipitate symptoms.
2. To prevent contamination, do not allow the dropper tip to touch the eyelids or surrounding areas.
3. Keep bottle tightly closed; do not use if the solution becomes discolored.
4. Avoid contact lens if eye irritated or red. Do not insert soft contact lens for 15 min after instilling drops (the preservative, benzalkonium chloride, may be absorbed.)

OUTCOMES/EVALUATE

- Relief of S&S allergic conjunctivitis
- ↓ Ocular itching

Enalapril maleate

(en-**AL**-ah-prill)

PREGNANCY CATEGORY: D

CLASSIFICATION(S):

Antihypertensive, ACE inhibitor

Rx: Vasotec, Vasotec I.V.

E

SEE ALSO *ANGIOTENSIN-CONVERTING ENZYME INHIBITORS.*

ACTION/KINETICS

Converted in the liver by hydrolysis to the active metabolite, enalaprilat. The parenteral product is enalaprilat injection. **Onset, PO:** 1 hr; **IV,** 15 min. **Time to peak action, PO:** 4–6 hr; **IV,** 1–4 hr. **Duration, PO:** 24 hr; **IV,** About 6 hr. Approximately 50%–60% is protein bound. **t½, enalapril, PO:** 1.3 hr; **IV,** 15 min. **t½, enalaprilat, PO:** 11 hr. Excreted through the urine (half unchanged) and feces; over 90% of enalaprilat is excreted through the urine.

USES

(1) Alone or in combination with other antihypertensives (e.g., a thiazide diuretic) for the treatment of hypertension. Hypertension in children. (2) As adjunct with digitalis and diuretic in acute and chronic CHF. (3) Asymptomatic left ventricular dysfunction in clinically stable asymptomatic clients. (4) IV for treatment of hypertension when PO is not practical. *Investigational:* Hypertension related to scleroderma renal crisis. Enalaprilat may be used for hypertensive emergencies (effect is variable).

SPECIAL CONCERNS

Use with caution during lactation. Safety and effectiveness have not been determined in children.

SIDE EFFECTS

CV: Palpitations, hypotension, chest pain, angina, ***CVA, MI,*** orthostatic hypotension, disturbances in rhythm, tachycardia, ***cardiac arrest,*** orthostatic effects, atrial fibrillation, tachycardia, bradycardia, Raynaud's phenomenon. **GI:** N&V, diarrhea, abdominal pain, alterations in taste, anorexia, dry mouth, constipation, dyspepsia, glossitis, ileus, melena, stomatitis. **CNS:** Insomnia, headache, fatigue, dizziness, paresthesias, nervousness, sleepiness, ataxia, confusion, depression, vertigo, abnormal dreams. **Hepatic:** Hepatitis, hepatocellular or cholestatic jaundice, pancreatitis, elevated liver enzymes, hepatic failure. **Respiratory:** Bronchitis, cough, dyspnea, bronchospasm, URI, pneumonia, pulmonary infiltrates, asthma, ***pulmonary embolism and infarction, pulmonary edema.*** **Renal:** Renal dysfunction, oliguria, UTI, transient increases in creatinine and BUN. **Hematologic:** Rarely, neutropenia, thrombocytopenia, bone marrow depression, decreased H&H in hypertensive or CHF clients. Hemolytic anemia, including hemolysis, in clients with G6PD deficiency. **Dermatologic:** Rash, pruritus, alopecia, flushing, erythema multiforme, exfoliative dermatitis, photosensitivity, urticaria, increased sweating, pemphigus, ***Stevens-Johnson syndrome,*** herpes zoster, toxic epidermal necrolysis. **Other:** Angioedema, asthenia, impotence, blurred vision, fever, arthralgia, arthritis, vasculitis, eosinophilia, tinnitus, syncope, myalgia, muscle cramps, rhinorrhea, sore throat, hoarseness, conjunctivitis, tearing, dry eyes, loss of sense of smell, hearing loss, peripheral neuropathy, anosmia, myositis, flank pain, gynecomastia.

ADDITIONAL DRUG INTERACTIONS

Rifampin may ↓ the effects of enalapril. Do not discontinue without first reporting to the provider.

HOW SUPPLIED

Tablet: 2.5 mg, 5 mg, 10 mg, 20 mg; *Injection:* 1.25 mg/mL (as enalaprilat)

DOSAGE

- **TABLETS (ENALAPRIL)**

Antihypertensive in clients not taking diuretics.

Initial: 5 mg/day; **then,** adjust dosage according to response (range: 10–40 mg/day in one to two doses).

Antihypertensive in clients taking diuretics.

Initial: 2.5 mg. Since hypotension may occur following the initiation of enalapril, the diuretic should be discontinued, if possible, for 2–3 days before initiating enalapril. If BP is not maintained with enalapril alone, diuretic therapy may be resumed.

Hypertension in children.

Initial: 0.08 mg/kg, up to 5 mg, once daily. Adjust dose depending on response. Do not give to neonates and children with a GFR <30 mL/min/1.73 m²

Adjunct with diuretics and digitalis in heart failure.

Initial: 2.5 mg 1–2 times/day; **then,** depending on the response, 2.5–20 mg/day in two divided doses. Dose should not exceed 40 mg/day. Dosage must be adjusted in clients with renal impairment or hyponatremia.

In clients with impaired renal function.

Initial: 5 mg/day if C_{CR} ranges between 30 and 80 mL/min and serum creatinine is less than 3 mg/dL; 2.5 mg/day if C_{CR} is less than 30 mL/min and serum creatinine is more than 3 mg/dL and in dialysis clients on dialysis days.

Renal impairment or hyponatremia.

Initial: 2.5 mg/day if serum sodium is less than 130 mEq/L and serum creatinine is more than 1.6 mg/dL. The dose may be increased to 2.5 mg b.i.d. and then 5 mg b.i.d. or higher if required; dose is given at intervals of 4 or more days. Maximum daily dose is 40 mg.

Asymptomatic LV dysfunction following MI.

2.5 mg b.i.d., titrated as tolerated to the daily dose of 20 mg in divided doses.

- **IV (ENALAPRILAT)**

Hypertension.

1.25 mg over a 5-min period; repeat q 6 hr.

Antihypertensive in clients taking diuretics.

Initial: 0.625 mg over 5 min; if an adequate response is seen after 1 hr, administer another 0.625-mg dose. Thereafter, 1.25 mg q 6 hr. In those taking diuretics, start with 0.625 mg enalaprilat over 5 min; if there is an inadequate effect after 1 hr, repeat the 0.625 mg dose. Give additional doses of 1.25 mg q 6 hr.

Clients with impaired renal function.

Give enalaprit, 1.25 mg q 6 hr for clients with a C_{CR} more than 30 mL/min and an initial dose of 0.625 mg for clients with a C_{CR} less than 30 mL/min. If there is an adequate response, an additional 0.625 mg may be given after 1 hr; thereafter, additional 1.25-mg doses can be given q 6 hr. For dialysis clients, the initial dose is 0.625 mg q 6 hr.

NURSING CONSIDERATIONS

SEE ALSO *NURSING CONSIDERATIONS* FOR *ACE INHIBITORS* AND *ANTIHYPERTENSIVE AGENTS*.

ADMINISTRATION/STORAGE

1. To convert from IV to PO therapy in clients on a diuretic, begin with 2.5 mg/day for clients responding to a 0.625-mg IV dose. Thereafter, 2.5 mg/day may be given.
2. Use lower dose if receiving diuretics or with impaired renal function.
3. A 1-mg/mL suspension may be prepared for use in children (see instructions in the labeling).

IV 4. To convert from PO to IV therapy in clients not on a diuretic, use the recommended IV dose (i.e., 1.25 mg/6 hr). To convert from IV to PO therapy, begin with 5 mg/day.

5. Following IV administration, first dose peak effect may take 4 hr (whether or not on a diuretic). For subsequent doses, the peak effect is usually within 15 min.
6. Give enalaprilat as a slow IV infusion (over 5 min) either alone or diluted up to 50 mL with an appropriate diluent. Any of the following can be used: D5W, D5/RL, Isolyte E, 0.9% NaCl, D5/0.9% NaCl.
7. When used initially for heart failure, observe for at least 2 hr after the initial dose and until BP has stabilized for an additional hour. If possible, reduce dose of diuretic.

ASSESSMENT

1. Document indications for therapy, presenting symptoms, other agents trialed, and the outcome.
2. Record ECG, VS, and weight.
3. Monitor CBC, electrolytes, liver and renal function studies. Reduce dose with impaired renal function.

CLIENT/FAMILY TEACHING

1. Use caution, may cause orthostatic effects and dizziness.
2. Maintain a healthy diet; limit intake of caffeine; avoid alcohol, salt substitutes, or high-Na and high-K foods.
3. Report any weight loss that may result from the loss of taste or rapid weight gain that may result from fluid overload.
4. Any flu-like symptoms should be reported immediately.

OUTCOMES/EVALUATE

- ↓ BP
- ↓ Preload and afterload with CHF

Enoxacin

(ee-**NOX**-ah-sin)

PREGNANCY CATEGORY: C
CLASSIFICATION(S):
Antibiotic, fluoroquinolone
Rx: Penetrex

SEE ALSO *FLUOROQUINOLONES*.

ACTION/KINETICS

Inhibits certain isozymes of the cytochrome P-450 hepatic microsomal enzyme system, resulting in alterations of metabolism of some drugs. **Peak plasma levels:** 0.83 mcg/mL 1–3 hr after a 200-mg dose and 2 mcg/mL 1–3 hr after a 400-mg dose. Mean peak plasma levels are 50% higher in geriatric clients than in young adults. Diffuses into the cervix, fallopian tubes, and myometrium at levels 1–2 times those seen in plasma and into kidney and prostate at levels 2–4 times those seen in plasma. **t½:** 3–6 hr. More than 40% excreted unchanged through the urine.

USES

(1) To treat uncomplicated urethral or cervical gonorrhea due to *Neisseria gonorrhoeae.* (2) To treat uncomplicated UTIs (e.g., cystitits) due to *Escherichia coli, Staphylococcus epidermidis,* or *S. saprophyticus;* for complicated UTIs due to *E. coli, Klebsiella pneumoniae, Proteus mirabilis, Pseudomonas aeruginosa, S. epidermidis,* or *Enterobacter cloacae.* Not effective for syphilis.

CONTRAINDICATIONS

Lactation.

SPECIAL CONCERNS
Safety and efficacy have not been determined in children less than 18 years of age. Dosage adjustment is not required in elderly clients with normal renal function. Not efficiently removed by hemodialysis or peritoneal dialysis.

ADDITIONAL SIDE EFFECTS
GI: Anorexia, bloody stools, gastritis, stomatitis. **CNS:** Confusion, nervousness, anxiety, tremor, agitation, myoclonus, depersonalization, hypertonia. **Dermatologic:** ***Toxic epidermal necrolysis, Stevens-Johnson syndrome,*** urticaria, hyperhidrosis, mycotic infection, erythema multiforme. **CV:** Palpitations, tachycardia, vasodilation. **Respiratory:** Dyspnea, cough, epistaxis. **GU:** Vaginal moniliasis, urinary incontinence, renal failure. **Hematologic:** Eosinophilia, leukopenia, increased or decreased platelets, decreased hemoglobin, leukocytosis. **Miscellaneous:** Glucosuria, pyuria, increased or decreased potassium, asthenia, back or chest pain, myalgia, arthralgia, purpura, vertigo, unusual taste, tinnitus, conjunctivitis.

LABORATORY TEST CONSIDERATIONS
↑ ALT, AST, alkaline phosphatase, bilirubin. Proteinuria, albuminuria.

ADDITIONAL DRUG INTERACTIONS
Bismuth subsalicylate / Enoxacin bioavailability is ↓ when bismuth subsalicylate is given within 1 hr; should not use together
Digoxin / ↓ Serum digoxin levels

HOW SUPPLIED
Tablet: 200 mg, 400 mg

DOSAGE

• **TABLETS**

Uncomplicated cervical or urethral gonorrhea.
Adults: 400 mg for one dose.

Uncomplicated UTIs (cystitis).
Adults: 200 mg q 12 hr for 7 days.

Complicated UTIs.
Adults: 400 mg q 12 hr for 14 days.

NURSING CONSIDERATIONS

SEE ALSO *GENERAL NURSING CONSIDERATIONS* FOR *ANTI-INFECTIVES* AND *FLUOROQUINOLONES.*

ADMINISTRATION/STORAGE
Adjust the dose if C_{CR} is 30 mL (or less)/min/1.73 m^2. After a normal initial dose, use a 12-hr interval and one-half the recommended dose.

ASSESSMENT
1. Note any sensitivity to quinolones.
2. Identify source of infection; obtain cultures.
3. List drugs prescribed noting those which utilize the P-450 system; drug may alter metabolism.
4. Obtain CBC, renal and LFTs; reduce dose with renal dysfunction.

CLIENT/FAMILY TEACHING
1. Take only as directed,1 hr before or 2 hr after meals. Report any adverse reactions or lack of response.
2. Increase fluid intake to 2L/day to prevent crystallization.
3. Avoid high intake of alkaline foods (dairy products) and drugs (antacids) or avoid for 2 hrs before drug ingestion.
4. With STDs, inform partners so they can receive treatment to prevent reinfections.
5. May cause photosensitivity reaction; wear sunscreen and avoid exposure.
6. Avoid hazardous activites until drug effects realized; may cause dizziness.

OUTCOMES/EVALUATE
• Resolution of infection
• Relief of pain and burning R/T UTI

Enoxaparin

(ee-**nox**-ah-**PAIR**-in)

PREGNANCY CATEGORY: B
CLASSIFICATION(S):
Anticoagulant, low molecular weight heparin
Rx: Lovenox

SEE ALSO *HEPARINS, LOW MOLECULAR WEIGHT.*

ACTION/KINETICS
t½, elimination: 4.5 hr after SC use. Elimination may be delayed in the elderly. **Duration:** 12 hr following a 40-mg dose. Excreted mainly through the urine.

USES

(1) Acute (in the hospital) and extended (at home for up to three weeks) prophylaxis of DVT, which may lead to pulmonary embolism, after hip or knee replacement surgery or abdominal surgery in those at risk for thromboembolic complications, including severely restricted mobility due to acute illness. (2) With warfarin for inpatient treatment of DVT with and without pulmonary embolism; with warfarin for outpatient treatment of DVT without pulmonary embolism. (3) With aspirin to prevent ischemic complications of unstable angina and non-Q-wave MI. Can be used in geriatric clients. *Investigational:* Systemic anticoagulation, secondary prophylaxis for thromboembolic recurrence.

SIDE EFFECTS

Hematologic: Thrombocytopenia, thrombocythemia, ***hemorrhage,*** hypochromic anemia, ecchymosis. **At Site of Injection:** Mild local irritation, pain, hematoma, erythema. **GI:** Nausea. **CNS:** Confusion. **Miscellaneous:** Fever, pain, edema, peripheral edema, spinal hematoma.

HOW SUPPLIED

Injection: 30 mg/0.3 mL, 40 mg/0.4 mL, 60 mg/0.6 mL, 80 mg/0.8 mL, 90 mg/0.6 mL, 100 mg/1 mL, 120 mg/0.8 mL, 150 mg/mL

DOSAGE

- **SC ONLY**

Prophylaxis of DVT in hip or knee replacement.

Adults: 30 mg b.i.d. with the initial dose given within 12–24 hr after surgery (providing hemostatsis has been established) for 7–10 days (usually), up to 14 days. For hip replacement, a dose of 40 mg once daily may be considered; give 9–15 hr before surgery and continue for 3 weeks.

Prophylaxis of DVT in abdominal surgery.

Adults: 40 mg once daily, with the initial dose given 2 hr prior to surgery. Give for 7–10 days, up to 12 days.

Treatment of DVT/pulmonary embolism for outpatients.

1 mg/kg SC q 12 hr.

Treatment of DVT/pulmonary embolism for inpatients.

1 mg/kg SC q 12 hr or 1.5 mg/kg SC once daily at the same time each day. *NOTE:* For both in- and outpatients, initiate warfarin within 72 hr of enoxaparin. Continue enoxaparin for a minimum of 5 days and until an INR of 2–3 is reached (average duration is 7 days; up to 17 days has been well tolerated).

Unstable angina/Non-Q-wave MI.

1 mg/kg q 12 hr with PO aspirin (100–325 mg once/day). Usual duration for enoxaparin is 2–8 days, up to 12.5 days.

NURSING CONSIDERATIONS

ADMINISTRATION/STORAGE

1. Consider adjusting dose for low weight (< 45 kg) clients and those with a C_{CR} < 30 mL/min.
2. Give only by deep SC when client is lying down; do *not* give IM.
3. Continue treatment throughout the postsurgical period until the risk of DVT has decreased.
4. Do not mix with other injections or infusions.
5. Discard any unused solution.
6. Do *not* interchange (unit for unit) with unfractionated heparin or other low molecular weight heparins.
7. The injection is clear colorless to pale yellow; store at temperatures < 25°C (< 77°F). Do not freeze.

ASSESSMENT

1. Note any history of heparin or pork product sensitivity or disorders that may preclude drug therapy.
2. Document baseline hematologic parameters, liver function, and coagulation studies and monitor. Drug may cause significant, nonsymptomatic increases in SGOT and SGPT.
3. Monitor VS; observe for early S&S of bleeding. Any unexplained fall in hematocrit or BP should lead to a search for a bleeding site.
4. Monitor clients with renal dysfunction and the elderly closely.
5. Report any evidence of a thromboembolic event.

CLIENT/FAMILY TEACHING

1. Lie down during self-administration; use prefilled syringes and administer at the same time each day.
2. Alternate administration between the left and right anterolateral and posterolateral abdominal wall.
3. Introduce the entire length of the needle into a skin fold held between the thumb and forefinger; hold throughout the injection. To minimize bruising, do not rub the site.
4. May experience mild discomfort, irritation, and hematoma at injection site. Report any unusual bruising, bleeding or weakness.
5. Avoid OTC agents that contain aspirin; use electric razor to shave, a soft toothbrush and a nightlight to prevent falls and potential bleeding.

OUTCOMES/EVALUATE

- DVT prophylaxis post surgery
- Thromboembolic occurrence/recurrence prophylaxis

Entacapone

(en-**TAH**-kah-pohn)

PREGNANCY CATEGORY: C
CLASSIFICATION(S):
Antiparkinson drug
Rx: Comtan

ACTION/KINETICS

A selective and reversible catechol-O-methyltransferase (COMT) inhibitor. COMT eliminates catechols (e.g., dopa, dopamine, norepinephrine, epinephrine) and in the presence of a decarboxylase inhibitor (e.g., carbidopa), COMT becomes the major metabolizing enzyme for dopa. Thus, in the presence of a COMT inhibitor, levels of dopa and dopamine increase. When entacapone is given with levodopa and carbidopa, plasma levels of levodopa are greater and more sustained than after levodopa/carbidopa alone. This leads to more constant dopaminergic stimulation in the brain resulting in improvement of the signs and symptoms of Parkinson's disease. Rapidly absorbed. High plasma protein binding (98%). Almost completely metabolized in the liver with most excreted in the feces. **$t^{1/2}$, elimination:** Biphasic 0.4–0.7 hr and 2.4 hr.

USES

As an adjunct to levodopa/carbidopa to treat idiopathic Parkinsonism clients who experience signs and symptoms of end-of-dose "wearing-off."

CONTRAINDICATIONS

Concomitant use with a nonselective MAO inhibitor (e.g., phenelzine, tranylcypromine).

SPECIAL CONCERNS

Use with caution during lactation and in clients with biliary obstruction. At the present, there is no potential use in children. Use with caution with drugs known to be metabolized by COMT (e.g., apomorphine, bitolterol, dobutamine, dopamine, epinephrine, isoetharine, isoproterenol, methyldopa, norepinephrine) due to the possibility of increased HR, arrhythmias, and excessive changes in BP.

SIDE EFFECTS

CNS: Dyskinesia, hyperkinesia, hypokinesia, dizziness, anxiety, somnolence, agitation, hallucinations. **GI:** Nausea, diarrhea, abdominal pain, constipation, vomiting, dry mouth, dyspepsia, flatulence, gastritis, GI disorder. **Body as a whole:** Fatigue, asthenia, increased sweating, bacterial infection. **Miscellaneous:** Urine discoloration, back pain, dsypnea, purpura, taste perversion, rhabdomyolysis.

OD OVERDOSE MANAGEMENT

Symptoms: Abdominal pain, loose stools. *Treatment:* Symptomatic with supportive care. Consider hospitalization. Monitor respiratory and circulatory systems. Review for possible drug interactions.

DRUG INTERACTIONS

Ampicillin / ↓ Entacapone biliary excretion
Apomorphine / Possible ↑ HR, arrhythmias, and excessive BP changes
Bitolterol / Possible ↑ HR, arrhythmias, and excessive BP changes
Chloramphenicol / ↓ Entacapone biliary excretion
Cholestyramine / ↓ Entacapone biliary excretion
Dobutamine / Possible ↑ HR, arrhythmias, and excessive BP changes

Dopamine / Possible ↑ HR, arrhythmias, and excessive BP changes
Epinephrine / Possible ↑ HR, arrhythmias, and excessive BP changes
Erythromycin / ↓ Entacapone biliary excretion
Isoetharine / Possible ↑ HR, arrhythmias, and excessive BP changes
Isoproterenol / Possible ↑ HR, arrhythmias, and excessive BP changes
MAO inhibitors (phenelzine, tranylcypromine) / Significant ↑ levels of catecholamines
Methyldopa / Possible ↑ HR, arrhythmias, and excessive BP changes
Norepinephrine / Possible ↑ HR, arrhythmias, and excessive BP changes
Probenecid / ↓ Entacapone biliary excretion
Rifampicin / ↓ Entacapone biliary excretion

HOW SUPPLIED

Tablets: 200 mg

DOSAGE

- **TABLETS**

Parkinsonism.

200 mg given concomitantly with each levodopa/carbidopa dose up to a maximum of 8 times/day (i.e., 1,600 mg/day).

NURSING CONSIDERATIONS

ADMINISTRATION/STORAGE

1. Always give entacapone in combination with levodopa/carbidopa; entacapone has no antiparkinson effect by itself.
2. Most clients required a decreased daily levodopa dose (about 25%) if their daily levodopa dose was 800 mg or more, or if they had moderate or severe dyskinesias prior to entacapone treatment.
3. Entacapone can be given with either immediate- or sustained-release levodopa/carbidopa formulations.
4. Rapid withdrawal or abrupt reduction in the entacapone dose can lead to emergence of S&S of Parkinsonism and could lead to a complex resembling neuroleptic malignant syndrome (hyperpyrexia and confusion).
5. If necessary to discontinue treatment, withdraw clients slowly from entacapone.

ASSESSMENT

1. Note onset of Parkinson's disease, levodopa/carbidopa dosage, and when symtoms occur in dosage cycle.
2. Determine any evidence of liver or biliary dysfunction.
3. List drugs prescribed to ensure none interact.

CLIENT/FAMILY TEACHING

1. Take as directed with levodopa/carbidopa.
2. Drug is used to prevent end-of-dose "wearing off" effects of Sinemet; alone it has no antiparkinson effect.
3. Never stop abruptly! Report any high fever or rigidity immediately.
4. Do not perform activities that require mental or physical alertness until drug effects realized.
5. May experience syncope, nausea, diarrhea, hallucinations, increase in dyskinesia, altered pulmonary or kidney function. Report if bothersome or persistent.
6. Urine may appear brownish-orange in color.
7. Rise slowly from a sitting or lying position to prevent postural hypotension or syncope.
8. Drug is not for use during pregnancy or breastfeeding. Report if pregnancy suspected or desired.

OUTCOMES/EVALUATE

Improved control of Parkinson's disease i.e.; ↓ stiffness, tremor and shuffling; ↑ coordination

Ephedrine sulfate

(eh-**FED**-rin)

PREGNANCY CATEGORY: C
CLASSIFICATION(S):

Sympathomimetic, direct- and indirect-acting
Rx: Systemic: Ephedrine Sulfate (Injection)
OTC: Systemic: Ephedrine Sulfate (oral dosage forms), **Nasal Decongestants:** Kondon's Nasal, Pretz-D

SEE ALSO *SYMPATHOMIMETIC DRUGS.*

ACTION/KINETICS

Releases norepinephrine from synaptic storage sites. Has direct effects on alpha, beta-1, and beta-2 receptors, causing increased BP due to arteriolar constriction and cardiac stimulation, bronchodilation, relaxation of GI tract smooth muscle, nasal decongestion, mydriasis, and increased tone of the bladder trigone and vesicle sphincter. It may also increase skeletal muscle strength, especially in myasthenia clients. Significant CNS effects include stimulation of the cerebral cortex and subcortical centers. Hepatic glycogenolysis is increased, but not as much as with epinephrine. More stable and longer-lasting than epinephrine. Rapidly and completely absorbed following parenteral use. **Onset, IM:** 10–20 min; **PO:** 15–60 min; **SC:** > 20 min. **Duration, IM, SC:** 30–60 min; **PO:** 3–5 hr. **t½, elimination:** About 3 hr when urine is at a pH of 5 and about 6 hr when urinary pH is 6.3. Excreted mostly unchanged through the urine (rate dependent on urinary pH—increased in acid urine).

USES

PO: Temporary relief of shortness of breath, tightness of chest, and wheezing due to bronchial asthma. **Parenteral:** Allergic disorders, including bronchial asthma. Vasopressor in shock. **Nasal:** Nasal congestion in vasomotor rhinitis, acute sinusitis, hay fever, and acute coryza.

ADDITIONAL CONTRAINDICATIONS

Angle closure glaucoma, anesthesia with cyclopropane or halothane, thyrotoxicosis, diabetes, obstetrics where maternal BP is greater than 130/80. Lactation.

SPECIAL CONCERNS

Geriatric clients may be at higher risk to develop prostatic hypertrophy. May cause hypertension resulting in intracranial hemorrhage or anginal pain in clients with coronary insufficiency or ischemic heart disease.

ADDITIONAL SIDE EFFECTS

CNS: Nervousness, shakiness, confusion, delirium, hallucinations. Anxiety and nervousness following prolonged use. **CV:** Precordial pain, ***excessive doses may cause hypertension sufficient to result in cerebral hemorrhage***. **GU:** Difficult and painful urination, urinary retention in males with prostatism, decrease in urine formation. **Miscellaneous:** Pallor, respiratory difficulty, hypersensitivity reactions. **Abuse:** Prolonged abuse can cause an anxiety state, including symptoms of paranoid schizophrenia, tachycardia, poor nutrition and hygiene, dilated pupils, cold sweat, and fever.

ADDITIONAL DRUG INTERACTIONS

Alpha-adrenergic blockers / Antagonism of vasoconstricting and hypertensive effects of ephedrine

Dexamethasone / ↓ Dexamethasone effect

Diuretics / Diuretics ↓ response to sympathomimetics

Furazolidone / ↑ Pressor effect → possible hypertensive crisis and intracranial hemorrhage

Guanethidine / ↓ Guanethidine effect by displacement from its action site

Halothane / Serious arrhythmias R/T sensitization of myocardium to sympathomimetics by halothane

MAO Inhibitors / ↑ Pressor effect → possible hypertensive crisis and intracranial hemorrhage

Methyldopa / Effect of ephedrine ↓ in methyldopa-treated clients

Oxytocic drugs / Severe persistent hypertension

HOW SUPPLIED

Capsule: 25 mg; *Injection:* 50 mg/mL; *Jelly:* 1%; *Spray:* 0.25%

DOSAGE

• **CAPSULES**

Bronchial asthma, systemic nasal decongestant.

Adults and children over 12 years of age: 12.5–25 mg 4 hr, not to exceed 150 mg in 24 hr. **Pediatric, under 12 years:** Consult a provider.

• **SC, IM, SLOW IV**

Bronchial asthma.

Adults: 25–50 mg SC or IM; or, 5–25 mg by slow IV repeated q 5–10 min, if needed. **Children:** 0.5 mg/kg or 16.7 mg/m[2] SC or IM q 4–6 hr.

Vasopressor.

Adults: 25–50 mg (IM or SC) or 5–25 mg (by slow IV push) repeated at 5- to 10-min intervals, if necessary. Absorption following IM is more rapid than following SC use. **Pediatric (IM):** 16.7 mg/m² q 4–6 hr.

• **TOPICAL (1% JELLY, 0.25% SPRAY)** *Nasal decongestant.*

Adults and children over 6 years: 2–3 gtt of solution or small amount of jelly in each nostril q 4 hr. Do not use topically for more than 3 or 4 consecutive days. Do not use in children under 6 years of age unless ordered by provider.

NURSING CONSIDERATIONS

SEE ALSO *NURSING CONSIDERATIONS* FOR *SYMPATHOMIMETIC DRUGS.*

ADMINISTRATION/STORAGE

1. Tolerance may develop; however, temporary cessation of therapy restores the original drug response.

IV 2. May administer 10 mg IV undiluted over at least 1 min.

3. Use only clear solutions and discard any unused solution with IV therapy. Protect against exposure to light; drug is subject to oxidation.

ASSESSMENT

1. Document indications for therapy, type and symptom characteristics.
2. Assess mental status and pulmonary function; monitor ECG and VS. If administered for hypotension, monitor BP until stabilized.
3. If used for prolonged periods, assess for drug resistance. Rest without medication for 3–4 days, then resume to regain response.

CLIENT/FAMILY TEACHING

1. Notify provider if SOB is unrelieved by medication and accompanied by chest pain, dizziness, or palpitations. Report any elevated or irregular pulse.
2. With males, report any difficulty or pain with voiding; may be drug-induced urinary retention.
3. Report any signs of depression, lack of interest in personal appearance, or complaints of insomnia or anorexia.
4. Avoid OTC drugs and alcohol.

OUTCOMES/EVALUATE

- Improved airway exchange
- ↓ Nasal congestion/mucus
- ↑ BP
- Control of narcolepsy

Epinephrine

(ep-ih-**NEF**-rin)

PREGNANCY CATEGORY: C
Rx: Adrenalin Chloride Solution, Ana-Guard, Epifrin, Sus-Phrine
OTC: Primatene Mist Solution

Epinephrine bitartrate

(ep-ih-**NEF**-rin)

PREGNANCY CATEGORY: C
OTC: Asthmahaler Mist

Epinephrine borate

(ep-ih-**NEF**-rin)

PREGNANCY CATEGORY: C
Rx: Epinal Ophthalmic Solution

Epinephrine hydrochloride

(ep-ih-**NEF**-rin)

PREGNANCY CATEGORY: C
Rx: AsthmaNefrin, Epinephrine Pediatric, Epipen, Epipen Jr., Glaucon, microNefrin, Nephron , Adrenalin Chloride
★**Rx:** Vaponefrin
OTC: S-2 Inhalant
CLASSIFICATION(S):
Sympathomimetic, direct-acting

SEE ALSO *SYMPATHOMIMETIC DRUGS.*

ACTION/KINETICS

Causes marked stimulation of alpha, beta-1, and beta-2 receptors, causing sympathomimetic stimulation, pressor effects, cardiac stimulation, bronchodilation, and decongestion. It crosses the placenta but not the blood-brain barrier. **Extreme caution must be taken never to inject 1:100 solution intended for inhalation—injection of this concentration has caused death. SC: Onset,** 5–10 min; **duration:** 4–6 hr. **Inhalation: Onset,** 1–5 min; **duration:** 1–3 hr. **IM, Onset:** variable; duration: 1–4 hr. Ineffective when given PO.

USES

Inhalation: (1) Temporary relief of shortness of breath, tightness of chest, and wheezing due to bronchial asthma. (2) Postintubation and infectious coup. (3) MicroNefrin is used for chronic obstructive lung disease, chronic bronchitis, broncheolitis, bronchial asthma, and other peripheral airway diseases.

Injection: (1) Relieve respiratory distress in bronchial asthma, during acute asthma attacks, and for reversible bronchospasm in chronic bronchitis, emphysema, and other obstructive pulmonary diseases. (2) Severe acute anaphylactic reactions, including anaphylactic shock and cardiac arrest, to restore cardiac rhythm. (3) Allergic reactions caused by bees, wasps, hornets, yellow jackets, bumble bees, and fire ants; severe allergic reactions or anaphylaxis caused by allergy injections; allergic reactions due to exposure to pollens, dusts, molds, foods, drugs, and exercise. (4) Severe, life-threatening asthma attacks with wheezing, dyspnea, and inability to breathe. (5) Vasopressor in shock. (6) Infiltration of tissue to delay absorption of drugs, including local anesthetics.

Ophthalmic: (1) Hemostatic during ocular surgery; treatment of conjunctival congestion during surgery; to induce mydriasis during surgery; treat ocular hypertension during surgery. (2) Adjunct in the treatment of open-angle glaucoma (may be used with miotics, beta blockers, hyperosmotic agents, or carbonic anhydrase inhibitors). (3) To produce mydriasis; to treat conjunctivitis.

Topical: Control bleeding.

NOTE: Autoinjectors are available for emergency self-administration of first aid for anaphylactic reactions due to insect stings or bites, foods, drugs, and other allergens as well as idiopathic or exercise-induced anaphylaxis.

ADDITIONAL CONTRAINDICATIONS

Narrow-angle glaucoma. Use when wearing soft contact lenses (may discolor lenses). Aphakia. Lactation.

SPECIAL CONCERNS

May cause anoxia in the fetus. Safety and efficacy of ophthalmic products have not been determined in children; administer parenteral epinephrine to children with caution. Syncope may occur if epinephrine is given to asthmatic children. Administration of the SC injection by the IV route may cause severe or fatal hypertension or cerebrovascular hemorrhage. Epinephrine may temporarily increase the rigidity and tremor of parkinsonism. Use with caution and in small quantities in the toes, fingers, nose, ears, and genitals or in the presence of peripheral vascular disease as vasoconstriction-induced tissue sloughing may occur.

ADDITIONAL SIDE EFFECTS

CV: ***Fatal ventricular fibrillation, cerebral or subarachnoid hemorrhage,*** obstruction of central retinal artery. ***A rapid and large increase in BP may cause aortic rupture, cerebral hemorrhage, or angina pectoris.*** **GU:** Decreased urine formation, urinary retention, painful urination. **CNS:** Anxiety, fear, pallor. Parenteral use may cause or aggravate disorientation, memory impairment, psychomotor agitation, panic, hallucinations, ***suicidal or homicidal tendencies,*** schizophrenic-type behavior. **Miscellaneous:** Prolonged use or overdose may cause elevated serum lactic acid with severe metabolic acidosis. **At injection site:** Bleeding, urticaria, wheal formation, pain. Repeated injections at the same site may cause necrosis from vascular constriction. **Ophthalmic:** Transient stinging or burning when administered, conjunctival hyperemia, brow ache, headache, blurred vision, photophobia, allergic lid reaction, ocular hypersensitivity, poor night vision, eye ache, eye pain. Prolonged ophthalmic use may cause deposits of pigment in the cornea, lids, or conjunctiva. When used for glaucoma in aphakic clients, reversible cystoid macular edema.

LABORATORY TEST CONSIDERATIONS

False + or ↑ BUN, fasting glucose, lactic acid, urinary catecholamines, glucose

(Benedict's). ↓ Coagulation time. The drug may affect electrolyte balance.

ADDITIONAL DRUG INTERACTIONS

Alpha-adrenergic blocking agents / Antagonism of vasocontricting and hypertensive effects

Antihistamines / Epinephrine effects potentiated

Beta-adrenergic blocking agents / Possible initial hypertension followed by bradycardia

Diuretics / ↓ Vascular response

Ergot alkaloids / Reversal of epinephrine pressor effects

General anesthetics (halothane, cyclopropane) / ↑ Sensitivity of myocardium to epinephrine → arrhythmias

Levothyroxine / Potentiation of epinephrine effects

Nitrites / Reversal of epinephrine pressor effects

Phenothiazines / Reversal of epinephrine pressor effects

HOW SUPPLIED

Epinephrine: *Aerosol:* 0.2 mg/inh; *Injection:* 1:200 (5 mg/mL), 1:1000 (1 mg/mL), 1:10,000 (0.1 mg/mL); *Kit:* 0.5 mg/mL, 1 mg/mL; *Solution, Topical:* 0.1%, 0.5%, 1%, 2%; *Solution for Inhalation (Racenephrine HCl):* 2.25%. **Epinephrine bitartrate:** *Metered dose inhaler:* 0.35 mg/inh. **Epinephrine borate:** *Solution:* 0.5%, 1%. **Epinephrine hydrochloride:** *Injection:* 1:1000 (1 mg/mL), 1:2000 (0.5 mg/mL), 1:10,000 (0.1 mg/mL as HCl), 1:100,000 (0.01 mg/mL as HCl); *Nasal Solution:* 0.1%; *Solution for Inhalation:* 1:100, 1:1000; *Ophthalmic solution:* 0.5%, 1%, 2%

DOSAGE

• **NEBULIZATION**

Bronchodilation.

Adults and children 4 years and older (for AsthmaNefrin, 12 years and older). *Hand pump nebulizer:* 0.5 mL (about 8–10 drops) of racemic epinephrine placed into the reservoir. Place the nebulizer nozzle into the partially opened mouth and squeeze the bulb 1–3 times. Inhale deeply. Give 2–3 additional inhalations if relief does not occur within 2–3 min. Can use 4–6 times/day but no more often than q 3 hr. *Aerosol nebulizer:* Add 0.5 mL (about 10 drops) of racemic epinephrine to 3 mL of diluent or 0.2–4 mL (about 4–8 drops) of MicroNefrin to 4.6–4.8 mL water. Give for 15 min q 3–4 hr.

• **SC, IM**

Bronchodilation

Adults, initial: 0.2–1 mL (0.2–1 mg) of the 1:1000 solution SC or IM q 4 hr. **Infants and children (except premature infants and full-term newborns):** 0.01 mL/kg or 0.3 mL/m² (0.1 mg/kg or 0.3 mg/m²) SC. Do not exceed 0.5 mL (0.5 mg) in a single pediatric dose. Can repeat q 20 min to 4 hr, if necessary.

The dose of Ana-Guard is as follows. **Adults and children over 12 years:** 0.3 mL; **6–12 years old:** 0.2 mL; **2–6 years old:** 0.15 mL; **infants to 2 years old:** 0.05–0.1 mL. Give a second dose after 10 min if symptoms are not noticeably improved.

• **IV**

Bronchodilation, hypersensitivity reactions.

Adults: 0.1–0.25 mg (1–2.5 mL) of the 1:10,000 solution injected slowly. **Infants:** 0.05 mg; may be repeated at 20–30 min intervals to manage asthma attacks. **Neonates:** 0.01 mg/kg. *NOTE:* If the client is intubated, the IV dose of epinephrine can be given via the endotracheal tube directly into the bronchial tree as it is rapidly absorbed through the lung capillary bed.

• **SC ONLY, 1:200 SUSPENSION**

Bronchodilation.

Adults: 0.1–0.3 mL (0.5–1.5 mg). **Children, less than 30 kg:** Maximum single dose is 0.15 mL (0.75 mg). **Infants and children, 1 month to 12 years old:** 0.005 mg/kg (0.025 mg/kg).

• **AUTOINJECTOR, IM**

First aid for anaphylaxis.

The autoinjectors deliver a single dose of either 0.3 mg or 0.15 mg (for children) of epinephrine. In cases of a severe reaction; repeat injections may be necessary.

Vasopressor.

Adults, IM or SC, initial: 0.5 mg repeated q 5 min if needed; **then,** give

0.025–0.050 mg IV q 5–15 min as needed. **Adults, IV, initial:** 0.1–0.25 mg given slowly. May be repeated q 5–15 min as needed. Or, use IV infusion beginning with 0.001 mg/min and increasing the dose to 0.004 mg/min if needed. **Pediatric, IM, SC:** 0.01 mg/kg, up to a maximum of 0.3 mg repeated q 5 min if needed. **Pediatric, IV:** 0.01 mg/kg/5–15 min if an inadequate response to IM or SC administration is observed.

Cardiac stimulant.

Adults, intracardiac or IV: 0.1–1 mg repeated q 5 min if needed. **Pediatric, intracardiac or IV:** 0.005–0.01 mg/kg (0.15–0.3 mg/m^2) repeated q 5 min if needed; this may be followed by IV infusion beginning at 0.0001 mg/kg/min and increased in increments of 0.0001 mg/kg/min up to a maximum of 0.0015 mg/kg/min.

Adjunct to local anesthesia.

Adults and children: 0.1–0.2 mg in a 1:200,000–1:20,000 solution.

Adjunct with intraspinal anesthetics.

Adults: 0.2–0.4 mg added to the anesthetic spinal fluid.

• **SOLUTION**

Antihemorrhagic, mydriatic.

Adults and children, intracameral or subconjunctival: 0.01%–0.1% solution.

Topical antihemorrhagic.

Adults and children: 0.002%–0.1% solution.

Nasal decongestant.

Adults and children over 6 years of age: Apply 0.1% solution as drops or spray or with a sterile swab as needed.

• **BORATE OPHTHALMIC SOLUTION, HYDROCHLORIDE OPHTHALMIC SOLUTION**

Glaucoma.

Adults: 1–2 gtt into affected eye(s) 1–2 times/day. Determine frequency of use by tonometry. Dosage has not been established in children.

NURSING CONSIDERATIONS

SEE ALSO *NURSING CONSIDERATIONS* FOR *SYMPATHOMIMETIC DRUGS*.

ADMINISTRATION/STORAGE

1. Briskly massage site of SC or IM injection to hasten drug action. Do not expose to heat, light, or air, as this causes deterioration of the drug.
2. Discard solution if reddish brown and after expiration date.
3. With sodium bisulfite as a preservative in the topical preparation, there may be slight stinging after administration.
4. Do not use the topical preparation in children under 6 years of age.
5. Ophthalmic use may result in discomfort, which decreases over time.
6. The ophthalmic preparation is not for injection.
7. If the ophthalmic glaucoma product is used with a miotic, instill miotic 2-10 min prior.
8. Keep the ophthalmic product tightly sealed and protected from light. Store at 2–4°C (36–75°F). Discard solution if it becomes discolored or contains a precipitate.
9. IV *Never administer* 1:100 solution IV, use the 1:1,000 solution.
10. Use a tuberculin syringe to measure; parenteral doses are small and drug is potent, errors in measurement may be disastrous.
11. For direct IV administration to adults, the drug must be well diluted as a 1:1,000 solution; inject quantities of 0.05–0.1 mL of solution cautiously taking about 1 min for each injection; note response (BP and pulse). Dose may be repeated several times if necessary. May be further diluted in D5W or NSS.

ASSESSMENT

1. Assess for sulfite sensitivity.
2. Document indications for therapy; describe type/onset of symptoms and anticipated results.
3. Assess cardiopulmonary function.
4. During IV therapy, continuously monitor ECG, BP, and pulse until desired effect achieved. Then take VS every 2–5 min until stabilized; once stable, monitor BP q 15–30 min.
5. Note any symptoms of shock such as cold, clammy skin, cyanosis, and loss of consciousness.

CLIENT/FAMILY TEACHING

1. Review method for administration carefully. When prescribed for anaphylaxis, administer autoinjector immedi-

ately and then seek further medical care.
2. Report any increased restlessness, chest pain, or insomnia as dosage adjustment may be necessary. May elevate blood sugar.
3. Limit intake of caffeine, as with colas, coffee, tea, and chocolate; avoid OTC drugs without approval.
4. Rinse mouth after MDI use.
5. Nasal application may sting slightly. Ophthalmic solution may burn initially and a brow/headache may occur; this should subside. Remove contact lens; may stain lens.
6. Use caution when performing activities that require careful vision; ophthalmic solution may diminish visual fields, cause double vision, and alter night vision.
7. Nasal OTC products may work initially but with prolonged use exacerbate symptoms.
8. Discard any discolored or precipitated solutions.

OUTCOMES/EVALUATE

- Restoration of cardiac activity
- Improved CO with EC bypass
- ↓ IOP
- Reversal of S&S of anaphylaxis
- Improved airway exchange
- Hemostasis with ocular surgery

Epirubicin hydrochloride

(ep-ee-**ROO**-bih-sin)

PREGNANCY CATEGORY: D
CLASSIFICATION(S):
Antineoplastic, antibiotic
Rx: Ellence
🍁**Rx:** Pharmorubicin PFS, Pharmorubicin RDF

SEE ALSO *ANTINEOPLASTIC AGENTS.*

ACTION/KINETICS

Cell cycle phase nonspecific anthracycline; has maximum cytotoxic effects on the S and G_2 phases. Precise mechanism of action is not known. It does form a complex with DNA by intercalation of its planar rings between nucleotide base pairs resulting in inhibition of DNA and RNA synthesis. Intercalation triggers DNA cleavage by topoisomerase II, resulting in cell death. The drug also inhibits DNA helicase activity which prevents enzymatic separation of double-stranded DNA and interferes with replication and transcription. The drug is also involved in oxidation-reduction reactions by generating cytotoxic free radicals. Following IV, it is rapidly and widely distributed; appears to concentrate in RBCs. Extensively and rapidly metabolized by the liver and RBCs. Parent drug and metabolites are excreted through both the feces and urine. **t½:** Triphasic with half-lives of about 3 min, 2.5 hr, and 33 hr.

USES

Adjunct to treat breast cancer in clients with evidence of axillary node tumor involvement after resection of primary breast cancer.

CONTRAINDICATIONS

Severe hepatic dysfunction; previous anthracycline treatment up to the maximum cumulative dose; severe myocardial insufficiency or recent MI; hypersensitivity to epirubicin, other anthracyclines, or anthracenediones; baseline neutrophil count < 1500 cells/mm³. Lactation.

SPECIAL CONCERNS

Use of epirubicin after previous radiation therapy may cause an inflammatory recall reaction at the site of irradiation. When used in combination with other cytotoxic drugs, additive hematologic and GI toxicity may occur. Safety and efficacy have not been determined in pediatric clients.

SIDE EFFECTS

GI: N&V, mucositis (oral stomatitis, esophagitis), diarrhea, anorexia. **CV: CHF**, sinus tachycardia, nonspecific ST-T wave changes, PVCs, ventricular tachycardia, bradycardia, AV and bundle branch block. **Dermatologic:** Alopecia, local toxicity, rash, itch, skin changes, flushes, skin and nail hyperpigmentation, photosensitivity, hypersensitivity to irradiated skin, urticaria, ***anaphylaxis***. **Hematologic:** Leukopenia, neutropenia, anemia, thrombocytopenia, secondary acute myelogenous leukemia, acute lymphoid leukemia. **Endocrine:** Amenorrhea, hot flashes. **Miscellaneous:** Lethargy, infection, febrile neutropenia, fever, conjunctivitis/keratitis, tumor lysis syndrome, injection site reactions (venous sclerosis, local pain, severe tissue lesions, necrosis).

E

DRUG INTERACTIONS

Cimetidine ↑ epirubicin blood levels by 50%; stop cimetidine therapy during use of epirubicin.

HOW SUPPLIED

Injection: 2 mg/mL

DOSAGE

• IV INFUSION

Breast cancer with evidence of axillary node tumor.

The following regimens are recommended: (1) Epirubicin, 100 mg/m²; 5-Fluorouracil, 500 mg/m²; and Cyclophosphamide, 500 mg/m². All drugs are given on day 1 and repeated q 21 days for 6 cycles. Clients are also given prophylactic antibiotic therapy with trimethoprim-sulfamethoxazole or fluoroquinolone. (2) Epirubicin, 60 mg/m² on days 1 and 8; 5-Fluorouracil, 500 mg/m² on days 1 and 8; and Cyclophosphamide, 75 mg/m² PO on days 1 and 14. The regimen is repeated q 28 days for 6 cycles.

NURSING CONSIDERATIONS

SEE ALSO *NURSING CONSIDERATIONS* FOR *ANTINEOPLASTIC AGENTS*.

ADMINISTRATION/STORAGE

1. Make dosage adjustments after the first treatment cycle based on hematologic and nonhematologic toxicity as follows:

• Reduce the day 1 dose in subsequent cycles to 75% of the day 1 dose given in the current cycle in clients experiencing cycle nadir platelet counts < 50,000/mm³, absolute neutrophil counts (ANC) < 250/mm³, neutropenic fever, or Grades 3/4 nonhematologic toxicity. Delay day 1 chemotherapy in subsequent courses of treatment until platelet counts are 100,000/mm³ or more, ANC is 1500/mm³ or more, and nonhematologic toxicities have recovered to Grade 1 or less.

• For clients receiving a divided dose of epirubicin on days 1 and 8, reduce the day 8 dose to 75% of day 1 if platelet counts are 75,000–100,000/mm³ and ANC is 1000–1499/mm³. Omit the day 8 dose, if day 8 platelet counts are < 75,000/mm³, ANC is < 1000/mm³, or Grade 3/4 nonhematologic toxicity has occurred.

2. Consider a lower starting dose (75–90 mg/m²) of epirubicin for heavily pretreated clients, those with preexisting bone marrow depression, or in the presence of neoplastic bone marrow infiltration.

3. For clients with elevated serum AST or serum total bilirubin levels, consider the following doses of epirubicin:

• Bilirubin, 1.2–3 mg/dL, or AST, 2–4 times ULN, give one-half the recommended starting dose.

• Bilirubin, > 3 mg/dL or AST > 4 times ULN, give one-fourth the recommended starting dose.

4. Consider lower doses of epirubicin in clients with severe renal impairment (serum creatinine > 5 mg/dL).

5. Clients given 120 mg/m² of epirubicin as part of combination therapy should receive prophylactic antibiotic therapy with a fluoroquinolone or trimethoprim-sulfamethoxazole.

6. Consider prophylactic use of antiemetics to reduce N&V, especially if epirubicin is given with other emetogenic drugs.

IV 7. Do not mix epirubicin with heparin or fluorouracil due to chemical incompatibility that may cause precipitation.

8. Avoid prolonged contact with any alkaline solution; hydrolysis of the drug will occur.

9. The solution is manufactured preservative-free and as a ready-to-use solution. Give over a 3–5 min period into the tubing of a freely flowing IV infusion (0.9% NaCl or D5W). Do not use a direct push injection due to the possbility of extravasation

10. Use within 24 hr of first penetration of the rubber stopper.

ASSESSMENT

1. Note disease onset, symptom characteristics, other medical conditions and other agents trialed.
2. Obtain baseline CBC, renal, LFTs, and LVEF; monitor carefully for anthracyline-induced cardiomyopathy by ECHO or MUGA determination of LVEF during therapy.
3. Assess IV site carefully; venous sclerosis at injection site or extravasation may occur which may cause pain and tissue necrosis. Give slowly over 3-5 min to prevent facial flushing or erythematous streaking along vein.
4. Give antiemetics 30-60 min before therapy to diminish N&V.
5. With 120 mg/m^2 regimen in combination therapy, also give ATX prophylaxis with trimethoprim-sulfamethoxazole or fluoroquinolone.
6. Lower dose with hematologic, renal or liver dysfunction. Follow dosing guidelines carefully.

CLIENT/FAMILY TEACHING

1. Therapy is usually given once every three weeks for 6 cycles for node positive resectable primary breast cancer.
2. May experience N&V, diarrhea, hair loss, and stomatitis.
3. Understand that there is a risk of irreversible myocardial damage and treatment related leukemia; need frequent echo or MUGA scans and blood work.
4. Report any increased SOB, lower extremity edema, vomiting, dehydration, fever, infection or injection site pain after therapy.
5. Urine may be red for several days after therapy; not worrisome.
6. If platelet counts, white count or nonhematologic toxicities occur the dosage will be reduced with the next dose or discontinued if prolonged.
7. Practice reliable birth control; men may experience chromosomal sperm damage and women may develop premature menopause or irreversible amenorrhea. Determine if sperm/egg harvesting indicated.
8. Avoid tagamet or cimetidine during therapy.
9. Avoid crowds, and persons with known infections as well as vaccinations during therapy.

OUTCOMES/EVALUATE

Control of malignant cell proliferation in breast cancer

Epoetin alfa recombinant

(ee-**POH**-ee-tin)

PREGNANCY CATEGORY: C
CLASSIFICATION(S):
Erythropoietin, human recombinant
Rx: Epogen, Procrit
✱**Rx:** Eprex

ACTION/KINETICS

A 165-amino-acid glycoprotein made by recombinant DNA technology; it has the identical amino acid sequence and same biologic effects as endogenous erythropoietin (which is normally synthesized in the kidney and stimulates RBC production). Epoetin alfa will elevate or maintain the RBC level, decreasing the need for blood transfusions. **t½:** 4–13 hr in clients with chronic renal failure. **Peak serum levels after SC:** 5–24 hr.

USES

(1) Treatment of anemia associated with chronic renal failure in adults and children, including clients on dialysis (end-stage renal disease) or adults not on dialysis. (2) Zidovudine-induced anemia in HIV-infected clients. (3) Treatment of anemia in clients with nonmyeloid malignancies (Procrit only). (4) Reduce allogeneic blood transfusions in surgery clients. *Investigational:* Pruritus associated with renal failure.

CONTRAINDICATIONS

Uncontrolled hypertension. Hypersensitivity to mammalian cell-derived products or to human albumin. Use in chronic renal failure clients who need severe anemia corrected. To treat anemia in HIV-infected or cancer clients due to factors such as iron or folate deficiences, hemolysis, or GI bleeding.

Anemic clients willing to donate autologous blood.

SPECIAL CONCERNS

Safety and efficacy have not been established in children or in clients with a history of seizures or underlying hematologic disease (e.g., hypercoagulable disorders, myelodysplastic syndromes, sickle cell anemia). Use with caution in clients with porphyria, during lactation, and preexisting vascular disease. Increased anticoagulation with heparin may be required in clients on epoetin alfa undergoing hemodialysis.

SIDE EFFECTS

In Chronic Renal Failure Clients (symptoms may be due to the disease).

CV: Hypertension, tachycardia, edema, ***MI, CV accident,*** TIA, clotted vascular access. **CNS:** Headache, fatigue, dizziness, ***seizures.*** **GI:** Nausea, diarrhea, vomiting, worsening of porphyria. **Allergic reactions:** Skin rashes, urticaria, ***anaphylaxis.*** **Miscellaneous:** SOB, hyperkalemia, arthralgias, myalgia, chest pain, skin reaction at administration site, asthenia.

In Zidovudine-Treated HIV-Infected Clients.

CNS: Pyrexia, fatigue, headache, dizziness, ***seizures.*** **Respiratory:** Cough, respiratory congestion, SOB. **GI:** Diarrhea, nausea. **Miscellaneous:** Rash, asthenia, reaction at injection site, allergic reactions.

In Cancer Clients.

CNS: Pyrexia, fatigue, dizziness. **GI:** Diarrhea, nausea, vomiting. **Musculoskeletal:** Asthenia, paresthesia, trunk pain. **Miscellaneous:** Edema, SOB, URI.

In Surgery Clients.

CNS: Pyrexia, insomnia, headache, dizziness, anxiety. **GI:** N&V, constipation, diarrhea, dyspepsia. **CV:** Hypertension, DVT, edema. **Miscellaneous:** Reaction at injection site, skin pain, pruritus, UTI.

OD OVERDOSE MANAGEMENT

Symptoms: Polycythemia. *Treatment:* Withhold drug until hematocrit returns to the target range.

HOW SUPPLIED

Injection: 2,000 U/mL, 3,000 U/mL, 4,000 U/mL, 10,000 U/mL, 20,000 U/mL

DOSAGE

• IV, SC

Chronic renal failure.

IV, initial (dialysis or nondialysis clients), SC (nondialysis clients), initial, adults: 50–100 U/kg 3 times/week. The rate of increase of hematocrit depends on both dosage and client variation. **Maintenance:** Individualize (usual: 25 U/kg 3 times/week). However, doses of 75–150 U/kg/week have maintained hematocrits of 36%–38% for up to 6 months in nondialysis clients.The median dose to achieve a hematocrit of 30%–36% in children on dialysis is 167units/kg/week.

Zidovudine-treated, HIV infections.

IV, SC, initial: 100 U/kg 3 times/week for 8 weeks (in clients with serum erythropoietin levels less than or equal to 500 mU/mL who are receiving less than or equal to 4,200 mg/week of Zidovudine). If a satisfactory response is obtained, the dose can be increased by 50–100 U/kg 3 times/week. Evaluate the response q 4–8 weeks thereafter with dosage adjusted by 50–100 U/kg increments 3 times/week. If clients have not responded to 300 U/kg 3 times/week, it is not likely they will respond to higher doses.

Cancer clients on chemotherapy (Procrit only).

Initial, SC: 150 units/kg 3 times/week. Treatment of clients with highly elevated erythropoetin levels (> 200 mU/mL) is not recommended. If response is not satisfactory after 8 wks, the dose may be increased up to 300 units/kg 3 times/week. Clients not responding at this level are not likely to respond at higher levels. If the hematocrit exceeds 40%, withhold the dose until the hematocrit falls to 36%. When treatment is resumed, reduce the dose by 25%.

NOTE: Individualize the dose for clients on dialysis. The median dose is 75 units/kg 3 times/week (range 12.5–525 units/kg 3 times/week).

Surgery to reduce allogeneic blood transfusions.
SC: 300 U/kg/day for 10 days before surgery, on the day of surgery, and for 4 days after surgery. Alternative: 600 U/kg SC once a week 21, 14, and 7 days before surgery plus a fourth dose on the day of surgery. Iron supplementation is required at the time of epoetin therapy and continuing throughout the course of therapy.

NURSING CONSIDERATIONS

ADMINISTRATION/STORAGE

1. During hemodialysis, clients may require increased anticoagulation with heparin to prevent clotting of the artificial kidney.
2. Determine hematocrit twice weekly until stabilized in the target range and the maintenance dose of epoetin alfa has been determined. Do not adjust more often than once a month, unless clinically indicated. Also, after any dosage adjustment, monitor the hematocrit twice weekly for 2–6 weeks.
3. If the hematocrit approaches 36%, decrease the dose to maintain the suggested target hematocrit range. If dose decrease does not stop the rise in hematocrit and it exceeds 35%, temporarily withhold doses until the hematocrit begins to decrease; then, reinitiate therapy at a lower dose. Then, determine maintenance doses individually.
4. If the hematocrit increases by more than 4 points in a 2-week period, decrease the dose by 25 U/kg. After reducing the dose, monitor the hematocrit twice weekly for 2–6 weeks; make further adjustments in dosage individually using the range outlined in the maintenance dose.
5. If the hematocrit does not increase by 5–6 points after 8 weeks of therapy and iron stores are adequate, increase the dose incrementally. Further increases may be made at 4–6-week intervals until a desired response is observed.
6. Do *not* shake; shaking will denature the glycoprotein, making it biologically inactive.
7. Do not use vials showing particulate matter or discoloration.
8. Withdraw only one dose per vial; discard any unused portion. The product contains no preservative.
9. Store at 2–8°C (36–46°F).
10. Do not give with any other drug solutions. However, at the time of SC administration, the drug may be admixed in a syringe with bacteriostatic 0.9% NaCl injection with benzyl alcohol, 0.9%, at a 1:1 ratio. The benzyl alcohol acts as a local anesthetic that may reduce discomfort at the SC injection site.

ASSESSMENT

1. Note any hypersensitivity to mammalian cell-derived products or human albumin.
2. Determine CBC and iron stores. Transferrin saturation should be at least 20% and serum ferritin should be at least 200 ng/mL. Provide supplemental iron to increase or maintain transferrin saturation to levels required to support stimulation of erythropoiesis by epoetin alfa.
3. With HIV, note when Zidovudine therapy was instituted, and anemia cause.
4. Assess BP; control hypertension.
5. Monitor renal function studies, I&O, electrolytes, phosphorous and uric acid levels; especially with CRF.
6. Assess for seizures if hematocrit increases by 4 points in 2 weeks.

CLIENT/FAMILY TEACHING

1. Do not shake vial; inactivates drug. Keep refrigerated.
2. Over 95% of clients with CRF manifested significant increases in hematocrit and nearly all were transfusion-independent within 2 mo after beginning therapy; drug does not cure renal disease and desired drug response may take up to 6 weeks.
3. Supplemental iron and vitamins are administered to enhance drug effects.
4. Report as scheduled for lab studies so drug can be adjusted.
5. Review list of drug side effects; report any persistent and/or bothersome

ones and practice contraception during therapy.
6. Must continue to follow prescribed dietary and dialysis recommendations; schedule activities to permit rest periods. Monitor BP and record.
7. Do not perform any tasks that require mental alertness until drug effects realized (especially during the first 3 mo of therapy).

OUTCOMES/EVALUATE

- ↑ Hematocrit
- Relief of symptoms of anemia
- ↓ Need for allogeneic blood transfusions

Epoprostenol sodium

(eh-poh-**PROST**-en-ohl)

PREGNANCY CATEGORY: B
CLASSIFICATION(S):
Vasodilator, peripheral
Rx: Flolan

SEE ALSO ANTIHYPERTENSIVE AGENTS.

ACTION/KINETICS

Acts by direct vasodilation of pulmonary and systemic arterial vascular beds and by inhibition of platelet aggregation. IV infusion in clients with pulmonary hypertension results in increases in cardiac index and SV and decreases in pulmonary vascular resistance, total pulmonary resistance, and mean systemic arterial pressure. Is rapidly hydrolyzed at the neutral pH of the blood as well as by enzymatic degradation. Metabolites are less active than the parent compound. **t½:** 6 min.

USES

Long-term IV treatment of primary pulmonary hypertension (including those with scleroderma spectrum of the disease who do not respond to conventional therapy) in New York Heart Association Class III and Class IV clients.

CONTRAINDICATIONS

Chronic use in those with CHF due to severe LV systolic dysfunction and in those who develop pulmonary edema during dosing.

SPECIAL CONCERNS

Abrupt withdrawal or sudden large decreases in the dose may cause rebound pulmonary hypertension. Use caution in dose selection in the elderly due to the greater frequency of decreased hepatic, renal, or cardiac function, as well as concomitant disease or other drug therapy. Use with caution during lactation. Safety and efficacy have not been determined in children.

SIDE EFFECTS

Side effects have been classified as those occurring during acute dosing, those as a result of the drug delivery system, and those occurring during chronic dosing.

Those occurring during acute dosing. **CV:** Flushing, hypotension, bradycardia, tachycardia. **GI:** N&V, abdominal pain, dyspepsia. **CNS:** Headache, anxiety, nervousness, agitation, dizziness, hypesthesia, paresthesia. **Miscellaneous:** Chest pain, musculoskeletal pain, dyspnea, back pain, sweating.

Those occurring as a result of the drug delivery system.

Due to the chronic indwelling catheter: Local infection, pain at the injection site, sepsis, infections.

Those occurring during chronic dosing.

CV: Flushing, tachycardia. **GI:** N&V, diarrhea. **CNS:** Headache, anxiety, nervousness, tremor, dizziness, hypesthesia, hyperesthesia, paresthesia. **Musculoskeletal:** Jaw pain, myalgia, nonspecific musculoskeletal pain. **Miscellaneous:** Flu-like symptoms, chills, fever, sepsis.

OD OVERDOSE MANAGEMENT

Symptoms: Flushing, headache, hypotension, tachycardia, nausea, vomiting, diarrhea. *Treatment:* Reduce dose of epoprostenol.

DRUG INTERACTIONS

Anticoagulants / Possible ↑ risk of bleeding
Antiplatelet drugs / Possible ↑ risk of bleeding
Diuretics / Additional ↓ in BP
Vasodilators / Additional ↓ in BP

HOW SUPPLIED

Powder for reconstitution: 0.5 mg, 1.5 mg

DOSAGE

• **CHRONIC IV INFUSION**

Pulmonary hypertension.

Acute dosing: The initial chronic infusion rate is first determined. The mean maximum dose that did not elicit dose-limiting pharmacologic effects was 8.6 ng/kg/min. **Continuous chronic infusion, initial:** 4 ng/kg/min less than the maximum-tolerated infusion rate determined during acute dosing. If the maximum-tolerated infusion rate is less than 5 ng/kg/min, start the chronic infusion at one-half the maximum-tolerated infusion rate. **Dosage adjustments:** Changes in the chronic infusion rate are based on persistence, recurrence, or worsening of the symptoms of primary pulmonary hypertension. If symptoms require an increase in infusion rate, increase by 1–2 ng/kg/min at intervals (at least 15 min) sufficient to allow assessment of the clinical response. If a decrease in infusion rate is necessary, gradually make 2-ng/kg/min decrements every 15 min or longer until the dose-limiting effects resolve. Avoid abrupt withdrawal or sudden large reductions in infusion rates.

NURSING CONSIDERATIONS

SEE ALSO *NURSING CONSIDERATIONS* FOR *ANTIHYPERTENSIVE AGENTS*.

ADMINISTRATION/STORAGE

IV 1. Chronic administration is delivered continuously by a permanent indwelling central venous catheter and an ambulatory infusion pump (see package insert for requirements for the infusion pump). Unless contraindicated, give anticoagulant therapy to decrease the risk of pulmonary thromboembolism or systemic embolism.

2. Do not dilute reconstituted solutions or administer with other parenteral solutions or medications.

3. Check package insert carefully to make 100 mL of a solution with the appropriate final concentration of drug and for infusion delivery rates for doses equal to or less than 16 ng/kg/min based on client weight, drug delivery rate, and concentration of solution to be used.

4. Protect unopened vials from light and store at 15–25°C (59–77°F). Protect reconstituted solutions from light and refrigerate at 2–8°C (36–46°F) for no more than 40 hr.

5. Do not freeze reconstituted solutions; discard any solution refrigerated for more than 48 hr.

6. A single reservoir of reconstituted solution can be given at room temperature for 8 hr; alternatively, it can be used with a cold pouch and given for up to 24 hr. Do not expose solution to sunlight.

ASSESSMENT

1. Perform a full cardiopulmonary assessment. Based on symptoms, determine New York Heart Association functional class (III or IV). Note other agents used and outcome.

2. Determine mental status and ability to handle medication preparation and IV administration; or identify someone in the home that can and is willing to perform this function on a regular basis and/or initiate home infusion referral.

3. Determine that a permanent indwelling central venous catheter is available for continuous ambulatory delivery once dosing completed.

4. Assess central venous access site for any evidence of infection, discharge, odor, erythema, or swelling.

5. Consult manufacturer's guidelines for dosage and delivery rate based on client weight for acute dosing.

CLIENT/FAMILY TEACHING

1. Drug helps reduce RV and LV afterload and increases CO and SV, improving symptoms of SOB, fatigue, and exercise intolerance.

2. Administered continously through an indwelling catheter to the heart by a portable external infusion pump; may be needed for years to help control symptoms.

3. Proper site care and pump maintenance as well as appropriate reconstitution for desired drug concentration, proper storage, protection from light, pouch filling, pump settings, and accessing VAD are imperative to safe therapy.

4. Review written guidelines for drug preparation, infusion, dose reduction, storage and administration and site inspection and care; pump maintenance, programming, trouble shooting, and care.
5. When drug is reconstituted and administered at room temperature, the pump must be programmed to administer pouch contents in 8 hr, whereas if drug is reconstituted and refrigerated at 2–8°C (36–46°F) may be administered in cold pouch over 24 hr.
6. Side effects that indicate excessive dosing and require a reduction in dosage and reporting include tachycardia, headache, N&V, diarrhea, hypotension.
7. Brief interruptions in therapy may cause rapid deterioration in condition.

OUTCOMES/EVALUATE

Improvement in exercise capacity; ↓ dyspnea and fatigue

Eprosartan mesylate

(eh-proh-**SAR**-tan)

PREGNANCY CATEGORY: C (FIRST TRIMESTER), D (SECOND AND THIRD TRIMESTERS)

CLASSIFICATION(S):

Antihypertensive, angiotensin II receptor blocker

Rx: Teveten

ACTION/KINETICS

Acts by blocking the vasoconstrictor and aldosterone-secreting effects of angiotensin II by blocking selectively the binding of angiotensin II to angiotensin II receptors located in the vascular smooth muscle and adrenal gland. **Peak plasma levels:** 1–2 hr. Food delays absorption. **t½, terminal:** 5–9 hr. Significantly bound (98%) to plasma protein. Excreted mostly unchanged in both the feces and urine.

USES

Used alone or with other antihypertensives (diuretics, calcium channel blockers) to treat hypertension.

SPECIAL CONCERNS

Drugs that act on the renin-angiotensin system directly during the second and third trimesters of pregnancy may cause fetal and neonatal injury. Symptomatic hypotension may be seen in clients who are volume- and/or salt-depleted (e.g., those taking diuretics). Safety and efficacy have not been determined in children.

SIDE EFFECTS

GI: Abdominal pain, diarrhea, dyspepsia, anorexia, constipation, dry mouth, esophagitis, flatulence, gastritis, gastroenteritis, gingivitis, nausea, periodontitis, toothache, vomiting. **CNS:** Depression, headache, dizziness, anxiety, ataxia, insomnia, migraine, neuritis, nervousness, paresthesia, somnolence, tremor, vertigo. **CV:** Angina pectoris, bradycardia, abnormal ECG, extrasystoles, atrial fibrillation, hypotension, tachycardia, palpitations, peripheral ischemia. **Respiratory:** URTI, sinusitis, bronchitis, chest pain, rhinitis, pharyngitis, coughing, asthma, epistaxis. **Musculoskeletal:** Arthralgia, myalgia, arthritis, aggravated arthritis, arthrosis, skeletal pain, tendonitis, back pain. **GU:** UTI, albuminuria, cystitis, hematuria, frequent micturition, polyuria, renal calculus, urinary incontinence. **Metabolic:** Diabetes mellitus, gout. **Body as a whole:** Viral infection, injury, fatigue, alcohol intolerance, asthenia, substernal chest pain, peripheral edema, dependent edema, fatigue, fever, hot flushes, flu-like symptoms, malaise, rigors, pain, leg cramps, herpes simplex. **Hematologic:** Anemia, purpura, leukopenia, neutropenia, thrombocytopenia. **Dermatologic:** Eczema, furunculosis, pruritus, rash, maculopapular rash, increased sweating. **Ophthalmic:** Conjunctivitis, abnormal vision, xerophthalmia. **Otic:** Otitis externa, otitis media, tinnitus.

LABORATORY TEST CONSIDERATIONS

↑ ALT, AST, creatine phosphokinase, BUN, creatinine, alkaline phosphatase. ↓ Hemoglobin. Glycosuria, hypercholesterolemia, hyperglycemia, hyperkalemia, hypokalemia, hyponatremia.

HOW SUPPLIED

Tablets: 400 mg, 600 mg

DOSAGE

- **TABLETS**

Hypertension.

Adults, initial: 600 mg once daily as monotherapy in clients who are not volume-depleted. Can be given once or twice daily with total daily doses ranging from 400–800 mg.

NURSING CONSIDERATIONS

SEE ALSO *NURSING CONSIDERATIONS* FOR *ANTIHYPERTENSIVE AGENTS*.

ADMINISTRATION/STORAGE

1. If the antihypertensive effect using once daily dosing is inadequate, a twice-a-day regimen at the same total daily dose or an increase in dose may be more effective.
2. Maximum BP reduction may not occur for 2–3 weeks.
3. May be used in combination with thiazide diuretics or calcium channel blockers if additional BP lowering effect is needed.
4. Discontinuing treatment does not lead to a rapid rebound increase in BP.

ASSESSMENT

1. Document disease onset, symptoms, and other agents trialed.
2. Correct volume depletion if evident. Monitor CBC, K^+, renal, and LFTs.

CLIENT/FAMILY TEACHING

1. Take as directed once or twice daily with or without food.
2. Continue life style modifications such as regular exercise, weight loss, smoking/alcohol cessation, low fat and low salt diet in the overall goal of BP control.
3. Practice reliable birth control. Report if pregnancy suspected or desired.
4. Keep a record of BP readings and bring to F/U visits.

OUTCOMES/EVALUATE

↓ BP; control of HTN

Eptifibatide

(**ep**-tih-**FY**-beh-tide)

PREGNANCY CATEGORY: B

CLASSIFICATION(S):

Antiplatelet drug, glycoprotein IIb/IIIa inhibitor

Rx: Integrilin

ACTION/KINETICS

Reversibly inhibits platelet aggregation by preventing the binding of fibrinogen, von Willebrand factor, and other adhesive ligands to GP IIb/IIIa. Immediately effective after IV use. **t½, elimination:** 2.5 hr. Drug and metabolites are excreted through kidneys.

USES

(1) Treatment of acute coronary syndrome (unstable angina or non-Q-wave MI), including those to be managed medically and those undergoing percutaneous coronary intervention. (2) Treatment of those undergoing percutaneous coronary intervention, including those undergoing intracoronary stenting.

CONTRAINDICATIONS

History of bleeding diathesis or evidence of active abnormal bleeding within the past 30 days. Severe hypertension (systolic BP > 200 mm Hg or diastolic BP > 110 mm Hg) inadequately controlled. Major surgery within the past 6 weeks, history of stroke within 30 days or any history of hemorrhagic stroke, current or planned use of another parenteral GP IIb/IIIa inhibitor, platelet count less than 100,000/mm^3, dependency on renal dialysis. Serum creatinine of 2.0 mg/dL or more (for the 180 mcg/kg bolus and the 2 mcg/kg/min infusion) or 4.0 mg/dL or more (for the 135 mcg/kg bolus and the 0.5 mcg/kg/min infusion). Lactation.

SPECIAL CONCERNS

Bleeding is the most common complication; there is a greater risk in older clients. Use with caution when used with other drugs that affect hemostasis, including thrombolytics, oral anticoagulants, NSAIDs, dipyridamole, ticlopidine, and clopidogrel. Use with caution during lactation. Safety and efficacy have not been determined in children.

SIDE EFFECTS

CV: Major bleeding, including ***intracranial hemorrhage,*** bleeding from the femoral artery access site, and bleeding that leads to decreases in hemoglobin greater than 5 g/dL. Minor bleeding, including spontaneous gross hematuria, spontaneous hematemesis, or blood loss with a hemoglobin decrease of more than 3 g/dL. Oropharyngeal (especially gingival), genitourinary, GI, and retroperitoneal bleeding. Hypotension. **Hypersenstivity/allergy:** ***Anaphylaxis,*** other allergic symptoms.

DRUG INTERACTIONS

Possible additive effects when used with thrombolytics, anticoagulants, or other antiplatelet drugs.

H *Evening primrose oil* / Potential for ↑ antiplatelet effect

H *Feverfew* / Potential for ↑ antiplatelet effect

H *Garlic* / Potential for ↑ antiplatelet effect

H *Ginger* / Potential for ↑ antiplatelet effect

H *Ginkgo biloba* / Potential for ↑ antiplatelet effect

H *Ginseng* / Potential for ↑ antiplatelet effect

H *Grapeseed extract* / Potential for ↑ antiplatelet effect

HOW SUPPLIED

Injection: 0.75 mg/mL, 2 mg/mL

DOSAGE

• IV

Acute coronary syndrome.

Adults, inital: IV bolus of 180 mcg/kg as soon as possible following diagnosis, followed by a continuous infusion of 2 mcg/kg/min until hospital discharge or initiation of coronary artery bypass surgery, up to 72 hr. If percutaneous coronary intervention will be undertaken, consider decreasing the infusion rate to 0.5 mcg/kg/min at the time of the procedure. Continue the infusion for an additional 20–24 hr after the procedure, allowing for up to 96 hr of therapy. Clients weighing > 121 kg have received a maximum bolus of 22.6 mg (11.3 mL of the 2 mg/mL injection) followed by a maximum rate of 15 mg (20 mL of the 0.75 mg/mL injection)/hr.

Percutaneous coronary intervention.

Adults, in those with a serum creatinine <2 mg/dL: IV bolus of 180 mcg/kg given immediately before initiation of PCI followed by a continuous infusion of 2 mcg/kg/min and a second bolus dose of 180 mcg/kg 10 min after the first bolus. This is followed by a continuous infusion until hospital discharge or for up to 18–24 hr, whichever comes first. A minimum of 12 hr of infusion is recommended. Give those weighing more than 121 kg a maximum of 22.6 mg/bolus followed by a maximum infusion rate of 7.5 mg/hr. **Adults, in those with a serum creatinine between 2 and 4 mg/dL:** IV bolus of 180 mcg/kg given immediately before initiation of PCI, immediately followed by a continuous infusion of 1 mcg/kg/min and a second 180 mcg/kg bolus given 10 min after the first. Give those weighing more than 121 kg a maximum of 22.6 mg/bolus followed by a maximum infusion rate of 7.5 mg/hr.

NURSING CONSIDERATIONS

ADMINISTRATION/STORAGE

IV 1. In those undergoing CABG surgery, discontinue prior to surgery.

2. Aspirin has been used with eptifibatide with the following possible doses. In acute coronary syndrome, aspirin, 160–325 mg initially and daily thereafter. In PCI, aspirin, 160–325 mg 1–24 hr prior to intervention and daily thereafter.

3. The following heparin doses are recommended. In acute coronary syndrome, achieve a target aPTT of 50–70 sec during medical management. If the weight is 70 or more kg, give a 5000 U heparin bolus followed by infusion of 1,000U/hr. If the weight is less than 70 kg, give a 60 U/kg bolus followed by infusion of 12 U/kg/hr. For PCI, achieve a target ACT of 200–300 sec. Give heparin, 60 U/kg as a bolus initially in those not treated with heparin within 6 hr prior to PCI. Give additional boluses during PCI to maintain ACT within target. Do not give heparin infusion after the PCI.

4. Inspect the vial for particulate matter or discoloration before use.
5. May be given in the same IV line as alteplase, atropine, dobutamine, heparin, lidocaine, meperidine, metoprolol, midazolam, morphine, nitroglycerin, or verapamil. Do not give in the same IV line as furosemide.
6. May be given in the same IV line with 0.9% NaCl or D5/NSS. These infusions may also contain up to 60 mEq/L of KCl.
7. Withdraw the bolus dose from the 10-mL vial and give by IV push over 1–2 min. Immediately following the bolus dose, start the continuous infusion. If using an infusion pump, give undiluted directly from the 100-mL vial by spiking the 100-mL vial with a vented infusion set. Center the spike within the circle on the stopper top.
8. Store vials at 2–8°C (36–46°F). Protect from light until use. Discard any portion left in the vial.

ASSESSMENT

1. Determine onset, duration, and characteristics of symptoms.
2. Note any conditions that would preclude therapy: recent CVA or surgery, platelets < 100,000/mm³, uncontrolled BP, abnormal bleeding or history of bleeding diathesis, hemorrhagic stroke, renal failure, or dialysis dependency.
3. Monitor ECG, bleeding times, liver and renal function studies.
4. Stop drug prior to CABG surgery.
5. Used in conjunction with aspirin and heparin; review dosing guidelines.
6. Assess femoral artery access site for evidence of bleeding. Stop heparin and eptifibatide therapy if unable to control bleeding with pressure.

CLIENT/FAMILY TEACHING

1. Review risks associated with therapy. Drug is used with unstable angina and non-Q-wave MI.
2. Bleeding is the most common side effect of drug therapy; usually occurs at graft site but may also occur as GU, GI, oropharyngeal, or retroperitoneal bleeding.
3. Family should learn CPR.

OUTCOMES/EVALUATE

- Inhibition of platelet aggregation
- ↓ Death/MI with acute coronary syndrome

Ertapenem for injection

(er-tah-**PEN**-em)

PREGNANCY CATEGORY: B
CLASSIFICATION(S):
Antibiotic, carbapenem
Rx: Invanz

SEE ALSO *ANTI-INFECTIVE DRUGS.*

ACTION/KINETICS

Almost completely absorbed following IM use. Highly bound to plasma proteins, primarily albumin. Metabolized in the liver. Unchanged drug and metabolites excreted primarily by the kidneys. **t½:** 4 hr. Excretion is decreased in those with renal insufficiency.

USES

(1) Complicated intra-abdominal infections due to *Escherichia coli, Clostridium clostridioforme, Eubacterium lentum, Peptostreptococcus* species, *Bacteroides fragilis, Bacteroides distasonis, Bacteroides ovatus, Bacteroides thetaiotaomicron,* or *Bacteroides uniformis.* (2) Complicated skin and skin structure infections due to *Staphylococcus aureus* (methicillin-susceptible strains only), *Streptococcus pyogenes, E. coli,* or *Peptostreptococcus* species. (3) Community acquired pneumonia due to *Streptococcus pneumoniae* (penicillin susceptible strains only) or *Moraxella catarrhalis.* (4) Complicated urinary tract infections, including pyelonephritis, due to *E. coli* (including cases with concurrent bacteremia) or *Klebsiella pneumoniae.* (5) Acute pelvic infections, including postpartum endomyometritis, septic abortion, and postsurgical gynecologic infections due to *Streptococcus agalactiae, E. coli, B. fragilis, Porphyromonas asaccharolytica, Peptostreptococcus* species, or *Prevotella bivia.*

CONTRAINDICATIONS
In known hypersensitvity to ertapenem or other drugs in the same class, in those who have shown anaphylactic reactions to beta-lactams. IM use in those hypersensitive to amide local anesthetics.

SPECIAL CONCERNS
Use with caution during lactation and in the elderly (use care in dose selection and monitor renal function). Safety and efficacy have not been determined in children less than 18 years of age.

SIDE EFFECTS
Listed are serious side effects and those with an incidence of 1% or more. **Hypersensitivity reactions: *Anaphylaxis.*** **GI:** Pseudomembranous colitis, antibiotic-associated colitis, diarrhea, N&V, abdominal pain, acid regurgitation, oral candidiasis, constipation, dyspepsia. **CNS:** Seizures (especially in those with brain lesions or a history of seizures and/or compromised renal function), headache, anxiety, altered mental status, dizziness, insomnia. **CV:** Hypertension, hypotension, tachycardia. **Injection site:** Extravasation, infused vein complication, phlebitis, thrombophlebitis. **Respiratory:** Cough, dyspnea, pharyngitis, rales/rhonchi, respiratory distress. **Dermatologic:** Erythema, pruritus, rash. **Body as a whole:** Asthenia, fatigue, edema, swelling, fever. **Miscellaneous:** Vaginitis, chest pain, leg pain, ***death.***

LABORATORY TEST CONSIDERATIONS
↑ ALT, AST, serum alkaline phosphatase, creatinine, glucose, serum bilirubin, esosinophils, prothrombin time, urine RBCs, urine WBCs. ↓ Serum albumin, hematocrit, hemoglobin, segmented neutrophils, WBCs. ↑ or ↓ Platelet count. Hypo- or hyperkalemia.

DRUG INTERACTIONS
Probenecid ↓ renal clearance of ertapenem.

HOW SUPPLIED
Powder, lyophilized for IM injection: 1 g, *Powder, lyophilized, for IV infusion:* 1 g

DOSAGE

• **IM, IV**

Complicated intra-abdominal infections.
Adults: 1 g for 5–14 days.

Complicated skin and skin structure infections.
Adults: 1 g for 7–14 days.

Communitiy acquired pneumonia, Complicated urinary tract infections (including pyelonephritis).
1 g for 10–14 days. Consider a switch to an appropriate PO therapy after at least 3 days of parenteral therapy once clinical improvement noted.

Acute pelvic infections.
1 g for 3–10 days.

NOTE: For all uses, if C_{CR} is 30 mL or less/min/1.73 m^2, give 0.5 g/day.

NURSING CONSIDERATIONS

SEE ALSO *NURSING CONSIDERATIONS* FOR *ANTI-INFECTIVE AGENTS.*

ADMINISTRATION/STORAGE

1. Can be given for up to 7 days IM.
2. When hemodialysis clients are given a dose of 0.5 g within 6 hr prior to dialysis, a supplementary dose of 150 mg is recommended following the hemodialysis session. No supplementary dose is needed if the drug is given at least 6 hr prior to hemodialysis.
3. Use the following procedure to prepare for IM use:
   - Reconstitute a 1 g vial with 3.2 mL of 1.0% lidocaine HCl injection (without epinephrine). Shake vial thoroughly to solubilize.
   - Immediately withdraw the contents of the vial and administer by deep IM injection into a large muscle mass (e.g., gluteal muscles or lateral part of the thigh).
   - Use the reconstituted IM solution within 1 hr of preparation.
   - **Do not give the reconstituted IM solution IV.**

IV 4. Can be given for up to 14 days IV.

5. Do not mix or co-infuse with other medications. Do not use diluents containing dextrose.
6. Use the following procedure to prepare for IV use:
   - Reconstitute a 1 g vial with 10 mL of either 0.9% NaCl injection, water, or bacteriostatic water for injection.
   - Shake well to dissolve and transfer contents of the reconstituted vial immediately to 50 mL of 0.9% NaCl injection.

• Complete infusion within 6 hr of reconstitution.
7. The reconstituted solution diluted in 0.9% NaCl injection may be stored at room temperature and used within 6 hr or stored for 24 hr in the refrigerator and used within 4 hr after removal from the refrigerator.
8. Do not freeze solutions of ertapenem.

ASSESSMENT

1. Document indications for therapy, onset, and characteristics of symptoms.
2. Assess for any history of sensitivity to multiple allergens or amide-type anesthetics, lidocaine HCl is used as diluent in IM preparation.
3. Adjust dosage with renal dysfunction and in those with uncontrolled seizures.
4. Monitor CBC, renal and LFTs. Review C&S to ensure organism susceptibility.

CLIENT/FAMILY TEACHING

1. Drug is administered once daily IV or IM for moderately severe infections.
2. It may alter normal flora in the colon and allow overgrowth of clostridia. Report any new onset diarrhea. May also experience N&V, headaches, pain/swelling at injection/infusion site, and vaginitis in females.
3. Any loss of effectiveness, adverse side effects, or worsening of condition warrant immediate reporting.

OUTCOMES/EVALUATE

Resolution of infection, symptomatic improvement

Erythromycin base

(eh-**rih**-throw-**MY**-sin)

PREGNANCY CATEGORY: B (A/T/S, ERYMAX, STATICIN, AND T-STAT ARE C)
CLASSIFICATION(S):
Antibiotic, macrolide
Rx: Capsules/Tablets: E-Base, E-Mycin, Eryc, Ery-Tab, Erythromycin Base Film-Tabs, PCE Dispertab, **Gel**: Emgel, Erygel, **Ointment**: Emgel, **Ophthalmic:** Ilotycin Ophthalmic **Pledgets:** Erythromycin Pledgets **Solution:** A/T/S, Del-Mycin, Erycette, Eryderm 2%, Erymax, Erythra-Derm, Staticin, Theramycin Z, T-Stat **Topical:** Akne-mycin, A/T/S
✱Rx: Capsules/Tablets: Apo-Erythro Base, Apo-Erythro E-C, Diomycin, Erybid, Erythromid, Novo–Rythro En-Cap, PMS-Erythromycin

SEE ALSO *ANTI-INFECTIVE AGENTS.*

ACTION/KINETICS

Erythromycins are macrolide antibiotics. They inhibit protein synthesis of microorganisms by binding reversibly to a ribosomal subunit (50S), thus interfering with the transmission of genetic information and inhibiting protein synthesis. The drugs are effective only against rapidly multiplying organisms. Absorbed from the upper part of the small intestine. Those for PO use are manufactured in enteric-coated or film-coated forms to prevent destruction by gastric acid. Erythromycin is approximately 70% bound to plasma proteins and achieves concentrations in body tissues about 40% of those in the plasma. Diffuses into body tissues; peritoneal, pleural, ascitic, and amniotic fluids; saliva; through the placental circulation; and across the mucous membrane of the tracheobronchial tree. Diffuses poorly into spinal fluid, although penetration is increased in meningitis. Alkalinization of the urine (to pH 8.5) increases the gram-negative antibacterial action. **Peak serum levels: PO,** 1–4 hr. **t½:** 1.5–2 hr, *but prolonged in clients with renal impairment.* Partially metabolized by the liver and primarily excreted in bile. Also excreted in breast milk.

USES

1. Mild to moderate upper respiratory tract infections due to *Streptococcus pyogenes* (group A beta-hemolytic streptococci), *Streptococcus pneumoniae,* and *Haemophilus influenzae* (combined with sulfonamides). 2. Mild to moderate lower respiratory tract infections due to *S. pyogenes* (group A beta-hemolytic streptococci) and *S. pneumoniae.* Respiratory tract infections due to *Mycoplasma pneumoniae.*

3. Pertussis (whooping cough) caused by *Bordetella pertussis;* may also be used as prophylaxis of pertussis in exposed individuals. 4. Mild to moderate skin and skin structure infections due to *S. pyogenes* and *Staphylococcus aureus.* Topically for acne vulgaris. 5. As an adjunct to antitoxin in diphtheria (caused by *Corynebacterium diphtheriae*), to prevent carriers, and to eradicate the organism in carriers. 6. Intestinal amebiasis due to *Entamoeba histolytica* (PO erythromycin only). 7. Acute pelvic inflammatory disease due to *Neisseria gonorrhoeae.* 8. Erythrasma due to *Corynebacterium minutissimum.* 9. *Chlamydia trachomatis* infections causing urogenital infections during pregnancy, conjunctivitis in the newborn, or pneumonia during infancy. Also, uncomplicated chlamydial infections of the urethra, endocervix, or rectum in adults (when tetracyclines are contraindicated or not tolerated). 10. Nongonococcal urethritis caused by *Ureaplasma urealyticum* when tetracyclines are contraindicated or not tolerated. 11. Legionnaires' disease due to *Legionella pneumophilia.* 12. PO as an alternative to penicillin (in penicillin-sensitive clients) to treat primary syphilis caused by *Treponema pallidum.* 13. Prophylaxis of initial or recurrent attacks of rheumatic fever in clients allergic to penicillin or sulfonamides. 14. Infections due to *Listeria monocytogenes.* 15. Bacterial endocarditis due to alpha-hemolytic streptococci, Viridans group, in clients allergic to penicillins.

Investigational: Severe or prolonged diarrhea due to *Campylobacter jejuni.* Genital, inguinal, or anorectal infections due to *Lymphogranuloma venereum.* Chancroid due to *Haemophilus ducreyi.* Primary, secondary, or early latent syphilis due to *T. pallidum.* Erythromycin base used with PO neomycin prior to elective colorectal surgery to reduce wound complications. As an alternative to penicillin to treat anthrax, Vincent's gingivitis, erysipeloid, actinomycosis, tetanus, with a sulfonamide to treat *Nocardia* infections, infections due to *Eikenella corrodens,* and *Borrelia* infections (including early Lyme disease). **Ophthalmic solution:** (1) Treatment of ocular infections (along with PO therapy) due to *Streptococcus pneumoniae, Staphylococcus aureus, S. pyogenes, Corynebacterium* species, *Haemophilus influenzae,* and *Bacteroides* infections. (2) Prophylaxis of ocular infections due to *Neisseria gonorrhoeae* and *Chlamydia trachomatis.* **Topical solution:** Acne vulgaris. **Topical ointment:** (1) Prophylaxis of infection in minor skin abrasions; treatment of superficial infections of the skin. (2) Acne vulgaris.

CONTRAINDICATIONS

Hypersensitivity to erythromycin; in utero syphilis. Use of topical preparations in the eye or near the nose, mouth, or any mucous membrane. Ophthalmic use in dendritic keratitis, vaccinia, varicella, myobacterial infections of the eye, fungal diseases of the eye. Use with steroid combinations following uncomplicated removal of a corneal foreign body.

SPECIAL CONCERNS

Use with caution in liver disease and during lactation. Use may result in bacterial and fungal overgrowth (i.e., superinfection). Use of other drugs for acne may result in a cumulative irritant effect. Although still recommended, use to treat whooping cough in newborns may cause pyloric stenosis.

SIDE EFFECTS

GI: Abdominal discomfort or pain, anorexia, diarrhea or loose stools, dyspepsia, flatulence, GI disorder, N&V, pseudomembranous colitis, hepatotoxicity. Possibility of hypertrophic pyloric stenosis in infants. **CV:** Ventricular arrhythmias, including ***ventricular tachycardia and torsades de pointes in clients with prolonged QT intervals***. After IV, increase in heart rate and prolongation of QT interval. **Dermatologic:** Pruritus, rash, urticaria, bullous eruptions, eczema, erythema multiforme, ***Stevens-Johnson syndrome, toxic epidermal necrolysis.*** **CNS:** Dizziness, headache, insomnia. **Miscellaneous:** Asthenia, dyspnea, increased cough, non-specific pain, vaginitis, allergic reaction, ***anaphylaxis.*** Reversible hearing loss in those with renal or hepatic insufficiency, in the elderly, and after doses greater than 4 g/day. **Following IV use:** Venous irritation, thrombophlebitis. **Following IM use:** Pain at the injection site, with development of necrosis or sterile abscesses. **Following topical use:** Itching, burning, irritation, stinging of skin; dry, scaly skin. **Also:** Erythema, desquamation, burning sensation, eye irritation, tenderness, dryness, pruritus, oily skin, generalized urticaria.

LABORATORY TEST CONSIDERATIONS

Interference with fluorometric assay for urinary catecholamines. ↑ Bicarbonate, eosinophils, platelet count, segmented neutrophils, serum CPK.

OD OVERDOSE MANAGEMENT

Symptoms: N&V, diarrhea, epigastric distress, acute pancreatitis (mild), hearing loss (with or without tinnitus and vertigo). *Treatment:* Induce vomiting. General supportive measures. Allergic reactions should be controlled with conventional therapy.

DRUG INTERACTIONS

Alfentanil / ↓ Alfentanil excretion → ↑ effect
Anticoagulants / ↑ Anticoagulant effects → possible hemorrhage
Antacids / Slight ↓ in elimination rate of erythromycin
Benzodiazepines (Alprazolam, Diazepam, Midazolam, Triazolam) / ↑ Plasma benzodiazepine levels → ↑ CNS depressant effects
Bromocriptine / ↑ Serum bromocriptine levels → ↑ pharmacologic and toxic effects
Buspirone / ↑ Plasma buspirone levels → ↑ pharmacologic and toxic effects
Carbamazepine / ↑ Carbamazepine effect (and toxicity requiring hospitalization and resuscitation) R/T ↓ liver breakdown
Clindamycin / Antagonism of effect if used together topically
Cyclosporine / ↑ Cyclosporine effect R/T ↓ excretion (possibly with renal toxicity)
Digoxin / ↑ Serum digoxin levels R/T effect on gut flora
Disopyramide / ↑ Plasma disopyramide levels → arrhythmias and ↑ QTc intervals
Ergot alkaloids / Acute ergotism manifested by peripheral ischemia and dysesthesia
Felodipine / ↑ Felodipine drug levels → ↑ pharmacologic and toxic effects
Grapefruit juice / ↑ Plasma erythromycin levels R/T ↓ metabolism in the small intestine
Grepafloxacin / ↑ Risk of life-threatening cardiac arrhythmias, including torsades de pointes
HMG-CoA Reductase inhibitors / ↑ Risk of myopathy or rhabdomyolysis; also ↑ plasma levels of atorvastatin, cerivastatin, lovastatin, or simvastatin R/T ↓ liver breakdown
Methylprednisolone / ↑ Methylprednisolone effect R/T ↓ liver breakdown
Penicillin / Either ↓ or ↑ effect of penicillins
Pimozide / Possibility of sudden death; do not use together
Rifabutin, Rifampin / ↓ Effect of erythromycin; ↑ risk of GI side effects
Sodium bicarbonate / ↑ Effect of erythromycin in urine due to alkalinization
Sparfloxacin / ↑ Risk of life-threatening cardiac arrhythmias, including torsades de pointes
Tacrolimus / ↑ Serum tacrolimus levels → ↑ risk of nephrotoxicity
Theophyllines / ↑ Theophylline effects R/T ↓ liver breakdown; ↓ erythromycin levels may also occur
Vinblastine / ↑ Risk of vinblastine toxicity (constipation, myalgia, neutropenia)

HOW SUPPLIED

Capsule, Delayed Release: 250 mg; *Gel/Jelly:* 2%; *Ointment:* 2%; *Ophthalmic ointment:* 5%; *Pledgets:* 2%; *Solution:* 1.5%, 2%; *Swab:* 2%; *Tablet:* 250 mg, 500 mg; *Tablet, Film Coated:* 250 mg, 500 mg; *Tablet, Polymer Coated Particles:* 333 mg, 500 mg; *Tablet, Enteric Coated:* 250 mg, 333 mg, 500 mg;

DOSAGE

Note: Doses are listed as erythromycin base.

• DELAYED-RELEASE CAPSULES, ENTERIC-COATED TABLETS, DELAYED-RELEASE TABLETS, FILM-COATED TABLETS, SUSPENSION

Respiratory tract infections due to Mycoplasma pneumoniae.

500 mg q 6 hr for 5–10 days (up to 3 weeks for severe infections).

Upper respiratory tract infections (mild to moderate) due to S. pyogenes *and S. pneumoniae.*

Adults: 250–500 mg q.i.d. for 10 days. **Children:** 20–50 mg/kg/day in divided doses, not to exceed the adult dose, for 10 days.

URTIs due to H. influenzae.

Erythromycin ethylsuccinate, 50 mg/kg/day for children, plus sulfisoxazole, 150 mg/kg/day, given together for 10 days.

Lower respiratory tract infections (mild to moderate) due to S. pyogenes *and S. pneumoniae.*

250–500 mg q.i.d. (or 20–50 mg/kg/day in divided doses) for 10 days.

Intestinal amebiasis due to Entamoeba histolytica.

Adults: 250 mg q.i.d. for 10–14 days; **pediatric:** 30–50 mg/kg/day in divided doses for 10 days.

Legionnaire's disease.

1–4 g/day in divided doses for 10–14 days.

Bordetella pertussis.

500 mg q.i.d. for 10 days (or for children, 40–50 mg/kg/day in divided doses for 5–14 days).

Infections due to Corynebacterium diphtheriae.

500 mg q 6 hr for 10 days.

Primary syphilis.

20–40 g in divided doses over 10 days.

Conjunctivitis of the newborn, pneumonia of infancy, urogenital infections during pregnancy due to Chlamydia trachomatis.

Infants: 50 mg/kg/day in four divided doses for 14 (conjunctivitis) to 21 (pneumonia) days; **adults:** 500 mg q.i.d. for 7 days or 250 mg q.i.d. for 14 days for urogenital infections.

Mild to moderate skin and skin structure infections due to S. pyogenes and *S. aureus.*

250–500 mg q 6 hr (or 20–50 mg/kg/day for children, in divided doses—to a maximum of 4 g/day) for 10 days.

Listeria monocytogenes infections.

Adults: 500 mg q 12 hr (or 250 mg q 6 hr), up to maximum of 4 g/day.

Pelvic inflammatory disease, acute due to N. gonorrhoeae.

Erythromycin lactobionate, 500 mg IV q 6 hr for 3 days; **then,** 250 mg erythromycin base 250 mg PO q 6 hr for 7 days. Alternatively for pelvic inflammatory disease, 500 mg PO q.i.d. for 10–14 days.

Prophylaxis of initial or recurrent rheumatic fever.

250 mg b.i.d.

Bacterial endocarditis due to alpha-hemolytic streptococcus.

Adults: 1 g 1–2 hr prior to the procedure; **then,** 500 mg 6 hr after the initial dose. **Pediatric,** 20 mg/kg 2 hr prior to the procedure; **then,** 10 mg/kg 6 hr after the initial dose.

Uncomplicated urethral, endocervical, or rectal infections due to C. trachomatis.

500 mg q.i.d. for 7 days (or 250 mg q.i.d. for 14 days).

Nongonococcal urethritis due to Ureaplasma urealyticum.

500 mg q.i.d. for at least 7 days or 250 mg q.i.d. for 14 days if client can not tolerate high doses of erythromycin.

Erythrasma due to Corynebacterium minutissimum.

250 mg t.i.d. for 21 days.

• **OPHTHALMIC OINTMENT**

Mild to moderate infections.

0.5-in. ribbon b.i.d.–t.i.d.

Acute infections.

0.5 in. ribbon q 3–4 hr until improvement is noted.

Prophylaxis of neonatal gonococcal or chlamydial conjunctivitis.

0.2–0.4 in. ribbon into each conjunctival sac.

• **TOPICAL GEL (2%), OINTMENT (2%), SOLUTION (2%)**

Clean the affected area and apply, using fingertips or applicator, morning and evening, to affected areas. If no improvement is seen after 6 to 8 weeks, discontinue therapy.

• **INVESTIGATIONAL USES.**

Diarrhea due to Campylobacter *enteritis or enterocolitis. Chancroid due to* Haemophilus ducreyi.

500 mg q.i.d. for 7 days.

Genital, inguinal, or anorectal infections due to Lymphogranuloma vener-

eum. *Early syphilis due to* Treponema pallidum.
500 mg q.i.d. for 14 days.

Tetanus due to Clostridium tetani.
500 mg q 6 hr for 10 days.

Granuloma inguinale due to Calymmatobacterium granulomatis.
500 mg PO q.i.d. for 21 or more days.

NURSING CONSIDERATIONS

SEE ALSO *GENERAL NURSING CONSIDERATIONS FOR ANTI-INFECTIVES*.

ADMINISTRATION/STORAGE

Topical gel is prepared by adding 3 mL of ethyl alcohol to the vial and immediately shaking to dissolve erythromycin. This solution is added to the gel and stirred until it appears homogenous (1–1.5 min). Refrigerate gel.

ASSESSMENT

1. Identify allergy to any antibiotics; note allergens. Assess for sensitivity reactions.
2. Document type, onset, and characteristics of symptoms, other agents used, and outcome.
3. Obtain cultures, CBC, wound documentation, and appropriate diagnostic studies.
4. Avoid if also prescribed (astemizole), digoxin, and theophyllines, because erythromycins can inhibit cytochrome P-450 and enhance effects of these drugs or cause lethal arrhythmias. Assess for hepatotoxicity and ototoxicity.

CLIENT/FAMILY TEACHING

1. Take on an empty stomach; the delayed-release forms of the base can be taken without regard for meals. Do not administer with or immediately prior to ingestion of fruit juice or other acidic drinks; acidity may decrease drug activity. Consume up to 8 oz of water with each dose and a fluid intake of 2.5 L/day.
2. May take with food to diminish GI upset; food decreases absorption of most erythromycins. Take only as directed and complete entire prescription despite feeling better.
3. If tablets are not coated, take them 2 hr after meals. Stomach acid destroys erythromycin base; must be administered with enteric coating.
4. Doses should be evenly spaced over 24 hr. Report any unusual or intolerable side effects or lack of response.
5. If nausea intolerable, report so the prescription can be changed to coated tablets that can be taken with meals.
6. Report symptoms of superinfection, i.e., furry tongue, vaginal itching, rectal itching, or diarrhea.
7. Any rash, yellow discoloration of skin or eyes, or irritation of the mouth or tongue should be reported.
8. Drug may increase GI motility with diabetic gastric paresis.
9. With topical use, clean affected area before applying ointment; wash hands before and after therapy.
10. A sterile bandage may be used with the topical ointment.
11. Instill ear solutions at room temperature. Pull ear lobe down and back for children under 3 years of age; pull ear lobe up and back when over 3 years of age.
12. Report any evidence of hearing loss, which is usually temporary.
13. Do not wash ophthalmic ointment from the eyes.
14. The topical and ophthalmic products are for external use only.

OUTCOMES/EVALUATE

- Resolution of infection (negative culture reports, ↓ temperature, wound healing, ↓ WBCs, improved appetite)
- Desired infection prophylaxis

Erythromycin estolate

(eh-**rih**-throw-**MY**-sin)

PREGNANCY CATEGORY: B
CLASSIFICATION(S):
Antibiotic, macrolide
Rx: Ilosone

SEE ALSO *ERYTHROMYCIN BASE*.

ACTION/KINETICS

Most active form of erythromycin, with relatively long-lasting activity.

USES

See Erythromycin Base.

ADDITIONAL CONTRAINDICATIONS
Cholestatic jaundice or preexisting liver dysfunction. Treatment of chronic disorders such as acne, furunculosis, or prophylaxis of rheumatic fever.
HOW SUPPLIED
Capsule: 250 mg; *Suspension:* 125 mg/5 mL, 250 mg/5 mL; *Tablet:* 500 mg

E

DOSAGE
• CAPSULES, SUSPENSION, TABLETS
See *Erythromycin base,*. Similar blood levels are achieved using erythromycin base, estolate, or stearate.

NURSING CONSIDERATIONS

SEE ALSO *NURSING CONSIDERATIONS FOR ERYTHROMYCIN BASE.*

ASSESSMENT
1. Document indications for therapy, onset and symptom characteristics.
2. Assess for evidence of liver failure.

CLIENT/FAMILY TEACHING
1. Shake suspension well before using; do not store for more than 2 weeks at room temperature.
2. Chew or crush chewable tablets.
3. Take without regard to meals.
4. Report lack of response or adverse drug effects.

OUTCOMES/EVALUATE
Resolution of infection

Erythromycin ethylsuccinate

(eh-**rih**-throw-**MY**-sin)

PREGNANCY CATEGORY: B
CLASSIFICATION(S):
Antibiotic, macrolide
Rx: E.E.S. 200 and 400, E.E.S. Granules, EryPed, EryPed 200, EryPed 400, EryPed Drops
✱Rx: Apo-Erythro-ES, EES 600

SEE ALSO *ERYTHROMYCIN BASE.*

USES
See *Erythromycin Base.*
ADDITIONAL CONTRAINDICATIONS
Preexisting liver disease.
HOW SUPPLIED
Chew Tablet: 200 mg; *Powder for Oral Suspension:* 200 mg/5 mL (when reconstituted); *Suspension:* 100 mg/2.5 mL, 200 mg/5 mL, 400 mg/5 mL; *Tablet:* 400 mg

DOSAGE
• ORAL SUSPENSION, TABLETS, CHEWABLE TABLETS
See *Erythromycin base. NOTE:* 400 mg of erythromycin ethylsuccinate will achieve the same blood levels of erythromycin as 250 mg of the base, estolate, or stearate forms.

Hemophilus influenzae *infections.*
Erythromycin ethylsuccinate, 50 mg/kg/day with sulfisoxazole, 150 mg/kg/day, both for a total of 10 days.

NURSING CONSIDERATIONS

SEE ALSO *NURSING CONSIDERATIONS FOR ERYTHROMYCIN BASE.*

CLIENT/FAMILY TEACHING
1. Take without regard to meals.
2. Chew or crush chewable tablets.
3. Refrigerate oral suspension; store for 1 week maximum.
4. Report lack of response or adverse drug effects.

OUTCOMES/EVALUATE
Resolution of infection

Erythromycin lactobionate

(eh-**rih**-throw-**MY**-sin)

PREGNANCY CATEGORY: B
CLASSIFICATION(S):
Antibiotic, macrolide
Rx: Erythrocin
✱Rx: Erythrocin I.V.

SEE ALSO *ERYTHROMYCIN BASE.*

USES
See *Erythromycin Base.*
ADDITIONAL DRUG INTERACTIONS
Do not add drugs to IV solutions of erythromycin lactobionate.
HOW SUPPLIED
Powder for injection: 500 mg, 1 g

DOSAGE
• IV
Adults and children: 15–20 mg/kg/day up to 4 g/day in severe infections.

Acute pelvic inflammatory disease caused by gonorrhea.

500 mg q 6 hr for 3 days followed by 250 mg erythromycin stearate, **PO,** q 6 hr for 7 days.

Legionnaire's disease.

1–4 g/day in divided doses. Change to PO therapy as soon as possible.

NURSING CONSIDERATIONS

SEE ALSO *NURSING CONSIDERATIONS* FOR *ERYTHROMYCIN BASE.*

ADMINISTRATION/STORAGE

IV 1. Sterile water for injection is the preferred diluent. However, D5W or D5/RL may also be used if buffered with 4% $NaHCO_3$ injection.
2. For intermittent IV administration, may be further diluted in 100 to 250 mL of D5W or NSS and infused over 20–60 min.
3. The initial reconstituted solution is stable for 2 weeks refrigerated or for 24 hr at room temperature if final diluted solution used within 8 hr. Use the reconstituted piggyback vial within 24 hr if refrigerated or 8 hr if stored at room temperature.
4. If reconstituted solution is frozen, may be stored for 30 days. Once thawed, use within 8 hr. Do not refreeze thawed solutions.

ASSESSMENT

1. Obtain CBC and cultures.
2. Assess for hearing deficits.

OUTCOMES/EVALUATE

Resolution of infection; negative cultures

Erythromycin stearate

(eh-**rih**-throw-**MY**-sin)

PREGNANCY CATEGORY: B
CLASSIFICATION(S):
Antibiotic, macrolide
Rx: Erythrocin Stearate
✱**Rx:** Apo-Erythro-S, Nu-Erythromycin-S

SEE ALSO *ERYTHROMYCIN BASE.*

USES

See *Erythromycin Base.*

ADDITIONAL SIDE EFFECTS

Causes more allergic reactions (e.g., skin rash and urticaria) than other erythromycins.

HOW SUPPLIED

Tablet film coated: 250 mg, 500 mg

DOSAGE

• TABLETS, FILM COATED

See *Erythromycin base.* Similar blood levels are achieved using erythromycin base, estolate, or stearate forms.

NURSING CONSIDERATIONS

SEE ALSO *NURSING CONSIDERATIONS* FOR *ERYTHROMYCIN BASE.*

CLIENT/FAMILY TEACHING

1. Take on an empty stomach; food decreases absorption.
2. Report lack of effect or evidence of allergic reaction, i.e., rash or itching.

OUTCOMES/EVALUATE

Resolution of infection

Esmolol hydrochloride

(**EZ**-moh-lohl)

PREGNANCY CATEGORY: C
CLASSIFICATION(S):
Beta-adrenergic blocking agent
Rx: Brevibloc

SEE ALSO *BETA-ADRENERGIC BLOCKING AGENTS.*

ACTION/KINETICS

Preferentially inhibits beta-1 receptors. Rapid onset (< 5 min) and a short duration of action. Has no membrane-stabilizing or intrinsic sympathomimetic activity. Low lipid solubility. **t½:** 9 min. Rapidly metabolized by esterases in RBCs.

USES

(1) Supraventricular tachycardia in those with atrial fibrillation or atrial flutter in perioperative, postoperative, or other emergent situations when short-term control is needed. (2) Noncompensatory sinus tachycardia when rapid heart rate requires intervention. (3) Tachycardia and hypertension during

induction and tracheal intubation, during surgery, on emergence from anesthesia, and postoperatively.

SPECIAL CONCERNS

Dosage has not been established in children.

ADDITIONAL SIDE EFFECTS

Dermatologic: Inflammation at site of infusion, flushing, pallor, induration, erythema, burning, skin discoloration, edema. **Other:** Urinary retention, midscapular pain, asthenia, changes in taste.

ADDITIONAL DRUG INTERACTIONS

Digoxin / ↑ Digoxin blood levels
Morphine / ↑ Esmolol blood levels

HOW SUPPLIED

Injection: 10 mg/mL, 250 mg/mL

DOSAGE

• **IV INFUSION**

SVT.

Initial: 500 mcg/kg/min for 1 min; **then,** 50 mcg/kg/min for 4 min. If after 5 min an adequate effect is not achieved, repeat the loading dose followed by a maintenance infusion of 100 mcg/kg/min for 4 min. This procedure may be repeated, increasing the maintenance infusion by 50 mcg/kg/min increments (for 4 min) until the desired HR or lowered BP is approached. **Then,** omit the loading infusion and reduce incremental infusion rate from 50 to 25 mcg/kg/min or less. The interval between titrations may be increased from 5 to 10 min.

Once the HR has been controlled, the client may be transferred to another antiarrhythmic agent. Reduce the infusion rate of esmolol by 50% 30 min after the first dose of the alternative antiarrhythmic agent. If satisfactory control is observed for 1 hr after the second dose of the alternative agent, the esmolol infusion may be stopped.

Intraoperative and postoperative tachycardia and hypertension.

Immediate control: 80 mg (about 1 mg/kg) bolus dose over 30 sec followed by 150 mcg/kg/min for 1 min followed by a 4-min maintenance infusion of 50 mcg/kg/min. If an adequate effect is not seen in 5 min, repeat the same loading dose and follow with a maintenance infusion of 100 mcg/kg/min. **Gradual control:** Dosing schedule is the same as for supraventricular tachycardia.

NURSING CONSIDERATIONS

SEE ALSO *NURSING CONSIDERATIONS* FOR *BETA-ADRENERGIC BLOCKING AGENTS.*

ADMINISTRATION/STORAGE

IV 1. Infusions may be necessary for 24–48 hr.

2. Not for direct IV push administration.

3. Do not dilute concentrate with sodium bicarbonate.

4. To minimize irritation and thrombophlebitis, do not infuse concentrations greater than 10 mg/mL.

5. Diluted esmolol (concentration of 10 mg/mL) is compatible with D5W, D5/RL, D5/Ringer's injection, D5/0.9% NaCl, D5/0.45% NaCl, 0.45% NaCl, RL, KCl (40 mEq/L) in D5W, 0.9% NaCl, and 0.45% NaCl.

ASSESSMENT

1. Note indications for therapy, type, onset, and characteristics of symptoms.

2. Document and monitor CP assessments, ECG, and VS. Assess for hypotension or bradycardia.

3. Administer in a monitored environment; wean using guidelines.

OUTCOMES/EVALUATE

• Suppression of SVT
• Restoration of stable rhythm

Esomeprazole magnesium

(**es**-oh-**MEP**-rah-zole)

PREGNANCY CATEGORY: B
CLASSIFICATION(S):
Proton pump inhibitor
Rx: Nexium

ACTION/KINETICS

Suppresses the final step in gastric acid production by inhibiting the H+/K+–ATPase in the gastric parietal cell. This decreases gastric acid secretion. **Peak plasma levels**:1.5 hr. Absorption is decreased by food. 97%

bound to plasma proteins. Extensively metabolized in the liver by the cytochrome P450 enzyme system. **t½, elimination**: 1–1.5 hr. About 80% excreted as inactive metabolites in the urine with 20% excreted in the feces.

USES

(1) Short-term treatment (4–8 weeks) in the healing and symptomatic resolution of diagnostically confirmed erosive esophagitis. To maintain symptom resolution and healing of erosive esophagitis. (2) Treatment of heartburn and other symptoms associated with GERD. (3) In combination with amoxicillin and clarithromycin to treat *H. pylori* infection and duodenal ulcer disease (active or history within the past 5 years) to eradicate *H. pylori*.

CONTRAINDICATIONS

Known hypersensitivity to any component of the formulation or to any macrolide antibiotic. Lactation.

SPECIAL CONCERNS

Symptomatic response does not preclude the presence of gastric malignancy. Safety and efficacy have not been determined in children.

SIDE EFFECTS

GI: Diarrhea, nausea, flatulence, abdominal pain, constipation, dry mouth, bowel irregularity, dyspepsia, dysphagia, GI dysplasia, epigastric pain, eructation, esophageal disorder, frequent stools, gastroenteritis, ***GI hemorrhage,*** hiccough, melena, mouth/pharynx/rectal/tongue disorder, tongue edema, ulcerative stomatitis, vomiting. **CNS**: Headache, anorexia, apathy, increased appetite, confusion, aggravated depression, dizziness, hypertonia, nervousness, hypoesthesia, impotence, insomnia, migraine, paresthesia, sleep disorder, somnolence, tremor, vertigo. **CV**: Hypertension, tachycardia. **Hematologic**: Anemia, hypochromic anemia, cervical lymphoadenopathy, leukocytosis, leukopenia, thrombocytopenia. **Respiratory**: Aggravated asthma, cough, dyspnea, epistaxis, ***larynx edema,*** pharyngitis, rhinitis, sinusitis. **Dermatologic**: Acne, angioedema, dermatitis, pruritus, pruritus ani, rash, erythematous/maculopapular rash, skin inflammation, increased sweating, urticaria. **Otic**: Earache, tinnitus, otitis media. **Ophthalmic**: Conjunctivitis, abnormal vision, visual field defect. **Musculoskeletal**: Arthralgia, aggravated arthritis, arthropathy, cramps, fibromyalgia syndrome, hernia, polymyalgia rheumatica. **GU**: Dysmenorrhea, menstrual disorder, vaginitis, abnormal urine, cystitis, dysuria, fungal infection, hematuria, frequent micturition, moniliasis, genital moniliasis, polyuria. **Body as a whole**: Enlarged abdomen, allergic reaction, asthenia, back/chest pain, substernal chest pain, facial/peripheral edema, hot flushes, fatigue, fever, flu-like symptoms, generalized/leg edema, malaise, pain, rigors. **Miscellaneous**: Goiter, abnormal hepatic function, thirst, increased/decreased weight, vitamin B_{12} deficiency, parosmia, taste loss/perversion.

LABORATORY TEST CONSIDERATIONS

↑ ALT, AST, alkaline phosphatase, serum gastrin, creatinine, uric acid, total bilirubin, WBC count, platelets, potassium, sodium, thyroxine, TSH. ↓ Hemoglobin, WBC count, platelets, potassium, sodium, thyroxine. Bilirubinemia, glycosuria, hyperuricemia, hyponatremia, albuminuria.

DRUG INTERACTIONS

Esomeprazole may interfere with the absorption of drugs where gasric pH is an important factor in bioavailability (e.g., digoxin, iron salts, ketoconazole).

HOW SUPPLIED

Capsules, delayed-release: 20 mg, 40 mg

DOSAGE

• **CAPSULES, DELAYED-RELEASE**

Healing of erosive esophagitis.

20 mg or 40 mg once daily for 4–8 weeks. For those who do not heal within 4–8 weeks, consider an additional 4–8 weeks of therapy.

Maintenance of healing of erosive esophagitis.

20 mg once daily, for up to 6 months.

Symptomatic GERD.

20 mg once daily for 4 weeks. If symptoms do not resolve completely, consider an additional 4 weeks of therapy.

Eradication of H. pylori *to reduce risk of duodenal ulcer recurrence.*
Use the following triple therapy. Esomeprazole, 40 mg once daily for 10 days; amoxicillin, 1,000 mg b.i.d. for 10 days; and, clarithromycin, 500 mg b.i.d. for 10 days. Do not exceed a dose of 20 mg daily in clients with severe hepatic insufficiency.

E

NURSING CONSIDERATIONS

ADMINISTRATION/STORAGE

1. For clients unable to swallow capsules, add one tablespoon of applesauce to an empty bowl. Empty the capsule and carefully empty the pellets onto the applesauce. Mix the pellets with the applesauce and swallow immediately. Do not use hot applesauce and do not chew or crush the pellets. Do not store the pellet/applesauce mixture for future use.
2. Store between 15–30°C (59–86°F) with container tightly closed.

ASSESSMENT

1. Document indications for therapy, type, onset, and characteristics of symptoms. List other agents prescribed.
2. Determine if pregnant.
3. Record abdominal assessments, radiographic/endoscopic findings, and *H. pylori* findings.
4. Monitor CBC and LFTs; note any liver dysfunction.

CLIENT/FAMILY TEACHING

1. Take the delayed release capsules whole at least 1 hr before meals. If unable to swallow whole may empty capsule onto one tablespoon of applesauce in a cup. Mix pellets into applesauce and swallow immediately taking care not to chew pellets.
2. May take antacids with esomeprazole.
3. Avoid alcohol and OTC products unless approved.
4. Drug is for short-term use only; it inhibits gastric acid secretion. Side effects of prolonged therapy and suppression of acid secretion alter bacterial colonization and lead to hypochlorhydria and hypergastrinemia, which may lead to an increased risk for gastric tumors.

OUTCOMES/EVALUATE

Promotion of ulcer healing; relief of pain; ↓ gastric acid production. Eradication of *H. pylori* with designated ATXs.

Estazolam

(es-**TAYZ**-oh-lam)

PREGNANCY CATEGORY: X
CLASSIFICATION(S):
Hypnotic, benzodiazepine
Rx: ProSom **C-IV**

SEE ALSO *TRANQUILIZERS, ANTIMANIC DRUGS, AND HYPNOTICS.*

ACTION/KINETICS

Peak plasma levels: 2 hr. **t½:** 10–24 hr. The clearance is increased in smokers compared with nonsmokers. Metabolized in the liver and excreted mainly in the urine. Two metabolites—4′-hydroxy estazolam and 1-oxo-estazolam—have minimal pharmacologic activity although at the levels present they do not contribute significantly to the hypnotic effect.

USES

Short-term use for insomnia characterized by difficulty in falling asleep, frequent awakenings, and/or early morning awakenings.

CONTRAINDICATIONS

Pregnancy. Use during labor and delivery and during lactation.

SPECIAL CONCERNS

Use with caution in geriatric or debilitated clients, in those with impaired renal or hepatic function, in those with compromised respiratory function, and in those with depression or who show suicidal tendencies. Safety and efficacy have not been determined in children less than 18 years of age.

HOW SUPPLIED

Tablet: 1 mg, 2 mg

DOSAGE

• **TABLETS**

Adults: 1 mg at bedtime (although some clients may require 2 mg). The initial dose in small or debilitated geriatric clients is 0.5 mg. Prolonged use is not recommended or necessary.

NURSING CONSIDERATIONS

SEE ALSO *NURSING CONSIDERATIONS* FOR *TRANQUILIZERS, ANTIMANIC DRUGS, AND HYPNOTICS.*

ASSESSMENT

1. Note history of depression, suicidal tendencies, or respiratory problems.
2. Monitor liver and renal function studies; reduce dose in geriatric and debilitated clients and those with impaired renal and hepatic function.
3. Identify underlying cause(s) for insomnia; investigate alternative nonpharmacologic methods for sleep inducement.
4. Drug may enhance the duration and quality of sleep for up to 12 weeks; assess need to continue.

CLIENT/FAMILY TEACHING

1. Identify symptoms that require immediate reporting.
2. Practice contraception; discontinue drug before becoming pregnant.
3. Do not perform tasks that require mental alertness until drug effects realized; ability to drive or operate machinery may be impaired.
4. Avoid alcohol and OTC drugs; smoking may alter drug absorption.
5. Take only as directed; may cause psychologic/physical dependence.
6. Do not stop abruptly; after prolonged treatment, withdraw slowly.
7. Identify any causative/contributing factors; review alternative methods for sleep induction.

OUTCOMES/EVALUATE

Enhanced duration and quality of sleep

Esterified estrogens

(es-**TER**-ih-fyd **ES**-troh-jens)

PREGNANCY CATEGORY: X
CLASSIFICATION(S):
Estrogen, natural
Rx: Estratab, Menest

SEE ALSO *ESTROGENS.*

ACTION/KINETICS

This product is a mixture of sodium salts of sulfate esters of natural estrogenic substances: 75%–85% estrone sodium sulfate and 6%–15% equilin sodium sulfate. Less potent than estrone.

USES

(1) Replacement therapy in primary ovarian failure, following castration, or hypogonadism. (2) Inoperable, progressing prostatic or breast carcinoma (in postmenopausal women and selected men). (3) Moderate to severe vasomotor symptoms, atrophic vaginitis, and kraurosis vulvae due to menopause. (4) Prophylaxis of osteoporosis (0.3 mg tablet).

HOW SUPPLIED

Tablet: 0.3 mg, 0.625 mg, 1.25 mg, 2.5 mg

DOSAGE

• TABLETS

Moderate to severe vasomotor symptoms, atrophic vaginitis, or kraurosis vulvae due to menopause.

0.3–1.25 mg/day given cyclically for short-term use. Adjust dose to the lowest effective level and discontinue as soon as possible.

Hypogonadism.

2.5–7.5 mg/day in divided doses for 20 days, followed by a 10-day rest period. If menses does not occur by the end of this period of time, repeat dosage schedule. The number of courses of estrogen required to produce bleeding varies, depending on the responsiveness of the endometrium. If bleeding occurs before the end of the 10-day period, a 20-day estrogen-progestin cycle should be started with 2.5–7.5 mg/day of estrogen with a progestin added the last 5 days. If bleeding occurs before the end of this regimen, discontinue therapy and resume on day 5 of bleeding.

Primary ovarian failure, castration.

1.25 mg/day given cyclically.

Prostatic carcinoma, inoperable and progressing.

1.25–2.5 mg t.i.d. Effectiveness can be determined using phosphatase determinations and symptomatic improvement.

Breast carcinoma, inoperable and progressing, in selected men and postmenopausal women.

10 mg t.i.d. for at least 3 months.

Prophylaxis of osteoporosis.

0.3 mg daily.

NURSING CONSIDERATIONS

SEE *NURSING CONSIDERATIONS* FOR *ESTROGENS*.

ASSESSMENT

Document indications for therapy; note type, onset, and characteristics of symptoms.

OUTCOMES/EVALUATE

- Stimulation of menses
- Relief of postmenopausal S&S
- Suppression of tumor growth/spread
- Osteoporosis prophylaxis

Estradiol hemihydrate

(ess-trah-**DYE**-ohl)

PREGNANCY CATEGORY: X
CLASSIFICATION(S):
Estrogen, semisynthetic
Rx: Vagifem

SEE ALSO *ESTROGENS*.

USES

Treatment of atrophic vaginitis.

HOW SUPPLIED

Tablets, Vaginal: 25 mcg

DOSAGE

- **VAGINAL TABLETS**

Atrophic vaginitis.

Initial: 1 tablet, inserted vaginally, once daily for 2 weeks; **maintenance:** 1 tablet, inserted vaginally, twice a week.

NURSING CONSIDERATIONS

SEE ALSO *NURSING CONSIDERATIONS* FOR *ESTROGENS*.

ADMINISTRATION/STORAGE

Attempt to discontinue or taper the drug at 3– to 6–month intervals.

ASSESSMENT

Note indications for therapy, age at onset and characteristics of symptoms.

CLIENT/FAMILY TEACHING

1. Gently insert the vaginal tablet into the vagina as far as it can comfortably go without force. Use the supplied applicator.
2. Insert the tablet at the same time each day.
3. Report any pain, odor, or increased discharge.

OUTCOMES/EVALUATE

Relief of S&S atrophic vaginitis

Estradiol transdermal system

(ess-trah-**DYE**-ohl)

PREGNANCY CATEGORY: X
CLASSIFICATION(S):
Estrogen, semisynthetic
Rx: Alora, Climara, Climara 25, E_2III, Esclim, Estraderm, FemPatch, Vivelle, Vivelle-Dot

SEE ALSO *ESTROGENS*.

ACTION/KINETICS

This transdermal system allows a constant low dose of estradiol to directly reach the systemic circulation. The system overcomes certain problems associated with PO use, including first-pass hepatic metabolism, GI upset, and induction of liver enzymes. The system is available in various surface areas, release rates, and total estradiol content (the package insert should be carefully consulted). The patches are made either with a reservoir and a rate-controlling membrane or using a matrix where estradiol is embedded in the adhesive, allowing for a translucent, small, thin patch.

USES

(1) Vasomotor symptoms (moderate to severe) due to menopause, including hot flashes, night sweats, and vaginal burning, itching, and dryness. (2) Female hypogonadism or castration; atrophic vaginitis or kraurosis vulvae due to deficient endogenous estrogen production; primary ovarian failure. (3) Prevention of osteoporosis in postmenopausal women. (4) Abnormal uterine bleeding due to hormonal imbalance in the absence of organic

pathology and only when associated with a hypoplastic or atrophic endometrium.

SIDE EFFECTS

Skin irritation, URTI, headache, breast tenderness.

HOW SUPPLIED

Film, Extended Release: 0.025 mg/24 hr, 0.0375 mg/24 hr, 0.05 mg/24 hr, 0.075 mg/24 hr, 0.1 mg/24 hr; *Insert, Controlled Release:* 0.0075 mg/24 hr

DOSAGE

• **TRANSDERMAL SYSTEM**

Menopausal symptoms.

Initial: Lowest dose needed to control symptoms: One 0.025- or 0.05-mg system applied to the skin twice weekly (if using Alora, Estraderm, Esclim, or Vivelle); one 0.025 mg system (Climara 25) daily; or, once a week (if using Climara or FemPatch). Adjust dose as necessary to control symptoms. Taper or discontinue dose at 3- to 6-month intervals. Alora is available in strengths to release 0.05-, 0.075-, and 0.1-mg/24 hr. Climara and Estraderm are available in strengths to release 0.05- or 0.1-mg/24 hr. Climara 25 releases 0.025 mg/24 hr. Esclim is available in strengths to release 0.025-, 0.0375-, 0.05-, 0.075-, or 0.1-mg/24 hr. FemPatch is available to release 0.025-mg/24 hr. Vivelle is available in strengths to release 0.0375-, 0.05-, 0.075-, or 0.1-mg/24 hr.

Prevention of osteoporosis.

Initial: 0.05 mg/day as soon as possible after menopause. Adjust dosage to control concurrent menopausal symptoms. For Climara 25, use 0.025 mg/day. For Vivelle, use 0.025 mg/day applied twice weekly.

NURSING CONSIDERATIONS

SEE ALSO *NURSING CONSIDERATIONS* FOR *ESTROGENS*.

ADMINISTRATION/STORAGE

Vivelle-Dot is 66% smaller than the original Vivelle and is applied twice weekly to the lower abdomen.

CLIENT/FAMILY TEACHING

1. If taking oral estrogens, stop pills and wait 1 week before applying the system.
2. Without a hysterectomy, the system is usually used for 3 weeks, followed by 1 week of rest. May be used continuously in those without an intact uterus.
3. Place the system on a clean, dry area of the skin on the trunk of the body (preferably the abdomen). Avoid using areas with excessive amounts of hair. Also may use on the hip or buttock. Do not apply to the breasts or the waistline.
4. Rotate application site; date patch. Allow one week intervals between reapplication to same site.
5. Apply system immediately after the pouch is opened and the protective liner is removed. Firmly press in place with the palm for approximately 10 sec. Ensure good contact, especially around the edges. If system falls, reapply the same system or place a new one and follow the same schedule.
6. Weight gain may occur; report if marked or if edema develops.
7. Stop smoking; smoking increases risk of thromboembolic problems.
8. Addition of a progestin for 7 or more days may reduce the incidence of endometrial hyperplasia.

OUTCOMES/EVALUATE

- Relief of menopausal symptoms
- Therapeutic estrogen levels

Estramustine phosphate sodium

(es-trah-**MUS**-teen)

CLASSIFICATION(S):

Antineoplastic, alkylating

Rx: Emcyt

SEE ALSO *ANTINEOPLASTIC AGENTS*.

ACTION/KINETICS

Water-soluble drug that combines estradiol and mechlorethamine (a nitrogen mustard). Estradiol facilitates uptake into cells containing the estrogen receptor while the nitrogen mustard acts as an alkylating agent. Chronic estramustine administration results in plasma levels and effects of estradiol similar to those of conventional estradiol therapy. Well absorbed from the GI tract and dephosphorylated before reaching the general circulation. Metabolites include estromustine, estrone, and estradiol. **t½:** 20 hr. Major route of excretion is in the feces.

USES

Palliative treatment of metastatic and/or progressive prostatic carcinoma.

CONTRAINDICATIONS

Active thrombophlebitis or thromboembolic disease unless the tumor mass is causing the thromboembolic disorder. Allergy to nitrogen mustard or estrogen.

SPECIAL CONCERNS

Use with caution in presence of cerebrovascular disease (e.g., thrombophlebitis, thrombosis, thromboembolic disease), CAD, diabetes, hypertension, CHF, impaired liver or kidney function, and metabolic bone diseases associated with hypercalcemia. Risk of thrombosis, including fatal or nonfatal MI, increases in men receiving estrogens for prostate cancer.

SIDE EFFECTS

CV: ***MI, CVA, cardiac arrest,*** thrombosis, CHF, hypertension, thrombophlebitis, leg cramps, edema. **Respiratory:** ***Pulmonary embolism,*** dyspnea, upper respiratory discharge, hoarseness. **GI:** Flatulence, N&V, diarrhea, minor GI upset, anorexia, GI bleeding, burning sensation of throat, thirst. **CNS:** Emotional lability, insomnia, anxiety, lethargy, depression, headache. **GU:** Breast tenderness/enlargement, impotence. **Dermatologic:** Easy bruising, flushing, peeling of skin or fingertips, pruritus, dry skin, rash, pigment changes, thinning hair. **Ophthalmic:** Tearing of eyes, pain in eyes. **Miscellaneous:** Chest pain, tinnitus, leg cramps, fluid retention, decreased glucose tolerance, night sweats, hot flashes.

LABORATORY TEST CONSIDERATIONS

↑ Bilirubin, AST, LDH. ↓ Glucose tolerance and testosterone. Abnormal hematologic tests for leukopenia and thrombocytopenia.

OD OVERDOSE MANAGEMENT

Symptoms: Extensions of the side effects. *Treatment:* Gastric lavage; treat symptoms. Monitor blood counts and liver profiles for at least 6 weeks.

DRUG INTERACTIONS

Drugs or food containing calcium may ↓ estramustine absorption.

HOW SUPPLIED

Capsule: Estramustine sodium phosphate equivalent to 140 mg estramustine phosphate

DOSAGE

• **CAPSULES**

14 mg/kg/day in three to four divided doses (range: 10–16 mg/kg/day) or 600 mg (base)/m² daily in three divided doses. One 140-mg capsule is taken for each 10 kg or 22 lb of body weight. Treat for 30–90 days before assessing beneficial effects; continue therapy as long as the drug is effective. Some clients have taken doses from 10 to 16 mg/kg/day for more than 3 years.

NURSING CONSIDERATIONS

SEE ALSO *NURSING CONSIDERATIONS* FOR *ANTINEOPLASTIC AGENTS*.

ADMINISTRATION/STORAGE

Store capsules in the refrigerator at 2–8°C (36–46°F), although may be kept at room temperature up to 48 hr without affecting potency.

ASSESSMENT

1. Note any allergy to nitrogen mustard or estrogen.
2. Assess diabetics for hyperglycemia, increased fatigue, weakness; glucose tolerance may be decreased.
3. Monitor CBC, electrolytes, liver and renal function studies.
4. Assess for symptoms of hypercalcemia: insomnia, lethargy, anorexia, N&V, coma, and vascular collapse.
5. Assess serum calcium levels (normal: 4.5–5.5 mEq/L). The effect of the steroid and osteolytic metastases may result in hypercalcemia.

CLIENT/FAMILY TEACHING

1. Take capsules with water 1 hr before or 2 hr after meals. Do not take milk, milk products, calcium-rich foods and drugs simultaneously with estramustine.

2. Referigerate capsules (may be at room temperature for 24-48 hr without losing potency).
3. Check BP and record; elevations may occur.
4. Monitor weight and check for signs of edema; may aggravate CHF; report breathing problems.
5. Consume 2–3 L/day of fluids to minimize hypercalcemia.
6. Report symptoms of hypercalcemia/CHF/PE (chest pain, SOB, swelling or redness and pain in an extremity).
7. Impotence resulting from previous estrogen therapy may be reversed.
8. Drug may cause genetic mutation; consider sperm/egg harvesting; practice contraceptive measures to prevent teratogenesis.

OUTCOMES/EVALUATE

↓ Size and spread of prostatic carcinoma

Estrogens conjugated, oral (conjugated estrogenic substances)

(**ES**-troh-jens)

PREGNANCY CATEGORY: X
Rx: Premarin
✱**Rx:** C.E.S., Congest, Conjugated Estrogens C.S.D., PMS-Conjugated Estrogens

Estrogens conjugated, parenteral

(**ES**-troh-jens)

PREGNANCY CATEGORY: X
Rx: Premarin IV

Estrogens conjugated, synthetic

(**ES**-troh-jens)

PREGNANCY CATEGORY: X
Rx: Cenestin

Estrogens conjugated, vaginal

(**ES**-troh-jens)

PREGNANCY CATEGORY: X
Rx: Premarin Vaginal Cream
CLASSIFICATION(S):
Estrogen, natural and Estrogen, synthetic

SEE ALSO *ESTROGENS* AND *ESTERIFIED ESTROGENS*.

ACTION/KINETICS

These products contain a blend of various estrogenic substances.

USES

PO: Moderate to severe vasomotor symptoms due to menopause, atrophic vaginitis, kraurosis vulvae, female hypogonadism, primary ovarian failure, female castration. Palliation in mammary cancer in men or postmenopausal women; prostatic carcinoma (inoperable and progressive). Prophylaxis of osteoporosis.

Parenteral: Abnormal bleeding due to imbalance of hormones and in the absence of disease.

Vaginal: Atrophic vaginitis and kraurosis vulvae associated with menopause.

SPECIAL CONCERNS

Use of estrogen replacement therapy for prolonged periods of time may increase the risk of fatal ovarian cancer, an increased risk of endometrial cancer, and possibly a higher risk of breast cancer.

HOW SUPPLIED

Estrogens conjugated, oral: *Tablet:* 0.3 mg, 0.625 mg, 0.9 mg, 1.25 mg, 2.5 mg. **Estrogens conjugated, parenteral:** *Powder for injection:* 25 mg. **Estrogens conjugated, synthetic:** *Tablet:* 0.625 mg, 0.9 mg, 1.25 mg. **Estrogens conjugated, vaginal:** *Cream:* 0.625 mg/g

DOSAGE

• **TABLETS (ESTROGENS CONJUGATED ORAL)**

Moderate to severe vasomotor symptoms due to menopause.

1.25 mg/day given cyclically. If the client has not menstruated in 2 or more months, begin therapy on any day; if, however, the client is menstruating, begin therapy on day 5 of bleeding.

Primary ovarian failure, female castration.

1.25 mg/day given cyclically (3 weeks on, 1 week off). Adjust dose to lowest effective level.

E

Atrophic vaginitis or kraurosis vulvae associated with menopause.

0.3–1.25 mg/day (higher doses may be necessary, depending on the response) given cyclically (3 weeks on, 1 week off).

Hypogonadism in females.

2.5–7.5 mg/day in divided doses for 20 days, followed by a 10-day rest period. If menses does not occur by the end of this period of time, repeat the dosage schedule. The number of courses of estrogen required to produce bleeding varies, depending on the responsiveness of the endometrium. If bleeding occurs before the end of the 10-day period, start a 20-day estrogen-progestin cycle with 2.5–7.5 mg/day of estrogen with a progestin added the last 5 days. If bleeding occurs before the end of this regimen, discontinue therapy and resume on day 5 of bleeding.

Palliation of mammary carcinoma in men or postmenopausal women.

10 mg t.i.d. for at least 90 days.

Palliation of prostatic carcinoma.

1.25–2.5 mg t.i.d. Effectiveness can be measured by phosphatase determinations and symptomatic improvement.

Prophylaxis of osteoporosis.

0.625 mg/day given cyclically (3 weeks on, 1 week off). Mainstays of therapy include calcium; exercise and nutrition may be important adjuncts.

• TABLETS (ESTROGENS CONJUGATED SYNTHETIC)

Moderate-to-severe vasomotor symptoms due to menopause.

Initial: 0.625 mg daily; **then,** titrate up to 1.25 mg daily. Discontinue as soon as possible. Attempt to discontinue or taper dosage at 3- to 6-month intervals.

• IM, IV

Abnormal bleeding.

25 mg; repeat after 6–12 hr if necessary.

• VAGINAL CREAM

½–2 g daily for 3 weeks on and 1 week off. Repeat as needed. Attempt to taper the dose or discontinue the medication at 3- to 6-month intervals.

NURSING CONSIDERATIONS

SEE ALSO *NURSING CONSIDERATIONS* FOR *ESTROGENS*.

ADMINISTRATION/STORAGE

1. For all uses, except palliation of mammary and prostatic carcinoma and prevention of postpartum breast engorgement, oral conjugated estrogens are best administered cyclically—3 weeks on and 1 week off.
2. When used vaginally, insert the cream high into the vagina (two-thirds the length of the applicator).
3. IV Administer IV Premarin slowly to prevent flushing.
4. Parenteral solutions of conjugated estrogens are compatible with NSS, invert sugar solutions, and dextrose solutions.
5. Parenteral solutions are incompatible with acid solutions, ascorbic acid solutions, and protein hydrolysates.
6. Use reconstituted parenteral solutions within a few hours after mixing if kept at room temperature. Put the date and time of reconstitution on the solution label.
7. IV use is preferred over IM as it induces a more rapid response.
8. Use the reconstituted solution within a few hours. If refrigerated, the reconstituted solution is stable for 60 days. Do not use if solution is dark or has a precipitate.

ASSESSMENT

1. Document indications for therapy, type, onset, and duration of symptoms.
2. Review potential risks R/T to the development of breast and fatal ovarian cancers with prolonged therapy.
3. Monitor serum phosphatase levels with prostatic cancer.

CLIENT/FAMILY TEACHING

1. Take cyclically as directed i.e., 3 weeks on, 1 week off.
2. Cenestin is the only plant derived form of estrogen.
3. Review potential risks of prolonged therapy i.e., endometrial cancer, abnormal blood clotting, gallbladder disease, and breast cancer.
4. If no hysterectomy has been performed remember to add progesterone to prevent cancer.

OUTCOMES/EVALUATE

- Control of abnormal uterine bleeding
- Osteoporosis prophylaxis
- Relief of menopausal symptoms
- Treatment of urogenital S&S R/T postmenopausal atrophy of vagina and lower urinary tract.

Estropipate (Piperazine estrone sulfate)

(es-troh-**PIE**-payt)

PREGNANCY CATEGORY: X
CLASSIFICATION(S):
Estrogen, semisynthetic
Rx: Ogen, Ogen Vaginal Cream, Ortho-Est

SEE ALSO *ESTROGENS*.

ACTION/KINETICS

Contains solubilized crystalline estrone stabilized with piperazine.

USES

PO: Moderate to severe vasomotor symptoms associated with menopause. Vulval and vaginal atrophy. Primary ovarian failure, female castration, female hypogonadism. Prevention of osteoporosis.

Vaginal: Atrophic vaginitis and kraurosis vulvae associated with menopause.

CONTRAINDICATIONS

Use during pregnancy.

HOW SUPPLIED

Vaginal cream: 1.5 mg/g; *Tablet:* 0.75 mg, 1.5 mg, 3 mg, 6 mg

DOSAGE

• TABLETS

Moderate to severe vasomotor symptoms; atrophic vaginitis or kraurosis vulvae due to menopause.

0.75–6 mg/day for short-term therapy (give cyclically). May also be used continuously. The lowest dose that will control symptoms should be selected. Attempt to discontinue or taper the dose at 3- to 6-month intervals.

Hypogonadism, primary ovarian failure, castration.

1.5–9 mg/day (calculated as 0.625 to 5 mg estrone sulfate) for first 3 weeks; **then,** rest period of 8–10 days. PO progestin can be given during the third week if withdrawal bleeding does not occur.

Prevention of osteoporosis.

0.625 mg/day for 25 days of a 31-day cycle per month. Mainstays of therapy include calcium; exercise and nutrition may be important adjuncts.

• VAGINAL CREAM

2–4 g (containing 3–6 mg estropipate) daily (depending on severity of condition) for 3 weeks followed by a 1-week rest period. Attempt to taper the dose or discontinue the medication at 3- to 6-month intervals.

NURSING CONSIDERATIONS

SEE ALSO *NURSING CONSIDERATIONS FOR ESTROGENS*.

ADMINISTRATION/STORAGE

1. Administration should be cyclic—3 weeks on and 1 week off medication.
2. When used to relieve vasomotor symptoms, cyclic administration is initiated on day 5 of bleeding if menstruating. If the client has not menstruated within the last 2 months (or more), cyclic administration may be initiated at any time.

CLIENT/FAMILY TEACHING

1. Take medications at the same time each day.
2. Relieve nausea during PO therapy by consuming solid foods.
3. Report any evidence of thromboembolic S&S (headache, blurred vision, pain, swelling or tenderness in the extremities); fluid retention (weight

gain, swelling of extremities); hepatic dysfunction (yellowing of skin or eyes, itching, dark urine, clay-colored stools); changes in mental status or any unusual bleeding.
4. With vaginal preparations, administer at bedtime, remaining recumbent for 30 min; protect clothing and bed linens by using a sanitary pad. Avoid tampons during therapy. To deliver cream, the end of the applicator (after the appropriate amount is introduced) should be inserted high into the vagina and the plunger pushed all the way down.
5. Between uses remove the plunger from the barrel and wash in warm, soapy water. Do not put in hot or boiling water.
6. Do not smoke.
7. Drug may cause increased pigmentation of skin. Wear protective clothing and sunscreens and avoid prolonged sun exposures.
8. Stop drug and report if pregnant.

OUTCOMES/EVALUATE

- Relief of menopausal symptoms
- Stimulation of menses
- Restoration of hormonal balance

Etanercept

(eh-**TAN**-er-sept)

PREGNANCY CATEGORY: B
CLASSIFICATION(S):
Immunomodulator
Rx: Enbrel

ACTION/KINETICS
Binds specifically to tumor necrosis factor (TNF) and blocks its interaction with cell surface TNF receptors. TNF is a cytokine that is involved in normal inflammatory and immune responses. Thus, the drug renders TNF biologically inactive. It is possible for etanercept to affect host defenses against infections and malignancies since TNF mediates inflammation and modulates cellular immune responses. It may also reverse CHF by decreasing inflammation in the heart. **t½:** 115 hr. Individual clients may undergo a two- to five-fold increase in serum levels with repeated dosing.

USES
(1) Reduce S&S and delays structural damage of moderately to severely active rheumatoid arthritis in adults who have had an inadequate response to one or more antirheumatic drugs. May be used in combination with methotrexate, in those who do not respond adequately to methotrexate alone. (2) Moderate to severe active polyarticular-course juvenile (ages 4–17 years) rheumatoid arthritis in those with inadequate response to at least one disease-modifying drug. *Investigational:* Psoriatic arthritis, psoriasis, ankylosing spondylitis, juvenile spondyloarthropathies.

CONTRAINDICATIONS
Sepsis. Use in any chronic or localized active infection. Concurrent administration of live vaccines. Use in those with preexisting or recent onset of CNS demyelinating disorders. Lactation.

SPECIAL CONCERNS
Use with caution with a history of recurring infections or with a condition that prediposes to infections (e.g., advanced or poorly controlled diabetes). Safety and efficacy have not been determined in those with immunosuppression, chronic infections, or in children less than 4 years of age.

SIDE EFFECTS
Injection site reactions: Erythema and/or itching, pain, swelling. **GI:** Abdominal pain, N&V, diarrhea, altered taste sense, mouth ulcer, dyspepsia, dry mouth, cholecystitis, pancreatitis, ***GI hemorrhage, intestinal perforation***. **CNS:** Headache, dizziness, depression, ***stroke, seizures,*** paresthesias. Rarely, demyelinating disorders (multiple sclerosis, myelitis, optic neuritis). **CV: *Heart failure, chest pain, flushing, MI,*** myocardial ischemia, cerebral ischemia, deep vein thrombosis, thrombophlebitis, hypertension, hypotension, vasodilation, cutaneous vasculitis. **Hematologic: *Pancytopenia, including aplastic anemia;*** adenopathy, anemia, leukopenia, thrombocytopenia. **Respiratory:** URI, non-URI, sinusitis, rhinitis, pharyngitis,

cough, pneumonitis, respiratory disorder, dyspnea, membranous glomerulonephropathy, interstitial lung disease, worsening of prior lung disorder, ***pulmonary embolism***. **Ophthalmic:** Ocular inflammation, dry eyes. **Dermatologic:** Urticaria, pruritus, rash, alopecia, cutaneous vasculitis, subcutaneous nodules. **Miscellaneous:** Formation of autoimmune antibodies, malignancies, asthenia, bursitis, ***serious infections and sepsis***, peripheral edema, malignancies, hypersensitivity reactions (including angioedema), polymyositis, joint pain, generalized pain, fatigue, anorexia, fever, flu-symptoms, angioedema, weight gain, chest pain.

HOW SUPPLIED

Lyophilized Powder for Injection, Single-Use Vial: 25 mg

DOSAGE

• SC

Moderate to severe active rheumatoid arthritis.

Adults: 25 mg twice weekly SC 72–96 hr apart.

Children with active polyarticular-course juvenile rheumatoid arthritis.

Children, 4–17 years: 0.4 mg/kg (maximum dose: 25 mg) twice weekly, 72–96 hr apart.

NURSING CONSIDERATIONS

ADMINISTRATION/STORAGE

1. Clients must enroll with the makers of etanercept so that pharmacies can obtain the product.
2. Methotrexate, glucocorticoids, salicylates, NSAIDs, or analgesics may be continued during therapy for rheumatoid arthritis. And, glucocorticoids, NSAIDs, or analgesics may be continued during treatment for polyarticular juvenile rheumatoid arthritis.
3. The needle cover of the diluent syringe contains latex; do not handle if sensitive to latex.
4. Reconstitute aseptically with 1 mL of the supplied sterile water for injection. Do not use other diluents. Slowly inject the diluent into the vial. Some foaming will occur. To avoid excessive foaming, do not shake or vigorously agitate. Swirl contents gently during dissolution, which takes less than 5 min. The reconstituted solution should be clear and colorless.
5. Before administration, visually inspect for particulate matter and discoloration. Do not use if discolored, cloudy, or if particulate matter remains after reconstitution.
6. Withdraw the solution into the syringe, removing as much liquid as possible from the vial. The final volume in the syringe will be about 1 mL.
7. Do not add other medications to solutions containing etanercept.
8. Do not filter reconstituted solution during preparation/administration.
9. Refrigerate etanercept sterile powder (do not freeze). Give reconstituted solutions as soon as possible. If not given immediately after reconstitution, solution may be stored in the vial at 2–8°C (36–46°F) for up to 6 hr.

ASSESSMENT

1. Note indications for therapy, joints affected, presenting characteristics, and other agents trialed/failed.
2. Observe client perform first injection after instruction.
3. Monitor closely if client develops a new infection during treatment. Discontinue if client develops a serious infection.
4. Ensure juvenile clients are brought up to date with all immunizations prior to starting etanercept therapy.

CLIENT/FAMILY TEACHING

1. Each tray contains all materials needed for administration. Do not use if breast feeding.
2. Review procedures for storage, reconstitution, inspection, withdraw, administration, site rotation and disposal of syringes.
3. If self-administering etanercept, the first injection will be performed by the client under the supervision of a qualified health care professional.
4. Always rotate sites for self-injection which include the thigh, abdomen, or upper arm. Give new injections at least one inch from the old site and never into areas where the skin is tender, bruised, red, or hard.

5. Report any abdominal pain, S&S of infection, dizziness, SOB, and chest pain.
6. Avoid immunizations with live vaccines.

OUTCOMES/EVALUATE

↓ Joint pain/swelling; delayed structural damage with RA

E

Ethacrynate sodium

(eth-ah-**KRIH**-nayt)

PREGNANCY CATEGORY: B
Rx: Edecrin Sodium

Ethacrynic acid

(eth-ah-**KRIH**-nik **AH**-sid)

PREGNANCY CATEGORY: B
Rx: Edecrin
CLASSIFICATION(S):
Diuretic, loop

SEE ALSO ***DIURETICS, LOOP.***

ACTION/KINETICS

Inhibits the reabsorption of sodium and chloride in the loop of Henle; it also decreases reabsorption of sodium and chloride and increases potassium excretion in the distal tubule. Also acts directly on the proximal tubule to enhance excretion of electrolytes. Large quantities of sodium and chloride and smaller amounts of potassium and bicarbonate ion are excreted during diuresis. **Onset: PO,** 30 min; **IV,** Within 5 min. **Peak: PO,** 2 hr; **IV,** 15–30 min. **Duration: PO,** 6–8 hr. **IV,** 2 hr. $\mathbf{t_{1/2}}$**, after PO:** 60 min. Metabolites are excreted through the urine. Diuresis and electrolyte loss are more pronounced with ethacrynic acid than with thiazide diuretics. Is often effective in clients refractory to other diuretics. Careful monitoring of the diuretic effects is necessary.

USES

Of value with resistance to less potent diuretics. (1) CHF, acute pulmonary edema, edema associated with nephrotic syndrome, ascites due to idiopathic edema, lymphedema, malignancy. (2) Short-term use for ascites as a result of malignancy, lymphedema, or idiopathic edema; also, for short-term use in pediatric clients (except infants) with congenital heart disease. *Investigational.* **Ethacrynic acid:** Single injection into the eye to treat glaucoma (effective for a week or more). **Ethacrynate sodium:** Hypercalcemia, bromide intoxication, and with mannitol in ethylene glycol poisoning.

CONTRAINDICATIONS

Pregnancy (usually), lactation, use in neonates. Anuria and severe renal damage.

SPECIAL CONCERNS

Geriatric clients may be more sensitive to the usual adult dose. Use with caution in diabetics and in those with hepatic cirrhosis (who are particularly susceptible to electrolyte imbalance). Monitor gout clients carefully. Safety and efficacy of oral use in infants and IV use in children have not been established.

SIDE EFFECTS

Electrolyte imbalance: Hypokalemia/natremia, hypochloremic alkalosis, hypomagnesemia/calcemia. **GI:** Anorexia, nausea, vomiting, diarrhea (may be sudden, watery, profuse diarrhea), acute pancreatitis, abdominal discomfort/pain, jaundice, ***GI bleeding or hemorrhage,*** dysphagia. **Hematologic:** Severe neutropenia, thrombocytopenia, ***agranulocytosis,*** rarely Henoch-Schoenlein purpura in clients with rheumatic heart disease. **CNS:** Apprehension, confusion, vertigo, headache. **Body as a whole:** Fever, chills, fatigue, malaise. **Otic:** Sense of fullness in the ears, tinnitus, irreversible hearing loss. **Miscellaneous:** Hematuria, acute gout, abnormal LFTs in seriously ill clients on multiple drug therapy including ethacrynic acid, blurred vision, rash, local irritation and pain following parenteral use, hyperuricemia/glycemia.

Ethacrynic acid may cause death in critically ill clients refractory to other diuretics. These include (a) clients with severe myocardial disease who also received digitalis and who developed acute hypokalemia with fatal arrhythmias and (b) those with severely decompensated hepatic cirrhosis with ascites, with or without encephalopathy, who had electrolyte imbalances. Death is due to intensification of the electrolyte effect.

OD OVERDOSE MANAGEMENT

Symptoms: Profound water loss, electrolyte depletion (causes dizziness, weakness, mental confusion, vomiting, anorexia, lethargy, cramps), dehydration, reduction of blood volume, ***circulatory collapse (possibility of vascular thrombosis and embolism).*** *Treatment:* Replace electrolytes and fluid and monitor urine output and serum electrolyte levels. Induce emesis or perform gastric lavage. Artificial respiration and oxygen may be needed. Treat other symptoms.

HOW SUPPLIED

Ethacrynate Sodium: *Powder for injection:* 50 mg/vial. **Ethacrynic Acid:** *Tablet:* 25 mg, 50 mg

DOSAGE

ETHACRYNATE SODIUM

• **IV**

Adults: 50 mg (base) (or 0.5–1 mg/kg); may be repeated in 2–4 hr, although only one dose is usually needed. A single 100-mg dose IV has also been used.

ETHACRYNIC ACID

• **TABLETS**

Adults, initial: 50–200 mg/day in single or divided doses to produce a gradual weight loss of 2.2–4.4 kg/day (1–2 lb/day). The dose can be increased by 25–50 mg/day if needed. **Maintenance:** Usually 50–200 mg (up to a maximum of 400 mg) daily may be required in severe, refractory edema. If used with other diuretics, the initial dose should be 25 mg with increments of 25 mg. **Pediatric, initial:** 25 mg/day; can increase by 25 mg/day if needed. **Maintenance:** Adjust dose to needs of client. Dosage for infants has not been determined.

NURSING CONSIDERATIONS

SEE ALSO *NURSING CONSIDERATIONS* FOR *DIURETICS, LOOP*.

ADMINISTRATION/STORAGE

1. Administer tablets after meals.
2. Due to local pain and irritation, do not give SC or IM.
3. Ammonium chloride or arginine chloride may be prescribed for those at a higher risk of developing metabolic acidosis.
4. IV Reconstitute powder for injection by adding 50 mL of D5W or NaCl injection.
5. Intermittent IV administration should be slowly over a 30-min period given either directly or through IV tubing. For direct IV, may give at a rate of 10 mg/min.
6. When reconstituted with D5W injection, the resulting solution may be hazy or opalescent; do not use. Do not mix solution with whole blood or its derivatives.
7. If a second IV injection is necessary, use a different site to prevent thrombophlebitis.
8. Use reconstituted solutions within 24 hr; discard any unused solution.

ASSESSMENT

1. Document indications for therapy, other agents trialed, and outcome.
2. Note any diabetes or cirrhosis.
3. Establish lack of anuria.
4. Monitor electrolytes, CBC, liver and renal function studies.
5. With prolonged therapy, obtain audiometric assessment.

INTERVENTIONS

1. Monitor VS, I&O, and weight. Note excessive diuresis or weight loss; electrolyte imbalance may develop quickly.
2. With rapid excessive diuresis, assess for pain in calves, pelvic area, or the chest; rapid hemoconcentration may cause thromboembolic effects.
3. Drug should be withdrawn if severe, watery diarrhea presents. Test for occult blood in urine and stools.
4. Observe for vestibular disturbances. Do not administer concomitantly with any other ototoxic agent. Hearing loss is most common following high dosing or rapid IV administration.
5. Monitor serum K^+ levels; assess need for supplemental potassium.

6. Since drug has such a profound effect on sodium excretion, dietary salt restriction is not necessary; if sodium is restricted, hyponatremia may result.

OUTCOMES/EVALUATE

- Enhanced diuresis
- ↓ Edema (↑ weight loss)
- ↓ Abdominal girth R/T ascites

E

Ethambutol hydrochloride

(eh-**THAM**-byou-tohl)

PREGNANCY CATEGORY: B
CLASSIFICATION(S):
Antitubercular drug
Rx: Myambutol
★**Rx:** Etibi

ACTION/KINETICS

Inhibits the synthesis of metabolites resulting in impairment of cell metabolism, arrest of multiplication, and ultimately cell death. Is active against *Mycobacterium tuberculosis,* but not against fungi, other bacteria, or viruses. Readily absorbed after PO administration. Widely distributed in body tissues except CSF. **Peak plasma concentration:** 2–5 mcg/mL after 2–4 hr. **t½:** 3–4 hr. About 65% of metabolized and unchanged drug excreted in urine and 20%–25% unchanged drug excreted in feces. Drug accumulates in clients with renal insufficiency.

USES

Pulmonary tuberculosis in combination with other tuberculostatic drugs. Use only in conjunction with at least one other antituberculostatic.

CONTRAINDICATIONS

Hypersensitivity to ethambutol, preexisting optic neuritis, and in children under 13 years of age.

SPECIAL CONCERNS

Use with caution and in reduced dosage in clients with gout and impaired renal function and in pregnant women.

SIDE EFFECTS

Ophthalmologic: Optic neuritis, decreased visual acuity, loss of color (green) discrimination, temporary loss of vision or blurred vision. **GI:** N&V, anorexia, abdominal pain. **CNS:** Fever, headache, dizziness, confusion, disorientation, malaise, hallucinations. **Allergic:** Pruritus, dermatitis, ***anaphylaxis.*** **Miscellaneous:** Peripheral neuropathy (numbness, tingling), precipitation of gout, thrombocytopenia, joint pain, toxic epidermal necrolysis. Renal damage. Also, hyperuricemia and decreased liver function. Adverse symptoms usually appear during the early months of therapy and disappear thereafter.

DRUG INTERACTIONS

Aluminum may delay and decrease the absorption of ethambutol.

HOW SUPPLIED

Tablet: 100 mg, 400 mg

DOSAGE

- **TABLETS**

Adults, initial treatment: 15 mg/kg/day until maximal improvement noted; **for retreatment:** 25 mg/kg/day as a single dose with at least one other tuberculostatic drug; **after 60 days:** 15 mg/kg/day.

NURSING CONSIDERATIONS

SEE ALSO GENERAL NURSING CONSIDERATIONS FOR ALL ANTI-INFECTIVES.

ASSESSMENT

1. Note indications for therapy, onset and symptom characteristics, other treatments/outcomes.
2. Obtain visual acuity test before therapy. Ensure no preexisting problems (especially if dose exceeds 15 mg/kg/day).
3. Monitor CBC, uric acid, cultures, liver and renal function studies.
4. With positive AFB cultures, report contacts and advise treatment.

CLIENT/FAMILY TEACHING

1. Take as prescribed to prevent any relapses or complications.
2. Consume 2–3 L/day of fluids to ensure adequate hydration.
3. Avoid aluminum-based antacids; may interfere with drug absorption.
4. Obtain periodic vision testing during therapy (q 1–2 months); report any vision changes that may indicate optic neuritis. Ocular side effects generally disappear within weeks to months after therapy completed .

5. Practice reliable birth control; stop drug and report if pregnancy is suspected.

OUTCOMES/EVALUATE

- Negative sputum cultures
- Resolution of infection (↓ fever, WBC, sputum; improved CXR)

Ethosuximide

(eth-oh-**SUCKS**-ih-myd)

PREGNANCY CATEGORY: C
CLASSIFICATION(S):
Anticonvulsant, succinimide
Rx: Zarontin

SEE ALSO *ANTICONVULSANTS* AND *SUCCINIMIDES*.

ACTION/KINETICS

Peak serum levels: 3–7 hr. **t½, adults:** 40–60 hr; **t½, children:** 30 hr. Steady serum levels reached in 7–10 days. **Therapeutic serum levels:** 40–100 mcg/mL. Not bound to plasma protein. Metabolized in the liver. Both inactive metabolites and unchanged drug are excreted in the urine.

USES

Absence (petit mal) seizures.

ADDITIONAL DRUG INTERACTIONS

Estrogens, Progestins / ↓ plasma hormone levels → ↓ effect
Isoniazid ↑ Ethosuximide effects
Valproic acid ↑ Ethosuximide effects

HOW SUPPLIED

Capsule: 250 mg; *Syrup:* 250 mg/5 mL

DOSAGE

- **CAPSULES, SYRUP**

Absence seizures.

Adults and children over 6 years, initial: 250 mg b.i.d.; the dose may be increased by 250 mg/day at 4–7-day intervals until seizures are controlled or until total daily dose reaches 1.5 g. **Children under 6 years, initial:** 250 mg/day; dosage may be increased by 250 mg/day every 4–7 days until control is established or total daily dose reaches 1 g.

NURSING CONSIDERATIONS

SEE ALSO *NURSING CONSIDERATIONS* FOR *ANTICONVULSANTS* AND *SUCCINIMIDES*.

ADMINISTRATION/STORAGE

May be given with other anticonvulsants when other forms of epilepsy are present.

CLIENT/FAMILY TEACHING

1. Take with meals to minimize GI upset.
2. Do not engage in hazardous activities while on drug therapy.
3. Do not stop abruptly; may precipitate withdrawal seizures.
4. Report significant weight loss or loss of seizure control.
5. Need lab studies q 3 mo to assess uric acid levels, hematologic, liver, and renal function.

OUTCOMES/EVALUATE

- Control of petit mal seizures
- Therapeutic serum drug levels (40–100 mcg/mL)

Etidronate disodium (oral)

(eh-tih-**DROH**-nayt)

PREGNANCY CATEGORY: B
Rx: Didronel

Etidronate disodium (parenteral)

(eh-tih-**DROH**-nayt)

PREGNANCY CATEGORY: B
Rx: Didronel IV
CLASSIFICATION(S):
Bone growth regulator, bisphosphonate

ACTION/KINETICS

Slows bone metabolism, thereby decreasing bone resorption, bone turnover, and new bone formation; it also reduces bone vascularization. Renal tubular reabsorption of calcium is not affected. **Absorption:** Dose-dependent; after 24 hr, one-half of absorbed drug is excreted unchanged. Absorption is affected by food or preparations containing divalent ions. **Onset:** 1 month for Paget's disease and within 24 hr for hypercalcemia. The drug remaining in the body is adsorbed to bone, where therapeutic effects for Paget's disease persist 3–12 months after discontinuation of the drug. **Plasma t½:** 6 hr; **bone t½:** Over 90 days. Approximately 50% excreted unchanged in the urine; unabsorbed drug is excreted through the feces.

USES

PO: (1) Paget's disease (osteitis deformans), especially of the polyostotic type accompanied by pain and increased urine levels of hydroxyproline and serum alkaline phosphatase. (2) Heterotopic ossification due to spinal cord injury or total hip replacement. **Parenteral:** Hypercalcemia of malignancy inadequately managed by dietary modification or oral hydration or which persists after adequate hydration is restored. *Investigational:* Postmenopausal osteoporosis and prevention of bone loss in early menopause.

CONTRAINDICATIONS

Enterocolitis, fracture of long bones, hypercalcemia of hyperparathyroidism. Serum creatinine greater than 5 mg/dL.

SPECIAL CONCERNS

Use with caution in the presence of renal dysfunction, in active UGI problems, and during lactation. Safety and efficacy have not been established in children.

SIDE EFFECTS

GI: Nausea, diarrhea, constipation, ulcerative stomatitis. **Bones:** Increased incidence of bone fractures and increased or recurrent bone pain. Drug should be discontinued if fracture occurs and not restarted until healing takes place. **Allergy:** Angioedema, rash, pruritus, urticaria. **Electrolytes:** Hypophosphatemia, hypomagnesemia. **Miscellaneous:** Metallic taste, chest pain, abnormal hepatic function, fever, fluid overload, dyspnea, convulsions. Symptoms of rachitic syndrome have been reported in children receiving 10 mg or more/kg daily for long periods (up to 1 year) to treat heterotopic ossification or soft tissue calcification.

LABORATORY TEST CONSIDERATIONS

Hypomagnesemia, hypophosphatemia.

OD OVERDOSE MANAGEMENT

Symptoms: Following PO ingestion, hypocalcemia may occur. Rapid IV administration may cause renal insufficiency. *Treatment:* Gastric lavage following PO ingestion. Treat hypocalcemia by giving calcium IV.

DRUG INTERACTIONS

Products containing calcium or other multivalent cations ↓ absorption of etidronate

HOW SUPPLIED

Etidronate disodium (oral): *Tablet:* 200 mg, 400 mg. **Etidronate disodium (parenteral):** *Injection:* 50 mg /mL

DOSAGE

• TABLETS

Paget's disease.

Adults, initial: 5–10 mg/kg/day for 6 months or less; or, 11–20 mg/kg for a maximum of 3 months. Reserve doses above 10 mg/kg when lower doses are ineffective, when there is a need for suppression of increased bone turnover, or when a prompt decrease in CO is needed. Do not exceed doses of 20 mg/kg/day. Another course of therapy may be instituted after rest period of 3 months if there is evidence of active disease process. Monitor every 3 to 6 months.

Heterotopic ossification due to spinal cord injury.

Adults: 20 mg/kg/day for 2 weeks; **then** 10 mg/kg/day for 10 weeks. Treatment should be initiated as soon as possible after the injury, preferably before evidence of heterotopic ossification.

Total hip replacement.

Initial: 20 mg/kg/day for 1 month preoperatively; **then,** 20 mg/kg/day for 3 months postoperatively for a total treatment duration of 4 months.

Heterotopic ossification complicating total hip replacement.

Adults: 20 mg/kg/day for 30 days preoperatively; **then,** 20 mg/kg/day for 90 days postoperatively.

• **IV INFUSION**

Hypercalcemia due to malignancy. 7.5 mg/kg/day for 3 successive days. If necessary, a second course of treatment may be instituted after a 7-day rest period. The safety and effectiveness of more than two courses of therapy has not been determined. Reduce the dose in those with renal impairment. Etidronate tablets may be started the day after the last infusion at a dose of 20 mg/kg/day for 30 days (treatment may be extended to 90 days if serum calcium levels are normal). Use for more than 90 days is not recommended.

NURSING CONSIDERATIONS

ADMINISTRATION/STORAGE

1. Administer PO as a single dose (if GI upset occurs, divide dose) with juice or water 2 hr before meals.
2. There are no indications to date that etidronate will affect mature heterotopic bone.
IV 3. Dilute IV dose in at least 250 mL of sterile NSS and administer over a 2-hr period.
4. May experience a metallic taste during IV administration.
5. The diluted solution shows no loss of drug for 48 hr if stored between 15–30°C (59–86°F).

ASSESSMENT

1. Note indications for therapy; rate pain level and note other agents trialed.
2. Assess for evidence of renal dysfunction. Monitor uric acid, alkaline phosphatase, urinary hydroxyproline excretion, electrolytes, magnesium, phosphate, calcium, and renal function studies.
3. Determine if pregnant.
4. Review xrays/bone density for evidence of bone loss.

CLIENT/FAMILY TEACHING

1. Maintain a well-balanced diet with adequate intake of calcium and vitamin D; see dietitian prn.
2. Do not eat for 2 hr after taking medication. Foods high in calcium (e.g., milk, milk products) and vitamins with mineral supplements (e.g., aluminum, calcium, iron, or magnesium) may decrease absorption. If GI upset with single dose, may divide dose.
3. Report any S&S of hypercalcemia, i.e., lethargy, N&V, anorexia, tremors, and bone pain.
4. Obtain lab studies as scheduled: with Paget's disease, levels of urinary hydroxyproline excretion and serum alkaline phosphatase reductions indicate a beneficial therapeutic response. Levels usually decrease 1–3 months after initiation of therapy.
5. With hypercalcemia, serum calcium levels show drug response and need for continued therapy. Reduction usually occurs in 2–8 days in hypercalcemia R/T bone metastasis. Therapy may be repeated only after 7 days of rest; risk for hypocalcemia greatest 3 days after IV therapy.

OUTCOMES/EVALUATE

- Suppression of bone resorption
- ↓ Serum calcium levels
- ↓ Bone pain with Paget's disease

Etodolac

(ee-toh-**DOH**-lack)

PREGNANCY CATEGORY: C
CLASSIFICATION(S):
Nonsteroidal anti-inflammatory drug
Rx: Lodine, Lodine XL
✱**Rx:** Apo-Etodolac, Gen-Etodolac, Ultradol

SEE ALSO *NONSTEROIDAL ANTI-INFLAMMATORY DRUGS.*

ACTION/KINETICS

Etodolac is a NSAID in a class called the pyranocarboxylic acids. **Time to peak levels:** 1–2 hr. **Onset of analgesic action:** 30 min; **duration:** 4–12 hr. **t½:** 7.3 hr. Over 99% protein bound. The drug is metabolized by the liver and metabolites are excreted through the kidneys.

USES

Acute and chronic treatment of osteoarthritis and rheumatoid arthritis. Mild to moderate pain (Lodine only).

CONTRAINDICATIONS
Clients in whom etodolac, aspirin, or other NSAIDs have caused asthma, rhinitis, urticaria, or other allergic reactions. Use during lactation, during labor and delivery, and in children.

SPECIAL CONCERNS
Use with caution in impaired renal or hepatic function, heart failure, those on diuretics, and in geriatric clients. Safety and effectiveness have not been determined in children.

ADDITIONAL SIDE EFFECTS
GI: Diarrhea, gastritis, thirst, ulcerative stomatitis, anorexia. **CNS:** Nervousness, depression. **CV:** Syncope. **Respiratory:** Asthma. **Dermatologic:** Angioedema, vesiculobullous rash, cutaneous vasculitis with purpura, hyperpigmentation. **Miscellaneous:** Jaundice, hepatitis.

LABORATORY TEST CONSIDERATIONS
False + reaction for urinary bilirubin and for urinary ketones (using the dipstick method). ↑ Liver enzymes, serum creatinine. ↑ Bleeding time.

OD OVERDOSE MANAGEMENT
Symptoms: N&V, drowsiness, lethargy, epigastric pain, ***anaphylaxis.*** Rarely, hypertension, acute renal failure, respiratory depression. *Treatment:* Since there are no antidotes, treatment is supportive and symptomatic. If discovered within 4 hr, emesis followed by activated charcoal and an osmotic cathartic may be tried.

ADDITIONAL DRUG INTERACTIONS
Cyclosporine / ↑ Serum cyclosporine levels R/T ↓ renal excretion; ↑ risk of cyclosporine-induced nephrotoxicity
Digoxin / ↑ Serum digoxin levels R/T ↓ renal excretion
Lithium / ↑ Serum lithium levels R/T ↓ renal excretion
Methotrexate / ↑ Serum methotrexate levels R/T ↓ renal excretion

HOW SUPPLIED
Capsule: 200 mg, 300 mg; *Tablet:* 400 mg, 500 mg; *Tablet, Extended Release:* 400 mg, 500 mg, 600 mg, 1,200 mg

DOSAGE

• **CAPSULES, TABLETS, EXTENDED RELEASE TABLETS**

Osteoarthritis, rheumatoid arthritis.
Adults, initial: 300 mg b.i.d. or t.i.d. or 400 mg or 500 mg b.i.d. using capsules or tablets. Dose may be adjusted up or down during long-term use, depending on the clinical response. *Extended-release tablets:* 400–1,000 mg given once daily. Doses above 1,000 mg/day have not been evaluated adequately.

Acute pain.
Adults: 200–400 mg q 6–8 hr, not to exceed 1,200 mg/day. Use capsules or tablets.
NOTE: Do not exceed 20 mg/kg in clients weighing 60 kg or less.

NURSING CONSIDERATIONS

SEE ALSO *NURSING CONSIDERATIONS FOR NONSTEROIDAL ANTI-INFLAMMATORY DRUGS*.

ADMINISTRATION/STORAGE
The capsules should be protected from moisture.

ASSESSMENT
1. Note any previous experience with NSAIDs or acetylsalicylic acid and the results.
2. Document indications for therapy (i.e., analgesic or anti-inflammatory), include onset and characteristics of symptoms, status of ROM and rate pain level.
3. With long-term therapy, monitor CBC, chemistry, liver and renal function studies periodically.
4. Determine any history of heart disease or cardiac failure.
5. Note age and weight of client and if currently prescribed diuretics.

CLIENT/FAMILY TEACHING
1. Take with food to decrease GI upset.
2. Report any unusual bruising/bleeding, rash, yellow skin discoloration, or lack of response.

OUTCOMES/EVALUATE
Control of pain and inflammation with improved joint mobility

Etomidate

(eh-**TOM**-ih-dayt)

PREGNANCY CATEGORY: C
CLASSIFICATION(S):
General anesthetic, induction
Rx: Amidate

ACTION/KINETICS
Is a hypnotic with no analgesic activity. Appears to act like GABA and is thought to exert its mechanism by depressing the activity of the brain stem reticular system. Minimal CV and respiratory depressant effects. **Onset:** 1 min. **Duration:** 3–5 min. **t½:** 75 min. Rapidly metabolized in the liver with inactive metabolites excreted mainly through the urine.
USES
Induction of general anesthesia. As a supplement to nitrous oxide during short surgical procedures. *Investigational:* Prolonged sedation of critically ill or ventilator-dependent clients (is an increased risk of acute insufficiency and mortality).
SPECIAL CONCERNS
Use with caution during lactation. Safety and efficacy have not been established in children less than 10 years of age.
SIDE EFFECTS
Skeletal muscle: Myoclonic skeletal muscle movements, tonic movements. **Respiratory:** Apnea of short duration, hyperventilation or hypoventilation, ***laryngospasm.*** **CV:** Either hypertension or hypotension; tachycardia or bradycardia; arrhythmias. **GI:** Postoperative N&V. **Miscellaneous:** Eye movements, averting movements, hiccoughs, snoring.
HOW SUPPLIED
Injection: 2 mg/mL

DOSAGE
• **IV ONLY**
Induction of anesthesia.
Adults and children over 10 years of age: 0.2–0.6 mg/kg (usual: 0.3 mg/kg) injected over 30–60 sec.

NURSING CONSIDERATIONS
ADMINISTRATION/STORAGE
IV 1. Lower doses may be used as adjuncts to supplement less potent general anesthetics (e.g., nitrous oxide.)
2. Etomidate may be used following preanesthetic medications.
3. Protect from extreme heat and freezing.

INTERVENTIONS
1. N&V are likely postoperatively; have equipment (e.g.; suction, basins, washcloths) to manage.
2. Monitor postoperatively for hypo/hypertension, tachy/bradycardia; treat symptomatically.
OUTCOMES/EVALUATE
Desired anesthetic level

Etoposide (VP-16–213)
(eh-**TOH**-poh-syd)

PREGNANCY CATEGORY: D
CLASSIFICATION(S):
Antineoplastic, miscellaneous
Rx: Etopophos, Toposar, VePesid

SEE ALSO *ANTINEOPLASTIC AGENTS.*
ACTION/KINETICS
Acts as a mitotic inhibitor at the G_2 portion of the cell cycle to inhibit DNA synthesis. At high doses, cells entering mitosis are lysed, whereas at low doses, cells will not enter prophase. **t½: biphasic, initial,** 1.5 hr; **final,** 4–11 hr. **Effective plasma levels:** 0.3–10 mcg/mL. Poor CNS penetration. Eliminated through both the urine and bile unchanged and as liver metabolites. Is water soluble.
USES
With combination therapy to treat refractory testicular tumors and small cell lung cancer. *Investigational:* Alone or in combination to treat acute monocytic leukemia, non-Hodgkin's lymphoma, Hodgkin's disease, AIDS-associated Kaposi's sarcoma, Ewing's sarcoma. Also, choriocarcinoma; hepatocellular carcinoma; nonsmall cell lung, breast, endometrial, and gastric cancers; acute lymphocytic leukemia; soft tissue carcinoma; rhabdomyosarcoma.
CONTRAINDICATIONS
Lactation.
SPECIAL CONCERNS
Safety and efficacy in children have not been established. Severe myelosuppression may occur.

ADDITIONAL SIDE EFFECTS
Anaphylactic-type reactions, hypotension, peripheral neuropathy, somnolence.

HOW SUPPLIED
Capsule: 50 mg; *Injection:* 20 mg/mL; *Powder for Injection:* 100 mg

DOSAGE

- **IV**

Testicular carcinoma.
50–100 mg/m²/day on days 1–5 or 100 mg/m²/day on days 1, 3, and 5 q 3–4 weeks (i.e., after recovery from toxic effects). Used in combination with other agents.

Small cell lung carcinoma.
35 mg/m²/day for 4 days to 50 mg/m²/day for 5 days, repeated q 3–4 weeks.

- **CAPSULES**

Small cell lung carcinoma.
70 mg/m² (rounded to the nearest 50 mg) daily for 4 days to 100 mg/m² (rounded to the nearest 50 mg) daily for 5 days; repeat q 3–4 weeks.

NOTE: Etopophos is given in higher concentrations than VePesid. Doses above are for VePesid.

NURSING CONSIDERATIONS

SEE ALSO *NURSING CONSIDERATIONS* FOR *ANTINEOPLASTIC AGENTS*.

ADMINISTRATION/STORAGE
1. Store capsules at 2–8°C (36–46°F); do not freeze.
IV 2. For IV use, dilute drug with either D5W or 0.9% NaCl for final concentration of 0.2 or 0.4 mg/mL (5-mL vial in 250 or 500 mL of IV solution).
3. A slow infusion over 30–60 min will decrease chance of hypotension. Do not give by rapid IV push; may give over a period of 5 min.
4. Wear gloves when preparing; if drug comes in contact with the skin or mucosa, wash immediately and thoroughly with soap and water.
5. Diluted solutions with a final concentration of 0.2 mg/mL are stable for 96 hr at room temperature; final concentrations of 0.4 mg/mL are stable for 48 hr at room temperature.

ASSESSMENT
1. Assess nutritional status. Pretreat with antiemetic; drug may cause N&V.
2. Monitor CBC, liver and renal function studies; may cause granulocyte and platelet suppression. Nadir: 14 days; recovery: 21 days.
3. Determine if pregnant.
4. May cause increased uric acid levels.
5. Assess for signs of infection and bleeding; occurs more often with this drug than with most antineoplastic agents.
6. With infusions, stress bed rest and supervise ambulation as orthostatic hypotension may occur. Record BP during infusions and at least twice a day with PO therapy; note any significant decreases.
7. Be prepared to treat anaphylactic reactions.

CLIENT/FAMILY TEACHING
1. Report any flu-like symptoms; drug combination therapy may cause severe myelosuppression.
2. Consume 2–3 L/day of fluids to prevent kidney damage.
3. May cause marked hair loss, and blood abnormalities.
4. Report sores in mouth so therapy may be initiated. Avoid irritant such as tobacco, alcohol, and hot spicy foods.
5. May cause postural hypotension, change postitions slowly.
6. May feel fatigued and sleepy during and after drug administration; schedule activities to ensure adequate rest.
7. Report any tingling sensations or numbness (S&S of peripheral neuropathy.)
8. Report if N&V impair intake.
9. Practice reliable contraception.

OUTCOMES/EVALUATE
- ↓ Malignant cell proliferation
- Improved hematologic parameters with leukemia

Exemestane

(ex-eh-**MESS**-tayn)

PREGNANCY CATEGORY: D
CLASSIFICATION(S):
Antineoplastic, hormone
Rx: Aromasin

ACTION/KINETICS

Irreversible, steroidal aromatase inactivator. Acts as a false substrate for the aromatase enzyme, which is the principal enzyme that converts androgens to estrogens. Drug is processed to an intermediate that binds irreversibly to the active enzyme site causing its inhibition (called "suicide inhibition"). Significantly lowers circulating estrogen levels in postmenopausal women; has no detectable effect on adrenal biosynthesis of corticosteroids or aldosterone. Rapidly absorbed. **t½, terminal:** About 24 hr. Metabolized in the liver and metabolites (some are active) excreted in both the urine and feces in equal amounts.

USES

Treatment of advanced breast cancer in postmenopausal women where the disease has progressed following tamoxifen therapy. *Investigational:* Prevention of prostate cancer.

CONTRAINDICATIONS

Administration to premenopausal women.

SPECIAL CONCERNS

Safety and efficacy have not been established in children.

SIDE EFFECTS

GI: N&V, abdominal pain, anorexia, constipation, diarrhea, increased appetite, dyspepsia. **CNS:** Depression, insomnia, anxiety, dizziness, headache, hypoesthesia, confusion. **Respiratory:** Dyspnea, coughing, bronchitis, sinusitis, chest pain, URTI, pharyngitis, rhinitis. **Body as a whole:** Fatigue, edema, fever, generalized weakness, paresthesia, asthenia, peripheal edema, leg edema, flu-like symptoms, increased sweating, rash, itching, infection. **Miscellaneous:** Hypertension, hot flashes, pain, pathological fracture, UTI, lymphedema, pain at tumor site, arthralgia, back pain, skeletal pain, alopecia, lymphocytopenia.

LABORATORY TEST CONSIDERATIONS

↑ AST, ALT, alkaline phosphatase, gamma glutamyl transferase. Slight ↑ serum LH and FSH. ↓ Sex hormone binding globulin.

HOW SUPPLIED

Tablets: 25 mg

DOSAGE

• **TABLETS**

Treatment of breast cancer.

25 mg once daily after a meal.

NURSING CONSIDERATIONS

ADMINISTRATION/STORAGE

Glucocorticoid and mineralocorticoid replacement therapy is not necessary.

ASSESSMENT

1. Note indications for therapy, disease onset, other therapies trialed and tamoxifen failure.
2. Drug is not for use in premenopausal women.
3. Monitor VS, CBC, chemistries, renal and LFT's.

CLIENT/FAMILY TEACHING

1. Take as directed once daily after a meal.
2. Drug will lower estrogen levels.
3. Report if GI upset, headaches, depression, fatigue or edema become intolerable.

OUTCOMES/EVALUATE

• Treatment of progressive breast cancer in postmenopausal women
• Prevention of prostate cancer

F 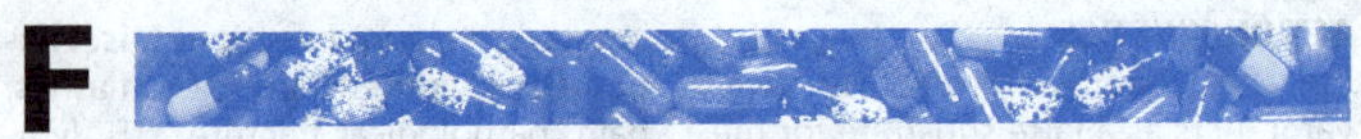

Factor IX Concentrates

(**FAK**-tor 9)

PREGNANCY CATEGORY: C
CLASSIFICATION(S):
Hemostatic, systemic
Rx: AlphaNine SD, Bebulin VH, Benefix, Mononine, Profilnine SD, Proplex T

ACTION/KINETICS
Causes an increase in factor IX levels, thus minimizing hemorrhage in those with factor IX deficiency. Factors II, VII, and X may also be increased. **t½:** 22 hr. The mean increase in circulating factor IX after IV infusion is 0.67–1.15 IU/dL rise per IU/kg body weight.
USES
To prevent or control bleeding in clients with factor IX deficiency, especially hemophilia B and Christmas disease. Hemarthroses in hemophiliacs with inhibitors to Factor VIII (Proplex T only).
CONTRAINDICATIONS
Factor VII deficiency, except for Proplex T. Use in mild Factor IX deficiency when fresh frozen plasma is effective. Liver disease with suspected intravascular coagulation or fibrinolysis. Hypersensitivity to mouse (Mononine) or hamster (Benefix) proteins.
SPECIAL CONCERNS
Assess benefit versus risk prior to use in liver disease or elective surgery. Factor IX products may be derived from pooled units of human plasma; although precautions are taken, the risk of viral infections from such products can not be eliminated completely.
SIDE EFFECTS
CV: ***DIC, thrombosis. High doses may cause MI, venous or pulmonary thrombosis.*** **Symptoms due to rapid infusion:** N&V, headache, fever, chills, tingling, flushing, urticaria, and changes in BP or pulse rate. Most of these side effects disappear when rate of administration is slowed. **Hypersensitivity:** Hives, generalized urticaria, angioedema, chest tightness, dyspnea, wheezing, faintness, hypotension, tachycardia, ***anaphylaxis.*** **GI:** Nausea, altered taste. **CNS:** Lightheadedness, headache, dizziness, drowsiness. **Miscellaneous:** Chills, fever, nephrotic syndrome, discomfort at IV site, burning sensation in jaw and skull, allergic rhinitis, tight chest, dry cough/sneeze, rash.

The preparation also contains trace amounts of blood groups A and B and isohemagglutinins, which may cause intravascular hemolysis when administered in large amounts to clients with blood groups A, B, and AB.

Although careful screening is undertaken, both hepatitis and AIDS may be transmitted using factor IX concentrates since it is derived from pooled human plasma.
DRUG INTERACTIONS
↑ Risk of thrombosis if administered with aminocaproic acid.
HOW SUPPLIED
Powder for injection

DOSAGE
• **IV**

Factor IX deficiency (hemophilia B [Christmas disease]).
Individualized, depending on severity of bleeding, degree of deficiency, body weight, and level of factor required. Minimum factor IX level required in surgery or following trauma is 25% of normal, which is maintained for 1 week after surgery. As a guide in determining the units required to raise blood level percentages of factor IX, use the following formula for human-derived factor IX:

1 unit/kg × body weight (kg) × desired increase (% of normal).
For recombinant factor IX, use the following formula:

1.2 IU/kg × body weight (kg) × desired increase (% of control).

Factor VII deficiency (Proplex T only).
To determine the units needed to raise blood level percentages, use the following:

0.5 unit/kg × body weight (kg) × desired increase (% of normal). The dose may be repeated q 4–6 hr. The package insert should be checked carefully as a guideline for doses for various factor deficiencies.

Factor VIII inhibitor (Proplex T only). Use dosage levels approximating 75 IU/kg.

NURSING CONSIDERATIONS

ADMINISTRATION/STORAGE

IV 1. The rate of administration varies with the product. As a general guideline, infuse about 100–200 IU/min at a rate of 2–3 mL/min, not to exceed 3 mL/min.
2. Store at 2–8°C (36–46°F).
3. Do not freeze provided diluent.
4. Discard 2 years after date of manufacture.
5. Before reconstitution, warm diluent to room temperature but not above 40°C (104°F).
6. Agitate the solution gently until powder is dissolved.
7. Administer within 3 hr of reconstitution to avoid incubation in case contamination occurred during preparation.
8. Do not refrigerate after reconstitution; active ingredient may precipitate out.

ASSESSMENT

1. Document any previous experience/treatment with factor replacement and outcome.
2. Obtain weight, height, and blood type. Dose must be individualized based on weight, degree of deficiency, and severity of bleed. Maintain plasma level at least 20% of normal until hemostasis achieved.
3. Note any S&S of liver disease (i.e., urticaria, fever, pruritus, anorexia, N&V); monitor LFTs.
4. Monitor VS, CBC, coagulation, and factor assay levels.
5. Assess carefully for abnormal bruising/bleeding, enlarged joints, restricted joint movement, oral mucosa for gingival bleeding, increased menses etc.

INTERVENTIONS

1. Monitor BP and pulse q 30 min during infusion.
2. Report increased bleeding and joint swelling; use rest, ice, and elevation with affected joints.
3. Reduce flow rate and report if a tingling sensation, headache, chills, or fever occur.
4. Avoid aminocaproic acid administration; may precipitate clot formation.
5. Assess for DIC if factor IX level is increased above 50% of normal. At 50% or greater, there is an increased risk for the development of a thromboembolic event and/or DIC.
6. Make sure client has received hepatitis B vaccine.
7. Monitor I&O; test urine for occult blood. Hemolytic reactions are more pronounced in clients with A, B, and AB type blood.

CLIENT/FAMILY TEACHING

1. Product is prepared from human plasma and carries potential risks (i.e., hepatitis, AIDS).
2. Avoid contact sports and any activities that may lead to injury or excessive jostling.
3. Use soft bristled tooth brush and electric razor to prevent unnecessary bleeding.
4. Report any uncontrolled bleeding, joint pain or swelling.
5. Ensure family members are screened and genetically counseled; disease is hereditary.
6. Avoid OTCs and aspirin-containing products.
7. Identify local support groups that may assist to cope with this disease.

OUTCOMES/EVALUATE

- Prevention of hemorrhage
- Factor levels within desired range

Famciclovir

(fam-**SY**-kloh-veer)

PREGNANCY CATEGORY: B
CLASSIFICATION(S):
Antiviral
Rx: Famvir

SEE ALSO *ANTIVIRAL AGENTS.*

ACTION/KINETICS
Undergoes rapid biotransformation to the active compound penciclovir. Inhibits viral DNA synthesis and therefore replication in HSV types 1 (HSV-1) and 2 (HSV-2) and varicella-zoster virus. Penciclovir is further metabolized to inactive compounds that are excreted through the urine. **t½, plasma:** 2 hr following IV administration of penciclovir and 2.3 hr following PO use of famciclovir. Half-life increased in renal insufficiency.

USES
Management of acute herpes zoster (shingles). Treatment of recurrent herpes simplex (genital herpes and cold sores), including those infected with HIV. To prevent outbreaks of recurrent genital herpes.

CONTRAINDICATIONS
Use during lactation.

SPECIAL CONCERNS
The dose should be adjusted in clients with C_{CR} less than 60 mL/min. Safety and efficacy have not been determined in children less than 18 years of age.

SIDE EFFECTS
GI: N&V, diarrhea, constipation, anorexia, abdominal pain, dyspepsia, flatulence. **CNS:** Headache, dizziness, paresthesia, somnolence, insomnia. **Body as a whole:** Fatigue, fever, pain, rigors. **Musculoskeletal:** Back pain, arthralgia. **Respiratory:** Pharyngitis, sinusitis, URI. **Dermatologic:** Pruritus; signs/symptoms/complications of zoster and genital herpes.

DRUG INTERACTIONS
Digoxin / ↑ Digoxin levels
Probenecid / ↑ Plasma penciclovir levels
Theophylline / ↑ Penciclovir levels

HOW SUPPLIED
Tablet: 125 mg, 250 mg, 500 mg

DOSAGE

• TABLETS

Herpes zoster infections.

500 mg q 8 hr for 7 days. Dosage reduction is recommended in clients with impaired renal function: for C_{CR} of 40–59 mL/min, the dose should be 500 mg q 12 hr; for C_{CR} of 20–39 mL/min, the dose should be 500 mg q 24 hr; for C_{CR} less than 20 mL/min, the dose should be 250 mg q 48 hr. For hemodialysis clients, the recommended dose is 250 mg given after each dialysis treatment.

Recurrent genital herpes.

125 mg b.i.d. for 5 days. Should be taken within 6 hr of symptoms or lesion onset. Dosage reduction is as follows for those with impaired renal function: for C_{CR} of 40 mL/min or greater, use the recommended dose of 125 mg b.i.d.; for C_{CR} of 20–39 mL/min, the dose should be 125 mg q 24 hr; for C_{CR} less than 20 mL/min, the dose should be 125 mg q 48 hr. For hemodialysis clients, the recommended dose is 125 mg given after each dialysis treatment.

Recurrent orolabial or genital herpes infection in HIV-infected clients.

500 mg b.i.d. for 7 days.

Prevent outbreaks of genital herpes.

250 mg b.i.d.

NURSING CONSIDERATIONS

SEE ALSO *NURSING CONSIDERATIONS* FOR *ANTIVIRAL AGENTS*.

ADMINISTRATION/STORAGE
1. Initiate therapy as soon as herpes zoster is diagnosed and at the first symptoms of genital herpes.
2. Therapy is most useful if started within first 48 hr of rash appearance.
3. Effect greatest in those over 50 years of age.
4. May be taken without regard for meals.

ASSESSMENT
1. Document onset of symptoms, location, extent of lesions; note duration and frequency of recurrence.
2. Initiate as soon as diagnosis is confirmed.
3. Monitor CBC and renal function studies. Anticipate reduced dosage with renal dysfunction; follow dosing guidelines.

CLIENT/FAMILY TEACHING
1. Review frequency, amount of drug to consume, and duration of therapy.
2. Side effects frequently associated with therapy include diarrhea, nausea, headaches, and fatigue; report if intolerable.

3. When lesions are open and draining, carrier is extremely contagious and should avoid any exposure or outside contact unless confirmed that the person(s) have had the chickenpox and are not pregnant.

OUTCOMES/EVALUATE

- Resolution of herpetic lesions
- ↓ Duration of neuralgia

Famotidine

(fah-**MOH**-tih-deen)

PREGNANCY CATEGORY: B
CLASSIFICATION(S):
Histamine H-2 receptor blocking drug
Rx: Pepcid, Pepcid RPD , Pepcid IV
OTC: Pepcid AC Acid Controller
✱OTC: Alti-Famotidine, Apo-Famotidine, Gen-Famotidine, Novo-Famotidine, Nu-Famotidine, Rhoxal-famotidine, Ulcidine

SEE ALSO ***HISTAMINE H_2 ANTAGONISTS.***

ACTION/KINETICS

Competitive inhibitor of histamine H_2 receptors leading to inhibition of gastric acid secretion. Both basal and nocturnal gastric acid secretion and secretion stimulated by food or pentagastrin are inhibited. **Peak plasma levels:** 1–3 hr. **t½:** 2.5–3.5 hr. **Onset:** 1 hr. **Duration:** 10–12 hr. Does not inhibit the cytochrome P-450 system in the liver; thus, drug interactions due to inhibition of liver metabolism are not expected to occur. From 25% to 30% of a PO dose is eliminated through the kidney unchanged; from 65% to 70% of an IV dose is excreted through the kidney unchanged.

USES

Rx: Treatment of active duodenal ulcers. Maintenance therapy for duodenal ulcer, at reduced dosage, after active ulcer has healed. Pathologic hypersecretory conditions such as Zollinger-Ellison syndrome or multiple endocrine adenomas. GERD, including erosive esophagitis. Treatment of benign gastric ulcer. *Investigational:* Prevent aspiration pneumonitis, for prophylaxis of stress ulcers, prevent acute upper GI bleeding, as part of multidrug therapy to eradicate *Helicobacter pylori*.

OTC: Relief of and prevention of the symptoms of heartburn, acid indigestion, and sour stomach.

CONTRAINDICATIONS

Cirrhosis of the liver, impaired renal or hepatic function, lactation.

SPECIAL CONCERNS

CNS side effects are possible in those with moderate to severe renal insufficiency. Safety and efficacy in children have not been established.

SIDE EFFECTS

GI: Constipation, diarrhea, N&V, anorexia, dry mouth, abdominal discomfort. **CNS:** Dizziness, headache, paresthesias, depression, anxiety, confusion, hallucinations, insomnia, fatigue, sleepiness, agitation, ***grand mal seizure,*** psychic disturbances. **Skin:** Rash, acne, pruritus, alopecia, urticaria, dry skin, flushing. **CV:** Palpitations. **Musculoskeletal:** Arthralgia, asthenia, musculoskeletal pain. **Hematologic:** Thrombocytopenia. **Other:** Fever, orbital edema, conjunctival injection, bronchospasm, tinnitus, taste disorders, decreased libido, impotence, pain at injection site (transient).

DRUG INTERACTIONS

Antacids / ↓ Famotidine absorption from the GI tract
Diazepam / ↓ Diazepam absorption from the GI tract

HOW SUPPLIED

Chewable Tablet: 10 mg; *Injection:* 10 mg/mL; *Injection Premixed:* 20 mg/50 mL; *Powder for Oral Suspension:* 40 mg/5 mL; *Tablet:* 10 mg, 20 mg, 40 mg; *Tablet, Oral Disintegrating:* 20 mg, 40 mg

DOSAGE

- **ORAL SUSPENSION, TABLETS**

Duodenal ulcer, acute therapy.

Adults: 40 mg once daily at bedtime or 20 mg b.i.d. Most ulcers heal within 4 weeks and it is rarely necessary to use the full dosage for 6–8 weeks.

Duodenal ulcer, maintenance therapy.

Adults: 20 mg once daily at bedtime.

Benign gastric ulcers, acute therapy. **Adults:** 40 mg at bedtime.

Hypersecretory conditions. **Adults, individualized, initial:** 20 mg q 6 hr; **then,** adjust dose to response, although doses of up to 160 mg q 6 hr may be required for severe cases.

Gastroesophageal reflux disease. **Adults:** 20 mg b.i.d. for 6 weeks. For esophagitis with erosions and ulcerations, give 20 or 40 mg b.i.d. for up to 12 weeks.

Prophylaxis of upper GI bleeding. **Adults:** 20 mg b.i.d.

Prophylaxis of stress ulcers. **Adults:** 40 mg/day.

Relief of and prevention of heartburn, acid indigestion, and sour stomach (OTC). **Adults and children over 12 years of age, for relief:** 10 mg (1 tablet) with water. **For prevention:** 10 mg 1 hr before eating a meal that may cause symptoms. **Maximum dose:** 20 mg/24 hr. Not to be used continuously for more than 2 weeks unless medically prescribed.

• **IM, IV, IV INFUSION**

Hospitalized clients with hypersecretory conditions, duodenal ulcers, gastric ulcers; clients unable to take PO medication. **Adults:** 20 mg IV q 12 hr.

Before anesthesia to prevent aspiration of gastric acid. **Adults:** 40 mg IM or PO.

NURSING CONSIDERATIONS

SEE ALSO *NURSING CONSIDERATIONS* FOR *HISTAMINE H_2 ANTAGONISTS*.

ADMINISTRATION/STORAGE

1. Use antacids concomitantly if needed.
2. Reduce the dose in moderate to severe renal impairment (C_{CR} < 50 mL/min. to half the usual dose at the usual dosage interval or the usual dose every 36–48 hr.
3. **IV** For IV injection, dilute 2 mL (containing 10 mg/mL) with 0.9% NaCl to a total volume of 5–10 mL; give over at least a 2-min period.
4. For IV infusion, dilute 2 mL (20 mg) with 100 mL of D5W and infuse over 15–30 min.
5. A solution is stable for 48 hr at room temperature when added to or diluted with water for injection, 0.9% NaCl, D5% or 10%, RL injection, or 5% $NaHCO_3$ injection.
6. Stable when mixed with various TPN solutions. Length of stability depends on the solution.

ASSESSMENT

1. Document reasons for therapy, type, onset, and duration of symptoms.
2. Note location, extent, and characteristics of abdominal pain.
3. Review UGI findings; note modifications trialed with GERD.
4. Assess mental status.
5. Check for occult blood in stools/GI secretions; note presence of *H. pylori* antibodies.
6. Assess for history of seizures.
7. If pregnant, list benefits versus risks.
8. Note hepatic/renal dysfunction; review CBC, assess for bleeding.

CLIENT/FAMILY TEACHING

1. Drug may cause dizziness, headaches, and anxiety; use caution and report if symptoms persist.
2. Increasing lack of concern for personal appearance, depression, or sleeplessness should be reported.
3. Report any diarrhea, constipation, appetite loss, easy bruising, or fatigue.
4. Avoid alcohol, aspirin-containing products, OTC cough and cold products, smoking, and foods that increase GI irritation (i.e., caffeine, black pepper, harsh spices).
5. Report a reduction in urinary output; may need a change in dosage.

OUTCOMES/EVALUATE

- ↓ Abdominal pain
- Prophylaxis of stress ulcers
- Control of hypersecretion of acid
- Duodenal ulcer healing
- Control of symptoms of GERD

Felbamate

(**FELL**-bah-mayt)

PREGNANCY CATEGORY: C

CLASSIFICATION(S):
Anticonvulsant, miscellaneous
Rx: Felbatol

SEE ALSO *ANTICONVULSANTS*.

NOTE: In August 1994 it was recommended that felbamate treatment be discontinued for epilepsy clients due to several cases of aplastic anemia. Revised labeling states, "...Felbatol should only be used in patients whose epilepsy is so severe that the risk of aplastic anemia is deemed acceptable in light of the benefits conferred by its use..."

ACTION/KINETICS
Mechanism not known. Felbamate may reduce seizure spread and increase seizure threshold. Has weak inhibitory effects on both GABA and benzodiazepine receptor binding. Well absorbed after PO use. **Terminal t½:** 20–23 hr. Trough blood levels are dose dependent. From 40% to 50% excreted unchanged in the urine.

USES
Alone or as part of adjunctive therapy for the treatment of partial seizures with and without generalization in adults with epilepsy. As an adjunct in the treatment of partial and generalized seizures associated with Lennox-Gastaut syndrome in children. The drug should be used only as second-line therapy.

CONTRAINDICATIONS
History of hepatic dysfunction or blood dyscrasia. Hypersensitivity to carbamates.

SPECIAL CONCERNS
Aplastic anemia and acute liver failure have been observed in a few clients. Use with caution during lactation. Safety and efficacy have not been established in children other than those with Lennox-Gastaut syndrome.

SIDE EFFECTS
May differ depending on whether the drug is used as monotherapy or adjunctive therapy in adults or for Lennox-Gastaut syndrome in children. **CNS:** Insomnia, headache, anxiety, somnolence, dizziness, nervousness, tremor, abnormal gait, depression, paresthesia, ataxia, stupor, abnormal thinking, emotional lability, agitation, psychologic disturbance, aggressive reaction, hallucinations, euphoria, ***suicide attempt,*** migraine. **GI:** Dyspepsia, vomiting, constipation, diarrhea, dry mouth, nausea, anorexia, abdominal pain, hiccoughs, esophagitis, increased appetite. **Respiratory:** Upper respiratory tract infection, rhinitis, sinusitis, pharyngitis, coughing. **CV:** Palpitation, tachycardia, SVT. **Body as a whole:** Fatigue, weight decrease or increase, facial edema, fever, chest pain, pain, asthenia, malaise, flu-like symptoms, ***anaphylaxis.*** **Ophthalmologic:** Miosis, diplopia, abnormal vision. **GU:** Urinary incontinence, intramenstrual bleeding, UTI. **Hematologic: *Aplastic anemia,*** purpura, leukopenia, lymphadenopathy, leukocytosis, thrombocytopenia, granulocytopenia, positive antinuclear factor test, ***agranulocytosis,*** qualitative platelet disorder. **Dermatologic:** Acne, rash, pruritus, urticaria, bullous eruption, buccal mucous membrane swelling, ***Stevens-Johnson syndrome.*** **Miscellaneous:** Otitis media, ***acute liver failure,*** taste perversion, hypophosphatemia, myalgia, photosensitivity, substernal chest pain, dystonia, allergic reaction.

LABORATORY TEST CONSIDERATIONS
↑ ALT, AST, gamma-glutamyl transpeptidase, LDH, alkaline phosphatase, CPK. Hypophosphatemia, hypokalemia, hyponatremia.

DRUG INTERACTIONS
Carbamazepine / ↓ Carbamazepine steady-state levels and ↑ steady-state carbamazepine epoxide (metabolite) levels. Also, drug → 50% ↑ in felbamate clearance
Methsuximide / ↑ Normethsuxide levels; decrease methsuximide dose
Phenobarbital / ↑ Phenobarbital plasma levels and ↓ in felbamate levels
Phenytoin / ↑ Phenytoin steady-state drug levels necessitating a 40% decrease in drug dose. Also, drug ↑ felbamate clearance
Valproic acid / ↑ Steady-state valproic acid levels

HOW SUPPLIED
Suspension: 600 mg/5 mL; *Tablet:* 400 mg, 600 mg

DOSAGE

- **SUSPENSION, TABLETS**

Monotherapy, initial therapy.

Adults over 14 years of age, initial: 1,200 mg/day in divided doses t.i.d.–q.i.d. The dose may be increased in 600-mg increments q 2 weeks to 2,400 mg/day based on clinical response and thereafter to 3,600 mg/day, if needed.

Conversion to monotherapy.

Adults: Initiate at 1,200 mg/day in divided doses t.i.d.–q.i.d. Reduce the dose of concomitant antiepileptic drugs by ⅓ at initiation of felbamate therapy. At week 2, the felbamate dose should be increased to 2,400 mg/day while reducing the dose of other antiepileptic drugs up to another ⅓ of the original dose. At week 3, increase the felbamate dose to 3,600 mg/day and continue to decrease the dose of other antiepileptic drugs as indicated by response.

Adjunctive therapy.

Adults: Add felbamate at a dose of 1,200 mg/day in divided doses t.i.d.–q.i.d. while reducing current antiepileptic drugs by 20%. Further decreases of concomitant antiepileptic drugs may be needed to minimize side effects due to drug interactions. The dose of felbamate can be increased by 1,200-mg/day increments at weekly intervals to 3,600 mg/day.

Lennox-Gastaut syndrome in children, aged 2–14 years.

As an adjunct, add felbamate at a dose of 15 mg/kg/day in divided doses t.i.d.–q.i.d. while decreasing present antiepileptic drugs by 20%. Further decreases in antiepileptic drug dosage may be needed to minimize side effects due to drug interactions. The dose of felbamate may be increased by 15-mg/kg/day increments at weekly intervals to 45 mg/kg/day.

NURSING CONSIDERATIONS

SEE ALSO *NURSING CONSIDERATIONS FOR ANTICONVULSANTS.*

ADMINISTRATION/STORAGE

1. Shake suspension well before use.
2. Store in a tightly closed container at room temperature away from heat, direct sunlight, or moisture and away from children.
3. Most side effects seen during adjunctive therapy are resolved as the dose of concomitant antiepileptic drugs is decreased.
4. For geriatric clients, start at the low end of the dosage range.

ASSESSMENT

1. Document type, location, duration, and characteristics of seizures.
2. Determine if monotherapy or adjunctive therapy is needed.
3. List drugs prescribed to ensure none interact unfavorably and to determine need for dosage change.
4. Inform of potentially lethal side effects R/T aplastic anemia.
5. Monitor CBC, renal and LFTs.

CLIENT/FAMILY TEACHING

1. Take only as prescribed; store appropriately to prevent loss of effectiveness.
2. Avoid activities that require mental alertness until drug effects realized.
3. Side effects include anorexia, vomiting, insomnia, nausea, and headaches; report if persistent.
4. Report any changes in mental status or loss of seizure control; clinical response determines dosage.
5. Do not stop taking; may increase seizure frequency.
6. Seizure control benefit should far outweigh the potential for development of aplastic anemia; assess risk.

OUTCOMES/EVALUATE

Control of seizures

Felodipine

(feh-**LOHD**-ih-peen)

PREGNANCY CATEGORY: C
CLASSIFICATION(S):
Calcium channel blocker
Rx: Plendil
★Rx: Renedil

SEE ALSO *CALCIUM CHANNEL BLOCKING AGENTS.*

ACTION/KINETICS
Onset after PO: 120–300 min. **Peak plasma levels:** 2.5–5 hr. Over 99% bound to plasma protein. **t½, elimination:** 11–16 hr. Metabolized in the liver.

USES
Treatment of mild to moderate hypertension, alone or with other antihypertensives. *Investigational:* Raynaud's syndrome, CHF.

CONTRAINDICATIONS
Lactation.

SPECIAL CONCERNS
Use with caution in clients with CHF or compromised ventricular function, especially in combination with a beta-adrenergic blocking agent. Use with caution in impaired hepatic function or reduced hepatic blood flow. May cause a greater hypotensive effect in geriatric clients. Safety and effectiveness have not been determined in children.

SIDE EFFECTS
CV: Significant hypotension, syncope, angina pectoris, peripheral edema, palpitations, AV block, ***MI, arrhythmias,*** tachycardia. **CNS:** Dizziness, lightheadedness, headache, nervousness, sleepiness, irritability, anxiety, insomnia, paresthesia, depression, amnesia, paranoia, psychosis, hallucinations. **Body as a whole:** Asthenia, flushing, muscle cramps, pain, inflammation, warm feeling, influenza. **GI:** Nausea, abdominal discomfort, cramps, dyspepsia, diarrhea, constipation, vomiting, dry mouth, flatulence. **Dermatologic:** Rash, dermatitis, urticaria, pruritus. **Respiratory:** Rhinitis, rhinorrhea, pharyngitis, sinusitis, nasal and chest congestion, SOB, wheezing, dyspnea, cough, bronchitis, sneezing, respiratory infection. **Miscellaneous:** Anemia, gingival hyperplasia, sexual difficulties, epistaxis, back pain, facial edema, erythema, urinary frequency or urgency, dysuria.

ADDITIONAL DRUG INTERACTIONS
Cimetidine / ↑ Bioavailability of felodipine
Digoxin / ↑ Peak plasma levels of digoxin
Fentanyl / Possible severe hypotension or ↑ fluid volume
Grapefruit juice / ↑ Plasma levels of felodipine R/T ↓ liver breakdown
Oxcarbazepine / ↓ Plasma felodipine levels
Ranitidine / ↑ Bioavailability of felodipine

HOW SUPPLIED
Tablet, Extended Release: 2.5 mg, 5 mg, 10 mg

DOSAGE

- **TABLETS, EXTENDED RELEASE**

Hypertension.

Initial: 5 mg once daily (2.5 mg in clients over 65 years of age and in those with impaired liver function); **then:** adjust dose according to response, usually at 2-week intervals with the usual dosage range being 2.5–10 mg once daily. Doses greater than 10 mg increase the rate of peripheral edema and other vasodilatory side effects.

NURSING CONSIDERATIONS

SEE ALSO *NURSING CONSIDERATIONS* FOR *CALCIUM CHANNEL BLOCKING AGENTS*.

ADMINISTRATION/STORAGE
Bioavailability is not affected by food. It is increased more than twofold when taken with doubly concentrated grapefruit juice as compared with water or orange juice.

ASSESSMENT
1. Document onset of symptoms, other agents used, and outcome.
2. Note history of heart failure or compromised ventricular function.
3. List drugs currently prescribed; note any potential interactions.
4. During dosage adjustments, monitor BP closely in clients over 65 or with impaired hepatic function.

CLIENT/FAMILY TEACHING
1. Swallow tablets whole; do not chew or crush. Avoid grapefruit juice.
2. Do not stop abruptly; abrupt withdrawal may increase frequency and duration of chest pain.
3. Avoid activities that require mental alertness until effects are realized.

4. Rise slowly from a lying position and dangle feet before standing to minimize postural effects.
5. Practice frequent oral hygiene to minimize incidence and severity of drug-induced gingival hyperplasia.

OUTCOMES/EVALUATE
Control of hypertension

Fenofibrate

(**fee**-noh-**FY**-brayt)

PREGNANCY CATEGORY: C
CLASSIFICATION(S):
Antihyperlipidemic
Rx: Tricor
✱Rx: Apo-Fenofibrate, Apo-Feno-Micro, Nu-Fenofibrate

ACTION/KINETICS
Is converted to the active fenofibric acid, which lowers plasma triglycerides. Probable mechanism is to inhibit triglyceride synthesis, resulting in a reduction of VLDL released into the circulation, and by stimulating catabolism of triglyceride-rich lipoprotein. Also increases urinary excretion of uric acid. Well absorbed; absorption is increased when given with food. **Peak plasma levels:** 6–8 hr; **steady-state plasma levels:** within 5 days. Highly bound to plasma proteins. **t½:** 20 hr with once daily dosing. Fenofibric acid and an inactive metabolite are excreted through the urine.

USES
(1) Adjunctive therapy to diet to reduce elevated LDL-C, total-C, triglycerides, and Apo B and to increase HDL-C in adults with primary hypercholesterolemia or mixed dyslipidemia (Fredrickson Types IIa and II b). (2) Adjunctive therapy to diet to treat adults with hypertriglyceridemia (Fredrickson Types IV and V hyperlipidemia). *Investigational:* Polymetabolic syndrome X.

CONTRAINDICATIONS
Hepatic or severe renal dysfunction (including primary biliary cirrhosis), those with unexplained, persistent abnormal liver function, and preexisting gallbladder disease. Lactation.

SPECIAL CONCERNS
Due to similarity to clofibrate and gemfibrozil, side effects, including death, are possible. Safety and efficacy have not been determined in children.

SIDE EFFECTS
GI: Pancreatitis, cholelithiasis, dyspepsia, N&V, diarrhea, abdominal pain, constipation, flatulence, eructation, hepatitis, cholecystitis, hepatomegaly. **CNS:** Decreased libido, dizziness, increased appetite, insomnia, paresthesia. **Respiratory:** Rhinitis, cough, sinusitis, allergic pulmonary alveolitis. **GU:** Polyuria, vaginitis. **Musculoskeletal:** Myopathy, myositis, arthralgia, myalgia, myasthenia, rhabdomyolysis. **Hypersensitivity:** Severe skin rashes, urticaria. **Ophthalmic:** Eye irritation, blurred vision, conjunctivitis, eye floaters. **Miscellaneous:** Infections, pain, headache, asthenia, fatigue, flu syndrome, arrhythmia, photosensitivity, eczema.

LABORATORY TEST CONSIDERATIONS
↑ AST, ALT, creatinine, blood urea. ↓ Hemoglobin, uric acid.

DRUG INTERACTIONS
Anticoagulants / Prolongation of PT
Bile acid sequestrants / ↓ Absorption of fenofibrate due to binding
Cyclosporine / ↑ Risk of nephrotoxicity
HMG-CoA reductase inhibitors / Possibility of rhabdomyolysis, myopathy, and acute renal failure

HOW SUPPLIED
Tablets: 54 mg, 160 mg

DOSAGE

• **TABLETS**

Hypertriglyceridemia.
Initial: 54–160 mg/day given with meals to optimize bioavailability. Then, individualize based on client response. Increase, if necessary, at 4– 8-week intervals. If C_{CR} is less than 50 mL/min, start with 54 mg/day; increase dose only after evaluation of effects on renal function and triglyceride levels. In the elderly, limit the initial dose to 54 mg/day.

Primary hypercholesterolemia or mixed hyperlipidemia.
Initial: 160 mg/day.

NURSING CONSIDERATIONS

ADMINISTRATION/STORAGE

1. Place clients on an appropriate triglyceride-lowering diet before starting fenofibrate and continue during treatment.
2. Withdraw therapy after 2 months if response is not adequate with the maximum daily dose.

ASSESSMENT

1. Note indications for therapy, other agents trialed, and cardiac risk factors.
2. Assess BS, renal and LFTs; avoid drug with severe dysfunction.
3. Monitor lipids, CBC, renal and LFTs; if ALT or AST > 3 times normal, discontinue therapy. Reduce dosage with C_{CR} < 50 mL/min.

CLIENT/FAMILY TEACHING

1. Take as directed with meals.
2. Continue to follow diet prescribed for triglyceride reduction as well as a regular exercise program, smoking cessation and alcohol reduction.
3. Report skin rash, GI upset, persistent abdominal pain, or muscle pain, tenderness, fatigue, or weakness.
4. Avoid therapy with pregnancy and breastfeeding.
5. Report as scheduled for regular liver function tests and triglyceride levels. Drug will be discontinued after 2 mo if desired lipid reduction is not evident with the maximum drug dose (201 mg/d).

OUTCOMES/EVALUATE

↓ Triglyceride levels

Fenoldopam mesylate

(feh-**NOL**-doh-pam)

PREGNANCY CATEGORY: B
CLASSIFICATION(S):
Treatment of hypertensive emergency
Rx: Corlopam

ACTION/KINETICS

Rapid-acting vasodilator that is an agonist for D_1-like dopamine receptors and α_2-adrenoreceptors. Causes vasodilation in coronary, renal, mesenteric, and peripheral arteries; vascular beds do not respond uniformly. **t½, elimination:** About 5 min in mild to moderate hypertensives. **Steady-state levels:** About 20 min. Metabolized in liver and most is excreted in urine.

USES

Hypertensive emergencies.

CONTRAINDICATIONS

Use with beta-blockers or in those with sulfite sensitivity.

SPECIAL CONCERNS

Use with caution during lactation and in those with glaucoma or intraocular hypertension. Safety and efficacy have not been determined in children.

SIDE EFFECTS

CV: Tachycardia, hypotension, flushing, ST-T abnormalities, postural hypotension, extrasystoles, palpitations, bradycardia, ***heart failure, ischemic heart disease, MI,*** angina pectoris. **Body as a whole:** Headache, sweating, back pain, non-specific chest pain, pyrexia, limb cramp. **CNS:** Nervousness, anxiety, insomnia, dizziness. **GI:** N&V, abdominal pain or fullness, constipation, diarrhea. **Respiratory:** Nasal congestion, dyspnea, upper respiratory disorder. **Hematologic:** Leukocytosis, bleeding. **Miscellaneous:** Reaction at injection site, UTI, oliguria.

LABORATORY TEST CONSIDERATIONS

↑ Creatinine, BUN, serum glucose, transaminase, LDH. Hypokalemia.

HOW SUPPLIED

Injection concentrate: 10 mg/mL

DOSAGE

- **CONSTANT IV INFUSION**

Hypertensive emergency.

Rate of infusion is individualized according to body weight and to desired speed and extent of effect. See package insert for table of infusion rates. Doses range from 0.025 mcg/kg/min–0.3 mcg/kg/min for a body weight of 40 kg to 0.094 mcg/kg/min–1.13mcg/kg/min for a body weight of 150 kg.

NURSING CONSIDERATIONS

ADMINISTRATION/STORAGE

IV 1. Do not use a bolus dose.

2. Most of the effect of a given infusion is reached in 15 min.
3. Initial dose is titrated up or down no more often than every 15 min, and less frequently as desired BP is approached. Recommended increments for titration are 0.05–0.1 mcg/kg/min.
4. Initial doses of 0.03–0.1 mcg/kg/min have been associated with less reflex tachycardia than higher doses (> 0.3 mcg/kg/min).
5. Administer using a calibrated mechanical infusion pump that can deliver desired infusion rate accurately.
6. Infusion may be discontinued abruptly or tapered gradually prior to discontinuation.
7. Transition to PO therapy can be started any time after BP is stablized during fenoldopam infusion.
8. Dilute ampule concentrate in 0.9% NaCl or D5W injection for a final concentration of 40 mcg/mL (i.e., add 4 mL of the concentrate to 1,000 mL; 2 mL of the concentrate to 500 mL; or, 1 mL of the concentrate to 250 mL). Each mL of concentrate contains 10 mg of drug. Each ampule is for single use only.
9. Store ampules at 2–30°C (36–86°F).
10. Diluted solution is stable under normal light and temperature for 24 hr or less. Discard any diluted solution that is not used within 24 hr.

ASSESSMENT

1. Document clinical presentation, onset, and characteristics of symptoms.
2. Note any glaucoma, sulfite sensitivity, or intraocular hypertension.
3. Monitor VS, ECG, electrolytes, liver and renal function studies. Obtain weight.
4. List drugs prescribed to ensure none interact unfavorably; avoid use with beta-blockers.
5. Assess for physical conditions that may have precipitated event; evaluate life-style changes needed.

OUTCOMES/EVALUATE

Reduction in BP with hypertensive crisis

Fenoprofen calcium

(fen-oh-**PROH**-fen)

PREGNANCY CATEGORY: B

CLASSIFICATION(S):
Nonsteroidal anti-inflammatory drug
Rx: Nalfon

SEE ALSO *NONSTEROIDAL ANTI-INFLAMMATORY DRUGS.*

ACTION/KINETICS

Peak serum levels: 1–2 hr. **Peak effect:** 2–3 hr. **Duration:** 4–6 hr. **t$^1/_2$:** 2–3 hr. **Onset, as antiarthritic:** Within 2 days; **maximum effect:** 2–3 weeks. Ninety-nine percent protein bound. Food (but not antacids) delays absorption and decreases the total amount absorbed. Eliminated through the kidneys.

USES

Rheumatoid arthritis, osteoarthritis, mild to moderate pain. *Investigational:* Juvenile rheumatoid arthritis, prophylaxis of migraine, migraine due to menses, sunburn.

CONTRAINDICATIONS

Use in pregnancy and children less than 12 years of age. Renal dysfunction.

SPECIAL CONCERNS

Safety and efficacy in children have not been established.

ADDITIONAL SIDE EFFECTS

GU: Dysuria, hematuria, cystitis, interstitial nephritis, nephrotic syndrome. Overdosage has caused tachycardia and hypotension.

HOW SUPPLIED

Capsule: 200 mg, 300 mg; *Tablet:* 600 mg

DOSAGE

• CAPSULES, TABLETS

Rheumatoid and osteoarthritis.

Adults: 300–600 mg t.i.d.–q.i.d. Adjust dose according to response of client. Two–three weeks may be needed for improvement.

Mild to moderate pain.

Adults: 200 mg q 4–6 hr. Maximum daily dose for all uses: 3,200 mg.

NURSING CONSIDERATIONS

SEE ALSO *NURSING CONSIDERATIONS FOR NONSTEROIDAL ANTI-INFLAMMATORY DRUGS.*

ADMINISTRATION/STORAGE

Those over 70 years of age generally require half the usual adult dose.

ASSESSMENT

1. Document indications for therapy, and symptom characteristics.
2. Assess joints for inflammation, swelling, deformities, and mobility; rate pain levels.
3. Perform periodic ophthalmic and auditory tests with chronic therapy.
4. Monitor CBC, PT/PTT, liver and renal function during chronic therapy.

CLIENT/FAMILY TEACHING

1. Take 30 min before or 2 hr after meals; food decreases absorption.
2. With swallowing difficulty, the tablets can be crushed and the contents mixed with applesauce or other similar foods.
3. Avoid aspirin, alcohol, and OTC agents.
4. If vomiting or diarrhea occurs, monitor appetite, and weight; report if persistent.
5. Report any unusual bruising/bleeding, blood oozing from gums/nose, sore throat, or fever.
6. Report increased headaches, sleepiness, dizziness, nervousness, weakness, or fatigue.
7. Report evidence of liver toxicity, such as jaundice, RUQ pain, or a change in the color/consistency of stools.

OUTCOMES/EVALUATE

↓ Joint pain and inflammation with ↑ mobility

Fentanyl citrate

(**FEN**-tah-nil)

PREGNANCY CATEGORY: C
Rx: Sublimaze **C-II**

Fentanyl transmucosal system

(**FEN**-tah-nil)

PREGNANCY CATEGORY: C
Rx: Actiq, Fentanyl Oralet **C-II**
CLASSIFICATION(S):
Narcotic analgesic

SEE ALSO *NARCOTIC ANALGESICS*.

ACTION/KINETICS

Similar to those of morphine and meperidine. **IV. Onset:** 7–8 min. **Peak effect:** Approximately 30 min. **Duration:** 1–2 hr. **t½:** 1.5–6 hr. When the oral lozenge (transmucosal administration) is sucked, fentanyl citrate is absorbed through the mucosal tissues of the mouth and GI tract. **Peak effect, transmucosal:** 20–30 min. Actiq resembles a lollipop; sucking provides a rapid onset of action. Faster-acting and shorter duration than morphine or meperidine.

USES

Parenteral: Preanesthetic medication, induction, and maintenance of anesthesia of short duration and immediate postoperative period. Supplement in general or regional anesthesia. Combined with droperidol for preanesthetic medication, induction of anesthesia, or as adjunct in maintenance of general or regional anesthesia. Combined with oxygen for anesthesia in high-risk clients undergoing open heart surgery, orthopedic procedures, or complicated neurologic procedures.

Oral (transmucosal): *Actiq:* Severe pain associated with cancer treatment in those tolerant to opiates and experience breakthrough pain. *Fentanyl Oralet:* Only for use in the hospital as an anesthetic premedication in the OR or to induce conscious sedation prior to a diagnostic or therapeutic procedure in monitored hospital settings.

CONTRAINDICATIONS

The transmucosal form is contraindicated in children who weigh less than 10 kg, for the treatment of acute or chronic pain (safety for this use not established), and for doses in excess of 15 mcg/kg in children and in excess of 5 mcg/kg (maximum of 400 mcg) in adults. Use outside the hospital setting is contraindicated. Myasthenia gravis and other conditions in which muscle relaxants should not be used. Clients particularly sensitive to respiratory depression. Use during labor. Lactation.

F

SPECIAL CONCERNS

Safety and effectiveness have not been determined in children less than 2 years of age. Use with caution and at reduced dosage in poor-risk clients, children, the elderly, and when other CNS depressants are used. Use of the transmucosal form carries a risk of hypoventilation that may result in death.

ADDITIONAL SIDE EFFECTS

Skeletal and thoracic muscle rigidity, especially after rapid IV administration. Bradycardia, ***seizures,*** diaphoresis. Transmucosal form may cause life-threatening hypoventilation.

ADDITIONAL DRUG INTERACTIONS

Diazepam / ↑ Risk of CV depression
Droperidol / Hypotension and ↓ pulmonary arterial pressure
Nitrous oxide / ↑ Risk of CV depression
Protease inhibitors / ↑ CNS and respiratory depression
Ritonavir / ↑ Fentanyl effect R/T ↓ liver metabolism

HOW SUPPLIED

Fentanyl Citrate: *Injection:* 0.05 mg/mL. **Fentanyl Transmucosal:** *Lozenge (Oralet):* 100 mcg, 200 mcg, 300 mcg, 400 mcg; *Lozenge on a stick (Actiq):* 200 mcg, 400 mcg, 600 mcg, 800 mcg, 1200 mcg, 1600 mcg

DOSAGE

• **IM, IV**

Preoperative medication.

Adults: 0.05–0.1 mg IM 30–60 min before surgery.

Adjunct to anesthesia, induction.

Adults: 0.002–0.05 mg/kg IV, depending on length and depth of anesthesia desired; **maintenance:** 0.025–0.1 mg/kg when indicated.

Adjunct to regional anesthesia.

Adults: 0.05–0.1 mg IM or IV over 1–2 min when indicated.

Postoperatively.

Adults: 0.05–0.1 mg IM q 1–2 hr for control of pain, tachypnea, and emergence delirium.

As general anesthetic with oxygen and a muscle relaxant.

0.05–0.1 mg/kg (up to 0.15 mg/kg may be required).

Children, induction and maintenance of anesthesia.

Pediatric, 2–12 years: 2–3 mcg/kg.

Children, general anesthetic, induction and maintenance.

2–3 mcg/kg. Safety and efficacy have not been determined in children less than 2 years of age.

• **TRANSMUCOSAL (ORAL LOZENGE)**

Individualize according to weight, age, physical status, general condition and medical status, underlying pathology, use of other drugs, type of anesthetic to be used, and the type and length of the surgical procedure. Doses of 5 mcg/kg are equivalent to IM fentanyl, 0.75–1.25 mcg/kg. Clients receiving more than 5 mcg/kg should be under the direct observation of medical personnel. Children may require up to 15 mcg/kg, provided their body weight is not less than 10 kg. Clients over 65 years of age should receive a dose from 2.5 to 5 mcg/kg. The maximum dose for adults and children, regardless of weight, is 400 mcg.

NURSING CONSIDERATIONS

SEE ALSO ***NURSING CONSIDERATIONS*** FOR ***NARCOTIC ANALGESICS.***

ADMINISTRATION/STORAGE

1. Protect drug from light. Protect transmucosal product from freezing and moisture; store below 30°C (86°F).
2. Consider lower doses of the transmucosal form with head injury, CV or pulmonary disease, liver dysfunction, or hepatic disease.
3. When using the transmucosal form, client must be attended to at all times by an individual skilled in airway management and resuscitative techniques. Have naloxone available in the event of an overdose.
4. IV Direct IV infusions may be given, undiluted, over a period of 1–3 min.

ASSESSMENT

1. Document indications for therapy, anticipated time frame, and any previous use. Have opiod antagonist (naloxone) available to reverse drug effect.
2. Monitor VS; assess for skeletal and thoracic muscle rigidity and weak-

ness. Respiratory depression may persist.

3. Note any neurovascular or pulmonary disease. Instruct in coughing and deep breathing exercises before therapy to ensure compliance.

CLIENT/FAMILY TEACHING

1. Rise slowly; may experience orthostatic hypotension. Drug causes dizziness and drowsiness.
2. Avoid alcohol and any other CNS depressant for at least 24 hr.
3. Reinforce that transmucosal agent is not candy with children; it is a very potent medication.
4. Recall or memory may be suppressed so may not fully recall events surrounding procedure. Assure that procedure was done, answer any questions; reassure that this is normal.

OUTCOMES/EVALUATE

- Desired analgesia/relaxation
- Conscious sedation

Fentanyl Transdermal System

(**FEN**-tah-nil)

PREGNANCY CATEGORY: C
CLASSIFICATION(S):
Narcotic analgesic
Rx: Duragesic-25, -50, -75, and -100

SEE ALSO *NARCOTIC ANALGESICS* AND *FENTANYL CITRATE*.

ACTION/KINETICS

The system provides continuous delivery of fentanyl for up to 72 hr. The amount of fentanyl released from each system each hour depends on the surface area (25 mcg/hr is released from each 10 cm^2). Each system also contains 0.1 mL of alcohol/10 cm^2; the alcohol enhances the rate of drug flux through the copolymer membrane and also increases the permeability of the skin to fentanyl. Following application of the system, the skin under the system absorbs fentanyl, resulting in a depot of the drug in the upper skin layers, which is then available to the general circulation. After the system is removed, the residual drug in the skin continues to be absorbed so that serum levels fall 50% in about 17 hr. Metabolized in the liver and excreted mainly in the urine.

USES

Restrict use for the management of severe chronic pain that cannot be managed with less powerful drugs. Only use 50, 75, and 100 mcg/hr doses on clients already on and tolerant to narcotic analgesics and who require continuous narcotic administration.

CONTRAINDICATIONS

Use for acute or postoperative pain (including out-patient surgeries). To manage mild or intermittent pain that can be managed by acetaminophen-opioid combinations, NSAIDs, or short-acting opioids. Hypersensitivity to fentanyl or adhesives. ICP, impaired consciousness, coma, medical conditions causing hypoventilation. Use during labor and delivery. Use of initial doses exceeding 25 mcg/hr, use in children less than 12 years of age and clients under 18 years of age who weigh less than 50 kg. Lactation.

SPECIAL CONCERNS

Use with caution in clients with brain tumors and bradyarrhythmias, as well as in elderly, cachectic, or debilitated individuals. Use Duragesic-50, -75, and -100 only in opioid-tolerant clients. Safety and efficacy have not been determined in children.

ADDITIONAL SIDE EFFECTS

Sustained hypoventilation.

HOW SUPPLIED

Film, Extended Release: 25 mcg/hr, 50 mcg/hr, 75 mcg/hr, 100 mcg/hr

DOSAGE

- **TRANSDERMAL SYSTEM**

Analgesia.

Adults, usual initial: 25 mcg/hr unless the client is tolerant to opioids (Duragesic-50, -75, and -100 are intended for use only in clients tolerant to opioids). Initial dose should be based on (1) the daily dose, potency, and characteristics (i.e., pure agonist, mixed agonist/antagonist) of the drug the client has been taking; (2) the reliability of the relative potency estimates used to calculate the dose as estimates vary depending on the route of administration; (3) the degree, if any, of tolerance to narcotics; and (4) the general condition and status of the client.

To convert clients from PO or parenteral opioids to the transdermal system, the following method should be used: (1) the previous 24-hr analgesic requirement should be calculated; (2) convert this amount to the equianalgesic PO morphine dose; (3) find the calculated 24-hr morphine dose and the corresponding transdermal fentanyl dose using the table provided with the product; and (4) initiate treatment using the recommended fentanyl dose. The dose may be increased no more frequently than 3 days after the initial dose or q 6 days thereafter. The ratio of 90 mg/24 hr of PO morphine to 25 mcg/hr increase in transdermal fentanyl dose should be used to base appropriate dosage increments on the daily dose of supplementary opioids.

If the dose of the fentanyl transdermal system exceeds 300 mcg/hr, it may be necessary to change clients to another narcotic analgesic. In such cases, the transdermal system should be removed and treatment initiated with one-half the equianalgesic dose of the new opioid 12–18 hr later. The dose of the new analgesic should be titrated based on the level of pain reported by the client.

NURSING CONSIDERATIONS

SEE ALSO *NURSING CONSIDERATIONS* FOR *NARCOTIC ANALGESICS* AND *FENTANYL CITRATE*.

ADMINISTRATION/STORAGE

1. Multiple systems may be used if the delivery rate needs to exceed 100 mcg/hr.
2. Do not undertake initial evaluation of the maximum analgesic effect until 24 hr after system applied.
3. If required, a short-acting analgesic may be used for the first 24 hr (i.e., until analgesic efficacy reached with transdermal system).
4. Clients may continue to require periodic supplemental doses of a short-acting analgesic to treat breakthrough pain.
5. If opioid therapy is to be discontinued, a gradual decrease in dose is recommended to minimize S&S of abrupt narcotic withdrawal.

ASSESSMENT

1. Document indications for therapy, previous agents used, and outcome.
2. Rate pain level at various times throughout the day to ensure adequate dosing. Determine that dose required is based on conversion guidelines provided by manufacturer.
3. It takes 17 or more hr for fentanyl serum levels to fall by 50% after system removal. Titrate the dose of the new analgesic based on client's report of pain until adequate analgesia is reached. If opioids are to be discontinued, titrate downward gradually since it is not known at what dose level the opiod may be discontinued without causing S&S of abrupt withdrawal.
4. Note ↑ ICP or brain tumors.

CLIENT/FAMILY TEACHING

1. Apply system to a nonirritated and nonirradiated fatty, flat surface of the skin, preferably on the upper torso. May clip hair (not shave) from site prior to application.
2. Use only clear water, if needed, to cleanse the site prior to application. Do not use soaps, oils, lotions, alcohol, or other agents that might irritate the skin. Allow the skin to dry completely prior to applying the system. If liquid comes in contact with the skin, use clear water only to remove.
3. Remove the system from the sealed package and apply immediately by pressing firmly in place (for 10–20 sec) with the palm of the hand. *Never cut or open the system.* Ensure complete contact of system, especially around the edges. Date and time patches and tape securely to avoid confusion or dislodgement.
4. Keep each system in place for 72 hr; if additional analgesia is required, use breakthrough analgesic and record. A new system can be applied to a different skin site after removal of the previous system.
5. Fold systems removed from a skin site so that the adhesive side adheres to

itself; flush down the toilet immediately after removal. Keep systems out of the reach of children.
6. Dispose of any unused systems as soon as they are no longer needed by removing them from their package and flushing down the toilet.
7. Note time and frequency of short-acting analgesic use for breakthrough pain. Report if use exceeds expected needs; transdermal dosage may require adjustment.
8. Use only as prescribed; do not stop suddenly.

OUTCOMES/EVALUATE
Desired pain control

Ferrous sulfate

(**FAIR**-us **SUL**-fayt)

OTC: ED-IN-SOL, Feosol, Fer-gen-sol, Fer-in-Sol, Fer-Iron
✱OTC: Apo-Ferrous Sulfate, Ferrodan

Ferrous sulfate, dried

(**FAIR**-us **SUL**-fayt)

OTC: Fe[50], Feosol, Feratab, Slow FE
CLASSIFICATION(S):
Antianemic, iron

ACTION/KINETICS
The normal daily iron intake for males is 12–20 mg and for females is 8–15 mg, although only about 10% (1–2 mg) of this iron is absorbed. Iron is absorbed from the duodenum and upper jejunum by an active mechanism through the mucosal cells where it combines with the protein transferrin. Iron is stored in the body as hemosiderin or aggregated ferritin which is found in reticuloendothelial cells of the liver, spleen, and bone marrow. About two-thirds of total body iron is in the circulating RBCs in hemoglobin. Absorption is enhanced when stored iron is depleted or when erythropoesis occurs at an increased rate. Food decreases iron absorption by up to two-thirds. The daily loss of iron through urine, sweat, and sloughing of intestinal mucosal cells is 0.5–1 mg in healthy men; in menstruating women, 1–2 mg is the normal daily loss. Least expensive, most effective iron salt for PO therapy. Ferrous sulfate products contain 20% elemental iron, whereas ferrous sulfate dried products contain 30% elemental iron. The exsiccated form is more stable in air.

USES
Prophylaxis and treatment of iron deficiency and iron-deficiency anemias. Dietary supplement for iron. Optimum therapeutic responses are usually noted within 2–4 weeks. *Investigational:* Clients receiving epoetin therapy (failure to give iron supplements either IV or PO can impair the hematologic response to epoetin).

CONTRAINDICATIONS
Hemosiderosis, hemochromatosis, peptic ulcer, regional enteritis, and ulcerative colitis. Hemolytic anemia, pyridoxine-responsive anemia, and cirrhosis of the liver. Use in those with normal iron balance.

SPECIAL CONCERNS
Allergic reactions may result due to certain products containing tartrazine and some products containing sulfites.

SIDE EFFECTS
GI: Constipation, gastric irritation, nausea, abdominal cramps, anorexia, vomiting, diarrhea, dark-colored stools. These effects may be minimized by administering preparations as a coated tablet. Soluble iron preparations may stain the teeth.

LABORATORY TEST CONSIDERATIONS
Iron may affect electrolyte balance determinations.

OD OVERDOSE MANAGEMENT
Symptoms: Symptoms occur in four stages—(1) Lethargy, N&V, abdominal pain, weak and rapid pulse, tarry stools, dehydration, acidosis, hypotension, and ***coma*** within 1–6 hr. (2) If client survives, symptoms subside for about 24 hr. (3) Within 24–48 hr symptoms return with ***diffuse vascular congestion, shock, pulmonary edema, acidosis, seizures, anuria, hyperthermia, and death.*** (4) If client sur-

vives, pyloric or antral stenosis, hepatic cirrhosis, and CNS damage are seen within 2–6 weeks. Toxic reactions are more likely to occur after parenteral administration.*Treatment (Iron Toxicity):*

- General supportive measures.
- Maintain a patent airway, respiration, and circulation.
- Induce vomiting with syrup of ipecac followed by gastric lavage using tepid water or 1%–5% sodium bicarbonate (to convert from ferrous sulfate to ferrous carbonate, which is poorly absorbed and less irritating). Saline cathartics can also be used.
- Deferoxamine is indicated for clients with serum iron levels greater than 300 mg/dL. Deferoxamine is usually given IM, but in severe cases of poisoning it may be given IV. Hydration should be maintained.
- It may be necessary to treat for shock, acidosis, renal failure, and seizures.

F

DRUG INTERACTIONS

Antacids, oral / ↓ Iron absorption from GI tract
Ascorbic acid / Ascorbic acid, 200 mg or more, ↑ iron absorption
Chloramphenicol / ↑ Serum iron levels
Cholestyramine / ↓ Iron absoprtion from GI tract
Cimetidine / ↓ Iron absorption from GI tract
Fluoroquinolones / ↓ Fluoroquinolone absorption from GI tract R/T formation of a ferric ion-quinolone complex
Levodopa / ↓ Levodopa absorption R/T formation of chelates with iron salts
Levothyroxine / ↓ Levothyroxine efficacy R/T ↓ absorption
Methyldopa / ↓ Methyldopa absorption from GI tract
Mycophenolate mofetil / ↓ GI absorption of mycophenolate R/T formation of a drug-iron complex in the GI tract
Pancreatic extracts / ↓ Iron absorption from GI tract
Penicillamine / ↓ Penicillamine absorption from GI tract due to chelation
H *St. John's wort* / May ↓ absorption of iron
Tetracyclines / ↓ Absorption of both tetracyclines and iron from GI tract
Vitamin E / ↓ Response to iron therapy

HOW SUPPLIED

Ferrous sulfate: *Elixir:* 220 mg/5 mL; *Liquid:* 75 mg/0.6 mL; *Syrup:* 90 mg/5 mL; *Tablet:* 324 mg, 325 mg. **Ferrous sulfate, dried:** *Capsule, Extended Release:* 160 mg; *Tablet:* 187 mg, 200 mg; *Tablet, Slow Release:* 160 mg

DOSAGE

FERROUS SULFATE

- **EXTENDED-RELEASE CAPSULES**

Adults: 150–250 mg 1–2 times/day. This dosage form is not recommended for children.

- **ELIXIR, ORAL SOLUTION, TABLETS, ENTERIC-COATED TABLETS**

Prophylaxis.
Adults: 300 mg/day. **Pediatric:** 5 mg/kg/day.

Anemia.
Adults: 300 mg b.i.d. increased to 300 mg q.i.d. as needed and tolerated. **Pediatric:** 10 mg/kg t.i.d. The enteric-coated tablets are not recommended for use in children.

- **EXTENDED-RELEASE TABLETS**

Adults: 525 mg 1–2 times/day. This dosage form is not recommended for use in children.

FERROUS SULFATE, DRIED

- **CAPSULES**

Prophylaxis.
Adults: 300 mg/day. **Pediatric:** 5 mg/kg/day.

Anemia.
Adults: 300 mg b.i.d. up to 300 mg q.i.d. as needed and tolerated. **Pediatric:** 10 mg/kg t.i.d.

- **TABLETS**

Prophylaxis.
Adults: 200 mg/day. **Pediatric:** 5 mg/kg/day.

Anemia.
Adults: 200 mg t.i.d. up to 200 mg q.i.d. as needed and tolerated. **Pediatric:** 10 mg/kg t.i.d.

- **EXTENDED-RELEASE TABLETS**

Adults: 160 mg 1–2 times/day. This dosage form is not recommended for use in children.

NURSING CONSIDERATIONS

ADMINISTRATION/STORAGE

1. For infants and young children, administer liquid preparation with a

dropper. Deposit liquid well back against the cheek.
2. Eggs and milk or coffee and tea consumed with a meal or 1 hr after may significantly inhibit absorption of dietary iron.
3. Ingestion of calcium and iron supplements with food can decrease iron absorption by one-third; iron absorption is not decreased if calcium carbonate is used and taken between meals.
4. Do not crush or chew sustained-release products.

ASSESSMENT

1. Take a drug history, including:
• Antacid use; any other drugs that may interact
• OTC drugs, i.e., iron compounds or vitamin E use
• Recent abdominal surgery; all currently prescribed drugs
• Allergy to sulfites or tartrazines (may be present in some products)
2. Note any GI bleeding; tarry stools or bright blood in stool or vomitus.
3. Assess for thalassemia; obtain hemoglobin electrophoresis, as iron administration could be lethal.
4. Note any complaints of fatigue, pallor, poor skin turgor, or change in mental status, especially in the elderly.
5. Assess nutritional status and diet history through questioning and intake if possible.
6. Review pregnancies and menstruation history; note frequency, amounts, and heavy or abnormal bleeding. Pregnancy is an indication for iron prophylactically.
7. Monitor VS, CBC, chemistry profile, stool for occult blood, reticulocytes, serum transferrin, and iron panel results. Discontinue if 500 mg of iron daily does not cause a 1 g-rise of hemoglobin in 1 mo. Note cause (i.e., iron-deficient or megaloblastic anemia) or if further workup is needed.

CLIENT/FAMILY TEACHING

1. Adhere to prescribed regimen; report any problems immediately. Coated tablets may diminish GI effects such as nausea, constipation or diarrhea, gastric irritation, and abdominal cramps.
2. Review the form of iron prescribed (bi- or trivalent) and frequency of administration.
3. Take with meals to reduce gastric irritation. Milk products, eggs, and antacids inhibit absorption so avoid unless taking ferrous lactate. Coffee and tea consumed within 1 hr of meals may inhibit absorption of dietary iron.
4. Taking with citrus juices enhances iron absorption.
5. May cause indigestion, change in stool color (black and tarry or dark green), abdominal cramps, diarrhea, or constipation; may be relieved by changing the med, dosage, or time of administration.
6. Increase intake of fruit, fiber, and fluids to minimize constipating effects. Eat a well-balanced diet with foods high in iron (i.e., meat proteins, dried fruits) and affordable foods (i.e., raisins, dark green leafy vegetables, and liver versus apricots or prunes).
7. Will reduce tetracycline absorption. If to receive both, allow at least 2 hr to elapse between doses.
8. Store out of reach of children as an overdosage can be fatal.
9. Dilute liquid preparations well with water or fruit juice and use a straw to minimize teeth staining.
10. Pregnant women need an iron-rich diet. The American Academy of Pediatrics recommends an iron supplement for infants during their first year of life.
11. Follow administration guidelines for each product to minimize side effects. Do not self-medicate with vitamin, mineral, and iron supplements.

OUTCOMES/EVALUATE

• Resolution of S&S of anemia; If hemoglobin has not increased 1 g in 4 weeks, then reconfirm diagnosis
• Restoration of serum iron levels
• Improvement in exercise tolerance and level of fatigue
• Improvement in skin pallor, color of nail beds, Hb and iron levels

Fexofenadine hydrochloride

(fex-oh-**FEN**-ah-deen)

PREGNANCY CATEGORY: C
CLASSIFICATION(S):
Antihistamine, second generation, piperidine
Rx: Allegra

F

SEE ALSO *ANTIHISTAMINES.*

ACTION/KINETICS
Fexofenadine, a metabolite of terfenadine, is an H_1-histamine receptor blocker. Low to no sedative or anticholinergic effects. **Onset:** Rapid. **Peak plasma levels:** 2.6 hr. **t½, terminal:** 14.4 hr. Approximately 90% of the drug is excreted through the feces (80%) and urine (10%) unchanged.

USES
(1) Seasonal allergic rhinitis, including sneezing; rhinorrhea; itchy nose, throat, or palate; and itchy, watery, and red eyes in adults and children 6 years of age and older. (2) Uncomplicated skin manifestations of chronic idiopathic urticaria in adults and children 6 years of age and older.

SPECIAL CONCERNS
Use with care during lactation. Safety and efficacy have not been determined in children less than 12 years of age.

SIDE EFFECTS
CNS: Drowsiness, fatigue, headache. **GI:** Nausea, dyspepsia. **Respiratory:** Sinusitis, throat irritation, pharyngitis. **Miscellaneous:** Viral infection (flu, colds), dysmenorrhea.

DRUG INTERACTIONS
No differences in side effects or the QTc interval were observed when fexofenadine was given with either erythromycin or ketoconazole.

HOW SUPPLIED
Capsule: 60 mg; *Tablet:* 30 mg, 60 mg, 180 mg

DOSAGE

• **CAPSULES, TABLETS**

Seasonal allergic rhinitis.

Adults and children over 12 years: 60 mg b.i.d. or 180 mg once daily. **Children, 6–11 years:** 30 mg b.i.d.

Chronic idiopathic urticaria.

Adults and children over 12 years: 60 mg b.i.d. **Children, 6–11 years:** 30 mg b.i.d.

NOTE: In adults and children over 12 years with decreased renal function, the initial dose should be 60 mg once daily; for children, 6–11 years with decreased renal function, use 30 mg once daily as the initial dose.

NURSING CONSIDERATIONS

SEE ALSO *NURSING CONSIDERATIONS FOR ANTIHISTAMINES.*

ASSESSMENT
1. Document onset, duration, and characteristics of symptoms; identify triggers if known.
2. Note other agents trialed, length of use, and outcome.
3. Assess for renal dysfunction; reduce dose if evident.

CLIENT/FAMILY TEACHING
1. Take exactly as directed; do not exceed prescribed dosage. Do not crush, break or chew caps or sustained release tabs.
2. May experience headaches, sore throat, nausea, and dysmenorrhea.
3. Avoid alcohol and other CNS depressants. Do not perform activities that require mental alertness until drug effects realized.
4. Report if symptoms intensify or don't improve after 48 hr.
5. Identify and avoid triggers.

OUTCOMES/EVALUATE
Control of symptoms of seasonal allergic rhinitis

Filgrastim

(fill-**GRASS**-tim)

PREGNANCY CATEGORY: C
CLASSIFICATION(S):
Granulocyte colony-stimulating factor, human
Rx: Neupogen

ACTION/KINETICS
Is a human granulocyte colony stimulating factor (G-CSF) produced by recombinant DNA technology by *Escherichia coli* that has been inserted with

the human G-CSF gene. Endogenous G-CSF is a glycoprotein that is produced by monocytes, fibroblasts, and other endothelial cells and that regulates the production of neutrophils in the bone marrow. Has minimal effects, either in vivo or in vitro, on the production of other hematopoietic cell types. Filgrastim has an amino acid sequence that is identical to the natural sequence predicted from human DNA sequence analysis except there is an N-terminal methionine that is required for expression in *E. coli.* IV infusion of 20 mcg/kg over 24 hr resulted in a mean serum level of 48 ng/mL, whereas SC administration of 11.5 mcg/kg resulted in a maximum serum level of 49 ng/mL within 2–8 hr. **t½, elimination:** 3.5 hr.

USES

To decrease the incidence of infection, as manifested by febrile neutropenia, in clients with nonmyeloid malignancies who are receiving myelosuppressive anticancer drugs, which are associated with severe neutropenia with fever. To reduce the duration of neutropenia in clients with nonmyeloid malignancies undergoing myeloablative chemotherapy followed by bone marrow transplantation. To reduce infection in severe chronic neutropenia (e.g., congenital, cyclical, or idiopathic neutropenia) after other diseases have been ruled out. For the mobilization of hematopoietic progenitor cells into the peripheral blood for leukapheresis collection. To reduce the time to neutrophil recovery and the duration of fever in clients being treated for acute myelogenous leukemia. *Investigational:* Use in AIDS, aplastic anemia, hairy cell leukemia, myelodysplasia, drug-induced and congenital agranulocytosis, and alloimmune neonatal neutropenia.

CONTRAINDICATIONS

Hypersensitivity to proteins derived from *E. coli.* The safety and effectiveness of filgrastim given simultaneously with cytotoxic chemotherapy have not been determined; thus, filgrastim should not be given 24 hr before to 24 hr after cytotoxic chemotherapy.

SPECIAL CONCERNS

Use with caution during lactation. Use with caution in any malignancy with myeloid characteristics since the drug may act as a growth factor for any tumor type. Filgrastim does not cause any greater incidence of toxicity in children than in adults. Safety and efficacy have not been determined in neonates and clients with autoimmune neutropenia of infancy. The safety and effectiveness of chronic filgrastim therapy have not been determined. Hypersensitivity reactions usually occur within 30 min after administration and are more frequent in clients receiving the drug IV.

SIDE EFFECTS

When used for myelosuppressive therapy.

Musculoskeletal: Medullary bone pain, skeletal pain. **GI:** N&V, diarrhea, anorexia, stomatitis, constipation, peritonitis. **Hypersensitivity:** Skin rash, facial edema, wheezing, dyspnea, hypotension, tachycardia. **Hematologic:** Leukocytosis; greater risk of thrombocytopenia and anemia. **Respiratory:** Dyspnea, cough, chest pain, sore throat. **Body as a whole:** Alopecia, neutropenic fever, fever, fatigue, headache, skin rash, mucositis, generalized weakness, unspecified pain. **CV:** Decreased BP (transient), cutaneous vasculitis, hypertension, ***arrhythmias, MI.***

When used for severe chronic neutropenia.

Musculoskeletal: Mild to moderate bone pain, abdominal/flank pain, arthralgia, osteoporosis. **Hematologic:** Thrombocytopenia, epistaxis (associated with thrombocytopenia), anemia, myelodysplasia or myeloid leukemia. **Dermatologic:** Exacerbation of certain skin conditions (e.g., psoriasis), rash, alopecia. **Miscellaneous:** Palpable splenomegaly, hepatomegaly, monosomy, reaction at injection site, cutaneous vasculitis, hematuria, proteinuria.

When used for bone marrow transplantation.

GI: N&V, stomatitis, peritonitis. **CV:** Hypertension, capillary leak syndrome (rare). **Miscellaneous:** Rash, renal insufficiency, erythema nodosum.

When used for peripheral blood progenitor cell collection.

Hematologic: Decreased platelet counts, anemia, increase in neutrophil count, WBC count greater than 100,000/mm^3. **Miscellaneous:** Mild to moderate musculoskeletal symptoms, medullary bone pain, headache, increases in alkaline phosphatase.

LABORATORY TEST CONSIDERATIONS

↑ Uric acid, LDH, alkaline phosphatase.

HOW SUPPLIED

Injection: 300 mcg/mL, 600 mcg/mL

DOSAGE

• **SC, IV**

Myelosuppressive chemotherapy.

Initial: 5 mcg/kg/day as a single injection, either as a SC bolus, by short IV infusion (15–30 min), or by continuous SC or IV infusion (over a 24-hr period). The dose may be increased in increments of 5 mcg/kg for each chemotherapy cycle depending on the duration and severity of the absolute neutrophil count (ANC) nadir. The dose should be given daily for up to 2 weeks, until ANC has reached 10,000/mm^3 following the expected chemotherapy-induced neutrophil nadir.

Severe chronic neutropenia.

5 mcg/kg/day SC for idiopathic and cyclic disease; 6 mcg/kg/day SC for congenital disease.

Bone marrow transplantation.

10 mcg/kg/day given as an IV infusion of 4 or 24 hr or as a continuous 24-hr SC infusion.

NOTE: During the period of neutrophil recovery, the daily dose should be titrated against the neutrophil response as follows:

1. When ANC is greater than 1,000/mm^3 for 3 consecutive days, reduce the dose of filgrastim to 5 mcg/kg/day. If ANC decreases to less than 1,000/mm^3 at any time during the 5-mcg/kg/day dosage, increase filgrastim to 10 mcg/kg/day.
2. If ANC remains greater than 1,000/mm^3 for 3 more consecutive days, discontinue filgrastim.
3. If ANC decreases to less than 1,000/mm^3, resume filgrastim at 5 mcg/kg/day.

Peripheral blood progenitor cell collection.

10 mcg/kg/day SC, either as a bolus or a continuous infusion. Filgrastim should be given at least 4 days before the first leukapheresis procedure and continued until the last leukapheresis.

NURSING CONSIDERATIONS

ADMINISTRATION/STORAGE

1. Discontinue therapy if ANC is greater than 10,000/mm^3 after chemotherapy-induced neutrophil nadir.
2. For myelosuppressive therapy or bone marrow transplantation, give no earlier than 24 hr after cytotoxic chemotherapy and in the 24 hr before administration of chemotherapy.
3. Discontinuing therapy usually results in a 50% decrease in circulating neutrophils within 1–2 days and return to pretreatment levels in 1–7 days.
4. Do not freeze; store in the refrigerator at 2–8°C (36–46°F). Prior to use, can be at room temperature for a maximum of 24 hr. Discard if left at room temperature more than 24 hr.
5. Solution should be clear and colorless.
6. Do not shake.
7. Use only one dose from each vial; do not reenter the vial.
8. Compatible with glass, PVC, or plastic syringes.
9. **IV** May be diluted in D5W. When diluted to concentrations between 5 and 15 mcg/mL, protect from adsorption to plastic materials by adding human albumin to a final concentration of 2 mg/mL.
10. The following drugs are incompatible as an admixture with filgrastim: amphotericin B, cefonicid, cefoperazone, cefotaxime, cefoxitin, ceftizoxime, ceftriaxone, cefuroxime clindamycin, dactinomycin, etoposide, fluorouracil, furosemide, heparin, mannitol, metronidazole, methylprednisolone,

mezlocillin, mitomycin, prochlorperazine, piperacillin, and thiotepa.

ASSESSMENT

1. Determine sensitivity to *E. coli*-derived products.
2. Document indications for therapy (i.e., chemotherapy-induced neutropenia, myelopsuppressive therapy for bone marrow transplantation, leukapheresis) and expected time frame.
3. Monitor CBC and platelet counts twice weekly during therapy.
4. Note last dose of cytotoxic agent and determine ANC nadir. Do not administer from 24 hr before to 24 hr after cytotoxic chemotherapy.

CLIENT/FAMILY TEACHING

1. Demonstrate appropriate technique for administration. Review written guidelines concerning dose, administration, drug storage/handling, and discarding syringes.
2. Do not shake container; only enter the vial once, then discard.
3. "Flu-like" symptoms (N&V and aching; bone pain) may be side effects of drug therapy. Take at bedtime, with prescribed analgesics.
4. Record temperatures; report unusual bruising/bleeding or infection.
5. Avoid crowds and persons with infectious diseases.

OUTCOMES/EVALUATE

- Prevention of infection
- ↓ Duration of neutropenia
- Improved neutrophil counts
- Mobilization of progenitor cells into peripheral blood

Finasteride

(fin-**AS**-teh-ride)

PREGNANCY CATEGORY: X
CLASSIFICATION(S):
Androgen hormone inhibitor
Rx: Propecia, Proscar

ACTION/KINETICS

Is a specific inhibitor of 5-α-reductase, the enzyme that converts testosterone to the active 5-α-dihydrotestosterone (DHT). Thus, there are significant decreases in serum and tissue DHT levels, resulting in rapid regression of prostate tissue and an increase in urine flow and symptomatic improvement. Also a decrease in scalp DHT levels. Well absorbed after PO administration. **Elimination t½:** 6 hr in clients 45–60 years of age and 8 hr in clients over 70 years of age. Slow accumulation after multiple dosing. Metabolized in the liver and excreted through both the urine and feces.

USES

Treatment of symptomatic benign prostatic hyperplasia to improve symptoms, reduce risk of acute urinary retention, and reduce risk for surgery and prostatectomy. Male pattern baldness (vertex and anterior midscalp). *Investigational:* In combination with flutamide following radical prostatectomy, prevention of the progression of first-stage prostate cancer, acne, and hirsutism.

CONTRAINDICATIONS

Hypersensitivity to finasteride or any excipient in the product. Use in women and in children. Lactation.

SPECIAL CONCERNS

Use with caution in clients with impaired liver function.

SIDE EFFECTS

GU: Impotence, decreased libido, decreased volume of ejaculate. **Miscellaneous:** Breast tenderness and enlargement, hypersensitivity reactions (including skin rash and lip swelling), testicular pain.

LABORATORY TEST CONSIDERATIONS

↓ Serum PSA levels.

DRUG INTERACTIONS

Significant ↑ plasma levels of finasteride when used with terazosin.

HOW SUPPLIED

Tablet: 1 mg, 5 mg

DOSAGE

- **TABLETS**

Benign prostatic hyperplasia.
5 mg/day, with or without meals.
Androgenetic alopecia.
Males: 1 mg once a day with or without meals.

NURSING CONSIDERATIONS

ADMINISTRATION/STORAGE

1. At least 6–12 months of therapy may be required in some to determine whether a beneficial response has been achieved for BPH.
2. Daily use for three months or longer is necessary to observe beneficial effects.
3. Continued use is required to sustain beneficial effects for hair growth. Withdrawal leads to reversal of effects within 12 months.
4. Women who are pregnant or may become pregnant should not handle crushed finasteride tablets as there is potential for drug absorption and subsequent potential risk to the male fetus. Also, when the male's sexual partner is or may become pregnant, exposure of semen to his partner should be avoided or drug use discontinued.
5. Do not adjust dosage in the elderly or in those with impaired renal function.

ASSESSMENT

1. Note indications for therapy, include onset, characteristics of clinical presentation, and any associated family history.
2. Review urologic exam to rule out other conditions similar to BPH (e.g., prostate cancer, infection, stricture, hypotonic bladder, neurogenic disorders).
3. Monitor LFTs and PSA. May cause a decrease in PSA levels (prostate-specific antigen: a blood screening study to detect prostate cancer) even in the presence of prostate cancer.
4. Schedule regular digital rectal exams to assess prostate gland.
5. Not for use in females.
6. With liver impairment monitor closely.
7. Not all clients show a response to finasteride. With a large residual urinary volume or severely diminished urinary flow assess for obstructive uropathy; may not be a finasteride candidate.
8. May obtain pre-treatment scalp photos to assess/gauge response.
9. Complete history/physical exam.

CLIENT/FAMILY TEACHING

1. The following symptoms of BPH should show improvement with continued drug therapy: hesitancy, feelings of incomplete bladder emptying, interruption of urinary stream, impairment of size and force of urinary stream, and terminal urinary dribbling. May take 6–12 months of continued therapy before a beneficial effect is evident.
2. Use barrier contraception; drug may cause male fetal abnormalities. If pregnancy occurs, either discontinue finasteride or avoid exposure of partner to semen (use a condom).
3. Take once a day with or without meals as directed. More than prescribed dose will not increase hair growth but may cause adverse symptoms. May take 3 mg or more before any response noted.
4. If partner is pregnant or may become pregnant, avoid exposure to semen. Drug may cause damage to male fetus; stop drug or use a condom to prevent exposure.
5. Decreased volume of ejaculate may occur but does not interfere with sexual function. Impotence and decreased libido may also occur.
6. Keep F/U lab, checkup, and prostate exams; report side effects.
7. Interruption of therapy will reverse effects within 12 mo and BPH symptoms will return.

OUTCOMES/EVALUATE

- ↓ Size of enlarged prostate gland
- Symptomatic improvement
- Regrowth of hair with male pattern baldness

Flavoxate hydrochloride

(flay-**VOX**-ayt)

PREGNANCY CATEGORY: B
CLASSIFICATION(S):
Urinary tract drug
Rx: Urispas

ACTION/KINETICS

Relieves muscle spasms of the urinary tract by relaxing the detrusor muscle by cholinergic blockade and also by a direct effect. Also has local anesthetic and analgesic effects. Well absorbed from GI tract; 10%–30% is excreted in urine.

USES

Symptomatic relief of urinary tract dysuria, urgency, frequency, nocturia, suprapubic pain, and incontinence associated with cystitis, prostatitis, urethritis, urethrocystitis, and urethrotrigonitis. Compatible for use with urinary tract germicides.

CONTRAINDICATIONS

Obstructive disorders of urinary tract, including pyloric or duodenal obstructions, obstructive intestinal lesions, ileus, achalasia, obstructive uropathies of the lower urinary tract, and GI hemorrhage.

SPECIAL CONCERNS

Use with caution in glaucoma and during lactation. Confusion is more likely to occur in geriatric clients. Safety and effectiveness have not been determined in children less than 12 years of age.

SIDE EFFECTS

GI: N&V, xerostomia. **CNS:** Drowsiness, headache, vertigo, nervousness, mental confusion (especially in the elderly). **CV:** Tachycardia, palpitations. **Hematologic:** Eosinophilia, leukopenia. **Ophthalmologic:** Blurred vision, increased ocular tension, accommodation disturbances. **Other:** Urticaria and other dermatoses, fever, dysuria.

HOW SUPPLIED

Tablet: 100 mg

DOSAGE

• TABLETS

Adults and children over 12 years:
100 or 200 mg t.i.d.–q.i.d. Reduce dose when symptoms improve.

NURSING CONSIDERATIONS

SEE ALSO *NURSING CONSIDERATIONS* FOR *CHOLINERGIC BLOCKING AGENTS.*

CLIENT/FAMILY TEACHING

1. May take with or without food.
2. Do not drive a car or operate hazardous machinery; may cause drowsiness and blurred vision.
3. Practice good oral hygiene. Relieve dryness of mouth with ice chips or hard candy. Ensure adequate hydration.
4. Avoid strenuous exercise; body's heat-regulating mechanism may be altered and sweating inhibited.
5. Report improvement of symptoms as well as any persistent, bothersome, or new symptoms.

OUTCOMES/EVALUATE

- Relief of urinary tract discomfort
- Normal elimination patterns

Flecainide acetate

(fleh-**KAY**-nyd)

PREGNANCY CATEGORY: C
CLASSIFICATION(S):
Antiarrhythmic, Class IC
Rx: Tambocor

SEE ALSO *ANTIARRHYTHMIC AGENTS.*

ACTION/KINETICS

The antiarrhythmic effect is due to a local anesthetic action, especially on the His-Purkinje system in the ventricle. Drug decreases single and multiple PVCs and reduces the incidence of ventricular tachycardia. **Peak plasma levels:** 3 hr.; **steady state levels:** 3–5 days. **Effective plasma levels:** 0.2–1 mcg/mL (trough levels). **t½:** 20 hr (12–27 hr). Forty percent is bound to plasma protein. Approximately 30% is excreted in urine unchanged. Impaired renal function decreases rate of elimination of unchanged drug. Food or antacids do not affect absorption.

USES

Life-threatening arrhythmias manifested as sustained ventricular tachycardia. Prevention of paroxysmal supraventricular tachycardias (PSVT) and paroxysmal atrial fibrillation or flutter (PAF) associated with disabling symptoms but not structural heart disease. Antiarrhythmic drugs have not been shown to improve survival in clients with ventricular arrhythmias.

CONTRAINDICATIONS
Cardiogenic shock, preexisting second- or third-degree AV block, RBBB when associated with bifascicular block (unless pacemaker is present to maintain cardiac rhythm). Recent MI. Cardiogenic shock. Chronic atrial fibrillation. Frequent PVCs and symptomatic nonsustained ventricular arrhythmias. Lactation.

SPECIAL CONCERNS
Use with caution in SSS, in clients with a history of CHF or MI, in disturbances of potassium levels, in clients with permanent pacemakers or temporary pacing electrodes, renal and liver impairment. Safety and efficacy in children less than 18 years of age are not established. The incidence of proarrhythmic effects may be increased in geriatric clients.

SIDE EFFECTS
CV: ***New or worsened ventricular arrhythmias, increased risk of death in clients with non-life-threatening cardiac arrhythmias,*** new or worsened CHF, palpitations, chest pain, sinus bradycardia, sinus pause, sinus arrest, ***ventricular fibrillation, ventricular tachycardia that cannot be resuscitated,*** second- or third-degree AV block, tachycardia, hypertension, hypotension, bradycardia, angina pectoris. **CNS:** Dizziness, faintness, syncope, lightheadedness, neuropathy, unsteadiness, headache, fatigue, paresthesia, paresis, hypoesthesia, insomnia, anxiety, malaise, vertigo, depression, ***seizures,*** euphoria, confusion, depersonalization, apathy, morbid dreams, speech disorders, stupor, amnesia, weakness, somnolence. **GI:** Nausea, constipation, abdominal pain, vomiting, anorexia, dyspepsia, dry mouth, diarrhea, flatulence, change in taste. **Ophthalmic:** Blurred vision, difficulty in focusing, spots before eyes, diplopia, photophobia, eye pain, nystagmus, eye irritation, photophobia. **Hematologic:** Leukopenia, thrombocytopenia. **GU:** Decreased libido, impotence, urinary retention, polyuria. **Musculoskeletal:** Asthenia, tremor, ataxia, arthralgia, myalgia. **Dermatologic:** Skin rashes, urticaria, exfoliative dermatitis, pruritus, alopecia. **Other:** Edema, dyspnea, fever, ***bronchospasm,*** flushing, sweating, tinnitus, swollen mouth, lips, and tongue.

OD OVERDOSE MANAGEMENT
Symptoms: Lengthening of PR interval; increase in QRS duration, QT interval, and amplitude of T wave; decrease in HR and contractility; conduction disturbances; hypotension; ***respiratory failure*** or ***asystole.*** *Treatment:* Charcoal will remove unabsorbed drug up to 90 min after drug ingestion. Administration of dopamine, dobutamine, or isoproterenol. Artificial respiration. Intra-aortic balloon pumping, transvenous pacing (to correct conduction block). Acidification of the urine may be beneficial, especially in those with an alkaline urine. Due to the long duration of action of the drug, treatment measures may have to be continued for a prolonged period of time.

DRUG INTERACTIONS
Acidifying agents / ↑ Renal excretion of flecainide
Alkalinizing agents / ↓ Renal excretion of flecainide
Amiodarone / ↑ Plasma levels of flecainide
Cimetidine / ↑ Bioavailability and renal excretion of flecainide
Digoxin / ↑ Digoxin plasma levels
Disopyramide / Additive negative inotropic effects
Propranolol / Additive negative inotropic effects; also, ↑ plasma levels of both drugs
Smoking (Tobacco) / ↑ Plasma clearance of flecainide
Verapamil / Additive negative inotropic effects

HOW SUPPLIED
Tablet: 50 mg, 100 mg, 150 mg

DOSAGE

• **TABLETS**

Sustained ventricular tachycardia.
Initial: 100 mg q 12 hr; **then,** increase by 50 mg b.i.d. q 4 days until effective dose reached. **Usual effective dose:** 150 mg q 12 hr, not to exceed 400 mg/day.

PSVT, PAF.
Initial: 50 mg q 12 hr; **then,** dose may be increased in increments of 50 mg b.i.d. q 4 days until effective dose

reached. Maximum recommended dose: 300 mg/day. *NOTE:* For PAF clients, increasing the dose from 50 to 100 mg b.i.d. may increase efficacy without a significant increase in side effects.

NOTE: For clients with a C_{CR} less than 35 mL/min/1.73 m², the starting dose is 100 mg once daily (or 50 mg b.i.d.). For less severe renal disease, the initial dose may be 100 mg q 12 hr.

NURSING CONSIDERATIONS

SEE ALSO *NURSING CONSIDERATIONS FOR ANTIARRHYTHMIC AGENTS.*

ADMINISTRATION/STORAGE

1. For most situations, start therapy in a hospital setting (especially in clients with symptomatic CHF, sustained ventricular arrhythmias, compensated clients with significant myocardial dysfunction, or sinus node dysfunction).
2. In renal impairment, increase the dose at intervals greater than 4 days. Monitor for adverse toxic effects.
3. The chance of toxic effects increases if the trough plasma levels exceed 1 mcg/mL.
4. If being transferred to flecainide from another antiarrhythmic, allow at least two to four plasma half-lives to elapse for the drug being discontinued before initiating flecainide therapy.
5. Dosing at 8-hr intervals may benefit some.
6. To minimize toxicity, reduce dose once arrhythmia controlled.

ASSESSMENT

1. Document physical assessment findings. Review history, echocardiograms, and ECGs for evidence of CHF, ventricular arrhythmias, sinus node dysfunction, or abnormal EF.
2. Monitor VS, ECG, CXR, electrolytes, renal and LFTs. Assess ECG for increased arrhythmias or AV block. Preexisting hypo- or hyperkalemia may alter drug effects; correct. Monitor for labile BP.
3. Concomitant administration with disopyramide, propranolol, or verapamil will promote negative inotropic (depressant) effects.
4. Check pacing thresholds of clients with pacemakers; adjust before and 1 week following drug therapy.

CLIENT/FAMILY TEACHING

1. Take at the dose and frequency prescribed. Report changes in elimination.
2. Report any bruising or increased bleeding tendencies, dyspnea, edema, or chest pain.
3. Keep appointments so that drug effectiveness can be monitored carefully.
4. Report adverse CNS effects, such as dizziness, visual disturbances, headaches, nausea, or depression.
5. Obtain urinary pH to detect alkalinity or acidity. Alkalinity decreases renal excretion and acidity increases renal excretion, affecting rate of drug elimination.

OUTCOMES/EVALUATE

- Termination of lethal ventricular arrhythmias; stable cardiac rhythm
- Therapeutic serum (trough) drug levels (0.2–1.0 mcg/mL)

Floxuridine

(flox-**YOUR**-ih-deen)

PREGNANCY CATEGORY: D
CLASSIFICATION(S):
Antineoplastic, antimetabolite
Rx: FUDR

SEE ALSO *ANTINEOPLASTIC AGENTS.*

ACTION/KINETICS

Cell-cycle specific for the S phase of cell division. Rapidly metabolized to fluorouracil. The drug inhibits DNA and RNA synthesis. Crosses blood-brain barrier. **t½:** 5–20 min. From 60% to 80% of fluorouracil is excreted as respiratory CO_2 (8–12 hr); small amount (15%) excreted in urine (1–6 hr).

USES

Intra-arterially as palliative treatment of GI adenocarcinoma metastatic to the liver (especially in clients incurable by surgery or other treatment). Used in clients with disease limited to an area capable of infusion by a single artery. *Investigational:* Cancer of the breast, ovaries, cervix, bladder, kidney, and prostate.

CONTRAINDICATIONS

If client is at poor risk, including depressed bone marrow function, nutritionally poor, or potentially serious infections. Lactation. Do not use during pregnancy unless benefits clearly outweigh risks.

ADDITIONAL SIDE EFFECTS

Esophagopharyngitis, myocardial ischemia, angina, acute cerebellar syndrome, photophobia, lacrimation, decreased vision. Complications of intra-arterial administration are arterial aneurysm, arterial ischemia, arterial thrombosis, bleeding at catheter site, occluded, displaced, or leaking catheters, embolism, fibromyositis, infection at catheter site, thrombophlebitis.

LABORATORY TEST CONSIDERATIONS

↑ Excretion of 5-hydroxyindoleacetic acid. ↑ Serum transaminase and bilirubin, LDH, alkaline phosphatase. ↓ Plasma albumin.

HOW SUPPLIED

Powder for injection: 0.5 g

DOSAGE

• **INTRA-ARTERIAL INFUSION ONLY**

0.1–0.6 mg/kg/day by continuous infusion over 24 hr. Infusion is continued as long as a response continues.

NURSING CONSIDERATIONS

SEE ALSO *NURSING CONSIDERATIONS* FOR *ANTINEOPLASTIC AGENTS*.

ADMINISTRATION/STORAGE

1. Higher doses (0.4–0.6 mg) best given by hepatic artery infusion; liver metabolizes drug, reducing the possibility of systemic toxicity.
2. Give until adverse effects are manifested. Resume therapy after effects have subsided. WBC nadir: 1 week; Platelet nadir: 10 days.
3. Use an infusion pump to overcome pressure in large arteries and to assure a uniform infusion rate.
4. Reconstitute each vial with 5 mL sterile water to yield a 100-mg/mL concentration. This may be further reconstituted in D5W or NSS and infused intra-arterially.
5. Store reconstituted vials in the refrigerator at 2–8°C (36–46°F) for no longer than 2 weeks.

ASSESSMENT

1. Note indications for therapy; monitor CBC, uric acid, creatinine and LFTs.
2. Assess carefully for bleeding at catheter site, S&S of infection and catheter displacement. Should be inserted under fluoro by trained individual.

CLIENT/FAMILY TEACHING

1. Drug may cause temporary thinning of hair.
2. Report any mouth lesions, diarrhea, intractable vomiting or infections.
3. Will premedicate for N&V, report recurrence so that therapy may be administered.

OUTCOMES/EVALUATE

Suppression of metastatic processes

Fluconazole

(flew-**KON**-ah-zohl)

PREGNANCY CATEGORY: C
CLASSIFICATION(S):
Antifungal
Rx: Diflucan
✱Rx: Apo-Fluconazole, Apo-Fluconazole-150, Difulcan-150

ACTION/KINETICS

Inhibits the enzyme cytochrome P-450 in the organism, which results in a decrease in cell wall integrity and extrusion of intracellular material, leading to death. Apparently does not affect the cytochrome P-450 enzyme in animals or humans. **Peak plasma levels:** 1–2 hr. **t½:** 30 hr, which allows for once daily dosing. Penetrates all body fluids at steady state. Bioavailability is not affected by agents that increase gastric pH. Eighty percent of the drug is excreted unchanged by the kidneys.

USES

Oropharyngeal and esophageal candidiasis. Serious systemic candidal infection (including UTIs, peritonitis, and pneumonia). Cryptococcal meningitis. Maintenance therapy to prevent cryptococcal meningitis in AIDS clients. Vaginal candidiasis. To decrease the incidence of candidiasis in clients undergoing a bone marrow transplant who receive cytotoxic chemotherapy or radiation therapy. Treatment of cryptococcal meningitis and candidal infections in children.

CONTRAINDICATIONS

Hypersensitivity to fluconazole.

SPECIAL CONCERNS

Use with caution during lactation and if client shows hypersensitivity to other azoles. Efficacy has not been adequately assessed in children.

SIDE EFFECTS

Following single doses.

GI: Nausea, abdominal pain, diarrhea, dyspepsia, taste perversion. **CNS:** Headache, dizziness. **Other:** Angioedema, ***anaphylaxis (rare).***

Following multiple doses.

Side effects are more frequently reported in HIV-infected clients than in non-HIV-infected clients. **GI:** N&V, abdominal pain, diarrhea, ***serious hepatic reactions***. **CNS:** Headache, ***seizures.*** **Dermatologic:** Skin rash, exfoliative skin disorders (including ***Stevens-Johnson syndrome,*** and toxic epidermal necrolysis), alopecia. **Hematologic:** Leukopenia, thrombocytopenia. **Other:** Hypercholesterolemia, hypertriglyceridemia, hypokalemia.

LABORATORY TEST CONSIDERATIONS

↑ AST, serum transaminase (especially if used with isoniazid, oral hypoglycemic agents, phenytoin, rifampin, valproic acid).

DRUG INTERACTIONS

Alfentanil / ↑ Pharmacologic and side effects R/T ↓ liver metabolism
Benzodiazepines / ↑ and Prolonged serum levels → CNS depression and psychomotor impairment
Buspirone / ↑ Plasma buspirone levels R/T ↓ metabolism
Cimetidine / ↓ Fluconazole plasma levels
Corticosteroids / ↑ Corticosteroid effects and toxicity R/T ↓ metabolism
Cyclosporine / ↑ Cyclosporine levels in renal transplant clients with or without impaired renal function
Glipizide / ↑ Plasma glipizide levels R/T ↓ liver breakdown
Glyburide / ↑ Plasma glyburide levels R/T ↓ liver breakdown
Hydrochlorothiazide / ↑ Plasma fluconazole levels R/T ↓ renal clearance
Losartan / ↑ Losartan effect/toxicity R/T ↓ metabolism
Nisoldipine / ↑ Effects/toxicity of nisoldipine levels R/T ↓ metabolism
Phenytoin / ↑ Plasma phenytoin levels
Rifabutin, Rifampin / ↓ Plasma fluconazole levels R/T ↑ liver breakdown
Tacrolimus / ↑ Plasma tacrolimus levels R/T ↓ gut metabolism
Theophylline / ↑ Plasma theophylline levels
Tolbutamide / ↑ Plasma tolbutamide levels R/T ↓ liver breakdown
Tricyclic antidepressants / ↑ TCA effects/toxicity R/T ↓ metabolism
Vinca alkaloids / ↑ Risk of vinca toxicity (constipation, myalgia, neutropenia)
Warfarin / ↑ PT
Zidovudine / ↑ Plasma zidovudine levels
Zolpidem / ↑ Zolpidem effects

HOW SUPPLIED

Injection: 2 mg/mL; *Powder for Oral Suspension:* 50 mg/5mL, 200 mg/5mL; *Tablet:* 50 mg, 100 mg, 150 mg, 200 mg

DOSAGE

- **TABLETS, ORAL SUSPENSION, IV**

Vaginal candidiasis.

150 mg as a single oral dose.

Oropharyngeal or esophageal candidiasis.

Adults, first day: 200 mg; **then,** 100 mg/day for a minimum of 14 days (for oropharyngeal candidiasis) or 21 days (for esophageal candidiasis). Up to 400 mg/day may be required for esophageal candidiasis. **Children, first day:** 6 mg/kg; **then,** 3 mg/kg once daily for a minimum of 14 days (for oropharyngeal candidiasis) or 21 days (for esophageal candidiasis).

Candidal UTI and peritonitis.

50–200 mg/day.

Systemic candidiasis (e.g., candidemia, disseminated candidiasis, and pneumonia).
Optimal dosage and duration in adults have not been determined although doses up to 400 mg/day have been used. **Children:** 6–12 mg/kg/day.

Acute cryptococcal meningitis.
Adults, first day: 400 mg; **then,** 200 mg/day (up to 400 mg may be required) for 10 to 12 weeks after CSF culture is negative. **Children, first day:** 12 mg/kg; **then,** 6 mg/kg once daily for 10 to 12 weeks after CSF culture is negative.

Maintenance to prevent relapse of cryptococcal meningitis in AIDS clients.
Adults: 200 mg once daily. **Pediatric:** 6 mg/kg once daily.

Prevention of candidiasis in bone marrow transplant.
400 mg once daily. In clients expected to have severe granulocytopenia (less than 500 neutrophils/mm^3), start fluconazole several days before the anticipated onset of neutropenia and continue for 7 days after the neutrophil count rises above 1,000 cells/mm^3. In clients with renal impairment, an initial loading dose of 50–400 mg can be given; then daily dose is based on C_{CR}.

NURSING CONSIDERATIONS

SEE ALSO *GENERAL NURSING CONSIDERATIONS* FOR *ANTI-INFECTIVES.*

ADMINISTRATION/STORAGE

1. The daily dose is the same for PO and IV administration.
2. Usually, a loading dose of twice the daily dose is recommended for the first day of therapy in order to obtain plasma levels close to the steady state by the second day of therapy.
3. Due to a long half-life, once daily dosing (either IV or PO) is possible.
4. To prevent relapse, maintenance therapy is usually required in clients with AIDS, cryptococcal meningitis, or recurrent oropharyngeal candidiasis.
5. Shake the oral suspension well before using. Store the reconstituted suspension at 5–30°C (4–86°F). Discard any unused drug after 2 weeks. Do not freeze suspension.

IV 6. Do not use IV solution if cloudy or precipitated or if seal not intact.
7. Do not exceed a continuous IV infusion rate of 200 mg/hr. Check site frequently for extravasation/necrosis.
8. Do not add supplementary medication to the IV bag.

ASSESSMENT

1. Note any sensitivity to azoles or similar drugs.
2. Determine if HIV infected; may increase risk for side effects.
3. Obtain baseline cultures, renal and LFTs. If abnormal LFTs, monitor closely for development of more serious liver toxicity.

CLIENT/FAMILY TEACHING

1. Review goals of therapy and appropriate method and schedule for medication administration and lab studies. Take as directed.
2. Report any rash, N&V, diarrhea, yellowing of skin, clay-colored stools, dark urine, or persistent side effects (especially if immunocompromised); drug may need to be discontinued.

OUTCOMES/EVALUATE

- Elimination of pathogenic fungi
- Candida prophylaxis in transplant recipients

Flucytosine

(flew-**SYE**-toe-seen)

PREGNANCY CATEGORY: C
CLASSIFICATION(S):
Antifungal
Rx: Ancobon

ACTION/KINETICS

May act directly on fungi to competitively inhibit purine and pyrimidine uptake and indirectly by intracellular metabolism to 5-fluorouracil. The FU is incorporated into fungal RNA inhibiting synthesis of DNA and RNA. Less toxic than amphotericin B. Well absorbed from the GI tract and distributed to the joints, aqueous humor, peritoneal and other body fluids and tissues. **Peak plasma concentration:** 2–6 hr. **Therapeutic serum concentration:** 20–25 mcg/mL. **t½:** 2–5 hr, higher in presence of impaired renal function. Eighty percent to 90% of the drug is excreted unchanged in urine.

USES

Serious systemic fungal infections by susceptible strains of *Candida* (e.g., endocarditis, septicemia, UTIs) or *Cryptococcus* (pulmonary or UTIs, meningitis, septicemia). *Investigational:* Treat chromomycosis.

CONTRAINDICATIONS

Hypersensitivity to drug. Lactation.

SPECIAL CONCERNS

Safety and effectiveness have not been determined in children. Use with extreme caution in clients with kidney disease or history of bone marrow depression. The bone marrow depressant effects may cause an increased incidence of microbial infection, gingival bleeding, and delayed healing.

SIDE EFFECTS

GI: N&V, diarrhea, abdominal pain, dry mouth, anorexia, duodenal ulcer, GI hemorrhage, ulcerative colitis. **Hematologic:** Anemia, leukopenia, thrombocytopenia, ***aplastic anemia, agranulocytosis,*** pancytopenia, eosinophilia. **CNS:** Headache, vertigo, confusion, sedation, hallucinations, paresthesia, parkinsonism, psychosis, pyrexia, convulsions. **CV: *Cardiac arrest,*** myocardial toxicity, ventricular dysfunction. **Hepatic:** Acute hepatic injury with ***possible death in debilitated clients,*** hepatic dysfunction, jaundice, elevation of hepatic enzymes, increase in bilirubin. **GU:** Increase in BUN and creatinine, azotemia, crystalluria, renal failure. **Respiratory:** Chest pain, dyspnea, ***respiratory arrest.*** **Dermatologic:** Pruritus, rash, urticaria, photosensitivity. **Other:** Ataxia, hearing loss, peripheral neuropathy, weakness, hypoglycemia, fatigue, hypokalemia, allergic reactions, Lyell's syndrome.

LABORATORY TEST CONSIDERATIONS

Interferes with creatinine determinations using the Kodak - Ektachem analyzer.

OD OVERDOSE MANAGEMENT

Symptoms (serum levels > 100 mcg/mL): N&V, diarrhea, leukopenia, thrombocytopenia, hepatitis. *Treatment:* Prompt induction of vomiting or gastric lavage. Adequate fluid intake (by IV if necessary). Monitor blood, liver, and kidney parameters frequently. Hemodialysis will quickly decrease serum levels.

DRUG INTERACTIONS

Amphotericin B / ↑ Effect/toxicity of flucytosine R/T kidney impairment
Cytosine / Inactivates antifungal effect of flucytosine

HOW SUPPLIED

Capsule: 250 mg, 500 mg

DOSAGE

• **CAPSULES**

Adults and children: 50–150 mg/kg/day in 6-hr intervals. Use lower doses in renal impairment.

NURSING CONSIDERATIONS

SEE ALSO *GENERAL NURSING CONSIDERATIONS* FOR *ANTI-INFECTIVES.*

ASSESSMENT

1. Obtain cultures, CBC, liver and renal function studies; reduce dose with impaired renal function
2. Describe clinical presentation.

CLIENT/FAMILY TEACHING

1. Reduce or avoid nausea by administering capsules a few at a time over a 15-min period.
2. Report for weekly cultures to determine that strains have not become resistant. A strain is considered resistant if the MIC is > 100.
3. Report any volume reduction, blood, sediment, or cloudiness in the urine.
4. Side effects that interfere with dosing should be reported.

OUTCOMES/EVALUATE

• Resolution of fungal infection
• Therapeutic drug levels (20–25 mcg/mL)

Fludarabine phosphate

(floo-**DAIR**-ah-bean)

PREGNANCY CATEGORY: D
CLASSIFICATION(S):
Antineoplastic, antimetabolite
Rx: Fludara

SEE ALSO *ANTINEOPLASTIC AGENTS.*

F

ACTION/KINETICS
Rapidly dephosphorylated to 2-fluoro-ara-A and then phosphorylated within the cell by the enzyme deoxycytidine kinase to the active 2-fluoro-ara-ATP. This compound inhibits DNA polymerase alpha, ribonucleotide reductase, and DNA primase, resulting in inhibition of DNA synthesis. **t½, 2-fluoro-ara-A:** About 10 hr. Approximately 23% of a dose of fludarabine is excreted in the urine as unchanged 2-fluoro-ara-A.

USES
Chronic lymphocytic leukemia in individuals who have not responded to at least one standard alkylating agent-containing regimen. *Investigational:* Non-Hodgkin's lymphoma, macroglobulinemic lymphoma, prolymphocytic leukemia or prolymphocytoid variant of chronic lymphocytic leukemia, mycosis fungoides, hairy cell leukemia, Hodgkin's disease.

CONTRAINDICATIONS
Lactation.

SPECIAL CONCERNS
Use with caution in clients with renal insufficiency. The safety and effectiveness of fludarabine in children and in previously untreated or nonrefractory chronic lymphocytic leukemia clients have not been established. Fludarabine produces dose-dependent toxic effects. An increased risk of toxicity is possible in geriatric clients, in renal insufficiency, and in bone marrow impairment.

SIDE EFFECTS
Hematologic: Neutropenia, thrombocytopenia, anemia. **Tumor lysis syndrome:** Hyperuricemia, hyperphosphatemia, hypocalcemia, hyperkalemia, hematuria, metabolic acidosis, urate crystalluria, renal failure. Flank pain and hematuria may signal the onset of the syndrome. **GI:** N&V, anorexia, stomatitis, diarrhea, GI bleeding. **CNS:** Malaise, fatigue, weakness, agitation, confusion, coma. **Neuromuscular:** Peripheral neuropathy, paresthesia, myalgia. **Respiratory:** Pneumonia, dyspnea, cough, interstitial pulmonary infiltrate. **GU:** Dysuria, urinary infection, hematuria. **Miscellaneous:** Edema (common), skin rashes, fever, chills, ***serious opportunistic infections,*** pain, visual disturbances, hearing loss.

OD OVERDOSE MANAGEMENT
Symptoms: Irreversible CNS toxicity including delayed blindness, ***coma, and death.*** Severe thrombocytopenia and neutropenia. *Treatment:* Discontinue administration of the drug and treat symptoms. Monitor the hematologic profile.

HOW SUPPLIED
Powder for reconstitution, lyophilized: 50 mg

DOSAGE
• **IV**
Adults, usual: 25 mg/m² given over a period of 30 min for 5 consecutive days. Initiate a 5-day course of therapy every 28 days.

NURSING CONSIDERATIONS

SEE ALSO *NURSING CONSIDERATIONS* FOR *ANTINEOPLASTIC AGENTS.*

ADMINISTRATION/STORAGE
IV 1. Dose may be decreased or delayed based on presence of hematologic or neurotoxicity.
2. After maximal response, give three additional cycles, then discontinue.
3. Reconstitute lyophilized product with 2 mL of sterile water for injection, USP. Each mL of the resulting solution will contain 25 mg fludarabine (final pH range: 7.2 to 8.2). This may then be diluted in 100 or 125 mL of D5W, or 0.9% NaCl, and administered over 30 min.
4. Use reconstituted drug within 8 hr; contains no preservatives.
5. If solution comes in contact with the skin or mucous membranes, wash thoroughly with soap and water. Rinse eyes thoroughly with plain water. Record exposure.
6. Store the product under refrigeration at 2–8°C (36–46°F).

ASSESSMENT
1. Document indications for therapy, previous agents used and outcome.
2. Document baseline CNS assessment, bone marrow impairment and renal dysfunction; high doses may precipitate toxicity.

3. Monitor hematologic and renal function studies. Nadir: 5–25 days.

CLIENT/FAMILY TEACHING

1. Report any evidence of flank pain or hematuria; may precede a tumor lysis syndrome.
2. Practice barrier contraception.
3. Report any evidence of infection (sore throat, fever) or any abnormal bruising or bleeding.

OUTCOMES/EVALUATE

Hematologic improvement; control of malignant process

Fludrocortisone acetate

(flew-droh-**KOR**-tih-sohn)

PREGNANCY CATEGORY: C
CLASSIFICATION(S):
Mineralocorticoid
Rx: Florinef

SEE ALSO *CORTICOSTEROIDS.*

ACTION/KINETICS

Produces marked sodium retention and inhibits excess adrenocortical secretion. Supplementary potassium may be indicated.

USES

Partial replacement therapy for primary and secondary adrenocortical insufficiency in Addison's disease. Treat salt-losing adrenogenital syndrome. *Investigational:* Severe orthostatic hypotension.

CONTRAINDICATIONS

Use systemically as an anti-inflammatory or for systemic fungal infections.

HOW SUPPLIED

Tablet: 0.1 mg

DOSAGE

• **TABLETS**

Addison's disease.

0.1 mg/day (range: 0.1 mg 3 times/week to 0.2 mg/day), usually in conjunction with hydrocortisone (10–30 mg/day) or cortisone (10–37.5 mg/day). Alternatively, for adults and children, can use 0.05–0.1 mg/24 hr.

Salt-losing adrenogenital syndrome.

0.1–0.2 mg/day.

Severe orthostatic hypotension.

0.1–0.4 mg/day.

NURSING CONSIDERATIONS

SEE *NURSING CONSIDERATIONS* FOR *CORTICOSTEROIDS.*

ASSESSMENT

1. Document clinical presentation and onset of symptoms.
2. Obtain baseline weight, VS, CXR, EKG, BS, Na and K levels.

CLIENT/FAMILY TEACHING

1. Addison's disease will require lifetime replacement therapy. Do not stop abruptly; may precipitate crisis. Always carry med ID.
2. Review dietary recommendations of high-potassium, low-sodium diet.
3. Report sudden weight gain, swelling of extremities, muscle cramps, fever, and headaches.
4. Severe trauma, stress, infection or surgery may require increased dosage.

OUTCOMES/EVALUATE

Control of symptoms during adrenal cortical hypofunction

Flumazenil

(floo-**MAZ**-eh-nill)

PREGNANCY CATEGORY: C
CLASSIFICATION(S):
Benzodiazepine receptor antagonist
Rx: Romazicon
♣**Rx:** Anexate

ACTION/KINETICS

Antagonizes the effects of benzodiazepines on the CNS by competitively inhibiting their action at the benzodiazepine recognition site on the GABA/benzodiazepine receptor complex. Does not antagonize the CNS effects of ethanol, general anesthetics, barbiturates, or opiates. Depending on the dose, there will be partial or complete antagonism of sedation, impaired recall, and psychomotor impairment. **Onset of reversal:** 1–2 min.

Peak effect: 6–10 min. The duration of reversal is related to the plasma levels of the benzodiazepine and the dose of flumazenil. **Distribution t½, initial:** 7–15 min; **terminal t½:** 41–79 min. Metabolized in the liver with 90%–95% excreted through the urine and 5%–10% excreted in the feces. Hepatic impairment prolongs the half-life of the drug. Ingestion of food results in a 50% increase in clearance of flumazenil.

USES

Complete or partial reversal of benzodiazepine-induced depression of the ventilatory responses to hypercapnia and hypoxia. Situations include cases where general anesthesia has been induced or maintained by benzodiazepines, where sedation has been produced by benzodiazepines for diagnostic and therapeutic procedures, and for the management of benzodiazepine overdosage.

CONTRAINDICATIONS

Use in clients given a benzodiazepine for control of intracranial pressure or status epilepticus. In clients manifesting signs of serious cyclic antidepressant overdose. Use during labor and delivery or in children as the risks and benefits are not known. To treat benzodiazepine dependence or for the management of protracted benzodiazepine abstinence syndrome. Use until the effects of neuromuscular blockade have been fully reversed.

SPECIAL CONCERNS

The reversal of benzodiazepine effects may be associated with the onset of seizures in certain high-risk clients (e.g., concurrent major sedative-hypnotic drug withdrawal, recent therapy with repeated doses of parenteral benzodiazepines, myoclonic jerking or seizure activity prior to administration of flumazenil in cases of overdose, and concurrent cyclic antidepressant overdosage). Use with caution in clients with head injury as the drug may precipitate seizures or alter cerebral blood flow in clients receiving benzodiazepines. Use with caution in clients with alcoholism and other drug dependencies due to the increased frequency of benzodiazepine tolerance and dependence. Use with caution during lactation.

Flumazenil may precipitate a withdrawal syndrome if the client is dependent on benzodiazepines. Flumazenil may cause panic attacks in clients with a history of panic disorder.

Use with caution in mixed-drug overdosage as toxic effects (e.g., cardiac dysrhythmias, convulsions) may occur (especially with cyclic antidepressants).

SIDE EFFECTS

Deaths have occurred in clients receiving flumazenil, especially in those with serious underlying disease or in those who have ingested large amounts of nonbenzodiazepine drugs (usually cyclic antidepressants) as part of an overdose. ***Seizures*** are the most common serious side effect noted.

CNS: Dizziness, vertigo, ataxia, anxiety, nervousness, tremor, palpitations, insomnia, dyspnea, hyperventilation, abnormal crying, depersonalization, euphoria, increased tears, depression, dysphoria, paranoia, delirium, difficulty concentrating, ***seizures,*** somnolence, stupor, speech disorder. **GI:** N&V, hiccoughs, dry mouth. **CV:** Sweating, flushing, hot flushes, ***arrhythmias (atrial, nodal, ventricular extrasystoles),*** bradycardia, tachycardia, hypertension, chest pain. **At injection site:** Pain, thrombophlebitis, rash, skin abnormality. **Body as a whole:** Headache, increased sweating, asthenia, malaise, rigors, shivering, paresthesia. **Ophthalmologic:** Abnormal vision including visual field defect and diplopia; blurred vision. **Otic:** Transient hearing impairment, tinnitus, hyperacusis.

HOW SUPPLIED

Injection: 0.1 mg/mL

DOSAGE

- **IV ONLY**

To reverse conscious sedation or in general anesthesia.

Adults, initial: 0.2 mg (2 mL) given IV over 15 sec. If the desired level of consciousness is not reached after waiting an additional 45 sec, a second dose of 0.2 mg (2 mL) can be given and repeated at 60-sec intervals, up to a maximum total dose of 1 mg (10 mL). Most clients will respond to doses of 0.6–1 mg. To treat resedation, give no more than 1 mg (given as 0.2 mg/min) at any one time and give no more than 3 mg in any 1 hr.

Management of suspected benzodiazepine overdose.
Adults, initial: 0.2 mg (2 mL) given IV over 30 sec; a second dose of 0.3 mg (3 mL) can be given over another 30 sec. Further doses of 0.5 mg (5 mL) can be given over 30 sec at 1-min intervals up to a total dose of 3 mg (although some clients may require up to 5 mg given slowly as described). If the client has not responded 5 min after receiving a cumulative dose of 5 mg, the major cause of sedation is probably not due to benzodiazepines and additional doses of flumazenil are likely to have no effect. For resedation, repeated doses may be given at 20-min intervals; no more than 1 mg (given as 0.5 mg/min) at any one time and no more than 3 mg in any 1 hr should be administered.

NURSING CONSIDERATIONS

ADMINISTRATION/STORAGE

IV 1. Must individualize dosage. Give only the smallest amount that is effective. The 1-min wait between individual doses in the dose-titration recommended for general uses may be too short for high-risk clients as it takes 6–10 min for any single dose of flumazenil to reach full effects. Thus, slow the rate of administration in high-risk clients.
2. A major risk is resedation; the duration of effect of a long-acting or a large dose of a short-acting benzodiazepine may exceed that of flumazenil. With resedation, give repeated doses at 20-min intervals as needed.
3. Best given as a series of small injections to allow the provider to control reversal of sedation to desired end point and to decrease possibility of side effects.
4. Reduce dose to 40%–60% of normal with severe hepatic dysfunction.
5. Give through a freely running IV infusion into a large vein to minimize pain at the injection site.
6. Doses larger than a total of 3 mg do not reliably produce additional effects.
7. Compatible with D5W, RL, and NSS solutions. If drawn into a syringe or mixed with any of these solutions, discard after 24 hr.
8. For optimum sterility, keep in the vial until just before use.
9. Before administering, have a secure airway and IV access; awaken clients gradually.

ASSESSMENT

1. Note any history of seizure disorder or panic attacks.
2. Determine type/time and amount of drug ingested; note any TCA or mixed-drug overdose.
3. Document liver dysfunction; subsequent doses require adjustment.
4. Assess for evidence of head injury or increased ICP.
5. Note evidence of sedative or benzodiazepine dependence, alcohol abuse, or any recent use; may precipitate withdrawal symptoms.

INTERVENTIONS

1. The effects of flumazenil usually wear off before the effects of many benzodiazepines. Observe closely for resedation, depressed respirations, or other benzodiazepine effects up to 2 hr after administration.
2. Flumazenil is intended as an adjunct to, not a substitute for, proper management of the airway, assisted breathing, circulatory access and support, use of lavage and charcoal, and adequate clinical evaluation. Prior to giving flumazenil, proper measures should be undertaken to secure an airway for ventilation and IV access. Be prepared for clients attempting to withdraw ET tubes or IV lines due to confusion and agitation following awakening; awakening should be gradual.
3. Drug should be used with caution in the ICU due to increased risk of unrecognized benzodiazepine dependence; may produce convulsions.

4. Not intended to be used to diagnose benzodiazepine-induced sedation in the ICU. Failure to respond may be masked by metabolic disorders, traumatic injury, or drugs.
5. Use seizure precautions; increased risk for seizures with large overdoses of cyclic antidepressants and with long-term benzodiazepine sedation.
6. Drug-associated convulsions may be treated with benzodiazepines, phenytoin, or barbiturates. (Higher doses of benzodiazepines may be needed).
7. Do not use until the effects of neuromuscular blockade have been fully reversed.
8. Flumazenil does not consistently reverse amnesia. Therefore, clients may not remember instructions during the postprocedure period; provide written instructions.

CLIENT/FAMILY TEACHING

1. Do not undertake any activities requiring complete alertness and do not operate hazardous machinery or a motor vehicle until at least 18–24 hr after discharge and until it has been determined that no residual sedative effects of benzodiazepines remain. Memory and judgment may be impaired.
2. Avoid alcohol or nonprescription drugs for 18–24 hr after administration of flumazenil or if the effects of the benzodiazepines persist.

OUTCOMES/EVALUATE

Reversal of benzodiazepine sedative/psychomotor effects

Flunisolide

(flew-**NISS**-oh-lyd)

PREGNANCY CATEGORY: C
CLASSIFICATION(S):
Glucocorticoid
Rx: Inhalation: AeroBid, AeroBid-M., **Intranasal:** Nasalide, Nasarel
✱Rx: Alti-Flunisolide, Apo-Flunisolide, Rhinalar

SEE ALSO *CORTICOSTEROIDS*.

ACTION/KINETICS

Minimal systemic effects with intranasal use. Significant first-pass after inhalation; rapidly metabolized by the liver. Several days may be required for full beneficial effects. **t½:** 1.8 hr. Metabolized in the liver and excreted by the feces (40%) and urine (50%).

USES

Inhalation: Prophylaxis of bronchial asthma in combination with other therapy. For asthma clients requiring systemic steroids where adding an inhaled steroid may decrease or eliminate the need for systemic steroids. **Intranasal:** Seasonal or perennial rhinitis, especially if other treatment has proven unsatisfactory.

CONTRAINDICATIONS

Active or quiescent TB, especially of the respiratory tract. Untreated fungal, bacterial, systemic viral infections. Ocular herpes simplex. Use until healing occurs following recent ulceration of nasal septum, nasal surgery, or trauma. Lactation.

SPECIAL CONCERNS

Safety and effectiveness in children less than 6 years of age have not been determined.

ADDITIONAL SIDE EFFECTS

Respiratory: Hoarseness, coughing, throat irritation; *Candida* infections of nose, larynx, and pharynx. **After intranasal use:** Nasopharyngeal irritation, stinging, burning, dryness, headache. **GI:** Dry mouth. Systemic corticosteroid effects, especially if recommended dose is exceeded.

HOW SUPPLIED

Metered Dose Inhaler: 250 mcg/inh; *Nasal Spray:* 25 mcg/inh

DOSAGE

• INHALATION

Bronchial asthma.

Adults: 2 inhalations (total of 500 mcg flunisolide) in a.m. and p.m., not to exceed 4 inhalations b.i.d. (i.e., total daily dose of 2,000 mcg). **Pediatric, 6–15 years:** 2 inhalations (250 mcg/inhalation) in the morning and evening (usual), with total daily dose not to exceed 1,250 mcg.

• INTRANASAL

Rhinitis.

Adults, initial: 50 mcg (2 sprays) in each nostril b.i.d.; may be increased to 2 sprays t.i.d., up to maximum daily dose of 400 mcg (i.e., 8 sprays in each nostril). **Pediatric, 6–14 years, initial:** 25 mcg (1 spray) in each nostril t.i.d. or 50 mcg (2 sprays) in each nostril b.i.d., up to maximum daily dose of 200 mcg (i.e., 4 sprays in each nostril). **Maintenance, adults, children:** Smallest dose necessary to control symptoms. Some clients (approximately 15%) are controlled on 1 spray in each nostril daily.

NURSING CONSIDERATIONS

SEE ALSO *NURSING CONSIDERATIONS* FOR *CORTICOSTEROIDS*.

ADMINISTRATION/STORAGE

1. When initiating the inhalant in clients receiving systemic corticosteroids, use aerosol concomitantly with the systemic steroid for 1 week. Then, slowly withdraw the systemic corticosteroid over several weeks.
2. If nasal congestion present, use a decongestant before administration to ensure drug reaches site of action.
3. If beneficial effects do not occur within 3 weeks, discontinue therapy. Improvement of symptoms usually is evident within a few days.

ASSESSMENT

Document baseline assessment of disease. When used chronically, monitor children for growth and effects on the HPA axis.

CLIENT/FAMILY TEACHING

1. Use a demonstrator and instruct client and family how to administer nasal spray or inhalant. If prescribed a bronchodilator instruct to use that first so steroid can better penetrate mucosa.
2. Clear nasal passages before using nasal spray. Gargle and rinse mouth with water after inhalation to prevent alterations in taste and to maintain adequate oral hygiene. Report any symptoms of irritation or fungal infections.
3. Mild nasal bleeding may occur; this is usually transient.
4. Instruct not to puncture the aerosol, store or administer near heat or open flame, or throw container into a fire or incinerator.

OUTCOMES/EVALUATE

- Improved airway exchange
- ↓ Allergic manifestations

Fluorouracil (5-Fluorouracil, 5-FU)

(flew-roh-**YOUR**-ah-sill)

PREGNANCY CATEGORY: X
CLASSIFICATION(S):
Antineoplastic, antimetabolite
Rx: Efudex, Fluoroplex (Abbreviation: 5-FU) , Adrucil

SEE ALSO *ANTINEOPLASTIC AGENTS*.

ACTION/KINETICS

Pyrimidine antagonist that inhibits the methylation reaction of deoxyuridylic acid to thymidylic acid. Thus, synthesis of DNA and, to a lesser extent, RNA is inhibited. Cell-cycle specific for the S phase of cell division. **t½, initial:** 5–20 min; **final:** 20 hr. From 60% to 80% eliminated as respiratory CO_2 (8–12 hr); small amount (15%) excreted unchanged in urine (1–6 hr). Highly toxic; initiate use in hospital. When used topically, the following response occurs:

- Early inflammation: erythema for several days (minimal reaction)
- Severe inflammation: burning, stinging, vesiculation
- Disintegration: erosion, ulceration, necrosis, pain, crusting, reepithelialization
- Healing: within 1–2 weeks with some residual erythema and temporary hyperpigmentation

USES

Systemic: Palliative management of certain cancers of the rectum, stomach, colon, pancreas, and breast. In combination with levamisole for Dukes' stage C colon cancer after surgical resection. In combination with leucovorin for metastatic colorectal cancer. *Investigational:* Cancer of the bladder, ovaries, prostate, cervix, endometrium, lung, liver, head, and neck. Also, malignant pleural, peritoneal, and pericardial effusions. **Topical (as solution or cream):** Multiple actinic or solar keratoses. Superficial basal cell carcinoma. *Investigational:* Condylomata acuminata (1% solution in 70% ethanol or the 5% cream).

ADDITIONAL CONTRAINDICATIONS

Systemic: Clients in poor nutritional state, with severe bone marrow depression, severe infection, or recent (4-week-old) surgical intervention. Lactation. To be used with caution in clients with hepatic or liver dysfunction.

F

SPECIAL CONCERNS

Safety and efficacy of topical products have not been established in children. Occlusive dressings may result in increased inflammation in adjacent normal skin when topical products are used.

ADDITIONAL SIDE EFFECTS

• **SYSTEMIC.**

Esophagopharyngitis, myocardial ischemia, angina, acute cerebellar syndrome, photophobia, lacrimation, decreased vision. Also, arterial thrombosis, arterial ischemia, arterial aneurysm, bleeding or infection at site of catheter, thrombophlebitis, embolism, fibromyositis, abscesses.

• **TOPICAL.**

Dermatologic: Pain, pruritus, hyperpigmentation, irritation, inflammation, burning at site of application, scarring, soreness, allergic contact dermatitis, tenderness, scaling, swelling, suppuration, alopecia, photosensitivity, urticaria. **CNS:** Insomnia, irritability. **GI:** Stomatitis, medicinal taste. **Miscellaneous:** Lacrimation, telangiectasia, toxic granulation.

LABORATORY TEST CONSIDERATIONS

↑ Alkaline phosphatase, LDH, serum bilirubin, and serum transaminase.

OD OVERDOSE MANAGEMENT

Symptoms: N&V, diarrhea, GI ulceration, GI bleeding, thrombocytopenia, ***agranulocytosis,*** leukopenia. *Treatment:* Monitor hematologically for at least 4 weeks.

DRUG INTERACTIONS

Leucovorin calcium ↑ toxicity of fluorouracil.

HOW SUPPLIED

Cream: 1%, 5%; *Injection:* 50 mg/mL; *Solution:* 1%, 2%, 5%

DOSAGE

• **IV**

Palliative management of selected carcinomas.

Individualize dosage. Initial: 12 mg/kg/day for 4 days, not to exceed 800 mg/day. If no toxicity seen, administer 6 mg/kg on days 6, 8, 10, and 12. Discontinue therapy on day 12 even if there are no toxic symptoms. **Maintenance:** Repeat dose of first course q 30 days or when toxicity from initial course of therapy is gone; or, give 10–15 mg/kg/week as a single dose. Do not exceed 1 g/week. **If client is debilitated or is a poor risk:** 6 mg/kg/day for 3 days; if no toxicity, give 3 mg/kg on days 5, 7, and 9 (daily dose should not exceed 400 mg).

Metastatic colorectal cancer.

Leucovorin, **IV,** 200 mg/m^2/day for 5 days followed by fluorouracil, **IV,** 370 mg/m^2/day for 5 days. Repeat q 28 days to maximize response and to prolong survival.

Dukes' stage C colon cancer after surgical resection.

See *Levamisole.*

• **CREAM, TOPICAL SOLUTION**

Actinic or solar keratoses.

Apply 1% or 5% cream or 1%–5% solution to cover lesion 1–2 times/day for 2–6 weeks.

Superficial basal cell carcinoma.

Apply 5% cream or solution to cover lesion b.i.d. for 3–6 weeks (up to 10–12 weeks may be required).

NURSING CONSIDERATIONS

SEE ALSO *NURSING CONSIDERATIONS* FOR *ANTINEOPLASTIC AGENTS.*

ADMINISTRATION/STORAGE

1. Apply with fingertips, nonmetallic applicator, or rubber gloves. Wash hands immediately thereafter.
2. Avoid contact with eyes, nose, and mouth.
3. Limit occlusive dressings to lesions; causes inflammatory reactions in normal skin.
4. Complete healing of keratoses may require 2 months.

IV 5. Further dilution not needed; solution may be injected directly into

the vein with a 25-gauge needle over 1–2 min.
6. Drug can be diluted in D5W or NSS and administered by IV infusion for periods of 30 min–8 hr. This method produces less systemic toxicity than rapid injection.
7. Do not mix with other drugs or IV additives.
8. If precipitate forms, resolubilize by heating to 60°C (140°F) with vigorous shaking. Allow to return to room temperature and allow air to settle out before withdrawing and administering medication.
9. Solution may discolor slightly during storage, but potency and safety are not affected.
10. Store in a cool place (10–27°C, or 50–80°F). Do not freeze. Excessively low temperature causes precipitation. Do not expose the solution to light.

ASSESSMENT

1. Observe for intractable vomiting, stomatitis, and diarrhea; early signs of toxicity requiring immediate withdrawal of drug.
2. Hydrate well before and after therapy. Give antiemetics 1 hr before therapy.
3. Protect and supervise ambulation if symptoms of cerebellar dysfunction occur (altered balance, dizziness, or weakness).
4. Prevent exposure to strong sunlight and other ultraviolet rays; these intensify skin reactions.
5. Hair loss and mouth lesions may occur but are usually transient.
6. Use precautions and strict asepsis when WBC count is below 2,000/mm^3.
7. Discontinue if WBC and platelet counts are depressed below 3,500/mm^3 and 100,000/mm^3, respectively. Nadir: 10–20 days; recovery: 30 days.

CLIENT/FAMILY TEACHING

1. Review appropriate method for topical application. Do not wear plastic eyeglass frames during treatment. Contact may cause severe skin burns. Apply at night when glasses may be removed.
2. Affected area may appear much worse before healing takes place in 1–2 months. If dressing is needed use only porous gauze; avoid occlusive dressings.
3. Drink plenty of fluids (2–3 L/day) during therapy.
4. Practice barrier contraception during systemic therapy.
5. Avoid exposure to sunlight. If exposed, wear protective clothing, sunglasses, and sunscreen.
6. Hair loss and mouth sores may occur but are usually transient with parenteral therapy.

OUTCOMES/EVALUATE

- Control of malignant process
- Reepithelialization of skin lesion

Fluoxetine hydrochloride

(flew-**OX**-eh-teen)

PREGNANCY CATEGORY: B
CLASSIFICATION(S):
Antidepressant, selective serotonin reuptake inhibitor
Rx: Prozac, Prozac Weekly, Sarafem
✱Rx: Alti-Fluoxetine Hydrochloride, Apo-Fluoxetine, Gen-Fluoxetine, Novo-Fluoxetine, Nu-Fluoxetine, PMS-Fluoxetine, Scheinpharm Fluoxetine

SEE ALSO *SELECTIVE SEROTONIN REUPTAKE INHIBITORS*.

ACTION/KINETICS

Metabolized in the liver to norfluoxetine, a metabolite with equal potency to fluoxetine. Norfluoxetine is further metabolized by the liver to inactive metabolites that are excreted by the kidneys. **Time to peak plasma levels:** 6–8 hr. **Peak plasma concentrations:** 15–55 ng/mL. **t½, fluoxetine:** 1–6 days; **t½, norfluoxetine:** 4–16 days. **Time to steady state:** 2–4 weeks. Active drug maintained in the body for weeks after withdrawal.

USES

Prozac: Depression in adults and geriatric (aged 65 and older) clients, obsessive-compulsive disorders (OCD; as defined in the DSM-III-R), bulimia nervosa. **Serafem:** Premenstrual dysphoric disorder. *Investigational:* Many (see *Dosage*).

SPECIAL CONCERNS

A lower initial dose may be necessary in geriatric clients. Use in hospitalized clients, use for longer than 5–6 weeks for depression, or use for more than 13 weeks for obsessive-compulsive disorder has not been studied adequately.

SIDE EFFECTS

A large number of side effects have been reported for this drug. Listed are those with a reported frequency of greater than 1%. **CNS:** Headache (most common), activation of mania or hypomania, insomnia, anxiety, nervousness, dizziness, fatigue, sedation, decreased libido, drowsiness, lightheadedness, decreased ability to concentrate, tremor, disturbances in sensation, agitation, abnormal dreams. Although less frequent than 1%, ***some clients may experience seizures or attempt suicide.*** **GI:** Nausea (most common), diarrhea, vomiting, constipation, dry mouth, dyspepsia, anorexia, abdominal pain, flatulence, alteration in taste, gastroenteritis, increased appetite. **CV:** Hot flashes, palpitations. **GU:** Sexual dysfunction, impotence, anorgasmia, frequent urination, UTI, dysmenorrhea. **Respiratory:** URTI, pharyngitis, cough, dyspnea, rhinitis, bronchitis, nasal congestion, sinusitis, sinus headache, yawn. **Skin:** Rash, pruritus, excessive sweating. **Musculoskeletal:** Muscle, joint, or back pain. **Miscellaneous:** Flu-like symptoms, asthenia, fever, chest pain, allergy, visual disturbances, blurred vision, weight loss, bacterial or viral infection, limb pain, chills.

ADDITIONAL DRUG INTERACTIONS

Alprazolam / ↑ Alprazolam levels and ↓ psychomotor performance
Buspirone / ↓ Buspirone effects; worsening of obsessive-compulsive disorder
Carbamazepine / ↑ Serum carbamazepine levels → toxicity
Clozapine / ↑ Serum clozapine levels
Cyproheptadine / ↓ or Reversal of fluoxetine effect
Dextromethorphan / Possibility of hallucinations
Diazepam / ↑ Diazepam half-life → excessive sedation or impaired psychomotor skills
Digoxin / ↓ Area under the curve of digoxin; use together with caution
Haloperidol / ↑ Serum haloperidol levels
Lithium / ↑ Serum lithium levels → possible neurotoxicity
Phenytoin / ↑ Phenytoin levels

HOW SUPPLIED

Capsule: 10 mg, 20 mg, 40 mg; *Capsule, Delayed Release:* 90 mg; *Oral Solution:* 20 mg/5 mL; *Tablet:* 10 mg

DOSAGE

• PROZAC: CAPSULES, DELAYED RELEASE CAPSULES, ORAL SOLUTION, TABLETS

Antidepressant.

Adults, initial: 20 mg/day in the morning. If clinical improvement is not observed after several weeks, the dose may be increased to a maximum of 80 mg/day in two equally divided doses. For weekly dosing for stablized clients requiring maintenance therapy, can use Prozac Weekly (90 mg delayed release capsule), given 7 days after the last 20 mg dose. If satisfactory response is not maintained, reestablish a daily dosing regimen.

OCD.

Initial: 20 mg/day in the morning. If improvement is not significant after several weeks, the dose may be increased. **Usual dosage range:** 20–60 mg/day; the total daily dosage should not exceed 80 mg.

Treatment of bulimia nervosa.

60 mg/day given in the morning. May be necessary to titrate up to this dose over several days.

Alcoholism.

40–80 mg/day.

Anorexia nervosa, bipolar II affective disorder, trichotillomania.

20–80 mg/day.

ADHD, schizophrenia.

20–60 mg/day.

Borderline personality disorder.

5–80 mg/day.

Cataplexy and narcolepsy, Tourette's syndrome.

20–40 mg/day.

Kleptomania.
60–80 mg/day.
Migraine, chronic daily headaches, tension headaches.
20 mg every other day to 40 mg/day.
PTSD.
10–80 mg/day.
PMS, recurrent syncope.
20 mg/day.
Levodopa-induced dyskinesia.
40 mg/day.
Social phobia.
10–60 mg/day.
Chronic rheumatoid pain.
20 mg/day.
Panic disorder.
10–70 mg/day.
Diabetic peripheral neuropathy.
5–40 mg/day.
Schizophrenia.
20–60 mg/day.

• **SERAFEM: CAPSULES**
Premenstrual dysphoric disorder.
Initial: 20 mg/day, not to exceed 80 mg/day; **maintenance:** 20 mg/day (efficacy maintained for 6 months or less). Not to be used PRN, but daily.

NURSING CONSIDERATIONS

SEE ALSO ***NURSING CONSIDERATIONS*** FOR ***SELECTIVE SEROTONIN REUPTAKE INHIBITORS.***

ADMINISTRATION/STORAGE

1. Divide doses greater than 20 mg/day and give in the morning and at noon.
2. If doses lower than 20 mg are necessary, the drug may be emptied from the capsule into cranberry, orange, or apple juice; this should not be refrigerated (is stable for 2 weeks). *NOTE:* A liquid preparation (20 mg/5 mL) is also available.
3. The maximum therapeutic effect may not be observed until 4 weeks after beginning therapy.
4. Elderly clients, clients taking multiple medications, and those with liver or kidney dysfunction should take lower or less frequent doses.
5. When used for obsessive-compulsive disorders and therapy has been continued for over 6 months, reassess periodically to determine if continued drug therapy is needed.
6. When given with tricyclic antidepressants or if fluoxetine has been recently discontinued, the dose of TCA may need to be reduced and plasma levels monitored temporarily.
7. Allow 14 days to elapse between discontinuing a MAOI and starting fluoxetine therapy; also, allow 5 weeks or more to elapse between stopping fluoxetine and starting a MAOI.

ASSESSMENT

1. Document indications for therapy, type and onset of symptoms.
2. Review drugs currently prescribed; note any that may interact unfavorably.
3. Determine if pregnant or lactating.
4. Obtain baseline liver and renal function studies; anticipate reduced dose with hepatic and/or renal insufficiency.
5. Periodically reassess client to determine need for continued therapy.

CLIENT/FAMILY TEACHING

1. Use caution when driving or performing tasks that require mental alertness; drug may cause drowsiness and/or dizziness. Change positions slowly to avoid orthostatic effects.
2. Report any side effects, especially rashes, hives, increased anxiety, and loss of appetite.
3. Take medication at the specific times designated as nervousness and insomnia may occur.
4. It usually takes 1 month to note any significant benefits from therapy. Do not become discouraged and discontinue the medication before benefits are attained.
5. Avoid alcohol; do not take any OTC medications without approval. Use sunscreen and avoid prolonged sun exposure.
6. Any thoughts of suicide or evidence of increased suicide ideations should be reported immediately.
7. Use reliable birth control during therapy.

OUTCOMES/EVALUATE

• ↓ Symptoms of depression, as evidenced by improved sleeping and

F

eating patterns, ↓ fatigue, and ↑ social involvement and activity
• Control of repetitive behavioral manifestations

Fluphenazine decanoate

(flew-**FEN**-ah-zeen)

Rx: Prolixin Decanoate
✱Rx: Modecate Concentrate, Modecate Decanoate, PMS-Fluphenazine, Rho-Fluphenazine Decanoate

Fluphenazine enanthate

(flew-**FEN**-ah-zeen)

Rx: Prolixin Enanthate
✱Rx: Moditen Enanthate

Fluphenazine hydrochloride

(flew-**FEN**-ah-zeen)

Rx: Permitil, Prolixin
✱Rx: Apo-Fluphenazine, Moditen HCl

CLASSIFICATION(S):
Antipsychotic, phenothiazine

SEE ALSO *ANTIPSYCHOTIC AGENTS, PHENOTHIAZINES*.

ACTION/KINETICS
High incidence of extrapyramidal symptoms and a low incidence of sedation, anticholinergic effects, antiemetic effects, and orthostatic hypotension. The enanthate and decanoate esters dramatically increase the duration of action. *Decanoate:* **Onset,** 24–72 hr; **peak plasma levels,** 24–48 hr; **t½** (approximate), 14 days; **duration,** up to 4 weeks. *Enanthate:* **Onset,** 24–72 hr; **peak plasma levels,** 48–72 hr; **t½** (approximate), 3.6 days; **duration,** 1–3 weeks.

Fluphenazine hydrochloride can be cautiously administered to clients with known hypersensitivity to other phenothiazines.

Fluphenazine enanthate may replace fluphenazine hydrochloride if desired response occurs with hypersensitivity reaction to fluphenazine.

USES
Psychotic disorders. Adjunct to tricyclic antidepressants for chronic pain states (e.g., diabetic neuropathy, and clients trying to withdraw from narcotics).

HOW SUPPLIED
Fluphenazine decanoate: *Injection:* 25 mg/mL **Fluphenazine enanthate:** *Injection:* 25 mg/mL **Fluphenazine hydrochloride:** *Concentrate:* 5 mg/mL; *Elixir:* 2.5 mg/5 mL; *Injection:* 2.5 mg/mL; *Tablet:* 1 mg, 2.5 mg, 5 mg, 10 mg

DOSAGE

Fluphenazine hydrochloride is administered **PO and IM.** Fluphenazine enanthate or decanoate are administered **SC and IM.**

HYDROCHLORIDE.

• **ELIXIR, ORAL SOLUTION, TABLETS**
Psychotic disorders.

Adults and adolescents, initial: 0.5–10 mg/day in divided doses q 6–8 hr; **then,** reduce gradually to maintenance dose of 1–5 mg/day (usually given as a single dose, not to exceed 20 mg/day). **Geriatric, emaciated, debilitated clients, initial:** 1–2.5 mg/day; **then,** dosage determined by response. **Pediatric:** 0.25–0.75 mg 1–4 times/day.

• **IM**
Psychotic disorders.

Adults and adolescents: 1.25–2.5 mg q 6–8 hr as needed. Maximum daily dose: 10 mg. Elderly, debilitated, or emaciated clients should start with 1–2.5 mg/day.

DECANOATE.

• **IM, SC**
Psychotic disorders.

Adults, initial: 12.5–25 mg; **then,** the dose may be repeated or increased q 1–3 weeks. The usual maintenance dose is 50 mg/1–4 weeks. Maximum adult dose: 100 mg/dose. **Pediatric, 12 years and older:** 6.25–18.75 mg/week; the dose can be increased to 12.5–25 mg given q 1–3 weeks. **Pediatric, 5–12 years:** 3.125–12.5 mg with this dose being repeated q 1–3 weeks.

ENANTHATE.

• **IM, SC**

Psychotic disorders.

Adults and adolescents: 12.5–25 mg; dose can be repeated or increased q 1–3 weeks. For doses greater than 50 mg, increases should be made in increments of 12.5 mg. Maximum adult dose: 100 mg.

NURSING CONSIDERATIONS

SEE ALSO *NURSING CONSIDERATIONS* FOR *ANTIPSYCHOTIC AGENTS, PHENOTHIAZINES.*

ADMINISTRATION/STORAGE

1. Protect all forms of medication from light.
2. Store at room temperature and avoid freezing the elixir.
3. Color of parenteral solution may vary from colorless to light amber. Do not use solutions that are darker than light amber.
4. Do not mix the hydrochloride concentrate with any beverage containing caffeine, tannates (e.g., tea), or pectins (e.g., apple juice) due to a physical incompatibility.
5. Give the short-acting form when beginning phenothiazine therapy. Consider the decanoate and enanthate forms after the response to the drug has been evaluated and for those who demonstrate compliance problems.

ASSESSMENT

1. Document indications for therapy, onset and characteristics of symptoms, other treatments utilized, and the outcome.
2. Note age, mental status, and physical condition. Elderly and debilitated clients are at increased risk for acute extrapyramidal symptoms.

CLIENT/FAMILY TEACHING

1. Review administration times; determine if client able to assume responsibility for self-medication. Many long term clients do better on the monthly injection.
2. Review written guidelines concerning side effects that should be reported and when to return for follow-up. Stress importance of regular psychotherapy.
3. Avoid hot tubs, hot shower and tub baths as low BP may occur; in hot weather, avoid strenuous activity, keep cool as heat stroke may occur.
4. Do not stop abruptly. Change positions slowly to avoid low BP effects.
5. Report any sore throat, bleeding, mouth sores, unusual fatigue or fever; need CBC drawn and drug withdrawn.
6. Wear sunscreen to prevent sunburns, increase fluids to prevent constipation and for dry mouth effects. Urine may turn pink-reddish brown.

OUTCOMES/EVALUATE

• Improved behavior patterns with ↓ agitation, ↓ paranoia and withdrawal
• Control of tics

Flurazepam hydrochloride

(flur-**AYZ**-eh-pam)

CLASSIFICATION(S):
Sedative-hypnotic, benzodiazepine
Rx: Dalmane **C-IV**
★**Rx:** Apo-Flurazepam, Somnol

SEE ALSO *TRANQUILIZERS, ANTIMANIC DRUGS, AND HYPNOTICS.*

ACTION/KINETICS

Combines with benzodiazepine receptors, which are part of the benzodiazepine-GABA receptor-chloride ionophore complex. Results in enhanced inhibitory action of GABA leading to interference of transmission of nerve impulses in the reticular activating system. **Onset:** 17 min. The major active metabolite, *N*-desalkyl-flurazepam, is active and has a **t½** of 47–100 hr. **Time to peak plasma levels, flurazepam:** 0.5–1 hr; **active metabolite:** 1–3 hr. **Duration:** 7–8 hr. **Maximum effectiveness:** 2–3 days (due to slow accumulation of active metabolite). Significantly bound to plasma protein. Elimination is slow because metabolites remain in the blood for several days. Exceeding the recommended dose may result in development of tolerance and dependence.

USES

Insomnia (all types). Is increasingly effective on the second or third night of consecutive use and for one or two nights after the drug is discontinued.

CONTRAINDICATIONS

Hypersensitivity. Pregnancy or in women wishing to become pregnant. Depression, renal or hepatic disease, chronic pulmonary insufficiency, children under 15 years.

SPECIAL CONCERNS

Use during the last few weeks of pregnancy may result in CNS depression of the neonate. Use during lactation may cause sedation and feeding problems in the infant. Geriatric clients may be more sensitive to the effects of flurazepam.

SIDE EFFECTS

CNS: Ataxia, dizziness, drowsiness/sedation, headache, disorientation. Symptoms of stimulation including nervousness, apprehension, irritability, and talkativeness. **GI:** N&V, diarrhea, gastric upset or pain, heartburn, constipation. **Miscellaneous:** Arthralgia, chest pains, or palpitations. Rarely, symptoms of allergy, SOB, jaundice, anorexia, blurred vision.

LABORATORY TEST CONSIDERATIONS

↑ Alkaline phosphatase, bilirubin, serum transaminases.

DRUG INTERACTIONS

Cimetidine / ↑ Flurazepam effect R/T ↓ liver breakdown
CNS depressants / Addition or potentiation of depression —drowsiness, lethargy, stupor, respiratory depression or collapse, coma, and possible death
Disulfiram / ↑ Flurazepam effect R/T ↓ liver breakdown
Ethanol / Additive depressant effects up to the day following flurazepam administration
Isoniazid / ↑ Flurazepam effect R/T ↓ liver breakdown
Oral contraceptives / Either ↑ or ↓ effect of benzodiazepines R/T effect on liver breakdown
Rifampin / ↓ Effect of benzodiazepines R/T ↑ liver breakdown

HOW SUPPLIED

Capsule: 15 mg, 30 mg

DOSAGE

• CAPSULES

Adults: 15–30 mg at bedtime; 15 mg for geriatric and/or debilitated clients.

NURSING CONSIDERATIONS

SEE ALSO NURSING CONSIDERATIONS FOR TRANQUILIZERS, ANTIMANIC DRUGS, AND HYPNOTICS.

ASSESSMENT

1. Document indications for therapy, symptom onset, other agents prescribed, and the results.
2. Anticipate short-term therapy. Attempt to identify and address causative factors.

CLIENT/FAMILY TEACHING

1. Use caution in driving or operating machinery until daytime sedative effects are evaluated. Report persistent morning "hangover."
2. With simple insomnia, try warm baths, warm drinks, soft music, white noise simulator, and other relaxation methods to induce sleep. No caffeine or caffeine containing products 10 hr before anticipated bedtime.
3. Avoid alcohol and CNS depressants.
4. Report tolerance and any symptoms of psychologic and/or physical dependence. For short-term therapy; continued use causes tolerance and decreased drug responsiveness.
5. Keep a diary of foods, activities, and events for at least 5 days to determine if there are any relationships to insomnia condition.

OUTCOMES/EVALUATE

Improved sleeping patterns and less frequent awakenings

Flurbiprofen

(flur-**BIH**-proh-fen)

PREGNANCY CATEGORY: B
Rx: Ansaid
★Rx: Alti-Flurbiprofen, Apo-Flurbiprofen, Froben, Novo-Flurprofen, Nu-Flurbiprofen

Flurbiprofen sodium

(flur-**BIH**-proh-fen)

PREGNANCY CATEGORY: C
Rx: Flurbiprofen Sodium Ophthalmic, Ocufen
CLASSIFICATION(S):
Nonsteroidal anti-inflammatory drug

SEE ALSO NONSTEROIDAL ANTI-INFLAMMATORY DRUGS.

ACTION/KINETICS
By inhibiting prostaglandin synthesis, flurbiprofen reverses prostaglandin-induced vasodilation, leukocytosis, increased vascular permeability, and increased intraocular pressure. Also inhibits miosis occurring during cataract surgery. **PO form, time to peak levels:** 1.5 hr; **t½:** 5.7 hr. More than 99% protein-bound. Over 70% excreted in the urine.

USES
Ophthalmic: Prevention of intraoperative miosis. **PO:** Rheumatoid arthritis, osteoarthritis. *Investigational:* Inflammation following cataract surgery, uveitis syndromes. Topically to treat cystoid macular edema. Primary dysmenorrhea, sunburn, mild to moderate pain.

CONTRAINDICATIONS
Dendritic keratitis.

SPECIAL CONCERNS
Use with caution in clients hypersensitive to aspirin or other NSAIDs and during lactation. Wound healing may be delayed with use of the ophthalmic product. Acetylcholine chloride and carbachol may be ineffective when used with ophthalmic flubiprofen. Safety and efficacy in children have not been established.

ADDITIONAL SIDE EFFECTS
Ophthalmic: Ocular irritation, transient stinging or burning following use, delay in wound healing. Increased bleeding of ocular tissues in conjunction with ocular surgery.

HOW SUPPLIED
Flurbiprofen: *Tablet:* 50 mg, 100 mg
Flurbiprofen sodium: *Ophthalmic solution:* 0.03%

DOSAGE
- **OPHTHALMIC DROPS**

Beginning 2 hr before surgery, instill 1 gtt q 30 min (i.e., total of 4 gtt of 0.03% solution).

- **TABLETS**

Rheumatoid arthritis, osteoarthritis.
Adults, initial: 200–300 mg/day in divided doses b.i.d.–q.i.d.; **then,** adjust dose to client response. Doses greater than 300 mg/day are not recommended.
Dysmenorrhea.
50 mg q.i.d.

NURSING CONSIDERATIONS

SEE ALSO NURSING CONSIDERATIONS FOR NONSTEROIDAL ANTI-INFLAMMATROY DRUGS.

ADMINISTRATION/STORAGE
Use a dose of 300 mg only for initiating therapy or for treating acute exacerbations of the disease.

ASSESSMENT
1. Document therapy indications. Rate pain level noting onset, location, and characteristics.
2. Assess ROM of involved extremity, noting any discoloration, swelling, crepitus, deformity, or warmth.
3. Prior to eye surgery, carefully follow the prescribed dosing intervals. Use care not to touch eye surface with dropper. Report any post-op tearing, dry eye, pain, and light sensitivity.

CLIENT/FAMILY TEACHING
1. May take tablets with food to decrease GI upset. Do not cut or chew tablets.
2. Review appropriate method of administering eye medication. Avoid rubbing eyes after medication administered; report any stinging, burning, or irritation immediately.
3. Report delays in wound healing.
4. Muscle-strengthening exercises should be performed daily.
5. Avoid alcohol and aspirin as this may increase GI upset.

OUTCOMES/EVALUATE
- ↓ Pain and inflammation with ↑ joint mobility
- ↓ Optic inflammation
- ↓ Abnormal pupillary contractions

Flutamide

(**FLOO**-tah-myd)

PREGNANCY CATEGORY: D
CLASSIFICATION(S):
Antineoplastic, hormone
Rx: Eulexin
★**Rx:** Apo-Flutamide, Euflex, Novo-Flutamide, PMS-Flutamide

F

SEE ALSO *ANTINEOPLASTIC AGENTS.*

ACTION/KINETICS

Acts either to inhibit uptake of androgen or to inhibit nuclear binding of androgen in target tissues. Thus, the effect of androgen is decreased in androgen-sensitive tissues. Rapidly metabolized to active (α-hydroxylated derivative) and inactive metabolites in the liver and mainly excreted in the urine. **t½ of active metabolite:** 6 hr (8 hr in geriatric clients). Ninety-four percent to 96% is bound to plasma proteins.

USES

In combination with leuprolide acetate (i.e., a LHRH agonist) to treat stage D_2 metastatic prostatic carcinoma as well as locally confined stage B_2-C prostate cancer. In combination with goserelin acetate depots (Zoladex) to treat locally confined early stage B_2-C prostate cancer before and during radiation therapy. *Investigational:* Treat hirsutism in women.

CONTRAINDICATIONS

Use during pregnancy or severe hepatic impairment (if baseline serum ALT values exceed twice ULN).

SPECIAL CONCERNS

Possible liver failure, especially within the first 3 months of therapy.

SIDE EFFECTS

Side effects are listed for treatment of flutamide with LHRH agonist. **GU:** Loss of libido, impotence. **CV:** Hot flashes, hypertension. **GI:** N&V, diarrhea, GI disturbances, anorexia. **CNS:** Confusion, depression, drowsiness, anxiety, nervousness. **Hematologic:** Anemia, leukopenia, thrombocytopenia, ***hemolytic anemia,*** macrocytic anemia, methemoglobinemia, sulfhemoglobinemia. **Hepatic:** Hepatitis, cholestatic jaundice, hepatic encephalopathy, jaundice, ***hepatic necrosis, liver failure.*** **Dermatologic:** Rash, injection site irritation, erythema, ulceration, bullous eruptions, photosensitivity, ***epidermal necrolysis***. **Miscellaneous:** Gynecomastia, edema, neuromuscular symptoms, pulmonary symptoms, GU symptoms, malignant breast tumors.

LABORATORY TEST CONSIDERATIONS

↑ AST, ALT, serum creatinine, SGGT, BUN, bilirubin. Urine may be colored amber or yellow-green due to the drug or its metabolites.

OD OVERDOSE MANAGEMENT

Symptoms: Breast tenderness, gynecomastia, increases in AST. Also possible are ataxia, anorexia, vomiting, decreased respiration, lacrimation, sedation, hypoactivity, and piloerection. *Treatment:* Induce vomiting if client is alert. Frequently monitor VS and observe closely.

HOW SUPPLIED

Capsule: 125 mg

DOSAGE

• CAPSULES

Locally confined stage B_2-C and stage D_2 metastatic cancer of the prostate.

250 mg (2 capsules) t.i.d. q 8 hr for a total daily dose of 750 mg.

Hirsutism in women.

250 mg/day.

NURSING CONSIDERATIONS

SEE ALSO *NURSING CONSIDERATIONS FOR ANTINEOPLASTIC AGENTS.*

ADMINISTRATION/STORAGE

1. For stage B_2-C prostatic cancer, start flutamide and the LHRH agonist 8 weeks prior to initiating and continue during radiation therapy.
2. For maximum benefit in stage D_2 metastatic prostatic cancer, start flutamide and the LHRH agonist together and continue until disease progression.

ASSESSMENT

1. Document indications for therapy, agents previously used, and the outcome.
2. Administer with an LHRH agonist (such as leuprolide acetate).

3. Monitor CBC and LFTs during therapy. Discontinue therapy if jaundice develops or ALT levels rise above two times the upper limit of normal.
4. Monitor liver function prior to therapy, monthly for the first 4 months, and periodically thereafter. Stop therapy (or do not start therapy) if ALT exceeds twice the normal limit.
5. Monitor methemoglobinemia in those susceptible to aniline toxicity (i.e., G-6-P dehydrogenase deficiency, hemoglobin M disease, smokers).

CLIENT/FAMILY TEACHING

1. Take flutamide and the LHRH agonist (leuprolide) at the same time.
2. Drug therapy should not be interrupted or discontinued without consulting the provider.
3. Hot flashes, impotence, and diarrhea are all potential side effects of drug therapy; report if persistent or bothersome.
4. Male sexual problems may be drug induced (impotence, decreased libido, gynecomastia). Counseling may be indicated.
5. Compliance may be a problem if diarrhea experienced. Manage diarrhea by cutting down on dairy products, drinking plenty of fluids, not using laxatives, using antidiarrheal products, and eating smaller, more frequent meals high in dietary fibers.

OUTCOMES/EVALUATE

- ↓ Production of testosterone
- ↓ Prostatic tumor size
- Control of metastatic processes

Fluticasone propionate

(flu-**TIH**-kah-sohn)

PREGNANCY CATEGORY: C
CLASSIFICATION(S):
Glucocorticoid
Rx: Cutivate, Flonase, Flovent, Flovent Rotadisk

SEE ALSO *CORTICOSTEROIDS*.

ACTION/KINETICS

Following intranasal use, a small amount is absorbed into the general circulation. **Onset:** Approximately 12 hr. **Maximum effect:** May take several days. **t½:** About 3.1 hr. Absorbed drug is metabolized in the liver and excreted in the urine.

USES

Nasal/Inhalation. Prevention and maintenance treatment of asthma in adults and children over four years of age (Flovent Rotadisk) or 12 years of age (Flovent). To manage seasonal and perennial allergic and nonallergic rhinitis in adults and children over four years of age. **Topical.** Relief of inflammatory and pruritic corticosteroid-responsive dermatoses in adults. Atopic dermatitis in clients as young as 3 months.

CONTRAINDICATIONS

Use for relief of acute bronchospasm. Use following nasal septal ulcers, nasal surgery, or nasal trauma until healing has occurred.

SPECIAL CONCERNS

Clients on immunosuppressant drugs, such as corticosteroids, are more susceptible to infections. Use with caution, if at all, in active or quiescent tuberculosis infections; untreated fungal, bacterial, or systemic viral infections; or ocular herpes simplex. Use with caution during lactation.

SIDE EFFECTS

Allergic: Rarely, immediate hypersensitivity reactions or contact dermatitis. **Respiratory:** Epistaxis, nasal burning, blood in nasal mucus, pharyngitis, irritation of nasal mucous membranes, sneezing, runny nose, nasal dryness, sinusitis, nasal congestion, bronchitis, nasal ulcer, nasal septum excoriation. **CNS:** Headache, dizziness. **Ophthalmologic:** Eye disorder, cataracts, glaucoma, increased intraocular pressure. **GI:** N&V, xerostomia. **Miscellaneous:** Unpleasant taste, urticaria. High doses have resulted in hypercorticism and adrenal suppression.

DRUG INTERACTIONS

Ketoconazole may ↑ fluticasone plasma levels due to ↓ liver breakdown.

HOW SUPPLIED

Aerosol (Flovent): 44 mcg/inh, 110 mcg/inh, 220 mcg/inh; *Cream:* 0.05%; *Nasal spray:* 50 mcg/inh; *Ointment:* 0.005%; *Powder for Inhalation (Flovent Rotadisk):* 50 mcg/inh, 100 mcg/inh, 250 mcg/inh;

DOSAGE

• **AEROSOL (FLOVENT)**

Treatment of asthma.

Adults and children over 4 years of age, initial: 88 mcg b.i.d. (maximum: 440 mcg b.i.d.) if previous therapy was bronchodilators alone; 88–220 mcg b.i.d. (maximum: 440 mcg b.i.d.) if previous therapy was inhaled corticosteroids; and, 880 mcg b.i.d. (maximum: 880 mcg b.i.d.) if previous therapy was oral corticosteroids.

• **POWDER (FLOVENT ROTADISK)**

Prevention of asthma.

Adults and adolescents: 100 mcg b.i.d. (maximum: 500 mcg b.i.d.) if previous therapy was bronchodilators alone; 100–250 mcg b.i.d. (maximum: 500 mcg b.i.d.) if previous therapy was inhaled corticosteroids; and, 1,000 mcg b.i.d. (maximum: 1,000 mcg b.i.d.) if previous therapy was oral corticosteroids. **Children, 4–11 years:** 50 mcg b.i.d. (maximum: 100 mcg b.i.d.) if previous therapy was bronchodilators alone or inhaled corticosteroids.

• **NASAL SPRAY**

Allergic rhinitis.

Adults and children over 4 years of age, initial: One 50-mcg spray in each nostril once a day, for a total daily dose of 100 mcg/day. Maximum dose is two sprays (200 mcg) in each nostril once a day.

• **OINTMENT, CREAM**

Apply sparingly to affected area 2–4 times daily. For Cutivate Cream, apply a thin film to the affected areas 1–2 times/day.

NURSING CONSIDERATIONS

SEE ALSO *NURSING CONSIDERATIONS* FOR *CORTICOSTEROIDS*.

ADMINISTRATION/STORAGE

1. Effectiveness depends on regular use.
2. For clients taking chronic oral steroids, reduce prednisone no faster than 2.5 mg/day on a weekly basis, beginning after 1 or more weeks of aerosol therapy. After prednisone reduction is complete, decrease fluticasone dosage to the lowest effective dose.
3. Store spray at 4–30°C (39–86°F). Store aerosol between 2–30°C (36–85°F) and the powder at 20–25°C (68–77°F) in a dry place.
4. Store aerosol canister with nozzle end down; protect from freezing and direct sunlight.
5. Use Rotadisk blisters within 2 months of opening the moisture-protective foil.

ASSESSMENT

1. Document indications for therapy, onset/characteristics of symptoms, and other agents trialed.
2. Examine for evidence of nasal septal ulcers; note turbinate findings.
3. Determine if immunocompromised or actively infected.

CLIENT/FAMILY TEACHING

1. Review technique for administration. With nasal spray, clear nasal passages before using. With inhalers, if others prescribed, use the bronchidilator first so steroid better permeates mucosa. Rinse mouth and inhaler with water after use to prevent infections.
2. Take at regular intervals to ensure effectiveness; do not exceed prescribed dose, it may take several days to achieve full benefits.
3. Do not interrupt therapy if side effects evident; notify provider as drug may require slow withdrawal. The dosage should also be slowly reduced if S&S of hypercorticism or adrenal suppression occur such as depression, lassitude, joint and muscle pain; report if evident, especially when replacing systemic corticosteroids with topical.
4. Use adequate humidity, especially during winter months when dry heat may aggravate mucosa.
5. Avoid persons with active infections. Report exposure to chicken pox or measles. (If not immunized or previously infected with the disease, Varicella or Immune Globulin prophylaxis may be given to high-risk clients on long-term therapy).

6. Height and weight will be monitored periodically in adolescents to detect any growth suppression.
7. Identify triggers that aggravate asthma (dust, pollen, smoke, chemicals, pets). Use peak flow meter to help manage asthma.

OUTCOMES/EVALUATE

- Control of asthma
- ↓ Symptoms of allergic rhinitis

Fluvastatin sodium

(flu-vah-**STAH**-tin)

PREGNANCY CATEGORY: X
CLASSIFICATION(S):
Antihyperlipidemic, HMG-CoA reductase inhibitor
Rx: Lescol, Lescol XL

SEE ALSO *ANTIHYPERLIPIDEMIC AGENTS—HMG-COA REDUCTASE INHIBITORS.*

ACTION/KINETICS
t½: 0.5–3.1 hr. Undergoes extensive first-pass metabolism. Significantly bound (greater than 98%) to plasma protein. Metabolized in the liver with 90% excreted through the feces and 5% through the urine.

USES
(1) Adjunct to diet for the reduction of elevated total and LDL cholesterol, apo-B, and triglyceride levels in clients with primary hypercholesterolemia and mixed dyslipidemia (Fredrickson type IIa and IIb) whose response to diet and other nondrug measures have been inadequate. The lipid-lowering effects of fluvastatin are enhanced when it is combined with a bile-acid binding resin or with niacin. (2) To slow the progression of coronary atherosclerosis in coronary heart disease.

SPECIAL CONCERNS
Use with caution in clients with severe renal impairment.

SIDE EFFECTS
Side effects listed are those most common with fluvastatin. A complete list of possible side effects is provided under *Antihyperlipidemic Agents—HMG-CoA Reductase Inhibitors.* **GI:** N&V, diarrhea, abdominal pain or cramps, constipation, flatulence, dyspepsia, tooth disorder. **Musculoskeletal:** Myalgia, back pain, arthralgia, arthritis. **CNS:** Headache, dizziness, insomnia. **Respiratory:** URI, rhinitis, cough, pharyngitis, sinusitis. **Miscellaneous:** Rash, pruritus, fatigue, influenza, allergy, accidental trauma.

LABORATORY TEST CONSIDERATIONS
↑ Serum transaminases.

ADDITIONAL DRUG INTERACTIONS
Alcohol / ↑ Fluvastatin absorbed
Digoxin / ↓ Bioavailability of fluvastatin
Rifampin / ↓ Fluvastatin clearance

HOW SUPPLIED
Capsule: 20 mg, 40 mg; *Tablet, Extended-Release:* 80 mg

DOSAGE

- **CAPSULES, TABLETS**

Hypercholesterolemia and mixed dyslipidemia. Antihyperlipidemic to slow progression of coronary atherosclerosis.
For those requiring LDL cholesterol reduction to 25% or more, **Adults, initial:** 40 mg as one capsule or 80 mg as one tablet once daily in the evening. Or, 80 mg in divided doses or the 40 mg capsule b.i.d. For those requiring LDL cholesterol reduction to less than 25%, **Adults, initial:** 20 mg. **Dose range:** 20–80 mg/day.

NURSING CONSIDERATIONS

SEE ALSO *NURSING CONSIDERATIONS FOR ANTIHYPERLIPIDEMIC AGENTS—HMG-COA REDUCTASE INHIBITORS.*

ADMINISTRATION/STORAGE
1. Maximum reductions of LDL cholesterol are usually seen within 4 weeks; order periodic lipid determinations during this time, with dosage adjusted accordingly.
2. To avoid fluvastatin binding to a bile-acid binding resin (if given together), give the fluvastatin at bedtime and the resin at least 2 hr before.

ASSESSMENT
1. Review risk factors. Attempt to change/modify as many as possible. Note total cholesterol profile.

2. Monitor LFTs prior to starting treatment, 6-8 weeks into therapy, 3 mo later, then yearly if stable; 12 weeks after a dose increase.
3. Evaluate on a standard cholesterol-lowering diet before giving fluvastatin. Continue diet during treatment.

CLIENT/FAMILY TEACHING

1. May be taken with or without food but is usually consumed with the evening meal.
2. Drugs are used to lower blood cholesterol and fat levels, which have been proven to promote CAD.
3. Must continue risk factor reduction, dietary restrictions of saturated fat and cholesterol and regular exercise programs in addition to drug therapy in the overall goal of lowering cholesterol levels and CHD.
4. Report any muscle pain or weakness especially with fever or severe fatigue; keep scheduled lab visits.

OUTCOMES/EVALUATE

↓ Triglycerides, LDL, and total cholesterol levels

Fluvoxamine maleate

(flu-**VOX**-ah-meen)

PREGNANCY CATEGORY: C
CLASSIFICATION(S):
Antidepressant, selective serotonin reuptake inhibitor
Rx: Luvox
✱Rx: Alti-Fluvoxamine, Apo-Fluvoxamine, Gen-Fluvoxamine, Novo-Fluvoxamine, Nu-Fluvoxamine, PMS-Fluvoxamine

SEE ALSO *SELECTIVE SEROTONIN REUPTAKE INHIBITORS.*

ACTION/KINETICS

Maximum plasma levels: 3–8 hr. About 80% if bound to plasma proteins. **t½:** 13.6–15.6 hr. **Peak plasma concentration:** 88–546 ng/mL. **Time to reach steady state:** About 7 days. Elderly clients manifest higher mean plasma levels and a decreased clearance. Metabolized in the liver and excreted through the urine.

USES

Obsessive-compulsive disorder (as defined in DSM-III-R) for adults, adolescents, and children. *Investigational:* Treatment of depression, autism, panic disorder, social phobia, generalized anxiety disorder, post-traumatic stress disorder, premenstrual dysphoric disorder.

ADDITIONAL CONTRAINDICATIONS

Alcohol ingestion.

SPECIAL CONCERNS

Use with caution in clients with a history of mania, seizure disorders, and liver dysfunction and in those with diseases that could affect hemodynamic responses or metabolism.

SIDE EFFECTS

Side effects listed occur at an incidence of 0.1% or greater. **CNS:** Somnolence, insomnia, nervousness, dizziness, tremor, anxiety, hypertonia, agitation, decreased libido, depression, CNS stimulation, amnesia, apathy, hyperkinesia, hypokinesia, manic reaction, myoclonus, psychoses, fatigue, malaise, agoraphobia, akathisia, ataxia, ***convulsion,*** delirium, delusion, depersonalization, drug dependence, dyskinesia, dystonia, emotional lability, euphoria, extrapyramidal syndrome, unsteady gait, hallucinations, hemiplegia, hostility, hypersomnia, hypochondriasis, hypotonia, hysteria, incoordination, increased libido, neuralgia, paralysis, paranoia, phobia, sleep disorders, stupor, twitching, vertigo, activation of mania/hypomania, seizures. **GI:** Nausea, dry mouth, diarrhea, constipation, dyspepsia, anorexia, vomiting, flatulence, toothache, tooth caries, dysphagia, colitis, eructation, esophagitis, gastritis, gastroenteritis, ***GI hemorrhage,*** GI ulcer, gingivitis, glossitis, hemorrhoids, melena, rectal hemorrhage, stomatitis. **CV:** Palpitations, hypertension, postural hypotension, vasodilation, syncope, tachycardia, angina pectoris, bradycardia, ***cardiomyopathy,*** CV disease, cold extremities, conduction delay, ***heart failure, MI,*** pallor, irregular pulse, ST segment changes. **Respiratory:** URI, dyspnea, yawn, increased cough, sinusitis, asthma, bronchitis, epistaxis, hoarseness, hyperventilation. **Body as a whole:** Headache, asthenia, flu syndrome, chills, malaise, edema, weight gain or loss, dehydration, hypercholesterolemia, allergic reaction, neck pain, neck rigidity, photosensitivity, ***suicide attempt.*** **Dermatologic:** Excessive sweating, acne, alopecia, dry skin, eczema, exfoliative dermatitis, furunculosis, seborrhea, skin discoloration, urticaria. **Musculoskeletal:** Arthralgia, arthritis, bursitis, generalized muscle spasm, myasthenia, tendinous contracture, tenosynovitis. **GU:** Delayed ejaculation, urinary frequency, impotence, anorgasmia, urinary retention, anuria, breast pain, cystitis, delayed menstruation, dysuria, female lactation, hematuria, menopause, menorrhagia, metrorrhagia, nocturia, polyuria, PMS, urinary incontinence, UTI, urinary urgency, impaired urination, ***vaginal hemorrhage,*** vaginitis. **Hematologic:** Anemia, ecchymosis, leukocytosis, lymphadenopathy, thrombocytopenia. **Ophthalmic:** Amblyopia, abnormal accommodation, conjunctivitis, diplopia, dry eyes, eye pain, mydriasis, photophobia, visual field defect. **Otic:** Deafness, ear pain, otitis media. **Miscellaneous:** Taste perversion or loss, parosmia, hypothyroidism, hypercholesterolemia, dehydration.

OD OVERDOSE MANAGEMENT

Treatment: Establish an airway and maintain respiration as needed. Monitor VS and ECG. Activated charcoal may be as effective as emesis or lavage in removing the drug from the GI tract. Since absorption in overdose may be delayed, measures to reduce absorption may be required for up to 24 hr.

ADDITIONAL DRUG INTERACTIONS

Beta-adrenergic blockers / Possible ↑ effects on BP and HR
Buspirone / ↓ Buspirone effects
Carbamazepine / ↑ Risk of carbamazepine toxicity
Cloxapine / ↑ Risk of orthostatic hypotension and seizures
Diazepam / ↑ Diazepam effect R/T ↓ clearance
Diltiazem / ↑ Risk of bradycardia
Haloperidol / ↑ Serum haloperidol levels
Lithium / ↑ Risk of seizures
Melatonin / ↑ Plasma melatonin levels
Methadone / ↑ Risk of methadone toxicity
Mexiletine / ↓ Mexiletine clearance R/T ↓ metabolism
Midazolam / ↑ Midazolam effect R/T ↓ clearance
Sumatriptan / ↑ Risk of weakness, hyperreflexia, incoordination
Theophylline / ↑ Risk of theophylline toxicity (decrease dose by one-third the usual daily maintenance dose)
Thioridazine / ↑ Plasma thioridazine levels
Tolbutamide / ↓ Tolbutamide clearance R/T ↓ metabolism
Triazolam / ↑ Triazolam effect R/T ↓ clearance

HOW SUPPLIED

Tablet: 25 mg, 50 mg, 100 mg

DOSAGE

- **TABLETS**

Obsessive-compulsive disorder.

Adults, initial: 50 mg at bedtime; **then,** increase the dose in 50-mg increments q 4–7 days, as tolerated, until a maximum benefit is reached, not to exceed 300 mg/day. **Children and adolescents, 8 to 17 years:** 25 mg at bedtime; **then,** increase the dose in 25-mg increments q 4–7 days until a maximum benefit is reached, not to exceed 200 mg/day up to 11 years and 300 mg/day up to 17 years. The therapeutic effect may be reached in female children with lower doses.

NURSING CONSIDERATIONS

SEE ALSO NURSING CONSIDERATIONS FOR SELECTIVE SEROTONIN REUPTAKE INHIBITORS.

ADMINISTRATION/STORAGE

1. If total daily dose exceeds 100 mg for adults or 50 mg in children, give in two divided doses. If the doses are unequal, give the larger dose at bedtime.
2. Initial and incremental doses may need to be lower in geriatric clients.
3. Use lowest effective dose; assess periodically to determine need for continued treatment.
4. Use for more than 10 weeks has not been evaluated.

ASSESSMENT

1. Document indications for therapy and presenting or described behavioral manifestations.
2. List agents currently prescribed to ensure none interact unfavorably.
3. Note history of mania, seizure disorders, or liver dysfunction.
4. Monitor ECG, CBC, and liver and renal function studies.

CLIENT/FAMILY TEACHING

1. Take only as directed, usually at bedtime, do not exceed dosage. May initially experience N&V; should subside.
2. May cause dizziness and drowsiness. Do not perform activities that require mental or physical alertness until drug effects realized.
3. Report any rash, hives, or unusual itching; increased depression or suicide ideations
4. Avoid alcohol and any other drugs or herbals without approval.
5. Practice reliable birth control.
6. Report for scheduled appointments so response to therapy, dosage, and need for continued therapy can be determined.

OUTCOMES/EVALUATE

- Reduction in excessive, repetitive behaviors
- ↓ Depression

Folic acid

(**FOH**-lik **AH**-sid)

PREGNANCY CATEGORY: A
CLASSIFICATION(S):
Vitamin B complex
Rx: Folvite
✱Rx: Apo-Folic

ACTION/KINETICS

Folic acid (which is converted to tetrahydrofolic acid) is necessary for normal production of RBCs and for synthesis of nucleoproteins. Tetrahydrofolic acid is a cofactor in the biosynthesis of purines and thymidylates of nucleic acids. Megaloblastic and macrocytic anemias in folic acid deficiency are believed to be due to impairment of thymidylate synthesis. Natural sources of folic acid include liver, dried beans, peas, lentils, whole-wheat products, asparagus, beets, broccoli, brussels sprouts, spinach, and oranges. Synthetic folic acid is absorbed from the GI tract even if the client suffers from malabsorption syndrome. **Peak plasma levels after an oral dose:** 1 hr. It is stored in the liver.

USES

Treatment of megaloblastic anemias due to folic acid deficiency (e.g., tropical and nontropical sprue, pregnancy, infancy or childhood, nutritional causes). Diagnosis of folate deficiency.

CONTRAINDICATIONS

Use in aplastic, normocytic, or pernicious anemias (is ineffective). Folic acid injection that contains benzyl alcohol should not be used in neonates or immature infants.

SPECIAL CONCERNS

Daily folic acid doses of 0.1 mg or greater may obscure pernicious anemia. Prolonged folic acid therapy may cause decreased vitamin B_{12} levels.

SIDE EFFECTS

Allergic: Skin rash, itching, erythema, general malaise, respiratory difficulty due to bronchospasm. **GI:** Nausea, anorexia, abdominal distention, flatulence, bitter or bad taste (in those taking 15 mg/day for 1 month). **CNS:** In doses of 15 mg daily, altered sleep patterns, irritability, excitement, difficulty in concentration, overactivity, depression, impaired judgment, confusion.

DRUG INTERACTIONS

Aminosalicylic acid / ↓ Serum folate levels
Corticosteroids (chronic use) / ↑ Folic acid requirements
Methotrexate / Folic acid antagonist
Oral contraceptives / ↑ Risk of folate deficiency
Phenytoin / ↑ Seizure frequency; ↓ serum folic acid levels.
Pyrimethamine / ↓ Pyrimethamine effect in toxoplasmosis; also, a folic acid antagonist
Sulfonamides / ↓ Absorption of folic acid
Triamterene / ↓ Utilization of folic acid as it is a folic acid antagonist

Trimethoprim / ↓ Utilization of folic acid as it is a folic acid antagonist

HOW SUPPLIED

Injection: 5 mg/mL; *Tablet:* 0.4 mg, 0.8 mg, 1 mg

DOSAGE

• TABLETS

Dietary supplement.

Adults and children: 100 mcg/day (up to 1 mg in pregnancy); may be increased to 500–1,000 mcg if requirements increase.

Treatment of deficiency.

Adults, initial: 250–1,000 mcg/day until a hematologic response occurs; **maintenance:** 400 mcg/day (800 mcg during pregnancy and lactation). **Pediatric, initial:** 250–1,000 mcg/day until a hematologic response occurs. **Maintenance, infants:** 100 mcg/day; **children up to 4 years:** 300 mcg/day; **children 4 years and older:** 400 mcg/day.

• IM, IV, DEEP SC

Treatment of deficiency.

Adults and children: 250–1,000 mcg/day until a hematologic response occurs.

Diagnosis of folate deficiency.

Adults, IM: 100–200 mcg/day for 10 days plus low dietary folic acid and vitamin B_{12}.

NURSING CONSIDERATIONS

ADMINISTRATION/STORAGE

1. Given PO; if there is severe malabsorption, give either IV or SC.
2. Regardless of age, the dosage should never be less than 0.1 mg/day.
IV 3. Folic acid will remain stable in solution if the pH is kept above 5.
4. May be administered IM, by direct IV push or added to infusions. When given IV, the rate should not exceed 5 mcg/min.
5. When parenteral forms are used, have drugs and equipment available to treat anaphylactic reactions.

ASSESSMENT

1. Document baseline CBC, reticulocytes, MCV, and serum folate and B_{12} levels. Assess for pernicious anemia with Shilling test and serum B_{12}level first to prevent permanent neurologic damage.
2. Review drugs prescribed; oral contraceptives, trimethoprim, hydantoins, and alcohol may cause increased body loss of folic acid.

CLIENT/FAMILY TEACHING

1. Take only as directed.
2. Dietary sources of folic acid include dark green leafy vegetables, beans, fortified breads, and cereals. Prolonged cooking destroys folate in vegetables.
3. Drug may discolor urine a deep yellow.
4. U.S. Public Health Service recommends that all women of childbearing age consume 0.4 mg of folic acid to reduce the risk of neural tube birth defects. Folic acid may prevent the development of spina bifida or anencephaly, which occur during the first month of pregnancy.

OUTCOMES/EVALUATE

• Desired hematologic response (↑ retic count in 5 days)
• Reversal in symptoms of folic acid deficiency and megaloblastic anemia
• Prophylaxis of newborn neural tube defects

Follitropin alfa

(fol-ih-**TROH**-pin **AL**-fah)

PREGNANCY CATEGORY: X
Rx: Gonal-F, Gonal-F Multi-Dose

Follitropin beta

(fol-ih-**TROH**-pin **BAY**-tah)

PREGNANCY CATEGORY: X
Rx: Follistim
✱**Rx:** Puregon
CLASSIFICATION(S):
Ovarian stimulant, gonadotropin

ACTION/KINETICS

Both products are human FSH prepared by recombinant DNA technology. When given with HCG, products stimulate ovarian follicular growth in women who do not have primary ovarian failure. Steady state plasma levels reached within 4 to 5 days. Increased body weight or body mass index (BMI) results in a decrease in rate of absorption. Increased risk of multiple births.

USES

(1) Induction of ovulation and pregnancy in anovulatory infertile clients where cause of infertility is functional. (2) Stimulate development of multiple follicles in ovulatory clients undergoing in-vitro fertilization. (3) Induce spermatogenesis in men with primary and secondary hypogonadotropic hypogonadism where failure is not due to primary testicular failure (use Gonal-F).

CONTRAINDICATIONS

Use in primary ovarian failure; uncontrolled thyroid or adrenal dysfunction; in presence of any cause of infertility other than anovulation; tumor of ovary, breast, uterus, hypothalamus, or pituitary gland; abnormal vaginal bleeding of undetermined origin; ovarian cysts or enlargement not due to polycystic ovary syndrome; pregnancy; use in children; hypersensitivity to products.

SPECIAL CONCERNS

Use with caution during lactation.

SIDE EFFECTS

CV: Intravascular thrombosis and embolism causing venous thrombophlebitis, ***pulmonary embolism,*** pulmonary infarction, stroke, arterial occlusion (leading to loss of limb). **Pulmonary:** Atelectasis, ARDS, exacerbation of asthma. **Ovarian hyperstimulation syndrome:** Ovarian enlargement, abdominal pain/distention, N&V, diarrhea, dyspnea, oliguria, ascites, pleural effusion, hypovolemia, electrolyte imbalance, hemoperitoneum, thromboembolic events. **Hypersensitivity:** Febrile reaction, chills, musculoskeletal aches, joint pains, malaise, headache, fatigue. **GI:** N&V, diarrhea, abdominal cramps, bloating. **Dermatologic:** Dry skin, body rash, hair loss, hives. **Miscellaneous:** Ovarian cysts, pain, swelling, headache, irritation at site of injection, breast tenderness.

HOW SUPPLIED

Follitropin alfa: *Powder for injection:* 37.5 IU, 75 IU, 150 IU. **Follitropin beta:** *Powder for injection:* 75 IU

DOSAGE

FOLLITROPIN ALFA

- **SC ONLY**

Ovulation induction.

Initial, first cycle: 75 IU/day. An incremental adjustment up to 37.5 IU may be considered after 14 days; further increases can be made, if needed, every 7 days. To complete follicular development and effect ovulation in absence of an endogenous LH surge, give 5,000 units of HCG 1 day after last dose of follitropin alfa. Withold HCG if serum estradiol is greater than 2,000 pg/mL. Base initial dose in subsequent cycles on response in the preceding cycle. Doses greater than 300 IU/day are not recommended routinely. As in initial cycle, HCG at a dose of 5,000 is given 1 day after last dose of follitropin alfa.

Follicle stimulation.

Initiate on day 2 or 3 of the follicular phase at a dose of 150 IU/day, until sufficient follicular development is achieved. Usually, therapy does not exceed 10 days. In those undergoing in vitro fertilization whose endogenous gonadotropin levels are suppressed, initiate follitropin alfa at a dose of 225 IU/day. Consider dosage adjustments after 5 days based on client response; adjust subsequent dosage every 3 to 4 days and by less than 75 to 150 IU additional drug at each adjustment, not to exceed 450 IU/day. Once follicular development is achieved, give HCG, 5,000–10,000 units, to cause final follicular maturation in preparation for oocyte retrieval.

FOLLITROPIN BETA

- **SC, IM**

Ovulation induction.

Use stepwise, gradually increasing dosage regimen. **Initial:** 75 IU/day for up to 14 days; increase by 37.5 IU at weekly intervals until follicular growth or serum estradiol levels indicate response. Maximum daily dose: 300 IU. Treat until ultrasonic visualization or serum estradiol levels indicate preovulatory conditions greater than or equal to normal values. Then, give HCG 5,000–10,000 IU.

Follicle stimulation.

Initial: 150–225 IU for first 4 days of treatment. Dose may be adjusted based on ovarian response. Daily maintenance doses from 75–300 IU (however, doses from 375–600 IU have been used) for 6 to 12 days are usually sufficient. Maximum daily dose: 600 IU. When sufficient number of follicles of adequate size are present, induce final maturation by giving HCG, 5,000–10,000 IU. Oocyte retrieval is undertaken 34–36 hr later.

NURSING CONSIDERATIONS

ADMINISTRATION/STORAGE

1. For follitropin alfa or follitropin beta:
• Store vials in refrigerator or at room temperature and protect from light.
• Use immediately after reconstitution; discard unused drug.
2. For follitropin alfa, dissolve powder from one or more vials in 0.5–1 mL of sterile water for injection. Concentration should not exceed 225 IU/0.5 mL.
3. For follitropin beta, inject 1 mL of 0.45% NaCl injection into the vial. Do not shake but gently swirl until the solution is clear. It usually dissolves immediately.
4. When using either drug, if ovaries are abnormally enlarged on last day of therapy, withhold HCG to reduce risk of ovarian hyperstimulation syndrome.
5. Gonal-F Multi-Dose is used to make several days worth of the formulation at one time. The new formulation is injected more comfortably and quickly due to decreased volume of doses.

ASSESSMENT

1. Document history and PE, including gynecologic (hysterosalpingogram) and endocrine evaluation, and indications for therapy.
2. Obtain serum hormonal levels, gonadotropin levels, pregnancy test, CBC, lytes, thyroid and adrenal function studies; document neurovascular assessments and peripheral pulses.
3. Determine partner's fertility potential.

INTERVENTIONS

1. Obtain urinary estrogen excretion levels daily. If greater than 100 mcg or if daily estriol excretion exceeds 50 mcg, *withhold HCG* and report; these signal impending hyperstimulation syndrome.
2. If hospitalized for hyperstimulation, perform the following:
• Place client on bed rest.
• Monitor I&O; weigh daily.
• Monitor urine sp. gravity, serum and urine lytes.
• Assess for hemoconcentration. May need heparin to prevent hypercoagulability.
• Increase fluid intake; replace lytes.
• Provide analgesics for comfort.
3. Monitor for respiratory distress or exacerbation of asthma.
4. Report any unexplained fever, ovarian enlargement, or complaints of abdominal pain.

CLIENT/FAMILY TEACHING

1. Dose is individualized. Alfa is given SC in the abdomen or upper thigh at 45° angle; beta is given SC or IM with IM administered in upper outer buttocks muscle at 90° angle.
2. Report any pain, coolness, or pale bluish color of an extremity (signs of arterial bloodclot).
3. Fever or development of lower abdominal pain may be result of overstimulation of ovaries that has caused cysts to form, loss of fluid into peritoneum, or bleeding; report immediately. Need exam for this at least every other day during drug therapy and for 2 weeks thereafter; hospitalize if evident.
4. Record temperatures.
5. Signs that indicate ovulation include increase in basal body temperature, and increase in appearance and volume of cervical mucus.
6. Engage in daily intercourse from day before HCG is administered until ovulation occurs.

7. If symptoms indicate overstimulation of ovaries, significant ovarian enlargement may have occurred. Report and abstain from intercourse; ↑ risk of ovarian cyst rupture.
8. Ultrasound is used to monitor for follicular maturization and serum estradiol levels.
9. Pregnancy usually occurs 4–6 weeks after completion of therapy. Multiple births may occur.

OUTCOMES/EVALUATE

Induction of ovulation; pregnancy

Fomivirsen sodium

(**foh**-mah-**VEER**-sin)

PREGNANCY CATEGORY: C
CLASSIFICATION(S):
Antiviral
Rx: Vitravene

SEE ALSO *ANTIVIRAL DRUGS.*

ACTION/KINETICS

A phosphorothioate oligonucleotide that inhibits cytomegalovirus (CMV) replication through an antisense mechanism. Binding of fomivirsen to the target mRNA causes inhibition of IE2 protein synthesis, thus inhibiting replication. CMV isolates that are resistant to fomivirsen may be sensitive to ganciclovir, foscarnet, or cidofovir. Levels of fomivirsen are highest in the retina and iris.

USES

Local treatment of CMV retinitis in AIDS clients who are intolerant of or have a contraindiction to other treatments of CMV retinitis, or who did not respond to other treatments.

CONTRAINDICATIONS

Use in those who have been treated with either IV or ophthalmic cidofovir in the past 2– 4–weeks, due to the risk of exaggerated ocular inflammation. Lactation.

SPECIAL CONCERNS

For ophthalmic (intravitreal injection) use only; does not provide treatment for systemic CMV disease. Safety and efficacy have not been determined in children.

SIDE EFFECTS

Ophthalmic: Ocular inflammation, including iritis and vitritis; abnormal vision, anterior chamber inflammation, blurred vision, cataract, conjunctival hemorrhage, decreased visual acuity, desaturation of color vision, eye pain, floaters, increased IOP, photophobia, retinal detachment, retinal edema, retinal hemorrhage, retinal pigment changes, application site reaction, conjunctival hyperemia, conjunctivitis, corneal edema, decreased peripheral vision, eye irritation, hypotony, keratic precipitates, optic neuritis, photopsia, retinal vascular disease, visual field defect, vitreous hemorrhage, vitreous opacity.

• **SYSTEMIC.**

GI: Abdominal pain, diarrhea, nausea, vomiting, abnormal liver function, anorexia, oral monilia, pancreatitis. **CNS:** Headache, abnormal thinking, depression, dizziness. **Respiratory:** Pneumonia, sinusitis, bronchitis, dyspnea, increased cough. **Hematologic:** Anemia, neutropenia, thrombocytopenia. **Whole body:** Asthenia, fever, infection, rash, ***sepsis,*** systemic CMV, allergic reactions, cachexia, decreased weight, dehydration, flu syndrome, lymphoma-like reaction, neuropathy, pain, sweating. **Miscellaneous:** Back pain, catheter infection, chest pain, kidney failure.

HOW SUPPLIED

Injection (as sodium): 6.6 mg/mL

DOSAGE

• **OPHTHALMIC INJECTION**

Treat ophthalmic CMV.

Induction dose: 330 mcg (0.05 mL) as a single intravitreal injection every other week for 2 doses; **maintenance:** 330 mcg (0.05 mL) once q 4 weeks.

NURSING CONSIDERATIONS

SEE ALSO *NURSING CONSIDERATIONS FOR ANTIVIRAL DRUGS.*

ADMINISTRATION/STORAGE

1. If inflammation of the face becomes unacceptable but the CMV retinitis is controlled, attempt interrupting therapy until inflammation decreases.

2. Prior to the injection, use a topical or local anesthetic and antimicrobial therapy.
3. For administration, use the following steps: using a 30–gauge needle on a low–volume (e.g., tuberculin) syringe.
• Attach a 5 micron filter needle to the injection syringe for solution withdrawal (to guard against introduction of stopper particulate); withdraw about 0.15 mL through the filter needle.
• Remove filter needle and attach a 30–gauge needle to drug syringe.
• Stabilize globe with cotton tip applicator and insert needle fully through an area 3.5 to 4 mm posterior to the lumbus (avoid horizontal meridian) aiming toward the center of the globe. Keep fingers off plunger until the needle has been completely inserted.
• Deliver 0.05 mL by slow injection. Roll cotton tip applicator over injection site as needle is withdrawn to reduce loss of eye fluid.
4. Store between 2–25°C (35–77°F). Protect from excessive heat and light.

ASSESSMENT

1. Note onset and duration of symptoms, and other therapies trialed/failed. If Cidofovir (IV or optic) used, determine last exposure.
2. Assess for systemic CMV infections (i.e., pneumonitis, colitis) as well as CMV infection in the other eye, if only one being treated.

CLIENT/FAMILY TEACHING

1. Drug is not a cure but controls symptoms; must be continued indefinitely.
2. Report as scheduled for injections and eye exams. Drug is administered by intravitreal injection into the infected eye after a local anesthetic is applied. Induction involves one injection every other week for two doses and then maintenance doses are administered every four weeks into the eye.
3. Irritation and inflammation may occur and is usually managed with topical corticosteroids. Once resolved, may resume intravitreal injections.
4. May require additional drugs to manage increased IOP which is measured at each visit and is usually transient.
5. Do not perform activities that require clear vision until effects realized; may cause blurring or decreased acuity.

OUTCOMES/EVALUATE

Treatment of CMV retinitis

Fondaparinux sodium

(**fon**-dah-**PAIR**-in-uks)

PREGNANCY CATEGORY: B
CLASSIFICATION(S):
Anticoagulant, antithrombin
Rx: Arixtra

ACTION/KINETICS

Antithrombotic action is due to antithrombin III (ATIII)-mediated selective inhibition of Factor Xa. By selectively binding to ATIII, fondaparinux potentiates the innate neutralization of Factor Xa by ATIII. Neutralization of Factor Xa interrupts the blood coagulation cascade and thus inhibits thrombin formation and thrombus development. Does not inactivate thrombin (activated Factor II), has no known effect on platelet function, and does not affect fibrinolytic activity or bleeding time. Rapidly and completely absorbed following SC administration. **Maximum levels:** 2 hr. Does not significantly bind to plasma proteins or RBCs. Excreted unchanged in the urine. **t½, elimination:** 17–21 hr. Elimination is prolonged in the elderly, in those with renal impairment, and in those weighing less than 50 kg. Anticoagulant effect may last for 2–4 days after discontinuation in clients with normal renal function and even longer in those with renal impairment.

USES

Prophylaxis of deep vein thrombosis in clients undergoing hip fracture surgery, hip replacement surgery, or knee replacement surgery.

CONTRAINDICATIONS

IM use. In those with severe renal impairment (C_{CR} <30 mL/min) or with body weight <50 kg (due to increased risk for major bleeding episodes). In those with active major bleeding, bacterial endocarditis, thrombocytopenia associated with a positive *in vitro* test for antiplatelet antibody in the presence of fondaparinux, or with known sensitivitiy to fondaparinux.

SPECIAL CONCERNS

The risk of hemorrhage increases with increasing renal impairment. Use with caution during lactation, in moderate renal impairment (C_{CR} 30–50 mL/min), in the elderly, in those with a history of heparin-induced thrombocytopenia, in those with a bleeding diathesis, uncontrolled arterial hypertension, history of recent GI ulceration, diabetic retinopathy, and hemorrhage. Use with extreme caution in conditions with increased risk of hemorrhage, including congenital or acquired bleeding disorders, active ulcerative and angiodysplastic GI disease, hemorrhagic stroke, in those treated concomitantly with platelet inhibitors, or shortly after brain, spinal, or ophthalmologic surgery. There is an increased risk of developing epidural or spinal hematoma which can cause long-term or permanent paralysis (risk is increased by use of indwelling epidural catheters for analgesia administration; by concomitant use of drugs such as NSAIDs, platelet inhibitors, or other anticoagulants; or, by traumatic or repeated epidural or spinal puncture). Safety and efficacy have not been determined in children.

SIDE EFFECTS

Bleeding.

The most common side effect is ***bleeding complications*** which include intracranial, cerebral, retroperitoneal, intra-ocular, pericardial, or spinal bleeding, bleeding in the adrenal gland, or reoperation due to bleeding. **CV:** Edema, hypotension, post-operative hemorrhage. **GI:** N&V, constipation, diarrhea, dyspepsia. **CNS:** Insomnia, dizziness, confusion, headache. **GU:** UTI, urinary retention. **Dermatologic:** Hematoma, purpura, rash, bullous eruption. **Miscellaneous:** Thrombocytopenia; injection site bleeding, rash, pruritus; anemia, fever, increased wound drainage, pain.

LABORATORY TEST CONSIDERATIONS

↑ AST, ALT. Hypokalemia.

HOW SUPPLIED

Injection: 2.5 mg/0.5 mL

DOSAGE

• **SC**

Hip fracture, hip or knee replacement surgery.

Adults, initial: 2.5 mg given 6–8 hr after surgery. **Duration:** Give 2.5 mg once daily for 5–9 days (up to 11 days has been tolerated).

NURSING CONSIDERATIONS

ADMINISTRATION/STORAGE

1. Is provided in a single dose, prefilled syringe affixed with an automatic needle protection system.
2. Can not be used interchangeably (unit for unit) with heparin, low molecular weight heparins, or heparinoids as they differ in the manufacturing process, anti-Xa and anti-IIa activity, units, and dosage.
3. To avoid loss of drug when using the prefilled syringe, do not expel the air bubble from the syringe before injection.
4. Do not mix with other injections or infusions.
5. Give in the fatty tissue, alternating injection sites (i.e., between the left and right anterolateral or the left and right posterolateral abdominal wall).
6. Store between 15–30°C (59–86°F). Keep out of the reach of children.

ASSESSMENT

1. Note condition(s) requiring therapy, onset, and estimated duration of therapy.
2. Assess for any conditions that may affect therapy (i.e age, weight, history of GI ulcerations, diabetic retinopathy, uncontrolled HTN, bleeding diathesis/disorders, hemorrhage, or heparin induced thrombocytopenia).
3. Monitor all sites, incisions, and orifices for bleeding. Assess mobility and adherence to exercise program.
4. Assess carefully for S&S of neurological impairment; anticoagulated clients undergoing epidural/spinal anesthesia may sustain a spinal/epidural hematoma which could result in paralysis.

5. Monitor CBC, INR, K+, renal and LFTs.

CLIENT/FAMILY TEACHING

1. Drug is used to prevent the formation of blood clots in those extremities that have compromised functioning due to a surgical procedure. Clots may get into the circulation and be transported to the lung causing a pulmonary embolus which can be lethal.
2. Review guidelines for the appropriate method of administration and demonstrate for provider. Start with proper skin prep, pinching and holding a fold of skin for the injection, injecting the solution, removing the syringe, and discarding into a designated container. The syringe has a retractable needle so that punctures can be prevented.
3. Store prefilled syringes and used syringes safely out of reach.
4. Report any adverse side effects as well as extremity pain, chest pain, SOB, or any other unusal symptoms.
5. Keep all F/U visits to evaluate incision site, response to therapy, recovery, and labs.

OUTCOMES/EVALUATE

DVT prevention in those undergoing hip fx repair or hip/knee replacements

Formoterol fumarate

(for-**MOH**-tur-all)

PREGNANCY CATEGORY: C
CLASSIFICATION(S):
Sympathomimetic, direct-acting
Rx: Foradil Aerolizer

SEE ALSO *SYMPATHOMIMETICS.*

ACTION/KINETICS

Long-acting selective $beta_2$-agonist. Acts locally in the lung as a bronchodilator. Acts in part by increasing cyclic AMP levels causing relaxation of bronchial smooth muscle and inhibition of release of mediators of immediate hypersensitivity, especially from mast cells. When inhaled, is rapidly absorbed into the plasma reaching maximum plasma levels within 5 min. From 61–64% bound to plasma proteins. Metabolized in the liver to inactive metabolites. Excreted in the urine and feces. **t½, terminal:** 10 hr.

USES

(1) Long-term maintenance treatment of asthma and to prevent bronchospasms in adults and children 5 years of age and older who have reversible obstructive airway disease, including nocturnal asthma, who require regular treatment with inhaled, short-acting, $beta_2$ agonists. (2) Acute prevention of exercise-induced bronchospasm in adults and children 12 years of age and older. Used on an occasional, as needed, basis. (3) Long-term use in the maintenance treatment of bronchoconstriction in those with COPD, including chronic bronchitis and emphysema.

CONTRAINDICATIONS

Use for those whose asthma can be controlled by occasional use of inhaled, short-acting, $beta_2$ agonists. Use to treat acute symptoms of asthma.

SPECIAL CONCERNS

May cause life-threatening, paradoxical bronchospasms. Use with extreme caution in clients treated with MAO inhibitors, tricyclic antidepressants, or drugs known to prolong the QTc interval (effect of adrenergic agonists may be prolonged). Use with caution during the co-administration of beta-agonists with nonpotassium sparing diuretics (loop or thiazide diuretics) since ECG changes and/or hypokalemia can be acutely worsened by beta-agonists. Use with caution in CV disorders (especially coronary insufficiency, cardiac arrhythmias, and hypertension), in convulsive disorders, in thyrotoxicosis, in those unusually responsive to sympathomimetics, and during lactation.

SIDE EFFECTS

See also *Sympathomimetics.*

CV: Increased pulse rate and BP, ECG changes (e.g., flattening of T wave, prolongation of QTc interval, and ST segment depression). **Body as a whole:** Immediate hypersensitivitiy reactions, including severe hypotension, ***anaphylaxis,*** and angioedema. Viral infection, fever, trauma. **Respiratory:** Worsening of asthma, bronchitis, chest infection, dyspnea, chest pain, tonsilitis, URTI, pharyngitis, sinusitis, increased sputum. **CNS:** Dizziness, insomnia, anxiety. **Musculoskeletal:** Back pain, leg/muscle cramps. **Miscellaneous:** Tremor, rash, dysphonia, pruritis, dry mouth.

LABORATORY TEST CONSIDERATIONS

Hypokalemia (transient and usually does not require supplementation).

HOW SUPPLIED

Capsules for use in Aerolizer: 12 mcg.

DOSAGE

• **CAPSULES FOR USE IN AEROLIZER**

Maintenance treatment of asthma.

Adults and children over 5 years: Inhale contents of one 12 mcg-capsule q 12 hr using the Aerolizer inhaler. Do not exceed 24 mcg/day.

Prevention of exercise-induced bronchospasm.

Adults and adolescents 12 years and older: Inhale contents of one 12 mcg-capsule at least 15 min before exercise. Give on an occasional, as needed, basis.

Maintenance treatment of COPD.

Inhale contents of one 12 mcg-capsule q 12 hr using the Aerolizer inhaler. Do not exceed 24 mcg/day.

NURSING CONSIDERATIONS

SEE ALSO *NURSING CONSIDERATIONS FOR SYMPATHOMIMETICS.*

ADMINISTRATION/STORAGE

1. Use only with the Aerolizer, do not take orally.
2. Can be used together with short-acting $beta_2$-agonists, inhaled or systemic corticosteroids, and theophylline.
3. If symptoms of asthma arise between doses, an inhaled short-acting, $beta_2$-agonist may be used for immediate relief.
4. If a previously used dose for asthma or COPD does not result in the usual response, seek medical advice immediately as this is often a sign of deteriorating asthma or COPD. Re-evaluate the therapeutic regimen and consider additional options such as systemic corticosteroids.
5. Clients taking formoterol in twice-daily doses for asthma should not take additional doses for exercise-induced bronchospasms.
6. A satisfactory response to formoterol does not eliminate the need for continued treatment with an anti-inflammatory drug.
7. Do not start formoterol therapy in clients with significantly worsening or acutely deteriorating asthma, which may be a life-threatening condition.
8. Formoterol is not a substitute for inhaled corticosteroids.
9. When starting formoterol therapy, instruct clients who have been taking inhaled, short-acting $beta_2$-agonists on a regular basis (q.i.d.) to discontinue the regular use of these drugs and use them only for symptomatic relief of acute asthma symptoms.
10. Store at 20–25°C (36–46°F).

ASSESSMENT

1. Note indications for therapy, symptom characteristics, and other agents trialed.
2. Assess for CAD, seizures, and HTN.
3. Monitor VS, electrolytes, PFTs, and lung sounds.

CLIENT/FAMILY TEACHING

1. Use only as directed, do not take orally. Demonstrate appropriate method for administration and storage. Review *Patient Instructions for Use.*
2. Use the capsules only with the Aerolizer inhaler provided. Do not use Aerolizer with any other capsules. Do not exceed dosage of 2 capsules per day.
3. Always store capsules in the blister package and remove from the blister immediately before use.
4. If symptoms of asthma arise between doses, an inhaled short-acting, $beta_2$-agonist may be used for immediate relief.
5. If a previously used dose for asthma or COPD does not result in the usual response, seek medical advice immediately as this is often a sign of deteriorating asthma or COPD. Use incentive spirometer to monitor breathing status. Not for use with marked re-

duction in spirometry readings or acute worsening of asthma condition.
6. Clients taking formoterol in twice-daily doses for asthma should not take additional doses for exercise-induced bronchospasms.
7. With exercise-induced asthma, use 15 min before exercise.
8. Do not expose capsules to moisture, handle with dry hands. Do not wet or wash the Aerolizer inhaler, keep dry. Always use the new aerolizer with each refill.
9. Do not use Aerolizer with a spacer and never exhale into the Aerolizer.
10. Store capsules as directed and only pierce once. If gelatin capsule breaks, the screen in the Aerolizer should retain it. Be aware that it may escape into the mouth or throat after inhalation.
11. Practice reliable contraception, report if pregnancy suspected.
12. Report any unusual side effects, loss of control of breathing patterns or intolerance to therapy. Keep F/U appointments to evaluate drug effects and prevent deterioration of lung function.

OUTCOMES/EVALUATE

Improved breathing patterns, ↓ bronchospasms

Foscarnet sodium

(fos-**KAR**-net)

PREGNANCY CATEGORY: C
CLASSIFICATION(S):
Antiviral
Rx: Foscavir

SEE ALSO *ANTIVIRAL AGENTS*.

ACTION/KINETICS

Inhibits replication of all known herpes viruses by selective inhibition at the pyrophosphate binding site on virus-specific DNA polymerases and reverse transcriptases at levels that do not affect cellular DNA polymerases. Active against herpes simplex virus mutants deficient in thymidine kinase. CMV strains resistant to ganciclovir may be sensitive to foscarnet; viral reactivation of CMV occurs after termination of foscarnet therapy. The latent state of any of the human herpes viruses is not sensitive to foscarnet. Believed to accumulate in human bone and has variable penetration into the CSF. **t½, plasma:** About 3 hr. Approximately 80%–90% of IV foscarnet is excreted unchanged through the urine.

USES

Treatment of CMV retinitis in clients with AIDS. Treatment of acyclovir-resistant HSV infections in immunocompromised clients. With ganciclorvir in those who have relapsed after monotherapy with either drug.

SPECIAL CONCERNS

Use with caution during lactation and in clients with impaired renal function (the effects of the drug have not been determined in clients with a C_{CR} < 50 mL/min or serum creatinine > 2.8 mg/dL). Use with caution with drugs that alter serum calcium levels as foscarnet decreases serum levels of ionized calcium. Safety and effectiveness have not been determined in children, for the treatment of other CMV infections such as pneumonitis or gastroenteritis, for congenital or neonatal CMV disease, and in nonimmunocompromised clients. Transient changes in electrolytes may increase the risk of cardiac disturbances and seizures. Side effects such as renal impairment, electrolyte abnormalities, and seizures may contribute to client death. The drug is not a cure for HSV infections and relapse occurs in most clients. Repeated treatment has led to the development of viral resistance.

SIDE EFFECTS

GU: Renal impairment (most common), albuminuria, dysuria, polyuria, urinary retention, urethral disorder, UTIs, ***acute renal failure,*** nocturia, hematuria, glomerulonephritis, urinary frequency, toxic nephropathy, nephrosis, urinary incontinence, pyelonephritis, renal tubular disorders, urethral irritation, uremia, perineal pain in women, penile inflammation.

F

Metabolic/Electrolyte: Hypocalcemia, hypokalemia, hypomagnesemia, hypophosphatemia, hyponatremia, hyperphosphatemia, hypercalcemia, acidosis, thirst, decreased weight, dehydration, glycosuria, diabetes mellitus, abnormal glucose tolerance, hypochloremia, hypervolemia, hypoproteinemia. **Hematologic:** Anemia (one-third of clients), granulocytopenia, neutropenia, leukopenia, thrombocytopenia, platelet abnormalities, thrombosis, WBC abnormalities, lymphadenopathy, coagulation disorders, decreased coagulation factors, decreased prothrombin, hypochromic anemia, pancytopenia, hemolysis, leukocytosis, cervical lymphadenopathy, lymphopenia. **Body as a whole:** Fever, fatigue, asthenia, pain, infection, rigors, malaise, sepsis, death, back or chest pain, cachexia, flu-like symptoms, edema, bacterial or fungal infections, abscess, moniliasis, leg edema, peripheral edema, hypothermia, syncope, substernal chest pain, ascites, ***malignant hyperpyrexia,*** herpes simplex, viral infections, toxoplasmosis. **CNS:** Headache, dizziness, ***seizures (including tonic-clonic),*** tremor, ataxia, dementia, stupor, meningitis, aphasia, abnormal coordination, EEG abnormalities, vertigo, coma, encephalopathy, dyskinesia, extrapyramidal disorders, hemiparesis, paraplegia, speech disorders, tetany, cerebral edema, depression, confusion, anxiety, insomnia, somnolence, amnesia, aggressive reaction, nervousness, agitation, hallucinations, impaired concentration, emotional lability, psychosis, ***suicide attempt,*** delirium, sleep disorders, personality disorders. **Peripheral nervous system:** Hypesthesia, neuropathy, sensory disturbances, generalized spasms, abnormal gait, hyperesthesia, hypertonia, hyperkinesia, vocal cord paralysis, hyporeflexia, hyperreflexia, neuralgia, neuritis, peripheral neuropathy. **Musculoskeletal:** Arthralgia, myalgia, involuntary muscle contractions, leg cramps, arthrosis, synovitis, torticollis. **GI:** N&V, diarrhea, anorexia, abdominal pain, dry mouth, dysphagia, dyspepsia, rectal hemorrhage, constipation, melena, flatulence, pancreatitis, ulcerative stomatitis, enteritis, glossitis, enterocolitis, proctitis, stomatitis, tenesmus, pseudomembranous colitis, gastroenteritis, oral leukoplakia, oral hemorrhage, rectal disorders, colitis, duodenal ulcer, hematemesis, paralytic ileus, ulcerative proctitis, tongue ulceration, esophageal ulceration. **Hepatic:** Abnormal hepatic function, cholecystitis, cholelithiasis, hepatitis, hepatosplenomegaly, cholestatic hepatitis, jaundice. **CV:** Hypertension, palpitations, sinus tachycardia, first degree AV block, nonspecific ST-T segment changes, hypotension, flushing, cerebrovascular disorder, ***cardiomyopathy, cardiac failure, cardiac arrest,*** bradycardia, arrhythmias, extrasystole, atrial fibrillation, phlebitis, superficial thrombophlebitis of arm, mesenteric vein thrombophlebitis. **Respiratory:** Cough, dyspnea, pneumonia, sinusitis, rhinitis, pharyngitis, respiratory insufficiency, pulmonary infiltration, ***pulmonary embolism,*** pneumothorax, hemoptysis, stridor, bronchospasm, laryngitis, bronchitis, respiratory depression, pleural effusion, ***pulmonary hemorrhage,*** pneumonitis. **Ophthalmic:** Visual field defects, nystagmus, periorbital edema, eye pain, conjunctivitis, diplopia, blindness, retinal detachment, mydriasis, photophobia. **Ear:** Deafness, earache, tinnitus, otitis. **Dermatologic:** Increased sweating, rash, skin ulceration, pruritus, seborrhea, erythematous rash, maculopapular rash, facial edema, skin discoloration, acne, alopecia, dermatitis, anal pruritus, genital pruritus, aggravated psoriasis, psoriaform rash, skin disorders, dry skin, urticaria, skin hypertrophy, verruca. **Miscellaneous:** Epistaxis, taste perversions, pain or inflammation at injection site, lymphoma-like disorder, sarcoma, ***malignant lymphoma,*** ADH disorders, decreased gonadotropins, gynecomastia.

LABORATORY TEST CONSIDERATIONS

↑ Alkaline phosphatase, AST, ALT, LDH, BUN, CPK, serum creatinine. ↓ C_{CR}. Abnormal X-ray. Abnormal A-G ratio.

OD OVERDOSE MANAGEMENT

Symptoms: Extensions of the preceding side effects. Of most concern are development of ***seizures,*** renal function impairment, paresthesias in limbs or periorally, and electrolyte disturbances especially involving calcium and phosphate. *Treatment:* Monitor the client for S&S of electrolyte imbalance and renal impairment. Symptomatic treatment. Hemodialysis and hydration may be of some benefit.

DRUG INTERACTIONS

Aminoglycosides / ↓ Elimination of foscarnet → ↑ risk of renal impairment
Amphotericin B / ↓ Elimination of foscarnet → ↑ risk of renal impairment
AZT / ↑ Risk of anemia
Didanosine / ↓ Elimination of foscarnet → ↑ risk of renal impairment
Pentamidine, IV / ↓ Elimination of foscarnet → ↑ risk of renal impairment; also, pentamidine causes hypocalcemia

HOW SUPPLIED

Injection: 24 mg/mL

DOSAGE

- **IV INFUSION**

CMV retinitis in AIDS.

Individualized, initial, normal renal function: Either 60 mg/kg over a minimum of 1 hr q 8 hr or 90 mg/kg q 12 hr for 2–3 weeks, depending on the response. **Maintenance:** 90–120 mg/kg/day (depending on renal function) given as an IV infusion over 2 hr. Start most clients on the 90-mg/kg/day dose; however, consider increasing the dose to 120 mg/kg/day due to progression of retinitis.

Acyclovir-resistant HSV infections in immunocompromised clients.

Initial: 40 mg/kg for clients with normal renal function given IV at a constant rate over a minimum of 1 hr q 8 or 12 hr for 2 to 3 weeks or until lesions are healed. **Maintenance:** See dose for CMV retinitis.

NURSING CONSIDERATIONS

ADMINISTRATION/STORAGE

IV 1. To avoid local irritation, infuse only into veins with adequate blood flow to allow rapid dilution and distribution.

2. The rate of infusion must be no more than 1 mg/kg/min using controlled IV infusion either by a central venous line or a peripheral vein. Do not give by rapid or bolus IV injection.

3. If using a central venous catheter for infusion, the standard 24-mg/mL solution may be used without dilution. However, if a peripheral vein catheter is used, dilute the 24-mg/mL solution to 12 mg/mL with D5W or NSS to avoid vein irritation. Use diluted solutions within 24 hr of first entry into sealed bottle.

4. To minimize potential for renal impairment, hydrate during drug administration; establish and maintain diuresis.

5. Adjust dose in renal impairment; use dosing guide.

6. Do not give any other drug or supplement through the same catheter. Foscarnet is incompatible with 30% dextrose, amphotericin B, and calcium-containing solutions (e.g., RL and TPN). Other incompatibilities include acyclovir sodium, diazepam, digoxin, diphenhydramine, dobutamine, droperidol, ganciclovir, gentamicin, haloperidol, isoethionate, leucovorin, midazolam, morphine sulfate, pentamidine, phenytoin, prochlorperazine, trimethoprim/sulfamethoxazole, trimetrexate, and vancomycin. A precipitate can result if foscarnet is given at the same time as divalent cations.

7. Store drug at room temperatures of 15–30°C (59–86°F). Do not freeze. Concentrations of 12 mg/mL in NSS are stable for 30 days at 5°C (41°F).

ASSESSMENT

1. Document indications for therapy.
2. Determine confirmation of CMV retinitis by indirect ophthalmoscopy.
3. Note any history of cardiac or neurologic dysfunction.
4. Monitor CBC, electrolytes, calcium, phosphorus, magnesium, and liver and renal function studies.

INTERVENTIONS

1. Hydrate to minimize potential for renal impairment; establish and maintain diuresis. Determine C_{CR} at 2–3 times/week during induction therapy,

and at least once every 1–2 weeks during maintenance therapy. Especially in geriatric clients who commonly have decreased GFRs.
2. Observe for possibility of chelation of divalent metal ions, which will alter serum levels of electrolytes.
3. Observe for any seizure activity; use seizure precautions.
4. Follow dilution and administration guidelines carefully. Ideally, product should be prepared daily, under a biologic hood, by the pharmacist. Refer to home infusion program for home therapy.

F

CLIENT/FAMILY TEACHING

1. Foscarnet is not a cure for CMV retinitis; may continue to experience progression of condition during or following treatment.
2. Report for ophthalmic exams.
3. Report any evidence of numbness of the extremities, paresthesias, or perioral tingling as these are symptoms of hypocalcemia. Stop infusion and notify provider to correct imbalance before resuming the infusion.

OUTCOMES/EVALUATE

Ophthalmic evidence of successful treatment of CMV retinitis

Fosfomycin tromethamine

(fos-foh-**MY**-sin)

PREGNANCY CATEGORY: B
CLASSIFICATION(S):
Antibiotic, miscellaneous
Rx: Monurol

SEE ALSO *ANTI-INFECTIVE AGENTS.*

ACTION/KINETICS

Bactericidal drug that inactivates enzyme enolpyruvyl transferase, irreversibly blocking condensation of uridine diphosphate-N-acetylglucosamine with p-enolpyruvate. This is one of first steps in bacterial wall synthesis. Also reduces adherence of bacteria to uroepithelial cells. Rapidly absorbed from GI tract and converted to fosfomycin. **Maximum serum levels:** 2 hr. **t$^1/_2$, elimination:** 5.7 hr. Excreted unchanged in both urine and feces.

USES

Treatment of uncomplicated urinary tract infections (acute cystitis) in women due to *Escherichia coli* and Enterococcus faecalis.

CONTRAINDICATIONS

Lactation.

SPECIAL CONCERNS

Safety and efficacy have not been determined in children 12 years and younger.

SIDE EFFECTS

GI: Diarrhea, nausea, dyspepsia, abdominal pain, abnormal stools, anorexia, constipation, dry mouth, flatulence, vomiting. **CNS:** Headache, dizziness, insomnia, migraine, nervousness, paresthesia, somnolence. **GU:** Vaginitis, dysmenorrhea, dysuria, hematuria, menstrual disorder. **Respiratory:** Rhinitis, pharyngitis. **Miscellaneous:** Asthenia, back pain, pain, rash, ear disorder, fever, flu syndrome, infection, lymphadenopathy, myalgia, pruritus, skin disorder.

LABORATORY TEST CONSIDERATIONS

↑ ALT, AST, eosinophil count, bilirubin, alkaline phosphatase. ↓ Hematocrit, hemoglobin. ↑ or ↓ WBC, platelet count.

DRUG INTERACTIONS

Metoclopramide / ↓ serum levels and urinary excretion of fosfomycin.

HOW SUPPLIED

Granules for Reconstitution: 3 g

DOSAGE

• **GRANULE**

Acute cystitis.

Women, 18 years and older: One packet of fosfomycin mixed with water before ingesting.

NURSING CONSIDERATIONS

SEE ALSO *NURSING CONSIDERATIONS FOR ANTI-INFECTIVE AGENTS.*

ADMINISTRATION/STORAGE

Store at controlled room temperature.

ASSESSMENT

1. Note onset, duration, frequency of occurrence, and symptoms.
2. Assess urine cultures.

CLIENT/FAMILY TEACHING

1. Pour entire contents of single-dose sachet into 3 to 4 oz water and stir to dissolve. Do not take dry, always mix with 3 to 4 oz water and stir to dis-

solve before ingesting. Do not use hot water. Take immediately after dissolving in water.
2. May be taken with or without food.
3. Use only one single dose to treat each episode of acute cystitis. Each packet contains 3 Gm of fosfomycin.
4. Symptoms should improve within 2 to 3 days; if not improved, contact health care provider.

OUTCOMES/EVALUATE

Resolution of UTI; symptomatic improvement

Fosinopril sodium

(foh-**SIN**-oh-prill)

PREGNANCY CATEGORY: D
CLASSIFICATION(S):
Antihypertensive, ACE inhibitor
Rx: Monopril

SEE ALSO *ANGIOTENSIN-CONVERTING ENZYME INHIBITORS.*

ACTION/KINETICS

Onset: 1 hr. **Time to peak serum levels:** About 3 hr. Metabolized in the liver to the active fosinoprilat. **Peak effect:** 2–6 hr. Over 99% bound to plasma proteins. **t½:** 12 hr for fosinoprilat (prolonged in impaired renal function) following IV administration. **Duration:** 24 hr. Approximately 50% excreted through the urine and 50% in the feces. Food decreases the rate, but not the extent, of absorption of fosinopril.

USES

Alone or in combination with other antihypertensive agents (especially thiazide diuretics) for the treatment of hypertension. Adjunct in treating CHF in clients not responding adequately to diuretics and digitalis. Diabetic hypertensive clients show a reduction in major CV events.

CONTRAINDICATIONS

Use during lactation.

SIDE EFFECTS

CV: Orthostatic hypotension, chest pain, hypotension, palpitations, angina pectoris, ***CVA, MI,*** rhythm disturbances, TIA, tachycardia, ***hypertensive crisis,*** claudication, bradycardia, hypertension, conduction disorder, ***sudden death, cardiorespiratory arrest, shock.*** **CNS:** Headache, dizziness, fatigue, confusion, memory disturbance, depression, behavior change, tremors, drowsiness, mood change, insomnia, vertigo, sleep disturbances. **GI:** N&V, diarrhea, abdominal pain, constipation, dry mouth, dysphagia, taste disturbance, abdominal distention, flatulence, heartburn, appetite changes, weight changes. **Hepatic:** Hepatitis, pancreatitis, hepatomegaly, ***hepatic failure.*** **Respiratory:** Cough, sinusitis, dyspnea, URI, ***bronchospasm,*** asthma, pharyngitis, laryngitis, tracheobronchitis, abnormal breathing, sinus abnormalities. **Hematologic:** Leukopenia, eosinophilia, decreases in hemoglobin (mean of 0.1 g/dL) or hematocrit, neutropenia. **Dermatologic:** Diaphoresis, photosensitivity, flushing, exfoliative dermatitis, pruritus, rash, urticaria. **Body as a whole:** Angioedema, muscle cramps, fever, syncope, influenza, cold sensation, pain, myalgia, arthralgia, arthritis, edema, weakness, musculoskeletal pain. **GU:** Decreased libido, sexual dysfunction, renal insufficiency, urinary frequency, abnormal urination, kidney pain. **Miscellaneous:** Paresthesias, tinnitus, gout, lymphadenopathy, rhinitis, epistaxis, vision disturbances, eye irritation, swelling/weakness of extremities, abnormal vocalization, pneumonia, muscle ache.

LABORATORY TEST CONSIDERATIONS

↑ Serum potassium. Transient ↓ H&H. False low measurement of serum digoxin levels with DigiTab RIA Kit for Digoxin.

HOW SUPPLIED

Tablet: 10 mg, 20 mg, 40 mg

DOSAGE

• **TABLETS**

Hypertension.

Initial: 10 mg once daily; **then,** adjust dose depending on BP response at peak (2–6 hr after dosing) and trough (24 hr after dosing) blood levels.

Maintenance: Usually 20–40 mg/day, although some clients manifest beneficial effects at doses up to 80 mg.

In clients taking diuretics.

Discontinue diuretic 2–3 days before starting fosinopril. If diuretic cannot be discontinued, use an initial dose of 10 mg fosinopril.

Congestive heart failure.

Initial: 10 mg once daily; **then,** following initial dose, observe the client for at least 2 hr for the presence of hypotension or orthostasis (if either is present, monitor until BP stabilizes). An initial dose of 5 mg is recommended in heart failure with moderate to severe renal failure or in those who have had significant diuresis. Increase the dose over several weeks, not to exceed a maximum of 40 mg daily (usual effective range is 20–40 mg once daily).

NURSING CONSIDERATIONS

SEE ALSO *NURSING CONSIDERATIONS* FOR *ANGIOTENSIN-CONVERTING ENZYME INHIBITORS* AND *ANTIHYPERTENSIVE AGENTS.*

ADMINISTRATION/STORAGE

1. If antihypertensive effect decreases at the end of the dosing interval with once-daily dosing, consider b.i.d. administration.
2. If also taking a diuretic, discontinue the diuretic 2–3 days prior to beginning fosinopril therapy. If BP is not controlled, reinstitute the diuretic. If the diuretic cannot be discontinued, give an initial dose of fosinopril of 10 mg.
3. Do not adjust the dose of fosinopril in renal insufficiency except as noted in Dosage.

CLIENT/FAMILY TEACHING

1. Take as directed. Control of BP does not exceed 24 hr therefore take at same time(s) each day.
2. May initially cause dizziness and light-headedness so use care. Monitor and record BP at different times during the day.
3. Avoid OTC agents with provider approval; also salt substitutes containing potassium should be avoided.
4. Change positions slowly to avoid low BP.
5. Use reliable contraception.
6. Report any adverse side effects especially sore throat, swelling of hands and feet, chest pain, mouth sores or irregular heart beat.

OUTCOMES/EVALUATE

- ↓ BP
- Control of symptoms of CHF

Fosphenytoin sodium

(**FOS**-fen-ih-toyn)

PREGNANCY CATEGORY: D
CLASSIFICATION(S):
Anticonvulsant, hydantoin
Rx: Cerebyx

SEE ALSO *ANTICONVULSANTS* AND *PHENYTOIN.*

ACTION/KINETICS

Fosphenytoin is a prodrug of phenytoin; thus, its anticonvulsant effects are due to phenytoin. For every millimole of fosphenytoin administered, 1 mmol of phenytoin is produced. **t½, fosphenytoin:** 15 min after IV infusion. **Peak plasma levels, after IM:** 30 min. Significantly bound (95% to 99%) to plasma protein. Fosphenytoin displaces phenytoin from plasma protein binding sites. Fosphenytoin is better tolerated at the infusion site than is phenytoin (i.e., pain and burning associated with IV phenytoin is decreased). The IV infusion rate for fosphenytoin is three times faster than for IV phenytoin. IM use results in systemic phenytoin concentrations that are similar to PO phenytoin, thus allowing interchangeable use. Phenytoin derived from fosphenytoin is extensively metabolized in the liver and excreted in the urine.

USES

Short-term parenteral use for the control of generalized convulsive status epilepticus and prophylaxis and treatment of seizures occurring during neurosurgery. It can be substituted, short term, for PO phenytoin when PO administration is not possible.

CONTRAINDICATIONS

Hypersensitivity to fosphenytoin, phenytoin, or other hydantoins. Use in clients with sinus bradycardia, SA block, second- and third-degree AV block, and Adams-Stokes syndrome. Use to treat absence seizures. Use during lactation.

SPECIAL CONCERNS

The safety and efficacy of fosphenytoin have not been determined for longer than 5 days. Safety has not been determined in pediatric clients. After administration of fosphenytoin to those with renal and/or hepatic dysfunction or in those with hypoalbuminemia, fosphenytoin clearance to phenytoin may be increased without a similar increase in phenytoin clearance, thus increasing the potential for serious side effects. Do not confuse Cerebyx (fosphenytoin sodium injection) with Celebrex (celecoxib) or Celexa (Citalopram hydrobromide) — read label carefully.

SIDE EFFECTS

See *Phenytoin*. The most common side effects include ataxia, dizziness, headache, nystagmus, paresthesia, pruritus, and somnolence.

LABORATORY TEST CONSIDERATIONS

See *Phenytoin*.

DRUG INTERACTIONS

See *Phenytoin*

HOW SUPPLIED

Injection: 75 mg/mL

DOSAGE

NOTE: Doses of fosphenytoin are expressed as phenytoin sodium equivalents (PE = phenytoin sodium equivalent). Thus, adjustments in the recommended doses should not be made when substituting fosphenytoin for phenytoin sodium or vice versa. Do not confuse the amount of fosphenytoin equivalents per mL with the total amount of equivalents in the vial.

- **IV**

Status epilepticus.

Loading dose: 15–20 mg PE/kg given at a rate of 100–150 mg PE/min. The loading dose is followed by maintenance doses of either fosphenytoin or phenytoin, either PO or parenterally.

- **IM, IV**

Nonemergency loading and maintenance dosing.

Loading dose: 10–20 mg PE/kg given at a rate of 100–150 mg PE/min. **Maintenance:** 4–6 mg PE/kg/day.

Temporary substitution for PO phenytoin.

Use the same daily PO dose of phenytoin in milligrams given at a rate not to exceed 150 mg PE/min.

NURSING CONSIDERATIONS

SEE ALSO *NURSING CONSIDERATIONS* FOR *ANTICONVULSANTS* AND *PHENYTOIN*.

ADMINISTRATION/STORAGE

1. Fosphenytoin can be substituted for PO phenytoin sodium therapy at the same total daily dose.
2. Phenytoin capsules as Dilantin are approximately 90% bioavailable by the PO route and fosphenytoin (available as Cerebyx) is 100% bioavailable by both the IM and IV routes. Plasma phenytoin may increase modestly when IM or IV fosphenytoin (as Cerebyx) is substituted for PO phenytoin sodium therapy.
3. Do not use IM fosphenytoin to treat status epilepticus because therapeutic phenytoin concentrations may not be reached as quickly as with IV administration.
4. Do not use vials that develop particulate matter.
5. Do not store at room temperature for more than 48 hr. Store under refrigeration at 2–8°C (36–46°F).
6. IV Prior to IV infusion fosphenytoin must be diluted in D5W or NSS solution to obtain a concentration ranging from 1.5 to 25 mg/PE (phenytoin sodium equivalents)/mL.
7. Due to risk of hypotension, do not administer at a rate greater than 150 PE/min.
8. Because the full antiepileptic effect of phenytoin (given as either fosphenytoin or parenteral phenytoin) is not known immediately, other measures to control status epilepticus (e.g., use of an IV benzodiazepine) will be necessary.

ASSESSMENT

1. Document type, onset, and characteristics of seizures; note other agents trialed and outcome.
2. Fosphenytoin converts to pheny-

F

toin and may be administered IV or IM; prescribed and dispensed in PE.
3. Monitor ECG, albumin, CBC, and liver and renal function studies. During IV administration, continously monitor ECG, BP, and respirations.
4. Do not use with bradycardia or heart block; may cause atrial and ventricular conduction depression.
5. The waiting period before ordering laboratory tests for phenytoin plasma levels: 2 hr following IV infusion and 4 hr following IM injection.

CLIENT/FAMILY TEACHING

1. Review goals of therapy; drug is generally for short-term use.
2. Report any fever, sore throat, bruising, rash, jaundice or swollen lymph glands.
3. May experience dizziness, drowsiness, itching, and tingling of groin and face. Presence of REMs, gait and speech impairment may indicate toxicity.
4. If rash appears, stop therapy and report. If mild, therapy may be resumed once rash has cleared. If rash recurs, do not reuse this class of drugs.

OUTCOMES/EVALUATE

- Control of convulsions
- Seizure prophylaxis with surgery
- Short-term substitution for PO phenytoin

Frovatriptan succinate

(**froh**-vah-**TRIP**-tan)

PREGNANCY CATEGORY: C
CLASSIFICATION(S):
Antimigraine drug
Rx: Frova

ACTION/KINETICS

Frovatriptan is a selective 5-$HT_{1B/1D}$ receptor agonist which binds with high affinity to 5-HT1B and 5-HT1D receptors. Believed to act on extracerebral, intracranial arteries to cause constriction and to inhibit excessive dilation of these vessels in migraine. **Maximum blood levels:** 2–4 hr. Food has no significant effect on bioavailability but delays the maximum levels by 1 hr. Metabolized in the liver with about ⅓ unchanged drug and metabolites excreted in the urine and ⅔ in the feces. **t½, mean terminal:** 26 hr.

USES

Acute treatment of migraine, with or without aura, in adults. Use only where a clear diagnosis of migraine has been established.

CONTRAINDICATIONS

Use for prophylaxis of migraine or use in management of hemiplegic or basilar migraine. Use in those with ischemic heart disease (e.g., angina pectoris, history of MI, documented silent ischemia) or in those who have symptoms or findings consistent with ischemic heart disease, coronary artery vasospasm (including Prinzmetal's variant angina), or other significant underlying CV disease. Use in those with CV syndromes, including (but not limited to) strokes of any type as well as TIAs. Use in those with peripheral vascular disease (including, but not limited to ischemic bowel disease), uncontrolled hypertension, use within 24 hr of treatment with another 5-HT_1 agonist or an ergotamine-containing or ergot-type medication (e.g., dihydroergotamine, methysergide), or in those hypersensitive to frovatriptan or any ingredients of the product. Use in those with documented ischemic or vasospastic CAD or in whom unrecognized CAD is predicted by the presence of risk factors (e.g., hypertension, hypercholesterolemia, smoking, obesity, diabetes, strong history of CAD, females with surgical or physiological menopause, or males over 40 years of age) unless a CV evaluation provides evidence that the client is reasonably free of CAD and ischemic myocardial disease. Use in children less than 18 years of age.

SPECIAL CONCERNS

Use with caution during lactation. Safety and efficacy have not been established for use in children less than 18 years of age or for cluster headaches (present in an older, predominately male population).

SIDE EFFECTS

CV: ***Acute MI, life-threatening disturbances of cardiac rhythm, death, cerebral hemorrhage, subarachnoid hemorrhage, stroke, ventricular fibrillation,*** coronary artery vasospasm, transient myocardial ischemia, ventricular tachycardia, peripheral vascular ischemia, colonic ischemia (with abdominal pain and bloody diarrhea), hypertension, palpitation, tachycardia, abnormal ECG. **CNS:** Dizziness, paresthesia, headache, dysesthesia, hypoesthesia, tremor, hyperesthesia, aggravated migraine, vertigo, ataxia, abnormal gait, speech disorder, insomnia, anxiety, confusion, nervousness, agitation, euphoria, impaired concentration, depression, emotional lability, amnesia, abnormal thinking, depersonalization. **GI:** Dry mouth, dyspepsia, vomiting, abdominal pain, diarrhea, dysphagia, flatulence, constipation, anorexia, esophagospasm, increased salivation. **Body as a whole:** Fatigue, flushing, hot or cold sensation, pain, asthenia, rigors, fever, hot flashes, malaise, dehydration, syncope. **Musculoskeletal:** Skeletal pain, involuntary muscle contraction, myalgia, back pain, arthralgia, arthrosis, leg cramps, muscle weakness. **Respiratory:** Sinusitis, rhinitis, pharyngitis, dyspnea, hyperventilation, laryngitis, epistaxis. **Dermatologic:** Increased sweating, pruritis, bullous eruption. **GU:** Frequent micturition, polyuria. **Ophthalmic:** Abnormal vision, eye pain, conjunctivitis, abnormal lacrimation. **Otic:** Tinnitus, ear ache, hyperacusis. **Miscellaneous:** Chest pain, thirst, taste perversion. Sensations of pain, tightness, pressure, and heaviness in the chest, throat, neck, and jaw.

DRUG INTERACTIONS

Dihydroergotamine/Prolonged vasospastic reaction; do not use within 24 hr of each other
Ergotamine / Frovatriptan maximum levels and AUC ↓ 25%
Methysergide / Prolonged vasospastic reaction; do not use within 24 hr of each other
Oral contraceptives / Frovatriptan maximum levels and AUC ↑30%
Propranolol / ↑ Frovatriptan maximum levels and AUC
Selective serotonin reuptake inhibitors / Possible weakness, hyperreflexia, incoordination

HOW SUPPLIED

Tablet: 2.5 mg

DOSAGE

• **TABLETS**

Migraine headache.

Adults: Single dose of 2.5 mg taken with fluids. If the headache recurs after initial relief, a second tablet (2.5 mg) may be taken provided there is an interval of at least 2 hr between doses. Do not exceed a total daily dose of 3 tablets (7.5 mg).

NURSING CONSIDERATIONS

ADMINISTRATION/STORAGE

1. If the first dose does not produce a response, reconsider the diagnosis of migraine before giving a second dose.
2. There is no evidence that a second dose is effective in clients who do not respond to a first dose.
3. The safety of treating an average of 4 migraine attacks in a 30-day period has not been determined.
4. Store at controlled room temperature of 15–30°C (59–86°F). Protect from moisture and light.

ASSESSMENT

1. Note indications for therapy, onset, family history, characteristics of symptoms, and ensure not hemiplegic or basilar type of migraine headaches.
2. List drugs currently prescribed to ensure none interact.
3. Assess for CAD, uncontrolled HTN, circulation problems, IBD, or history of CVA/TIAs. With increased CAD risk factors give first dose in the office and assess client for adverse effects.
4. Determine renal and LFT's; evaluate for dysfunction.

CLIENT/FAMILY TEACHING

1. Take only as directed for migraine headaches; do not use for other types of headaches. Never share meds with

another person no matter what the symptoms.
2. If headache returns may repeat dose in two hr; do not exceed 3 tabs (7.5 mg) in 24 hr.
3. Use caution if driving or performing activities that require mental alertness; may cause dizziness, fatigue, or drowsiness.
4. Store in a safe place and away from heat, light, and moisture.
5. Drug acts to shrink swollen blood vessels surrounding the brain that cause migraine headaches. Keep a headache diary and identify factors/foods/events that surround migraine headaches.
6. Avoid known triggers, i.e. chocolate, cheese, citrus fruit, caffeine, alcohol, missing sleep/meals etc.
7. Report any chest pain, SOB, palpitations, rash/itching, or unusual side effects, intolerance, or lack of response.

OUTCOMES/EVALUATE

Resolution of acute migraine attack

Furosemide

(fur-**OH**-seh-myd)

PREGNANCY CATEGORY: C
CLASSIFICATION(S):
Diuretic, loop
Rx: Lasix
✱Rx: Apo-Furosemide, Lasix Special

SEE ALSO *DIURETICS, LOOP.*

ACTION/KINETICS

Inhibits the reabsorption of sodium and chloride in the proximal and distal tubules as well as the ascending loop of Henle; this results in the excretion of sodium, chloride, and, to a lesser degree, potassium and bicarbonate ions. The resulting urine is more acid. Diuretic action is independent of changes in clients' acid-base balance. Has a slight antihypertensive effect. **Onset: PO, IM:** 30–60 min; **IV:** 5 min. **Peak: PO, IM:** 1–2 hr; **IV:** 20–60 min. **t½:** About 2 hr after PO use. **Duration: PO, IM:** 6–8 hr; **IV:** 2 hr. Metabolized in the liver and excreted through the urine. May be effective for clients resistant to thiazides and for those with reduced GFRs.

USES

Edema associated with CHF, nephrotic syndrome, hepatic cirrhosis, and ascites. IV for acute pulmonary edema. PO to treat hypertension in conjunction with spironolactone, triamterene, and other diuretics *except* ethacrynic acid. *Investigational:* Hypercalcemia.

CONTRAINDICATIONS

Never use with ethacrynic acid. Anuria, hypersensitivity to drug, severe renal disease associated with azotemia and oliguria, hepatic coma associated with electrolyte depletion. Lactation.

SPECIAL CONCERNS

Use with caution in premature infants and neonates due to prolonged half-life in these clients (dosing interval must be extended). Geriatric clients may be more sensitive to the usual adult dose. Allergic reactions may be seen in clients who show hypersensitivity to sulfonamides.

SIDE EFFECTS

Electrolyte and fluid effects: Fluid and electrolyte depletion leading to dehydration, hypovolemia, thromboembolism. Hypokalemia and hypochloremia may cause metabolic alkalosis. Hyperuricemia, azotemia, hyponatremia. **GI:** Nausea, oral and gastric irritation, vomiting, anorexia, diarrhea (especially in children) or constipation, cramps, pancreatitis, jaundice, ischemic hepatitis. **Otic:** Tinnitus, hearing impairment (may be reversible or permanent), reversible deafness. Usually following rapid IV or IM administration of high doses. **CNS:** Vertigo, headache, dizziness, blurred vision, restlessness, paresthesias, xanthopsia. **CV:** Orthostatic hypotension, thrombophlebitis, chronic aortitis. **Hematologic:** Anemia, thrombocytopenia, neutropenia, leukopenia, ***agranulocytosis,*** purpura. ***Rarely, aplastic anemia.*** **Allergic:** Rashes, pruritus, urticaria, photosensitivity, exfoliative dermatitis, vasculitis, erythema multiforme. **Miscellaneous:** Interstitial nephritis, fever, weakness, hyperglycemia, glycosuria, exacerbation of, aggravation of or worsening of SLE, increased perspiration, muscle spasms, urinary bladder spasm, urinary frequency.

Following IV use.

Thrombophlebitis, ***cardiac arrest.*** *Following IM use:* Pain and irritation at injection site, ***cardiac arrest.*** Because this drug is resistant to the effects of pressor amines and potentiates the effects of muscle relaxants, it is recommended that the PO drug be discontinued 1 week before surgery and the IV drug 2 days before surgery.

OD OVERDOSE MANAGEMENT

Symptoms: Profound water loss, electrolyte depletion (manifested by weakness, anorexia, vomiting, lethargy, cramps, mental confusion, dizziness), decreased blood volume, ***circulatory collapse (possibly vascular thrombosis and embolism).*** *Treatment:* Replace fluid and electrolytes. Monitor urine electrolyte output and serum electrolytes. Induce emesis or perform gastric lavage. Oxygen or artificial respiration may be needed. Treat symptoms.

ADDITIONAL DRUG INTERACTIONS

Charcoal / ↓ Absorption of furosemide from GI tract
Clofibrate / Enhanced diuretic effect
Hydantoins / ↓ Diuretic effect of furosemide
Propranolol / ↑ Plasma propranolol levels

HOW SUPPLIED

Injection: 10 mg /mL; *Oral Solution:* 10 mg/ mL, 40 mg/5 mL; *Tablet:* 20 mg, 40 mg, 80 mg

DOSAGE

• **ORAL SOLUTION, TABLETS**

Edema.

Adults, initial: 20–80 mg/day as a single dose. For resistant cases, dosage can be increased by 20–40 mg q 6–8 hr until desired diuretic response is attained. Maximum daily dose should not exceed 600 mg. **Pediatric, initial:** 2 mg/kg as a single dose; **then,** dose can be increased by 1–2 mg/kg q 6–8 hr until desired response is attained (up to 5 mg/kg may be required in children with nephrotic syndrome; maximum dose should not exceed 6 mg/kg). A dose range of 0.5–2 mg/kg b.i.d. has also been recommended.

Hypertension.

Adults, initial: 40 mg b.i.d. Adjust dosage depending on response.

CHF and chronic renal failure.

Adults: 2–2.5 g/day.

Antihypercalcemic.

Adults: 120 mg/day in one to three doses.

• **IV, IM**

Edema.

Adults, initial: 20–40 mg; if response inadequate after 2 hr, increase dose in 20-mg increments. **Pediatric, initial:** 1 mg/kg given slowly; if response inadequate after 2 hr, increase dose by 1 mg/kg. Doses greater than 6 mg/kg should not be given.

Antihypercalcemic.

Adults: 80–100 mg for severe cases; dose may be repeated q 1–2 hr if needed.

• **IV**

Acute pulmonary edema.

Adults: 40 mg slowly over 1–2 min; if response inadequate after 1 hr, give 80 mg slowly over 1–2 min. Concomitant oxygen and digitalis may be used.

CHF, chronic renal failure.

Adults: 2–2.5 g/day. For IV bolus injections, the maximum should not exceed 1 g/day given over 30 min.

Hypertensive crisis, normal renal function.

Adults: 40–80 mg.

Hypertensive crisis with pulmonary edema or acute renal failure.

Adults: 100–200 mg.

NURSING CONSIDERATIONS

SEE ALSO *NURSING CONSIDERATIONS* FOR *DIURETICS, LOOP.*

ADMINISTRATION/STORAGE

1. Give 2–4 days/week.
2. Food decreases the bioavailability of furosemide and ultimately the degree of diuresis.
3. Slight discoloration resulting from light does not affect potency. However, do not dispense discolored tablets or injection.

4. If used with other antihypertensives, reduce the dose of other agents by at least 50% when furosemide is added in order to prevent an excessive drop in BP.
5. Store in light-resistant containers at room temperature (15–30°C, or 59–86°F).
6. In CHF or chronic renal failure, oral and parenteral doses of 2–2.5 g/day (or higher) are well tolerated.
IV 7. Give IV injections slowly over 1–2 min.
8. If used IV, do not mix with solutions with a pH below 5.5. After pH adjustment, furosemide can be mixed with NaCl injection, RL injection, and D5W and infused at a rate not to exceed 4 mg/min, to prevent ototoxicity.
9. A precipitate may form if mixed with gentamicin, netilmicin, or milrinone in either D5W or NSS.

ASSESSMENT

1. When more than 40 mg/day is required, give in divided doses, i.e., 40 mg PO b.i.d. (7am and 3 pm)
2. With renal impairment or if receiving other ototoxic drugs, observe for ototoxicity.
3. Assess closely for signs of vascular thrombosis and embolism, particularly in the elderly.
4. Monitor electrolytes; observe for S&S of hypokalemia.
5. With rapid diuresis, observe for dehydration and circulatory collapse; monitor BP and pulse.
6. With chronic use, assess for thiamine deficiency; when used with zaroxlyn assess for low phosphate levels.

CLIENT/FAMILY TEACHING

1. Take in the morning on an empty stomach to enhance absorption and to avoid interruption of sleep. Time administration to participate in social activities and not have to get up during the night to void frequently.
2. Immediately report any muscle weakness, dizziness, numbness, or tingling.
3. Drug may cause orthostatic hypotension.
4. Sorbitol in the solution vehicle may result in diarrhea, especially in children.
5. Monitor weights; report any gains of > 2 lb/day or > 10 lb/week.
6. Consult provider before taking aspirin for any reason. Salicylate intoxication occurs at lower levels than normal because of competition at the renal excretory sites.
7. Use sunscreens and protective clothing when sun exposed to minimize the effects of drug-induced photosensitivity.
8. Supplement diet with vegetables and fruits high in potassium if oral supplements are not prescribed. Those on a salt-restricted diet should not increase salt intake; NSAIDs and alpha blockers may also cause sodium retention with resultant edema.

OUTCOMES/EVALUATE

- Enhanced diuresis
- Resolution of pulmonary edema
- ↓ Dependent edema
- ↓ Serum calcium levels

G

Gabapentin
(**gab**-ah-**PEN**-tin)

PREGNANCY CATEGORY: C
CLASSIFICATION(S):
Anticonvulsant, miscellaneous
Rx: Neurontin

SEE ALSO *ANTICONVULSANTS*.

ACTION/KINETICS
Anticonvulsant mechanism is not known. Food has no effect on the rate and extent of absorption; however, as the dose increases, the bioavailability decreases. **t½:** 5–7 hr. Excreted unchanged through the urine.

USES
Treatment of partial seizures with and without secondary generalization in clients 12 years and older. Adjunct to

treat partial seizures in children 3–12 years of age. *Investigational:* Neuropathic pain, bipolar disorder, prevent migraine, tremors associated with multiple sclerosis.

SPECIAL CONCERNS

Use during lactation only if benefits outweigh risks. Plasma clearance is reduced in geriatric clients and in those with impaired renal function. Use in children 3–12 years of age is associated with various neuropsychiatric side effects.

SIDE EFFECTS

Side effects listed are those with an incidence of 0.1% or greater. **CNS:** Most common: somnolence, ataxia, dizziness, and fatigue. Also, nystagmus, tremor, nervousness, dysarthria, amnesia, depression, abnormal thinking, twitching, abnormal coordination, headache, ***convulsions (including the possibility of precipitation of status epilepticus),*** confusion, insomnia, emotional lability, vertigo, hyperkinesia, paresthesia, decreased/increased/absent reflexes, anxiety, hostility, CNS tumors, syncope, abnormal dreaming, aphasia, hypesthesia, ***intracranial hemorrhage,*** hypotonia, dysesthesia, paresis, dystonia, hemiplegia, facial paralysis, stupor, cerebellar dysfunction, positive Babinski sign, decreased position sense, subdural hematoma, apathy, hallucinations, decreased or loss of libido, agitation depersonalization, euphoria, "doped-up" sensation, ***suicidal tendencies, sudden unexplained deaths,*** psychoses.

Neuropsychiatric effects in children:

Emotional lability (behavioral problems), hostility (aggressive behavior), thought disorder (concentration problems and change in school performance), restlessness, hyperactivity.

GI: Most common is: N&V. Also, dyspepsia, dry mouth and throat, constipation, dental abnormalities, increased appetite, abdominal pain, diarrhea, anorexia, flatulence, gingivitis, glossitis, gum hemorrhage, thirst, stomatitis, taste loss, unusual taste, increased salivation, gastroenteritis, hemorrhoids, bloody stools, fecal incontinence, hepatomegaly. **CV:** Hypertension, vasodilation, hypotension, angina pectoris, peripheral vascular disorder, palpitation, tachycardia, migraine, murmur. **Musculoskeletal:** Myalgia, fracture, tendinitis, arthritis, joint stiffness or swelling, positive Romberg test. **Respiratory:** Rhinitis, pharyngitis, coughing, pneumonia, epistaxis, dyspnea, apnea. **Dermatologic:** Pruritus, abrasion, rash, acne, alopecia, eczema, dry skin, increased sweating, urticaria, hirsutism, seborrhea, cyst, herpes simplex. **Body as a whole:** Weight increase, back pain, peripheral edema, asthenia, facial edema, allergy, weight decrease, chills. **GU:** Hematuria, dysuria, frequent urination, cystitis, urinary retention, urinary incontinence, vaginal hemorrhage, amenorrhea, dysmenorrhea, menorrhagia, breast cancer, inability to climax, abnormal ejaculation, impotence. **Hematologic:** Leukopenia, decreased WBCs, purpura, anemia, thrombocytopenia, lymphadenopathy. **Ophthalmologic:** Diplopia, amblyopia, abnormal vision, cataract, conjunctivitis, dry eyes, eye pain, visual field defect, photophobia, bilateral or unilateral ptosis, eye hemorrhage, hordeolum, eye twitching. **Otic:** Hearing loss, earache, tinnitus, inner ear infection, otitis, ear fullness.

LABORATORY TEST CONSIDERATIONS

False + reading with Ames N-Multistix SG dipstick test for urinary protein.

OD OVERDOSE MANAGEMENT

Symptoms: Double vision, slurred speech, drowsiness, lethargy, diarrhea. *Treatment:* Hemodialysis.

DRUG INTERACTIONS

Antacids / ↓ Bioavailability of gabapentin

Cimetidine / ↓ Renal excretion of gabapentin

HOW SUPPLIED

Capsule: 100 mg, 300 mg, 400 mg; *Solution, Oral:* 250 mg/5 mL; *Tablet:* 600 mg, 800 mg

DOSAGE

• CAPSULES, ORAL SOLUTION, TABLETS

Partial seizures with and without secondary generalization.

Clients 12 years and older: Dose range of 900–1,800 mg/day in three divided doses using 300 or 400 mg capsules or 600 or 800 mg tablets. **Initial dose:** 300 mg t.i.d.; dose may be increased, as needed, up to 1800 mg/day. Doses up to 2,400 and 3,600 mg/day have been well tolerated for short periods. In clients with a C_{CR} of 30–60 mL/min, the dose is 300 mg b.i.d.; if the C_{CR} is 15–30 mL/min, the dose is 300 mg/day; if the C_{CR} is less than 15 mL/min, the dose is 300 mg every other day.

Adjunctive therapy for partial seizures in children.
Initial: 10–15 mg/kg/day in 3 divided doses. Attain effective dose by titration over 3 days. Effective dose in clients 5 years and older is 25–35 mg/kg/day and in clients 3 and 4 years of age is 40 mg/kg/day; give in divided doses t.i.d. May use capsules, oral solution or tablets.

NURSING CONSIDERATIONS

SEE ALSO *NURSING CONSIDERATIONS* FOR *ANTICONVULSANTS*.

ADMINISTRATION/STORAGE

1. Do not exceed 12 hr between doses using the t.i.d. daily regimen.
2. If gabapentin is discontinued or an alternate anticonvulsant is added to the regimen, do gradually over a 1-week period.
3. The first dose on day 1 may be taken at bedtime to minimize somnolence, dizziness, fatigue, and ataxia.

ASSESSMENT

1. Document onset, frequency, and characteristics of symptoms, any other agents prescribed, and the outcome. With chronic pain, rate pain level.
2. List other drugs prescribed to ensure that none interact unfavorably.
3. Obtain baseline renal function studies; reduce dose in the elderly and with impaired renal function.
4. When drug therapy is discontinued or supplemental therapy is added, do so gradually over at least 1 week.

CLIENT/FAMILY TEACHING

1. May be taken with or without food. Do not stop abruptly.
2. Avoid antacids 1 hr before or 2 hr after taking drug.
3. Drug may cause dizziness, fatigue, drowsiness, ataxia, and nystagmus. Do not perform any activities that require mental alertness until full drug effects are realized.
4. Report any new/unusual S&S.

OUTCOMES/EVALUATE

- Control of seizure activity
- Chronic pain control

Galantamine hydrobromide

PREGNANCY CATEGORY: B
CLASSIFICATION(S):
Treatment of Alzheimer's disease
Rx: Reminyl

ACTION/KINETICS

The drug is a competitive and reversible inhibitor of acetylcholinesterase. It is believed the drug enhances cholinergic function, which is believed to be impaired in Alzheimer's disease. The drug's effect may lessen as the disease process advances and as fewer cholinergic neurons remain functionally intact. There is no evidence the drug alters the course of the underlying dementing process. Well absorbed; **time to peak levels:** About 1 hr. Food does not affect the amount absorbed but does delay the maximum time by 1.5 hr. Metabolized by hepatic cytochrome P450 enzymes. **t½, terminal:** 7 hr. Excreted in the urine.

USES

Treatment of mild to moderate dementia of the Alzheimer's type.

CONTRAINDICATIONS

Hypersensitivity to galantamine or any components of the product. Use in those with severe renal impairment (C_{CR} less than 9 mL/min). Lactation, use in children.

SPECIAL CONCERNS

Use with caution in those with severe asthma, obstructive pulmonary disease, or moderately impaired renal function.

SIDE EFFECTS

GI: N&V, anorexia, diarrhea, abdominal pain, dyspepsia, constipation, active/occult GI bleeding, peptic ulcer disease, flatulence. **CNS:** Dizziness, headache, tremor, depression, insomnia, somnolence, agitation, confusion, anxiety, hallucination. **CV:** Bradycardia, AV block, syncope, hypertension. **GU:** UTI, hematuria, urinary incontinence. **Respiratory:** Rhinitis, URTI, bronchitis, coughing. **Body as a whole:** Weight decrease, fatigue, anemia, peripheral edema, asthenia. **Miscellaneous:** Injury, back/chest pain, fall, purpura.

OD OVERDOSE MANAGEMENT

Symptoms: Severe N&V, GI cramping, salivation, lacrimation, urination, defecation, sweating, bradycardia, hypotension, respiratory depression, ***collapse, convulsions.*** Also, increasing muscle weakness which may result in death if respiratory muscles are involved. *Treatment:* IV atropine sulfate at an initial dose of 0.5–1 mg with subsequent doses based on clinical response.

DRUG INTERACTIONS

Amitriptyline / ↓ Galantamine clearance R/T ↓ liver metabolism
Bethanecol / Synergistic effects
Cimetidine / ↑ Galantamine bioavailability
Erythromycin / ↓ Galantamine clearance R/T ↓ liver metabolism
Fluoxetine / ↓ Galantamine clearance R/T ↓ liver metabolism
Fluvoxamine / ↓ Galantamine clearance R/T ↓ liver metabolism
Ketoconazole / ↑ Blood levels R/T ↓ liver metabolism
Paroxetine / ↑ Galantamine bioavailability R/T ↓ liver metabolism
Quinidine / ↓ Galantamine clearance R/T ↓ liver metabolism
Succinylcholine-type drugs. Exaggeration of neuromuscular blocking effects

HOW SUPPLIED

Oral Solution: 4 mg/mL; *Tablet:* 4 mg, 8 mg, 12 mg

DOSAGE

• **ORAL SOLUTION, TABLETS**

Dementia of the Alzheimer's type.

Initial: 4 mg b.i.d. After a minimum of 4 weeks if this dose is well tolerated, increase to 8 mg b.i.d.. Attempt a further increase to 12 mg b.i.d. only after a minimum of 4 weeks. Although a dosage range of 16–32 mg/day given as twice daily dosing is possible, due to side effects the recommended dose range is 16–24 mg/day given as b.i.d. dosing. Do not exceed 16 mg/day in those with moderately impaired hepatic function or moderate renal impairment.

NURSING CONSIDERATIONS

ASSESSMENT

1. Document onset/duration of behavioral changes, other agents trialed, and the outcome.
2. Describe clinical presentation.
3. Note any history of asthma, COPD, or renal dysfunction.
4. Monitor ECG and labs.

CLIENT/FAMILY TEACHING

1. Take twice daily, with the morning and evening meals.
2. If therapy is interrupted for several days or longer, must restart at the lowest dose and increase back up to the current dose.
3. Most side effects occur during periods of increasing dosage. Take with food, use prescribed anti-emetic medication, and ensure adequate fluid intake to reduce impact of such side effects.
4. Report any irregular pulse or dizzy spells, lack of response, or worsening of symptoms.

OUTCOMES/EVALUATE

Improved cognitive functioning with Alzheimer's disease

Ganciclovir sodium (DHPG)

(gan-**SYE**-kloh-veer)

PREGNANCY CATEGORY: C
CLASSIFICATION(S):
Antiviral
Rx: Vitrasert , Cytovene

SEE ALSO *ANTIVIRAL AGENTS.*

G

ACTION/KINETICS

Upon entry into viral cells infected by CMV, ganciclovir is converted to ganciclovir triphosphate by the CMV. Ganciclovir triphosphate inhibits viral DNA synthesis by competitive inhibition of viral DNA polymerases and direct incorporation into viral DNA; this results in eventual termination of viral DNA elongation. Ganciclovir is active against CMV, herpes simplex virus-1 and -2, Epstein-Barr virus, and varicella zoster virus. Use of the intraocular implant causes a significantly slower disease progression than did those treated with IV ganciclovir. **t½:** Approximately 2.9 hr. Believed to cross the blood-brain barrier. Most excreted unchanged through the urine. Renal impairment increases the t½ of the drug; make dosage adjustments based on C_{CR}.

USES

IV: (1) Treatment of CMV retinitis in immunocompromised clients, including those with AIDS. Diagnosis may be confirmed by culture of CMV from the blood, urine, or throat; note that a negative CMV culture does not rule out CMV retinitis. (2) Prevention of CMV disease in transplant clients at risk; duration of treatment depends on duration and degree of immunosuppression.

PO: (1) Alternative to IV for maintenance treatment of CMV retinitis in immunocompromised (including AIDS) clients. (2) Prevention of CMV disease in solid organ transplant clients and in those with advanced HIV infection at risk for developing CMV pneumonitis. *Investigational:* CMV pneumonia in organ transplants, CMV gastroenteritis in those with irritable bowel disease, and CMV pneumonitis.

Intraocular implant: CMV retinitis in those with AIDS.

CONTRAINDICATIONS

Hypersensitivity to acyclovir or ganciclovir. Lactation. Use when the absolute neutrophil count is less than 500/mm³ or the platelet count is less than 25,000/mm³.

SPECIAL CONCERNS

Safety and effectiveness of ganciclovir have not been established for nonimmunocompromised clients, treatment of other CMV infections such as pneumonitis or colitis, or congenital or neonatal CMV disease. Use with caution in impaired renal function, in elderly clients, or with preexisting cytopenias or with a history of cytopenic reactions to other drugs, chemicals, or irradiation. Use in children only if potential benefits outweigh potential risks, including carcinogenicity and reproductive toxicity. Not a cure for CMV retinitis and progression of the disease may continue in immunocompromised clients. Treatment with zidovudine and ganciclovir (e.g., in AIDS clients) will likely not be tolerated and lead to severe granulocytopenia.

SIDE EFFECTS

Hematologic: Granulocytopenia, thrombocytopenia, neutropenia (may be irreversible), eosinophilia, leukopenia, anemia, hypochromic anemia, bone marrow depression, pancytopenia, ***leukemia, lymphoma***. **CNS:** Ataxia, ***coma,*** neuropathy, confusion, abnormal dreams or thoughts, dizziness, headache, paresthesia, psychosis, nervousness, somnolence, tremor, agitation, amnesia, anxiety, depression, euphoria, hypertonia, hypesthesia, insomnia, manic reaction, ***seizures,*** trismus, emotional lability. **GI:** N&V, aphthous stomatitis, diarrhea, anorexia, dry mouth, ***GI hemorrhage, pancreatitis,*** abdominal pain, flatulence, dyspepsia, constipation, dysphagia, esophagitis, eructation, fecal incontinence, melena, mouth ulceration, tongue disorder, hepatitis, weight loss. **CV:** Hypertension or hypotension, arrhythmias, phlebitis, deep thrombophlebitis, ***cardiac arrest, intracranial hypertension, MI, stroke,*** pericarditis, vasodilation, migraine. **Body as a whole:** Fever (most common), chills, edema, infections, malaise, ***sepsis, multiple organ failure,*** asthenia, enlarged abdomen, abscess, back pain, cellulitis, chest pain, facial edema, neck pain or rigidity. **Dermatologic:** Rash (most common), alopecia, pruritus, urticaria, sweating, acne, dry skin, fixed eruption, herpes simplex, maculopapular rash, skin discoloration, vesiculobullous rash, photosensitivity, phototoxicity. **GU:** Hematuria, breast pain, kidney failure, abnormal kidney function, urinary frequency, UTI. **At injection site:** Catheter infection, catheter sepsis, inflammation or pain, abscess, edema, hemorrhage, phlebitis. **Musculoskeletal:** Arthralgia, bone pain, leg cramps, myalgia, myasthenia. **Ophthalmologic:** Abnormal vision, amblyopia, blindness, conjunctivitis, eye pain, glaucoma, retinitis, photophobia, cataracts, vitreous disorder. **Respiratory:** Dyspnea, increased cough, pneumonia. **Hepatic:** Cholestasis, cholangitis. **Miscellaneous:** Abnormal gait, decreased libido, deafness, ***anaphylaxis,*** taste perversion, tinnitus, acidosis, congenital anomaly, encephalopathy, impotence, transverse myelitis, infertility, splenomegaly, ***Stevens-Johnson syndrome, unexplained death,*** retinal detachment in CMV retinitis clients.

LABORATORY TEST CONSIDERATIONS

↑ Serum creatinine, BUN, alkaline phosphatase, CPK, LDH, AST, ALT. ↓ Blood glucose. Abnormal LFT. Hypokalemia, hyponatremia.

OD OVERDOSE MANAGEMENT

Symptoms: Neutropenia. Possibility of hypersalivation, anorexia, vomiting, bloody diarrhea, inactivity, cytopenia, testicular atrophy, increased BUN and LFT results. *Treatment:* Hydration, hemodialysis.

DRUG INTERACTIONS

Adriamycin / Additive cytotoxicity in rapidly dividing cells
Amphotericin B / Additive cytotoxicity in rapidly dividing cells; also, ↑ serum creatinine levels
Cyclosporine / ↑ Serum creatinine levels
Cytotoxic drugs / Additive cytotoxicity
Dapsone / Additive cytotoxicity in rapidly dividing cells
Didanosine: ↑ Didanosine area under the curve.
Dapsone / Additive cytotoxicity in rapidly dividing cells
Flucytosine / Additive cytotoxicity in rapidly dividing cells
Imipenem/Cilastatin combination / Possibility of seizures
Nephrotoxicity / ↑ Serum creatinine
Pentamidine / Additive cytotoxicity in rapidly dividing cells
Probenecid / ↑ Effect of ganciclovir R/T ↓ renal excretion
Sulfamethoxazole/Trimethoprim combinations / Additive cytotoxicity in rapidly dividing cells
Vinblastine / Additive cytotoxicity in rapidly dividing cells
Vincristine / Additive cytotoxicity in rapidly dividing cells
Zidovudine / ↑ Risk of neutropenia and anemia

HOW SUPPLIED

Capsules: 250 mg, 500 mg; *Ocular implant:* 4.5 mg; *Powder for injection:* 500 mg/vial

DOSAGE

• **IV INFUSION, CAPSULES**

CMV retinitis.

Induction treatment: 5 mg/kg IV over 1 hr q 12 hr for 14–21 days in clients with normal renal function. Do not use PO treatment for induction. **Maintenance, IV:** 5 mg/kg over 1 hr by IV infusion daily for 7 days or 6 mg/kg/day for 5 days each week. Dosage must be reduced in clients with renal impairment. **Maintenance, PO:** 1,000 mg t.i.d. with food. Or, 500 mg 6 times/day q 3 hr with food during waking hours.

Prevention of CMV retinitis in those with advanced HIV infection and normal renal function.

1,000 mg t.i.d. with food.

Prophylaxis of CMV disease in transplant clients.

Initial dose, IV: 5 mg/kg over 1 hr q 12 hr for 7–14 days in those with normal renal function. **Maintenance:** 5 mg/kg/day on 7 days each week (or 6 mg/kg/day on 5 days each week). The PO prophylactic dose is 1,000 mg t.i.d. with food.

In renal impairment, the following dosages are recommended. **IV. C_{CR} 50–69 mL/min:** Induction dose of 2.5 mg/kg q 12 hr and maintenance dose of 2.5 mg/kg q 24 hr; **C_{CR} 25–49 mL/min:** Induction dose of 2.5 mg/kg q 24 hr and maintenance dose of 1.25

mg/kg q 24 hr; **C_{CR} 10–24 mL/min:** Induction dose of 1.25 mg/kg q24 hr and maintenance dose of 0.625 mg/kg q 24 hr; **C_{CR} less than 10 mL/min:** Induction dose of 1.25 mg/kg three times/week following hemodialysis and maintenance dose of 0.625 mg/kg three times/week following hemodialysis. **PO. C_{CR} 50–69 mL/min:** 1,500mg once daily or 500 mg t.i.d.; **C_{CR} 25–49 mL/min:** 1,000 mg once daily or 500 mg b.i.d.; **C_{CR} 10–24 mL/min:** 500 mg once daily; **C_{CR} less than 10 mL/min:** 500 mg 3 times/week after hemodialysis.

G

NURSING CONSIDERATIONS

SEE ALSO *NURSING CONSIDERATIONS* FOR *ANTIVIRAL AGENTS*.

ADMINISTRATION/STORAGE

1. Use capsules only for whom the risk of a more rapid progression of the disease is offset by the benefit of avoiding daily IV infusions.

IV 2. Reconstitute by injecting 10 mL sterile water for injection followed by shaking. Discard if particulate matter or discoloration is noted. Parabens is incompatible with ganciclovir; do not use bacteriostatic water for injection for reconstitution.

3. IV infusion concentrations greater than 10 mg/mL are not recommended. Further reconstitute ganciclovir with 100 mL of any of the following solutions: D5W, RL or Ringer's solution, 0.9% NaCl. Infuse over 1 hr. Doses greater than 6 mg/kg infused over 1 hr may result in increased toxicity.

4. Due to the high pH (9–11) of reconstituted ganciclovir, do not give IM or SC. Do not give by IV bolus or rapid IV injection.

5. To minimize phlebitis or pain at the injection site, give into veins with an adequate blood flow to allow rapid dilution and distribution.

6. Do not exceed 1.25 mg/kg/day in clients undergoing hemodialysis.

7. The reconstituted solution is stable for 12 hr at room temperature.

8. Follow guidelines for handling and disposal of cytotoxic drugs. Avoid inhalation and contact with skin. Wear latex gloves and safety glasses and mix under a biologic hood.

ASSESSMENT

1. Document onset, characteristics of symptoms, and any treatments.

2. Determine CMV retinitis by indirect ophthalmoscopy.

3. Assess orientation and mentation levels.

4. Monitor CBC and renal function studies; reduce dose with impaired renal function. Granulocytopenia and thrombocytopenia are side effects of drug therapy; do not administer if neutrophil count drops below 500 cells/mm^3 or the platelet count falls below 25,000/mm^3. Concomitant therapy with zidovudine may increase neutropenia.

5. Monitor I&O. Ensure adequate hydration before/during IV therapy.

6. May experience pain/phlebitis at infusion site because pH of *diluted* solution is high (pH 9–11). Follow administration guidelines carefully.

7. Review list of drug interactions; some may induce renal failure and have additive toxicity if given during ganciclovir therapy.

CLIENT/FAMILY TEACHING

1. Drug is not a cure; is used to control symptoms.

2. Drug therapy should not be interrupted unless deemed necessary by provider; a relapse may occur.

3. Take PO ganciclovir with food to increase bioavailability.

4. Report any dizziness, confusion, and/or seizures immediately.

5. Use protection (sunglasses, clothing/hat, sunscreen) with sun exposure to prevent photosensitivity reaction.

6. Report for scheduled labs; results may require adjustment of dose or discontinuation of therapy.

7. Have regular ophthalmologic examinations because retinitis may progress to blindness (retinal detachment). With intraocular implant identify side effects that require immediate reporting.

8. May impair fertility; determine if candidate for sperm/egg harvesting.

9. During and for 90 days following drug therapy, women of childbearing age should use safe contraception and men should practice barrier contraception.

10. Report any unusual behavior or altered thought processes.

OUTCOMES/EVALUATE

• CMV prophylaxis in transplant and at-risk clients
• ↓ Progression of CMV retinitis
• Prevention of CMV retinitis in those with advanced HIV infection

Ganirelix acetate

(**gan**-ih-**REL**-icks)

PREGNANCY CATEGORY: X
CLASSIFICATION(S):
Gonadotropin-releasing hormone antagonist
Rx: Antagon

ACTION/KINETICS

Synthetic decapeptide that antagonizes gonadotropin-releasing hormone (GnRH). Acts by competitively blocking GnRH receptors in the pituitary gland leading to a rapid, reversible suppression of gonadotropin secretion. When discontinued, pituitary LH and FSH levels fully recover within 48 hr. **Steady state:** Within 3 days. Metabolized to peptides. Excreted in both the feces and urine. **t½, elimination:** 16.2 hr after multiple doses.

USES

Infertility treatment to inhibit premature LH surges in women undergoing controlled ovarian stimulation.

CONTRAINDICATIONS

Hypersensitivity to ganirelix or any of its components, hypersensitivity to GnRH or GnRH analogs, known or suspected pregnancy. Lactation.

SPECIAL CONCERNS

Use with caution in hypersensitivity to GnRH. Packaging of the product contains natural rubber latex, which may cause allergic reactions.

SIDE EFFECTS

Abdominal pain (gynecological), fetal death, headache, ovarian hyperstimulation syndrome, vaginal bleeding, injection site reaction, nausea, abdominal pain (GI).

LABORATORY TEST CONSIDERATIONS

↑ Neutrophils. ↓ Hematocrit, total bilirubin.

DRUG INTERACTIONS

Because ganirelix suppresses secretion of pituitary gonadotropins, dosage adjustments of exogenous gonadotropins may be necessary when used during controlled ovarian hyperstimulation.

HOW SUPPLIED

Injection: 250 mcg/0.5 mL

DOSAGE

• **SC ONLY**

Infertility treatment.

Initiate FSH therapy on day 2 or 3 of the cycle (may reduce exogenous FSH requirement). Give ganirelix, 250 mcg, SC once daily during the early to mid follicular phase. Continue ganirelix treatment daily until the day of chorionic gonadotropion (HCG) treatment. When a sufficient number of follicles of adequate size are present (assess by ultrasound), give HCG to finalize maturation of follicles.

NURSING CONSIDERATIONS

ADMINISTRATION/STORAGE

1. The most convenient sites for SC administration are in the upper thigh or in the abdomen around the navel.
2. Swab the injection site with disinfectant. Clean about 2 inches around the point where the needle will be inserted. Let the disinfectant dry a minute or more before proceeding.
3. Pinch up a large area of skin between the finger and thumb. Insert the needle at the base of the pinched-up skin at a 45–90° angle to the skin surface.
4. When the needle is positioned correctly, it will be difficult to draw back on the plunger. If the needle tip penetrates a vein (if blood is drawn into the syringe), withdraw the needle slightly and reposition the needle without removing it from the skin. Alternatively, remove the needle and use a new, sterile, prefilled syringe.
5. Once the needle is positioned correctly, depress the plunger slowly and

steadily so the solution is correctly injected and the skin is not damaged.
6. Pull the syringe out quickly and apply pressure to the site with a swab containing disinfectant. The site should stop bleeding within 1 or 2 min.
7. Use the sterile, prefilled syringe only once and dispose of it correctly.
8. Store the syringes at 25°C (77°F). Protect from light.

ASSESSMENT

1. Note indications for therapy, other medical conditions and duration of infertility.
2. Use cautiously in gonadotropin-releasing hormone (GnRH) hypersensitivity.
3. Ensure not pregnant.
4. Product packaging contains latex.

CLIENT/FAMILY TEACHING

1. Therapy requires SC administration daily during early to mid follicular phases after initial FSH therapy or day 2 or 3 of cycle. It must be continued until day of HCG administration.
2. Follows guidelines for administration under administration/storage and/or review package insert for proper administration procedure.
3. An ultrasound is used to check for sufficient number and size of follicles.
4. May experience abdominal pain, fetal death, headache, ovarian hyperstimulation syndrome, vaginal bleeding, nausea and injection site pain.
5. Not for use in pregnancy as may cause fetal loss.
6. Therapy requires a long term committment for F/U and medical visits from user.

OUTCOMES/EVALUATE

Inhibition of premature LH surges during controlled ovarian stimulation, desired pregnancy

Gatifloxacin

(**gat**-ih-**FLOX**-ah-sin)

PREGNANCY CATEGORY: C
CLASSIFICATION(S):
Antibiotic, quinolone
Rx: Tequin

SEE ALSO *ANTI-INFECTIVE DRUGS.*

ACTION/KINETICS

Well absorbed after PO use. **Peak plasma levels:** 1–2 hr after PO. The PO and IV routes are interchangeable. Steady-state levels are reached by the third daily PO or IV dose. **Mean steady-state peak and trough plasma levels after 400 mg once daily:** About 4.2 mcg/mL and 0.4 mcg/mL, respectively after PO and 4.6 mcg/mL and 0.4 mcg/mL, respectively, after IV. Widely distributed throughout the body. **t½, PO:** 7.1 hr after multiple doses of 400 mg; **t½, IV:** 13.9 hr after multiple doses of 400 mg. Excreted primarily unchanged by the kidneys.

USES

(1) Acute bacterial exacerbation of chronic bronchitis due to *Streptococcus pneumoniae, Haemophilus influenzae, Haemophilus parainfluenzae, Moraxella catarrhalis,* or *Staphylococcus aureus.* (2) Acute sinusitis due to *S. pneumoniae* or *H. influenzae.* (3) Community-acquired pneumonia due to *S. pneumoniae, H. influenze, H. parainfluenzae, M. catarrhalis, S. aureus, Mycoplasma pneumoniae, Chlamydia pneumoniae,* or *Legionella pneumoniae.* (4) Uncomplicated UTIs (cystitis) or complicated UTIs due to *Escherichia coli, Klebsiella pneumoniae,* or *Proteus mirabilis.* (5) Pyelonephritis due to *E. coli.* (6) Uncomplicated urethral and cervical gonorrhea due to *Neisseria gonorrhoeae.* (7) Acute, uncomplicated rectal infections in women due to *N. gonorrhoeae. Investigational:* Atypical pneumonia, uncomplicated skin and soft tissue infections, chronic prostatitis.

CONTRAINDICATIONS

Use with drugs that prolong the QTc interval, in clients with uncorrected hypokalemia, and in those receiving Class IA (e.g., quinidine, procainamide) or Class III (e.g., amiodarone, sotalol) antiarrhythmics.

SPECIAL CONCERNS

Reduce dosage in clients with a C_{CR} less than 40 mL/min, including those requiring hemodialysis or continuous ambulatory peritoneal dialysis. Use with caution with antidepressants, antipsychotics, or erythromycin or in those with bradycardia or acute myocardial ischemia. Safety and efficacy in children, adolescents (less than 18 years of age), pregnant women, and lactating women have not been established.

SIDE EFFECTS

CNS: Tremors, restlessness, lightheadedness, confusion, hallucinations, paranoia, depression, nightmares, insomnia, paresthesia, vertigo. **GI:** Abdominal pain, constipation, dyspepsia, glossitis, oral moniliaisis, stomatitis, mouth ulcer, vomiting, pseudomembranous colitis, hepatitis, jaundice, ***acute hepatic necrosis or failure.*** **Body as a whole:** Fever, chills, back pain, chest pain. **CV:** Vasculitis, palpitation, vasodilation. **Respiratory:** Dyspnea, pharyngitis, allergic pneumonitis. **Hypersensitivity:** ***Anaphylaxis, CV collapse, angioedema, acute respiratory distress, bronchospasm, shock,*** hypotension, seizure, loss of consciousness, tingling, shortness of breath, dyspnea, urticaria, itching, serious skin reactions. **Hematologic:** Hemolytic or aplastic anemia, thrombotic thrombocytopenic purpura, leukopenia, agranulocytosis, pancytopenia. **Dermatologic:** Rash, sweating, ***toxic epidermal necrolysis, Stevens-Johnson syndrome.*** **Musculoskeletal:** Arthralgia, myalgia. **GU:** Dysuria, hematuria, interstitial nephritis, acute renal insufficiency or failure. **Miscellaneous:** Serum sickness, peripheral edema, abnormal vision, taste perversion, tinnitus.

LABORATORY TEST CONSIDERATIONS

Hyper- or hypoglycemia, especially in diabetics receiving an oral hypoglycemic or insulin.

DRUG INTERACTIONS

Aluminum- or magnesium-containing antacids / ↓ Absorption of gatifloxacin
Digoxin / ↑ Risk of digoxin toxicity
Ferrous sulfate / ↓ Bioavailability of gatifloxacin
NSAIDs / ↑ Risk of CNS stimulation and convulsions
Probenecid / ↓ Bioavailability of gatifloxacin

HOW SUPPLIED

Solution for Injection, Premix Bags: 200 mg/100 mL, 400 mg/200 mL; *Solution for Injection, Single-use vial:* 200 mg/20 mL, 400 mg/40 mL; *Tablets:* 200 mg, 400 mg

DOSAGE

• IV INFUSION, TABLETS

Acute bacterial exacerbation of chronic bronchitis, complicated UTIs, acute pyelonephritis. A five-day course of therapy may be used for acute bacterial exacerbation of chronic bronchitis.

Adults: 400 mg once daily for 7–10 days.

Acute sinusitis.

Adults: 400 mg once daily for 10 days.

Community-acquired pneumonia.

Adults: 400 mg once daily for 7–14 days.

Uncomplicated UTIs (cystitis).

Adults: 400 mg as a single dose or 200 mg daily for 3 days.

Uncomplicated urethral gonorrhea in men, endocervical and rectal gonorrhea in women.

Single dose of 400 mg.

Atypical pneumonia.

400 mg/day for 14 days.

Uncomplicated skin and soft tissue infections.

400 mg/day for 7–10 days.

Chronic prostatitis.

200 mg PO b.i.d. for 14 days.

Adjust dosage as follows in clients with impaired renal function. **C_{CR} less than 40 mL/min: Initial,** 400 mg; **then,** 200 mg every day. **Hemodialysis: Initial,** 400 mg; **then,** 200 mg every day. **Continuous peritoneal dialysis: Initial,** 400 mg; **then,** 200 mg every day.

NURSING CONSIDERATIONS

SEE ALSO *NURSING CONSIDERATIONS FOR ANTI-INFECTIVE DRUGS.*

ADMINISTRATION/STORAGE

IV 1. Further dilute single-use vials with appropriate solution (see package insert) prior to IV administration.

2. Give by IV infusion over 60 min. Not to be given IM, IP, SC, or intrathecally.

3. Do not add additives or other medications to single-use gatifloxacin vials or through the same IV line. If the same IV line is used for sequential drug infusions, flush the line before and after infusion of gatifloxacin.

4. When diluted with compatible IV fluid to 2 mg/mL, solution is stable for 14 days when stored between 20–26°C (68–79°F) or when stored under refrigeration.
5. No dosage adjustment is needed when switching from IV to PO.

ASSESSMENT

1. Note indications for therapy, onset and characteristics of symptoms.
2. Assess for sensitivity to quinolones.
3. Note any congenital prolongation of the QTc interval.
4. Determine if prescribed therapy for heart rhythm disturbance; monitor digoxin levels if prescribed.
5. Assess electrolytes; avoid with hypokalemia and report if taking diuretics. Obtain C&S and CBC and monitor.

CLIENT/FAMILY TEACHING

1. Take as directed once daily at the same time each day.
2. Can take without regard for food, including milk and calcium-containing dietary supplements.
3. Take at least 4 hr before the administration of ferrous sulfate; dietary supplements containing zinc, magnesium, or iron; aluminum/magnesium-containing antacids; or didanosine buffered tablets, buffered solution, or buffered powder for oral suspension.
4. Complete prescription despite feeling better; report if S&S do not improve with therapy.
5. Avoid activities that require mental alertness until drug effects realized.
6. May cause GI upset, dizziness, and headaches.
7. Report any heart palpitations or fainting spells immediately.
8. Use reliable birth control.
9. Store away from children in a tightly sealed container at room temperature.

OUTCOMES/EVALUATE

Resolution of infection; symptomatic improvement

Gemcitabine hydrochloride

(jem-**SIGHT**-ah-been)

PREGNANCY CATEGORY: D

CLASSIFICATION(S):

Antineoplastic, miscellaneous

Rx: Gemzar

SEE ALSO *ANTINEOPLASTIC AGENTS.*

ACTION/KINETICS

A nucleoside analog that kills cells undegoing DNA synthesis (S-phase) and by blocking the progression of cells through the G1/S-phase boundary. Metabolized within cells by nucleoside kinases to the active gemcitabine diphosphate and triphosphate nucleosides. The diphosphate inhibits ribonucleotide reductase, which is responsible for catalyzing reactions that generate the deoxynucleoside triphosphate for DNA synthesis. Inhibition of the reductase enzyme causes a decrease in the levels of deoxynucleotides. The triphosphate competes with triphosphate nucleosides for incorporation into DNA, resulting in inhibition of DNA synthesis. DNA polymerase is not able to remove the gemcitabine nucleoside and repair the growing DNA strands. The metabolite of gemcitabine nucleoside is excreted through the urine.

USES

First-line treatment for locally advanced (nonresectable Stage II or Stage III) or metastatic (Stage IV) adenocarcinoma of the pancreas. Indicated for those who have been treated previously with 5-fluorouracil. First-line therapy, with cisplatin, for treatment of inoperable, locally advanced (Stage IIIA or IIIB), or metastatic (Stage IV) non-small cell lung cancer.

CONTRAINDICATIONS

Lactation.

SPECIAL CONCERNS

Use with caution in those with preexisting renal impairment or hepatic insufficiency. Safety and efficacy have not been determined in children.

SIDE EFFECTS

GI: N&V, diarrhea, constipation, stomatitis. **CNS:** Somnolence, mild to severe paresthesias, insomnia. **CV:** Arrhythmia, hypertension, ***MI, CVA.*** **Hematologic:** Anemia, leukopenia, neutropenia, thrombocytopenia, platelet transfusions. **Respiratory:** Dyspnea, bronchospasm, cough, rhinitis, parenchymal lung toxicity (rare). **Dermatologic:** Alopecia, macular or finely granular maculopapular pruritic eruptions, pruritus, hair loss (minimal). **Body as a whole:** Pain, fever, peripheral edema, flu syndrome (including fever), asthenia, chills, myalgia, sweating, malaise. **Miscellaneous:** ***Hemorrhage, sepsis,*** hemolytic uremic syndrome, infections, petechiae, ***anaphylaxis (rare).***

LABORATORY TEST CONSIDERATIONS

↑ ALT, AST, alkaline phosphatase, bilirubin, BUN, creatinine. Proteinuria, hematuria.

OD OVERDOSE MANAGEMENT

Symptoms: Myelosuppression, paresthesias, severe rash. *Treatment:* Monitor with appropriate blood counts. Supportive therapy as needed.

HOW SUPPLIED

Powder for injection, lyophilized: 20 mg/mL

DOSAGE

• **IV ONLY**

Adenocarcinoma of the pancreas.

Adults: 1,000 mg/m^2 given over 30 min once a week for up to 7 weeks (or until toxicity necessitates reducing or holding a dose). This is followed by a 1-week rest period. Subsequent cycles should consist of infusions once a week for 3 consecutive weeks out of 4. Those who complete the entire 7 weeks of initial therapy or a subsequent 3-week cycle at the 1,000-mg/m^2 dose may have the dose for subsequent cycles increased by 25% to 1,250 mg/m^2 provided that the absolute neutrophil count nadir exceeds 1,500 X 10^6/L and the platlet nadir exceeds 100,000 X 10^6/L and if nonhematologic toxicity has not been greater than World Health Organization Grade 1. If clients tolerate a dose of 1,250 mg/m^2 once weekly, the dose for the next cycle can be increased to 1,500 mg/m^2 provided the absolute neutrophil count and platelet nadirs are as defined above.

The dose should be reduced to 75% of the full dose if the absolute granulocyte count is 500–999 × 10^6/L and the platelet count is 50,000–99,000 × 10^6/L. The dose should be held if the absolute granulocyte count falls below 500 × 10^6/L and the platelet count falls below 50,000 × 10^6/L.

Non-small cell lung cancer.

Two schedules are used. (1) Four-week schedule: Gemcitabine, 1,000 mg/m^2 over 30 min on days 1, 8, and 15 of each 28-day cycle. Give cisplatin, IV, 100 mg/m^2 on day 1 after gemcitabine. (2) Three-week schedule: Gemcitabine, 1,250 mg/m^2 over 30 min on days 1 and 8 of each 21-day cycle. Give cisplatin, IV, 100 mg/m^2 after gemcitabine on day 1.

G

NURSING CONSIDERATIONS

SEE ALSO *NURSING CONSIDERATIONS* FOR *ANTINEOPLASTIC AGENTS*.

ADMINISTRATION/STORAGE

IV 1. To reconstitute the drug, use 0.9% NaCl injection without preservatives. The maximum concentration upon reconstitution is 40 mg/mL; greater concentrations may cause incomplete dissolution.

2. Give over 30 min; prolonging the infusion time beyond 60 min and more frequent administration than once weekly increases toxicity.

3. To reconstitute, add 5 mL of 0.9% NaCl to the 200-mg vial or 25 mL to the 1-g vial. Shake to dissolve. This results in a concentration of 40 mg/mL which may be further diluted, if needed, with 0.9% NaCl to concentrations as low as 0.1 mg/mL.

4. Do not refrigerate reconstituted drug as crystallization may occur. Store diluted product at controlled room temperatures of 20–25°C (68–77°F). Reconstituted solutions are stable at these temperatures for 24 hr.

ASSESSMENT

1. Document disease stage, onset, duration of symptoms, organ(s) involved, and other agents trialed.

2. Obtain CBC, liver and renal function studies. Monitor CBC prior to each dose and liver and renal function tests periodically; causes thrombocytopenia and myelosuppression. Nadir: 1 week.

CLIENT/FAMILY TEACHING

1. Anticipate IV therapy once weekly over 30 min for up to 7 weeks; then weekly for 3 out of every 4 weeks.
2. May experience fever and flu-like symptoms as well as a rash involving trunk and extremities.
3. Report any evidence of blood or pain with voiding.
4. Use reliable birth control during and for several months following therapy; can cause fetal harm.

OUTCOMES/EVALUATE

Suppression of malignant cell proliferation

G

Gemfibrozil

(jem-**FIH**-broh-zill)

PREGNANCY CATEGORY: C
CLASSIFICATION(S):
Antihyperlipidemic, fibric acid derivative
Rx: Lopid
🍁**Rx:** Apo-Gemfibrozil, Gen-Gemfibrozil, Novo-Gemfibrozil, Nu-Gemfibrozil, PMS-Gemfibrozil

ACTION/KINETICS

Gemfibrozil, a fibric acid derivative, decreases triglycerides, cholesterol, and VLDL and increases HDL; LDL levels either decrease or do not change. Also, decreases hepatic triglyceride production by inhibiting peripheral lipolysis and decreasing extraction of free fatty acids by the liver. Also, gemfibrozil decreases VLDL synthesis by inhibiting synthesis of VLDL carrier apolipoprotein B as well as inhibits peripheral lipolysis and decreases hepatic extraction of free fatty acids (thus decreasing hepatic triglyceride production). May be beneficial in inhibiting development of atherosclerosis. **Onset:** 2–5 days. **Peak plasma levels:** 1–2 hr; **t½:** 1.5 hr. Metabolized in the liver with nearly 70% excreted in the urine.

USES

(1) Hypertriglyceridemia (type IV and type V hyperlipidemia) unresponsive to dietary control or in clients who are at risk of pancreatitis and abdominal pain. (2) Reduce risk of coronary heart disease in clients with type IIb hyperlipidemia who have not responded to diet, weight loss, exercise, and other drug therapy.

CONTRAINDICATIONS

Gallbladder disease, primary biliary cirrhosis, hepatic or renal dysfunction. Lactation.

SPECIAL CONCERNS

Safety and efficacy have not been established in children. The dose may have to be reduced in geriatric clients due to age-related decreases in renal function.

SIDE EFFECTS

GI: Cholelithiasis, abdominal or epigastric pain, N&V, diarrhea, dyspepsia, constipation, acute appendicitis, colitis, pancreatitis, cholestatic jaundice, hepatoma. **CNS:** Dizziness, headache, fatigue, vertigo, somnolence, paresthesia, hypesthesia, depression, confusion, syncope, peripheral neuritis, ***seizures.*** **CV:** Atrial fibrillation, extrasystole, peripheral vascular disease, ***intracerebral hemorrhage.*** **Hematopoietic:** Anemia, leukopenia, eosinophilia, thrombocytopenia, bone marrow hypoplasia. **Musculoskeletal:** Painful extremities, arthralgia, myalgia, myopathy, myositis, myasthenia, rhabdomyolysis, synovitis. **Allergic:** Urticaria, lupus-like syndrome, angioedema, ***laryngeal edema,*** vasculitis, ***anaphylaxis.*** **Dermatologic:** Eczema, dermatitis, pruritus, skin rashes, exfoliative dermatitis, alopecia. **GU:** Impotence, decreased libido, decreased male fertility, impaired renal function, UTI. **Ophthalmic:** Blurred vision, retinal edema, cataracts. **Miscellaneous:** Increased chance of viral and bacterial infections, taste perversion, weight loss.

LABORATORY TEST CONSIDERATIONS

↑ AST, ALT, LDH, CPK, alkaline phosphatase, bilirubin. Hypokalemia, hyperglycemia. Positive antinuclear antibody. ↓ Hemoglobin, WBCs, hematocrit.

DRUG INTERACTIONS

Anticoagulants, oral / ↑ Anticoagulant effects; adjust dosage

Cyclosporine / ↓ Cyclosporine effect
Lovastatin / Possible rhabdomyolysis
Simvastatin / Possible rhabdomyolysis
Sulfonylureas / ↑ Hypoglycemic effect

HOW SUPPLIED

Tablet: 600 mg

DOSAGE

• **TABLETS**

Adults: 600 mg b.i.d. 30 min before the morning and evening meal. Dosage has not been established in children. Discontinue if significant improvement not observed within 3 months.

NURSING CONSIDERATIONS

SEE ALSO *NURSING CONSIDERATIONS* FOR *CLOFIBRATE*.

ASSESSMENT

1. Document serum levels and note any previous therapy utilized. (Drug usually reserved until triglycerides greater than 500 mg/dL).
2. Assess compliance with therapeutic regimens and life-style changes including restriction of fat in diet, weight reduction, regular exercise, and avoidance of alcohol.

CLIENT/FAMILY TEACHING

1. Take 30 min before meals.
2. Take as directed; continue to follow prescribed dietary guidelines and regular exercise program to reduce risk factors.
3. Use caution when driving or performing other dangerous tasks until drug effects realized; may experience dizziness or blurred vision.
4. Report any unusual bruising or bleeding. If also on anticoagulant therapy, a reduction in anticoagulant is indicated with this therapy.
5. Limit intake of alcohol.
6. Report any muscle pain/cramps, RUQ abdominal pain or change in stool color or consistency.
7. Report any S&S of gallstones, such as abdominal pain and vomiting.

OUTCOMES/EVALUATE

↓ Serum cholesterol and triglyceride levels

Gemtuzumab ozogamicin

(gem-**TOO**-zeh-mab oh-zoh-**GAM**-ih-sin)

PREGNANCY CATEGORY: D
CLASSIFICATION(S):
Antineoplastic, monoclonal antibody
Rx: Mylotarg

ACTION/KINETICS

Composed of a recombinant humanized IgG_4 kappa antibody conjugated with a cytotoxic antitumor antibiotic (calicheamicin). Binding of the anti-CD33 antigen forms a complex that is internalized. Upon internalization, the calicheamicin derivative is released inside the lysosomes of the myeloid cell. The released calicheamicin derivative binds to DNA in the minor groove resulting in DNA double strand breaks and cell death. The drug is cytotoxic to the CD33 positive HL-60 human leukemia cell line. There is significant myelosuppression but this is reversible because pluripotent hematopoietic stem cells are spared. **t½, elimination, after first dose:** About 45 hr for total and 100 hr for unconjugated calicheamicin. **t½, elimination, after second dose:** About 60 hr for total calicheamicin, while t½ for unconjugated did not change from the first dose. Appears to be metabolized by liver microsomes.

USES

Treatment of CD33 positive acute myeloid leukemia in first relapse in those 60 years or older who are not candidates for cytotoxic chemotherapy.

CONTRAINDICATIONS

Hypersensitivity to gemtuzumab ozogamicin or any of its components: anti-CD33 antibody, calicheamicin derivatives, or inactive ingredients. Lactation.

SPECIAL CONCERNS

Severe myelosuppression will occur in all clients given the recommended dose. Use with caution in hepatic impairment. Clients with a WBC count of

>30,000/µL may be at an increased risk of a drug-related severe pulmonary event. Safety and efficacy have not been determined in children.

SIDE EFFECTS

Myelosuppression: Grade 3 or 4 neutropenia, anemia, and/or thrombocytopenia. **GI:** Mucositis, stomatitis, hepatotoxicity, N&V, diarrhea, anorexia, constipation, dyspepsia. **CV:** Bleeding, including epistaxis; ***hemorrhage***, hyper/hypotension, tachycardia. **CNS:** Depression, dizziness, insomnia. **Respiratory:** Dyspnea, increased cough, pharyngitis, pneumonia, rales, rhonchi, change in breath sounds, rhinitis. **Dermatologic:** Herpes simplex, rash, local reaction, peripheral edema, ecchymosis, petechiae. **GU:** Hematuria, vaginal hemorrhage. **Infusion reactions: *Severe hypersensitivity, anaphylaxis, fatal pulmonary events,*** tumor lysis syndrome. **Body as a whole:** Infections (grade 3 or 4), including opportunistic infections; arthralgia, asthenia, chills, fever, neutropenic fever, pain, ***sepsis.*** **Miscellaneous:** Enlarged abdomen, abdominal pain, back pain, headache.

LABORATORY TEST CONSIDERATIONS

↑ ALT, AST, bilirubin, LDH. Hypokalemia, hypomagnesemia. Changes in hemoglobin, total absolute neutrophils, WBCs, lymphocytes, platelet count, PT/PTT.

HOW SUPPLIED

Powder for injection, lyophilized: 5 mg

DOSAGE

• **IV**

Acute myeloid leukemia.

9 mg/m² as a 2-hr infusion. Give the following prophylactic medications 1-hr before gemtuzumab: diphenhydramine, 50 mg PO and acetaminophen, 650–1000 mg PO. Thereafter, 2 additional doses of acetaminophen, 650–1000 mg PO q 4 hr as needed. The recommended treatment course for gemtuzumab is a total of 2 doses, 14 days apart.

NURSING CONSIDERATIONS

ADMINISTRATION/STORAGE

IV 1. Full recovery from hematologic toxicity is not a requirement for administration of a second dose of gemtuzumab.

2. Protect from direct and indirect sunlight and unshielded fluorescent light during preparation and administration of the infusion.

3. Prepare in a biologic safety hood with the flourescent light off.

4. Prior to reconstitution, allow the drug vials to come to room temperature.

5. Reconstitute each vial with 5 mL sterile water for injection, using sterile syringes. Gently swirl each vial. The final concentration is 1 mg/mL.

6. Inspect visually for particulate matter and discoloration following reconstitution and prior to administration.

7. Withdraw the desired volume from each vial and inject into a 100 mL IV bag of 0.9% NaCl injection. Place the 100 mL bag into a UV protectant bag. Use the resulting drug solution in the IV bag immediately.

8. Do not give as an IV push or bolus.

9. Give over 2-hr. Use a separate IV line equipped with a low protein-binding 1.2 micron terminal filter. May be given peripherally or through a central line.

10. To reduce the risk of a severe pulmonary event, consider reducing the peripheral WBC count with hydroxyurea therapy or leukapheresis before giving gemtuzumab.

11. Store refrigerated at 2–8°C (36–46°F) and protect from light. While in the vial, the reconstituted drug may be stored refrigerated and protected from light for 8 hr or less.

ASSESSMENT

1. Note indications for therapy, date of first treatment for CD33 AML, and why client is not candidate for cytotoxic chemotherapy.

2. Remember to premedicate with diphenhydramine and acetaminophen to help control side effects.

3. Monitor CBC, lytes, uric acid, and LFTs; use cautiously with any liver impairment.

4. Ensure adequate hydration and medication (allopurinol) to prevent hyperuricemia.

5. Assess for myelosuppression and thrombocytopenia; nadir day 35-45.

CLIENT/FAMILY TEACHING

1. Report any fever, sore throat, or S&S infections.
2. Avoid hazardous activities and tasks; may experience dizziness and confusion. Protect from injury during bone marrow suppression.
3. Report any unusual bruising or bleeding or dark tarry stools.
4. Avoid immunizations during therapy as drug lowers body resistance. Avoid persons with disease and those who have recently received live virus vaccines (polio).

OUTCOMES/EVALUATE

Hematologic improvement/recovery with AML

Gentamicin sulfate

(jen-tah-**MY**-sin)

PREGNANCY CATEGORY: C
CLASSIFICATION(S):
Antibiotic, aminoglycoside
Rx: Garamycin Cream or Ointment, Garamycin IV Piggyback, Garamycin Ophthalmic Ointment, Garamycin Ophthalmic Solution, Genoptic Ophthalmic Liquifilm, Genoptic S.O.P. Ophthalmic, Gentacidin Ophthalmic, Gentak Ophthalmic, Gentamicin, Gentamicin Ophthalmic, G-myticin Cream or Ointment , Garamycin, Gentamicin Sulfate IV Piggyback, Pediatric Gentamicin Sulfate
✱Rx: Alcomicin, Diogent, Garatec, Minims Gentamcin, Scheinpharm Gentamicin

SEE ALSO *AMINOGLYCOSIDES*.

ACTION/KINETICS

Therapeutic serum levels: IM, 4–8 mcg/mL. **Toxic serum levels:** >12 mcg/mL (peak) and >2 mcg/mL (trough). Prolonged serum levels above 12 mcg/mL should be avoided. **t½:** 2 hr. Can be used with carbenicillin to treat serious *Pseudomonas* infections; do not mix these drugs in the same flask as carbenicillin will inactivate gentamicin.

USES

Systemic: Serious infections caused by *Pseudomonas aeruginosa, Proteus, Klebsiella, Enterobacter, Serratia, Citrobacter,* and *Staphylococcus*. Infections include bacterial neonatal sepsis, bacterial septicemia, and serious infections of the skin, bone, soft tissue (including burns), urinary tract, GI tract (including peritonitis), and CNS (including meningitis). Should be considered as initial therapy in suspected or confirmed gram-negative infections. In combination with carbenicillin for treating life-threatening infections due to *P. aeruginosa*. In combination with penicillin for treating endocarditis caused by group D streptococci. In combination with penicillin for treating suspected bacterial sepsis or staphylococcal pneumonia in the neonate. Intrathecal administration is used in combination with systemic gentamicin for treating meningitis, ventriculitis, or other serious CNS infections due to *Pseudomonas*. *Investigational:* Pelvic inflammatory disease.

Ophthalmic: Ophthalmic infections due to *Staphylococcus, S. aureus, Streptococcus pneumoniae,* beta-hemolytic streptococci, *Corynebacterium* species, *Streptococcus pyogenes, Escherichia coli, Haemophilus influenzae, H. aegyptius, H. ducreyi, Klebsiella pneumoniae, Neisseria gonorrhoeae, Proteus* species, *Acinetobacter calcoaceticus, Enterobacter aerogenes, P. aeruginosa, Serratia marcescens, Moraxella lacunata.*

Topical: Prevention of infections following minor cuts, wounds, burns, and skin abrasions. Treatment of primary or secondary skin infections. Treatment of infected skin cysts and other skin abscesses when preceded by incision and drainage to permit adequate contact between the drug and the infecting bacteria, infected stasis and other skin ulcers, infected superficial burns, paronychia, infected insect bites and stings, infected lacerations and abrasions and wounds from minor surgery.

CONTRAINDICATIONS

Ophthalmic use to treat dendritic keratitis, vaccinia, varicella, mycobacterial infections of the eye, fungal diseases of the eye, use with steroids after uncomplicated removal of a corneal foreign body.

SPECIAL CONCERNS

Use with caution in premature infants and neonates. Ophthalmic ointments may retard corneal epithelial healing.

ADDITIONAL SIDE EFFECTS

Muscle twitching, numbness, ***seizures,*** increased BP, alopecia, purpura, pseudotumor cerebri. Photosensitivity when used topically. **After ophthalmic use:** Transient irritation, burning, stinging, itching, inflammation, angioneurotic edema, urticaria, vesicular and maculopapular dermatitis, mydriasis, conjunctival paresthesia, conjunctival hyperemia, nonspecific conjunctivitis, conjunctival epithelial defects, lid itching and swelling, bacterial/fungal corneal ulcers.

ADDITIONAL DRUG INTERACTIONS

With carbenicillin or ticarcillin, gentamicin may result in increased effect when used for *Pseudomonas* infections.

HOW SUPPLIED

Cream, Topical: 0.1%; *Injection:* 10 mg/mL, 40 mg/mL; *Ointment, Ophthalmic:* 3 mg/g; *Ointment, Topical:* 1%; *Solution, Ophthalmic:* 3 mg/mL

DOSAGE

• IM (USUAL), IV

Adults with normal renal function.

Infections.

1 mg/kg q 8 hr, up to 5 mg/kg/day in life-threatening infections; **children:** 2–2.5 mg/kg q 8 hr; **infants and neonates:** 2.5 mg/kg q 8 hr; **premature infants or neonates less than 1 week of age:** 2.5 mg/kg q 12 hr. Therapy may be required for 7–10 days.

Prevention of bacterial endocarditis, dental or respiratory tract procedures.

Adults: 1.5 mg/kg gentamicin (not to exceed 80 mg) plus 1 g ampicillin, each IM or IV, 30–60 min before the procedure; one additional dose of each can be given 8 hr later (alternative: penicillin V, 1 g PO, 6 hr after initial dose).

Prophylaxis of bacterial endocarditis in GI or GU tract procedures or surgery.

Adults: 1.5 mg/kg gentamicin (not to exceed 80 mg) plus 2 g ampicillin, each IM or IV, 30–60 min before procedure; dose should be repeated 8 hr later. **Children:** 2 mg/kg gentamicin plus penicillin G, 30,000 units/kg, or ampicillin, 50 mg/kg in same dosage interval as for adults. Pediatric dosage should not exceed single or 24-hr adult doses.

NOTE: In clients allergic to penicillin, vancomycin, 1 g IV given slowly over 1 hr, may be substituted; the dose of vancomycin should be repeated 8–12 hr later. **Adults with impaired renal function:** To calculate interval (hr) between doses, multiply serum creatinine level (mg/100 mL) by 8.

• IV

Septicemia.

Initially: 1–2 mg/kg infused over 30–60 min; **then,** maintenance doses may be administered.

• INTRATHECAL

Meningitis.

Use only the intrathecal preparation. Adults, usual: 4–8 mg/day; **children and infants 3 months and older:** 1–2 mg/day

Pelvic inflammatory disease.

Initial: 2 mg/kg IV; **then,** 1.5 mg/kg t.i.d. plus clindamycin, 500 mg IV q.i.d. Continue for at least 4 days and at least 48 hr after client improves. Continue clindamycin, 450 mg PO q.i.d. for 10–14 days.

• OPHTHALMIC SOLUTION (0.3%)

Acute infections.

Initially: 1–2 gtt in conjunctival sac q 15–30 min; **then,** as infection improves, reduce frequency.

Moderate infections.

1–2 gtt in conjunctival sac 4–6 times/day.

Trachoma.

2 gtt in each eye b.i.d.–q.i.d.; treatment should be continued for up to 1–2 months.

• OPHTHALMIC OINTMENT (0.3%)

Depending on the severity of infection, ½-in. ribbon from q 3–4 hr to 2–3 times/day.

• TOPICAL CREAM/OINTMENT (0.1%)

Apply 3–4 times/day to affected area. The area may be covered with a sterile bandage.

NURSING CONSIDERATIONS

SEE ALSO *NURSING CONSIDERATIONS* FOR *AMINOGLYCOSIDES*.

ADMINISTRATION/STORAGE

1. When used intrathecally, the usual site is the lumbar area.

IV 2. For intermittent IV administration, dilute adult dose in 50–200 mL of NSS or D5W and administer over a 30–120-min period; use less volume for infants and children.

3. Do not mix with other drugs for parenteral use.

4. For parenteral use, the duration of treatment is 7–10 days; a longer course may be required for severe or complicated infections.

ASSESSMENT

1. Document type, onset and characteristics of symptoms.

2. Obtain renal function studies, CBC, and appropriate specimens for culture.

3. With eye disorders, note baseline ophthalmologic assessments.

4. Assess for tinnitus, vertigo, or hearing losses during therapy. Persistently increased gentamicin levels have been associated with 8th CN dysfunction. Monitor levels and ensure adequate hydration.

CLIENT/FAMILY TEACHING

1. Review the appropriate method and frequency for administration. Wash hands before and after treatment; prepare site and apply as directed.

2. With topical administration:

- Remove crusts of impetigo contagiosa before applying the cream or ointment to permit maximum contact between antibiotic and infection.
- Apply cream or ointment gently and cover with gauze dressing if desirable or as ordered.
- Avoid direct exposure to sunlight as photosensitivity reaction may occur.
- Avoid further contamination of infected skin.

3. Identify symptoms and wound changes that require medical attention; i.e., pain, redness, swelling, increased drainage or odor.

4. Report any evidence of visual impairment, vertigo, dizziness, hearing impairment, or worsening of symptoms.

5. Avoid vaccinia during treatment.

OUTCOMES/EVALUATE

- Resolution of infection
- Therapeutic serum drug levels 4–8 mcg/mL; (peak 5–10 mcg/mL trough 1–2 mcg/mL)

Glatiramer acetate

(glah-**TER**-ah-mer)

PREGNANCY CATEGORY: B
CLASSIFICATION(S):
Immunosuppressant
Rx: Copaxone

ACTION/KINETICS

May act by modifying immune processes responsible for pathology of multiple sclerosis. Some of drug enters lymphatic circulation reaching regional lymph nodes. MRI gadolinium-enhanced lesions are reduced following treatment.

USES

Reduce frequency of relapsing-remitting multiple sclerosis.

CONTRAINDICATIONS

Hypersensitivity to glatiramer or mannitol.

SPECIAL CONCERNS

Use with caution during lactation. Safety and efficacy have not been determined in children less than 18 years of age. May interfere with useful immune function.

SIDE EFFECTS

Side effects listed are those with incidence of 1% or more. **Immediate-post injection reaction:** Flushing, chest pain, palpitations, anxiety, dyspnea, laryngeal constriction, urticaria. **CNS:** Anxiety, hypertonia, tremor, vertigo, agitation, foot drop, nervousness, nystagmus, speech disorder, confusion, abnormal dreams, emotional lability, stupor, migraine. **GI:** Nausea, diarrhea, anorexia, vomiting, GI disorder, abdominal pain, gastroenteritis, bowel urgency, oral moniliasis, salivary gland enlargement, tooth caries, ulcerative stomatitis. **CV:** Vasodilation, palpitations, tachycardia, syncope, hypertension. **Body as a whole:** Infection, asthenia, pain, transient chest pain, flu syndrome, back pain, fever, neck pain, face edema, bacterial infection, chills, cyst, headache, injection site ecchymosis, accidental injury, neck rigidity, malaise, injection site edema or atrophy, abscess, peripheral edema, edema, weight gain. **Dermatologic:** Rash, pruritus, sweating, herpes simplex, erythema, urticaria, skin nodule, eczema, herpes zoster, pustular rash, skin atrophy and warts. **GU:** Urinary urgency, vaginal monoliasis, dysmenorrhea, amenorrhea, hematuria, impotence, menorrhagia, suspicious Pap smear, vaginal hemorrhage. **Hematologic:** Ecchymosis, lymphadenopathy. **Respiratory:** Dyspnea, allergic rhinitis, bronchitis, laryngismus, hyperventilation.**At injection site:** Pain, erythema, inflammation, pruritus, mass, induration, welt, hemorrhage, urticaria. **Miscellaneous:** Ear pain, eye disorder, arthralgia.

DRUG INTERACTIONS

H Do not give echinacea with glatiramer.

HOW SUPPLIED

Powder for Injection: 20 mg

DOSAGE

• **SC**

Multiple sclerosis.

Adults: 20 mg/day SC.

NURSING CONSIDERATIONS

ADMINISTRATION/STORAGE

1. SC sites include arms, abdomen, hips, and thighs.
2. Reconstitute with diluent provided (sterile water for injection). Gently swirl vial after diluent is added. Let stand at room temperature until solid material is dissolved.
3. Use reconstituted drug immediately; contains no preservative. Before reconstitution store at 2–8°C (36–46°F).

ASSESSMENT

1. Document age at onset, frequency of exacerbations, degree of physical disability, and other treatments.
2. RRMS is characterized by recurrent attacks of neurologic dysfunction followed by complete or incomplete recovery; assess frequency.

CLIENT/FAMILY TEACHING

1. Use exactly as directed, do not stop without consulting provider.
2. Reconstitute with diluent provided and gently swirl vial. Let stand at room temperature until solid material is dissolved. Administer SC into arms, abdomen, hips or thighs, rotating sites.
3. Patient Information booklet is enclosed with drug for review of self–injection procedure.
4. Drug is used to slow accumulation of physical disablilty and to decrease frequency of clinical exacerbations with MS. Continue to use aids i.e., cane, brace, walker, etc. for ambulation.
5. May experience pain, itching, swelling, and hardening of skin at injection site.
6. Chest tightness, flushing, SOB, and anxiety may occur within minutes of injection and last up to 30 min.
7. Practice reliable contraception.

OUTCOMES/EVALUATE

↓ Frequency and severity of MS exacerbations

Glimepiride

(**GLYE**-meh-pye-ride)

PREGNANCY CATEGORY: C

CLASSIFICATION(S):

Antidiabetic, oral; second generation sulfonylurea

Rx: Amaryl

SEE ALSO *HYPOGLYCEMIC AGENTS.*

ACTION/KINETICS

Lowers blood glucose by stimulating the release of insulin from functioning pancreatic beta cells and by increasing the sensitivity of peripheral tissues to insulin. Completely absorbed from the GI tract within 1 hr. **Onset:** 2–3 hr. **t½, serum:** About 9 hr. **Duration:** 24 hr. Completely metabolized in the liver and metabolites are excreted through both the urine and feces.

USES

(1) As an adjunct to diet and exercise to lower blood glucose in non-insulin-dependent diabetes mellitus (Type II diabetes mellitus). (2) In combination with insulin to decrease blood glucose in those whose hyperglycemia cannot be controlled by diet and exercise in combination with an oral hypoglycemic drug. (3) In combination with metformin (Glucophage) if control is not reached with diet, exercise, and either hypoglycemic alone.

CONTRAINDICATIONS

Diabetic ketoacidosis with or without coma. Use during lactation.

SPECIAL CONCERNS

The use of oral hypoglycemic drugs has been associated with increased CV mortality compared with treatment with diet alone or diet plus insulin. Safety and efficacy have not been determined in children.

SIDE EFFECTS

The most common side effect is hypoglycemia. **GI:** N&V, GI pain, diarrhea, cholestatic jaundice (rare). **CNS:** Dizziness, headache. **Dermatologic:** Pruritus, erythema, urticaria, morbilliform or maculopapular eruptions. **Hematologic:** Leukopenia, agranulocytosis, thrombocytopenia, hemolytic anemia, aplastic anemia, pancytopenia. **Miscellaneous:** Hyponatremia, increased release of ADH, changes in accommodation and/or blurred vision.

DRUG INTERACTIONS

See *Hypoglycemic Agents.*

HOW SUPPLIED

Tablet: 1 mg, 2 mg, 4 mg

DOSAGE

• **TABLETS**

Non-insulin-dependent diabetes mellitus (Type II diabetes).

Adults, initial: 1–2 mg once daily, given with breakfast or the first main meal. The initial dose should be 1 mg in those sensitive to hypoglycemic drugs, in those with impaired renal or hepatic function, and in elderly, debilitated, or malnourished clients. The maximum initial dose is 2 mg or less daily. **Maintenance:** 1–4 mg once daily up to a maximum of 8 mg once daily. After a dose of 2 mg is reached, increase the dose in increments of 2 mg or less at 1- to 2-week intervals (determined by the blood glucose response). **When combined with insulin therapy:** 8 mg once daily with the first main meal with low-dose insulin. The fasting glucose level for beginning combination therapy is greater than 150 mg/dL glucose in the plasma or serum.

Type II diabetes—transfer from other hypoglycemic agents

When transferring clients to glimipiride, no transition period is required. However, observe clients closely for 1 to 2 weeks for hypoglycemia when being transferred from longer half-life sulfonylureas (e.g., chlorpropamide) to glimepiride.

NURSING CONSIDERATIONS

SEE ALSO NURSING CONSIDERATIONS FOR HYPOGLYCEMIC AGENTS.

ADMINISTRATION/STORAGE

1. Dispense tablets in well-closed containers with safety caps.
2. Store tablets at 15–30°C (59–86°F).

ASSESSMENT

1. Note indications for therapy, if newly diagnosed or transferred therapy, glycemic control and characteristics of disease.
2. List other agents trialed and drugs currently taking to ensure none interact unfavorably.
3. Assess lifestyle and diet, identify changes needed and list risk factors.
4. Obtain and monitor electrolytes, BS, HbA1-C, Ca, Mg, urinalysis, liver and renal function studies.

CLIENT/FAMILY TEACHING

1. Review dose and frequency for administration. Usually once a day with first main meal of day.
2. Record finger sticks, include 1 or 2 hr post meal FS; record for provider evaluation.
3. Continue regular exercise and dietary restrictions in addition to drug therapy.

G

4. Avoid alcohol and prolonged sun exposure. Report any adverse drug effects.
5. Report as scheduled for teaching reinforcement, follow-up labs, foot exams, and medication evaluation.

OUTCOMES/EVALUATE

Blood sugar and HbA1-C within desired range

Glipizide

(**GLIP**-ih-zyd)

PREGNANCY CATEGORY: C
CLASSIFICATION(S):
Antidiabetic, oral; second generation sulfonylurea
Rx: Glucotrol, Glucotrol XL

SEE ALSO *ANTIDIABETIC AGENTS.*

ACTION/KINETICS

Also has mild diuretic effects. **Onset:** 1– 3 hr. **t½:** 2–4 hr. **Duration:** 10–24 hr. Metabolized in liver to inactive metabolites, which are excreted through the kidneys.

USES

Adjunct to diet for control of hyperglycemia in clients with non-insulin-dependent diabetes.

ADDITIONAL DRUG INTERACTIONS

Cimetidine may ↑ effect of glipizide due to ↓ breakdown by liver.

HOW SUPPLIED

Tablet: 5 mg, 10 mg; *Tablet, Extended Release:* 2.5 mg, 5 mg, 10 mg

DOSAGE

• **TABLETS, IMMEDIATE RELEASE**

Diabetes.

Adults, initial: 5 mg 30 min before breakfast; **then,** adjust dosage by 2.5–5 mg every few days, depending on the blood glucose response, until adequate control is achieved. **Maintenance:** 15–40 mg/day. Older clients should begin with 2.5 mg.

• **TABLETS, EXTENDED RELEASE**

Diabetes.

Adults, initial: 5 mg with breakfast. Monitor response to therapy by measuring HbA1c at 3-month intervals. Dose can be increased to 10 mg if response is inadequate. **Maintenance:** 5 or 10 mg once daily; some may require 20 mg/day (maximum).

NURSING CONSIDERATIONS

SEE ALSO *NURSING CONSIDERATIONS FOR ANTIDIABETIC AGENTS.*

ADMINISTRATION/STORAGE

1. Some clients are better controlled on once daily dosing while others are better controlled with divided dosing.
2. Divide maintenance doses greater than 15 mg/day; give before the morning and evening meals. Total daily doses of 30 mg or more may be given safely on twice daily dosing.
3. Clients on immediate release glipizide can be safely switched to the extended release tablets once a day at the nearest equivalent total daily dose. They can also be titrated to the appropriate dose of extended release tablets starting with 5 mg once daily.
4. No transition period is needed when transferring clients to extended release tablets from other oral antidiabetic drugs. Observe for 1–2 weeks if transferred from long half-life sulfonylureas (e.g., chlorpropamide) to extended release glipizide due to overlapping effects.
5. When transferring from an insulin dose of < 20 units/day, insulin may be discontinued abruptly. When transferring from an insulin dose of > 20 units/day, reduce the insulin dose by 50%; further reduce depending on response. The initial glipizide dose when transferring from insulin is 5 mg/day.
6. Assess lifestyle to ensure that maximal changes in the areas of diet and exercise have been taken before increasing dosage. Once maximum dosage attained, if renal function is normal, consider adding metformin, pioglitazone, or rosiglitazone for better control.

ASSESSMENT

1. Note indications for therapy, if newly diagnosed or transferred therapy; glycemic control and characteristics of disease.
2. List other agents trialed and drugs currently taking to ensure none interact unfavorably.

3. Assess lifestyle and diet, identify changes needed and list risk factors.
4. Obtain and monitor electrolytes, BS, HbA1-C, Ca, Mg, urinalysis, liver and renal function studies.

CLIENT/FAMILY TEACHING

1. For greatest effect, take 20 min before or with meals.
2. Report CNS side effects such as drowsiness or headache; check fingerstick.
3. May experience anorexia, constipation or diarrhea, vomiting, and stomach pain. Report if severe, record weight, I&O.
4. Skin reactions may occur and should be reported. Avoid sun exposure; use sunscreen, sunglasses and protective clothing when out.
5. Assess lifestyle and diet, identify changes needed and list risk factors.
6. Avoid alcohol in any form.
7. Practice barrier contraception.
8. Continue prescribed diet and regular exercise program. Record FS, also obtain FS 1-2 hr after eating; report loss of control.

OUTCOMES/EVALUATE

BS and HbA1-C (< 7) within desired range

Glucagon

(**GLOO**-kah-gon)

PREGNANCY CATEGORY: B
CLASSIFICATION(S):
Insulin antagonist
Rx: Glucacon Diagnostic Kit, Glucagon Emergency Kit

ACTION/KINETICS

Produced by the alpha islet cells of the pancreas, glucagon accelerates liver glycogenolysis by stimulating synthesis of cyclic AMP and increasing phosphorylase kinase activity. Increased blood glucose levels result from increased breakdown of glycogen to glucose and inhibition of glycogen synthetase. Is effective only with sufficient liver glycogen. Glucagon stimulates hepatic gluconeogenesis by increasing the uptake of amino acids and converting them to glucose precursors. Also, lipolysis is increased, resulting in free fatty acids and glycerol for gluconeogenesis. Effective in overcoming hypoglycemia only if the liver has a glycogen reserve. Also relaxes smooth muscle of the GI tract and decreases gastric and pancreatic secretions; increases myocardial contractility. Glucagon for injection is of rDNA origin and is identical to human glucacon. **Maximum plasma levels of glucagon:** About 20 min following SC injection and about 13 min after IM injection. **Peak glucose levels:** 30 min after 1 mg glucagon SC and 26 min after 1 mg glucacon IM. **Duration:** 1–2 hr. **t½:** 8–18 min. Metabolized in the liver, kidney, and plasma.

USES

Treatment of severe hypoglycemia. Diagnostic aid in radiologic exams of the stomach, duodenum, small bowel, and colon where decreased intestinal motility is desired. Use only under medical supervision or in accordance with strict instructions received from the physician. *Investigational:* Treatment of propranolol overdose and in CV emergencies.

CONTRAINDICATIONS

Use in pheochromocytoma.

SPECIAL CONCERNS

Use with caution during lactation, in clients with renal or hepatic disease, in those who are undernourished and emaciated, and in clients with a history of insulinoma. Safety and efficacy have not been determined for use in children as a diagnostic aid.

SIDE EFFECTS

GI: N&V. **Allergy:** Respiratory distress, urticaria, hypotension. ***Stevens-Johnson syndrome when used as diagnostic aid.***

OD OVERDOSE MANAGEMENT

Symptoms: N&V, gastric hypotonicity, diarrhea, hypokalemia. Possible transient ↑ BP and pulse rate. *Treatment:* Symptomatic.

DRUG INTERACTIONS

Anticoagulants, oral / ↑ Anticoagulant effects by ↑ hypoprothrombinemia

Antidiabetic agents / Hyperglycemia due to glucagon antagonizes hypoglycemic drug effect
Corticosteroids, Epinephrine, Estrogens, Phenytoin / Additive hyperglycemic effect of drugs listed

HOW SUPPLIED

Powder for Injection: 1 mg (1 unit)

DOSAGE

- **IM, IV, SC**

Severe hypoglycemia.

Adults and children > 20 kg: 1 mg (1 unit); if the response is delayed, give an additional dose of glucagon. **Children < 20 kg:** 0.5 mg (0.5 unit) or a dose equivalent to 20–30 mcg/kg.

Diagnostic aid for GI tract.

Dose dependent on desired onset of action and duration of effect necessary for the examination. **IV:** 0.25–0.5 mg (onset: 1 min; duration: 9–17 min); 2 mg (onset: 1 min; duration 22–25 min). **IM:** 1 mg (onset: 8–10 min; duration: 12–27 min); 2 mg (onset: 4–7 min; duration: 21–32 min). Because the stomach is less sensitive to glucagon, give 0.5 mg IV or 2 mg IM.

For colon examination.

IM: 2 mg 10 min prior to procedure.

Treatment of toxicity of beta-adrenergic blocking agents.

Adults, IV, initial: 2–3 mg given over 30 sec; may be repeated at the rate of 5 mg/hr until client is stabilized.

NURSING CONSIDERATIONS

ADMINISTRATION/STORAGE

1. Treat severe hypoglycemia first with IV glucose, if possible. If parenteral glucose cannot be used, administer glucagon. After client responds, give supplemental carbohydrate to restore liver glycogen and to prevent secondary hypoglycemia.

IV 2. Before reconstituting, store powder at room temperature.

3. Use only the diluent in reconstituting. Do not use glucagon at concentrations > 1 mg/mL (1 unit/mL).

4. Following reconstitution, use the solution immediately and only if clear and of water-like consistency. Inspect for particulate matter and discoloration prior to use. Discard any unused portion.

5. With direct IV administration, inject at a rate not exceeding 1 mg/min.

6. Administer with dextrose solutions. A precipitate may form if saline solutions are used.

CLIENT/FAMILY TEACHING

1. Instruct family in the administration of glucagon SC or IM in the event of hypoglycemic reaction, loss of consciousness, or inability to swallow.

2. Following administration of glucagon, keep client on side and administer a CHO once awake.

3. Have rapidly available sugar, such as orange juice and Karo syrup in water (or Lifesavers®) to administer. If the shock was caused by a long-acting medication, administer slowly digestible carbohydrates, such as bread with honey.

4. Do not try to administer fluids by mouth if client has a reaction and is not fully conscious; could aspirate fluids into lungs.

5. Record time of day and activity and report all hypoglycemic reactions so that insulin dosage can be adjusted.

OUTCOMES/EVALUATE

- Reversal of S&S of hypoglycemia
- Termination of insulin-induced shock
- Inhibition of bowel peristalsis with small muscle relaxation during radiologic imaging of the GI tract

Glyburide

(**GLYE**-byou-ryd)

PREGNANCY CATEGORY: B

CLASSIFICATION(S):

Antidiabetic, oral; second generation sulfonylurea

Rx: Diabeta, Glynase PresTab, Micronase

✱Rx: Albert Glyburide, Apo-Glyburide, Euglucon, Gen-Glybe, Novo-Glyburide, Nu-Glyburide, PMS-Glyburide

SEE ALSO *ANTIDIABETIC AGENTS.*

ACTION/KINETICS

Has a mild diuretic effect. **Onset, nonmicronized:** 2–4 hr; **micronized:** 1 hr. **t½, nonmicronized:** 10 hr; **micron-**

ized: Approximately 4 hr. **Time to peak levels:** 4 hr. **Duration, nonmicronized:** 16–24 hr; **micronized:** 12–24 hr. Metabolized in liver to weakly active metabolites. Excreted in bile (50%) and through the kidneys (50%). Micronized glyburide (3 mg tablets) produces serum levels that are not bioequivalent to those from nonmicronized glyburide (5 mg tablets).

USES

May be used with metformin when diet and glyburide or diet and metformin alone do not provide adequate control.

ADDITIONAL DRUG INTERACTIONS

Anticoagulants / Either ↑ or ↓ anticoagulant effect

Ciprofloxacin / Potentiation of hypoglycemic effect

HOW SUPPLIED

Tablet, micronized: 1.5 mg, 3 mg, 4.5 mg, 6 mg; *Tablet, nonmicronized:* 1.25 mg, 2.5 mg, 5 mg

DOSAGE

• TABLETS, NONMICRONIZED (DIABETA/MICRONASE)

Diabetes.

Adults, initial: 2.5–5 mg/day given with breakfast (or the first main meal); **then,** increase by 2.5 mg at weekly intervals to achieve the desired response. **Maintenance:** 1.25–20 mg/day. Clients sensitive to sulfonylureas should start with 1.25 mg/day.

• TABLETS, MICRONIZED (GLYNASE PRESTAB)

Diabetes.

Adults, initial: 1.5–3 mg/day given with breakfast (or the first main meal). Those sensitive to sulfonylureas should start with 0.75 mg/day. Increase by no more than 1.5 mg at weekly intervals to achieve the desired response. **Maintenance:** 0.75–12 (maximum) mg/day.

NURSING CONSIDERATIONS

SEE ALSO *NURSING CONSIDERATIONS* FOR *ANTIDIABETIC AGENTS* AND *GLIPIZIDE*.

ADMINISTRATION/STORAGE

1. For best results, administer 30 min prior to meals.
2. Do not exceed 20 mg/day of the nonmicronized product and 12 mg/day of the micronized product.
3. If daily dosage of the nonmicronized product exceeds 15 mg or the micronized product exceeds 6 mg, divide the dose and give before the morning and evening meals.
4. When transferring from oral hypoglycemics, other than chlorpropamide, no transition and no initial priming dose is required. When transferring from chlorpropamide, use caution for the first 2 weeks due to the long duration of action of chlorpropamide and possible overlapping drug effects.
5. Use the following guidelines when transferring from insulin to glyburide:
   - Insulin dose < 20 units/day, start with 1.5–3 mg/day micronized or 2.5–5 mg/day nonmicronized glyburide. Insulin may be discontinued abruptly.
   - Insulin dose from 20–40 units/day, start with 3 mg/day micronized or 5 mg/day nonmicronized glyburide. Insulin may be discontinued abruptly.
   - Insulin dose > 40 units/day, start with 3 mg/day micronized or 5 mg/day nonmicronized glyburide. Reduce insulin dose by 50%; reduce further as determined by response. Consider hospitalization during the transition.

CLIENT/FAMILY TEACHING

1. Review dose and frequency for administration.
2. Record finger sticks at various times (i.e., fasting, 1 or 2 hr after meal, bedtime).
3. Continue regular daily exercise, life-style changes, and dietary restrictions in addition to drug therapy.
4. Report as scheduled for teaching reinforcement, F/U labs, foot/eye exams, and medication evaluation.

OUTCOMES/EVALUATE

BS and HbA1-C (< 7) within desired range

Goserelin acetate

(**GO**-seh-rel-in)

PREGNANCY CATEGORY: X (WHEN USED FOR ENDOMETRIOSIS); D (WHEN USED FOR BREAST CANCER)
CLASSIFICATION(S):
Antineoplastic, hormone
Rx: Zoladex
✱Rx: Zoladex LA

SEE ALSO *ANTINEOPLASTIC AGENTS.*

G

ACTION/KINETICS
Synthetic decapeptide analog of LHRH (or GnRH) which is a potent inhibitor of gonadotropin secretion from the pituitary gland. Initially, there is actually an increase in serum luteinizing hormone and FSH. This is followed by a long-term suppression of pituitary gonadotropins with serum levels of testosterone decreasing to those seen in surgically castrated males. When used for endometriosis, the drug controls the secretion of hormones required for the ovary to synthesize estrogen resulting in plasma estrogen levels seen in menopause. **Peak serum levels after SC implantation of 3.6 mg:** 12–15 days. **Mean peak serum levels:** Approximately 2.5 ng/mL. Available as an implant in a preloaded syringe. For the first 8 days of the treatment cycle, the rate of absorption of the 3.6 mg implant is slower than for the remainder of the period. For the 10.8 mg depot, mean levels increase to a peak within the first 24 hr and then decline rapidly until day 4; thereafter, mean levels remain constant until the end of the treatment period. **t½, elimination:** 4.2 hr for normal renal function and 12.1 hr for C_{CR} less than 20 mL/min. Rapidly cleared by a combination of hepatic metabolism and urinary excretion.

USES
Implant, 3.6 mg or 10.8 mg: (1) Palliative treatment of advanced prostatic carcinoma as an alternative to orchiectomy or estrogen administration when these are either unacceptable to the client or not indicated. (2) With flutamide (Eulexin) prior to (start 8 weeks before) and during radiation therapy to treat early stage B2-C prostatic carcinoma. **Implant, 3.6 mg only:** (1) Endometriosis, including pain relief and reduction of endometriotic lesions. Use limited to women 18 years and older who have been treated for 6 months. (2) Palliative treatment of advanced breast cancer in pre- and postmenopausal women. (3) For endometrial thinning prior to ablation for dysfunctional uterine bleeding.

CONTRAINDICATIONS
Pregnancy, lactation, nondiagnosed vaginal bleeding, hypersensitivity to LHRH or LHRH agonist analogs. Use of the 10.8-mg implant in women.

SPECIAL CONCERNS
Safety and effectiveness have not been determined in clients less than 18 years of age. There may be transient worsening of symptoms during the first few weeks of therapy. Use with caution in males who are at particular risk of developing ureteral obstruction or spinal cord compression.

SIDE EFFECTS
In males.
GU: Sexual dysfunction, decreased erections, lower urinary tract symptoms, gynecomastia, renal insufficiency, urinary obstruction, UTI, bladder neoplasm, hematuria, impotence, urinary frequency, incontinence, urinary tract disorder, impaired urination. **CV:** CHF, ***CVA, MI, heart failure, pulmonary embolus,*** arrhythmia, hypertension, peripheral vascular disorder, chest pain, angina pectoris, cerebral ischemia, varicose veins. **CNS:** Lethargy, dizziness, insomnia, asthenia, anxiety, depression, headache, paresthesia. **GI:** N&V, diarrhea, constipation, ulcer, anorexia, hematemesis. **Respiratory:** URI, COPD, increased cough, dyspnea, pneumonia. **Metabolic:** Gout, hypercalcemia, weight increase, diabetes mellitus. **Miscellaneous:** Pelvic or bone pain, anemia, chills, fever, breast pain, breast swelling or tenderness, abdominal or back pain, flu syndrome, sepsis, aggravation reaction, herpes simplex, pruritus, peripheral edema, injection site reaction, hot flashes, rash, sweating, complications of surgery, hypersensitivity, pain, edema.

In females.
GU: Vaginitis, decreased or increased libido, pelvic symptoms, dyspareunia, dysmenorrhea, urinary frequency, UTI, vaginal bleeding (during the first 2 months) of varying duration and intensity. **CV:** ***Hemorrhage,*** hypertension, palpitations, migraine, tachycardia. **CNS:** Emotional lability, depression, headache, insomnia, dizziness, nervousness, anxiety, paresthesia, somnolence, abnormal thinking, malaise, fatigue, lethargy. **GI:** N&V, abdominal pain, increased appetite, anorexia, constipation, diarrhea, dry mouth, dyspepsia, flatulence. **Musculoskeletal:** Asthenia, back pain, myalgia, hypertonia, arthralgia, joint disorder, decrease of vertebral trabecular bone mineral density. **Dermatologic:** Sweating, acne, seborrhea, hirsutism, pruritus, alopecia, dry skin, ecchymosis, rash, skin discoloration, hair disorders. **Respiratory:** Pharyngitis, bronchitis, increased cough, epistaxis, rhinitis, sinusitis. **Ophthalmic:** Amblyopia, dry eyes. **Miscellaneous:** Hot flashes, breast atrophy or enlargement, breast pain, tumor flare, pain, infection, application site reaction, flu syndrome, voice alterations, weight gain, allergic reaction, chest pain, fever, peripheral edema, hypercalcemia, osteoporosis, hypersensitivity.

LABORATORY TEST CONSIDERATIONS
↑ LDL and HDL cholesterol, triglycerides, AST, ALT. Misleading results of pituitary-gonadotropic and gonadal function tests that are conducted during treatment.

HOW SUPPLIED
Implant: 3.6 mg, 10.8 mg

DOSAGE

- **SC IMPLANT, 3.6 MG**

Prostatic carcinoma, endometriosis, advanced breast cancer, thinning prior to endometrial ablation for dysfunctional uterine bleeding.
3.6 mg q 28 days into the upper abdominal wall using sterile technique under the direction of a physician.

- **SC IMPLANT, 10.8 MG**

Advanced prostatic carcinoma.
10.8 mg q 12 weeks into the upper abdominal wall using sterile technique under the direction of a physician.

With flutamide to treat Stage B2-C prostatic carcinoma.
One goserelin 3.6 mg depot followed in 28 days by one 10.8 mg depot.

NURSING CONSIDERATIONS

SEE ALSO *NURSING CONSIDERATIONS* FOR *ANTINEOPLASTIC AGENTS.*

ADMINISTRATION/STORAGE

1. Do not remove the sterile syringe containing the drug until immediately before use. Examine syringe for damage and to ensure drug is visible in the translucent chamber.
2. Administer drug under physician supervision/orders.
3. Clean the area with an alcohol swab; a topical (i.e., ethyl chloride) or a local anesthetic may be used prior to the injection.
4. To administer, stretch the skin with one hand and grip the needle with the fingers around the barrel of the syringe. Insert needle into the SC fat; do not aspirate. If a large vessel is penetrated, blood will be seen immediately in the syringe; withdraw needle and make injection elsewhere with a new syringe.
5. The direction of the needle is changed so it parallels the abdominal wall. The needle is then pushed in until the barrel hub touches the skin and then withdrawn approximately 1 cm to create a space to inject the drug. The plunger is depressed to deliver the drug. The needle is then withdrawn and the area bandaged.
6. To confirm the drug has been delivered, ensure that the tip of the plunger is visible within the tip of the needle.
7. If there is need to remove goserelin surgically, it can be located by ultrasound.
8. Adhere to the 28-day and 12-week schedules as closely as possible.
9. Store at room temperatures not exceeding 25°C (77°F).
10. There is no evidence the drug accumulates with either hepatic and/or renal dysfunction.
11. Duration of treatment for endometriosis is 6 months.

12. Males with ureteral obstruction or spinal cord compression should have appropriate treatment prior to initiating goserelin therapy.

CLIENT/FAMILY TEACHING

1. Drug will be implanted into abdomen with a syringe every 28 days to 3 mo as prescribed. Be sure not to miss scheduled administration days.
2. The most common side effects (e.g.; hot flashes, decreased erections, and sexual dysfunction) R/T ↓ testosterone levels.
3. There may be initial worsening of symptoms; results of transient increases of testosterone.
4. May experience increased bone pain and develop spinal cord compression or ureteral obstruction; usually only temporary but must be reported promptly so that appropriate treatment may be initiated. Report all unusual/adverse side effects.
5. Not for use in women who are likely to become pregnant or who are pregnant. Drug may harm fetus and may impair fertility; identify for sperm or egg harvesting.
6. Clients with prostate cancer who decide against surgery (orchiectomy), for medication therapy, must come in regularly for abdominal implants for the rest of their lives.
7. Identify appropriate resources and support groups.

OUTCOMES/EVALUATE

- Symptom control; ↑ comfort
- ↓ Tumor size and spread
- ↓ Testosterone levels

Granisetron hydrochloride

(gran-**ISS**-eh-tron)

PREGNANCY CATEGORY: B
CLASSIFICATION(S):
Antiemetic, 5-HT3 receptor antagonist
Rx: Kytril

ACTION/KINETICS

Selective $5\text{-}HT_3$ (serotonin) receptor antagonist with little or no affinity for other 5-HT, beta-adrenergic, dopamine, or histamine receptors. During chemotherapy-induced vomiting, mucosal enterochromaffin cells release serotonin, which stimulates $5\text{-}HT_3$ receptors. The stimulation of $5\text{-}HT_3$ receptors by serotonin causes vagal discharge resulting in vomiting. Granisetron blocks serotonin stimulation and subsequent vomiting. In adult cancer clients undergoing chemotherapy, infusion of a single 40-mcg/kg dose over 5 min produced the following data. **Peak plasma level:** 63.8 ng/mL. **Plasma t½, terminal:** 5–9 hr, depending on age and disease state. Metabolized in the liver with unchanged drug (12%) and metabolites excreted through both the urine and feces.

USES

Prevention of N&V associated with initial and repeat cancer chemotherapy, including high-dose cisplatin. Prevention of N&V associated with radiation, including total body irradiation and fractionated abdominal radiation. *Investigational:* Acute N&V following surgery.

CONTRAINDICATIONS

Known hypersensitivity to the drug.

SPECIAL CONCERNS

Use with caution during lactation. Safety and efficacy in children less than 2 years of age have not been established.

SIDE EFFECTS

- **AFTER IV USE**

CNS: Headache, somnolence, agitation, anxiety, CNS stimulation, insomnia, extrapyramidal syndrome. **GI:** Diarrhea, constipation, taste disorder. **CV:** Hypertension, hypotension, arrhythmias (e.g., sinus bradycardia, atrial fibrillation, ***AV block,*** ventricular ectopy including nonsustained tachycardia, ECG abnormalities). **Allergic:** ***Hypersensitivity reactions (anaphylaxis),*** skin rashes. **Miscellaneous:** Asthenia, fever.

- **AFTER PO USE**

CNS: Headache, dizziness, insomnia, anxiety, somnolence. **GI:** N&V, diarrhea, constipation, abdominal pain. **CV:** Hypertension, hypotension, angina, atrial fibrillation, syncope (rare). **Hypersensitivity:** Rarely, hypersensitivity reactions; ***severe anaphylaxis,*** shortness of breath, hypotension, urticaria. **Miscellaneous:** Fever, leukopenia, decreased appetite, anemia, alopecia, thrombocytopenia.

LABORATORY TEST CONSIDERATIONS

↑ AST, ALT.

DRUG INTERACTIONS

Because granisetron is metabolized by hepatic cytochrome P-450 drug-metabolizing enzymes, agents that induce or inhibit these enzymes may alter the clearance (and thus the half-life) of granisetron.

HOW SUPPLIED

Injection: 1 mg/mL; *Tablet:* 1 mg

DOSAGE

• **IV**

Antiemetic during cancer chemotherapy.

Adults and children over 2 years of age: 10 mcg/kg within 30 min before initiation of chemotherapy either undiluted over 30 seconds, or diluted and infused over 5 min.

• **TABLETS**

Protection from chemotherapy-induced N&V.

Adults: 2 mg once daily or 1 mg twice daily. In the 2 mg once daily regime, two 1 mg tablets are given up to 1 hr before chemotherapy. In the 1 mg twice daily regime, the first 1 mg tablet is given up to 1 hr before chemotherapy and the second tablet is given 12 hr after the first. Either regimen is administered only on the day(s) chemotherapy is given. Data are not available for PO use in children.

Protection from radiation-induced N&V.

Adults: 2 mg once daily taken within 1 hr of radiation.

Investigational: Antiemetic following surgery.

1–3 mg.

NURSING CONSIDERATIONS

ADMINISTRATION/STORAGE

1. Give drug only on the day chemotherapy is given.
2. Dosage adjustment is not necessary for geriatric clients or with impaired renal or hepatic function.
3. IV Administer either undiluted over 30 seconds or diluted with NSS or D5W to a total volume of 20 to 50 mL and infused over 5 minutes. Drug is stable for at least 24 hr when diluted in NSS or D5W and stored at room temperature under normal lighting.
4. Do not mix in solution with other drugs.
5. Do not freeze vial; protect from light.

ASSESSMENT

1. Note indications for therapy; chemotherapy or postop N&V.
2. Anticipate administration 30 min before the start of emetogenic cancer chemotherapy.

CLIENT/FAMILY TEACHING

1. Review the appropriate method and frequency of dosing.
2. May be given IV or orally to help decrease chemotherapy-induced N&V.
3. May experience headaches; usually relieved with Tylenol.

OUTCOMES/EVALUATE

- Prevention of N&V
- Protection from chemotherapy-induced nausea and vomiting

G

Griseofulvin microsize

(griz-ee-oh-**FULL**-vin)

PREGNANCY CATEGORY: C

Rx: Fulvicin-U/F, Grifulvin V, Grisactin 250 and 500

Griseofulvin ultramicrosize

(griz-ee-oh-**FULL**-vin)

PREGNANCY CATEGORY: C

Rx: Fulvicin-P/G, Grisactin Ultra, Gris-PEG, Ultramicrosize Griseofulvin

CLASSIFICATION(S):

Antibiotic, antifungal

SEE ALSO *ANTI-INFECTIVES.*

ACTION/KINETICS

Derived from a species of *Penicillium.* Is deposited in keratin precursor cells which are exfoliated gradually and replaced by noninfected tissue. Believed to interfere with cell division (metaphase) or DNA replication. Is tightly bound to the new keratin which becomes highly resistant to fungal infection. Absorbed from the duodenum. **Peak plasma concentration:** 0.5–2 mcg/mL after 4 hr. **t½:** 9–24 hr. Levels may be increased by giving the drug with a high-fat diet. GI absorption of the ultramicrosize products is about 1.5 times that of the microsize products; no evidence that this causes any difference in the safety and effectiveness of the drug compared with the microsize form.

USES

Tinea (ringworm) infections of skin (including athlete's foot), scalp, groin, and nails. Effective against tinea corporis, tinea pedis, tinea barbae, tinea unguium, tinea cruris, tinea capitis due to *Trichophyton* species, *Microsporum audouinii, M. canis, M. gypseum,* and *Epidermophyton floccosum*. It is the only PO drug effective against dermatophytid (tinea ringworm) infections. Not effective against *Candida.* Establish susceptibility of the infectious agent before treatment is begun.

CONTRAINDICATIONS

Pregnancy. Porphyria or history thereof, hepatocellular failure, and hypersensitivity to drug. Exposure to artificial light or sunlight. Use for infections due to bacteria, candidiasis, actinomycosis, sporotrichosis, tinea versicolor, histoplasmosis, chromoblastomycosis, coccidioidomycosis, cryptococcosis, and North American blastomycosis.

SPECIAL CONCERNS

Cross sensitivity with penicillin is possible. Safety and efficacy for prophylaxis of fungal infections not determined.

SIDE EFFECTS

Hypersensitivity: Rashes, urticaria, ***angioneurotic edema,*** allergic reactions, erythema multiforme-like reactions. **GI:** N&V, diarrhea, epigastric pain, ***GI bleeding***. **CNS:** Dizziness, headache, confusion, mental fatigue, insomnia, impaired performance of routine activities. **GU:** Proteinuria, menstrual irregularities, nephrosis. **Miscellaneous:** Oral thrush, acute intermittent porphyria, paresthesias of extremities after long-term therapy, leukopenia, photosensitivity, worsening of lupus erythematosus, hepatic toxicity, granulocytopenia.

LABORATORY TEST CONSIDERATIONS

↑ ALT, AST, alkaline phosphatase, BUN, and creatinine level values.

DRUG INTERACTIONS

Alcohol, ethyl / Tachycardia and flushing
Anticoagulants, oral / ↓ Anticoagulant effect R/T ↑ liver breakdown
Barbiturates / ↓ Effect of griseofulvin R/T ↓ GI tract absorption
Cyclosporine / ↓ Plasma cyclosporine levels → ↓ pharmacologic effect
Oral contraceptives / ↓ Oral contraceptive effect → breakthrough bleeding, pregnancy, or amenorrhea
Salicylates / ↓ Serum salicylate levels

HOW SUPPLIED

Griseofulvin microsize: *Capsule:* 250 mg; *Suspension:* 125 mg/5 mL; *Tablet:* 250 mg, 500 mg. **Griseofulvin ultramicrosize:** *Tablet:* 125 mg; 165 mg; 250 mg; 330 mg

DOSAGE

• CAPSULES, ORAL SUSPENSION, TABLETS

Tinea corporis, cruris, or capitis.

Adults: 0.5 g griseofulvin microsize daily in a single dose or divided dose (or 330–375 mg ultramicrosize).

Tinea pedis or unguium.

Adults: 0.75–1 g/day of griseofulvin microsize (or 660–750 mg ultramicrosize). After response, decrease dose of microsize to 0.5 g/day. **Pediatric, 13.6–22.6 kg:** 125–250 mg griseofulvin microsize daily (or 82.5–165 mg ultramicrosize); **pediatric, over 22.6 kg:** 250–500 mg microsize daily (or 165–330 mg ultramicrosize). *NOTE:* Dose has not been determined in children less than 2 years of age.

NURSING CONSIDERATIONS

SEE ALSO *GENERAL NURSING CONSIDERATIONS* FOR *ANTI-INFECTIVES*.

ADMINISTRATION/STORAGE

Assure sufficient length of treatment; i.e., treatment for tinea capitis: 4 to 6 weeks; 2 to 4 weeks for tinea corporis; 4 to 8 weeks for tinea pedis; and 4 to 6 months (fingernails) and 6 to 18 months (toe nails) for tinea unguium.

ASSESSMENT

1. Document location, size, and characteristics of skin infection.
2. Obtain baseline CBC, renal and LFTs and monitor with prolonged therapy. Obtain cultures and scrapings as needed.
3. May not be the drug of choice with CAD and hyperlipidemia due to the high-fat consumption necessary to enhance absorption.

CLIENT/FAMILY TEACHING

1. Eat high-fat food with drug (i.e., ice cream, bread and butter, gravy, fried chicken); fat enhances absorption of griseofulvin from the intestines.
2. Take all medication as prescribed to prevent any recurrence of infection. If the course of therapy is interrupted or not completed, therapy may have to be started all over again.
3. Practice appropriate hygiene to prevent reinfection.
4. Avoid exposure to intense natural and artificial light because photosensitivity reactions may occur. Wear protective clothing, sunglasses, and a sunscreen if exposure is necessary.
5. Report any fever, sore throat, and malaise, (all symptoms of leukopenia).
6. Use a nonhormonal form of birth control.
7. To be considered cured, repeated cultures and scrapings of affected sites must be negative.
8. Persistent N&V and diarrhea and any mental confusion should be immediately reported.
9. Avoid alcohol during therapy.
10. Anticipate long-term therapy, i.e., 2 weeks to 18 months depending on location of infection. Usual duration of treatment for tinea capitis (scalp ringworm), 2-4 weeks; tinea corporis (body ringworm), 2-4 weeks; tinea pedis (athletes foot), 4-8 weeks; tinea unguium (nail fungus), at least 4 weeks for fingernails, and 6 or more mo for toenails depending on rate of growth.

OUTCOMES/EVALUATE

- Improvement in symptoms
- Clearing of rash
- Negative cultures and scrapings

Guaifenesin (Glyceryl guaiacolate)

(gwye-**FEN**-eh-sin)

PREGNANCY CATEGORY: C
CLASSIFICATION(S):
Expectorant
Rx: Sinumist-SR Capsulets
OTC: Anti-Tuss, Breonesin, Diabetic Tussin EX, Gee-Gee, Genatuss, GG-Cen, Glyate, Glycotuss, Glytuss, Guiatuss, Hytuss, Hytuss-2X, Mytussin, Naldecon Senior EX, Robitussin, Scottussin, Siltussin, Siltussin SA, Tusibron, Tussin, Uni-tussin
✱OTC: Balminil Expectorant, Benylin-E Extra Strength, Koffex Expectorant

ACTION/KINETICS

May increase the output of fluid of the respiratory tract by reducing the viscosity and surface tension of respiratory secretions, thereby facilitating their expectoration. Data on efficacy are lacking.

USES

Dry, nonproductive cough due to colds and minor upper respiratory tract infections when there is mucus in the respiratory tract.

CONTRAINDICATIONS

Chronic cough (e.g., due to smoking, asthma, or emphysema), cough accompanied by excess secretions. Use in children under age 12 for persistent or chronic cough due to asthma or cough accompanied by excessive mucus (unless prescribed by a provider).

SPECIAL CONCERNS

Persistent cough may indicate a serious infection, thus, the provider should be consulted if cough lasts for more than 1 week, is recurring, or is accompanied by high fever, rash, or persistent headache.

SIDE EFFECTS
GI: N&V, GI upset. **CNS:** Dizziness, headache. **Dermatologic:** Rash, urticaria.

LABORATORY TEST CONSIDERATIONS
False + urinary 5-hydroxyindoleacetic acid. Color interference with determination of urinary vanillylmandelic acid.

OD OVERDOSE MANAGEMENT
Symptoms: N&V. *Treatment:* Treat symptomatically.

DRUG INTERACTIONS
Inhibition of platelet adhesiveness by guaifenesin may result in bleeding tendencies.

HOW SUPPLIED
Caplet, Sustained Release: 600 mg; *Capsule:* 200 mg; *Capsule, Extended Release:* 300 mg; *Liquid:* 100 mg/5 mL, 200 mg/5 mL; *Syrup:* 100 mg/5 mL; *Tablet:* 100 mg, 200 mg, 1200 mg; *Tablet, Extended Release:* 600 mg

DOSAGE

• **CAPSULES, TABLETS, ORAL LIQUID, SYRUP**

Expectorant.

Adults and children over 12 years: 100–400 mg q 4 hr, not to exceed 2.4 g/day, **pediatric, 6–12 years:** 100–200 mg q 4 hr, not to exceed 1.2 g/day, **pediatric, 2–6 years:** 50–100 mg q 4 hr, not to exceed 600 mg/day. If less than 2 years of age, individualize the dosage.

• **SUSTAINED-RELEASE CAPSULES, EXTENDED-RELEASE TABLETS**

Expectorant.

Adults and children over 12 years: 600–1,200 mg q 12 hr, not to exceed 2.4 g/day, **pediatric, 6–12 years:** 600 mg q 12 hr, not to exceed 1.2 g/day, **pediatric, 2–6 years:** 300 mg q 12 hr, not to exceed 600 mg/day. *NOTE:* The liquid dosage forms may be more suitable for children less than 6 years of age.

NURSING CONSIDERATIONS

ASSESSMENT
1. Document pulmonary assessment findings, CXR.
2. Note type, frequency, duration, and characteristics of cough and sputum production.
3. Assess for tobacco/nasal drug use, fever/chills, loss of appetite, or increased fatigue.

CLIENT/FAMILY TEACHING
1. Take only as directed and do not exceed prescribed dose.
2. If symptoms persist more than 1 week, recur, or are accompanied by a persistent headache, fever, or rash, notify provider.
3. Report any evidence of increased bruising/bleeding or lack or response.
4. Do not perform activities that require mental alertness, may cause drowsiness.
5. Increase fluids to 2.5 L/day to decrease secretion viscosity.
6. Avoid triggers: dust, chemicals, cleansers, cigarette smoke, environmental pollutants, and perfumes.

OUTCOMES/EVALUATE
- Control of coughing episodes
- Mobilization of mucus

Guanabenz acetate

(**GWON**-ah-benz)

PREGNANCY CATEGORY: C
CLASSIFICATION(S):
Antihypertensive, centrally-acting
Rx: Wytensin

SEE ALSO *ANTIHYPERTENSIVE AGENTS*.

ACTION/KINETICS
Stimulates alpha-2-adrenergic receptors in the CNS, resulting in a decrease in sympathetic impulses and in sympathetic tone. It also decreases the pulse rate, but postural hypotension has not been manifested. **Onset:** 60 min. **Peak effect:** 2–4 hr. **Peak plasma levels:** 2–5 hr. **t½:** 6 hr. **Duration:** 8–12 hr.

USES
Hypertension, alone or as adjunct with thiazide diuretics.

CONTRAINDICATIONS
Lactation, children under 12 years of age.

SPECIAL CONCERNS
Use with caution in severe coronary insufficiency, cerebrovascular disease, recent MI, hepatic or renal disease. Geriatric clients may be more sensitive to the hypotensive and sedative effects; dose reduction may be necessary due to age-related decreases in

renal function. Sudden cessation may result in an increase in catecholamines and, rarely, "overshoot" hypertension.

SIDE EFFECTS

CNS: Drowsiness and sedation (common), dizziness, weakness, headache, ataxia, depression, disturbances in sleep, excitement. **GI:** Dry mouth (common), N&V, diarrhea, constipation, abdominal discomfort, epigastric pain. **CV:** Palpitations, chest pain, arrhythmias, AV dysfunction or block. **Dermatologic:** Rash, pruritus. **Miscellaneous:** Edema, blurred vision, muscle aches, dyspnea, nasal congestion, urinary frequency, gynecomastia, disturbances of sexual function, taste disorders, aches in extremities.

OD OVERDOSE MANAGEMENT

Symptoms: Hypotension, sleepiness, irritability, miosis, lethargy, bradycardia. *Treatment:* Supportive treatment. VS and fluid balance should be monitored. Syrup of ipecac or gastric lavage followed by activated charcoal; administration of fluids, pressor agents, and atropine. Maintain an adequate airway; artificial respiration may be required.

DRUG INTERACTIONS

Additive sedation with CNS depressants.

HOW SUPPLIED

Tablet: 4 mg, 8 mg

DOSAGE

• **TABLETS**

Hypertension.

Adults, initial: 4 mg b.i.d. alone or with a thiazide diuretic; **then,** increase by 4–8 mg/day q 1–2 weeks until control achieved. Maximum recommended dose: 32 mg b.i.d.

NURSING CONSIDERATIONS

SEE ALSO *NURSING CONSIDERATIONS FOR ANTIHYPERTENSIVE AGENTS.*

ADMINISTRATION/STORAGE

The drug should be kept tightly closed and protected from light.

CLIENT/FAMILY TEACHING

1. Take exactly as prescribed. Do not skip doses or stop suddenly.
2. Do not drive or operate machinery until the drug's sedative effect assessed.
3. Report severe dry mouth effects; sleep disturbances may indicate a depressive episode.
4. Avoid tobacco, alcohol, and other CNS depressants.
5. Continue prescribed dietary and exercise recommendations.

OUTCOMES/EVALUATE

↓ BP

Guanadrel sulfate

(**GWON**-ah-drell)

PREGNANCY CATEGORY: B
CLASSIFICATION(S):
Antihypertensive, peripherally-acting antiadrenergic
Rx: Hylorel

G

SEE ALSO *ANTIHYPERTENSIVE AGENTS.*

ACTION/KINETICS

Similar to that of guanethidine. Inhibits vasoconstriction by blocking efferent, peripheral sympathetic pathways by depleting norepinephrine reserves and inhibiting norepinephrine release. Causes increased sensitivity to norepinephrine. **Onset:** 2 hr. **Peak plasma levels:** 1.5–2 hr. **Peak effect:** 4–6 hr. **t½:** Approximately 10 hr. **Duration:** 4–14 hr. Excreted through the urine as unchanged drug (40%) and metabolites.

USES

Hypertension in those not responding to a thiazide diuretic.

CONTRAINDICATIONS

Pheochromocytoma, CHF, within 1 week of MAO drug use, within 2–3 days of elective surgery, lactation.

SPECIAL CONCERNS

Use with caution in bronchial asthma and peptic ulcer. Safety and efficacy not established in children. Geriatric clients may be more sensitive to the hypotensive effects.

SIDE EFFECTS

CNS: Fainting, fatigue, headache, drowsiness, paresthesias, confusion, psychological problems, depression, syncope, sleep disorders, visual disturbances. **CV:** Chest pain, orthostatic hypotension, palpitations, peripheral edema. **Respiratory:** Exertional or resting SOB, coughing. **GI:** Increase in number of bowel movements, constipation, anorexia, indigestion, flatus, glossitis, N&V, dry mouth and throat, abdominal distress or pain. **GU:** Difficulty in ejaculation, impotence, nocturia, hematuria, urinary urgency or frequency. **Miscellaneous:** Leg cramps during both the day and night, excessive weight gain or loss, backache, neckache, joint pain or inflammation, aching limbs.

G

OD OVERDOSE MANAGEMENT

Symptoms: Postural hypotension, syncope, dizziness, blurred vision. *Treatment:* Administration of a vasoconstrictor (e.g., phenylephrine) if hypotension persists. If used, monitor carefully as client may be hypersensitive.

DRUG INTERACTIONS

Beta-adrenergic blocking agents / Excessive hypotension, bradycardia
Phenothiazines / Reverses effect of guanadrel
Phenylpropanolamine / ↓ Effect of guanadrel
Reserpine / Excessive hypotension, bradycardia
Sympathomimetics / Hypotensive effect of guanadrel may be reversed; also, guanadrel may ↑ the effects of directly acting sympathomimetics
Tricyclic antidepressants / Reverses effect of guanadrel
Vasodilators / ↑ Risk of orthostatic hypotension

HOW SUPPLIED

Tablet: 10 mg, 25 mg

DOSAGE

• **TABLETS**

Hypertension.

Individualized. Initial: 5 mg b.i.d.; **then,** increase dosage to maintenance level of 20–75 mg/day in two to four divided doses. With a C_{CR} of 30–60 mL/min, use an initial dose of 5 mg q 24 hr. If the C_{CR} is less than 30 mL/min, increase the dosing interval to q 48 hr. Make dose changes carefully q 7 or more days for moderate renal insufficiency and q 14 or more days for severe insufficiency.

NURSING CONSIDERATIONS

SEE ALSO *NURSING CONSIDERATIONS FOR ANTIHYPERTENSIVE AGENTS.*

ADMINISTRATION/STORAGE

1. Tolerance may occur with long-term therapy, necessitating a dosage increase.
2. While adjusting dosage, monitor both supine and standing BP.

CLIENT/FAMILY TEACHING

1. May develop a dry mouth and become drowsy. Do not perform tasks that require mental alertness, such as driving, until drug effects realized and when dosage is adjusted.
2. Diarrhea may occur; report if persistant as a severe electrolyte imbalance may occur (particularly with the elderly) requiring cessation of drug therapy.
3. Stop drug 48-72 hr prior to surgery to reduce risk of vascular collapse and cardiac arrest during anesthesia.

OUTCOMES/EVALUATE

Control of hypertension

Guanfacine hydrochloride

(**GWON**-fah-seen)

PREGNANCY CATEGORY: B
CLASSIFICATION(S):
Antihypertensive, centrally-acting
Rx: Tenex

SEE ALSO *ANTIHYPERTENSIVE AGENTS.*

ACTION/KINETICS

Thought to act by central stimulation of alpha-2 receptors. Causes a decrease in peripheral sympathetic output and HR resulting in a decrease in BP. May also manifest a direct peripheral alpha-2 receptor stimulant action. **Onset:** 2 hr. **Peak plasma levels:** 1–4 hr. **Peak effect:** 6–12 hr. **t½:** 12–23 hr. **Duration:** 24 hr. Approximately 50% excreted through the kidneys unchanged.

USES

Hypertension alone or with a thiazide diuretic. *Investigational:* Withdrawal from heroin use, to reduce the frequency of migraine headaches.

CONTRAINDICATIONS

Hypersensitivity to guanfacine. Acute hypertension associated with toxemia. Children less than 12 years of age.

SPECIAL CONCERNS

Use with caution during lactation and in clients with recent MI, cerebrovascular disease, chronic renal or hepatic failure, or severe coronary insufficiency. Geriatric clients may be more sensitive to the hypotensive and sedative effects. Safety and efficacy in children less than 12 years of age have not been determined.

SIDE EFFECTS

GI: Dry mouth, constipation, nausea, abdominal pain, diarrhea, dyspepsia, dysphagia, taste perversion or alterations in taste. **CNS:** Sedation, weakness, dizziness, headache, fatigue, insomnia, amnesia, confusion, depression, vertigo, agitation, anxiety, malaise, nervousness, tremor. **CV:** Bradycardia, substernal pain, palpitations, syncope, chest pain, tachycardia, cardiac fibrillation, CHF, heart block, MI (rare), cardiovascular accident (rare). **Ophthalmic:** Visual disturbances, conjunctivitis, iritis, blurred vision. **Dermatologic:** Pruritus, dermatitis, purpura, sweating, skin rash with exfoliation, alopecia, rash. **GU:** Decreased libido, impotence, urinary incontinence or frequency, testicular disorder, nocturia, acute renal failure. **Musculoskeletal:** Leg cramps, hypokinesia, arthralgia, leg pain, myalgia. **Other:** Rhinitis, tinnitus, dyspnea, paresthesias, paresis, asthenia, edema, abnormal LFTs.

OD OVERDOSE MANAGEMENT

Symptoms: Drowsiness, bradycardia, lethargy, hypotension. *Treatment:* Gastric lavage. Supportive therapy, as needed. The drug is not dialyzable.

DRUG INTERACTIONS

Additive sedative effects when used concomitantly with CNS depressants.

HOW SUPPLIED

Tablet: 1 mg, 2 mg

DOSAGE

• **TABLETS**

Hypertension.

Initial: 1 mg/day alone or with other antihypertensives; if satisfactory results are not obtained in 3–4 weeks, dosage may be increased by 1 mg at 1–2-week intervals up to a maximum of 3 mg/day in one to two divided doses.

Heroin withdrawal.

0.03–1.5 mg/day.

Reduce frequency of migraine headaches.

1 mg/day for 12 weeks.

NURSING CONSIDERATIONS

SEE ALSO *NURSING CONSIDERATIONS* FOR *ANTIHYPERTENSIVE AGENTS*.

ADMINISTRATION/STORAGE

1. Divide the daily dose if a decrease in BP is not maintained for over 24 hr; however, the incidence of side effects increases.
2. Adverse effects increase significantly when dose exceeds 3 mg/day.
3. Initiate antihypertensive therapy in clients already taking a thiazide diuretic.
4. Abrupt cessation may result in increases in plasma and urinary catecholamines, symptoms of nervousness and anxiety, and BPs greater than those prior to therapy.

ASSESSMENT

1. Document indications for therapy, onset of symptoms, and any previous agents used and the outcome.
2. Determine the extent of CAD, and note any evidence of renal or liver dysfunction.

CLIENT/FAMILY TEACHING

1. To minimize daytime drowsiness, take at bedtime. Do not perform activities that require mental alertness until drug effects realized.
2. Do not stop drug abruptly; may experience rebound effect.
3. Avoid alcohol. May use sugarless gum, ice chips, or sips of water for dry mouth effects.
4. May cause skin rash; report if persistent or severe.
5. Avoid OTC cough/cold remedies.

OUTCOMES/EVALUATE

- ↓ BP
- ↓ S&S of heroin withdrawal
- ↓ Migraine headaches

G

H 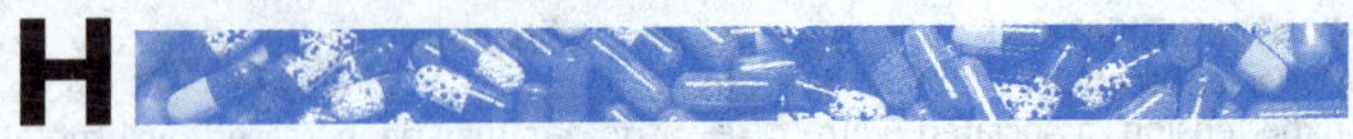

Halofantrine hydrochloride

(**hal**-oh-**FAN**-treen)

PREGNANCY CATEGORY: C
CLASSIFICATION(S):
Antimalarial
Rx: Halfan

ACTION/KINETICS
Blood schizonticide. Exact mechanism is unknown. At therapeutic doses, it prolongs QTc interval. The primary metabolite, n–butyl halofantrine, and the parent compound are equally active. Has wide interindividual variability in pharmacokinetics; probably due to erratic GI absorption. **Peak plasma levels:** 5–7 hr. When given with high fat foods, there is a 7–fold increase in peak plasma levels; a 3– to 5–fold increase in absorption seen if given 2 hr after a meal. **t½, distribution:** 16 hr; **t½, terminal elimination:** 6–10 days. Excreted through the feces.

USES
Mild to moderate (100,000 or less parasites/mm³) malaria due to *Plasmodium falciparum* or *P. vivax*.

CONTRAINDICATIONS
Use in combination with drugs or clinical situations known to prolong QTc interval, family history of congenital QTc prolongation, in those who previously received mefloquine, or in those with known or suspected ventricular dysrhythmias, AV conduction disorders, or unexplained syncopal attacks. Lactation.

SPECIAL CONCERNS
The safety and efficacy in children, for use in prophylaxis of malaria, in cerebral malaria, or other complicated malaria forms have not been established. Clients with acute *P. vivax* are at risk of relapse because the drug does not eliminate the exoerythrocytic form; to eliminate the exoerythrocytic phase and avoid relapse, give the client an 8–aminoquinoline after initial halofantrine therapy. Prolongation of QTc interval can cause serious ventricular dysrhythmias with death (may be sudden).

SIDE EFFECTS
GI: Abdominal pain, diarrhea, N&V, anorexia, abdominal distention, constipation, dyspepsia, stomatitis. **CNS:** Dizziness, headache, asthenia, confusion, depression, paresthesia, sleep disorder, ***convulsions***. **CV:** Chest pain, palpitations, postural hypotension, ***serious ventricular dysrhythmias***. **Musculoskeletal:** Rigors, myalgias, arthralgia, back pain. **Miscellaneous:** Cough, pruritus, fatigue, malaise, rash, urinary frequency, abnormal vision, tinnitus, decreased consciousness.

LABORATORY TEST CONSIDERATIONS
↑ Hepatic transaminases. ↓ Hematocrit and platelet counts. ↑ and ↓ WBC counts.

OD OVERDOSE MANAGEMENT
Symptoms: GI distress with abdominal pain, vomiting, cramping, diarrhea, palpitations, dehydration. *Treatment:* Induce vomiting and institute supportive treatment, including ECG monitoring. Treat dehydration with IV fluids.

DRUG INTERACTIONS
Use with drugs known to prolong the QTc interval → further prolongation of the QTc interval due to the possibility of a fatal reaction.

HOW SUPPLIED
Tablets: 250 mg, 500 mg

DOSAGE
• **TABLETS**
P. falciparum or *P. vivax malaria. Non–immune clients:* 500 mg q 6 hr for 3 doses, followed by a repeat course given 7 days after the first. *Semi–immune clients:* Consider omitting the second course of therapy.

NURSING CONSIDERATIONS

ADMINISTRATION/STORAGE
Give on an empty stomach as increased absorption, and thus increased toxicity, may result if taken with food.

ASSESSMENT

1. Note onset, duration, and characteristics of symptoms of mild to moderate malaria (equal to or less than 100,000 parasites/mm³).
2. Determine any previous treatment with mefloquine.
3. Treatment of acute *P. vivax* malaria requires subsequent treatment with an aminoquinolone (i.e., primaquine) to prevent relapse (to eradicate the exoerythrocytic parasites).
4. Note any ventricular arrhythmias, AV conduction disorders, family history of congenital QTc prolongation, or unexplained syncopal attacks.
5. List drugs currently prescribed to ensure none interact or prolong the QTc interval.
6. Obtain ECG and assess QT interval; monitor cardiac rhythm for 8-12 hr following therapy.

CLIENT/FAMILY TEACHING

1. Take as directed on an empty stomach at least one hr before or two hr after meals. Dosing with food may result in increased absorption and toxicity.
2. Report any unusual or adverse side effects. Transient abdominal pain, N&V, diarrhea, headache, and dizziness may occur.
3. Practice reliable contraception and avoid prolonged sun exposure.

OUTCOMES/EVALUATE

Treatment of malaria infection

Haloperidol

(hah-low-**PAIR**-ih-dohl)

PREGNANCY CATEGORY: C
Rx: Haldol
✱**Rx:** Apo-Haloperidol, Novo–Peridol, Peridol, PMS Haloperidol LA

Haloperidol decanoate

(hah-low-**PAIR**-ih-dohl)

PREGNANCY CATEGORY: C
Rx: Haldol Decanoate 50 and 100
✱**Rx:** Rho-Haloperidol Decanoate

Haloperidol lactate

(hah-low-**PAIR**-ih-dohl)

PREGNANCY CATEGORY: C
Rx: Haldol Lactate
CLASSIFICATION(S):
Antipsychotic

ACTION/KINETICS

Precise mechanism not known. Competitively blocks dopamine receptors in the tuberoinfundibular system to cause sedation. Also causes alpha-adrenergic blockade, decreases release of growth hormone, and increases prolactin release by the pituitary. Causes significant extrapyramidal effects, as well as a low incidence of sedation, anticholinergic effects, and orthostatic hypotension. Narrow margin between the therapeutically effective dose and that causing extrapyramidal symptoms. Also has antiemetic effects. **Peak plasma levels: PO,** 3–5 hr; **IM,** 20 min; **IM, decanoate:** approximately 6 days. **Therapeutic serum levels:** 3–10 ng/mL. **t½, PO:** 12–38 hr; **IM:** 13–36 hr; **IM, decanoate:** 3 weeks; **IV:** approximately 14 hr. **Plasma protein binding:** 90%. Metabolized in liver, slowly excreted in urine and bile.

USES

(1) Psychotic disorders including manic states, drug-induced psychoses, and schizophrenia. (2) Severe behavior problems in children (those with combative, explosive hyperexcitability not accounted for by immediate provocation). (3) Short-term treatment of hyperactive children who show excessive motor activity with accompanying conduct consisting of impulsivity, poor attention, aggression, mood lability, or poor frustration tolerance. (4) Control of tics and vocal utterances associated with Tourette's syndrome in adults and children. The decanoate is used for prolonged therapy in chronic schizophrenia.

Investigational: Antiemetic for cancer chemotherapy, phencyclidine (PCP) psychosis, intractable hiccoughs, infantile autism. IV for acute psychiatric conditions.

CONTRAINDICATIONS

Use with extreme caution, or not at all, in clients with parkinsonism. Lactation.

SPECIAL CONCERNS

PO dosage has not been determined in children less than 3 years of age; IM dosage is not recommended in children. Geriatric clients are more likely to exhibit orthostatic hypotension, anticholinergic effects, sedation, and extrapyramidal side effects (such as parkinsonism and tardive dyskinesia).

SIDE EFFECTS

Extrapyramidal symptoms, especially akathisia and dystonias, occur more frequently than with the phenothiazines. Overdosage is characterized by severe extrapyramidal reactions, hypotension, or sedation. The drug does not elicit photosensitivity reactions like those of the phenothiazines.

LABORATORY TEST CONSIDERATIONS

↑ Alkaline phosphatase, bilirubin, serum transaminase; ↓ PT (clients on coumarin), serum cholesterol.

OD OVERDOSE MANAGEMENT

Symptoms: CNS depression, hypertension or hypotension, extrapyramidal symptoms, agitation, restlessness, fever, hypothermia, hyperthermia, ***seizures, cardiac arrhythmias,*** changes in the ECG, autonomic reactions, ***coma.*** *Treatment:* Treat symptomatically. Antiparkinson drugs, diphenhydramine, or barbiturates can be used to treat extrapyramidal symptoms. Fluid replacement and vasoconstrictors (either norepinephrine or phenylephrine) can be used to treat hypotension. Ventricular arrhythmias can be treated with phenytoin. To treat seizures, use pentobarbital or diazepam. A saline cathartic can be used to hasten the excretion of sustained-release products.

DRUG INTERACTIONS

Amphetamine / ↓ Amphetamine effect by ↓ uptake of drug at its site of action
Anticholinergics / ↓ Effect of haloperidol
Antidepressants, tricyclic / ↑ TCA effects R/T ↓ liver breakdown
Barbiturates / ↓ Effect of haloperidol R/T ↑ liver breakdown
Guanethidine / ↓ Guanethidine effect by ↓ uptake of drug at site of action
Lithium / ↑ Toxicity of haloperidol
Methyldopa / ↑ Toxicity of haloperidol
Phenytoin / ↓ Effect of haloperidol due to ↑ liver breakdown

HOW SUPPLIED

Haloperidol: *Tablet:* 0.5 mg, 1 mg, 2 mg, 5 mg, 10 mg, 20 mg. **Haloperidol decanoate:** *Injection:* 50 mg/mL, 100 mg/mL. **Haloperidol lactate:** *Concentrate:* 2 mg/mL; *Injection:* 5 mg/mL

DOSAGE

• ORAL SOLUTION, TABLETS

Psychoses.

Adults: 0.5–2 mg b.i.d.–t.i.d. up to 3–5 mg b.i.d.–t.i.d. for severe symptoms; **maintenance:** reduce dosage to lowest effective level. Up to 100 mg/day may be required in some. **Geriatric or debilitated clients:** 0.5–2 mg b.i.d.–t.i.d. **Pediatric, 3–12 years or 15–40 kg:** 0.5 mg/day in two to three divided doses; if necessary the daily dose may be increased by 0.5-mg increments q 5–7 days for a total of 0.15 mg/kg/day for psychotic disorders.

Tourette's syndrome.

Adults, initial: 0.5–1.5 mg t.i.d., up to 10 mg daily. Adjust dose carefully to obtain the optimum response. **Children, 3 to 12 years:** 0.05–0.075 mg/kg/day. Higher doses may be needed for those severely disturbed.

Behavioral disorders/hyperactivity in children.

Children, 3 to 12 years: 0.05–0.075 mg/kg/day. Higher doses may be needed for those severely disturbed.

Intractable hiccoughs (investigational).

1.5 mg t.i.d.

Infantile autism (investigational).

0.5–4 mg/day.

• IM, LACTATE

Acute psychoses.

Adults and adolescents, initial: 2–5 mg to control acute agitation; may be repeated if necessary q 4–8 hr to a total of 100 mg/day. Switch to **PO** therapy as soon as possible.

- **IM, DECANOATE**

Chronic therapy.

Adults, initial dose: 10–15 times the daily PO dose, not to exceed 100 mg initially, regardless of the previous oral antipsychotic dose; **then,** repeat q 4 weeks (decanoate is not to be given IV).

NURSING CONSIDERATIONS

SEE ALSO *NURSING CONSIDERATIONS* FOR *ANTIPSYCHOTIC AGENTS*.

ADMINISTRATION/STORAGE

1. Give the decanoate by deep IM injection using a 21-gauge needle. Do not exceed a volume of 3 mL/site.
2. Do not give decanoate IV.

ASSESSMENT

1. Document behavior, appearance, response to environment and questions, and characteristics of symptoms; note S&S parkinsonism and tardive dyskinesias.
2. Use with caution in the elderly; they tend to exhibit toxicity more frequently; may also benefit from a periodic "drug holiday."
3. Document evidence of new onset of extrapyramidal symptoms; may be drug induced.
4. Assess CBC, lytes, liver and renal function.

CLIENT/FAMILY TEACHING

1. Take exactly as prescribed. Do not stop abruptly with long term therapy.
2. Avoid activities that require mental alertness until drug effects realized.
3. Avoid alcohol. May use sugarless gum, ice chips or sips of water for dry mouth effects.
4. Report muscle weakness/stiffness. Avoid prolonged sun exposure, may cause a photosensitivity reaction.
5. May take up to 6 weeks for full benefits to occur.

OUTCOMES/EVALUATE

- Improved behavior patterns: ↓ agitation, hostility, psychosis, delusions
- Control of tics/vocal utterances
- ↓ Hyperactive behaviors

Heparin sodium injection

(**HEP**-ah-rin)

PREGNANCY CATEGORY: C

★Rx: Hepalean, Hepalean-Lok, Heparin Leo

Heparin sodium and sodium chloride

(**HEP**-ah-rin)

PREGNANCY CATEGORY: C

Rx: Heparin Sodium and 0.45% Sodium Chloride, Heparin Sodium and 0.9% Sodium Chloride

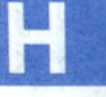

Heparin sodium lock flush solution

(**HEP**-ah-rin)

PREGNANCY CATEGORY: C

Rx: Heparin Lock Flush, Hep-Lock, Hep-Lock U/P

CLASSIFICATION(S):

Anticoagulant, heparin

ACTION/KINETICS

Anticoagulants do not dissolve previously formed clots, but they do forestall their enlargement and prevent new clots from forming. Heparin potentiates the inhibitory action of antithrombin III on various coagulation factors including factors IIa, IXa, Xa, XIa, and XIIa. This occurs due to the formation of a complex with and causing a conformational change in the antithrombin III molecule. Inhibition of factor Xa results in interference with thrombin generation; thus, the action of thrombin in coagulation is inhibited. Heparin also increases the rate of formation of antithrombin III–thrombin complex causing inactivation of thrombin and preventing the conversion of fibrinogen to fibrin. By inhibiting the activation of fibrin-stabilizing factor by thrombin, heparin also prevents formation of a stable fibrin clot. Therapeutic doses of heparin prolong thrombin time, whole blood clotting time, activated clotting time, and PTT. Heparin also decreases the levels of triglycerides by releasing lipoprotein lipase from tissues; the resultant hydrolysis of triglycerides causes increased blood levels of free fatty acids. **Onset: IV,** immediate; **deep SC:** 20–60 min. **Peak plasma levels, after SC:** 2–4 hr. **t½:** 30–180 min in healthy persons. t½ increases with dose, severe renal disease, and cirrhosis and in anephric clients and decreases with pulmonary embolism and liver impairment other than cirrhosis. *Metabolism:* Probably by reticuloendothelial system, although up to 50% is excreted unchanged in the urine. Clotting time returns to normal within 2–6 hr.

USES

Pulmonary/peripheral arterial embolism, prophylaxis, and treatment of venous thrombosis and its extension. Atrial fibrillation with embolization. Diagnosis and treatment of DIC. Low doses to prevent DVT and PE in pregnant clients with a history of thromboembolism, urology clients over 40 years of age, clients with stroke or heart failure, AMI or pulmonary infection, high-risk surgery clients, moderate and high-risk gynecologic clients with no malignancy, neurology clients with extracranial problems, and clients with severe musculoskeletal trauma. Prophylaxis of clotting in blood transfusions, extracorporeal circulation, dialysis procedures, blood samples for lab tests, and arterial and heart surgery. *Investigational:* Prophylaxis of post-MI, CVAs, and LV thrombi. By continuous infusion to treat myocardial ischemia in unstable angina refractory to usual treatment. Adjunct to treat coronary occlusion with AMI. Prophylaxis of cerebral thrombosis in evolving stroke.

Heparin lock flush solution: Dilute solutions are used to maintain patency of indwelling catheters used for IV therapy or blood sampling. Not to be used therapeutically.

CONTRAINDICATIONS

Active bleeding, blood dyscrasias (or other disorders characterized by bleeding tendencies such as hemophilia), clients with frail or weakened blood vessels, purpura, thrombocytopenia, liver disease with hypoprothrombinemia, suspected intracranial hemorrhage, suppurative thrombophlebitis, inaccessible ulcerative lesions (especially of the GI tract), open wounds, extensive denudation of the skin, and increased capillary permeability (as in ascorbic acid deficiency). IM use.

Do not administer during surgery of the eye, brain, or spinal cord or during continuous tube drainage of the stomach or small intestine. Use is also contraindicated in subacute endocarditis, shock, threatened abortion, severe hypertension, diverticulitis, colitis, SBE, or hypersensitivity to drug. Premature neonates due to the possibility of a fatal "gasping syndrome." Also, regional anesthesia and lumbar block, vitamin K deficiency, leukemia with bleeding tendencies, open wounds or ulcerations, acute nephritis, impaired hepatic or renal function, or severe hypertension. In the presence of drainage tubes in any orifice. Alcoholism.

SPECIAL CONCERNS

Use with caution in menstruation, in pregnant women (because they may cause hypoprothrombinemia in the infant), during lactation, during the postpartum period, and following cerebrovascular accidents. Geriatric clients may be more susceptible to developing bleeding complications, unusual hair loss, and itching.

SIDE EFFECTS

CV: ***Hemorrhage ranging from minor local ecchymoses to major hemorrhagic complications from any organ or tissue.*** Higher incidence is seen in women over 60 years of age. Hemorrhagic reactions are more likely to occur in prophylactic administration during surgery than in the treatment of thromboembolic disease. White clot syndrome. **Hematologic:** Thrombocytopenia (both early and late). **Hypersensitivity:** Chills, fever, urticaria are the most common. Rarely, asthma, lacrimation, headache, N&V, rhinitis, ***shock, anaphylaxis.*** Allergic vasospastic reaction within 6–10 days after initiation of therapy (lasts 4–6 hr) including painful, ischemic, cyanotic limbs. Use a test dose of 1,000 units in clients with a history of asthma or allergic disease. **Miscellaneous:** Hyperkalemia, cutaneous necrosis, osteoporosis (after long-term high doses), delayed transient alopecia, priapism, suppressed aldosterone synthesis. Discontinuance of heparin has resulted in rebound hyperlipemia. **Following IM (usual), SC:** Local irritation, erythema, mild pain, ulceration, hematoma, and tissue sloughing.

LABORATORY TEST CONSIDERATIONS

↑ AST and ALT.

OD OVERDOSE MANAGEMENT

Symptoms: Nosebleeds, hematuria, tarry stools, petechiae, and easy bruising may be the first signs. *Treatment:* Drug withdrawal is usually sufficient to correct heparin overdosage. Protamine sulfate (1%) solution; each mg of protamine neutralizes about 100 USP heparin units.

DRUG INTERACTIONS

Alteplase, recombinant / ↑ Risk of bleeding, especially at arterial puncture sites
Anticoagulants, oral / Additive ↑ PT
Antihistamines / ↓ Effect of heparin
Aspirin / Additive ↑ PT
H *Bromelain* / ↑ Tendency for bleeding
Cephalosporins / ↑ Risk of bleeding R/T additive effect
H *Cinchona bark* / ↑ Anticoagulant effect
Dextran / Additive ↑ PT
Digitalis / ↓ Effect of heparin
Dipyridamole / Additive ↑ PT
H *Feverfew* / Possible additive antiplatelet effect
H *Ginger* / Possible additive antiplatelet effect
H *Ginkgo biloba* / ↑ Effect on blood coagulation
H *Ginseng* / Potential for ↓ effect on platelet aggregation
H *Goldenseal* / Antagonizes action of heparin
Hydroxychloroquine / Additive ↑ PT
Ibuprofen / Additive ↑ PT
Indomethacin / Additive ↑ PT
Insulin / Heparin antagonizes insulin effect
Nicotine / ↓ Effect of heparin
Nitroglycerin / ↓ Effect of heparin
NSAIDs / Additive ↑ PT
Penicillins / ↑ Risk of bleeding R/T possible additive effects
Salicylates / ↑ Risk of bleeding
Streptokinase / Relative resistance to effects of heparin
Tetracyclines / ↓ Effect of heparin
Ticlopidine / Additive ↑ PT

HOW SUPPLIED

Heparin sodium injection: *Injection:* 1,000 U/mL, 2,000 U/mL, 2,500 U/mL, 5,000 U/mL, 7,500 U/mL, 10,000 U/mL, 20,000 U/mL, 40,000 U/mL. **Heparin sodium and sodium chloride:** *Injection:* 200 U/100 mL-0.9%, 5,000 U/100 mL-0.45%, 10,000 U/100 mL-0.45%. **Heparin sodium lock flush solution:** *Kit:* 10 U/mL, 100 U/mL

DOSAGE

NOTE: Adjusted for each client on the basis of laboratory tests.

- **DEEP SC**

General heparin dosage.

Initial loading dose: 10,000–20,000 units; **maintenance:** 8,000–10,000 units q 8 hr or 15,000–20,000 units q 12 hr. *Use concentrated solution.*

Prophylaxis of postoperative thromboembolism.

5,000 units of concentrated solution 2 hr before surgery and 5,000 units q 8–12 hr thereafter for 7 days or until client is ambulatory.

- **INTERMITTENT IV**

General heparin dosage.

Initial loading dose: 10,000 units undiluted or in 50–100 mL saline; **then,** 5,000–10,000 units q 4–6 hr undiluted or in 50–100 mL saline.

- **CONTINUOUS IV INFUSION**

General heparin dosage.

Initial loading dose: 20,000–40,000 units/day in 1,000 mL saline (preceded initially by 5,000 units IV).

- **SPECIAL USES**

Surgery of heart and blood vessels.

Initial, 150–400 units/kg to clients undergoing total body perfusion for open heart surgery. *NOTE:* 300 units/

kg may be used for procedures less than 60 min while 400 units/kg is used for procedures lasting more than 60 min. To prevent clotting in the tube system, add heparin to fluids in pump oxygenator.

Extracorporeal renal dialysis.
See instructions on equipment.

Blood transfusion.
400–600 units/100 mL whole blood. 7,500 units should be added to 100 mL 0.9% sodium chloride injection; from this dilution, add 6–8 mL/100 mL whole blood.

Laboratory samples.
70–150 units/10- to 20-mL sample to prevent coagulation.

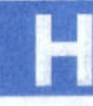

Heparin lock sets.
To prevent clot formation in a heparin lock set, inject 10–100 units/mL heparin solution through the injection hub in a sufficient quantity to fill the entire set to the needle tip.

NURSING CONSIDERATIONS

ADMINISTRATION/STORAGE

1. Do *not* administer IM.
2. Administer by deep SC injection to minimize local irritation, hematoma, and tissue sloughing and to prolong action of drug.
   - Z-track method: Use any fat roll, but abdominal fat rolls are preferred. Use a ½-in. or ⅝-in. 25- or 27-gauge needle. Grasp the skin layer of the fat roll and lift it up. Insert the needle at about a 45° angle to the skin's fat layer and then administer the medication. It is not necessary to aspirate to check if needle is in a blood vessel. Rapidly withdraw the needle while releasing the skin.
   - "Bunch technique" method: Grasp tissue around the injection site, creating a tissue roll of about ½ in. in diameter. Insert needle into the tissue roll at a 90° angle to the skin surface and inject the medication. Again, it is not necessary to aspirate. Withdraw the needle rapidly when the skin is released.
   - Do not administer within 2 in. of the umbilicus (due to increased vascularity of area).
3. Do not massage site.
4. Rotate sites of administration.
5. Slight discoloration does not affect potency.

IV 6. Hospitalize for IV therapy.
7. May be diluted in dextrose, NSS, or Ringer's solution and administered over 4–24 hr with an infusion pump.
8. Protect solutions from freezing.
9. Have protamine sulfate, a heparin antagonist, available should excessive bleeding occur.
10. NaCl, 0.9%, is effective in maintaining patency of peripheral (noncentral) intermittent infusion devices and in reducing added medical costs. The following procedure has been recommended:
   - Determine patency by aspirating lock.
   - Flush with 2 mL NSS.
   - Administer medication therapy. (Flush between drugs.)
   - Flush with 2 mL NSS.
   - Frequency of flushing to maintain patency when not actively in use varies from every 8 hr to every 24–48 hr.
   - This does *NOT* apply to any central venous access devices.

ASSESSMENT

1. Identify any bleeding incidents, i.e., bleeding tendencies, family history, or any other incidents of unexplained or active bleeding.
2. Perform test dose (1,000 units SC) to clients with multiple allergies or asthma history.
3. Review drug profile to ensure none interact unfavorably; otherwise, anticipate heparin dosage adjustment.
4. Assess for defects in clotting mechanism or any capillary fragility.
5. Note indications for therapy, time frame (i.e., DVT [initial] 6 months; valve replacement—lifetime), and desired INR, PT/PTT and record.
6. Review PMH for conditions that may preclude therapy: alcoholic, chronic GI tract ulcerations, severe renal or liver dysfunction, infections of the endocardium, or PUD which may be a potential site of bleeding. Note any evidence of intracranial hemorrhage.
7. Monitor CBC, PT, PTT, renal, and LFTs.

INTERVENTIONS

1. Post/advise client receiving anticoagulant therapy.
2. Monitor PT/INR or PTT levels closely.

3. Question about bleeding (gums, urine, stools, vomit, bruises). If urine discolored, determine cause, i.e., from drug therapy or hematuria. Indanedione-type anticoagulants turn alkaline urine a red-orange color; acidify urine or test for occult blood.
4. Sudden lumbar pain may indicate retroperitoneal hemorrhage.
5. GI dysfunction may indicate intestinal hemorrhage. Test for blood in urine and feces; check H&H to assess for abnormal bleeding.
6. Have protamine sulfate for heparin overdose available (generally for every 100 U of heparin administer 1 mg protamine sulfate IV).
7. Apply pressure to all venipuncture and injection sites to prevent bleeding and hematoma formation.
8. In heparin lock devices, the presence of heparin or NSS may cause lab test interferences.
• To clear flush solution: aspirate and discard 1 mL of fluid from device before withdrawing blood sample.
• Inject 1 mL of flush solution into lock after blood samples are drawn.
• With excessively abnormal results, obtain a repeat sample from another site before altering treatment.
9. With SC administration, do not aspirate or massage; administer in lower abdomen and rotate sites.

For Heparin Lock Flush Solution:

1. Aspirate lock to determine patency. Maintain patency: inject 1 mL of flush solution into device diaphragm after each use (maintains catheter patency for up to 24 hr).
2. If administering a drug incompatible with heparin, flush with 0.9% NaCl injection or sterile water for injection before and immediately after incompatible drug administered. Inject another dose of heparin lock flush solution after the final flush.
3. Observe coagulation times carefully with underlying bleeding disorders; ↑ risk for hemorrhage.
4. The presence of heparin or NSS may cause lab test interferences. To clear flush solution:
• Aspirate and discard 1 mL of fluid from device before withdrawing blood sample.
• Inject 1 mL of flush solution into lock after blood samples are drawn.
• With excessively abnormal results, obtain a repeat sample from another site before initiating treatment.
5. Monitor for allergic reactions due to various biologic sources of heparin.

CLIENT/FAMILY TEACHING

1. Review administration technique. Can only be given parenterally.
2. Report signs of active bleeding or any excessive menstrual flow; may need to withhold/reduce dosage.
3. Alopecia is generally temporary.
4. Report alterations in GU function, urine color, or any injury.
5. Use an electric razor for shaving and a soft-bristle toothbrush to decrease gum irritation.
6. Arrange furniture to allow open space for unimpeded ambulation and to diminish chances of bumping into objects that may cause bruising/bleeding. Always wear shoes or slippers.
7. Use a night light to illuminate trips to the bathroom.
8. Avoid contact sports and any activities where excessive bumping, bruising or injury may occur.
9. Eat potassium-rich foods (e.g., baked potato, orange juice, bananas, beef, flounder, haddock, sweet potato, turkey, raw tomato).
10. Avoid eating large amounts of vitamin K foods; mostly yellow and dark green vegetables.
11. Report increased bruising, bleeding of nose, mouth, gums, mucus or oral secretions, tarry stools, or GI upset.
12. Avoid alcohol, aspirin, tobacco, and NSAIDs; increase anticoagulant response.
13. Alert all providers of therapy and wear/carry drug identification.

OUTCOMES/EVALUATE

• PTT: 2–2.5 times the control/normal
• Prevention of thrombus formation
• Clot prophylaxis/treatment
• Indwelling catheter patency

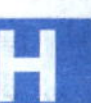

Histrelin acetate

(hiss-**TREL**-in)

PREGNANCY CATEGORY: X
CLASSIFICATION(S):
Gonadotropion-releasing hormone
Rx: Supprelin, Synarel

ACTION/KINETICS
Histrelin contains a synthetic nonapeptide agonist of the naturally occurring GnRH. Initially the drug stimulates release of GnRH; however, chronic use desensitizes responsiveness of the pituitary gonadotropin, causing a reduction in ovarian and testicular steroidogenesis. Decreases in LH, FSH, and sex steroid levels are observed within 3 months of initiation of therapy.

USES
To control the biochemical and clinical symptoms of central precocious puberty (either idiopathic or neurogenic) occurring before 8 years of age in girls or 9.5 years of age in boys.

CONTRAINDICATIONS
Hypersensitivity to the product or any of its components. Lactation.

SPECIAL CONCERNS
Acute, serious hypersensitivity reactions may occur that require emergency medical treatment. Safety and efficacy in children less than 2 years of age have not been determined.

SIDE EFFECTS
Acute hypersensitivity reaction: Angioedema, urticaria, ***CV collapse,*** hypotension, tachycardia, loss of consciousness, ***bronchospasm,*** dyspnea, flushing, pruritus. **CV:** Vasodilation (common), edema, palpitations, tachycardia, epistaxis, hypertension, migraine headache, pallor. **GI:** GI or abdominal pain, N&V, diarrhea, flatulence, decrease appetite, dyspepsia, GI cramps or distress, constipation, decreased appetite, thirst, gastritis. **CNS:** Headache (common), nervousness, dizziness, depression, changes in libido, mood changes, insomnia, anxiety, paresthesia, syncope, somnolence, cognitive changes, lethargy, impaired consciousness, tremor, hyperkinesia, convulsions (increased frequency), hot flashes or flushes, conduct disorder. **Endocrine:** Vaginal dryness, leukorrhea, metrorrhagia, breast pain, breast edema, decreased breast size, breast discharge, tenderness of female genitalia, anemia, goiter, hyperlipidemia, glycosuria. **Musculoskeletal:** Arthralgia, joint stiffness, muscle cramp or stiffness, myalgia, hypotonia, pain. **Respiratory:** Cough, URI, pharyngitis, respiratory congestion, asthma, breathing disorder, rhinorrhea, bronchitis, sinusitis, hyperventilation. **Dermatologic:** Commonly, redness, itching, and swelling at the injection site. Also, urticaria, sweating, keratoderma, pruritus, pain, dyschromia, alopecia, erythema. **Ophthalmologic:** Visual disturbances, abnormal pupillary function, polyopia, photophobia. **Otic:** Otalgia, hearing loss. **GU:** Vaginal bleeding (most often one episode within 1–3 weeks after starting therapy and lasting several days). Also, vaginitis, dysmenorrhea, and problems of the female genitalia including pruritus, irritation, odor, pain, infections, and hypertrophy. Dyspareunia, polyuria, dysuria, incontinence, urinary frequency, hematuria, nocturia. **Miscellaneous:** Pyrexia (common), weight gain, fatigue, viral infection, chills, various body pains, malaise, purpura.

HOW SUPPLIED
Kit: 120 mcg/0.6 mL (200 mcg/mL peptide base), 300 mcg/0.6 mL (500 mcg/mL peptide base), 600 mcg/0.6 mL (1000 mcg/mL peptide base)

DOSAGE
- **SC**

Central precocious puberty.
10 mcg/kg given as a single, daily SC injection. Doses greater than 10 mcg/kg/day have not been evaluated.

NURSING CONSIDERATIONS

ADMINISTRATION/STORAGE
1. Reevaluate if prepubertal levels of sex hormones or a prepubertal gonadotropin response to GnRH administration are not achieved within the first 3 months of therapy.
2. Rotate injection site daily.

3. Contains no preservative; store vials at 2–8°C (36–46°F) and protect from light.
4. Use vials only once; discard any unused solution.
5. Remove vial from the packaging only at the time of use. Allow vial to reach room temperature before using.

ASSESSMENT

1. Assess for histrelin-related hypersensitivity reactions.
2. Note results of physical and endocrinologic evaluation. This should include:
• Baseline height and weight
• Baseline hand and wrist X rays to determine bone age
• Sex steroid level (estradiol or testosterone)
• Adrenal steroid level (to R/O congenital hyperplasia)
• Beta-human chorionic gonadotropin level (to R/O chorionic gonadotropin-secreting tumor)
• GnRH stimulation test (to document activation of HPG [hypothalamic-pituitary-gonadal] axis)
• Pelvic ultrasound (adrenal, testicular) to R/O steroid-secreting tumor and to obtain baseline gonadal size
• CT of head (to R/O any undiagnosed intracranial tumor)

CLIENT/FAMILY TEACHING

1. Review instructions provided with 7-day kit. Drug contains no preservative; once vials entered, discard any unused solution.
2. Administer at room temperature.
3. Establish a daily administration schedule; rotate injection sites. If not administered daily, the pubertal process may be reactivated.
4. Compliance with therapy and scheduled clinical evaluations to assess progress and perform height measurements are important. Yearly bone growth determinations and serial GnRH testing document that gonadotropin responsiveness of the pituitary remains prepubertal during therapy.
5. Report any sudden swelling, dyspnea, dysphagia, rash, itching, and/or rapid heartbeat.
6. Hypogonadism may result if HPG axis reactivation fails after discontinuation of drug.
7. Drug should be discontinued when onset of puberty is desired; need F/U to assess menstrual cyclicity, reproductive function, and adult height attained.

OUTCOMES/EVALUATE

Control of biochemical/physical manifestations of puberty

Hydrochlorothiazide

(**hy**-droh-klor-oh-**THIGH**-ah-zyd)

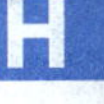

PREGNANCY CATEGORY: B
CLASSIFICATION(S):
Diuretic, thiazide
Rx: Esidrex, Ezide, HydroDIURIL, Hydro-Par, Microzide Capsules, Oretic
★**Rx:** Apo-Hydro

SEE ALSO *DIURETICS, THIAZIDE.*

ACTION/KINETICS

Onset: 2 hr. **Peak effect:** 4–6 hr. **Duration:** 6–12 hr. **t½:** 5.6–14.8 hr.

ADDITIONAL USES

Microzide is available for once-daily, low-dose treatment for hypertension.

SPECIAL CONCERNS

Geriatric clients may be more sensitive to the usual adult dose.

ADDITIONAL SIDE EFFECTS

CV: Allergic myocarditis, hypotension. **Dermatologic:** Alopecia, exfoliative dermatitis, ***toxic epidermal necrolysis,*** erythema multiforme, ***Stevens-Johnson syndrome.*** **Miscellaneous:** ***Anaphylactic reactions, respiratory distress including pneumonitis and pulmonary edema.***

HOW SUPPLIED

Capsule: 12.5 mg; *Solution:* 50 mg/5 mL; *Tablet:* 25 mg, 50 mg, 100 mg

DOSAGE

• **CAPSULES, ORAL SOLUTION, TABLETS**

Diuretic.

Adults, initial: 25–200 mg/day for several days until dry weight is reached; **then,** 25–100 mg/day or intermittently.

Some clients may require up to 200 mg/day.

Antihypertensive.

Adults, initial: 25 mg/day as a single dose. The dose may be increased to 50 mg/day in one to two doses. Doses greater than 50 mg may cause significant reductions in serum potassium. **Pediatric, under 6 months:** 3.3 mg/kg/day in two doses; **up to 2 years of age:** 12.5–37.5 mg/day in two doses; **2–12 years of age:** 37.5–100 mg/day in two doses.

NURSING CONSIDERATIONS

H

SEE ALSO *NURSING CONSIDERATIONS* FOR *DIURETICS, THIAZIDE.*

ADMINISTRATION/STORAGE

1. Divide daily doses in excess of 100 mg.
2. Give b.i.d. at 6–12-hr intervals.
3. When used with other antihypertensives, hydrochlorothiazide dose is usually not more than 50 mg.

ASSESSMENT

Assess for glucose intolerance; monitor electrolytes and replace potassium as needed.

CLIENT/FAMILY TEACHING

1. Take once daily in the morning as directed, usually with a glass of orange juice. Report any unusual side effects.
2. May cause dizziness, change positions slowly.
3. Report any swelling of extremities or weight gain of > 3 lb/day.
4. Avoid prolonged sun exposure; may cause delayed (10-14 day) photosensitivity reaction.
5. With diabetes, monitor BS and potassium closely, may cause glucose intolerance.

OUTCOMES/EVALUATE

- ↓ BP
- ↑ Urine output; ↓ edema

—COMBINATION DRUG—

Hydrocodone bitartrate and Acetaminophen

(**high**-droh-**KOH**-dohn, ah-**seat**-ah-**MIN**-oh-fen)

PREGNANCY CATEGORY: C

CLASSIFICATION(S):

Analgesic

Rx: Anexia 10/660, Anexia 5/500, Anexia 7.5/650, Bancap HC, Ceta-Plus, Co-Gesic, Dolacet, Duocet, Hydrocet, Hydrogesic, Hy-Phen, Lorcet Plus, Lorcet-10/650, Lorcet-HD, Lortab 10/500, Lortab 5/500, Lortab 7.5/500, Margesic H, Maxidone, Norco, Norco 5/325, Norco 7.5/325, Panacet 5/500, Stagesic, T-Gesic, Vicodin, Vicodin ES, Vicodin HP, Zydone **C-III**

SEE ALSO *NARCOTIC ANALGESICS* AND *ACETAMINOPHEN.*

CONTENT

Several possible combinations of hydrocodone bitartrate (narcotic analgesic) and acetaminophen (nonnarcotic analgesic)—amount of hydrocodone listed first: 5 mg/325 mg, 7.5/325, 10/325, 5 mg/500 mg, 7.5 mg/400 mg, 7.5 mg/500 mg, 7.5 mg/650 mg, 7.5 mg/750 mg, 10 mg/325 mg, 10 mg/400 mg, 10 mg/500 mg, 10 mg/650 mg, 10 mg/660 mg, 10 mg/750 mg.

ACTION/KINETICS

Hydrocodone produces its analgesic activity by an action on the CNS via opiate receptors. The analgesic action of acetaminophen is produced by both peripheral and central mechanisms.

USES

Relief of moderate to moderately severe pain.

CONTRAINDICATIONS

Hypersensitivity to acetaminophen or hydrocodone. Lactation.

SPECIAL CONCERNS

Use with caution, if at all, in clients with head injuries as the CSF pressure may be increased further. Use with caution in geriatric or debilitated clients; in those with impaired hepatic or renal function; in hypothyroidism, Addison's disease, prostatic hypertrophy, or urethral stricture; and in clients with pulmonary disease. Use shortly before delivery may cause respiratory depression in the newborn. Safety and efficacy have not been determined in children.

SIDE EFFECTS

CNS: Lightheadedness, dizziness, sedation, drowsiness, mental clouding, lethargy, impaired mental and physical performance, anxiety, fear, dysphoria, psychologic dependence, mood changes. **GI:** N&V. **Respiratory:** Respiratory depression (dose-related), irregular and periodic breathing. **GU:** Ureteral spasm, spasm of vesical sphincters, urinary retention.

OD OVERDOSE MANAGEMENT

Symptoms: ***Acetaminophen overdose may result in potentially fatal hepatic necrosis.*** Also, renal tubular necrosis, hypoglycemic coma, and thrombocytopenia. Symptoms of hepatotoxic overdose include N&V, diaphoresis, and malaise. Symptoms of hydrocodone overdose include respiratory depression, somnolence progressing to stupor or ***coma,*** skeletal muscle flaccidity, cold and clammy skin, bradycardia, and hypotension. ***Severe overdose may cause apnea, circulatory collapse, cardiac arrest, and death.***

Treatment (Acetaminophen):

- Empty stomach promptly by lavage or induction of emesis with syrup of ipecac.
- Serum acetaminophen levels should be determined as early as possible but no sooner than 4 hr after ingestion.
- Determine liver function initially and at 24-hr intervals.
- The antidote, *N*-acetylcysteine, should be given within 16 hr of overdose for optimal results.

Treatment (Hydrocodone):

- Reestablish adequate respiratory exchange with a patent airway and assisted or controlled ventilation.
- Respiratory depression can be reversed by giving naloxone IV.
- Oxygen, IV fluids, vasopressors, and other supportive measures may be instituted as required.

DRUG INTERACTIONS

Anticholinergics / ↑ Risk of paralytic ileus

CNS depressants, including other narcotic analgesics, antianxiety agents, antipsychotics, alcohol / Additive CNS depression

MAO inhibitors / ↑ Effect of either the narcotic or the antidepressant

Tricyclic antidepressants / ↑ Effect of either the narcotic or the antidepressant

HOW SUPPLIED

See Content

DOSAGE

- **CAPSULES, TABLETS**

Analgesia.

For 5/500 products, the dose is 1 or 2 q 4–6 hr, up to 8/day. For 5/325, 7.5/325, 10/325, and 7.5/400, the dose is 1 q 4–6 hr, up to 6/day. For 7.5/500 and 7.5/650, the dose is 1 q 4–6 hr. For 7.5/750, the dose is 1 q 4–6 hr, up to 5/day. For 10/325, 10/400, 10/500, and 10/650, the dose is 1 q 4–6 hr, up to 6/day. For 10/650, 10/660, and 10/750, the dose is 1 q 4–6 hr.

NURSING CONSIDERATIONS

SEE ALSO *NURSING CONSIDERATIONS* FOR *NARCOTIC ANALGESICS* AND *ACETAMINOPHEN*.

ASSESSMENT

1. Note onset, location, and characteristics of symptoms, other agents prescribed, and the outcome. Determine if pain is acute or chronic; rate pain level.
2. Note history of hypothyroidism, BPH, urethral stricture, Addison's, or pulmonary disease.
3. Monitor renal and LFTs.
4. Coadministration of an NSAID may reduce the dosage required for pain relief.

CLIENT/FAMILY TEACHING

1. Take only as prescribed.
2. Do not perform activities that require mental alertness; causes dizziness, lethargy, and impaired physical and mental performance.
3. Report any evidence of abnormal bleeding or bruising, respiratory difficulties, N&V, urinary difficulty, or excessive sedation.
4. Avoid alcohol and any other medications without approval.
5. Store drug appropriately, away from the bedside and safely out of the reach of children.
6. Drug is for short term use; may be habit forming.

OUTCOMES/EVALUATE

Desired pain control; ↓ Cough

H

Hydrocortisone (Cortisol)

(hy-droh-**KOR**-tih-zohn)

PREGNANCY CATEGORY: C (TOPICAL AND DENTAL PRODUCTS)
Rx: Parenteral: Sterile Hydrocortisone Suspension; **Rectal:** Dermolate Anal-Itch, Proctocort, Procto-Cream.HC 2.5%; **Retention Enema:** Colocort; **Roll-on Applicator:** Cortaid FastStick; **Tablets:** Cortef, Hydrocortone; **Topical Cream:** Ala-Cort, Alphaderm, Cort-Dome, Cortifair, Dermacort, DermiCort, H_2Cort, Hi-Cor 1.0 and 2.5, Hytone, Nutracort, Penecort., Synacort; **Topical Lotion:** Acticort 100, Ala-Cort, Ala-Scalp, Allercort, Cetacort, Cort-Dome, Delacort, Dermacort, Gly-Cort, Hytone, LactiCare-HC, Lemoderm, Lexocort Forte, My Cort, Nutracort, Pentacort, Rederm, S-T Cort; **Topical Ointment:** Allercort, Cortril, Hytone, Lemoderm, Penecort; **Topical Solution:** Emo-Cort Scalp Solution, Penecort, Texacort Scalp Solution; **Topical Spray:** Cortenema
★Rx: Rectal: Cortenema, Rectocort; **Retention Enema:** Hycort, Rectocort; **Topical Lotion:** Aquacort, Cortate, Emo-Cort, Sarna HC; **Topical Cream:** Cortate, Emo-cort Prevex HC; **Topical Oinment:** Cortoderm
OTC: Roll-on Applicator: Maximum Strength Cortaid Faststick; **Topical Cream:** Allercort, Bactine, Dermolate Anti-Itch, Dermtex HC, Hydro-Tex; **Topical Gel:** Extra Strength CortaGel; **Topical Liquid:** T/Scalp, Scalpicin; **Topical Lotion:** Dermolate Scalp-Itch; **Topical Spray:** Cortaid, Dermolate Anti-Itch, Maximum Strength Coraid, Procort

Hydrocortisone acetate

(hy-droh-**KOR**-tih-zohn)

PREGNANCY CATEGORY: C (TOPICAL AND DENTAL PRODUCTS)
Rx: Dental Paste: Orabase-HCA; **Intrarectal Foam:** Cortifoam; **Parenteral:** Hydrocortone Acetate; **Rectal:** Cort-Dome High Potency, Cortenema, Corticaine, Cortifoam; **Topical Cream/Ointment:** Maximum Strength Hydrocortisone Acetate; **Topical Cream:** CaldeCORT Light, Carmol-HC, Gynecort, Lanacort, Pharma-Cort; **Topical Ointment:** Nov–Hydrocort.
★Rx: Ophthalmic/Optic: Cortamed; **Suppository:** Cortiment, Rectocort; **Topical Cream:** Corticreme, Hyderm; **Topical Ointment:** DermaPlex HC1%
OTC: Topical Cream: Cortaid, Cortef Feminine Itch, Corticaine, FoilleCort, Gynecort Female Cream, Lanacort 10, Lanacort 5, Maximum Strength Cortaid, Rhulicort; **Topical Lotion:** Cortaid, Rhulicort; **Topical Ointment:** Cortef Acetate, Lanacort, Lanacort 5, Maximum Strength Cortaid

Hydrocortisone buteprate

(hy-droh-**KOR**-tih-zohn)

PREGNANCY CATEGORY: C
Rx: Topical Cream: Pandel

Hydrocortisone butyrate

(hy-droh-**KOR**-tih-zohn)

PREGNANCY CATEGORY: C (TOPICAL PRODUCTS)
Rx: Topical Cream, Ointment, Solution: Locoid

Hydrocortisone cypionate

(hy-droh-**KOR**-tih-zohn)

PREGNANCY CATEGORY: C
Rx: Oral Suspension: Cortef

Hydrocortisone sodium phosphate

(hy-droh-**KOR**-tih-zohn)

PREGNANCY CATEGORY: C
Rx: Parenteral: Hydrocortone Phosphate

Hydrocortisone sodium succinate

(hy-droh-**KOR**-tih-zohn)

PREGNANCY CATEGORY: C
Rx: Parenteral: A-Hydrocort, Solu-Cortef

Hydrocortisone valerate

(hy-droh-**KOR**-tih-zohn)

PREGNANCY CATEGORY: C (TOPICAL PRODUCTS)
Rx: Topical Cream/Ointment: Westcort
CLASSIFICATION(S):
Glucocorticoid

SEE ALSO *CORTICOSTEROIDS*.

ACTION/KINETICS
Short-acting. **t½:** 80–118 min. Topical products are available without a prescription in strengths of 0.5% and 1%.

HOW SUPPLIED
Hydrocortisone (Cortisol): *Balm:* 1%; *Cream:* 0.5%, 1%, 2.5%; *Enema:* 100 mg/60 mL; *Gel/jelly:* 1%; *Liquid:* 1%; *Lotion:* 0.25%, 0.5%, 1%, 2%, 2.5%; *Ointment:* 0.5%, 1%, 2.5%; *Pad:* 0.5%, 1%; *Solution:* 1%, 2.5%; *Spray:* 1%; *Tablet:* 5 mg, 10 mg, 20 mg. **Hydrocortisone acetate:** *Cream:* 0.5%, 1%; *Foam:* 10%; *Injection:* 25 mg/mL, 50 mg/mL; *Ointment:* 0.5%, 1%; *Spray:* 0.5%; *Suppository:* 25 mg, 30 mg. **Hydrocortisone buteprate:** *Cream:* 0.1%, 1%. **Hydrocortisone butyrate:** *Cream:* 0.1%; *Ointment:* 0.1%; *Solution:* 0.1%. **Hydrocortisone cypionate:** *Suspension:* 10 mg/5 mL. **Hydrocortisone sodium phosphate:** *Injection:* 50 mg/mL. **Hydrocortisone sodium succinate:** *Powder for injection:* 100 mg, 250 mg, 500 mg, 1 g. **Hydrocortisone valerate:** *Cream:* 0.2%; *Ointment:* 0.2%.

DOSAGE

HYDROCORTISONE

• **TABLETS**
20–240 mg/day, depending on disease.

• **IM ONLY**
One-third to one-half the PO dose q 12 hr.

• **RECTAL**
100 mg in retention enema nightly for 21 days (up to 2 months of therapy may be needed; discontinue gradually if therapy exceeds 3 weeks).

• **TOPICAL OINTMENT, CREAM, GEL, LOTION, SOLUTION, SPRAY**
Apply sparingly to affected area and rub in lightly t.i.d.–q.i.d.

HYDROCORTISONE ACETATE

• **INTRALESIONAL, INTRA-ARTICULAR, SOFT TISSUE**
5–50 mg, depending on condition.

• **INTRARECTAL FOAM**
1 applicatorful (90 mg) 1–2 times/day for 2–3 weeks; **then** every second day.

• **TOPICAL**
See *Hydrocortisone*.

HYDROCORTISONE BUTEPRATE

• **TOPICAL CREAM**
Apply a thin film to the affected area 1–2 times/day.

HYDROCORTISONE BUTYRATE

• **TOPICAL CREAM, OINTMENT, SOLUTION**
Apply a thin film to the affected area b.i.d.–t.i.d.

HYDROCORTISONE CYPIONATE

• **SUSPENSION**
20–240 mg/day, depending on the severity of the disease.

HYDROCORTISONE SODIUM PHOSPHATE

• **IV, IM, SC**
General uses.
Initial: 15–240 mg/day depending on use and on severity of the disease. Usually, one-half to one-third of the PO dose is given q 12 hr.

Adrenal insufficiency, acute.
Adults, initial: 100 mg IV; **then,** 100 mg q 8 hr in an IV fluid; **older children, initial:** 1–2 mg/kg by IV bolus; **then,** 150–250 mg/kg/day **IV** in divided doses; **infants, initial:** 1–2 mg/kg by IV bolus; **then,** 25–150 mg/kg/day in divided doses.

H

HYDROCORTISONE SODIUM SUCCINATE
• **IM, IV**
Initial: 100–500 mg; **then,** may be repeated at 2-, 4-, and 6-hr intervals depending on response and severity of condition.
HYDROCORTISONE VALERATE
• **TOPICAL CREAM**
See *Hydrocortisone.*

NURSING CONSIDERATIONS

SEE ALSO *NURSING CONSIDERATIONS* FOR *CORTICOSTEROIDS*.

ADMINISTRATION/STORAGE

IV 1. Check label of parenteral hydrocortisone because IM and IV preparations are not necessarily interchangeable.
2. Give reconstituted direct IV solution at a rate of 100 mg over 30 sec. Doses larger than 500 mg should be infused over 10 min. Drug may be further diluted in 50–100 mL of dextrose or saline solutions and administered as ordered within 24 hr.

ASSESSMENT

1. Document indications for therapy, type, location, onset, and characteristics of symptoms.
2. List other agents used and the outcome.
3. Assess weight, VS, CBC, BS, chemistry profile, liver and renal function studies. Note findings of xray, TB skin test, EKG.

CLIENT/FAMILY TEACHING

1. When using topical products, wash area prior to application or shower/bathe first, to increase drug penetration. Use only a small amount and rub into area thoroughly. Do not allow topical product to come in contact with the eyes.
2. Avoid prolonged use of topical products near the genital/rectal areas and eyes, on the face, and in creases of the skin.
3. For the butyrate topical products, use an occlusive dressing only on advice of the provider if used to treat psoriasis or other deep-seated dermatoses.
4. Do not use buteprate products in the diaper area. With the buteprate products, do not use tight-fitting diapers or plastic pants (occlusive).
5. No part of the intrarectal foam aerosol container should be inserted into the anus. With the suspension, shake well. Lie on left side with left leg extended and the right leg forward and flexed. Insert applicator tip of the suspension into the rectum pointed towards the navel and slowly instill medication as directed.
6. Report worsening of condition or lack of improvement; may need dosage adjustment. Report any fever, sore throat, muscle aches, or sudden weight gain or swelling of extremities.
7. With prolonged use of oral products, do not stop suddenly. Drug must be weaned/tapered down to prevent adrenal crisis. Cushingoid S&S of adrenal insufficiency include fatigue, dizziness, nausea, lack of appetitie, weakness, SOB, joint pain.
8. Avoid all OTC agents without approval.

OUTCOMES/EVALUATE

• Replacement of adrenocortical deficiency
• Restoration of skin integrity
• Relief of allergic manifestations
• ↓ Inflammation

Hydromorphone hydrochloride

(hy-droh-**MOR**-fohn)

PREGNANCY CATEGORY: C
CLASSIFICATION(S):
Narcotic analgesic
Rx: Dilaudid, Dilaudid-5, Dilaudid-HP
✱Rx: PMS-Hydromorphone, Dilaudid Sterile Powder, Dilaudid-HP-Plus, Dilaudid-XP, Hydromorph Contin **C-II**

SEE ALSO *NARCOTIC ANALGESICS*.

ACTION/KINETICS

Hydromorphone is 7–10 times more analgesic than morphine, with a shorter duration of action. It manifests less sedation, less vomiting, and less nausea than morphine, although it induces pronounced respiratory depression. **Onset:** 15–30 min. **Peak effect:** 30–60 min. **Duration:** 4–5 hr. **t½:** 2–3 hr. Give rectally for prolonged activity.

USES

Analgesia for moderate to severe pain (e.g., surgery, cancer, biliary colic, burns, renal colic, MI, bone trauma). Dilaudid-HP is a concentrated solution intended for those tolerant to narcotics.

ADDITIONAL CONTRAINDICATIONS

Migraine headaches. Use in children or during labor. Status asthmaticus, obstetrics, respiratory depression in absence of resuscitative equipment. Lactation.

SPECIAL CONCERNS

Do not confuse Dilaudid-HP with standard parenteral solutions of Dilaudid or with other narcotics as overdose and death can result. Use Dilaudid-HP with caution in clients with circulatory shock.

ADDITIONAL SIDE EFFECTS

Nystagmus.

ADDITIONAL DRUG INTERACTIONS

↑ CNS and respiratory depression when used with protease inhibitors.

HOW SUPPLIED

Injection: 1 mg/mL, 2 mg/mL, 4 mg/mL, 10 mg/mL; *Liquid, Oral:* 1 mg/mL; *Powder for injection, lyophilized:* 250 mg/vial; *Suppository:* 3 mg; *Tablet:* 1 mg, 2 mg, 3 mg, 4 mg, 8 mg

DOSAGE

• **LIQUID**

Analgesia.

Adults: 2.5–10 mg q 4–6 hr as necessary.

• **SUPPOSITORIES**

Analgesia.

Adults: 3 mg q 6–8 hr or as directed by physician.

• **TABLETS**

Analgesia.

Adults: 2–4 mg q 4–6 hr; for more severe pain, 4 or more mg q 4–6 hr.

• **SC, IM, IV**

Analgesia.

Adults: 1–2 mg IM or SC q 4–6 hr. For severe pain, 3–4 mg q 4–6 hr. May be given by slow IV over 2–3 min.

NURSING CONSIDERATIONS

SEE ALSO *NURSING CONSIDERATIONS* FOR *NARCOTIC ANALGESICS.*

ADMINISTRATION/STORAGE

1. Refrigerate suppositories.

IV 2. May be given by slow IV injection. Administer slowly to minimize hypotensive effects and respiratory depression. Dilute with 5 mL of sterile water or NSS and administer at a rate of 2 mg over 5 min.

ASSESSMENT

1. Document type, location, onset, and characteristics of symptoms. Use a rating scale to rate pain.

2. Assess for respiratory depression; more profound with hydromorphone than with other narcotic analgesics. Encourage to turn, cough, deep breathe or use incentive spirometry every 2 hr to prevent atelectasis.

3. Drug may mask symptoms of acute pathology; assess abdomen carefully.

CLIENT/FAMILY TEACHING

1. Use exactly as directed at the onset of pain and in the dose prescribed. Report any unusual or intolerable side effects or difficulty breathing.

2. May be given as Dilaudid brand cough syrup. Be alert to an allergic response in those sensitive to yellow dye number 5.

3. Store away from bedside.

4. Increase intake of fluids and fiber to offset constipating effects.

5. Do not perform activities that require mental alertness or coordination. Change positions slowly to avoid dizziness.

6. Do not stop suddenly with long term use; drug dependence occurs.

OUTCOMES/EVALUATE

Relief of pain; Control of cough

Hydroxyurea

(hy-**DROX**-ee-you-**ree**-ah)

PREGNANCY CATEGORY: D

CLASSIFICATION(S):

Antineoplastic, antimetabolite

H

Rx: Droxia, Hydrea (Abbreviation: HYD), Mylocel

SEE ALSO *ANTINEOPLASTIC AGENTS*.

ACTION/KINETICS

Inhibits DNA synthesis but not synthesis of RNA or protein. As an antimetabolite, it interferes with the conversion of ribonucleotides to deoxyribonucleotides due to blockade of the ribonucleotide reductase system. May also inhibit incorporation of thymidine into DNA. Effectiveness in sickle cell anemia may be due to increases in hemoglobin F levels in RBCs, decrease in neutrophils, increases in the water content of RBCs, increases the deformability of sickled cells, and altered adhesion of RBCs to the endothelium. Rapidly absorbed from GI tract. **Peak serum concentration:** 1–2 hr. **t½:** 3–4 hr. Crosses the blood-brain barrier. Degraded in liver; 80% excreted through the urine with 50% unchanged; also excreted as respiratory CO_2.

USES

(1) Chronic, resistant, myelocytic leukemia. (2) Carcinoma of the ovary (recurrent, inoperable, or metastatic). (3) Melanoma. (4) With irradiation to treat primary squamous cell carcinoma of the head and neck (but not the lip). (5) Droxia: Reduce frequency of painful crises and reduce need for blood transfusions in adults with sickle cell anemia. *Investigational:* Thrombocytopenia, HIV, refractory psoriasis.

CONTRAINDICATIONS

Leukocyte count less than 2,500/mm³ or thrombocyte count less than 100,000/mm³. Severe anemia.

SPECIAL CONCERNS

Use during pregnancy only if benefits clearly outweigh risks. Give with caution to clients with marked renal dysfunction. Geriatric clients may be more sensitive to the effects of hydroxyurea necessitating a lower dose. Dosage has not been established in children.

ADDITIONAL SIDE EFFECTS

Erythrocyte abnormalities including megaloblastic erythropoiesis. Constipation, redness of the face, maculopapular rash.

LABORATORY TEST CONSIDERATIONS

↑ Serum uric acid, BUN, and creatinine.

HOW SUPPLIED

Droxia: *Capsule:* 200 mg, 300 mg, 400 mg. **Hydrea:** *Capsule:* 500 mg. **Mylocel:** *Tablet:* 1000 mg.

DOSAGE

• CAPSULES

Solid tumors, intermittent therapy or when used together with irradiation.

Dose individualized. Usual: 80 mg/kg as a single dose every third day. Intermittent dosage offers advantage of reduced toxicity. If effective, maintain client on drug indefinitely unless toxic effects preclude such a regimen.

Solid tumors, continuous therapy.

20–30 mg/kg/day as a single dose.

Resistant chronic myelocytic leukemia.

20–30 mg/kg/day in a single dose or two divided daily doses.

Concomitant therapy with irradiation for cacinoma of the head and neck.

80 mg/kg as a single dose every third day.

Reduce platelet count and prevent thrombosis in essential thrombocytopenia.

About 15 mg/kg/day.

Refractory psoriasis.

0.5–1.5 g/day.

Sickle cell anemia (Use Droxia).

Base dose on the smaller of ideal or actual body weight. **Initial:** 15 mg/kg/day as a single dose. If blood counts are acceptable, may increase dose by 5 mg/kg/day q 12 weeks until a maximum tolerated dose (highest dose that does not produce toxic blood counts over 24 consecutive weeks) or 35 mg/kg/day is reached.

NURSING CONSIDERATIONS

SEE ALSO *NURSING CONSIDERATIONS* FOR *ANTINEOPLASTIC AGENTS*.

ADMINISTRATION/STORAGE

1. Calculate dosage based on actual or ideal weight (whichever is less).

2. Start hydroxyurea at least 7 days before initiation of irradiation; continue through irradiation and indefinitely afterward as long as the client can tolerate the dose. The dosage of radia-

tion is not usually adjusted with concomitant usage of hydroxyurea.
3. Do not store in excessive heat.

ASSESSMENT

1. Assess for exacerbation of postirradiation erythema.
2. Monitor uric acid, liver and renal function studies. With sickle cell anemia, monitor blood count q 2 weeks; adjust dosage to keep neutrophil, platelet, hemoglobin, and reticulocyte counts within acceptable ranges.
3. Initially, obtain hematologic profiles weekly. Drug may cause severe granulocyte and platelet suppression. Nadir: 7 days; recovery: 14 days.

CLIENT/FAMILY TEACHING

1. Take as directed; continue therapy for at least 6 weeks before efficacy is assessed.
2. If unable to swallow a capsule, contents may be given in glass of water and drunk immediately; some material may not dissolve and may float on top of glass.
3. Consume 8—10 glasses of fluids per day.
4. Report any S&S of infection: fever, chills, sore throat, flu like symptoms, N&V, loss of appetite, unusual bruising or bleeding, or sores in the mouth.
5. Practice reliable contraception.

OUTCOMES/EVALUATE

- Suppression of malignant process
- ↓ Tumor size and spread
- ↓ Occurrence of sickle cell crisis

Hydroxyzine hydrochloride

(hy-**DROX**-ih-zeen)

Rx: Atarax, Atarax 100, Vistaril, Vistazine 50
Rx: Apo-Hydroxyzine, Novo-Hydroxyzide, PMS Hydroxyzine

Hydroxyzine pamoate

(hy-**DROX**-ih-zeen)

Rx: Vistaril
CLASSIFICATION(S):
Antianxiety drug, nonbenzodiazepine

ACTION/KINETICS

Manifests anticholinergic, antiemetic, antispasmodic, local anesthetic, antihistaminic, and skeletal relaxant effects. Has mild antiarrhythmic activity and mild analgesic effects. High sedative and antiemetic effects and moderate anticholinergic activity. **Onset:** 15–30 min. **t½:** 3 hr. **Duration:** 4–6 hr. Metabolized by the liver and excreted through the urine. The pamoate salt is believed to be converted to the hydrochloride in the stomach.

USES

PO: (1) Sedative when used as premedication and following general anesthesia. (2) Management of pruritus caused by allergies, including chronic urticaria, atopic and contact dermatoses, and in histamine-mediated pruritus. **IM:** (1) Acutely disturbed or hysterical client. (2) Treat acute or chronic alcoholism with anxiety withdrawal symptoms or delirium tremens. (3) As pre- and postoperative and pre- and postpartum adjunctive therapy to control anxiety. (4) To control nausea and vomiting (except that due to pregnancy). (5) As pre- and postoperative and pre- and postpartum adjunctive therapy to control emesis. (6) As pre- and postoperative and pre- and postpartum adjunctive therapy to allow a reduction in dosage of narcotics.

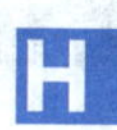

CONTRAINDICATIONS

Hypersensitivity to hydroxyzine or cetirizine. Pregnancy (especially early) or lactation. Treatment of morning sickness during pregnancy or as sole agent for treatment of psychoses or depression. Use in porphyria. IV, SC, or intra-arterial use.

SPECIAL CONCERNS

Possible increased anticholinergic and sedative effects in geriatric clients.

SIDE EFFECTS

Low incidence at recommended dosages. Drowsiness, dryness of mouth, involuntary motor activity (rarely, tremors and convulsions), ECG abnormalities (e.g., alterations in T-waves), dizziness, urticaria, skin reactions, hypersensitivity. Worsening of porphyria. Marked discomfort, induration, and even gangrene at site of IM injection.

OD OVERDOSE MANAGEMENT

Symptoms: Oversedation. *Treatment:* Immediate induction of vomiting or performance of gastric lavage. General supportive care with monitoring of VS. Control hypotension with IV fluids and either norepinephrine or metaraminol (epinephrine should not be used).

DRUG INTERACTIONS

Additive effects when used with other CNS depressants. See *Drug Interactions* for *Tranquilizers*.

HOW SUPPLIED

Hydroxyzine hydrochloride: *Injection:* 25 mg/mL, 50 mg/mL; *Syrup:* 10 mg/5 mL; *Tablet:* 10 mg, 25 mg, 50 mg, 100 mg. **Hydroxyzine pamoate:** *Capsule:* 25 mg, 50 mg, 100 mg; *Suspension, Oral:* 25 mg/5 mL

DOSAGE

HYDROXYZINE HYDROCHLORIDE AND HYDROXYZINE PAMOATE

• **CAPSULES, ORAL SUSPENSION, SYRUP, TABLETS.**

Antianxiety.

Adults: 50–100 mg q.i.d.; **pediatric under 6 years:** 50 mg/day in divided doses; **over 6 years:** 50–100 mg/day in divided doses.

Pruritus.

Adults: 25 mg t.i.d.–q.i.d.; **children under 6 years:** 50 mg/day in divided doses; **children over 6 years:** 50–100 mg/day in divided doses.

Preoperative or post-operative general anesthetic sedative.

Adults: 50–100 mg; **children:** 0.6 mg/kg.

HYDROXYZINE HYDROCHLORIDE

• **IM.**

Anxiety.

Adults: 50–100 mg q.i.d.

Antiemetic/analgesia, adjunctive therapy.

Adults: 25–100 mg; **pediatric,** 1.1 mg/kg. Switch to **PO** as soon as possible.

Pruritus.

Adults: 25 mg t.i.d.-q.i.d.

Sedative, as premedication and following general anesthesia.

Adults: 50–100 mg. **Children:** 0.6 mg/kg.

NURSING CONSIDERATIONS

SEE ALSO *NURSING CONSIDERATIONS FOR TRANQUILIZERS*.

ADMINISTRATION/STORAGE

1. Inject IM only. Make injection into the upper, outer quadrant of the buttocks or the midlateral muscles of the thigh. In children inject into the midlateral muscles of the thigh. In infants and small children, to minimize sciatic nerve damage, use the periphery of the upper outer quadrant of the gluteal region only when necessary (e.g., burn clients).
2. Shake suspension vigorously until it is completely resuspended.

ASSESSMENT

Document indications for therapy, type, onset, and characteristics of symptoms. Note any associated contributing factors i.e., dehydration, sweating, hives, areas of pruritus.

CLIENT/FAMILY TEACHING

1. Take only as directed, do not exceed dosing guidelines.
2. Frequent mouth rinsing, sucking hard candy, chewing sugarless gums, and increased fluid intake may relieve symptoms of dry mouth.
3. Wait and evaluate sedative effects of drug before performing tasks that require mental alertness.
4. Avoid alcohol or any other CNS depressants or OTC agents.
5. Drug is only for short-term management; report adverse effects or lack of response.

OUTCOMES/EVALUATE

- ↓ Anxiety and agitation
- Relief of itching/allergic S&S
- Control of N&V

Hylan G-F 20

(**HIGH**-lan)

Rx: Synvisc

SEE *SODIUM HYALURONATE*.

Hyoscyamine sulfate

(high-oh-**SIGH**-ah-meen)

PREGNANCY CATEGORY: C

CLASSIFICATION(S):

Cholinergic blocking drug

Rx: Anaspaz, A-Spas S/L, Cystospaz-M, Cytospaz, Donnamar, ED-SPAZ, Gastrosed, Levbid, Levsin/SL, Levsinex, NuLev , Levsin

SEE ALSO *CHOLINERGIC BLOCKING AGENTS.*

ACTION/KINETICS

One of the belladonna alkaloids; acts by blocking the action of acetylcholine at the postganglionic nerve endings of the parasympathetic nervous system. **t½:** 3½ hr for tablets, 7 hr for extended-release capsules, and 9 hr for extended-release tablets. Majority of the drug is excreted in the urine unchanged.

USES

(1) To control gastric secretion, visceral spasm, and hypermotility in spastic colitis, spastic bladder, cystitis, pylorospasm, and associated abdominal cramps. (2) Adjunctive therapy to treat irritable bowel syndrome and functional GI disorders. (3) Adjunctive therapy in neurogenic bladder and neurogenic bowel disturbances. (4) Treat infant colic (use elixir or solution). Use with morphine or other narcotics for symptomatic relief of biliary and renal colic. (5) In Parkinsonism to reduce rigidity and tremors and to control sialorrhea and hyperhidrosis. (6) To treat poisoning by anticholinesterase agents. (7) To reduce GI motility to facilitate diagnostic procedures, such as endoscopy or hypersecretion in pancreatitis. (8) To treat selected cases of partial heart block associated with vagal activity. (9) Used as a preoperative medication to reduce salivary, tracheobronchial, and pharyngeal secretions. (10) Adjunctive therapy to treat peptic ulcer.

SPECIAL CONCERNS

Heat prostration may occur if the drug is taken in the presence of high environmental temperatures. Use with caution during lactation.

SIDE EFFECTS

See *Cholinergic Blocking Agents.*

HOW SUPPLIED

Capsule, Extended Release: 0.375 mg; *Elixir:* 0.125 mg/5 mL; *Injection:* 0.5 mg/mL; *Liquid:* 0.125 mg/mL; *Tablet:* 0.125 mg, 0.15 mg; *Tablet, Extended Release:* 0.375 mg; *Tablet, Oral Disintegrating:* 0.125 mg; *Tablet, Sublingual:* 0.125 mg

DOSAGE

• **EXTENDED-RELEASE CAPSULES (0.375 MG) OR EXTENDED-RELEASE TABLETS (0.375 MG)**

Adults and children over 12 years of age: 0.375–0.750 mg q 12 hr, not to exceed 1.5 mg in 24 hr.

• **TABLETS (0.125 MG)**

Adults and children over 12 years of age: 0.125–0.25 mg q 4 hr or as needed, not to exceed 1.5 mg in 24 hr.

• **TABLETS, ORAL DISINTEGRATING**

Adults and children over 12 years: 1 or 2 q 4 hr, up to 12/day. **Children, 2–less than 12 years:** ½–1 q 4 hr, up to 6/day.

• **ELIXIR (0.125 MG/5 ML)**

Adults and children over 12 years of age: 0.125 mg–0.25 mg (5–10 mL) q 4 hr, not to exceed 1.5 mg (60 mL) in 24 hr. **Children, 2 to 12 years of age: 10 kg:** 1.25 mL (0.031 mg) q 4 hr; **20 kg:** 2.5 mL (0.062 mg) q 4 hr; **40 kg:** 3.75 mL (0.093 mg) q 4 hr; **50 kg:** 5 mL (0.125 mg) q 4 hr.

• **DROPS (0.125 MG/ML)**

Adults and children over 12 years of age: 0.125–0.25 mg (5–10 mL) q 4 hr, not to exceed 1.5 mg (12 mL) in 24 hr. **Children, 2 to 12 years of age:** 0.031–0.125 mg (0.251 mL)q 4 hr or as needed, not to exceed 0.75 mg (6 mL) in 24 hr. **Children, under 2 years of age: 3.4 kg:** 4 drops q 4 hr, not to exceed 24 drops in 24 hr; **5 kg:** 5 drops q 4 hr, not to exceed 30 drops in 24 hr; **7 kg:** 6 drops q 4 hr, not to exceed 36 drops in 24 hr; **10 kg:** 8 drops q 4 hr, not to exceed 48 drops in 24 hr.

• **INJECTION (0.5 MG/ML)**

GI disorders.

Adults: 0.25–0.5 mg (0.5–1 mL). Some clients need only one dose while others require doses 2, 3, or 4 times a day at 4 hr intervals.

Diagnostic procedures.

Adults: 0.25–0.5 mg (0.5–1 mL) given IV 5 to 10 min prior to the procedure.

Preanesthetic medication.

Adults and children over 2 years of age: 0.005 mg/kg 30–60 min prior to the time of induction of anesthesia. May also be given at the time the preanesthetic sedative or narcotic is given.

During surgery to reduce drug-induced bradycardia.

Adults and children over 2 years of age: Increments of 0.125 mg (0.25 mL) IV repeated as needed.

Reverse neuromuscular blockade.

Adults and children over 2 years of age: 0.2 mg (0.4 mL) for every 1 mg neostigmine or equivalent dose of physostigmine or pyridostigmine.

NURSING CONSIDERATIONS

SEE ALSO *NURSING CONSIDERATIONS* FOR *CHOLINERGIC BLOCKING AGENTS.*

ADMINISTRATION/STORAGE

1. May take hyoscyamine SL tablets sublingually, PO, or chewed. May take hyoscyamine tablets PO or SL.
2. Depending on the use, may give injection SC, IM, or IV.
3. IV Visually inspect the injectable form for particulate matter/discoloration.

ASSESSMENT

1. Document indications for therapy, type, onset, and characteristics of symptoms.
2. List other agents trialed and the outcome.
3. Determine any evidence of glaucoma, bladder neck or GI tract obstruction.
4. Assess abdomen, UGI, CT/US abdomen to R/O pathology.

CLIENT/FAMILY TEACHING

1. Take as prescribed; avoid antacids within 1 hr of taking drug (decreases effectiveness).
2. Do not perform activities that require mental alertness until drug effects realized; dizziness, drowsiness, and blurred vision may occur.
3. Report any loss of symptom control so provider can adjust dose and frequency of administration. Report diarrhea as it may be symptom of intestinal obstruction, esp. with a colostomy or ileostomy.
4. Avoid excessive temperatures and activity; drug may decrease perspiration, which may cause fever, heat prostration, or stroke.
5. Stop drug and report any mental confusion, impaired gait, disorientation, or hallucinations.

OUTCOMES/EVALUATE

- ↓ GI motility
- Control of epigastric pain/spasm

I

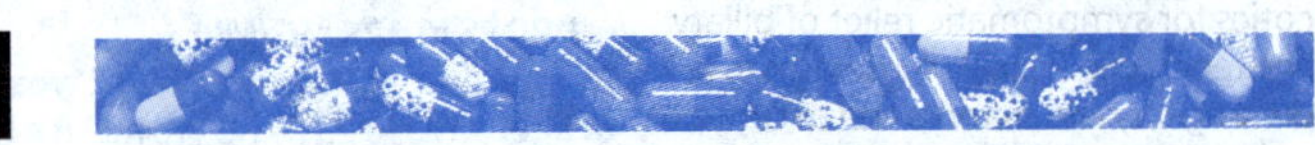

Ibuprofen

(eye-byou-**PROH**-fen)

PREGNANCY CATEGORY: B (FIRST TWO TRIMESTERS), D (THIRD TRIMESTER)

CLASSIFICATION(S):

Nonsteroidal anti-inflammatory drug

Rx: Motrin

★Rx: Apo-Ibuprofen, Novo&-Profen, Nu-Ibuprofen

OTC: Advil Tablets, Advil Liqui-Gels, Advil Migraine, Children's Advil, Children's Advil Chewable Tablets, Children's Motrin Chewable Tablets and Suspension, Genpril Tablets, Haltran, Infants' Motrin Drops, Junior Strength Advil, Junior Strength Motrin Tablets, Menadol, Midol Maximum Strength Cramp Formula, Migraine Pain, Motrin Junior Strength, Motrin Migraine Pain, Motrin-IB Tablets, Nuprin Tablets, PediaCare Fever Drops and Oral Suspension, Pediatric Advil Drops

SEE ALSO *NONSTEROIDAL ANTI-INFLAMMATORY DRUGS.*

ACTION/KINETICS

Time to peak levels: 1–2 hr. **Onset:** 30 min for analgesia and approximately 1 week for anti-inflammatory effect. **Peak serum levels:** 1–2 hr. **Duration:** 4–6 hr for analgesia and 1–2 weeks for anti-inflammatory effect. Food delays absorption rate but not total amount of drug absorbed. **t½:** 1.8–2 hr. 99% protein-bound. 45–70% excreted in the urine.

USES

Rx: (1) Analgesic for mild to moderate pain. (2) Primary dysmenorrhea, rheumatoid arthritis, osteoarthritis, antipyretic. *Investigational:* Resistant acne *vulgaris* (with tetracyclines); inflammation due to ultraviolet-B exposure (sunburn), juvenile rheumatoid arthritis. High doses to treat progressive lung deterioration in cystic fibrosis. Prophylactically to lower the risk of Alzheimer's disease. **OTC:** Relief of fever and minor aches and pains due to colds, flu, sore throats, headaches, and toothaches. Treat pain of migraine headaches.

CONTRAINDICATIONS

Pregnancy, especially during the last trimester.

SPECIAL CONCERNS

Individualize dosage for children less than 12 years of age as safety and effectiveness have not been established. May cause stomach bleeding in individuals who consume large amounts of alcohol regularly.

ADDITIONAL SIDE EFFECTS

Dermatitis (maculopapular type), rash. Hypersensitivity reaction consisting of abdominal pain, fever, headache, ***meningitis,*** N&V, signs of liver damage; especially seen in clients with SLE.

ADDITIONAL DRUG INTERACTIONS

Furosemide / ↓ Diuretic effect R/T ↓ renal prostaglandin synthesis
Lithium / ↑ Plasma lithium levels
Thiazide diuretics / See furosemide

HOW SUPPLIED

Capsule: 200 mg; *Chew Tablet:* 50 mg, 100 mg; *Oral Drops:* 40 mg/mL; *Suspension:* 50 mg/1.25 mL, 100 mg/5 mL; *Tablet:* 100 mg, 200 mg, 400 mg, 600 mg, 800 mg

DOSAGE

• **CAPSULES, ORAL DROPS, SUSPENSION, CHEWABLE TABLETS, TABLETS**

Rheumatoid arthritis, osteoarthritis.

Either 300 mg q.i.d. or 400, 600, or 800 mg t.i.d.–q.i.d.; adjust dosage according to client response. Full therapeutic response may not be noted for 2 or more weeks.

Juvenile arthritis.

30–40 mg/kg/day in three to four divided doses (20 mg/kg/day may be adequate for mild cases). Do not exceed 50 mg/kg/day.

Mild to moderate pain.

Adults: 400 mg q 4–6 hr, as needed.

Antipyretic.

Pediatric, 6 months–12 years of age: 5 mg/kg if baseline temperature is 102.5°F (39.1°C) or below or 10 mg/kg if baseline temperature is greater than 102.5°F (39.1°C). Maximum daily dose: 40 mg/kg.

Primary dysmenorrhea.

Adults: 400 mg q 4 hr, as needed.

• **TABLETS FOR OTC USE**

Mild to moderate pain, antipyretic, dysmenorrhea.

200 mg q 4–6 hr; dose may be increased to 400 mg if pain or fever persist. Dose should not exceed 1,200 mg/day.

• **SUSPENSION FOR OTC USE**

Pain, fever.

Children, 2–11 years: 7.5 mg/kg, up to q.i.d., to a maximum of 30 mg/kg/day.

NURSING CONSIDERATIONS

SEE ALSO *NURSING CONSIDERATIONS* FOR *NONSTEROIDAL ANTI-INFLAMMATORY DRUGS.*

ADMINISTRATION/STORAGE

1. Do not use OTC ibuprofen as an antipyretic for more than 3 days or as an analgesic for more than 10 days, unless medically cleared.
2. Do not take more than 3.2 g/day of prescription products and no more than 1.2 g/day of OTC products.

ASSESSMENT

1. Document indications for therapy, onset, location, and characteristics of symptoms. With pain, rate level and evaluate for effectiveness.

2. Review history for any conditions that may preclude drug therapy i.e., PUD, lupus, ASA intolerance, heavy alcohol intake.
3. Obtain/monitor CBC, liver and renal function studies (X rays and eye exam) prior to initiating long-term therapy.

CLIENT/FAMILY TEACHING

1. Take with a snack, milk, antacid, or meals to decrease GI upset. Report any N&V, diarrhea, or constipation.
2. Take the dosage prescribed for best results; report lack of response.
3. May cause dizziness and drowsiness, perform activities that require mental alertness after drug response evaluated.
4. With history of CHF or compromised cardiac function, keep weight records, report swelling; drug causes sodium retention.
5. Report blurred vision; obtain periodic eye exams with chronic therapy.
6. Avoid alcohol, NSAIDS, and ASA as bleeding may occur.
7. Report as scheduled for follow-up evaluations: ROM, CBC, renal function, X rays, and stool for blood.

OUTCOMES/EVALUATE

- ↓ Joint pain and ↑ mobility
- ↓ Fever, ↓ Inflammation
- ↓ Uterine cramping

Ibutilide fumarate

(ih-**BYOU**-tih-lyd)

PREGNANCY CATEGORY: C
CLASSIFICATION(S):
Antiarrhythmic
Rx: Corvert

ACTION/KINETICS

Class III antiarrhythmic agent. Delays repolarization by activation of a slow, inward current (mostly sodium), rather than by blocking outward potassium currents (the way other class III antiarrhythmics act). This results in prolongation in the duration of the atrial and ventricular action potential and refractoriness. Also a dose-related prolongation of the QT interval. High systemic plasma clearance that approximates liver blood flow; protein binding is less than 40%. **t½, terminal:** 6 hr. Over 80% is excreted in the urine (with 7% excreted unchanged) and approximately 20% is excreted through the feces.

USES

For rapid conversion of atrial fibrillation or atrial flutter of recent onset to sinus rhythm. Determination of clients to receive ibutilide should be based on expected benefits of maintaining sinus rhythm and whether this outweighs both the risks of the drug and of maintenance therapy. Is used in post-cardiac surgery clients.

CONTRAINDICATIONS

Use of certain class Ia antiarrhythmic drugs (e.g., disopyramide, quinidine, procainamide) and certain class III drugs (e.g., amiodarone and sotalol) concomitantly with ibutilide or within 4 hr of postinfusion.

SPECIAL CONCERNS

May cause potentially fatal arrhythmias, especially sustained polymorphic ventricular tachycardia, usually in association with QT prolongation (torsades de pointes). Effectiveness has not been determined in clients with arrhythmias of more than 90 days in duration. Breast feeding should be discouraged during therapy. Safety and efficacy have not been determined in children less than 18 years of age.

SIDE EFFECTS

CV: ***Life-threatening arrhythmias, either sustained or nonsustained polymorphic ventricular tachycardia (torsades de pointes).*** Induction or worsening of ventricular arrhythmias. Nonsustained monomorphic ventricular extrasystoles, nonsustained monomorphic ventricular tachycardia, sinus tachycardia, SVT, hypotension, postural hypotension, bundle branch block, AV block, bradycardia, QT-segment prolongation, hypertension, palpitation, supraventricular extrasystoles, nodal arrhythmia, CHF, ***idioventricular rhythm, sustained monomorphic VT***. **Miscellaneous:** Headache, nausea, syncope, renal failure.

OD OVERDOSE MANAGEMENT
Symptoms: Increased ventricular ectopy, monomorphic ventricular tachycardia, AV block, nonsustained polymorphic VT. *Treatment:* Treat symptoms.

DRUG INTERACTIONS
Amiodarone / ↑ Risk of prolonged refractoriness
Antidepressants, tricyclic and tetracyclic / ↑ Risk of proarrhythmias
Digoxin / Supraventricular arrhythmias due to ibutilide, may mask cardiotoxicity R/T high digoxin levels
Disopyramide / ↑ Risk of prolonged refractoriness
Histamine H_1 receptor antagonists / ↑ Risk of proarrhythmias
Phenothiazines / ↑ Risk of proarrhythmias
Procainamide / ↑ Risk of prolonged refractoriness
Quinidine / ↑ Risk of prolonged refractoriness
Sotalol / ↑ Risk of prolonged refractoriness

HOW SUPPLIED
IV Solution: 0.1 mg/mL.

DOSAGE

• **IV INFUSION**

Atrial fibrillation or atrial flutter of recent onset.

Clients weighing 60 kg or more, initial: 1 mg (one vial) infused over 10 min. **Clients weighing less than 60 kg, initial:** 0.01 mg/kg infused over 10 min. If the arrhythmia does not terminate within 10 min after the end of the initial infusion (regardless of the body weight), a second 10-min infusion of equal strength may be given 10 min after completion of the first infusion.

NURSING CONSIDERATIONS

ADMINISTRATION/STORAGE

IV 1. Anticoagulate clients with atrial fibrillation (>2–3 days duration) for at least 2 weeks.
2. May give undiluted or diluted in 50 mL of 0.9% NaCl or D5W. One vial (1 mg) mixed with 50 mL of diluent forms an admixture of approximately 0.017 mg/mL of ibutilide; administer infusion over 10 min.
3. Either PVC or polyolefin bags are compatible with drug admixtures.
4. Admixtures with approved diluents are chemically and physically stable for 24 hr at room temperature and for 48 hr if refrigerated.

ASSESSMENT

1. Document onset of arrhythmia and any associated symptoms. Those with AF > 2-3 days require anticoagulation for at least 2 weeks prior to ibutilide therapy.
2. List drugs currently prescribed to ensure none interact unfavorably.
3. Monitor VS, I&O, Mg, and electrolytes, and ECG.
4. Ibutilide must be given in a setting with continuous ECG monitoring and by those trained in the identification and treatment of acute ventricular arrhythmias, especially polymorphic ventricular tachycardia.
5. Document conversion to NSR (usually within 30–90 min). Stop drug infusion when arrhythmia is terminated or in the event of sustained or nonsustained ventricular tachycardia or marked prolongation of QT interval.
6. Observe for at least 4 hr following infusion or until QT interval has returned to baseline. Monitor longer if arrhythmic activity observed.

CLIENT/FAMILY TEACHING

1. Explain the reasons for dosing and why new-onset atrial fibrillation should be terminated (to prevent embolus formation).
2. Review the benefits and possible adverse side effects. Drug can only be given IV, may experience rapid irregular heart beat, headache, and other arrhythmias. Report any chest pain, SOB, numbness or tingling in extremities.
3. Stress the importance of close medical follow-up to determine stability of rhythm.

OUTCOMES/EVALUATE

Conversion of atrial fibrillation to sinus rhythm

Idarubicin hydrochloride

(eye-dah-**ROOB**-ih-sin)

PREGNANCY CATEGORY: D
CLASSIFICATION(S):
Antineoplastic, antibiotic
Rx: Idamycin For Injection, Idamycin PFS
✱Rx: Idamycin

SEE ALSO *ANTINEOPLASTIC AGENTS.*

ACTION/KINETICS
Inhibits nucleic acid synthesis and interacts with the enzyme topoisomerase II. Rapidly taken up into cells due to significant lipid solubility. **t½ (terminal):** 22 hr when used alone and 20 hr when used with cytarabine. Metabolized in the liver to the active idarubicinol, which is excreted through both the bile and urine. Both idarubicin and idarubicinol are significantly bound (97% and 94%, respectively) to plasma proteins.

USES
In combination with other drugs (often cytarabine) to treat AML in adults, including French-American-British classifications M1–M7. Comparison with daunorubicin indicates that idarubicin is more effective in inducing complete remissions in clients with AML.

CONTRAINDICATIONS
Lactation. Preexisting bone marrow suppression induced by previous drug therapy or radiotherapy (unless benefit outweighs risk). Administration by the IM or SC routes.

SPECIAL CONCERNS
Safety and effectiveness have not been demonstrated in children. Skin reactions may occur if the powder is not handled properly.

SIDE EFFECTS
GI: N&V, mucositis, diarrhea, abdominal pain, abdominal cramps, ***hemorrhage.*** **Hematologic:** ***Severe myelosuppression.*** **Dermatologic:** Alopecia, generalized rash, urticaria, bullous erythrodermatous rash of the palms and soles, hives at injection site. **CNS:** Headache, ***seizures,*** altered mental status. **CV:** CHF, ***serious arrhythmias including atrial fibrillation, chest pain, MI, cardiomyopathies,*** decrease in LV ejection fraction. *NOTE:* Cardiac toxicity is more common in clients who have received anthracycline drugs previously or who have preexisting cardiac disease. **Miscellaneous:** Altered hepatic and renal function tests, infection (95% of clients), fever, pulmonary allergy, neurologic changes in peripheral nerves.

OD OVERDOSE MANAGEMENT
Symptoms: Severe GI toxicity, myelosuppression. *Treatment:* Supportive treatment including antibiotics and platelet transfusions. Treat mucositis.

HOW SUPPLIED
Injection: 1 mg/mL; *Powder for Injection, Lyophilized:* 5 mg, 10 mg, 20 mg

DOSAGE
• **IV**

Induction therapy in adults with AML.

12 mg/m²/day for 3 days by slow (10–15 min) IV injection in combination with cytarabine, 100 mg/m²/day given by continuous infusion for 7 days or as a 25-mg/m² IV bolus followed by 200 mg/m²/day for 5 days by continuous infusion. A second course may be given if there is evidence of leukemia after the first course. Delay the second course in those with severe mucositis until recovery occurs; a dosage reduction of 25% is recommended. The drug should not be given if the bilirubin level is greater than 5 mg/dL.

NURSING CONSIDERATIONS

SEE ALSO *NURSING CONSIDERATIONS FOR ANTINEOPLASTIC AGENTS.*

ADMINISTRATION/STORAGE
IV 1. Reconstitute the 5-, 10-, and 20-mg vials with 5, 10, and 20 mL, respectively, of 0.9% NaCl injection to give a final concentration of 1 mg/mL. Do not use diluents containing bacteriostatic agents.
2. Vial contents are under negative pressure. To minimize aerosol formation during reconstitution use care when

the needle is inserted. Avoid inhalation of any aerosol formed.
3. Give slowly into a freely flowing IV infusion over 10–15 min.
4. If extravasation suspected/evident, keep extremity elevated and apply intermittent ice packs (immediately for ½ hr, then 4 times/day at ½-hr intervals for 3 days) over area.
5. Do not mix IV solution with any other drugs.
6. Reconstituted solutions are stable for 7 days if refrigerated and 3 days at room temperature. Discard unused solution.
7. If drug comes in contact with the skin, wash area thoroughly with soap and water. Use goggles, gloves, and protective gowns to prepare and administer.

ASSESSMENT

1. Document any preexisting cardiac disease.
2. Note any previous radiation therapy or treatment with anthracyclines.
3. Monitor CBC, platelets, and liver and renal function studies. Reduce dose with impaired hepatic or renal function; hold If bilirubin levels > 5 mg/dL.

CLIENT/FAMILY TEACHING

1. Nausea and diarrhea are frequent side effects of drug therapy; take antiemetic 1 hr before drug therapy.
2. Hair loss may occur.
3. Report any evidence of SOB or chest pain as drug may cause myocardial toxicity.
4. Report any S&S of anemia, i.e., dyspnea, fatigue, or faintness. Severe myelosuppression may occur; report any abnormal bruising/bleeding or infection.
5. Complaints of severe abdominal pain should be reported.
6. Use reliable contraception before, during, and for several months after therapy.
7. Avoid all OTC products without provider approval; avoid vaccinia, crowds and those with infections during therapy.
8. Encourage a high fluid intake, and keep the urine slightly alkaline to prevent the formation of uric acid stones. Clients with gout may require therapy.

OUTCOMES/EVALUATE

• Presence of leukemia cells (second course of therapy may be indicated after hematologic recovery)
• Complete remission; improved hematologic parameters

Idoxuridine (IDU)

(eye-dox-**YOUR**-ih-deen)

PREGNANCY CATEGORY: C
CLASSIFICATION(S):
Antiviral
Rx: Herplex Liquifilm
🍁**Rx:** Herplex-D

SEE ALSO *ANTIVIRAL AGENTS.*

ACTION/KINETICS

Resembles thymidine; inhibits thymidylic phosphorylase and specific DNA polymerases required for incorporation of thymidine into viral DNA. Idoxuridine, instead of thymidine, is incorporated into viral DNA, resulting in faulty DNA and the inability of the virus to infect tissue or reproduce. May also be incorporated into mammalian cells. Does not penetrate the cornea well. Rapidly inactivated by nucleotidases or deaminases.

USES

Herpes simplex keratitis, especially for initial epithelial infections characterized by the presence of thread-like extensions. *NOTE:* Idoxuridine will control infection but will not prevent scarring, loss of vision, or vascularization. Alternative form of therapy must be instituted if no improvement is noted after 7 days or if complete reepithelialization fails to occur after 21 days of therapy.

CONTRAINDICATIONS

Hypersensitivity; deep ulcerations involving stromal layers of cornea. Lactation. Concomitant use of corticosteroids in herpes simplex keratitis (corticosteroids may accelerate the spread of the viral infection).

SPECIAL CONCERNS
May be sensitizing, especially with dermal use. Safety and efficacy have not been determined in children.

SIDE EFFECTS
Localized to eye. Temporary visual haze, irritation, pain, pruritus, inflammation, sensitivity to bright light, follicular conjunctivitis with preauricular adenopathy, mild edema of eyelids and cornea, allergic reactions (rare), photosensitivity, corneal clouding and stippling, small punctate defects. *NOTE:* Squamous cell carcinoma has been reported at the site of application.

OD OVERDOSE MANAGEMENT
Symptoms (frequent administration): Defects on corneal epithelium. *Treatment:* If an excess amount of drug is instilled in the eye, flush with water or normal saline.

DRUG INTERACTIONS
Concurrent use of boric acid may cause irritation.

HOW SUPPLIED
Ophthalmic Solution: 0.1%

DOSAGE

• **OPHTHALMIC (0.1%) SOLUTION.**
Initially: 1 gtt every hour during the day and q 2 hr during the night until definite improvement is noted (usually within 7 days). **Following improvement:** 1 gtt q 2 hr during the day and q 4 hr at night. Continue for 3–7 days after healing is complete. Alternate dosing schedule: 1 gtt q min for 5 min; repeat q 4 hr, day and night.

NURSING CONSIDERATIONS

SEE ALSO GENERAL NURSING CONSIDERATIONS FOR ALL ANTI-INFECTIVES.

ADMINISTRATION/STORAGE

1. For best results, keep the infected tissues saturated with idoxuridine.
2. Store solution at 2–8°C (36–46°F); protect from light.
3. Do not mix with other meds.
4. Store ointment at 2–15°C (36–59°F).
5. Do not use drug that was improperly stored because of loss of activity and increased toxic effects.
6. Topical corticosteroids may be used with idoxuridine in the treatment of herpes simplex with corneal edema, stromal lesions, or iritis.
7. To control secondary infections, antibiotics may be used with drug.
8. Atropine may be used concomitantly with idoxuridine, if appropriate.
9. Improvement usually observed within 7–8 days; if there is continuous improvement, continue therapy for 21 days.
10. Some strains of herpes simplex may be resistant to idoxuridine; if there is no decrease in fluorescein staining after 14 days of use, another form of therapy should be used.

CLIENT/FAMILY TEACHING

1. Review method and frequency for instillation, and proper storage. Use as scheduled ATC, even during the night (q1h during day and q2h at night); do not exceed amount, frequency, and duration of therapy.
2. Report any symptoms of vision loss. Hazy vision following instillation will be of short duration.
3. *Do not* apply boric acid to the eye during idoxuridine therapy; boric acid may cause irritation.
4. Avoid using eye makeup; sharing towels and washcloths during therapy; wash hands frequently.
5. Wear dark glasses if photophobia occurs.
6. Store drug exactly as directed to prevent loss of effectiveness and toxicity. (Drops refrigerated in a tight, light-resistant container and ointment refrigerated).
7. If used concurrently with corticosteroids, the idoxuridine will be continued longer than the steroid, to prevent reinfection.
8. Report for scheduled ophthalmic exams to determine drug response and to assess application site.

OUTCOMES/EVALUATE

• Control of ophthalmic infection
• Reepithelialization of eye lesions

Ifosfamide

(eye-**FOS**-fah-myd)

PREGNANCY CATEGORY: D

CLASSIFICATION(S):
Antineoplastic, alkylating
Rx: Ifex

SEE ALSO *ANTINEOPLASTIC AGENTS* AND *ALKYLATING AGENTS.*

ACTION/KINETICS
Synthetic analog of cyclophosphamide that must be converted in the liver to active metabolites. The alkylated metabolites of ifosfamide then interact with DNA. **t½, elimination:** 7 hr. Excreted in the urine both as unchanged drug and metabolites.

USES
As third-line therapy, in combination with other antineoplastic drugs, for germ cell testicular cancer. Always give with mesna to prevent ifosfamide-induced hemorrhagic cystitis. *Investigational:* Cancer of the breast, lung, pancreas, ovary, and stomach. Also for sarcomas, acute leukemias (except AML), malignant lymphomas.

CONTRAINDICATIONS
Severe bone marrow depression. Lactation.

SPECIAL CONCERNS
Use with caution in clients with compromised bone marrow reserve, impaired renal function, and during lactation. Safety and efficacy have not been established in children. May interfere with wound healing.

ADDITIONAL SIDE EFFECTS
GU: ***Hemorrhagic cystitis,*** hematuria, dysuria, urinary frequency. **CNS:** Confusion, depressive psychosis, somnolence, hallucinations. Less frequently: dizziness, disorientation, cranial nerve dysfunction, ***seizures, coma.*** **GI:** Salivation, stomatitis. **Miscellaneous:** Myelosuppression, alopecia, infection, liver dysfunction, phlebitis, FUO, dermatitis, fatigue, hyper/hypotension, polyneuropathy, pulmonary symptoms, ***cardiotoxicity,*** interference with normal wound healing.

LABORATORY TEST CONSIDERATIONS
↑ Liver enzymes, bilirubin.

OD OVERDOSE MANAGEMENT
Symptoms: See *Additional Side Effects.*
Treatment: General supportive measures.

HOW SUPPLIED
Powder for Injection: 1 g, 3 g

DOSAGE

• **IV**

Testicular cancer.

1.2 g/m²/day for 5 consecutive days. Treatment may be repeated q 3 weeks or if platelet counts are at least 100,000/mm³ and WBCs are at least 4,000/mm³.

NURSING CONSIDERATIONS

SEE ALSO *NURSING CONSIDERATIONS* FOR *ANTINEOPLASTIC AGENTS.*

ADMINISTRATION/STORAGE
IV 1. To prevent bladder toxicity, give with at least 2 L/day of PO or IV fluid as well as with mesna.
2. Reconstitute by adding either sterile or bacteriostatic water for injection for a final concentration of 50 mg/mL. Solutions may be further diluted to achieve concentrations from 0.6 to 20 mg/mL by adding D5W, 0.9% NaCl, RL, or sterile water for injection. Infuse slowly over 30 min.
3. Reconstituted solutions (50 mg/mL) are stable for 1 week at 30°C (86°F) or 3 weeks at 5°C (41°F).
4. Refrigerate dilutions of ifosfamide not prepared with bacteriostatic water for injection; use within 6 hr.

ASSESSMENT
1. Anticipate concomitant administration with mesna to minimize hemorrhagic cystitis.
2. Send urine for analysis prior to each dose of ifosfamide. If hematuria occurs (>10 RBCs per HPF) hold therapy until clears.
3. Monitor CBC; immunosuppression may activate latent infections such as herpes.

CLIENT/FAMILY TEACHING
1. Hair loss and N&V are frequent side effects of drug therapy.
2. Hyperpigmentation of skin and mucous membranes may occur; report any injury or interference with normal wound healing.
3. Report confusion, hallucinations, or marked drowsiness.

4. Females should practice contraceptive measures during and for at least 4 months following treatments. Infertility may result if treatment lasts 6 months.
5. Consume 2 L/day of fluids. Report presence of frothy dark urine, jaundice, or light-colored stools; S&S of hepatotoxicity requiring dosage adjustments.
6. Joint or flank pain may be caused by the increase in uric acid that results from the rapid cytolysis of tumor and RBCs.
7. Report symptoms of neurotoxicity (numbness, tingling). Elicit family support in making observations/evaluations and recording.
8. Do not take salicylates or alcohol.
9. Avoid crowds, vaccinations, and persons with known infections.

OUTCOMES/EVALUATE

- ↓ Tumor size and spread
- Desired hematologic parameters

Imatinib mesylate

(eh-**MAT**-eh-nib)

PREGNANCY CATEGORY: D
CLASSIFICATION(S):
Antineoplastic, miscellaneous
Rx: Gleevec

ACTION/KINETICS

Imatinib is a protein-tyrosine kinase inhibitor that inhibits the Bcr-Abl tyrosine kinase which is the abnormal form of tyrosine kinase created by the Philadelphia chromosome abnormality in chronic myeloid leukemia (CML). Imatinib inhibits proliferation and causes apoptosis in Bcr-Abl positive cell lines, as well as fresh leukemic cells from Philadelphia chromosome positive CML. The drug may also inhibit receptor tyrosine kinases for platelet-derived growth factor and stem cell factor, c-Kit; inhibits platelet-derived growth factor and stem cell factor cellular events. Well absorbed after PO administration; **maximum levels:** 2–4 hr. **t½, terminal, imatinib and N-desmethyl derivative (active metabolite):** About 18 and 40 hr, respectively. Metabolized in the liver by the CYP3A4 enzyme. Excretion is mainly through the feces.

USES

Treatment of CML in blast crisis, accelerated phase, or chronic phase after failure of interferon-alpha therapy.

CONTRAINDICATIONS

Lactation.

SPECIAL CONCERNS

Safety and efficacy have not been determined in children.

SIDE EFFECTS

GI: N&V, diarrhea, ***GI hemorrhage,*** dyspepsia, abdominal pain, constipation, hepatotoxicity (may be severe). **CNS:** Headache, ***CNS hemorrhage.*** **Musculoskeletal:** Musculoskeletal pain, muscle cramps, arthralgia, myalgia. **Dermatologic:** Skin rash, pruritus, night sweats, petechiae. **Respiratory:** Cough, dyspnea, pneumonia, epistaxis, nasopharyngitis, pleural effusion, pulmonary edema. **Hematologic:** Neutropenia, thrombocytopenia. **Miscellaneous:** Fluid retention, superficial edema, ascites, pericardial effusion, anasarca, ***hemorrhage,*** fatigue, increased weight, pyrexia, anorexia, weakness, hypokalema.

LABORATORY TEST CONSIDERATIONS

↑ Liver transaminases, bilirubin.

DRUG INTERACTIONS

Calcium channel blockers / ↑ Plasma levels of calcium channel blockers
Carbamazepine / ↓ Imatinib plasma levels R/T ↑ metabolism
Clarithromycin / ↑ Imatinib levels R/T ↓ metabolism
Dexamethasone / ↓ Imatinib plasma levels R/T ↑ metabolism
Dihydropyridine / ↑ Plasma levels of dihydropyridine
Erythromycin / ↑ Imatinib levels R/T ↓ metabolism
Itraconazole / ↑ Imatinib levels R/T ↓ metabolism
Ketoconazole / ↑ Imatinib levels R/T ↓ metabolism
Phenobarbital / ↓ Imatinib plasma levels R/T ↑ metabolism
Phenytoin / ↓ Imatinib plasma levels R/T ↑ metabolism
Rifampicin / ↓ Imatinib plasma levels R/T ↑ metabolism

Simvastastin / ↑ Simvastatin AUC and maximum concentration R/T ↓ metabolism
H *St. John's wort* / ↓ Imatinib plasma levels R/T ↑ metabolism
Warfarin / Possible ↑ warfarin effect (use low molecular weight heparins or standard heparin)

HOW SUPPLIED

Capsule: 100 mg

DOSAGE

• CAPSULES

Chronic myeloid leukemia.

400 mg/day for those in chronic phase of CML and 600 mg/day for those in accelerated phase or blast crisis. Increases in dose from 400 mg to 600 mg in those with chronic phase disease or from 600 mg to 800 mg (400 mg b.i.d.) in those with accelerated phase or blast crisis may be considered if there are no severe side effects, severe non-leukemia-related neutropenia, or thrombocytopenia in the following situations: disease progression, failure to achieve a satisfactory hematologic response after 3 or more months of treatment, or loss of a previously achieved hematologic response.

NURSING CONSIDERATIONS

ADMINISTRATION/STORAGE

1. If severe hepatotoxicity or fluid retention occurs, withhold imatinib until event is resolved. Treatment can be resumed depending on the initial severity of the event.
2. If elevations in bilirubin > 3 times institutional upper limit of normal (IULN) or in liver transaminases > 5 IULN occur, withhold imatinib until bilirubin levels have returned to <1.5 times IULN and transaminase levels to < 2.5 times IULN. Treatment with imatinib may be continued at a reduced daily dose (400 mg reduced to 300 mg or 600 mg reduced to 400 mg).
3. Use the following guidelines to adjust dose for neutropenia and thrombocytopenia:

• For chronic phase CML (starting dose 400 mg). If ANC is < 1 x 10^9/L and/or platelets are < 50 x 10^9/L, stop imatinib until ANC is 1.5 or more x 10^9/L and platelets are 75 or more x 10^9/L. Resume treatment with a dose of 400 mg. If recurrence of ANC and/or platelets occur at levels indicated above, withhold until levels return to those indicated above and resume imatinib at reduced dose of 300 mg.

• For accelerated phase of CML and blast crisis (starting dose 600 mg). If ANC is < 0.5 x 10^9/L and/or platelets are < 10 x 10^9/L (after 1 month or more of treatment), check if cytopenia is related to leukemia. If cytopenia is unrelated to leukemia, reduce dose of imatinib to 400 mg. If cytopenia persists 2 weeks, reduce further to 300 mg. If cytopenia persists 4 weeks and is still unrelated to leukemia, stop imatinib until ANC is 1 or more x 10^9/L and platelets are 20 or more x 10^9/L and resume treatment at 300 mg.

ASSESSMENT

1. Note disease onset, phase of disease, and other therapies trialed/failed. Document last interferon-alpha therapy and failure date.
2. List drugs prescribed to ensure none interact unfavorably.
3. Monitor CBC, LFTs, and renal function studies.
4. Follow administration guidelines carefully as dose is adjusted for various phases of disease as well as altered renal/liver function and neutropenia/thrombocytopenia.

CLIENT/FAMILY TEACHING

1. Take with food and a large glass of water to minimize GI irritation.
2. Drug is given once daily initially and may be increased to twice daily.
3. Monitor weight and report any significant increases/decreases.
4. May experience N&V, diarrhea, swelling of extremities/around the eyes, skin rash, and muscle cramps. Report as well as increased SOB, changes in urinary output, ↑ bruising/bleeding, and increased exercise intolerance. Keep all F/U visits so drug may be adjusted as needed.

OUTCOMES/EVALUATE

Hematologic stabilization of CML

—*COMBINATION DRUG*—

Imipenem-Cilastatin sodium

(em-ee-**PEN**-em, sigh-lah-**STAT**-in)

PREGNANCY CATEGORY: C
CLASSIFICATION(S):
Antibiotic, carbapenem
Rx: Primaxin I.M., Primaxin I.V.

SEE ALSO *ANTI-INFECTIVES.*

CONTENT
The powder for IM injection contains: imipenem, 500 mg, and cilastatin, 500 mg, or imipenem, 750 mg, and cilastatin, 750 mg. The powder for IV injection contains: imipenem, 250 mg, and cilastatin, 250 mg, or imipenem, 500 mg, and cilastatin, 500 mg.

ACTION/KINETICS
Inhibits cell wall synthesis. Is bactericidal against a wide range of gram-positive and gram-negative organisms. Stable in the presence of beta-lactamases. Addition of cilastatin prevents the metabolism of imipenem in the kidneys by dehydropeptidase I, thus ensuring high levels of the imipenem in the urinary tract. **t½, after IV:** 1 hr for each component. **Peak plasma levels of imipenem, after 20 min IV infusion:** 14–24 mcg/mL for the 250-mg dose, 21–58 mcg/mL for the 500-mg dose, and 41–83 mcg/mL for the 1-g dose. **Peak plasma levels, after IM:** 10–12 mcg/mL within 2 hr. Compared with IV administration, imipenem is approximately 75% bioavailable after IM use with cilastatin being 95% bioavailable. **t½, imipenem:** 2–3 hr. About 70% of imipenem and cilastin is recovered in the urine within 10 hr of administration.

USES
IV: To treat the following serious infections: lower respiratory tract, urinary tract (complicated and uncomplicated), gynecologic, skin and skin structures, bone and joint, endocarditis, intra-abdominal, bacterial septicemia, and infections caused by more than one agent. Infections resistant to aminoglycosides, cephalosporins, or penicillins have responded to imipenem. Bacterial eradication may not be achieved in clients with cystic fibrosis, chronic pulmonary disease, and lower respiratory tract infections caused by *Pseudomonas aeruginosa.*

IM: This route of administration is not intended for severe or life-threatening infections (including endocarditis, or bacterial sepsis). Used for lower respiratory tract infections (including pneumonia and bronchitis), intra-abdominal infections, skin and skin structure infections, gynecologic infections.

CONTRAINDICATIONS
IM use in clients allergic to local anesthetics of the amide type and use in clients with heart block (due to the use of lidocaine HCl diluent) or severe shock. Use in clients with a C_{CR} of less than or equal to 5 mL/min/1.73 m², unless hemodialysis is begun within 48 hr. IV use in children with CNS infections due to the risk of seizures and in children less than 30 kg with impaired renal function.

SPECIAL CONCERNS
Use with caution in pregnancy and lactation. Due to cross sensitivity, use with caution in clients with penicillin allergy. Safety and effectiveness have not been determined for use IM in children less than 12 years of age.

SIDE EFFECTS
GI: ***Pseudomembranous colitis,*** nausea, diarrhea, vomiting, abdominal pain, heartburn, increased salivation, ***hemorrhagic colitis,*** gastroenteritis, glossitis, pharyngeal pain, tongue papillar hypertrophy, hepatitis, jaundice, staining of the teeth or tongue. **CNS:** Fever, confusion, ***seizures,*** dizziness, sleepiness, myoclonus, headache, vertigo, paresthesia, encephalopathy, tremor, psychic disturbances (including hallucinations). **CV:** Hypotension, tachycardia, palpitations. **Dermatologic:** Rash, urticaria, pruritus, flushing, cyanosis, facial edema, erythema multiforme, skin texture changes, hyperhidrosis, angioneurotic edema, ***toxic epidermal necrolysis, Stevens-Johnson syndrome.*** **CV:** Hypotension, palpitations, tachycardia. **Respiratory:** Chest discomfort, dyspnea, hyper-

ventilation. **GU:** Pruritus vulvae, anuria/oliguria, acute renal failure, polyuria, urine discoloration. **Hematologic:** Pancytopenia, bone marrow depression, thrombocytopenia, neutropenia, leukopenia, hemolytic anemia. **Miscellaneous:** Candidiasis, superinfection, tinnitus, polyarthralgia, asthenia, muscle weakness, transient hearing loss in clients with existing hearing impairment, taste perversion, thoracic spine pain.

Children, 3 months and older: Diarrhea, rash, phlebitis, gastroenteritis, vomiting, IV site irritation, urine discoloration. **Children, newborn to 3 months:** Convulsions, diarrhea, oliguria, anuria, oral candidiasis, rash, tachycardia.

The following side effects may occur at the injection site: Thrombophlebitis, phlebitis, pain, erythema, vein induration, infused vein infection.

LABORATORY TEST CONSIDERATIONS

IV: ↑ AST, ALT, alkaline phosphatase, bilirubin, LDH, BUN, creatinine, eosinophils, monocytes, lymphocytes, basophils, potassium, chloride. ↓ Neutrophils, hemoglobin, hematocrit. ↑ or ↓ WBCs, platelets. Positive Coombs' test and abnormal PT. Presence of protein, RBCs, WBCs, casts, bilirubin, or urobilinogen in the urine.

IM: ↑ AST, ALT, alkaline phosphatase, bilirubin, BUN, creatinine, PT. ↓ Hemoglobin, hematocrit, erythrocytes. ↑ or ↓ WBCs and platelets. Presence of RBCs, WBCs, casts, and bacteria in urine.

DRUG INTERACTIONS

Cyclosporine / ↑ CNS side effects of both drugs

Ganciclovir / ↑ Risk of generalized seizures

Probenecid / ↑ Imipenem levels and half-life; do not use together

HOW SUPPLIED

See Content

DOSAGE

• **IV**

Fully susceptible gram-positive organisms, gram-negative organisms, anaerobes.

Mild: 250 mg q 6 hr; **moderate:** 500 mg q 6 hr or q 8 hr; **severe/life-threatening:** 500 mg q 6 hr.

Urinary tract infections due to fully susceptible organisms.

Uncomplicated: 250 mg q 6 hr; **complicated:** 500 mg q 6 hr.

Moderately susceptible organisms (especially some strains of P. aeruginosa*).*

Mild: 500 mg q 6 hr; **moderate,** 500 mg q 6 hr to 1 g q 6 hr; **severe/life-threatening,** 1 g q 6 or 8 hr.

Urinary tract infections due to moderately susceptible organisms.

Uncomplicated: 250 mg q 6 hr; **complicated:** 500 mg q 6 hr.

The total daily dose should not exceed 50 mg/kg or 4 g, whichever is lower.

Pediatric, non-CNS infections.

Children, 3 months of age or older: 15–25 mg/kg/dose q 6 hr, up to a maximum dose of 2 g/day for treating infections with fully susceptible organisms and up to a maximum of 4 g/day for infections with moderately susceptible organisms. Doses as high as 90 mg/kg/day have been used in older children with cystic fibrosis. **Children, three months of age or less (weighing 1,500 g or more):** Less than 1 week of age, 25 mg/kg q 12 hr; 1–4 weeks of age, 25 mg/kg q 8 hr; 4 weeks to 3 months of age, 25 mg/kg q 6 hr. Give doses less than or equal to 500 mg by IV infusion over 15 to 20 min; give doses greater than 500 mg by IV infusion over 40 to 60 min.

• **IM**

Lower respiratory tract, skin and skin structure, or gynecologic infections: mild to moderate.

500 or 750 mg q 12 hr depending on severity.

Intra-abdominal infections: mild to moderate.

750 mg q 12 hr. The total daily dose should not exceed 1.5 g.

Pediatric, 3 months to 3 years, all uses: 15–25 mg/kg q 6 hr, to a maximum of 2 g/day. **Pediatric, over 3 years, all uses:** 15 mg/kg q 6 hr.

NURSING CONSIDERATIONS

SEE ALSO *GENERAL NURSING CONSIDERATIONS* FOR *ANTI-INFECTIVES*.

ADMINISTRATION/STORAGE

1. When used IM, give in a large muscle mass with a 21-gauge 2-in. needle.
2. For IM use, prepare with 1% lidocaine HCl solution without epinephrine. The 500-mg vial is prepared with 2 mL and the 750-mg vial with 3 mL of lidocaine HCl. Use reconstituted IM solutions within 1 hr of preparation.
3. Continue IM use for at least 2 days after S&S of infection are absent. Safety and effectiveness have not been established for use for more than 14 days.
4. Reduce dosage with a C_{CR} of 70 mL/min/1.73 m^2 or less. Check package insert for specific dosage information.

IV 5. Reconstitute for IV use by mixing with 100 mL of diluent.

6. Base initial dose on the type and severity of infection. Give doses between 250 and 500 mg by IV infusion over 20–30 min. Give doses of 1 g by IV infusion over 40–60 min. If nausea develops, decrease infusion rate.
7. The following solutions can be used as diluents: 0.9% NaCl, 5% or 10% dextrose injection, D5/0.9% NaCl, D5% with either 0.225% or 0.45% saline solution, D5% with 0.15% KCl solution, mannitol (2.5%, 5%, or 10%).
8. Reconstituted IV solutions vary from colorless to yellow while reconstituted IM solutions vary from white to light tan in color. Color variations do not affect potency.
9. Do not mix with other antibiotics; however, may be administered with other antibiotics, if necessary.
10. Most reconstituted IV solutions can be stored at room temperature for 4 hr and, if refrigerated, for 24 hr. The exception is imipenem-cilastatin reconstituted with 0.9% NaCl solution, which is stable at room temperature for 10 hr and, if refrigerated, for 48 hr.

ASSESSMENT

1. Document indications for therapy, onset, duration, and characteristics of symptoms. Check culture reports.
2. Do not use in clients allergic to local anesthetics of the amide type or in clients with heart block (due to the use of lidocaine HCl diluent) or severe shock. Use cautiously with penicillin, beta-lactams or cephalosporin allergy. Assess for seizure history. The cilastatin component prevents renal metabolism of imipenem.
3. Monitor renal function; avoid if C_{CR} of less than or equal to 5 mL/min/1.73 m^2, unless hemodialysis is begun within 48 hr. See administration guidelines.
4. Avoid IV use in children with CNS infections due to the risk of seizures and in children less than 30 kg with impaired renal function.
5. Assess IV site for phlebitis, pain or erythema.

OUTCOMES/EVALUATE

- Resolution of infection
- Symptomatic improvement

Imipramine hydrochloride

(im-**IHP**-rah-meen)

PREGNANCY CATEGORY: B
Rx: Tofranil
✱**Rx:** Apo-Imipramine

Imipramine pamoate

(im-**IHP**-rah-meen)

PREGNANCY CATEGORY: B
Rx: Tofranil-PM
CLASSIFICATION(S):
Antidepressant, tricyclic

SEE ALSO *ANTIDEPRESSANTS, TRICYCLIC*.

ACTION/KINETICS

Moderate anticholinergic and sedative effects; high orthostatic hypotensive effects. Biotransformed into its active metabolite, desmethylimipramine (desipramine). **Effective plasma level of imipramine and desmethylimipramine:** 200–350 ng/mL. **t½:** 11–25 hr. **Time to reach steady state:** 2–5 days.

USES

(1) Symptoms of depression; endogenous depression is more likely to be

helped. (2) Enuresis in children 6 years or older.

ADDITIONAL SIDE EFFECTS

High therapeutic dosage may increase frequency of seizures in epileptic clients and cause seizures in nonepileptic clients. Elderly and adolescent clients may have low tolerance to the drug.

LABORATORY TEST CONSIDERATIONS

↑ Metanephrine (Pisano test); ↓ Urinary 5-HIAA.

ADDITIONAL DRUG INTERACTIONS

H Possible ↓ imipramine plasma levels when taken with St. John's wort; R/T ↑ metabolism

HOW SUPPLIED

Imipramine hydrochloride: *Tablet:* 10 mg, 25 mg, 50 mg. **Imipramine pamoate:** *Capsule:* 75 mg, 100 mg, 125 mg, 150 mg

DOSAGE

- **TABLETS, CAPSULES**

Depression.

Hospitalized clients: 50 mg b.i.d.–t.i.d. Can be increased by 25 mg every few days up to 200 mg/day. After 2 weeks, dosage may be increased gradually to maximum of 250–300 mg/day at bedtime. **Outpatients, initial:** 75 mg/day, increased to 150 mg/day. Maximum dose for outpatients is 200 mg/day. Decrease when feasible to maintenance dosage: 50–150 mg/day at bedtime. **Adolescent and geriatric clients, initial:** 30–40 mg/day up to maximum of 100 mg/day.

Childhood enuresis.

Age 6 years and over: 25 mg/day 1 hr before bedtime. If satisfactory effect is not seen in 1 week, increase dose to 50 mg/day up to 12 years of age and to 75 mg/day in children over 12 years of age. Dose should not exceed 2.5 mg/kg/day.

NURSING CONSIDERATIONS

SEE ALSO *NURSING CONSIDERATIONS* FOR *ANTIDEPRESSANTS, TRICYCLIC.*

ADMINISTRATION/STORAGE

1. Total daily dose can be given once daily at bedtime.
2. In early night bed wetters, the drug may be more effective if given in doses of 25 mg in midafternoon and 25 mg at bedtime.
3. Children who relapse after discontinuing the drug may not respond to a subsequent course. Gradually tapering the dose may decrease tendency to relapse.

CLIENT/FAMILY TEACHING

1. Review appropriate times and methods for administration.
2. Report any increase in frequency of seizures in epileptics and any occurrence of seizures in nonepileptics.
3. Children may experience mild N&V, unusual tiredness, nervousness, or insomnia; report if pronounced.
4. Do not perform activities that require mental alertness until drug effects realized; may cause sedation.
5. With enuresis, refer parents to regional centers with incontinence programs if bed-wetting persists.

OUTCOMES/EVALUATE

- Improved S&S of depression
- Prevention of bed-wetting
- Control of severe neurogenic pain
- Therapeutic serum drug levels (200–350 ng/mL)

Imiquimod

(ih-**MIH**-kwih-mod)

PREGNANCY CATEGORY: B

CLASSIFICATION(S):

Immunomodulator

Rx: Aldara

ACTION/KINETICS

May induce cytokines, including interferon-alpha and others, to modify immune response. Minimal percutaneous absorption.

USES

External genital and perianal warts/condyloma acuminata in adults.

CONTRAINDICATIONS

Use in urethral, intravaginal, cervical, rectal, or intra-anal human papilloma viral disease.

SPECIAL CONCERNS

Safety and efficacy have not been determined in clients less than 18 years of age. Use with caution during lactation.

SIDE EFFECTS

Dermatologic: Erythema, itching, erosion, burning, excoriation/flaking, edema, pain, induration, ulceration, scabbing, vesicles, soreness. **Systemic:** Fungal infection, fatigue, fever, flu-like symptoms, headache, diarrhea, myalgia.

HOW SUPPLIED

Topical Cream: 5%

DOSAGE

- **CREAM**

Genital/perianal warts.

Adults: Apply 3 times/week prior to normal sleeping hours; leave on skin for 6–10 hr. Following treatment, remove by washing the area with mild soap and water. Continue treatment until there is total clearance of warts (16 weeks or less).

NURSING CONSIDERATIONS

ADMINISTRATION/STORAGE

1. Wash hands before and after application.
2. Apply a thin layer to the wart area and rub in until cream is not visible.
3. Avoid using excessive amounts of cream; single-use packets contain sufficient cream to cover up to 20 cm^2.
4. Due to skin reactions, rest period of several days may be necessary. Treatment may resume once reactions subside.
5. May weaken condoms or vaginal diaphragms; do not use together.
6. For external use only. Avoid contact with eyes.
7. Do not occlude treatment area with bandages or other covers/wraps. Non-occlusive dressings (e.g., cotton gauze or underwear) can be used to manage skin reactions.
8. Do not store at temperatures greater than 30°C (86°F). Avoid freezing.

ASSESSMENT

Describe clinical presentation noting number and size of warts/condyloma, location, and condition of pretreatment area. Photographs may be useful in assessing response to therapy.

CLIENT/FAMILY TEACHING

1. Apply a thin layer of cream to completely cover each wart at bedtime, after bathing. Usually prescribed three times per week. Do not cover area with occlusive bandages or wraps.
2. Wash hands before and after treatment, avoid eye contact.
3. Not a cure for genital warts but helps clear and diminish wart area. New warts may occur during therapy.
4. Avoid sexual contact (genital, rectal, oral) while cream is on skin. Wash off before sexual activity; may also weaken condoms and diaphragms. Use extra protection and practice safe sex to avoid infecting and/or acquiring from partners.
5. May experience redness, peeling, burning, itching, and swelling in treatment area; report if severe skin reaction occurs as rest period may be needed before continuing therapy once subsided.
6. Wash area with mild soap and water 6 to 10 hr after application.
7. Uncircumcised males treating warts under foreskin should retract foreskin and clean area daily.

OUTCOMES/EVALUATE

Clearing of genital and perianal warts/condyloma

Immune globulin IV (Human)

(im-**MYOUN GLOH**-byou-lin)

PREGNANCY CATEGORY: C

CLASSIFICATION(S):

Immune globulin

Rx: Gamimune N 5% and 10%, Gammagard S/D, Gammar-P I.V., Iveegam, Polygam, Polygam S/D, Sandoglobulin, Venoglobulin-I, Venoglobulin-S Solvent Detergent Treated

★Rx: Baygam, Iveegam Immuno

ACTION/KINETICS

Derived from a human volunteer pool. Contains the various IgG antibodies normally occurring in humans. The products may also contain traces of IgA and IgM. Plasma in the manufacturing pool has been found nonreactive for hepatitis B antigen. No documented cases of viral transmission. Antibodies present in the products will cause both opsonization and neutralization of microbes and toxins. Reconstituted products may contain sucrose, maltose, protein, and/or small amounts of sodium chloride. Immune globulin IV provides immediate antibody levels. The percentage of IgG in the products is over 90%. **t½:** Gamimune N and Sandoglobulin, 3 weeks; Venoglobulin-I, 29 days.

USES

All products: Severe combined immunodeficiency and primary immunoglobulin deficiency syndromes, including congenital agammaglobulinemia, X-linked agammaglobulinemia with or without hyper IgM, combined immunodeficiency, and Wiskott-Aldrich syndrome. *Investigational:* Chronic fatigue syndrome, quinidine-induced thrombocytopenia.

Gamimune N, Gammagard S/D, Polygam S/D, Sandoglobulin, Venoglobulin-I and Venoglobulin-S: Acute and chronic ITP in both children and adults.

Gammagard S/D, Polygam S/D: B-cell CLL in those with hypogammaglobulinemia or recurrent associated bacterial infections.

Gammagard S/D, Iveegam: Kawasaki syndrome (given with aspirin within 10 days of onset of the disease).

Gamimune N: Prophylactic use to decrease infections and the incidence of graft-versus-host-disease in bone marrow clients and in HIV-infected children to prevent bacterial infections.

Gammar-P: Primary immune deficiency in adolescents and children who are at increased risk of infection. Not for use in those with isolated immunoglobulin (IgA) deficiency.

CONTRAINDICATIONS

Clients with selective IgA deficiency who have antibodies to IgA (the products contain IgA). Sensitivity to human immune globulin.

SPECIAL CONCERNS

The various products are used for different conditions and at different doses; thus, check information carefully. Products containing sucrose (Gammar-P I.V., Sandoglobulin) may be more likely to cause acute renal failure than sucrose-free products.

SIDE EFFECTS

CNS: Headache, malaise, feeling of faintness. Aseptic meningitis syndrome, including symptoms of severe headache, nuchal rigidity, drowsiness, fever, photophobia, painful eye movements, N&V. **Allergic:** Hypersensitivity or ***anaphylactic reactions.*** **Body as a whole:** Fever, chills. **GI:** Headache, nausea, vomiting. **Miscellaneous:** Chest tightness, dyspnea; chest, back, or hip pain; mild erythema following infiltration; burning sensation in the head; tachycardia, renal insufficiency and acute renal failure.

Agammaglobulinemic and hypogammaglobulinemic clients never having received immunoglobulin therapy or where the time from the last treatment is more than 8 weeks may manifest side effects if the infusion rate exceeds 1 mL/min. Symptoms include flushing of the face, hypotension, tightness in chest, chills, fever, dizziness, diaphoresis, and nausea.

HOW SUPPLIED

Injection: 50 mg/mL, 100 mg/mL; *Powder for injection:* 50 mg/mL; *Powder for injection, freeze-dried:* 50 mg/mL; *Powder for injection, lyophilized:* 50 mg/mL, 5 %, 1 g, 3 g, 6, g, 12 g; *Solution for injection:* 5%, 10%

DOSAGE

NOTE: Due to differences in products, dosage must be listed separately for each product.

- **IV ONLY FOR ALL PRODUCTS**

GAMIMUNE N

Immunodeficiency syndrome.

100–200 mg/kg given once a month; if response is satisfactory, dose can be increased to 400 mg/kg or infusion may be repeated more frequently than once a month. Rate of infusion for all uses: 0.01–0.02 mL/kg/min for

30 min; if no discomfort is experienced, the rate can be increased up to 0.08 mL/kg/min.

ITP.

400 mg/kg for 5 consecutive days or 1,000 mg/kg/day for 1 day or 2 consecutive days. **Maintenance:** If platelet count falls to less than 30,000/mm³ or if bleeding occurs, 400 mg/kg may be given as a single infusion. If an adequate response is not seen, the dose can be increased to 800–1,000 mg/kg given as a single infusion. Maintenance infusions are given, as needed, to maintain platelet counts greater than 30,000/mm³.

Bone marrow transplantation.

500 mg/kg beginning on days 7 and 2 pretransplant or at the time conditioning therapy for transplantation is initiated; then, give weekly throughout the 90-day post-transplant period.

Pediatric HIV infection.

400 mg/kg q 28 days.

GAMMAGARD S/D

Immunodeficiency syndrome.

200–400 mg/kg (minimum of 100 mg/kg/month).

B-cell CLL.

400 mg/kg q 3–4 weeks.

ITP.

1,000 mg/kg; additional doses depend on platelet count (up to three doses can be given on alternate days). Rate of infusion: 0.5 mL/kg/min initially; may be increased gradually, not to exceed 4 mL/kg/hr if there is no client distress.

GAMMAR-P I.V.

Immunodeficiency syndrome.

200–400 mg/kg q 3–4 weeks. An alternative is a loading dose of at least 200 mg/kg at more frequent intervals and then 200–600 mg/kg at 3-week intervals once a therapeutic plasma level has been reached. Rate of infusion: 0.01 mL/kg/min, increasing to 0.02 mL/kg/min after 15 to 30 min. Most clients will tolerate a gradual increase to 0.03–0.06 mL/kg/min.

IVEEGAM

Immunodeficiency syndrome.

200 mg/kg/month. If desired effect not achieved, the dose may be increased up to fourfold (i.e., up to 800 mg/kg/month) or the intervals between doses shortened. Rate of infusion for all uses: 1 mL/min to a maximum of 2 mL/min of the 5% solution. The product may be further diluted with saline or 5% dextrose.

Kawasaki syndrome.

400 mg/kg/day for 4 consecutive days or a single dose of 2,000 mg/kg given over a 10-hr period. Treatment should be initiated within 10 days of onset and should include aspirin, 100 mg/kg each day through the 14th day of illness; then, aspirin is given at a dose of 3–5 mg/kg/day for 5 weeks.

POLYGAM S/D

Immunodeficiency syndrome.

Initial: 200–400 mg/kg may be given; **then,** 100 mg/kg/month. Rate of administration for all uses: Initially, 0.5 mL/kg/hr. If there is no distress, the rate can be gradually increased, not to exceed 4 mL/kg/hr. Those who tolerate the 5% solution at a rate of 4 mL/kg/hr can receive the 10% solution starting at 0.5 mL/kg/hr.

B-cell CLL.

400 mg/kg q 3 to 4 weeks.

ITP.

1 g/kg. Depending on response, additional doses can be given—three separate doses on alternate days can be given, if needed.

SANDOGLOBULIN

Immunodeficiency syndrome.

200 mg/kg/month; increase to 300 mg/kg if client response satisfactory (i.e., IgG serum level of 300 mg/dL). Rate of administration for all uses: 3% solution at an initial rate of 0.5–1 mL/min; after 15–30 min can increase to 1.5–2.5 mL/min (subsequent infusions at a rate of 2–2.5 mL/min). If the 6% solution is used, the initial infusion rate should be 1–1.5 mL/min and increased after 15–30 min to a maximum of 2.5 mL/min.

ITP.

400 mg/kg for 2–5 consecutive days.

VENOGLOBULIN-I

Immunodeficiency disease.

200 mg/kg/month by IV infusion; can increase to 300–400 mg/kg if response is insufficient or can repeat infusion more frequently than once monthly. Rate of infusion for all uses: 0.01 to 0.02 mL/kg/min for the first 30 min; if no

distress is noted, the rate may be increased to 0.04 mL/kg/min. Higher rates may be used if tolerated. The drug can be given sequentially into a primary IV line containing normal saline; it is not compatible with 5% dextrose solution.

ITP.

Induction: Up to 2,000 mg/kg for 2 to 7 consecutive days; those who respond to induction therapy (platelet count of 30,000/mm^3–50,000/mm^3) may be discontinued after two to seven daily doses. **Maintenance:** Single infusion of 2,000 mg/kg q 2 weeks, as needed to maintain a platelet count of 30,000/mm^3 in children and 20,000/mm^3 in adults or to prevent bleeding episodes between infusions.

VENOGLOBULIN-S

Immunodeficiency disease.

200 mg/kg/month; can increase to 300–400 mg/kg if response is insufficient or can repeat infusion more frequently than once monthly. Rate of infusion for all uses: Initially, 0.01–0.02 mL/kg/min or 1.2 mL/kg/hr for the first 30 min. If no discomfort is noted, the rate for the 5% solution may be increased to 0.04 mL/kg/min or 2.4 mL/kg/hr and the rate for the 10% solution may be increased to 0.05 mL/kg/min or 3 mL/kg/hr.

ITP.

Induction: 2,000 mg/kg over a maximum of 5 days. **Maintenance:** 1,000 mg/kg as needed to maintain platelet counts of 30,000/mm^3 for children and 20,000/mm^3 for adults or to prevent bleeding episodes between infusions.

NURSING CONSIDERATIONS

ADMINISTRATION/STORAGE

IV 1. Follow administration guidelines explicitly and the manufacturer's directions carefully for reconstitution of either the 5% or 10% solution.

2. In agamma- or hypogammaglobulinemic clients, use the 3% solution. Initially, administer at a rate of 10–20 gtt/min (0.5–1 mL/min). After 15–30 min the rate may be increased to 30–50 gtt/min (1.5–2.5 mL/min). Subsequent infusions may be given at a rate of 40–50 gtt/min (2–2.5 mL/min). If the first bottle of the 3% solution is given with good tolerance, subsequent infusions may be given using the 6% solution.

3. Do not shake the solutions because excessive foaming will occur.

4. Infuse only if the solution is clear and at room temperature.

5. Give only IV ; the IM or SC routes have not been evaluated.

6. Give by a separate IV line; do not mix with other fluids or medications.

7. A rapid decrease in serum IgG level in the first week postinfusion will be observed; this is expected and due to the equilibration of IgG between the plasma and extravascular space.

8. Use a pump to administer.

9. Have epinephrine readily available in the event of an acute anaphylactic reaction.

ASSESSMENT

1. Document indications for therapy; for passive immunization note date and type of exposure; assess closely for anaphylaxis.

2. Administer within 2 weeks of exposure to hepatitis A, within 6 days after measles exposure, and within 7 days after hepatitis B exposure.

3. Any history of ITP warrants close hematologic monitoring. Monitor CBC and determine if pregnant; this requires close observation and management.

4. Monitor VS; if hypotension occurs, decrease or interrupt infusion rate until hypotension subsides.

5. Administer in a closely monitored environment and away from persons with active infections if immunocompromised.

6. Monitor LFTs, hematologic parameters, IgG levels, and appropriate blood and urine chemistries.

7. To reduce the risk of IGIV-associated acute renal failure,

- Ensure client is adequately hydrated before infusing IgIV.
- Be especially cautious when giving IgIV to those at increased risk for acute renal failure (renal insufficiency, diabetes mellitus, those over 65 years of

age, volume depletion, sepsis, paraproteinemia, or clients taking nephrotoxic drugs).
• Do not exceed the recommended dose. For those at risk of acute renal failure, dilute or reconstitute the product so the IgIV concentration is as low and the infusion rate as slow as is practical. Do not exceed a sucrose infusion rate of 3 mg/kg/min).
• Assess renal function before infusing IgIV and at regular intervals.

CLIENT/FAMILY TEACHING

1. Immunoglobulin helps to prevent and/or reduce intensity of various infectious diseases. With thrombocytopenia, expect increased platelets and enhanced clotting.
2. Once-monthly therapy is needed to maintain IgG serum levels.
3. Drug may cause N&V, fever, chills, flushing, lightheadedness, and tightness in the chest; report immediately, may be dosage and rate related.
4. Close observation and frequent labs are essential with pregnancy to improve chances of a healthy baby and to ensure maternal safety.
5. Warm soaks to injection site and PO Tylenol may relieve discomfort.
6. Drug is derived from human plasma (except for those engineered genetically); be aware of potential risks.

OUTCOMES/EVALUATE

• IgG levels within normal range
• ↑ Antibody titer; passive immunity
• ↑ Platelets; ↓ hemorrhaging

Inamrinone lactate

(in-**AM**-rih-nohn)

PREGNANCY CATEGORY: C
CLASSIFICATION(S):
Inotropic drug
Rx:

ACTION/KINETICS

Causes an increase in CO by increasing the force of contraction of the heart, probably by inhibiting cyclic AMP phosphodiesterase, thereby increasing cellular levels of c-AMP. It reduces afterload and preload by directly relaxing vascular smooth muscle. **Time to peak effect:** 10 min. **t½, elimination, after rapid IV:** 3.6 hr; **after IV infusion:** 5.8 hr. **Steady-state plasma levels:** 2.4 mcg/mL by maintaining an infusion of 5–10 mcg/kg/min. **Duration:** 30 min–2 hr, depending on the dose. Excreted primarily in the urine both unchanged and as metabolites. Children have a larger volume of distribution and a decreased elimination half-life.

NOTE: Due to medication errors and confusion with amiodarone, the generic name for amrinone was changed to inamrinone.

USES

Congestive heart failure (short-term therapy in clients unresponsive to digitalis, diuretics, and/or vasodilators). Can be used in digitalized clients.

CONTRAINDICATIONS

Hypersensitivity to inamrinone or bisulfites. Severe aortic or pulmonary valvular disease in lieu of surgery. Acute MI.

SPECIAL CONCERNS

Safety and efficacy have not been established in children. Use with caution during lactation.

SIDE EFFECTS

GI: N&V, abdominal pain, anorexia. **CV:** Hypotension, ***supraventricular and ventricular arrhythmias.*** **Allergic:** Pericarditis, pleuritis, ascites, allergic reaction to sodium bisulfite present in the product, vasculitis with nodular pulmonary densities, hypoxemia, jaundice. **Other:** Thrombocytopenia, ***hepatotoxicity,*** fever, chest pain, burning at site of injection.

OD OVERDOSE MANAGEMENT

Symptoms: Hypotension. *Treatment:* Reduce or discontinue drug administration and begin general supportive measures.

DRUG INTERACTIONS

Excessive hypotension when used with disopyramide.

HOW SUPPLIED

Injection: 5 mg/mL

DOSAGE

• **IV**

CHF.

Initial: 0.75 mg/kg as a bolus given slowly over 2–3 min; may be repeated after 30 min if necessary. **Maintenance, IV infusion:** 5–10 mcg/kg/min. Do not exceed a daily dose of 10 mg/kg, although up to 18 mg/kg/day has been used in some clients for short periods.

NURSING CONSIDERATIONS

ADMINISTRATION/STORAGE

IV 1. Administer undiluted or diluted in 0.9% or 0.45% saline to a concentration of 1–3 mg/mL. Use diluted solutions within 24 hr.
2. Do not dilute with solutions containing dextrose (glucose) prior to injection. However, the drug may be injected into running dextrose (glucose) infusions through a Y connector or directly into the tubing.
3. Administer loading dose over 2–3 min; may be repeated in 30 min.
4. Solutions should be clear yellow.
5. Do not administer with furosemide; precipitate will form.
6. Protect from light and store at room temperature.

ASSESSMENT

1. Obtain baseline VS, CXR, and ECG.
2. Assess electrolytes and CBC; report any unusual bruises or bleeding.
3. Document cardiac and pulmonary assessments, noting any new-onset S_3, rales, or edema.
4. Monitor VS, I&O, weights, and urine output. Document CVP, CO, and PA pressures if catheter in place.
5. Observe for any hypersensitivity reactions, including pericarditis, pleuritis, or ascites.
6. Identify previous pharmacologic agents used and results.

CLIENT/FAMILY TEACHING

1. Drug is used IV for congestive heart failure in clients who have not responded to the normal treatment with digoxin, diuretics or vasodilators.
2 Expect frequent monitoring of ECG, BP and heart rate as well as weights. Drug may cause more frequent voiding.
3. Report any increased dizziness, weakness, fatigue, numbness, tingling or swelling of extremities, or pain at IV site.

OUTCOMES/EVALUATE

- ↓ Preload and afterload; ↑ CO
- Improvement in S&S of CHF

Indapamide

(in-**DAP**-ah-myd)

PREGNANCY CATEGORY: B
Rx: Lozol
✱Rx: Apo-Indapamide, Novo-Indapamide, PMS-Indapamide

Indapamide Hemihydrate

(in-**DAP**-ah-myd)

PREGNANCY CATEGORY: B
✱Rx: Gen-Indapamide, Nu-Indapamide
CLASSIFICATION(S):
Diuretic, thiazide

SEE ALSO ***DIURETICS, THIAZIDE.***

ACTION/KINETICS
Onset: 1–2 weeks after multiple doses. **Peak levels:** 2 hr. **Duration:** Up to 8 weeks with multiple doses. **t½:** 14 hr. Nearly 100% is absorbed from the GI tract. Excreted through the kidneys (70% with 7% unchanged) and the GI tract (23%).

USES
Alone or in combination with other drugs for treatment of hypertension. Edema in CHF.

SPECIAL CONCERNS
Dosage has not been established in children. Geriatric clients may be more sensitive to the hypotensive and electrolyte effects.

HOW SUPPLIED
Tablet: 1.25 mg, 2.5 mg

DOSAGE

- **TABLETS**

Edema of CHF.

Adults: 2.5 mg as a single dose in the morning. If necessary, may be increased to 5 mg/day after 1 week.

Hypertension.

Adults: 1.25 mg as a single dose in the morning. If the response is not satisfactory after 4 weeks, the dose may be increased to 2.5 mg taken once daily. If the response to 2.5 mg is not satisfactory after 4 weeks, the dose may be increased to 5 mg taken once daily (however, consideration should be given to adding another antihypertensive).

NURSING CONSIDERATIONS

SEE ALSO *NURSING CONSIDERATIONS* FOR *DIURETICS* AND *ANTIHYPERTENSIVE AGENTS*.

ADMINISTRATION/STORAGE

1. May be combined with other antihypertensive agents if response inadequate. Initially, reduce the dose of other agents by 50%.
2. Doses greater than 5 mg/day do not increase effectiveness but may increase hypokalemia.

ASSESSMENT

Document indications for therapy, type, onset, and characteristics of symptoms. Note other agents trialed and the outcome.

OUTCOMES/EVALUATE

- ↓ BP
- ↑ Urinary output with ↓ edema

Indinavir sulfate

(in-**DIN**-ah-veer)

PREGNANCY CATEGORY: C
CLASSIFICATION(S):
Antiviral, protease inhibitor
Rx: Crixivan

SEE ALSO *ANITIVIRAL DRUGS*.

ACTION/KINETICS

Binds to active sites on the HIV protease enzyme resulting in inhibition of enzyme activity. Inhibition prevents cleavage of the viral polyproteins resulting in the formation of immature noninfectious viral particles. Varying degrees of cross resistance have been noted between indinavir and other HIV-protease inhibitors. Rapidly absorbed in fasting clients; **time to peak plasma levels:** Approximately 0.8 hr. Administration with a meal high in calories, fat, and protein results in a significant decrease in the amount absorbed and in the peak plasma concentration. Approximately 60% bound to plasma proteins. **t½:** 1.8 hr. Metabolized in the liver with both parent drug and metabolites excreted through the feces (over 80%) and the urine.

USES

Treatment of HIV infection in adults when antiretroviral therapy is indicated. May be used with other anti-HIV drugs.

CONTRAINDICATIONS

Lactation. Use with astemizole, midazolam, rifampin, terfenadine, and triazolam. Mild to moderate liver or kidney disease.

SPECIAL CONCERNS

Not a cure for HIV infections; clients may continue to develop opportunistic infections and other complications of HIV disease. Not been shown to reduce the risk of transmission of HIV through sexual contact or blood contamination. No data on the effect of indinavir therapy on clinical progression of HIV infection, including survival or the incidence of opportunistic infections. Hemophiliacs treated for HIV infections with protease inhibitors may manifest spontaneous bleeding episodes. Safety and efficacy have not been determined in children.

SIDE EFFECTS

GI: N&V, diarrhea, abdominal pain/distention, acid regurgitation, anorexia, dry mouth, aphthous stomatitis, cheilitis, cholecystitis, cholestasis, constipation, dyspepsia, eructation, flatulence, gastritis, gingivitis, glossodynia, gingival hemorrhage, increased appetite, infectious gastroenteritis, jaundice, liver cirrhosis. **CNS:** Headache, insomnia, dizziness, somnolence, agitation, anxiety, bruxism, decreased mental acuity, depression, dream abnormality, dysesthesia, excitement, fasciculation, hypesthesia, nervousness, neuralgia, neurotic disorder, paresthesia, peripheral neuropathy, sleep disorder, tremor, vertigo. **CV:** CV disorder, palpitation. **Musculoskeletal:** Back pain, arthralgia, leg pain, myalgia, muscle cramps, muscle weakness, musculoskeletal pain, shoulder pain, stiffness. **Body as a whole:** Asthenia, fatigue, flank pain, malaise, chest pain, chills, fever, flu-like illness, fungal infection, malaise, pain, syncope. **Hematologic:** Anemia, lymphadenopathy, spleen disorder. **Respiratory:** Cough, dyspnea, halitosis, pharyngeal hyperemia, pharyngitis, pneumonia, rales, rhonchi, ***respiratory failure,*** sinus disorder, sinusitis, URI. **Dermatologic:** Body odor, contact dermatitis, dermatitis, dry skin, flushing, folliculitis, herpes simplex, herpes zoster, night sweats, pruritus, seborrhea, skin disorder, skin infection, sweating, urticaria. **GU:** Nephrolithiasis, dysuria, hematuria, hydronephrosis, nocturia, PMS, proteinuria, renal colic, urinary frequency, UTI, uterine abnormality, urine sediment abnormality, urolithiasis. **Ophthalmic:** Accommodation disorder, blurred vision, eye pain, eye swelling, orbital edema. **Miscellaneous:** Asymptomatic hyperbilirubinemia, food allergy, taste disorder.

LABORATORY TEST CONSIDERATIONS

↑ Serum transaminases (ALT, AST), total serum bilirubin, serum amylase. ↓ Hemoglobin, platelet count, neutrophils. Hyperbilirubinemia.

DRUG INTERACTIONS

Aldesleukin / ↑ Plasma indinavir levels R/T ↓ liver metabolism

Amiodarone / Possible ↑ amiodarone plasma levels R/T ↓ liver metabolism

Clarithromycin / ↑ Plasma levels of both indinavir and clarithromycin

Didanosine / pH Dependent ↓ in absorption

Fluconazole / ↓ Plasma levels of indinavir

Grapefruit juice / Slight delay in absorption of indinavir; no effect on bioavailability

Isoniazid / ↑ Plasma isoniazid levels

Ketoconazole / ↑ Plasma levels of indinavir

Midazolam / ↓ Midazolam metabolism → possibility of cardiac arrhythmias and prolonged sedation

Oral contraceptives / ↑ Plasma levels of both estrogen and progestin components of product

Quinidine / ↑ Plasma indinavir levels

Rifabutin / ↑ Plasma rifabutin levels; ↓ dose by 50%

Rifampin / ↓ Plasma levels of indinavir

H *St. John's wort* / Significant ↓ in indinavir plasma levels R/T ↑ liver metabolism

Stavudine / ↑ Plasma stavudine levels

Triazolam / ↓ Triazolam metabolism → possibility of cardiac arrhythmias and prolonged sedation

Trimethoprim/Sulfamethoxazole / ↑ Plasma levels of trimethoprim (no change in sulfamethoxazole levels)

Zidovudine / ↑ Plasma levels of both indinavir and zidovudine

HOW SUPPLIED

Capsules: 200 mg, 333 mg, 400 mg.

DOSAGE

• **CAPSULES**

HIV infections.

Adults: 800 mg (two 400-mg capsules) q 8 hr ATC. The dosage is the same whether the drug is used alone or in combination with other retroviral agents. Reduce the dose to 600 mg q 8 hr with mild to moderate hepatic insufficiency due to cirrhosis.

NURSING CONSIDERATIONS

SEE ALSO NURSING CONSIDERATIONS FOR ANTIVIRAL DRUGS.

ADMINISTRATION/STORAGE

1. Capsules are moisture sensitive. Store in original container; keep desiccant in the bottle. Keep tightly closed, protected from moisture and at a room temperature of 15–30°C (59–86°F).
2. If indinavir and didanosine are given together, give at least 1 hr apart on an empty stomach.
3. If indinavir is taken with rifabutin, reduce the dose of rifabutin to one-half the standard dose.
4. When indinavir is taken with ketoconazole, reduce the dose of indinavir to 600 mg q 8 hr.

ASSESSMENT

1. Document symptom onset, confirmation of HIV, other agents trialed with the outcome.
2. Monitor CD4 cell count, viral load, and LFTs. Anticipate reduced dosage

with impaired liver function; drug is hepatically metabolized.
3. Review list of drugs currently prescribed to ensure that none interact.

CLIENT/FAMILY TEACHING

1. Take as prescribed at 8-hr intervals ATC with water 1 hr before or 2 hr after meals for optimal absorption. May be taken with other liquids, such as skim milk, juice, coffee, or tea, or with a light meal (e.g., dry toast with jelly, juice, and coffee with skim milk and sugar; or corn flakes, skim milk, and sugar). Avoid grapefruit juice, foods high in calories, fat , or protein.
2. If a dose is missed by more than 2 hr, wait and take the next dose at the regularly scheduled time. If a dose is missed by less than 2 hr, take immediately.
3. Must adequately hydrate. To ensure adequate hydration, drink at least 1.5 L of liquids during a 24-hr period.
4. Report any symptoms of nephrolithiasis (e.g., flank pain with or without hematuria, including microscopic hematuria); therapy should be interrupted for 1–3 days.
5. Drug is not a cure for HIV, continue to take precautions with disease transmission; opportunistic infections may occur.
6. Use reliable birth control and barrier protection; drug does not decrease the risk of transmitting disease through sexual contact or blood contamination.
7. Report severe, N&V, diarrhea, fever, chills, personality changes or changes in the color of urine or stool.
8. The original desiccant must be dispensed with the medication. Counsel to store the drug at room temperature away from moisure.

OUTCOMES/EVALUATE

Treatment of HIV infection progression

Indomethacin

(in-doh-**METH**-ah-sin)

Rx: Indochron E-R, Indocin, Indocin SR, Indomethacin SR
✱Rx: Apo-Indomethacin, Indocid, Indocid Ophthalmic Suspension, Indocid SR, Indotec, Novo–Methacin, Nu-Indo, Rhodacine

Indomethacin sodium trihydrate

(in-doh-**METH**-ah-sin)

Rx: Indocin I.V.
✱Rx: Indocid P.D.A.
CLASSIFICATION(S):
Nonsteroidal anti-inflammatory drug

SEE ALSO *NONSTEROIDAL ANTI-INFLAMMATORY DRUGS.*

ACTION/KINETICS

PO. Onset: 30 min for analgesia and up to 1 week for anti-inflammatory effect. **Peak plasma levels:** 1–2 hr (2–4 hr for sustained-release). **Peak action for gout:** 24–36 hr; swelling gradually disappears in 3–5 days. **Peak activity for antirheumatic effect:** About 4 weeks. **Duration:** 4–6 hr for analgesia and 1–2 weeks for anti-inflammatory effect. **Therapeutic plasma levels:** 10–18 mcg/mL. **t½:** Approximately 5 hr (up to 6 hr for sustained-release). **Plasma t½ following IV in infants:** 12–20 hr, depending on age and dose. Approximately 90% plasma protein bound. Metabolized in the liver and excreted in both the urine and feces.

USES

Not a simple analgesic; use only for the conditions listed. Moderate to severe rheumatoid arthritis (including acute flares of chronic disease), osteoarthritis, and ankylosing spondylitis (drug of choice). Acute gouty arthritis and acute painful shoulder (tendinitis, bursitis). *IV:* Pharmacologic closure of persistent patent ductus arteriosus in premature infants. *Investigational:* Topically to treat cystoid macular edema (0.5% and 1% drops), sunburn, primary dysmenorrhea, prophylaxis of migraine, cluster headache, polyhydramnios.

ADDITIONAL CONTRAINDICATIONS

Pregnancy and lactation. PO indomethacin in children under 14 years of age. GI lesions or history of recurrent GI lesions. *IV use:* GI or intracranial bleeding, thrombocytopenia, renal disease, defects of coagulation, necrotizing enterocolitis. *Suppositories:* Recent rectal bleeding, history of proctitis.

SPECIAL CONCERNS
Restrict use in children to those unresponsive to or intolerant of other antiinflammatory agents; efficacy has not been determined in children less than 14 years of age. Geriatric clients are at greater risk of developing CNS side effects, especially confusion. Use with caution in clients with history of epilepsy, psychiatric illness, or parkinsonism and in the elderly. Use with extreme caution in the presence of existing, controlled infections.

ADDITIONAL SIDE EFFECTS
Reactivation of latent infections may mask signs of infection. More marked CNS manifestations than for other drugs of this group. Aggravation of depression or other psychiatric problems, epilepsy, and parkinsonism.

ADDITIONAL DRUG INTERACTIONS
Captopril / ↓ Captopril effect, probably R/T inhibition of prostaglandin synthesis
Diflunisal / ↑ Plasma levels of indomethacin; also, possible fatal GI hemorrhage
Diuretics (loop, potassium-sparing, thiazide) / May reduce antihypertensive and natriuretic action of diuretics
Lisinopril / Possible ↓ lisinopril effect
Losartan / ↓ Antihypertensive effect of losartan
Prazosin / ↓ Antihypertensive drug effects

HOW SUPPLIED
Indomethacin: *Capsule:* 25 mg, 50 mg; *Capsule, Extended Release:* 75 mg; *Suppository:* 50 mg; *Suspension, Oral:* 25 mg/5 mL **Indomethacin sodium trihydrate:** *Powder for injection:* 1 mg

DOSAGE

• **CAPSULES, ORAL SUSPENSION**

Moderate to severe arthritis, osteoarthritis, ankylosing spondylitis.

Adults, initial: 25 mg b.i.d.–t.i.d.; may be increased by 25–50 mg at weekly intervals, according to condition and, if tolerated, until satisfactory response is obtained. With persistent night pain or morning stiffness, a maximum of 100 mg of the total daily dose can be given at bedtime. **Maximum daily dosage:** 150–200 mg. In acute flares of chronic rheumatoid arthritis, the dose may need to be increased by 25–50 mg/day until the acute phase is under control.

Acute gouty arthritis.

Adults, initial: 50 mg t.i.d. until pain is tolerable; **then,** reduce dosage rapidly until drug is withdrawn. Pain relief usually occurs within 2–4 hr, tenderness and heat subside in 24–36 hr, and swelling disappears in 3–4 days.

Acute painful shoulder (bursitis/tendinitis).

75–150 mg/day in three to four divided doses for 1–2 weeks.

• **SUSTAINED-RELEASE CAPSULES**

Antirheumatic, anti-inflammatory.

Adults: 75 mg, of which 25 mg is released immediately, 1–2 times/day.

• **SUPPOSITORIES**

Anti-inflammatory, antirheumatic, antigout.

Adults: 50 mg up to q.i.d. **Pediatric:** 1.5–2.5 mg/kg/day in three to four divided doses (up to a maximum of 4 mg/kg or 250–300 mg/day, whichever is less).

• **IV ONLY**

Patent ductus arteriosus.

3 IV doses, depending on age of the infant, are given at 12–24-hr intervals. **Infants less than 2 days:** first dose, 0.2 mg/kg, followed by two doses of 0.1 mg/kg each; **infants 2–7 days:** three doses of 0.2 mg/kg each; **infants more than 7 days:** first dose, 0.2 mg/kg, followed by two doses of 0.25 mg/kg each. If patent ductus arteriosus reopens, a second course of one to three doses may be given. Surgery may be required if there is no response after two courses of therapy.

NURSING CONSIDERATIONS

SEE ALSO NURSING CONSIDERATIONS FOR NONSTEROIDAL ANTI-INFLAMMATORY DRUGS.

ADMINISTRATION/STORAGE

1. Do not crush the sustained-release form; do not use for acute gouty arthritis.
2. With dysphagia, the capsule contents may be emptied into apple-

sauce, food, or liquid to ensure that client receives the prescribed dose.
3. Suppositories (50 mg) may be used if unable to take PO medication. Store below 30°C (86°F).
4. Use the smallest effective dose, based on individual need. Adverse reactions are dose related.
IV 5. Store in amber-colored containers.
6. Prepare the IV solution with 1–2 mL of preservative-free NaCl or sterile water for injection. Prepare just prior to use.
7. Reconstitute to 0.1 mg/mL or 0.05 mg/mL immediately before use and infuse over 5–10 sec.

ASSESSMENT

1. Note indications for therapy, onset, and characteristics of symptoms.
2. Note agents currently prescribed.
3. Assess and document characteristics of involved joint(s), including goniometric measurements, ROM, functional ability, and rate pain levels.
4. Monitor U/A, CBC, liver and renal function studies. Avoid with severe renal impairment.

CLIENT/FAMILY TEACHING

1. Take with food or milk to decrease GI upset. Do not crush or break capsules; may sprinkle capsule contents on food if unable to swallow.
2. Use caution when operating potentially hazardous equipment; may cause lightheadedness and decreased alertness.
3. Withhold drug and report if adverse side effects occur since many may be serious enough to stop therapy.
4. Record weights, especially if N or V occur; report any abdominal pain or diarrhea.
5. Indomethacin masks infections; report any S&S of infection or fever.
6. Report for scheduled ophthalmologic exams and lab studies.
7. It will take from 2 to 4 weeks of therapy before significant improvement evident in arthritic conditions. Follow prescribed dosing regimen carefully and refrain from becoming discouraged.

OUTCOMES/EVALUATE

- ↓ Pain and inflammation; ↑ joint mobility
- Closure of patent ductus arteriosus
- Therapeutic serum drug levels (10–18 mcg/mL)

Infliximab

(in-**FLIX**-ih-mab)

PREGNANCY CATEGORY: C
CLASSIFICATION(S):
Treatment of Crohn's disease
Rx: Remicade

ACTION/KINETICS

Chimeric $IgG1_K$ monoclonal antibody produced by a recombinant cell line to treat Crohn's disease. Acts by neutralizing the biological activity of TNFα by high-affinity binding to its soluble and transmembrane forms and inhibits TNFα receptor binding. **t½, terminal:** 8–9.5 days.

USES

(1) Reduce S&S of moderate to severe Crohn's disease unresponsive to conventional therapy. (2) To reduce the number of draining enterocutaneous fistulas in fistulizing Crohn's disease. (3) With methotrexate for inhibition of structural damage progression in those with moderate-to-severe rheumatoid arthritis who do not respond adequately to methotrexate alone.

CONTRAINDICATIONS

Hypersensitivity to murine proteins. Lactation. Use in CHF or in those with a clinically important, active infection. Concurrent use with live vaccines.

SPECIAL CONCERNS

Safety and efficacy have not been determined for use in children or beyond a single dose in moderate to severe Crohn's disease or beyond three doses in fistulizing Crohn's disease. Use with caution in the elderly.

Serious infections, including sepsis and death, have occurred in those treated with TNF-blocking agents. Thus, use with caution in clients with a chronic infection or a history of recurrent infection. May worsen CHF. Clients beginning therapy may develop signs and symptoms of tuberculosis, including tissues other than the lungs.

VISUAL IDENTIFICATION GUIDE

Use this section to quickly verify the identity of a capsule, tablet, or other solid oral medication. More than 300 leading tablets and capsules are shown in actual size and color, organized alphabetically by generic name. Each is labeled with its brand name, if applicable, as well as its strength and the name of its supplier.

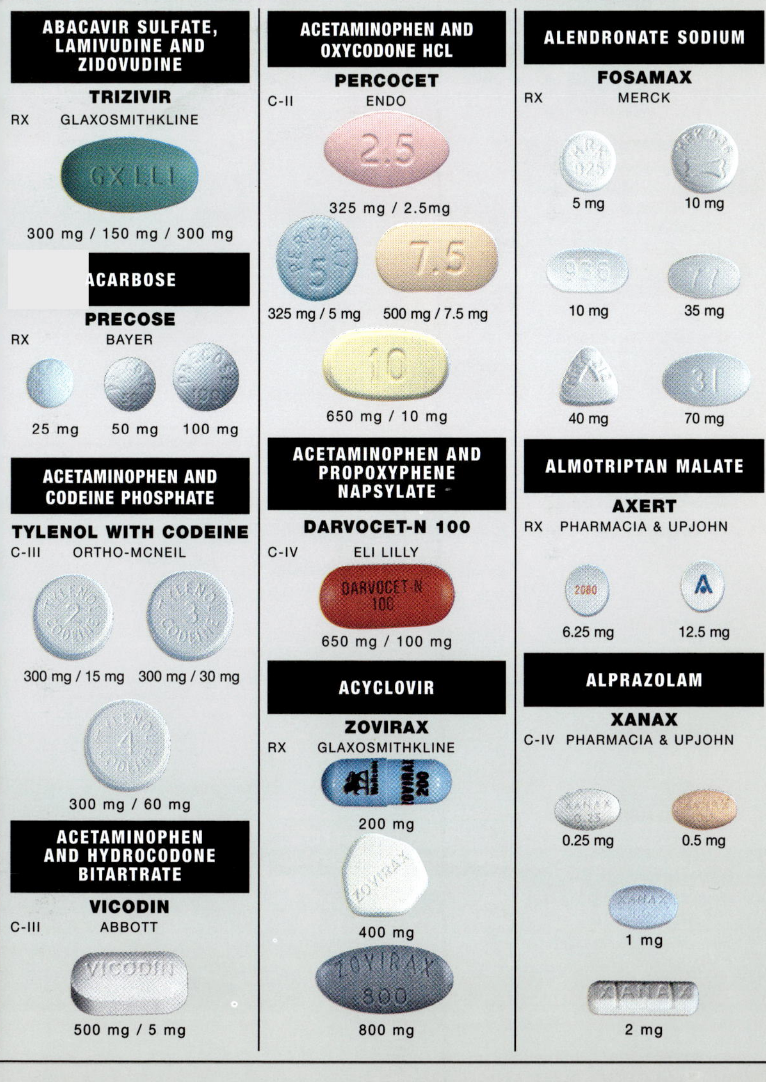

AMLODIPINE BESYLATE

NORVASC
RX PFIZER

2.5 mg 5 mg 10 mg

AMOXICILLIN

AMOXIL
RX GLAXOSMITHKLINE

250 mg

500 mg

AMOXICILLIN AND CLAVULANATE POTASSIUM

AUGMENTIN
RX GLAXOSMITHKLINE

125 mg / 31.25 mg

200 mg / 28.5 mg

250 mg / 62.5 mg

400 mg / 57.0 mg

Chewable Tablets

250 mg / 125 mg

500 mg / 125 mg

875 mg / 125 mg

ASPIRIN AND DIPYRIDAMOLE ER

AGGRENOX
RX BOEHRINGER INGELHEIM

25 mg / 200 mg

ATENOLOL

TENORMIN
RX ASTRAZENECA

25 mg 50 mg 100 mg

AZITHROMYCIN

ZITHROMAX
RX PFIZER

250 mg

600 mg

BENAZEPRIL HCL

LOTENSIN
RX NOVARTIS

5 mg 10 mg

20 mg 40 mg

CANDESARTAN CILEXETIL

ATACAND
RX ASTRAZENECA LP

4 mg 8 mg

16 mg 32 mg

CANDESARTAN CILEXETIL AND HYDROCHLOROTHIAZIDE

ATACAND HCT
RX ASTRAZENECA LP

16 mg / 12.5 mg

32 mg / 12.5 mg

CAPECITABINE

XELODA
RX ROCHE

150 mg

500 mg

CARBAMAZEPINE

TEGRETOL
RX NOVARTIS

200 mg

CEFADROXIL MONOHYDRATE

DURICEF
RX BRISTOL-MYERS SQUIBB

500 mg

1 g

CEFIXIME

SUPRAX
RX LEDERLE

200 mg

400 mg

CELECOXIB

CELEBREX
RX PFIZER

100 mg

200 mg

CILOSTAZOL

PLETAL
RX OTSUKA

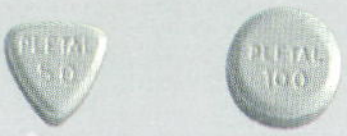

50 mg 100 mg

CIMETIDINE

TAGAMET
RX GLAXOSMITHKLINE

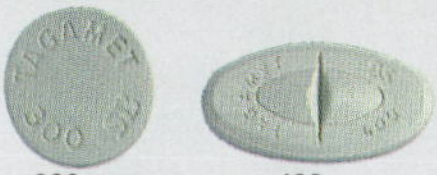

300 mg 400 mg

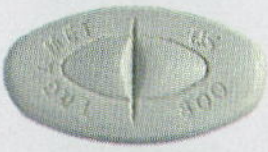

800 mg

CIPROFLOXACIN HCL

CIPRO
RX BAYER

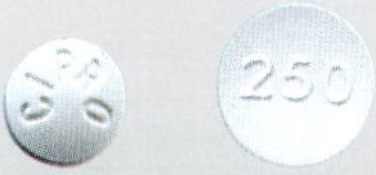

100 mg 250 mg

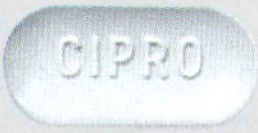

500 mg

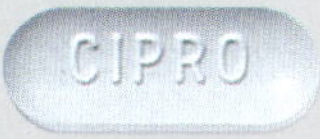

750 mg

CITALOPRAM HYDROBROMIDE

CELEXA
RX FOREST

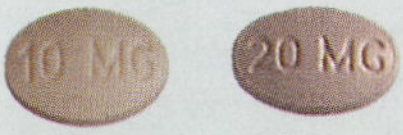

10 mg 20 mg

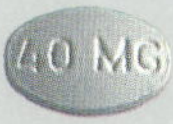

40 mg

CLARITHROMYCIN

BIAXIN FILMTAB
RX ABBOTT

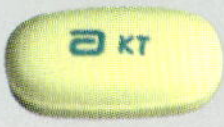

250 mg

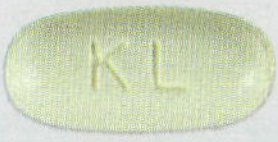

500 mg

CLONAZEPAM

KLONOPIN
C-IV ROCHE

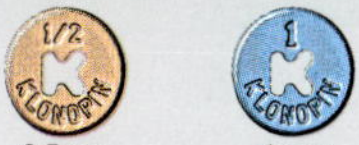

0.5 mg 1 mg

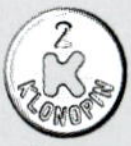

2 mg

CLOPIDOGREL BISULFATE

PLAVIX
RX SANOFI-SYNTHELABO

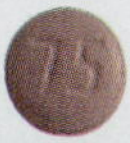

75 mg

CYCLOBENZAPRINE HCL

FLEXERIL
RX MERCK

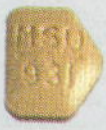

10 mg

DESLORATADINE

CLARINEX
RX SCHERING

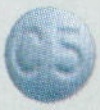

5 mg

DEXMETHYLPHENIDATE HCL

FOCALIN
C-II NOVARTIS

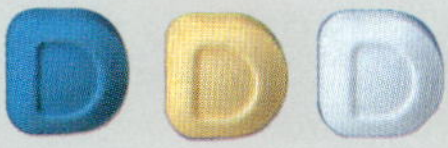

2.5 mg 5 mg 10 mg

DIAZEPAM

VALIUM
C-IV ROCHE

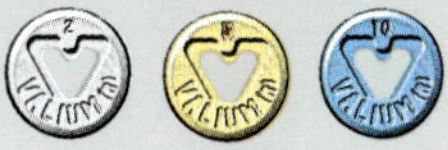

2 mg 5 mg 10 mg

DICLOFENAC SODIUM

VOLTAREN
RX NOVARTIS

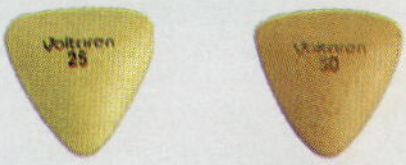

25 mg 50 mg

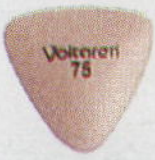

75 mg

DICLOFENAC SODIUM AND MISOPROSTOL

ARTHROTEC
RX G.D. SEARLE

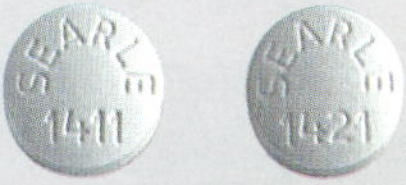

50 mg / 200 mcg 75 mg / 200 mcg

DIGOXIN

LANOXIN
RX GLAXOSMITHKLINE

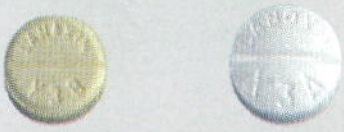

0.125 mg 0.25 mg

DIVALPROEX SODIUM

DEPAKOTE
RX ABBOTT

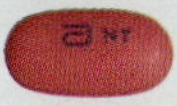

125 mg

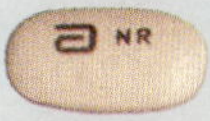

250 mg

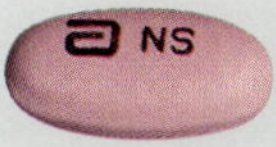

500 mg

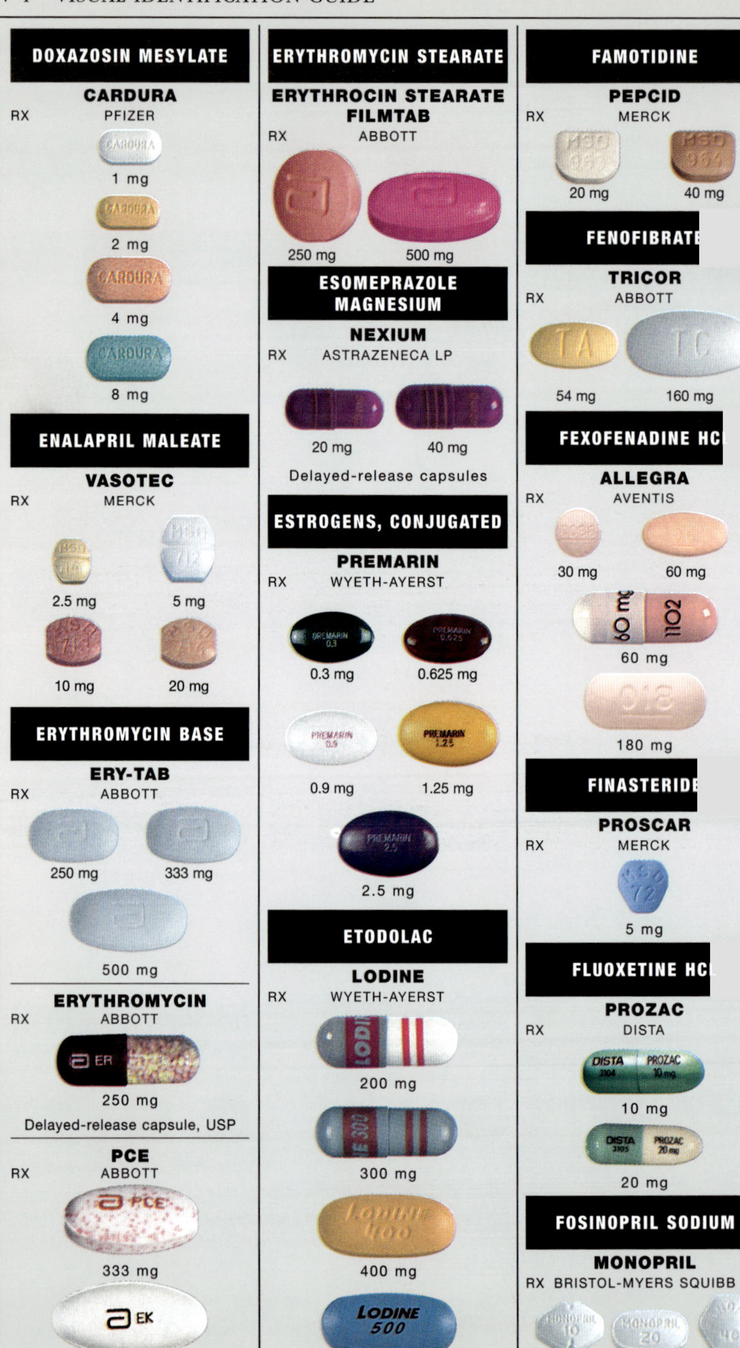
DOXAZOSIN MESYLATE
CARDURA
RX PFIZER
1 mg
2 mg
4 mg
8 mg
ENALAPRIL MALEATE
VASOTEC
RX MERCK
2.5 mg
5 mg
10 mg
20 mg
ERYTHROMYCIN BASE
ERY-TAB
RX ABBOTT
250 mg
333 mg
500 mg
ERYTHROMYCIN
RX ABBOTT
250 mg
Delayed-release capsule, USP
PCE
RX ABBOTT
333 mg
500 mg
ERYTHROMYCIN STEARATE
ERYTHROCIN STEARATE FILMTAB
RX ABBOTT
250 mg
500 mg
ESOMEPRAZOLE MAGNESIUM
NEXIUM
RX ASTRAZENECA LP
20 mg
40 mg
Delayed-release capsules
ESTROGENS, CONJUGATED
PREMARIN
RX WYETH-AYERST
0.3 mg
0.625 mg
0.9 mg
1.25 mg
2.5 mg
ETODOLAC
LODINE
RX WYETH-AYERST
200 mg
300 mg
400 mg
500 mg
FAMOTIDINE
PEPCID
RX MERCK
20 mg
40 mg
FENOFIBRATE
TRICOR
RX ABBOTT
54 mg
160 mg
FEXOFENADINE HCL
ALLEGRA
RX AVENTIS
30 mg
60 mg
60 mg
180 mg
FINASTERIDE
PROSCAR
RX MERCK
5 mg
FLUOXETINE HCL
PROZAC
RX DISTA
10 mg
20 mg
FOSINOPRIL SODIUM
MONOPRIL
RX BRISTOL-MYERS SQUIBB
10 mg
20 mg
40 mg

GATIFLOXACIN

TEQUIN
RX BRISTOL-MYERS SQUIBB

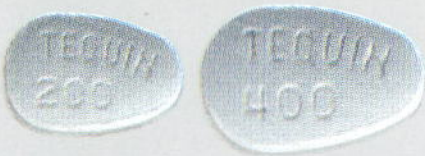

200 mg 400 mg

GEMFIBROZIL

LOPID
RX PARKE-DAVIS

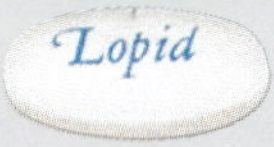

600 mg

GLIMEPIRIDE

AMARYL
RX AVENTIS

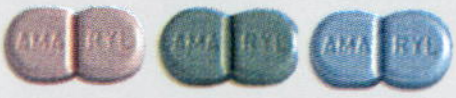

1 mg 2 mg 4 mg

GLIPIZIDE

GLUCOTROL
RX PFIZER

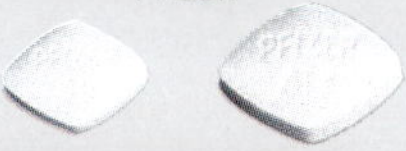

5 mg 10 mg

GLYBURIDE

DIABETA
RX AVENTIS

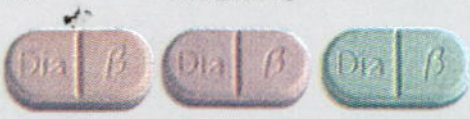

1.25 mg 2.5 mg 5 mg

GLYBURIDE AND METFORMIN HCL

GLUCOVANCE
RX BRISTOL-MYERS SQUIBB

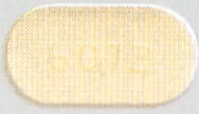

1.25 mg / 250 mg

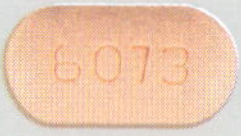

2.5 mg / 500 mg

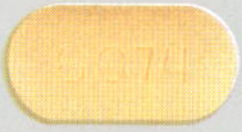

5 mg / 500 mg

IRBESARTAN

AVAPRO
RX BRISTOL-MYERS SQUIBB

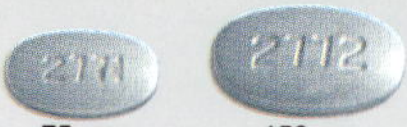

75 mg 150 mg

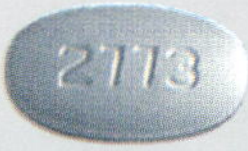

300 mg

KETOCONAZOLE

NIZORAL
RX JANSSEN

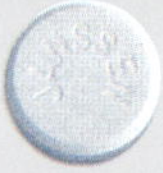

200 mg

KETOROLAC TROMETHAMINE

TORADOL
RX ROCHE

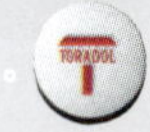

10 mg

LEFLUNOMIDE

ARAVA
RX AVENTIS

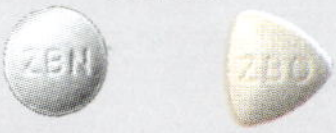

10 mg 20 mg

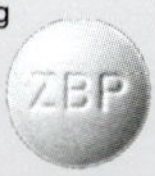

100 mg

LEVOTHYROXINE SODIUM

SYNTHROID
RX ABBOTT

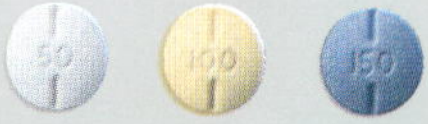

50 mcg 100 mcg 150 mcg

LINEZOLID

ZYVOX
RX PHARMACIA & UPJOHN

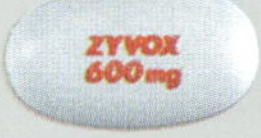

600 mg

LISINOPRIL

PRINIVIL
RX MERCK

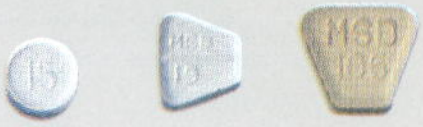

2.5 mg 5 mg 10 mg

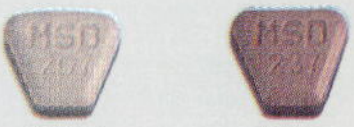

20 mg 40 mg

ZESTRIL
RX ASTRAZENECA

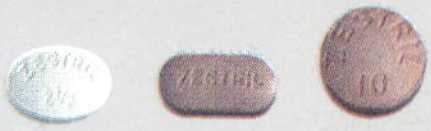

2.5 mg 5 mg 10 mg

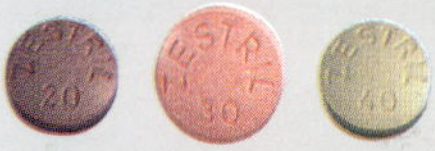

20 mg 30 mg 40 mg

LOPINAVIR/RITONAVIR

KALETRA
RX ABBOTT

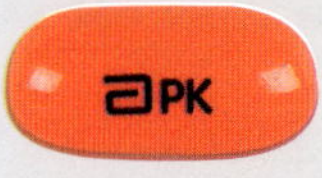

133.3 mg / 33.3 mg

LORATADINE

CLARITIN
RX SCHERING

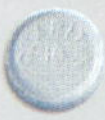

10 mg

LORAZEPAM

ATIVAN
C-IV WYETH-AYERST

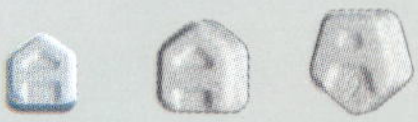

0.5 mg 1 mg 2 mg

LOSARTAN POTASSIUM

COZAAR
RX MERCK

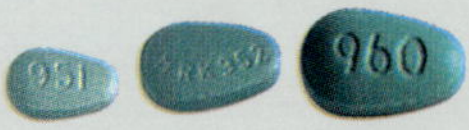

25 mg 50 mg 100 mg

LOVASTATIN

MEVACOR

RX MERCK

10 mg 20 mg 40 mg

MEDROXYPROGESTERONE ACETATE

PROVERA

RX PHARMACIA & UPJOHN

2.5 mg 5 mg 10 mg

MELOXICAM

MOBIC

RX BOEHRINGER INGELHEIM

7.5 mg 15 mg

METFORMIN HYDROCHLORIDE ER

GLUCOPHAGE XR

RX BRISTOL-MYERS SQUIBB

500 mg

Extended Release Tablet

METHYLPHENIDATE HCL

RITALIN

C-II NOVARTIS

5 mg 10 mg 20 mg

METOPROLOL TARTRATE

LOPRESSOR

RX NOVARTIS

50 mg 100 mg

MISOPROSTOL

CYTOTEC

RX G. D. SEARLE

100 mcg 200 mcg

MOXIFLOXACIN HCL

AVELOX

RX BAYER

400 mg

NAPROXEN

NAPROSYN

RX ROCHE

250 mg 375 mg

500 mg

NAPROXEN SODIUM

ANAPROX

RX ROCHE

275 mg

ANAPROX DS

RX ROCHE

550 mg

NEFAZODONE HCL

SERZONE

RX BRISTOL-MYERS SQUIBB

50 mg

100 mg 150 mg

200 mg 250 mg

NIFEDIPINE

PROCARDIA XL

RX PFIZER

30 mg 60 mg

90 mg

Extended Release Tablets

NIZATIDINE

AXID

RX RELIANT

150 mg

300 mg

OFLOXACIN

FLOXIN

RX ORTHO-MCNEIL

200 mg

300 mg

400 mg

OMEPRAZOLE

PRILOSEC

RX ASTRAZENECA LP

10 mg

20 mg

40 mg

Delayed-Release capsules

OSELTAMIVIR PHOSPHATE

TAMIFLU
RX ROCHE

75 mg

PAROXETINE HCL

PAXIL
RX GLAXOSMITHKLINE

10 mg 20 mg

30 mg 40 mg

PENTOXIFYLLINE

TRENTAL
RX AVENTIS

400 mg

PHENYTOIN SODIUM, EXTENDED

DILANTIN KAPSEALS
RX PARKE-DAVIS

30 mg

100 mg

PIOGLITAZONE HCL

ACTOS
RX TAKEDA

15 mg 30 mg 45 mg

PRAVASTATIN SODIUM

PRAVACHOL
RX BRISTOL-MYERS SQUIBB

10 mg 20 mg 40 mg

PROPRANOLOL HCL

INDERAL
RX WYETH-AYERST

10 mg 20 mg 40 mg

QUINAPRIL HCL

ACCUPRIL
RX PARKE-DAVIS

5 mg 10 mg

20 mg 40 mg

QUINAPRIL HCL AND HYDROCHLOROTHIAZIDE

ACCURETIC
RX PARKE-DAVIS

10 mg / 12.5 mg 20 mg / 12.5 mg

20 mg / 25 mg

RANITIDINE HCL

ZANTAC
RX GLAXOSMITHKLINE

150 mg 300 mg

RISEDRONATE SODIUM

ACTONEL
RX PROCTOR & GAMBLE

5 mg 30 mg

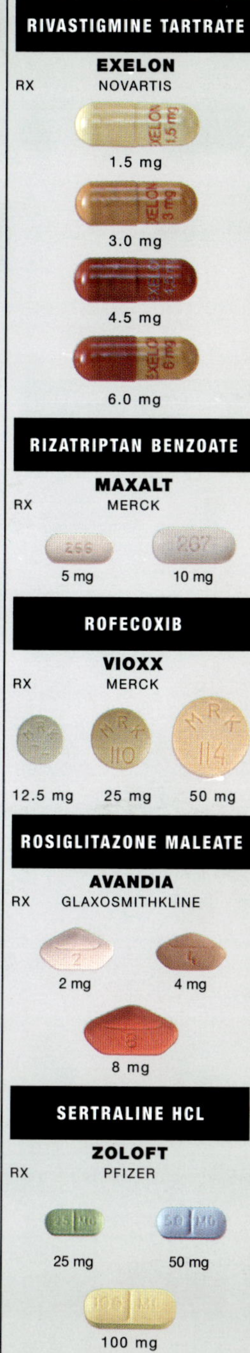

RIVASTIGMINE TARTRATE

EXELON
RX NOVARTIS

1.5 mg

3.0 mg

4.5 mg

6.0 mg

RIZATRIPTAN BENZOATE

MAXALT
RX MERCK

5 mg 10 mg

ROFECOXIB

VIOXX
RX MERCK

12.5 mg 25 mg 50 mg

ROSIGLITAZONE MALEATE

AVANDIA
RX GLAXOSMITHKLINE

2 mg 4 mg

8 mg

SERTRALINE HCL

ZOLOFT
RX PFIZER

25 mg 50 mg

100 mg

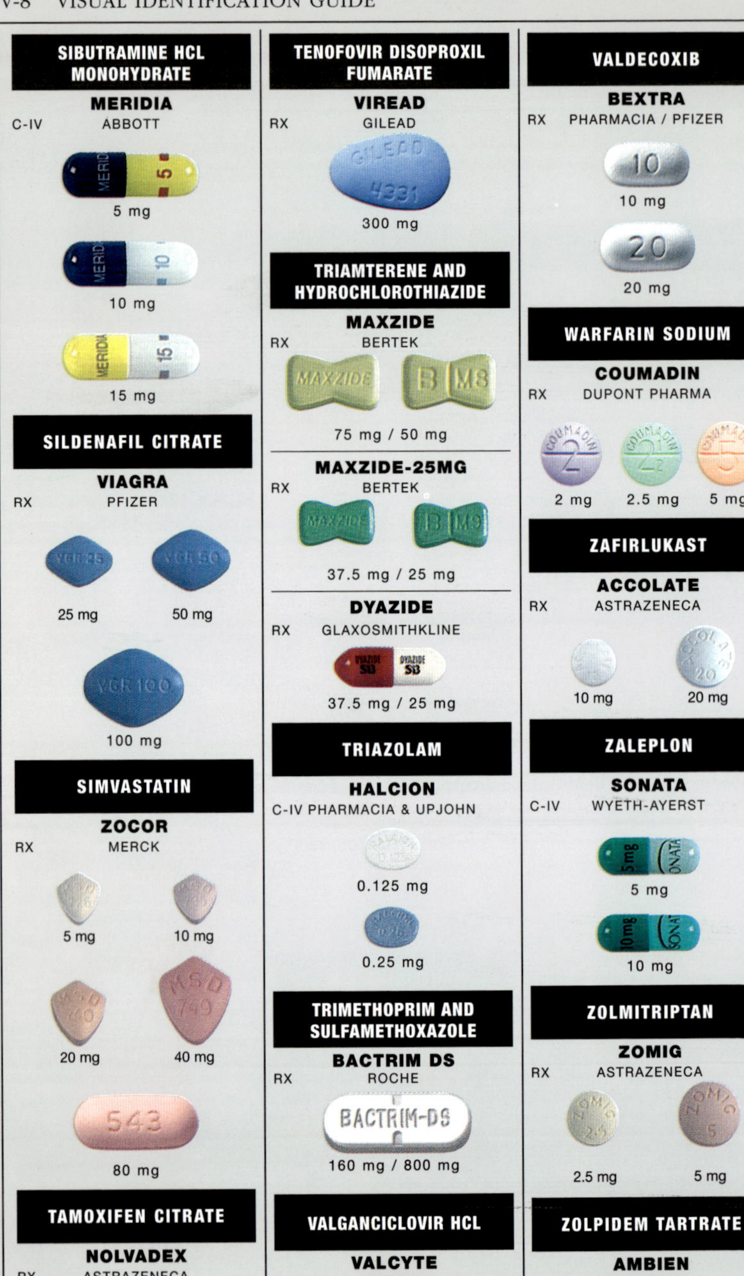
SIBUTRAMINE HCL MONOHYDRATE
MERIDIA
C-IV ABBOTT
5 mg
10 mg
15 mg
SILDENAFIL CITRATE
VIAGRA
RX PFIZER
25 mg
50 mg
100 mg
SIMVASTATIN
ZOCOR
RX MERCK
5 mg
10 mg
20 mg
40 mg
80 mg
TAMOXIFEN CITRATE
NOLVADEX
RX ASTRAZENECA
10 mg
20 mg
TENOFOVIR DISOPROXIL FUMARATE
VIREAD
RX GILEAD
300 mg
TRIAMTERENE AND HYDROCHLOROTHIAZIDE
MAXZIDE
RX BERTEK
75 mg / 50 mg
MAXZIDE-25MG
RX BERTEK
37.5 mg / 25 mg
DYAZIDE
RX GLAXOSMITHKLINE
37.5 mg / 25 mg
TRIAZOLAM
HALCION
C-IV PHARMACIA & UPJOHN
0.125 mg
0.25 mg
TRIMETHOPRIM AND SULFAMETHOXAZOLE
BACTRIM DS
RX ROCHE
160 mg / 800 mg
VALGANCICLOVIR HCL
VALCYTE
RX ROCHE
450 mg
VALDECOXIB
BEXTRA
RX PHARMACIA / PFIZER
10 mg
20 mg
WARFARIN SODIUM
COUMADIN
RX DUPONT PHARMA
2 mg
2.5 mg
5 mg
ZAFIRLUKAST
ACCOLATE
RX ASTRAZENECA
10 mg
20 mg
ZALEPLON
SONATA
C-IV WYETH-AYERST
5 mg
10 mg
ZOLMITRIPTAN
ZOMIG
RX ASTRAZENECA
2.5 mg
5 mg
ZOLPIDEM TARTRATE
AMBIEN
C-IV G.D.SEARLE
5 mg
10 mg

SIDE EFFECTS

Infusion-related (during infusion or within 2 hr post-infusion): Fever, chills, pruritus, urticaria, chest pain, hypo/hypertension, dyspnea. **Hypersensitivity:** Urticaria, dyspnea, hypotension. **Infections:** Pneumonia, cellulitis, infection at CNS venous catheter, sepsis, cholecystitis, endophthalmitis, furunculosis. **GI:** N&V, diarrhea, abdominal pain, constipation, dyspepsia, flatulence, intestinal obstruction, oral pain, ulcerative stomatitis, toothache. **CNS:** Dizziness, paresthesia, vertigo, anxiety, depression, insomnia. **CV:** Hypotension, hypertension, tachycardia. **Dermatologic:** Rash, pruritus, acne, alopecia, fungal dermatitis, eczema, erythema, erythematous/maculopapular rash, pruritus, papular rash, dry skin, increased sweating, urticaria, ecchymoses, flushing, hematoma. **GU:** Dysuria, micturition frequency, UTIs. **Musculoskeletal:** Myalgia, back pain, arthralgia, arthritis. **Respiratory:** URTI, pharyngitis, bronchitis, rhinitis, coughing, sinusitis, dyspnea, laryngitis, respiratory tract allergic reaction. **Miscellaneous:** Fatigue, fever, pain, moniliasis, chest pain, chills, peripheral edema, fall, hot flashes, malaise, anemia, abscess, flu syndrome, herpes simplex/zoster, conjunctivitis, malignancies, lymphoproliferative disorders, lupus-like syndrome.

NOTE: Possible formation of autoimmune antibodies (anti-dsDNA antibodies); development of lupus-like syndrome.

Retreatment after an extended treatment-free period may cause delayed, potentially serious side effects. Symptoms include fever, myalgia, polyarthralgia, pruritus, rash and, less frequently, facial or hand edema, dysphagia, urticaria, sore throat, and headache. Use of acetaminophen, antihistamines, corticosteroids, or epinephrine helps the symptoms.

DRUG INTERACTIONS

When used with clients also taking immunosuppressants, there were fewer infusion reactions compared with those taking no immunosuppressants.

HOW SUPPLIED

Powder for injection: 100 mg

DOSAGE

• **IV**

Moderate to severe Crohn's disease
5 mg/kg as a single IV dose.

Fistulizing Crohn's disease.
Initial: 5 mg/kg IV followed by additional doses of 5 mg/kg at 2 and 6 weeks after the initial infusion.

With methotrexate to treat rheumatoid arthritis.
Infliximab, 3 mg/kg at 2 and 6 weeks; then, q 8 weeks thereafter. If response is incomplete, may adjust the dose up to 10 mg/kg or treat as often as q 4 weeks.

NURSING CONSIDERATIONS

ADMINISTRATION/STORAGE

IV 1. Use vials immediately after reconstitution; no preservative.
2. Infliximab solution is incompatible with PVC equipment or devices. Prepare only in glass infusion bottles or polypropylene or polyolefin infusion bags. Infuse through polyethylene-lined infusion sets.
3. Calculate the total amount of reconstituted solution required. Reconstitute each vial with 10 mL sterile water for injection using a syringe equipped with a 21-gauge or smaller needle. Direct the stream of water to the glass wall of the vial. Gently swirl the solution by rotating the vial to dissolve the contents. Do not shake; some foaming is usual. Allow the reconstituted solution to stand for 5 min. The solution should be colorless to light yellow and opalescent; a few translucent particles (protein) may develop. Do not use if opaque particles, discoloration, or other foreign bodies are present.
4. Dilute reconstituted infliximab dose to a total of 250 mL with 0.9% NaCl injection. Slowly add the reconstituted solution to the 250 mL infusion bag or bottle. Mix gently.
5. Administer for 2 or more hours using an in-line, sterile, nonpyrogenic, low protein-binding filter (1.2 µm or less pore size).

6. Do not reuse or store any unused portion of the infusion solution.
7. Do not infuse concomitantly in the same IV line with other agents.
8. Store the lyophilized product at 2–8°C (36–46°F). Do not freeze.

ASSESSMENT

1. Note disease onset, surgeries, and previous treatments trialed.
2. Determine stool frequency and consistency. Assess abdomen and note pain levels, and with fistulas assess number, size, and amount and type of drainage.
3. List medical conditions that may preclude this therapy. In those with worsening CHF, stop infliximab.
4. Evaluate for latent tuberculosis as the drug quadruples the risk of TB.

CLIENT/FAMILY TEACHING

1. Drug is for short term therapy. Infusion-related symptoms, i.e. headache, fever, itching, nausea, and pain may be managed with antihistamines, acetaminophen, corticosteroids and/or epinephrine.
2. With prolonged symptoms and diffuse disease, surgical intervention may improve quality of life and prevent increased mortality.

OUTCOMES/EVALUATE

↓ Number of draining enterocutaneous fistulas

Insulin aspart

(**IN**-sue-lin **AS**-part)

PREGNANCY CATEGORY: C
CLASSIFICATION(S):
Insulin, rDNA origin
Rx: NovoLog

SEE ALSO *ANTIDIABETIC AGENTS: INSULINS.*

ACTION/KINETICS

Rapid-acting. Is homologous with regular human insulin except for a single substitution of the amino acid proline by aspartic acid in position B28. This reduces the tendency of the molecule to form hexamers as with regular human insulin. Has a faster absorption (40–50 min), faster onset, and shorter duration (3–5 hr) than regular human insulin after SC use. **t½:** 81 min (compared with 141 min for regular human insulin).

USES

Treat diabetes mellitus in adults. Due to the short duration of action, use with an intermediate or long-acting insulin.

SPECIAL CONCERNS

Use with caution during lactation.

SIDE EFFECTS

See *Antidiabetic Agents: Insulins.*

LABORATORY TEST CONSIDERATIONS

Small, but persistent ↑ in alkaline phosphatase.

DRUG INTERACTIONS

ACE inhibitors / ↑ Blood glucose lowering effect and susceptibility to hypoglycemia
Clonidine / Either potentiate or weaken blood-glucose lowering effect of insulin
Danazol / ↓ Blood glucose lowering effect
Disopyramide / ↑ Blood glucose lowering effect and susceptibility to hypoglycemia
Diuretics / ↓ Blood glucose lowering effect
Fluoxetine / ↑ Blood glucose lowering effect and susceptibility to hypoglycemia
Isoniazid / ↓ Blood glucose lowering effect
Lithium salts / Either potentiate or weaken blood-glucose lowering effect of insulin
MAO inhibitors / ↑ Blood glucose lowering effect and susceptibility to hypoglycemia
Niacin / ↓ Blood glucose lowering effect
Octreotide / ↑ Blood glucose lowering effect and susceptibility to hypoglycemia
Propoxyphene / ↑ Blood glucose lowering effect and susceptibility to hypoglycemia
Salicylates / ↑ Blood glucose lowering effect and susceptibility to hypoglycemia
Somatropin / ↓ Blood glucose lowering effect
Sulfonamides / ↑ Blood glucose lowering effect and susceptibility to hypoglycemia

ADDITIONAL DRUG INTERACTIONS

ACE inhibitors / ↑ Blood glucose lowering effect and susceptibility to hypoglycemia
Clonidine / Either potentiate or weaken blood glucose lowering effect of insulin
Danazol / ↓ Blood glucose lowering effect
Disopyramide / ↑ Blood glucose lowering effect and susceptibility to hypoglycemia
Diuretics / ↓ Blood glucose lowering effect
Fluoxetine / ↑ Blood glucose lowering effect and susceptibility to hypoglycemia
Isoniazid / ↓ Blood glucose lowering effect
Lithium salts / Either potentiate or weaken blood glucose lowering effect of insulin
Niacin / ↓ Blood glucose lowering effect
Octreotide / ↑ Blood glucose lowering effect and susceptibility to hypoglycemia
Propoxyphene / ↑ Blood glucose lowering effect and susceptibility to hypoglycemia
Somatropin / ↓ Blood glucose lowering effect
Sulfonamides / ↑ Blood glucose lowering effect and susceptibility to hypoglycemia

HOW SUPPLIED

Injection: 100 units/mL

DOSAGE

• **SC ONLY**

Diabetes mellitus.

Individualized. The total daily individual insulin dosage requirement is usually between 0.5–1 unit/kg/day. About 50–70% may be provided by insulin aspart and the rest by an intermediate- or long-acting insulin.

NURSING CONSIDERATIONS

SEE ALSO *NURSING CONSIDERATIONS FOR ANTIDIABETIC AGENTS: INSULINS.*

ADMINISTRATION/STORAGE

1. If used with NPH human insulin immediately before injection, there is some attenuation in the peak level of insulin aspart but the time to peak and the total bioavailability are not affected significantly.
2. If insulin aspart is mixed with NPH human insulin, draw insulin aspart into the syringe first. Make the injection immediately upon mixing.
3. Do not mix insulin aspart with crystalline zinc insulin products.
4. *Do not give IV.*
5. Never use if the product has become viscous or cloudy. Do not use after the expiration date.
6. Store between 2–8°C (36–46°F). Do not freeze and do not use if the product has been frozen. Vials may be kept at room temperature below 30°C (86°F) for up to 28 days but should never be exposed to excessive heat or sunlight.

ASSESSMENT

1. Note indications for therapy, onset of diabetes, other agents used and the outcome.
2. Monitor BS, electrolytes, HbA1c, U/A: microalbumin, liver and renal function.
3. Adjust dosage with impaired hepatic or renal function.

CLIENT/FAMILY TEACHING

1. This insulin is of rapid onset (1-3 hr) and short duration (3-5 hr) and should be used with an intermediate or long acting insulin to maintain glucose control.
2. Due to the fast onset of action, immediately follow the insulin aspart injection by a meal.
3. Monitor BS; adjust dosage with any change in physical activity or usual meal plan. Illness, emotional disturbances, and stress may alter insulin requirements.
4. Continue diet, exercise, and behaviors to enhance blood sugar control.
5. May initially experience local itching, swelling or redness; report if persistent. SOB, wheezing, diffuse rash, ↑ heart rate , and ↓ BP are S&S of shock.
6. Avoid pregnancy; if desired notify provider.

OUTCOMES/EVALUATE

Glycemic control; HbA1c < 7

Insulin glargine

(**IN**-sue-lin **GLAR**-jeen)

PREGNANCY CATEGORY: C
CLASSIFICATION(S):
Insulin, rDNA origin
Rx: Lantus

SEE ALSO *ANTIDIABETIC AGENTS: INSULINS*

ACTION/KINETICS

Long-acting recombinant human insulin analog. Differs from human insulin in that the amino acid asparagine at position A21 is replaced by glycine and two arginines are added to the C-terminus of the B-chain. Is designed to have low aqueous solubility at neutral pH while at pH 4, it is completely soluble. After injection into SC tissue, the acidic solution is neutralized, leading to formation of microprecipitates from which small amounts of insulin glargine are slowly released. This allows a relatively constant concentration/time profile over 24 hr with no pronounced peak. Duration is prolonged (up to 24 hr) when compared with NPH human insulin (about 14.5 hr). Metabolized in the liver. Dosage adjustment may be necessary in impaired renal or hepatic function.

USES

Once daily (at bedtime) treatment of adult and pediatric clients with type 1 diabetes mellitus or adults with type 2 diabetes mellitus who require long-acting insulin to control hyperglycemia.

CONTRAINDICATIONS

IV use.

SPECIAL CONCERNS

The long duration of insulin glargine may delay recovery from hypoglycemia. Use with caution during lactation. Not the drug of choice for diabetic ketoacidosis (use a short-acting insulin). Safety and efficacy have not been determined in children from 6–15 years of age with type 1 diabetes.

ADDITIONAL SIDE EFFECTS

Higher incidence of treatment-emergent injection site pain compared with NPH insulin-treated clients.

DRUG INTERACTIONS

ACE inhibitors / ↑ Blood glucose lowering effect and susceptibility to hypoglycemia
Clonidine / Either potentiate or weaken blood-glucose lowering effect of insulin
Danazol / ↓ Blood glucose lowering effect
Disopyramide / ↑ Blood glucose lowering effect and susceptibility to hypoglycemia
Diuretics / ↓ Blood glucose lowering effect
Fluoxetine / ↑ Blood glucose lowering effect and susceptibility to hypoglycemia
Isoniazid / ↓ Blood glucose lowering effect
Lithium salts / Either potentiate or weaken blood-glucose lowering effect of insulin
MAO inhibitors / ↑ Blood glucose lowering effect and susceptibility to hypoglycemia
Niacin / ↓ Blood glucose lowering effect
Octreotide / ↑ Blood glucose lowering effect and susceptibility to hypoglycemia
Propoxyphene / ↑ Blood glucose lowering effect and susceptibility to hypoglycemia
Salicylates / ↑ Blood glucose lowering effect and susceptibility to hypoglycemia
Somatropin / ↓ Blood glucose lowering effect
Sulfonamides / ↑ Blood glucose lowering effect and susceptibility to hypoglycemia

HOW SUPPLIED

Injection: 100 units/mL

DOSAGE

- **SC ONLY**

Diabetes mellitus.

Dose individualized. Give once daily at bedtime. **Initial:** Average of 10 units once daily; **then,** adjust according to client need to a total daily dose ranging from 2–100 units.

NURSING CONSIDERATIONS

SEE ALSO *NURSING CONSIDERATIONS FOR ANTIDIABETIC AGENTS: INSULINS.*

ADMINISTRATION/STORAGE

1. Do not dilute or mix with any other insulin or solution as the mixture may become cloudy and the properties of either insulin glargine or other insulins may be altered.
2. Use only if the solution is clear and colorless with no visible particles.
3. Syringes must not contain any other medicinal product or residue.
4. If changing from an intermediate- or long-acting insulin to insulin glargine, the amount and timing of the short-acting insulin or fast-acting insulin analog may need to be adjusted.
5. Store unopened product in a refrigerator at 2–8°C (36–46°F). Do not store in the freezer and do not allow product to freeze. If refrigeration is not possible, 10 mL vials/cartridges can be kept unrefrigerated for up to 28 days and 5 mL vials/cartridges can be kept unrefrigerated for up to 14 days, away from direct heat and light, as long as the temperature does not exceed 30°C (86°F).
6. Once the cartridge is placed in an OptiPen One, do not put in the refrigerator.

ASSESSMENT

1. Note disease onset, other agents trialed and the outcome.
2. Monitor BS, electrolytes, HbA1c, U/A: microalbumin, liver and renal function.
3. Adjust dosage with hepatic or renal dysfunction.

CLIENT/FAMILY TEACHING

1. Insulin glargine is given once daily at bedtime.
2. Do not dilute or mix with any other insulin solution.
3. Monitor FS and assess for hypo/hyperglycemia S&S.
4. Report any systemic rash, cough or dizziness.
5. Continue life style changes necessary to control blood sugar with diabetes.
6. Avoid pregnancy; consult provider if desired.
7. Store in refrigerator. If not available can keep unrefrigerated away from direct heat or light <86°F (30°C) and use within 28 days. Once placed in OptiPen One do not put in refrigerator.

OUTCOMES/EVALUATE

Glycemic control; HbA1c <7

Insulin injection (regular insulin)

(**IN**-sue-lin)

CLASSIFICATION(S):
Insulin product
Rx: Human: Humulin-R, Novolin R, Velosulin Human BR; **Pork:** Regular Iletin II.
✱**Rx: Human:** Novolinge Toronto
Pork: Iletin II Pork Regular
OTC: Human: Novolin R PenFill, Novolin R Prefilled

SEE ALSO *INSULINS.*

ACTION/KINETICS

Rarely administered as the sole agent due to its short duration of action. Injections of 100 units/mL are clear; cloudy, colored solutions should not be used. Regular insulin is the only preparation suitable for IV administration. Available only as 100 units/mL. **Onset, SC:** 30–60 min; **IV:** 10–30 min. **Peak, SC:** 2–4 hr; **IV:** 15–30 min. **Duration, SC:** 6–8 hr; **IV:** 30–60 min. *NOTE:* Regular beef/pork insulins are being phased out.

USES

Suitable for treatment of diabetic coma, diabetic acidosis, or other emergency situations. Especially suitable for the client suffering from labile diabetes. During acute phase of diabetic acidosis or for the client in diabetic crisis, client is monitored by serum glucose and serum ketone levels.

Velosulin BR is used in external insulin infusion pumps and with U-100 insulin syringes.

HOW SUPPLIED

Injection: 100 U/mL

DOSAGE

• **SC**

Diabetes.

Adults, individualized, usual, initial: 5–10 units; **pediatric:** 2–4 units. Injection is given 15–30 min before meals and at bedtime.

Diabetic ketoacidosis.

Adults: 0.1 unit/kg/hr given by continuous IV infusion.

NURSING CONSIDERATIONS

SEE ALSO *NURSING CONSIDERATIONS* FOR *INSULINS*.

ADMINISTRATION/STORAGE

IV 1. When used IV, reduce rate or stop insulin infusion when plasma glucose levels reach 250 mg/dL.
2. Due to the short half-life of regular insulin, avoid large single IV doses.

OUTCOMES/EVALUATE

Control of hyperglycemia

Insulin injection, concentrated

(**IN**-sue-lin)

PREGNANCY CATEGORY: C
CLASSIFICATION(S):
Insulin product
Rx: Regular (Concentrated) Iletin II U-500

SEE ALSO *INSULINS*.

ACTION/KINETICS
Concentrated insulin injection (500 U/mL). Depending on response, may be given SC or IM as a single or as two or three divided doses.

USES
Insulin resistance requiring more than 200 units insulin/day.

CONTRAINDICATIONS
Allergy to pork or mixed pork/beef insulin (unless client has been desensitized). IV use due to possible allergic or anaphylactoid reactions.

SPECIAL CONCERNS
Use with caution during lactation.

ADDITIONAL SIDE EFFECTS
Deep secondary hypoglycemia 18–24 hr after administration.

DRUG INTERACTIONS
Do not use together with PO hypoglycemic agents.

HOW SUPPLIED
Injection: 500 U/mL

DOSAGE

• **SC, IM**

Individualized, depending on severity of condition. Clients must be kept under close observation until dosage is established.

NURSING CONSIDERATIONS

SEE ALSO *NURSING CONSIDERATIONS* FOR *INSULINS*.

ADMINISTRATION/STORAGE

1. Administer only water/clear solutions (concentrated insulin may appear straw-colored).
2. Use small-caliber syringe for accuracy of measurement.
3. Deep secondary hypoglycemia may occur 18–24 hr after administration; monitor closely and have 10–20% dextrose solution available.
4. Keep insulin cool or refrigerated.

ASSESSMENT

1. Observe closely for S&S of hyper- or hypoglycemia until dosage established.
2. Monitor BS frequently and HbA1-C q 3 mo.

CLIENT/FAMILY TEACHING

1. Review technique for self-administration.
2. Be alert for signs of hypoglycemia, which may indicate that responsiveness to insulin has been regained and that a reduction in dosage is warranted.
3. Record FS especially 2 hr PP to assess response.

OUTCOMES/EVALUATE

BS and HbA1-C within desired range

Insulin lispro injection (rDNA origin)

(**IN**-sue-lin **LYE**-sproh)

PREGNANCY CATEGORY: B
CLASSIFICATION(S):
Insulin, $_R$DNA origin
Rx: Humalog

SEE ALSO *INSULINS*.

ACTION/KINETICS
Rapid-acting insulin derived from *Escherichia coli* that has been genetically

altered by the addition of the gene for insulin lispro. Is a human insulin analog created when the amino acids at positions 28 and 29 on the insulin B-chain are reversed. Absorbed faster than regular human insulin. Compared to regular insulin, has a more rapid onset of glucose-lowering activity, an earlier peak for glucose lowering, and a shorter duration of glucose-lowering activity. However, is equipotent to human regular insulin (i.e., one unit of insulin lispro has the same glucose-lowering capacity as one unit of regular insulin). May lower the risk of nocturnal hypoglycemia in clients with type I diabetes. **Onset:** 15 min. **Peak effect:** 30–90 min. **t½:** 1 hr. **Duration:** 5 hr or less.

USES

Type 1 diabetes mellitus. In combination with sulfonylureas to treat high blood sugar in children over 3 years of age and adults over 65 years of age. In combination with sulfonylureas in type 2 diabetes.

CONTRAINDICATIONS

Use during episodes of hypoglycemia. Hypersensitivity to insulin lispro.

SPECIAL CONCERNS

Since insulin lispro has a more rapid onset and shorter duration of action than regular insulin, clients with type I diabetes also require a longer acting insulin to maintain glucose control. Requirements may be decreased in impaired renal or hepatic function. Use with caution during lactation. Safety and efficacy have not been determined in children less than 12 years of age.

SIDE EFFECTS

See *Insulins.*

DRUG INTERACTIONS

See *Insulins.*

HOW SUPPLIED

Injection: 100 U/mL

DOSAGE

• **SC**

Diabetes.

Individualized, depending on severity of the condition.

NURSING CONSIDERATIONS

SEE ALSO *NURSING CONSIDERATIONS* FOR *INSULINS*.

ADMINISTRATION/STORAGE

1. When used as a mealtime insulin, give within 15 min before a meal or 15 min of finishing a meal, as compared with human regular insulin, which is best given 30–60 min before a meal.
2. May be mixed with Humulin N, Humulin L, or Humulin U. A decrease in the rate of absorption (but not the total bioavailability) was seen when Humalog was mixed with Humulin N.
3. When Humalog is mixed with either Humulin U or Humulin N, give mixture within 15 min before a meal and immediately after mixing.
4. If Humalog is mixed with a longer acting insulin, Humalog should be drawn into the syringe first to prevent clouding of the Humalog by the longer-acting insulin.
5. Do not give mixtures IV.
6. Store in the refrigerator at 2–8°C (36–46°F). Do not freeze. If refrigeration not possible, can store unrefrigerated for up to 28 days, provided it is kept as cool as possible and away from direct heat and light.

ASSESSMENT

1. Document indications for therapy, disease onset, previous agents trialed, and the outcome.
2. Monitor CBC, HbA1-C, U/A: microalbumin, and liver and renal function studies.

CLIENT/FAMILY TEACHING

1. Review method for preparation, storage, and administration; rotate sites.
2. Drug has a more rapid onset of action and a shorter duration of action than regular insulin.
3. Take within 15 min of meals and immediately after mixing, with combined therapy.
4. Monitor/record FS, especially 2 hr PP until response evident. Review S&S of hypoglycemia and appropriate management.

5. Clients with type I diabetes also require a longer-acting insulin preparation for adequate glucose control.
6. Report as scheduled for follow-up labs, reinforcement of teaching, and evaluation of response to medication.

OUTCOMES/EVALUATE

BS/HbA1-C within desired range

Insulin zinc suspension (Lente)

(**IN**-sue-lin)

CLASSIFICATION(S):
Insulin product
OTC: Human: Humulin L, Novolin L
Pork: Lente Iletin II.
✱**OTC: Human:** Novolinge NPH
Pork: Iletin II Pork NPH

SEE ALSO *INSULINS.*

ACTION/KINETICS

Contains 70% crystalline and 30% amorphous insulin suspension. Considered intermediate-acting. Principal advantage is the absence of a sensitizing agent such as protamine. **Onset:** 1–2.5 hr. **Peak:** 7–15 hr. **Duration:** About 22 hr. *NOTE:* Lente beef/pork insulins are being phased out.

USES

Allergy to other types of insulin and in clients disposed to thrombotic phenomena in which protamine may be a factor. Not a replacement for regular insulin and is not suitable for emergency use.

HOW SUPPLIED

Injection: 100 U/mL

DOSAGE

• **SC**

Diabetes.

Adults, initial: 7–26 units 30–60 min before breakfast. Dosage is then increased by daily or weekly increments of 2–10 units until satisfactory readjustment is established. A second smaller dose may be given prior to the evening meal or at bedtime. Clients on NPH can be transferred to insulin zinc suspension on a unit-for-unit basis. Clients being transferred from regular insulin should begin zinc insulin at two-thirds to three-fourths the regular insulin dosage. If the client is being transferred from protamine zinc insulin, the dose of zinc insulin should be about 50% of that required for protamine zinc insulin.

NURSING CONSIDERATIONS

SEE *NURSING CONSIDERATIONS* FOR *INSULINS.*

OUTCOMES/EVALUATE

Normalization of BS; HbA1-C < 7

Insulin zinc suspension, extended (Ultralente)

(**IN**-sue-lin)

CLASSIFICATION(S):
Insulin product
OTC: Humulin U Ultralente
✱**OTC:** Humulin-U, Novolin ge Ultralente

SEE ALSO *INSULINS.*

ACTION/KINETICS

Large crystals of insulin and a high content of zinc are responsible for the slow-acting properties of this preparation. **Onset:** 4–8 hr. **Peak:** 10–30 hr. **Duration:** 36 hr or longer.

USES

Mild to moderate hyperglycemia in stabilized diabetics.

CONTRAINDICATIONS

Use to treat diabetic coma or emergency situations

HOW SUPPLIED

Injection: 100 U/mL

DOSAGE

• **SC**

Individualized.

Usual, initial: 7–26 units as a single dose 30–60 min before breakfast. **Do not administer IV.**

NURSING CONSIDERATIONS

SEE *NURSING CONSIDERATIONS* FOR *INSULINS.*

OUTCOMES/EVALUATE

Normalization of BS; HbA1C < 7

Interferon alfa-2a recombinant (rl FN-A; IFLrA)

(in-ter-**FEER**-on **AL**-fah)

PREGNANCY CATEGORY: C
CLASSIFICATION(S):
Antineoplastic, miscellaneous
Rx: Roferon-A

ACTION/KINETICS
Interferon alfa-2a is the product of recombinant DNA technology using strains of genetically engineered *Escherichia coli.* Activity is expressed as International Units, which are determined by comparing the antiviral activity of recombinant interferons with the activity of the international reference standard of human leukocyte interferon. Interferons bind to specific receptors on the cell surface, resulting in inhibition of virus replication in virus-infected cells, suppression of cell proliferation, increase in the phagocytic activity of macrophages, and enhancement of the toxic effects of leukocytes for target cells. **Peak serum levels:** 3.8–7.3 hr. **t½:** 3.7–8.5 hr. Metabolized by the kidney.

USES
(1) Hairy cell leukemia in clients older than 18 years of age. Can be used in splenectomized and nonsplenectomized clients. (2) AIDS-related Kaposi's sarcoma in clients older than 18 years of age. (3) Chronic myelogenous leukemia. (4) Chronic hepatitis C. *Investigational:* The drug has been used for a large number of other conditions. Significant activity has been noted against the following neoplastic diseases: locally for superficial bladder tumors, carcinoid tumor, cutaneous T-cell lymphoma, essential thrombocythemia, low-grade non-Hodgkin's lymphoma. Limited activity has been noted in acute leukemias, cervical carcinoma, chronic lymphocytic leukemia, Hodgkin's disease, malignant gliomas, melanoma, multiple myeloma, mycosis fungoides/Sézary syndrome, nasopharyngeal carcinoma, osteosarcoma, ovarian carcinoma, renal carcinoma. Interferon alfa-2a also has significant activity against the following viral infections: chronic non-A, non-B hepatitis, *Condylomata acuminata,* cutaneous warts, cytomegaloviruses, herpes keratoconjunctivitis; limited activity is seen against herpes simplex, papillomaviruses, rhinoviruses, vaccinia virus, varicella zoster, and viral hepatitis B.

CONTRAINDICATIONS
Lactation.

SPECIAL CONCERNS
Use with caution in clients with a history of unstable angina, uncontrolled CHF, COPD, diabetes mellitus prone to ketoacidosis, thrombophlebitis, pulmonary embolism, seizure disorders, severe renal and hepatic disease, compromised CNS function, and severe myelosuppression. Safety and efficacy in individuals less than 18 years of age have not been established.

SIDE EFFECTS
Flu-like symptoms: Fever, headache, fatigue, arthralgia, myalgias, chills, weight loss, dizziness. **CV:** Hypo/hypertension, ***arrhythmias,*** syncope, edema, palpitations, TIAs, pulmonary edema, CHF, cardiac murmur, ***MI, stroke, cardiomyopathy,*** hot flashes, Raynaud's phenomenon, thrombophlebitis. **Respiratory:** Coughing, dyspnea, dryness or inflammation of oropharynx, chest pain or congestion, ***bronchospasm,*** pneumonia, tachypnea, rhinitis, rhinorrhea, sinusitis. **CNS:** Depression, confusion, dizziness, headache, paresthesia, anxiety, ataxia, aphasia, aphonia, dysarthria, amnesia, weakness, nervousness, emotional lability, impotence, numbness, lethargy, sleep disturbances, visual disturbances, vertigo, decreased mental status, memory loss, disturbances of libido, involuntary movements, ***suicidal ideation, seizures,*** forgetfulness, neuropathy, tremor. **GI:** Anorexia, N&V, diarrhea, emesis, abdominal pain, hypermotility, abdominal fullness/pain, flatulence, constipation, gastric distress. **Hematologic:** Throm-

bocytopenia, neutropenia, leukopenia, decreased hemoglobin, ***severe anemia, severe cytopenias***, coagulopathy, Coombs' positive hemolytic anemia, ***aplastic anemia.*** **Musculoskeletal:** Joint/bone pain, arthritis, polyarthritis, poor coordination, muscle contractions, gait disturbances. **Dermatologic:** Rash, pruritus, dry skin, ecchymosis, petechiae, skin flushing, alopecia, urticaria, diaphoresis, cyanosis, bruising. **Miscellaneous:** Generalized pain, back pain, inflammation at injection site, epistaxis, bleeding gums, weight loss, alteration of taste, altered hearing, edema, night sweats, earache, eye irritation, hypothyroidism, hypertriglyceridemia.

LABORATORY TEST CONSIDERATIONS

↑ AST, ALT, LDH, BUN, serum creatinine, alkaline phosphatase, bilirubin, uric acid, serum glucose, serum phosphorus. ↓ H&H. Hypocalcemia, proteinuria.

DRUG INTERACTIONS

Interleukin-2 / ↑ Risk of renal failure
Theophylline / ↓ Theophylline clearance

HOW SUPPLIED

Injection Solution: 3 million IU/mL, 6 million IU/0.5 mL, 6 million IU/mL, 9 million IU/0.5 mL, 9 million IU/0.9 mL, 36 million IU/mL; *Powder for Injection:* 6 million IU/mL

DOSAGE

• **IM, SC**

Hairy cell leukemia.

Induction: 3 million IU/day for 16–24 weeks; **maintenance,** 3 million IU 3 times/week. Doses higher than 3 million IU are not recommended.

AIDS-related Kaposi's sarcoma.

Induction: 36 million IU/day for 10–12 weeks; or, 3 million IU/day on days 1–3; 9 million IU/day on days 4–6; and 18 million IU/day on days 7–9 followed by 36 million IU/day for the remainder of the 10 to 12-week induction period. **Maintenance:** 36 million IU 3 times/week. If severe side effects occur, the dose can be withheld or reduced by one-half.

Chronic myelogenous leukemia.

Induction: 9 million IU/day. The dose can be graded during the first week of therapy to improve short-term tolerance by giving 3 million IU/day for 3 days to 6 million IU/day for 3 days and then to the target dose of 9 million IU/day. **Maintenance:** Optimal dose and duration of therapy have not been determined. Continue the regimen until the disease progresses.

Chronic hepatitis C.

3 million IU, SC or IM, 3 times/week for 12 months.

NURSING CONSIDERATIONS

ADMINISTRATION/STORAGE

1. Discontinue treatment if leukemia does not respond within 6 mo.
2. If severe reactions occur, reduce dose of drug by one-half or withhold individual doses. Assess effect on bone marrow of previous radiation or chemotherapy.
3. Although optimal treatment duration has not been established, clients have been treated for up to 20 consecutive months. Nadir: leukocytes, 20–40 days; platelets, 15–20 days.
4. Consider SC route with a platelet count less than 50,000/mm^3.
5. Although not approved by the FDA, interferon alfa-2a has been given by continuous or intermittent IV infusion as well as ophthalmically and intravaginally.
6. The reconstituted solution is stable for 30 days when stored at 2–8°C (36–46°F) and for 24 hr when stored at room temperature. The undiluted drug is not stable in syringes due to adhesion to syringe surfaces.

CLIENT/FAMILY TEACHING

1. Review appropriate method for administration, care and safe storage of drug and equipment.
2. Most common side effects are flu-like symptoms, such as fever, fatigue, headache, chills, nausea, and loss of appetite; may be minimized by taking at bedtime.
3. Flu-like symptoms usually diminish in severity as treatment continues. Acetaminophen/ibuprofen may be used for fever and headache.
4. Drink 2–3 L/day of fluids
5. Hypotension may occur up to 2 days following drug therapy; sit before standing and rise slowly.

6. Do not change brands of interferon without approval; changes in dosage may occur with different brands.
7. Report for CBC, electrolytes, and LFTs as scheduled.
8. Report any evidence of neurologic or psychologic disturbances.
9. Hair loss may occur.
10. Practice safe sex and birth control.
11. Avoid alcohol and any other unprescribed CNS depressants.

OUTCOMES/EVALUATE

- ↓ Tumor size and spread
- Inhibition of viral replication
- ↓ Lesions with Kaposi's sarcoma

Interferon alfa-2b recombinant (rl FN-α2; α-2-interferon)

(in-ter-**FEER**-on **AL**-fah)

PREGNANCY CATEGORY: C
CLASSIFICATION(S):
Antineoplastic, miscellaneous
Rx: Intron A

ACTION/KINETICS

A product of recombinant DNA technology using strains of genetically engineered *Escherichia coli.* The activity is expressed as International Units, which are determined by comparing the antiviral activity of the recombinant interferon with the activity of the international reference standard of human leukocyte interferon. Interferons bind to specific receptors on the cell surface, resulting in inhibition of virus replication in virus-infected cells, suppression of cell proliferation, increase in the phagocytic activity of macrophages, and enhancement of the toxic effects of leukocytes for target cells. **Peak serum levels after IM, SC:** 18–116 IU/mL after 3–12 hr. **t½, IM, SC:** 2–3 hr. **Peak serum levels after IV infusion:** 135–270 IU/mL at the end of the infusion. **t½, IV:** 2 hr. The main site of metabolism may be the kidney.

USES

(1) Hairy cell leukemia in clients older than 18 years of age (in both splenectomized and nonsplenectomized clients). (2) Intralesional use for genital or venereal warts (*Condylomata acuminata.*) (3) AIDS-related Kaposi's sarcoma in clients over 18 years of age. (4) Chronic hepatitis C in clients at least 18 years of age with compensated liver disease and a history of blood or blood product exposure or who are HCV antibody positive. (5) Chronic hepatitis B in clients over 18 years of age with compensated liver disease and HBV replication (clients must be serum HBsAg positive for at least 6 months and have HBV replication with elevated serum ALT). Chronic hepatitis B in pediatric clients 1 year of age and older. (6) Adjunct therapy for malignant melanoma in those who are 18 years of age or older who are free of the disease but at a high risk for recurrence within 56 days of surgery. (7) With an anthracycline drug for the initial treatment of clinically aggressive non-Hodgkin's lymphoma.

Investigational: The drug has been used for a large number of conditions. Significant activity has been noted against the following neoplastic diseases: locally for superficial bladder tumors, carcinoid tumor, chronic myelogenous leukemia, cutaneous T-cell lymphoma, essential thrombocythemia, low-grade non-Hodgkin's lymphoma, and chronic granulocytic leukemia. Limited activity has been noted in acute leukemias, cervical carcinoma, chronic lymphocytic leukemia, Hodgkin's disease, malignant gliomas, melanoma, multiple myeloma, nasopharyngeal carcinoma, osteosarcoma, ovarian carcinoma, renal carcinoma, and chronic granulomatous disease. Interferon alfa-2b has also been used to treat the following viral infections: Significant activity has been seen against cutaneous warts, CMVs, herpes keratoconjunctivitis, and herpes simplex. Limited activity has been noted against papillomaviruses, rhinoviruses, vaccinia virus, varicella zos-

I

ter, and HIV (used with foscarnet/zidovudine). It has also been used to treat multiple sclerosis.

CONTRAINDICATIONS

Lactation. Use to treat rapidly progressive visceral disease in AIDS-related Kaposi's sarcoma. Use in clients with decompensated liver disease, autoimmune hepatitis, history of autoimmune disease, or immunosuppressed transplant clients.

SPECIAL CONCERNS

Use with caution in clients with a history of unstable angina, uncontrolled CHF, COPD, diabetes mellitus prone to ketoacidosis, thrombophlebitis, pulmonary embolism, seizure disorders, severe renal and hepatic disease, compromised CNS function, and severe myelosuppression. Safety and efficacy in individuals less than 18 years of age have not been established.

SIDE EFFECTS

Flu-like symptoms: Fever, headache, fatigue, myalgia, chills. **CV:** Hypo/hypertension, ***arrhythmias,*** tachycardia, syncope, coagulation disorders, chest pain, palpitations, flushing, atrial fibrillation, bradycardia, ***cardiac failure, cardiomyopathy,*** extrasystoles, postural hypotension. **CNS:** Depression, confusion, somnolence, migraine, dizziness, ataxia, insomnia, irritability, paresthesia, anxiety, nervousness, emotional lability, amnesia, impaired concentration, weakness, tremor, syncope, abnormal coordination, hypesthesia, abnormal coordination, aggravated depression, aggressive reaction, hypertonia, impaired consciousness, neuropathy, agitation, apathy, aphasia, dysphonia, extrapyramidal disorder, hot flashes, hyper/hypoesthesia, hypo/hyperkinesia, neurosis, paresis, paroniria, parosmia, personality disorder, ***seizures, coma,*** polyneuropathy, ***suicide attempt.*** **GI:** N&V, diarrhea, stomatitis, weight loss, anorexia, flatulence, thirst, dehydration, constipation, eructation, loose stools, abdominal distention/pain, dysphagia, esophagitis, gastric ulcer, ***GI hemorrhage,*** GI mucosal discoloration, gum hyperplasia, gingival bleeding, gingivitis, increased saliva, increased appetite, melena, oral leukoplakia, rectal bleeding after stool, ***rectal hemorrhage,*** ulcerative stomatitis, ascites, gallstones, gastroenteritis, halitosis. **Hematologic:** Thrombocytopenia, granulocytopenia, anemia, ***hemolytic anemia,*** leukopenia. **Musculoskeletal:** Arthralgia, leg cramps, asthenia, arthrosis, arthritis, muscle pain or weakness, back pain, bone pain, rigors, CTS. **Respiratory:** Pharyngitis, coughing, dyspnea, sinusitis, rhinitis, epistaxis, nasal congestion, dry mouth, ***bronchospasm,*** pleural pain, pneumonia, rhinorrhea, sneezing, wheezing, bronchitis, cyanosis, lung fibrosis. **EENT:** Alteration or loss of taste, tinnitus, hearing disorders, conjunctivitis, photophobia, vision disorders, eye pain, diplopia, dry eyes, earache, lacrimal gland disorder, periorbital edema, vertigo, speech disorder. **Dermatologic:** Rash, pruritus, alopecia, urticaria, dry skin, dermatitis, purpura, photosensitivity, acne, nail disorder, facial edema, moniliasis, reaction at injection site, abnormal hair texture, cold/clammy skin, cyanosis of the hand, epidermal necrolysis, dermatitis lichenoides, furunculosis, increased hair growth, erythema, melanosis, nonherpetic cold sores, peripheral ischemia, skin depigmentation or discoloration, vitiligo, folliculitis, lipoma, psoriasis. **GU:** Amenorrhea, hematuria, impotence, leukorrhea, menorrhagia, urinary frequency, nocturia, polyuria, uterine bleeding, increased BUN, incontinence, pelvic pain. **Endocrine:** Gynecomastia, thyroid disorder, aggravation of diabetes mellitus, virilism. **Hepatic:** Jaundice, upper right quadrant pain, ***hepatic encephalopathy, hepatic failure.*** **Other:** Pain, increased sweating, malaise, decreased libido, herpes simplex, lymphadenopathy, chest pain, abscess, cachexia, hypercalcemia, peripheral edema, stye, substernal chest pain, weakness, sepsis, dehydration, fungal infection, herpes zoster, viral infection, trichomoniasis.

LABORATORY TEST CONSIDERATIONS

↑ AST, ALT, LDH, BUN, serum creatinine, alkaline phosphatase. ↓ H&H. Abnormal hepatic function tests, bilirubinemia.

DRUG INTERACTIONS

Aminophylline / ↓ Aminophylline clearance R/T ↓ liver breakdown
Zidovudine/ ↑ Risk of neutropenia

HOW SUPPLIED

Powder for injection: 3 million IU/vial, 5 million IU/vial, 10 million IU/vial, 18 million IU, 25 million IU; *Solution for Injection:* 3 million IU/vial, 5 million IU/vial, 10 million IU/vial, 18 million IU/vial, 25 million IU/vial, 50 million IU/vial

DOSAGE

- **IM, SC**

Hairy cell leukemia.

2 million IU/m² 3 times/week. Higher doses are not recommended. May require 6 or more months of therapy for improvement. Do not use the 50 million-IU strength of the powder for injection for treating hairy cell leukemia.

AIDS-related Kaposi's sarcoma

30 million IU/m² 3 times/week SC or IM using only the 50 million-IU vial. Using this dose, clients should tolerate an average dose of 110 million IU/week at the end of 12 weeks of therapy and 75 million IU/week at the end of 24 weeks of therapy.

Chronic hepatitis C.

3 million IU 3 times/week for 16 weeks. At 16 weeks, extend treatment to 18 to 24 months at 3 million IU 3 times/week to improve the sustained response of normalization of ALT. Discontinue therapy if there is no response after 16 weeks.

Chronic hepatitis B.

30–35 million IU/week SC or IM, given as either 5 million IU/day or 10 million IU 3 times/week for 16 weeks. If serious side effects occur, the dose may be decreased by 50%.

- **IV**

Malignant melanoma.

20 million IU/m² IV on 5 consecutive days/week for 4 weeks. **Maintenance:** 10 million IU/m² SC 3 times/week for 48 weeks.

- **INTRALESIONAL**

Condylomata acuminata (genital or venereal warts).

1 million IU/lesion 3 times/week for 3 weeks. For this purpose, use only the vial containing 10 million units and reconstitute using no more than 1 mL diluent. To reduce side effects, give in the evening with acetaminophen. Maximum response usually occurs within 4–8 weeks. If results are unsatisfactory after 12–16 weeks, a second course may be started.

NURSING CONSIDERATIONS

SEE ALSO *NURSING CONSIDERATIONS* FOR *INTERFERON ALFA-2A RECOMBINANT* AND *INTERFERON ALFA-N3.*

ADMINISTRATION/STORAGE

1. Prior to administration, reconstitute drug with bacteriostatic water for injection, which is provided. Consult enclosed chart to prepare powder for injection based on use. Client may self-administer dose at bedime.
2. If severe side effects occur, dose may be reduced as much as 50% or therapy can be discontinued until side effects subside. For example, if the granulocyte count is less than 750/mm³ and the platelet count is less than 50,000/mm³, reduce the dose by 50%; if the granulocyte count is less than 500/mm³ and the platelet count is less than 30,000/mm³, interrupt drug therapy until counts return to normal or baseline levels. Nadir: 3–5 days.
3. Discontinue treatment for leukemia if no response within 6 mo.
4. When used for venereal or genital warts, maximum response usually occurs 4–8 weeks after therapy is initiated. If results not satisfactory after 12–16 weeks, a second course of therapy may be undertaken.
5. Although the optimal duration of treatment has not been established, clients have been treated for up to 20 consecutive months.
6. If the platelet count is less than 50,000/mm³, give SC rather than IM.
7. Use a Tuberculin type syringe with a 25- to 30-gauge needle for intralesion administration. Do not give beneath the lesion too deeply or inject too superficially. As many as five lesions can be treated at one time.
8. Store powder from 2–8°C (36–46°F). The reconstituted solution is stable for 30 days when stored from 2°–8°C (36°–46°F). The solution for injection is stable at 35°C (95°F) for up to 7 days and at 30°C (86°F) for up to 14

days. The undiluted drug is not stable in syringes due to adhesion to syringe surfaces.

IV 9. Although not approved by the FDA, interferon alfa-2a has been given by continuous or intermittent IV infusion as well as ophthalmically and intravaginally.

10. For infusion solutions, after reconstitution, withdraw the appropriate dose and inject into a 100-mL bag of 0.9% NaCl injection. The final concentration should be 10 million IU/10 mL or more. Infuse over a 20-min period. Prepare solution immediately prior to use.

CLIENT/FAMILY TEACHING

1. Flu-like symptoms may be minimized by administering the drug at bedtime. Use acetaminophen/ibuprofen for fever and headache.
2. Consume 2–3 L/day of fluids.
3. May cause dizziness/confusion, avoid hazardous tasks until drug effects realized.
4. Fatigue may be experienced. Report if depression, hallucinations, or suicide ideations occur.
5. Report for labs and bone marrow hairy cell determinations as ordered.

OUTCOMES/EVALUATE

- Improved hematologic response
- ↓ Size/number of genital/venereal warts
- ↓ Viral load

Interferon alfacon-1

(in-ter-**FEER**-on **AL**-fah-kon)

PREGNANCY CATEGORY: C
CLASSIFICATION(S):
Immunomodulator
Rx: Infergen

SEE ALSO *INTERFERON ALFA-2A* AND *INTERFERON ALFA-2B*.

ACTION/KINETICS

Prepared by recombinant technology. Has antiviral, antiproliferative, and immunomodulatory effects. Plasma levels are too small to measure.

USES

Treatment of chronic hepatitis C infections in those over 18 years of age with compensated liver disease. *Investigational:* With G-CSF therapy to treat hairy-cell leukemia.

CONTRAINDICATIONS

Hypersensitivity to alpha interferons or to products derived from *E. coli*. Use in autoimmune hepatitis or in decompensated hepatic disease.

SPECIAL CONCERNS

Use with caution during lactation and in preexisting cardiac disease, in depression, in those with abnormally low peripheral blood cell counts, in those receiving myelosuppressive agents, and in autoimmune disorder. Safety and efficacy have not been determined in children less than 18 years of age.

SIDE EFFECTS

Flu-like symptoms: Headache, fatigue, fever, myalgia, rigors, arthralgia, increased sweating. **Body as a whole:** Body pain, hot flushes, non-cardiac chest pain, malaise, asthenia, peripheral edema, access pain, allergic reactions, weight loss. **Hypersensitivity:** Urticaria, angioedema, bronchoconstriction, ***anaphylaxis.*** **CNS:** Insomnia, dizziness, paresthesia, amnesia, hypoesthesia, hypertonia, nervousness, depression, anxiety, emotional lability, abnormal thinking, agitation, decreased libido. **GI:** Abdominal pain, N&V, diarrhea, anorexia, dyspepsia, constipation, flatulence, toothache, hemorrhoids, decreased saliva, tender liver. **CV:** Hypertension, palpitation. **Hematologic:** Granulocytopenia, thrombocytopenia, leukopenia, ecchymosis, lymphadenopathy, lymphocytosis. **Respiratory:** Pharyngitis, URI, cough, sinusitis, rhinitis, respiratory tract congestion, upper respiratory tract congestion, epistaxis, dyspnea, bronchitis. **Dermatologic:** Alopecia, pruritus, rash, erythema, dry skin. **Musculoskeletal:** Back, limb, neck, or skeletal pain. **GU:** Dysmenorrhea, vaginitis, menstrual disorder. **Ophthalmic:** Conjunctivitis, eye pain. **Otic:** Tinnitus, earache. **At injection site:** Erythema, pain, ecchymosis.

LABORATORY TEST CONSIDERATIONS

↑ TSH, triglycerides. ↓ H&H. Abnormal thyroid tests.

HOW SUPPLIED

Injection: 9 mcg, 15 mcg; *Prefilled syringes:* 9 mcg, 15 mcg

DOSAGE

- **SC INJECTION**

Chronic hepatitis C infection.

Adults over 18 years of age: 9 mcg SC as a single injection three times a week for 24 weeks. At least 48 hr should elapse between doses. Those who tolerate therapy but did not respond or relapsed following discontinuation may be subsequently treated with 15 mcg three times a week for 6 months.

NURSING CONSIDERATIONS

SEE ALSO *NURSING CONSIDERATIONS* FOR *INTERFERON ALFA-2A* AND *INTERFERON ALFA-2B*.

ADMINISTRATION/STORAGE

1. Do not give 15 mcg three times a week if not received or not tolerated at initial course of therapy.
2. Reduce dose to 7.5 mcg following an intolerable adverse reaction. If adverse effects continue at reduced dosage, discontinue therapy or reduce dose further.
3. Store refrigerated but do not freeze. Avoid vigorous shaking.

ASSESSMENT

1. Determine indications for therapy, onset, other therapies trialed, and disease characteristics.
2. Note any cardiac disease, hypertension, or severe psychiatric disorders as these preclude drug therapy.
3. Monitor CBC, TSH, HCV RNA, liver and renal function studies.

CLIENT/FAMILY TEACHING

1. Review dose and method of administration (SC); usually administered 3 times per week with 48 hr between doses.
2. May experience flu-like symptoms, including headache, fatigue, fever, muscle/joint pain, rigors, and increased sweating.
3. Stop drug and report any S&S of depression, suicide thoughts/attempt.
4. Report as scheduled for F/U labs, evaluations. Do not change brands of interferon without provider approval.

OUTCOMES/EVALUATE

Improvement in LFTs; ↓ viral load

Interferon alfa-n3

(in-ter-**FEER**-on **AL**-fah)

PREGNANCY CATEGORY: C
CLASSIFICATION(S):
Antineoplastic
Rx: Alferon N

ACTION/KINETICS

Made from pooled human leukocytes induced by incomplete infection with Sendai (avian) virus. Is a sterile, aqueous formulation of purified, natural, human interferon alpha proteins. Binds to receptors on cell surfaces leading to a sequence of events including inhibition of virus replication and suppression of cell proliferation. Also, causes immunomodulation characterized by enhanced phagocytosis by macrophages, augmentation of the cytotoxicity of lymphocytes, and enhancement of human leukocyte antigen expression. Intralesional use of interferon alfa-n3 does not result in detectable plasma levels of the drug.

USES

Intralesional treatment of refractory or recurring external condylomata acuminata (genital or venereal warts) in clients 18 years of age or older. *Investigational:* Alpha interferons are being tested for use in a large number of neoplastic diseases and viral infections.

CONTRAINDICATIONS

Hypersensitivity to human interferon alpha; clients who are allergic to mouse immunoglobulin (IgG), egg protein, or neomycin (the production process involves a nutrient medium containing neomycin although it has not been detected in the final product). Lactation. Use in clients less than 18 years of age.

SPECIAL CONCERNS

Due to fever and flu-like symptoms with use of interferon alfa-n3, use with caution in clients with debilitating diseases, including unstable angina, uncontrolled CHF, COPD, diabetes mellitus with ketoacidosis, thrombophlebitis, pulmonary embolism, hemophilia, severe myelosuppression, or seizure disorders. Use with caution in fertile men. Since the drug is made from human blood, it may carry a risk of transmitting infections. Safety and effectiveness have not been determined in children less than 18 years of age.

SIDE EFFECTS

Flu-like symptoms: Commonly, fever, headache, myalgias which decrease with repeated doses. Also, chills, fatigue, malaise. **Hypersensitivity reaction:** Urticaria, angioedema, bronchoconstriction, ***anaphylaxis.*** **CNS:** Dizziness, headache, lightheadedness, insomnia, depression, nervousness, decreased ability to concentrate. **GI:** N&V, heartburn, dyspepsia, heartburn, diarrhea, tongue hyperesthesia, thirst, altered taste, increased salivation. **Musculoskeletal/Skin:** Arthralgia, myalgia, back pain, hot sensation at bottom of feet, tingling of legs/feet, muscle cramps. **Respiratory:** Nose or sinus drainage, nose bleed, throat tightness, pharyngitis. **Miscellaneous:** Pruritus, swollen lymph nodes, heat intolerance, visual disturbances, sensitivity to allergens, papular rash on neck, hot flashes, herpes labialis, dysuria, photosensitivity, sweating, vasovagal reaction.

NOTE: When used for treatment of cancer, the incidence of many of the preceding side effects was increased. Additional side effects were noted including: **GI:** Constipation, anorexia, stomatitis, dry mouth, mucositis, sore mouth. **Miscellaneous:** Insomnia, blurred vision, ocular rotation pain, sore injection site, chest pains, low BP.

LABORATORY TEST CONSIDERATIONS

↓ WBC. The following may be affected in cancer clients: Hemoglobin levels, WBC and platelet count, GGT, AST, alkaline phosphatase, and total bilirubin.

HOW SUPPLIED

Injection: 5 million IU/mL

DOSAGE

- **INTRALESIONAL INJECTION**

Condylomata acuminata.

0.05 mL (250,000 IU)/wart twice a week for up to 8 weeks. The maximum recommended dose per treatment session is 0.5 mL (2.5 million IU). The safety and effectiveness of a second course of treatment have not been determined.

NURSING CONSIDERATIONS

SEE ALSO *NURSING CONSIDERATIONS* FOR *INTERFERON ALFA-2A* AND *INTERFERON ALFA-2B RECOMBINANT.*

ADMINISTRATION/STORAGE

1. Inject drug into the base of the wart using a 30-gauge needle.
2. For large warts, inject at several points around the wart periphery using a total of 0.05 mL/wart.
3. Do not give further drug or conventional therapy for 3 months after the initial 8-week course of treatment unless the warts enlarge or new warts appear.
4. Store drug at 2–8°C (36–46°F). Do not freeze or shake.

ASSESSMENT

1. Note any allergic reactions to egg protein or neomycin; may have increased sensitivity to drug.
2. Determine any preexisting debilitating diseases; note functional level.
3. For condylomata therapy, measure and document size and number of lesions.

CLIENT/FAMILY TEACHING

1. Intralesional treatment should be continued for 8 weeks.
2. Genital warts may disappear both during and after treatment has been completed. When this occurs, unless new warts appear or warts become enlarged, there should be a 3-month waiting period after the first 8-week course of therapy.
3. Do not change brands without approval; manufacturing process, strength, and type of interferon may vary.
4. Practice reliable contraception.
5. Report early signs of hypersensitivity reactions (e.g., hives, chest tightness, generalized urticaria, hypotension, wheezing, anaphylaxis).

OUTCOMES/EVALUATE

- ↓ Pain, number of genital warts
- Suppression of malignant cell proliferation

Interferon beta-1a Interferon beta-1b (r1FN-B)

(in-ter-**FEER**-on **BAY**-tah)

PREGNANCY CATEGORY: C
CLASSIFICATION(S):
Immunomodulator
Rx: Interferon beta-1b: Betaseron.
✱**Rx: Interferon beta-1a:** Avonex, Rebif.

ACTION/KINETICS
Interferon beta-1a is produced by mammalian cells into which the human interferon beta gene has been introduced. Interferon beta-1b is made by bacterial fermentation of a strain of *Escherichia coli* that is a genetically engineered plasmid containing the gene for human interferon $beta_{ser17}$. Interferon betas have antiviral, antiproliferative, and immunoregulatory effects. Mechanism for the beneficial effect in MS is unknown, although the effects are mediated through combination with specific cell receptors located on the cell membrane. The receptor-drug complex induces the expression of a number of interferon-induced gene products that are thought to be the mediators of the biologic effects of interferon beta-1a and beta-1b. **t½, interferon beta-1a:** 10 hr. Kinetic information is not available for interferon beta-1b since serum levels are low or not detectable following SC administration to MS clients. **Peak serum levels of beta-1b:** Within 1–8 hr with a mean serum concentration of 40 IU/mL. Mean terminal half-lives ranged from 8 min to 4.3 hr.

USES
Interferon beta-1a: Treatment of relapsing forms of MS to slow the appearance of physical disability (and possibly mental decline) and decrease the frequency of clinical exacerbations. **Interferon beta-1b:** Treatment of ambulatory clients with relapsing-remitting MS to reduce the frequency of clinical exacerbations. Remitting-relapsing MS is manifested by recurrent attacks of neurologic dysfunction followed by complete or incomplete recovery. *Investigational:* Treatment of AIDS, AIDS-related Kaposi's sarcoma, metastatic renal cell carcinoma, herpes of the lips or genitals, malignant melanoma, cutaneous T-cell lymphoma, and acute non-A/non-B hepatitis.

CONTRAINDICATIONS
Hypersensitivity to natural or recombinant interferon beta or human albumin. Lactation.

SPECIAL CONCERNS
The safety and efficacy for use in chronic progressive MS and in children less than 18 years of age have not been studied. Depression and attempted suicide and suicide have occurred. Potential to be an abortifacient. Use with caution in those with preexisting seizure disorder.

SIDE EFFECTS
• **SIDE EFFECTS COMMON TO INTERFERON BETA-1A AND -1B.**
Body as a whole: Headache, fever, flu-like symptoms, pain, asthenia, chills, reaction at injection site (including necrosis/inflammation), malaise. **GI:** Abdominal pain, diarrhea, dry mouth, ***GI hemorrhage,*** gingivitis, hepatomegaly, intestinal obstruction, periodontal abscess, proctitis. **CV:** Arrhythmia, hypotension, postural hypotension. **CNS:** Dizziness, speech disorder, convulsion, ***suicide attempt***, abnormal gait, depersonalization, facial paralysis, hyperesthesia, neurosis, psychosis. **Respiratory:** Sinusitis, dyspnea, hemoptysis, hyperventilation. **Musculoskeletal:** Myalgia, arthritis. **Dermatologic:** Contact dermatitis, furunculosis, seborrhea, skin ulcer. **GU:** Epididymitis, gynecomastia, hematuria, kidney calculus, nocturia, ***vaginal hemorrhage***, ovarian cyst. **Miscellaneous:** Abscess, ascites, cellulitis, hernia, hypothyroidism, ***sepsis,*** hiccoughs, thirst, leukorrhea.
• **INTERFERON BETA-1A.**
Body as a whole: Infection. **GI:** Nausea, dyspepsia, anorexia, blood in stool,

I

colitis, constipation, diverticulitis, gall bladder disorder, gastritis, gum hemorrhage, hepatoma, increased appetite, ***intestinal perforation,*** periodontitis, tongue disorder. **CV:** Syncope, vasodilation, arteritis, ***heart arrest, hemorrhage, pulmonary embolus,*** palpitation, pericarditis, peripheral ischemia, peripheral vascular disorder, spider angioma, telangiectasia. **CNS:** Sleep difficulty, muscle spasm, ataxia, amnesia, Bell's palsy, clumsiness, drug dependence, increased libido. **Respiratory:** URTI, emphysema, laryngitis, pharyngeal edema, pneumonia. **Musculoskeletal:** Arthralgia, bone pain, myasthenia, osteonecrosis, synovitis. **Dermatologic:** Urticaria, alopecia, nevus, herpes zoster/simplex, basal cell carcinoma, blisters, cold clammy skin, erythema, genital pruritus, skin discoloration. **GU:** Vaginitis, breast fibroadenosis, breast mass, dysuria, fibrocystic change of the breast, fibroids, kidney pain, menopause, PID, penis disorder, Peyronie's disease, polyuria, postmenopausal hemorrhage, prostatic disorder, pyelonephritis, testis disorder, urethral pain, urinary urgency/retention/incontinence. **Hematologic:** Anemia, ecchymosis at injection site, eosinophils > 10%, hematocrit < 37%, increased coagulation time, ecchymosis, lymphadenopathy, petechia. **Metabolic:** Dehydration, hypoglycemia/magnesemia/kalemia. **Ophthalmic:** Abnormal vision, conjunctivitis, eye pain, vitreous floaters. **Miscellaneous:** Otitis media, decreased hearing, facial edema, fibrosis at injection site, hypersensitivity at injection site, lipoma, neoplasm, photosensitivity, toothache, sinus headache, chest pain.

• **INTERFERON BETA-1B.**

Body as a whole: Generalized edema, hypothermia, ***anaphylaxis, shock,*** adenoma, sarcoma. **GI:** Constipation, vomiting, GI disorder, aphthous stomatitis, cardiospasm, cheilitis, cholecystitis, cholelithiasis, duodenal ulcer, enteritis, esophagitis, fecal impaction or incontinence, flatulence, gastritis, glossitis, hematemesis, hepatic neoplasia, hepatitis, ileus, increased salivation, melena, nausea, oral leukoplakia, oral moniliasis, ***pancreatitis, rectal hemorrhage,*** salivary gland enlargement, stomach ulcer, peritonitis, tenesmus. **CV:** Migraine, palpitation, hypertension, tachycardia, peripheral vascular disorder, ***hemorrhage,*** angina pectoris, atrial fibrillation, cardiomegaly, ***cardiac arrest, cerebral hemorrhage, heart failure, MI, pulmonary embolus, ventricular fibrillation*** cerebral ischemia, endocarditis, pericardial effusion, spider angioma, subarachnoid hemorrhage, syncope, thrombophlebitis, thrombosis, varicose veins, vasospasm, venous pressure increase, ventricular extrasystoles. **CNS:** Mental symptoms, hypertonia, somnolence, hyperkinesia, acute/chronic brain syndrome, agitation, apathy, aphasia, ataxia, brain edema, ***coma,*** delirium, delusions, dementia, dystonia, encephalopathy, euphoria, hallucinations, hemiplegia, hypalgesia, incoordination, intracranial hypertension, decreased libido, manic reaction, meningitis, neuralgia, neuropathy, paralysis, paranoid reaction, decreased reflexes, stupor, subdural hematoma, torticollis, tremor. **Respiratory:** Laryngitis, apnea, asthma, atelectasis, lung carcinoma, hypoventilation, interstitial pneumonia, lung edema, pleural effusion, pneumothorax. **Musculoskeletal:** Myasthenia, arthrosis, bursitis, leg cramps, muscle atrophy, myopathy, myositis, ptosis, tenosynovitis. **Dermatologic:** Sweating, alopecia, erythema nodosum, exfoliative dermatitis, hirsutism, leukoderma, lichenoid dermatitis, maculopapular rash, photosensitivity, psoriasis, benign skin neoplasm, skin carcinoma, skin hypertrophy/necrosis, urticaria, vesiculobullous rash. **GU:** Dysmenorrhea, menstrual disorder, metrorrhagia, cystitis, breast pain, menorrhagia, urinary urgency, fibrocystic breast, breast neoplasm, urinary retention, anuria, balanitis, breast engorgement, cervicitis, impotence, kidney failure, tubular disorder, nephritis, oliguria, polyuria, salpingitis, urethritis, urinary incontinence, enlarged uterine fibroids, uterine neoplasm. **Hematologic:** Lymphocytes < 1500/mm^3, active neutrophil count < 1500/mm^3,

WBCs < 3000/mm³, lymphadenopathy, chronic lymphocytic leukemia, petechia, hemoglobin < 9.4 g/dL, platelets < 75,000/mm³, splenomegaly. **Metabolic:** Weight gain/loss, goiter, glucose < 55 mg/dL or > 160 mg/dL, AST or ALT > 5 times baseline, total bilirubin > 2.5 times baseline, urine protein > 1+, alkaline phosphatase > 5 times baseline, BUN > 40 mg/dL, calcium > 11.5 mg/dL, cyanosis, edema, glycosuria, hypoglycemic reaction, hypoxia, ketosis. **Ophthalmic:** Conjunctivitis, abnormal vision, diplopia, nystagmus, oculogyric crisis, papilledema, blepharitis, blindness, dry eyes, iritis, keratoconjunctivitis, mydriasis, photophobia, retinitis, visual field defect. **Miscellaneous:** Pelvic pain, hydrocephalus, alcohol intolerance, otitis externa, otitis media, parosmia, taste loss/perversion.

LABORATORY TEST CONSIDERATIONS

↑ ALT, total bilirubin, AST, BUN, urine protein. Hypoglycemia or hyperglycemia. Ketosis.

HOW SUPPLIED

Interferon Beta-1a: *Powder for Injection, lyophilized:* 33 mcg (6.6 million IU). **Interferon Beta-1b:** *Powder for Injection, lyophilized:* 0.3 mg (9.6 million IU)

DOSAGE

- **INTERFERON BETA-1A: IM**

  Relapsing forms of MS.

30 mcg IM once a week.

- **INTEFERON BETA-1B: SC**

  Relapsing-remitting MS clients.

0.25 mg (8 mIU) every other day.

NURSING CONSIDERATIONS

ADMINISTRATION/STORAGE

1. Effectiveness beyond 2 years of use is not known.
2. To reconstitute and use interferon beta-1a, use the following process:
   • Reconstitute with 1.1 mL of diluent and swirl gently to dissolve.
   • Vials must be stored in a refrigerator at 2–8°C (36–46°F).
   • Following reconstitution, use within 6 hr; store at same temperatures as unreconstituted drug.
3. To reconstitute and use interferon beta-1b, use the following process:
   • Using a sterile syringe and needle, inject 1.2 mL of diluent provided (0.54% NaCl) into the vial. Swirl gently to dissolve the drug completely. (Do not shake.)
   • Visually inspect reconstituted product; discard if it contains particulate matter or is discolored.
   • Withdraw 1 mL of the reconstituted solution from the vial into a sterile syringe fitted with a 27-gauge needle and inject SC. Injection sites include the arms, abdomen, hips, and thighs.
   • Since the reconstituted product contains no preservative, discard any unused portions after one use.
   • Before and after reconstitution with diluent, store the drug at 2–8°C (36–46°F). Use the product within 3 hr of reconstitution.

ASSESSMENT

1. Document age of diagnosis, frequency of exacerbations, other therapies prescribed and the outcome.
2. Note any hypersensitivity to human albumin or interferon beta.
3. Determine if pregnant; drug has abortifacient properties.
4. Monitor hematologic profile and hepatic enzyme levels q 3 mo.

CLIENT/FAMILY TEACHING

1. Review guidelines for drug reconstitution, proper dose, administration, and care and disposal of equipment.
2. Do not change dose or administration schedule without approval.
3. Flu-like symptoms are common; acetaminophen may help.
4. Report any mental changes, depression, or suicide thoughts.
5. Practice reliable birth control; drug may harm fetus.
6. May cause photosensitivity reactions; wear protective clothing, sunscreen, sun glasses, and a hat.
7. Avoid alcohol in any form.
8. With diabetes, monitor FS and report any overt changes.
9. Identify support groups that may assist to cope with chronic diseases.

OUTCOMES/EVALUATE

↓ Frequency and severity of MS exacerbations

Interferon gamma-1b

(in-ter-**FEER**-on **GAM**-uh)

PREGNANCY CATEGORY: C
CLASSIFICATION(S):
Immunomodulator
Rx: Actimmune

ACTION/KINETICS

Consists of a single-chain polypeptide of 140 amino acids. Produced by fermentation of a genetically engineered *Escherichia coli* bacterium containing the DNA that encodes for the human protein. Manifests potent phagocyte-activating effects including generation of toxic oxygen metabolites within phagocytes. Such metabolites result in the death of microorganisms such as *Staphylococcus aureus, Toxoplasma gondii, Leishmania donovani, Listeria monocytogenes,* and *Mycobacterium avium intracellulare.* Since interferon gamma regulates activity of immune cells, it is characterized as a lymphokine of the interleukin type. Interferon gamma interacts functionally with other interleukin molecules (e.g., interleukin-2) and all interleukins form part of a complex, lymphokine regulatory network. As an example, interferon gamma and interleukin-4 may interact reciprocally to regulate murine IgE levels; interferon gamma can suppress IgE levels and inhibit the production of collagen at the transcription level in humans. Slowly absorbed after SC injection. **$t^1/_2$, elimination: SC,** 5.9 hr. **Peak plasma levels:** 7 hr after SC.

USES

(1) Decrease the frequency and severity of serious infections associated with chronic granulomatous disease. (2) Delay time to disease progression in severe, malignant osteoporosis.

CONTRAINDICATIONS

Hypersensitivity to interferon gamma or *E. coli*-derived products. Lactation.

SPECIAL CONCERNS

Safety and effectiveness have not been determined in children less than 1 year of age. Use with caution in clients with preexisting cardiac disease, including symptoms of ischemia, arrhythmia, or CHF, and in clients with myelosuppression or taking other potentially myelosuppressive drugs, seizure disorders, or compromised CNS function.

SIDE EFFECTS

The following side effects were noted in clients with chronic granulomatous disease or severe, malignant osteoporosis receiving the drug SC.

GI: Diarrhea, N&V, abdominal pain, anorexia. **CNS:** Fever (over 50%), headache, fatigue, depression. **Miscellaneous:** Rash, chills, erythema or tenderness/pain at injection site, weight loss, myalgia, arthralgia, back pain, myelosuppression, hypersensitivity reactions.

When used in clients other than those with chronic granulomatous disease, in addition to the preceding, the following side effects were reported.

GI: ***GI bleeding,*** pancreatitis, hepatic insufficiency. **CV:** Hypotension, heart block, ***heart failure,*** syncope, ***tachyarrhythmia, MI.*** **CNS:** Confusion, disorientation, symptoms of parkinsonism, gait disturbance, ***seizures,*** hallucinations, TIAs. **Hematologic:** ***DVT, pulmonary embolism.*** **Respiratory:** ***Bronchospasm,*** tachypnea, interstitial pneumonitis. **Metabolic:** Hyperglycemia, hyponatremia. **Miscellaneous:** Reversible renal insufficiency, worsening of dermatomyositis.

HOW SUPPLIED

Injection: 2 million IU/0.5 mL, 3 million IU/0.5 mL

DOSAGE

• **SC**

Chronic granulomatous disease. Severe, malignant osteoporosis.

50 mcg/m² (1 million units/m²) for clients whose body surface is greater than 0.5 m². If the body surface is less than 0.5 m², the dose of interferon gamma should be 1.5 mcg/kg/dose. The drug is given 3 times/week (e.g., Monday, Wednesday, Friday).

NURSING CONSIDERATIONS

ADMINISTRATION/STORAGE

1. Preferred injection sites: right and left deltoid; anterior thigh.

2. Does not contain a preservative. Use the vial only for a single dose and discard any unused portion.
3. Safety and effectiveness have not been determined for doses greater or less than 50 mcg/m^2.
4. If severe side effects occur, dose can be reduced by 50% or therapy can be discontinued until these subside.
5. May be administered using either sterilized glass or plastic disposable syringes.
6. Do not shake the vial; avoid vigorous agitation.
7. Vials must be stored at 2–8°C (36–46°F) to assure optimal retention of activity. Do not freeze vial.
8. Discard vials stored at room temperature for more than 12 hr.
9. Do not store undiluted drug in syringes due to syringe adhesion.
IV 10. Although not FDA approved, the drug has been given by continuous (10 days to 8 weeks) or intermittent (at 1, 6, or 24 hr) IV infusion as well as by IM injection.

ASSESSMENT

1. Determine age of onset, any treatments used in the past to reduce frequency and severity of infections, and note DEXA scan results.
2. Note history of CAD or CNS disorders; assess for symptoms.
3. Monitor urinalysis, CBC, liver and renal function studies q 3 mo.

CLIENT/FAMILY TEACHING

1. Review reconstitution, method for administration, storage (keep vial refrigerated), and disposal of drug/equipment.
2. Keep drug in the refrigerator; do *not* shake container.
3. Take at bedtime with acetaminophen to minimize flu-like symptoms (fever and headaches).
4. Consume 2–3 L/day of fluids.
5. Avoid alcohol and any other CNS depressants.
6. Avoid activities that require mental alertness until drug effects realized.
7. Close medical supervision is imperative with this disease and genetically engineered drug therapy as dosage may require frequent adjustments. Report concerns and adverse effects.

OUTCOMES/EVALUATE

- Suppression of infective organisms associated with chronic granulomatous disease
- Control of malignant osteoporosis progression

Ipecac syrup

(**IP**-eh-kak)

PREGNANCY CATEGORY: C
CLASSIFICATION(S):
Agent to induce vomiting (emesis)

ACTION/KINETICS

Acts both locally on the gastric mucosa as an irritant and centrally to stimulate the CTZ. The central effect is caused by emetine and cephaeline, which are two alkaloids in the product. **Onset:** 20 min. **Duration:** 20–25 min. In contrast to apomorphine, a second dose may be given if necessary. **Ipecac syrup must not be confused with ipecac fluid extract, which is 14 times as potent.** Syrup of ipecac can be purchased without a prescription.

USES

To empty the stomach promptly and completely after oral poisoning or drug overdose.

CONTRAINDICATIONS

With corrosives or petroleum distillates, in individuals who are unconscious or semicomatose, severely inebriated, or in shock. Infants under 6 months of age.

SPECIAL CONCERNS

Use with caution during lactation. If used in children less than 12 months of age, there is an increased risk of aspiration of vomitus. Abuse may occur in anorexic or bulemic clients and its use in these groups has been associated with severe cardiomyopathies and death.

SIDE EFFECTS

Diarrhea, drowsiness, coughing, or choking with emesis, mild CNS depression, GU upset (may last several hours) after emesis. Can be cardiotoxic if not vomited and allowed to be absorbed. ***Cardiotoxic effects include heart conduction disturbances, atrial fibrillation, or fatal myocarditis.***

OD OVERDOSE MANAGEMENT

Symptoms: If absorbed into the general circulation, symptoms may include cardiac conduction disturbances, bradycardia, atrial fibrillation, hypotension, or ***fatal myocarditis.*** *Treatment:* Activated charcoal to absorb ipecac syrup. Gastric lavage. Support the CV system with symptomatic treatment.

DRUG INTERACTIONS

Activated charcoal adsorbs ipecac syrup, thus decreasing its effect.

HOW SUPPLIED

Syrup

DOSAGE

- **SYRUP**

Emetic.

Adults and children over 12 years: 15–30 mL followed by 240 mL of water; **infants up to 1 year:** 5–10 mL followed by one-half to one glass of water; **pediatric, 1–12 years:** 15 mL followed by one to two glasses of water.

NURSING CONSIDERATIONS

ADMINISTRATION/STORAGE

1. Check label of medication closely so that the syrup and the fluid extract are not confused.
2. Dosage may be repeated once in children over 1 year of age and adults if vomiting does not occur within 30 min. Consider gastric lavage if vomiting does not occur within 15 min of second dose.
3. Administer ipecac syrup with 200–300 mL of water.
4. There is controversy as to whether ipecac should be given to children less than 1 year old. It appears to be both safe and effective.

ASSESSMENT

1. Estimate amount and time of ingestion and compare with plasma level of agent ingested.
2. Do not use if intoxicant is a convulsant (i.e., TCAs); may trigger seizures abruptly.
3. Do not use for petroleum-based or caustic substances such as kerosene, lye, Drano, or gasoline.
4. Assess respiratory status and level of consciousness; do not use if there is no gag reflex or if semicomatose.

CLIENT/FAMILY TEACHING

1. For use in the event of accidental poisoning. Available in premeasured doses for home emergency use.
2. Before administering ipecac syrup, contact regional poison control center, provider, or local hospital ER.
3. Store in a locked closet, out of the reach of children. Check expiration date periodically and always before use.
4. Review abuse potential, such as to induce vomiting after meals for weight reduction and its potential cardiac toxic effects. (Some states have banned OTC sales.)
5. Give to conscious persons only with adequate amounts of water to induce vomiting.

OUTCOMES/EVALUATE

Inducement of vomiting following drug overdose or poisoning

Ipratropium bromide

(eye-prah-**TROH**-pee-um)

PREGNANCY CATEGORY: B

CLASSIFICATION(S):

Cholinergic blocking drug

Rx: Atrovent

✱Rx: Alti-Ipratropium Bromide, Apo-Ipravent, Gen-Ipratropium, Novo-Ipramide, Nu-Ipratropium, PMS-Ipratropium

SEE ALSO *CHOLINERGIC BLOCKING AGENTS.*

ACTION/KINETICS

Chemically related to atropine. Antagonizes the action of acetylcholine. Prevents the increase in intracellular levels of cyclic guanosine monophosphate, which is caused by the interaction of acetylcholine with muscarinic receptors in bronchial smooth muscle; this leads to bronchodilation which is primarily a local, site-specific effect. Poorly absorbed into the systemic circulation. About 50% of unchanged drug excreted through the urine. **t½, elimination:** 2 hr after inhalation.

USES

Aerosol or solution: Bronchodilation in COPD, including chronic bronchitis and emphysema. **Nasal spray:** (1) Symptomatic relief (using 0.03%) of rhinorrhea associated with allergic and nonallergic perennial rhinitis in clients over 6 years of age. (2) Symptomatic relief (using 0.06%) of rhinorrhea associated with the common cold in those aged 5 and older. *NOTE:* The use of ipratropium with sympathomimetic bronchodilators, methylxanthines, steroids, or cromolyn sodium (all of which are used in treating COPD) are without side effects.

CONTRAINDICATIONS

Hypersensitivity to atropine, ipratropium, or derivatives. Hypersensitivity to soy lecithin or related food products, including soy bean or peanut (inhalation aerosol). Use for initial treatment of acute bronchospasms.

SPECIAL CONCERNS

Use with caution in clients with narrow-angle glaucoma, prostatic hypertrophy, or bladder neck obstruction and during lactation. Safety and efficacy of the aerosol and solution have not been determined in children less than 12 years of age, of the nasal spray, 0.03%, in children less than 6 years of age, and of the nasal spray, 0.06%, in children less than 5 years of age. Use of ipratropium as a single agent for the relief of bronchospasm in acute COPD has not been studied adequately.

SIDE EFFECTS

• INHALATION AEROSOL.

CNS: Cough, nervousness, dizziness, headache, fatigue, insomnia, drowsiness, difficulty in coordination, tremor. **GI:** Dryness of oropharynx, GI distress, dry mouth, nausea, constipation. **CV:** Palpitations, tachycardia, flushing. **Dermatologic:** Itching, hives, alopecia. **Miscellaneous:** Irritation from aerosol, worsening of symptoms, rash, hoarseness, blurred vision, difficulty in accommodation, drying of secretions, urinary difficulty, paresthesias, mucosal ulcers.

• INHALATION SOLUTION.

CNS: Dizziness, insomnia, nervousness, tremor, headache. **GI:** Dry mouth, nausea, constipation. **CV:** Hypertension, aggravation of hypertension, tachycardia, palpitations. **Respiratory:** Worsening of COPD symptoms, coughing, dyspnea, bronchitis, ***bronchospasm***, increased sputum, URI, pharyngitis, rhinitis, sinusitis. **Miscellaneous:** Urinary retention, UTIs, urticaria, pain, flu-like symptoms, back/chest pain, arthritis.

• NASAL SPRAY.

CNS: Headache, dizziness. **GI:** Nausea, dry mouth, taste perversion. **CV:** Palpitation, tachycardia. **Respiratory:** URI, epistaxis, pharyngitis, nasal dryness, miscellaneous nasal symptoms, nasal irritation, blood-tinged mucus, dry throat, cough, nasal congestion/burning, coughing. **Ophthalmic:** Ocular irritation, blurred vision, conjunctivitis. **Miscellaneous:** Hoarseness, thirst, tinnitis, urinary retention.

• ALL PRODUCTS.

Allergic: Skin rash; angioedema of the tongue, throat, lips, and face; urticaria, ***laryngospasm***, oropharyngeal edema, ***bronchospasm, anaphylaxis.*** **Anticholinergic reactions:** Precipitation or worsening of narrow angle glaucoma, prostatic disorders, tachycardia, urinary retention, constipation, bowel obstruction, blurred vision, difficulty in accommodation.

HOW SUPPLIED

Aerosol: 0.018 mg/inh; *Nasal Spray:* 0.03% (21 mcg/spray), 0.06% (42 mcg/spray); *Solution for Inhalation:* 0.02% (500 mcg/vial)

DOSAGE

• RESPIRATORY AEROSOL

Treat bronchospasms.

Adults: 2 inhalations (36 mcg) q.i.d. Additional inhalations may be required but should not exceed 12 inhalations/day.

• SOLUTION FOR INHALATION

Treat bronchospasms.

Adults: 500 mcg (1-unit-dose vial)

given t.i.d.–q.i.d. by oral nebulization with doses 6–8 hr apart.

• **NASAL SPRAY, 0.03%**

Perennial rhinitis.

Children, 6 years and older: 2 sprays (42 mcg) per nostril b.i.d.–t.i.d. for a total daily dose of 168–252 mcg/day. Optimum dose varies.

• **NASAL SPRAY, 0.06%**

Rhinitis due to the common cold.

Children, 5 years and older: 2 sprays (84 mcg) per nostril t.i.d.–q.i.d. for a total daily dose of 504–672 mcg/day. The safety and efficacy for use for the common cold for more than 4 days have not been determined.

NURSING CONSIDERATIONS

SEE ALSO *NURSING CONSIDERATIONS* FOR *CHOLINERGIC BLOCKING AGENTS.*

ADMINISTRATION/STORAGE

1. If also taking albuterol, ipratropium may be mixed in the nebulizer with albuterol if used within 1 hr.
2. Store the aerosol between 15 and 30°C (59 and 86°F); avoid excessive humidity.
3. Store solution between 15–30°C (59–86°F); protect from light. Store unused vials in the foil pouch.
4. Store nasal spray tightly closed between 15–30°C (59–86°F). Avoid freezing.

ASSESSMENT

1. Document type, onset, characteristics of symptoms, any other agents used and the results.
2. Perform full pulmonary assessment; review PFTs and X-rays.
3. Note any prostate enlargement or difficulty urinating.

CLIENT/FAMILY TEACHING

1. Take only as directed; shake well before using. Review administration technique and rinse mouth and equipment after use.
2. If using more than one inhalation per dose, wait 3 min before administering the second inhalation.
3. Drug is not for use in terminating an acute attack; effects take up to 15 min. Have another prescribed agent readily available in this event.
4. Avoid contact with the eyes. A spacer may be useful with the inhaler and a mouthpiece with the nebulizer to help prevent solution (mist) contact with the eyes.
5. May experience a bitter taste and dry mouth; use frequent mouth rinses and hard candy to relieve.
6. Transient dizziness, insomnia, blurred vision, or excessive weakness may occur.
7. Stop smoking now to preserve current level of lung function and to prevent further damage; utilize smoking cessation program.

OUTCOMES/EVALUATE

• Improved airway exchange and breathing patterns
• ↓ Wheezing, dyspnea
• Relief of rhinorrhea

—COMBINATION DRUG—

Ipratropium bromide and Albuterol sulfate

(eye-prah-**TROH**-pee-um/ al-**BYOU**-ter-ohl)

PREGNANCY CATEGORY: C
CLASSIFICATION(S):
Cholinergic blocking drug and Sympathomimetic
Rx: Combivent, DuoNeb

SEE ALSO *IPRATROPIUM BROMIDE* AND *ALBUTEROL SULFATE.*

CONTENT

Each actuation of metered dose inhaler delivers: *Cholinergic blocking drug:* Ipratropium bromide, 18 mcg; and *Sympathomimetic:* Albuterol sulfate, 103 mcg.

USES

Treatment of COPD (including bronchospasms) in those who are on regular aerosol bronchodilator therapy and who require a second bronchodilator.

CONTRAINDICATIONS

History of hypersensitivity to soya lecithin or related food products, such as soybean and peanuts. Lactation.

SPECIAL CONCERNS

Use with caution in CV disorders, especially coronary insufficiency, cardiac arrhythmias, and hypertension. Use with caution in narrow-angle glaucoma, prostatic hypertrophy, bladder-neck obstruction, convulsive disorders, hyperthyroidism, diabetes mellitus, in those unusually responsive to sympathomimetic amines, and renal or hepatic disease. Safety and efficacy have not been determined in children.

SIDE EFFECTS

Respiratory: ***Paradoxical bronchospasm,*** bronchitis, dyspnea, coughing, respiratory disorders, pneumonia, URTI, pharyngitis, sinusitis, rhinitis. **CV:** ECG changes including flattening of T wave, prolongation of QTc interval, and ST segment depression. Also, arrhythmias, palpitation, tachycardia, angina, hypertension. **Hypersensitivity, immediate:** Urticaria, ***angioedema, bronchospasm, anaphylaxis, oropharyngeal edema.*** **Body as a whole:** Headache, pain, flu, chest pain, edema, fatigue. **GI:** N&V, dry mouth, diarrhea, dyspepsia. **CNS:** Dizziness, nervousness, paresthesia, tremor, dysphonia, insomnia. **Miscellaneous:** Arthralgia, increased sputum, taste perversion, UTI, dysuria.

DRUG INTERACTIONS

See individual drugs.

HOW SUPPLIED

See Content

DOSAGE

• **INHALATION**

COPD.

2 inhalations q 6 hr not to exceed 12 inhalations/24-hr.

NURSING CONSIDERATIONS

SEE ALSO *NURSING CONSIDERATIONS* FOR *IPRATROPIUM BROMIDE* AND *ALBUTEROL SULFATE.*

ADMINISTRATION/STORAGE

1. Canister provides sufficient medication for 200 inhalations.
2. Discard canister after labeled number of inhalations used.
3. Store between 15–30°C (59–86°F).

ASSESSMENT

1. Assess for any soybean or peanut allergy.
2. Note indications for therapy, characteristics and frequency of symptoms, other agents trialed, and outcome.
3. Assess breath sounds, CXR, and PFTs.

CLIENT/FAMILY TEACHING

1. Use as directed; do not increase dose or frequency of administration unless specifically directed.
2. Avoid excessive humidity. For best results, have canister at room temperature before use.
3. Shake canister well before using. Rinse mouth and equipment after each use.
4. Test spray 3 times before first use and again if the canister has not been used for 24 hr.
5. Report any loss of effectiveness.
6. Avoid eye contact; report any visual disturbances or eye irritation.
7. Drug is not for use in terminating an acute attack; effects take up to 15 min. Have another prescribed agent readily available in this event.
8. Stop smoking now to preserve current level of lung function and to prevent further damage; utilize smoking cessation program.

OUTCOMES/EVALUATE

Improved airway exchange

Irbesartan

(ihr-beh-**SAR**-tan)

PREGNANCY CATEGORY: C (FIRST TRIMESTER), D (SECOND AND THIRD TRIMESTERS)

CLASSIFICATION(S):

Antihypertensive, angiotensin II receptor blocker

Rx: Avapro

SEE ALSO *ANGIOTENSIN II RECEPTOR ANTAGONISTS* AND *ANTIHYPERTENSIVE DRUGS.*

ACTION/KINETICS

Rapid absorption after PO use. **Peak plasma levels:** 1.5–2 hr. Food does not affect bioavailability. Effect somewhat less in Blacks. **t½, terminal elimination:** 11–15 hr. Over 90% bound to plasma proteins. Metabolized in liver and both unchanged drug and metabolites excreted through urine (20%) and feces (80%).

ADDITIONAL USES
Investigational: Heart failure, reduce rate of progression of renal disease and adverse clinical sequelae in hypertensives with diabetic nephropathy.

SIDE EFFECTS
GI: Diarrhea, dyspepsia, heartburn, abdominal distension/pain, N&V, constipation, oral lesion, gastroenteritis, flatulence. **CV:** Tachycardia, syncope, orthostatic hypotension, hypotension (especially in volume- or salt-depletion), flushing, hypertension, cardiac murmur, ***MI, cardio-respiratory arrest, heart failure, hypertensive crisis, CVA,*** angina pectoris, arrhythmias, conduction disorder, TIA. **CNS:** Sleep disturbance, anxiety, nervousness, dizziness, numbness, somnolence, emotional disturbance, depression, paresthesia, tremor. **Musculoskeletal:** Extremity swelling, muscle cramp/ache/weakness, arthritis, musculoskeletal pain, musculoskeletal chest pain, joint stiffness, bursitis. **Respiratory:** Epistaxis, tracheobronchitis, congestion, pulmonary congestion, dyspnea, wheezing, URI, rhinitis, pharyngitis, sinus abnormality. **GU:** Abnormal urination, prostate disorder, UTI, sexual dysfunction, libido change. **Dermatologic:** Pruritus, dermatitis, ecchymosis, facial erythema, urticaria. **Ophthalmic:** Vision disturbance, conjunctivitis, eyelid abnormality. **Otic:** Hearing abnormality, ear infection/pain/abnormality. **Miscellaneous:** Gout, fever, fatigue, chills, facial edema, upper extremity edema, headache, influenza, rash, chest pain.

LABORATORY TEST CONSIDERATIONS
↑ BUN (minor), serum creatinine. ↓ Hemoglobin. Neutropenia.

HOW SUPPLIED
Tablet: 75 mg, 150 mg, 300 mg

DOSAGE

• TABLETS

Hypertension.

150 mg once daily, up to 300 mg once daily. Lower initial dose of 75 mg is recommended for clients with depleted intravascular volume or salt. If BP is not controlled by irbesartan alone, hydrochlorothiazide may have an additive effect. Clients not adequately treated by 300 mg irbesartan are unlikely to get benefit from higher dose or b.i.d. dosing.

NURSING CONSIDERATIONS

SEE ALSO *NURSING CONSIDERATIONS* FOR *ANTIHYPERTENSIVE DRUGS.*

ADMINISTRATION/STORAGE
1. Adjustment of dose is not required in geriatric clients or in hepatic or renal impairment.
2. May be given with other antihypertensive drugs.

ASSESSMENT
1. Document indications for therapy, onset, duration, characteristics of symptoms, and other agents trialed.
2. Observe infants exposed to an angiotensin II inhibitor in utero for hypotension, oliguria, and ↑ K.

CLIENT/FAMILY TEACHING
1. Take only as directed. May take with or without food.
2. Avoid tasks that require mental alertness until drug effects realized; change positions slowly to prevent sudden drop in BP.
3. Continue low-fat, low-cholesterol diet, regular exercise, tobacco cessation, salt restriction and lifestyle changes necessary to maintain lowered BP.
4. Practice reliable contraception. Stop drug and report if pregnancy suspected.

OUTCOMES/EVALUATE
↓ BP

Irinotecan hydrochloride

(**eye**-rih-noh-**TEE**-kan)

PREGNANCY CATEGORY: D
CLASSIFICATION(S):
Antineoplastic, hormone
Rx: Camptosar

SEE ALSO *ANTINEOPLASTIC AGENTS.*

ACTION/KINETICS
The cytotoxic effect is due to double-strand DNA damage produced during DNA synthesis when replication enzymes interact with the ternary complex

formed by topoisomerase I, DNA, and either irinotecan or SN-38 (its active metabolite). Conversion of irinotecan to SN-38 occurs in the liver. **t½, terminal, irinotecan:** About 6 hr; **t½, terminal, SN-38:** About 10 hr. SN-38 is 95% bound to plasma proteins.

USES

First-line therapy with 5-fluorouracil and leucovorin for metastatic colon or rectal carcinomas. Metastatic carcinoma of the colon or rectum in those whose disease has recurred or progressed following 5-fluorouracil therapy.

CONTRAINDICATIONS

Lactation.

SPECIAL CONCERNS

Clients who have previously received pelvic or abdominal irradiation are at an increased risk for severe myelosuppression when treated with irinotecan. Safety and efficacy have not been determined in children.

SIDE EFFECTS

GI: Diarrhea, N&V, anorexia, abdominal cramping or pain, constipation, flatulence, stomatitis, dyspepsia. **Hematologic:** Leukopenia, anemia, neutropenia, serious thrombocytopenia (rare). **CNS:** Insomnia, dizziness. **Respiratory:** Dyspnea, increased coughing, rhinitis, severe pulmonary events (rare). **CV:** Vasodilation, flushing. **Body as a whole:** Asthenia, fever, pain, headache, back pain, chills, minor infections (usually UTI), edema, abdominal enlargement. **Dermatologic:** Alopecia, sweating, rashes. **Metabolic/nutritional:** Decreased body weight, dehydration.

LABORATORY TEST CONSIDERATIONS

↑ AST, alkaline phosphatase.

OD OVERDOSE MANAGEMENT

Symptoms: Extension of side effects. *Treatment:* Maximum supportive care to prevent dehydration due to diarrhea. Treat any infections.

DRUG INTERACTIONS

Antineoplastic agents / ↑ Risk of myelosuppression and diarrhea
Dexamethasone / ↑ Risk of lymphocytopenia and hyperglycemia
Prochlorperazine / ↑ Risk of akathisia

HOW SUPPLIED

Injection: 20 mg/mL

DOSAGE

• **IV INFUSION**

Metastatic carcinoma of the colon or rectum.

Initial: 125 mg/m² given as an IV infusion over 90 min once weekly for 4 weeks. This is followed by a 2-week rest period. **Subsequent dosing:** Additional courses of treatment may be repeated q 6 weeks (4 weeks on therapy, 2 weeks off therapy). Doses can be adjusted to as high as 150 mg/m² or as low as 50 mg/m² in 25- to 50-mg/m² increments, depending on the client's tolerance. If intolerable toxicity does not occur, courses of treatment may be continued indefinitely. *NOTE:* Modifications of the dosage are based on the degree of neutropenia, neutropenic fever, diarrhea, and other toxicities. Consult the package insert for specific dosage modifications.

NURSING CONSIDERATIONS

SEE ALSO *NURSING CONSIDERATIONS* FOR *ANTINEOPLASTIC AGENTS.*

ADMINISTRATION/STORAGE

IV 1. Avoid extravasation. If extravasation occurs, flush site with sterile water and apply ice.

2. Causes vomiting; thus, give clients antiemetic therapy. Antiemetic therapy includes dexamethasone, 10 mg, and a 5-HT_3 blocker such as granisetron or ondansetron; give 30 min before giving irinotecan.

3. Prepare the infusion solution by diluting in D5W (preferred) or 0.9% NaCl to a final concentration of 0.12–1.1 mg/mL; administer over 90 min.

4. Solutions diluted in D5W, stored in the refrigerator, and protected from light are stable for 48 hr. However, due to possible microbial contamination during dilution, use refrigerated admixtures within 24 hr or, if kept at room temperature, use within 6 hr. Do not refrigerate admixtures containing 0.9% NaCl. Freezing irinotecan or admixtures may cause drug precipitation.

ASSESSMENT

1. Document indications for therapy; note history of pelvic/abdominal irradiation and last 5-FU therapy.
2. List all drugs currently prescribed to ensure none exacerbate side effects.
3. Drug is emetogenic; administer antiemetics 30 min prior to therapy.
4. May need IV atropine for those who experience early-onset abdominal cramps, diarrhea, or diaphoresis.
5. Assess infusion site carefully; flush site with sterile water and apply ice with extravasation.
6. Obtain CBC before each treatment. Hold if ANC below 500/mm^3 or neutropenic fever occurs. Any significant reduction in WBC (less then 2,000/mm^3), neutrophil count (less than 1,000/mm^3), or platelet count (below 100,000 mm^3) warrants a dose reduction.

CLIENT/FAMILY TEACHING

1. Diarrhea may occur within 24 hr of therapy; is cholinergic in nature and usually transient.
2. Report if temperature is over 101°F or diarrhea, vomiting, or dehydration develop.
3. With late-onset diarrhea (usually 10 days after therapy) take 4 mg of loperamide, followed by 2 mg q 2 h for 12 hr until diarrhea free. Consume extra fluids to prevent dehydration.
4. Avoid laxatives unless approved.
5. Practice birth control during and for several months following therapy.
6. Avoid crowds, those with active infections, and immunizations during drug therapy.

OUTCOMES/EVALUATE

Inhibition of malignant cell proliferation

Iron dextran parenteral

PREGNANCY CATEGORY: C
CLASSIFICATION(S):
Antianemic, iron
Rx: DexFerrum, InFeD
✱**Rx:** Dexiron, Infufur

ACTION/KINETICS

A complex of ferric hydroxide and dextran that is removed from the plasma by the reticuloendothelial system which splits the complex into iron and dextran. The iron is bound to protein to form hemosiderin or ferritin, which replenishes hemoglobin and depleted iron stores. After IM, most absorbed within 72 hr and the rest over 3–4 weeks. **t½:** From 5 hr (circulating iron dextran) to more than 20 hr (total iron, both circulating and bound). Negligible amounts of iron in iron dextran are lost via the urine and feces.

USES

Treatment of documented iron deficiency where oral use is unsatisfactory or impossible. *Investigational:* Iron supplementation in clients receiving epoetin therapy.

CONTRAINDICATIONS

All anemias not associated with iron deficiency. Acute phase of infectious kidney disease. Use in infants less than 4 months of age.

SPECIAL CONCERNS

Use with extreme caution in seriously impaired liver function. Use with caution during lactation and in clients with a history of significant allergies/asthma. Rheumatoid arthritis clients may have an acute exacerbation of joint pain and swelling after iron dextran. Side effects may exacerbate CV complications in clients with preexisting CV disease. Unwarranted therapy will cause excess storage of iron with the possibility of exogenous hemosiderosis.

Large IV or IM doses may cause arthralgia, backache, chills, dizziness, moderate to high fever, headache, malaise, myalgia, N&V (onset is 24–48 hr; symptoms usually subside within 3–4 days after IV and within 3–7 days after IM).

SIDE EFFECTS

Delayed reactions: Arthralgia, backache, chills, dizziness, fever, headache, malaise, myalgia, N&V. **Hypersensitivity:** ***Anaphylaxis.*** **GI:** Abdominal pain, N&V, diarrhea. **CNS:** Convulsions, syncope, headache, weakness, unresponsiveness, paresthesia, febrile episodes, chills, dizziness, disorientation, numbness, unconsciousness. **CV:** Chest pain, chest tightness, shock,

cardiac arrest, hypotension, hypertension, tachycardia, bradycardia, flushing, arrhythmias. Also, flushing and hypotension from too rapid IV injection. **Respiratory:** Dyspnea, bronchospasm, wheezing, ***respiratory arrest.*** **Musculoskeletal:** Arthralgia, arthritis (including reactivation), myalgia, backache, sterile abscess, atrophy/fibrosis (at IM injection site), soreness or pain at or near IM injection site, cellulitis, swelling, inflammation, local phlebitis at or near IV injection site. **Hematologic:** Leukocytosis, lymphadenopathy. **Dermatologic:** Urticaria, pruritus, purpura, rash, cyanosis. **Miscellaneous:** Hematuria, febrile episodes, sweating, shivering, chills, malaise, altered taste.

DRUG INTERACTIONS

If taken with chloramphenicol, may see ↑ serum iron levels R/T ↓ iron clearance and erythropoiesis due to direct bone marrow toxicity.

HOW SUPPLIED

Injection: 50 mg iron/mL (as dextran)

DOSAGE

Dosage is based on results of hematology data. The table in the package insert must be used to estimate the total iron required to restore hemoglobin to normal or near normal levels plus an additional allowance to replenish iron stores. The information in the table is to be used only in clients with iron deficiency anemia; they are not to be used to determine dosage in those needing iron replacement for blood loss.

IV injection. Prior to the first therapeutic dose, give an IV test dose of 0.5 mL slowly (over 30 seconds for InFeD or 5 minutes or more for DexFerrum). To ensure the client does not experience an anaphylactic reaction, allow 1 hr or more to elapse before the remainder of the initial therapeutic dose is given. Individual doses of 2 mL or less may be given daily until the calculated total amount of iron required has been administered. Give undiluted and slowly 50 mg or less/min (1 mL or less/min).

IM injection. As with IV administration, give a 0.5 mL test dose as described above. If no side effects occur, give injections as follows until the calculated total amount of iron has been administered. Do not exceed a daily dose of 25 mg iron (i.e., 0.5 mL) for infants less than 5 kg, 50 mg iron (i.e., 1 mL) for children less than 10 kg, and 100 mg iron (i.e., 2 mL) for all others.

NURSING CONSIDERATIONS

ADMINISTRATION/STORAGE

1. For IM, inject into the upper outer quadrant of the buttock; never inject into the arm or other exposed areas. Inject deeply with a 2 or 3 inch 19 or 20 gauge needle.
2. If the client is standing, have them bear weight on the leg opposite the injection site. If in bed, have them lie in a lateral position with injection site uppermost.
3. To avoid leakage or injection into SC tissue, use a Z-track technique.
4. IV Do not mix iron dextran with other drugs or add to parenteral nutrition solutions for IV infusion.

ASSESSMENT

1. Document indications for therapy (ensure iron deficieny anemia), onset, reason oral replacement not used and previous therapies trialed.
2. Assess for any CAD, significant allergies or asthma.
3. Those with rheumatoid arthritis may experience acute exacerbation of joint swelling /pain after dosing.
4. Ensure that test dose performed as directed.
5. Serum iron levels not useful until 3 weeks, ferritin peaks in 7-9 days and reliable at 3 weeks.
6. May alter bone scans and discolor blood brown in samples drawn 4 hr after treatment.
7. May falsely elevate bilirubin and decrease calcium. Keep this in mind when monitoring lab values.

CLIENT/FAMILY TEACHING

1. May notice pain and brown staining at injection site.
2. Do not consume oral iron or vitamins when receiving injections. Iron poisoning may occur if intake excessive.

3. Stools usually appear black to dark green in color during therapy.
4. Therapy may end once anemia corrected.

OUTCOMES/EVALUATE

Iron replacement with iron deficiency anemia

Isoetharine hydrochloride

(eye-so-**ETH**-ah-reen)

PREGNANCY CATEGORY: C
CLASSIFICATION(S):
Sympathomimetic
Rx:

SEE ALSO *SYMPATHOMIMETIC DRUGS.*

ACTION/KINETICS

Has a greater stimulating activity on beta-2 receptors of the bronchi than on beta-1 receptors of the heart. Causes relief of bronchospasms. **Inhalation: Onset,** within 5 min; **peak effect:** 15–60 min; **duration:** 2–3 hr. Partially metabolized; excreted in urine.

USES

Bronchial asthma, bronchospasms due to chronic bronchitis or emphysema, bronchiectasis, pulmonary obstructive disease.

SPECIAL CONCERNS

Safety and efficacy have not been established in children less than 12 years of age.

HOW SUPPLIED

Solution for Inhalation: 1%

DOSAGE

- **INHALATION SOLUTION, 1%**

Hand nebulizer.

Adults: 3–7 inhalations of the undiluted solution.

Oxygen aerosolization.

Adults, usual: 0.5 mL (range: 1–2 mL of 1:3 dilution). Give with oxygen flow adjusted to 4–6 L/min over 15–20 min.

IPPB.

Adults, usual: 0.5 mL (range: 1–4 mL of 1:3 dilution). Usual inspiratory flow rate is 15 L/min at a cycling pressure of 15 cm H_2O. May be necessary (depending on client and type of IPPB apparatus) to adjust flow rate to 6–30 L/min and cycling pressure to 10–15 cm H_2O (further dilution may also be required).

NURSING CONSIDERATIONS

SEE SPECIAL *NURSING CONSIDERATIONS* FOR *ADRENERGIC BRONCHODILATORS* UNDER *SYMPATHOMIMETIC DRUGS.*

ADMINISTRATION/STORAGE

1. One or 2 inhalations are usually sufficient; wait 1 min after initial dose to determine if another dose needed.
2. Usually does not need to be repeated more than q 4 hr.
3. Do not use if solution contains a precipitate or is brown.

ASSESSMENT

Document indications for therapy, pulmonary assessments, oxygen saturation, X-rays and review PFTs. Note any allergy to sulfites.

CLIENT/FAMILY TEACHING

1. Review proper technique for administration.
2. Rinse mouth and equipment after each use.
3. Increase fluid intake to help liquify secretions.
4. Stop smoking; enroll in smoking cessation program. Avoid triggers.

OUTCOMES/EVALUATE

Improved airway exchange; ↓ airway resistance

Isoniazid (INH, Isonicotinic acid hydrazide)

(eye-so-**NYE**-ah-zid)

PREGNANCY CATEGORY: C
CLASSIFICATION(S):
Antitubercular drug
Rx: Laniazid, Nydrazid Injection
✱Rx: Isotamine, PMS-Isoniazid

ACTION/KINETICS

The most effective tuberculostatic agent. Probably interferes with lipid and nucleic acid metabolism of growing bacteria, resulting in alteration of the bacterial wall. Is tuberculostatic.

Readily absorbed after PO and parenteral (IM) administration and widely distributed in body tissues, including cerebrospinal, pleural, and ascitic fluids. **Peak plasma concentration: PO,** 1–2 hr. **t½, fast acetylators:** 0.5–6 hr; **t½, slow acetylators:** 2–5 hr. Liver and kidney impairment increase these values. Metabolized in liver and excreted primarily in urine.

The metabolism of isoniazid is genetically determined. Clients fall into two groups, depending on the rapidity with which they metabolize isoniazid. As a rule, 50% of whites and Blacks inactivate the drug slowly, whereas the majority of American Indians, Eskimos, Japanese, and Chinese are rapid acetylators (inactivators).

1. **Slow acetylators:** These clients show earlier, favorable response but have more toxic reactions (e.g., neuropathies because of higher blood levels of drug).
2. **Rapid acetylators:** These clients have possible poor clinical response due to rapid inactivation, which is 5–6 times faster than slow acetylators. This group requires an increased daily dose of the drug. They are more likely to develop hepatitis.

USES

(1) Tuberculosis caused by human, bovine, and BCG strains of *Mycobacterium tuberculosis.* Not to be used as the sole tuberculostatic agent. (2) Prophylaxis of tuberculosis in the following: HIV, close contacts with those newly diagnosed with infectious tuberculosis, recent converters, abnormal chest radiographs, IV drug users, those with increased risk of tuberculosis, those less than 35 years of age with tuberculin skin test reaction 10 mm or greater, and children less than 4 years of age if they have greater than 10 mm induration from a purified protein derviative Mantoux tuberculin skin test. *Investigational:* To improve severe tremor in clients with multiple sclerosis.

CONTRAINDICATIONS

Severe hypersensitivity to isoniazid or in clients with previous isoniazid-associated hepatic injury or side effects.

SPECIAL CONCERNS

Severe and sometimes fatal hepatitis may occur even after several months of therapy; incidence is age-related and current alcohol use increases the risk. Increased risk of fatal hepatitis in minority women, especially Blacks and Hispanics; also increased risk postpartum. Extreme caution should be exercised in clients with convulsive disorders, in whom the drug should be administered only when the client is adequately controlled by anticonvulsant medication. Also, use with caution for the treatment of renal tuberculosis and, in the lowest dose possible, in clients with impaired renal function and in alcoholics.

SIDE EFFECTS

Neurologic: Peripheral neuropathy characterized by symmetrical numbness and tingling of extremities (dose-related). Rarely, toxic encephalopathy, optic neuritis, optic atrophy, ***seizures,*** impaired memory, toxic psychosis. **GI:** N&V, epigastric distress, xerostomia. **Hypersensitivity:** Fever, skin rashes and eruptions, vasculitis, lymphadenopathy. **Hepatic:** Liver dysfunction, jaundice, bilirubinemia, bilirubinuria, ***serious and sometimes fatal hepatitis*** (especially in clients over 50 years of age). Increases in serum AST and ALT. **Hematologic:** ***Agranulocytosis,*** eosinophilia, thrombocytopenia, ***hemolytic, sideroblastic, or aplastic anemia.*** **Metabolic/Endocrine:** Metabolic acidosis, pyridoxine deficiency, pellagra, hyperglycemia, gynecomastia. **Miscellaneous:** Tinnitus, urinary retention, rheumatic syndrome, lupus-like syndrome, arthralgia.

NOTE: Pyridoxine, 10–50 mg/day, may be given concomitantly with isoniazid to decrease CNS side effects. Ophthalmologic and liver function tests are recommended periodically.

LABORATORY TEST CONSIDERATIONS

Altered liver function tests. False + or ↑ potassium, AST, ALT, urine glucose (Benedict's test, Clinitest).

OD OVERDOSE MANAGEMENT

Symptoms: N&V, dizziness, blurred vision, slurred speech, visual hallucinations within 30–180 min. Severe overdosage may cause respiratory distress, ***CNS depression (coma can occur), severe seizures,*** metabolic acidosis, acetonuria, hyperglycemia. *Treatment:* Maintain respiration and undertake gastric lavage (within first 2–3 hr providing seizures are not present). To control seizures, give diazepam or a short-acting IV barbiturate followed by pyridoxine (1 mg IV/1 mg isoniazid ingested). Sodium bicarbonate IV to correct metabolic acidosis. Forced osmotic diuresis; monitor fluid I&O. For severe cases, consider hemodialysis or peritoneal dialysis.

DRUG INTERACTIONS

Aluminum salts / ↓ Effect of isoniazid R/T ↓ GI tract absorption
Anticoagulants, oral / ↓ Anticoagulant effect
Atropine / ↑ Side effects of isoniazid
Benzodiazepines / ↑ Effect of benzodiazepines that undergo oxidative metabolism (e.g., diazepam, triazolam)
Carbamazepine / ↑ Risk of carbamazepine and isoniazid toxicity
Chlorzoxazone / ↑ Chlorzoxazone peak levels and plasma elimination t½ R/T ↓ liver metabolism
Cycloserine / ↑ Risk of cycloserine CNS side effects
Disulfiram / ↑ Risk of acute behavioral and coordination changes
Enflurane / May → high levels of hydrazine → ↑ defluorination of enflurane
Ethanol / ↑ Chance of isoniazid-induced hepatitis
Halothane / ↑ Risk of hepatotoxicity and hepatic encephalopathy
Hydantoins (phenytoin) / ↑ Hydantoins effect R/T ↓ liver breakdown
Ketoconazole / ↓ Serum ketoconazole levels → ↓ effect
Meperidine / ↑ Risk of hypotension or CNS depression
Niacin / Possible ↑ of niacin requirements
Amino salicylate / ↑ Effect of isoniazid by ↑ blood levels
Pyridoxine / Possible ↑ of pyridoxine requirements
Rifampin / Additive liver toxicity

HOW SUPPLIED

Injection: 100 mg/mL; *Syrup:* 50 mg/5 mL; *Tablet:* 50 mg, 100 mg, 300 mg

DOSAGE

• **SYRUP, TABLETS**

Active tuberculosis.

Adults: 5 mg/kg/day (up to 300 mg/day) as a single dose; **children and infants:** 10–20 mg/kg/day (up to 300 mg total) in a single dose.

Prophylaxis.

Adults: 300 mg/day in a single dose; **children and infants:** 10 mg/kg/day (up to 300 mg total) in a single dose.

• **IM**

Active tuberculosis.

Adults: 5 mg/kg (up to 300 mg) once daily. **Pediatric:** 10–20 mg/kg (up to 300 mg) once daily.

Prophylaxis.

Adults/adolescents: 300 mg/day. **Pediatric:** 10 mg/kg/day.

NOTE: Pyridoxine, 6–50 mg/day, is recommended in the malnourished and those prone to neuropathy (e.g., alcoholics, diabetics).

NURSING CONSIDERATIONS

ADMINISTRATION/STORAGE

1. Store in dark, tightly closed containers.
2. Solutions for IM injection may crystallize at low temperature; warm to room temperature if precipitation is evident.
3. Anticipate a slight local irritation at the site of injection. Rotate and document injection sites.
4. Administer with pyridoxine, 10–50 mg/day, in malnourished, alcoholic, or diabetic clients to prevent symptoms of peripheral neuropathy.

ASSESSMENT

1. Document indications for therapy, type/onset of symptoms and note if travel outside of country. List other therapies used and outcome.
2. Obtain baseline labs, CXR, and AFB sputums; note date of PPD conversion. Monitor renal and LFTs; reduce dose with dysfunction.
3. New PPD converters without symptoms still require treatment and then yearly CXR. +AFB clients require treatment and isolation initially and

tracking/treatment of contacts if +AFB or PPD converters.

4. Perform pulmonary assessment; note cough/sputum characteristics.

CLIENT/FAMILY TEACHING

1. Take on an empty stomach 1 hr before or 2 hr after meals.
2. Consume 2–3 L/day of fluids to ensure adequate hydration.
3. Pyridoxine is given to prevent neurotoxic drug effects (peripheral neuritis).
4. Avoid alcohol to prevent hepatic toxicity.
5. Withhold drug and report fatigue, weakness, malaise, and anorexia (S&S of hepatitis).
6. Report any visual disturbances; may precede optic neuritis.
7. With diabetes, monitor FS closely.
8. Take drugs as ordered, missing doses may require retreatment; report for periodic lab and eye exams.

OUTCOMES/EVALUATE

- Negative sputum cultures for AFB
- ↓ Neurotoxic drug effects
- Symptomatic improvement (↓ fever, ↓ secretions, ↑ appetite)

Isophane insulin suspension (NPH)

(**EYE**-so-fayn **IN**-sue-lin)

CLASSIFICATION(S):
Insulin product
★**Rx: Pork:** Iletin II Pork NPH
Human: Novolin ge NPH
OTC: Human: Humulin N, Novolin N, Novolin N PenFill, Novolin N Prefilled,
Pork: NPH Iletin II

SEE ALSO *INSULINS*.

ACTION/KINETICS

Contains zinc insulin crystals modified by protamine, appearing as a cloudy or milky suspension. Not recommended for emergency use. Not suitable for IV administration or in the presence of ketosis. **Onset:** 1–1.5 hr. **Peak:** 4–12 hr. **Duration:** Up to 24 hr. *NOTE:* NPH beef/pork insulins are being phased out.

HOW SUPPLIED

Injection: 100 U/mL

DOSAGE

- **SC**

Diabetes.

Adult, individualized, usual, initial: 7–26 units as a single dose 30–60 min before breakfast. A second smaller dose may be given, if needed, prior to the evening meal or at bedtime. If necessary, the daily dose may be increased in increments of 2–10 units at daily or weekly intervals until desired control is achieved.

Clients on insulin zinc may be transferred directly to isophane insulin on a unit-for-unit basis. If client is being transferred from regular insulin, the initial dose of isophane should be from two-thirds to three-fourths the dose of regular insulin.

NURSING CONSIDERATIONS

SEE *NURSING CONSIDERATIONS* FOR *INSULINS*.

OUTCOMES/EVALUATE

- Control of BS; HbA1-C < 7
- ↓ Target organ damage

COMBINATION DRUG

Isophane insulin suspension and Insulin injection

(**EYE**-so-fayn **IN**-sue-lin)

CLASSIFICATION(S):
Insulin product
★ **OTC:** Humulin 10/90, Humulin 20/80, Humulin 30/70, Humulin 40/60, Humulin ge 10/90, Humulin ge 20/80, Humulin ge 30/60, Humulin ge 40/60, Humulin ge 50/50
OTC: Human: Humulin 50/50, Humulin 70/30, Novolin 70/30, Novolin 70/30 PenFill, Novolin 70/30 Prefilled

SEE ALSO *INSULINS*.

CONTENT

Contains from 10% to 50% insulin injection and from 50% to 70% isophane insulin. Except for Humulin 50/50 and

Novolin ge 50/50, the larger number in the product refers to the percentage of isophane insulin suspension.

ACTION/KINETICS

This combination allows for a rapid onset (30–60 min) due to insulin injection and a long duration (24 hr) due to isophane insulin. **Peak effect:** 4–8 hr.

HOW SUPPLIED

See Content

DOSAGE

- **SC**

Diabetes.

Adults: Individualized and given once daily 15–30 min before breakfast, or as directed. **Children:** Individualized according to client size.

NURSING CONSIDERATIONS

SEE *NURSING CONSIDERATIONS* FOR *INSULINS*.

OUTCOMES/EVALUATE

Control of BS; HbA1-C < 7

Isoproterenol hydrochloride

PREGNANCY CATEGORY: C

Rx: Isuprel Mistometer , Isuprel

Isoproterenol sulfate

PREGNANCY CATEGORY: C

Rx: Medihaler-Iso

CLASSIFICATION(S):

Sympathomimetic

SEE ALSO *SYMPATHOMIMETIC DRUGS*.

ACTION/KINETICS

Produces pronounced stimulation of both beta-1 and beta-2 receptors of the heart, bronchi, skeletal muscle vasculature, and the GI tract. Has both positive inotropic and chronotropic activity; systolic BP may increase while diastolic BP may decrease. Thus, mean arterial BP may not change or may be decreased. Causes less hyperglycemia than epinephrine, but produces bronchodilation and the same degree of CNS excitation. **Inhalation: Onset,** 2–5 min; **peak effect:** 3–5 min; **duration:** 1–3 hr. **IV: Onset,** immediate; **duration:** less than 1 hr. Partially metabolized; excreted in urine.

USES

Inhalation: Relief of bronchospasms associated with acute and chronic asthma, chronic bronchitis, or emphysema. **Injection:** Bronchospasm during anesthesia. As an adjunct to fluid and electrolyte replacement therapy to treat hypovolemic and septic shock, low cardiac output states, CHF, and cardiogenic shock. Mild or transient heart block that does not require electric shock or pacemaker therapy. For serious episodes of heart block and Adams-Stokes attacks, except when caused by ventricular tachycardia or fibrillation. Use in cardiac arrest until electric shock or pacemaker therapy is available.

CONTRAINDICATIONS

Tachyarrhythmias, tachycardia, or heart block caused by digitalis intoxication, ventricular arrhythmias that require inotropic therapy, and angina pectoris.

SPECIAL CONCERNS

Use with caution during lactation and in the presence of tuberculosis. Safety and effectiveness have not been determined in children less than 12 years of age.

ADDITIONAL SIDE EFFECTS

CV: ***Cardiac arrest,*** Adams-Stokes attack, hypotension, precordial pain or distress. **CNS:** Hyperactivity, hyperkinesia. **Respiratory:** Wheezing, bronchitis, increase in sputum, ***bronchial edema and inflammation, pulmonary edema, paradoxical airway resistance.*** Excessive inhalation causes refractory bronchial obstruction. **Miscellaneous:** Flushing, sweating, swelling of the parotid gland. Sublingual administration may cause buccal ulceration. Side effects of drug are less severe after inhalation.

DRUG INTERACTIONS

Bretylium / Possibility of arrhythmias

Guanethidine / ↑ Pressor response of isoproterenol

Halogenated hydrocarbon anesthetics / Sensitization of the heart to catecholamines → serious arrhythmias

Oxytocic drugs / Possibility of severe, persistent hypertension

Tricyclic antidepressants / Potentiation of pressor effect

HOW SUPPLIED

Isoproterenol Hydrochloride: *Metered dose inhaler (Aerosol):* 103 mcg/inh; *Injection:* 0.02 mg/mL (1:50,000), 0.2 mg/mL (1:5000); *Solution for Inhalation:* 0.5% (1:200), 1% (1:100). **Isoproterenol Sulfate:** *Metered dose inhaler:* 80 mcg/inh

DOSAGE

ISOPROTERENOL HYDROCHLORIDE

• **INHALATION**

Acute bronchial asthma.

Hand bulb nebulizer. **Adults and children:** Give 5–15 deep inhalations of the 1:200 solution. Alternatively, in adults, give 3–7 deep inhalations of the 1:100 solution. If no relief occurs after 5–10 min, repeat doses once more. If acute attack recurs, can repeat treatment up to 5 times/day, if necessary. *Metered dose inhaler.* One inhalation (103 mcg). Wait 1 min to determine effect before considering a second inhalation. Repeat up to 5 times/day, if necessary.

Bronchospasm in COPD.

Hand bulb nebulizer. Give 5–15 deep inhalations using the 1:200 solution. Severe attacks may require 3–7 inhalations using the 1:100 solution. Wait at least 3–4 hr between doses. *Nebulization by compressed air or oxygen.* Dilute 0.5 mL of the 1:200 solution to 2–2.5 mL with appropriate diluent for a concentration of 1:800 to 1:1000. Deliver the solution over 10–20 min. May repeat up to 5 times/day. *Intermittent positive pressure breathing.* Dilute 0.5 mL of the 1:200 solution to 2–2.5 mL with water or isotonic saline. Deliver over 15–20 min. May repeat up to 5 times/day. *Metered dose inhaler.* 1 or 2 inhalations repeated at no less than 3–4 hr intervals (6–8 times/day). **Children:** For acute bronchospasms, use the 1:200 solution. Do not use more than 0.25 mL of the 1:200 solution for each 10–15 min programmed treatment.

• **IV**

Bronchospasms during anesthesia.

Dilute 1 mL of a 1:5000 solution to 10 mL with NaCl injection or D5W. **Initial dose:** 0.01–0.02 mg (0.5–1 mL of diluted solution). Repeat when necessary.

Hypovolemic and septic shock.

Start the 1:50,000 solution at the lowest recommended dose and increase the rate of administration gradually, while carefully monitoring.

Heart block, Adams-Stokes attacks, cardiac arrest.

IV injection. Dilute 1 mL of the 1:5000 solution (0.2 mg) to 10 mL with NaCl or D5W. **Initial dose:** 0.02–0.06 mg (1–3 mL of diluted solution); **then,** 0.01–0.2 mg (0.5–10 mL of diluted solution). *IV infusion.* Dilute 10 mL of the 1:5000 solution (2 mg) in 500 mL of D5W or dilute 5 mL of the 1:5000 solution (1 mg) in 250 mL of D5W. **Initial dose:** 5 mcg/min (1.25 mL/min of diluted solution).

• **IM**

Heart block, Adams-Stokes attacks, cardiac arrest.

Initial: 0.2 mg (1 mL) of undiluted 1:5000 solution; **then,** 0.02–1 mg (0.1–5 mL) of undiluted 1:5000 solution.

• **SC**

Heart block, Adams-Stokes attacks, cardiac arrest.

Initial: 0.2 mg (1 mL) of undiluted 1:5000 solution; **then,** 0.15–0.2 mg (0.75–1 mL) of undiluted 1:5000 solution.

• **INTRACARDIAC**

Emergency use in heart block, Adams-Stokes attacks, cardiac arrest.

Give 0.02 mg (0.1 mL) of the undiliuted 1:5000 solution.

ISOPROTERENOL SULFATE

• **INHALATION**

Acute bronchial asthma.

Initial: 1 inhalation (80 mcg). If no relief is evident after 2–5 min, a second inhalation may be given. **Maintenance:** 1–2 inhalations 4–6 times/day. Do not give more than 2 inhalations at any one time and no more than 6 inhalations/hr.

NURSING CONSIDERATIONS

SEE ALSO *SPECIAL NURSING CONSIDERATIONS FOR ADRENERGIC BRONCHODILATORS* UNDER *SYMPATHOMIMETIC DRUGS*.

ADMINISTRATION/STORAGE

1. Administration to children, except where noted, is the same as that for adults; their smaller ventilatory exchange capacity will permit a proportionally smaller aerosol intake. For their acute bronchospasms, use 1:200 solution.
2. In children, no more than 0.25 mL of the 1:200 solution should be used for each 10–15 min of programmed treatment.
3. Elderly clients usually receive a lower dose.

IV 4. Do not use the injection if it is pinkish to brownish in color. Protect from light and store at 15–30°C (59–86°F).

ASSESSMENT

1. Document indications for therapy, triggers, characteristics of symptoms.
2. Perform pulmonary assessment; note PFTs and CXRs. Report respiratory problems that worsen after administration; refractory reactions may necessitate drug withdrawal.
3. Identify arrhythmias (especially ventricular) and angina; may preclude drug therapy.

CLIENT/FAMILY TEACHING

1. Review method for inhaler use; a spacer enhances dispersion.
2. Rinse mouth and equipment with water; removes drug residue and minimizes dryness after inhalation.
3. Maintain fluid intake of 2–3 L/day to help liquefy secretions.
4. Sputum and saliva may appear pink after inhalation therapy; do not become alarmed.
5. When also taking inhalant glucocorticoids, take isoproterenol first and wait 15 min before using the second inhaler.
6. Do not use more often than prescribed; over use can cause severe cardiac and respiratory problems.
7. Identify parotid gland; withhold drug and report if enlarged.
8. Stop smoking now to preserve current level of lung function; enroll in smoking cessation program.

OUTCOMES/EVALUATE

- Improved airway exchange
- ↓ Bronchoconstriction/spasms
- Stable cardiac rhythm

Isosorbide dinitrate

(eye-so-**SOR**-byd)

PREGNANCY CATEGORY: C
CLASSIFICATION(S):
Coronary vasodilator
Rx: Dilatrate-SR, Isordil, Isordil Tembids, Isordil Titradose, Sorbitrate
✱Rx: Apo-ISDN, Cedocard-SR

SEE ALSO *ANTIANGINAL DRUGS, NITRATES/NITRITES*.

ACTION/KINETICS

Sublingual, chewable. Onset: 2–5 min; **duration:** 1–3 hr. **Oral Capsules/Tablets. Onset:** 20–40 min; **duration:** 4–6 hr. **Extended-release. Onset:** up to 4 hr; **duration:** 6–8 hr.

ADDITIONAL USES

Diffuse esophageal spasm. Oral tablets are only for prophylaxis while sublingual and chewable forms may be used to terminate acute attacks of angina.

ADDITIONAL CONTRAINDICATIONS

Use to abort acute anginal attacks.

SPECIAL CONCERNS

Use with caution during lactation. Safety and efficacy have not been established in children.

ADDITIONAL SIDE EFFECTS

Vascular headaches occur especially frequently.

ADDITIONAL DRUG INTERACTIONS

Acetylcholine / Acetylcholine effect antagonized
Norepinephrine / Norepinephrine effect antagonized

HOW SUPPLIED

Chew Tablet: 5 mg, 10 mg; *Capsule, Extended Release:* 40 mg; *Tablet:* 5 mg, 10 mg, 20 mg, 30 mg, 40 mg; *Tablet, Extended Release:* 40 mg; *Tablet, Sublingual:* 2.5 mg, 5 mg, 10 mg

DOSAGE

- **TABLETS**

Antianginal.

Initial: 5–20 mg q 6 hr; **maintenance:** 10–40 g q 6 hr (usual: 20–40 mg q.i.d.

- **CHEWABLE TABLETS**

Antianginal, acute attack.

Initial: 5 mg q 2–3 hr. The dose can be titrated upward until angina is relieved or side effects occur.

Prophylaxis.
5–10 mg q 2–3 hr.

• **EXTENDED-RELEASE CAPSULES**
Antianginal.
Initial: 40 mg; **maintenance:** 40–80 mg q 8–12 hr.

• **EXTENDED-RELEASE TABLETS**
Antianginal.
Initial: 40 mg; **maintenance:** 40–80 mg q 8–12 hr.

• **SUBLINGUAL**
Acute attack.
2.5–5 mg q 2–3 hr as required. The dose can be titrated upward until angina is relieved or side effects occur.
Prophylaxis.
5–10 mg q 2–3 hr.

NURSING CONSIDERATIONS

SEE ALSO *NURSING CONSIDERATIONS* FOR *ANTIANGINAL DRUGS, NITRATES/NITRITES*.

ASSESSMENT

1. Note onset, location, and characteristics of pain. Rate pain levels.
2. Assess ECG; note stress thallium or catherization findings as well as CAD history.

CLIENT/FAMILY TEACHING

1. Administer with meals to eliminate or reduce headaches; otherwise, take on an empty stomach to facilitate absorption. Leave product in original container.
2. Tolerance may develop. Short-acting products can be given b.i.d.–t.i.d. with the last dose no later than 7:00 p.m. The extended-release products can be given once or twice daily at 8:00 a.m. and 2:00 p.m.
3. Review method for administration; do not chew SL tablets. None of the products should be crushed or chewed, unless ordered.
4. Hold chewable tablets in the mouth for 1–2 min; allows absorption through buccal membranes.
5. May take before any stressful activity (sexual activity, exercise).
6. Avoid hazardous activity if dizziness occurs and all forms of alcohol.
7. Acetaminophen may assist to relieve drug-induced headaches.

OUTCOMES/EVALUATE

- ↓ Frequency/severity of attacks
- ↑ Exercise tolerance
- Resolution of esophageal spasm

Isosorbide mononitrate

(eye-so-**SOR**-byd)

PREGNANCY CATEGORY: C
CLASSIFICATION(S):
Coronary vasodilator
Rx: Imdur, ISMO, Monoket

SEE ALSO *ANTIANGINAL DRUGS, NITRATES/NITRITES*, AND *ISOSORBIDE DINITRATE*.

ACTION/KINETICS

Isosorbide mononitrate is the major metabolite of isosorbide dinitrate. The mononitrate is not subject to first-pass metabolism. Bioavailability is nearly 100%. **Onset:** 30–60 min. **t½:** About 5 hr.

USES

Prophylaxis and treatment of angina pectoris.

CONTRAINDICATIONS

To abort acute anginal attacks. Use in acute MI or CHF.

SPECIAL CONCERNS

Use with caution during lactation and in clients who may be volume depleted or who are already hypotensive. Safety and effectiveness have not been determined in children. The benefits have not been established in acute MI or CHF.

SIDE EFFECTS

CV: Hypotension (may be accompanied by paradoxical bradycardia and increased angina pectoris). **CNS:** Headache, lightheadedness, dizziness. **GI:** N&V. **Miscellaneous:** Possibility of methemoglobinemia.

OD OVERDOSE MANAGEMENT

Symptoms: Increased intracranial pressure manifested by throbbing headache, confusion, moderate fever. Also, vertigo, palpitations, visual disturbances, N&V, syncope, air hunger, dyspnea (followed by reduced ventilatory effort), diaphoresis, skin either flushed or cold and clammy, heart block, bradycardia, paralysis, ***coma, seizures, death.*** *Treatment:* Direct therapy toward an increase in central fluid volume. Do *not* use vasoconstrictors.

DRUG INTERACTIONS

Ethanol / Additive vasodilation
Calcium channel blockers / Severe orthostatic hypotension
Organic nitrates / Severe orthostatic hypotension

HOW SUPPLIED

Tablet: 10 mg, 20 mg; *Tablet, Extended Release:* 30 mg, 60 mg, 120 mg

DOSAGE

TABLETS

Prophylaxis of angina.

20 mg b.i.d. with the two doses given 7 hr apart, with the first dose upon awakening. A starting dose of 5 mg (½ tablet of the 10 mg tablet) may be appropriate for clients of particularly small stature; however, increase to at least 10 mg by the second or third day.

TABLETS, EXTENDED RELEASE

Prophylaxis of angina.

Initial: 30 mg (given as one-half of the 60-mg tablet) or 60 mg once daily; **then,** after several days dosage may be increased to 120 mg given as 2–60-mg tablets once daily. Rarely, 240 mg daily may be needed.

NURSING CONSIDERATIONS

SEE ALSO *NURSING CONSIDERATIONS FOR ANTIANGINAL DRUGS, NITRATES/NITRITES,* AND *ISOSORBIDE DINITRATE.*

ADMINISTRATION/STORAGE

The treatment regimen minimizes the development of refractory tolerance.

CLIENT/FAMILY TEACHING

1. Consume 1–2 L/day of fluids to ensure adequate hydration.
2. Take the extended-release tablet in the morning upon arising. Do not crush or chew; take with a half glass of water.
3. May cause marked hypotension.
4. Report if angina persists/recurs.

OUTCOMES/EVALUATE

Angina prophylaxis

Isotretinoin

(eye-so-**TRET**-ih-noyn)

PREGNANCY CATEGORY: X
CLASSIFICATION(S):
Retinoid
Rx: Accutane
★Rx: Accutane Roche, Isotrex

ACTION/KINETICS

Reduces sebaceous gland size, decreases sebum secretion, and inhibits abnormal keratinization. Approximately 25% of the PO dosage form is bioavailable. **Peak plasma levels:** 3 hr. **Steady-state blood levels following 80 mg/day:** 160 ng/mL. Nearly 100% bound to plasma protein. **t½:** 10–20 hr. Metabolized in the liver to 4-oxo-isotretinoin, which is also active. Approximately equal amounts are excreted through the urine and in the feces.

USES

Severe recalcitrant nodular acne unresponsive to standard therapies. *Investigational:* Treat premalignant lesions and reduce incidence of second primary tumors in clients with prior head and neck, lung, or liver cancers.

CONTRAINDICATIONS

Due to the possibility of fetal abnormalities or spontaneous abortion at any dose, women who are pregnant or intend to become pregnant should not use the drug. Certain conditions for use should be met in women with childbearing potential (see package insert). Use during lactation and in children.

SPECIAL CONCERNS

Intolerance to contact lenses may develop. Increased risks for birth defects and psychiatric disorders (including suicidal tendencies).

SIDE EFFECTS

Skin: Cheilitis, skin fragility, pruritus, dry skin, desquamation of facial skin, drying of mucous membranes, brittle nails, photosensitivity, rash, hypo- or hyperpigmentation, urticaria, erythema nodosum, hirsutism, excess granulation of tissues as a result of healing, petechiae, peeling of palms and soles, skin infections, paronychia, thinning of hair, nail dystrophy, pyogenic granuloma, bruising, acne fulminans, sweating. **CNS:** Headache, fatigue, pseudotumor cerebri (i.e., headaches, papilledema, disturbances in vision, dizziness), depression, psychosis, suicidal ideation, ***suicide attempts, suicide,*** drowsiness, insomnia, lethargy, malaise, nervousness, paresthesias, ***seizures, stroke,*** syncope, weakness, emotional instability. **Hematologic:** Neutropenia, thrombocytopenia, anemia, ***agranulocytosis.*** **Ocular:** Conjunctivitis, optic neuritis, corneal opacities, dry eyes, decrease in acuity of night vision, photophobia, eyelid inflammation, cataracts, visual disturbances, color vision disorder, keratitis. **GI:** Dry mouth, N&V, abdominal pain, nonspecific GI symptoms, hepatitis, hepatotoxicity, inflammatory bowel disease (including regional enteritis), anorexia, weight loss, ***acute pancreatitis,*** inflammation and bleeding of gums, colitis, ileitis. **Neuromuscular:** Arthralgia, muscle pain, bone and joint pain and stiffness, skeletal hyperostosis, calcification of tendons and ligaments, premature epiphyseal closure, arthritis, tendonitis. **CV:** Flushing, palpitation, tachycardia, vascular thrombotic disease. **GU:** White cells in urine, proteinuria, nonspecific urogenital findings, microscopic or gross hematuria, abnormal menses, glomerular nephritis. **Respiratory:** Bronchospasms with or without a history of asthma, respiratory infections, voice alterations, epistaxis, dry nose. **Other:** Dry mouth, disseminated herpes simplex, edema, transient chest pain, development of diabetes, vasculitis, lymphadenopathy, flushing, impaired hearing, tinnitus, severe allergic reactions (including ***anaphylaxis,*** cutaneous allergic reactions, allergic vasculitis, purpura).

LABORATORY TEST CONSIDERATIONS

↑ Plasma triglycerides, sedimentation rate, platelet counts, alkaline phosphatase, AST, ALT, GGTP, LDH, fasting blood glucose, uric acid in blood, cholesterol, CPK levels in clients who exercise vigorously. ↓ HDL, RBC parameters, WBC counts.

OD OVERDOSE MANAGEMENT

Symptoms: Abdominal pain, ataxia, cheilosis, dizziness, facial flushing, headache, vomiting. Symptoms are transient. *Treatment:* Symptoms are quickly resolved with drug cessation or decrease in dose.

DRUG INTERACTIONS

Alcohol / Potentiation of ↑ serum triglycerides
Benzoyl peroxide / ↑ Drying effects of isotretinoin
Carbamazepine / ↓ Plasma carbamazepine levels
Minocycline / ↑ Risk of developing pseudotumor cerebri or papilledema
Tetracycline / ↑ Risk of developing pseudotumor cerebri or papilledema
Tretinoin / ↑ Drying effects of isotretinoin
Vitamin A / ↑ Risk of toxicity

HOW SUPPLIED

Capsule: 10 mg, 20 mg, 40 mg

DOSAGE

• CAPSULES

Recalcitrant cystic acne.

Adults, individualized, initial: 0.5–1 mg/kg/day (range: 0.5–2 mg/kg/day) divided in two doses for 15–20 weeks. Adjust dose based on toxicity and clinical response; if cyst count decreases by 70% or more, drug may be discontinued. If necessary, a second course of therapy may be instituted after a rest period of 2 months. Doses of 0.05–0.5 mg/kg/day are effective but result in higher frequency of relapses.

Keratinization disorders.

Doses up to 4 mg/kg/day have been used.

Prevent second tumors in squamous-cell carcinoma of the head and neck.

50–100 mg/m^2.

NURSING CONSIDERATIONS

ADMINISTRATION/STORAGE

1. Before using drug, have client complete consent form included with the package insert.
2. A rest period of 2 months is recommended if a second course of therapy is needed.

ASSESSMENT

1. Document clinical presentation; photos may help.
2. Perform a pregnancy test on all potentially fertile females.
3. Determine other agents used and the outcome.
4. Monitor serum glucose levels, chemistry, CBC, urinalysis, and LFTs, especially lipoprotein, cholesterol, and triglycerides.

CLIENT/FAMILY TEACHING

1. Before receiving isotretinoin, clients must sign an informed consent form that details the risks associated with isotretinoin use. Clients will also receive a medication guide and must have watched the videotape that gives information about contraceptive methods. Females must confirm they have a negative result for the second urine pregnancy request, conducted on the second day of the next menstrual period or 11 days or more after the last unprotected act of sexual intercourse, whichever is later.
2. Do not crush capsules. Food or milk will increase the absorption of isotretinoin
3. Avoid donating blood for 30 days after discontinuing drug therapy.
4. Drug is teratogenic; perform monthly pregnancy test. Females of childbearing age should practice reliable birth control 1 mo before, during, and 1 mo following therapy; severe fetal damage may occur.
5. A 30-day prescription will be dispensed to ensure compliance.
6. Report if persistent headache, N&V, or visual disturbances occur. Lubricants may help diminish symptoms of dry, chapped skin and lips.
7. Contact lens wearers may develop sensitivity to contacts during and after therapy. Excessively dry eyes may require an eye lubricant.
8. Condition may become worse before healing starts.
9. Avoid OTC meds, especially vitamin A, without consent.
10. Eliminate or markedly reduce consumption of alcohol; may increase triglyceride levels.
11. Avoid prolonged sunlight exposure; may cause photosensitivity. Wear protective clothing, sunscreen, and sunglasses when exposed.
12. Possible decreased tolerance to contact lenses.

OUTCOMES/EVALUATE

↓ Number and severity of cystic acne lesions

Isradipine

(iss-**RAD**-ih-peen)

PREGNANCY CATEGORY: C

CLASSIFICATION(S):

Antihypertensive, calcium channel blocking drug

Rx: DynaCirc, DynaCirc CR

SEE ALSO *CALCIUM CHANNEL BLOCKING AGENTS.*

ACTION/KINETICS

Binds to calcium channels resulting in the inhibition of calcium influx into cardiac and smooth muscle and subsequent arteriolar vasodilation. Reduced systemic resistance leads to a decrease in BP with a small increase in resting HR. In clients with normal ventricular function, the drug reduces afterload leading to some increase in CO. Well absorbed from the GI tract, although it undergoes significant first-pass metabolism. **Peak plasma levels:** 1 ng/mL after 1.5 hr. **Onset:** 2–3 hr. Food increases the time to peak effect by about 1 hr, although the total bioavailability does not change. **t½, initial:** 1.5–2 hr; **terminal,** 8 hr. Completely metabolized in the liver with 60%–65% excreted through the kidneys and 25%–30% through the feces. Maximum effect may not be observed for 2–4 wks.

USES

Alone or with thiazide diuretics in the management of essential hypertension. *Investigational:* Chronic stable angina.

CONTRAINDICATIONS

Lactation.

SPECIAL CONCERNS

Safety and effectiveness have not been determined in children. Use with caution in clients with CHF, especially those taking a beta-adrenergic blocking agent. Bioavailability increases in those over 65 years of age, in impaired hepatic function, and in mild renal impairment.

SIDE EFFECTS

CV: Palpitations, edema, flushing, tachycardia, SOB, hypotension, transient ischemic attack, ***stroke,*** atrial fibrillation, ***ventricular fibrillation, MI,*** CHF, angina. **CNS:** Headache, dizziness, fatigue, drowsiness, insomnia, lethargy, nervousness, depression, syncope, amnesia, psychosis, hallucinations, weakness, jitteriness, paresthesia. **GI:** Nausea, abdominal discomfort, diarrhea, vomiting, constipation, dry mouth. **Respiratory:** Dyspnea, cough. **Dermatologic:** Pruritus, urticaria. **Miscellaneous:** Chest pain, rash, pollakiuria, cramps of the legs and feet, nocturia, polyuria, hyperhidrosis, visual disturbances, numbness, throat discomfort, leukopenia, sexual difficulties.

LABORATORY TEST CONSIDERATIONS

↑ LFTs.

DRUG INTERACTIONS

Severe hypotension possible during fentanyl anesthesia with concomitant use of a beta-blocker and a calcium channel blocker.

HOW SUPPLIED

Capsule: 2.5 mg, 5 mg; *Tablet, Controlled Release:* 5 mg, 10 mg

DOSAGE

• **CAPSULES**

Hypertension.

Adults, initial: 2.5 mg b.i.d. alone or in combination with a thiazide diuretic. If BP is not decreased satisfactorily after 2–4 weeks, the dose may be increased in increments of 5 mg/day at 2 *to* 4-week intervals up to a maximum of 20 mg/day. Adverse effects increase at doses above 10 mg/day.

• **TABLETS, CONTROLLED-RELEASE**

Hypertension.

Adults: 5–10 mg once daily.

NURSING CONSIDERATIONS

SEE *NURSING CONSIDERATIONS* FOR *CALCIUM CHANNEL BLOCKING AGENTS.*

ADMINISTRATION/STORAGE

Store in a tight container protected from light.

CLIENT/FAMILY TEACHING

1. Use caution, may cause dizziness and confusion; assess drug effects.
2. Report any SOB, swelling of extremities, irregular heart beat, or prolonged dizziness.
3. Change positions slowly to prevent rapid drop in BP.
4. Report for scheduled lab tests: liver and renal function studies every 3–6 months.

OUTCOMES/EVALUATE

Control of HTN

Itraconazole

(**ih**-trah-**KON**-ah-zohl)

PREGNANCY CATEGORY: C
CLASSIFICATION(S):
Antifungal
Rx: Sporanox

ACTION/KINETICS

Believed to inhibit cytochrome P-450-dependent synthesis of ergosterol, a necessary component of fungal cell membranes. Absorption appears to increase when taken with a cola beverage. Concentrates in fatty tissues, omentum, liver, kidney, and skin. **t½ at steady-state:** 30–40 hr. Extensively metabolized by the liver; the major metabolite is hydroxyitraconazole, which also has antifungal activity. The drug and major metabolite are extensively bound (over 99%) to plasma proteins. Metabolites are excreted in both the urine and feces.

USES

Capsules: For the following fungal infections in normal, predisposed, or immunocompromised clients: (1) Chronic pulmonary histoplasmosis; (2) Chromomycosis; (3) Blastomycosis; (4) Dermatomycoses due to tinea corporis, tinea cruris, tinea pedis, and pityriasis versicolor when PO therapy is warranted; (5) Onychomycosis; (6) Invasive and noninvasive pulmonary aspergillosis; (7) Oral and oral/esophageal candidiasis; (8) Cutaneous and lymphatic sporotrichosis; (9) Paracoccidioidomycosis.

Oral Solution: Oropharyngeal and esophageal candidiasis in adult HIV-positive or other immunocompromised clients.

Injection: For the following fungal infections in immunocompromised and nonimmunocompromised clients: (1) Pulmonary and extrapulmonary blastomycosis; (2) Histoplasmosis, including chronic cavitary pulmonary disease and dissemintated, nonmeningeal histoplasmosis; (3) Pulmonary and extrapulmonary aspergillosis in those who are intolerant of or refractory to amphotericin B.

Investigational: (1) Superficial mycoses including dermatophytoses (tinea capitis, tinea manuum, tinea pedis) and sebopsoriasis. (2) Systemic mycoses including dimorphic infections (coccidioidomycosis) and cryptococcal infections (meningitis, disseminated). (3) Miscellaneous mycoses including fungal keratitis, alternariosis, leishmaniasis (cutaneous), and zygomycosis.

CONTRAINDICATIONS

Concomitant use of dofetilide, pimozide, quinidine, triazolam, or oral midazolam due to possible serious CV events. Hypersensitivity to the drug or its excipients. Lactation. Use for the treatment of onychomycosis in pregnant women or in women wishing to become pregnant. Use with severe renal dysfunction (C_{CR} less than 30 mL/min) or in clients with a history of cardiac dysfunction (e.g., CHF or a history of CHF) or other ventricular dysfuction. Use with HMG-CoA reductase inhibitors metabolized by the P450 3A enzyme system (i.e., lovastatin, simvastatin).

SPECIAL CONCERNS

Use with caution in clients with hypersensitivity to other azoles. Safety and efficacy have not been determined in children although pediatric clients have been treated for systemic fungal infections. Liver enzymes may be elevated more than twice that of normal.

SIDE EFFECTS

GI: N&V, diarrhea, abdominal pain, anorexia, taste perversion, flatulence, general GI disorders, constipation, dyspepsia, gingivitis, ulcerative stomatitis, gastritis, gastroenteritis, increased appetite, dyspepsia, dysphagia, hemorrhoids, abnormal hepatic function, ***liver failure,*** jaundice. **CNS:** Headache, anxiety, depression, vertigo, dizziness, somnolence, decreased libido, abnormal dreaming, insomnia. **CV:** Hypertension, orthostatic hypotension, vasculitis, congestive heart failure. **Respiratory:** URTI, rhinitis, sinusitis, pharyngitis, coughing, dyspnea, pneumonia, increased sputum. **Dermatologic:** Increased sweating, skin disorders, hot flushes, rash, pruritus. **GU:** UTI, impotence, cystitis, menstrual disorders, abnormal renal function, gynecomastia, hematuria. **Allergic:** Rash, pruritus, urticaria, angioedema, ***anaphylaxis*** (rare). **Body as a whole:** Edema, fatigue, pain, fever, malaise, myalgia, asthenia, tremor, dehydration, infection. **Miscellaneous:** Bursitis, injury, herpes zoster, chest pain, *Pneumocystis carinii* infection, vein disorder, reaction at injection site, adrenal insufficiency, back pain, male breast pain, rigors, tinnitus, abnormal vision, weight loss.

LABORATORY TEST CONSIDERATIONS

↑ ALT, AST, alkaline phosphatase, BUN, serum creatinine. Hypertriglyceridemia, hypokalemia, hypomagnesemia, albuminuria, bilirubinemia. Abnormal hepatic function.

OD OVERDOSE MANAGEMENT

Symptoms: Extension of side effects. *Treatment:* Use supportive measures, including gastric lavage and sodium bicarbonate. Dialysis will not remove itraconazole.

DRUG INTERACTIONS

Alfentanil / ↑ Alfentanil effect and toxicity due to inhibition of metabolism

Amphotericin B / ↓ Activity of amphotericin B

Antacids / ↓ Itraconazole absorption R/T ↓ gastric acidity

Benzodiazepines (Alprazolam, PO Midazolam, Triazolam) / ↑ & Prolonged

serum levels $\rightarrow$ CNS depression and psychomotor impairment
Buspirone / $\uparrow$ Plasma buspirone levels $\rightarrow$ $\uparrow$ effects and toxicity
Calcium blockers / Inhibition of metabolism of felodipine, nifedipine, nisoldipine, and verapamil; also $\uparrow$ negative inotropic effects and possible edema
Carbamazepine / $\uparrow$ Plasma carbamazepine levels $\rightarrow$ clinical and adverse effects
Clarithromycin / $\uparrow$ Plasma itraconazole levels
Corticosteroids / Enhanced corticosteroid effects $\rightarrow$ $\uparrow$ toxicity
Cyclosporine / $\uparrow$ Cyclosporine levels (dose of cyclosporine should be $\downarrow$ by 50% if itraconazole doses are much greater than 100 mg/day)
Didanosine / $\downarrow$ Effects of itraconazole
Digoxin / $\uparrow$ Digoxin levels
Dofetilide / $\uparrow$ Dofetilide levels $\rightarrow$ possible serious CV events; **Do not use together**
Erythromycin / $\uparrow$ Plasma levels of itraconazole $\rightarrow$ serious side effects
Felodipine / $\uparrow$ Serum felodipine levels (possible edema)
Grapefruit juice / $\downarrow$ Itraconazole bioavailability R/T inhibition of absorption
Haloperidol / $\uparrow$ Haloperidol levels $\rightarrow$ $\uparrow$ risk of side effects
H_2 Antagonists / $\downarrow$ Itraconazole absorption R/T $\downarrow$ gastric acidity
HMG-CoA Reductase Inhibitors / $\uparrow$ Plasma levels and side effects of reductase inhibitors; possibility of rhabdomyolysis
Indinavir / $\downarrow$ Itraconazole bioavailability
Losartan / $\uparrow$ Losartan antihypertensive effect
Lovastatin / $\uparrow$ Plasma lovastatin levels $\rightarrow$ possible rhabdomyolysis
Midazolam, oral / $\uparrow$ Levels of oral midazolam $\rightarrow$ potentiation of sedative and hypnotic effects
Nisoldipine / $\uparrow$ Nisoldipine levels
Isoniazid / $\downarrow$ Plasma levels of itraconazole
Oral Contraceptives / $\downarrow$ Oral contraceptive effect
Phenytoin / $\downarrow$ Effect of itraconazole and $\uparrow$ effect of phenytoin (do not use together)
Pimozide / Possible serious CV events, including QT prolongation, torsade de pointes, ventricular tachycardia, cardiac arrest and/or sudden death
Quinidine / Possible serious CV events, including QT prolongation, torsade de pointes, ventricular tachycardia, cardiac arrest and/or sudden death
Protease inhibitors / $\uparrow$ Levels of protease inhibitors $\rightarrow$ $\uparrow$ toxicity
Proton pump inhibitors / $\downarrow$ Itraconazole absorption R/T $\downarrow$ gastric acidity
Quinidine / $\uparrow$ Quinidine levels $\rightarrow$ toxicity
Rifampin, Rifabutin, Rifapentine / $\downarrow$ Itraconazole plasma levels; possible $\uparrow$ rifabutin plasma levels
Simvastatin / $\uparrow$ Plasma simvastatin levels $\rightarrow$ possible rhabdomyolysis
Ritonavir / $\downarrow$ Bioavailability of itraconazole
Sulfonylureas / $\uparrow$ Risk of hypoglycemia
Tacrolimus / $\uparrow$ Tacrolimus levels
Tolterodine / $\uparrow$ Plasma tolterodine levels
Triazolam / $\uparrow$ Drug levels $\rightarrow$ potentiation of sedative and hypnotic effects
Vinca alkaloids / $\uparrow$ Risk of vinca alkaloid toxicity due to inhibition of metabolism
Warfarin / $\uparrow$ Anticoagulant drug effect
Zolpidem / $\uparrow$ Zolpidem effects due to inhibition of metabolism

HOW SUPPLIED

Capsule: 100 mg; *Injection:* 10 mg/mL; *Oral Solution:* 10 mg/mL

DOSAGE

• CAPSULES

Blastomycosis or chronic pulmonary histoplasmosis.

Adults: 200 mg once daily. If there is no improvement or the disease is progressive, the dose may be increased in 100-mg increments to a maximum of 400 mg/day. Give doses greater than 200 mg/day in 2 divided doses.

Oral and oral/esophageal candidiasis.
100 mg/day for 2 weeks (4 weeks for oral/esophageal candidiasis). Increase dose to 200 mg/day in those with AIDS and neutropenia.

Aspergillosis, pulmonary.
200 mg/day for 3–4 months.

Aspergillosis, invasive pulmonary.
200 mg b.i.d. for 3–4 months.

Sporotrichosis, Paracoccidioidomycosis.
100 mg/day for 3 months (sporotrichosis) or 6 months (paracoccidioidomycosis).

Chromomycosis.
If due to *Cladosporium carrioni:* 100 mg/day for 3 months. If due to *Fonsecaea pedrosoi*: 200 mg/day for 6 months.

Dermatomycoses.
For *Tinea corporis/Tinea cruris:* 100 mg once daily for 14 consecutive days. Alternatively, 200 mg/day for 7 consecutive days. For *Tinea pedis:* 100 mg once daily for 28 consecutive days. Alternatively, 200 mg b.i.d. for 7 consecutive days. For *Pityriasis versicolor:* 200 mg once daily for 7 consecutive days.

Onychomycosis.
For a 1-week treatment course, give 200 mg b.i.d. Treatment with 2 one-week courses is recommended for fingernail infections and 3 one-week courses for toenail infections. One-week courses are always separated by a 3-week drug-free interval.

• **ORAL SOLUTION**

Oropharyngeal candidiasis.
200 mg/day (20 mL) in single or divided doses for 1–2 weeks.

Esophageal candidiasis.
100 mg/day (10 mL) for a minimum of 3 weeks. Continue for 2 weeks following resolution of symptoms.

• **IV**

Blastomycosis, histoplasmosis, aspergillosis.
200 mg IV b.i.d. for 4 doses, followed by 200 mg/day. Infuse each IV dose over 1 hr.

NURSING CONSIDERATIONS

ADMINISTRATION/STORAGE

1. Take capsules, but not the oral solution, after a full meal to ensure maximal absorption. Swallow capsules whole. Swish solution in oral cavity and swallow; do not rinse after swallowing.
2. Give daily doses greater than 200 mg in two divided doses.
3. Continue treatment for a minimum of 3 mo until symptoms and lab tests indicate the active fungal infection has subsided. Recurrence of active infection may occur with inadequate treatment period.
4. Do not use capsules and oral solution interchangeably.
5. Absorption from capsules is impaired when gastric acidity is decreased (e.g., use of antacids, proton pump inhibitors, H_2 histamine blockers). Thus, give such drugs at least 2 hr after itraconazole.
6. Plasma levels using capsules are lower in neutropenic and AIDS clients than in healthy subjects. However, the bioavailability of the oral solution in AIDS clients is not different from healthy subjects.
7. Protect capsules from light and moisture. Discard any unused oral solution 3 months after opening.

IV 8. To prepare, add the full contents (25 mL) of the ampule into the infusion bag provided (contains 50 mL of 0.9% NaCl injection). Mix gently. Do not dilute with D5W or lactated Ringer's.

9. Using a flow control device, infuse 60 mL of the dilute solution (which contains 3.33 mg/mL; therefore total dose will be 200 mg) over 60 min, using an extension line and the infusion set provided. After administration, flush the infusion set with 15–20 mL of 0.9% NaCl injection over 0.5–15 min via the 2-way stopcock. Discard the entire infusion line.
10. Do not introduce any other medication through the same bag or same line. Other drugs may be given after flushing the line/catheter with 0.9% NaCl injection, and removing and replacing the entire infusion line.
11. Do not use IV if C_{CR} is less than 30 mL/min.
12. Store the injection at 25°C or less (77°F) and protect from light and freezing after reconstitution, refrigerate

the diluted drug at 2–8°C (36–46°F) or store at room temperature from 15–25°C (59–77°F) for up to 48 hr. Protect from direct light.

ASSESSMENT

1. Document indications for therapy, location, onset, characteristics of symptoms, and other agents prescribed, noting compliance and outcome. Drug is extremely expensive and should not be used as first-line therapy with typical fungal infections.
2. Due to the possibility of liver failure, confirm diagnosis of onychomycosis through scrapings/lab tests.
3. If symptoms of CHF develop, discontinue the drug.
4. List drugs currently prescribed to prevent any unfavorable effects.
5. Monitor CBC, electrolytes, fungal cultures/scrapings, renal and LFTs.
6. Drug is not intended for pregnant or nursing mothers.
7. The response rate of histoplasmosis in HIV-infected clients is similar to non-HIV-infected clients, although the clinical course in HIV-infected clients is more severe and usually requires maintenance therapy to prevent relapse.
8. Absorption may be decreased in HIV-infected clients with hypochlorhydria.

CLIENT/FAMILY TEACHING

1. Take capsules with food to enhance absorption and only as directed (usually for 3 months). Do not take the oral solution with food. Noncompliance or inadequate treatment period may lead to recurrence of active infection.
2. Practice reliable hygiene measures to prevent spread of infection and reinfection.
3. Report S&S suggesting liver dysfunction; i.e., anorexia, unusual fatigue, N&V, diarrhea, yellow skin/eyes, or dark urine. Avoid alcohol during therapy.
4. Report symptoms that may indicate reactivation of histoplasmosis, such as weight loss, chest pain, SOB, fever, rales, and pain.
5. S&S of blastomycosis include SOB, rales, hemoptysis, chest pain, fever, cough, skin lesions, rashes, and weight loss; requires immediate attention.

OUTCOMES/EVALUATE

Eradication of infecting organisms; symptom relief

Ivermectin

(eye-ver-**MEK**-tin)

PREGNANCY CATEGORY: C
CLASSIFICATION(S):
Anthelmintic
Rx: Stromectol

ACTION/KINETICS

Binds selectively to glutamate-gated chloride channels that occur in invertebrate nerve and muscle cells. This leads to increase in permeability of cell membrane to chloride ions and hyperpolarization of nerve or muscle cell, resulting in paralysis and death of parasite. The drug may also interact with other ligand-gated chloride channels (e.g., those gated by GABA). **Peak plasma levels:** About 4 hr. **t½:** About 19 hr. Metabolized in liver and excreted through feces.

USES

(1) Intestinal strongyloidiasis due to *Strongyloides stercoralis.* (2) Onchocerciasis due to *Onchocerca volvulus.* The drug has no effect against adult *Onchocerca volvulus. Investigational:* Prophylaxis and treatment of infections due to Loa loa, *Wucheria bancrofti,* scabies, and human cutaneous larva migrans.

SPECIAL CONCERNS

Use during lactation only if benefits outweigh risks. Those with hyperreactive onchodermatitis (sowdah) may be more likely to have severe side effects. Control of extraintestinal strongyloidiasis is difficult in immunocompromised clients. Clients may develop cutaneous or systemic reactions of varying severity, called the Mazzotti reaction, as well as ophthalmologic reactions in those with onchocercia-

I

sis. Safety and efficacy have not been determined in children weighing less than 15 kg.

SIDE EFFECTS

When used to treat strongyloidiasis.
GI: Diarrhea, nausea, anorexia, constipation, vomiting, abdominal pain. **CNS:** Dizziness, somnolence, tremor, vertigo. **Dermatologic:** Pruritus, rash, urticaria. **Miscellaneous:** Asthenia, fatigue.

When used to treat onchocerciasis. *Mazzotti reaction:* Pruritus, edema, papular and pustular or frank urticarial rash, fever, inguinal lymph node enlargement and tenderness, axillary lymph node enlargement and tenderness, arthralgia, synovitis, cervical lymph node enlargement and tenderness. **Ophthalmic:** Limbitis, punctate opacity, abnormal sensation in the eyes, anterior uveitis, chorioretinitis, choroiditis, conjunctivitis, eyelid edema, keratitis. **Miscellaneous:** Tachycardia, peripheral edema, facial edema, orthostatic hypotension, headache, myalgia, worsening of bronchial asthma, serious or ***fatal encephalopathy*** in those who are also heavily infected with Loa loa.

LABORATORY TEST CONSIDERATIONS

When used to treat strongyloidiasis: ↑ ALT, AST, hemoglobin. ↓ Leukocyte count. **When used to treat onchocerciasis:** ↑ Hemoglobin. Eosinophilia.

OD OVERDOSE MANAGEMENT

Symptoms: Asthenia, diarrhea, dizziness, edema, headache, nausea, rash, vomiting, abdominal pain, ataxia, dyspnea, paresthesia, seizure, urticaria. *Treatment:* Supportive therapy, including parenteral fluids and electrolytes, respiratory support, and pressor agents (if significant hypotension). Induce emesis or gastric lavage as soon as possible, followed by laxatives and other anti-poison measures.

HOW SUPPLIED

Tablet: 3 mg, 6 mg

DOSAGE

• **TABLETS**

Strongyloidiasis.

Single oral dose to provide about 200 mcg/kg: **15–24 kg:** One 3-mg tablet or one-half 6-mg tablet; **25–35 kg:** Two 3- mg tablets or one 6-mg tablet; **36–50 kg:** Three 3-mg tablets or 1.5 6-mg tablets; **51–65 kg:** Four 2-mg tablets or two 6-mg tablets; **66–79 kg:** Five 3-mg tablets or 2.5 6-mg tablets. **80 kg or more:** 200 mcg/kg.

Onchocerciasis.

Single oral dose to provide about 150 mcg/kg: **15–25 kg:** One 3-mg tablet or one-half 6-mg tablet; **26–44 kg:** Two 3-mg tablets or one 6-mg tablet; **45–64 kg:** Three 3-mg tablets or 1.5 6-mg tablets; **65–84 kg:** Four 3-mg tablets or two 6-mg tablets. **85 kg or more:** 150 mcg/kg.

NURSING CONSIDERATIONS

ADMINISTRATION/STORAGE

1. For either use, take with water.
2. For strongyloidiasis, perform follow-up stool examinations to verify eradication of infection.
3. For onchocerciasis, may retreat at intervals as short as 3 mo.

ASSESSMENT

Determine dates of exposure, onset, duration, and characteristics of symptoms, and lab confirmation of parasitic nematode.

CLIENT/FAMILY TEACHING

1. Take as directed with a full glass of water.
2. Report if abdominal pain, chest discomfort, severe rash, joint inflammation, or vision alterations occur.
3. Must bring consecutive F/U stool specimens to lab to verify eradication of strongyloides parasite. With onchocerciasis, the adult parasite is not killed, thus retreatment is usually required.

OUTCOMES/EVALUATE

Control/eradication of extraintestinal strongyloidiasis/onchocerciasis

K 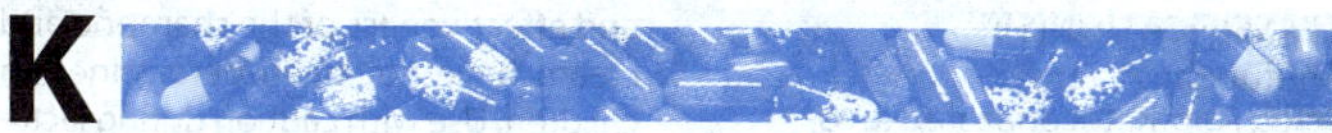

Kanamycin sulfate

(kan-ah-**MY**-sin)

PREGNANCY CATEGORY: D
CLASSIFICATION(S):
Aminoglycoside antibiotic and antitubercular agent (tertiary)
Rx: Kantrex

SEE ALSO *ANTI-INFECTIVES* AND *AMINOGLYCOSIDES*.

ACTION/KINETICS
Activity resembles that of neomycin and streptomycin. **Peak therapeutic serum levels: IM,** 15–40 mcg/mL. **t$^{1}/_{2}$:** 2–3 hr. Toxic serum levels: >35 mcg/mL (peak) and >10 mcg/mL (trough).

USES
Parenteral: Initial therapy for infections due to *Escherichia coli, Proteus, Enterobacter aerogenes, Klebsiella pneumoniae, Serratia marcescens,* and *Acinetobacter.* May be combined with a penicillin or cephalosporin before knowing results of susceptibility tests. *Investigational:* As part of a multiple-drug regimen for *Mycobacterium avium* complex in AIDS clients.

PO: Adjunct to mechanical cleansing of large bowel for suppression of intestinal bacteria; hepatic coma.

SPECIAL CONCERNS
Use with caution in premature infants and neonates.

ADDITIONAL SIDE EFFECTS
Sprue-like syndrome with steatorrhea, malabsorption, and electrolyte imbalance.

ADDITIONAL DRUG INTERACTIONS
Procainamide ↑ muscle relaxation.

HOW SUPPLIED
Capsule: 500 mg; *Injection:* 1 g/2 mL, 1 g/3 mL, 75 mg/2 mL, 500 mg/2 mL

DOSAGE

- **CAPSULES**

Intestinal bacteria suppression.
1 g every hour for 4 hr; **then,** 1 g q 6 hr for 36–72 hr.

Hepatic coma.
8–12 g/day in divided doses.

- **IM, IV**

Adults and children: 15 mg/kg/day in two to three equal doses. Maximum daily dose should not exceed 1.5 g regardless of route of administration.

For calculating dosage interval (in hr) in clients with impaired renal function, multiply serum creatinine (mg/100 mL) by 9.

- **IM**

Tuberculosis.
Adults: 15 mg/kg/day. Not recommended for use in children.

- **INTRAPERITONEAL**

500 mg diluted in 20 mL sterile distilled water.

- **INHALATION**

250 mg in saline—nebulize b.i.d.–q.i.d.
Irrigation of abscess cavities, pleural space, ventricular cavities.
0.25% solution.

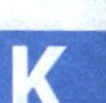

NURSING CONSIDERATIONS

SEE ALSO *GENERAL NURSING CONSIDERATIONS FOR ANTI-INFECTIVES* AND *AMINOGLYCOSIDES*.

ASSESSMENT
Document indications for therapy, onset, duration, and characteristics of symptoms. Reduce dose with renal dysfunction. Obtain baseline culture results.

CLIENT/FAMILY TEACHING
1. Take exactly as directed and complete the full course of therapy.
2. Report any loss of hearing, headaches, dizziness, ringing or noise in the ears, N&V, severe diarrhea or loss of appetite.

OUTCOMES/EVALUATE
- Negative culture reports
- Desired bowel cleansing

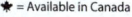

Ketoconazole

(kee-toe-**KON**-ah-zohl)

PREGNANCY CATEGORY: C

CLASSIFICATION(S):
Antifungal
✱Rx: Apo-Ketoconazole, Novo-Ketoconazole
OTC: Nizoral

SEE ALSO *ANTI-INFECTIVES*.

ACTION/KINETICS
Inhibits synthesis of ergosterol (the main sterol of fungal cell membranes), damaging the cell membrane and resulting in loss of essential intracellular material. Also inhibits biosynthesis of triglycerides and phospholipids and inhibits oxidative and peroxidative enzyme activity. When used to treat *Candida albicans,* it inhibits transformation of blastospores into the invasive mycelial form. Inhibits growth of *Pityrosporum ovale* when used to treat dandruff. Use in Cushing's syndrome is due to its ability to inhibit adrenal steroidogenesis. **Peak plasma levels:** 3.5 mcg/mL after 1–2 hr after a 200-mg dose. **t½, biphasic:** first, 2 hr; second, 8 hr. Requires acidity for dissolution. Metabolized in liver to inactive metabolites and most excreted through feces.

USES
PO: Candidiasis, chronic mucocutaneous candidiasis, candiduria, histoplasmosis, chromomycosis, oral thrush, blastomycosis, coccidioidomycosis, paracoccidioidomycosis. Recalcitrant cutaneous dermatophyte infections not responding to other therapy. *Investigational:* Onychomycosis due to *Trichophyton* and *Candida.* CNS fungal infections (high doses). Cushing's syndrome. **Cream:** Tinea pedis, tinea corporis and tinea cruris due to *Trichophyton rubrum, T. mentagrophytes,* and *Epidermophyton floccosum.* Tinea versicolor caused by *Microsporum furfur;* cutaneous candidiasis caused by *Candida* species; seborrheic dermatitis. **Shampoo:** To reduce scaling due to dandruff and tinea versicolor.

CONTRAINDICATIONS
Hypersensitivity, fungal meningitis. Topical product not for ophthalmic use. Use during lactation.

SPECIAL CONCERNS
Use tablets with caution in children less than 2 years of age. The safety and effectiveness of the shampoo and cream have not been determined in children. Use with caution during lactation.

SIDE EFFECTS
GI: N&V, abdominal pain, diarrhea. **CNS:** Headache, dizziness, somnolence, fever, chills, suicidal tendencies, depression (rare). **Hematologic:** Thrombocytopenia, leukopenia, ***hemolytic anemia.*** **Miscellaneous:** Hepatotoxicity, photophobia, pruritus, gynecomastia, impotence, bulging fontanelles, urticaria, decreased serum testosterone levels, anaphylaxis (rare).

- **TOPICAL CREAM.**
  Stinging, irritation, pruritus.
- **SHAMPOO.**
  Increased hair loss, irritation, abnormal hair texture, itching, oiliness or dryness of the scalp and hair, scalp pustules.

LABORATORY TEST CONSIDERATIONS
Transient ↑ serum liver enzymes. ↓ Serum testosterone.

DRUG INTERACTIONS
Antacids / ↓ Absorption of ketoconazole R/T ↑ pH
Anticoagulants / ↑ Anticoagulant effect
Benzodiazepines / ↑ Prolonged serum levels → ↑ CNS depression and psychomotor impairment
Buspirone / ↑ Plasma buspirone levels
Carbamazepine / ↑ Plasma carbamazepine levels
Corticosteroids / ↑ Risk of drug toxicity R/T ↑ bioavailability
Cyclosporine / ↑ Cyclosporine levels (ketaconazole may be used therapeutically to decrease cyclosporine dose) due to inhibition of metabolism
Didanosinse / ↓ Ketoconazole effect due to ↓ absorption
Donepezil / ↑ Plasma levels of donepezil R/T ↓ liver metabolism
Histamine H_2 antagonists / ↓ Ketoconazole absorption R/T ↑ gastric pH
Isoniazid / ↓ Bioavailability of ketoconazole
Nisoldipine / ↑ Nisoldipine plasma levels R/T ↓ liver metabolism
Oral Contraceptives / Possible ↓ effect of contraceptive

Protease inhibitors (Indinavir, Ritonavir, Saquinavir) / ↑ Serum levels of protease inhibitor
Proton pump inhibitors / ↓ Ketoconazole effect due to ↓ bioavailability
Quinidine / ↑ Quinidine serum levels
Rifampin / ↓ Serum levels of either drug
Sucralfate / ↓ Ketoconazole effect due to ↓ bioavailabilitiy
Sulfonylureas / ↑ Hypoglycemic effect due to ↑ serum levels
Theophyllines / ↓ Serum theophylline levels due to ↓ absorption
Tolterodine / ↑ Tolterodine t½ and area under the curve in those deficient in CYP2D6 enzymes
Tricyclic antidepressants / ↑ TCA serum levels
Vinca alkaloids / ↑ Risk of vinca toxicity due to inhibition of metabolism
Zolpidem / ↑ Half-life of zolpidem R/T ↓ liver metabolism

HOW SUPPLIED

Cream: 2%; *Shampoo:* 2%; *Tablet:* 200 mg

DOSAGE

• **TABLETS**

Fungal infections.

Adults: 200 mg once daily; in serious infections or if response is not sufficient, increase to 400 mg once daily. **Pediatric, over 2 years:** 3.3–6.6 mg/kg once daily. Dosage has not been established for children less than 2 years of age.

CNS fungal infections.

Adults: 800–1,200 mg/day.

Cushing's syndrome.

800–1,200 mg/day.

• **TOPICAL CREAM (2%)**

Tinea corporis, tinea cruris, tinea versicolor, tinea pedis, cutaneous candidiasis.

Cover the affected and immediate surrounding areas once daily (twice daily for more resistant cases). Duration of treatment is usually 2 weeks.

Seborrheic dermatitis.

Apply to affected area b.i.d. for 4 weeks or until symptoms clear.

• **SHAMPOO (2%)**

Use twice a week for 4 weeks with at least 3 days between each shampooing. **Then,** use as required to maintain control.

NURSING CONSIDERATIONS

SEE ALSO *GENERAL NURSING CONSIDERATIONS* FOR *ANTI-INFECTIVES*.

ADMINISTRATION/STORAGE

1. Give a minimum of 2 hr before administration of drugs that increase gastric pH (such as antacids, anticholinergics, or H_2 blockers). Delay any antacid administration by 2 hr.
2. The minimum treatment for candidiasis (using tablets) is 1–2 weeks; for other systemic mycoses 6 mo. The minimum treatment for recalcitrant dermatophyte infections is 4 weeks in cases involving glabrous skin; palmar and plantar infections may respond more slowly.

CLIENT/FAMILY TEACHING

1. Take tablets with food to decrease GI upset. Take 2 hr before drugs (antacids) that change gastric pH.
2. Apply shampoo to wet hair in sufficient quantities to cover the entire scalp for 1 min. Rinse with warm water; repeat, leaving shampoo on the scalp for 3 min. After the second washing, rinse thoroughly and dry hair with towel or warm air flow. Use twice a week for 4 weeks with at least 3 days between treatments.
3. Report persistent fever, pain, rash, severe N&V, unusual bruising/bleeding, yellow skin or eyes, dark urine, pale stools or diarrhea.
4. With lack of stomach acid, may dissolve each tablet in 4 mL aqueous solution of 0.2 N HCl; use a straw to avoid contact with teeth. Follow by drinking a glass of tap water.
5. Use caution when driving or performing hazardous tasks; tablets may cause headaches, dizziness, and drowsiness.
6. Avoid all forms of alcohol. Report lack of desired response.
7. Wear sunglasses, sunscreen, and protective clothing to prevent photosensitivity reactions.
8. Complete the full course of therapy. Long-term therapy is needed and

K

beneficial effects may not be evident for several weeks.

OUTCOMES/EVALUATE

- Eradication of fungal infections
- Clearing of skin lesions
- Control of dandruff with ↓ scaling

Ketoprofen

(kee-toe-**PROH**-fen)

PREGNANCY CATEGORY: B
CLASSIFICATION(S):
Nonsteroidal anti-inflammatory drug
Rx: Orudis, Oruvail
✱Rx: Apo-Keto, Apo-Keto-E, Apo-Keto-SR, Novo-Keto, Novo-Keto-EC, Nu-Ketoprofen, Nu-Ketoprofen-E, Nu-Ketoprofen-SR, Orafen, Orudis-SR, Rhodis, Rhodis SR, Rhodis-EC, Rhovail
OTC: Orudis KT

K

SEE ALSO ***NONSTEROIDAL ANTI-INFLAMMATORY DRUGS.***

ACTION/KINETICS

Possesses anti-inflammatory, antipyretic, and analgesic properties. Known to inhibit both prostaglandin and leukotriene synthesis, to have antibradykinin activity, and to stabilize lysosomal membranes. **Onset:** 15–30 min. **Peak plasma levels:** 0.5–2 hr. **Duration:** 4–6 hr. **t½:** 2–4 hr. **t½, geriatrics:** Approximately 5 hr. For Ketoprofen ER: **Peak:** 6–7 hr; **t½:** 5.4 hr. Is 99% bound to plasma proteins. Food does not alter the bioavailability; however, the rate of absorption is reduced.

USES

Rx: Acute or chronic rheumatoid arthritis and osteoarthritis (both capsules and sustained-release capsules). Primary dysmenorrhea and analgesic for mild to moderate pain (capsule only).

OTC: Temporary relief of aches and pains associated with the common cold, toothache, headache, muscle aches, backache, menstrual cramps, reduction of fever, and minor arthritic pain.

Investigational: Juvenile rheumatoid arthritis, sunburn, prophylaxis of migraine, migraine due to menses.

CONTRAINDICATIONS

Use during late pregnancy, in children, and during lactation. Use of the extended-release product for acute pain in any client or for initial therapy in clients who are small, elderly, or who have renal or hepatic impairment.

SPECIAL CONCERNS

Safety and effectiveness have not been established in children. Geriatric clients may manifest increased and prolonged serum levels due to decreased protein binding and clearance. Use with caution in clients with a history of GI tract disorders, in fluid retention, hypertension, and heart failure.

ADDITIONAL SIDE EFFECTS

GI: Peptic ulcer, ***GI bleeding,*** dyspepsia, nausea, diarrhea, constipation, abdominal pain, flatulence, anorexia, vomiting, stomatitis. **CNS:** Headache. **CV:** Peripheral edema, fluid retention.

ADDITIONAL DRUG INTERACTIONS

Acetylsalicylic acid / ↑ Plasma ketoprofen levels due to ↓ plasma protein binding
Hydrochlorothiazide / ↓ Chloride and potassium excretion
Methotrexate / Concomitant use → toxic plasma levels of methotrexate
Probenecid / ↓ Plasma clearance of ketoprofen and ↓ plasma protein binding
Warfarin / Additive effect to cause bleeding

HOW SUPPLIED

Capsule: 25 mg, 50 mg, 75 mg; *Capsule, Extended Release:* 100 mg, 150 mg, 200 mg; *Tablet:* 12.5 mg

DOSAGE

- **RX: EXTENDED RELEASE CAPSULES, CAPSULES**

Rheumatoid arthritis, osteoarthritis.

Adults, initial: 75 mg t.i.d. or 50 mg q.i.d.; **maintenance:** 150–300 mg in three to four divided doses daily. Doses above 300 mg/day are not recommended. Alternatively, 200 mg once daily using the sustained-release formulation (Oruvail). Decrease dose by one-half to one-third in clients with impaired renal function or in geriatric clients.

Mild to moderate pain, dysmenorrhea.
Adults: 25–50 mg q 6–8 hr as required, not to exceed 300 mg/day. Reduce dose in smaller or geriatric clients and in those with liver or renal dysfunction. Doses greater than 75 mg do not provide any added therapeutic effect.
• **OTC: TABLETS**
Adults, over 16 years of age: 12.5 mg with a full glass of liquid every 4 to 6 hr. If pain or fever persists after 1 hr follow with an additional 12.5 mg. Experience may determine that an initial dose of 25 mg gives a better effect. Do not exceed a dose of 25 mg in a 4- to 6-hr period or 75 mg in a 24-hr period.

NURSING CONSIDERATIONS

SEE ALSO *NURSING CONSIDERATIONS* FOR *NONSTEROIDAL ANTI-INFLAMMATORY DRUGS.*

ASSESSMENT
1. Document indications for therapy, type, onset, location, pain level, and symptom characteristics.
2. Note history of GI disorders, cardiac failure, hypertension, or edema.
3. Determine if pregnant. Not for children under age 12.
4. Monitor hematologic profiles, renal and LFTs. In high doses, may prolong bleeding times by decreasing platelet aggregation. Reduce dose in the elderly and those with impaired renal function.

CLIENT/FAMILY TEACHING
1. GI side effects may be minimized by taking with antacids, milk, or food.
2. Avoid alcohol. Report lack of desired response.
3. Do not take any aspirin products unless specifically prescribed.
4. Report any new symptoms such as rash, headaches, black stools, disturbances in vision, unexplained bruising, bleeding from the gums, or nose bleeds.
5. Report any S&S of liver dysfunction such as fatigue, upper right quadrant pain, clay-colored stools, or yellowing of the skin and sclera.

OUTCOMES/EVALUATE
• ↓ Joint pain/swelling; ↑ mobility
• ↓ Uterine cramping

Ketorolac tromethamine

(kee-toh-**ROH**-lack)

PREGNANCY CATEGORY: C
CLASSIFICATION(S):
Nonsteroidal anti-inflammatory drug
Rx: Acular, Acular PF, Toradol
★Rx: Apo-Ketorolac, Novo-Ketorolac

SEE ALSO *NONSTEROIDAL ANTI-INFLAMMATORY DRUGS.*

ACTION/KINETICS
Possesses anti-inflammatory, analgesic, and antipyretic effects. Completely absorbed following IM use. **Onset:** Within 30 min. **Maximum effect:** 1–2 hr after IV or IM dosing. **Duration:** 4–6 hr. **Peak plasma levels:** 2.2–3.0 mcg/mL 50 min after a dose of 30 mg. **t½, terminal:** 3.8–6.3 hr in young adults and 4.7–8.6 hr in geriatric clients. Over 99% is bound to plasma proteins. Metabolized in the liver with over 90% excreted in the urine and the remainder excreted in the feces.

USES
PO: Short-term (up to 5 days) management of severe, acute pain that requires analgesia at the opiate level. Always initiate therapy with IV or IM followed by PO only as continuation treatment, if necessary. **IM/IV:** Ketorolac has been used with morphine and meperidine and shows an opioid-sharing effect. The combination can be used for break through pain. **Ophthalmic:** Relieve itching caused by seasonal allergic conjunctivitis. Treat postoperative inflammation following cataract surgery.

CONTRAINDICATIONS
Hypersensitivity to the drug or allergic symptoms (angioedema, bronchospasm) to aspirin or other NSAIDs. Active peptic ulcer disease, recent GI bleeding or perforation, history of peptic ulcer disease or GI bleeding.

K

Advanced renal impairment and in those at risk for renal failure due to volume depletion. Suspected or confirmed cerebrovascular bleeding, hemorrhagic diathesis, or incomplete hemostasis and in those with a high risk of bleeding. As prophylactic analgesic before any major surgery or intraoperatively when hemostasis is critical (due to increased risk of bleeding). Intrathecal or epidural administration (due to alcohol content of product). Use in labor, delivery, or during lactation. Use with aspirin or other NSAIDs. Use of the ophthalmic solution in clients wearing soft contact lenses.

SPECIAL CONCERNS

Use with caution in impaired hepatic or renal function, during lactation, in geriatric clients, and in clients on high-dose salicylate regimens. The age, dosage, and duration of therapy should receive special consideration when using this drug. Safety and effectiveness have not been determined in children.

ADDITIONAL SIDE EFFECTS

CV: Vasodilation, pallor. **GI:** GI pain, peptic ulcers, nausea, dyspepsia, flatulence, GI fullness, stomatitis, excessive thirst, GI bleeding (higher risk in geriatric clients), ***perforation***. **CNS:** Headache, nervousness, abnormal thinking, depression, euphoria. **Hypersensitivity:** ***Bronchospasm, anaphylaxis.*** **Miscellaneous:** Purpura, asthma, abnormal vision, abnormal liver function.

- **OPHTHALMIC SOLUTION.**

Transient stinging and burning following instillation, ocular irritation, allergic reactions, superficial ocular infections, superficial keratitis.

DRUG INTERACTIONS

Ketorolac may ↑ plasma levels of salicylates due to ↓ plasma protein binding.

HOW SUPPLIED

Injection: 15 mg/mL, 30 mg/mL; *Ophthalmic solution:* 0.5%; *Tablet:* 10 mg

DOSAGE

- **IM**

Analgesic, single dose.

Adults: less than 65 years of age: One 60-mg dose. **Adults, over 65 years of age, in renal impairment, or weight less than 50 kg:** One 30-mg dose.

- **IM/IV**

Analgesic, multiple dose.

Adults, less than 65 years of age: 30 mg q 6 hr, not to exceed 120 mg daily. **Adults, over 65 years of age, in renal impairment, or weight less than 50 kg:** 15 mg q 6 hr, not to exceed 60 mg daily.

- **IV**

Analgesic, single dose.

Adults, less than 65 years of age: One 30-mg dose. **Adults, over 65 years of age, in renal impairment, or weight less than 50 kg:** One 15-mg dose.

- **TABLETS**

Transition from IV/IM to PO.

Adults less than 65 years of age: 20 mg as a first PO dose for clients who received 60 mg IM single dose, 30 mg IV single dose, or 30 mg multiple dose IV/IM; **then,** 10 mg q 4–6 hr, not to exceed 40 mg in a 24-hr period. **Adults, over 65 years of age, in renal impairment, or weight less than 50 kg:** 10 mg as a first PO dose for those who received a 30-mg IM single dose, a 15-mg IV single dose, or a 15-mg multiple dose IV/IM; **then,** 10 mg q 4–6 hr, not to exceed 40 mg in a 24-hr period.

- **OPHTHALMIC SOLUTION**

Seasonal allergic conjunctivitis.

1 gtt (0.25 mg) q.i.d. Efficacy has not been determined beyond 1 week of use.

Following cataract extraction.

1 gtt to the affected eye(s) q.i.d. beginning 24 hr after surgery and continuing for 2 weeks postoperatively.

NURSING CONSIDERATIONS

SEE ALSO *NURSING CONSIDERATIONS* FOR *NONSTEROIDAL ANTI-INFLAMMATORY DRUGS.*

ADMINISTRATION/STORAGE

1. Use as part of a regular analgesic schedule rather than on an as needed basis.
2. If given on p.r.n. basis, base the size of a repeat dose on the duration of pain relief from the previous dose. If the pain returns within 3–5 hr, the next dose can be increased by up to

50% (as long as the total daily dose is not exceeded). If the pain does not return for 8–12 hr, the next dose can be decreased by as much as 50% or the dosing interval can be increased to q 8–12 hr.

3. Shortening the dosing intervals recommended will lead to an increased frequency and duration of side effects.

4. Correct hypovolemia prior to administering.

IV 5. Do not mix IV/IM ketorolac in a small volume (i.e., a syringe) with morphine sulfate, meperidine HCl, promethazine HCl, or hydroxyzine HCl; will precipitate from solution.

6. When used IM/IV, the IV bolus must be given over no less than 15 sec. Give IM slowly and deeply into the muscle.

7. Protect the injection from light.

ASSESSMENT

1. Document indications for therapy, onset, location, pain intensity/level, and characteristics of symptoms.

2. Note any previous experience with NSAIDs and the results.

3. Determine any liver or renal dysfunction; assess hydration.

CLIENT/FAMILY TEACHING

1. Take only as directed; do not exceed prescribed dosage. May take with food/milk if GI upset occurs. Report if symptoms unrelieved.

2. Drug may cause drowsiness and dizziness; avoid activities that require mental alertness until drug effects realized.

3. Avoid alcohol, ASA, and all OTC agents without approval.

4. Report any unusual bruising/bleeding, weight gain, swelling of feet or ankles, increased joint pain, or change in urine patterns.

5. With eye drops, transient stinging or burning may occur. Do not wear soft contact lens. Report ocular reactions that do not subside with therapy.

OUTCOMES/EVALUATE

- Effective pain control
- ↓ Ocular allergic manifestations
- ↓ Ocular pain/photophobia

Ketotifen fumarate

(kee-**TOHT**-ih-fen)

PREGNANCY CATEGORY: C
CLASSIFICATION(S):
Ophthalmic decongestant
Rx: Zaditor
★Rx: Apo-Ketotifen, Novo-Ketotifen, Zaditen

ACTION/KINETICS

Selective, non-competitive histamine H_1 receptor antagonist and mast cell stabilizer. Inhibits release of mediators from cells involved in hypersensitivity reactions. Decreased chemotaxis and activation of eosinophils. Rapid acting; effect seen within minutes of administration.

USES

Temporary prophylaxis of itching of the eye due to allergic conjunctivitis.

CONTRAINDICATIONS

Use orally or by injection. Use to treat contact lens-related irritation.

SPECIAL CONCERNS

Use with caution during lactation. Safety and efficacy have not been determined in children less than 3 years of age.

SIDE EFFECTS

Ophthalmic: Burning, stinging, conjunctivitis, conjunctival injection, discharge, dry eyes, eye pain, eyelid disorder, itching, keratitis, lacrimation disorder, mydriasis, photophobia. **Miscellaneous:** Headache, rhinitis, allergic reactions, rash, flu syndrome, pharyngitis.

HOW SUPPLIED

Solution: 0.025%

DOSAGE

- **SOLUTION, OPHTHALMIC**
  Allergic conjunctivitis.

1 gtt in the affected eye(s) q 8–12 hr.

NURSING CONSIDERATIONS

ASSESSMENT

1. Document indications for therapy, onset, and characteristics of symptoms.

2. Assist to identify triggers; teach avoidance.

CLIENT/FAMILY TEACHING

1. To prevent contaminating the dropper tip and solution, do not touch the eyelids or surrounding areas with the dropper tip.
2. For topical use only. Keep bottle tightly closed when not in use.
3. Not for use with contact lens/related irritation; do not wear contact lenses if eyes are red.
4. Benzalkonium chloride, the preservative in the product, may be absorbed by soft contact lenses. For those who wear soft contact lenses and whose eyes are not red, wait 10 min or longer after instilling ketotifen before inserting contact lenses.
5. May experience burning, stinging and inflammation with instillation; notify provider if persistent.

OUTCOMES/EVALUATE

Relief of S&S allergic conjunctivitis

L

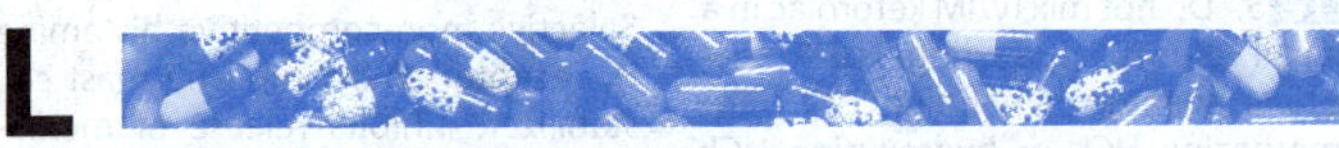

Labetalol hydrochloride

(lah-**BET**-ah-lohl)

PREGNANCY CATEGORY: C
CLASSIFICATION(S):
Alpha-beta adrenergic blocking agent
Rx: Normodyne, Trandate

SEE ALSO *BETA-ADRENERGIC BLOCKING AGENTS* AND *ANTIHYPERTENSIVE AGENTS*.

ACTION/KINETICS

Decreases BP by blocking both alpha- and beta-adrenergic receptors. Standing BP is lowered more than supine. Significant reflex tachycardia and bradycardia do not occur although AV conduction may be prolonged. **Onset: PO,** 2–4 hr; **IV,** 5 min. **Peak plasma levels, PO:** 1–2 hr. **Peak effects, PO:** 2–4 hr. **Duration: PO,** 8–12 hr. **t½: PO,** 6–8 hr; **IV,** 5.5 hr. Significant first-pass effect; metabolized in liver. Food increases bioavailability of the drug.

USES

PO: Hypertension, alone or in combination with other drugs (especially thiazide and loop diuretics). **IV:** Severe hypertension. *Investigational:* Pheochromocytoma, clonidine withdrawal hypertension.

CONTRAINDICATIONS

Cardiogenic shock, cardiac failure, bronchial asthma, bradycardia, greater than first-degree heart block.

SPECIAL CONCERNS

Use with caution during lactation, in impaired renal and hepatic function, in chronic bronchitis and emphysema, and in diabetes (may prevent premonitory signs of acute hypoglycemia). Safety and efficacy in children have not been established.

SIDE EFFECTS

See also *Beta-Adrenergic Blocking Agents.*

After PO Use.
GI: Diarrhea, cholestasis with or without jaundice. **CNS:** Fatigue, drowsiness, paresthesias, headache, syncope (rare). **GU:** Impotence, priapism, ejaculation failure, difficulty in micturition, Peyronie's disease, acute urinary bladder retention. **Respiratory:** Dyspnea, ***bronchospasm***. **Musculoskeletal:** Muscle cramps, asthenia, toxic myopathy. **Dermatologic:** Generalized maculopapular, lichenoid, or urticarial rashes; bullous lichen planus, psoriasis, facial erythema, reversible alopecia. **Ophthalmic:** Abnormal vision, dry eyes. **Miscellaneous:** SLE, positive antinuclear factor, antimitochondrial antibiodies, fever, edema, nasal stuffiness.

After parenteral use. CV: Ventricular arrhythmias. **CNS:** Numbness, somnolence, yawning. **Miscellaneous:** Pruritus, flushing, wheezing.

After PO or parenteral use. GI: N&V, dyspepsia, taste distortion. **CNS:** Dizziness, tingling of skin or scalp, vertigo. **Miscellaneous:** Postural hypotension, increased sweating.

LABORATORY TEST CONSIDERATIONS

False + increase in urinary catecholamines. Transient ↑ serum transaminases, BUN, serum creatinine.

OD OVERDOSE MANAGEMENT

Symptoms: Excessive hypotension and bradycardia. *Treatment:* Induce vomiting or perform gastric lavage. Place clients in a supine position with legs elevated. If required, the following treatment can be used:

- Epinephrine or a beta-2 agonist (aerosol) to treat bronchospasm.
- Atropine or epinephrine to treat bradycardia.
- Digitalis glycoside and a diuretic for cardiac failure; dopamine or dobutamine may also be used.
- Diazepam to treat seizures.
- Norepinephrine (or another vasopressor) to treat hypotension.
- Administration of glucagon (5–10 mg rapidly over 30 sec), followed by continuous infusion of 5 mg/hr, may be effective in treating severe hypotension and bradycardia.

DRUG INTERACTIONS

Beta-adrenergic bronchodilators / ↓ Bronchodilator drug effects
Cimetidine / ↑ Bioavailability of PO labetalol
Glutethimide / ↓ Labetalol effects R/T ↑ liver breakdown
Halothane / ↑ Risk of severe myocardial depression → hypotension
Nitroglycerin / Additive hypotension
Tricyclic antidepressants / ↑ Risk of tremors

HOW SUPPLIED

Injection: 5 mg/mL; *Tablet:* 100 mg, 200 mg, 300 mg

DOSAGE

- **TABLETS**

Hypertension.

Individualize. Initial: 100 mg b.i.d. alone or with a diuretic. After 2 or 3 days, using BP as a guide, titrate dosage in increments of 100 mg b.i.d., q 2–3 days. **Maintenance:** 200–400 mg b.i.d. up to 1,200–2,400 mg/day for severe cases.

- **IV**

Hypertension.

Individualize. Initial: 20 mg slowly over 2 min; **then,** 40–80 mg q 10 min until desired effect occurs or a total of 300 mg has been given.

- **IV INFUSION**

Hypertension.

Initial: 2 mg/min; **then,** adjust rate according to response. **Usual dose range:** 50–300 mg.

Transfer from IV to PO therapy.

Initial: 200 mg; **then,** 200–400 mg 6–12 hr later, depending on response. Thereafter, dosage based on response.

NURSING CONSIDERATIONS

SEE ALSO *NURSING CONSIDERATIONS* FOR *BETA-ADRENERGIC BLOCKING AGENTS* AND *ANTIHYPERTENSIVE AGENTS*.

ADMINISTRATION/STORAGE

1. When transferring to PO labetalol from other antihypertensive therapy, slowly reduce dosage of current therapy.
2. Full antihypertensive effect is usually seen within the first 1–3 hr after the initial dose or dose increment.
3. IV To transfer from IV to PO therapy in hospitalized clients, begin when supine BP begins to increase.
4. Not compatible with 5% sodium bicarbonate injection.
5. May give IV undiluted (20 mg over 2 min) or reconstituted with dextrose or saline solutions (infuse at a rate of 2 mg/min). When given by IV infusion, use a device that allows precise control of dose/flow rate.

ASSESSMENT

1. Note indications for therapy, other agents trialed and the outcome.
2. Assess effect of labetalol tablets on standing BP before hospital discharge. Obtain standing BP at different times during the day to assess full effects.
3. To reduce chance of orthostatic hypotension, keep supine for 3 hr after receiving parenteral labetalol.

CLIENT/FAMILY TEACHING

1. Take as directed with meals. Do not stop taking abruptly; may cause chest pain.
2. Use caution; may precipitate orthostatic hypotension and cause diz-

ziness. Report any low heart rate, confusion, fever, swelling of extremities, difficulty breathing, or night cough. Record heart rate and BP for provider review.

3. May cause increased sensitivity to cold; dress appropriately.
4. Avoid alcohol, OTC products especially cold remedies, high sodium intake and tobacco.

OUTCOMES/EVALUATE

↓ BP

Lamivudine (3TC)

(lah-**MIH**-vyou-deen)

PREGNANCY CATEGORY: C
CLASSIFICATION(S):
Antiviral, nucleoside reverse transcriptase inhibitor
Rx: Epivir, Epivir HBV
✱**Rx:** 3TC

SEE ALSO *ANTIVIRAL DRUGS*.

ACTION/KINETICS

Synthetic nucleoside analog effective against HIV. Converted to active 5′-triphosphate (L-TP) metabolite which inhibits HIV reverse transcription via viral DNA chain termination. L-TP also inhibits the RNA- and DNA-dependent DNA polymerase activities of reverse transcriptase. Rapidly absorbed after PO administration. Most eliminated unchanged through the urine.

USES

Epivir. In combination with other antiretroviral drugs for the treatment of HIV infection. **Epivir-HBV.** Chronic hepatitis B associated with evidence of hepatitis B replication and active liver inflammation. Hepatitis B in children 2–17 years of age.

CONTRAINDICATIONS

Lactation. Use of Epivir-HBV tablets or oral solution to treat HIV infections (due to the lower amount of lamivudine compared with Epivir).

SPECIAL CONCERNS

Clients taking lamivudine and zidovudine may continue to develop opportunistic infections and other complications of HIV infection. Use with caution and at a reduced dose in those with impaired renal function. Data on the use of lamivudine and zidovudine in pediatric clients are lacking; however, use the combination with extreme caution in children with pancreatitis.

Epivir-HBV contains a lower dose of lamivudine than Epivir. If Epivir-HBV is used for chronic hepatitis B in a client with unrecognized or untreated HIV infection, rapid emergence of HIV resistance is likely due to subtherapeutic amounts of the drug given.

Safety and efficacy of Epivir-HBV have not been determined in those with decompensated liver disease or organ transplants or in clients dually infected with HBV and HCV, hepatitis delta, or HIV.

SIDE EFFECTS

Side effects include those when lamivudine is taken alone or with other antiretroviral drugs.

GI: N&V, diarrhea, anorexia or decreased appetite, abdominal pain/cramps, dyspepsia, stomatitis, lactic steatosis, severe hepatomegaly with steatosis, pancreatitis, posttreatment worsening of hepatitis B. **CNS:** Neuropathy, insomnia or other sleep disorders, dizziness, depressive disorders, paresthesias, peripheral neuropathies. **Hematologic:** Neutropenia, anemia, thrombocytopenia. **Respiratory:** Nasal S&S, cough, abnormal breath sounds/wheezing. **Musculoskeletal:** Musculoskeletal pain, myalgia, arthralgia, muscle weakness with CPK elevation. **Dermatologic:** Alopecia, pruritus, rash, urticaria. **Body as a whole:** Headache, malaise, fatigue, fever or chills, skin rashes, weakness. **Miscellaneous:** ENT infections; sore throat, lactic acidosis, hyperglycemia, ***anaphylaxis,*** rhabdomyolysis, lymphadenopathy, splenomegaly. *NOTE:* Pediatric clients have an increased risk to develop ***pancreatitis.***

LABORATORY TEST CONSIDERATIONS

↑ ALT, AST, amylase, bilirubin, serum lipase, CPK.

DRUG INTERACTIONS

Trimethoprim-Sulfamethoxazole Significant ↑ in lamivudine level
Zidovudine / ↑ Zidovudine levels

HOW SUPPLIED
Epivir. *Oral Solution:* 10 mg/mL; *Tablet:* 150 mg. **Epivir-HBV.** *Oral solution:* 5 mg/mL; *Tablet:* 100 mg

DOSAGE

• **ORAL SOLUTION, TABLETS**

HIV infection.

Epivir. Adults: 150 mg b.i.d. in combination with other antiretroviral drugs. For adults with low body weight (less than 50 kg), the recommended dose is 2 mg/kg b.i.d. in combination with other antiretroviral drugs. **Children, 3 months to 16 years of age:** 4 mg/kg b.i.d. (up to a maximum of 150 mg b.i.d.) in combination with other antiretroviral drugs. In clients over 16 years of age, adjust the dose as follows in impaired renal function: C_{CR} 50 mL/min or more: 150 mg b.i.d.; C_{CR} 30–49 mL/min: 150 mg once daily; C_{CR} 15–29 mL/min: 150 mg for the first dose followed by 100 mg once daily; C_{CR} 5–14 mL/min: 150 mg for the first dose followed by 50 mg once daily; C_{CR} less than 5 mL/min: 50 mg for the first dose followed by 25 mg once daily.

Chronic hepatitis.

Epivir-HBV. Adults: 100 mg once daily. **Children, 2–17 years:** 3 mg/kg once daily, not to exceed 100 mg daily. Adjust the dose in adults as follows in impaired renal function: C_{CR} 50 mL/min or more: 100 mg once daily; C_{CR} 30–49 mL/min: 100 mg for the first dose followed by 50 mg once daily; C_{CR} 15–29 mL/min: 100 mg for the first dose followed by 25 mg once daily; C_{CR} 5–14 mL/min: 35 mg for the first dose followed by 15 mg once daily; C_{CR} Less than 5 mL/min: 35 mg for the first dose followed by 10 mg once daily.

NURSING CONSIDERATIONS

SEE ALSO ***NURSING CONSIDERATIONS FOR ANTIVIRAL DRUGS.***

ADMINISTRATION/STORAGE

1. Consult zidovudine or other antiviral drug prescribing information before using with lamivudine.
2. Store PO solution at 2–25°C (36–77°F).

ASSESSMENT

1. Note disease confirmation, other agents trialed, and the outcome.
2. Monitor children for clinical symptoms of pancreatitis.
3. Assess for HIV, HCV, and hepatitis delta when treating hepatitis B.
4. Monitor liver, renal, and hematologic parameters, including CD_4 and viral load. Adjust dose with impaired renal function.

CLIENT/FAMILY TEACHING

1. Take exactly as prescribed with other antiretroviral drug(s) twice a day.
2. May be taken without regard to food.
3. Drug is not a cure; may continue to experience illnesses and opportunistic infections associated with HIV.
4. Use barrier protection with sexual partners to prevent HIV transmission.
5. May experience fainting or dizziness; GI upset, and insomnia may resolve after 3-4 week of therapy.
6. With children especially, report symptoms of pancreatitis (i.e., abdominal pain, N&V, fever, loss of appetite, yellow skin discoloration).

OUTCOMES/EVALUATE

Control of HIV disease progression with zidovudine; stabilization of hepatitis B disease

COMBINATION DRUG

Lamivudine/ Zidovudine

(lah-**MIH**-vyou-deen, zye-**DOH**-vyou-deen)

PREGNANCY CATEGORY: C
CLASSIFICATION(S):
Antiviral, nucleoside reverse transcriptase inhibitor
Rx: Combivir

SEE ALSO ***LAMIVUDINE, ZIDOVUDINE, AND ANTIVIRAL DRUGS.***

CONTENT
Each Combivir tablet contains: *Antiviral:* Lamivudine, 150 mg and *Antiviral:* Zidovudine, 300 mg.

L

ACTION/KINETICS
Both drugs are reverse transcriptase inhibitors with activity against HIV. Combination results in synergistic antiretroviral effect. Each drug is rapidly absorbed. **t½, lamivudine:** 5–7 hr; **t½, zidovudine:** 0.5–3 hr.
USES
Treatment of HIV infection in combination with other antiretrovirals.
CONTRAINDICATIONS
Use in clients requiring dosage reduction, children less than 12 years of age, C_{CR} less than 50 mL/min, body weight less than 50 kg, and in those experiencing dose-limiting side effects.
SIDE EFFECTS
See individual drugs. Note especially, possibility of hematologic toxicity, lactic acidosis, and severe hepatomegaly with steatosis.
HOW SUPPLIED
See Content

DOSAGE
• **TABLETS**
HIV infection.
Adults and children over 12 years of age: One combination tablet—150 mg lamivudine/300 mg zidovudine—b.i.d.

NURSING CONSIDERATIONS

SEE ALSO *NURSING CONSIDERATIONS* FOR *LAMIVUDINE, ZIDOVUDINE,* AND *ANTIVIRAL DRUGS*.
ADMINISTRATION/STORAGE
May be taken without regard to food.
ASSESSMENT
1. Document disease onset, clinical characteristics, other agents trialed, and outcome.
2. Weigh client; not for use in those with low body weight or $C_{CR} < 50$ mL/min.
3. Monitor CBC, renal and LFTs; report dysfunction.
4. Assess for hepatomegaly and lactic acidosis (pH < 7.35 or serum lactate > 5-6 mEq/L).
CLIENT/FAMILY TEACHING
1. Take as directed, with or without food, twice daily.
2. Report any severe fatigue, SOB, dizziness, or muscle pain; drug may cause neutropenia and anemia.
3. Drug is not a cure; may experience opportunistic infections.
4. Practice safe sex; drug does not prevent disease transmission.
OUTCOMES/EVALUATE
Control of HIV; ↓ viral load

Lamotrigine

(lah-**MAH**-trih-jeen)

PREGNANCY CATEGORY: C
CLASSIFICATION(S):
Anticonvulsant, miscellaneous
Rx: Lamictal, Lamictal Chewable Dispersible Tablets

SEE ALSO *ANTICONVULSANTS*.
ACTION/KINETICS
Mechanism of anticonvulsant action not known. May act to inhibit voltage-sensitive sodium channels. This effect stabilizes neuronal membranes and modulates presynaptic transmitter release of excitatory amino acids such as glutamate and aspartate. Rapidly and completely absorbed after PO use. **Peak plasma levels:** 1.4–4.8 hr. **t½, after repeated doses:** Depends on whether taken alone or with other anticonvulsant drugs; ranges from about 12 to 70 hr in adults. Metabolized by the liver with metabolites and unchanged drug excreted mainly through the urine (94%). Lamotrigine induces its own metabolism. Eliminated more rapidly in clients who have been taking antiepileptic drugs that induce liver enzymes. However, valproic acid decreases the clearance of lamotrigine.
USES
(1) Adjunct in the treatment of partial seizures in adults with epilepsy. (2) As an adjunct in treating of generalized seizures in adults and children with Lennox-Gastaut syndrome. (3) Conversion to monotherapy in adults with partial seizures who are receiving a single enzyme-inducing anticonvulsant drug. *Investigational:* Adults with generalized tonic-clonic, absence, atypical absence, myoclonic seizures, and drug-resistant seizures in epilepsy syndromes with multiple seizures types.

Central poststroke pain. Acute management of bipolar I depression and as a mood stabilizer in rapid-cycling bipolar II disorder.

CONTRAINDICATIONS

Lactation and in children less than 16 years of age, other than as adjunctive therapy for generalized seizures of Lennox-Gastaut syndrome.

SPECIAL CONCERNS

Use with caution in clients with diseases or conditions that could affect metabolism or elimination of the drug, such as in impaired renal, hepatic, or cardiac function. Sudden unexplained death has occurred, rarely.

Serious rashes requiring hospitalization have been noted, especially in children. Risk of rash may be increased by giving lamotrigine with valproic acid, exceeding the recommended initial dose, and exceeding the recommended dose escalation for lamotrigine. Most rashes occur within 2–8 weeks of starting treatment but some rashes are seen after chronic treatment (e.g., 6 months).

SIDE EFFECTS

Side effects listed are those with an incidence of 0.1% or greater.

CNS: Dizziness, ataxia, somnolence, headache, incoordination, insomnia, tremor, depression, anxiety, irritability, decreased memory, speech/sleep disorder, confusion, disturbed concentration, emotional lability, vertigo, mind racing, amnesia, nervousness, abnormal thinking/dreams, agitation, akathisia, aphasia, CNS depression, depersonalization, dyskinesia, dysphoria, euphoria, faintness, hallucinations, hostility, hyperkinesia, hypesthesia, myoclonus, panic attack, paranoid reaction, personality disorder, psychosis, stupor. **GI:** N&V, diarrhea, dyspepsia, constipation, tooth disorder, anorexia, dry mouth, abdominal pain, dysphagia, flatulence, gingivitis, gum hyperplasia, increased appetite, increased salivation, abnormal LFTs, mouth ulceration, stomatitis, thirst. **CV:** Hot flashes, palpitations, flushing, migraine, syncope, tachycardia, vasodilation. **Musculoskeletal:** Arthralgia, joint disorder, myasthenia, dysarthria, muscle spasm, twitching. **Hematologic:** Anemia, ecchymosis, leukocytosis, leukopenia, lymphadenopathy, petechiae. **Hypersensitivity:** Fever, lymphadenopathy, rash, multiorgan dysfunction, ***DIC.*** **Respiratory:** Rhinitis, pharyngitis, increased cough, dyspnea, epistaxis, hyperventilation. **Dermatologic:** Serious rashes, including ***Stevens-Johnson syndrome, toxic epidermal necrolysis,*** pruritus, alopecia, acne, dry skin, eczema, erythema, hirsutism, maculopapular rash, sweating, urticaria, photosensitivity. **Ophthalmologic:** Diplopia, blurred vision, nystagmus, abnormal vision/accommodation, conjunctivitis, oscillopsia, photophobia. **GU:** Dysmenorrhea, vaginitis, amenorrhea, female lactation, hematuria, polyuria, urinary frequency or incontinence, UTI, vaginal moniliasis. **Body as a whole: *Possibility of sudden unexplained death in epilepsy,*** flu syndrome, fever, infection, neck pain, malaise, ***seizure exacerbation,*** chills, halitosis, facial edema, weight gain or loss, peripheral edema, hyperglycemia. **Miscellaneous:** Ear pain, tinnitus, taste perversion.

OD OVERDOSE MANAGEMENT

Symptoms: Possibility of dizziness, headache, somnolence, coma. *Treatment:* Hospitalization with general supportive care. If indicated, induce emesis or perform gastric lavage. Protect the airway.

DRUG INTERACTIONS

Acetaminophen / ↓ Serum lamotrigine levels
Carbamazepine / 40% ↓ in lamotrigine levels
Folate inhibitors / Lamotrigine inhibits dihydrofolate reductase
Oxcarbazepine / ↓ Lamotrigine serum levels due to ↑ liver metabolism
Phenobarbital / 40% ↓ in lamotrigine levels
Phenytoin / 45%–54% ↓ in lamotrigine levels
Primidone / 40% ↓ in lamotrigine levels
Rifamycins (e.g., Rifampin) / ↓ Lamotrigine levels due to ↑ liver metabolism

L

Succinimide / ↓ Serum lamotrigine levels
Valproic acid / Twofold ↑ in lamotrigine levels; 25% ↓ in valproic acid levels

HOW SUPPLIED

Tablet, Chewable Dispersible: 2 mg, 5 mg, 25 mg; *Tablet:* 25 mg, 100 mg, 150 mg, 200 mg

DOSAGE

• TABLETS

Treatment of partial seizures, lamotrigine added to valproic acid.

Adults and children over 12 years of age: Weeks 1 and 2, 25 mg q other day. **Weeks 3 and 4,** 25 mg/day. **Maintenance:** To achieve maintenance doses of lamotrigine of 100–200 mg/day, increase dose by 25–50 mg/day q 1–2 weeks. **Children, 2–12 years: Weeks 1 and 2,** 0.15 mg/kg/day in 1 or 2 divided doses, rounded down to the nearest whole tablet. **Weeks 3 and 4,** 0.3 mg/kg/day in 1 or 2 divided doses; round down to the nearest whole tablet. **Maintenance:** 1–5 mg/kg/day, not to exceed 200 mg/day in 1 or 2 divided doses. To reach maintenance dose, increase dose as follows q 1–2 weeks: Calculate 0.3 mg/kg/day and round this down to the nearest whole tablet; add this amount to the previously administered daily dose.

Partial seizures, lamotrigine added to enzyme-inducing antiepileptic drugs (e.g., carbamazepine, phenobarbital, phenytoin, primidone) without valproic acid.

Adults and children over 12 years: Weeks 1 and 2, 50 mg/day. **Weeks 3 and 4,** 100 mg/day in 2 divided doses. **Maintenance:** To achieve maintenance doses of 300–500 mg/day (in 2 divided doses), increase dose by 100 mg/day q 1–2 weeks. **Children, 2–12 years: Weeks 1 and 2,** 0.6 mg/kg/day in 2 divided doses, rounded down to the nearest whole tablet. **Weeks 3 and 4,** 1.2 mg/kg/day in 2 divided doses, rounded down to the nearest whole tablet. **Maintenance:** 5–15 mg/kg/day, to a maximum of 400 mg/day in 2 divided doses. To reach maintenance doses, increase the dose as follows q 1–2 weeks: Calculate 1.2 mg/kg/day and round down to the nearest whole tablet; add this amount to the previously administered daily dose.

Conversion from a single enzyme-inducing antiepileptic drug to lamotrigine alone.

Clients 16 years and older: 500 mg/day (maintenance dose) in 2 divided doses. To convert, titrate lamotrigine to 500 mg/day in 2 divided doses while maintaining the dose of the enzyme-inducing drug at a fixed level. Withdraw the enzyme-inducing drug by 20% decrements each q week over a 4-week period.

NURSING CONSIDERATIONS

SEE ALSO *NURSING CONSIDERATIONS* FOR *ANTICONVULSANTS*.

ADMINISTRATION/STORAGE

1. Base dose on the therapeutic response since a therapeutic plasma level has not been determined.
2. If a change in seizure control or worsening of side effects is noted in clients receiving lamotrigine in combination with other antiepileptic drugs, reevaluate all drugs in the regimen.
3. Discontinuing an enzyme-inducing antiepileptic drug should prolong the drug half-life, whereas discontinuing valproic acid should shorten the half-life of lamotrigine.
4. If it is decided to discontinue lamotrigine therapy, a stepwise reduction of dose over 2 weeks (about 50% per week) is recommended unless safety concerns mandate a more rapid withdrawal.

ASSESSMENT

1. Document type, onset, and characteristics of seizures, previous agents used, and the outcome.
2. If also prescribed other anticonvulsant agents (i.e., valproate, carbamazepine), monitor closely for adverse effects.
3. Monitor CBC, renal and LFTs; reduce dose with dysfunction.
4. Discontinue drug at first sign of rash.

CLIENT/FAMILY TEACHING

1. Swallow chewable dispersible tablets whole, chewed, or dispersed in water or

diluted fruit juice. If chewed, drink a small amount of water or diluted fruit juice to help in swallowing. To disperse chewable tablets, add the tablets to 5 mL (or enough to cover the drug) of liquid. About 1 min later, when tablets are completely dispersed, swirl the solution and consume the entire amount immediately. Do not give partial amounts of the dispersed tablets.
2. Do not stop abruptly; may cause increased seizure frequency. Drug should be gradually decreased over at least 2 weeks unless safety concerns require rapid withdrawal.
3. Do not perform activities that require mental alertness and/or coordination until drug effects realized; may cause dizziness, ataxia, somnolence, headache, and blurred vision.
4. Report loss of seizure control or if a rash occurs.
5. Photosensitization may occur; wear protective clothing, sunscreen, and sunglasses until tolerance determined.

OUTCOMES/EVALUATE

Control of seizures

Lansoprazole

(lan-**SAHP**-rah-zohl)

PREGNANCY CATEGORY: B
CLASSIFICATION(S):
Proton pump inhibitor
Rx: Prevacid

ACTION/KINETICS

Suppresses gastric acid secretion by inhibition of the (H^+, K^+)-ATPase system located at the secretory surface of the parietal cells in the stomach. Drug is a gastric acid (proton) pump inhibitor in that it blocks the final step of acid production. Both basal and stimulated gastric acid secretion are inhibited, regardless of the stimulus. May have antimicrobial activity against *Helicobacter pylori*. Absorption begins only after lansoprazole granules leave the stomach, but absorption is rapid. **Peak plasma levels:** 1.7 hr. **Mean plasma t½:** 1.5 hr. Over 97% bound to plasma proteins. **Duration:** Over 24 hr. Food does not appear to affect the rate of absorption, if given before meals. Metabolized in the liver with metabolites excreted through both the urine (33%) and feces (66%).

USES

(1) Short-term treatment (up to 4 weeks) for healing and symptomatic relief of active duodenal ulcer. (2) Maintain healing of duodenal ulcer. (3) With clarithromycin and/or amoxicillin to eradicate *Helicobacter pylori* infection in active or recurrent duodenal ulcers. (4) Short-term treatment (up to 8 weeks) for healing and symptomatic relief of benign gastric ulcer. (5) Treatment of NSAID-associated gastric ulcer in those who continue NSAID use. Reduce the risk of NSAID-associated gastric ulcer in those with a history of documented gastric ulcer who required a NSAID. (6) Short-term treatment (up to 8 weeks) for healing and symptomatic relief of all grades of erosive esophagitis. Maintain healing of erosive esophagitis. (7) Long-term treatment of pathologic hypersecretory conditions, including Zollinger-Ellison syndrome. (8) Heartburn and other symptoms of GERD.

CONTRAINDICATIONS

Lactation. Use with rabeprazole.

SPECIAL CONCERNS

Reduce dosage in impaired hepatic function. Symptomatic relief does not preclude the presence of gastric malignancy. Safety and efficacy have not been determined in children less than 18 years of age.

SIDE EFFECTS

GI: Diarrhea, abdominal pain, nausea, melena, anorexia, bezoar, cardiospasm, cholelithiasis, constipation, dry mouth, thirst, dyspepsia, dysphagia, eructation, esophageal stenosis/ulcer, esophagitis, fecal discoloration, flatulence, gastric nodules, fundic gland polyps, gastroenteritis, ***GI hemorrhage, rectal hemorrhage,*** hematemesis, increased appetite/salivation, stomatitis, tenesmus, vomiting, ulcerative colitis.

L

CV: Angina, hyper- or hypotension, ***CVA, MI, shock,*** palpitations, vasodilation. **CNS:** Headache, agitation, amnesia, anxiety, apathy, confusion, depression, syncope, dizziness, hallucinations, hemiplegia, aggravated hostility, decreased libido, nervousness, paresthesia, abnormal thinking. **GU:** Abnormal menses, breast enlargement/tenderness, gynecomastia, hematuria, albuminuria, glycosuria, impotence, kidney calculus. **Respiratory:** Asthma, bronchitis, increased cough, dyspnea, epistaxis, hemoptysis, hiccoughs, pneumonia, URI/inflammation. **Endocrine:** Diabetes mellitus, goiter, hypo- or hyperglycemia. **Hematologic:** Anemia, eosinophilia, hemolysis. **Musculoskeletal:** Arthritis, arthralgia, musculoskeletal pain, myalgia. **Dermatologic:** Acne, alopecia, pruritus, rash, urticaria. **Ophthalmologic:** Amblyopia, eye pain, visual field defect. **Otic:** Deafness, otitis media, tinnitus. **Miscellaneous:** Gout, weight loss/gain, taste perversion, asthenia, candidiasis, chest pain, edema, fever, flu syndrome, halitosis, infection, malaise.

LABORATORY TEST CONSIDERATIONS

Abnormal LFTs. ↑ AST, ALT, creatinine, alkaline phosphatase, globulins, GGTP, glucocorticoids, LDH, gastrin. ↑ or ↓ of abnormal WBC and platelets. Abnormal AG ratio, RBC. Bilirubinemia, hyperlipemia. ↑ or ↓ Electrolytes or cholesterol.

DRUG INTERACTIONS

Ampicillin / ↓ Ampicillin effect R/T ↓ absorption
Digoxin / ↓ Digoxin effect R/T ↓ absorption
Iron salts / ↓ Effect of iron salts R/T ↓ absorption
Ketoconazole / ↓ Ketoconazole effect R/T ↓ absorption
Sucralfate / Delayed absorption of lansoprazole

HOW SUPPLIED

Capsule, delayed-release: 15 mg, 30 mg

DOSAGE

- **CAPSULES, DELAYED RELEASE**

Treatment of duodenal ulcer.

Adults: 15 mg once daily before breakfast for 4 weeks.

Maintenance of healed duodenal ulcer.

Adults: 15 mg once daily.

H. pylori *infections.*

The following regimens may be used. (1) *Triple therapy.* Lansoprazole, 30 mg b.i.d., plus clarithromycin, 500 mg b.i.d., plus amoxicillin, 1 g, b.i.d. for 10 or 14 days. (2) *Dual Therapy.* Lansoprazole, 30 mg plus amoxicillin, 1 g, t.i.d. for 14 days (for clients intolerant or resistant to clarithromycin). (3) Lansoprazole, 30 mg b.id., plus clarithromycin, 500 mg b.i.d., plus metronidazole, 500 mg b.i.d. for 14 days. (4) Lansoprazole, 30 mg b.i.d., plus tetracycline, 500 mg q.i.d., plus metronidazole, 500 mg t.i.d. or 250 mg q.i.d. plus bismuth subsalicylate, 525 mg q.i.d. for 14 days.

Treatment of gastric ulcer.

30 mg once daily for up to 8 weeks.

Reduce risk of NSAID-associated gastric ulcer.

15 mg once daily for up to 12 weeks.

Treatment of NSAID-associated gastric ulcer

30 mg once daily for 8 weeks.

Treatment of erosive esophagitis.

30 mg before eating for up to 8 weeks. If the client does not heal in 8 weeks, an additional 8 weeks of therapy may be given. If there is a recurrence, an additional 8-week course may be considered.

Maintenance of healed erosive esophagitis.

15 mg once daily for up to 12 months.

Pathologic hypersecretory conditions.

Initial: 60 mg once daily. Adjust the dose to client need. Dosage may be continued as long as necessary. Doses up to 90 or 120 mg (in divided doses) daily have been given.

Treatment of GERD.

15 mg once daily for up to 8 weeks.

NURSING CONSIDERATIONS

ADMINISTRATION/STORAGE

1. Consider dosage reduction in those with severe liver disease.
2. For those unable to swallow capsules, open the delayed-release capsule and sprinkle the contents on a

tablespoon of applesauce, *Ensure* pudding, cottage cheese, yogurt, or strained pears and swallow immediately. Alternatively, contents of the capsule can be mixed with about 2 oz of either orange or tomato juice, mixed briefly, and swallowed immediately. Do not chew or crush the granules.
3. To give with a NG tube in place, open the capsule and mix intact granules with 40 mL of apple juice. Instill through the NG tube into the stomach, flushing with additional apple juice to clear the tube.
4. Adjust dosage in severe liver disease.
5. Store in a tight container protected from moisture. Store between 15–30°C (59–86°F).

ASSESSMENT

1. Document indications for therapy, onset, duration, characteristics of and what triggers symptoms, and any other agents trialed.
2. Note findings of US, UGI, barium swallow, or endoscopy. Check *H. pylori* results.
3. Monitor CBC, electrolytes, triglycerides, renal and LFTs; reduce dose with severe liver disease.

CLIENT/FAMILY TEACHING

1. Take before meals exactly as prescribed; do not exceed dose or share meds.
2. Swallow capsules whole, do not open. chew, or crush. Those who have difficulty swallowing capsules may open capsule and sprinkle the contents onto apple sauce, *Ensure*, yogurt, cottage cheese or strained pairs or into juices.
3. Follow prescribed diet and activities to control S&S of GERD. Drug should be withdrawn once condition cleared/resolved.
4. Keep scheduled appointments. Drug is generally for short-term therapy and discontinued once condition is healed. Long-term effects are not known; users should be assessed periodically for gastric malignancy.
5. Report any severe headaches, worsening of symptoms, fever, chills or diarrhea as drug may have to be stopped.
6. Avoid hazardous activities until drug effects realized as dizziness many occur.
7. Avoid alcohol, ASA, NSAIDS and OTC agents; may increase GI irritation.

OUTCOMES/EVALUATE

- Suppression of acid secretion
- Healing of ulcer/erosive esophagitis
- ↓ Pain; relief of heartburn

Leflunomide

(leh-**FLOON**-oh-myd)

PREGNANCY CATEGORY: X
CLASSIFICATION(S):
Antiarthritic drug
Rx: Arava

ACTION/KINETICS

Inhibits dihydroorotate dehydrogenase, an enzyme involved in de novo pyrimidine synthesis; has antiproliferative activity and anti-inflammatory and uricosuric effects. After PO, is metabolized to an active metabolite (M1). **Peak levels, M1:** 6–12 hr. **t½, M1:** About 2 weeks. M1 is extensively bound to albumin. M1 is further metabolized and excreted through the kidney (more significant over the first 96 hr) and bile.

USES

Treatment of active rheumatoid arthritis in adults, including to retard structural damage.

CONTRAINDICATIONS

Use in pregnancy, lactation, in children less than 18 years of age, in hepatic insufficiency, or positive hepatitis B or C. Also, use in those with severe immunodeficiency, bone marrow dysplasia, severe uncontrolled infections, or vaccination with live vaccines.

SPECIAL CONCERNS

Use with caution in those with renal insufficiency.

SIDE EFFECTS

GI: Diarrhea, N&V, dyspepsia, abnormal liver enzymes, abdominal pain, anorexia, dry mouth, gastroenteritis, mouth ulcer, cholelithiasis, colitis, constipation, esophagitis, flatulence, gastritis, gingivitis, melena, oral moniliasis, pharyngitis, enlarged salivary gland, stomatitis or aphthous stomatitis, tooth disorder. **CNS:** Headache, dizziness, paresthesia, anxiety, depression, insomnia, neuralgia, neuritis, sleep disorder, sweat, vertigo. **CV:** Hypertension (as pre-existing condition was over represented in drug treatment groups), chest pain, angina pectoris, migraine, palpitation, tachycardia, vasculitis, vasodilation, varicose vein. **Dermatologic:** Alopecia, rash, pruritus, eczema, dry skin, acne, contact dermatitis, fungal dermatitis, hair discoloration, hematoma, herpes simplex/zoster, nail disorder, skin/subcutaneous nodule, maculopapular rash, skin disorder/discoloration/ulcer. **Musculoskeletal:** Joint disorder, tenosynovitis, synovitis, arthralgia, leg/muscle cramps, arthrosis, bursitis, myalgia, bone pain/ necrosis, tendon rupture. **Respiratory:** Respiratory infection, bronchitis, increased cough, pharyngitis, pneumonia, rhinitis, sinusitis, asthma, dyspnea, epistaxis, lung disorder. **GU:** Albuminuria, cystitis, dysuria, hematuria, menstrual disorder, vaginal moniliasis, prostate disorder, urinary frequency, UTI. **Hematologic:** Anemia, including iron deficiency anemia; ecchymosis. **Metabolic:** Weight loss, hypokalemia, peripheral edema, hyperglycemia, hyperlipidemia. **Ophthalmic:** Blurred vision, cataract, conjunctivitis, eye disorder. **Miscellaneous:** Diabetes mellitus, hyperthyroidism, taste perversion, back pain, injury accident, infection, asthenia, allergic reaction, flu syndrome, pain, abscess, cyst, fever, hernia, malaise, neck/pelvic pain.

LABORATORY TEST CONSIDERATIONS

↑ ALT, AST, creatine phosphokinase. Uricosuric effect, hypophosphatemia.

OD OVERDOSE MANAGEMENT

Symptoms: See Side Effects. *Treatment:* Give cholestyramine or charcoal. Dose of cholestyramine is 8 g t.i.d. PO for 24 hr. Dose of charcoal is 50 g made into a suspension for PO or NGT given q 6 hr for 24 hr.

DRUG INTERACTIONS

Charcoal / Rapid/significant ↓ in leflunomide active M1 metabolite
Cholestyramine / Rapid/significant ↓ in leflunomide active M1 metabolite
Hepatotoxic drugs / ↑ Side effects
Rifampin / ↑ M1 peak levels

HOW SUPPLIED

Tablets: 10 mg, 20 mg, 100 mg

DOSAGE

• **TABLETS**

Rheumatoid arthritis.

Loading dose: 100 mg/day PO for 3 days. **Maintenance:** 20 mg/day; if this dose is not well tolerated, decrease to 10 mg/day. Doses greater than 20 mg/day are not recommended due to increased risk of side effects.

NURSING CONSIDERATIONS

ADMINISTRATION/STORAGE

1. Aspirin, NSAIDs, or low dose corticosteroids may be continued during leflunomide therapy.
2. To achieve nondetectable plasma levels (less than 0.02 mcg/mL) after stopping treatment, give cholestyramine, 8 g t.i.d. for 11 days (do not need to be consecutive unless there is a need to lower plasma levels rapidly). Verify plasma levels by 2 separate tests at least 14 days apart. Without the drug elimination procedure, it may taken 2 years or less to reach plasma M1 levels of 0.02 mcg/mL due to variations in drug clearance.

ASSESSMENT

1. Note indications for therapy, severity of joint disease and limitations, joint(s) characteristics, and other agents trialed.
2. Assess for liver dysfunction and hepatitis B or C; as this precludes therapy.
3. Obtain negative pregnancy test.
4. Monitor SGPT (ALT) and AST monthly and adjust dosage with elevations. If elevations persist 2-3x ULN and continued therapy is desired, may consider liver biopsy.
5. Drug metabolite M1 has an extremely long half-life (up to 2 years). Cholestyramine may accelerate drug elimination. Women of childbearing

age desiring pregnancy should undergo the drug elimination procedure that has been established to prevent fetal death or damage.

CLIENT/FAMILY TEACHING

1. Therapy consists of a three day loading dose and then a daily maintenance dose.
2. May take with or without food. May take up to 8 weeks to see desired effects.
3. Drug will cause fetal damage. Practice reliable birth control. If pregnancy desired or suspected in females or males wish to father a child, report so drug elimination procedure can be initiated.
4. Avoid live vaccines.
5. May experience diarrhea, nausea, GI upset, URI, headache and rash; report if persistent or intolerable.
6. Report as scheduled for monthly liver function studies.

OUTCOMES/EVALUATE

- ↓ Bone erosion/joint narrowing
- Slowed RA disease progression

Lepirudin

(leh-**PEER**-you-din)

PREGNANCY CATEGORY: B
CLASSIFICATION(S):
Anticoagulant, thrombin inhibitor
Rx: Refludan

SEE ALSO *ANTICOAGULANTS.*

ACTION/KINETICS

Recombinant hirudin from yeast cells; highly specific direct inhibitor of thrombin. One antithrombin unit (ATU) is the amount of lepirudin that neutralizes one unit of World Health Organization preparation 89/588 of thrombin. One molecule of lepirudin binds to one molecule of thrombin, blocking the thrombogenic activity of thrombin. Thus, all thrombin-dependent assays are affected (i.e., activated partial thromboplastin time—aPTT), resulting in an increase in aPTT. **t½, distribution:** About 10 min; **t½, elimination:** About 1.3 hr. Systemic clearance is dependent on glomerular filtration rate. About half is excreted in the urine as unchanged drug and other fragments. Dose must be adjusted based on C_{CR}.

USES

Treat heparin-induced thrombocytopenia and associated thromboembolic disease to prevent further complications.

CONTRAINDICATIONS

Hypersensitivity to hirudins. Lactation.

SPECIAL CONCERNS

Assess risk of therapy in those with an increased risk of bleeding, including recent puncture of large vessels or organ biopsy; anomaly of vessels or organs; recent CVA, stroke, intracerebral surgery or other neuraxial procedures; severe uncontrolled hypertension; bacterial endocarditis; advanced renal impairment; hemorrhagic diathesis; recent major surgery; recent intracranial, GI, intraocular, or pulmonary major bleeding. Formation of antihirudin antibodies or serious hepatic injury may increase the anticoagulant effect. Increased risk of allergic reactions in those also receiving thrombolytic therapy (e.g., streptokinase) for acute MI or contrast media for coronary angiography. Safety and efficacy have not been determined in children.

SIDE EFFECTS

Hemorrhagic events: Bleeding from puncture sites and wounds, anemia or isolated drop in hemoglobin, hematoma, hematuria, GI and rectal bleeding, epistaxis, hemothorax, vaginal bleeding, intracranial bleeding, hemoperitoneum, hemoptysis, liver bleeding, lung bleeding, mouth bleeding, retroperitoneal bleeding.
CV: ***Heart failure, pericardial effusion, ventricular fibrillation.*** **Allergic reactions:** Cough, ***bronchospasms,*** stridor, dyspnea, pruritus, urticaria, rash, flushes, chills, ***anaphylaxis,*** angioedema, ***facial/tongue/larynx edema.*** **Miscellaneous:** Fever, abnormal liver function, pneumonia, sepsis, allergic skin reactions, abnormal kidney

function, unspecified infections, ***multi-organ failure***.

OD OVERDOSE MANAGEMENT

Symptoms: Bleeding. *Treatment:* Immediately stop administration. Determine aPTT and other coagulation levels as appropriate. Determine hemoglobin and prepare for blood transfusion. Follow guidelines for treatment of shock. Hemofiltration or hemodialysis may be helpful.

DRUG INTERACTIONS

Coumarin derivatives / ↑ Risk of bleeding

Thrombolytics (streptokinase, tPA) / ↑ Risk of bleeding complications and ↑ effect on aPTT prolongation

HOW SUPPLIED

Powder for Injection: 50 mg

DOSAGE

• **IV**

Heparin-induced thrombocytopenia and associated thromboembolic disease.

Adults, initial: 0.4 mg/kg given slowly over 15–20 seconds as a bolus dose followed by 0.15 mg/kg/hr as a continuous IV infusion for 2–10 days or longer if needed. The maximum bolus dose is 44 mg and the maximal initial infusion dose is 16.5 mg/hr. Adjust dose according to the aPTT ratio (client aPTT at a given time over an aPTT reference value, usually median of the lab normal range for aPTT).

The bolus and infusion doses must be reduced in known or suspected renal insufficiency (C_{CR} less than 60 mL/min or serum creatinine greater than 1.5 mg/dL).

Concomitant use with thrombolytics.

Initial IV bolus: 0.2 mg/kg; **continuous IV infusion:** 0.1 mg/kg/hr.

NURSING CONSIDERATIONS

SEE ALSO NURSING CONSIDERATIONS FOR ANTICOAGULANTS.

ADMINISTRATION/STORAGE

IV 1. If client is to receive coumarin derivatives for PO anticoagulation after lepirudin, gradually reduce the dose of lepirudin to reach an aPTT ratio just above 1.5 before initiating PO anticoagulation. As soon as an INR of 2 is reached, stop drug.

2. Do not mix with other drugs except water for injection, 0.9% NaCl, or D5W injection.

3. Reconstitution and further dilution are to be done under sterile conditions as follows:

• Use D5W or water for injection for reconstitution

• For further dilution, 0.9% NaCl injection or D5W injection is suitable.

• For rapid, complete reconstitution, inject 1 mL of diluent into the vial and shake gently. A clear, colorless solution is usually obtained in a few seconds, but less than 3 min.

• Do not use solutions that are cloudy or contain particles.

• Use reconstituted solution immediately; it is stable for 24 hr or less at room temperature (i.e., during infusion).

• Warm the product to room temperature before administration.

• Discard any unused solution.

4. For the initial IV bolus, use a 5 mg/mL solution. Prepare as follows:

• Reconstitute one vial (50 mg) with 1 mL of 0.9% NaCl or water for injection.

• To obtain a final concentration of 5 mg/mL, transfer the contents of the vial into a sterile, single-use syringe (10 mL or greater capacity) and dilute the solution to a total volume of 10 mL using water for injection, 0.9% NaCl, or D5W.

5. For continuous IV infusion, use a concentration of 0.2 or 0.4 mg/mL. Prepare as follows:

• Reconstitute two vials (50 mg each) with 1 mL each using either 0.9% NaCl or water for injection.

• To obtain a final concentration of 0.2 or 0.4 mg/mL, transfer the contents of both vials into an infusion bag containing 500 or 250 mL of 0.9% NaCl or D5W.

• The infusion rate (mL/hr) is determined according to body weight).

ASSESSMENT

1. Assess for conditions that preclude therapy. Note allergic reactions with thrombolytic therapy.

2. Monitor LFTs, CBC, bleeding parameters, and renal function studies; reduce dosage with dysfunction.
3. If weight is more than 110 kg, do not increase dosage beyond that weight dose.
4. Monitor carefully at all sites for evidence of excessive bleeding. Have RBCs available for transfusion.
5. Get PTT 4 hr after first dose and at least daily during therapy (more frequently with liver/renal impairment). If PTT ratio >2.5 stop infusion for 2 hr and report.

CLIENT/FAMILY TEACHING

1. Drug is used to anticoagulate those with heparin-induced-thrombocytopenia(HIT).
2. Report any evidence of bleeding or oozing from catheter sites, under skin or gums, in urine or stools.
3. Use soft bristled tooth brush, electric razor, night light, and slippers to prevent injury; avoid contact sports or aggressive hugging, juggling or wrestling.

OUTCOMES/EVALUATE

- Inhibition of thromboembolic complications
- PTT ratio 1.5 to 2.5

Letrozole

(**LET**-roh-zohl)

PREGNANCY CATEGORY: D
CLASSIFICATION(S):
Antineoplastic, hormone
Rx: Femara

SEE ALSO *ANTINEOPLASTIC AGENTS.*

ACTION/KINETICS

A nonsteroidal competitive inhibitor of aromatase, resulting in inhibition of conversion of androgens to estrogens. It acts by competitively binding to heme of cytochrome P450 subunit of aromatase, leading to decreased biosynthesis of estrogen in all tissues. Does not cause increase in serum FSH and does not affect synthesis of adrenocorticosteroids, aldosterone, or thyroid hormones. **t½, elimination:** About 2 days. Steady state plasma levels after daily doses of 2.5 mg reached in 2 to 6 weeks. Inactive liver metabolites are excreted in urine.

USES

Advanced or metastatic breast cancer in postmenopausal women who are hormone-receptor positive disease or hormone-receptor unknown and where there is progression following antiestrogen therapy.

SPECIAL CONCERNS

Use with caution during lactation and in those with severely impaired hepatic function. Safety and efficacy have not been determined in children.

SIDE EFFECTS

CNS: Headache, somnolence, dizziness, vertigo, depression, anxiety. **GI:** N&V, constipation, diarrhea, abdominal pain, anorexia, dyspepsia. **Body as a whole:** Fatigue, viral infections, peripheral edema, asthenia, increased weight. **Dermatologic:** Hot flashes, rash, pruritus, alopecia, increased sweating. **Respiratory:** Dyspnea, coughing, pleural effusion. **Miscellaneous:** Chest pain, hypertension, arthralgia, fracture, hypercholesterolemia, hypercalcemia, vertigo.

LABORATORY TEST CONSIDERATIONS

↑ AST, ALT, GGT. ↓ Lymphocyte counts. Hypercholesterolemia, hypercalcemia.

HOW SUPPLIED

Tablet: 2.5 mg

DOSAGE

- **TABLETS**

Advanced breast cancer.

Adults and elderly: 2.5 mg once/day. Continue until tumor progression is evident. Dosage adjustment is not needed in renal impairment if C_{CR} is greater than or equal to 10 mL/min.

NURSING CONSIDERATIONS

SEE ALSO *NURSING CONSIDERATIONS FOR ANTINEOPLASTIC AGENTS.*

ASSESSMENT

1. Note disease onset, clinical findings, previous antiestrogen therapy, and response.
2. Monitor renal and LFTs.

CLIENT/FAMILY TEACHING

1. Take as directed; may take without regard to meals.
2. Report any severe rash, diarrhea, pain, dyspnea, or chest pain.
3. May experience drowsiness; use caution.
4. Practice reliable contraception; may cause serious fetal harm.

OUTCOMES/EVALUATE

↓ Tumor mass; ↓ malignant cell proliferation

Leucovorin calcium (Citrovorum factor, Folinic acid)

(loo-koh-**VOR**-in)

PREGNANCY CATEGORY: C
CLASSIFICATION(S):
Folic acid derivative
Rx: Wellcovorin

L

ACTION/KINETICS

Derivative of folic acid; is a mixture of the diasterioisomers of the 5-formyl derivative of tetrahydrofolic acid. Does not require reduction by dihydrofolate reductase to be active in intracellular metabolism; thus, it is not affected by dihydrofolate inhibitors. Rapidly absorbed following PO administration. Quickly metabolized to 1,5-methyltetrahydrofolate, which is then metabolized by other pathways back to 5,10-methylene-tetrahydrofolate and then converted to 5-methyltetrahydrofolate using the cofactors $FADH_2$ and NADPH. Leucovorin can counteract the therapeutic and toxic effects of methotrexate (acts by inhibiting dihydrofolate reductase) but can enhance the effects of 5-fluorouracil (5-FU). Is rapidly absorbed. **Peak serum levels, PO:** Approximately 2.3 hr; **after IM:** 52 min; **after IV:** 10 min. **Onset, PO:** 20–30 min; **IM:** 10–20 min; **IV:** < 5 min. **Terminal t½:** 5.7 hr (PO), 6.2 hr (IM and IV). **Duration:** 3–6 hr. Excreted by the kidney.

USES

PO and Parenteral: Prophylaxis and treatment of toxicity due to methotrexate and folic acid antagonists (e.g., pyrimethamine and trimethoprim). Leucovorin rescue following high doses of methotrexate for osteosarcoma. **Parenteral:** Megaloblastic anemias due to nutritional deficiency, sprue, pregnancy, and infancy when oral folic acid is not appropriate. Adjunct with 5-FU to prolong survival in the palliative treatment of metastatic colorectal carcinoma. *Note:* It is recommended for megaloblastic anemia caused by pregnancy even though the drug is pregnancy category C.

CONTRAINDICATIONS

Pernicious anemia or megaloblastic anemia due to vitamin B_{12} deficiency.

SPECIAL CONCERNS

Use with caution during lactation. May increase the frequency of seizures in susceptible children. When leucovorin is used with 5-FU for advanced colorectal cancer, the dosage of 5-FU must be lower than usual as leucovorin enhances the toxicity of 5-FU. The benzyl alcohol in the parenteral form may caues a fatal gasping syndrome in premature infants.

SIDE EFFECTS

Leucovorin alone. Allergic reactions, including urticaria and ***anaphylaxis.***

Leucovorin and 5-FU. **GI:** N&V, diarrhea, stomatitis, constipation, anorexia. **Hematologic:** Leukopenia, thrombocytopenia. **CNS:** Fatigue, lethargy, malaise. **Miscellaneous:** Infection, alopecia, dermatitis.

DRUG INTERACTIONS

5-FU / ↑ 5-FU toxicity
Methotrexate / High doses ↓ effect of intrathecal methotrexate
PAS / ↓ Serum folate levels → folic acid deficiency
Phenobarbital / ↓ Phenobarabital effect → ↑ seizure frequency, especially in children
Phenytoin / ↓ Phenytoin effect R/T ↑ rate of liver breakdown; also, drug may ↓ plasma folate levels
Primidone / ↓ Primidone effect → ↑ seizure frequency, especially in children
Sulfasalazine / ↓ Serum folate levels → folic acid deficiency

HOW SUPPLIED

Injection: 3 mg/mL; *Powder for injection:* 50 mg, 100 mg, 350 mg; *Tablet:* 5 mg, 15 mg, 25 mg

DOSAGE

• **IM, IV, TABLETS**

Advanced colorectal cancer.

Either leucovorin, 200 mg/m² by slow IV over a minimum of 3 min followed by 5-FU, 370 mg/m² IV **or** leucovorin 20 mg/m² IV followed by 5-FU, 425 mg/m² IV. Treatment is repeated daily for 5 days with the 5-day treatment course repeated at 28-day intervals for two courses and then repeated at 4- to 5-week intervals as long as the client has recovered from the toxic effects.

Leucovorin rescue after high-dose methotrexate therapy.

The dose of leucovorin is based on a methotrexate dose of 12–15 mg/m² given by IV infusion over 4 hr. The dose of leucovorin is 15 mg (10 mg/m²) PO, IM, or IV q 6 hr for 10 doses starting 24 hr after the start of the methotrexate infusion. Give leucovorin parenterally if there is nausea, vomiting, or GI toxicity. If serum methotrexate levels are greater than 0.2 μM at 72 hr and greater than 0.05 μM at 96 hr after administration, leucovorin should be continued at a dose of 15 mg PO, IM, or IV q 6 hr until methotrexate levels are less than 0.05 μM. If serum methotrexate levels are equal to or greater than 50 μM at 24 hr or equal to or greater than 5 μM at 48 hr after administration or if there is a 100% or greater increase in serum creatinine levels at 24 hr after methotrexate administration, the dose of leucovorin should be 150 mg IV q 3 hr until methotrexate levels are less than 1 μM; **then,** give leucovorin, 15 mg IV q 3 hr until methotrexate levels are less than 0.05 μM. If significant clinical toxicity is seen following methotrexate, leucovorin rescue should total 14 doses over 84 hr in subsequent courses of methotrexate therapy.

Impaired methotrexate elimination or accidental overdose.

Start leucovorin rescue as soon as the overdose is discovered and within 24 hr of methotrexate administration when excretion is impaired. Give leucovorin, 10 mg/m² PO, IM, or IV q 6 hr until serum methotrexate levels are less than 10^{-8} M. If the 24-hr serum creatinine has increased 50% over baseline or if the 24- or 48-hr methotrexate level is more than 5×10^{-6} M or greater than 9×10^{-7} M, respectively, the dose of leucovorin should be increased to 100 mg/m² IV q 3 hr until the methotrexate level is less than 10^{-8} M. Urinary alkalinization with sodium bicarbonate solution (to maintain urine pH at 7 or greater) and hydration with 3 L/day should be undertaken at the same time.

Overdosage of folic acid antagonists.

5–15 mg/day.

Megaloblastic anemia due to folic acid deficiency.

Adults and children: Up to 1 mg/day.

NURSING CONSIDERATIONS

ADMINISTRATION/STORAGE

1. Oral solution stable for 14 days refrigerated or 7 days stored at room temperature.

IV 2. If used for methotrexate rescue, hydrate well and alkalinize urine to reduce nephrotoxicity.

3. Dilute with 5 mL bacteriostatic water for injection and use within 1 week. If sterile water for injection is added, use the solution immediately.

4. Give doses higher than 25 mg parenterally because PO absorption is saturated.

5. Do not use leucovorin calcium injection containing benzyl alcohol in doses greater than 10 mg/m².

6. Parenteral use is preferred if there is a possibility client may vomit or not absorb leucovorin.

7. In treating overdosage due to folic acid antagonists, give as soon as possible. As the time interval between the overdosage and administration of leucovorin increases, the effectiveness of leucovorin decreases.

8. Protect from light.

ASSESSMENT

1. Document indications for therapy: replacement or rescue. If for rescue

therapy, administer promptly (first dose within 1 hr) following a high dose of folic acid antagonists; follow dosage exactly to be effective.
2. Note history of B_{12} deficiency that has resulted in pernicious or megaloblastic anemia. Leucovorin may obscure the diagnosis of pernicious anemia if previously undiagnosed.
3. Determine any history of seizure disorders; assess for recurrence.
4. Monitor renal, B_{12}, folic acid, and hematologic values. Creatinine increases of 50% over pretreatment levels indicate severe renal toxicity.
5. Urine pH should be greater than 7.0; monitor q 6 hr during therapy. Urine alkalinization with $NaHCO_3$ or acetazolamide may be necessary to prevent nephrotoxic effects.

CLIENT/FAMILY TEACHING

1. This drug is used to save or "rescue" normal cells from the damaging effects of chemotherapy allowing them to survive while the cancer cells die.
2. Report immediately any skin rash, itching, malaise, or difficulty breathing.
3. Parenteral therapy generally is used following chemotherapy; N&V may prevent oral absorption.
4. When high-dose therapy is used, be alert for mental confusion and impaired judgment. Safety measures and supervision help to ensure safety and protection.
5. Consume at least 3 L/day of fluids with rescue therapy.

OUTCOMES/EVALUATE

- Symptom improvement (↓ fatigue, ↑ weight, improved mentation)
- ↑ Normoblasts (with anemia)
- Prevention/reversal of GI, renal, and bone marrow toxicity in methotrexate therapy or during overdosage of folic acid antagonists

Leuprolide acetate

(loo-**PROH**-lyd)

PREGNANCY CATEGORY: X
CLASSIFICATION(S):
Antineoplastic, hormone

Rx: Lupron, Lupron Depot, Lupron Depot - 3 month, Lupron Depot—4 Month, Lupron Depot-Ped, Lupron for Pediatric Use, Viadur
✱**Rx:** Lupron Depot 3.75 mg/11.25 mg, Lupron/Lupron Depot 3.75 mg/7.5 mg, Lupron/Lupron Depot 7.5 mg/22.5 mg/30 mg

SEE ALSO *ANTINEOPLASTIC AGENTS.*

ACTION/KINETICS

Related to the naturally occurring GnRH. By desensitizing GnRH receptors, gonadotropin secretion is inhibited. Initially, however, LH and FSH levels increase, leading to increases of sex hormones. However, decreases in these hormones will be observed within 2–4 weeks. **Peak plasma levels:** 4 hr for various doses. **t½:** 3 hr. Chronic use results in a measureable increase in body length, return to prepubertal state of reproductive organs, and cessation of menses (if present). A miniature titanium implant is available which releases leuprolide over one year and provides an alternative to frequent injections.

USES

(1) Palliative treatment in advanced prostatic cancer when orchiectomy or estrogen treatment are not appropriate (use injection, implant, or depot 7.5, 22.5, and 30 mg). (2) Viadur is used as a once yearly implant for advanced prostate cancer. (3) Endometriosis (use depot 3.75 and 11.25 mg). (4) Central precocious puberty (use pediatric injection or Depot-Ped). (5) In combination with iron supplements for the presurgical treatment of anemia caused by uterine fibroid tumors (use depot form, 3.75 and 11.25 mg). *Investigational:* With flutamide for metastatic prostatic cancer.

CONTRAINDICATIONS

Pregnancy, in women who may become pregnant while receiving the drug, and during lactation. Sensitivity to benzyl alcohol (found in leuprolide injection). Undiagnosed abnormal vaginal bleeding. Hypersensitivity to GnRH or GnRH agonist analogs. The 30-mg depot in women and the implant in women and children.

SPECIAL CONCERNS

Safety and efficacy have not been determined in children (except depot-PED). May cause increased bone pain and difficulty in urination during the first few weeks of therapy for prostatic cancer.

SIDE EFFECTS

Injection and Depot.

GI: N&V, anorexia, diarrhea, constipation, taste disorders/perversion, gingivitis, dysphagia, hepatic dysfunction, GI bleeding. **CNS:** Pain, depression, mood swings, hearing disorder, peripheral neuropathy, spinal fracture/paralysis, emotional lability, insomnia, headache, dizziness, nervousness, paresthesias, anxiety, memory disorder, syncope, personality disorder, somnolence. **CV:** Peripheral edema, angina, ***cardiac arrhythmias, TIA/stroke, pulmonary embolism,*** hypotension, vasodilation, pulmonary infiltrates. **GU:** Hematuria, urinary frequency or urgency, dysuria, testicular pain, incontinence, cervix disorder, penile swelling, prostate pain, accelerated sexual maturity. **Respiratory:** Dyspnea, hemoptysis, pneumonia, epistaxis, pulmonary infiltrates. **Endocrine:** Gynecomastia, breast tenderness, impotency, hot flashes, sweating, decreased testicular size, increased or decreased libido. **Musculoskeletal:** Myalgia, bone pain, pelvic fibrosis, ankylosing spondylosis, fibromyalgia, tenosynovitis-like symptoms. **Dermatologic:** Dermatitis, skin reactions, acne, seborrhea, hair growth, ecchymosis, hair loss, skin striae, erythema multiforme and other rashes, androgen-like effects. **Ophthalmic:** Ophthalmic disorder, abnormal vision. **Hypersensitivity:** Rash, urticaria, photosensitivity, ***anaphylaxis.*** **Other:** Asthenia, diabetes, fever, chills, tinnitus, infection, body odor, hard nodule in throat, accelerated sexual maturation, decreased WBCs, hemoptysis, weight gain, hair growth, increased libido.

Injection. CV: ***MI, pulmonary embolism,*** CHF, phlebitis, thrombosis. **GI:** ***GI bleeding,*** rectal polyps, peptic ulcer. **CNS:** Lethargy, mood swings, numbness, blackouts, fatigue. **Respiratory:** Cough, ***pulmonary fibrosis***, pleural rub, pneumonia. **Dermatologic:** Carcinoma of the skin/ear, itching, dry skin, pigmentation, skin lesions. **GU:** Bladder spasms, urinary obstruction. **Miscellaneous:** Enlarged thyroid, inflammation, temporal bone swelling, blurred vision.

Depot. CV: Tachycardia, bradycardia, ***heart failure***, varicose vein, palpitations, hypertension, atrial fibrillation, ***deep thrombophlebitis,*** hypotension. **CNS:** Delusions, confusion, hypesthesia, abnormal thinking, amnesia, convulsions, dementia, depression. **GI:** Dysphagia, gingivitis, duodenal ulcer, dry mouth, thirst, appetite changes, thirst, eructation, ***GI hemorrhage,*** gum hemorrhage, hepatomegaly, intestinal obstruction, periodontal abscess. **Respiratory:** Rhinitis, pharyngitis, pleural effusion, asthma, bronchitis, hiccough, lung disorder, sinusitis, voice alteration, hypoxia. **Endocrine:** Lactation, menstrual disorder. **GU:** Penis disorder, testis disorder, ***bladder carcinoma,*** epididymitis, prostate disorder, menstrual disorder, androgen-like effects. **Ophthalmic:** Conjunctivitis, amblyopia, dry eyes, ptosis. **Miscellaneous:** Nail/hair disorder, flu syndrome, enlarged abdomen, lymphedema, dehydration, lymphadenopathy, abscess, accidental injury, allergic reaction, cyst, hernia, neck pain, neoplasm, abnormal healing, leg cramps, pathological fracture, herpes zoster, melanosis, tinnitus, lactation.

Implant. CNS: Amnesia, anxiety. **Dermatologic:** Pruritus, rash, hirsutism. **GU:** Prostatic disorder, dysuria, urinary incontinence, urinary retention. **Miscellaneous:** Chills, abdominal pain, malaise, dry mucous membranes, iron deficiency, anemia, arthritis.

LABORATORY TEST CONSIDERATIONS

Injection and Depot. ↑ Calcium. ↓ WBC. Hypoproteinemia. **Injection:** ↑ BUN, creatinine. **Depot:** ↑ LDH, alkaline phosphatase, AST, uric acid, cholesterol, LDL, triglycerides, PT, PTT, glucose, WBC. ↓ Platelets, potassium. Hyperphosphatemia, abnormal LFTs. Misleading results from tests of pituitary gonadotropic and gonadal function up to 4–8 weeks after discontinuing depot therapy.

HOW SUPPLIED

Implant: 72 mg; *Injection:* 5 mg/mL; *Microspheres for injection, lyophilized:* 3.75 mg, 7.5 mg. 11.25 mg, 15 mg, 22.5 mg, 30 mg

DOSAGE

• DEPOT, INJECTION, IMPLANT

Advanced prostatic cancer.

Injection: 1 mg/day SC using the syringes provided. Depot (IM): 7.5 mg monthly, 22.5 mg q 3 months, or 30 mg q 4 months. Implant: One implant q 12 months. The implant delivers 120 mcg/day.

Central precocious puberty.

Individualize based on a mg/kg ratio of drug to body weight. Injection: **Initial:** 50 mcg/kg/day SC as a single dose. Dose may increased by 10 mcg/kg/day, which is the maintenance dose. Depot-Ped: **Initial:** 0.3 mg/kg/4 weeks (minimum 7.5 mg) as a single IM dose. If total down regulation is not reached, titrate upward in 3.75 mg increments q 4 weeks (which will be the maintenance dose).

Endometriosis, uterine fibroids.

3.75 mg IM once a month or 11.25 mg IM q 3 months for at least 6 months for endometriosis. If further treatment is contemplated, assess bone density prior to beginning therapy.

Uterine leiomyomata.

Use 3.75 mg of the depot only IM monthly or one 11.25 mg IM injection for three months with concomitant iron therapy. Duraiton of therapy is 3 months or less. If further treatment is contemplated, assess bone density prior to beginning therapy.

NURSING CONSIDERATIONS

SEE ALSO *NURSING CONSIDERATIONS FOR ANTINEOPLASTIC AGENTS.*

ADMINISTRATION/STORAGE

1. Follow manufacturer's guidelines carefully to prepare the depot form. Reconstitute only with the diluent provided; after reconstitution, the preparation is stable for 24 hr. There is no preservative so discard if not used immediately.
2. Due to different release properties, a fractional dose of the 3-month and 4-month depot formulations is not equivalent to the same dose of the monthly product; thus, do not interchange.
3. When injecting depot form, do not use needles smaller than 22 gauge.
4. Give the injection using only the syringes provided.
5. Injection: Store below room temperature at 25°C (77°F) or less. Avoid freezing and protect from light. Store vial in carton until use.
6. Depot may be stored at room temperature.
7. The titanium implant is placed under the skin in the inner aspects of the arm.

ASSESSMENT

Document indications for therapy, onset of symptoms, other agents trialed, and the outcome.

CLIENT/FAMILY TEACHING

1. Hot flashes may occur with drug therapy.
2. Record weight; report gains of more than 2 lb/day.
3. Immediately report any weakness, numbness, respiratory difficulty, or impaired urination.
4. Altered sexual effects (impotence, decreased testes size) may occur; identify appropriate resources for counseling and support.
5. Increased bone pain may be evident at the start of therapy; analgesics may be used for pain control.

OUTCOMES/EVALUATE

- ↓ Tumor size and spread
- Improved symptoms with endometriosis

Levalbuterol hydrochloride

(lehv-al-**BYOU**-ter-all)

CLASSIFICATION(S):
Sympathomimetic
Rx: Xopenex

SEE ALSO *SYMPATHOMIMETICS.*

USES

Treatment or prevention of bronchospasms in adults and adolescents 12 years and older with reversible obstructive airway disease.

HOW SUPPLIED

Inhalation Solution: 0.63 mg/3 mL, 1.25 mg/3 mL

DOSAGE

- **INHALATION SOLUTION: NEBULIZATION**

  Bronchospasms.

Adults and adolescents over 12 years of age, initial: 0.63 mg t.i.d. (q 6–8 hr) by nebulization. Those with severe asthma or who do not respond to the 0.63 mg dose may benefit from a dose of 1.25 mg t.i.d.

NURSING CONSIDERATIONS

SEE ALSO *NURSING CONSIDERATIONS* FOR *SYMPATHOMIMETICS.*

ADMINISTRATION/STORAGE

1. Continue the drug as necessary to control recurring bronchospasms. Most clients gain optimal benefit from regular use of the inhalation solution.
2. Store the inhalation solution in the protective foil pouch between 15–25°C (59–77°F). Protect from light and excessive heat. Keep unopened vials in the foil pouch.
3. Once the foil pouch is opened, use the vials within 2 weeks.
4. Once an individual vial is removed from the foil pouch and is not used immediately, protect from light and use within 1 week. Discard if the solution is not colorless.

ASSESSMENT

1. Note indications for therapy, onset and characteristics of symptoms, other medical conditions and current drugs prescribed.
2. Obtain and monitor ECG, VS, CXR, PFTs, and lab values.

CLIENT/FAMILY TEACHING

1. Review technique for administration and demonstrate at each visit. Remind to rinse mouth and equipment following each treatment.
2. Record peak flow readings and identify what to do in each zone i.e. green, yellow and red zone (good, fair, poor).
3. Increase fluid consumption to help thin secretions.
4. This is a pure isomer form of albuterol and thus the frequently untolerated effects i.e insomnia, palpitations etc. are minimal.
5. Report any unusual side effects as well as S&S URIs.
6. Stop smoking. Identify triggers and practice avoidance.

OUTCOMES/EVALUATE

Improved breathing patterns; ↓ S&S asthma

Levarterenol bitartrate (Norepinephrine bitartrate)

(lee-var-**TER**-ih-nohl)

PREGNANCY CATEGORY: C

CLASSIFICATION(S):

Sympathomimetic

Rx: Levophed

SEE ALSO *SYMPATHOMIMETIC DRUGS.*

ACTION/KINETICS

Produces vasoconstriction (increase in BP) by stimulating alpha-adrenergic receptors. Also causes a moderate increase in contraction of heart by stimulating beta-1 receptors. Minimal hyperglycemic effect. **Onset:** immediate; **duration:** 1–2 min. Metabolized in liver and other tissues by the enzymes MAO and catechol-O-methyltransferase; however, the pharmacologic activity is terminated by uptake and metabolism in sympathetic nerve endings. Metabolites excreted in urine.

USES

(1) Hypotensive states caused by trauma, septicemia, blood transfusions, drug reactions, spinal anesthesia, poliomyelitis, central vasomotor depression, and MI. (2) Adjunct to treatment of cardiac arrest and profound hypotension.

ADDITIONAL CONTRAINDICATIONS
Hypotension due to blood volume deficiency (except in emergencies), mesenteric or peripheral vascular thrombosis, in halothane or cyclopropane anesthesia (due to possibilities of fatal arrhythmias). Pregnancy (may cause fetal anoxia or hypoxia).

SPECIAL CONCERNS
Use with caution in clients taking MAO inhibitors or tricyclic antidepressants.

ADDITIONAL SIDE EFFECTS
Bradycardia that can be abolished by atropine.

HOW SUPPLIED
Injection: 1 mg/mL

DOSAGE

- **IV INFUSION ONLY**

Effect on BP determines dosage, initial: 8–12 mcg/min or 2–3 mL of a 4-mcg/mL solution/min; **maintenance,** 2–4 mcg/min with the dose determined by client response.

NURSING CONSIDERATIONS

SEE ALSO *NURSING CONSIDERATIONS FOR SYMPATHOMIMETIC DRUGS.*

ADMINISTRATION/STORAGE

IV 1. Discard solutions that are brown or that have a precipitate.
2. Do not administer through the same tube as blood products.
3. Continue the infusion until BP is maintained without therapy. Avoid abrupt withdrawal of levarterenol.
4. Dilute in either D5W or 5% dextrose in saline.
5. For IV administration, use a large vein (preferably the antecubital or subclavian). Avoid veins with poor circulation.
6. Administer IV solutions with an electronic infusion device. Monitor the rate of flow constantly.
7. Have phentolamine available for use at the site of extravasation to dilate local blood vessels and to minimize local necrosis.

ASSESSMENT

1. Ensure adequately hydrated.
2. Administer in a monitored environment.
3. Monitor BP by arterial line or electronically. Assess I&O, ECG, VS, CVP, and PA wedge pressures.
4. Observe infusion site frequently for extravasation; ischemia and sloughing may occur. Blanching along the course of the vein may indicate permeability of the vein wall, which could allow leakage to occur. If evident, change IV site and give phentolamine at extravasation site.
5. Withdraw drug gradually; may experience an initial rebound drop in BP. Extra fluids parenterally may diminish rebound hypotension and help stabilize BP during withdrawal.

OUTCOMES/EVALUATE

- ↑ BP
- Improved tissue perfusion
- Urinary output > 30 mL/hr

Levetiracetam

(**lehv**-ah-ter-**ASS**-ah-tam)

PREGNANCY CATEGORY: C
CLASSIFICATION(S):
Anticonvulsant, miscellaneous
Rx: Keppra

ACTION/KINETICS
Prescise mechanism unknown. May act in synaptic plasma membranes in the CNS to inhibit burst firing without affecting normal neuronal excitability. Thus, it may selectively prevent hypersynchronization of epileptiform burst firing and propagation of seizure activity. Rapidly absorbed. **Peak plasma levels:** 1 hr during fasting. Metabolized in the liver. **t½:** 7 hr. Excreted through the urine as metabolites and unchanged drug.

USES
Adjunctive treatment of partial onset seizures in adults with epilepsy.

SPECIAL CONCERNS
Reduce dosage in clients with impaired renal function. Clearance is increased in children. Half-life is prolonged in the elderly. Use with caution during lactation. Safety and efficacy have not been determined in children less than 16 years of age.

SIDE EFFECTS
CNS: Somnolence, dizziness, depression, nervousness, ataxia, vertigo, am-

nesia, anxiety, hostility, paresthesia, emotional lability, psychotic symptoms, withdrawal seizures. **Respiratory:** Pharyngitis, rhinitis, sinusitis, increased cough. **GI:** Abdominal pain, constipation, diarrhea, dyspepsia, gastroenteritis, gingivitis, N&V. **Miscellaneous:** Asthenia, headache, infection, pain, anorexia, diplopia, coordination difficulties.

LABORATORY TEST CONSIDERATIONS

Infrequent abnormalities in hematologic parameters and LFTs.

OD OVERDOSE MANAGEMENT

Symptom: Drowsiness. *Treatment:* Emesis or gastric lavage; maintain airway. General supportive care. Monitor VS. Hemodialysis may be beneficial.

HOW SUPPLIED

Tablets: 250 mg, 500 mg, 750 mg

DOSAGE

• **TABLETS**

Partial onset seizures in adults.

Initial: 500 mg b.i.d. Can increase dose by 1,000 mg/day q 2 weeks up to a maximum daily dose of 3,000 mg. For impaired renal function, use the following doses: **C_{CR}, 50–80 mL/min:** 500–1,000 mg q 12 hr; **C_{CR}, 30–50 mL/min:** 250–750 mg q 12 hr; **C_{CR}, less than 30 mL/min:** 250–500 mg q 12 hr.

NURSING CONSIDERATIONS

ASSESSMENT

1. Document history and characteristics of seizures.
2. Monitor CBC, renal and LFTs; with impaired renal function, drug dose based on creatinine clearance.

CLIENT/FAMILY TEACHING

1. Take exactly as directed. May take with food to ↓ GI upset.
2. May cause dizziness and sleepiness. Do not engage in activities that require mental alertness until drug effects realized.
3. Use reliable birth control. Notify provider if pregnant or planning to become pregnant.
4. Report any unusual side effects or loss of seizure control.

OUTCOMES/EVALUATE

Control of seizures

Levobetaxolol hydrochloride

(**lee**-voh-bay-**TAX**-oh-lohl)

PREGNANCY CATEGORY: C

CLASSIFICATION(S):

Beta-adrenergic blocking agent

Rx: Betaxon

ACTION/KINETICS

A cardioselective (beta-1-adrenergic) receptor blocking agent. No significant membrane-stabilizing (i.e., local anesthetic) activity and is devoid of sympathomimetic activity. Reduces IOP probably by decreasing aqueous humor production. **Onset:** 30 min. **Maximum effect:** 2 hr. **Duration:** 12 hr.

USES

Decrease IOP in chronic open-angle glaucoma or ocular hypertension.

CONTRAINDICATIONS

Use with sinus bradycardia, greater than first degree AV block, cardiogenic shock, or overt cardiac failure.

SPECIAL CONCERNS

May be absorbed systemically leading to respiratory and cardiac effects. Use with caution in those with a history of cardiac failure or heart block; in those subject to spontaneous hypoglycemia or in diabetics receiving insulin or oral hypoglycemic drugs; in those with excessive restriction of pulmonary function; and during lactation. Safety and efficacy have not been determined in children.

SIDE EFFECTS

Ophthalmic: Transient blurred vision, cataracts, vitreous disorders. **CV:** Bradycardia, heart block, hypertension, hypotension, tachycardia, vascular anomaly. **CNS:** Anxiety, dizziness, hypertonia, vertigo. **GI:** Constipation, dyspepsia. **Musculoskeletal:** Arthritis, tendonitis. **Respiratory:** Bronchitis, dyspnea, pharyngitis, pneumonia, rhinitis, sinusitis. **Metabolic/Endocrine:** Gout, hypercholesterolemia, hyperlipidemia, diabetes, hypothyroidism. **Dermato-**

logic: Alopecia, dermatitis, psoriasis. **GU:** Breast abscess, cystitis. **Miscellaneous:** Accidental injury, headache, infection.

HOW SUPPLIED

Ophthalmic suspension: 0.5% (as base)

DOSAGE

- **OPHTHALMIC SUSPENSION**

Lower IOP.

1 gtt in affected eye(s) b.i.d. In some, a few weeks may be needed to stabilize.

NURSING CONSIDERATIONS

ADMINISTRATION/STORAGE

1. The use of two topical beta-adrenergic agents is not recommended.
2. Protect from light.
3. Shake well before using.

ASSESSMENT

1. Note indications for therapy and other agents prescribed.
2. Assess for any restrictive airway disease, diabetes or severe CAD.
3. Monitor EKG and VS; periodically assess cholesterol panel, TSH and BS.

CLIENT/FAMILY TEACHING

1. Use drops as directed do not skip therapy.
2. Drug is used to lower pressures in the eye with ocular hypertension or chronic open-angle glaucoma to help prevent optic nerve damage and visual field loss.
3. When instilling, do not touch dropper tip to any surface, as this may result in contamination.
4. Do not use with contact lenses in the eyes.
5. Report any increased SOB, edema, or eye irritation, pain, swelling, or itching.

OUTCOMES/EVALUATE

↓ IOP

L

Levobunolol hydrochloride

(lee-voh-**BYOU**-no-lohl)

PREGNANCY CATEGORY: C

CLASSIFICATION(S):

Beta-adrenergic blocking agentb

Rx: AKBeta, Betagan Liquifilm

★**Rx:** Betagan, Novo-Levobunolol, Ophtho-Bunolol, PMS-Levobunolol

SEE ALSO *BETA-ADRENERGIC BLOCKING AGENTS.*

ACTION/KINETICS

Both beta-1- and beta-2-adrenergic receptor agonist. May act by decreasing the formation of aqueous humor. **Onset:** < 60 min. **Peak effect:** 2–6 hr. **Duration:** 24 hr.

USES

To decrease intraocular pressure in chronic open-angle glaucoma or ocular hypertension.

CONTRAINDICATIONS

Use of 2 or more topical ophthalmic beta-adrenergic blocking agents simultaneously.

SPECIAL CONCERNS

Safety and effectiveness have not been determined in children. Significant absorption in geriatric clients may result in myocardial depression. Also, use with caution in angle-closure glaucoma (use with a miotic), in clients with muscle weaknesses, and in those with decreased pulmonary function.

ADDITIONAL SIDE EFFECTS

Ophthalmic: Stinging and burning (transient), decreased corneal sensitivity, blepharoconjunctivitis. **Dermatologic:** Urticaria, pruritus.

HOW SUPPLIED

Ophthalmic Solution: 0.25%, 0.5%

DOSAGE

- **OPHTHALMIC SOLUTION (0.25%, 0.5%)**

Adults, usual: 1–2 gtt of 0.25% solution in affected eye(s) b.i.d. or 1–2 gtt of 00.5% solution in affected eye(s) once a day (use b.i.d. in more severe or uncontrolled glaucoma).

NURSING CONSIDERATIONS

SEE ALSO *NURSING CONSIDERATIONS* FOR *BETA-ADRENERGIC BLOCKING AGENTS.*

ADMINISTRATION/STORAGE

1. If IOP is not decreased sufficiently, pilocarpine, epinephrine, or systemic carbonic anhydrase inhibitors may be used.

2. Due to diurnal IOP variations, a satisfactory response to twice daily therapy is best determined by measuring IOP at different times during the day.
3. Do not give two or more ophthalmic beta-adrenergic blocking agents simultaneously.

CLIENT/FAMILY TEACHING

1. Used to lower pressures in the eye and to prevent vision loss.
2. Apply gentle pressure to the inside corner of the eye for approximately 60 sec following instillation.
3. When instilling, do not touch dropper tip to any surface, as this may result in contamination.
4. Wait at least 5 min before instilling other eye drops.
5. Do not close the eyes tightly or blink more frequently than usual after instillation of the drug.
6. Return for evaluation of intraocular pressure and drug's effectiveness.

OUTCOMES/EVALUATE

↓ IOP

Levodopa

(lee-voh-**DOH**-pah)

CLASSIFICATION(S):
Antiparkinson drug
Rx: Dopar, Larodopa, L-Dopa

ACTION/KINETICS

Depletion of dopamine in the striatum of the brain is thought to cause the symptoms of Parkinson's disease. Levodopa, a dopamine precursor, is able to cross the blood-brain barrier to enter the CNS. It is decarboxylated to dopamine in the basal ganglia, thus replenishing depleted dopamine stores. **Peak plasma levels:** 0.5–2 hr (may be delayed if ingested with food). **t½, plasma:** 1–3 hr. **Onset:** 2–3 weeks, although some clients may require up to 6 months. Extensively metabolized both in the GI tract and the liver; metabolites are excreted in the urine.

USES

Idiopathic, arteriosclerotic, or postencephalitic parkinsonism due to carbon monoxide or manganese intoxication and in the elderly associated with cerebral arteriosclerosis. Not effective in drug-induced extrapyramidal symptoms. Levodopa only provides symptomatic relief and does not alter the course of the disease. When effective, it relieves rigidity, bradykinesia, tremors, dysphagia, seborrhea, sialorrhea, and postural instability. Used in combination with carbidopa. *Investigational:* Pain from herpes zoster; restless legs syndrome.

CONTRAINDICATIONS

Concomitant use with MAO inhibitors, except MAO-B inhibitors (e.g., selegiline). History of melanoma or in clients with undiagnosed skin lesions. Lactation. Hypersensitivity to drug, narrow-angle glaucoma, blood dyscrasias, hypertension, coronary sclerosis.

SPECIAL CONCERNS

Use with extreme caution in clients with history of MIs, convulsions, arrhythmias, bronchial asthma, emphysema, active peptic ulcer, psychosis or neurosis, wide-angle glaucoma, and renal, hepatic, or endocrine diseases. Use during pregnancy only if benefits clearly outweigh risks. Safety has not been established in children less than 12 years of age. Geriatric clients may require a lower dose as they have a reduced tolerance for the drug and its side effects (including cardiac effects). Clients may experience an "on-off" phenomenon in which they experience an improved clinical status followed by loss of therapeutic effect.

SIDE EFFECTS

The side effects of levodopa are numerous and usually dose related. Some may abate with usage.

CNS: Choreiform and/or dystonic movements, sudden sleep attacks, paranoid ideation, psychotic episodes, depression (with possibility of suicidal tendencies), dementia, ***seizures*** (rare), dizziness, headache, faintness, confusion, insomnia, nightmares, hallucinations, delusions, agitation, anxiety, malaise, fatigue, euphoria. **GI:** N&V, anorexia, abdominal pain, dry mouth, sialorrhea, dysphagia, dysgeusia, hiccups, diarrhea, constipation, burning sensation of tongue, bitter taste, flatulence, weight gain/loss, GI bleeding (rare), duodenal ulcer (rare). **CV:** Cardiac irregularities, palpitations, orthostatic hypotension, hypertension, phlebitis, hot flashes. **Ophthalmologic:** Diplopia, dilated pupils, blurred vision, development of Horner's syndrome, oculogyric crisis. **Hematologic: Hemolytic anemia, agranulocytosis,** leukopenia. **Musculoskeletal:** Muscle twitching (early sign of overdose), tonic contraction of the muscles of mastication, increased hand tremor, ataxia. **Miscellaneous:** Blepharospasm (early sign of overdose), urinary retention/incontinence, increased sweating, unusual breathing patterns, weakness, numbness, bruxism, alopecia, priapism, hoarseness, edema, dark sweat/urine, flushing, skin rash, sense of stimulation. Levodopa interacts with many other drugs (see what follows) and must be administered cautiously.

L

LABORATORY TEST CONSIDERATIONS

↑ BUN, AST, LDH, ALT, bilirubin, alkaline phosphatase, protein-bound iodine, uric acid (with colorimetric test). ↓ H&H, WBCs. False + Coombs' test. Interference with tests for urinary glucose and ketones.

OD OVERDOSE MANAGEMENT

Symptoms: Muscle twitching, blepharospasm. Also see *Side Effects*. *Treatment:* Immediate gastric lavage for acute overdose. Maintain airway and give IV fluids carefully. General supportive measures.

DRUG INTERACTIONS

Antacids / ↑ Effect of levodopa R/T ↑ absorption from GI tract
Anticholinergic drugs / Possible ↓ levodopa effect R/T ↑ levodopa breakdown in stomach (R/T delayed gastric emptying time)
Antidepressants, tricyclic / ↓ Levodopa effect R/T ↓ GI tract absorption; also, ↑ risk of hypertension
Benzodiazepines / ↓ Levodopa effect
Clonidine / ↓ Levodopa effect
Digoxin / ↓ Digoxin effect
Furazolidone / ↑ Levodopa effect R/T ↓ liver breakdown
Guanethidine / ↑ Hypotensive drug effect
Hypoglycemic drugs / Levodopa upsets diabetic control with hypoglycemic agents
H *Indian snakeroot* / ↓ Effect of levodopa but ↑ extrapyramidal symptoms
MAO inhibitors / Concomitant administration may result in hypertension, lightheadedness, and flushing R/T ↓ breakdown of dopamine and norepinephrine formed from levodopa
Methionine / ↓ Levodopa effect
Methyldopa / Additive effects including hypotension
Metoclopramide / ↑ Bioavailability of levodopa; ↓ metoclopramide effect
Papaverine / ↓ Levodopa effect
Phenothiazines / ↓ Levodopa effect R/T ↓ uptake of dopamine into neurons
Phenytoin / Antagonizes levodopa effect
Propranolol / May antagonize the hypotensive and positive inotropic effect of levodopa
Pyridoxine / Reverses levodopa-induced improvement in Parkinson's disease
Thioxanthines / ↓ Levodopa effect in Parkinson clients
Tricyclic antidepressants / ↓ Levodopa absorption → ↓ effect

HOW SUPPLIED

Capsule: 100 mg, 250 mg, 500 mg; *Tablet:* 100 mg, 250 mg, 500 mg

DOSAGE

• **CAPSULES, TABLETS**

Parkinsonism.

Adults, initial: 250 mg b.i.d.–q.i.d. taken with food; **then,** increase total daily dose by 100–750 mg/3–7 days until optimum dosage reached (should not exceed 8 g/day). Up to 6 months may be required to achieve a significant therapeutic effect.

NURSING CONSIDERATIONS

SEE ALSO NURSING CONSIDERATIONS FOR CHOLINERGIC BLOCKING AGENTS.

ADMINISTRATION/STORAGE

1. If unable to swallow tablets or capsules, crush tablets or empty the capsule into a small amount of fruit juice at the time of administration.

2. Often administered together with an anticholinergic agent.

ASSESSMENT

1. Review medical history for any contraindications to therapy. Stop drug 24 hr before surgery and note when drug is to be restarted.
2. Document baseline rigidity, tremors, motor function, and involuntary movements. Note mental status.
3. Note adverse side effects that may require ↓ drug dose or "drug holiday".
4. Monitor ECG, CBC, liver/renal function studies, and protein bound iodine tests.

CLIENT/FAMILY TEACHING

1. Take exactly as prescribed; may take with food to decrease GI upset.
2. Report headaches; may indicate drug-induced glaucoma. Twitching or eye spasms may indicate toxicity.
3. Dosage should not exceed 8 g/day; do not stop abruptly.
4. Avoid taking multivitamin preparations containing 10–25 mg of B_6; reverses the antiparkinson effect. *Larobec* is a form that does not contain pyridoxine.
5. Significant results may take up to 6 months to be realized.
6. May cause dizziness or drowsiness. Do not perform tasks that require mental alertness until drug effects realized.
7. Sweat and urine may appear dark; this is not harmful.
8. Sustained erection may occur; report immediately.
9. Report any evidence of depression or psychosis or other unusual mental or behavioral changes.
10. Report for all scheduled visits so that drug effectiveness can be evaluated and dosage adjusted as needed.
11. Identify local support groups/services.

OUTCOMES/EVALUATE

Improvement in motor function, reflexes, gait, strength of grip, and amount of tremor

Levofloxacin

(**lee**-voh-**FLOX**-ah-sin)

PREGNANCY CATEGORY: C

CLASSIFICATION(S):
Antibiotic, fluoroquinolone
Rx: Quixin, Levaquin

SEE ALSO *FLUOROQUINOLONES*.

USES

Systemic. (1) Acute maxillary sinusitis due to *Streptococcus pneumoniae, Haemophilus influenzae,* or *Moraxella catarrhalis.* (2) Acute bacterial exacerbation of chronic bronchitis due to *Staphylococcus aureus, S. pneumoniae, H. influenzae, Haemophilus parainfluenzae,* or *M. catarrhalis.* (3) Community acquired pneumonia due to *S. aureus, S. pneumoniae* (including penicillin-resistant *S. pneumoniae*), *H. influenzae, H. parainfluenzae, Klebsiella pneumoniae, M. catarrhalis, Chlamydia pneumoniae, Legionella pneumophila* or *Mycoplasma pneumoniae.* (4) Uncomplicated mild to moderate infections of the skin and skin structures, including abscesses, cellulitis, furuncies, impetigo, pyoderma, and wound infections due to *S. aureus* or *Streptococcus pyogenes.* (5) Complicated skin and skin structure infections, including surgical incisions, infected bites and lacerations, major abscesses, and infected ulcers due to methicillin-sensitive *S. aureus, Enterococcus faecalis, S. pyogenes,* or *Proteus mirabilis.* (6) Mild to moderate complicated UTIs due to *Enterococcus faecalis, Enterobacter cloacae, Escherichia coli, Klebsiella pneumoniae, P. mirabilis,* or *Pseudomonas aeruginosa.* (7) Uncomplicated UTIs due to *E. coli, K. pneumoniae,* or *Staphylococcus saprophyticus.* (8) Acute mild to moderate pyelonephritis due to *E. coli.* **Ophthalmic.** (1) Bacterial conjunctivitis caused by *Staphylococcus aureus* (methicillin-susceptible strains only), *Corynebacterium* species, *Staphylococcus epidermidis* (methicillin-susceptible strains only), *Streptococcus pneumoniae, Streptococcus* (Groups C/F and G), Viridans Group streptococci, *Acinetobacter lwoffi, Haemophilus influenzae, Serratia marcescens.* (2) Corneal ulcers caused by *S. aureus, S. epidermidis, S. pneumoniae, P. aeruginosa, S. marcescens.*

L

CONTRAINDICATIONS
Lactation. IM, intrathecal, intraperitoneal, or SC administration.

SPECIAL CONCERNS
The dose must be reduced with impaired renal function. (See *Administration/Storage.*) Safety and efficacy have not been determined in those less than 18 years of age.

SIDE EFFECTS
See *Fluoroquinolones*.

HOW SUPPLIED
Injection: 500 mg (25 mg/mL), 750 mg (25 mg/mL); *Injection (premix):* 250 mg (5 mg/mL), 500 mg (5 mg/mL), 750 mg (5 mg/mL); *Ophthalmic Solution:* 0.5%; *Tablets:* 250 mg, 500 mg, 750 mg.

DOSAGE

- **SLOW IV INFUSION, TABLETS**

Acute maxillary sinusitis.
500 mg once daily for 10–14 days.

Acute bacterial exacerbation of chronic bronchitis.
500 mg once daily for 7 days.

Community acquired pneumonia.
500 mg once daily for 7–14 days.

Uncomplicated skin and skin structure infections.
500 mg once daily for 7–10 days.

Complicated skin/skin structure infections.
750 mg once daily for 7–14 days.

Complicated UTIs.
250 mg once daily for 10 days.

Uncomplicated UTIs.
250 mg once daily for 3 days.

Acute pyelonephritis.
250 mg once daily for 10 days.

- **OPHTHALMIC SOLUTION**

Bacterial conjunctivitis.
Days 1 and 2: 1–2 gtt in the affected eye(s) q 2 hr while awake, up to 8 times/day; **Days 3 through 7:** 1–2 gtt in the affected eye(s) q 4 hr while awake, up to q.i.d.

Bacterial corneal ulcer.
Days 1 and 2: 1–2 gtt in the affected eye(s) q 30 min while awake. Awaken at about 4 and 6 hr after retiring and instill 1–2 gtt. **Days 3 through 7 to 9:** Instill 1–2 gtt hourly while awake. **Days 7 to 9 to treatment completion:** 1–2 gtt q.i.d.

NURSING CONSIDERATIONS

SEE ALSO *NURSING CONSIDERATIONS FOR FLUOROQUINOLONES.*

ADMINISTRATION/STORAGE

1. Reduce dose with impaired renal function as follows when used for *acute maxillary sinusitis, acute bacterial exacerbation of chronic bronchitis, community acquired pneumonia,* and *uncomplicated skin and skin structure infections.* If C_{CR} is between 20 and 49 mL/min, the initial dose is 500 mg and subsequent doses are 250 mg q 24 hr. If C_{CR} is between 10 and 19 mL/min, the initial dose is 500 mg and subsequent doses are 250 mg q 48 hr. If the client is on hemodialysis or chronic ambulatory peritoneal dialysis, the initial dose is 500 mg and subsequent doses are 250 mg q 48 hr.
2. Reduce dose, as follows, with impaired renal function when used for *complicated UTI* or *acute pyelonephritis*: If C_{CR} is 20 mL/min or more, no dosage adjustment is needed. If the C_{CR} is between 10 and 19 mL/min, the initial dose is 250 mg and subsequent doses are 250 mg q 48 hr.
3. Reduce dose, as follows, with impaired renal function when used for *complicated skin and skin structure infections*: If C_{CR} is from 20–49 mL/min, the initial dose is 750 mg and subsequent doses are 750 mg q 48 hr; if C_{CR} is from 10–10 mL/min, the initial dose is 750 mg and subsequent doses are 500 mg q 48 hr. If on hemodialysis, the initial dose is 750 mg and subsequent doses are 500 mg q 48 hr.
4. Oral doses are given at least 2 hr before or 2 hr after antacids containing Mg or Al, as well as sucralfate, iron products, multivitamin preparations containing zinc, and didanosine (chewable/buffered tablets or pediatric powder for PO solution).
5. Store tablets in a tight container at 15–30°C (59–85°F).
6. **IV** The injectable form may be mixed with 0.9% NaCl, D5W, D5/0.9% NaCl, D5/RL, Plasma-Lyte 56/5% dextrose, D5/0.45% NaCl, 0.15% KCl injection, or M/6 sodium lactate injection.

7. Give my IV infusion only, slowly over a period of 60–90 min. Avoid rapid or bolus IV infusion.
8. Diluted solutions for IV use are stable for 72 hr up to a concentration of 5 mg/mL when stored in IV containers at 25°C or less (77°F or less). Such solutions stable for 14 days when stored under refrigeration at 5°C (41°F). Diluted solutions that are frozen in glass bottles or plastic IV containers are stable for 6 months when stored at -20°C (-4°F).
9. Thaw frozen solutions at room temperature or in a refrigerator. Do not thaw in a microwave or by bath immersion. After initial thawing, do not refreeze.

ASSESSMENT

1. Note indications for therapy, onset, and characteristics of illness.
2. Obtain baseline cultures, liver, and renal function studies. Follow manufacturers guidelines for reduced dosage with renal impairment.

CLIENT/FAMILY TEACHING

1. Take only as directed on an empty stomach; complete entire prescription. Consume plenty of fluids.
2. Avoid multivitamins with zinc, iron products, sucralfate, and Mg- or aluminum-containing antacids 2 hr before and after dose.
3. Practice reliable birth control.
4. Use caution until drug effects realized; may experience dizziness, drowsiness or visual changes. May also experience N&V, abdominal pain, diarrhea/constipation, and photosensitivity.
5. Report if S&S do not improve or worsen after 72 hr of therapy.

OUTCOMES/EVALUATE

- Symptomatic improvement
- Resolution of infective organism

Levomethadyl acetate hydrochloride

(lee-voh-**METH**-ah-dill)

PREGNANCY CATEGORY: C

CLASSIFICATION(S):
Narcotic analgesic
Rx: ORLAAM **C-II**

SEE ALSO *NARCOTIC ANALGESICS.*

ACTION/KINETICS

Onset: 2–4 hr. **Peak:** 1.5–2 hr. **Duration:** 48–72 hr. **t½:** 2–6 days.

USES

Treatment of opiate dependence in those who do not show an acceptable response to other treatments for dependence. *NOTE:* This drug can be dispensed only by treatment programs approved by the FDA, DEA, and the designated state authority. The drug can be dispensed only in the oral form and according to treatment requirements stated in federal regulations. The drug has no approved uses outside of the treatment of opiate dependence.

CONTRAINDICATIONS

Pregnancy. Use during labor and delivery unless potential benefits outweight potential hazards.

SPECIAL CONCERNS

Usual dose must not be given on consecutive days due to the risk of fatal overdosage. Use with extreme caution in those at risk for development of prolonged QT syndrome (e.g., CHF, bradycardia, use of a diuretic, cardiac hypertrophy, hypokalemia, hypomagnesemia).

SIDE EFFECTS

See *Narcotic Analgesics*. Induction with levomethadyl that is too rapid for the level of tolerance of the client may result in overdosage, including symptoms of both ***respiratory and CV depression.*** CV side effects include QT prolongation and ***severe cardiac arrhythmias (torsades de pointes).*** Withdrawal symptoms (nasal congestion, abdominal symptoms, diarrhea, muscle aches, anxiety) may be seen over the 72-hr dosing period if the dose is too low.

ADDITIONAL DRUG INTERACTIONS

Levomethadyl is metabolized to active metabolites by the cytochrome P450 system. Thus, concomitant use

L

of drugs that induce the enzyme (e.g., phenobarbital, phenytoin, rifampin) or inhibit the enzyme (e.g., erythromycin, ketoconazole, saquinavir) could → levomethadyl levels and precipitate serious arrhythymias, including torsades de pointes.

HOW SUPPLIED

Oral Solution: 10 mg/mL

DOSAGE

• ORAL SOLUTION

Induction.

Initial: 20–40 mg administered at 48–72-hr intervals; **then,** dose may be increased in increments of 5–10 mg until steady state is reached (usually within 1–2 weeks). Clients dependent on methadone may require higher initial doses of levomethadyl; the suggested initial 3-times/week dose for such clients is 1.2–1.3 times the daily methadone maintenance dose being replaced. This initial dose should not exceed 120 mg with subsequent doses given at 48- or 72-hr intervals, depending on the response. If additional opioids are required, supplemental amounts of methadone should be given rather than giving levomethadyl on 2 consecutive days.

Maintenance.

Most clients are stabilized on doses of 60–90 mg 3 times/week although the dose may range from 10 to 140 mg 3 times/week. The maximum *total* amount of levomethadyl recommended for any client is either 140, 140, 140 mg or 130, 130, 180 mg on a thrice-weekly schedule.

Reinduction after an unplanned lapse in dosing: following a lapse of one levomethadyl dose.

If the client comes to the clinic the day following a missed scheduled dose (e.g., misses Monday and arrives at clinic on Tuesday), the regular Monday dose is given, with the scheduled Wednesday dose given on Thursday and the Friday dose given on Saturday. The client's regular schedule can be resumed the following Monday. If the client misses one dose and comes to the clinic the day of the next scheduled dose (i.e., misses Monday, comes to clinic on Wednesday), the usual dose will be well tolerated in most cases although some clients will need a reduced dose.

Reintroduction after a lapse of more than one levomethadyl dose.

Restart the client at an initial dose of 50%–75% of the previous dose, followed by increases of 5–10 mg every dosing day (i.e., intervals of 48–72 hr) until the previous maintenance dose is reached.

Transfer from levomethadyl to methadone.

Transfer can be done directly, although the dose of methadone should be 80% of the levomethadyl dose being replaced. The first methadone dose should not be given sooner than 48 hr after the last levomethadyl dose. Increases or decreases of 5–10 mg may be made in the daily methadone dose to control symptoms of withdrawal or symptoms of excessive sedation.

Detoxification from levomethadyl.

Both gradual reduction (i.e., 5%–10% a week) and abrupt withdrawal have been used successfully.

NURSING CONSIDERATIONS

ADMINISTRATION/STORAGE

1. The drug is usually given 3 times/week—either on Monday, Wednesday, and Friday or on Tuesday, Thursday, and Saturday. If withdrawal is a problem with this interval, the preceding dose may be increased.
2. If the degree of tolerance is not known, may start on methadone to facilitate more rapid titration to an effective dose. Then can be converted to levomethadyl after a few weeks. The cross-over from methadone to levomethadyl should be accomplished in a single dose.
3. During maintenance therapy, if, e.g., those on a Monday, Wednesday, and Friday schedule complain of withdrawal symptoms on Sunday, the Friday dose may be increased in 5- to 10-mg increments up to 40% over the Monday/Wednesday dose up to a maximum of 140 mg.
4. Levomethadyl take-home doses are not permitted. If a situation arises

where the client cannot come to the clinic for a regular dose of levomethadyl, they may be switched to receive one or more doses of methadone. These should be 80% of the client's Monday/Wednesday levomethadyl dose; the first dose of methadone should be taken no sooner than 48 hr after the last dose of levomethadyl. The number of take-home doses of methadone should be two less than the number of days expected absence and should not exceed the number of take-home doses allowed in the methadone regulations. Upon return to clinic, client should resume levomethadyl maintenance following the same dosage schedule prior to the temporary interruption. If more than 48 hr has elapsed since the last methadone dose, reintroduce on levomethadyl at a dose determined by the clinical evaluation.
5. If transferring from levomethadyl to methadone, wait 48 hr after the last dose of levomethadyl before giving the first dose of methadone.

ASSESSMENT

1. Document that client is opiate dependent, length of dependence, method and type of drugs used.
2. Determine methadone usage as drug requirements may be higher.
3. Confirm acceptance/approval for drug through federally approved treatment protocol.
4. In clients who have missed scheduled doses, follow administration guidelines carefully.

CLIENT/FAMILY TEACHING

1. Must comply with regularly scheduled doses of levomethadyl. Skipped doses or use of street drugs can cause serious complications/death.
2. Drug must be given in an approved opiate withdrawal clinic that have control over the drug delivery. Although the program does not require daily dosing, it does require that the client physically come to clinic for scheduled dosing (usually every other day).
3. Report any severe N&V, heart palpitations, difficulty breathing or increased shortness of breath.
4. Identify additional support groups/persons who may assist in their goal of freedom from addiction.
5. Determine other resources (child care, job retraining, food stamps, etc.) that would support them in their goal to live drug free.

OUTCOMES/EVALUATE

Freedom from drug (opiate) dependence

Levonorgestrel Implants

(**lee**-voh-nor-**JES**-trel)

PREGNANCY CATEGORY: X
CLASSIFICATION(S):
Progestin contraceptive system
Rx: Norplant System

SEE ALSO *PROGESTERONE AND PROGESTINS.*

ACTION/KINETICS

Levonorgestrel implants are marketed in a set of six flexible Silastic capsules each containing 36 mg of levonorgestrel (Norplant System); an insertion kit is provided to the provider to assist with implantation. Small amounts of the drug slowly diffuse through the wall of each capsule resulting in blood levels of levonorgestrel that are lower than those seen when levonorgestrel or norgestrel is taken as oral contraceptive. The dose released is initially 85 mcg/day, followed by a decrease to approximately 50 mcg/day after 9 months, to 35 mcg/day after 18 months, and then leveling off to 30 mcg/day thereafter. Blood levels of levonorgestrel vary over a wide range and cannot be used as the sole measure of the risk of pregnancy. If used properly, the risk of pregnancy is less than 1 for every 100 users. Does not have any estrogenic effects. The implant system lasts up to 5 years and the contraceptive effect is rapidly reversed if the system is removed from the body.

USES

Prevention of pregnancy (system lasts for up to 5 years). A new system may be

L

inserted after 5 years if continuing contraception is desired.

CONTRAINDICATIONS

Active thrombophlebitis, thromboembolic disorders, undiagnosed abnormal genital bleeding, acute liver disease, benign or malignant liver tumors, known or suspected breast carcinoma, confirmed or suspected pregnancy.

SPECIAL CONCERNS

Menstrual bleeding irregularities are commonly observed. Monitor carefully women who have a family history of breast cancer or who have breast nodules. Monitor closely women being treated for hyperlipidemias because an increase in LDL levels may occur. Use with caution in individuals in whom fluid retention might be dangerous and in those with a history of depression. Do not insert until 6 weeks after parturition in women who are breast-feeding. Women whose implants were manufactured prior to October 20, 1999, should use a back-up method of contraception due to lower than expected release rates from implants.

SIDE EFFECTS

Menstrual irregularities: Prolonged menses, spotting, irregular onset of menses, frequent menses, amenorrhea, scanty bleeding, cervicitis, vaginitis. **At implant site:** Pain or itching, infection, bruising following insertion or removal, hyperpigmentation (reversible upon removal).
GI: Abdominal discomfort, nausea, change of appetite, weight gain. **CNS:** Headache, nervousness, dizziness. **Dermatologic:** Dermatitis, acne, hirsutism, scalp hair loss, excess hair growth. **Miscellaneous:** Breast discharge, breast pain, leukorrhea, musculoskeletal pain, fluid retention, possibility of ectopic pregnancy in long-term users, delayed follicular atresia.

LABORATORY TEST CONSIDERATIONS

↓ Sex hormone binding globulin levels, T_4 levels (slight). ↑ Uptake of T_3.

OD OVERDOSE MANAGEMENT

Symptoms: Overdosage can result if more than six capsules are inserted. Symptoms include fluid retention and uterine bleeding irregularities. *Treatment:* All capsules should be removed.

DRUG INTERACTIONS

Carbamazepine / ↓ Effectiveness → ↑ risk of pregnancy
Phenobarbital / ↓ Effectiveness → ↑ risk of pregnancy
Phenytoin / ↓ Effectiveness → ↑ risk of pregnancy

HOW SUPPLIED

Kit: 6 capsules each containing 36 mg

DOSAGE

- **SILASTIC CAPSULES**

Six Silastic capsules (36 mg levonorgestrel each) implanted subdermally in the midportion of the upper arm (8–10 cm above the elbow crease). Capsules are distributed in a fan-like pattern 15° apart (total of 75°).

NURSING CONSIDERATIONS

SEE ALSO *NURSING CONSIDERATIONS* FOR *PROGESTERONE AND PROGESTINS*.

ADMINISTRATION/STORAGE

1. To ensure effectiveness and to be sure not pregnant at the time of capsule implantation, implant during the first 7 days of the cycle or immediately after an abortion.
2. The system should be inserted only by individuals instructed on the proper procedure for insertion. If capsules are placed too deeply, they may be more difficult to remove.
3. If all capsules cannot be removed at the first attempt, allow the site to heal before another attempt is made.
4. Expulsion is not common but may occur if capsules are placed too shallow/too close to the incision or if infection occurs.
5. If infection occurs, treat and cure before replacing capsules.
6. After 5 years, remove capsules; if additional contraception desired, a new system can be inserted.

ASSESSMENT

1. A complete medical history, physical and gynecologic exam should be performed prior to implantation or reimplantation and annually during use.
2. Ensure not pregnant at the time of implantation.

3. Determine if breast-feeding; do not insert until 6 weeks after delivery.
4. Note any history of thromboembolic disorders or depression.
5. Assess liver function and for evidence of hyperlipidemia.
6. Assess for family history of breast cancer. Note presence of breast nodules; monitor carefully.
7. Obtain weight; effectiveness of levonorgestrel may be decreased with weights exceeding 70.5 kg.

CLIENT/FAMILY TEACHING

1. Review procedure for wound care postinsertion and report symptoms of infection/rejection. A small scar may be evident at insertion site.
2. Expect some irregularity with the menstrual cycle such as longer periods, missed periods, and spotting in between during the first year of implantation.
3. Report for regularly scheduled F/U visits so that therapy can be carefully evaluated.
4. The system may be removed at any time if necessary; pregnancy can occur after the next menstrual cycle.
5. Additional protection must be used to prevent STDs.

OUTCOMES/EVALUATE

Effective contraception

Levothyroxine sodium (T_4)

(lee-voh-thigh-**ROX**-een)

PREGNANCY CATEGORY: A
CLASSIFICATION(S):
Thyroid product
Rx: Eltroxin, Levo-T, Levothroid, Levoxyl, L-Thyroxine Sodium, Unithroid (formerly Thyrox), Levoxine, Synthroid

SEE ALSO *THYROID DRUGS*.

ACTION/KINETICS

Levothyroxine is the synthetic sodium salt of the levoisomer of T_4 (tetraiodothyronine). Levothyroxine, 0.05–0.6 mg equals approximately 60 mg (1 grain) of thyroid. Absorption from the GI tract is incomplete and variable, especially when taken with food. Has a slower onset but a longer duration than sodium liothyronine. More active on a weight basis than thyroid. Is usually the drug of choice. Effect is predictable as thyroid content is standard. **Time to peak therapeutic effect:** 3–4 weeks. **t$^1/_2$:** 6–7 days in a euthyroid person, 9–10 days in a hypothyroid client, and 3–4 days in a hyperthyroid client. Is 99% protein bound. **Duration:** 1–3 weeks after withdrawal of chronic therapy. *NOTE:* All levothyroxine products are not bioequivalent; thus, changing brands is not recommended.

DRUG INTERACTIONS

Aluminum hydroxide / Adsorption of levothyroxine to the aluminum and increased fecal elmination of levothyroxine
Carbamazepine / ↑ Levothyroxine elimination due to ↑ liver metabolism
Cholestyramine / ↓ Absorption of thyroxine due to binding to cholestyramine in the GI tract
Digoxin / ↓ Digoxin serum levels and therapeutic effect
Iron salts / ↓ Absorption of levothyroxine due to complex formation with iron in the GI tract
Sucralfate / ↓ Absorption of thyroxine due to binding to cholestyramine in the GI tract
Theophylline / ↓ Theophylline effect due to ↑ elimination
Warfarin / ↑ Risk of bleeding

HOW SUPPLIED

Powder for injection, lyophilized: 0.2 mg, 0.5 mg; *Tablet:* 0.025 mg, 0.05 mg, 0.075 mg, 0.088 mg, 0.1 mg, 0.112 mg, 0.125 mg, 0.137 mg, 0.15 mg, 0.175 mg, 0.2 mg, 0.3 mg

DOSAGE

• **TABLETS**

Mild hypothyroidism.

Adults, initial: 50 mcg once daily; **then,** increase by 25–50 mcg q 2–3 weeks until desired clinical response is attained; **maintenance, usual:** 75–125 mcg/day (although doses up to 200 mcg/day may be required in some clients).

L

Severe hypothyroidism.

Adults, initial: 12.5–25 mcg once daily; **then,** increase dose, as necessary, in increments of 25 mcg at 2- to 3-week intervals.

Congenital hypothyroidism.

Pediatric, 12 years and older: 2–3 mcg/kg once daily until the adult daily dose (usually 150 mcg) is reached. **6–12 years of age:** 4–5 mcg/kg/day or 100–150 mcg once daily. **1–5 years of age:** 5–6 mcg/kg/day or 75–100 mcg once daily. **6–12 months of age:** 6–8 mcg/kg/day or 50–75 mcg once daily. **Less than 6 months of age:** 8–10 mcg/kg/day or 25–50 mcg once daily.

• **IM, IV**

Myxedematous coma.

Adults, initial: 400 mcg by rapid IV injection, even in geriatric clients; **then,** 100–200 mcg/day, IV. **Maintenance:** 100–200 mcg/day, IV. Smaller daily doses should be given until client can tolerate PO medication.

Hypothyroidism.

Adults: 50–100 mcg once daily; **pediatric, IV, IM:** A dose of 75% of the usual PO pediatric dose should be given.

NURSING CONSIDERATIONS

SEE ALSO *NURSING CONSIDERATIONS* FOR *THYROID DRUGS*.

ADMINISTRATION/STORAGE

1. In infants and children who cannot swallow tablets, the correct dosage tablet may be crushed and suspended in a small amount of formula or water and given by dropper or spoon. The crushed tablet may also be sprinkled over cooked cereal or applesauce.
2. Transfer from liothyronine to levothyroxine: administer replacement drug for several days before discontinuing liothyronine. Transfer from levothyroxine to liothyronine: discontinue levothyroxine before starting low daily dose of liothyronine.
3. IV Prepare solution for injection immediately before administration. Reconstitute by adding 5 mL of 0.9% NaCl or bacteriostatic NaCl injection and shake vial to ensure complete mixing.
4. Discard any unused portion of the IV medication.
5. Do not mix with other IV infusion solutions.

ASSESSMENT

1. Elderly clients are likely to have undetected cardiac problems. Obtain ECG prior to initiating therapy.
2. Monitor response, cardiac status and adjust dose based on regular thyroid panels.
3. If pregnant, must continue taking thyroid preparations throughout the pregnancy.
4. Note height, weight, and psychomotor development in child.
5. List drugs currently consumed to ensure none interact unfavorably.

CLIENT/FAMILY TEACHING

1. This drug is prescribed to replace a hormone that is low in the body causing hypothyroidism. Drug is not a cure for hypothyroidism; must be taken for life to control symptoms.
2. Take first thing in the morning before breakfast. Do not take with food unless specifically instructed; may interfere with absorption. Avoid iodine-rich foods.
3. Do not switch brands; bioavailability may change.
4. Report any severe headache, palpitations, chest pain, diarrhea, irritability, excitability, insomnia, intolerance to heat, significant weight loss, and/or excessive sweating.

OUTCOMES/EVALUATE

- Promotion of normal metabolism
- ↑ Levels of T_3 and T_4, ↓ TSH

Lidocaine hydrochloride

(**LYE**-doh-kayn)

PREGNANCY CATEGORY: B
CLASSIFICATION(S):
Antiarrhythmic, Class IB
Rx: IM: LidoPen Auto-Injector , Xylocaine HCl IV for Cardiac Arrhythmias; **Direct IV or IV Admixtures:** Lidocaine HCl for Cardiac Arrhythmias; **IV Infusion:** Lidocaine HCl in 5% Dextrose
✱**Rx:** Xylocard

SEE ALSO *ANTIARRHYTHMIC AGENTS*.

ACTION/KINETICS

Shortens the refractory period and suppresses the automaticity of ectopic foci without affecting conduction of impulses through cardiac tissue. Increases the electrical stimulation threshold of the ventricle during diastole. It does not affect BP, CO, or myocardial contractility. **IV: Onset,** 45–90 sec; **duration:** 10–20 min. **IM, Onset,** 5–15 min; **duration,** 60–90 min. **t¹/₂:** 1–2 hr. **Therapeutic serum levels:** 1.5–6 mcg/mL. **Time to steady-state plasma levels:** 3–4 hr (8–10 hr in clients with AMI). **Protein-binding:** 40–80%. Ninety percent is rapidly metabolized in the liver to active metabolites. Since lidocaine has little effect on conduction at normal antiarrhythmic doses, use in acute situations (instead of procainamide) in instances in which heart block might occur.

USES

IV: Treatment of acute ventricular arrhythmias such as those following MIs or occurring during surgery. The drug is ineffective against atrial arrhythmias. **IM:** Certain emergency situations (e.g., ECG equipment not available; mobile coronary care unit, under advice of a physician).

Investigational: IV in children who develop ventricular couplets or frequent premature ventricular beats.

CONTRAINDICATIONS

Hypersensitivity to amide-type local anesthetics, Stokes-Adams syndrome, Wolff-Parkinson-White syndrome, severe SA, AV, or intraventricular block (when no pacemaker is present). Use of the IM autoinjector for children.

SPECIAL CONCERNS

Use with caution during labor and delivery, during lactation, and in the presence of liver or severe kidney disease, CHF, marked hypoxia, digitalis toxicity with AV block, severe respiratory depression, or shock. In geriatric clients, the rate and dose for IV infusion should be decreased by one-half and slowly adjusted. Safety and efficacy have not been determined in children.

SIDE EFFECTS

Body as a whole: Malignant hyperthermia characterized by tachycardia, tachypnea, labile BP, metabolic acidosis, temperature elevation. **CV:** Precipitation or aggravation of arrhythmias (following IV use), hypotension, bradycardia ***(with possible cardiac arrest), CV collapse.*** **CNS:** Dizziness, apprehension, euphoria, lightheadedness, nervousness, drowsiness, confusion, changes in mood, hallucinations, twitching, "doom anxiety," ***convulsions,*** unconsciousness. **Respiratory:** Difficulties in breathing or swallowing, ***respiratory depression or arrest.*** **Allergic:** Rash, cutaneous lesions, urticaria, edema, ***anaphylaxis.*** **Other:** Tinnitus, blurred/double vision, vomiting, numbness, sensation of heat or cold, twitching, tremors, soreness at IM injection site, fever, ***venous thrombosis or phlebitis (extending from site of injection),*** extravasation. During anesthesia, CV depression may be the first sign of lidocaine toxicity. During other usage, *convulsions are the first sign of lidocaine toxicity.*

LABORATORY TEST CONSIDERATIONS

↑ CPK following IM use.

OD OVERDOSE MANAGEMENT

Symptoms: Dependent on plasma levels. If plasma levels range from 4 to 6 mcg/mL, mild CNS effects are observed. Levels of 6 to 8 mcg/mL may result in significant CNS and CV depression while levels greater than 8 mcg/mL cause hypotension, decreased CO, respiratory depression, obtundation, ***seizures, and coma.*** *Treatment:* Discontinue the drug and begin emergency resuscitative procedures. Seizures can be treated with diazepam, thiopental, or thiamylal. Succinylcholine, IV, may be used if the client is anesthetized. IV fluids, vasopressors, and CPR are used to correct circulatory depression.

DRUG INTERACTIONS

Aminoglycosides / ↑ Neuromuscular blockade

Beta-adrenergic blockers / ↑ Lidocaine levels with possible toxicity

Cimetidine / ↓ Clearance of lidocaine → possible toxicity
Phenytoin / IV phenytoin → excessive cardiac depression
Procainamide / Additive cardiodepressant effects
Succinylcholine / ↑ Succinylcholine action by ↓ plasma protein binding
Tocainide / ↑ Risk of side effects
Tubocurarine / ↑ Neuromuscular blockade

HOW SUPPLIED

IM Injection: 300 mg/3 mL; *Direct IV Injection:* 1%, 2%; *For IV Admixture:* 4%, 10%, 20%; *For IV Infusion:* 0.2%, 0.4%, 0.8%

DOSAGE

- **IV BOLUS**

Antiarrhythmic.

Adults: 50–100 mg at rate of 25–50 mg/min. Bolus is used to establish rapid therapeutic plasma levels. Repeat if necessary after 5-min interval. Onset of action is 10 sec. **Maximum dose/hr:** 200–300 mg.

- **INFUSION**

Antiarrhythmic.

20–50 mcg/kg at a rate of 1–4 mg/min. No more than 200–300 mg/hr should be given. **Pediatric, loading dose:** 1 mg/kg IV or intratracheally q 5–10 min until desired effect reached (maximum total dose: 5 mg/kg).

- **IV CONTINUOUS INFUSION**

Maintain therapeutic plasma levels following loading doses.

Adults: Give at a rate of 1–4 mg/min (20–50 mcg/kg/min). Reduce the dose in clients with heart failure, with liver disease, or who are taking drugs that interact with lidocaine. **Pediatric:** 20–50 mcg/kg/min (usual is 30 mcg/kg/min).

- **IM**

Antiarrhythmic.

Adults: 4.5 mg/kg (approximately 300 mg for a 70-kg adult). Switch to IV lidocaine or oral antiarrhythmics as soon as possible although an additional IM dose may be given after 60–90 min.

NURSING CONSIDERATIONS

SEE ALSO *NURSING CONSIDERATIONS* FOR *ANTIARRHYTHMIC AGENTS*.

ADMINISTRATION/STORAGE

IV 1. *Do not add lidocaine to blood transfusion assembly.*
2. Do not use lidocaine solutions that contain epinephrine to treat arrhythmias. Make certain that vial states, "For Cardiac Arrhythmias." Check prefilled syringes closely to ensure appropriate dose has been obtained. (Lidocaine prefilled syringes come in both milligrams and grams.)
3. Use D5W to prepare solution; this is stable for 24 hr. Administer with an electronic infusion device.
4. Reduce IV bolus dosage in clients over 70 years old, with CHF or liver disease, and if taking cimetidine or propranolol (i.e., where metabolism of lidocaine is reduced).

ASSESSMENT

1. Note any hypersensitivity to amide-type local anesthetics.
2. Elderly clients who have hepatic or renal disease or who weigh less than 45.5 kg will need to be watched especially closely for adverse side effects; adjust dosage as directed.
3. Document CNS status; report sudden changes in mental status, dizziness, visual disturbances, twitching, and tremors. These symptoms may precede convulsions. Note pulmonary findings; assess for respiratory depression, characterized by slow, shallow respirations. Monitor liver and renal function studies, electrolytes, and ECG; assess for hypotension and cardiac collapse.
4. View monitor strips for myocardial depression, variations of rhythm, or aggravation of arrhythmia.

OUTCOMES/EVALUATE

- Control of ventricular arrhythmias
- Therapeutic serum drug levels (1.5–6 mcg/mL)

Lincomycin hydrochloride

(link-oh-**MY**-sin)

PREGNANCY CATEGORY: B

CLASSIFICATION(S):
Antibiotic, lincosamide
Rx: Lincocin, Lincorex

SEE ALSO *ANTI-INFECTIVES.*

ACTION/KINETICS
Isolated from *Streptomyces lincolnensis.* Suppresses protein synthesis by microorganisms by binding to ribosomes (50S subunit), which is essential for transmittal of genetic information. Both bacteriostatic and bactericidal. Rapidly absorbed from the GI tract and is widely distributed. **Peak serum levels: PO,** 1.8–5.3 mcg/mL after 500 mg; **IM,** 9.3–18.5 mcg/mL after 600 mg; **IV,** 15.9–20.9 mcg/mL after 600 mg. **t½:** 4.4–6.4 hr. Metabolized by the liver; about 60% excreted through the urine and 40% in the feces. Do not use for trivial infections.

USES
Not a first-choice drug but useful for clients allergic to penicillin. Spectrum resembles that of the erythromycins. Used for serious respiratory tract, skin, and soft tissue infections due to staphylococci, streptococci, or pneumococci and some gram-negative organisms. Septicemia. In conjunction with diphtheria antitoxin in the treatment of diphtheria.

CONTRAINDICATIONS
Hypersensitivity to drugs. Use in pre-existing liver disease, in infants up to 1 month of age, or in treating viral and minor bacterial infections.

SPECIAL CONCERNS
Safe use during pregnancy has not been established. Use with caution in clients with GI disease, liver or renal disease, or a history of allergy or asthma.

SIDE EFFECTS
GI: N&V, diarrhea (may be severe), abdominal pain, tenesmus, flatulence, bloating, anorexia, weight loss, esophagitis, pruritus ani. Nonspecific colitis, pseudomembranous colitis (may be severe). **Allergic:** Morbilliform rash (most common). Also, maculopapular rash, urticaria, pruritus, fever, hypotension. Rarely, polyarteritis, ***anaphylaxis,*** erythema multiforme. **Hematologic:** Leukopenia, neutropenia, eosinophilia, thrombocytopenia, ***agranulocytosis.*** **Miscellaneous:** Superinfection.

Following IV use: Thrombophlebitis, erythema, pain, swelling. IV lincomycin may cause hypotension, syncope, and ***cardiac arrest*** (rare). *Following IM use:* Pain, induration, sterile abscesses. *Following topical use:* Erythema, irritation, dryness, peeling, itching, burning, oiliness. Also, sore throat, fatigue, urinary frequency, headache.

NOTE: The injection contains benzyl alcohol, which has been associated with a fatal gasping syndrome in infants.

LABORATORY TEST CONSIDERATIONS
↓ Levels of AST, ALT, NPN, alkaline phosphatase, bilirubin, BSP retention, and ↓ platelet count.

DRUG INTERACTIONS
Antiperistaltic antidiarrheals (opiates, Lomotil) / ↑ Diarrhea due to ↓ removal of toxins from colon
Erythromycin / Cross-interference → ↓ effect of both drugs
Kaolin (e.g., Kaopectate) / ↓ Effect due to ↓ absorption from GI tract
Neuromuscular blocking agents / ↑ Effect of blocking agents; possible severe respiratory depression

HOW SUPPLIED
Capsule: 500 mg; *Injection:* 300 mg/mL

DOSAGE

• **CAPSULES**

Infections.

Adults: 500 mg t.i.d. for serious infections. **Adults:** 500 mg or more q 6 hr for more severe infections. Continue treatment for at least 10 days with β–hemolytic streptococcal infections. **Children over 1 month of age:** 30–60 mg/kg/day in three to four divided doses, depending on severity of infection.

• **IM**

Infections.

Adults: 600 mg q 24 hr for serious infections and every 12 hr or more for more severe infections. **Children over 1 month of age:** 10 mg/kg q 12–24 hr, depending on severity of infection.

• **IV**

Infections.

Adults: 0.6–1.0 g q 8–12 hr up to 8 g/day, depending on severity of infection. **Children over 1 month of age:** 10–20 mg/kg/day, depending on severity of infection.

NOTE: In impaired renal function, reduce dosage by 70%–75%.

• **SUBCONJUNCTIVAL INJECTION**
0.75 mg/0.25 mL.

NURSING CONSIDERATIONS

SEE ALSO *GENERAL NURSING CONSIDERATIONS* FOR *ANTI-INFECTIVES*.

ADMINISTRATION/STORAGE

1. Prepare drug for administration as directed on package insert.
2. Administer slowly IM to minimize pain.

IV 3. For IV use, carefully follow concentration and recommended rate for administration to prevent severe cardiopulmonary reactions. Usually reconstituted and placed in 250-500 mL D5/W or NSS and infused over 1-4 h.

4. Injection contains benzyl alcohol; may cause fatal gasping syndrome in infants.

ASSESSMENT

1. Note indications for therapy, onset and characteristics of symptoms, if PCN allergy and culture results.
2. Manage colitis by providing fluids, electrolytes, protein supplements, systemic corticosteroids, and vancomycin (may occur 2–9 days to several weeks after therapy).
3. Assess for transient flushing, sensations of warmth and cardiac disturbances, with IV infusions.
4. Monitor VS, CBC, and LFTs. Note asthma, any liver dysfunction/disease.

CLIENT/FAMILY TEACHING

1. Take on an empty stomach between meals and not with a sugar substitute, to ensure optimum absorption. Report GI disturbances, including abdominal pain, diarrhea, anorexia, N&V, bloody or tarry stools, and excessive flatulence.
2. Do not use antiperistaltic agents if diarrhea occurs; may prolong or aggravate condition.
3. Avoid acne or topical mercury preparations containing a peeling agent in area affected by medication; severe irritation can occur.
4. Do not take kaolin concomitantly; will reduce absorption of lincomycin. If kaolin is required, administer 3 hr before.

OUTCOMES/EVALUATE

- Negative culture reports
- Resolution of infection

Linezolid

(lih-**NAY**-zoh-lid)

PREGNANCY CATEGORY: C
CLASSIFICATION(S):
Antibiotic, oxazolidinone
Rx: Zyvox

ACTION/KINETICS

Binds to a site on the bacterial 23S ribosomal RNA of the 50S subunit thus preventing the formation of a functional 70S initiation complex (is an essential component of the bacterial translational process). Is bacteriostatic against *Enterococci* and *Staphylococci* and bactericidal for most strains of *Streptococci.* Rapidly and extensively absorbed after PO use. Metabolized in the liver and both parent drug and metabolites are primarily excreted in the urine. **t½, after IV or PO:** 4.7–5.4 hr.

USES

(1) Vancomycin-resistant *Enterococcus faecium* infections, including cases with concurrent bacteremia. (2) Nosocomial pneumonia due to *Staphylococcus aureus* (methicillin-susceptible and resistant strains) or *Streptococcus pneumoniae* (penicillin-susceptible strains only). Combination therapy may be used if pathogens include gram-negative organisms. (3) Complicated skin and skin structure infections due to *Staphylococcus aureus* (methicillin-susceptible and resistant strains), *Streptococcus pyogenes,* or *Streptococcus agalactiae.* Combination therapy may be used if pathogens include gram-negative organisms. (4) Uncomplicated skin and skin structure infections due to *S. aureus* (methicillin-susceptible strains only) and *S. pyogenes.* (5) Community acquired pneumonia due to *S. pneumoniae* (penicillin-susceptible strains

only), including cases with concurrent bacteremia and *S. aureus* (methicillin-susceptible strains only). *NOTE:* Due to concerns of inappropriate use of antibiotics causing resistant organisms, consider alternatives before starting treatment with linezolid in the outpatient setting.

SPECIAL CONCERNS

Pseudomembranous colitis may occur; severity ranges from mild to life-threatening. Use with caution during lactation. Drug clearance is increased in pediatric clients resulting in a shorter half-life; however, pediatric dosing regimens have not been determined. The resistance rate for linezolid may be higher than anticipated. Safety and efficacy have not been evaluated for use over 28 days.

SIDE EFFECTS

Hematologic: Myelosuppression, including anemia, leukopenia, pancytopenia, and thrombocytopenia. **GI:** N&V, diarrhea, taste alteration, tongue discoloration, ***pseudomembranous colitis***. **CNS:** Headache, dizziness. **Miscellaneous:** Vaginal moniliasis, fungal infection, oral moniliasis.

LABORATORY TEST CONSIDERATIONS

The following lab values may be abnormal: Hemoglobin, platelet count, WBCs, neutrophils, AST, ALT, LDH, alkaline phosphatase, lipase, amylase, total bilirubin, BUN, creatinine.

DRUG INTERACTIONS

Adrenergic agents / Possible enhancement of pressor response to indirect-acting sympathomimetics (e.g., pseudoephedrine)

Monoamine oxidase inhibitors / Linezolid is a reversible, nonselective MAO inhibitor → ↑ potential for interaction with adrenergic and serotonergic drugs

Serotonergic drugs (e.g., fluoxetine, paroxetine, sertraline) / Possible serotonin sydrome, including hyperpyrexia and cognitive dysfunction.

HOW SUPPLIED

Injection: 2 mg/mL; *Powder for reconstitution, oral:* 100 mg/5 mL; *Tablet:* 400 mg, 600 mg

DOSAGE

- **IV, ORAL SOLUTION, TABLETS**

Vancomycin-resistant Enterococcus faecium *infections, including concurrent bacteremia.*

600 mg q 12 hr for 14–28 days.

Nosocomial pneumonia, complicated skin and skin structure infections, community-acquired pneumonia including concurrent bacteremia.

600 mg q 12 hr for 10–14 days.

Uncomplicated skin and skin structure infections.

400 mg q 12 hr for 10–14 days.

NURSING CONSIDERATIONS

ADMINISTRATION/STORAGE

1. Store the reconstituted oral suspension at room temperature and use within 21 days of reconstitution.

IV 2. Dosage adjustment is not necessary when switching from IV to PO administration. Those started on IV therapy may be switched to either tablets or oral suspension when indicated.

3. The drug is compatible with D5W, saline injection, and lactated Ringer's injection.

4. Administer over a 30–120 min period.

5. Do not use IV infusion bag in series connections and do not introduce additives into the solution.

6. Do not administer together with another drug; give each drug separately. Physical incompatibility was noted with : amphotericin B, chlorpromazine HCl, diazepam, erythromycin lactobionate, pentamidine isothionate, phenytoin sodium, and trimethoprim-sulfamethoxazole. Chemical incompatibility was noted when mixed with ceftriaxone sodium.

7. If the same line is used for sequential infusion of two or more drugs, flush the line before and after infusion of IV linezolid with a compatible solution.

8. Keep the infusion bags in the overwrap until ready for use and store at room temperature. Protect from freezing.

9. The IV injection may exhibit a yellow color that may intensify over time; this does not affect the potency adversely.

L

ASSESSMENT

1. Document indications for therapy, onset, location and characteristics of symptoms.
2. Monitor CBC weekly in those taking the drug for over 2 weeks. Discontinue drug if clients develop or have worsening myelosuppression.
3. Note any history of hypertension and record readings. List drugs consuming to ensure none interact.
4. Assess for diarrhea and culture for *C. difficile* if evident.
5. Oral suspension contains phenylalanine; assess for contraindications.

CLIENT/FAMILY TEACHING

1. May take with or without food. Taking with food may help with gi upset.
2. Avoid foods high in tyramine such as fermented, pickled, or smoked foods during therapy.
3. Do not take OTC decongestants or cold remedies which contain pseudoephedrine during therapy.
4. Notify provider if taking anti-depressants or SSRIs.
5. Report any loss of effectiveness or adverse side effects, as well as rash, tremors, weakness, anxiety, increased bleeding or severe gi side effects.

OUTCOMES/EVALUATE

Resolution of infection; symptomatic relief

Liothyronine sodium (T_3)

(lye-oh-**THIGH**-roh-neen)

PREGNANCY CATEGORY: A
CLASSIFICATION(S):
Thyroid product
Rx: Cytomel, Sodium-L-Triiodothyronine, Triostat

SEE ALSO *THYROID DRUGS*.

ACTION/KINETICS

Synthetic sodium salt of levoisomer of T_3. Has more predictable effects due to standard hormone content. From 15 to 37.5 mcg is equivalent to about 60 mg of desiccated thyroid. May be preferred when a rapid effect or rapidly reversible effect is required. Has a rapid onset, which may result in difficulty in controlling the dosage as well as the possibility of cardiac side effects and changes in metabolic demands. However, its short duration allows quick adjustment of dosage and helps control overdosage. **t½:** 24 hr for euthyroid clients, approximately 34 hr in hypothyroid clients, and approximately 14 hr in hyperthyroid clients. **Duration:** Up to 72 hr. Is 99% protein bound.

ADDITIONAL CONTRAINDICATIONS

Use in children with cretinism because there is some question about whether the hormone crosses the blood-brain barrier.

HOW SUPPLIED

Injection: 10 mcg/mL; *Tablet:* 5 mcg, 25 mcg, 50 mcg

DOSAGE

• **TABLETS**

Mild hypothyroidism.

Adults, individualized, initial: 25 mcg/day. Increase by 12.5–25 mcg q 1–2 weeks until satisfactory response has been obtained. **Usual maintenance:** 25–75 mcg/day (100 mcg may be required in some clients). Use lower initial dosage (5 mcg/day) for the elderly, children, and clients with CV disease. Increase only by 5-mcg increments.

Myxedema.

Adults, initial: 5 mcg/day increased by 5–10 mcg/day q 1–2 weeks until 25 mcg/day is reached; **then,** increase q 1–2 weeks by 12.5–50 mcg. **Usual maintenance:** 50–100 mcg/day.

Simple (nontoxic) goiter.

Adults, initial: 5 mcg/day; **then,** increase q 1–2 weeks by 5–10 mcg until 25 mcg/day is reached; **then,** dose can be increased by 12.5–25 mcg/week until the maintenance dose of 50–100 mcg/day is reached (usual is 75 mcg/day).

T_3 suppression test.

75–100 mcg/day for 7 days followed by a repeat of the I^{131} thyroid uptake test (a 50% or greater suppression of uptake indicates a normal thyroid-pituitary axis).

Congenital hypothyroidism.
Adults and children, initial: 5 mcg/day; **then,** increase by 5 mcg/day q 3–4 days until the desired effect is achieved. Approximately 20 mcg/day may be sufficient for infants a few months of age while children 1 year of age may require 50 mcg/day. Children above 3 years may require the full adult dose.

• **IV ONLY**
Myxedema coma, precoma.
Adults, initial: 25–50 mcg. Base subsequent doses on continuous monitoring of client's clinical status and response. Doses should be given at least 4 hr, and no more than 12 hr, apart. Total daily doses of 65 mcg in initial days of therapy are associated with a lower incidence of mortality. In cases of known CV disease, give an initial dose of 10–20 mcg.

NURSING CONSIDERATIONS

SEE ALSO *NURSING CONSIDERATIONS FOR THYROID DRUGS* AND *LEVOTHYROXINE.*

ADMINISTRATION/STORAGE

1. *Transfer from other thyroid preparations to liothyronine:* Discontinue old preparation before starting on low daily dose of liothyronine. *Transfer from liothyronine to another thyroid preparation:* Start therapy with replacement drug several days prior to complete withdrawal of sodium liothyronine.
2. If symptoms of hyperthyroidism noted, the drug can be withdrawn for 2–3 days and can be reinstituted at a lower dose.
IV 3. A *Cytomel* injection kit is available for the emergency treatment of myxedema coma.

CLIENT/FAMILY TEACHING

1. Take once a day as directed before breakfast.
2. This drug is used to control symptoms of hypothyroidism and will require replacement for life.
3. Report any chest pain, palpitations, fever, insomnia, irritability, unusual sweating, heat intolerance, diarrhea, weight loss and headaches.
4. Report as scheduled for physical exam and blood work.

OUTCOMES/EVALUATE

Desired thyroid hormone replacement

Liotrix

(**LYE**-oh-trix)

PREGNANCY CATEGORY: A
CLASSIFICATION(S):
Thyroid product
Rx: Thyrolar

SEE ALSO *THYROID DRUGS.*

ACTION/KINETICS

Mixture of synthetic levothyroxine sodium (T_4) and liothyronine (T_3) in a 4:1 ratio by weight and in a 1:1 ratio by biologic activity.

HOW SUPPLIED

Tablet: 15 mg, 30 mg, 60 mg, 120 mg, 180 mg

DOSAGE

• **TABLETS**
Hypothyroidism.
Adults and children, initial: 50 mcg levothyroxine and 12.5 mcg liothyronine (Thyrolar); **then,** at monthly intervals, increments of like amounts can be made until the desired effect is achieved. **Usual maintenance:** 50–100 mcg of levothyroxine and 12.5–25 mcg liothyronine daily.

Congenital hypothyroidism.
Children, 0–6 months: 8–10 mcg T_4/kg/day (25–50 mcg/day); **6–12 months:** 6–8 mcg T_4/kg/day (50–75 mcg/day); **1–5 years:** 5–6 mcg T_4/kg/day (75–100 mcg/day); **6–12 years:** 4–5 mcg T_4/kg/day (100–150 mcg/day); **over 12 years:** 2–3 mcg T_4/kg/day (over 150 mcg/day).

NURSING CONSIDERATIONS

SEE ALSO *NURSING CONSIDERATIONS FOR THYROID DRUGS* AND *INDIVIDUAL AGENTS.*

ADMINISTRATION/STORAGE

1. The initial dose for geriatric clients is ½ the usual adult dose; this can be

L

doubled q 6–8 weeks until desired effect is attained.
2. In children, make dosing increments q 2 weeks until desired response attained.
3. Always do thyroid function tests before initiating dosage changes.
4. Administer as a single dose before breakfast.
5. Protect tablets from light, heat, and moisture.
6. Due to differences in the amounts of hormones between Euthroid and Thyrolar, do not switch brands once started on a particular brand.

CLIENT/FAMILY TEACHING
1. Take once a day as directed before breakfast. May split dose if nausea and diarrhea persist.
2. This drug is used to control symptoms of hypothyroidism and will require replacement for life.Do not stop suddenly.
3. Report any chest pain, palpitations, fever, insomnia, irritability, unusual sweating, heat intolerance, diarrhea, weight loss and headaches.
4. Report as scheduled for physical exam and blood work.

OUTCOMES/EVALUATE
Thyroid hormone replacement

L

Lisinopril

(lie-**SIN**-oh-prill)

PREGNANCY CATEGORY: C
CLASSIFICATION(S):
Antihypertensive, ACE inhibitor
Rx: Prinivil, Zestril
✱Rx: Apo-Lisinopril

SEE ALSO *ANGIOTENSIN-CONVERTING ENZYME INHIBITORS.*

ACTION/KINETICS
Both supine and standing BPs are reduced, although the drug is less effective in blacks than in Caucasians. Although food does not alter the bioavailability of lisinopril, only 25% of a PO dose is absorbed. **Onset:** 1 hr. **Peak serum levels:** 7 hr. **Duration:** 24 hr. **t½:** 12 hr. 100% of the drug is excreted unchanged in the urine.

USES
(1) Alone or in combination with a diuretic (usually a thiazide) to treat hypertension. (2) In combination with digitalis and a diuretic for treating CHF not responding to other therapy. (3) Use within 24 hr of acute MI to improve survival in hemodynamically stable clients (clients should receive the standard treatment, including thrombolytics, aspirin, and beta blockers).

SPECIAL CONCERNS
Use with caution during lactation. Safety and efficacy have not been established in children. Geriatric clients may manifest higher blood levels. Reduce the dosage in clients with impaired renal function.

SIDE EFFECTS
CV: Hypotension, orthostatic hypotension, angina, tachycardia, palpitations, rhythm disturbances, ***stroke,*** chest pain, orthostatic effects, peripheral edema, ***MI, CVA,*** worsening of heart failure, chest sound abnormalities, PVCs, TIAs, decreased blood pressure, atrial fibrillation. **CNS:** Dizziness, headache, fatigue, vertigo, insomnia, depression, sleepiness, paresthesias, malaise, nervousness, confusion, ataxia, impaired memory, tremor, irritability, hypersomnia, peripheral neuropathy, spasm. **GI:** Diarrhea, N&V, dyspepsia, anorexia, constipation, dysgeusia, dry mouth, abdominal pain, flatulence, dry mouth, gastritis, heartburn, GI cramps, weight loss/gain, taste alterations, increased salivation. **Respiratory:** Cough, dyspnea, bronchitis, upper respiratory symptoms, nasal congestion, sinusitis, pharyngeal pain, bronchospasm, asthma, pulmonary edema, ***pulmonary embolism, pulmonary infarction,*** PND, chest discomfort, common cold, nasal congestion, pulmonary infiltrates, pleural effusion, wheezing, painful respiration, epistaxis, laryngitis, pharyngitis, rhinitis, rhinorrhea, orthopnea. **Musculoskeletal:** Asthenia, muscle cramps, neck/hip/leg/knee/arm/joint/shoulder/back/pelvic/flank pain, myalgia, arthralgia, arthritis, lumbago. **Hepatic:** Hepatitis, hepatocellular/cholestatic jaundice, pancreatitis, hepatomegaly. **Dermato-**

logic: Rash, pruritus, flushing, increased sweating, urticaria, alopecia, erythema multiforme, photophobia. **GU:** Impotence, oliguria, progressive azotemia, acute renal failure, UTI, anuria, uremia, renal dysfunction, pyelonephritis, dysuria. **Ophthalmic:** Blurred vision, visual loss, diplopia. **Miscellaneous:** ***Angioedema (may be fatal if laryngeal edema occurs),*** hyperkalemia, neutropenia, anemia, ***bone marrow depression,*** decreased libido, fever, syncope, vasculitis of the legs, gout, eosinophilia, fluid overload, dehydration, diabetes mellitus, chills, virus infection, edema, ***anaphylactoid reaction,*** malignant lung neoplasms, hemoptysis, breast pain.

LABORATORY TEST CONSIDERATIONS

↑ Serum potassium, BUN, serum creatinine. ↓ H&H.

OD OVERDOSE MANAGEMENT

Symptoms: Hypotension. *Treatment:* Supportive. To correct hypotension, IV normal saline is treatment of choice. Lisinopril may be removed by hemodialysis.

DRUG INTERACTIONS

Diuretics / Excess ↓ BP
Indomethacin / Possible ↓ lisinopril effect
Potassium-sparing diuretics / Significant ↑ serum potassium

HOW SUPPLIED

Tablet: 2.5 mg, 5 mg, 10 mg, 20 mg, 40 mg

DOSAGE

• **TABLETS**

Essential hypertension, used alone.

Initial: 10 mg once daily. Adjust dosage depending on response (range: 20–40 mg/day given as a single dose). Doses greater than 80 mg/day do not give a greater effect.

Essential hypertension in combination with a diuretic.

Initial: 5 mg. The BP-lowering effects of the combination are additive. Reduce dosage in renal impairment as follows: C_{CR}, 10–30 mL/min; give an initial dose of 5 mg /day for hypertension. C_{CR}, less than 10 mL/min; give an initial dose of 2.5 mg/day and adjust dose depending on BP response.

CHF.

Initial: 5 mg once daily (2.5 mg/day in clients with hyponatremia) in combination with diuretics and digitalis. **Dosage range:** 5–20 mg/day as a single dose.

Acute MI.

First dose: 5 mg; **then,** 5 mg after 24 hr, 10 mg after 48 hr, and then 10 mg daily. Continue dosing for 6 weeks. In clients with a systolic pressure less than 120 mm Hg when treatment is started or within 3 days after the infarct should be given 2.5 mg. If hypotension occurs (systolic BP less than 100 mm Hg), the dose may be temporarily reduced to 2.5 mg. If prolonged hypotension occurs, withdraw the drug.

NURSING CONSIDERATIONS

SEE ALSO *NURSING CONSIDERATIONS* FOR *ANGIOTENSIN-CONVERTING ENZYME INHIBITORS* AND *ANTIHYPERTENSIVE AGENTS.*

ADMINISTRATION/STORAGE

1. When considering use of lisinopril in a client taking diuretics, discontinue the diuretic, if possible, 2–3 days before beginning lisinopril therapy. If the diuretic cannot be discontinued, the initial dose of lisinopril should be 5 mg; observe closely for at least 2 hr.
2. Maximum antihypertensive effects may not be observed for 2–4 weeks in some.
3. When starting treatment for CHF, give under medical supervision, especially if SBP less than 100 mm Hg.
4. With clients whose BP is controlled with lisinopril, 20 mg plus hydrochlorothiazide 25 mg, given separately should trial Prinzide 12.5 mg or Zestoretic 20–12.5 mg before Prinzide 25 mg or Zestoretic 20–25 mg is used.
5. The maximum recommended daily dose of lisinopril is 80 mg in a single daily dose. Clients usually do not require hydrochlorothiazide in doses exceeding 50 mg/day, especially if combined with other antihypertensives.
6. Use of potassium supplements, potassium-sparing diuretics, or potassium salt substitutes with Prinzide or Zestoretic may lead to increases in serum potassium.

7. Prinzide or Zestoretic is recommended for those with a C_{CR} greater than 30 mL/min.
8. Anticipate reduced dosage with renal insufficiency—initial dose of 10 mg/day if C_{CR} is greater than 30 mL/min, 5 mg/day if C_{CR} is between 10 and 30 mL/min, and 2.5 mg/day in dialysis clients (i.e., C_{CR} less than 10 mL/min).

ASSESSMENT

1. Document indications for therapy, agents trialed and the outcome,
2. Perform physical exam noting cardio-pulmonary status, review history for any existing conditions, and labs for any organ dysfunction.
3. Obtain ECG, CXR, and baseline labs. Reduce dose with renal dysfunction.
4. Identify risk factors and those that are modifiable to reduce CHD.
5. Start within 24 hr of AMI in addition to ASA, beta blockers and thrombolytics to reduce mortality.

CLIENT/FAMILY TEACHING

1. Must be taken as directed at least once a day to control BP.
2. Avoid symptoms of orthostatic hypotension (i.e., rise slowly from sitting or lying position and wait until symptoms subside).
3. Avoid all potassium supplements as well as foods high in potassium, unless otherwise directed.
4. Review drug side effects; report for BP check, ECG, and lab studies.
5. Report any new or unusual side effects or any aggravation of existing conditions, as well as sore throat, hoarseness, chest pain, difficulty breathing or swelling of hands or feet or face.

OUTCOMES/EVALUATE

- ↓ BP
- Improved survival with acute MI

Lithium carbonate

(**LITH**-ee-um)

PREGNANCY CATEGORY: D
Rx: Eskalith, Eskalith CR, Lithobid, Lithonate, Lithotabs, PMS-Lithium Carbonate
✱Rx: Carbolith, Duralith, Lithane

Lithium citrate

(**LITH**-ee-um)

PREGNANCY CATEGORY: D
✱Rx: PMS-Lithium Citrate
CLASSIFICATION(S):
Antipsychotic

ACTION/KINETICS

Mechanism for the antimanic effect of lithium is unknown. Various hypotheses include: (a) a decrease in catecholamine neurotransmitter levels caused by lithium's effect on Na^+–K^+ ATPase to improve transneuronal membrane transport of sodium ion; (b) a decrease in cyclic AMP levels caused by lithium which decreases sensitivity of hormonal-sensitive adenyl cyclase receptors; or (c) interference by lithium with lipid inositol metabolism ultimately leading to insensitivity of cells in the CNS to stimulation by inositol.

Affects the distribution of calcium, magnesium, and sodium ions and affects glucose metabolism. **Peak serum levels** (regular release): 1–4 hr; (slow-release): 4–6 hr. **Onset:** 5–14 days. **Therapeutic serum levels:** 0.4–1.0 mEq/L (must be carefully monitored because toxic effects may occur at these levels and significant toxic reactions occur at serum lithium levels of 2 mEq/L). **t½ (plasma):** 24 hr (longer in presence of renal impairment and in the elderly). Lithium and sodium are excreted by the same mechanism in the proximal tubule. Thus, to reduce the danger of lithium intoxication, sodium intake must remain at normal levels.

USES

Control of mania in manic-depressive clients. *Investigational:* To reverse neutropenia induced by cancer chemotherapy, in children with chronic neutropenia, and in AIDs clients receiving zidovudine. Prophylaxis of cluster headaches. Also for premenstrual tension, alcoholism accompanied by depression, tardive dyskinesia, bulimia, hyperthyroidism, excess ADH secretion, postpartum affective psychosis, corticosteroid-induced psychosis.

Lithium succinate, in a topical form, has been used for the treatment of genital herpes and seborrheic dermatitis.

CONTRAINDICATIONS

Cardiovascular or renal disease. Brain damage. Dehydration, sodium depletion, clients receiving diuretics. Lactation.

SPECIAL CONCERNS

Safety and efficacy have not been established for children less than 12 years of age. Use with caution in geriatric clients because lithium is more toxic to the CNS in these clients; also, geriatric clients are more likely to develop lithium-induced goiter and clinical hypothyroidism and are more likely to manifest excessive thirst and larger volumes of urine.

SIDE EFFECTS

Due to initial therapy: Fine hand tremor, polyuria, thirst, transient and mild nausea, general discomfort. The following side effects are dependent on the serum level of lithium.

CV: Arrhythmia, hypotension, ***peripheral circulatory collapse,*** bradycardia, sinus node dysfunction with ***severe bradycardia causing syncope***; reversible flattening, isoelectricity, or inversion of T waves. **CNS:** Blackout spells, epileptiform seizures, slurred speech, dizziness, vertigo, somnolence, psychomotor retardation, restlessness, sleepiness, confusion, stupor, ***coma,*** acute dystonia, startled response, hypertonicity, slowed intellectual functioning, hallucinations, poor memory, tics, cog wheel rigidity, tongue movements. Pseudotumor cerebri leading to increased intracranial pressure and papilledema; if undetected may cause enlargement of the blind spot, constriction of visual fields, and eventual blindness. Diffuse slowing of EEG; widening of frequency spectrum of EEG; disorganization of background rhythm of EEG. **GI:** Anorexia, N&V, diarrhea, dry mouth, gastritis, salivary gland swelling, abdominal pain, excessive salivation, flatulence, indigestion, incontinence of urine or feces, dysgeusia/taste distortion, salty taste, swollen lips, dental caries. **Dermatologic:** Drying and thinning of hair, anesthesia of skin, chronic folliculitis, xerosis cutis, alopecia, exacerbation of psoriasis, acne, angioedema. **Neuromuscular:** Tremor, muscle hyperirritability (fasciculations, twitching, clonic movements), ataxia, choreo-athetotic movements, hyperactive DTRs, polyarthralgia. **GU:** Albuminuria, oliguria, polyuria, glycosuria, decreased C_{CR}, symptoms of nephrogenic diabetes, impotence/sexual dysfunction. **Thyroid:** Euthyroid goiter or hypothyroidism, including myxedema, accompanied by lower T_3 and T_4. **Miscellaneous:** Fatigue, lethargy, dehydration, weight loss, transient scotomata, tightness in chest, hypercalcemia, hyperparathyroidism, thirst, swollen painful joints, fever.

The following symptoms are unrelated to lithium dosage. Transient EEG and ECG changes, leukocytosis, headache, diffuse nontoxic goiter with or without hypothyroidism, transient hyperglycemia, generalized pruritus with or without rash, cutaneous ulcers, albuminuria, worsening of organic brain syndrome, excessive weight gain, edematous swelling of ankles or wrists, thirst or polyuria (may resemble diabetes mellitus), metallic taste, symptoms similar to Raynaud's phenomenon.

LABORATORY TEST CONSIDERATIONS

False + urinary glucose test (Benedict's), ↑ serum glucose, creatinine kinase. False – or ↓ serum PBI, uric acid; ↑ TSH, I^{131} uptake; ↓ T_3, T4

OD OVERDOSE MANAGEMENT

Symptoms: Symptoms dependent on serum lithium levels. Levels less than 2 mEq/L: N&V, diarrhea, muscle weakness, drowsiness, loss of coordination.

Levels of 2–3 mEq/L: Agitation, ataxia, blackouts, blurred vision, choreoathetoid movements, confusion, dysarthria, fasciculations, giddiness, hyperreflexia, hypertonia, agitation or manic-like behavior, myoclonic twitching or movement of entire limbs, slurred speech, tinnitus, urinary or fecal incontinence, vertigo.

Levels over 3 mEq/L: Complex clinical picture involving multiple organs and organ systems. ***Arrhythmias, coma,*** hypotension, ***peripheral vascular collapse, seizures (focal and generalized),*** spasticity, stupor, twitching of muscle groups.

Treatment: Early symptoms are treated by decreasing the dose or stopping treatment for 24–48 hr:

- Use gastric lavage.
- Restore fluid and electrolyte balance (can use saline) and maintain kidney function.
- Increase lithium excretion by giving aminophylline, mannitol, or urea.
- Prevent infection. Maintain adequate respiration.
- Monitor thyroid function.
- Institute hemodialysis.

DRUG INTERACTIONS

Acetazolamide / ↓ Lithium effect by ↑ renal excretion
Bumetanide / ↑ Lithium toxicity R/T ↓ renal clearance
Carbamazepine / ↑ Risk of lithium toxicity
Diazepam / ↑ Risk of hypothermia
Ethacrynic acid / ↑ Lithium toxicity R/T ↓ renal clearance
Fluoxetine / ↑ Serum lithium levels
Furosemide / ↑ Lithium toxicity R/T ↓ renal clearance
Haloperidol / ↑ Risk of neurologic toxicity
Iodide salts / Additive effect to cause hypothyroidism
Mannitol / ↓ Lithium effect by ↑ renal excretion
Mazindol / ↑ Chance of lithium toxicity R/T ↑ serum levels
Methyldopa / ↑ Chance of neurotoxic effects with or without ↑ lithium serum levels
Neuromuscular blocking agents / Lithium ↑ neuromuscular blockade → severe respiratory depression and apnea
NSAIDs / ↓ Lithium renal clearance, possibly R/T inhibition of renal prostaglandin synthesis
Phenothiazines / ↓ Phenothiazine levels or ↑ lithium levels
Phenytoin / ↑ Risk of lithium toxicity
Probenecid / ↑ Risk of lithium toxicity R/T ↑ serum levels
Sibutramine / Additive serotonergic effectgs → possible serotonin syndrome
Sodium chloride / Excretion of lithium is proportional to amount of sodium chloride ingested; if client is on salt-free diet, may develop lithium toxicity since less lithium excreted
Sympathomimetics / ↓ Drug pressor effects
Theophyllines, including Aminophylline / ↓ Lithium effect R/T ↑ renal excretion
Thiazide diuretics, triamterene / ↑ Risk of lithium toxicity R/T ↓ renal clearance
Tricyclic antidepressants / ↑ TCA effects
Urea / ↓ Lithium effect by ↑ renal excretion
Urinary alkalinizers / ↓ Lithium effect by ↑ renal excretion
Verapamil / ↓ Lithium levels and toxicity

HOW SUPPLIED

Lithium carbonate: *Capsule:* 150 mg, 300 mg, 600 mg; *Tablet:* 300 mg; *Tablet, Extended Release:* 300 mg, 450 mg; **Lithium citrate:** *Syrup:* 300 mg/5 mL

DOSAGE

• CAPSULES, TABLETS, EXTENDED-RELEASE TABLETS, SYRUP

Acute mania.

Adults: Individualized and according to lithium serum level (not to exceed 1.4 mEq/L) and clinical response. **Usual initial:** 300–600 mg t.i.d. or 600–900 mg b.i.d. of slow-release form; **elderly and debilitated clients:** 0.6–1.2 g/day in three doses. **Maintenance:** 300 mg t.i.d.–q.i.d.

Administration of drug is discontinued when lithium serum level exceeds 1.2 mEq/L and resumed 24 hr after it has fallen below that level.

To reverse neutropenia.

300–1,000 mg/day (to achieve serum levels of 0.5–1.0 mEq/L) for 7–10 days.

Prophylaxis of cluster headaches.

600–900 mg/day.

NURSING CONSIDERATIONS

ADMINISTRATION/STORAGE

1. To prevent toxic serum levels, determine blood levels 1–2 times/week

during initiation of therapy, and monthly thereafter, on blood drawn 8–12 hr after dosage.
2. Full beneficial drug effects may not be noted for 6–10 days.

ASSESSMENT

1. Conduct a drug history; determine if taking other medications likely to interact i.e thiazide diuretics which may induce dehydration.
2. With arthritic conditions, document anti-inflammatory agent use.
3. Monitor thyroid function studies; assess for decreased function.
4. Document mental status; monitor CV function, chemistry, urinalysis, weight, and ECG.

CLIENT/FAMILY TEACHING

1. Take with food or immediately after meals. Avoid any caffeinated beverages/foods because these may aggravate mania.
2. Report persistent diarrhea; may need supplemental fluids or salt.
3. Maintain a constant level of salt intake to avoid fluctuations in lithium activity. Weight gain and edema may be related to sodium retention; report if excessive.
4. Drink 10–12 glasses of water each day; avoid dehydration (e.g., vigorous exercise, sunbathing, sauna) to prevent increased concentrations of lithium in urine.
5. Review goals of therapy, drug interactions/side effects. Report diarrhea, vomiting, drowsiness, muscular weakness, or lack of coordination.
6. Do not engage in physical activities that require alertness or physical coordination until drug effects are realized; may cause drowsiness.
7. Will take several weeks to realize a behavioral benefit from therapy.
8. Do not change brands of drug. Avoid all OTCs unless prescribed.
9. Lithium works well in the manic phase; concomitant antidepressant use may be necessary during depressive phases.
10. Transient acneiform eruptions, folliculitis, and altered sexual function in men may occur.
11. Carry name and telephone number of persons to contact if needed or if family members note behavioral changes or physical changes contrary to expectations. Carry ID, noting diagnosis and prescribed meds.

OUTCOMES/EVALUATE

- Stabilization of mood swings
- ↓ Symptoms of mania (↓ hyperactivity, ↓ sleeplessness, and improved judgment)
- Therapeutic serum drug levels (0.4–1.0 mEq/L)

Lomefloxacin hydrochloride

(**loh**-meh-**FLOX**-ah-sin)

PREGNANCY CATEGORY: C
CLASSIFICATION(S):
Antibiotic, fluoroquinolone
Rx: Maxaquin

SEE ALSO *FLUOROQUINOLONES*.

ACTION/KINETICS

Mean peak plasma levels: 4.2 mcg/mL after a 400-mg dose. The rate and extent of absorption are decreased if taken with food. **t½:** 8 hr. Metabolized in the liver with 65% excreted unchanged through the urine and 10% excreted unchanged in the feces.

USES

(1) Acute bacterial exacerbation of chronic bronchitis caused by *Haemophilus influenzae* or *Morazella catarrhalis.* (Not to be used for empiric treatment of acute bacterial exacerbation of chronic bronchitis due to *Streptococcus pneumoniae.* (2) Uncomplicated UTIs (cystitis) due to *Escherichia coli, Klebsiella pneumoniae, Proteus mirabilis,* or *Staphylococcus saprophyticus.* (3) Complicated UTIs due to *E. coli, K. pneumoniae, P. mirabilis, Pseudomonas aeruginosa, Citrobacter diversus,* or *Enterobacter cloacae.* (4) Preoperatively to decrease the incidence of UTIs 3–5 days and 3–4 weeks after surgery in clients undergoing transrectal prostate biopsy. (5)

Reduce the incidence of UTIs in the early postoperative period (3–5 days postsurgery). (6) Uncomplicated gonococcal infections.

CONTRAINDICATIONS

Use in minor urologic procedures for which prophylaxis is not indicated (e.g., simply cystoscopy, retrograde pyelography). Use for the empiric treatment of acute bacterial exacerbation of chronic bronchitis due to *Streptococcus pneumoniae*. Lactation.

SPECIAL CONCERNS

Plasma clearance is reduced in the elderly. Safety and efficacy have not been determined in children less than 18 years of age. Serious hypersensitivity reactions that are occasionally fatal have occurred, even with the first dose. No dosage adjustment is needed for elderly clients with normal renal function. Not efficiently removed from the body by hemodialysis or peritoneal dialysis.

ADDITIONAL SIDE EFFECTS

CNS: Confusion, tremor, vertigo, nervousness, anxiety, hyperkinesia, anorexia, agitation, increased appetite, depersonalization, paranoia, ***coma***. **GI:** GI inflammation or bleeding, dysphagia, tongue discoloration, bad taste in mouth. **GU:** Dysuria, hematuria, micturition disorder, anuria, strangury, leukorrhea, intermenstrual bleeding perineal pain, vaginal moniliasis, orchitis, epididymitis, proteinuria, albuminuria. **Hypersensitivity Reactions:** Urticaria, itching, pharyngeal or facial edema, ***CV collapse,*** tingling, loss of consciousness, dyspnea. **CV:** Hypotension, tachycardia, bradycardia, extrasystoles, cyanosis, ***arrhythmia, cardiac failure,*** angina pectoris, ***MI, pulmonary embolism, cardiomyopathy,*** phlebitis, cerebrovascular disorder. **Respiratory:** Dyspnea, respiratory infection, epistaxis, ***bronchospasm,*** cough, increased sputum, respiratory disorder, stridor. **Hematologic:** Eosinophilia, leukopenia, increase or decrease in platelets, increase in ESR, lymphocytopenia, decreased hemoglobin, anemia, bleeding, increased PT, increase in monocytes. **Dermatologic:** Urticaria, eczema, skin exfoliation, skin disorder. **Ophthalmologic:** Conjunctivitis, eye pain. **Otic:** Earache, tinnitus. **Musculoskeletal:** Back or chest pain, asthenia, leg cramps, arthralgia, myalgia. **Miscellaneous:** Increase or decrease in blood glucose, flushing, increased sweating, facial edema, influenza-like symptoms, decreased heat tolerance, purpura, lymphadenopathy, increased fibrinolysis, thirst, gout, hypoglycemia, phototoxicity.

LABORATORY TEST CONSIDERATIONS

↑ ALT, AST, alkaline phosphatase, bilirubin, BUN, gamma-glutamyltransferase. ↑ or ↓ Potassium. Abnormalities of urine specific gravity or serum electrolytes.

HOW SUPPLIED

Tablet: 400 mg

DOSAGE

• TABLETS

Acute bacterial exacerbation of chronic bronchitis. Uncomplicated cystitis.

Adults: 400 mg once daily for 10 days.

Complicated UTIs.

Adults: 400 mg once daily for 14 days.

Uncomplicated cystitis in females due to E. coli.

400 mg once daily for 3 days.

Prophylaxis of infection before surgery for transurethral procedures.

Single 400-mg dose 2–6 hr before surgery.

Transrectal prostate biopsy.

Single 400 mg dose 1–6 hr prior to the procedure.

Uncomplicated gonococcal infections.

Single 400 mg dose (as an alternative to ciprofloxacin or ofloxacin).

NURSING CONSIDERATIONS

SEE ALSO *GENERAL NURSING CONSIDERATIONS* FOR *ANTI-INFECTIVES* AND *FLUOROQUINOLONES*.

ADMINISTRATION/STORAGE

1. May take without regard for meals.
2. Dosage modification is required for clients with C_{CR} less than 40 mL/min/1.73 m^2 and more than 10 mL/min/1.73 m^2. Following an initial loading dose of 40 mg, give daily maintenance doses of 200 mg for the duration of treatment. Assess lomefloxacin levels to determine any need to alter

dosing interval. Follow this same regimen for clients on hemodialysis.

ASSESSMENT

1. Note indications for therapy, type and characteristics of symptoms.
2. Obtain cultures and renal function studies; modify dosage with renal dysfunction.

CLIENT/FAMILY TEACHING

1. May take without regard to food. Increase fluid intake to 2L/day.
2. Avoid antacids for 2h surrounding drug dose.
3. May experience dizziness and lightheadedness; use caution until drug effects realized.
4. Avoid prolonged sunlight exposure; may experience photosensitivity.
5. Report any rash, severe GI upset, diarrhea, weakness, tremors, visual changes or seizures.

OUTCOMES/EVALUATE

- Prostate/bladder/UTI prophylaxis
- Resolution of infective organism

Lomustine

(loh-**MUS**-teen)

PREGNANCY CATEGORY: D
CLASSIFICATION(S):
Antineoplastic, alkylating
Rx: CeeNu (Abbreviation: CCNU)

SEE ALSO *ANTINEOPLASTIC AGENTS* AND *ALKYLATING AGENTS*.

ACTION/KINETICS

Alkylating agent that inhibits DNA and RNA synthesis through DNA alkylation. It also affects other cellular processes, including RNA, protein synthesis and the processing of ribosomal and nucleoplasmic messenger RNA; DNA base component structure; the rate of DNA synthesis and DNA polymerase activity. Is cell cycle nonspecific. Rapidly absorbed from the GI tract; crosses the blood-brain barrier resulting in concentrations higher than in plasma. **Peak plasma level:** 1–6 hr; **t½:** biphasic; **initial,** 6 hr; **postdistribution:** 1–2 days. From 15% to 20% of drug remains in body after 5 days. Fifty percent of drug excreted within 12 hr through the kidney, 75% within 4 days. Small amounts are excreted through the lungs and feces. Metabolites present in milk.

USES

(1) Used alone or in combination to treat primary and metastatic brain tumors. (2) Secondary therapy in Hodgkin's disease (in combination with other antineoplastics).

CONTRAINDICATIONS

Lactation.

ADDITIONAL SIDE EFFECTS

High incidence of N&V 3–6 hr after administration and lasting for 24 hr. Renal and pulmonary toxicity. Dysarthria. Delayed bone marrow suppression may occur due to cumulative bone marrow toxicity. ***Thrombocytopenia and leukopenia may lead to bleeding and overwhelming infections.*** Secondary malignancies.

LABORATORY TEST CONSIDERATIONS

↑ LFTs (reversible).

HOW SUPPLIED

Capsule: 10 mg, 40 mg, 100 mg; *Dose Pack:* 2-100 mg capsules, 2-40 mg capsules, and 2-10 mg capsules

DOSAGE

- **CAPSULES**

Adults and children, initial: 130 mg/m² as a single dose q 6 weeks. If bone marrow function is reduced, decrease dose to 100 mg/m² q 6 weeks. Subsequent dosage based on blood counts of clients (platelet count above 100,000/mm³ and leukocyte count above 4,000/mm³). Undertake weekly blood tests and do not repeat therapy before 6 weeks.

NURSING CONSIDERATIONS

SEE ALSO *NURSING CONSIDERATIONS FOR ANTINEOPLASTIC AGENTS*.

ADMINISTRATION/STORAGE

1. Store below 40°C (104°F).
2. Given alone or in combination with other drugs, surgery, or XRT.
3. Causes platelet and leukocyte suppression. Nadir: 3–7 weeks.

CLIENT/FAMILY TEACHING

1. Medication comes in capsules of three strengths and a combination of capsules will make up the correct dose; take all at one time.
2. May have N&V up to 36 hr after treatment; may be followed by 2–3 days of anorexia. Take antiemetics as prescribed. GI distress may be reduced by taking antiemetics before drug administration or by taking the drug after fasting.
3. Report feelings of depression caused by prolonged N&V so that various antiemetics can be tried and to ensure that psychological support is available as needed.
4. Report abnormal bruising or bleeding, sore throat or flu S&S.
5. Avoid all OTC agents.
6. 6 week intervals are needed between doses for optimum effect with minimal toxicity; hematologic profiles should be assessed weekly.

OUTCOMES/EVALUATE

Control/remission of metastatic processes

Loperamide hydrochloride

(loh-**PER**-ah-myd)

PREGNANCY CATEGORY: B
CLASSIFICATION(S):
Antidiarrheal
Rx: Imodium
OTC: Diar-aid Caplets, Imodium A-D Caplets, Kaopectate II Caplets, Maalox Anti-Diarrheal Caplets, Neo-Diaral, Pepto Diarrhea Control
✱**OTC:** Apo-Loperamide, Diarr-Eze, Loperacap, Novo-Loperamide, PMS-Loperamide Hydrochloride, Rho-Loperamide, Riva-Loperamide

ACTION/KINETICS

Slows intestinal motility by acting on the nerve endings and/or intramural ganglia embedded in the intestinal wall. The prolonged retention of the feces in the intestine results in reducing the volume of the stools, increasing viscosity, and decreasing fluid and electrolyte loss. Reportedly more effective than diphenoxylate. **Time to peak effect, capsules:** 5 hr; **PO solution:** 2.5 hr. **t½:** 9.1–14.4 hr. Twenty-five percent excreted unchanged in the feces.

USES

Rx: (1) Symptomatic relief of acute nonspecific diarrhea and of chronic diarrhea associated with inflammatory bowel disease. (2) Decrease the volume of discharge from ileostomies.

OTC: Control symptoms of diarrhea, including traveler's diarrhea. *Investigational:* With trimethoprim-sulfamethoxazole to treat traveler's diarrhea.

CONTRAINDICATIONS

In clients in whom constipation should be avoided. OTC if body temperature is over 101°F (38°C) and in presence of bloody diarrhea. Use in acute diarrhea associated with organisms that penetrate the intestinal mucosa, such as *E. coli, Salmonella,* and Shigella.

SPECIAL CONCERNS

Safe use in children under 2 years of age and during lactation has not been established. Fluid and electrolyte depletion may occur in clients with diarrhea. Children less than 3 years of age are more sensitive to the narcotic effects of loperamide.

SIDE EFFECTS

GI: Abdominal pain, distention, or discomfort. Constipation, dry mouth, N&V, epigastric distress. Toxic megacolon in clients with acute colitis. **CNS:** Drowsiness, dizziness, fatigue. **Other:** Allergic skin rashes.

OD OVERDOSE MANAGEMENT

Symptoms: Constipation, CNS depression, GI irritation. *Treatment:* Give activated charcoal (it will reduce absorption up to ninefold). If vomiting has not occurred, perform gastric lavage followed by activated charcoal, 100 g, through a gastric tube. Give naloxone for respiratory depression.

HOW SUPPLIED

Capsule: 2 mg; *Liquid:* 1 mg/1 mL, 1 mg/5 mL; *Tablet:* 2 mg

DOSAGE

• RX CAPSULES, LIQUID

Acute diarrhea.

Adults, initial: 4 mg, followed by 2 mg after each unformed stool, up to maximum of 16 mg/day. **Pediatric:** *Day 1 doses:* **8–12 years:** 2 mg t.i.d.; **6–8 years:** 2 mg b.i.d.; **2–5 years:** 1 mg t.i.d. using only the liquid. *After day 1:* 1 mg/10 kg after a loose stool (total daily dosage should not exceed day 1 recommended doses).

Chronic diarrhea.

Adults: 4–8 mg/day as a single or divided dose. Dosage not established for chronic diarrhea in children.

- **OTC ORAL SOLUTION, TABLETS**

Acute diarrhea.

Adults: 4 mg after the first loose bowel movement followed by 2 mg after each subsequent bowel movement to a maximum of 8 mg/day for no more than 2 days. **Pediatric, 9–11 years:** 2 mg after the first loose bowel movement followed by 1 mg after each subsequent loose bowel movement, not to exceed 6 mg/day for no more than 2 days. **Pediatric, 6–8 years:** 1 mg after the first bowel movement followed by 1 mg after each subsequent loose bowel movement, not to exceed 4 mg/day for no more than 2 days.

NURSING CONSIDERATIONS

ASSESSMENT

1. Note any allergy to piperidine derivatives.
2. Document indications for therapy, onset, frequency, and characteristics of symptoms. Identify any contributing causative factors.
3. Discontinue drug promptly and report if abdominal distention develops in clients with acute ulcerative colitis.

CLIENT/FAMILY TEACHING

1. May cause a dry mouth; try ice, sugarless gum, and candy to alleviate.
2. Use caution while driving or performing tasks requiring alertness; may cause dizziness/drowsiness.
3. OTC products are not intended for use in children less than 6 years of age unless physician prescribed.
4. Record the number, frequency, and consistency of stools per day and the amount of medication consumed. Report if diarrhea lasts up to 5 days without relief.
5. In *acute diarrhea,* discontinue after 48 hr and report if ineffective.
6. If no improvement within 10 days after using up to 16 mg/day for *chronic diarrhea,* symptoms are not likely to improve with further use. Seek medical intervention.
7. Report if fever, nausea, abdominal pain, or abdominal distention occurs; may require dosage adjustment.
8. Dietary treatment of diarrhea is preferred, if possible, in children (avoid apple juices, high-fat and highly spiced foods).

OUTCOMES/EVALUATE

↓ Diarrhea

Loracarbef

(**lor**-ah-**KAR**-bef)

PREGNANCY CATEGORY: B
CLASSIFICATION(S):
Antibiotic, beta-lactam
Rx: Lorabid

SEE ALSO *ANTI-INFECTIVES.*

ACTION/KINETICS

Related chemically to cephalosporins. Acts by inhibiting cell wall synthesis. Stable in the presence of certain bacterial beta-lactamases. **Average peak plasma levels:** 8 mcg/mL following a single 200-mg dose in a fasting subject after 90 min and 14 mcg/mL following a single 400-mg dose in a fasting subject after 90 min. Following doses of 7.5 mg/kg and 15 mg/kg of the oral suspension to children, average peak plasma levels were 13 and 19 mcg/mL, respectively, within 40–60 min. **Elimination t½:** 1 hr (increased to 5.6 hr in clients with a C_{CR} from 10 to 50 mL/min/1.73 m² and to 32 hr in clients with a C_{CR} of less than 10 mL/min/1.73 m²). Over 90% excreted unchanged in the urine.

USES

(1) Secondary bacterial infections of acute bronchitis and acute bacterial exacerbations of chronic bronchitis caused by *Streptococcus pneumoniae, Haemophilus influenzae,* or *Morazella*

catarrhalis (including beta-lactamase-producing strains of both organisms). (2) Pneumonia caused by *S. pneumoniae* or *H. influenzae* (only non-beta-lactamase-producing strains). (3) Otitis media caused by *S. pneumoniae, Streptococcus pyogenes, H. influenzae,* or *M. catarrhalis* (including beta-lactamase-producing strains of both organisms). (4) Acute maxillary sinusitis caused by *S. pneumoniae, H. influenzae* (only non-beta-lactamase-producing strains), or *M. catarrhalis* (including beta-lactamase-producing strains). (5) Pharyngitis and tonsillitis caused by *S. pyogenes.* (6) Uncomplicated skin and skin structure infections caused by *Staphylococcus aureus* (including penicillinase-producing strains) or *S. pyogenes.* (7) Uncomplicated UTIs caused by *Escherichia coli* or *Staphylococcus saprophyticus.* Uncomplicated pyelonephritis caused by *E. coli.*

CONTRAINDICATIONS

Hypersensitivity to loracarbef or cephalosporin-class antibiotics.

SPECIAL CONCERNS

Use during labor and delivery only if clearly needed. Pseudomembranous colitis is possible with most antibacterial agents. Use with caution and at reduced dosage in clients with impaired renal function, in those with a history of colitis, in clients receiving concurrent treatment with potent diuretics, during lactation, and in clients with known penicillin allergies. Safety and efficacy in children less than 6 months of age have not been determined.

SIDE EFFECTS

The incidence of certain side effects is different in the pediatric population compared with the adult population. **GI:** Diarrhea, N&V, abdominal pain, anorexia, pseudomembranous colitis. **Hypersensitivity:** Skin rashes, urticaria, pruritus, erythema multiforme. **CNS:** Headache, somnolence, nervousness, insomnia, dizziness. **Hematologic:** Transient thrombocytopenia, leukopenia, eosinophilia. **Miscellaneous:** Vasodilation, vaginitis, vaginal moniliasis, rhinitis.

OD OVERDOSE MANAGEMENT

Symptoms: N&V, epigastric distress, diarrhea. *Treatment:* Hemodialysis may be effective in increasing the elimination of loracarbef from plasma from clients with chronic renal failure.

DRUG INTERACTIONS

Diuretics, potent / ↑ Risk of renal dysfunction

Probenecid / ↓ Renal excretion → ↑ plasma loracarbef levels

HOW SUPPLIED

Capsule: 200 mg, 400 mg; *Powder for Oral Suspension:* 100 mg/5 mL, 200 mg/5 mL

DOSAGE

• CAPSULES, ORAL SUSPENSION

Secondary bacterial infection of acute bronchitis.

Adults 13 years of age and older: 200–400 mg q 12 hr for 7 days.

Acute bacterial exacerbation of chronic bronchitis.

Adults 13 years of age and older: 400 mg q 12 hr for 7 days.

Pneumonia.

Adults 13 years of age and older: 400 q 12 hr for 14 days.

Pharyngitis, tonsillitis.

Adults 13 years of age and older: 200 mg q 12 hr for 10 days (longer for *S. pyogenes* infections). **Infants and children, 6 months–12 years:** 15 mg/kg/day in divided doses q 12 hr for 10 days (longer for *S. pyogenes* infections).

Sinusitis.

Adults 13 years of age and older: 400 mg q 12 hr for 10 days.

Acute otitis media, Acute maxillary sinusitis.

Infants and children, 6 months–12 years: 30 mg/kg/day in divided doses q 12 hr for 10 days. Use the suspension as it is more rapidly absorbed than the capsules, resulting in higher peak plasma levels when given at the same dose.

Skin and skin structure infections (impetigo).

Adults: 200 mg q 12 hr for 7 days. **Infants and children, 6 months–12 years:** 15 mg/kg/day in divided doses q 12 hr for 7 days.

Uncomplicated cystitis.

Adults 13 years of age and older: 200 mg q 24 hr for 7 days.

Uncomplicated pyelonephritis.
Adults 13 years of age and older: 400 mg q 12 hr for 14 days.

NURSING CONSIDERATIONS

SEE ALSO *GENERAL NURSING CONSIDERATIONS* FOR *ANTI-INFECTIVES*.

ADMINISTRATION/STORAGE

1. The manufacturer provides a chart to assist with establishing the dosage regimen for pediatric clients.
2. Clients with C_{CR} levels of 10–49 mL/min may be given one-half the recommended dose at the usual dosage interval. Clients with C_{CR} less than 10 mL/min may be treated with the recommended dose given every 3–5 days. Clients on hemodialysis should receive another dose following dialysis.
3. Reconstitute the oral suspension by adding 30 mL water to the 50-mL bottle or 60 mL water to the 100-mL bottle. After mixing, the suspension may be kept at room temperature for 14 days without significant loss of potency. Keep tightly closed and discard any unused portion after 14 days.

ASSESSMENT

1. Note indications for therapy and any sensitivity to cephalosporins and penicillin derivatives.
2. List drugs currently prescribed to ensure none interact unfavorably.
3. Obtain baseline cultures and renal function studies. Adjust dosage with dysfunction.

CLIENT/FAMILY TEACHING

1. Take at least 1 hr before or at least 2 hr after meals. Complete entire prescription.
2. Report persistent diarrhea, which may be secondary to pseudomembranous colitis and requires medical intervention.
3. Lack of response or worsening of symptoms as well as any unusual side effects (rash, allergic reaction) should be reported.

OUTCOMES/EVALUATE

- Negative C&S reports
- Relief of ear/throat pain
- Improved breathing patterns
- Evidence of wound healing

Loratidine

(loh-**RAH**-tih-deen)

PREGNANCY CATEGORY: B
CLASSIFICATION(S):
Antihistamine, second generation, piperidine
Rx: Claritin, Claritin Reditabs

SEE ALSO *ANTIHISTAMINES*.

ACTION/KINETICS

Metabolized in the liver to active metabolite descarboethoxyloratidine. Low to no sedative and anticholinergic effects. Does not alter cardiac repolarization and has not been linked to development of torsades de pointes as seen with astemizole and terfenadine. **Onset:** 1–3 hr. **Maximum effect:** 8–12 hr. Food delays absorption. **t½, loratidine:** 8.4 hr; **t½, descarboethoxyloratidine:** 28 hr. **Duration:** 24 hr. Excreted through both the urine and feces.

USES

Relief of nasal and nonnasal symptoms of seasonal allergic rhinitis, including runny nose, itchy and watery eyes, itchy palate, and sneezing and treatment of chronic idiopathic urticaria in clients 2 years of age and older.

SPECIAL CONCERNS

Use with caution, if at all, during lactation. Give a lower initial dose in liver impairment. Safety and efficacy have not been determined in children less than 2 years of age.

SIDE EFFECTS

Most commonly, headache, somnolence, fatigue, and dry mouth. **GI:** Altered salivation, gastritis, dyspepsia, stomatitis, tooth ache, thirst, altered taste, flatulence. **CNS:** Hypoesthesia, hyperkinesia, migraine, anxiety, depression, agitation, paroniria, amnesia, impaired concentration. **Ophthalmologic:** Altered lacrimation, conjunctivitis, blurred vision, eye pain, blepharospasm. **Respiratory:** URI, epistaxis, pharyngitis, dyspnea, coughing, rhinitis, sinusitis, sneezing, bronchitis, ***bronchospasm,*** hemoptysis,

L

laryngitis. **Body as a whole:** Asthenia, increased sweating, flushing, malaise, rigors, fever, dry skin, aggravated allergy, pruritus, purpura. **Musculoskeletal:** Back/chest pain, leg cramps, arthralgia, myalgia. **GU:** Breast pain, menorrhagia, dysmenorrhea, vaginitis. **Miscellaneous:** Earache, dysphonia, dry hair, urinary discoloration.

HOW SUPPLIED

Syrup: 1 mg/mL; *Tablet:* 10 mg; *Tablet, Rapidly Disintegrating:* 10 mg

DOSAGE

• SYRUP, TABLETS

Allergic rhinitis, chronic idiopathic urticaria.

Adults and children, 6 and older: 10 mg once daily. **Children, 2–5 years of age:** 5 mg syrup once daily. *In clients with impaired liver function (GFR less than 30 mL/min):* **Adults and children 6 years and older:** 10 mg every other day initially. **Children, 2–5 years:** 5 mg every other day initially.

L

NURSING CONSIDERATIONS

SEE ALSO *NURSING CONSIDERATIONS* FOR *ANTIHISTAMINES.*

ADMINISTRATION/STORAGE

1. Use the syrup or rapid-distintegrating tablets for children 6 to 11 years of age.
2. Use caution. The concentration of the syrup is 10 mg/10 mL.

ASSESSMENT

1. Document indications for therapy, type, onset, and characteristics of symptoms. List other agents trialed and the outcome.
2. Monitor LFTs; reduce dose with dysfunction. Assess the elderly and clients with hepatic and renal impairment for increasing somnolence.
3. Document pulmonary findings; assess throat, cervical nodes, turbinates and skin testing when necessary.
4. Identify triggers that may contribute to allergic symptoms. Advise to remove carpet, enclose mattress and pillows in plastic, control dust, and remove pets and plants from sleeping area.
5. Review drug profile. Cautiously coadminister with drugs that inhibit hepatic metabolism (i.e., macrolide antibiotics, cimetidine, ranitidine, ketoconazole, or theophylline).

CLIENT/FAMILY TEACHING

1. Take on an empty stomach; food may delay absorption.
2. If using rapid-disintegrating tablets, place under the tongue. Disintegration occurs within seconds, after which the tablet contents may be swallowed with or without water.
3. Use rapid-disintegrating tablets within 6 months of opening the foil pouch and immediately after opening the individual tablet blister.
4. Do not perform activities that require mental alertness until drug effects realized; should not cause drowsiness.
5. Identify triggers, i.e., foods, detergents, or materials that may have induced urticarial response.

OUTCOMES/EVALUATE

- Relief of nasal congestion and seasonal allergic manifestations
- Control of skin eruption R/T antigenic offender

Lorazepam

(lor-**AYZ**-eh-pam)

PREGNANCY CATEGORY: D

CLASSIFICATION(S):

Antianxiety drug, benzodiazepine

Rx: Lorazepam Intensol, Ativan **C-IV**

✱Rx: Apo-Lorazepam, Novo-Lorazem, Nu-Loraz, Riva-Lorazepam

SEE ALSO *TRANQUILIZERS, ANTIMANIC DRUGS, AND HYPNOTICS.*

ACTION/KINETICS

Absorbed and eliminated faster than other benzodiazepines. **Peak plasma levels: PO,** 1–6 hr; **IM,** 1–1.5 hr. **$t^1/_2$:** 10–20 hr. Metabolized to inactive compounds, which are excreted through the kidneys.

USES

PO: Anxiety, tension, anxiety with depression, insomnia, acute alcohol withdrawal symptoms. **Parenteral:** Amnesic agent, anticonvulsant, antitremor drug, adjunct to skeletal muscle relaxants, preanesthetic medication, adjunct prior to endoscopic procedures, treatment of status epilepticus, relief of acute alcohol withdrawal symptoms. *Investigational:* Antiemetic in cancer chemotherapy.

ADDITIONAL CONTRAINDICATIONS

Narrow-angle glaucoma. Parenterally in children less than 18 years.

SPECIAL CONCERNS

PO dosage has not been established in children less than 12 years of age and IV dosage has not been established in children less than 18 years of age. Use cautiously in presence of renal and hepatic disease.

ADDITIONAL DRUG INTERACTIONS

With parenteral lorazepam, scopolamine → sedation, hallucinations, and behavioral abnormalities.

HOW SUPPLIED

Concentrate, Oral Solution: 2 mg/mL; *Injection:* 2 mg/mL, 4 mg/mL; *Tablet:* 0.5 mg, 1 mg, 2 mg

DOSAGE

- **TABLETS, CONCENTRATE**

Anxiety.

Adults: 1–3 mg b.i.d.–t.i.d.

Hypnotic.

Adults: 2–4 mg at bedtime. **Geriatric/debilitated clients, initial:** 0.5–2 mg/day in divided doses. Dose can be adjusted as required.

- **IM**

Preoperatively.

Adults: 0.05 mg/kg up to maximum of 4 mg 2 hr before surgery for maximum amnesic effect.

- **IV**

Preoperatively.

Adults, initial: 0.044 mg/kg or a total dose of 2 mg, whichever is less.

Amnesic effect.

Adults: 0.05 mg/kg up to a maximum of 4 mg administered 15–20 min prior to surgery.

Antiemetic in cancer chemotherapy.

Initial: 2 mg 30 min before beginning chemotherapy; **then,** 2 mg q 4 hr as needed.

NURSING CONSIDERATIONS

SEE ALSO *NURSING CONSIDERATIONS FOR TRANQUILIZERS, ANTIMANIC DRUGS, AND HYPNOTICS.*

ADMINISTRATION/STORAGE

1. If higher doses are required, increase the evening dose before the daytime doses.

IV 2. For IV use, dilute just before use with equal amounts of either sterile water, NaCl, or 5% dextrose injection.

3. Do not exceed 2 mg/min IV.

4. Do not use if solution is discolored or contains a precipitate.

ASSESSMENT

1. Document indications for therapy, onset, and characteristics of symptoms. Assess mental status; describe characteristics of anxiety, any associated factors/triggers.

2. List other agents used to treat this condition and the outcome.

3. Determine if psychological evaluation/counselling has been initiated.

CLIENT/FAMILY TEACHING

1. Take only as directed; report loss of effectiveness and do not share.

2. Drug may cause dizziness and drowsiness; use with caution until drug effects realized.

3. Report any increased depression or suicidal ideations.

4. Avoid alcohol and any other CNS depressants.

5. With long-term therapy, do not stop suddenly; must be tapered to prevent withdrawal symptoms.

OUTCOMES/EVALUATE

- ↓ Levels of anxiety, tension, and depression
- Control of alcohol withdrawal
- Muscle relaxation/amnesia

Losartan potassium

(loh-**SAR**-tan)

PREGNANCY CATEGORY: C (FIRST TRIMESTER), D (SECOND AND THIRD TRIMESTERS)

CLASSIFICATION(S):

Antihypertensive, angiotensin II receptor blocker

Rx: Cozaar

SEE ALSO *ANGTIOTENSIN II RECEPTOR ANTAGONISTS AND ANTIHYPERTENSIVE AGENTS.*

L

ACTION/KINETICS
Undergoes significant first-pass metabolism in the liver, where it is converted to an active carboxylic acid metabolite that is responsible for most of the angiotensin receptor blockade. Rapidly absorbed after PO administration, although food slows absorption. **Peak plasma levels of losartan and metabolite:** 1 hr and 3–4 hr, respectively. When used alone, decease in BP in blacks was less than in non-blacks. **t½, losartan:** 2 hr; **t½, metabolite:** 6–9 hr. The drug and metabolite are highly bound to plasma proteins. **Maximum effects:** 1 week (3 to 6 weeks in some clients). Drug and metabolites are excreted through both the urine (35%) and feces (60%).

USES
Antihypertensive, alone or in combination with other antihypertensive drugs.

SPECIAL CONCERNS
In severe CHF there is a risk of oliguria and/or progressive azotemia with acute renal failure and/or death (which are rare). In those with unilateral or bilateral renal artery stenosis, there is a risk of increased serum creatinine or BUN. Lower doses are recommended in those with hepatic insufficiency.

SIDE EFFECTS
GI: Diarrhea, dyspepsia, anorexia, constipation, dental pain, dry mouth, flatulence, gastritis, vomiting, taste perversion. **CV:** Angina pectoris, second-degree AV block, ***CVA, MI, ventricular tachycardia, ventricular fibrillation,*** hypotension, palpitation, sinus bradycardia, tachycardia, orthostatic effects. **CNS:** Dizziness, insomnia, anxiety, anxiety disorder, ataxia, confusion, depression, abnormal dreams, hypesthesia, decreased libido, impaired memory, migraine, nervousness, paresthesia, peripheral neuropathy, panic disorder, sleep disorder, somnolence, tremor, vertigo. **Respiratory:** URI, cough, nasal congestion, sinus disorder, sinusitis, dyspnea, bronchitis, pharyngeal discomfort, epistaxis, rhinitis, respiratory congestion. **Musculoskeletal:** Muscle cramps, myalgia, joint swelling, musculoskeletal pain, stiffness, arthralgia, arthritis, fibromyalgia, muscle weakness; pain in the back, legs, arms, hips, knees, shoulders. **Dermatologic:** Alopecia, dermatitis, dry skin, ecchymosis, erythema, flushing, photosensitivity, pruritus, rash, sweating, urticaria. **GU:** Impotence, nocturia, urinary frequency, UTI. **Ophthalmologic:** Blurred vision, burning/stinging in the eye, conjunctivitis, decrease in visual acuity. **Miscellaneous:** Gout, anemia, tinnitus, facial edema, fever, syncope.

LABORATORY TEST CONSIDERATIONS
Minor ↑ BUN, serum creatinine. Occasional ↑ liver enzymes and/or serum bilirubin. Small ↓ H&H.

OD OVERDOSE MANAGEMENT
Symptoms: Hypotension, tachycardia, bradycardia (due to vagal stimulation). *Treatment:* Supportive treatment. Hemodialysis is not indicated.

DRUG INTERACTIONS
Grapefruit juice / ↓ Liver metabolism of losartan to its active form
Indomethacin / ↓ Antihypertensive effect of losartan
Phenobarbital / ↓ Plasma losartan levels (20%)

HOW SUPPLIED
Tablet: 25 mg, 50 mg, 100 mg

DOSAGE

• TABLETS

Hypertension.

Adults: 50 mg once daily with or without food. Total daily doses range from 25 to 100 mg. In those with possible depletion of intravascular volume (e.g., clients treated with a diuretic), use 25 mg once daily. If the antihypertensive effect (measured at trough) is inadequate, a twice-a-day regimen, using the same dose, may be tried; or an increase in dose may give a more satisfactory result. If BP is not controlled by losartan alone, a diuretic (e.g., hydrochlorothiazide) may be added.

NURSING CONSIDERATIONS

SEE ALSO *NURSING CONSIDERATIONS FOR ANGIOTENSIN II RECEPTOR ANTAGONISTS* AND *ANTIHYPERTENSIVE AGENTS*.

ADMINISTRATION/STORAGE
May be given with other antihypertensive drugs.

ASSESSMENT
1. Document indications for therapy, onset, other agents used and outcome.
2. Monitor CBC, renal and LFTs. Correct any volume depletion prior to using to prevent sympathomimetic hypotension. Reduce starting dose with volume depletion or hepatic impairment. Observe for S&S of fluid or electrolyte imbalance.

CLIENT/FAMILY TEACHING
1. Take only as directed with or without food.
2. Regular exercise, proper low-salt diet, and life-style changes (i.e., no smoking, low alcohol, low-fat diet, low stress, adequate rest) may also contribute to enhanced BP control.
3. Do not change positions suddenly, dangle before rising, and rest until symptoms subside to prevent postural symptoms.
4. Avoid any OTC agents.
5. May cause photosensitivity reaction; use precautions.
6. Use effective contraception; report immediately if pregnancy is suspected because drug during second and third trimesters is associated with fetal injury and morbidity.

OUTCOMES/EVALUATE
Decreased BP

Loteprednol etabonate

(**loh**-teh-**PRED**-nohl)

PREGNANCY CATEGORY: C
CLASSIFICATION(S):
Glucocorticoid
Rx: Alrex, Lotemax

SEE ALSO ***CORTICOSTEROIDS***.

ACTION/KINETICS
Rapidly metabolized to inactive compounds by eye esterases. After ocular use, minimal amounts are absorbed.

USES
0.2% Suspension: Seasonal allergic conjunctivitis. **0.5% Suspension:** (1) Steroid-responsive inflammatory conditions of the conjunctiva, cornea, and anterior segment of the globe (e.g., allergic conjunctivitis, superficial punctate keratitis, herpes zoster keratitis, acne rosacea, iritis) cyclitis, certain infective conjunctivitis. (2) Treatment of postoperative inflammation after ocular surgery.

CONTRAINDICATIONS
Bacterial, fungal, or viral eye infection.

SPECIAL CONCERNS
Use with caution with cataracts, diabetes mellitus, glaucoma, intraocular hypertension, use beyond 10 days. Safety and efficacy have not been determined in children.

SIDE EFFECTS
Ophthalmic: Increased IOP, thinning of sclera or cornea, blurred vision, discharge, dry eyes, burning on instillation.

HOW SUPPLIED
Ophthalmic Suspension: 0.2%, 0.5%

DOSAGE
- **SUSPENSION, 0.2%**

Seasonal allergic conjunctivitis.
1 gtt in the affected eye(s) q.i.d.

- **SUSPENSION, 0.5%**

Steroid-responsive disease.
1–2 gtt into the conjunctival sac of the affected eye q.i.d. For the first week, dose may be increased to 1 gtt every hour.

Postoperative inflammation.
1–2 gtt into the conjunctival sac of the operated eye(s) q.i.d. beginning 24 hr after surgery and continuing for 2 weeks.

NURSING CONSIDERATIONS
SEE ALSO ***NURSING CONSIDERATIONS*** FOR ***CORTICOSTEROIDS***.

ADMINISTRATION/STORAGE
Re-evaluate if symptoms do not improve after 2 days of treatment.

ASSESSMENT
Note indications for therapy, symptoms, and related factors (triggers).

CLIENT/FAMILY TEACHING

1. Shake well before use. Instill as directed.
2. Contact lenses may continue to be worn if the drug is used to treat lens-associated giant papillary conjunctivitis. Remove lens prior to each instillation; reinsert 10–15 min later.
3. Report if symptoms do not improve after 2 days of treatment.
4. When used for steroid responsive disease, do *not* discontinue therapy prematurely.

OUTCOMES/EVALUATE

↓ Eye irritation, inflammation, and allergic S&S

Lovastatin (Mevinolin)

(**LOW**-vah-**STAT**-in, me-**VIN**-oh-lin)

L

PREGNANCY CATEGORY: X
CLASSIFICATION(S):
Antihyperlipidemic, HMG-CoA reductase inhibitor
Rx: Mevacor
🍁**Rx:** Apo-Lovastatin

SEE ALSO ANTIHYPERLIPIDEMIC AGENTS—HMG-COA REDUCTASE INHIBITORS.

ACTION/KINETICS

Isolated from a strain of *Aspergillus terreus.* Approximately 35% of a dose is absorbed. Extensive first-pass effect—less than 5% reaches the general circulation. Absorption is decreased by about one-third if the drug is given on an empty stomach rather than with food. **Onset:** within 2 weeks using multiple doses. **Time to peak plasma levels:** 2–4 hr. **Time to peak effect:** 4–6 weeks using multiple doses. **t½, elimination:** 1.1–1.7 hr. **Duration:** 4–6 weeks after termination of therapy. Over 95% is bound to plasma proteins. Metabolized in the liver (its main site of action) to active metabolites. Over 80% of a PO dose is excreted in the feces, via the bile, and approximately 10% is excreted through the urine.

USES

(1) As an adjunct to diet to reduce elevated total and LDL cholesterol in primary hypercholesterolemia (types IIa and IIb) in clients with a significant risk of CAD and who have not responded to diet or other measures. May also be useful in clients with combined hypercholesterolemia and hypertriglyceridemia. (2) To slow the progression of coronary atherosclerosis in clients with CAD in order to lower total and LDL cholesterol levels. (3) Primary prevention of risk of first heart attack, unstable angina, and coronary revascularization procedures in those with average to moderately elevated total cholesterol and LDL-cholesterol and below average HDL-cholesterol. *Investigational:* Diabetic dyslipidemia, nephrotic hyperlipidemia, familial dysbetalipoproteinemia, and familial combined hyperlipidemia.

ADDITIONAL CONTRAINDICATIONS

Use with mibefradil (Posicor).

SPECIAL CONCERNS

Carefully monitor clients with impaired renal function.

SIDE EFFECTS

See *Antihyperlipidemic Agents—HMG-COA Reductase Inhibitors.*

CNS: Headache, dizziness, insomnia, paresthesia, insomnia. **GI:** Flatus (most common), abdominal pain, cramps, diarrhea, constipation, dyspepsia, N&V, heartburn, dysgeusia, acid regurgitation, dry mouth. **Musculoskeletal:** Myalgia, muscle cramps, pain, arthralgia, leg pain, shoulder pain, localized pain. **Miscellaneous:** Blurred vision, eye irritation, rash, pruritus, chest pain, alopecia.

LABORATORY TEST CONSIDERATIONS

↑ Risk of elevated serum transaminases in clients with homozygous familial hypercholesterolemia.

ADDITIONAL DRUG INTERACTIONS

Grapefruit juice / ↑ Lovastatin plasma levels R/T ↓ liver metabolism; ↑ risk of myopathy and rhabdomyolysis
Isradipine / ↑ Clearance of lovastatin

HOW SUPPLIED

Tablet: 10 mg, 20 mg, 40 mg

DOSAGE

• **TABLETS**

Adults/adolescents, initial: 20 mg once daily with the evening meal. Initiate at 10 mg/day in clients on immunosuppressants. Dose range: 10–80 mg/day in single or two divided doses, not to exceed 20 mg/day if given with immunosuppressants. Adjust dose at intervals of every 4 weeks, if necessary. If C_{CR} is less than 30 mL/min, use doses greater than 20 mg/day with caution.

NURSING CONSIDERATIONS

SEE ALSO *NURSING CONSIDERATIONS* FOR *ANTIHYPERLIPIDEMIC AGENTS—HMG-COA REDUCTASE INHIBITORS.*

ADMINISTRATION/STORAGE

1. Place on standard cholesterol-lowering diet before starting lovastatin; continue during therapy.
2. Dosage modification is not necessary with renal insufficiency.

ASSESSMENT

1. Document serum cholesterol profile, other therapies and the outcome.
2. Note hepatic disease and any heavy consumption of alcohol.
3. Determine if pregnant.
4. Request recent eye exam; slight changes have been noted in the lenses of some clients.
5. Assess LFTs q 4–6 weeks for the first 12 mo of therapy. A threefold increase in serum transaminase or new-onset abnormal LFTs is an indication to stop therapy.
6. Assess life-style, including weight, diet (intake of fats, CHOs, and proteins), activity (regular exercise), alcohol consumption, and smoking history. Identify areas that may contribute to increased cholesterol levels.

CLIENT/FAMILY TEACHING

1. Take with meals. Avoid coadministration with grapefruit juice due to increased serum levels of lovastatin. Continue cholesterol-lowering diet and exercise program as prescribed. Cholesterol production by the liver is highest in the evening; drug usually taken with the evening meal.
2. Adhere to dietary restrictions, daily exercise, and weight loss in the overall management and control of hypercholesterolemia/hyperlipidemia.
3. Practice reliable birth control; drug is pregnancy category X.
4. Report malaise, muscle spasms, or fever. These may be mistaken for the flu, but could be serious side effects of drug therapy.
5. Any RUQ abdominal pain or change in color and consistency of stools should be reported.
6. Periodic LFTs and eye exams are mandatory; report any early visual disturbances.

OUTCOMES/EVALUATE

• ↓ Cholesterol/triglyceride levels
• ↓ progression of coronary atherosclerosis

Lymphocyte immune globulin, anti-thymocyte globulin sterile solution (equine)

(**LIM**-foh-sight im-**MYOUN GLOH**-byou-lin an-tih-**THIGH**-moh-sight **GLOH**-byou-lin, **EE**-kwine)

PREGNANCY CATEGORY: C
CLASSIFICATION(S):
Immunosuppressant
Rx: Atgam

ACTION/KINETICS

Obtained from hyperimmune serum of horses immunized with human thymus lymphocytes. Reduces the number of circulating, thymus-dependent lymphocytes that form rosettes from sheep erythrocytes. Antilymphocytic effect may be due to alteration of the function of T-lymphocytes, which are responsible, in part, for cell-mediated immunity. **t½, serum:** 5.7 days when the drug is given with other immunosuppressants and measured as horse IgG.

USES

(1) Management of allograft rejection in renal transplant clients, given either at the time of rejection or as an adjunct with other immunosuppressants to delay onset of the first rejection episode. (2) Treatment of moderate to severe aplastic anemia in those who are unsuitable for bone marrow transplantation. *Investigational:* As an immunosuppressant in liver, bone-marrow, heart, or other organ transplants. Treatment of multiple sclerosis, pure red-cell aplasia, and scleroderma. *Note:* Only physicians with experience in immunosuppressive therapy in treating renal transplant or aplastic anemia should use this drug.

CONTRAINDICATIONS

In those who have demonstrated a severe systemic reaction during prior administration of the drug or any other equine gamma globulin preparation.

SPECIAL CONCERNS

A systemic reaction, such as a generalized rash, tachycardia, dyspnea, hypotension, or anaphylaxis, precludes any further administration of the drug. Potency may vary from lot to lot. The possibility of transmission of infectious agents exists. Use with caution during lactation.

SIDE EFFECTS

General side effects.* Whole body:** Fever, chills, systemic or localized infection, malaise, serum sickness, edema, sweating. **GI:** N&V, diarrhea, ***GI bleeding or perforation, sore mouth or throat, epigastric or stomach pain, abdominal pain. **CNS:** Headache, ***seizures,*** confusion, disorientation, dizziness, faintness, paresthesias. **CV:** Hypertension or hypotension, tachycardia, deep vein thrombosis, thrombophlebitis, CHF, vasculitis, renal artery thrombosis. **Hematologic:** Thrombocytopenia, leukopenia, eosinophilia, neutropenia, granulocytopenia, anemia, lymphadenopathy, aplasia, pancytopenia, hemolysis, hemolytic anemia. **Dermatologic:** Rashes. **Respiratory:** Dyspnea, apnea, cough, ***pulmonary edema,*** nosebleed. **Musculoskeletal:** Chest, back, or flank pain; arthralgia, myalgias, leg pains, abnormal involuntary movement or tremor, rigidity. **Miscellaneous:** Herpes simplex infection, swelling or redness at infusion site, swelling, ***anaphylaxis, laryngospasm/edema,*** hyperglycemia, ***acute renal failure,*** viral hepatitis, enlarged or ruptured kidney.

When used for renal transplantation with other immunosuppressants. Whole body: Fever, chills, weakness or faintness. **CNS:** Headache, dizziness, paresthesia, ***seizures.*** **GI:** Diarrhea, nausea and/or vomiting, stomatitis, hiccoughs, epigastric pain, malaise. **Hematologic:** Leukopenia, thrombocytopenia. **Dermatologic:** Rash, pruritus, urticaria, wheal, flare. **CV:** Hypotension, peripheral thrombophlebitis, edema, hypertension, renal artery stenosis, tachycardia. **Musculoskeletal:** Arthralgia, chest or back pain (or both), myalgia. **Respiratory:** Dyspnea, laryngospasm, pulmonary edema. **Miscellaneous:** Clotted arteriovenous fistula, pain at infusion site, night sweats, ***anaphylaxis,*** herpes simplex reactivation, hyperglycemia, iliac vein obstruction, localized infection, lymphadenopathy, serum sickness, systemic infection, ***toxic epidermal necrosis,*** wound dehiscence.

When used for aplastic anemia with support therapy. Whole body: Fever, chills, diaphoresis, aches. **GI:** N&V, diarrhea. **CNS:** Headache, agitation, lethargy, listlessness, lightheadedness, ***seizures,*** encephalitis or postviral encephalopathy. **CV:** Chest pain, phlebitis, bradycardia, myocarditis, cardiac irregularity, hypotension, CHF, hypertension. **Hematologic:** Lymphadenopathy, postcervical lymphadenopathy, tender lymph nodes. **Respiratory:** Bilateral pleural effusion, respiratory distress. **Musculoskeletal:** Arthralgia, myalgia, joint stiffness, muscle aches. **Miscellaneous:** Periorbital edema, edema, hepatosplenomegaly, burning soles/palms, foot sole pain, proteinuria, ***anaphylaxis.***

LABORATORY TEST CONSIDERATIONS

↑ SGOT, SGPT, alkaline phosphatase, serum creatinine.

DRUG INTERACTIONS

Previously masked reactions to Atgam may appear when the drug is given concomitantly with corticosteroids or other immunosuppressants.

HOW SUPPLIED

Injection: 50 mg horse gamma globulin/mL

DOSAGE

• IV ONLY

Renal allograft recipients.

Adults: 10–20 mg/kg daily. **Children:** 5–25 mg/kg daily. Usually used concomitantly with azathioprine and corticosteroids. When used to delay the onset of allograft rejection, a fixed dose of 15 mg/kg for 14 days is used; then, the dose is given every other day for 14 days for a total of 21 doses in 28 days. Give the first dose within 24 hr before or after the transplant. When used to treat allograft rejection, the first dose can be delayed until the first rejection episode is diagnosed. **Recommended dose:**10–15 mg/kg daily for 14 days; additional alternate day therapy can be given for a total of 21 doses.

Aplastic anemia.

10–20 mg/kg daily for 8–14 days; additional alternate day therapy may be given for a total of 21 doses.

NURSING CONSIDERATIONS

ADMINISTRATION/STORAGE

IV 1. Recommended that clients be skin tested with an intradermal injection of 0.1 mL of a 1:1,000 dilution (5 mg horse IgG) of Atgam in NaCl and a contralateral NaCl injection. Observe for the first hour after intradermal injection. A local reaction of 10 mm or greater with a wheal or erythema (or both) with or without pseudopod formation and itching or a marked local swelling should be considered a positive test.

NOTE: Anaphylaxis has occurred following negative skin tests.

2. Dilution of Atgam with dextrose injection is not recommended, as low salt concentrations may cause precipitation.

3. Avoid highly acidic infusion solutions due to the possibility of physical instability over time.

4. The product can be transparent to slightly opalescent, colorless to faintly pink or brown. A slight granular or flaky deposit may form during storage.

5. To avoid excessive foaming and/or denaturation of protein, do not shake either diluted or undiluted Atgam.

6. For IV infusion, dilute in an inverted bottle of sterile vehicle so the undiluted drug does not come in contact with the air inside. Do not exceed a 4 mg/mL concentration; gently rotate or swirl the diluted solution so it is thoroughly mixed. Allow diluted drug to come to room temperature before administration.

7. Administer drug into a vascular shunt, arterial venous fistula, or a high-flow central vein through an in-line filter with a pore size of 0.2–1.0 micron. The filter prevents administration of any insoluble material that may develop during product storage. Use of high-flow veins will minimize development of phlebitis and thrombosis.

8. Do not administer in less than 4 hr.

9. Diluted Atgam is stable for up to 24 hr at concentrations up to 4 mg/mL in 0.9% NaCl, D5/0.25% NaCl, and D5/0.45% NaCl. Store diluted solution in the refrigerator.

ASSESSMENT

1. Document type of symptoms, date of transplant, and/or hematologic profile.

2. Administer concomitantly with corticosteroids, antihistamines, and antipyretics to help control drug-induced side effects.

3. With repeated treatments, exclude those exhibiting any evidence of a systemic reaction.

4. Monitor ECG, electrolytes, hematologic profile, liver and renal function studies.

5. Assess for S&S infection, liver/renal function studies, and pregnancy. Determine that skin testing has been completed prior to treatment.

INTERVENTIONS

1. Only those experienced with immunosuppressive therapy in treating

L

aplastic anemia or renal transplant should use the drug.
2. Observe for evidence of concurrent infection, thrombocytopenia, or leukopenia.
3. Discontinue if any of the following occurs: (a) symptoms of anaphylaxis, (b) severe and unremitting thrombocytopenia or leukopenia.
4. Continuously observe for possible allergic reactions. Respiratory distress and pain in the chest, back, or flank may indicate anaphylactoid reaction; stop drug and report.
5. Clients with aplastic anemia may require platelet transfusions during therapy to maintain acceptable platelet levels.

CLIENT/FAMILY TEACHING

1. Drug is used to prevent transplant rejection; close followup is required.
2. Report any fever, chills, fatigue, sore throat, chest, flank or back pain or night sweats or unusual side effects.
3. Use effective contraception during treatment and for 12 wks after completing therapy.

OUTCOMES/EVALUATE

- Interruption of cell-mediated renal allograft rejection
- ↓ Rejection and graft loss
- Hematologic remission

M

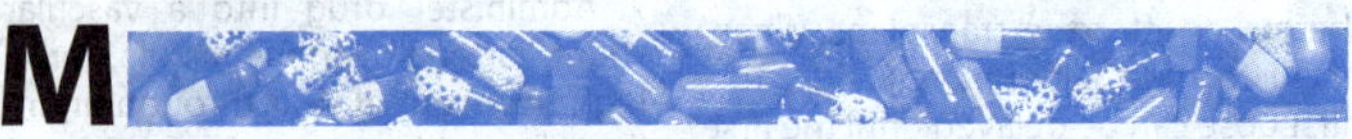

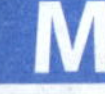

Mafenide acetate

(**MAH**-fen-eyed)

PREGNANCY CATEGORY: C
CLASSIFICATION(S):
Sulfonamide, topical
Rx: Sulfamylon

SEE ALSO *SULFONAMIDES.*

ACTION/KINETICS

Active against many gram-positive and gram-negative organisms and in the presence of serum and pus. When applied topically, it diffuses through devascularized areas, is absorbed, and is rapidly metabolized.

USES

Topical application to prevent infections in second- and third-degree burns. To control bacterial infections when used under moist dressing over meshed autografts on excised burn wounds.

CONTRAINDICATIONS

Use for established infections or in infants less than 1 month of age.

SPECIAL CONCERNS

Use with caution during lactation and in those with acute renal failure.

SIDE EFFECTS

Allergic: Rash, itching, swelling, hives, blisters, facial edema, erythema, eosinophilia. **Dermatologic:** Pain or burning (common) on application; excoriation of new skin, bleeding (rare). **Respiratory:** Hyperventilation or tachypnea, decrease in arterial pCO_2. **Metabolic:** Acidosis, increase in serum chloride. **Miscellaneous:** ***Fatal hemolytic anemia with DIC,*** diarrhea.

HOW SUPPLIED

Cream: 85 mg (as acetate)/g; *Topical Solution:* 5% (as acetate)

DOSAGE

- **CREAM**

1/16-in.-thick film applied over entire surface of burn with gloves once or twice daily until healing is progressing satisfactorily or until site is ready for grafting.

NURSING CONSIDERATIONS

SEE ALSO *GENERAL NURSING CONSIDERATIONS* FOR *ANTI-INFECTIVES* AND FOR *SULFONAMIDES.*

ADMINISTRATION/STORAGE

1. Continue until healing is progressing well or until the burn site is ready for grafting. Do not withdraw if there is still possibility of infections.
2. Avoid exposure to excessive heat.

CLIENT/FAMILY TEACHING

1. Apply cream to a cleansed, debrided, burn site using a gloved hand.
2. Undertake daily bathing to assist in wound debridement.

3. Cover treated burns with only a thin dressing.
4. Causes pain on application; use analgesics as prescribed.
5. Report any abnormal odor/drainage or fever; reactions including rashes, bruising, bleeding, swelling, or breathing difficulty.

OUTCOMES/EVALUATE

Readiness for grafting at burn site; infection prophylaxis

Magnesium sulfate

(mag-**NEE**-see-um **SUL**-fayt)

PREGNANCY CATEGORY: A
CLASSIFICATION(S):
Anticonvulsant, miscellaneous; and Laxative, saline

SEE ALSO *ANTICONVULSANTS* AND *LAXATIVES*.

ACTION/KINETICS

Magnesium is an essential element for muscle contraction, certain enzyme systems, and nerve transmission. Extracellular fluid levels: 1.5–2.5 mEq/L. Mg depresses the CNS and controls convulsions by blocking release of acetylcholine at the myoneural junction. Also, Mg decreases the sensitivity of the motor end plate to acetylcholine and decreases the excitability of the motor membrane. **Therapeutic serum levels:** 4–6 mEq/L (normal Mg levels: 1.5–3.0 mEq/L). **Onset: IM,** 1 hr; **IV,** immediate. **Duration: IM,** 3–4 hr; **IV,** 30 min. Excreted by the kidneys.

USES

(1) Seizures associated with toxemia of pregnancy, epilepsy, or when abnormally low levels of magnesium may be a contributing factor in convulsions, such as in hypothyroidism or glomerulonephritis. For eclampsia, IV use is restricted to control of life-threatening seizures. (2) Acute nephritis in children to control hypertension, encephalopathy, and seizures. (3) Replacement therapy in magnesium deficiency. (4) Adjunct in TPN. (5) Laxative. *Investigational:* Inhibit premature labor (not a first-line agent). IV use as an adjunct to treat acute exacerbations of moderate to severe asthma in clients who respond poorly to beta agonists. IV use to reduce early mortality in clients with acute MI (is given as soon as possible and continued for 24–48 hr).

CONTRAINDICATIONS

In the presence of heart block or myocardial damage. In toxemia of pregnancy during the 2 hr prior to delivery.

SPECIAL CONCERNS

Use with caution in clients with renal disease because magnesium is removed from the body solely by the kidneys.

SIDE EFFECTS

Magnesium intoxication.
CNS: Depression. **CV:** Flushing, hypotension, ***circulatory collapse, depression of the myocardium.*** **Other:** Sweating, hypothermia, muscle paralysis, CNS depression, ***respiratory paralysis.*** Suppression of knee jerk reflex can be used to determine toxicity. ***Respiratory failure may occur if given after knee jerk reflex disappears.*** Hypocalcemia with signs of tetany secondary to magnesium sulfate when used for eclampsia.

OD OVERDOSE MANAGEMENT

Symptoms: Serum levels can predict symptoms of toxicity. Symptoms include ***sharp decrease in BP and respiratory paralysis,*** changes in ECG (increased PR interval, increased QRS complex, prolonged QT interval), ***asystole, heart block.*** At serum levels of 7–10 mEq/L there is hypotension, narcosis, and loss of DTRs. ***Levels of 12–15 mEq/L result in respiratory paralysis; greater than 15 mEq/L cause cardiac conduction problems. Levels greater than 25 mEq/L cause cardiac arrest.***

Treatment:
- Use artificial ventilation immediately.
- Have 5–10 mEq of calcium (e.g., 10–20 mL of 10% calcium gluconate) readily available for IV injection to reverse heart block and respiratory depression.

• Hemodialysis and peritoneal dialysis are effective.

DRUG INTERACTIONS

CNS depressants (general anesthetics, sedative-hypnotics, narcotics) / Additive CNS depression
Digitalis / Heart block when Mg intoxication is treated with calcium in digitalized clients
Neuromuscular blocking agents / Possible additive neuromuscular blockade

HOW SUPPLIED

Injection: 10% (0.8 mEq/mL), 12.5% (1 mEq/mL), 50% (4 mEq/mL)

DOSAGE

• **IM**

Anticonvulsant.

Adults: 1–5 g of a 25%–50% solution up to 6 times/day. **Pediatric:** 20–40 mg/kg using the 20% solution (may be repeated if necessary).

• **IV**

Anticonvulsant.

Adults: 1–4 g using 10%–20% solution, not to exceed 1.5 mL/min of the 10% solution.

Hypomagnesemia, mild.

Adults: 1 g as a 50% solution q 6 hr for 4 times (or total of 32.5 mEq/24 hr).

Hypomagnesemia, severe.

Adults: Up to 2 mEq/kg over 4 hr.

• **IV INFUSION**

Anticonvulsant.

Adults: 4–5 g in 250 mL 5% dextrose at a rate not to exceed 3 mL/min.

Hypomagnesemia, severe.

Adults: 5 g (40 mEq) in 1,000 mL dextrose 5% or sodium chloride solution by **slow** infusion over period of 3 hr.

Hyperalimentation.

Adults: 8–24 mEq/day; **infants:** 2–10 mEq/day.

• **ORAL SOLUTION**

Laxative.

Adults: 10–15 g; **pediatric:** 5–10 g.

NURSING CONSIDERATIONS

SEE ALSO *NURSING CONSIDERATIONS* FOR *ANTICONVULSANTS* AND *LAXATIVES*.

ADMINISTRATION/STORAGE

1. When used as a laxative, dissolve in a glassful of ice water or other chilled fluid to lessen the disagreeable taste.
2. Dilutions for IM: deep injection of 50% concentrate for adults. Use a 20% solution for children.
IV 3. For IV injections, administer undiluted only 1.5 mL of 10% solution per minute; discontinue when convulsions cease.
4. For IV infusion, dilute 4 g in 250 mL of D5W or NSS; do not exceed 3 mL/min.

ASSESSMENT

1. Document indications for therapy, onset and characteristics of symptoms.
2. Evaluate cardiac status and ECG.
3. Note any kidney disease. Assess Mg levels and renal function.
4. With premature labor, continually assess fetal heart rate and intensity and timing of contractions.

INTERVENTIONS

1. Before administering IV check for the following conditions:
• Absent patellar reflexes
• Respirations below 16/min
• Urine output < 100 mL in past 4 hr
• Early signs of hypermagnesemia: flushing, sweating, hypotension, or hypothermia
• Past history of heart block or myocardial damage; prolonged PR and widened QRS intervals
2. Adjust dose of CNS depressants.
3. Digitalis toxicity treated with calcium is extremely dangerous and may result in heart block.
4. With acute MI, administer immediately and continue for 24–48 hr.
5. Do not administer for 2 hr preceding delivery.
6. If mother received continuous IV Mg therapy 24 hr prior to delivery, assess newborn for neurologic and respiratory depression.

CLIENT/FAMILY TEACHING

Do not exceed prescribed dose. Ensure well balanced diet, with increased bulk, increased water intake, and regular daily exercise to promote bowel motility.

OUTCOMES/EVALUATE

• Control of seizures
• Magnesium levels (1.8–3 mEq/L)
• Successful evacuation of stool

Mannitol

(**MAN**-nih-tol)

PREGNANCY CATEGORY: C
CLASSIFICATION(S):
Diuretic, osmotic
Rx: Resectisol, Osmitrol

ACTION/KINETICS

Increases the osmolarity of the glomerular filtrate, which decreases the reabsorption of water and increases excretion of sodium and chloride. It also increases the osmolarity of the plasma, which causes enhanced flow of water from tissues into the interstitial fluid and plasma. Thus, cerebral edema, increased ICP, and CSF volume and pressure are decreased. **Onset, IV:** 30–60 min for diuresis and within 15 min for reduction of cerebrospinal and intraocular pressures. **Peak:** 30–60 min. **Duration:** 6–8 hr diuresis and 4–8 hr for reduction of intraocular pressure. **t½:** 15–100 min. Over 90% excreted through the urine unchanged. A test dose is given in clients with impaired renal function or oliguria.

USES

(1) Diuretic to prevent or treat the oliguric phase of acute renal failure before irreversible renal failure occurs. (2) Decrease ICP and cerebral edema by decreasing brain mass. (3) Decrease elevated intraocular pressure when the pressure cannot be lowered by other means. (4) To promote urinary excretion of toxic substances. (5) As a urinary irrigant to prevent hemolysis and hemoglobin buildup during transurethral prostatic resection or other transurethral surgical procedures. *Investigational:* Prevent hemolysis during cardiopulmonary bypass surgery.

CONTRAINDICATIONS

Anuria, pulmonary edema, severe dehydration, active intracranial bleeding except during craniotomy, progressive heart failure or pulmonary congestion after mannitol therapy, progressive renal damage following mannitol therapy.

SPECIAL CONCERNS

Use with caution during lactation. If blood is given simultaneously with mannitol, add at least 20 mEq of sodium chloride to each liter of mannitol solution to avoid pseudoagglutination. Sudden expansion of the extracellular volume that occurs after rapid IV mannitol may lead to fulminating CHF. Mannitol may obscure and intensify inadequate hydration or hypovolemia.

SIDE EFFECTS

Electrolyte: Fluid and electrolyte imbalance, acidosis, loss of electrolytes, dehydration. **GI:** Nausea, vomiting, dry mouth, thirst, diarrhea. **CV:** Edema, hypotension or hypertension, increase in heart rate, angina-like chest pain, CHF, thrombophlebitis. **CNS:** Dizziness, headaches, blurred vision, ***seizures.*** **Miscellaneous:** Pulmonary congestion, marked diuresis, rhinitis, chills, fever, urticaria, pain in arms, skin necrosis.

LABORATORY TEST CONSIDERATIONS

↑ or ↓ Inorganic phosphorus. ↑ Ethylene glycol values because mannitol also is oxidized to an aldehyde during test.

OD OVERDOSE MANAGEMENT

Symptoms: Increased electrolyte excretion, especially sodium, chloride, and potassium. Sodium depletion results in orthostatic tachycardia or hypotension and decreased CVP. Potassium loss can impair neuromuscular function and cause intestinal dilation and ileus. If urine flow is inadequate, pulmonary edema or water intoxication may occur. Other symptoms include hypotension, polyuria that rapidly becomes oliguria, stupor, ***seizures,*** hyperosmolality, and hyponatremia. *Treatment:* Discontinue the infusion immediately and begin supportive measures to correct fluid and electrolyte imbalances. Hemodialysis is effective.

DRUG INTERACTIONS

May cause deafness when used in combination with kanamycin.

HOW SUPPLIED

Injection: 5%, 10%, 15%, 20%, 25%; *Irrigation solution:* 5%

M

DOSAGE

- **IV INFUSION ONLY**

Test dose (oliguria or reduced renal function).

Either 50 mL of a 25% solution, 75 mL of a 20% solution, or 100 mL of a 15% solution infused over 3–5 min. If urine flow is 30–50 mL/hr, therapeutic dose can be given. If urine flow does not increase, give a second test dose; if still no response, client must be reevaluated.

Prevention of acute renal failure (oliguria).

Adults: 50–100 g, as a 5%–25% solution, given at a rate to maintain urine flow of at least 30–50 mL/hr.

Treatment of oliguria.

Adults: 50–100 g of a 15%–25% solution.

Reduction of intracranial pressure and brain mass.

Adults: 1.5–2 g/kg as a 15%–25% solution, infused over 30–60 min.

Reduction of intraocular pressure.

Adults: 1.5–2 g/kg as a 20% solution (7.5–10 mL/kg) or as a 15% solution (10–13 mL/kg) given over 30–60 min. When used preoperatively, the dose should be given 1–1.5 hr before surgery to maintain the maximum effect.

Antidote to remove toxic substances.

Adults: Dose depends on the fluid requirement and urinary output. IV fluids and electrolytes are given to replace losses. If a beneficial effect is not seen after 200 g mannitol, the infusion should be discontinued.

- **IRRIGATION SOLUTION**

Urologic irrigation.

Adults: Use as a 2.5% irrigating solution for the bladder (this concentration minimizes the hemolytic effect of water alone).

NURSING CONSIDERATIONS

SEE ALSO *NURSING CONSIDERATIONS* FOR *DIURETICS, THIAZIDES*.

ADMINISTRATION/STORAGE

IV 1. Use a filter with concentrated mannitol (15%, 20%, and 25%).

2. Concentrations greater than 15% may crystallize. To redissolve, warm the bottle in a hot water bath or autoclave; cool to body temperature before administering.

3. Do not add to other IV solutions or mix with other medications.

4. If blood is administered concurrently, add 20 mEq of NaCl to each liter of mannitol to prevent pseudoagglutination.

ASSESSMENT

1. Document indications for therapy, type and onset of symptoms.

2. List other meds prescribed to ensure none alter drug effects.

3. Document neurologic findings.

4. When used to reduce ICP and brain mass, evaluate the circulatory and renal reserve, fluid and electrolyte balance, body weight, and total I&O before and after infusion.

5. Assess for S&S of electrolyte imbalances and dehydration; replace as needed. If renal failure or oliguria present, perform test dose.

6. Monitor VS and I&O. Slow infusion and report S&S of pulmonary edema manifested by dyspnea, cyanosis, rales, or frothy sputum.

OUTCOMES/EVALUATE

- Desired diuresis with ↓ edema
- ↓ ICP, intraocular pressures

Mebendazole

(meh-**BEN**-dah-zohl)

PREGNANCY CATEGORY: C
CLASSIFICATION(S):
Anthelmintic
Rx: Vermox

ACTION/KINETICS

Anthelmintic effect occurs by blocking the glucose uptake of the organisms, thereby reducing their energy until death results. It also inhibits the formation of microtubules in the helminth. **Peak plasma levels:** 2–4 hr. Poorly absorbed from the GI tract. Excreted in feces as unchanged drug or metabolites.

USES

Whipworm, pinworm, roundworm, common and American hookworm infections; in single or mixed infections. Mebendazole is not effective for hydatid disease.

CONTRAINDICATIONS
Hypersensitivity to mebendazole.
SPECIAL CONCERNS
Use with caution in children under 2 years of age and during lactation.
SIDE EFFECTS
GI: Transient abdominal pain and diarrhea. **Hematologic:** Reversible neutropenia. **Miscellaneous:** Fever.
DRUG INTERACTIONS
Carbamazepine and hydantoin may ↓ effect due to ↓ plasma levels of mebendazole.
HOW SUPPLIED
Chew Tablet: 100 mg

DOSAGE

• **TABLETS, CHEWABLE**

Whipworm, roundworm, and hookworm.

Adults and children: 1 tablet morning and evening on 3 consecutive days.

Pinworms.

1 tablet, one time. All treatments can be repeated after 3 weeks if the client is not cured.

NURSING CONSIDERATIONS

CLIENT/FAMILY TEACHING

1. Tablets may be chewed, swallowed, or crushed and mixed with food. Fasting or purging are not required.
2. Pinworms may be highly contagious:
• Carefully wash hands with soap and water before and after eating and toileting; clean nails and keep out of mouth.
• Advise school nurse of treatment.
• Do not share washcloths and towels. Wear tight underpants; change daily. Sleep alone; wear shoes during waking hours.
• Do not shake or share linens/clothing; wash in hot water.
• Clean toilet and seats with disinfectant daily; vacuum or wet mop bedroom floors daily.
• All family members should be treated simultaneously
3. Wash all fruits and vegetables. Thoroughly cook all meats and vegetables.
4. Immobilization followed by death of parasites is slow. Complete clearance from the GI tract may take up to 3 days after initiation of treatment.

OUTCOMES/EVALUATE

• Three consecutive negative stool and/or perianal swabs
• Organism expulsion/destruction

Mechlorethamine hydrochloride (Nitrogen mustard)

(meh-klor-**ETH**-ah-meen)

PREGNANCY CATEGORY: D
CLASSIFICATION(S):
Antineoplastic, alkylating
Rx: Mustargen

SEE ALSO *ANTINEOPLASTIC AGENTS* AND *ALKYLATING AGENTS*.

ACTION/KINETICS
Cell-cycle nonspecific. Forms an unstable ethylenimmonium ion, which then alkylates or binds with various compounds, including nucleic acids. Cytotoxic activity is due to cross-linking of DNA and RNA strands and protein synthesis. When used for intracavitary tumors, exerts both an inflammatory reaction and sclerosis on serous membranes, which causes adherence of the drug to serosal surfaces. Reacts rapidly with tissues and within minutes after administration the active drug is no longer present. Metabolites are excreted through the urine.
USES
IV: Bronchogenic carcinoma; CLL and CML; palliative treatment of stages III and IV of Hodgkin's disease, polycythemia vera, mycosis fungoides, lymphosarcoma. **Intracavity:** Intrapericardial, intraperitoneal, or intrapleural: Metastatic carcinoma resulting in effusion. *Investigational:* **Topical:** Cutaneous mycosis fungoides.
CONTRAINDICATIONS
Lactation. During infectious disease.

M

SPECIAL CONCERNS
Extravasation into SC areas causes painful inflammation and induration. Use in children has been limited although the drug has been used in MOPP (mechlorethamine, Oncovin, procarbazine, prednisone) therapy.

ADDITIONAL SIDE EFFECTS
High incidence of N&V. Amyloidosis, hyperuricemia, petechiae, SC hemorrhages, tinnitus, deafness, herpes zoster, or temporary amenorrhea. Extravasation into SC tissue causes painful inflammation.

DRUG INTERACTIONS
Amphotericin B: Combination ↑ possibility of blood dyscrasias.

HOW SUPPLIED
Powder for injection: 10 mg

DOSAGE

• **IV**

Adults, children: a total dose of 0.4 mg/kg per course of therapy given as a single dose or in two to four divided doses of 0.1–0.2 mg/kg over 2–4 days. Depending on blood cell count, a second course may be given after 3 weeks.

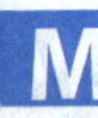

• **INTRAPLEURAL, INTRAPERITONEAL, INTRAPERICARDIAL**

0.4 mg/kg (0.2 mg/kg has been used intrapericardially).

• **TOPICAL OINTMENT, SOLUTION**

Apply to entire skin surface once daily until 6–12 months after a complete response is obtained; **then,** use once to several times a week for up to 3 years.

NURSING CONSIDERATIONS

SEE ALSO *NURSING CONSIDERATIONS FOR ANTINEOPLASTIC AGENTS.*

ADMINISTRATION/STORAGE

1. For intracavitary administration, may be further diluted in 100 mL of NSS; turn client every 60 sec for 5 min to the following positions: prone, supine, right side, left side, and knee-chest. Lack of effect often results from failure to move client often enough. Remaining fluid may be removed after 24–36 hr.

IV 2. Drug is highly irritating; avoid skin contact. Wear gloves during preparation.

3. Best administered through tubing of a rapidly flowing IV saline infusion.

4. Prepare solution immediately before administration because it decomposes on standing.

5. Drug is available in a rubber-stoppered vial to which 10 mL of either NaCl or sterile water for injection is added to give a concentration of 1 mg/mL; administer over 3–5 min.

6. Insert the needle and keep it inserted until the medication is dissolved and the required dose withdrawn. Carefully discard the vial with the remaining solution so that no one will come in contact with it.

7. Use aqueous solution of equal parts 5% sodium thiosulfate and 5% $NaHCO_3$ to clean glassware, tubings, and other articles after drug administration. Soak for 45 min.

8. Monitor IV closely because extravasation causes swelling, erythema, induration, and sloughing. In case of extravasation, remove IV, infuse area with isotonic sodium thiosulfate (4.14% solution of USP salt), and apply cold compresses. If sodium thiosulfate is not available, use isotonic NaCl solution or 1% lidocaine. Apply ice for 6–12 hr.

ASSESSMENT

1. Document indications for therapy and route of administration. Note any agents used previously.

2. Monitor I&O, uric acid, renal and hematologic function. Assess for dehydration, anemia, infection, and gout (allopurinol may help lower uric acid levels). Drug causes granulocyte and platelet suppression. Nadir: 7–14 days; recovery 21 days.

INTERVENTIONS

1. Administer phenothiazine and/or a sedative as ordered (30–45 min prior to medication and RTC as needed) to control severe N&V that usually occurs 1–3 hr after administration.

2. Administer late afternoon or early evening; follow with a sedative (sleeping pill) to control adverse symptoms and induce sleep.

3. If drug comes in contact with the eye, irrigate with copious amounts of saline solution and consult opthal-

mologist. Irrigate skin with water for 15 min and then with 2% sodium thiosulfate solution in the event of accidental contact.

CLIENT/FAMILY TEACHING

1. Drug may be administered either IV or directly into a body cavity.
2. Medications will be given to control N&V and to help you relax and sleep.
3. Hair loss may occur.
4. Avoid vaccinia and exposure to infections or infected persons.
5. Drug may cause irreversible gonadal suppression.
6. Practice birth control during and for 4 months following therapy.

OUTCOMES/EVALUATE

- ↓ Tumor size/spread
- Improved hematologic profile
- Resolution of effusion

Meclizine hydrochloride

(**MEK**-lih-zeen)

PREGNANCY CATEGORY: B
CLASSIFICATION(S):
Antiemetic
Rx: Antivert, Antivert/25 and /50, Antrizine, Meni-D
OTC: Bonine, Dramamine Less Drowsy Formula, Vergon
✱OTC: Bonamine

SEE ALSO *ANTIHISTAMINES* AND *ANTIEMETICS*.

ACTION/KINETICS

Mechanism for the antiemetic effect may be due to a central anticholinergic effect to decrease vestibular stimulation and depress labyrinthine activity. May also act on the CTZ to decrease vomiting. **Onset:** 30–60 min; **Duration:** 8–24 hr. **t½:** 6 hr.

USES

Prevention and treatment of nausea, vomiting, and dizziness of motion sickness. Possibly effective for vertigo associated with diseases of the vestibular system.

SPECIAL CONCERNS

Safety for use during lactation and in children less than 12 years of age has not been determined. Use with caution in glaucoma, obstrucvtive disease of the GI or GU tract, and in prostatic hypertrophy. Pediatric and geriatric clients may be more sensitive to the anticholinergic effects of meclizine.

SIDE EFFECTS

CNS: Drowsiness, excitation, nervousness, restlessness, insomnia, euphoria, vertigo, hallucinations (auditory or visual). **GI:** N&V, diarrhea, constipation, dry mouth, anorexia. **GU:** Urinary frequency or retention; difficulty in urination. **CV:** Hypotension, tachycardia, palpitations. **Miscellaneous:** Dry nose and throat, blurred or double vision, tinnitus, rash, urticaria.

HOW SUPPLIED

Capsule: 25 mg, 30 mg; *Chew Tablet:* 25 mg; *Tablet:* 12.5 mg, 25 mg, 50 mg

DOSAGE

• CAPSULES, TABLETS, CHEWABLE TABLETS

Motion sickness.

Adults: 25–50 mg 1 hr before travel; may be repeated q 24 hr during travel.

Vertigo.

Adults: 25–100 mg/day in divided doses.

NURSING CONSIDERATIONS

SEE ALSO *NURSING CONSIDERATIONS* FOR *ANTIHISTAMINES* AND *ANTIEMETICS*.

ASSESSMENT

1. Document onset, duration, and characteristics of symptoms.
2. Assess for other adverse symptoms; drug may mask signs of drug overdose or pathology such as increased ICP or intestinal obstruction.

CLIENT/FAMILY TEACHING

1. Take only as directed and report if condition does not improve.
2. Antiemetics tend to cause drowsiness and dizziness. Do not drive or perform other hazardous tasks until drug response evident.

3. With motion sickness, take 1 hr before departure to ensure best results.
4. Avoid alcohol; markedly increases sedative effects.

OUTCOMES/EVALUATE

- Prevention of motion sickness
- Control of vertigo

Meclofenamate sodium

(me-kloh-fen-**AM**-ayt)

PREGNANCY CATEGORY: B (D IF USED DURING THIRD TRIMESTER OR NEAR DELIVERY)

CLASSIFICATION(S):

Nonsteroidal anti-inflammatory drug

Rx: Meclomen

SEE ALSO *NONSTEROIDAL ANTI-INFLAMMATORY DRUGS.*

ACTION/KINETICS

Peak effect: 30–120 min. **t½:** 1.3 hr. Peak anti-inflammatory activity may not be observed for 2–3 weeks. More than 99% protein-bound. Excreted through urine (70%) and feces (30%).

USES

(1) Acute and chronic rheumatoid arthritis and osteoarthritis. Not indicated as the initial drug for rheumatoid arthritis due to GI side effects. Has been used in combination with gold salts or corticosteroids. (2) Mild to moderate pain. (3) Primary dysmenorrhea, idiopathic excessive menstrual blood loss. *Investigational:* Sunburn, prophylaxis of migraine, migraine due to menses.

ADDITIONAL CONTRAINDICATIONS

Use during pregnancy, lactation, or in children less than 14 years of age.

SPECIAL CONCERNS

Safe use during lactation not established. Safety and efficacy not established in functional class IV rheumatoid arthritis or in children less than 14 years old.

ADDITIONAL SIDE EFFECTS

Severe diarrhea, nausea, headache, rash, dermatitis, abdominal pain, pyrosis, flatulence, malaise, fatigue, paresthesia, insomnia, depression, taste disturbances, nocturia, blood loss (through feces: 2 mL/day).

LABORATORY TEST CONSIDERATIONS

↑ Serum transaminase, alkaline phosphatase; rarely, ↑ serum creatinine or BUN.

DRUG INTERACTIONS

Aspirin / ↓ Plasma levels of meclofenamate
Warfarin / ↑ Effect of warfarin

HOW SUPPLIED

Capsule: 50 mg, 100 mg

DOSAGE

- **CAPSULES**

Rheumatoid arthritis, osteoarthritis.

Adults, usual: 200–400 mg/day in three to four equal doses. Initiate at lower dose and increase to maximum of 400 mg/day if necessary. After initial satisfactory response, lower dosage to decrease severity of side effects.

Mild to moderate pain.

Adults: 50 mg q 4–6 hr (100 mg may be required in some clients), not to exceed 400 mg/day.

Excessive menstrual blood loss and primary dysmenorrhea.

Adults: 100 mg t.i.d. for up to 6 days, starting at the onset of menses.

NURSING CONSIDERATIONS

SEE ALSO *NURSING CONSIDERATIONS FOR NONSTEROIDAL ANTI-INFLAMMATORY DRUGS.*

ADMINISTRATION/STORAGE

1. Lower doses may be effective for chronic use.
2. Reduce dose or discontinue temporarily if diarrhea occurs.

ASSESSMENT

Note indications for therapy, onset, and characteristics of symptoms. List other agents trialed and outcome. Assess baseline CBC, LFTs, and renal function.

CLIENT/FAMILY TEACHING

1. May take with food or milk to diminish GI upset.
2. Report any changes in stool color or diarrhea, visual changes, weight gain, or other unusual side effects.
3. Take as ordered and do not become discouraged; may take 2–3 weeks to see improvement in arthritic conditions.
4. Practice reliable birth control.

OUTCOMES/EVALUATE

- Improvement in joint pain and mobility with ↓ inflammation
- Relief of pain and dysmenorrhea

Medroxyprogesterone acetate

(meh-**drox**-see-proh-**JESS**-ter-ohn)

PREGNANCY CATEGORY: X
CLASSIFICATION(S):
Progestin
Rx: Amen, Curretab, Cycrin, Depo-Provera, Depo-Provera C-150, Provera
✱Rx: Alti-MPA, Gen-Medroxy, Novo-Medrone

SEE ALSO *PROGESTERONE AND PROGESTINS* AND *ANTINEOPLASTIC AGENTS*.

ACTION/KINETICS
Synthetic progestin devoid of estrogenic and androgenic activity. Prevents stimulation of endometrium by pituitary gonadotropins. Priming with estrogen is necessary before response is noted. Rapidly absorbed from GI tract. **Maximum levels:** 1–2 hr. **$t^{1/2}$, after PO:** 2–3 hr for first 6 hr; then, 8–9 hr. **$t^{1/2}$, long-acting forms IM:** About 10 weeks with maximum levels within 24 hr.

USES
(1) Secondary amenorrhea. (2) Abnormal uterine bleeding due to hormonal imbalance (no organic pathology). (3) Adjunct in palliative treatment of inoperable, recurrent, or metastatic endometrial or renal carcinoma. (4) Long-acting contraceptive (injectable form given q 3 months). (5) Reduce endometrial hyperplasia in postmenopausal women receiving 0.625 mg conjugated estrogen for 12 to 14 days/month; can begin on the 1st or 16th day of the cycle. *Investigational:* Polycystic ovary syndrome, precocious puberty. With estrogen to treat menopausal symptoms and hypermenorrhea. To stimulate respiration in obesity-hypoventilation syndrome (oral).

CONTRAINDICATIONS
Clients with or a history of thrombophlebitis, thromboembolic disease, cerebral apoplexy. Liver dysfunction. Known or suspected malignancy of the breasts or genital organs. Missed abortion; as a diagnostic for pregnancy. Undiagnosed vaginal bleeding. Use during the first 4 months of pregnancy.

SPECIAL CONCERNS
The overall risk of breast, liver, ovarian, endometrial, and cervical cancer is not thought to increase with use of the injectable long-acting contraceptive preparation. Possibility of ectopic pregnancy. Use with caution with a history of depression. Due to the possibility of fluid retention, use with caution in clients with epilepsy, migraine, asthma, or cardiac or renal dysfunction.

SIDE EFFECTS
GU: Amenorrhea or infertility for up to 18 months. **CV:** Thrombophlebitis, ***pulmonary embolism.*** **GI:** Nausea (rare), jaundice. **CNS:** Nervousness, drowsiness, insomnia, fatigue, dizziness, headache (rare). **Dermatologic:** Pruritus, urticaria, rash, acne, hirsutism, alopecia, angioneurotic edema. **Miscellaneous:** ***Hyperpyrexia, anaphylaxis,*** decrease in glucose tolerance, weight gain, fluid retention.

DRUG INTERACTIONS
Aminoglutethimide may ↑ metabolism of medroxyprogesterone → ↓ effect.

HOW SUPPLIED
Injection: 150 mg/mL, 400 mg/mL; *Tablet:* 2.5 mg, 5 mg, 10 mg

DOSAGE

- **TABLETS**

Secondary amenorrhea.
5–10 mg/day for 5–10 days, with therapy beginning at any time during the menstrual cycle. If endometrium has been estrogen primed: 10 mg medroxyprogesterone/day for 10 days beginning any time.

Abnormal uterine bleeding with no pathology.
5–10 mg/day for 5–10 days, with therapy beginning on day 16 or 21 of the

menstrual cycle. If endometrium has been estrogen primed: 10 mg/day for 10 days, beginning on day 16 of the menstrual cycle. Bleeding usually begins within 3–7 days.

• **IM**

Endometrial or renal carcinoma.

Initial: 400–1,000 mg/week; **then,** if improvement noted, 400 mg/month. Medroxyprogesterone is not intended to be the primary therapy.

Long-acting contraceptive.

150 mg of depot form q 3 months by deep IM injection given only during the first 5 days after the onset of a normal menstrual period, within 5 days postpartum if not breastfeeding, or 6 weeks postpartum if breastfeeding.

NURSING CONSIDERATIONS

SEE ALSO *NURSING CONSIDERATIONS* FOR *ANTINEOPLASTIC AGENTS* AND *PROGESTERONE AND PROGESTINS.*

ASSESSMENT

1. Document type, onset, and characteristics of symptoms.
2. Note any thromboembolic disease.
3. Monitor calcium levels and LFTs. With severe hypercalcemia, have IV fluids, diuretics, corticosteroids, and phosphate supplements available; monitor closely once corrected.

CLIENT/FAMILY TEACHING

1. With oral administration mark calendar to ensure dosing. IM injection may be painful. After repeated injections infertility and amenorrhea may last as long as 18 mo.
2. With cancer therapy, the combined effect of the drug and osteolytic metastases may result in hypercalcemia. Report insomnia, lethargy, anorexia, and N&V. Increase fluids to minimize hypercalcemia.
3. Keep scheduled appointments for contraceptive evaluation and regular GYN exams. Additional barrier protection is necessary to prevent STDs and HIV transmission. Practice regular breast exams.
4. Report pain or swelling in calves, sudden chest pain or shortness of breath as well as any other unusual side effects.

OUTCOMES/EVALUATE

• Prevention of pregnancy
• Control of tumor size and spread
• Regular menses; normal hormone levels
• ↓ Endometrial hyperplasia in postmenopausal women receiving estrogen

Mefenamic acid

(meh-fen-**NAM**-ick **AH**-sid)

PREGNANCY CATEGORY: C
CLASSIFICATION(S):
Nonsteroidal anti-inflammatory drug
Rx: Ponstel
★Rx: Apo-Mefenamic, Nu-Mefenamic, PMS-Mefenamic Acid, Ponstan

SEE ALSO *NONSTEROIDAL ANTI-INFLAMMATORY DRUGS.*

ACTION/KINETICS

Inhibits prostaglandin synthesis. Is an anti-inflammatory, antipyretic, and analgesic. **Peak:** 2–4 hr; **t½:** 2 hr; **duration:** 4–6 hr. Over 90% protein-bound. Slowly absorbed from the GI tract, metabolized by the liver, and excreted in the urine and feces.

USES

(1) Short-term relief (< 1 week) of mild to moderate pain (e.g., pain associated with tooth extraction and musculoskeletal disorders) in those over 14 years old. (2) Primary dysmenorrhea. *Investigational:* PMS, sunburn.

CONTRAINDICATIONS

Ulceration or chronic inflammation of the GI tract, pregnancy or possibility thereof, children under 14, and hypersensitivity to the drug.

SPECIAL CONCERNS

Dosage has not been established in children less than 14 years of age. Use with caution in clients with impaired renal or hepatic function, asthma, or clients on anticoagulant therapy.

ADDITIONAL SIDE EFFECTS

Autoimmune hemolytic anemia if used more than 12 months. Diarrhea may be significant. Rash (maculopapular type).

LABORATORY TEST CONSIDERATIONS
False + test for urinary bile using diazo tablets.

DRUG INTERACTIONS
Anticoagulants / ↑ Hypoprothrombinemia R/T ↓ plasma protein binding
Insulin / ↑ Insulin requirement
Lithium / ↑ Lithium plasma levels

HOW SUPPLIED
Capsule: 250 mg

DOSAGE

• **CAPSULES**

Analgesia, primary dysmenorrhea.

Adults and children over 14 years of age, initial: 500 mg; **then,** 250 mg q 6 hr, not to exceed 1 week for acute pain and 2–3 days for dysmenorrhea.

NURSING CONSIDERATIONS

SEE ALSO *NURSING CONSIDERATIONS* FOR *NONSTEROIDAL ANTI-INFLAMMATORY DRUGS.*

ADMINISTRATION/STORAGE
Do not use for more than a week at a time.

CLIENT/FAMILY TEACHING
1. Take with food to minimize GI upset.
2. Use caution when driving or operating machinery; drug may cause dizziness or confusion.
3. Report any unusual bleeding, rashes, itching, diarrhea, lightheadedness, or increased sweating.

OUTCOMES/EVALUATE
- Relief of pain
- Control of uterine cramping

Mefloquine hydrochloride

(meh-**FLOH**-kwin)

PREGNANCY CATEGORY: C
CLASSIFICATION(S):
Antimalarial
Rx: Lariam

ACTION/KINETICS
Related chemically to quinine and acts as a blood schizonticide. It may increase intravesicular pH in acid vesicles of parasite. Mefloquine is a mixture of enantiomeric molecules that results in differences in the rates of release, absorption, distribution, metabolism, elimination, and activity of the drug. It shows myocardial depressant activity with about 20% of the antifibrillatory activity of quinidine and 50% of the increase in the PR interval noted with quinine. **t½:** 13–24 days (average 3 weeks). Is 98% bound to plasma proteins and is concentrated in blood erythrocytes (i.e., the target cells in treatment of malaria).

USES
(1) Mild to moderate acute malaria caused by mefloquine-susceptible strains of *Plasmodium falciparum* (both chloroquine susceptible and resistant strains) or *P. vivax*. Data are not available regarding effectiveness in treating *P. ovale* or *P. malariae.* (2) Prophylaxis of *P. falciparum* and *P. vivax* infections, including prophylaxis of chloroquine-resistant strains of *P. falciparum. NOTE:* Clients with acute *P. vivax* malaria are at a high risk for relapse as mefloquine does not eliminate the exoerythrocytic (hepatic) parasites. Thus, these clients should also be treated with primaquine. *NOTE:* Strains of *P. falciparum* are reported to be resistant to mefloquine.

CONTRAINDICATIONS
Hypersensitivity to mefloquine or related compounds.

SPECIAL CONCERNS
Use with caution during lactation and in those with psychiatric disturbances due to the possibility of emotional reactions. Safety and effectiveness have not been determined in children.

SIDE EFFECTS
NOTE: At the doses used, it is difficult to distinguish side effects due to the drug from symptoms attributable to the disease itself. ***When used for treatment of acute malaria.*** **GI:** N&V, diarrhea, abdominal pain, loss of appetite. **CNS:** Dizziness, fever, headache, fatigue, emotional problems, ***seizures.*** **Miscellaneous:** Myalgia, chills, skin rash, tinnitus, bradycardia, hair loss, pruritus, asthenia. ***When used for prophylaxis of malaria.***

M

CNS: Dizziness, syncope, encephalopathy of unknown etiology. **Miscellaneous:** Vomiting, extrasystoles. ***Postmarketing surveillance.*** **CNS:** Vertigo, psychoses, confusion, anxiety, depression, ***seizures,*** hallucinations, insomnia, abnormal dreams, forgetfulness, motor and sensory neuropathy. **CV:** Hypertension, hypotension, tachycardia, palpitations. **Dermatologic:** Flushing, urticaria, Stevens-Johnson syndrome, erythema multiforme. **Miscellaneous:** Visual disturbances.

LABORATORY TEST CONSIDERATIONS

When used for prophylaxis: Transient ↑ transaminases, leukocytosis, thrombocytopenia. **When used for treatment of acute malaria:** ↓ Hematocrit, transient ↑ transaminases, leukocytosis, thrombocytopenia.

OD OVERDOSE MANAGEMENT

Symptoms: Cardiotoxic effects, vomiting, diarrhea. *Treatment:* Induce vomiting and administer fluid therapy to treat vomiting and diarrhea.

DRUG INTERACTIONS

Beta-adrenergic blocking agents / ECG abnormalities or cardiac arrest
Chloroquine / ↑ Risk of seizures
Quinidine / ↑ Risk of ECG abnormalities or cardiac arrest
Quinine / ↑ Risk of seizures, ECG abnormalities, or cardiac arrest
Valproic acid / Loss of seizure control and ↓ valproic acid blood levels

HOW SUPPLIED

Tablet: 250 mg

DOSAGE

- **TABLETS**

Mild to moderate malaria caused by susceptible strains of P. falciparum *or* P. vivax.

1,250 mg (5 tablets) as a single dose with at least 8 oz of water (not to be taken on an empty stomach).

Prophylaxis of malaria.

250 mg (1 tablet) once a week for 4 weeks; **then,** 1 tablet every other week. The CDC recommends a single dose taken weekly starting 1 week before travel, continued weekly during travel, and for 4 weeks after leaving malarious areas. **Pediatric, 15–19 kg:** ¼ tablet (62.5 mg) weekly; **20–30 kg:** ½ tablet (125 mg) weekly; **31–45 kg:** ¾ tablet (187.5 mg) weekly; **over 45 kg:** 1 tablet (250 mg) weekly. The CDC recommends a similar dosing schedule for children as for adults.

NURSING CONSIDERATIONS

SEE ALSO *GENERAL NURSING CONSIDERATIONS* FOR *ANTI-INFECTIVES.*

ADMINISTRATION/STORAGE

Store tablets at 15–30°C (59–86°F).

ASSESSMENT

1. Determine if for prophylaxis or treatment of malaria as dosages differ.
2. Obtain lab confirmation of causative organism; monitor LFTs.
3. Note any psychiatric disturbances or severe emotional lability.
4. With life-threatening *P. falciparum* infection, treat with an IV antimalarial and follow with mefloquine, to complete therapy.
5. To reduce cardiotoxic effects, induce vomiting with overdose.

CLIENT/FAMILY TEACHING

1. Do not take on an empty stomach; take with at least 8 oz of water.
2. Report any visual disturbance; obtain periodic eye exams.
3. For prophylaxis, the CDC recommends a single dose taken weekly starting 1 week before travel, continued weekly during travel, and for 4 weeks after leaving malarious areas.

OUTCOMES/EVALUATE

Treatment/prophylaxis of malaria (with drug-sensitive malarial parasites)

Megestrol acetate

(meh-**JESS**-trohl)

PREGNANCY CATEGORY: D
CLASSIFICATION(S):
Progestin
Rx: Megace
Rx: Apo-Megestrol, Lin-Megestrol, Megace OS, Nu-Megestrol

SEE ALSO *PROGESTERONE AND PROGESTINS* AND *ANTINEOPLASTIC AGENTS.*

ACTION/KINETICS

Antineoplastic activity is due to suppression of gonadotropins (antiluteinizing effect). Has appetite-enhancing properties (mechanism unknown). Contains tartrazine, which can cause allergic-type reactions, including asthma, often occurring in aspirin sensitivity.

USES

Tablets: Palliative treatment of advanced endometrial or breast cancer. Do not use in place of chemotherapy, radiation, or surgery. **Oral suspension:** Treatment of anorexia, cachexia, or an unexplained, significant weight loss in clients with a diagnosis of AIDS.

CONTRAINDICATIONS

Use as a diagnostic aid test for pregnancy, in known or suspected pregnancy, or for prophylaxis to avoid weight loss. Use during the first 4 months of pregnancy. Use for other types of neoplasms.

SPECIAL CONCERNS

Use with caution in clients with a history of thromboembolic disease. Use in HIV-infected women with endometrial or breast cancer has not been widely studied. Long-term use may increase the risk of respiratory infections and may cause secondary adrenal suppression. Safety and efficacy in children have not been determined.

SIDE EFFECTS

GI: Diarrhea, flatulence, nausea, dyspepsia, vomiting, constipation, dry mouth, hepatomegaly, increased salivation, abdominal pain, oral moniliasis. **CV:** Hypertension, ***cardiomyopathy,*** palpitation. **CNS:** Insomnia, headache, paresthesia, confusion, ***seizures,*** depression, neuropathy, hypesthesia, abnormal thought process. **Respiratory:** Pneumonia, dyspnea, cough, pharyngitis, chest pain, lung disorder, increased risk of respiratory infection with chronic use. **Dermatologic:** Rash, alopecia, herpes, pruritus, vesiculobullous rash, sweating, skin disorder. **GU:** Impotence, decreased libido, urinary frequency, albuminuria, urinary incontinence, UTI, gynecomastia. **Body as a whole:** Asthenia, anemia, fever, pain, moniliasis, infection, sarcoma. **Miscellaneous:** Leukopenia, edema, peripheral edema, amblyopia.

LABORATORY TEST CONSIDERATIONS

Hyperglycemia, ↑ LDH.

HOW SUPPLIED

Suspension: 40 mg/mL; *Tablet:* 20 mg, 40 mg

DOSAGE

- **ORAL SUSPENSION**

Appetite stimulant in AIDS clients.

Adults, initial: 800 mg/day (20 mL/day). The dose should be adjusted to 400 mg/day (10 mL/day) after 1 month.

- **TABLETS**

Breast cancer.

40 mg q.i.d.

Endometrial cancer.

40–320 mg/day in divided doses. To determine efficacy, treatment should be continued for at least 2 months.

NURSING CONSIDERATIONS

SEE ALSO *NURSING CONSIDERATIONS* FOR *ANTINEOPLASTIC AGENTS* AND *PROGESTERONE AND PROGESTINS.*

ADMINISTRATION/STORAGE

The oral suspension is available in a lemon-lime flavor that contains 40 mg of micronized megestrol acetate/mL; shake well before using.

ASSESSMENT

1. Document indications for therapy, symptom onset and weight history.
2. Note any thromboembolic disease.
3. Determine if pregnant.
4. Note sensitivity to tartrazines.
5. With long-term therapy, assess for respiratory infections and adrenal suppression.

CLIENT/FAMILY TEACHING

1. Take exactly as prescribed; do not skip or double up doses. May take with meals if GI upset occurs.
2. Report vaginal bleeding, headaches, breast tenderness, or pain/weakness in thumb (CTS).
3. Practice reliable birth control.
4. Report any pain, swelling or warmth in calves (S&S DVT); as well as any other unusual side effects.

OUTCOMES/EVALUATE

- ↓ Tumor size and spread
- Stimulation of appetite in HIV-related cachexia

M

Meloxicam

(meh-**LOX**-ih-kam)

PREGNANCY CATEGORY: C
CLASSIFICATION(S):
Nonsteroidal anti-inflammatory drug
Rx: Mobic

NONSTEROIDAL ANTI-INFLAMMATORY DRUGS

ACTION/KINETICS
Prolonged drug absorption. Steady state reached in 5 days. Over 99% plasma protein bound. Metabolized in the liver by P450 mediated metabolism. **Peak:** 4–5 hr. **t½, elimination:** 15–20 hr. Excreted in about equal amounts in the urine and feces.

USES
Treat signs and symptoms of osteoarthritis.

CONTRAINDICATIONS
Use in those who have exhibited asthma, urticaria, or allergic-type reactions after taking aspirin or other NSAIDs (anaphylaxis is possible). Use in advanced renal disease or late pregnancy (may cause premature closure of the ductus arteriosus). Lactation.

SPECIAL CONCERNS
Use in clients with severe hepatic or renal failure has not been studied. Use with caution in those 65 years of age and older. Safety and efficacy have not been determined in children less than 18 years of age.

SIDE EFFECTS
Side effects listed are those with an incidence of 2% or greater. See also *Nonsteroidal Anti-Inflammatory Drugs*. **GI:** Abdominal pain, diarrhea, dyspepsia, constipation, flatulence, N&V. **CNS:** Dizziness, headache, insomnia. **Respiratory:** Pharyngitis, URTI, coughing. **GU:** Renal papillary necrosis, micturition frequency, UTI. **Hematologic:** Anemia. **Musculoskeletal:** Arthralgia, back pain. **Dermatologic:** Pruritus, rash. **Body as a whole:** Fluid retention, edema, pain, flu-like symptoms, accidents.

LABORATORY TEST CONSIDERATIONS
Elevation of LFTs.

DRUG INTERACTIONS
ACE Inhibitors / ↓ Antihypertensive effect of ACE inhibitors
Aspirin / ↑ Risk of GI side effects, including GI ulceration or other complications
Cholestyramine / ↑ Meloxicam clearance
Lithium / ↑ Plasma lithium levels
Warfarin / ↑ Risk of bleeding

HOW SUPPLIED
Tablet: 7.5 mg, 15 mg

DOSAGE

- **TABLETS**

Osteoarthritis.

Initial and maintenance: 7.5 mg once daily. Some may gain additional benefit from 15 mg once daily. Maximum recommended daily dose: 15 mg.

NURSING CONSIDERATIONS

ADMINISTRATION/STORAGE
Store at 15–30°C (59–86°F). Keep in a dry place in a tight container.

ASSESSMENT
1. Document indications for therapy, onset and characteristics of disease, ROM, deformity/loss of function, level of pain, other agents trialed and the outcome.
2. Determine any GI bleed or ulcer history, aspirin or other NSAID-induced asthma, urticaria, or allergic-type reactions.
3. List drugs prescribed to ensure none interact.
4. Assess for liver/renal dysfunction; monitor lytes, renal and LFTs. Avoid with dysfunction.

CLIENT/FAMILY TEACHING
1. Take exactly as directed and at the same time each day. May take with or without food.
2. The lowest dose for symptom control will be used. Take only the prescribed dose.
3. Avoid activites that require mental alertness until drug effects realized; may cause dizziness or drowsiness.
4. Report any unusual or persistent side effects including dyspepsia, abdominal pain, dizziness, and changes in stool or skin color.
5. Avoid therapy during pregnancy; may cause premature closure of babys' heart duct.

6. Report weight gain, skin rash, swelling of ankles, chest pain, SOB, or lack of effect.

OUTCOMES/EVALUATE

• Relief of joint pain and inflammation with improved mobility

Melphalan (L-PAM, L-Phenylalanine mustard, L-Sarcolysin, MPL)

(**MEL**-fah-lan)

PREGNANCY CATEGORY: D
CLASSIFICATION(S):
Antineoplastic, alkylating
Rx: Alkeran

SEE ALSO *ANTINEOPLASTIC AGENTS* AND *ALKYLATING AGENTS*.

ACTION/KINETICS

A bifunctional alkylating agent that forms an unstable ethylenimmonium ion that binds to or alkylates various intracellular substances including nucleic acids. It produces a cytotoxic effect by cross-linking of DNA and RNA strands as well as inhibition of protein synthesis. Absorption from GI tract is variable and incomplete. **t½ after PO:** 90 min. Inactivated in tissues and body fluids although it will remain active in the blood for approximately 6 hr. Within 24 hr, 10% is excreted unchanged in the urine.

USES

Multiple myeloma. Epithelial carcinoma of ovary (nonresectable). Use IV only when PO therapy is not appropriate. *Investigational:* Cancer of the breast and testes.

CONTRAINDICATIONS

Lactation. Known resistance to drug.

SPECIAL CONCERNS

Safety and efficacy have not been determined in children less than 12 years of age. Use with extreme caution in those with compromised bone marrow function due to prior chemotherapy or radiation. Reduce IV dosage in impaired renal function. Use caution not to confuse Alkeran (melphalan), Leukeran (chlorambucil), and Myleran (busulfan).

ADDITIONAL SIDE EFFECTS

Severe bone marrow depression (especially after IV use), chromosomal aberrations (may be mutagenic), ***leukemia (acute, nonlymphatic) in clients with multiple myeloma.*** Also, hypersensitivity reactions including ***anaphylaxis, pulmonary fibrosis,*** interstitial pneumonia, vasculitis, ***hemolytic anemia.***

LABORATORY TEST CONSIDERATIONS

↑ Uric acid and urinary 5-HIAA levels.

OD OVERDOSE MANAGEMENT

Symptoms: Severe N&V, decreased consciousness, ***seizures,*** muscle paralysis, cholinomimetic symptoms, diarrhea, severe mucositis, stomatitis, colitis, ***hemorrhage of GI tract, bone marrow toxicity.*** *Treatment:* General supportive treatment, blood transfusions, antibiotics. Monitor hematology for up to 6 weeks. Use of filgrastim or sargramostim may decrease the period of pancytopenia.

DRUG INTERACTIONS

Carmustine / ↑ Risk of lung toxicity
Cisplatin / Drug-induced renal dysfunction → ↓ melphalan excretion
Cyclosporine / ↑ Risk of nephrotoxicity
Interferon alfa / ↓ Levels of melphalan
Nalidixic acid / ↑ Risk of severe hemorrhagic necrotic enterocolitis in pediatric clients

HOW SUPPLIED

Powder for injection: 50 mg; *Tablet:* 2 mg

DOSAGE

• **TABLETS**

Multiple myeloma.

One of the following regimens may be used. (1) 6 mg given once daily for 2–3 weeks (adjust dose based on weekly blood counts). Drug is then discontinued for up to 4 weeks with blood count being monitored. When WBC and platelet counts are increasing, a maintenance dose of 2 mg/day can be started. (2) 10 mg/day for 7–10 days. Maximum leukocyte and platelet suppression occurs within 3–5 weeks with recovery within 4–8 weeks. When the

M

WBC exceeds 4,000/mm³ and the platelet count is greater than 100,000/mm³, a maintenance dose of 2 mg/day can be started. Dose is then adjusted to 1–3 mg/day, depending on the hematologic response. Keep leukocytes in the range of 3,000–3,500 cells/mm³. (3) 0.15 mg/kg/day for 7 days followed by a rest period of at least 2 weeks (up to 5 weeks may be needed). During the rest period, the leukocyte count will decrease; when WBC and platelet counts are increasing, a maintenance dose of 0.05 mg/kg/day may be given. (4) 0.25 mg/kg/day for 4 consecutive days (or 0.2 mg/kg/day for 5 consecutive days) for a total dose of 1 mg/kg/course of therapy. The 4- to 5-day courses can be repeated q 4–6 weeks if the granulocyte and platelet counts have returned to normal.

Epithelial ovarian cancer.

0.2 mg/kg/day for 5 days repeated q 4–5 weeks (as long as blood counts return to normal).

• **IV**

Multiple myeloma.

Adults, usual: 16 mg/m² as a single infusion over 15–20 min. Give this dose at 2-week intervals for a total of four doses. Reduce the dose up to 50% in clients with a BUN less than or equal to 30 mg/dL.

M

NURSING CONSIDERATIONS

SEE ALSO *NURSING CONSIDERATIONS* FOR *ANTINEOPLASTIC AGENTS.*

ADMINISTRATION/STORAGE

IV 1. About one-third to one-half of clients with multiple myeloma show a favorable response to IV melphalan.
2. For IV use, reconstitute powder with 10 mL of the supplied diluent for a concentration of 5 mg/mL. Then shake vial vigorously until a clear solution is obtained. Immediately dilute the dose to be given with 0.9% NaCl injection to a concentration of less than or equal to 0.45 mg/mL.
3. Complete administration within 60 min after reconstitution. After dilution, about 1% label strength of melphalan hydrolyzes every 10 min.
4. Protect from light and dispense in glass.
5. A precipitate forms if the reconstituted IV product is stored at 5°C (41°F).

ASSESSMENT

1. Document any previous radiation or chemotherapy treatments. Do not give full dosage until 4 wk after chemo of XRT due to risk of severe bone marrow depression.
2. Monitor CBC, uric acid levels; also liver and renal function studies- reduce dose with dysfunction. Drug causes granulocyte and platelet suppression. Nadir: 14 days; recovery: 28–40 days.

CLIENT/FAMILY TEACHING

1. Take once a day as directed. May divide dose if nausea and vomiting severe.
2. Use reliable birth control; may cause severe birth defects.
3. Increase fluid intake to protect against hyperuricemia. Avoid crowds and those with infections.
4. Report any unusual bruising, bleeding, fever, chills, SOB, sore throat, stomach, flank, or joint pains, or black tarry stools. Expect to lose hair; will grow back.

OUTCOMES/EVALUATE

- ↓ Malignant cell proliferation
- Improved hematologic profile

Menotropins

(men-oh-**TROH**-pinz)

PREGNANCY CATEGORY: X
CLASSIFICATION(S):
Ovarian stimulant
Rx: Humegon, Pergonal, Repronex

ACTION/KINETICS

Menotropins are a mixture of FSH and LH extracted from the urine of postmenopausal women. Causes growth and maturation of ovarian follicles. For ovulation to occur, HCG is administered the day following menotropins. **Time to peak effect, females:** 18 hr. In men, menotropins with HCG given for a minimum of 3 months induce spermatogenesis. Eliminated through the kidneys.

USES

Females: In combination with HCG to induce ovulation in clients with anovulatory cycles not due to primary ovarian failure. Use Repronex in conjunction with HCG for multiple follicular development and induction of ovulation in clients who have previously received pituitary suppression. **Males:** In combination with HCG to induce spermatogenesis in clients with primary or secondary hypogonadotrophic hypogonadism.

CONTRAINDICATIONS

Women: Pregnancy. Primary ovarian failure as indicated by high levels of urinary gonadotropins, ovarian cysts, intracranial lesions, including pituitary tumors. Overt thyroid and adrenal dysfunction. Any cause of infertility other than anovulation. Abnormal bleeding of undetermined origin. Ovarian cysts or enlargement of the ovaries not due to polycystic ovarian syndrome. **Men:** Normal gonadotropin levels, primary testicular failure, disorders of fertility other than hypogonadotrophic hypogonadism. Thyroid or adrenal dysfunction. Absence of neoplastic disease should be established before treatment is initiated.

SIDE EFFECTS

Women. GU: Ovarian overstimulation, hyperstimulation syndrome (maximal 7–10 days after discontinuation of drug), ovarian enlargement (20% of clients), adnexal torsion, ***ruptured ovarian cysts, ectopic pregnancy,*** multiple births (20%). **CV:** ***Hemoperitoneum, thromboembolism,*** tachycardia, pulmonary and vascular complications. **Hypersensitivity:** Generalized urticaria, angioneurotic edema, facial edema, ***dysnpea indicating laryngeal edema.*** **CNS:** Headaches, malaise, dizziness. **GI:** N&V, abdominal pain, diarrhea, abdominal cramps, bloating. **At injection site:** Pain, rash, swelling, irritation. **Miscellaneous:** Fever, chills, musculoskeletal aches, joint pains, body rashes, dyspnea, tachypnea.

Men. Gynecomastia, breast pain, mastitis, nausea, abnormal lipoprotein fraction, abnormal AST and ALT.

HOW SUPPLIED

Powder for injection, lyophilized: 75 IU FSH/75 IU LH, 150 IU FSH/150 IU LH

DOSAGE

- **IM**

Induction of ovulation.

Individualized, initial: 75 IU of FSH and 75 IU of LH for 7–12 days (maximum), followed by 10,000 USP units of HCG 1 day after last dose of menotropins. **Subsequent courses:** Same dosage schedule for two more courses, if ovulation has occurred. **Then,** dose may be increased to 150 IU of FSH and 150 IU of LH for 7–12 days, followed by HCG as in the preceding for two or more courses. *Note:* Repronex can also be given or self-administered SC.

Induction of spermatogenesis.

It may be necessary to give HCG alone, 5,000 IU 3 times/week, for 4–6 months prior to menotropins; **then,** 75 IU FSH and 75 IU LH IM 3 times/week and HCG 2,000 IU 2 times/week for at least 4 months. If no response after 4 months, double each dose of menotropins with the HCG dose unchanged.

NURSING CONSIDERATIONS

ADMINISTRATION/STORAGE

1. Administer parenterally; menotropins are destroyed in the GI tract.
2. To prepare solution, dissolve contents of one ampule in 1–2 mL sterile saline. Use reconstituted solutions immediately; discard unused portions.
3. Store the lyophilized powder at room temperature or in the refrigerator (3–25°C or 37–77°F).

ASSESSMENT

1. Document indications for therapy and other therapy or drugs used.
2. Assess for high levels of urinary gonadotropins or presence of ovarian cysts; drug contraindicated.
3. Obtain CBC, electrolytes, urinary gonadotropin levels, thyroid and adrenal function studies; assess neuro status, check peripheral pulses.

INTERVENTIONS

1. If urinary estrogen excretion levels greater than 100 mcg or if daily estriol

M

excretion exceeds 50 mcg, *withhold HCG* and report; impending hyperstimulation syndrome.
2. If hospitalized for hyperstimulation, perform the following:
• Place client on bed rest.
• Monitor I&O; weigh daily.
• Monitor urine sp. gravity, serum and urine lytes.
• Assess for hemoconcentration; heparin may ↓ hypercoagulability.
• Increase fluid intake; replace electrolytes.
• Provide analgesics for comfort.
3. Monitor CBC; an occasional client will develop erythrocytosis.

CLIENT/FAMILY TEACHING

1. Drug is used to help women become pregnant and/or to help men produce sperm.
2. Report any pain, coolness, or pale bluish color of an extremity (signs of arterial bloodclot). Fever or lower abdominal pain may be the result of overstimulation of the ovaries that has caused cysts to form, a loss of fluid into the peritoneum, or bleeding. Need exam every other day with this during drug therapy and for 2 weeks thereafter; hospitalization may be necessary.
3. Need a daily 24-hr urine for estrogen.
4. Graph basal body temperature.
5. Signs of ovulation include an increase in the basal body temperature, and an increase in the appearance and volume of cervical mucus.
6. Engage in daily intercourse from the day before HCG administration until ovulation occurs. Support male partner as this may require long term therapy, regular sperm counts, and also masculinizing effects of HCG.
7. If symptoms indicate overstimulation of the ovaries, a significant ovarian enlargement may have occurred. Report and abstain from intercourse because of increased risk of ovarian cyst rupture.
8. Pregnancy usually occurs 4–6 weeks after completion of therapy. Multiple births may occur.
9. For men receiving drug, if no evidence of increased sperm production after 4 mo, may continue therapy at an increased dosage.

OUTCOMES/EVALUATE

• Ovulation evidenced by ↑ estrogen levels and desired pregnancy
• Male spermatogenesis evidenced by ↑ testosterone levels

Meperidine hydrochloride (Pethidine hydrochloride)

(meh-**PER**-ih-deen)

PREGNANCY CATEGORY: C
CLASSIFICATION(S):
Narcotic analgesic
Rx: Demerol Hydrochloride, **C-II**

SEE ALSO *NARCOTIC ANALGESICS*.

ACTION/KINETICS

One-tenth as potent an analgesic as morphine. Its analgesic effect is only one-half when given PO rather than parenterally. Has no antitussive effects and does not produce miosis. Less smooth muscle spasm, constipation, and antitussive effect than equianalgesic doses of morphine. **Duration:** Less than that of most opiates; keep in mind when establishing a dosing schedule. Produces both psychologic and physical dependence; overdosage causes severe respiratory depression (see *Narcotic Overdose*). **Onset:** 10–45 min. **Peak effect:** 30–60 min. **Duration:** 2–4 hr. **t½:** 3–4 hr.

USES

PO, Parenteral: (1) Analgesic for moderate to severe pain. Particularly useful for minor surgery, as in orthopedics, ophthalmology, rhinology, laryngology, and dentistry. (2) For diagnostic procedures such as cystoscopy, retrograde pyelography, and gastroscopy. (3) Spasms of GI tract, uterus, urinary bladder. Anginal syndrome and distress of CHF. **Parenteral:** Preoperative medication, adjunct to anesthesia, obsetrical analgesia.

ADDITIONAL CONTRAINDICATIONS

Hypersensitivity to drug, convulsive states as in epilepsy, tetanus and strychnine poisoning, children under

6 months, diabetic acidosis, head injuries, shock, liver disease, respiratory depression, increased cranial pressure, and before labor during pregnancy. Use with sibutramine.

SPECIAL CONCERNS

Use with caution during lactation, in older, or debilitated clients. Use with extreme caution in clients with asthma. Atropine-like effects may aggravate glaucoma, especially when given with other drugs used with caution in glaucoma.

ADDITIONAL SIDE EFFECTS

Transient hallucinations, transient hypotension (high doses), visual disturbances. Active metabolite may accumulate in renal dysfunction, leading to an increased risk of CNS toxicity.

OD OVERDOSE MANAGEMENT

Symptoms: Severe respiratory depression. See *Narcotic Analgesics. Treatment:* Naloxone 0.4 mg IV is effective in the treatment of acute overdosage. In PO overdose, gastric lavage and induced emesis are indicated. Treatment, however, is aimed at combating the progressive respiratory depression usually through artificial ventilation.

ADDITIONAL DRUG INTERACTIONS

Antidepressants, tricyclic / Additive anticholinergic side effects
Cimetidine / ↑ Respiratory and CNS depression
Hydantoins / ↓ Meperidine effect R/T ↑ liver breakdown
MAO inhibitors / ↑ Risk of severe symptoms including hyperpyrexia, restlessness, hyper- or hypotension, convulsions, or coma
Protease inhibitors / Avoid combination
Sibutramine / Possibility of life-threatening serotonin syndrome

HOW SUPPLIED

Injection: 25 mg/mL, 50 mg/mL, 75 mg/mL, 100 mg/mL; *Syrup:* 50 mg/5 mL; *Tablet:* 50 mg, 100 mg

DOSAGE

• **IM, SC, SYRUP, TABLETS**

Analgesic.

Adults: 50–100 mg q 3–4 hr as needed; **pediatric:** 1.1–1.75 mg/kg, up to adult dosage, q 3–4 hr as needed. **Adults, PCA dosage, initial:** 10 mg with a range of 1–5 mg per incremental dose. Recommended lock-out interval is 6–10 min (minimum of 5 min).

Preoperatively.

Adults, IM, SC: 50–100 mg 30–90 min before anesthesia; **pediatric, IM, SC:** 1.1–2.2 mg/kg (up to adult dose) 30–90 min before anesthesia.

Obstetrical analgesia.

Adults, IM, SC: 50–100 mg q 1–3 hr when pains become regular.

• **IV**

Analgesic.

Adults: 15–35 mg/hr by continuous IV.

Support of anesthesia.

IV infusion: 1 mg/mL or **slow IV injection:** 10 mg/mL until client needs met.

NURSING CONSIDERATIONS

SEE ALSO *NURSING CONSIDERATIONS FOR NARCOTIC ANALGESICS.*

ADMINISTRATION/STORAGE

1. For repeated doses, IM administration is preferred over SC use.
2. More effective when given parenterally than when given PO.
3. Take the syrup with ½ glass of water to minimize anesthetic effect on mucous membranes.
4. If used concomitantly with phenothiazines or antianxiety agents, reduce the dose by 25%–50%.
IV 5. Meperidine for IV use is incompatible with the following drugs: aminophylline, barbiturates, heparin, iodide, methicillin, morphine sulfate, phenytoin, sodium bicarbonate, sulfadiazine, and sulfisoxazole.
6. The following IV solutions are compatible with meperidine: D5W and lactated Ringer's, Dextrose-saline combinations, dextrose (2.5%, 5%, 10%) in water; Ringer's, Lactated Ringer's, 0.45% or 0.5% NaCl, or 1/6 M sodium lactate.

ASSESSMENT

1. Document intensity, location, onset, characteristics and pain level (use a pain rating scale).

M

2. Note any head injury, seizure disorder, or conditions that compromise respirations.
3. Assess renal function and for glaucoma.

CLIENT/FAMILY TEACHING

1. Take drug within ordered intervals to prevent pain recurring; report pain levels and lack of effectiveness.
2. Drug causes dizziness and drowsiness; do not engage in activities that require mental alertness.
3. Rise slowly, do not to change positions abruptly; postural effects.
4. Increase fluid intake and bulk; report constipation so it can be treated early.
5. Store safely away from bedside; record dose and time of administration. Drug causes dependence.

OUTCOMES/EVALUATE

Desired level of analgesia

Mephentermine sulfate

(meh-**FEN**-ter-meen)

PREGNANCY CATEGORY: C
CLASSIFICATION(S):
Sympathomimetic, indirect-acting
Rx: Wyamine Sulfate

SEE ALSO *SYMPATHOMIMETIC DRUGS.*

ACTION/KINETICS

Acts indirectly by releasing norepinephrine from its storage sites and directly by exerting a slight effect on alpha and beta-1 receptors and a moderate effect on beta-2 receptors mediating vasodilation. Causes increased CO; also elicits slight CNS effects. **IV: Onset,** immediate; **duration:** 15–30 min. **IM: Onset,** 5–15 min; **duration:** 1–2 hr. Metabolized in liver. Excreted in urine within 24 hr (rate increased in acidic urine).

USES

Hypotension due to anesthesia, ganglionic blockade, or hemorrhage (only as emergency treatment until blood or blood substitutes can be given).

CONTRAINDICATIONS

To treat hypotension caused by chlorpromazine. In combination with MAO inhibitors.

SPECIAL CONCERNS

Use with caution in CV disease, in chronically ill clients, and in treating shock secondary to hemorrhage. Safety and efficacy have not been demonstrated in children.

SIDE EFFECTS

Anxiety, cardiac arrhythmias, increased BP (especially in those with heart disease).

ADDITIONAL DRUG INTERACTIONS

Mephentermine will potentiate hypotensive effects of phenothiazines.

HOW SUPPLIED

Injection: 15 mg/mL, 30 mg/mL

DOSAGE

• **IV, IM**

Hypotension during spinal anesthesia.

IV, Adults: 30–45 mg; 30-mg doses may be repeated as required; or, **IV infusion, Adults and children:** 0.1% (1 mg/mL) mephentermine in D5W with the rate of infusion and duration dependent on client response. **IV, Pediatric:** 0.4 mg/kg (12 mg/m^2) as a single dose.

Prophylaxis of hypotension in spinal anesthesia.

IM, Adults: 30–45 mg 10–20 min before anesthesia. **IM, Pediatric:** 0.4 mg/kg (12 mg/m^2) as a single dose.

Shock following hemorrhage.

Not recommended, but IV infusion of 0.1% in D5W may maintain BP until blood volume is replaced.

NURSING CONSIDERATIONS

SEE ALSO *NURSING CONSIDERATIONS FOR SYMPATHOMIMETIC DRUGS.*

ADMINISTRATION/STORAGE

IV 1. For shock, the preferred method of administration is either injection of the undiluted solution containing 30 mg/mL or a continuous infusion of a 1-mg/mL solution in D5W directly into the vein.
2. Prepare the 0.1% solution by adding 10 or 20 mL of mephentermine (the

30-mg/mL strength) to either 250 or 500 mL of D5W, respectively.

ASSESSMENT

Determine cause of hypotensive episode; note CV disease, hemorrhage, or chronic illness.

INTERVENTIONS

Record BP q 5 min until stable; once stabilized, check q 15–30 min beyond duration of action (IM 1–4 hr; IV 5–15 min).

OUTCOMES/EVALUATE

Stabilization of BP

Meprobamate

(meh-proh-**BAM**-ayt)

PREGNANCY CATEGORY: D
CLASSIFICATION(S):
Antianxiety drug, nonbenzodiazepine
Rx: Equanil, Miltown
✱**Rx:** Apo-Meprobamate **C-IV**

SEE ALSO *TRANQUILIZERS, ANTIMANIC DRUGS, AND HYPNOTICS.*

ACTION/KINETICS

Carbamate that possesses antianxiety, muscle relaxant, and anticonvulsant effects. Acts on the limbic system and the thalamus, as well as inhibits polysynaptic spinal reflexes. **Onset:** 1 hr. **Blood levels, chronic therapy:** 5–20 mcg/mL. **t½:** 6–17 hr. Extensively metabolized in liver and inactive metabolites and some unchanged drug (8%–19%) are excreted in the urine (90%) and feces (less than 10%).

USES

Short-term treatment (no more than 4 months) of anxiety disorders.

CONTRAINDICATIONS

Hypersensitivity to meprobamate or carisoprodol. Porphyria. Children less than 6 years of age.

SPECIAL CONCERNS

Use with caution in pregnancy, lactation, epilepsy, liver and kidney disease. Geriatric clients may be more sensitive to the depressant effects of meprobamate; also, due to age-related impaired renal function, the dose of meprobamate may have to be reduced.

SIDE EFFECTS

CNS: Ataxia, drowsiness, dizziness, weakness, headache, paradoxical excitement, overstimulation, fast EEG activity, euphoria, slurred speech, vertigo. **GI:** N&V, diarrhea. **CV:** Palpiations, tachycardia, various arrhythmias, transient ECG changes, syncope, ***hypotensive crisis.*** **Hematologic:** Agranulocytosis, aplastic anemia (rarely fatal). **Miscellaneous:** Impairment of visual accommodation, allergic reactions (usually between the first and fourth doses) including hematologic and dermatologic symptoms, paresthesias, worsening of porphyria.

LABORATORY TEST CONSIDERATIONS

With test methods: ↑ 17-Hydroxycorticosteroids, 17-ketogenic steroids, and 17-ketosteroids. *Pharmacologic effects:* ↑ Alkaline phosphatase, bilirubin, serum transaminase, urinary estriol (calorimetric tests), porphobilinogen. ↓ PT in clients on Coumarin.

OD OVERDOSE MANAGEMENT

Symptoms: Drowsiness, stupor, lethargy, ataxia, ***shock, coma, respiratory collapse, death.*** Also, arrhythmias, tachycardia or bradycardia, reduced venous return, ***profound hypotension, CV collapse.*** Excessive oronasal secretions, ***relaxation of pharyngeal wall leading to obstruction of airway.*** *Treatment:* Induction of vomiting or gastric lavage if detected shortly after ingestion. It is imperative that gastric lavage be continued or gastroscopy be performed as incomplete gastric emptying can cause relapse and death.

- Give fluids to treat hypotension. Avoid fluid overload.
- Institute artificial respiration.
- Use care in treating seizures due to combined CNS depressant effects.
- Use forced diuresis and vasopressors followed by hemodialysis or hemoperfusion if condition deteriorates.

DRUG INTERACTIONS

Additive depressant effects when used with CNS depressants (alcohol, barbiturates, narcotics), MAO inhibitors, and tricyclic antidepressants.

M

HOW SUPPLIED

Tablet: 200 mg, 400 mg

DOSAGE

- **TABLETS**

Anxiety.

Adults: 400 mg t.i.d.–q.i.d., up to a maximum of 2.4 g/day. **Pediatric, 6–12 years of age:** 100–200 mg b.i.d.–t.i.d.

NURSING CONSIDERATIONS

SEE ALSO *NURSING CONSIDERATIONS* FOR *TRANQUILIZERS, ANTIMANIC DRUGS, AND HYPNOTICS.*

ADMINISTRATION/STORAGE

Do not crush or chew tablets.

ASSESSMENT

1. Document onset and characteristics of symptoms; identify causes. Assess mental status and note behavioral manifestations.
2. Monitor VS, EKG, CBC, renal and LFTs.

CLIENT/FAMILY TEACHING

1. Take exatly as prescribed. Do not crush or chew sustained release products. Report any loss of effectiveness after several mo of therapy.
2. Avoid activities that require mental alertness until drug effects realized; may cause dizziness or drowsiness.
3. Avoid alcohol, anti-insomnia agents, or OTC drugs as adverse side effects may occur.
4. Practice reliable contraception.
5. Report any skin rash, sore throat, fever, unusual bruising or bleeding. Keep all F/U visits.

OUTCOMES/EVALUATE

↓ Symptoms of anxiety

Mercaptopurine (6-Mercaptopurine, 6-MP)

(mer-kap-toe-**PYOUR**-een)

PREGNANCY CATEGORY: D

CLASSIFICATION(S):

Antineoplastic, antimetabolite

Rx: Purinethol

SEE ALSO *ANTINEOPLASTIC AGENTS.*

ACTION/KINETICS

Cell-cycle specific for the S phase of cell division. Converted to thioinosinic acid by the enzyme hypoxanthine-guanine phosphoribosyltransferase. Thioinosinic acid then inhibits reactions involving inosinic acid. Also, both thioinosinic acid and 6-methylthioinosinate (also formed from mercaptopurine) inhibit RNA synthesis. About 50% absorbed from GI tract. **Plasma t½:** 47 min in adults and 21 min in children. Metabolites are excreted in urine with up to 39% excreted unchanged. Cross-resistance with thioguanine has been observed.

USES

Acute lymphocytic or myelocytic leukemia. Lymphoblastic leukemia, especially in children. Acute myelogenous and myelomonocytic leukemia. Effectiveness varies depending on use. The drug is not effective for leukemia of the CNS, solid tumors, lymphomas, or chronic lymphatic leukemia. *Investigational:* Inflammatory bowel disease, chronic myelocytic leukemia, polycythemia vera, non-Hodgkin's lymphoma, psoriatic arthritis.

CONTRAINDICATIONS

Use in resistance to mercaptopurine or thioguanine. To treat CNS leukemia, chronic lymphatic leukemia, lymphomas (including Hodgkin's disease), solid tumors. Lactation.

SPECIAL CONCERNS

Use with caution in clients with impaired renal function. Use during lactation only if benefits clearly outweigh risks. Severe bone marrow depression (anemia, leukopenia, thrombocytopenia) may occur. There is an increased risk of pancreatitis when used for inflammatory bowel disease.

ADDITIONAL SIDE EFFECTS

Hepatotoxicity, oral lesions, drug fever, hyperuricemia. Produces less GI toxicity than folic acid antagonists, and side effects are less frequent in children than in adults. *Pancreatitis* (when used for inflammatory bowel disease).

OD OVERDOSE MANAGEMENT

Symptoms: Immediate symptoms include N&V, diarrhea, and anorexia while delayed symptoms include myelosuppression, gastroenteritis, and liver dysfunction. *Treatment:* Induction of emesis if detected soon after ingestion. Supportive measures.

DRUG INTERACTIONS

Allopurinol / ↑ Methotrexate effect R/T ↓ liver breakdown (reduce methotrexate dose by 25%–33%)
Trimethoprim–Sulfamethoxazole / ↑ Risk of bone marrow suppression

HOW SUPPLIED

Tablet: 50 mg

DOSAGE

• **TABLETS**

Highly individualized: 2.5 mg/kg/day. **Adults, usual:** 100–200 mg; **pediatric:** 50 mg. Dosage may be increased to 5 mg/kg/day after 4 weeks if beneficial effects are not noted. Dosage is increased until symptoms of toxicity appear. **Maintenance after remission:** 1.5–2.5 mg/kg/day.

NURSING CONSIDERATIONS

SEE ALSO *NURSING CONSIDERATIONS FOR ANTINEOPLASTIC AGENTS.*

ADMINISTRATION/STORAGE

Since the maximum effect on the blood count may be delayed and the count may drop for several days after drug has been discontinued, stop therapy at first sign of abnormally large drop in leukocyte count. Nadir: 14 days.

ASSESSMENT

1. Document indications for therapy, onset of symptoms, and other treatments prescribed.
2. Obtain liver and renal function studies, uric acid, and hematologic profile. Drug causes granulocyte and platelet suppression. Nadir: 10–14 days; recovery: 21–28 days.

CLIENT/FAMILY TEACHING

1. Take drug in one dose daily as directed.
2. Drink 8-10 glasses of water/fluids each day. Avoid alcoholic beverages.
3. Reports and S&S of infection, anemia, mouth sores, fever, chills, unusual bruising, bleeding, or pain.
4. Practice reliable contraception.

OUTCOMES/EVALUATE

• Improved hematologic profile
• ↓ Malignant cell proliferation
• Symptoms of disease remission

Meropenem

(**mer**-oh-**PEN**-em)

PREGNANCY CATEGORY: B
CLASSIFICATION(S):
Antibiotic, miscellaneous
Rx: Merrem IV
★**Rx:** Merrem

SEE ALSO *ANTI-INFECTIVES.*

ACTION/KINETICS

Broad-spectrum carbapenem antibiotic. Acts by inhibiting cell wall synthesis in gram-positive and gram-negative bacteria. **t½, elimination:** About 1 hr. Both unchanged drug (65% to 83%) and the inactive metabolite (20% to 32%) are excreted through the urine. Adjust dosage in impaired renal function.

USES

(1) Complicated appendicitis and peritonitis caused by *Escherichia coli, Klebsiella pneumoniae, Pseudomonas aeruginosa, Bacteroides fragilis, Bacteroides thetaiotaomicron, Peptostreptococcus* species, and viridans group streptococci. (2) Bacterial meningitis (in clients 3 months and older only) caused by *Streptococcus pneumoniae, Haemophilus influenzae* (β-lactamase- and non-β-lactamase-producing strains), and *Neisseria meningitidis.*

CONTRAINDICATIONS

Hypersensitivity to meropenem or other drugs in the same class. Those who have had anaphylactic reactions to β-lactams.

SPECIAL CONCERNS

Use with caution during lactation. Heart failure, kidney failure, seizures, and shock seen more frequently in those with a C_{CR} between 10–26 mL/min. Safety and efficacy have not been determined for children less than 3 months of age.

M

SIDE EFFECTS

GI: Diarrhea, N&V, constipation, abdominal pain, ***GI hemorrhage,*** pseudomembranous colitis, abdominal pain, melena, oral moniliasis, anorexia, cholestatic jaundice, jaundice, flatulence, ileus. **CNS:** Insomnia, agitation, headache, delirium, confusion, dizziness, nervousness, paresthesia, hallucinations, somnolence, anxiety, depression, ***seizures.*** **CV:** ***Heart failure, cardiac arrest, MI, pulmonary embolus,*** tachycardia, hypertension, bradycardia, hypotension, syncope. **Dermatologic:** Rash, pruritus, urticaria, sweating. **Body as a whole:** Pain, chest pain, ***sepsis, shock, hepatic failure,*** fever, abdominal enlargement, back pain. **GU:** Dysuria, kidney failure, presence of urine RBCs. **Respiratory:** Respiratory disorder, dyspnea. **At injection site:** Inflammation, phlebitis, thrombophlebitis, pain, edema. **Miscellaneous:** Anemia, peripheral edema, hypoxia, epistaxis, hemoperitoneum.

In children, the drug may cause diarrhea, rash, and vomiting when used for bacterial infections. Also, when used for meningitis in children, rash (diaper area moniliasis), diarrhea, oral moniliasis, and glossitis have been noted.

LABORATORY TEST CONSIDERATIONS

↑ Eosinophils, ALT, AST, alkaline phosphatase, LDH, bilirubin, creatinine, BUN. ↓ Hemoglobin, hematocrit, WBCs. ↑ or ↓ platelets. Prolonged or shortened PT, PTT. Positive direct or indirect Coombs' test.

HOW SUPPLIED

Powder for injection: 500 mg, 1 g

DOSAGE

• **IV**

Bacterial infections, meningitis.

Adults: 1 g IV q 8 hr given over 15–30 min or as an IV bolus injection (5–20 mL) over 3–5 min. In clients with impaired renal function, the dose is reduced as follows: C_{CR} 26–50 mL/min, 1 g q 12 hr; C_{CR} 10–25 mL/min, one-half the recommended dose q 12 hr; C_{CR} less than 10 mL/min, one-half the recommended dose q 24 hr. **Children, 3 months or older:** 20 or 40 mg/kg (depending on the type of infection) q 8 hr, up to a maximum of 2 g q 8 hr. For pediatric clients weighing 50 kg or more, administer 1 g q 8 hr for intra-abdominal infections and 2 g q 8 hr for meningitis given over 15–30 min or as an IV bolus injection (5–20 mL) over 3–5 min.

NURSING CONSIDERATIONS

SEE ALSO GENERAL ***NURSING CONSIDERATIONS*** FOR ***ANTI-INFECTIVES.***

ADMINISTRATION/STORAGE

IV 1. For IV use only. Do not mix with solutions containing other drugs.
2. Stability varies depending on the solution used to prepare the injection; consult package insert.
3. May give infusion over 15-30 min or by direct IV injection over 3-5 min.
4. Store at controlled room temperature of 20–25°C (68–77°F).

ASSESSMENT

1. Document onset, duration, and characteristics of symptoms.
2. Note any drug or PCN sensitivity.
3. Monitor CBC, cultures, liver and renal function studies.
4. Determine CNS disorders (i.e., brain lesions, seizure history or bacterial meningitis); monitor closely.
5. Reduce dose with renal dysfunction and in the elderly; monitor for seizures.
6. Do not administer with probenecid; may cause toxic drug blood levels.

OUTCOMES/EVALUATE

Resolution of infection

Mesalamine (5-Aminosalicylic acid)

(mes-**AL**-ah-meen)

PREGNANCY CATEGORY: B
CLASSIFICATION(S):
Anti-inflammatory drug
Rx: Asacol, Canasa, Pentasa, Rowasa
✱**Rx:** Mesasal, Novo-5 ASA, Quintasa, Salofalk

ACTION/KINETICS

Chemically related to acetylsalicylic acid. Acts locally in the colon to inhibit cyclo-oxygenase and therefore prostaglandin synthesis, resulting in a reduction of inflammation of colitis. Following PR administration, between 10% and 30% is absorbed and is excreted through the urine as the N-acetyl-5-aminosalicylic acid metabolite; the remainder is excreted in the feces. PO tablets are coated with an acrylic-based resin that prevents release of mesalamine until it reaches the terminal ileum and beyond. Approximately 28% of the drug found in tablets is absorbed with the remaining drug available for action in the colon. Capsules are ethylcellulose coated, controlled release designed to release the drug throughout the GI tract; from 20% to 30% is absorbed. **t½, mesalamine:** 0.5–1.5 hr; **t½, N-acetyl mesalamine:** 5–10 hr. **Time to reach maximum plasma levels:** 4–12 hr for both mesalamine and metabolite. Excreted mainly through the kidneys.

USES

PO: Maintaining remission and treatment of mild to moderate active ulcerative colitis. **Rectal:** Treatment of active mild to moderate distal ulcerative colitis, proctosigmoiditis, or proctitis.

CONTRAINDICATIONS

Hypersensitivity to salicylates.

SPECIAL CONCERNS

Use with caution in clients with sulfasalazine sensitivity, in those with impaired renal function, and during lactation. Safety and efficacy have not been established in children. Pyloric stenosis may delay the drug in reaching the colon.

SIDE EFFECTS

Sulfite sensitivity: Hives, wheezing, itching, ***anaphylaxis.*** **Intolerance syndrome:** Acute abdominal pain, cramping, bloody diarrhea, rash, fever, headache.

GI: Abdominal pain or discomfort, flatulence, cramps, dyspepsia, nausea, diarrhea, hemorrhoids, rectal pain/burning/urgency, constipation, bloating, worsening of colitis, eructation, pain following insertion of enema, vomiting (after PO use). **CNS:** Headache, dizziness, insomnia, fatigue, malaise, chills, fever, asthenia. **Respiratory:** Cold, sore throat; increased cough, pharyngitis, rhinitis following PO use. **Dermatologic:** Acne, pruritus, itching, rash. **Musculoskeletal:** Back pain, hypertonia, arthralgia, myalgia, leg/joint pain, arthritis. **Miscellaneous:** Flu-like symptoms, hair loss, anorexia, peripheral edema, urinary burning, sweating, pain, chest pain, conjunctivitis, dysmenorrhea, pancreatitis.

In addition to the preceding, PO use may result in the following side effects. **GI:** Anorexia, gastritis, gastroenteritis, cholecystitis, dry mouth, increased appetite, oral ulcers, tenesmus, perforated peptic ulcer, bloody diarrhea, duodenal ulcer, dysphagia, esophageal ulcer, fecal incontinence, GI bleeding, oral moniliasis, rectal bleeding, abnormal stool color and texture. **CNS:** Anxiety, depression, hyperesthesia, nervousness, confusion, peripheral neuropathy, somnolence, emotional lability, vertigo, paresthesia, migraine, tremor, transverse myelitis, Guillain-Barré syndrome. **Dermatologic:** Dry skin, psoriasis, pyoderma gangrenosum, urticaria, erythema nodosum, eczema, photosensitivity, lichen planus, nail disorder. **CV:** Pericarditis, myocarditis, vasodilation, palpitations, ***fatal myocarditis,*** chest pain, T-wave abnormalities. **GU:** Nephropathy, interstitial nephritis, urinary urgency, dysuria, hematuria, menorrhagia, epididymitis, amenorrhea, hypomenorrhea, metrorrhagia, nephrotic syndrome, urinary frequency, albuminuria, nephrotoxicity. **Hematologic:** ***Agranulocytosis,*** anemia, eosinophilia, leukopenia, thrombocytopenia, lymphadenopathy, thrombocythemia, ecchymosis. **Respiratory:** Worsening of asthma, sinusitis, interstitial pneumonitis, pulmonary infiltrates, fibrosing alveolitis. **Ophthalmologic:** Eye pain, blurred vision. **Miscellaneous:** Ear pain, tinnitus, taste perversion, neck pain, enlargement of abdomen, facial edema, gout, hypersensitivity pneumonitis, breast pain, Kawasaki-like syndrome.

M

LABORATORY TEST CONSIDERATIONS

↑ AST, ALT, BUN, LDH, alkaline phosphatase, serum creatinine, amylase, lipase, GTTP.

OD OVERDOSE MANAGEMENT

Symptoms: Salicylate toxicity manifested by tinnitus, vertigo, headache, confusion, drowsiness, sweating, hyperventilation, vomiting, and diarrhea. Severe toxicity results in disruption of electrolyte balance and blood pH, ***hyperthermia,*** and ***dehydration.*** *Treatment:* Therapy to treat salicylate toxicity, including emesis, gastric lavage, fluid and electrolyte replacement (if necessary), maintenance of adequate renal function.

HOW SUPPLIED

Capsule, Extended Release: 250 mg; *Rectal Suspension:* 4 g/60 mL; *Suppository:* 500 mg; *Tablet, Delayed Release:* 400 mg

DOSAGE

- **SUPPOSITORY**

One suppository (500 mg) b.i.d.

- **RECTAL SUSPENSION ENEMA**

4 g in 60 mL once daily for 3–6 weeks, usually given at bedtime. For maintenance, the drug can be given every other day or every third day at doses of 1–2 g.

- **CAPSULES, EXTENDED-RELEASE**

1 g (4 capsules) q.i.d. for a total daily dose of 4 g for up to 8 weeks.

- **TABLETS, ENTERIC-COATED**

800 mg t.i.d. for a total dose of 2.4 g/day for 6 weeks.

NURSING CONSIDERATIONS

ADMINISTRATION/STORAGE

1. Shake the bottle well to ensure suspension is homogeneous.
2. Beneficial effects using the suppository or enema may be seen within 3–21 days, with a full course of therapy lasting up to 6 weeks.

ASSESSMENT

1. Determine any sulfite sensitivity.
2. Document character/frequency of stools. Assess abdomen for bowel sounds, distension, pain/tenderness.
3. Monitor chemistries, liver and renal function studies, and abdominal films.

CLIENT/FAMILY TEACHING

1. Do not chew, take tablets whole, being careful not to break the outer coating.
2. Review technique for enema/suppository administration.
   - Prior to use, shake bottle until all contents are thoroughly mixed. Remove cap, insert tip into rectum, and squeeze steadily to completely discharge contents.
   - Lie on the left side with the lower leg extended and the upper right leg flexed forward. The knee-chest position may also be used for suppository administration.
   - Retain the enema for 8 hr to ensure proper absorption; may best be accomplished by administering at bedtime, after bowel movement, and retaining throughout the sleep cycle.
   - Remove the foil wrapper from the suppository and avoid excess handling as the suppository will melt at body temperature
   - Insert the pointed end first into the rectum
   - For maximal effect, retain suppository for 1–3 hr or more.
   - Protect bed linens with towels or rubber pads.
3. Hold drug and report severe abdominal pain, cramping, bloody diarrhea, rash, fever, or headache.
4. Avoid smoking and cold foods; increases bowel motility.
5. The therapy may last 3–6 weeks; follow as prescribed.

OUTCOMES/EVALUATE

- Relief of pain and diarrhea
- Normalization of bowel patterns

Mesna

(**MEZ**-nah)

PREGNANCY CATEGORY: B
CLASSIFICATION(S):
Antidote for ifosfamide toxicity
Rx: Mesnex
✱Rx: Uromitexan

ACTION/KINETICS

Ifosfamide is metabolized to products that cause hemorrhagic cystitis. In the kidney, mesna reacts chemically with these ifosfamide metabolites to cause their detoxification. Following IV use, mesna is rapidly oxidized to mesna disulfide (dimesna), which is eliminated by the kidneys. **t½ in blood, mesna:** 0.36 hr; **dimesna:** 1.17 hr. **t½, terminal:** 7 hr.

USES

Prophylactically to reduce the incidence of hemorrhagic cystitis caused by ifosfamide. *Investigational:* Reduce incidence of hemorrhagic cystitis caused by cyclophosphamide.

CONTRAINDICATIONS

Hypersensitivity to thiol compounds. Lactation.

SPECIAL CONCERNS

This product contains benzyl alcohol, which may cause a fatal "gasping syndrome" in infants.

SIDE EFFECTS

Since mesna is used with ifosfamide and other antineoplastic agents, it is difficult to identify those side effects due to mesna. The following symptoms are believed possible. **GI:** Bad taste in mouth (100%), soft stools, diarrhea, limb pain, headache, fatigue, nausea, hypotension, and allergy.

LABORATORY TEST CONSIDERATIONS

False + test for urinary ketones.

HOW SUPPLIED

Injection: 100 mg/mL

DOSAGE

• **IV BOLUS**

Prophylaxis of ifosfamide-induced hemorrhagic cystitis.

Dosage of mesna equal to 20% of the ifosfamide dose given at the time of ifosfamide and at 4 and 8 hr after each dose of ifosfamide. Thus, the total daily dose of mesna is 60% of the ifosfamide dose (e.g., an ifosfamide dose of 1.2 g/m² would mean doses of mesna would be 240 mg/m² at the time the ifosfamide dose was given, 240 mg/m² after 4 hr, and 240 mg/m² after 8 hr). This dosage should be given on each day that ifosfamide is administered.

NURSING CONSIDERATIONS

ADMINISTRATION/STORAGE

IV 1. If the dosage of ifosfamide is increased or decreased, adjust mesna dosage accordingly.

2. Reconstitute to a final concentration of 20 mg mesna/mL fluid by adding D5W, D5/0.2% NaCl, D5/0.33% NaCl, D5/0.45% NaCl, 0.9% NaCl, or RL injection.

3. Diluted solutions are stable for 24 hr at 25°C (77°F). However, when mesna is exposed to oxygen, dimesna is formed; use a new ampule for each administration.

4. Mesna is not compatible with cisplatin.

ASSESSMENT

1. Drug must be administered with each dose of ifosfamide and at 4- and 8-hr intervals following the initial dose to be effective against drug-induced hemorrhagic cystitis.

2. Analyze morning urine specimen each day before ifosfamide therapy.

3. Note age and any sensitivity to benzyl alcohol.

CLIENT/FAMILY TEACHING

1. Drug is used to prevent ifosfamide-induced hemorrhagic cystitis; will not prevent any other drug associated adverse reactions of toxicities.

2. May experience a bad taste in the mouth during drug therapy; use hard candy to mask taste.

3. N&V and diarrhea are frequent side effects of drug therapy; report those and headaches if persistent or bothersome.

OUTCOMES/EVALUATE

Prevention of ifosfamide-induced hemorrhagic cystitis

Metaproterenol sulfate (Orciprenaline sulfate)

(met-ah-proh-**TER**-ih-nohl)

PREGNANCY CATEGORY: C

CLASSIFICATION(S):

Sympathomimetic, direct-acting

Rx: Alupent

✱**Rx:** Alti-Orciprenaline, Apo-Orciprenaline, Tanta Orciprenaline

SEE ALSO *SYMPATHOMIMETIC DRUGS*.

M

ACTION/KINETICS

Markedly stimulates beta-2 receptors, resulting in relaxation of smooth muscles of the bronchial tree, as well as peripheral vasodilation. Minimal effects on beta-1 receptors. Similar to isoproterenol but with a longer duration of action and fewer side effects. **Onset, aerosol, hand bulb nebulizer or IPPB:** 5–30 min; **duration:** 1–6 or more hr after repeated doses. **PO: Onset,** 15–30 min; **peak effect:** 1 hr. **Duration:** 4 hr. Marked first-pass effect after PO use. Metabolized in the liver and excreted through the kidney.

USES

(1) Bronchodilator in asthma, bronchitis, emphysema, and other conditions associated with reversible bronchospasms. (2) Treatment of acute asthmatic attacks in children over 6 years of age (use only 5% solution for inhalation).

ADDITIONAL CONTRAINDICATIONS

PO in children less than 6 years old.

SPECIAL CONCERNS

Dosage of syrup or tablets not determined in children less than 6 years of age.

ADDITIONAL SIDE EFFECTS

GI: Diarrhea, bad taste or taste changes. **Respiratory:** Worsening of asthma, nasal congestion, hoarseness. **Miscellaneous:** Hypersensitivity reactions, rash, fatigue, backache, skin reactions.

DRUG INTERACTIONS

Possible potentiation of adrenergic effects if used before or after other sympathomimetic bronchodilators.

HOW SUPPLIED

Metered dose inhaler (MDI): 0.65 mg/inh; *Solution for Inhalation:* 0.4%, 0.6%, 5%; *Syrup:* 10 mg/5 mL; *Tablet:* 10 mg, 20 mg

DOSAGE

• SYRUP, TABLETS

Bronchodilation.

Adults and children over 27.2 kg or 9 years: 20 mg t.i.d.–q.i.d.; **children under 27.2 kg or 6–9 years of age:** 10 mg t.i.d.–q.i.d.; **children less than 6 years of age:** 1.3–2.6 mg/kg/day of the syrup has been studied.

• INHALATION USING HAND BULB NEBULIZER

Bronchodilation.

Usual dose is 10 inhalations (range: 5–15 inhalations) of undiluted 5% solution.

• NEBULIZER

Bronchodilation.

0.1 mL (0.1–0.2 mL) diluted in saline to 3 mL.

• IPPB

Bronchodilation.

0.3 mL (range: 0.2–0.3 mL) of 5% solution diluted to 2.5 mL saline or other diluent. Give the unit-dose vial as follows: **Adults:** 1 vial/nebulization treatment. Each 0.4% vial is equal to 0.2 mL of the 5% solution diluted to 2.5 mL with normal saline. Each 0.5% vial is equal to 0.3 mL of the 5% solution diluted to 2.5 mL with normal saline.

• MDI

Bronchodilation.

2–3 inhalations (1.30–2.25 mg) q 3–4 hr. Do not exceed a total daily dose of 12 inhalations (9 mg).

NURSING CONSIDERATIONS

SEE ALSO *ADRENERGIC BRONCHODILATORS* UNDER *SYMPATHOMIMETIC DRUGS*.

ADMINISTRATION/STORAGE

Refrigerate unit dose vials at 2–8°C (35–46°F).

CLIENT/FAMILY TEACHING

1. Review appropriate method for administration. Shake container before each use.
2. Report loss of effectiveness with prescribed dosage and frequency.
3. Store the inhalant solution at room temperature, but avoid excessive heat and light.
4. Do not use the solution if it is brown or shows a precipitate.
5. Do not use inhalant solutions more often than q 4 hr to relieve acute bronchospasms. In chronic bronchospastic disease, the dose can be given t.i.d.–q.i.d. A single dose of nebulized drug may not completely abort acute asthma attack. Allow 2 or more min between inhalations; rinse mouth with water after each use.
6. Stop smoking to help preserve lung function.

OUTCOMES/EVALUATE

- Improved airway exchange; ↑ oxygen saturation levels
- Relief of respiratory distress

Metaraminol bitartrate

(met-ah-**RAM**-ih-nohl)

PREGNANCY CATEGORY: C
CLASSIFICATION(S):
Sympathomimetic, indirect and direct-acting
Rx: Aramine

SEE ALSO *SYMPATHOMIMETIC DRUGS.*

ACTION/KINETICS
Indirectly releases norepinephrine from storage sites and directly stimulates primarily alpha receptors and, to a slight extent, beta-1 receptors. Causes marked increases in BP due primarily to vasoconstriction and to a slight increase in CO. Reflex bradycardia is also manifested. Increases venous tone, causes pulmonary vasoconstriction, and increases pulmonary pressure, even if CO is decreased. CNS stimulation usually does not occur. **Onset: IV:** 1–2 min; **IM:** 10 min; **SC:** 5–20 min. **Duration, IV:** 20 min; **IM, SC:** About 60 min. Metabolized in the liver and excreted through the urine and feces. Enhance urinary excretion of unchanged drug by acidifying the urine.

USES
(1) Hypotension associated with surgery, spinal anesthesia, hemorrhage, trauma, infections, tumors, and adverse drug reactions. (2) Adjunct to the treatment of either septicemia or cardiogenic shock. *Investigational:* Injected intracavernosally to treat priapism due to phentolamine, papaverine, or other causes.

CONTRAINDICATIONS
Use with cyclopropane or halothane anesthesia (unless clinical conditions mandate such use). As a substitute for blood or fluid replacement.

SPECIAL CONCERNS
Use with caution in cirrhosis, malaria, heart or thyroid disease, hypertension, diabetes, or during lactation. Hypertension and ischemic ECG changes may occur when used to treat priapism. Use is not a substitute for the replacement of blood, plasma, fluids, and electrolytes.

ADDITIONAL SIDE EFFECTS
Rapidly induced hypertension may cause acute pulmonary edema, arrhythmias, and ***cardiac arrest.*** Due to its long duration of action, cumulative effects are possible with prolonged increases in BP.

DRUG INTERACTIONS
Digitalis glycosides / ↑ Risk of ectopic arrhythmias
Furazolidone / Possible hypertensive crisis and IC hemorrhage
Guanethidine / Antihypertensive drug effects may be partially or totally reversed
Halogenated hydrocarbons / Sensitization of the heart to catecholamines; use of metaraminol may cause serious arrhythmias
MAO Inhibitors / Possible hypertensive crisis and IC hemorrhage
Oxytocic drugs / Possiblity of severe, persistent hypertension
Tricyclic antidepressants / ↓ Pressor effect of metaraminol

HOW SUPPLIED
Injection: 10 mg/mL

DOSAGE

- **IM, SC**

Prophylaxis of hypotension.

Adults: 2–10 mg given IM or SC; **pediatric:** 0.01 mg/kg (3 mg/m²) IM or SC.

- **IV INFUSION**

Hypotension.

Adults: 15–100 mg in 250–500 mL of 0.9% NaCl injection or 5% dextrose injection by IV infusion at a rate to maintain desired BP (up to 500 mg/500 mL has been used). **Pediatric:** 0.4 mg/kg (12 mg/m²) by IV infusion in a solution containing 1 mg/25 mL 0.9% NaCl injection or 5% dextrose injection.

M

• **DIRECT IV**

Severe shock.

Adults: 0.5–5.0 mg by direct IV followed by IV infusion of 15–100 mg in 250–500 mL fluid. **Pediatric:** 0.01 mg/kg (0.3 mg/m²) by direct IV.

• **ENDOTRACHEAL TUBE**

If IV access is not possible, metaraminol may be given by an ET tube. Perform five quick insufflations; forcefully expel 5 mg diluted to 10 mL into the ET tube and follow with five quick insufflations.

NURSING CONSIDERATIONS

SEE ALSO *NURSING CONSIDERATIONS* FOR *SYMPATHOMIMETIC DRUGS*.

ADMINISTRATION/STORAGE

IV 1. Administer with an infusion device during IV therapy for accurate drug control and titration.
2. The following solutions may be used to dilute metaraminol: NaCl, D5W, Ringer's injection, RL injection, 5% dextran in saline, Normosol-R pH 7.4, and Normosol-M in 5% dextrose injection.
3. Avoid storage at temperatures below -20°C (-4°F).
4. Use infusion solutions within 24 hr.
5. Have phentolamine in case of extravasation (5-10 mg in 10-15 mL NSS used to infiltrate affected area to prevent necrosis).

ASSESSMENT

1. Document type and onset of symptoms and precipitating factors.
2. Take BP every 15 min. Monitor ECG, I&O, and VS. Ensure adequate hydration.
3. Assess IV site frequently; extravasation may result in tissue necrosis.
4. Acidifying the urine enhances urinary drug excretion.

OUTCOMES/EVALUATE

↑ BP with hypotensive episode

Metformin hydrochloride

(met-**FOR**-min)

PREGNANCY CATEGORY: B
CLASSIFICATION(S):
Antidiabetic, oral; biguanide

Rx: Glucophage, Glucophage XR
✱Rx: Apo-Metformin, Gen-Metformin, Glycon, Novo-Metformin, Nu-Metformin, Rho-Metformin

ACTION/KINETICS
Decreases hepatic glucose production, decreases intestinal absorption of glucose, and increases peripheral uptake and utilization of glucose. Does not cause hypoglycemia in either diabetic or nondiabetic clients, and it does not cause hyperinsulinemia. Insulin secretion remains unchanged, while fasting insulin levels and day-long plasma insulin response may decrease. In contrast to sulfonylureas, the body weight of clients treated with metformin remains stable or may decrease somewhat. Food decreases and slightly delays the absorption of metformin. Negligibly bound to plasma protein; steady-state plasma levels (less than 1 mcg/mL) are reached within 24–48 hr. Excreted unchanged in the urine; no biliary excretion. **t½, plasma elimination:** 6.2 hr. The plasma and blood half-lives are prolonged in decreased renal function.

USES
(1) Alone as an adjunct to diet to lower blood glucose in clients having NIDDM whose blood glucose cannot be managed satisfactorily via diet alone. (2) Metformin may be used concomitantly with a sulfonylurea when diet and metformin or a sulfonylurea alone do not result in adequate control of blood glucose. Use with insulin in type 2 diabetes.

CONTRAINDICATIONS
Renal disease or dysfunction (serum creatinine levels greater than 1.5 mg/dL in males and greater than 1.4 mg/dL in females) or abnormal C_{CR} due to cardiovascular collapse, acute MI, or septicemia. In clients undergoing radiologic studies using iodinated contrast media, because use of such products may cause alteration of renal function, leading to acute renal failure and lactic acidosis. Acute or chronic metabolic acidosis, including diabetic ketoacidosis, with or without coma. Lactation.

SPECIAL CONCERNS
Cardiovascular collapse, acute CHF, acute MI, and other conditions characterized by hypoxia have been associated with ***lactic acidosis,*** which may also be caused by metformin. Use of oral hypoglycemic agents may increase the risk of ***cardiovascular mortality.*** Although hypoglycemia does not usually occur with metformin, it may result with deficient caloric intake, with strenuous exercise not supplemented by increased intake of calories, or when metformin is taken with sulfonylureas or alcohol. Because of age-related decreases in renal function, use with caution as age increases. Safety and efficacy have not been determined in children.

SIDE EFFECTS
Metabolic: ***Lactic acidosis*** (fatal in approximately 50% of cases). **GI:** Diarrhea, N&V, abdominal bloating, flatulence, anorexia, unpleasant or metallic taste. **Hematologic:** Asymptomatic subnormal serum vitamin B_{12} levels.

OD OVERDOSE MANAGEMENT
Symptoms: Lactic acidosis.

DRUG INTERACTIONS
Alcohol / ↑ Metformin effect on lactate metabolism
Cimetidine / ↑ (by 60%) Peak metformin plasma and whole blood levels
Furosemide / ↑ Metformin plasma and blood levels; also, metformin ↓ the half-life of furosemide
Iodinated contrast media / ↑ Risk of acute renal failure and lactic acidosis
Nifedipine / ↑ Absorption of metformin, leading to ↑ plasma metformin levels
Propantheline / ↑ Absorption of metformin R/T slowed GI motility

HOW SUPPLIED
Tablet: 500 mg, 850 mg, 1,000 mg; *Tablet, Extended-Release:* 500 mg

DOSAGE

• **TABLETS**
NIDDM.

Adults, using 500-mg tablet: Starting dose is one 500-mg tablet b.i.d. given with the morning and evening meals. Dosage increases may be made in increments of 500 mg every week, given in divided doses, up to a maximum of 2,500 mg/day. If a 2,500-mg daily dose is required, it may be better tolerated when given in divided doses t.i.d. with meals. The extended-release tablet is given once daily. **Adults, using 850-mg tablet:** Starting dose is 850 mg once daily given with the morning meal. Dosage increases may be made in increments of 850 mg every other week, given in divided doses, up to a maximum of 2,550 mg/day. **Usual maintenance dose:** 850 mg b.i.d. with the morning and evening meals. However, some clients may require 850 mg t.i.d. with meals.

NURSING CONSIDERATIONS

ADMINISTRATION/STORAGE

1. Individualize dosage based on tolerance and effectiveness.
2. Give with meals starting at a low dose with gradual escalation. This will reduce GI side effects and allow determination of the minimal dose necessary for adequate control of blood glucose.
3. No transition period is required when transferring from standard oral hypoglycemic drugs (other than chlorpropamide) to metformin. When transferring from chlorpropamide, exercise caution during the first 2 weeks because of chlorpropamide's long duration of action.
4. If the maximum dose of metformin for 4 weeks does not provide adequate control of blood glucose, gradual addition of an oral sulfonylurea (data are available for glyburide, chlorpropamide, tolbutamide, and glipizide) may be considered, while maintaining the maximum dose of metformin. The desired control of blood glucose may be attained by adjusting the dose of each drug.
5. If no response to 1–3 months of concomitant metformin and oral sulfonylurea therapy, consider initiating insulin therapy and discontinuing the oral agents.
6. The initial and maintenance doses of metformin in geriatric and debilitated

M

clients should be conservative because of the potential for decreased renal function. Do not titrate these clients to the maximum dose.

ASSESSMENT

1. Document age at diabetes onset, previous therapies utilized, and the outcome.
2. Monitor CBC, BS, electrolytes, HbA1-C, urinalysis, liver and renal function studies. Assess for liver or renal failure; may precipitate lactic acidosis (i.e., serum lactate levels greater than 5 mmol/L, decreased blood pH, increased anion gap).
3. Withhold for surgery and iodinated procedures; administer when normal diet resumed or the day after the procedure. (usually 48 hr before and 48 hr after)
4. If anemia develops, exclude vitamin B_{12} deficiency; may interfere with B_{12} absorption.
5. A small dose with insulin therapy may enhance glucose control.

CLIENT/FAMILY TEACHING

1. Take with food to diminish GI upset.
2. May cause a metallic taste; should subside.
3. Regular exercise, decreased caloric intake, and weight loss are required to reduce blood glucose levels; medication neither replaces nor excuses compliance with these modalities.
4. Inadequate caloric intake or strenuous exercise without caloric replacement may precipitate hypoglycemia.
5. Do regular blood sugar monitoring (fingersticks), especially 1-2 hr after meals and maintain record for provider review.
6. Avoid alcohol and any situations that may precipitate dehydration.
7. Consume plenty of fluids; report when illnesses with fever, vomiting, and diarrhea are persistent/severe.
8. Stop drug and immediately report any symptoms of difficulty breathing, severe weakness, muscle pain, increased sleepiness, or sudden increased abdominal distress.

OUTCOMES/EVALUATE

- Control of BS; prevention of microvascular complications
- HbA1-C < 7%

M

Methadone hydrochloride

(METH-ah-dohn)

PREGNANCY CATEGORY: C
CLASSIFICATION(S):
Narcotic analgesic
Rx: Dolophine, Methadone HCl Diskets, Methadone HCl Intensol, Methadose
✱Rx: Metadol **C-II**

SEE ALSO *NARCOTIC ANALGESICS*.

ACTION/KINETICS

Produces only mild euphoria, which is the reason it is used as a heroin withdrawal substitute and for maintenance programs. Produces physical dependence; withdrawal symptoms develop more slowly and are less intense but more prolonged than those associated with morphine. Does not produce sedation or narcosis. Not effective for preoperative or obstetric anesthesia. Only one-half as potent PO as when given parenterally. **Onset:** 30–60 min. **Peak effects:** 30–60 min. **Duration:** 4–6 hr. **t½:** 15–30 hr. Both the duration and half-life increase with repeated use due to cumulative effects.

USES

Severe pain. Detoxification and maintenance of narcotic dependence.

ADDITIONAL CONTRAINDICATIONS

IV use, liver disease, during pregnancy, in children, or in obstetrics (due to long duration of action and chance of respiratory depression in the neonate). Use to relieve general anxiety.

SPECIAL CONCERNS

Use with caution during lactation.

ADDITIONAL SIDE EFFECTS

Marked constipation, excessive sweating, pulmonary edema, choreic movements.

LABORATORY TEST CONSIDERATIONS

↑ Immunoglobulin G.

ADDITIONAL DRUG INTERACTIONS

Cimetidine / ↑ Respiratory and CNS depression
Desipramine / ↑ Desipramine blood levels
Nelfinavir / ↓ Methadone plasma levels

Phenytoin / ↓ Methadone effect R/T ↑ liver metabolism
Protease inhibitors / ↑ Respiratory and CNS depression
Ritonavir / ↓ Methadone plasma levels
Rifampin / ↓ Methadone effect R/T ↑ liver metabolism; may precipitate withdrawal

HOW SUPPLIED

Injection: 10 mg/mL; *Oral Concentrate:* 10 mg/mL; *Oral Solution:* 5 mg/5 mL, 10 mg/5 mL; *Tablet:* 5 mg, 10 mg; *Tablet, Dispersable:* 40 mg

DOSAGE

• TABLETS, DISPERSABLE TABLETS, ORAL SOLUTION, ORAL CONCENTRATE, INJECTION

Analgesia.

Adults, individualized: 2.5–10 mg q 3–4 hr, although higher doses may be necessary for severe pain or due to development of tolerance.

Narcotic withdrawal.

Initial: 15–20 mg/day PO (some may require 40 mg/day); **then,** depending on need of the client, slowly decrease dosage.

Maintenance following narcotic withdrawal.

Adults, individualized, initial: 20–40 mg PO 4–8 hr after heroin is stopped; **then,** adjust dosage as required up to 120 mg/day.

NURSING CONSIDERATIONS

SEE ALSO *NURSING CONSIDERATIONS* FOR *NARCOTIC ANALGESICS*.

ADMINISTRATION/STORAGE

1. Dilute solution in at least 90 mL of water prior to administration.
2. If taking dispersible tablets, dilute in 120 mL of water, orange juice, citrus-flavored drink, or other acidic fruit drink. Allow at least 1 min for complete drug dispersion.
3. For repeated analgesic doses, IM administration is preferred over SC administration due to local irritation. Inspect sites for signs of irritation.
4. Duration of treatment for detoxification purposes is no longer than 21 days. Do not repeat treatment for 4 weeks.
5. If transferring from levomethadyl to methadone, wait 48 hr after the last dose of levomethadyl before starting methadone.

CLIENT/FAMILY TEACHING

1. If ambulatory and not suffering acute pain, side effects may be more pronounced.
2. Avoid alcohol. Do not perform activites that require mental alertness until drug effects realized; causes sedation, drowsiness, impaired vision.
3. Report N&V; a lower drug dose may relieve symptoms. Practice reliable contraception.
4. To minimize constipation, exercise regularly and increase intake of fluids, fruit, and bulk.
5. For chronic pain control, use as directed. May adversely affect employment R/T type of drug consumed and drug association. Do not stop suddenly. Drug causes tolerance and dependence; must be weaned slowly.
6. For clients on narcotic withdrawal therapy, store drug out of the reach of children. Continue to attend group therapy as with Narcotics Anonymous. Identify social service groups for assistance in child care, food and living arrangements, and expenses.

OUTCOMES/EVALUATE

- Control of severe pain
- Detoxification and maintenance in narcotic-dependent individual

Methenamine hippurate

(meh-**THEEN**-ah-meen)

PREGNANCY CATEGORY: C
Rx: Hiprex, Urex

Methenamine mandelate

(meh-**THEEN**-ah-meen)

PREGNANCY CATEGORY: C
🍁**Rx:** Mandelamine
CLASSIFICATION(S):
Urinary anti-infective

M

ACTION/KINETICS

Converted in an acid medium into ammonia and formaldehyde (the active principle), which denatures protein. Formaldehyde levels in the urine may be bacteriostatic or bactericidal, depending on the pH; it is most effective when the urine has a pH value of 5.5 or less, which is maintained by using the hippurate or mandelate salt. Readily absorbed from GI tract, but up to 60% may be hydrolyzed by gastric acid if tablets are not enteric-coated. To be effective, urinary formaldehyde concentration must be greater than 25 mcg/mL. **Peak levels of formaldehyde:** 2 hr if using hippurate and 3–8 hr if using mandelate (if urinary pH is 5.5 or less) **t½:** 3–6 hr. Seventy to 90% of drug and metabolites excreted in urine within 24 hr.

USES

Acute, chronic, and recurrent UTIs by susceptible organisms, especially gram-negative organisms including *Escherichia coli.* As a prophylactic before urinary tract instrumentation. Never used as sole agent in the treatment of acute infections.

M

CONTRAINDICATIONS

Renal insufficiency, severe liver damage, severe dehydration. Concurrent use of sulfonamides as an insoluble precipitate may form with formaldehyde.

SPECIAL CONCERNS

Use with caution in gout (methenamine may cause urate crystals to precipitate in the urine).

SIDE EFFECTS

GI: N&V, diarrhea, anorexia, cramps, stomatitis. **GU:** Hematuria, albuminuria, crystalluria, dysuria, urinary frequency or urgency, bladder irritation. **Dermatologic:** Skin rashes, urticaria, pruritus, erythematous eruptions. **Other:** Headache, dyspnea, edema, lipoid pneumonitis.

LABORATORY TEST CONSIDERATIONS

False + urinary glucose with Benedict's solution. Drug interferes with determination of urinary catecholamines and estriol levels by acid hydrolysis technique (enzymatic techniques not affected). False + catecholamines, hydroxycorticosteroids, vanillylmandelic acid; false – 5-hydroxyindoleacetic acid.

OD OVERDOSE MANAGEMENT

Treatment: Absorption following overdose may be minimized by inducing vomiting or by gastric lavage, followed by activated charcoal. Fluids should be forced.

DRUG INTERACTIONS

Acetazolamide / ↓ Methenamine effect R/T inhibition of conversion to formaldehyde
Sodium bicarbonate / ↓ Methenamine effect R/T inhibition of conversion to formaldehyde
Sulfonamides / ↑ Chance of sulfonamide crystalluria R/T acid urine produced by methenamine
Thiazide diuretics / ↓ Methenamine effect R/T ↑ urine alkalinity produced by thiazides

HOW SUPPLIED

Methenanamine hippurate: *Tablet:* 1 g **Methenamine mandelate:** *Tablet, Enteric Coated:* 0.5 g, 1 g; *Suspension:* 0.5 g/5 mL

DOSAGE

HIPPURATE

• **TABLETS**

Adults and children over 12 years: 1 g b.i.d. in the morning and evening; **children, 6–12 years:** 0.5 g b.i.d.

MANDELATE

• **ORAL SUSPENSION, ENTERIC-COATED TABLETS**

Adults: 1 g q.i.d. after meals and at bedtime; **children 6–12 years:** 0.5 g q.i.d.; **children under 6 years:** 0.25 g/13.6 kg q.i.d.

NURSING CONSIDERATIONS

SEE ALSO *GENERAL NURSING CONSIDERATIONS* FOR *ANTI-INFECTIVES*.

ASSESSMENT

1. Document indications for therapy, onset and characteristics of symptoms.
2. Note any history of gout.
3. List other agents prescribed. Urine may become turbid and full of sediment when administered with sulfamethizole; avoid co-administration. Monitor urine pH- a pH of 5 or less is required for optimum drug response. (May use ascorbic acid or ammonium chloride to lower pH).

4. Obtain baseline C&S. Monitor urine for evidence of hematuria and/or albuminuria.
5. Maintain acidic urine when treating *Proteus* or *Pseudomonas* infections.
6. Ensure adequate hydration; monitor renal and LFTs.
7. Oral suspensions have a vegetable oil base; take particular care with the elderly or debilitated to prevent lipid pneumonia.

CLIENT/FAMILY TEACHING

1. May take with food if GI upset occurs.
2. Consume 1.5–2 L/day of fluids.
3. To maintain an acidic urine, alkalizing foods (e.g., milk products) or medication (e.g., acetazolamide, bicarbonate) should be avoided.
4. Foods (such as prunes, plums, and cranberry juice) may help maintain acid urine. Drugs such as ascorbic acid, methionine, ammonium chloride, or sodium diphosphate may additionally be required.
5. Test urine pH; keep at 5.5 or lower.
6. With high dosage, report any evidence of bladder irritation or painful and frequent micturition.
7. Report adverse effects of N&V, skin rash, tinnitus, and muscle cramps as these may require termination of drug therapy.

OUTCOMES/EVALUATE

- Resolution of UTI
- Negative urine C&S results

Methocarbamol

(meth-oh-**KAR**-bah-mohl)

CLASSIFICATION(S):
Skeletal muscle relaxant, centrally-acting
Rx: Robaxin-750, Robaxin

SEE ALSO SKELETAL MUSCLE RELAXANTS, CENTRALLY ACTING.

ACTION/KINETICS
Beneficial effect may be related to the sedative properties of the drug. Has no direct effect on the contractile mechanism of striated muscle, the motor endplate, or the nerve fiber and it does not directly relax tense skeletal muscles. Of limited usefulness. May be given IM or IV in polyethylene glycol 300 (50% solution). PO therapy should be initiated as soon as possible. **Onset:** 30 min. **Peak plasma levels:** 2 hr after 2 g. **$t^{1/2}$:** 1–2 hr. Inactive metabolites are excreted in the urine.

USES
Adjunct for the relief of acute, painful musculoskeletal conditions (e.g., sprains, strains). Adjunct in tetanus.

CONTRAINDICATIONS
Hypersensitivity, when muscle spasticity is required to maintain upright position, seizure disorders, pregnancy, lactation, children under 12 years. Renal disease (parenteral dosage form only since it contains polyethylene glycol 300).

SPECIAL CONCERNS
Use with caution in epilepsy and during lactation. Use the injectable form with caution in suspected or known epileptics.

SIDE EFFECTS

- **FOLLOWING PO USE.**

CNS: Dizziness, drowsiness, lightheadedness, vertigo, lassitude, headache. **GI:** Nausea. **Miscellaneous:** Allergic symptoms including rash, urticaria, pruritus, conjunctivitis, nasal congestion, blurred vision, fever.

- **FOLLOWING IV USE (IN ADDITION TO THE PRECEDING).**

CV: Hypotension, bradycardia, syncope. **CNS:** Fainting, mild muscle incoordination. **Miscellaneous:** Metallic taste, GI upset, flushing, nystagmus, double vision, thrombophlebitis, sloughing or pain at injection site, ***anaphylaxis.***

LABORATORY TEST CONSIDERATIONS
Color interference in 5-HIAA and VMA.

OD OVERDOSE MANAGEMENT
Symptoms: CNS depression, including coma, is often seen when methocarbamol is used with alcohol or other CNS depressants. *Treatment:* Supportive, depending on the symptoms.

DRUG INTERACTIONS
Central nervous system depressants (including alcohol) may ↑ the effect of methocarbamol.

M

HOW SUPPLIED
Injection: 100 mg/mL; *Tablet:* 500 mg, 750 mg

DOSAGE

• **TABLETS**

Skeletal muscle disorders.

Adults, initial: 1.5 g q.i.d. for the first 2–3 days (for severe conditions, 8 g/day may be given); **maintenance:** 1 g q.i.d., 0.75 g q 4 hr, or 1.5 g t.i.d.

• **IM, IV**

Skeletal muscle disorders.

Adults, usual initial: 1 g; in severe cases, up to 2–3 g may be necessary. **IV administration should not exceed 3 days.**

Tetanus.

Adults: 1–2 g IV, initially, into tube of previously inserted indwelling needle. An additional 1–2 g may be added to the infusion for a total initial dose of 3 g. May be given q 6 hr (up to 24 g/day may be needed) until PO administration is feasible. **Pediatric, initial:** 15 mg/kg given into tube of previously inserted indwelling needle. Dose may be repeated q 6 hr.

M

NURSING CONSIDERATIONS

SEE ALSO NURSING CONSIDERATIONS FOR SKELETAL MUSCLE RELAXANTS.

ADMINISTRATION/STORAGE

1. With IM, inject no more than 5 mL into each gluteal region.
2. When administering IM to a child, use the vastus lateralis; with adults, select a large muscle mass. Document and rotate sites.
IV 3. If administered IV, do not exceed a rate of 3 mL/min.
4. For IV drip, one ampule may be added to no more than 250 mL of NaCl or D5W.
5. With IV, check frequently for infiltration. Extravasation of fluid may cause sloughing/thrombophlebitis.
6. Before removing IV, clamp off the tubing to prevent extravasation of the hypertonic solution, which may cause thrombophlebitis.

ASSESSMENT

Note indications for therapy, onset and characteristics of symptoms. Review xray if indicated and note assessment findings.

INTERVENTIONS

1. Monitor VS. Maintain a recumbent position during IV administration for 10–15 min after injection to minimize side effects of postural hypotension.
2. Keep side rails up and supervise ambulation of elderly clients or those who have been immobilized prior to drug therapy.
3. Observe seizure precautions.

CLIENT/FAMILY TEACHING

1. Take exactly as directed. Do not exceed dosage parameters. Drugs is usually tapered off over 1-2 weeks with extended use.
2. Drug causes drowsiness; do not operate dangerous machinery and equipment or drive a car.
3. Rise slowly from a recumbent position and dangle legs before standing up to minimize hypotensive effects.
4. Diplopia, blurred vision, and nystagmus may occur; report if persistent.
5. Report any skin eruptions/rash, or itching; allergic responses which may require drug withdrawal.
6. Nausea, anorexia, and a metallic taste may occur; report if severe or interferes with nutrition.
7. Avoid alcohol/CNS depressants.
8. Urine may turn black, brown, or green upon standing; will resolve once drug stopped.
9. Drug is for short term use during acute sprain/strain. Use as needed and perform exercises/stretching as directed. Complete PT if ordered.

OUTCOMES/EVALUATE

• Improvement in muscle spasticity, pain, and mobility
• Control of tetanus-induced neuromuscular manifestations

Methotrexate, Methotrexate sodium (MTX)

(meth-oh-**TREKS**-ayt)

PREGNANCY CATEGORY: D (X FOR PREGNANT PSORIATIC OR RHEUMATOID ARTHRITIS CLIENTS)

CLASSIFICATION(S):
Antineoplastic, antimetabolite
Rx: Amethopterin, Rheumatrex Dose Pack, Trexall, Methotrexate LPF, Rheumatrex

SEE ALSO *ANTINEOPLASTIC AGENTS*.

ACTION/KINETICS
Cell-cycle specific for the S phase of cell division. Acts by inhibiting dihydrofolate reductase, which prevents reduction of dihydrofolate to tetrahydrofolate; this results in decreased synthesis of purines and consequently DNA. The most sensitive cells are bone marrow, fetal cells, dermal epithelium, urinary bladder, buccal mucosa, intestinal mucosa, and malignant cells. When used for rheumatoid arthritis it may affect immune function. Variable absorption from GI tract. **Peak serum levels, IM:** 30–60 min; **PO:** 1–2 hr. **t½:** initial, 1 hr; intermediate, 2–3 hr; final, 8–12 hr. May accumulate in the body. Excreted by kidney (55%–92% in 24 hr). Renal function tests are recommended before initiation of therapy; perform daily leukocyte counts during therapy.

USES
(1) Certain carcinomas including, uterine choriocarcinoma (curative), chorioadenoma destruens, hydatidiform mole, acute lymphocytic and lymphoblastic leukemia, lymphosarcoma, and other disseminated neoplasms in children. (2) Meningeal leukemia. (3) Some beneficial effect in regional chemotherapy of head and neck tumors, breast tumors, and lung cancer. (4) In combination for advanced stage non-Hodgkin's lymphoma. (5) Advanced mycosis fungoides. (6) High doses followed by leucovorin rescue in combination with other drugs for prolonging relapse-free survival in nonmetastatic osteosarcoma in individuals who have had surgical resection or amputation for the primary tumor. (7) Severe, recalcitrant, disabling psoriasis. (8) Rheumatoid arthritis (severe, active, classical, or definite) in clients who have had inadequate response to NSAIDs and at least one or more antirheumatic drugs (disease modifying). *Investigational:* Severe corticosteroid-dependent asthma to reduce corticosteroid dosage; adjunct to treat osteosarcoma. Psoriatic arthritis and Reiter's disease.

CONTRAINDICATIONS
Psoriasis clients with kidney or liver disease; blood dyscrasias as hypoplasia, thrombocytopenia, anemia, or leukopenia. Alcoholism, alcoholic liver disease, or other chronic liver disease. Immunodeficiency syndromes. Pregnancy and lactation.

SPECIAL CONCERNS
Use with caution in impaired renal function and elderly clients. Use with extreme caution in the presence of active infection and in debilitated clients. Safety and efficacy have not been established for juvenile rheumatoid arthritis.

ADDITIONAL SIDE EFFECTS
Severe bone marrow depression. Hepatotoxicity, fibrosis, cirrhosis. ***Hemorrhagic enteritis, intestinal ulceration or perforation,*** acne, ecchymosis, hematemesis, melena, increased pigmentation, diabetes, leukoencephalopathy, chronic interstitial obstructive pulmonary disease, acute renal failure. Intrathecal use may result in chemical arachnoiditis, transient paresis, or ***seizures.*** Concomitant exposure to sunlight may aggravate psoriasis; painful plaque erosions when used to treat psoriasis. Bone and soft tissue necrosis following radiation therapy.

OD OVERDOSE MANAGEMENT
Symptoms: See *Antineoplastic Agents*. *Treatment:* Leucovorin, given as soon as possible, may decrease toxic effects. The dose used is 10 mg/m² PO or parenterally followed by 10 mg/m² PO q 6 hr for 72 hr. Charcoal hemoperfusion or high-flux dialysis will reduce serum levels. In massive overdosage, routine hemodialysis and hemoperfusion are ineffective. Hydration and urinary alkalinization are needed to prevent precipitation of methotrexate and metabolites in the renal tubules.

DRUG INTERACTIONS
Alcohol, ethyl / Additive hepatotoxicity; combination can → coma

M

Aminoglycosides, oral / ↓ Absorption of PO methotrexate
Anticoagulants, oral / Additive hypoprothrombinemia
Azathioprine / ↑ Risk of hepatotoxicity; monitor closely
Chloramphenicol / ↑ Methotrexate effect by ↓ plasma protein binding
Doxycycline / GI and hematologic toxicity after high dose methotrexate
Etretinate / Possible hepatotoxicity if used together for psoriasis; monitor closely
Folic acid–containing vitamin preparations / ↓ Methotrexate response
Ibuprofen / ↑ Methotrexate effect by ↓ renal secretion
NSAIDs / Possible fatal interaction
PABA / ↑ Methotrexate effect by ↓ plasma protein binding
Phenytoin / ↑ Methotrexate effect by ↓ plasma protein binding
Probenecid / ↑ Methotrexate effect by ↓ renal clearance
Procarbazine / Possible ↑ nephrotoxicity
Pyrimethamine / ↑ Methotrexate toxicity
Salicylates (aspirin) / ↑ Methotrexate effect by ↓ plasma protein binding; also, salicylates ↓ methotrexate renal excretion
Smallpox vaccination / Methotrexate impairs immunologic response to smallpox vaccine
Sulfasalazine / ↑ Risk of hepatotoxicity; monitor closely
Sulfonamides / ↑ Methotrexate effect by ↓ plasma protein binding
Tetracyclines / ↑ Methotrexate effect by ↓ plasma protein binding
Thiopurines / ↑ Plasma drug levels

HOW SUPPLIED

Injection: 2.5 mg/mL, 25 mg/mL; *Powder for injection, lyophilized:* 20 mg/vial, 50 mg/vial, 1 g/vial; *Tablet:* 2.5 mg, 5 mg, 7.5 mg, 10 mg, 15 mg

DOSAGE

• TABLETS (METHOTREXATE). IM, IV, IA, INTRATHECAL (METHOTREXATE SODIUM)

Choriocarcinoma and similar trophoblastic diseases.

Dose individualized. PO, IM: 15–30 mg/day for 5 days. May be repeated 3–5 times with 1-week rest period between courses.

Acute lymphatic (lymphoblastic) leukemia.

Initial: 3.3 mg/m² (with 60 mg/m² prednisone daily); **maintenance: PO, IM,** 30 mg/m² 2 times/week or **IV,** 2.5 mg/kg q 14 days.

Meningeal leukemia.

Intrathecal: 12 mg/m² q 2–5 days until cell count returns to normal.

Lymphomas.

PO: 10–25 mg/day for 4–8 days for several courses of treatment with 7- to 10-day rest periods between courses.

Mycosis fungoides.

PO: 2.5–10 mg/day for several weeks or months; **alternatively, IM:** 50 mg once weekly or 25 mg twice weekly.

Lymphosarcoma.

0.625–2.5 mg/kg/day in combination with other drugs.

Osteosarcoma.

Used in combination with other drugs, including doxorubicin, cisplatin, bleomycin, cyclophosphamide, and dactinomycin. **Usual IV starting dose for methotrexate:** 12 g/m²; dose may be increased to 15 g/m² to achieve a peak serum level of 10^{-3} mol/L at the end of the methotrexate infusion.

Psoriasis.

Adults, usual: PO, IM, IV, 10–25 mg/week, continued until beneficial response observed. Weekly dose should not exceed 50 mg. **Alternate regimens: PO,** 2.5 mg q 12 hr for three doses or q 8 hr for four doses each week (not to exceed 30 mg/week); or **PO,** 2.5 mg daily for 5 days followed by 2 days of rest (dose should not exceed 6.25 mg/day). Once beneficial effects are noted, reduce dose to lowest possible level with longest rest periods between doses.

Rheumatoid arthritis.

Initial: Single PO doses of 7.5 mg/week or divided PO doses of 2.5 mg at 12-hr intervals for three doses given once a week; **then,** adjust dosage to achieve optimum response, not to exceed a total weekly dose of 20 mg. Once response has been reached, reduce the dose to the lowest possible effective dose.

NURSING CONSIDERATIONS

SEE ALSO *NURSING CONSIDERATIONS FOR ANTINEOPLASTIC AGENTS*.

ADMINISTRATION/STORAGE

1. Use only sterile, preservative-free NaCl injection to reconstitute powder for intrathecal administration.
2. Prevent inhalation of medication particles and skin exposure.
3. When used for rheumatoid arthritis, improvement is thought to be maintained for up to 2 years with continuous therapy. When discontinued, the arthritis usually worsens within 3–6 weeks.

IV 4. Six hours prior to initiation of a methotrexate infusion, hydrate with 1 L/m^2 of IV fluid. Continue hydration at 125 mL/m^2/hr during the methotrexate infusion and for 2 days after infusion completed.

5. Alkalinize urine (see *Sodium Bicarbonate*) to a pH > 7 during infusion.
6. Follow guidelines provided for leucovorin rescue schedule following high doses of methotrexate.

ASSESSMENT

1. Note indications for therapy, onset, and characteristics of symptoms; other agents trialed and outcome.
2. List drugs client currently prescribed. Determine if receiving other organic acids, such as aspirin, phenylbutazone, probenecid, and/or sulfa drugs; these affect renal clearance of methotrexate and increase thrombocytopenia and GI side effects. Note any acute infections.
3. Monitor CBC, uric acid, liver and renal function studies; report oliguria, Drug causes granulocyte and platelet suppression. Nadir: 10 days; recovery: 14 days.
4. Have calcium leucovorin—a potent antidote for folic acid antagonists—readily available in case of overdosage. Antidotes are ineffective if not administered within 4 hr of overdosage; may give corticosteroids concomitantly with initial dose of methotrexate. Allow maximum rest between doses.

CLIENT/FAMILY TEACHING

1. Take tablets at bedtime with an antacid to minimize GI upset. Prepare calendar to ensure correct dosage days.
2. Avoid salicylates and alcohol as liver toxicity/bleeding may result.
3. Report oral ulcerations, one of the first signs of toxicity.
4. Avoid vaccinations (especially for smallpox) because the impaired immunologic response may result in vaccinia.
5. Consume 2–3 L/day of fluids to prevent renal damage and facilitate drug excretion.
6. Test urine pH and report if less than 6.5; bicarbonate tablets may be prescribed to assist in alkalizing the urine.
7. Drug may precipitate gouty arthritis; allopurinol may be prescribed to reduce uric acid levels.
8. Avoid sun exposure and use sunscreens, sunglasses, and appropriate clothing when necessary.
9. Practice reliable contraception during and for at least 8 weeks following therapy.

OUTCOMES/EVALUATE

- Suppression of malignant cell proliferation, ↓ tumor size/spread
- Improvement in skin lesions
- ↓ Joint swelling/pain; ↑ mobility

Methsuximide

(meth-**SUCKS**-ih-myd)

PREGNANCY CATEGORY: C
CLASSIFICATION(S):
Anticonvulsant, succinimide
Rx: Celontin Kapseals

SEE ALSO *ANTICONVULSANTS* AND *SUCCINIMIDES*.

ACTION/KINETICS

Peak levels: 1–4 hr. **t½:** 1–3 hr for methsuximide and 36–45 hr for the active metabolite. **Therapeutic serum levels:** 10–40 mcg/mL.

M

USES
Treat absence seizures refractory to other drugs. May be given with other anticonvulsants when absence seizures coexist with other types of epilepsy.
ADDITIONAL SIDE EFFECTS
Most common are ataxia, dizziness, and drowsiness.
ADDITIONAL DRUG INTERACTIONS
Methsuximide may ↑ the effect of primidone.
HOW SUPPLIED
Capsule: 150 mg, 300 mg

DOSAGE
• **CAPSULES**
Absence seizures.
Determine dosage by trial. **Adults and children, initial:** 300 mg/day for first week; **then,** if necessary, increase dosage by 300 mg/day at weekly intervals until control established. **Maximum daily dose:** 1.2 g in divided doses.

NURSING CONSIDERATIONS

SEE ALSO NURSING CONSIDERATIONS FOR ANTICONVULSANTS AND SUCCINIMIDES.

ADMINISTRATION/STORAGE
The 150-mg dosage form can be used for children.
ASSESSMENT
1. Document type and frequency of seizures, noting characteristics, other drugs prescribed, and the outcome.
2. Note baseline level of consciousness and balance; drug may impair.
CLIENT/FAMILY TEACHING
1. Take exactly as prescribed to ensure seizure free. May take with food or milk for GI upset. Do not stop abruptly/change dosage without approval.
2. Report any rash, fever, sore throat, joint pain, unusual bruising/bleeding, pregnancy, or seizures.
3. Avoid alcohol and all OTC agents without approval.
4. Do not perform activities that require mental alertness until drug effects realized. May cause dizziness, drowsiness, blurred vision or confusion.
OUTCOMES/EVALUATE
• Control of seizures
• Therapeutic drug levels (10–40 mcg/mL)

Methyldopa
(meth-ill-**DOH**-pah)

PREGNANCY CATEGORY: B (PO)
Rx: Aldomet
✱**Rx:** Apo-Methyldopa, Novo-Medopa, Nu-Medopa

Methyldopate hydrochloride
(meth-ill-**DOH**-payt)

PREGNANCY CATEGORY: B (PO), C (IV)
Rx: Aldomet Hydrochloride
CLASSIFICATION(S):
Antihypertensive, centrally-acting

SEE ALSO ANTIHYPERTENSIVE AGENTS.

ACTION/KINETICS
The active metabolite, alpha-methylnorepinephrine, lowers BP by stimulating central inhibitory alpha-adrenergic receptors, false neurotransmission, and/or reduction of plasma renin. Little change in CO. **PO: Onset:** 7–12 hr. **Duration:** 12–24 hr. All effects terminated within 48 hr. Absorption is variable. **IV: Onset:** 4–6 hr. **Duration:** 10–16 hr. Seventy percent of drug excreted in urine. **Full therapeutic effect:** 1–4 days. **t½:** 1.7 hr. Metabolites excreted in the urine.
USES
Moderate to severe hypertension. Particularly useful for clients with impaired renal function, renal hypertension, resistant cases of hypertension complicated by stroke, CAD, or nitrogen retention, and for hypertensive crisis (parenterally).
CONTRAINDICATIONS
Sensitivity to drug (including sulfites), labile and mild hypertension, pregnancy, active hepatic disease, use with MAO inhibitors, or pheochromocytoma.
SPECIAL CONCERNS
Use with caution in clients with a history of liver or kidney disease. A decrease in dose in geriatric clients may prevent syncope.

SIDE EFFECTS

CNS: Sedation (transient), weakness, headache, asthenia, dizziness, paresthesias, Parkinson-like symptoms, psychic disturbances, symptoms of CV impairment, choreoathetotic movements, Bell's palsy, decreased mental acuity, verbal memory impairment. **CV:** Bradycardia, orthostatic hypotension, hypersensitivity of carotid sinus, worsening of angina, paradoxical hypertensive response (after IV), myocarditis, CHF, pericarditis, vasculitis. **GI:** N&V, abdominal distention, diarrhea or constipation, flatus, colitis, dry mouth, sore or "black tongue," pancreatitis, sialoadenitis. **Hematologic:** ***Hemolytic anemia,*** leukopenia, granulocytopenia, thrombocytopenia, ***bone marrow depression.*** **Endocrine:** Gynecomastia, amenorrhea, galactorrhea, lactation, hyperprolactinemia. **GU:** Impotence, failure to ejaculate, decreased libido. **Dermatologic:** Rash, ***toxic epidermal necrolysis.*** **Hepatic:** Jaundice, hepatitis, liver disorders, abnormal LFTs. **Miscellaneous:** Edema, fever, lupus-like symptoms, nasal stuffiness, arthralgia, myalgia, ***septic shock-like syndrome.***

LABORATORY TEST CONSIDERATIONS

False + or ↑: Alkaline phosphatase, bilirubin, BUN, BSP, cephalin flocculation, creatinine, AST, ALT, uric acid, Coombs' test, PT. Positive LE cell preparation and ANA.

OD OVERDOSE MANAGEMENT

Symptoms: CNS, GI, and CV effects including sedation, weakness, lightheadedness, dizziness, coma, bradycardia, acute hypotension, impairment of AV conduction, constipation, diarrhea, distention, flatus, N&V. *Treatment:* Induction of vomiting or gastric lavage if detected early. General supportive treatment with special attention to HR, CO, blood volume, urinary function, electrolyte imbalance, paralytic ileus, and CNS activity. In severe cases, hemodialysis is effective.

DRUG INTERACTIONS

Anesthetics, general / Additive hypotension
Antidepressants, tricyclic / May block methyldopa hypotensive effects
Haloperidol / ↑ Haloperidol toxic effects
Levodopa / ↑ Effect of both drugs
Lithium / ↑ Possibility of lithium toxicity
MAO inhibitors / Accumulation of methyldopa metabolites may → excessive sympathetic stimulation
Methotrimeprazine / Additive hypotensive effect
Phenothiazines / Possible ↑ BP
Propranolol / Paradoxical hypertension
Sympathomimetics / Potentiation of hypertensive drug effects
Thiazide diuretics / Additive hypotensive effect
Thioxanthenes / Additive hypotensive effect
Tolbutamide / ↑ Hypoglycemia R/T ↓ liver breakdown
Tricyclic antidepressants / ↓ Methyldopa effect
Vasodilator drugs / Additive hypotensive effect
Verapamil / ↑ Methyldopa effect

HOW SUPPLIED

Methyldopa: *Oral Suspension:* 50 mg/mL *Tablet:* 125 mg, 250 mg, 500 mg. **Methyldopate hydrochloride:** *Injection:* 50 mg/mL

DOSAGE

• METHYLDOPA TABLETS, ORAL SUSPENSION

Hypertension.

Initial: 250 mg b.i.d.–t.i.d. for 2 days. Adjust dose q 2 days. If increased, start with evening dose. **Usual maintenance:** 0.5–3.0 g/day in two to four divided doses; **maximum:** 3 g/day. Gradually transfer to and from other antihypertensive agents, with initial dose of methyldopa not exceeding 500 mg. *NOTE:* Do not use combination medication to initiate therapy. **Pediatric, initial:** 10 mg/kg/day in two to four divided doses, adjusting maintenance to a maximum of 65 mg/kg/day (or 3 g/day, whichever is less).

M

• **METHYLDOPATE HCL, IV INFUSION**

Hypertension.

Adults: 250–500 mg q 6 hr; **maximum:** 1 g q 6 hr for hypertensive crisis. Switch to PO methyldopa, at same dosage level, when BP is brought under control. **Pediatric:** 20–40 mg/kg/day in divided doses q 6 hr; **maximum:** 65 mg/kg/day (or 3 g/day, whichever is less).

NURSING CONSIDERATIONS

SEE ALSO *NURSING CONSIDERATIONS* FOR *ANTIHYPERTENSIVE AGENTS*.

ADMINISTRATION/STORAGE

1. Tolerance may occur following 2–3 months of therapy. Increasing the dose or adding a diuretic often restores effect on BP.

IV 2. For IV, mix with 100 mL of D5W or administer in D5W at a concentration of 10 mg/mL. Infuse over 30–60 min.

ASSESSMENT

1. Document indications for therapy, onset of symptoms, other agents prescribed and the outcome.
2. Monitor CBC, LFTs, and Coombs' test. If blood transfusion required, obtain both direct and indirect Coombs' tests; if positive, consult hematologist.
3. Avoid during pregnancy. Note any jaundice; contraindicated with active hepatic disease.
4. Assess for drug tolerance; may occur during the second or third month of therapy.

CLIENT/FAMILY TEACHING

1. To prevent dizziness and fainting, rise slowly to a sitting position and dangle legs over the bed edge.
2. Sedation may occur initially; should disappear once maintenance dose established.
3. In rare cases, may darken or turn urine blue; not harmful.
4. Withhold and report any of the following symptoms: tiredness, fever, or yellowing of eyes/skin.
5. Continue to follow prescribed diet and exercise program in the overall goal of BP control.
6. Do not take any other medications or remedies unless appoved.

OUTCOMES/EVALUATE

↓ BP

Methylergonovine maleate

(meth-ill-er-**GON**-oh-veen)

PREGNANCY CATEGORY: C
CLASSIFICATION(S):
Oxytocic drug
Rx: Methergine

ACTION/KINETICS

Synthetic drug related to ergonovine. Methylergonovine stimulates the rate, tone, and amplitude of uterine contractions. The uterus becomes more sensitive to the drug toward the end of pregnancy. **Onset** (uterine contractions): **PO,** 5–10 min; **IM,** 2–5 min; **IV,** immediate. **t½, IV:** 2–3 min (initial) and 20–30 min (final). **Duration, PO, IM:** 3 hr; **IV:** 45 min.

USES

Management and prevention of postpartum and postabortal hemorrhage by producing firm uterine contractions and decreasing uterine bleeding. During the second stage of labor following delivery of the anterior shoulder, but only under full obstetric supervision. *Investigational:* Ergonovine has been used to diagnose Prinzmetal's angina (variant angina).

CONTRAINDICATIONS

Pregnancy, toxemia, hypertension. Ergot hypersensitivity. To induce labor or threatened spontaneous abortions. Administration before delivery of the placenta.

SPECIAL CONCERNS

Use with caution in sepsis, obliterative vascular disease, impaired renal or hepatic function, and during lactation.

SIDE EFFECTS

CV: Hypertension that may be associated with ***seizure*** or headache; hypotension, thrombophlebitis, palpitation. **GI:** N&V, diarrhea, foul taste. **CNS:** Dizziness, headache, tinnitus, hallucinations. **Miscellaneous:** Sweating, chest pain, dyspnea, hematuria, water intoxication, leg cramps, nasal congestion. *NOTE:* ***Use of methylergonovine during labor may result in uterine tetany with rupture, cervical and perineal***

lacerations, embolism of amniotic fluid as well as hypoxia and intracranial hemorrhage in the infant.

OD OVERDOSE MANAGEMENT

Symptoms: Initially, N&V, abdominal pain, increase in BP, tingling of extremities, numbness. Symptoms of severe overdose include hypotension, hypothermia, ***respiratory depression, seizures, coma.*** *Treatment:* Induce vomiting or perform gastric lavage. Administer a cathartic; institute diuresis. Maintain respiration, especially if seizures or coma occur. Treat seizures with anticonvulsant drugs. Warm extremities to control peripheral vasospasm.

DRUG INTERACTIONS

Hypertension may occur if methylergonovine is used with vasoconstrictors.

HOW SUPPLIED

Injection: 0.2 mg /mL; *Tablet:* 0.2 mg

DOSAGE

• **IM, IV (EMERGENCIES ONLY)**

0.2 mg q 2–4 hr following delivery of placenta, of the anterior shoulder, or during the puerperium.

• **TABLETS**

0.2 mg t.i.d.–q.i.d. until danger of hemorrhage and uterine atony is over (usually within 2 days, but no more than 1 week).

NURSING CONSIDERATIONS

ADMINISTRATION/STORAGE

IV 1. Administer slowly over 1 min; check VS for evidence of shock or hypertension after IV administration. Have emergency drugs available.

2. Discard ampules if discolored.

ASSESSMENT

1. Document indications for therapy, onset and characteristics of symptoms. Avoid with liver or renal dysfunction.

2. List drugs prescribed to ensure none interact.

3. Document fundal tone and nonphasic contractures; massage to check for relaxation or severe cramping.

4. Monitor baseline calcium; correct if low to improve drug effectiveness. Monitor prolactin levels; assess for decreased milk production.

CLIENT/FAMILY TEACHING

1. Take only as directed; do not exceed dosage.

2. Avoid smoking; nicotine constricts blood vessels.

3. Report any S&S of ergotism (cold/numb fingers/toes, N&V, headache, muscle or chest pain, weakness).

4. Abdominal cramps may be experienced; report any severe cramping or increased bleeding.

5. Follow up with provider to ensure no complications.

OUTCOMES/EVALUATE

Improved uterine tone; control of postpartum hemorrhage

Methylphenidate hydrochloride

(meth-ill-**FEN**-ih-dayt)

PREGNANCY CATEGORY: C

CLASSIFICATION(S):

CNS stimulant

Rx: Concerta, Metadate CD, Metadate ER, Methylin, Methylin ER, Ritalin, Ritalin-SR

★**Rx:** PMS-Methylphenidate, Riphenidate **C-II**

ACTION/KINETICS

May act by blocking the reuptake mechanism of dopaminergic neurons. In children with attention-deficit disorders, methylphenidate causes decreases in motor restlessness with an increased attention span. In narcolepsy the drug acts on the cerebral cortex and subcortical structures (e.g., thalamus) to increase motor activity and mental alertness and decrease fatigue. **Peak blood levels, children:** 1.9 hr for tablets and 4.7 hr for extended-release tablets. **Duration:** 4–6 hr. **t½:** 1–3 hr. Metabolized by the liver and excreted by the kidney.

USES

(1) Attention-deficit disorders (ADD) and attention deficit hyperactivity disorders (ADHD) in children as part of overall treatment regimen. (2) Narcolepsy (Ritalin, Ritalin SR). *Investigational:* Depression in elderly, cancer, brain in-

M

jury, HIV, and poststroke clients. Anesthesia-related hiccups.

CONTRAINDICATIONS

Marked anxiety, tension and agitation, glaucoma. Severe depression, to prevent normal fatigue, diagnosis of Tourette's syndrome, motor tics. In children who manifest symptoms of primary psychiatric disorders (psychoses) or acute stress. Concurrent treatment with monoamine oxidase inhibitors and within a minimum of 14 days after stopping MAOI therapy (hypertensive crisis may occur).

SPECIAL CONCERNS

Use with caution during lactation. Use with great caution in clients with history of hypertension or convulsive disease. Safety and efficacy in children less than 6 years of age have not been established.

SIDE EFFECTS

CNS: Nervousness, insomnia, headaches, dizziness, drowsiness, chorea, depressed mood (transient). Toxic psychoses, dyskinesia, Tourette's syndrome. Psychologic dependence. **CV:** Palpitations, tachycardia, angina, arrhythmias, hyper/hypotension, cerebral arteritis or occlusion. **GI:** Nausea, anorexia, abdominal pain, weight loss (chronic use). **Allergic:** Skin rashes, fever, urticaria, arthralgia, exfoliative dermatitis, erythema multiforme with necrotizing vasculitis, erythema. **Hematologic:** Thrombocytopenic purpura, leukopenia, anemia. **Miscellaneous:** Hair loss, abnormal liver function.

In children, the following side effects are more common: anorexia, abdominal pain, weight loss (chronic use), tachycardia, insomnia.

LABORATORY TEST CONSIDERATIONS

↑ Urinary excretion of epinephrine.

OD OVERDOSE MANAGEMENT

Symptoms: Characterized by CV symptoms (hypertension, cardiac arrhythmias, tachycardia), mental disturbances, agitation, headaches, vomiting, hyperreflexia, ***hyperpyrexia, convulsions, and coma.*** *Treatment:* Symptomatic. Treat excess CNS stimulation by keeping the client in quiet, dim surroundings to reduce external stimuli. Protect the client from self-injury. A short-acting barbiturate may be used. Undertake emesis or gastric lavage if the client is conscious. Adequate circulatory and respiratory function must be maintained. Hyperpyrexia may be treated by cooling the client (e.g., cool bath, hypothermia blanket).

DRUG INTERACTIONS

Anticoagulants, oral / ↑ Anticoagulant effect R/T ↓ liver breakdown
Anticonvulsants (phenobarbital, phenytoin, primidone) / ↑ Anticonvulsant effect R/T ↓ liver breakdown
Carbamazepine / ↓ Methylphenidate levels
Guanethidine / ↓ Guanethidine effect by displacement from its action site
MAO inhibitors / Possibility of hypertensive crisis, hyperthermia, convulsions, coma
Selective serotonin reuptake inhibitors / ↑ Serum levels of SSRIs
Tricyclic antidepressants / ↑ TCA effect R/T ↓ liver breakdown

HOW SUPPLIED

Capsule, Extended Release: 20 mg; *Tablet:* 5 mg, 10 mg, 20 mg; *Tablet, Extended Release:* 10 mg, 18 mg, 20 mg, 36 mg, 54 mg; *Tablet, Sustained Release:* 20 mg

DOSAGE

- **TABLETS**

Narcolepsy.

Adults: 5–20 mg b.i.d.–t.i.d. preferably 30–45 min before meals.

Attention-deficit disorders.

Pediatric, 6 years and older, initial: 5 mg b.i.d. before breakfast and lunch; **then,** increase by 5–10 mg/week to a maximum of 60 mg/day.

NOTE: See *Administration/Storage* for additional dosing information.

NURSING CONSIDERATIONS

SEE ALSO *NURSING CONSIDERATIONS* FOR *PEMOLINE*.

ADMINISTRATION/STORAGE

1. If receiving for ADD and no improvement noticed in 1 mo, or if stimulation occurs, stop drug.
2. Discontinue periodically to assess condition as drug therapy is not indefinite; discontinue at puberty.
3. Sustained-release tablets are effective for 8 hr and may be substituted

for regular-release tablets if the 8-hr dosage of the sustained-release tablets is the same as the titrated 8-hr dosage of regular tablets.
4. Give Concerta once daily in the a.m. with or without food. Swallow capsules whole with liquids; do not chew, divide, or crush them.
5. The recommended starting dose for Concerta is 18 mg/day for those not currently taking methylphenidate or for clients on stimulants other than methylphenidate. Dose may be adjusted in 18 mg increments at weekly intervals up to a maximum of 54 mg/day taken once in the a.m.
6. The recommended dose for Concerta for clients currently taking methylphenidate b.i.d., t.i.d., or SR at doses from 10–60 mg/day is:
- 18 mg every a.m. if previously taking methylphenidate 5 mg b.i.d. or t.i.d. or methylphenidate-SR, 20 mg/day.
- 36 mg every a.m. if previously taking methylphenidate 10 mg b.i.d. or t.i.d. or methylphenidate-SR, 40 mg/day.
- 54 mg every a.m. if previously taking methylphenidate 15 mg b.i.d. or t.i.d. or methylphenidate-SR, 60 mg/day.

7. For Metadate CD, give once daily in the a.m. before breakfast. Swallow capsules whole with liquids; do not chew, divide, or crush them.
8. For Metadate CD, the dose is 20 mg once daily. Thirty % is rapidly released and the remaining 70% is released continuously permitting once daily dosage. Adjust dose in weekly 20 mg increments up to a maximum of 60 mg/day taken once daily in the a.m.

ASSESSMENT

1. Document indications for therapy, onset and characteristics of symptoms. Note other drugs prescribed that may interact unfavorably.
2. Ensure psychologic evaluations show no evidence of psychotic disorder or severe stress.
3. Obtain baseline CBC, CNS evaluation, and ECG.
4. Assess growth (Ht and Wt) and provide periodic "drug holiday" to determine need for continued therapy.

CLIENT/FAMILY TEACHING

1. Take before breakfast and lunch to avoid interference with sleep.
2. Use caution when driving or operating hazardous machinery as drug may mask fatigue and/or cause physical incoordination, dizziness, or drowsiness.
3. Record weight 2 times/week and report any significant loss as weight loss may occur.
4. Report any overt changes in client mood or attention span.
5. Skin rashes, fever, or joint pains should be reported immediately.
6. Therapy may be interrupted every few months ("drug holiday") to determine if still necessary in those responsive to therapy.
7. Avoid caffeine in any form.
8. Swallow extended-release forms whole with a liquid; do not cut, chew, or crush.

OUTCOMES/EVALUATE

- ↑ Ability to sit quietly/concentrate
- ↓ Daytime sleeping

Methylprednisolone

(meth-ill-pred-**NISS**-oh-lohn)

PREGNANCY CATEGORY: C
Rx: Tablets: Medrol

Methylprednisolone acetate

(meth-ill-pred-**NISS**-oh-lohn)

PREGNANCY CATEGORY: C
Rx: Enema: Medrol Enpak **Parenteral:** depMedalone-40 and -80, Depoject 40 and 80, Depo-Medrol, Depopred-40 and -80, Duralone-40 and -80, Medralone-40 and -80, M-Prednisol-40 and -80

M

Methylprednisolone sodium succinate

(meth-ill-pred-**NISS**-oh-lohn)

PREGNANCY CATEGORY: C
Rx: Parenteral: A-methaPred, Solu-Medrol
CLASSIFICATION(S):
Glucocorticoid

SEE ALSO *CORTICOSTEROIDS*.

ACTION/KINETICS
Low incidence of increased appetite, peptic ulcer, psychic stimulation, and sodium and water retention. May mask negative nitrogen balance. **Onset:** Slow, 12–24 hr. **t½, plasma:** 78–188 min. **Duration:** Long, up to 1 week. Rapid onset of sodium succinate by both IV and IM routes. Long duration of action of the acetate.

ADDITIONAL USES
Severe hepatitis due to alcoholism. Within 8 hr of severe spinal cord injury (to improve neurologic function). Septic shock (controversial).

SPECIAL CONCERNS
Use during pregnancy only if benefits outweigh risks.

LABORATORY TEST CONSIDERATIONS
↓ Immunoglobulins A, G, M.

ADDITIONAL DRUG INTERACTIONS
Erythromycin / ↑ Methylprednisolone effect R/T ↓ liver metabolism
Grapefruit juice / ↑ AUC, peak levels, and t½ of methylprednisolone R/T ↓ liver metabolism
Troleandomycin / ↑ Methylprednisolone effect R/T ↓ liver metabolism

HOW SUPPLIED
Methylprednisolone: *Tablet:* 2 mg, 4 mg, 8 mg, 16 mg, 24 mg, 32 mg. **Methylprednisolone acetate:** *Injection:* 20 mg/mL, 40 mg/mL, 80 mg/mL. **Methylprednisolone sodium succinate:** *Powder for injection:* 40 mg, 125 mg, 500 mg, 1 g, 2 g

DOSAGE

METHYLPREDNISOLONE

• **TABLETS**

Rheumatoid arthritis.

Adults: 6–16 mg/day. Decrease gradually when condition is under control. **Pediatric:** 6–10 mg/day.

SLE.

Adults, acute: 20–96 mg/day; **maintenance:** 8–20 mg/day.

Acute rheumatic fever.

1 mg/kg body weight daily. Drug is always given in four equally divided doses after meals and at bedtime.

METHYLPREDNISOLONE ACETATE

• **IM**

Adrenogenital syndrome.

40 mg q 2 weeks.

Rheumatoid arthritis.

40–120 mg/week.

Dermatologic lesions, dermatitis.

40–120 mg/week for 1–4 weeks; for severe cases, a single dose of 80–120 mg should provide relief.

Seborrheic dermatitis.

80 mg/week.

Asthma, rhinitis.

80–120 mg.

• **INTRA-ARTICULAR, SOFT TISSUE AND INTRALESIONAL INJECTION**

4–80 mg, depending on site.

• **RETENTION ENEMA**

40 mg 3–7 times/week for 2 or more weeks.

METHYLPREDNISOLONE SODIUM SUCCINATE

• **IM, IV**

Most conditions.

Adults, initial: 10–40 mg, depending on the disease; **then,** adjust dose depending on response, with subsequent doses given either **IM, IV.**

Severe conditions.

Adults: 30 mg/kg infused IV over 10–20 min; may be repeated q 4–6 hr for 2–3 days only. **Pediatric:** not less than 0.5 mg/kg/day.

NURSING CONSIDERATIONS

SEE ALSO *NURSING CONSIDERATIONS FOR CORTICOSTEROIDS*.

ADMINISTRATION/STORAGE

1. Dosage must be individualized.
2. Methylprednisolone acetate is not for IV use.
3. Use sodium succinate solutions within 48 hr after preparation.
4. For alternate day therapy, twice the usual PO dose is given every other morning (client receives beneficial effect while minimizing side effects).

ASSESSMENT

1. Document indications for treatment; describe clinical presentation.
2. Note any aspirin allergy; the 24 mg tablets distributed as Medrol contain tartrazine which may cause allergic reaction.
3. Monitor CBC, HbA1C, glucose, renal/LFTs, and electrolytes.

CLIENT/FAMILY TEACHING

1. Take exactly as directed. Do not ↑, ↓, or stop taking suddenly after prolonged use without provider consent; may cause rebound symptoms/adrenal crisis. Usually if administered before 9 am may mimic normal peak body corticosteroid levels and also prevent insomnia.
2. Report any ususual weight gain, extremitiy swelling, fatigue, nausea, anorexia, joint pain, muscle weakness,dizziness, fever, black or tarry stools, prolonged sore throat/colds, infections or worsening of problem.
3. May take with food or milk to diminish GI upset.
4. Avoid live vaccines and persons with infections or diseases.
5. Severe stress or trauma may require increased dosage.
6. Prolonged use may cause glucose intolerance requiring treatment with insulin or oral agents.

OUTCOMES/EVALUATE

- Relief of allergic manifestations
- ↓ Pain/inflammation; ↑ mobility
- ↓ Nerve fiber destruction in spinal cord injury (SCI)

Methysergide maleate

(meth-ih-**SIR**-jyd)

PREGNANCY CATEGORY: X
CLASSIFICATION(S):
Antimigraine drug
Rx: Sansert

ACTION/KINETICS

Semisynthetic ergot alkaloid derivative. May act by directly stimulating smooth muscle leading to vasoconstriction. Blocks the effects of serotonin, a powerful vasodilator believed to play a role in vascular headaches; it also inhibits the release of histamine from mast cells and prevents the release of serotonin from platelets. Has weak emetic and oxytocic activity. **Onset:** 1–2 days. **Peak plasma levels:** 60 ng/mL. **Duration:** 1–2 days. Excreted through the urine as unchanged drugs and metabolites.

USES

Prevention or reduction of the intensity and frequency of vascular headache (in clients having one or more per week or in cases where headaches are so severe preventive therapy is indicated). Prophylaxis of vascular headache.

CONTRAINDICATIONS

Severe renal or hepatic disease, severe hypertension, CAD, peripheral vascular disease, tendency toward thromboembolic disease, cachexia (profound ill health or malnutrition), severe arteriosclerosis, pulmonary disease, phlebitis or cellulitis of lower limbs, collagen diseases or fibrotic processs, debilitated states, valvular heart disease, infectious disease, or peptic ulcer. Use to terminate acute attacks. Pregnancy, lactation, use in children.

SPECIAL CONCERNS

Geriatric clients may be more affected by peripheral vasoconstriction leading to the possibility of hypothermia.

SIDE EFFECTS

The drug is associated with a high incidence of side effects. **Fibrosis:** ***Retroperitoneal fibrosis, cardiac fibrosis, pleuropulmonary fibrosis,*** Peyronie's-like disease. The fibrotic condition may result in vascular insufficiency in the lower legs. **CV:** Vasoconstriction of arteries leading to paresthesia, chest pain, abdominal pain, or extremities that are cold, numb, or painful. Tachycardia, postural hypotension. **CNS:** Dizziness, ataxia, drowsiness, vertigo, insomnia, euphoria, lightheadedness, and psychic reactions such as depersonalization, depression, and hallucinations. **GI:** N&V, diarrhea, heartburn, abdominal pain, increased gastric acid, constipation. **Hematologic:** Eosinophilia, neu-

M

tropenia. **Other:** Peripheral edema, flushing of face, skin rashes, transient alopecia, myalgia, arthralgia, weakness, weight gain, telangiectasia.

DRUG INTERACTIONS

Methysergide inhibits narcotic analgesics.

HOW SUPPLIED

Tablet: 2 mg

DOSAGE

• **TABLETS**

Adults: Administer 4–8 mg/day in divided doses. Continuous administration should not exceed 6 months. May be readministered after a 3- to 4-week rest period.

NURSING CONSIDERATIONS

ADMINISTRATION/STORAGE

If drug is not effective after 3 weeks, it is not likely to be beneficial and should be discontinued.

ASSESSMENT

1. Note frequency and severity of headaches and efforts made in the past to control or prevent them.
2. Obtain CBC, liver and renal function studies; assess for dysfunction.
3. Determine behavior prior to therapy. Review diet (tyramine foods, additives, preservatives, colorings), activity, substance use (including caffeine and nicotine), OTC medications, and stress levels; may have precipitated event.
4. Review medical history/exam. Do not use with severe HTN, CAD, PVD, cellulitis, or thromboembolic disease.

CLIENT/FAMILY TEACHING

1. Take with meals or milk to minimize GI irritation R/T increased hydrochloric acid production.
2. Discontinue gradually to avoid headache rebound.
3. Report symptoms of nervousness, weakness, insomnia, rashes, alopecia, or peripheral edema.
4. Report any unusual weight gain; check extremities for swelling. If weight gain excessive, adjust caloric intake; maintain a low-salt diet.
5. Keep a diary noting any events, foods, or activities that may relate to the onset of headaches.
6. Administration should not be continued on a regular basis for longer than 6 months without a 3- to 4-week rest.
7. General malaise, fatigue, weight loss, low-grade fever, or urinary tract problems may be symptoms of fibrosis (cardiac or pleuropulmonary); report immediately.
8. Do not drive or engage in other hazardous tasks until drug effects are realized; may cause drowsiness.
9. If dizziness or lightheadedness occurs upon arising, rise slowly from a supine position and dangle legs for a few minutes before standing erect. If feeling faint, lie down with the legs elevated.
10. Avoid alcohol, caffeine, nicotine, and cannabis, as these may precipitate vascular headaches.
11. Report if psychologic changes occur, especially hallucinations.

OUTCOMES/EVALUATE

↓ Frequency/intensity of vascular headaches; Headache prophylaxis

Metipranolol hydrochloride

(met-ih-**PRAN**-oh-lohl)

PREGNANCY CATEGORY: C

CLASSIFICATION(S):

Beta-adrenergic blocking agent

Rx: OptiPranolol

SEE ALSO *BETA-ADRENERGIC BLOCKING AGENTS.*

ACTION/KINETICS

Blocks both beta-1- and beta-2-adrenergic receptors. Reduction in intraocular pressure may be related to a decrease in production of aqueous humor and a slight increase in the outflow of aqueous humor. A decrease from 20% to 26% in intraocular pressure may be seen if the intraocular pressure is greater than 24 mm Hg at baseline. May be absorbed and exert systemic effects. When used topically, has no local anesthetic effect and exerts no action on pupil size or accommodation. **Onset:** 30 min. **Maximum effect:** 1–2 hr. **Duration:** 12–24 hr.

USES
Reduce IOP in ocular hypertension or chronic open-angle glaucoma.

SPECIAL CONCERNS
Use with caution during lactation. Safety and effectiveness have not been determined in children.

SIDE EFFECTS
Ophthalmologic: Local discomfort, dermatitis of the eyelid, blepharitis, conjunctivitis, browache, tearing, blurred/abnormal vision, photophobia, edema. Due to absorption, the following systemic side effects have been reported. **CV:** Hypertension, ***MI***, atrial fibrillation, angina, bradycardia, palpitation. **CNS:** Headache, dizziness, anxiety, depression, somnolence, nervousness. **Respiratory:** Dyspnea, rhinitis, bronchitis, coughing. **Miscellaneous:** Allergic reaction, asthenia, nausea, epistaxis, arthritis, myalgia, rash.

HOW SUPPLIED
Ophthalmic solution: 0.3%

DOSAGE

• **OPHTHALMIC SOLUTION (0.3%)**

Adults: 1 gtt in the affected eye(s) b.i.d. Increasing the dose or more frequent administration does not increase the beneficial effect.

NURSING CONSIDERATIONS

SEE ALSO *NURSING CONSIDERATIONS* FOR *BETA-ADRENERGIC BLOCKING AGENTS*.

ADMINISTRATION/STORAGE

1. May be used concomitantly with other drugs to lower IOP.
2. Due to diurnal variation in response, measure IOP at different times during the day.

ASSESSMENT

1. Note ocular condition and record pretreatment pressures.
2. Document baseline ECG and VS.

CLIENT/FAMILY TEACHING

1. Transient burning or stinging is common during administration; report if severe.
2. Take only as directed; report any persistent bothersome side effects or symptoms of intolerance.
3. Report for F/U visits to assess for systemic effects, measure intraocular pressures, and determine drug effectiveness.

OUTCOMES/EVALUATE
↓ IOP

Metoclopramide

(meh-toe-kloh-**PRAH**-myd)

PREGNANCY CATEGORY: B
CLASSIFICATION(S):
Gastrointestinal stimulant
Rx: Maxolon, Metoclopramide Intensol, Octamide PFS, Reglan
🍁**Rx:** Apo-Metoclop, Nu-Metoclopramide

ACTION/KINETICS
Dopamine antagonist that acts by increasing sensitivity to acetylcholine; results in increased motility of the upper GI tract and relaxation of the pyloric sphincter and duodenal bulb. Gastric emptying time and GI transit time are shortened. No effect on gastric, biliary, or pancreatic secretions. Facilitates intubation of the small bowel and speeds transit of a barium meal. Produces sedation, induces release of prolactin, increases circulating aldosterone levels (is transient), and is an antiemetic. **Onset, IV:** 1–3 min; **IM,** 10–15 min; **PO,** 30–60 min. **Duration:** 1–2 hr. **t½:** 5–6 hr. Significant first-pass effect following PO use; unchanged drug and metabolites excreted in urine. Renal impairment decreases clearance of the drug.

USES
PO: Acute and recurrent diabetic gastroparesis, gastroesophageal reflux. **Parenteral:** (1) Facilitate small bowel intubation, stimulate gastric emptying, and increase intestinal transit of barium to aid in radiologic examination of stomach and small intestine. (2) Prophylaxis of N&V in cancer chemotherapy and following surgery (when nasogastric suction is not desired). *Investigational:* To improve lactation. N&V due to various causes, including vomiting

M

during pregnancy and labor, gastric ulcer, anorexia nervosa. Improve client response to ergotamine, analgesics, and sedatives when used to treat migraine (may increase absorption). Postoperative gastric bezoars. Atonic bladder. Esophageal variceal bleeding.

CONTRAINDICATIONS

Gastrointestinal hemorrhage, obstruction, or perforation; epilepsy; clients taking drugs likely to cause extrapyramidal symptoms, such as phenothiazines. Pheochromocytoma.

SPECIAL CONCERNS

Use with caution during lactation and in hypertension. Extrapyramidal effects are more likely to occur in children and geriatric clients.

SIDE EFFECTS

CNS: Restlessness, drowsiness, fatigue, lassitude, akathisia, anxiety, insomnia, confusion. Headaches, dizziness, extrapyramidal symptoms (especially acute dystonic reactions), Parkinson-like symptoms (including cogwheel rigidity, mask-like facies, bradykinesia, tremor), dystonia, myoclonus, ***depression (with suicidal ideation),*** tardive dyskinesia (including involuntary movements of the tongue, face, mouth, or jaw), ***seizures,*** hallucinations. **GI:** Nausea, bowel disturbances (usually diarrhea). **CV:** Hypertension (transient), hypotension, SVT, bradycardia. **Hematologic: *Agranulocytosis,*** leukopenia, neutropenia. Methemoglobinemia in premature and full-term infants at doses of 1–4 mg/kg/day IM, IV, or PO for 1–3 or more days. **Endocrine:** Galactorrhea, amenorrhea, gynecomastia, impotence (due to hyperprolactinemia), fluid retention (due to transient elevation of aldosterone). ***Neuroleptic malignant syndrome: Hyperthermia, altered consciousness, autonomic dysfunction, muscle rigidity, death.*** **Miscellaneous:** Incontinence, urinary frequency, porphyria, visual disturbances, flushing of the face and upper body, hepatotoxicity.

OD OVERDOSE MANAGEMENT

Symptoms: Agitation, irritability, hypertonia of muscles, drowsiness, disorientation, extrapyramidal symptoms. *Treatment:* Treat extrapyramidal effects by giving anticholinergic drugs, anti-Parkinson drugs, or antihistamines with anticholinergic effects. General supportive treatment. Reverse methemoglobinemia by giving methylene blue.

DRUG INTERACTIONS

Acetaminophen / ↑ Acetaminophen absorption
Anticholinergics / ↓ Metoclopramide effect
Cimetidine / ↓ Cimetidine effect R/T ↓ GI tract absorption
CNS depressants / Additive sedative effects
Cyclosporine / ↑ Cyclosporine absorption → ↑ immunosuppressive and toxic effects
Digoxin / ↓ Digoxin effect R/T ↓ GI tract absorption
Ethanol / ↑ Ethanol GI absorption
Levodopa / ↑ Levodopa GI absorption and ↓ metoclopramide effects on gastric emptying and lower esophageal pressure
MAO inhibitors / ↑ Release of catecholamines → toxicity
Narcotic analgesics / ↓ Metoclopramide effect
Succinylcholine / ↑ Succinylcholine effect R/T plasma cholinesterase inhibition
Tetracyclines / ↑ Tetracycline GI absorption

HOW SUPPLIED

Concentrate: 10 mg/mL; *Injection:* 5 mg/mL; *Syrup:* 5 mg/5 mL, *Tablet:* 5 mg, 10 mg

DOSAGE

• **TABLETS, SYRUP, CONCENTRATE**

Diabetic gastroparesis.

Adults: 10 mg 30 min before meals and at bedtime for 2–8 weeks (therapy should be reinstituted if symptoms recur).

Gastroesophageal reflux.

Adults: 10–15 mg q.i.d. 30 min before meals and at bedtime. If symptoms occur only intermittently, single doses up to 20 mg prior to the provoking situation may be used.

To enhance lactation.

Adults: 30–45 mg/day.

• **IM, IV**

Prophylaxis of vomiting due to chemotherapy.

Initial: 1–2 mg/kg IV q 2 hr for two doses, with the first dose 30 min before chemotherapy; **then,** 10 mg or more q 3 hr for three doses. Inject slowly IV over 15 min.

Prophylaxis of postoperative N&V.

Adults: 10–20 mg IM near the end of surgery.

Facilitate small bowel intubation.

Adults: 10 mg given over 1–2 min; **pediatric, 6–14 years:** 2.5–5 mg; **pediatric, less than 6 years:** 0.1 mg/kg.

Radiologic examinations to increase intestinal transit time.

Adults: 10 mg as a single dose given IV over 1–2 min.

NURSING CONSIDERATIONS

ADMINISTRATION/STORAGE

1. After PO use, absorption of certain drugs from the GI tract may be affected (see *Drug Interactions*).

IV 2. Inject slowly IV over 1–2 min to prevent transient feelings of anxiety and restlessness.

3. Metoclopramide is physically and/or chemically incompatible with a number of drugs; check package insert if drug is to be admixed.

4. For IV use, dilute doses greater than 10 mg in 50 mL of D5W, D5/0.45% NaCl, RL, Ringer's injection, or NaCl; infuse over 15 min.

ASSESSMENT

1. Document indications for therapy, type and onset of symptoms. List drugs prescribed, ensuring none interact unfavorably.

2. Assess abdomen for bowel sounds and distention; note any N&V.

CLIENT/FAMILY TEACHING

1. Do not operate a car or hazardous machinery until drug effects realized; drug has a sedative effect.

2. Report any persistent side effects so they can be properly evaluated and counteracted.

3. Avoid alcohol and any other CNS depressants.

4. Extrapyramidal effects (trembling hands, facial grimacing) should be reported; may be treated with IM diphenhydramine.

OUTCOMES/EVALUATE

- Prevention of N&V
- Enhanced gastric motility
- Promotion of gastric emptying
- Prophylaxis of gastric bezoars

Metolazone

(meh-**TOH**-lah-zohn)

PREGNANCY CATEGORY: B

CLASSIFICATION(S):

Diuretic, thiazide

Rx: Mykrox, Zaroxolyn

SEE ALSO *DIURETICS, THIAZIDE.*

ACTION/KINETICS

Onset: 1 hr. **Peak blood levels, rapid availability tablets:** 2–4 hr; **t½, elimination:** About 14 hr. **Peak blood levels, slow availability tablets:** 8 hr. **Duration, rapid or slow availablity tablets:** 24 hr or more. Most excreted unchanged through the urine.

USES

Slow availability tablets: (1) Edema accompanying CHF; edema accompanying renal diseases, including nephrotic syndrome and conditions of reduced renal function. (2) Alone or in combination with other drugs for the treatment of hypertension.

Rapid availability tablets: Treatment of newly diagnosed mild to moderate hypertension alone or in combination with other drugs. The rapid availability tablets are not to be used to produce diuresis.

Investigational: Alone or as an adjunct to treat calcium nephrolithiasis, premanagement of menstrual syndrome, and adjunct treatment of renal failure.

CONTRAINDICATIONS

Anuria, prehepatic and hepatic coma, allergy or hypersensitivity to metolazone. Routine use during pregnancy. Lactation.

SPECIAL CONCERNS

Use with caution in those with severely impaired renal function. Safety and ef-

M

fectiveness have not been determined in children.

SIDE EFFECTS

See *Diuretics, Thiazide.* The most commonly reported side effects are dizziness, headache, muscle cramps, malaise, lethargy, lassitude, joint pain/swelling, and chest pain.

ADDITIONAL DRUG INTERACTIONS

Alcohol / ↑ Hypotensive effect
Barbiturates / ↑ Hypotensive effect
Narcotics / ↑ Hypotensive effect
NSAIDs / ↓ Hypotensive effect of metolazone
Salicylates / ↓ Hypotensive effect of metolazone

HOW SUPPLIED

Tablets: 0.5 mg, 2.5 mg, 5 mg, 10 mg.

DOSAGE

• SLOW AVAILABILITY TABLETS (ZAROXOLYN)

Edema due to cardiac failure or renal disease.

Adults: 5–20 mg once daily. For those who experience paroxysmal nocturnal dyspnea, a larger dose may be required to ensure prolonged diuresis and saluresis for a 24-hr period.

Mild to moderate essential hypertension.

Adults: 2.5–5 mg once daily.

• RAPID AVAILABILITY TABLETS (MYKROX)

Mild to moderate essential hypertension.

Adults, initial: 0.5 mg once daily, usually in the morning. If inadequately controlled, the dose may be increased to 1 mg once a day. Increasing the dose higher than 1 mg does not increase the effect.

NURSING CONSIDERATIONS

SEE ALSO *NURSING CONSIDERATIONS* FOR *DIURETICS, THIAZIDE*.

ADMINISTRATION/STORAGE

1. Formulations of slow availability tablets should not be interchanged with formulations of rapid availability tablets as they are not therapeutically equivalent.
2. The antihypertensive effect may be observed from 3 to 4 days to 3 to 6 weeks.
3. If BP is not controlled with 1 mg of the rapid availability tablets, add another antihypertensive drug, with a different mechanism of action, to the therapy.
4. Store tablets at room temperature in a tight, light-resistant container.

ASSESSMENT

1. Document indications for therapy, noting onset, duration, and clinical characteristics.
2. Monitor BP, ECG, CBC, electrolytes, liver and renal function studies; assess for symptoms of electrolyte imbalance (i.e., ↓ Na/K/Mg/P and hypochloremic alkalosis).

CLIENT/FAMILY TEACHING

1. May take with food. Take exactly as directed; early in the day to prevent nighttime awakening for urination.
2. May cause orthostatic hypotension and syncope; use caution.
3. Weigh self regularly; report increases of more than 3 lb/day.
4. Avoid exposure to sun or bright lights; may cause photosensitivity.
5. May cause potassium depletion; eat a K rich diet (whole grain cereals, legumes, meat, bananas, apricots, orange juice, potatoes, raisins) and report as scheduled for regular lab test evaluations.
6. Report any muscle weakness/cramps, fatigue, nausea, or dizziness.

OUTCOMES/EVALUATE

↓ Edema; ↓ BP

Metoprolol succinate

(me-toe-**PROH**-lohl)

PREGNANCY CATEGORY: C
Rx: Toprol XL

Metoprolol tartrate

(me-toe-**PROH**-lohl)

PREGNANCY CATEGORY: B
Rx: Lopressor
✱Rx: Apo-Metoprolol, Apo-Metoprolol (Type L), Betaloc, Betaloc Durules, Gen-Metoprolol, Gen-Metoprolol (Type L), Novo–Metoprol, Nu-Metop, PMS-Metoprolol-B, PMS-Metoprolol-L

CLASSIFICATION(S):
Beta-adrenergic blocking agent

SEE ALSO *BETA-ADRENERGIC BLOCKING AGENTS*.

ACTION/KINETICS
Exerts mainly beta-1-adrenergic blocking activity although beta-2 receptors are blocked at high doses. Has no membrane stabilizing or intrinsic sympathomimetic effects. Moderate lipid solubility. **Onset:** 15 min. **Peak plasma levels:** 90 min. **t½:** 3–7 hr. Effect of drug is cumulative. Food increases bioavailability. Exhibits significant first-pass effect. Metabolized in liver and excreted in urine.

USES
Metoprolol Succinate: (1) Alone or with other drugs to treat hypertension. (2) Chronic management of angina pectoris. (3) Treatment of stable, symptomatic (NYHA Class II or III) heart failure of ischemic, hypertensive, or cardiomyopathic origin.

Metoprolol Tartrate: (1) Hypertension (either alone or with other antihypertensive agents, such as thiazide diuretics). (2) Acute MI in hemodynamically stable clients. (3) Angina pectoris. *Investigational:* IV to suppress atrial ectopy in COPD, aggressive behavior, prophylaxis of migraine, ventricular arrhythmias, enhancement of cognitive performance in geriatric clients, essential tremors.

ADDITIONAL CONTRAINDICATIONS
Myocardial infarction in clients with a HR of less than 45 beats/min, in second- or third-degree heart block, or if SBP is less than 100 mm Hg. Moderate to severe cardiac failure.

SPECIAL CONCERNS
Safety and effectiveness have not been established in children. Use with caution in impaired hepatic function and during lactation.

LABORATORY TEST CONSIDERATIONS
↑ Serum transaminase, LDH, alkaline phosphatase.

ADDITIONAL DRUG INTERACTIONS
Cimetidine / May ↑ plasma metoprolol levels
Contraceptives, oral / May ↑ metoprolol effects
Diphenhydramine / ↓ Metoprolol clearance → prolonged negative chronotropic and inotropic effects in extensive metabolizers
Hydroxychloroquine / ↑ Bioavailability of metoprolol in homozygous extensive metabolizers
Methimazole / May ↓ metoprolol effects
Phenobarbital / ↓ Metoprolol effect R/T ↑ liver metabolism
Propylthiouracil / May ↓ metoprolol effects
Quinidine / May ↑ metoprolol effects
Rifampin / ↓ Metoprolol effect R/T ↑ liver metabolism

HOW SUPPLIED
Metoprolol succinate: *Tablet, Extended Release:* 25 mg, 50 mg, 100 mg, 200 mg. **Metoprolol tartrate:** *Injection:* 1 mg/mL; *Tablet:* 50 mg, 100 mg

DOSAGE

• METOPROLOL SUCCINATE TABLETS

Angina pectoris.

Individualized. Initial: 100 mg/day in a single dose. Dose may be increased slowly, at weekly intervals, until optimum effect is reached or there is a pronounced slowing of HR. Doses above 400 mg/day have not been studied.

Hypertension.

Initial: 50–100 mg/day in a single dose with or without a diuretic. Dosage may be increased in weekly intervals until maximum effect is reached. Doses above 400 mg/day have not been studied.

CHF.

Individualize dose. **Initial:** 25 mg once daily for 2 weeks in clients with NYHA Class II heart failure and 12.5 mg once daily in those with more severe heart failure. Double the dose q 2 weeks to the highest dose level tolerated or up to 200 mg.

• METOPROLOL TARTRATE TABLETS

Hypertension.

Initial: 100 mg/day in single or divided doses; **then,** dose may be increased

M

weekly to maintenance level of 100–450 mg/day. A diuretic may also be used.

Angina pectoris.

Initial: 100 mg/day in 2 divided doses. Dose may be increased gradually at weekly intervals until optimum response is obtained or a pronounced slowing of HR occurs. Effective dose range: 100–400 mg/day. If treatment is to be discontinued, reduce dose gradually over 1–2 weeks.

Aggressive behavior.

200–300 mg/day.

Essential tremors.

50–300 mg/day.

Prophylaxis of migraine.

50–100 mg b.i.d.

Ventricular arrhythmias.

200 mg/day.

• **METOPROLOL TARTRATE INJECTION (IV) AND TABLETS**

Early treatment of MI.

3 IV bolus injections of 5 mg each at approximately 2-min intervals. If clients tolerate the full IV dose, give 50 mg q 6 hr PO beginning 15 min after the last IV dose (or as soon as client's condition allows). This dose is continued for 48 hr followed by **late treatment:** 100 mg b.i.d. as soon as feasible; continue for 1–3 months (although data suggest treatment should be continued for 1–3 years). In clients who do not tolerate the full IV dose, begin with 25–50 mg q 6 hr PO beginning 15 min after the last IV dose or as soon as the condition allows.

NURSING CONSIDERATIONS

SEE ALSO *NURSING CONSIDERATIONS FOR BETA-ADRENERGIC BLOCKING AGENTS* AND *ANTIHYPERTENSIVE AGENTS.*

ADMINISTRATION/STORAGE

1. If transient worsening of heart failure occurs, may be treated with increased doses of diuretics. May be necessary to lower the dose of metoprolol or temporarily discontinue.
2. For CHF, do not increase dose until symptoms of worsening have been stabilized. Initial difficulty with titration should not preclude attempts later to use metoprolol.
3. If CHF clients experience symptomatic bradycardia, reduce the dose.

ASSESSMENT

1. Document indications for therapy; note any CAD and NYHA class.
2. Monitor liver and renal function studies, ECG, and VS.

CLIENT/FAMILY TEACHING

1. Take doses at the same time each day.
2. Continue with diet, regular exercise, and weight loss in the overall plan to control BP.
3. Report any symptoms of fluid overload such as sudden weight gain, edema, or dyspnea.
4. Dress appropriately; may cause an increased sensitivity to cold.
5. Keep a log of symptoms, BP and HR readings for provider review.

OUTCOMES/EVALUATE

• ↓ BP; ↓ anginal attacks
• Prevention of myocardial reinfarction and associated mortality

Metronidazole

(meh-troh-**NYE**-dah-zohl)

PREGNANCY CATEGORY: B
CLASSIFICATION(S):
Trichomonacide - amebicide
Rx: Flagyl, Flagyl 375, Flagyl ER, Metric 21, Metro I.V., MetroGel Topical, MetroGel-Vaginal, MetroLotion, Noritate Cream 1%, Protostat, Satric, Satric 500, Flagyl I.V., Flagyl I.V. RTU, Metronidazole Redi-Infusion
✱Rx: Apo-Metronidazole, Metro-Cream, NidaGel, Novo–Nidazol

SEE ALSO *ANTI-INFECTIVES.*

ACTION/KINETICS

Effective against anaerobic bacteria and protozoa. Specifically inhibits growth of trichomonae and amoebae by binding to DNA, resulting in loss of helical structure, strand breakage, inhibition of nucleic acid synthesis, and cell death. Well absorbed from GI tract and widely distributed in body tissues. **Peak serum concentration: PO,** 6–40 mcg/mL, depending on the dose, after 1–2 hr. **t½: PO,** 6–12 hr; average: 8 hr. Eliminated primarily in

M

urine (20% unchanged), which may be red-brown in color following either PO or IV use. The mechanism for its effectiveness in reducing the inflammatory lesions of acne rosacea is not known.

USES

Systemic: (1) Amebiasis. Symptomatic and asymptomatic trichomoniasis; to treat asymptomatic partner. Amebic dysentery and amebic liver abscess. (2) To reduce postoperative anaerobic infection following colorectal surgery, elective hysterectomy, and emergency appendectomy. (3) Anaerobic bacterial infections of the abdomen, female genital system, skin or skin structures, bones and joints, lower respiratory tract, and CNS. Also, septicemia, endocarditis, hepatic encephalopathy. (4) PO for Crohn's disease and pseudomembranous colitis. (5) As part of the regimen to eradicate *Helicobacter pylori* infections. *Investigational:* Giardiasis, *Gardnerella vaginalis.*

Topical: Inflammatory papules, pustules, and erythema of rosacea. *Investigational:* Infected decubitus ulcers (use 1% solution prepared from oral tablets).

Vaginal: Bacterial vaginosis.

CONTRAINDICATIONS

Blood dyscrasias, active organic disease of the CNS, trichomoniasis during the first trimester of pregnancy, lactation. Topical use if hypersensitive to parabens or other ingredients of the formulation. Consumption of alcohol during use.

SPECIAL CONCERNS

Safety and efficacy have not been established in children.

SIDE EFFECTS

• **SYSTEMIC USE.**

GI: Nausea, dry mouth, metallic taste, vomiting, diarrhea, abdominal discomfort, constipation. **CNS:** Headache, dizziness, vertigo, incoordination, ataxia, confusion, irritability, depression, weakness, insomnia, syncope, ***seizures***, peripheral neuropathy including paresthesias. **Hematologic:** Leukopenia, ***bone marrow aplasia.*** **GU:** Burning, dysuria, cystitis, polyuria, incontinence, dryness of vagina or vulva, dyspareunia, decreased libido. **Allergic:** Urticaria, pruritus, erythematous rash, flushing, nasal congestion, fever, joint pain. **Miscellaneous:** Furry tongue, glossitis, stomatitis (due to overgrowth of *Candida*) ECG abnormalities, thrombophlebitis.

• **TOPICAL USE.**

Watery eyes if gel applied too closely to this area; transient redness; mild burning, dryness, and skin irritation.

• **VAGINAL USE.**

Symptomatic *Candida vaginitis,* N&V.

OD OVERDOSE MANAGEMENT

Symptoms: Ataxia, N&V, peripheral neuropathy, ***seizures*** up to 5–7 days. *Treatment:* Supportive treatment.

DRUG INTERACTIONS

Barbiturates / Possible therapeutic failure of metronidazole
Cimetidine / ↑ Serum metronidazole levels R/T ↓ clearance
Disulfiram / Concurrent use may cause confusion or acute psychosis
Ethanol / Possible disulfiram-like reaction, including flushing, palpitations, tachycardia, and N&V
Hydantoins / ↑ Hydantoins effect R/T ↓ clearance
Lithium / ↑ Lithium toxicity
Warfarin / ↑ Anticoagulant effect

HOW SUPPLIED

Capsule: 375 mg; *Cream:* 1%; *Gel:* 0.75%; *Injection:* 500 mg/100 mL (ready-to-use); *Injection, lyophilized:* 500 mg; *Tablet:* 250 mg, 500 mg; *Tablet, Extended-Release:* 750 mg

DOSAGE

• **CAPSULES, TABLETS**

Amebiasis: Acute amebic dysentery or amebic liver abscess.

Adult: 500–750 mg t.i.d. for 5–10 days; **pediatric:** 35–50 mg/kg/day in three divided doses for 10 days.

Trichomoniasis, female.

250 mg t.i.d. for 7 days, 2 g given on 1 day in single or divided doses, or 375 mg b.i.d. for 7 days. **Pediatric:** 5 mg/kg t.i.d. for 7 days. An interval of 4–6 weeks should elapse between courses of therapy. *NOTE:* Do not treat preg-

M

nant women during the first trimester. **Male:** Individualize dosage; usual, 250 mg t.i.d. for 7 days.

Treat Helicobacter pylori *infections.*

One of the following regimens may be used: (1) Metronidazole, 500 mg b.i.d.; clarithromycin, 500 mg b.i.d.; and, either lansoprazole, 30 mg b.i.d. or omeprazole, 20 mg b.i.d. All drugs given for 2 weeks. (2) Metronidazole, 500 mg b.i.d. for 2 weeks, or amoxicillin, 1 g b.i.d. for 2 weeks, or tetracycline, 500 mg b.i.d. for 2 weeks; plus, clarithromycin, 500 mg b.i.d. for 2 weeks and ranitidine bismuth citrate, 400 mg b.i.d. for 4 weeks. (3) Tetracycline, 500 mg q.i.d.; metronidazole, 500 mg t.i.d.; bismuth subsalicylate, 525 mg q.i.d; and, either lansoprazole, 30 mg once daily or omeprazole, 20 mg once daily. All drugs given for 2 weeks. (4) Tetracycline, 500 mg q.i.d.; metronidazole, 250 mg q.i.d.; bismuth subsalicylate, 525 mg q.i.d.; and, a H2-receptor antagonist. Drugs are given for 2 weeks except for the H2-receptor antagonist which is given for 4 weeks.

M

Giardiasis.

250 mg t.i.d. for 7 days.

G. vaginalis.

500 mg b.i.d. for 7 days.

• **TABLETS, EXTENDED-RELEASE**

Bacterial vaginosis.

One 750-mg tablet per day for 7 days.

• **IV**

Anaerobic bacterial infections.

Adults, initially: 15 mg/kg infused over 1 hr; **then,** after 6 hr, 7.5 mg/kg q 6 hr for 7–10 days (daily dose should not exceed 4 g). Treatment may be necessary for 2–3 weeks, although PO therapy should be initiated as soon as possible.

Prophylaxis of anaerobic infection during surgery.

Adults: 15 mg/kg given over a 30- to 60-min period, with completion 1 hr prior to surgery and 7.5 mg/kg infused over 30–60 min 6 and 12 hr after the initial dose.

• **TOPICAL CREAM, GEL, LOTION**

Rosacea.

After washing, apply a thin film and rub in well either once daily or b.i.d. in the morning and evening for 4–9 weeks.

• **VAGINAL (0.75%)**

Bacterial vaginosis.

One applicatorful (5 g) in the morning and evening for 5 days. Metro-Gel Vaginal allows for once-daily dosing at bedtime.

NURSING CONSIDERATIONS

SEE ALSO *GENERAL NURSING CONSIDERATIONS* FOR *ANTI-INFECTIVES*.

ADMINISTRATION/STORAGE

1. For topical use, therapeutic results should be seen within 3 weeks with continuing improvement through 9 weeks of therapy.
2. Cosmetics may be used after application of topical metronidazole.
3. IV Do not give by IV bolus. Administer each single dose over 1 hr.
4. Do not use syringes with aluminum needles or hubs.
5. Discontinue primary IV infusion during infusion of metronidazole.
6. The order of mixing to prepare powder for injection is important:
   - Reconstitute.
   - Dilute in IV solutions in glass or plastic containers.
   - Neutralize pH with $NaHCO_3$ solution. Do not refrigerate neutralized solutions.
7. Premixed, ready to use Flagyl comes 5 mg/mL (500 mg metronidazole in 100 mL of solution) in plastic bags; administer over 1 hr.
8. Drug has a high sodium content.

ASSESSMENT

1. Document indications for therapy and symptom characteristics.
2. Monitor CBC, LFTs, and cultures.

CLIENT/FAMILY TEACHING

1. Take with food or milk to reduce GI upset; may cause a metallic taste.
2. Report any symptoms of CNS toxicity, such as ataxia or tremor and any unusual bruising or bleeding.
3. Do not perform tasks that require mental alertness until drug effects are realized; dizziness may occur.
4. During treatment for trichomoniasis, partner should also have therapy since organisms may be in the male urogenital tract and reinfect partner. Use condom to prevent reinfections.
5. Do not engage in intercourse while using the vaginal gel.

6. With topical preparation, cleanse area and then apply a thin film into affected area. Avoid eye contact. May apply cosmetics after application and area dry.
7. Drug may turn urine brown; do not be alarmed.
8. No alcohol; a disulfiram-like reaction may occur. Symptoms include abdominal cramps, vomiting, flushing, and headache.

OUTCOMES/EVALUATE

- Symptomatic improvement
- Negative culture reports

Mexiletine hydrochloride

(mex-**ILL**-eh-teen)

PREGNANCY CATEGORY: C
CLASSIFICATION(S):
Antiarrhythmic, Class IB
Rx: Mexitil
✱**Rx:** Novo-Mexiletine

SEE ALSO *ANTIARRHYTHMIC DRUGS.*

ACTION/KINETICS

Similar to lidocaine but is effective PO. Inhibits the flow of sodium into the cell, thereby reducing the rate of rise of the action potential. The drug decreases the effective refractory period in Purkinje fibers. BP and pulse rate are not affected following use, but there may be a small decrease in CO and an increase in peripheral vascular resistance. Also has both local anesthetic and anticonvulsant effects. **Onset:** 30–120 min. **Peak blood levels:** 2–3 hr. **Therapeutic plasma levels:** 0.5–2 mcg/mL. **Plasma t½:** 10–12 hr. Approximately 10% excreted unchanged in the urine; acidification of the urine enhances excretion, whereas alkalinization decreases excretion.

USES

Documented life-threatening ventricular arrhythmias (such as ventricular tachycardia). *Investigational:* Prophylactically to decrease the incidence of ventricular tachycardia and other ventricular arrhythmias in the acute phase of MI. To reduce pain, dysesthesia, and paresthesia associated with diabetic neuropathy.

CONTRAINDICATIONS

Cardiogenic shock, preexisting second- or third-degree AV block (if no pacemaker is present). Use with lesser arrhythmias. Lactation.

SPECIAL CONCERNS

There is the possibility of increased risk of death when used in clients with non-life-threatening cardiac arrhythmias. Use with caution in hypotension, severe CHF, or known seizure disorders. Dosage has not been established in children.

SIDE EFFECTS

CV: ***Worsening of arrhythmias,*** palpitations, chest pain, increased ventricular arrhythmias (PVCs), CHF, angina or angina-like pain, hypotension, bradycardia, syncope, ***AV block or conduction disturbances,*** atrial arrhythmias, hypertension, ***cardiogenic shock,*** hot flashes, edema. **GI:** High incidence of UGI distress, N&V, heartburn. Also, diarrhea/constipation, changes in appetite, dry mouth, abdominal cramps/pain/discomfort, salivary changes, dysphagia, altered taste, pharyngitis, changes in oral mucous membranes, UGI bleeding, peptic ulcer, esophageal ulceration. **CNS:** High incidence of lightheadedness, dizziness, tremor, coordination difficulties, and nervousness. Also, changes in sleep habits, headache, fatigue, weakness, tinnitus, paresthesias, numbness, depression, confusion, difficulty with speech, short-term memory loss, hallucinations, malaise, psychosis, ***seizures,*** loss of consciousness. **Hematologic:** Leukopenia, neutropenia, agranulocytosis, thrombocytopenia. **GU:** Decreased libido, impotence, urinary hesitancy/retention. **Dermatologic:** Rash, dry skin. Rarely, exfoliative dermatitis, and ***Stevens-Johnson syndrome.*** **Miscellaneous:** Blurred vision, visual disturbances, dyspnea, arthralgia, fever, diaphoresis, loss of hair, hiccoughs, laryngeal or pharyngeal changes, syndrome of SLE, myelofibrosis.

M

LABORATORY TEST CONSIDERATIONS
↑ AST. Positive ANA. Abnormal LFTs.

OD OVERDOSE MANAGEMENT
Symptoms: Nausea. CNS symptoms (dizziness, drowsiness, paresthesias, seizures) usually precede CV symptoms (hypotension, sinus bradycardia, intermittent left bundle branch block (LBBB), ***temporary asystole). Massive overdoses cause coma and respiratory arrest.*** *Treatment:* General supportive treatment. Give atropine to treat hypotension or bradycardia. Acidification of the urine may increase rate of excretion.

DRUG INTERACTIONS
Aluminum hydroxide / ↓ Mexiletine absorption
Atropine / ↓ Mexiletine absorption
Caffeine / ↓ Drug clearance (50%)
Cimetidine / ↑ or ↓ Plasma mexiletine levels
Fluvoxamine / ↓ Oral clearance and ↑ in AUC and peak serum levels of mexiletine R/T ↓ liver metabolism
Magnesium hydroxide / ↓ Mexiletine absorption
Metoclopramide / ↑ Mexiletine absorption
Narcotics / ↓ Mexiletine absorption
Phenobarbital / ↓ Plasma mexiletine levels
Phenytoin / ↑ Clearance → ↓ plasma mexiletine levels
Propafenone / ↓ Metabolic clearance of mexiletine in extensive metabolizers → no differences between extensive and poor metabolizers
Rifampin / ↑ Clearance → ↓ plasma mexiletine levels
Theophylline / ↑ Drug effect R/T ↑ serum levels
Urinary acidifiers / ↑ Rate of mexiletine excretion
Urinary alkalinizers / ↓ Rate of mexiletine excretion

HOW SUPPLIED
Capsule: 150 mg, 200 mg, 250 mg

DOSAGE
- **CAPSULES**

Antiarrhythmic.
Adults, individualized, initial: 200 mg q 8 hr if rapid control of arrhythmia not required; dosage adjustment may be made in 50- or 100-mg increments q 2–3 days, if required. **Maintenance:** 200–300 mg q 8 hr, depending on response and tolerance of client. If adequate response is not achieved with 300 mg or less q 8 hr, 400 mg q 8 hr may be tried although the incidence of CNS side effects increases. If the drug is effective at doses of 300 mg or less q 8 hr, the same total daily dose may be given in divided doses q 12 hr (e.g., 450 mg q 12 hr). Maximum total daily dose: 1,200 mg.

Rapid control of arrhythmias.
Initial loading dose: 400 mg followed by a 200-mg dose in 8 hr.

Diabetic neuropathy.
Initial: 150 mg/day for 3 days; **then,** 300 mg/day for 3 days. **Maintenance:** 10 mg/kg/day.

NURSING CONSIDERATIONS

SEE ALSO *NURSING CONSIDERATIONS FOR ANTIARRHYTHMIC DRUGS.*

ADMINISTRATION/STORAGE
1. If transferring to mexiletine from other class I antiarrhythmics, initiate mexiletine at a dose of 200 mg and then titrate according to the response at the following times: 6–12 hr after the last dose of quinidine sulfate, 3–6 hr after the last dose of procainamide, 6–12 hr after the last dose of disopyramide, or 8–12 hr after the last dose of tocainide.
2. Hospitalize client when transferring to mexiletine if there is a chance that withdrawal of the previous antiarrhythmic may produce life-threatening arrhythmias.

ASSESSMENT
1. Document indications for therapy; list any other agents trialed and the outcome.
2. Note evidence of CHF; assess ECG for AV block.
3. Document pulmonary assessment findings; note SaO_2/PO_2.
4. Monitor ECG, CXR, CBC, electrolytes, renal and LFTs.
5. Reduce dose with severe liver disease and marked right-sided CHF.
6. Assess urinary pH; alkalinity decreases and acidity increases renal drug excretion.

CLIENT/FAMILY TEACHING

1. Take with food or an antacid to ↓ GI upset.
2. Do not stop drug suddenly; maintain acidity level in urine by not changing dietary patterns.
3. Report any bruising, bleeding, fevers, or sore throat or adverse CNS effects such as dizziness, tremor, impaired coordination, N&V.
4. Immediately report any increase in heart palpitations, irregularity, or rate less than 50 beats/min.
5. Do not perform tasks that require mental alertness until drug effects are realized.
6. Carry identification that lists drugs currently prescribed. Keep regularly scheduled appointments

OUTCOMES/EVALUATE

- Control of ventricular arrhythmias
- Therapeutic drug levels (0.5–2 mcg/mL)
- ↓ S&S of diabetic neuropathy

Mezlocillin sodium

(mez-low-**SILL**-in)

PREGNANCY CATEGORY: B
CLASSIFICATION(S):
Antibiotic, penicillin
Rx: Mezlin

SEE ALSO *ANTI-INFECTIVES* AND *PENICILLINS.*

ACTION/KINETICS

Broad-spectrum (gram-negative and gram-positive organisms, including aerobic and anaerobic strains) antibiotic used parenterally. **Therapeutic serum levels:** 35–45 mcg/mL. **t½: IV,** 55 min. Excreted mostly unchanged by the kidneys. Penetration to CSF is poor unless meninges are inflamed.

USES

(1) Lower respiratory tract infections, including pneumonia and lung abscess, due to *Haemophilus influenzae, Klebsiella pneumoniae, Proteus mirabilis, Pseudomonas aeruginosa, E. coli,* and *Bacteroides fragilis.* (2) Intra-abdominal infections, including acute cholecystitis, cholangitis, peritonitis, hepatic abscess, and intra-abdominal abscess due to *E. coli, P. mirabilis, Klebsiella* species (sp.), *Pseudomonas* sp., *Streptococcus faecalis, Bacteroides* sp., *Peptococcus* sp., and *Peptostreptococcus* sp. (3) UTIs due to *E. coli, P. mirabilis, Proteus* sp. (indole-positive), *Morganella morganii, Klebsiella* sp., *Enterobacter* sp., *Serratia* sp., *Pseudomonas* sp., and *S. faecalis.* (4) Uncomplicated gonorrhea due to *Neisseria gonorrhoeae.* (5) Gynecologic infections, including endometritis, pelvic cellulitis, and PID due to *N. gonorrhoeae, Peptococcus* sp., *Peptostreptococcus* sp., *Bacteroides* sp., *E. coli, P. mirabilis, Klebsiella* sp., and *Enterobacter* sp. (6) Skin and skin structure infections due to *S. faecalis, E. coli, P. mirabilis, Proteus* sp. (indole-positive), *P. vulgaris, Providencia rettgeri, Klebsiella* sp., *Enterobacter* sp., *Pseudomonas* sp., *Peptococcus* sp., and *Bacteroides* sp. (7) Septicemia, including bacteremia, due to *E. coli, Klebsiella* sp., *Enterobacter* sp., *Pseudomonas* sp., *Bacteroides* sp., and *Peptococcus* sp. (8) Streptococcal infections due to *Streptococcus* sp., including group A beta-hemolytic streptococcus and *S. pneumoniae.* However, these infections are usually treated with more narrow spectrum penicillins. (9) Use in certain severe infections when the causative organisms are not known; give in conjunction with an aminoglycoside or a cephalosporin. (10) In combination with an aminoglycoside to treat life-threatening *P. aeruoginosa* infections. (11) Perioperative use to decrease incidence of infection in clients undergoing surgical procedures that are classified as contaminated or potentially contaminated (e.g., vaginal hysterectomy, colorectal surgery). (12) Caesarean section intraoperative after clamping the umbilical cord and postoperative to reduce postoperative infections.

ADDITIONAL SIDE EFFECTS

Bleeding abnormalities. Decreased hemoglobin or hematocrit values.

LABORATORY TEST CONSIDERATIONS

↑ AST, ALT, serum alkaline phosphatase, serum bilirubin, serum creatinine, and/or BUN. ↓ Serum potassium.

M

HOW SUPPLIED
Powder for injection: 1 g, 2 g, 3 g, 4 g, 20 g

DOSAGE

• **IV, IM**

Serious infections.

Adults: 200–300 mg/kg/day in four to six divided doses; **usual:** 3 g q 4 hr or 4 g q 6 hr. **Infants and children, 1 month–12 years:** 50 mg/kg q 4 hr given **IM** or **IV** over 30 min; **infants more than 2 kg and less than 1 week of age or less than 2 kg and less than 1 week of age:** 75 mg/kg q 12 hr; **infants less than 2 kg and more than 1 week of age:** 75 mg/kg q 8 hr; **infants more than 2 kg and more than 1 week of age:** 75 mg/kg q 6 hr.

Life-threatening infections.

Adults: Up to 350 mg/kg/day, not to exceed 24 g/day. If C_{CR} is 10 to 30 mL/min, give 3 g q 8 hr; if C_{CR} is less than 10 mL/min, give 2 g q 8 hr.

Uncomplicated UTIs.

100–125 mg/kg/day (6 to 8 g/day); 1.5–2 g q 6 hr. If there is renal impairment, give 1.5 g q 8 hr.

Complicated UTIs.

150–200 mg/kg/day (12 g/day); 3 g q 6 hr IV. If C_{CR} is 10 to 30 mL/min, give 1.5 g q 6 hr; if C_{CR} is less than 10 mL/min, give 1.5 g q 8 hr.

Lower respiratory tract infection, intra-abdominal infection, gynecologic infection, skin and skin structure infections, septicemia.

225–300 mg/kg/day (16 to 18 g/day); 4 g q 6 hr or 3 g q 4 hr IV. If C_{CR} is 10 to 30 mL/min, give 3 g q 8 hr; if C_{CR} is less than 10 mL/min, give 2 g q 8 hr. For serious systemic infections in those undergoing hemodialysis for renal failure or peritoneal dialysis: 3–4 g after each dialysis; then q 12 hr.

Gonococcal urethritis.

Adults: Single dose of 1–2 g IV or IM with probenecid, 1 g given at time of dosing or up to 30 min before.

Prophylaxis of postoperative infection.

Adults: 4 g 30–90 min prior to start of surgery; **then,** 4 g, IV, 6 and 12 hr later.

Prophylaxis of infection in clients undergoing cesarean section.

First dose: 4 g IV when cord is clamped; **second and third doses:** 4 g IV 4 and 8 hr after the first dose.

NURSING CONSIDERATIONS

SEE ALSO *NURSING CONSIDERATIONS* FOR *PENICILLINS*.

ADMINISTRATION/STORAGE

1. IM doses should not exceed 2 g/injection. Continue for at least 2 days after symptoms of infection have disappeared.
2. For group A beta-hemolytic streptococcus, continue therapy for at least 10 days.
3. **IV** With IV infusion (including piggyback), do not administer other drugs during mezlocillin infusion.
4. Drug is very irritating to veins. Direct IV administration should be slow to prevent phlebitis; 1 g over 3–5 min. May further dilute in 50–100 mL of dextrose or saline solution and administer over 30 min.
5. For pediatric IV administration, infuse over 30 min.
6. Store vials and infusion bottles at temperatures below 30°C (86°F).
7. The powder and reconstituted solution may darken slightly, but potency is not affected.

ASSESSMENT

1. Note any sensitivity to penicillin or cephalosporins.
2. Monitor cultures, CBC, PT, PTT, electrolytes, and renal function studies. Reduce dose with impaired renal function.

CLIENT/FAMILY TEACHING

1. Drug is given IV or IM for severe infections.
2. Immediately report any evidence of increased bruising and/or bleeding, difficulty breathing, rashes, severe diarrhea, mouth sores, or severe pain at injection site.
3. Report symptoms of drug-induced anemia manifested by fatigue, pallor, weakness, vertigo, headache, dyspnea, and palpitations.

OUTCOMES/EVALUATE

• Negative culture reports
• Therapeutic serum drug levels (35–45 mcg/mL)

M

Miconazole

(my-**KON**-ah-zohl)

PREGNANCY CATEGORY: C
CLASSIFICATION(S):
Antifungal
Rx: Topical: Monistat-Derm, **Vaginal:** Monistat 3, Monistat 3 Combination Pack, Monistat Dual-Pak, M-Zole 3 Combination Pack
✱Rx: Micozole, Monazole 7
OTC: Topical: Absorbine Antifungal Foot Powder, Breezee Mist Antifungal, Fungoid Creme, Fungoid Tincture, Lotrimin AF, Maximum Strength Desenex Antifungal, Micatin, Ony-Clear, Prescription Strength Desenex, Tetterine, Zeasorb-AF; **Vaginal:** Monistat 7, Monistat 7 Combination Pack, M-Zole 7 Dual Pack, Femizol-M

SEE ALSO *ANTI-INFECTIVES*.

ACTION/KINETICS
Broad-spectrum fungicide that alters the permeability of the fungal membrane by inhibiting synthesis of sterols; thus, essential intracellular materials are lost. The drug also inhibits biosynthesis of triglycerides and phospholipids and also inhibits oxidative and peroxidative enzyme activity. May be fungistatic or fungicidal, depending on the concentration.

USES
Topical: Tinea pedis, tinea cruris, tinea corporis caused by *Trichophyton rubrum, T. mentagrophytes,* and *Epidermophyton floccosum* (both OTC and Rx). **Vaginal:** Vulvovaginal candidiasis (suppositories). Relief of external vulvar itching and irritation associated with a yeast infection (cream).

CONTRAINDICATIONS
Hypersensitivity. Use of topical products in or around the eyes.

SPECIAL CONCERNS
Safe use in children less than 1 year of age has not been established.

SIDE EFFECTS
Following topical use: Vulvovaginal burning, pelvic cramps, hives, skin rash, headache, itching, irritation, maceration, and allergic contact dermatitis.

HOW SUPPLIED
Topical. *Cream:* 2%; *Ointment:* 2%; *Powder:* 2%; *Solution:* 2%; *Spray, Spray Powder:* 2%; *Spray Liquid:* 2%. **Vaginal.** *Cream:* 2%; *Dual-Pak or Combination Pack:* Suppository, 100 mg and Topical Cream, 2%; Suppository, 200 mg and Topical Cream, 2%; Suppository, 1,200 mg and Topical Cream, 2%; *Suppositories:* 100 mg, 200 mg

DOSAGE
• TOPICAL, AEROSOL POWDER, AEROSOL SOLUTION, CREAM, LOTION, POWDER

Apply to cover affected areas in morning and evening (once daily for tinea versicolor) for 7 days.

• VAGINAL CREAM OR SUPPOSITORY

Suppositories: One suppository daily at bedtime for 7 days (100-mg suppositories), 3 consecutive days (200-mg suppositories), or 1 day (1,200 mg). Cream: 1 applicatorful intravaginally once daily at bedtime for 3–7 days. For topical use, apply cream to affected areas b.i.d. (morning and evening) for up to 7 days or as needed. Repeat course, if needed, after ruling out other pathogens.

NURSING CONSIDERATIONS

SEE ALSO *GENERAL NURSING CONSIDERATIONS* FOR *ANTI-INFECTIVES*.

ADMINISTRATION/STORAGE
1. The lotion is preferred for intertriginous areas.
2. To reduce recurrence of symptoms, tinea cruris, tinea corporis, and candida should be treated for 2 weeks; tinea pedis should be treated for 1 month.
3. Refrigerate vaginal products below 15–30°C (59–86°F).

ASSESSMENT
1. Determine any previous experience with this drug, any sensitivity, and response obtained.
2. Monitor cultures, CBC, electrolytes, and LFTs.
3. Document clinical presentation, noting size, number, and extent of lesions.

M

CLIENT/FAMILY TEACHING

1. Review technique for administration; use only as directed. Complete full course of therapy despite symptom improvement.
2. Use sanitary pads to protect clothing and linens when using cream or suppositories.
3. When used for vaginal infections, refrain from intercourse or use a condom to prevent reinfection.
4. When used vaginally, continue treatment during menses.
5. Report if exposed to HIV and recurrent vaginal infections occur.
6. Report lack of response or persistent N&V, diarrhea, dizziness, and itching.

OUTCOMES/EVALUATE

- Negative culture reports
- Resolution of vaginitis evidenced by ↓ itching/burning; ↓ discharge
- ↓ Size and number of lesions

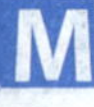

Midazolam hydrochloride

(my-**DAYZ**-oh-lam)

PREGNANCY CATEGORY: D
CLASSIFICATION(S):
Benzodiazepine, adjunct to general anesthesia
Rx: Versed, **C-IV**

SEE ALSO *TRANQUILIZERS, ANTIMANIC DRUGS, AND HYPNOTICS*.

ACTION/KINETICS

Short-acting benzodiazepine with sedative–general anesthetic properties. Depresses the response of the respiratory system to carbon dioxide stimulation, which is more pronounced in clients with COPD. Possible mild to moderate decreases in CO, mean arterial BP, SV, and systemic vascular resistance. HR may rise somewhat in those with slow HRs (< 65/min) and decrease in others (especially those with HRs > 85/min). **Onset, IM:** 15 min; **IV:** 2–2.5 min for induction (if combined with a preanesthetic narcotic, induction is about 1.5 min). If preanesthetic medication (morphine) is given, the **Peak plasma levels, IM:** 45 min. **Maximum effect:** 30–60 min. **Time to recovery:** Usually within 2 hr, although up to 6 hr may be required. About 97% bound to plasma protein. **$t^{1/2}$, elimination:** 1.2–12.3 hr. Rapidly metabolized in the liver to inactive compounds; excreted through the urine.

USES

IV, IM: Preoperative sedation, anxiolysis, and amnesia. **IV:** (1) Sedation, anxiolysis, and amnesia prior to or during short diagnostic, therapeutic, or endoscopic procedures (either alone or with other CNS depressants). (2) Induction of general anesthesia before administration of other anesthetics. Supplement to nitrous oxide and oxygen in balanced anesthesia. (3) Sedation of intubated and mechanically ventilated clients as a component of anesthesia or during treatment in a critical care setting. **PO:** In children to help alleviate anxiety before a diagnostic or therapeutic procedure or before anesthesia induction. Also to reduce ability to recall events that occurred during sedation. *Investigational:* Treat epileptic seizures. Alternative to terminate refractory status epilepticus.

CONTRAINDICATIONS

Hypersensitivity to benzodiazepines. Acute narrow-angle glaucoma. Use in obstetrics, coma, shock, or acute alcohol intoxication where VS are depressed. IA injection.

SPECIAL CONCERNS

Use with caution during lactation. Pediatric clients may require higher doses than adults. Hypotension may be more common in conscious sedated clients who have received a preanesthetic narcotic. Geriatric and debilitated clients require lower doses to induce anesthesia and they are more prone to side effects. Use IV with extreme caution in severe fluid or electrolyte disturbances.

SIDE EFFECTS

Fluctuations in VS, including decreased respiratory rate and tidal volume, apnea, variations in BP and pulse rate are common. The following are general side effects regardless of the route of administration. **CV:** Hypotension, ***cardiac arrest.*** **CNS:** Oversedation, headache, drowsiness, grogginess, confusion, retrograde amnesia, euphoria, nervousness, agitation, anxiety, argumentativeness, restlessness, emergence delirium, increased time for emergence, dreaming during emergence, nightmares, insomnia, tonic-clonic movements, ataxia, muscle tremor, involuntary or athetoid movements, dizziness, dysphoria, dysphonia, slurred speech, paresthesia. **GI:** Hiccoughs, N&V, acid taste, retching, excessive salivation. **Ophthalmologic:** Double/blurred vision, nystagmus, pinpoint pupils, visual disturbances, cyclic eyelid movements, difficulty in focusing. **Dermatologic:** Hives, swelling or feeling of burning, warmth or cold feeling at injection site, hive-like wheal at injection site, pruritus, rash. **Miscellaneous:** Blocked ears, loss of balance, chills, weakness, faint feeling, lethargy, yawning, toothache, hematoma.

• **MORE COMMON FOLLOWING IM USE.**

Pain at injection site, headache, induration and redness, muscle stiffness.

• **MORE COMMON FOLLOWING IV USE:**

Respiratory: ***Bronchospasm,*** coughing, dyspnea, ***laryngospasm,*** hyperventilation, shallow respirations, tachypnea, ***airway obstruction***, wheezing, respiratory depression and ***respiratory arrest*** when used for conscious sedation. **CV:** PVCs, bigeminy, bradycardia, tachycardia, vasovagal episode, nodal rhythm. **At injection site:** Tenderness, pain, redness, induration, phlebitis.

DRUG INTERACTIONS

Alcohol / ↑ Risk of apnea, airway obstruction, desaturation or hypoventilation
Anesthetics, inhalation / ↓ Dose if midazolam used as an induction agent
Antifungals, azole / ↑ Effect of midazolam R/T ↓ liver metabolism
Cimetidine / ↑ Sedation
Clarithromycin / ↑ Effect of midazolam R/T ↓ liver metabolism
CNS Depressants / ↑ Risk of apnea, airway obstruction, desaturation or hypoventilation
Contraceptives, oral / Prolongation of midazolam half-life
Droperidol / ↑ Hypnotic effect of midazolam when used as a premedication
Erythromycin / ↑ Effect of midazolam R/T ↓ liver metabolism
Fentanyl / ↑ Hypnotic effect of midazolam when used as a premedication
Fluvoxamine / ↑ Serum midazolam levels, reduced clearance, and prolonged half-life
Indinavir / Possible prolonged sedation and respiratory depression
Meperidine / See *Narcotics;* also, ↑ Risk of hypotension
Narcotics / ↑ Hypnotic effect of midazolam when used as premedications
Propofol / ↑ Effect of propofol
Protease inhibitors / ↑ Effect of midazolam R/T ↓ liver metabolism
Rifamycins / Possible pharmacokinetic chagnes of midazolam
Ritonavir / Possible prolonged sedation and respiratory depression
Selective serotonin reuptake inhibitors / ↑ Effect of midazolam R/T ↓ liver metabolism
Theophyllines / Antagonism of midazolam's sedative effects
Thiopental / ↓ Dose if midazolam used as an induction agent
Valproic acid / Possible ↓ liver metabolism of midazolam
Verapamil / Possible ↑ CNS depression and prolonged midazolam effects

HOW SUPPLIED

Injection: 1 mg/mL, 5 mg/mL; *Syrup:* 2 mg/mL

DOSAGE

• **IM**

Preoperative sedation, anxiolysis, amnesia.

Adults: 0.07–0.08 mg/kg IM (average: 5 mg) 1 hr before surgery. **Children:** 0.1–0.15 mg/kg (up to 0.5 mg/kg may be needed for more anxious clients).

• **IV**

Conscious sedation, anxiolysis, amnesia for endoscopic or CV procedures in healthy adults less than 60 years of age.

M

Using the 1 mg/mL (can be diluted with 0.9% sodium chloride or D5W) product, titrate slowly to the desired effect (usually slurred speech); initial dose should be no higher than 2.5 mg IV (may be as low as 1 mg IV) within a 2-min period; wait an additional 2 min to evaluate the sedative effect. If additional sedation is necessary, give small increments waiting an additional 2 min or more after each increment to evaluate the effect. Total doses greater than 5 mg are usually not required. **Children:** Dosage must be individualized by the physician.

Conscious sedation for endoscopic or CV procedures in debilitated or chronically ill clients or clients aged 60 or over.

Slowly titrate to the desired effect using no more than 1.5 mg initially IV (may be as little as 1 mg IV) given over a 2-min period; wait an additional 2 min or more to evaluate the effect. If additional sedation is needed, no more than 1 mg should be given over 2 min; wait an additional 2 min or more after each increment in dose. Total doses greater than 3.5 mg are usually not needed.

Induction of general anesthesia, before use of other general anesthetics, in unmedicated clients.

Adults, unmedicated clients up to 55 years of age, IV, initial: 0.3–0.35 mg/kg given over 20–30 sec, waiting 2 min for effects to occur. If needed, increments of about 25% of the initial dose can be used to complete induction; or, induction can be completed using a volatile liquid anesthetic. Up to 0.6 mg/kg may be used but recovery will be prolonged. **Adults, unmedicated clients over 55 years of age who are good risk surgical clients, initial IV:** 0.15–0.3 mg/kg given over 20–30 sec. **Adults, unmedicated clients over 55 years of age with severe systemic disease or debilitation, initial IV:** 0.15–0.25 mg/kg given over 20–30 sec. **Pediatric:** 0.05–0.2 mg/kg IV.

Induction of general anesthesia, before use of other general anesthetics, in medicated clients.

Adults, premedicated clients up to 55 years of age, IV, initial: 0.15–0.35 mg/kg. If less than 55 years of age, 0.25 mg/kg may be given over 20–30 sec, allowing 2 min for effect. **Adults, premedicated clients over 55 years of age who are good risk surgical clients, initial, IV:** 0.2 mg/kg. **Adults, premedicated clients over 55 years of age with severe systemic disease or debilitation, initial, IV:** 0.15 mg/kg may be sufficient.

Maintenance of balanced anesthesia for short surgical procedures.

IV: Incremental injections about 25% of the dose used for induction when signs indicate anesthesia is lightening.

NOTE: Narcotic preanesthetic medication may include fentanyl, 1.5–2 mcg/kg IV 5 min before induction; morphine, up to 0.15 mg/kg IM; meperidine, up to 1 mg/kg IM; or, Innovar, 0.02 mL/kg IM. Sedative preanesthetic medication may include secobarbital sodium, 200 mg PO or hydroxyzine pamoate, 100 mg PO. Except for fentanyl, give all preanesthetic medications 1 hr prior to midazolam. Always individualize doses.

NURSING CONSIDERATIONS

SEE ALSO *NURSING CONSIDERATIONS FOR TRANQUILIZERS, ANTIMANIC DRUGS, AND HYPNOTICS.*

ADMINISTRATION/STORAGE

1. When used for procedures via the mouth, use a topical anesthetic.
2. Give IM doses in a large muscle mass.
3. IV When used for conscious sedation, do not give by rapid or single bolus IV; may cause respiratory depression.
4. When used for induction of general anesthesia, give the initial dose over 20–30 sec.
5. If preanesthetic medications with a depressant component are given (e.g., narcotic analgesics or CNS depressants), reduce the midazolam dosage by 50% compared with healthy, young unmedicated clients.
6. Give maintenance doses to all clients in increments of 25% of the dose first required to achieve the sedative endpoint.

7. Give a narcotic preanesthetic for bronchoscopic procedures.
8. Carefully monitor all IV doses with the immediate availability of oxygen, resuscitative equipment, and personnel who are skilled in maintaining a patent airway and for support of ventilation; continue monitoring during recovery period.
9. May be mixed in the same syringe with atropine, meperidine, morphine, or scopolamine
10. At a concentration of 0.5 mg/mL midazolam is compatible with D5W and 0.9% NaCl for up to 24 hr and with RL solution for up to 4 hr.

CLIENT/FAMILY TEACHING

1. Drug may cause dizziness and drowsiness. Avoid alcohol, CNS depressants, and activities that require mental alertness for 24-48 hr following drug administration.
2. Repeat postprocedure instructions and obtain in writing as may not fully recall instructions; transient amnesia is normal and memory of procedure may be minimal.

OUTCOMES/EVALUATE

Desired level of sedation and amnesia; ↓ anxiety

Midodrine hydrochloride

(**MIH**-doh-dreen)

PREGNANCY CATEGORY: C
CLASSIFICATION(S):
Vasopressor
Rx: ProAmatine
✱**Rx:** Amatine

ACTION/KINETICS

Midodrine, a prodrug, is converted to an active metabolite—desglymidodrine—that is an alpha-1 agonist. Desglymidodrine produces an increase in vascular tone and elevation of BP by activating alpha-adrenergic receptors of the arteriolar and venous vasculature. No effect on cardiac beta-adrenergic receptors. The active metabolite does not cross the blood-brain barrier; thus, there are no CNS effects. Standing systolic BP is increased by approximately 15–30 mm Hg at 1 hr after a 10-mg dose; duration: 2–3 hr. Rapidly absorbed from the GI tract. **Peak plasma levels, midodrine:** 30 min; **t½:** 25 min. **Peak plasma levels, desglymidodrine:** 1–2 hr; **t½:** 3–4 hr. The bioavailability of the active metabolite is not affected by food. Desglymidodrine is eliminated in the urine.

USES

Orthostatic hypotension in those whose lives are significantly impaired despite standard clinical care. *Investigational:* Management of urinary incontinence.

CONTRAINDICATIONS

Use in severe organic heart disease, acute renal disease, urinary retention, pheochromocytoma, thyrotoxicosis, persistent and excessive supine hypertension.

SPECIAL CONCERNS

Use with caution in impaired renal or hepatic function, during lactation, in orthostatic hypotensive clients who are also diabetic, or in those with a history of visual problems or who are also taking fludrocortisone acetate. Safety and efficacy have not been determined in children.

SIDE EFFECTS

CNS: Paresthesia, pain, headache, feeling of pressure or fullness in the head, confusion, abnormal thinking, nervousness, anxiety. Rarely, dizziness, insomnia, somnolence. **GI:** Dry mouth. Rarely, canker sore, nausea, GI distress, flatulence. **Dermatologic:** Piloerection, pruritus, rash, vasodilation, flushed face. Rarely, erythema multiforme, dry skin. **Miscellaneous:** Dysuria, supine hypertension. Rarely, visual field defect, skin hyperesthesia, impaired urination, asthenia, backache, pyrosis, leg cramps.

OD OVERDOSE MANAGEMENT

Symptoms: Hypertension, piloerection, sensation of coldness, urinary retention. *Treatment*: Emesis and administration of an alpha-adrenergic blocking agent (e.g., phentolamine).

DRUG INTERACTIONS
Alpha-adrenergic agonists / ↑ Pressor effects of midodrine
Alpha-adrenergic antagonists / Antagonism of the effects of midodrine
Beta-adrenergic blockers / ↑ Risk of bradycardia, AV block, or arrhythmias
Cardiac glycosides / ↑ Risk of bradycardia, AV block, or arrhythmias
Fludrocortisone / ↑ Intraocular pressure and glaucoma
Psychopharmacologic drugs / ↑ Risk of bradycardia, AV block, or arrhythmias

HOW SUPPLIED
Tablet: 2.5 mg, 5 mg

DOSAGE

• **TABLETS**

Orthostatic hypotension.

10 mg t.i.d. given during the daytime hours when the client is upright and pursuing daily activities (e.g., shortly before or upon arising in the morning, midday, and late afternoon–not later than 6:00 p.m.). To control symptoms, dosing may be q 3 hr. Initial dose in impaired renal function: 2.5 mg t.i.d.

Urinary incontinence.

2.5–5 mg b.i.d.–t.i.d.

M

NURSING CONSIDERATIONS

ASSESSMENT

1. Document onset, duration, and characteristics of symptoms. Note other nonpharmacologic treatments (i.e., support stockings, increased salt in diet, fluid expansion, sleeping with head of bed raised) trialed.
2. Orthostatic hypotension is defined as SBP reductions > 20 mm Hg or DBP of over 10 mm Hg reduction within 3 min of standing; assess carefully on several occasions.
3. Document any acute renal disease, urinary retention, pheochromocytoma, severe organic heart disease, or thyrotoxicosis, as these preclude drug therapy. Assess for liver and renal dysfunction.

CLIENT/FAMILY TEACHING

1. Take during the day while up and around. Do not take after the evening meal or within 4 hr of bedtime.
2. Use OTC products containing phenylephrine (e.g.; cold/allergy remedies/ diet aids) cautiously; may increase supine BP.
3. May experience supine hypertension; check BP regularly while lying and sitting and keep a record. Stop drug and report blurred vision, pounding in ears, headache, cardiac awareness, increased dizziness/syncope.

OUTCOMES/EVALUATE

Relief of symptomatic orthostatic hypotension: ↓ dizziness, ↓ lightheadedness, ↓ unsteadiness

Mifepristone

(mih-feh-**PRIS**-tohn)

CLASSIFICATION(S):
Abortifacient
Rx: Mifeprex

ACTION/KINETICS
Competes with progesterone at progesterone-receptor sites, thus inhibiting the activity of endogenous or exogenous progesterone. During pregnancy, the drug sensitizes the myometrium to the contraction-inducing activity of prostaglandins. Termination of pregnancy results. Also exhibits antiglucocorticoid and weak antiandrogenic activity. Rapidly absorbed. **Peak plasma levels:** 1.98 mg/L after 90 min. Is 98% plasma protein bound. **t½, elimination:** 50% eliminated between 12 and 72 hr followed by a more rapid phase with a terminal **t½** of 18 hr. Metabolized in the liver by CYP450 3A4 with most eliminated in the feces.

USES
Medical termination of intrauterine pregnancy through day 49 of pregnancy. Pregnancy is dated from the first day of the last menstrual period in a presumed 28-day cycle with ovulation occurring at mid-cycle. When mifepristone and misoprostol fail to cause termination of intrauterine pregnancy, pregnancy termination by surgery is recommended.

CONTRAINDICATIONS
Use for termination of pregnancy in any one of the following conditions: confirmed or suspected ectopic pregnancy or undiagnosed adnexal mass;

IUD in place; chronic adrenal failure; concurrent long-term corticosteroid therapy; history of allergy to mifepristone, misoprostol, or other prostaglandins; hemorrhagic disorders or concurrent anticoagulant therapy; pregnancy termination > 49 days; inherited porphyrias. Use if client does not have adequate access to medical facilities equipped to provide emergency treatment of incomplete abortion, blood transfusions, and emergency resuscitation during the period from the first visit until discharged by the administering physician. Use in those who can not understand the effects of the treatment procedure or comply with its regimen.

SPECIAL CONCERNS

Clients should expect vaginal bleeding or spotting for an average of 9–16 days. Safety and efficacy have not been determined for use in cardiovascular, hypertensive, hepatic, respiratory, or renal disease; insulin-dependent diabetes mellitus; severe anemia; heavy smoking; or, pediatric clients. Use with caution during lactation; decision may be made to discard breast milk for a few days following use.

SIDE EFFECTS

NOTE: Bleeding and cramping are expected results of therapy. Only side effects with an incidence of 1% or greater are listed. **GI:** N&V, diarrhea, abdominal pain, dyspepsia. **GU:** Uterine cramping, uterine hemorrhage, vaginitis. **CNS:** Headache, dizziness, insomnia, anxiety. **Body as a whole:** Asthenia, fatigue, fever, viral infection, chills/shaking. **Miscellaneous:** Fainting, pelvic pain, back pain, leg pain, anemia, leukorrhea, sinusitis.

LABORATORY TEST CONSIDERATIONS

Rarely, ↑ AST, ALT, alkaline phosphatase, gamma-glutamyltransferase. ↓ Hemoglobin, hematocrit, RBCs in women who bleed heavily.

DRUG INTERACTIONS

Carbamazepine / Possible ↓ mifepristone serum levels R/T ↑ liver metabolism
Dexamethasone / Possible ↓ mifepristone serum levels R/T ↑ liver metabolism
Erythromycin / Possible ↑ mifepristone serum levels R/T ↓ liver metabolism
Grapefruit juice / Possible ↑ mifepristone serum levels R/T ↓ liver metabolism
Itraconazole / Possible ↑ mifepristone serum levels R/T ↓ liver metabolism
Ketoconazole / Possible ↑ mifepristone serum levels R/T ↓ liver metabolism
Phenobarbital / Possible ↓ mifepristone serum levels R/T ↑ liver metabolism
Phenytoin / Possible ↓ mifepristone serum levels R/T ↑ liver metabolism
Rifampin / Possible ↓ mifepristone serum levels R/T ↑ liver metabolism
H *St. John's wort* / Possible ↓ mifepristone serum levels R/T ↑ liver metabolism

NOTE: When used with mifepristone, possible increase in serum levels of drugs that are **CYP 3A4** substrates. Use with caution with such drugs that have a narrow therapeutic range (e.g., some agents used during general anesthesia).

HOW SUPPLIED

Tablets: 200 mg

DOSAGE

• **TABLET**

Termination of intrauterine pregnancy.

Treatment includes both mifepristone and misoprostol and requires three office visits. **Day 1:** Three-200 mg tablets (600 mg) of mifepristone taken as a single dose. **Day 3:** Unless abortion has occurred and has been confirmed by clinical examination or ultrasonographic scan, clients must take misoprostol, 400 mcg PO. **Day 14:** Client returns for follow-up visit to confirm by clinical examination or ultrasonographic scan that complete termination of pregnancy has occurred.

NURSING CONSIDERATIONS

ADMINISTRATION/STORAGE

1. The drug is supplied only to licensed physicians who sign and return a Prescriber's Agreement. It is not

M

available to the public through licensed pharmacies.
2. Remove any intrauterine device before beginning mifepristone treatment.
3. Available only in single dose packaging.
4. Administration must be under the supervision of a qualified physician.
5. Clients must read the Medication Guide and read and sign the Patient Agreement before mifepristone is given.
6. Mifepristone may be less effective if misoprostol is given more than 2 days after mifepristone use.

ASSESSMENT

1. The duration of pregnancy can be determined from menstrual history and clinical examination. Use an ultrasonographic scan if the duration of pregnancy is uncertain or if ectopic pregnancy is suspected.
2. Ensure client fully understands the results of treatment and is in concurrence. Provide a copy of the Medication Guide and the Patient Agreement. May obtain by contacting Danco-Laboratories.
3. List drugs prescribed to ensure none interact unfavorably (CYP 3A4 metabolism).
4. Obtain history to assess for CAD, HTN, IDDM, smoking, hepatic/respiratory/renal disease, or severe anemia as drug has not been studied in these groups.

CLIENT/FAMILY TEACHING

1. Review Medication Guide and Patient Agreement to understand the treatment procedure and its effects. Request clarification or pose questions as needed and sign agreement.
2. The treatment consists of three (3) visits to the provider. On day one a dose of mifepristone (600 mg) po is administered. Return on day 3 to determine if abortion has occurred by clinical exam or by ultrasound. If not, misoprostol 400 mcg will be administered orally. Finally, must return on day 14-16 to confirm termination of pregnancy.
3. Onset of action usually occurrs between 2 and 24 hrs of initial treatment. Menses should begin within 5 days of treatments and will last 1-2 weeks.
4. May experience vaginal bleeding and uterine cramping, nausea, vomiting, diarrhea, and headache.
5. Prolonged, heavy bleeding, does not confirm a complete expulsion. With treatment failure, there is an increased risk of fetal malformation.
6. If medical treatment fails, these cases are managed by surgical termination (D&C).
7. Contraception must be initiated as soon as the termination of pregnancy has been confirmed or before sexual intercourse is resumed as pregnancy can occur before resumption of normal menses.
8. In addition to uterine bleeding and cramping, may experience N&V, pelvic pain, diarrhea, fainting, headaches, and dizziness. Bleeding and spotting may occur for over 2 weeks after treatment. Report immediately if persistent or significant side effects.

OUTCOMES/EVALUATE

Termination of pregnancy

Miglitol

(**MIG**-lih-tohl)

PREGNANCY CATEGORY: B
CLASSIFICATION(S):
Antidiabetic, oral; alpha-glucosidase inhibitor
Rx: Glyset

SEE ALSO *ANTIDIABETIC AGENTS.*

ACTION/KINETICS

Acts by delaying digestion of ingested carbohydrates resulting in smaller rise in blood glucose levels after meals. Effect is due to reversible inhibition of membrane-bound intestinal glucoside hydrolase enzymes which hydrolyze oligosaccharides and disaccharides to glucose and other monosaccharides. Reduces levels of glycosylated hemoglobin in type II diabetes. Does not enhance insulin secretion or increase insulin sensitivity. Does not cause hypoglycemia when given in fasted state. Absorption is saturable at high doses (i.e., only 50% to 70% of 100 mg dose is absorbed while 25 mg dose is 100% absorbed). **Peak levels:** 2–3 hr. Drug is not metabolized and is eliminated unchanged in urine. Reduce dose in impaired renal function.

USES

Alone as adjunct to diet to treat non-insulin-dependent diabetes. With sulfonylurea when diet plus either miglitol or a sulfonylurea alone do not result in adequate control (effects of sulfonylurea and miglitol are additive).

CONTRAINDICATIONS

Lactation, diabetic ketoacidosis, inflammatory bowel disease, colonic ulceration, partial intestinal obstruction, those predisposed to intestinal obstruction, chronic intestinal diseases associated with marked disorders of digestion or absorption, conditions that may deteriorate due to increased gas formation in the intestine, hypersensitivity to drug.

SPECIAL CONCERNS

When given with sulfonylurea or insulin, miglitol causes further decrease in blood sugar and increased risk of hypoglycemia. Safety and efficacy have not been determined in children.

SIDE EFFECTS

GI: Flatulence, diarrhea, abdominal pain, soft stools, abdominal discomfort. **Dermatologic:** Skin rash (transient).

DRUG INTERACTIONS

Amylase / ↓ Miglitol effect
Charcoal / ↓ Miglitol effect
Digestive enzymes / ↓ Miglitol absorption
Digoxin / May ↓ plasma digoxin levels
Pancreatin / ↓ Miglitol effect
Propranolol / Significant ↓ propranolol bioavailability
Ranitidine / Significant ↓ ranitidine bioavailability

HOW SUPPLIED

Tablets: 25 mg, 50 mg, 100 mg

DOSAGE

• **TABLETS**

Type II diabetes.

Individualize dosage. **Initial:** 25 mg t.i.d. with first bite of each main meal (some may benefit from starting with 25 mg once daily to minimize GI side effects). After 4 to 8 weeks of 25 mg t.i.d. dose, increase dosage to 50 mg t.i.d. for about 3 months. Measure glycosylated hemoglobin; if not satisfactory, increase dose to 100 mg t.i.d. **Maintenance:** 50 mg t.i.d., up to 100 mg t.i.d. (maximum).

NURSING CONSIDERATIONS

SEE ALSO *NURSING CONSIDERATIONS* FOR *ANTIDIABETIC AGENTS.*

ASSESSMENT

1. Document indications, other agents trialed, and outcome.
2. Determine any IBD, colonic ulceration, intestinal obstruction, or severe digestion/absorption problems.
3. Monitor BS, HbA1-C, and renal function; reduce dose with impaired function and avoid if creatinine > 2 mg/dL.

CLIENT/FAMILY TEACHING

1. Take with first bite of each meal, 3 x per day.
2. Attend diabetic education program to enhance understanding of disease, diet control, weight loss, foot care, eye care, hygiene, and exercise as it relates to overall health.
3. May experience abdominal pain and diarrhea which should diminish with continued treatment.
4. Any stress, fever, trauma, infection, or surgery may alter glucose control; monitor FS regularly.
5. Drug inhibits breakdown of table sugar; have glucose available for episodes of marked hypoglycemia.
6. Continue prescribed diet and regular exercise. Report for F/U as scheduled.

OUTCOMES/EVALUATE

↓ BS; HbA1-C < 7

Milrinone lactate

(**MILL**-rih-nohn)

PREGNANCY CATEGORY: C
CLASSIFICATION(S):
Inotropic drug
Rx: Primacor

M

ACTION/KINETICS

Selective inhibitor of peak III cyclic AMP phosphodiesterase isozyme in cardiac and vascular muscle, resulting in a direct inotropic effect and a direct arterial vasodilator activity. Also improves diastolic function as manifested by improvements in LV diastolic relaxation. In clients with depressed myocardial function, produces a prompt increase in CO and a decrease in pulmonary wedge pressure and vascular resistance, without a significant increase in HR or myocardial oxygen consumption. Causes an inotropic effect in clients who are fully digitalized without causing signs of glycoside toxicity. Also, LV function has improved in clients with ischemic heart disease. **Therapeutic plasma levels:** 150–250 ng/mL. **t½:** 2.3 hr following doses of 12.5–125 mcg/kg to clients with CHF. Metabolized in the liver and excreted primarily through the urine.

USES

Short-term IV treatment of CHF, usually in clients receiving digoxin and diuretics.

CONTRAINDICATIONS

Hypersensitivity to the drug. Use in severe obstructive aortic or pulmonary valvular disease in lieu of surgical relief of the obstruction.

SPECIAL CONCERNS

Use with caution during lactation. Safety and efficacy have not been determined in children.

SIDE EFFECTS

CV: ***Ventricular and supraventricular arrhythmias, including ventricular ectopic activity, nonsustained ventricular tachycardia, sustained ventricular tachycardia, and ventricular fibrillation. Infrequently, life-threatening arrhythmias associated with preexisting arrhythmias,*** metabolic abnormalities, abnormal digoxin levels, and catheter insertion. Also, hypotension, angina, chest pain. **Miscellaneous:** Mild to moderately severe headaches, hypokalemia, tremor, thrombocytopenia, bronchospasm (rare).

OD OVERDOSE MANAGEMENT

Symptoms: Hypotension. *Treatment:* If hypotension occurs, reduce or temporarily discontinue administration of milrinone until the condition of the client stabilizes. Use general measures to support circulation.

HOW SUPPLIED

Injection: 1 mg/mL; *Injection, premixed:* 200 mcg/mL in D5W

DOSAGE

• IV INFUSION

Adults, loading dose: 50 mcg/kg administered slowly over 10 min. **Maintenance, minimum:** 0.59 mg/kg/24 hr (infused at a rate of 0.375 mcg/kg/min); **maintenance, standard:** 0.77 mg/kg/24 hr (infused at a rate of 0.5 mcg/kg/min); **maintenance, maximum:** 1.13 mg/kg/24 hr (infused at a rate of 0.75 mcg/kg/min).

NURSING CONSIDERATIONS

ADMINISTRATION/STORAGE

IV 1. Give IV infusions at rates described in the package insert.

2. Adjust rate depending on the hemodynamic and clinical response.

3. Prepare dilutions using 0.45% or 0.9% NaCl or 5% dextrose injection.

4. Reduce rate in renal impairment (see package insert for chart).

5. Do not give furosemide in IV lines containing milrinone as a precipitate will form.

6. Store at room temperatures of 15–30°C (59–86°F).

ASSESSMENT

1. Document indications, onset and characteristics of symptoms. Identify other meds used and the outcome.

2. Monitor CBC, lytes, liver/renal function studies. Document ECG, CO, CVP, and PAWP; rule out acute MI.

INTERVENTIONS

1. Monitor I&O, electrolyte levels, and renal function. Potassium loss due to excessive diuresis may cause arrhythmias in digitalized clients; correct hypokalemia.

2. Monitor VS; review parameters for interruption of infusion (e.g., SBP < 80; HR < 50).

3. Observe for increased supraventricular and ventricular arrhythmias on monitor.

OUTCOMES/EVALUATE

- ↑ CO and ↓ PACWP
- Resolution of S&S of CHF
- Drug levels (150–250 ng/mL)

Minocycline hydrochloride

(mih-no-**SYE**-kleen)

PREGNANCY CATEGORY: D
CLASSIFICATION(S):
Antibiotic, tetracycline
Rx: Arestin, Dynacin, Minocin, Vectrin
✱Rx: Alti-Minocycline, Apo-Minocycline, Gen-Minocycline, Novo-Minocycline, Rhoxal-minocycline, Scheinpharm Minocycline

SEE ALSO *ANTI-INFECTIVES* AND *TETRACYCLINES.*

ACTION/KINETICS

In fasting adults, 90% to 100% of an oral dose is absorbed. **Peak plasma levels:** 1–4 hr. Absorption is less affected by milk or food than for other tetracyclines. **t½, elimination:** 11–26 hr. Metabolized in the liver.

USES

See also *Tetracyclines.* To eliminate meningococci from the nasopharynx of asymptomatic *Neisseria meningitidis* carriers in which the risk of meningococcal meningitis is high. *NOTE:* Due to adverse CNS effects, use rifampin to treat meningococcus carriers when the drug susceptibility is not known or when the organism is sulfa-resistant. Use minocycline only when rifampin is contraindicated.

(1) Granulomas of the skin caused by *Mycobacterium marinum.* (2) In combination with gonococcal regimens for presumptive treatment of coexisting chlamydial infections. (3) Uncomplicated gonogoccal urethritis in adult males. (4) Treatment of uncomplicated urethral, endocervical, or rectal infections caused by *Chlamydia trachomatis* or *Ureaplasma urealyticum* in adults. (5) Intrapleurally as a sclerosing agent to control pleural effusions assocated with metastatic tumors. (6) Treatment of cholera and nocardiosis. (7) Adjunctive treatment of inflammatory acne unresponsive to oral tetracycline HCl or oral erythromycin. (7) Adjunctive treatment of adult periodontitis (Arestin).

ADDITIONAL SIDE EFFECTS

Blue-gray pigmentation areas of cutaneous inflammation, vertigo, ataxia, drowsiness, ***Stevens-Johnson syndrome*** (rare).

HOW SUPPLIED

Capsules: 50 mg, 100 mg; *Capsules, pellet filled:* 50 mg, 100 mg; *Powder for Injection:* 100 mg; *Oral Suspension:* 50 mg/5 mL

DOSAGE

• CAPSULES, INJECTION, ORAL SUSPENSION, TABLETS

Infections against which effective, including asymptomatic meningococcus carriers.

Adults, initial: 200 mg; **then,** 100 mg q 12 hr. An alternative regimen is 100–200 mg initially followed by 50 mg q 6 hr. The length of treatment is 5 days for meningococcus carriers. **Children over 8 years of age, initial:** 4 mg/kg; **then,** 2 mg/kg q 12 hr.

Mycobacterial infections.

100 mg PO b.i.d. for 6–8 weeks.

Uncomplicated gongococcal urethritis in adult males.

100 mg b.i.d. for 5 days.

Uncomplicated urethral, endocervical, or rectal infections due to Chlamydia trachomatis *or* Ureaplasma urealyticum.

100 mg PO b.i.d. for at least 7 days.

Nongonococcal urethritis caused by C. trachomatis *or* Mycoplasma.

100/day PO in 1 or 2 divided doses for 1 to 3 weeks.

Sclerosing agent to control pleural effusions associated with metastatic cancer.

300 mg diluted with 40–50 mL of 0.9% NaCl injection and instilled into the pleural space through a thoracostomy tube.

Cholera in conjunction with fluid and electrolyte replacement.

Initial: 200 mg PO; **then,** 100 mg PO 12 hr for 48–72 hr.

Adjunct to treat inflammatory acne unresponsive to PO tetracycline HCl or erythromycin.

50 mg PO 1–3 times/day.

NURSING CONSIDERATIONS

SEE ALSO *NURSING CONSIDERATIONS FOR ANTI-INFECTIVES* AND *TETRACYCLINES*.

ADMINISTRATION/STORAGE

(1) Minocycline microspheres (Arestin) are delivered directly into the infected periodontal pocket after scaling and root planing. No refrigeration or mixing is needed and the product does not require removal.

IV (2) Do not dissolve in solutions containing calcium; forms a precipitate.

(3) After dissolving medication in the vial, further dilute to 500–1,000 mL with any of the following: dextrose, dextrose and NaCl, NaCl, RL, Ringer's injection.

(4) Start administration of the final dilution immediately.

(5) Discard reconstituted solutions after 24 hr at room temperature.

ASSESSMENT

1. Document onset, location, and characteristics of S&S.
2. Monitor C&S, renal and LFTs, and CBC; identify contacts when treating contagious diseases. Ensure ID referral.

CLIENT/FAMILY TEACHING

1. Take complete prescription; may take with meals if GI upset occurs.
2. With STDs, use condoms during therapy to prevent reinfections and obtain periodic cultures.
3. Practice reliable non-hormonal birth control; drug may cause fetal harm.
4. Avoid prolonged sunlight exposure; may cause photosensitivity reaction.
5. Report any unusual bruising or bleeding, severe rash or diarrhea, difficulty breathing, dark urine or light stools, severe cramps, and lack of improvement after 72 hr.

OUTCOMES/EVALUATE

Symptomatic improvement; resolution of infection

Minoxidil, oral

(mih-**NOX**-ih-dil)

PREGNANCY CATEGORY: C

CLASSIFICATION(S):
Antihypertensive, peripheral vasodilator
Rx: Loniten

SEE ALSO *ANTIHYPERTENSIVE AGENTS*.

ACTION/KINETICS

Decreases elevated BP by decreasing peripheral resistance by a direct effect. Causes increase in renin secretion, increase in cardiac rate and output, and salt/water retention. Does not cause orthostatic hypotension. **Onset:** 30 min. **Peak plasma levels:** reached within 60 min; **plasma t½:** 4.2 hr. **Duration:** 24–48 hr. Ninety percent absorbed from GI tract; excretion: renal (90% metabolites). The time needed to reach the maximum effect is inversely related to the dose.

USES

Severe hypertension not controllable by the use of a diuretic plus two other antihypertensive drugs. Usually taken with at least two other antihypertensive drugs (a diuretic and a drug to minimize tachycardia such as a beta-adrenergic blocking agent). Can produce severe side effects; reserve for resistant cases of hypertension. Close medical supervision required, including possible hospitalization during initial administration.

CONTRAINDICATIONS

Pheochromocytoma. Within 1 month after a MI. Dissecting aortic aneurysm.

SPECIAL CONCERNS

Safe use during lactation not established. Use with caution and at reduced dosage in impaired renal function. Geriatric clients may be more sensitive to the hypotensive and hypothermic effects of minoxidil; also, may be necessary to decrease the dose due to age-related decreases in renal function. BP controlled too rapidly may cause syncope, stroke, MI, and ischemia of affected organs. Experience with use in children is limited.

SIDE EFFECTS

CV: Edema, ***pericardial effusion that may progress to tamponade*** (acute compression of heart caused by fluid or blood in pericardium), CHF, angina pectoris, changes in direction of T waves, increased HR. In children, rebound hypertension following slow withdrawal. **GI:** N&V. **CNS:** Headache, fatigue. *Hypersensitivity:* Rashes, including bullous eruptions and ***Stevens-Johnson syndrome.*** **Hematologic:** Initially, decrease in hematocrit, hemoglobin, and erythrocyte count but all return to normal. Rarely, thrombocytopenia and leukopenia. **Other:** Hypertrichosis (enhanced hair growth, pigmentation and thickening of fine body hair 3–6 weeks after initiation of therapy), breast tenderness, darkening of skin.

LABORATORY TEST CONSIDERATIONS

Nonspecific changes in ECG. ↑ Alkaline phosphatase, serum creatinine, and BUN.

OD OVERDOSE MANAGEMENT

Symptoms: Excessive hypotension. *Treatment:* Give NSS IV (to maintain BP and urine output). Vasopressors, such as phenylephrine and dopamine, can be used but only in underperfusion of a vital organ.

DRUG INTERACTIONS

Concomitant use with guanethidine may result in severe hypotension.

HOW SUPPLIED

Tablet: 2.5 mg, 10 mg

DOSAGE

• **TABLETS**

Hypertension.

Adults and children over 12 years, Initial: 5 mg/day. For optimum control, dose can be increased to 10, 20, and then 40 mg in single or divided doses/day. Do not exceed 100 mg/day. **Children under 12 years: Initial,** 0.2 mg/kg/day. Effective dose range: 0.25–1.0 mg/kg/day. Dosage must be titrated to individual response. Do not exceed 50 mg/day.

NURSING CONSIDERATIONS

SEE ALSO *NURSING CONSIDERATIONS* FOR *ANTIHYPERTENSIVE AGENTS.*

ADMINISTRATION/STORAGE

1. Give once daily if supine DBP has been reduced less than 30 mm Hg and twice daily (in two equal doses) if it has been reduced more than 30 mm Hg.
2. Wait at least 3 days between dosage adjustments as the full response is not obtained until then. However, if more rapid control is required, may adjust q 6 hr but with careful monitoring.

ASSESSMENT

1. Anticipate BP decreases within 30 min.
2. List other agents trialed and the outcome. Note if diuretic prescribed.
3. Assess cardiopulmonary status.
4. Monitor CBC, glucose, electrolytes, and renal function studies.

CLIENT/FAMILY TEACHING

1. Can be taken with fluids and without regard to meals.
2. Record weight daily; report any S&S of fluid overload (gain of 6 lb/week; edema of extremities, face, and abdomen; or dyspnea).
3. Report any symptoms of angina, fainting, dizziness, or dyspnea that occurs, especially when lying down.
4. Drug may cause elongation, thickening, and increased pigmentation of body hair; should resolve once discontinued.

OUTCOMES/EVALUATE

↓ BP; control of hypertension

Minoxidil, topical solution

(mih-**NOX**-ih-dill)

PREGNANCY CATEGORY: C
CLASSIFICATION(S):
Hair growth stimulant
OTC: Minoxidil for Men, Rogaine, Rogaine Extra Strength for Men
✱**OTC:** Apo-Gain, Minox

ACTION/KINETICS

The topical solution stimulates vertex hair growth in clients with male pattern baldness or in women with androgenetic alopecia. Mechanism may be related to dilation of arterioles and stimulation of resting hair follicles into active growth. Following topical administration, approximately 1.4% is absorbed into the systemic circula-

M

tion. **Onset:** 4 months but is variable. **Duration:** New hair growth may be lost 3–4 months after withdrawal of therapy. Minoxidil and its inactive metabolites are excreted in the urine. Also, see *Minoxidil, oral*.

USES

To treat male and female pattern baldness (alopecia androgenetica). Extra Strength (5%) is only for treatment of hereditary male pattern baldness. *Investigational:* Alopecia areata.

CONTRAINDICATIONS

Lactation. Use of 5% solution in women.

SPECIAL CONCERNS

Use with caution in clients with hypertension, coronary heart disease, or predisposition to heart failure. Safety and efficacy in clients under 18 years of age have not been determined. Increased systemic absorption may occur if the scalp is irritated or there are abrasions.

SIDE EFFECTS

Dermatologic: Allergic contact dermatitis, irritant dermatitis, pruritus, dry skin, flaking of scalp, alopecia, hypertrichosis, erythema, eczema, worsening of hair loss. **Allergic:** Hives, facial swelling, allergic rhinitis, nonspecific allergic reactions. **GI:** N&V, diarrhea. **CNS:** Dizziness, lightheadedness, headache, faintness, anxiety, depression, fatigue. **CV:** Edema, chest pain, BP increase or decrease, palpitations, increase/decrease in pulse rate. **Respiratory:** Sinusitis, bronchitis, URTI. **Endocrine:** Menstrual changes, breast symptoms. **GU:** UTI, renal calculi, urethritis, prostatitis, epididymitis, vaginitis, vulvitis, vaginal discharge, itching. **Hematologic:** Lymphadenopathy, thrombocytopenia, anemia. **Musculoskeletal:** Fractures, back pain, tendinitis, aches and pains. **Ophthalmic:** Conjunctivitis, visual disturbances, decreased visual acuity. **Miscellaneous:** Vertigo, ear infections, edema, weight gain. *NOTE:* The incidence of side effects due to placebos is often similar to the incidence of side effects due to the drug itself.

DRUG INTERACTIONS

Corticosteroids, topical / Enhance absorption of topical minoxidil
Guanethidine / Possible ↑ risk of orthostatic hypotension
Petrolatum / Enhances absorption of topical minoxidil
Retinoids / Enhance absorption of topical minoxidil

HOW SUPPLIED

Solution: 2%, 5%

DOSAGE

- **TOPICAL SOLUTION: 2%, 5%**
  Stimulate hair growth.

Adults: Apply 1 mL b.i.d. directly onto the scalp in the hair loss area. 5% solution not to be used on women.

NURSING CONSIDERATIONS

ADMINISTRATION/STORAGE

1. Use only in clients with normal, healthy scalps. Dermatitis, scalp abrasions, scalp psoriasis, or severe sunburn may increase the absorption of topical minoxidil and lead to systemic side effects (See *Minoxidil, oral*).
2. Hair may be shampooed before treatment, but dry the hair and scalp prior to topical application.
3. The product comes with a metered spray attachment (for application to large areas of the scalp), extender spray attachment (for application to small scalp areas or under the hair), and a rub-on applicator tip (to spread the solution on the scalp). Follow the directions on the package insert carefully for each of these methods of application. Warn not to inhale the spray mist.
4. If the fingertips are used to apply the drug, wash the hands thoroughly after application.
5. At least 4 months of continuous therapy is necessary before evidence of hair growth can be expected. Further hair growth continues through 1 year of treatment.
6. The alcohol base in topical minoxidil will cause irritation and burning of the eyes, abraded skin, or mucous membranes. If contact with any of these areas, wash the site with copious amounts of water.
7. Avoid inhaling the spray mist.

CLIENT/FAMILY TEACHING

1. Review appropriate method and frequency for application; solution

may dry and leave a residue on the hair, this is harmless.
2. May permanently discolor linens, hats and pillows with prolonged use/contact.
3. More frequent than prescribed applications will not enhance hair growth but will increase systemic side effects. Review info booklet.
4. New hair growth will be soft and hard to see and is not permanent. Drug is a treatment, not a cure; cessation of therapy will lead to hair loss within a few months. Topical minoxidil must be used indefinitely to sustain the effect.
5. Treatment has positive benefits for only approximately one-half the population. May take up to 4 months of continuous therapy before any response is noted.
6. Report any evidence of irritation or rash.
7. Do not apply any other topical products to the scalp without approval.
8. Consult provider before using if no family history of gradual hair loss, if hair loss is sudden or patchy, if hair loss is accompanied by other symptoms, or if the reasons for hair loss are not clear.

OUTCOMES/EVALUATE

Stimulation of hair growth

Mirtazapine

(mir-**TAZ**-ah-peen)

PREGNANCY CATEGORY: C
CLASSIFICATION(S):
Antidepressant, tetracyclic
Rx: Remeron, Remeron SolTab

SEE ALSO *ANTIDEPRESSANTS*.

ACTION/KINETICS

Enhances central noradrenergic and serotonergic activity, perhaps by antagonism at central presynaptic alpha-2 adrenergic inhibitory autoreceptors and heteroreceptors. Also a potent antagonist of 5-HT_2, 5-HT_3, and histamine H_1 receptors. Moderate antagonist of peripheral alpha-1 adrenergic receptors and muscarinic receptors. Rapidly and completely absorbed from the GI tract. **Peak plasma levels:** Within 2 hr. **t½:** 20–40 hr. Extensively metabolized in the liver and excreted in both the urine (75%) and feces (15%). Females exhibit significantly longer elimination half-lives than males.

USES

Treatment of depression.

CONTRAINDICATIONS

Use in combination with a MAO inhibitor or within 14 days of initiating or discontinuing therapy with a MAO inhibitor. Known or suspected seizure disorders. During acute phase of MI.

SPECIAL CONCERNS

Use with caution in those with impaired renal or hepatic disease, in geriatric clients, during lactation, in CV or cerebrovascular disease that can be exacerbated by hypotension (e.g., history of MI, angina, ischemic stroke), and in conditions that would predispose to hypotension (e.g., dehydration, hypovolemia, treatment with antihypertensive medications). The effect of mirtazapine for longer than 6 weeks has not been evaluated, although treatment is indicated for 6 months or longer. Safety and efficacy have not been determined in children.

SIDE EFFECTS

Side effects with an incidence of 0.1% or greater are listed. **CNS:** Somnolence, dizziness, activation of mania or hypomania, ***suicidal ideation***, sedation, drowsiness, abnormal dreams, abnormal thinking, tremor, confusion, hypesthesia, apathy, depression, hypokinesia, vertigo, twitching, agitation, anxiety, amnesia, hyperkinesia, paresthesia, ataxia, delirium, delusions, depersonalization, dyskinesia, extrapyramidal syndrome, increased libido, abnormal coordination, dysarthria, hallucinations, neurosis, dystonia, hostility, increased reflexes, emotional lability, euphoria, paranoid reaction. **GI:** N&V, anorexia, dry mouth, constipation, ulcer, eructation, glossitis, cholecystitis, gum hemorrhage,

M

stomatitis, colitis, abnormal LFTs. **CV:** Hypertension, vasodilation, angina pectoris, ***MI,*** bradycardia, ventricular extrasystoles, syncope, migraine, orthostatic hypotension. **Hematologic:** Agranulocytosis. **Body as a whole:** Asthenia, flu syndrome, back pain, malaise, abdominal pain, acute abdominal syndrome, chills, fever, facial edema, photosensitivity reaction, neck rigidity, neck pain, enlarged abdomen. **Respiratory:** Dyspnea, increased cough, sinusitis, epistaxis, bronchitis, asthma, pneumonia. **GU:** Urinary frequency, UTI, kidney calculus, cystitis, dysuria, urinary incontinence, urinary retention, vaginitis, hematuria, breast pain, amenorrhea, dysmenorrhea, leukorrhea, impotence. **Musculoskeletal:** Myalgia, myasthenia, arthralgia, arthritis, tenosynovitis. **Dermatologic:** Pruritus, rash, acne, exfoliative dermatitis, dry skin, herpes simplex, alopecia. **Metabolic/nutritional:** Increased appetite, weight gain, peripheral edema, edema, thirst, dehydration, weight loss. **Ophthalmic:** Eye pain, abnormal accommodation, conjunctivitis, keratoconjunctivitis, lacrimation disorder, glaucoma. **Miscellaneous:** Deafness, hyperacusis, ear pain.

LABORATORY TEST CONSIDERATIONS

↑ ALT and nonfasting cholesterol and triglycerides.

OD OVERDOSE MANAGEMENT

Symptoms: Disorientation, drowsiness, impaired memory, tachycardia. *Treatment:* General supportive measures. If the client is unconscious, establish and maintain an airway. Consider induction of emesis or gastric lavage and administration of activated charcoal. Monitor cardiac and vital signs.

DRUG INTERACTIONS

Clonidine / Possible ↓ clonidine's hypertensive effect
CNS depressants / Enhanced CNS depressant effect
Diazepam / Additive impairment of motor skills

HOW SUPPLIED

Tablet: 15 mg, 30 mg, 45 mg; *Tablet, Oral Disintegrating:* 15 mg, 30 mg, 45 mg

DOSAGE

• ORAL DISINTEGRATING TABLETS, TABLETS

Treatment of depression.

Initial: 15 mg/day given as a single dose, preferably in the evening before sleep. Those not responding to the 15-mg dose may respond to doses up to a maximum of 45 mg/day. Do not make dose changes at intervals of less than 1 to 2 weeks. Consider treatment for up to 6 months.

NURSING CONSIDERATIONS

SEE ALSO *NURSING CONSIDERATIONS* FOR *ANTIDEPRESSANTS*.

ADMINISTRATION/STORAGE

1. The oral disintegrating tablet (SolTab) can be swallowed with or without water, chewed, or allowed to disintegrate.
2. At least 2 weeks should elapse between discontinuing an MAOI and starting mirtazapine therapy. Also, 14 or more days should elapse after stopping mirtazapine and starting an MAOI.

ASSESSMENT

1. Document indications, onset, triggers, and symptom characteristics.
2. Note precipitating events that may relate to depression, i.e., death, divorce, illness, or job loss.
3. List drugs currently and previously prescribed; ensure no MAO inhibitor use within past 2 weeks.
4. Monitor ECG, CBC, LFTs, cholesterol, and triglyceride levels.

CLIENT/FAMILY TEACHING

1. Take as directed; do not exceed prescribed dosing schedule.
2. For the orally disintegrating tablet, open tablet blister pack with dry hands and place tablet on the tongue. It will disintegrate within 30 seconds and can be swallowed with saliva or chewed. Do not split the tablet and do not open the blister pack until just before use.
3. Report any S&S of infection or flu (fever, sore throat, stomatitis, etc.); drug may cause (a lack of WBC's) agranulocytosis.
4. Do not engage in activities that require mental alertness until drug ef-

fects realized; dizziness and drowsiness may occur.
5. Avoid alcohol and OTC agents; may potentiate drug's cognitive and motor skill impairment.
6. Report as scheduled for follow-up labs, counselling, and evaluation of clinical response to drug therapy.

OUTCOMES/EVALUATE

Improved sleeping and eating patterns; improved mood, ↑ interest in social activities

Misoprostol

(my-soh-**PROST**-ohl)

PREGNANCY CATEGORY: X
CLASSIFICATION(S):
Prostaglandin
Rx: Cytotec

ACTION/KINETICS

Synthetic prostaglandin E_1 analog that inhibits gastric acid secretion, protects the gastric mucosa by increasing bicarbonate and mucous production, and decreases pepsin levels during basal conditions. May also stimulate uterine contractions that may endanger pregnancy. Rapidly converted to the active misoprostol acid. **Time for peak levels of misoprostol acid:** 12 min. **t½, misoprostol acid:** 20–40 min. Misoprostol acid is less than 90% bound to plasma protein. *NOTE:* Misoprostol does not prevent development of duodenal ulcers in clients on NSAIDs.

USES

Prevention of aspirin and other nonsteroidal anti-inflammatory-induced gastric ulcers in clients with a high risk of gastric ulcer complications (e.g., geriatric clients with debilitating disease) or in those with a history of ulcer. *Investigational:* Treat duodenal ulcers including those unresponsive to histamine H_2 antagonists. With cyclosporine and prednisone to decrease the incidence of acute graft rejection in renal transplant clients (the drug improves renal function). With methotrexate to induce abortion.

CONTRAINDICATIONS

Allergy to prostaglandins, pregnancy, during lactation (may cause diarrhea in nursing infants). Use to induce labor or abortion (may cause fetal/maternal death; uterine hyperstimulation, rupture, or perforation; amniotic fluid embolism, severe vaginal bleeding, shock, or fetal bradycardia).

SPECIAL CONCERNS

Use with caution in clients with renal impairment and in clients older than 64 years of age. Safety and efficacy have not been established in children less than 18 years of age. May cause miscarriage with potentially serious bleeding.

SIDE EFFECTS

GI: Diarrhea, abdominal pain, nausea, dyspepsia, flatulence, vomiting, constipation. **Gynecologic:** Spotting, cramps, dysmenorrhea, hypermenorrhea, menstrual disorders, postmenopausal vaginal bleeding. **Miscellaneous:** Headache.

OD OVERDOSE MANAGEMENT

Symptoms: Abdominal pain, diarrhea, dyspnea, sedation, tremor, fever, palpitations, bradycardia, hypotension, ***seizures.*** *Treatment:* Use supportive therapy.

HOW SUPPLIED

Tablet: 100 mcg, 200 mcg

DOSAGE

• **TABLETS**

Adults: 200 mcg q.i.d. with food. Dose can be reduced to 100 mcg if the larger dose cannot be tolerated. In renal impairment, the 200-mcg dose can be reduced if necessary.

NURSING CONSIDERATIONS

ADMINISTRATION/STORAGE

1. Reduce diarrhea by giving after meals and at bedtime; avoid magnesium-containing antacids. Diarrhea is usually self-limiting.
2. Maximum plasma levels are decreased if drug is taken with food.
3. Take for the duration of NSAID therapy.
4. Drug may increase gastric bicarbonate and mucous production.

M

ASSESSMENT

1. Document any ulcer disease; assess GI symptoms, clinical presentation and indications.
2. Obtain a negative pregnancy test unless being used with methotrexate to induce abortion.

CLIENT/FAMILY TEACHING

1. Do not share medications.
2. Avoid foods/spices that may aggravate condition: caffeine, alcohol, and black pepper.
3. Take misoprostol exactly as prescribed for the duration of aspirin or NSAID therapy to prevent ulcer formation.
4. May experience abdominal discomfort and/or diarrhea; take misoprostol after meals and at bedtime to minimize these side effects. Avoid magnesium-containing antacids.
5. Report persistent diarrhea, postmenopausal bleeding, or increased menstrual bleeding.
6. All women of childbearing age must practice effective contraceptive measures; drug has abortifacient properties.
7. With abortion, report any increased bleeding, pain, or fever.

OUTCOMES/EVALUATE

Prevention of drug-induced gastric ulcers

Mitomycin (MTC)

(my-toe-**MY**-sin)

CLASSIFICATION(S):
Antineoplastic, antibiotic
Rx: Mutamycin

SEE ALSO *ANTINEOPLASTIC AGENTS.*

ACTION/KINETICS

Antibiotic produced by *Streptomyces caespitosus* that inhibits DNA synthesis. At high doses both RNA and protein synthesis are inhibited. Most active during late G_1 and early S stages. **t½, initial:** 5–15 min; **final:** 50 min. Metabolized in liver; 10% excreted unchanged in urine, more when dose is increased.

USES

Palliative treatment and adjunct to surgical or radiologic treatment of disseminated adenocarcinoma of the stomach and pancreas. Used in combination with other agents (not recommended as a single agent for primary treatment or in place of surgery and/or radiotherapy). *Investigational:* Superficial bladder cancer; cancer of the breast, head and neck, lung, cervix; colorectal cancer; biliary cancer; chronic myelocytic leukemia. Ophthalmic solution used as an adjunct to surgical excision to treat primary or recurrent pterygia.

CONTRAINDICATIONS

Pregnancy and lactation. Thrombocytopenia, coagulation disorders, increase in bleeding tendency due to other causes. In clients with a serum creatinine level greater than 1.7 mg/dL.

SPECIAL CONCERNS

Use with extreme caution in presence of impaired renal function.

ADDITIONAL SIDE EFFECTS

Severe bone marrow depression, especially leukopenia and thrombocytopenia. Pulmonary toxicity including dyspnea with nonproductive cough. ***Microangiopathic hemolytic anemia with renal failure and hypertension (hemolytic uremic syndrome),*** especially when used long-term in combination with fluorouracil. Cellulitis. Extravasation causes severe necrosis of surrounding tissue. ***Respiratory distress syndrome in adults, especially when used with other chemotherapy.***

DRUG INTERACTIONS

Severe bronchospasm and SOB when used with vinca alkaloids.

HOW SUPPLIED

Powder for injection: 5 mg, 20 mg, 40 mg

DOSAGE

• IV ONLY

10–20 mg/m² as a single dose via infusion q 6–8 wk. Subsequent courses of treatment are based on hematologic response; do not repeat until leukocyte count is at least 4,000/mm³ and platelet count is at least 100,000/mm³.

NURSING CONSIDERATIONS

SEE ALSO *NURSING CONSIDERATIONS* FOR *ANTINEOPLASTIC AGENTS.*

ADMINISTRATION/STORAGE

IV 1. Drug is toxic; avoid extravasation. Observe infusion site closely for evidence of erythema or complaints of discomfort. Apply ice and use thiosulfate for infiltrate.

2. Reconstitute 5-, 20-, or 40-mg vial with 10, 40, or 80 mL sterile water for injection, respectively, as indicated and administer over 5–10 min; will dissolve if allowed to remain at room temperature.

3. Drug concentration of 0.5 mg/mL is stable for 14 days under refrigeration or 7 days at room temperature.

4. Diluted concentrations of 20–40 mcg/mL, are stable for 3 hr in D5W, for 12 hr in isotonic saline, and for 24 hr in sodium lactate injection.

5. Mitomycin (5–15 mg) and heparin (1,000–10,000 units) in 30 mL of isotonic saline is stable for 48 hr at room temperature.

ASSESSMENT

1. Document pulmonary function. Obtain CXR; pulmonary infiltrates and fibrosis can occur with cumulative doses. Observe closely for early evidence of pulmonary complications, such as dyspnea, nonproductive cough, and abnormal ABGs/lung sounds.

2. Obtain baseline CBC, PT, PTT, and renal function; do not initiate if serum creatinine level is >1.7 mg/dL. Drug may cause platelet and granulocyte suppression. Nadir: 28 days; recovery: 40–55 days.

OUTCOMES/EVALUATE

↓ Tumor size/spread

Mitotane (O,P'-DDD)

(**MY**-toe-tayn)

PREGNANCY CATEGORY: C
CLASSIFICATION(S):
Antineoplastic, miscellaneous
Rx: Lysodren

SEE ALSO *ANTINEOPLASTIC AGENTS*.

ACTION/KINETICS

Directly suppresses activity of adrenal cortex and changes the peripheral metabolism of corticosteroids, resulting in a decrease in 17-hydroxycorticosteroids. About 40% absorbed from GI tract; detectable in serum for 6–9 weeks after administration. Mostly stored in adipose tissue. **t½:** After therapy terminated, 18–159 days. Unchanged drug is excreted in the feces while metabolites are excreted in the urine. Steroid replacement therapy may have to be instituted (i.e., increased) to correct adrenal insufficiency. Therapy is continued as long as drug seems effective. Beneficial results may not become apparent until after 3 months of therapy.

USES

Inoperable carcinoma (both functional and nonfunctional) of the adrenal cortex. *Investigational:* Cushing's syndrome.

CONTRAINDICATIONS

Hypersensitivity to drug. Discontinue temporarily after shock or severe trauma. Lactation.

SPECIAL CONCERNS

Use with caution in the presence of liver disease other than metastatic lesions. Long-term usage may cause brain damage and functional impairment.

SIDE EFFECTS

CNS: Continuous doses may result in brain damage and impairment of function. Depression, lethargy, somnolence, dizziness, vertigo. **GI:** N&V, anorexia, diarrhea. **CV:** Hypertension, orthostatic hypotension, flushing. **Dermatologic:** Transient skin rashes. **Ophthalmic:** Visual blurring, diplopia, lens opacity, toxic retinopathy. **GU:** Hematuria, hemorrhagic cystitis, albuminuria. **Miscellaneous:** Adrenal insufficiency, generalized aching, hyperpyrexia.

LABORATORY TEST CONSIDERATIONS

↓ PBI and urinary 17-hydroxycorticosteroids.

DRUG INTERACTIONS

Corticosteroids / ↑ Corticosteroid metabolism → need for ↑ doses
Warfarin / ↑ Rate of warfarin metabolism → need for ↑ dosage

M

HOW SUPPLIED
Tablet: 500 mg

DOSAGE

• **TABLETS**

Carcinoma of the adrenal cortex.

Adults, initial: 2–6 g/day in three to four equally divided doses; increase dose incrementally to 9–10 g/day (maxiumum tolerated dose: 2–16 g/day). Adjust dosage upward or downward according to severity of side effects or lack thereof. **Pediatric, initial:** 1–2 g/day in divided doses; **then,** dose can be increased gradually to 5–7 g/day.

Cushing's syndrome.

Initial: 3–6 g/day in three to four divided doses; **then,** 0.5 mg 2 times/week to 2 g/day.

NURSING CONSIDERATIONS

SEE ALSO *NURSING CONSIDERATIONS FOR ANTINEOPLASTIC AGENTS.*

ADMINISTRATION/STORAGE

1. Initiate in hospital until stable dosage schedule is achieved.
2. Continue treatment for 3 mo. If no beneficial effects noted after 3 mo at the maximum tolerated dose, a clinical failure can be concluded.
3. Discontinue immediately following shock or severe trauma. To counteract shock or trauma, be prepared to administer steroid medications in high doses; depressed adrenals may not produce sufficient steroids.

ASSESSMENT

1. Note indications for therapy and other agents trialed. Assess for any sensitivity to mitotane; document any episodes of shock or severe trauma that would necessitate discontinuation of drug therapy.
2. Assess for evidence of brain damage or impairment of function by performing behavioral and neurologic assessments.
3. To minimize possibility of infarction and hemorrhage in the tumor due to the rapid cytotoxic effect, ensure all possible tumor tissue is removed surgically before giving mitotane.

CLIENT/FAMILY TEACHING

1. Report any symptoms of adrenal insufficiency, such as weakness, increased fatigue, lethargy, and GI effects (including weight loss, N&V, and anorexia).
2. Always wear identification in case of trauma or shock; carry list of drugs currently prescribed.
3. Avoid tasks that require mental alertness until drug effects realized. Avoid situations that may cause injury or exposure to infections.
4. Desired effects may not be evident for 3 mo. If none noted after 3 mo at maximum tolerated dosage, drug will be stopped and a clinical failure concluded.
5. Use reliable contraception; drug may cause fetal abnormalities/death.

OUTCOMES/EVALUATE

• ↓ Tumor size and spread
• Desired cortisol levels

Mitoxantrone hydrochloride

(my-toe-**ZAN**-trohn)

PREGNANCY CATEGORY: D
CLASSIFICATION(S):
Antineoplastic, antibiotic
Rx: Novantrone

SEE ALSO *ANTINEOPLASTIC AGENTS.*

ACTION/KINETICS

Most active in the late S phase of cell division but is not cell-cycle specific. Appears to bind to DNA by intercalation between base pairs and a nonintercalative electrostatic interaction, causing an inhibition of DNA and RNA synthesis. Low distribution to the brain, spinal cord, spinal fluid, and eyes. **t½:** Approximately 6 days. Highly bound to plasma proteins. Excreted through both the feces (via the bile) and the urine (up to 65% unchanged).

USES

(1) In combination with other drugs, for the initial treatment of acute nonlymphocytic leukemias, including monocytic, promyelocytic, myelocytic, and acute erythroid leukemias. (2) In combination with steroids to treat pain from advanced hormone-refractory prostate cancer. (3) Treat secon-

dary progressive, progressive relapsing, or worsening relapsing-remitting multiple sclerosis. *Investigational:* Alone or in combination with other drugs to treat breast and liver cancer; non-Hodgkin's lymphomas.

CONTRAINDICATIONS

Preexisting myelosuppression (unless benefits outweigh risks). Use with baseline neutrophil counts less than 1,500 cells/mm³ (except for treatment of acute nonlymphocytic leukemia). Lactation. Intrathecal use.

SPECIAL CONCERNS

Safety and efficacy have not been established in children. May be mutagenic.

SIDE EFFECTS

Hematologic: Severe myelosuppression, ecchymosis, petechiae, secondary acute myelogenous leukemia. **GI:** N&V, diarrhea, stomatitis, mucositis, abdominal pain, GI bleeding. **CNS:** Headache, seizures. **CV:** CHF (***potentially fatal***), decreases in LV ejection fraction, arrhythmias, tachycardia, chest pain, hypotension. **Respiratory:** Cough, dyspnea. **Miscellaneous:** Conjunctivitis, urticaria, rashes, renal failure, hyperuricemia, alopecia, fever, phlebitis (at infusion site), tissue necrosis (as a result of extravasation), jaundice. In addition, there is an increased risk of pneumonia, urinary tract and fungal infections, and sepsis.

LABORATORY TEST CONSIDERATIONS

Transient ↑ AST and ALT.

OD OVERDOSE MANAGEMENT

Symptoms: Severe leukopenia with infection. *Treatment:* Antibiotic therapy. Monitor hematology.

HOW SUPPLIED

Injection: 2 mg (base)/mL

DOSAGE

• **IV INFUSION**

Initial therapy for acute nonlymphocytic leukemia, induction.

Mitoxantrone, 12 mg/m²/day on days 1–3 combined with cytosine arabinoside, 100 mg/m² as a continuous 24-hr infusion on days 1–7. If the response is incomplete, a second induction course may be given using the same daily dosage, but giving mitoxantrone for 2 days and cytosine arabinoside for 5 days. *Consolidation therapy, approximately 6 weeks after final induction therapy.* Mitoxantrone, 12 mg/m²/day on days 1 and 2 combined with cytosine arabinoside, 100 mg/m² as a continuous 24-hr infusion on days 1–5. A second consolidation course of therapy may be given 4 weeks after the first.

Secondary progressive multiple sclerosis.

12 mg/m² q 3 months. Due to the risk of cardiotoxicity, no more than 8–12 doses can be given over 2–3 years.

NURSING CONSIDERATIONS

SEE ALSO *NURSING CONSIDERATIONS* FOR *ANTINEOPLASTIC AGENTS*.

ADMINISTRATION/STORAGE

IV 1. Do not mix in the same infusion with other drugs.
2. Must be diluted prior to use with at least 50 mL of either D5W or 0.9% NaCl injection.
3. Give diluted solution into a freely running IV infusion of either D5W or 0.9% NaCl slowly over at least 3 min.
4. Avoid extravasation at the injection site. Do not allow contact with the eyes, mucous membranes, or skin.
5. Do not freeze.
6. Closely follow hospital procedures for the handling and disposal of antineoplastic drugs.

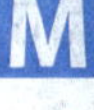

ASSESSMENT

1. Note indications for therapy, other agents trialed and any cardiac disease. Perform baseline ECG and assess for symptoms of cardiotoxicity.
2. Anticipate N&V, mucositis/stomatitis; initiate appropriate protocol. Assess need for allopurinol therapy with rapid tumor lysis.
3. Monitor VS, CBC, uric acid, liver and renal function studies. Drug may cause granulocyte and platelet suppression. Nadir: 10–14 days; recovery: 21 days.

CLIENT/FAMILY TEACHING

1. Drug is usually given for 3 days IV with cytosine or other drug therapy; freq lab tests will be done to eval drug effects.

2. May temporarily discolor urine and/or sclera greenish blue for 24 hr after therapy.
3. Report any persistent diarrhea, N&V, abnormal bruising and bleeding, sore throat, severe dyspnea, swelling of extremities, severe joint pain, or any S&S of infection.
4. Consume 2–3 L/day of fluids to prevent hyperuricemia.
5. Avoid vaccinia, persons with infections and crowds, especially during flu season.
6. Practice reliable contraception.
7. May experience stomatitis/mucositis within one week of therapy.

OUTCOMES/EVALUATE

Improved hematologic parameters; suppression of malignant cell proliferation

Mivacurium chloride

(**mih**-vah-**KYOUR**-ee-um)

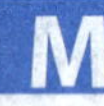

PREGNANCY CATEGORY: C
CLASSIFICATION(S):
Neuromuscular blocking drug
Rx: Mivacron

SEE ALSO ***NEUROMUSCULAR BLOCKING AGENTS.***

ACTION/KINETICS

Competitively inhibits the action of acetylcholine on the motor end plate, resulting in a block of neuromuscular transmission. Time to maximum neuromuscular blockade is similar to atracurium (2.3–4.9 min in adults depending on the dose and 1.6–2.8 min in children depending on the dose). **Clinically effective neuromuscular block, adults:** 15–20 min after 0.15 mg/kg; **children:** 6–15 min after 0.2 mg/kg. Spontaneous recovery may be 95% complete in 25–30 min after an initial dose of 0.15 mg/kg in adults during opioid/nitrous oxide/oxygen anesthesia. Repeated administration or continuous infusion (for up to 2.5 hr) does not cause tachyphylaxis or cumulative neuromuscular blockade. Higher doses may cause transient decreases in mean arterial BP (especially seen in obese clients) and increases in HR in some clients within 1–3 min following the dose (can be minimized by giving the drug over 30–60 sec). The product is actually a mixture of isomers with varying elimination half-lives. Inactivated by plasma cholinesterase with metabolites excreted in the urine and bile.

USES

Adjunct to general anesthesia to facilitate tracheal intubation and to provide relaxation of skeletal muscle during surgery or mechanical ventilation.

CONTRAINDICATIONS

Sensitivity to mivacurium or other similar agents. Use of multidose vials in clients with allergy to benzyl alcohol.

SPECIAL CONCERNS

Use with caution during lactation, in clients with significant CV disease, and in those with any history of a greater sensitivity to the release of histamine or related mediators such as asthma. Volatile anesthetics may decrease the dosing requirement and prolong the duration of action. Duration may be prolonged in clients with decreased plasma cholinesterase. Reduced clearance of one or more isomers is observed in clients with end-stage kidney or liver disease. Geriatric clients show a longer duration of neuromuscular blockade. Acid-base or serum electrolyte abnormalities may potentiate or antagonize the action of neuromuscular blocking agents. Antagonism of neuromuscular blockade may be delayed in the presence of debilitation, carcinomatosis, and concomitant use of certain broad-spectrum antibiotics, anesthetic agents, and other drugs that enhance neuromuscular blockade. In children 2–12 years of age, mivacurium has a faster onset, shorter duration, and a faster recovery following reversal than adults. The drug has not been studied in children less than 2 years of age.

SIDE EFFECTS

Neuromuscular: Prolonged neuromuscular blockade, muscle spasms. **CV:** Flushing of face, neck, or chest; hypotension, tachycardia, bradycardia, cardiac arrhythmias, phlebitis. **Respiratory: *Bronchospasm,*** wheezing, hypoxemia. **Dermatologic:** Rash, urticaria, erythema, reaction at injection site. **CNS:** Dizziness.

OD OVERDOSE MANAGEMENT

Symptoms: Neuromuscular blockade beyond the time needed for surgery and anesthesia. Increased risk of hemodynamic side effects such as hypotension. *Treatment:*

- Primary treatment is maintenance of a patent airway and controlled ventilation until there is recovery of normal neuromuscular function.
- Neostigmine (0.03–0.064 mg/kg) or edrophonium (0.5 mg/kg) can be given once there is evidence of recovery from neuromuscular blockade.
- A peripheral nerve stimulator can be used to assess recovery and antagonism of neuromuscular block.

DRUG INTERACTIONS

SEE *NEUROMUSCULAR BLOCKING AGENTS.*

Also, there is enhanced neuromuscular blockade when magnesium is given to pregnant women for toxemia.

HOW SUPPLIED

Injection: 0.5 mg/mL, 2 mg/mL

DOSAGE

- **IV ONLY**

Facilitation of tracheal intubation.

Adults: 0.15 mg/kg given over 5–15 sec. Maintenance doses of 0.1 mg/kg provide about 15 min of additional clinically effective blockade. **Children, 2–12 years:** The dosage requirements on a mg/kg basis are higher in children and onset and recovery occur more rapidly. **Initial:** 0.2 mg/kg given over 5–15 sec.

Facilitation of tracheal intubation using continuous IV infusion.

Continuous IV infusion may be used to maintain neuromuscular block. **Adults:** On evidence of spontaneous recovery from an initial dose, an initial infusion rate of 9–10 mcg/kg/min is recommended. If continuous infusion is started at the same time as the administration of an initial dose, use a lower initial infusion rate (such as 4 mcg/kg/min). In either case, adjust the initial infusion rate according to the response to peripheral nerve stimulation and to clinical criteria. An average infusion rate of 6–7 mcg/kg/min will maintain neuromuscular block within the range of 89%–99% for extended periods of time in adults receiving opioid/nitrous oxide/oxygen anesthesia. **Children:** Require higher infusion rates. During opioid/nitrous oxide/oxygen anesthesia, the infusion rate needed to maintain 89%–99% blockade averages 14 mcg/kg/min (range: 5–31 mcg/kg/min).

Tracheal intubation in clients with renal or hepatic impairment.

0.15 mg/kg. Infusion rates should be decreased by as much as 50% in these clients depending on the degree of renal or hepatic impairment.

Use in clients with reduced cholinesterase activity.

Initial doses greater than 0.03 mg/kg are not recommended.

Use in clients who are cachectic, are debilitated, or have carcinomatosis or neuromuscular disease.

A test dose of 0.015–0.02 mg/kg is recommended.

Use with isoflurane or enflurane anesthesia.

An initial dose of 0.15 mg/kg may be used for intubation prior to administration of the isoflurane or enflurane. If mivacurium is given after establishment of anesthesia, reduce the initial dose by as much as 25% and decrease the infusion rate by as much as 35%–40%. When used with halothane, no adjustment of the initial dose is necessary but decrease the infusion rate by as much as 20%.

Use in burn clients.

A test dose of not more than 0.015–0.02 mg/kg is recommended, followed by additional dosing guided by the use of a neuromuscular block monitor.

Use in obese clients weighing equal to or greater than 30% more than their ideal body weight (IBW).

The initial dose is calculated using the IBW according to the following formulas:

M

Men: IBW in kg = (106 + [6 × height in inches above 5 ft])/2.2

Women: IBW in kg = (100 + [5 × height in inches above 5 ft])/2.2

Use in clients with clinically significant CV disease or in those with any history of a greater sensitivity to the release of histamine or related mediators (asthma).

An initial dose less than or equal to 0.15 mg/kg given over 60 sec.

NURSING CONSIDERATIONS

SEE ALSO *NURSING CONSIDERATIONS* FOR *NEUROMUSCULAR BLOCKING AGENTS*.

ADMINISTRATION/STORAGE

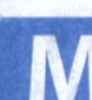

IV 1. Give only in carefully adjusted dosage under the supervision of trained clinicians who know the action of the drug as well as possible complications from its use. Have resuscitative equipment available.

2. For adults and children, the amount of infusion solution required per hour depends on the clinical requirements, the concentration of mivacurium in the solution, and client weight. Consult tables provided by the manufacturer to determine the infusion rates using either the premixed infusion of 0.5 mg/mL or the injection containing 2 mg/mL. Clients 64–86 years old require 38% less mivacurium during a 2–3 hr infusion than do those 18–41 years old.

3. Dosage adjustment may be necessary with significant liver, kidney, or CV disease; in obese clients weighing more than 30% of their ideal body weight for height; asthma; those with reduced plasma cholinesterase activity; and the use of inhalation general anesthetics.

4. Do not introduce additives into mivacurium premixed infusion in flexible plastic containers.

5. Ensure the premixed infusion is clear and the container undamaged. For single-client use only; discard any unused portion.

6. Vials (2 mg/mL) may be diluted to 0.5 mg/mL with D5W, D5/0.9% NaCl, 0.9% NaCl, RL injection, or D5/RL and then given by Y-site injection and titrated to desired response. The dilution is stable when stored in PVC bags at 5–25°C (41–77°F). Use the dilution within 24 hr; for single-client use only; discard unused portions.

7. Injection is compatible with sufentanil citrate injection, alfentanil hydrochloride injection, fentanyl citrate injection, midazolam hydrochloride injection, and droperidol injection. May not be compatible with alkaline solutions having a pH greater than 8.5 (e.g., barbiturate solutions).

8. The injection and premixed infusion are stored at 15–25°C (59–77°F). Avoid exposure to direct UV light; do not freeze or expose to excessive heat.

ASSESSMENT

1. Note indications for therapy. Review conditions/drugs that antagonize and enhance neuromuscular blockade; assess for presence.

2. Note any CV disease or asthma.

3. Monitor ABGs, electrolytes, liver and renal function studies; reduce dose with dysfunction.

4. Multidose vials contain benzyl alcohol; assess for intolerance.

5. Clients homozygous for the atypical plasma cholinesterase gene are sensitive to drugs' blocking effects.

6. Burn clients may show resistance depending on the time elapsed since the burn and the size of the burn; however, clients with burns may have decreased plasma cholinesterase, which offsets the resistance.

INTERVENTIONS

1. Administer in a carefully monitored environment by persons specially trained in the use of neuromuscular blocking agents.

2. Ensure client is unconscious/sedated before administering.

3. Use a peripheral nerve stimulator to measure neuromuscular function (assess response), adjust dosage, and confirm recovery (5-sec head lift and grip strength).

4. The elderly show a longer duration of neuromuscular blockade.

5. Monitor VS. Mivacurium will not counteract the bradycardia produced by many anesthetic agents or by vagal stimulation.

6. Transient flushing, wheezing, and tachycardia may be experienced.

OUTCOMES/EVALUATE

- Skeletal muscle relaxation
- Suppression of twitch response

Modafinil

(moh-**DEH**-fin-ill)

PREGNANCY CATEGORY: C
CLASSIFICATION(S):
Analeptic
Rx: Provigil
✱**Rx:** Alertec

ACTION/KINETICS
Precise mechanism unknown. Has wake-promoting effects similar to amphetamine and methylphenidate. Produces psychoactive and euphoric effects; alterations in mood, perception, and thinking; and, feelings typical of other CNS stimulants. Rapidly absorbed. **Peak plasma levels:** 2–4 hr. Absorption may be delayed by about 1 hr if taken with food. Metabolized by the liver and excreted in the urine. After chronic use, may induce its own metabolism. Clearance may be decreased in the elderly.

USES
Improve wakefulness in clients with excessive daytime sleepiness associated with narcolepsy.

SPECIAL CONCERNS
Use with caution, and at reduced doses, in severe hepatic impairment. Safety and efficacy in clients over 65 years of age or in children less than 16 years of age have not been determined. Use with caution during lactation. Is a reinforcing drug; use may lead to abuse/dependence. Thus, use with caution in those with a history of drug or stimulant abuse. Use with caution when coadministered with drugs that depend on CYP1A2, CYP2B6, or CYP3A4 for their clearance as lower blood levels of such drugs could result.

SIDE EFFECTS
CNS: Headache, nervousness, dizziness, depression, anxiety, cataplexy, insomnia, paresthesia, oro-facial dyskinesia, hypertonia, confusion, amnesia, emotional lability, ataxia, tremor. **GI:** N&V, diarrhea, dry mouth, anorexia, mouth ulcer, gingivitis, thirst. **CV:** Hypotension, hypertension, vasodilation, arrhythmia, syncope. **Dermatologic:** Herpes simplex, dry skin. **GU:** Abnormal urine, urinary retention, abnormal ejaculation. **Respiratory:** Rhinitis, pharyngitis, lung disorder, dyspnea, asthma, epistaxis. **Ophthalmic:** Amblyopia, abnormal vision. **Miscellaneous:** Infection, chest pain, neck pain, eosinophilia, rigid neck, fever, chills, joint disorder.

LABORATORY TEST CONSIDERATIONS
↑ Liver enzymes, GGT. Albuminuria, hyperglycemia.

OD OVERDOSE MANAGEMENT
Symptoms: Excitation, agitation, insomnia, slight to moderate increases in hemodynamic parameters. *Treatment:* Supportive care, including CV monitoring. Consider inducing emesis or gastric lavage.

DRUG INTERACTIONS
Cyclosporine / Possible ↓ blood levels of modafinil
MAO inhibitors / Use caution when taken together
Methylphenidate / Delayed absorption (by 1 hr) of modafinil
Oral contraceptives / Possible ↓ effectiveness of oral contraceptives
Phenytoin / Possible phenytoin toxicity
Tricyclic antidepressants / Possible ↑ plasma levels of clomipramine or desipramine
Warfarin / Possible ↑ effects of warfarin

HOW SUPPLIED
Tablets: 100 mg, 200 mg

DOSAGE

- **TABLETS**

Narcolepsy.

Adults: 200 mg/day as a single dose in the morning. Doses of 400 mg/day are well tolerated but no data to indicate increased beneficial effect. In clients with impaired hepatic function reduce the dose by 50%. Consider lower doses in elderly clients.

NURSING CONSIDERATIONS

ASSESSMENT

1. Note onset, duration, and characteristics of narcolepsy episodes.Identify how often it interferes with normal functioning.
2. Reduce dose with liver dysfunction and in the elderly.
3. Obtain ECG and monitor BP; do not use with LVH, ischemic ECG changes, chest pain, or arrhythmias.
4. Observe for S&S of abuse (e.g.,drug seeking behaviors, increased useage).

CLIENT/FAMILY TEACHING

1. Drug is used to promote wakefulness. It can cause psychoactive and euphoric effects similar to those with other controlled substances.
2. May alter judgement, thinking, and motor skills. Do not engage in activities that require mental alertness until drug effects realized.
3. Increased risk of pregnancy with oral, depot, or implantable agents with and for one mo after drug therapy; use additional protection.
4. Avoid alcohol; do not take any OTC agents unless cleared.

OUTCOMES/EVALUATE

↑ Wakefulness with narcolepsy

M

Moexipril hydrochloride

(moh-**EX**-ih-prill)

PREGNANCY CATEGORY: C (FIRST TRIMESTER), D (SECOND AND THIRD TRIMESTERS)
CLASSIFICATION(S):
Antihypertensive, ACE inhibitor
Rx: Univasc

SEE ALSO ANGIOTENSIN-CONVERTING ENZYME INHIBITORS.

ACTION/KINETICS
Converted in the liver to the active moexiprilat. **Onset:** 1–2 hr. **Peak effect:** 3–6 hr. **Duration:** 24 hr. Food decreases absorption of the drug. **t½, moexiprilat:** 2–9 hr. About 50% is bound to plasma protein. Active metabolite is excreted through both the urine and feces.

USES
Treatment of hypertension alone or in combination with thiazide diuretics.

CONTRAINDICATIONS
In those with a history of angioedema as a result of previous treatment with ACE inhibitors.

SPECIAL CONCERNS
Use with caution during lactation, in clients with impaired renal function or renal artery stenosis, hyperkalemia, CHF, severe hepatic impairment, and volume depletion. Those who are salt or volume depleted are at a greater risk of developing hypotension. Safety and efficacy have not been determined in children.

SIDE EFFECTS
GI: Abdominal pain, N&V, diarrhea, dysgeusia, constipation, dry mouth, dyspepsia, pancreatitis, hepatitis, changes in appetite, weight changes. **CNS:** Insomnia, sleep disturbances, headache, dizziness, fatigue, drowsiness/sleepiness, malaise, nervousness, anxiety, mood changes. **CV:** Chest pain, hypotension, palpitations, angina pectoris, ***CVA, MI,*** orthostatic hypotension, rhythm disturbances, peripheral edema. **Respiratory:** Cough, bronchospasm, dyspnea, URI, pharyngitis, rhinitis. **GU:** Oliguria, urinary frequency, renal insufficiency. **Dermatologic:** Flushing, rash, diaphoresis, photosensitivity, pruritus, urticaria, pemphigus, alopecia. **Musculoskeletal:** Myalgia, arthralgia. **Miscellaneous:** Angioedema, neutropenia, syncope, anemia, tinnitus, flu syndrome, pain, hyponatremia, hyperkalemia.

DRUG INTERACTIONS
Diuretics / Excessive hypotension
Lithium / ↑ Serum lithium levels → lithium toxicity
Potassium-sparing diuretics / ↑ Hyperkalemic effect of moexipril
Potassium supplements / ↑ Hyperkalemic effect of moexipril

HOW SUPPLIED
Tablet: 7.5 mg, 15 mg

DOSAGE

• **TABLETS**

Hypertension.

Initial, adults not receiving diuretics: 7.5 mg 1 hr before meals once daily. Dose is adjusted depending on response. **Maintenance:** 7.5–30 mg daily in one or two divided doses 1 hr before meals. **Initial, adults receiving diuretics:** Discontinue diuretic 2–3 days before beginning moexipril at a dose of 7.5 mg. If BP is not controlled, diuretic therapy can be resumed. If diuretic cannot be discontinued, give moexipril in an initial dose of 3.75 mg once daily 1 hr before meals. In those with impaired renal function, start with 3.75 mg once daily if C_{CR} is less than 40 mL/min/1.73 m^2. The dose may be increased to a maximum of 15 mg/day.

NURSING CONSIDERATIONS

SEE ALSO *NURSING CONSIDERATIONS FOR ANGIOTENSIN-CONVERTING ENZYME INHIBITORS.*

ASSESSMENT

1. Document indications for therapy, onset of disease, other agents trialed and the outcome.
2. Assess for dehydration, CHF, or hyperkalemia. Monitor ECG, electrolytes, renal and LFTs; reduce dose with renal impairment.

CLIENT/FAMILY TEACHING

1. Take on an empty stomach 1 hr before meals.
2. Rise slowly from a sitting or lying position; report persistent dizziness/lightheadedness, or fainting.
3. Seek help if angioedema (respiratory difficulty or swelling of lips, eyes, tongue, face) or neutropenia (fever, sore throat) occurs.
4. Use reliable contraception; stop drug and report if pregnancy is suspected, as drug is harmful to fetus.
5. Do not take potassium supplements or potassium-containing salt substitutes; drug may increase potassium levels.

OUTCOMES/EVALUATE

↓ BP

Mometasone furoate monohyrate

(moh-**MET**-ah-sohn)

PREGNANCY CATEGORY: C

CLASSIFICATION(S):
Glucocorticoid
Rx: Nasonex

SEE ALSO *CORTICOSTEROIDS.*

ACTION/KINETICS

Anti-inflammatory corticosteroid. Undetected in plasma although some may be swallowed after use. No effect on adrenal function.

USES

(1) Prophylaxis and treatment of the nasal symptoms of seasonal allergic rhinitis and perennial allergic rhinitis in adults and children 12 years and older. (2) Treat seasonal or perennial allergic rhinitis in children 3 years and older.

CONTRAINDICATIONS

Use in those with recent nasal septum ulcers, nasal surgery, or nasal trauma until healing has occurred.

SPECIAL CONCERNS

Use with caution, if at all, in those with active or quiescent tuberculosis infection of the respiratory tract, or in untreated fungal, bacterial, systemic viral infections, or ocular herpes simplex. Use with caution during lactation. Safety and efficacy have not been determined in children less than 12 years of age.

SIDE EFFECTS

Respiratory: Pharyngitis, epistaxis, blood-tinged mucus, coughing, URI, sinusitis, rhinitis, asthma, bronchitis. Rarely, nasal ulcers and nasal and oral candidiasis. **GI:** Diarrhea, dyspepsia, nausea. **Miscellaneous:** Headache, viral infection, dysmenorrhea, musculoskeletal pain, arthralgia, chest pain, conjunctivitis, earache, flu-like symptoms, myalgia, increased IOP.

HOW SUPPLIED

Nasal spray: 50 mcg/actuation

DOSAGE

• **NASAL SPRAY**

Seasonal/perennial allergic rhinitis.

Adults and children over 12 years: 2 sprays (50 mcg in each spray) in each nostril once daily (i.e., total daily dose: 200 mcg). In those with a known seasonal allergen that precipitates sea-

M

sonal allergic rhinitis, give prophylactically, 200 mcg/day, 2 to 4 weeks prior to the anticipated start of the pollen season. **Children over 3 years of age:** One spray (50 mcg) in each nostril once daily.

NURSING CONSIDERATIONS

SEE ALSO *NURSING CONSIDERATIONS* FOR *CORTICOSTEROIDS*.

ADMINISTRATION/STORAGE

Improvement is usually seen within 2 days after the first dose. Maximum benefit: within 1 to 2 weeks.

ASSESSMENT

Note onset, duration, and characteristics of symptoms. Attempt to identify triggers.

CLIENT/FAMILY TEACHING

1. Review enclosed instructions to ensure proper use.
2. Prior to initial use, prime the pump by actuating ten times or until a fine spray appears.
3. The pump may be stored, unused, for up to 1 week without repriming. If more than one week has elasped between use, reprime by actuating 2 times, or until a fine spray appears.
4. Use regularly as directed. Do not increase dose or frequency as this does not increase effectiveness.
5. Identify triggers and practice avoidance.
6. Report if condition does not improve or worsens after 3-5 days of therapy.

OUTCOMES/EVALUATE

Relief of allergic rhinitis

Montelukast sodium

(mon-teh-**LOO**-kast)

PREGNANCY CATEGORY: B
CLASSIFICATION(S):
Antiasthmatic, leukotriene receptor antagonist
Rx: Singulair

ACTION/KINETICS

Cysteinyl leukotrienes and leukotriene receptor occupation are associated with symptoms of asthma, including airway edema, smooth muscle contraction, and inflammation. Montelukast binds with cysteinyl leukotriene receptors thus preventing the action of cysteinyl leukotrienes. Rapidly absorbed after PO use. **Time to peak levels:** 3–4 hr for 10 mg tablet, 2–2.5 hr for 5 mg tablet, and 2 hr for 4 mg tablet. Metabolized in liver and mainly excreted in feces. **t½:** 2.7–5.5 hr for healthy, young adults.

USES

Prophylaxis and chronic treatment of asthma in adults and children 2 years of age and older. *Investigational:* With loratidine for hayfever.

CONTRAINDICATIONS

Use to reverse bronchospasm in acute asthma attacks, including status asthmaticus. Use to abruptly substitute for inhaled or oral corticosteroids. Use as monotherapy to treat and manage exercise-induced bronchospasm. Use with known aspirin or NSAID sensitivity.

SPECIAL CONCERNS

Use with caution during lactation. Safety and efficacy have not been determined for children less than 2 years of age.

SIDE EFFECTS

Adolescents and adults aged 15 and older: GI: Dyspepsia, infectious gastroenteritis, abdominal pain, dental pain. **CNS:** Headache, dizziness. **Body as a whole:** Asthenia, fatigue, trauma. **Respiratory:** Influenza, fever, cough, nasal congestion. **Dermatologic:** Rash. **Miscellaneous:** Pyuria.

Children, aged 6 to 14 years. GI: Nausea, diarrhea. **Respiratory:** Pharyngitis, laryngitis, otitis, sinusitus. **Miscellaneous:** Viral infection, eosinophilic conditions consistent with Churg-Strauss syndrome.

Children, aged 2 to 5 years: Rhinorrhea, otitis, ear pain, bronchitis, leg pain, thirst, sneezing, rash, urticaria.

LABORATORY TEST CONSIDERATIONS

↑ ALT, AST.

HOW SUPPLIED

Tablets: 10 mg. *Chewable Tablets:* 4 mg, 5 mg.

DOSAGE

- **TABLETS**

Asthma.

Adolescents and adults age 15 years and older: One 10 mg once daily taken in evening.

- **CHEWABLE TABLETS**

Asthma.

Pediatric clients aged 6 to 14 years: One 5 mg chewable tablet once daily taken in evening. **Pediatric clients aged 2 to 5 years:** One 4 mg chewable tablet taken once daily in the evening.

NURSING CONSIDERATIONS

ADMINISTRATION/STORAGE

Take daily as prescribed, even when client is asymptomatic. Contact provider if asthma is not well controlled.

ASSESSMENT

1. Document indications for therapy, onset, triggers, and characteristics of disease. List other agents trialed and outcome.
2. Note other agents prescribed for asthma and reinforce which should be continued.
3. Document lung assessments, PFTs, and x-rays.
4. Chewable 5 mg tablet contains 0.842 mg of phenylalanine and 4 mg tablet contains 0.674 mg phenylalanine; not to be used with phenylketonurics.
5. Assist to identify and eliminate/minimize triggers.

CLIENT/FAMILY TEACHING

1. Take once daily in evening.
2. Drug should be continued during acute attacks as well as during symptom free periods.
3. Use short-acting prescribed β-agonist inhalers to treat acute asthma attacks. Report if increased use/frequency of inhalers needed for symptom control.
4. Continue other prescribed anti-asthma meds during this therapy.
5. With exercise-induced asthma, must continue to use prescribed inhaler for prophylaxis.
6. Report any unusual side effects, changes in disease, or significant drop in peak flow readings.
7. Notify provider if pregnancy suspected or planned.
8. Ensure that environment is assessed for triggers and that appropriate steps are taken to minimize or avoid exposures.

OUTCOMES/EVALUATE

Asthma prophylaxis; ↑ FEV1

Moricizine hydrochloride

(mor-**IS**-ih-zeen)

PREGNANCY CATEGORY: B
CLASSIFICATION(S):
Antiarrhythmic, Class IA
Rx: Ethmozine

SEE ALSO *ANTIARRHYTHMIC AGENTS.*

ACTION/KINETICS

Causes a stabilizing effect on the myocardial membranes as well as local anesthetic activity. Shortens phase II and III repolarization leading to a decreased duration of the action potential and an effective refractory period. Also, there is a decrease in the maximum rate of phase O depolarization and a prolongation of AV conduction in clients with ventricular tachycardia. Whether the client is at rest or is exercising, has minimal effects on cardiac index, stroke index volume, systemic or pulmonary vascular resistance or ejection fraction, and pulmonary capillary wedge pressure. There is a small increase in resting BP and HR. The time, course, and intensity of antiarrhythmic and electrophysiologic effects are not related to plasma levels of the drug. **Onset:** 2 hr. **Peak plasma levels:** 30–120 min. **t½:** 1.5–3.5 hr (reduced after multiple dosing). **Duration:** 10–24 hr. 95% is protein bound. Significant first-pass effect. Metabolized almost completely by the liver with metabolites excreted through both the urine and feces; the drug induces its own metabolism. Food de-

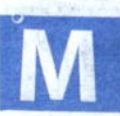

lays the rate of absorption resulting in lower peak plasma levels; however, the total amount absorbed is not changed.

USES

Documented life-threatening ventricular arrhythmias (e.g., sustained VT) where benefits of the drug are determined to outweigh the risks. *Investigational:* Ventricular premature contractions, couplets, and nonsustained VT.

CONTRAINDICATIONS

Preexisting second- or third-degree block, right bundle branch block when associated with bifascicular block (unless the client has a pacemaker), cardiogenic shock. Lactation.

SPECIAL CONCERNS

There is the possibility of increased risk of death when used in clients with non-life-threatening cardiac arrhythmias. Safety and effectiveness in children less than 18 years of age have not been determined. Geriatric clients have a higher rate of side effects. Increased survival rates following use of antiarrhythmic drugs have not been proven in clients with ventricular arrhythmias. Use with caution in clients with sick sinus syndrome due to the possibility of sinus bradycardia, sinus pause, or sinus arrest. Use with caution in clients with CHF.

SIDE EFFECTS

CV: ***Proarrhythmias, including new rhythm disturbances or worsening of existing arrhythmias;*** ECG abnormalities, including conduction defects, sinus pause, junctional rhythm, AV block; palpitations, ***sustained VT,*** cardiac chest pain, CHF, ***cardiac death,*** hypotension, hypertension, atrial fibrillation, atrial flutter, syncope, bradycardia, ***cardiac arrest, MI, pulmonary embolism,*** vasodilation, thrombophlebitis, ***cerebrovascular events.*** **CNS:** Dizziness (common), anxiety, headache, fatigue, nervousness, paresthesias, sleep disorders, tremor, anxiety, hypoesthesias, depression, euphoria, somnolence, agitation, confusion, ***seizures,*** hallucinations, loss of memory, vertigo, coma. **GI:** Nausea, dry mouth, abdominal pain, vomiting, diarrhea, dyspepsia, anorexia, ileus, flatulence, dysphagia, bitter taste. **Musculoskeletal:** Asthenia, abnormal gait, akathisia, ataxia, abnormal coordination, dyskinesia, pain. **GU:** Urinary retention, dysuria, urinary incontinence, urinary frequency, impotence, kidney pain, decreased libido. **Respiratory:** Dyspnea, apnea, asthma, hyperventilation, pharyngitis, cough, sinusitis. **Ophthalmologic:** Nystagmus, diplopia, blurred vision, eye pain, periorbital edema. **Dermatologic:** Rash, pruritus, dry skin, urticaria. **Miscellaneous:** Sweating, drug fever, hypothermia, temperature intolerance, swelling of the lips and tongue, speech disorder, tinnitus, jaundice.

LABORATORY TEST CONSIDERATIONS

↑ Bilirubin and liver transaminases.

OD OVERDOSE MANAGEMENT

Symptoms: Vomiting, hypotension, lethargy, worsening of CHF, ***MI, conduction disturbances, arrhythmias (e.g., junctional bradycardia, VT, ventricular fibrillation, asystole), sinus arrest, respiratory failure.*** *Treatment:* In acute overdose, induce vomiting, taking care to prevent aspiration. Hospitalize and closely monitor for cardiac, respiratory, and CNS changes. Provide life support, including an intracardiac pacing catheter, if necessary.

DRUG INTERACTIONS

Cimetidine / ↑ Plasma moricizine levels R/T ↓ excretion
Digoxin / Additive prolongation of the PR interval (but no significant increase in the rate of second- or third-degree AV block)
Propranolol / Additive prolongation of the PR interval
Theophylline / ↓ Plasma theophylline levels R/T ↑ rate of clearance

HOW SUPPLIED

Tablet: 200 mg, 250 mg, 300 mg

DOSAGE

- **TABLETS**

Antiarrhythmic.

Adults: 600–900 mg/day in equally divided doses q 8 hr. If needed, the dose can be increased in increments of 150 mg/day at 3-day intervals until the desired effect is obtained. In clients with hepatic or renal impairment, the initial dose should be 600 mg or less with close monitoring and dosage adjustment.

NURSING CONSIDERATIONS

SEE ALSO *NURSING CONSIDERATIONS* FOR *ANTIARRHYTHMIC AGENTS*.

ADMINISTRATION/STORAGE

1. When transferring clients from other antiarrhythmics to moricizine, withdraw the previous drug for one to two plasma half-lives before starting moricizine. For example, when transferring from quinidine or disopyramide, moricizine can be started 6–12 hr after the last dose; when transferring from procainamide, moricizine can be initiated 3–6 hr after the last dose; when transferring from mexiletine, propafenone, or tocainide, start 8–12 hr after the last dose; and, when transferring from flecainide, start moricizine 12–24 hr after the last dose.
2. If clients are well controlled on an 8-hr regimen, they might be given the same total daily dose q 12 hr to increase compliance.

ASSESSMENT

1. Document cardiac history, note preexisting conditions and ECG abnormalities.
2. Monitor ECG, electrolytes, CXR, PFTs, liver and renal function studies; correct any electrolyte disturbance and reduce dose with liver or renal dysfunction.
3. Monitor cardiac rhythm closely to observe for drug-induced rhythm disturbances.
4. Hospitalize clients for initial dosing. Antiarrhythmic response may be determined by ECG, exercise testing, or programmed electrical stimulation testing.
5. Assess pacing parameters with pacemakers.
6. Monitor VS and report any persistent temperature elevations.

CLIENT/FAMILY TEACHING

1. Drug is used to terminate life threatening ventricular arrhythmias.
2. Take before meals; food delays rate of absorption.
3. Drug may cause dizziness. Use care when rising from a lying or sitting position. Report any unusual or new side effects.
4. Advise family member or significant other to learn CPR.

OUTCOMES/EVALUATE

Termination of life-threatening ventricular arrhythmias

Morphine hydrochloride

(**MOR**-feen)

PREGNANCY CATEGORY: C

✱Rx: M.O.S., M.O.S.-S.R., Morphitec-1, -5, -10, -20, **C-II**

Morphine sulfate

(**MOR**-feen **SUL**-fayt)

PREGNANCY CATEGORY: C

Rx: Kadian, MS Contin, MSIR, Oramorph SR, RMS Rectal Suppositories, Roxanol, Roxanol 100, Roxanol-T, Astramorph PF, Duramorph, Infumorph 200 or 500

✱Rx: M.O.S.-Sulfate, M-Eslon, Morphine HP, Statex, **C-II**

CLASSIFICATION(S):

Narcotic analgesic

M

SEE ALSO *NARCOTIC ANALGESICS*.

ACTION/KINETICS

Morphine is the prototype for opiate analgesics. **Onset:** approximately 15–60 min, based on epidural or intrathecal use. **Peak effect:** 30–60 min. **Duration:** 3–7 hr. **t½:** 1.5–2 hr. Oral morphine is only one-third to one-sixth as effective as parenteral products.

USES

Oral: (1) Relief of moderate to severe pain (immediate-release tablets/solution). (2) Relief of moderate to severe pain in those requiring narcotic analgesia for more than a few days (controlled/extended/sustained-release tablets). **IV:** (1) Relief of severe pain. Pain from MI. (2) Preoperatively for sedation and to reduce apprehension. (3) Facilitate induction of anesthesia and reduce anesthetic dose. (4) Control postoperative pain. (5) Relieve anxiety and reduce left ventricular work by reducing preload pressure. (6) Treat dyspnea associated with acute left ventricular failure and pulmonary edema. (7) Anesthesia for open-heart surgery. **SC, IM:** (1) Relief of severe pain. (2) Reduce preoperative apprehension and produce sedation. (3) Control postoperative pain. (4) Supplement to anesthesia. (5) Analagesia during labor. (6) Acute pulmonary edema. (7) Allay anxiety. **IV, Epidural, Intrathecal:** (1) Treat pain not responsive to nonnarcotic analgesics (use Astramorph PF or Duramorph). (2) Use Infumorph for continuous epidural/intrathecal use). **Rectal:** Severe acute and chronic pain.

ADDITIONAL CONTRAINDICATIONS

Epidural or intrathecal morphine: If infection is present at injection site, anticoagulant therapy, bleeding diathesis, if client has received parenteral corticosteroids within the past 2 weeks. **Morphine injection:** Heart failure secondary to chronic lung disease, cardiac arrhythmias, brain tumor, acute alcoholism, delirium tremens, convulsive states. **Immediate release oral solution of morphine:** Respiratory insufficiency, severe CNS depression, heart failure secondary to chronic lung disease, cardiac arrhythmias, increased intracranial or CSF pressure, head injuries, brain tumor, acute alcoholism, delirium tremens, after biliary tract surgery, suspected surgical abdomen, convulsive disorders, surgical anastomosis, with MAO inhibitors or within 14 days of these drugs.

SPECIAL CONCERNS

May increase the length of labor. Clients with known seizure disorders may be at greater risk for morphine-induced seizure activity. Respiratory depression may be delayed up to 24 hr after epidural or intrathecal use.

ADDITIONAL DRUG INTERACTIONS

Amitriptyline / ↑ CNS and respiratory depression
Cimetidine / ↑ CNS and respiratory depression
Clomipramine / ↑ CNS and respiratory depression
Nortriptyline / ↑ CNS and respiratory depression
Warfarin / ↑ Warfarin anticoagulant effect

HOW SUPPLIED

Morphine hydrochloride: *Syrup:* 1 mg/mL, 5 mg/mL, 10 mg/mL, 20 mg/mL; *Concentrate:* 20 mg/mL, 50 mg/mL; *Suppository:* 10 mg, 20 mg, 30 mg; *Tablets:* 10 mg, 20 mg, 40 mg, 60 mg; *Slow-release tablets:* 30 mg, 60 mg. **Morphine sulfate:** *Capsule:* 15 mg, 30 mg; *Capsule, Sustained Release Pellets:* 20 mg, 30 mg, 50 mg, 60 mg, 100 mg; *Injection:* 0.5 mg/mL, 1 mg/mL, 2 mg/mL, 4 mg/mL, 5 mg/mL, 8 mg/mL, 10 mg/mL, 15 mg/mL, 25 mg/mL, 50 mg/mL; *Oral Solution:* 10 mg/5 mL, 20 mg/5 mL, 20 mg/mL, 100 mg/5 mL; *Suppository, Rectal:* 5 mg, 10 mg, 20 mg, 30 mg; *Tablet:* 15 mg, 30 mg; *Tablet, Controlled Release:* 15 mg, 30 mg, 60 mg, 100 mg, 200 mg; *Tablets, Extended Release:* 15 mg, 30 mg, 60 mg, 100 mg; *Tablets, Soluble:* 10 mg, 15 mg, 30 mg

DOSAGE

• **CAPSULES, TABLETS, ORAL SOLUTION, SOLUBLE TABLETS, SYRUP**

Analgesia.

5–30 mg (solution or tablets) q 4 hr, or as directed by prescriber.

• **SUSTAINED-RELEASE TABLETS**

Analgesia.

Titrate first to analgesia using an immediate release product and then transfer to a long-acting product. To convert from immediate release PO morphine to controlled release PO morphine, give the total daily PO morphine dose q 24 hr if using Kadian; or, ½ the total daily PO morphine dose q 12 hr if using Oramorph SR, Kadian, or MS Contin; or, ⅓ the total daily PO morphine dose q 8 hr if using MS Contin. If Kadian is selected as the initial product, start with either 20 mg q 12 hr or 40 mg once daily. The MS Contin 200 mg tablet is only for narcotic tolerant clients requiring daily morphine equivalent doses of 400 or more mg.

• **IM, SC**

Analgesia.

Adults: 10 mg (range: 5–20 mg)/70 kg q 4 hr as needed. **Pediatric:** 50–200 mcg/kg q 4 hr, up to a maximum of 10–15 mg/dose.

MI.
8–15 mg. For very severe pain, give additional smaller amounts q 3–4 hr.
• **IV INFUSION**
Analgesia.
Adults: 2–10 mg/70 kg. A strength of 2.5–15 mg can be used in 4–5 mL of water for injection (administer slowly over 4–5 min).
• **IV INFUSION, CONTINUOUS**
Analgesia.
Adults: 0.1–1 mg/mL in D5W by a controlled-infusion pump.
Chronic severe pain associated with terminal cancer.
Initial: Loading dose of 15 mg or more of morphine by IV push followed by the infusion of 0.2–1 mg/mL. Infusion amount may range from 0.8–80 mg/hr, up to 160 mg/hr.
• **IV**
Open-heart surgery.
0.5–3 mg/kg as the sole anesthetic or with a suitable anesthetic. Give oxygen and adequate ventilation.
• **RECTAL SUPPOSITORIES**
Adults: 10–30 mg q 4 hr or as directed by prescriber.
• **INTRATHECAL**
Adults: 0.2–1 mg as a single daily injection. Usually use 1/10 epidural dose.
• **EPIDURAL**
Initial: 5 mg/day in the lumbar region; if analgesia is not manifested in 1 hr, increasing doses of 1–2 mg can be given, not to exceed 10 mg/day. For continuous infusion, 2–4 mg/day with additional doses of 1–2 mg if analgesia is not satisfactory. Usual starting dose of those not tolerate to opiates ranges from 2.5–7.5 mg/day whereas the usual starting dose for continuous epidural infusion in those who have some degree of opiate tolerance is 4.5–10 mg/day. Dose requirements may increases significantly (i.e., up to 20–30 mg/day) during treatment.

NURSING CONSIDERATIONS

SEE ALSO *NURSING CONSIDERATIONS* FOR *NARCOTIC ANALGESICS*.

ADMINISTRATION/STORAGE

1. The contents of the immediate release capsule may be delivered through a NG or a gastric tube.
2. For intrathecal use, do not give more than 2 mL of the 5-mg/10-mL preparation or 1 mL of the 10-mg/10-mL product.
3. Give intrathecally only in the lumbar region; repeated injections are not recommended.
4. To reduce the chance of side effects with intrathecal administration, a constant IV infusion of naloxone (0.6 mg/hr for 24 hr after intrathecal injection) is recommended.
5. For Infumorph, Duramorph, and Astromorph PF use epidural doses of 20 mg or more with caution due to the increased possibility of serious side effects.
6. In certain circumstances (e.g., tolerance, severe pain), the physician may prescribe doses higher than those listed under *Dosage*.
7. Dose may be lower in geriatric clients or those with respiratory disease.
8. Intraventricular administration may be effective in select clients with a short life expectancy and recalcitrant pain due to head and neck malignancies and tumors and breast cancer that affects the brachial plexus. Only 1–2 doses/day are usually used.
IV 9. For IV use, dilute 2–10 mg with at least 5 mL sterile water or NSS and administer over 4–5 min. For continous infusions, reconstitute to a concentration of 0.1–1 mg/mL and administer as prescribed to control symptoms.
10. Rapid IV administration increases the risk of adverse effects; have a narcotic antagonist (e.g., naloxone) available.

ASSESSMENT

1. Document location and characteristics of pain. Rate utilizing a pain-rating scale.
2. List other agents prescribed and the outcome.
3. Note any seizure disorder.

CLIENT/FAMILY TEACHING

1. May be administered with food to diminish GI upset. Do not crush or chew controlled-release tablets.
2. Immediate-release capsules may be swallowed intact or the contents of the capsule may be sprinkled on food

M

or stirred in juice to avoid the bitter taste.
3. Drug may cause dizziness and drowsiness; avoid activities that require mental alertness.
4. Practice cough and deep-breathing exercises and incentive spirometry to decrease risk of atelectasis.
5. Record drug use for breakthrough pain when SR therapy prescribed, to ensure adequate dosage.
6. Avoid alcohol/CNS depressants OTC agents.

OUTCOMES/EVALUATE

- ↓ Rating/ ↑ control of pain
- Control of respirations during mechanical ventilation

Moxifloxacin hydrochloride

(**mox**-ee-**FLOX**-ah-sin)

PREGNANCY CATEGORY: C
CLASSIFICATION(S):
Antibiotic, fluoroquinolone
Rx: Avelox

M

SEE ALSO *FLUOROQUINOLONES.*

ACTION/KINETICS
Well absorbed from the GI tract (about 90% bioavailable). A high fat meal does not affect absorption. **t½, elimination:** About 12 hr. Steady state is reached in 3 days (400 mg/day). Widely distributed in the body. Metabolized in the liver; metabolites and unchanged drug are excreted in the feces and urine.

USES
(1) Acute bacterial sinusitis due to *Streptococcus pneumoniae, Haemophilus influenzae,* or *Moraxella catarrhalis.* (2) Acute bacterial exacerbation of chronic bronchitis due to *S. pneumoniae, H. influenzae, Haemophilus parainfluenzae, Klebsiella pneumoniae, Staphylococcus aureus,* or *M. catarrhalis.* (3) Mild to moderate community acquired pneumonia due to *S. pneumoniae, H. influenzae, Mycoplasma pneumoniae, Chlamydia pneumoniae,* or *M. catarrhalis.* (4) Uncomplicated skin and skin structure infections due to *S. aureus* or *Streptococcus pyogenes.*

CONTRAINDICATIONS
Hypersensitivitiy to moxifloxacin or any quinolone antibiotic. Use with moderate to severe hepatic insufficiency. Use in clients with known prolongation of the QT interval (the drug prolongs the QT interval in some), with uncorrected hypokalemia, and in those receiving class IA (e.g., quinidine, procainamide) or Class III (e.g., amiodarone, sotalol) antiarrhythmic drugs. Lactation.

SPECIAL CONCERNS
Use with caution in those with clinically significant bradycardia or acute myocardial ischemia, in clients with known or suspected CNS disorders (e.g., severe cerebral arteriosclerosis, epilepsy), or in the presence of risk factors that predispose to seizures or lower the seizure threshold. Safety and efficacy have not been determined in children, adolescents less than 18 years of age, in pregnancy, and during lactation.

SIDE EFFECTS
Hypersensitivity: ***Anaphylaxis after the first dose, CV collapse,*** loss of consciousness, tingling, pharyngeal or facial edema, dyspnea, urticaria, itching. **CNS:** Dizziness, headache, convulsions, confusion, tremors, hallucinations, depression, insomnia, nervousness, anxiety, depersonalization, hypertonia, incoordination, somnolence, vertigo, paresthesia, suicidal thoughts/acts (rare). **GI:** N&V, diarrhea, abdominal pain, taste perversion, dyspepsia, dry mouth, constipation, oral moniliasis, anorexia, stomatitis, gastritis, glossitis, GI disorder, pseudomembranous colitis, cholestatic jaundice. **CV:** Palpitation, vasodilatation, tachycardia, hypertension, peripheral edema, hypotension. **Body as a whole:** Asthenia, moniliasis, pain, malaise, allergic reaction, leg pain, pelvic pain, back pain, chills, infection, chest pain, hand pain. **Hematologic:** Thrombocytopenia, thrombocythemia, eosinophilia, leukopenia. **Respiratory:** Asthma, dyspnea, increased cough, pneumonia, pharyngitis, rhinitis, sinusitis. **Musculoskeletal:** Arthralgia, myalgia. **Dermatologic:** Rash, pruritus, sweating, urticaria, dry skin. **GU:**

Vaginal moniliasis, vaginitis, cystitis. **Miscellaneous:** Tinnitus, amblyopia.

LABORATORY TEST CONSIDERATIONS

↑ GGTP, lactic dehydrogenase, MCH, WBCs, PT ratio, ionized calcium, chloride, albumin, globulin, bilirubin. ↓ Hemoglobin, RBCs, eosinophils, basophils, glucose, pO_2. Either ↑ or ↓ Amylase, PT, bilirubin, neutrophils. Hyperglycemia, hyperlipidemia. Abnormal LFTs and kidney function.

DRUG INTERACTIONS

Antacids / Significant ↓ bioavailability of moxifloxacin
Antidepressants, tricyclic / Potential to add to the QTC prolonging effect of moxifloxacin
Antipsychotics / Potential to add to the QTC prolonging effect of moxifloxacin
Didanosine / ↓ Absorption of moxifloxacin
Erythromycin / Potential to add to the QTC prolonging effect of moxifloxacin
Iron products / Significant ↓ bioavailabilitiy of moxifloxaicn
NSAIDs / ↑ Risk of CNS stimulation and convulsions
Sucralfate / ↓ Absorption of moxifloxacin

HOW SUPPLIED

Tablets: 400 mg

DOSAGE

• **TABLETS**

Acute bacterial sinusitis, community acquired pneumonia.

Adults: 400 mg q 24 hr for 10 days.

Acute bacterial exacerbation of chronic bronchitis.

Adults: 400 mg q 24 hr for 5 days.

Uncomplicated skin and skin structure infections.

Adults: 400 mg q 24 hr for 7 days.

NURSING CONSIDERATIONS

ASSESSMENT

1. Determine onset, location, and characteristics of symptoms.
2. List drugs prescribed to ensure none interact.
3. Avoid with uncorrected hypokalemia, prolonged QT intervals and if receiving class 1A or III antiarrhythmic agents.
4. Monitor C&S, ectrolytes, CBC, renal and LFTs; avoid with moderate-severe liver dysfunction.

CLIENT/FAMILY TEACHING

1. Take once a day at the same time, as directed.
2. May take with or without meals. Drink fluids liberally.
3. Take at least 4 hr before or 8 hr after multivitamins containing iron or zinc, antacids containing magnesium/calcium/aluminum, sucralfate, or didanosine (chewable/buffered tablets or the pediatric powder for PO solution).
4. Do not perform activities that require mental alertness until drug effects realized.
5. May cause GI upset, dizziness, and headaches.
6. Stop drug and report any skin rash immediately.
7. Report any adverse effects, lack of effectiveness or worsening of condition.

OUTCOMES/EVALUATE

Resolution of infection; symptomatic improvement

Mupirocin

(myou-**PEER**-oh-sin)

PREGNANCY CATEGORY: B
Rx: Bactroban

Mupirocin Calcium

PREGNANCY CATEGORY: B
Rx: Bactroban Cream, Bactroban Nasal

CLASSIFICATION(S):
Antibiotic, topical

ACTION/KINETICS

Binds to bacterial isoleucyl transfer RNA synthetase, which results in inhibition of protein synthesis by the organism. Not absorbed into the systemic circulation. Serum present in exudative wounds decreases the antibacterial activity. Metabolized to the inactive monic acid in the skin which is removed by normal skin desquamation.

No cross resistance with other antibiotics such as chloramphenicol, erythromycin, gentamicin, lincomycin, methicillin, neomycin, novobiocin, penicillin, streptomycin, or tetracyclines.

USES

Topical: To treat impetigo and secondarily infected traumatic skin lesions due to *Staphylococcus aureus, Streptococcus pyogenes,* and beta-hemolytic streptococcus. **Nasal:** Eradication of nasal colonization with methicillin-resistant *S. aureus* in adult clients and health care workers.

CONTRAINDICATIONS

Ophthalmic use. Lactation. Use if absorption of large quantities of polyethylene glycol is possible (i.e., large, open wounds). Use with other nasal products.

SPECIAL CONCERNS

Superinfection may result from chronic use. Safety and efficacy have not been established in children for mupirocin nasal.

SIDE EFFECTS

• **TOPICAL USE.**

Superinfection, rash, burning, stinging, pain, nausea, tenderness, erythema, swelling, dry skin, contact dermatitis, and increased exudate.

• **NASAL USE.**

Headache, rhinitis, respiratory disorder (including upper respiratory tract congestion), pharyngitis, taste perversion, burning, stinging, cough, pruritus, blepharitis, diarrhea, dry mouth, ear pain, epistaxis, nausea, rash.

HOW SUPPLIED

Nasal Ointment: 2%; *Ointment:* 2%; *Topical Cream:* 2%

DOSAGE

• **TOPICAL CREAM**

Apply to affected area t.i.d. for 10 days.

• **TOPICAL OINTMENT**

Children, over 2 months of age: A small amount of ointment is applied to the affected area t.i.d. If no response is seen after 3–5 days, the client should be reevaluated.

• **NASAL OINTMENT**

Divide about one-half of the ointment from the single-use tube between the nostrils and apply in the morning and evening for 5 days.

NURSING CONSIDERATIONS

ADMINISTRATION/STORAGE

1. A gauze dressing may be used if desired.
2. After application in the nose, close the nostrils by pressing them together for about 1 min.
3. Store the topical ointment between 15–30°C (59–86°F); store nasal ointment below 25°C (77°F).

ASSESSMENT

Document type, onset, duration, and characteristics of symptoms.

CLIENT/FAMILY TEACHING

1. Review technique for administering topical and/or nasal medications; use aseptic measures and hand washing before and after therapy to prevent contamination.
2. Report any symptoms of chemical irritation or hypersensitivity such as increased rash, itching, pain at site, or lack of healing.
3. Do not use other nasal products during nasal therapy.
4. Report if no improvement in skin infection after 3–5 days.
5. Notify school nurse to ensure appropriate screening is performed when treating school-aged children with impetigo.

OUTCOMES/EVALUATE

• Healing of lesions; symptomatic improvement
• Eradication of nasal colonization MRSA

Muromonab-CD3

(myour-oh-**MON**-ab)

PREGNANCY CATEGORY: C
CLASSIFICATION(S):
Immunosuppressant
Rx: Orthoclone OKT 3

ACTION/KINETICS

A murine monoclonal antibody that is a purified IgG_{2a} immunoglobulin. Acts to prevent rejection of transplanted kidney tissue by blocking the action of T cells, which play a significant role in acute rejection. Specifically, the CD3 molecule in the membrane of T cells is blocked; this molecule is necessary for signal transduction. Does not cause myelosuppression. Antibodies to muromonab-CD3 have been observed after approximately 20 days. **Average serum levels after 3 days:** 0.9 mcg/mL. **Time to steady-state trough levels:** 3 days. **Duration:** 1 week for return of circulating CD3 positive T cells to pretreatment levels.

USES

To reverse acute allograft rejection in kidney transplant clients; used in combination with azathioprine, cyclosporine, corticosteroids. Treatment of steroid-resistant acute allograft rejection in cardiac and hepatic transplant clients.

CONTRAINDICATIONS

Hypersensitivity to drug (or any product of murine origin), clients with antimouse titers greater than or equal to 1:1,000. Clients with fluid overload or uncompensated CHF as confirmed by CXR or more than a 3% weight gain within the week prior to treatment. History of seizures or predisposition to seizures. Use during pregnancy (IgG antibody potentially hazardous to the fetus) and lactation.

SPECIAL CONCERNS

Although used in children, safety and effectiveness have not been assessed. Following the first two to three doses, a cytokine release syndrome due to the release of cytokines by activated lymphocytes or monocytes may occur. Clients at greatest risk for cytokine release syndrome are those with unstable angina, recent MI, symptomatic ischemic heart disease, heart failure, pulmonary edema, COPD, intravascular volume overload or depletion, cerebrovascular disease, advanced symptomatic vascular disease or neuropathy, history of seizures, or septic shock.

SIDE EFFECTS

Cytokine release syndrome (CRS).

Flu-like symptoms, such as pyrexia, chills, dyspnea, N&V, chest pain, diarrhea, tremor, wheezing, headache, tachycardia, rigor, and hypertension. ***Rarely, severe, life-threatening shock-like syndrome including serious CV and CNS effects.***

Within the first 45 days of therapy for renal transplants.

Infections (which may be life-threatening) due to CMV, HSV, *Staphylococcus epidermidis, Pneumocystis carinii, Legionella, Cryptococcus, Serratia,* and other gram-negative bacteria.

Within the first 45 days of therapy for liver transplants.

CMV, fungal infections, HSV, Legionella, and other severe, life-threatening gram-positive, gram-negative, and viral infections.

Within the first 45 days of therapy for heart transplants.

Most commonly herpes simplex, fungal, and CMV infections. *Hypersensitivity reactions:* ***Cardiovascular collapse, cardiorespiratory arrest, shock,*** loss of consciousness, hypotension, tachycardia, tingling, angioedema, ***airway obstruction, bronchospasm,*** dyspnea, urticaria, pruritus. *Neuropsychiatric:* ***Seizures,*** encephalopathy, cerebral edema, ***aseptic meningitis,*** headaches. **CV:** ***Cardiac arrest, shock, heart failure, CV collapse, MI,*** hypotension, angina, tachycardia, bradycardia, hemodynamic instability, hypertension, LV dysfunction, arrhythmias, chest pain or tightness. **Respiratory:** ***Respiratory arrest, ARDS, respiratory failure, cardiogenic or noncardiogenic pulmonary edema, apnea,*** dyspnea, ***bronchospasm,*** wheezing, SOB, hypoxemia, tachypnea, hyperventilation, abnormal chest sounds, pneumonia, pneumonitis. **Dermatologic:** Rash, urticaria, pruritus, erythema, flushing, diaphoresis, ***Stevens-Johnson syndrome.*** **GI:** N&V, diarrhea, abdominal pain, ***bowel infarction, GI hemorrhage.*** **Hematologic:** Pancytopenia, ***aplastic anemia,*** neutropenia, leukopenia, thrombocytopenia, lymphopenia, leukocytosis, lymphadenopathy, ***arterial and venous thrombosis of allografts and other vascular beds (heart, lung, brain, bowel), disturbances of coag-***

M

ulation. **Musculoskeletal:** Arthralgia, arthritis, myalgia, stiffness, aches and pain. **Hepatic:** Hepatomegaly, splenomegaly, hepatitis (usually secondary to viral infection or lymphoma). **GU:** Anuria, oliguria, delayed graft function, abnormal urinary cytology (including exfoliation of damaged lymphocytes, collecting ducts, and cellular casts). **Ophthalmic:** Blindness, blurred vision, diplopia, photophobia, conjunctivitis. **Otic:** Hearing loss, otitis media, tinnitus, vertigo, nasal and ear stuffiness. **Body as a whole:** Fever, chills, rigors, flu-like syndrome, fatigue, malaise, generalized weakness, anorexia. **Miscellaneous:** Palsy of cranial nerve VI, ***increased risk of developing neoplasms.***

LABORATORY TEST CONSIDERATIONS

↑ AST, ALT. Transient and reversible ↑ in BUN and serum creatinine.

OD OVERDOSE MANAGEMENT

Symptoms: Hyperthermia, myalgia, severe chills, diarrhea, vomiting, edema, oliguria, pulmonary edema, acute renal failure. *Treatment:* Observe client carefully and provide symptomatic and supportive treatment.

DRUG INTERACTIONS

Azathioprine, corticosteroids, cyclosporine / Psychosis, infections, malignancies, seizures, encephalopathy, and thrombosis when taken with muromonab-CD3

H *Echinacea* / Do not give with muromonab-CD3

Indomethacin / Encephalopathy and other CNS effects

HOW SUPPLIED

Injection: 1 mg/mL

DOSAGE

• **IV BOLUS**

Reverse acute allograft rejection in kidney transplants.

Adults: 5 mg/day for 10–14 days, beginning treatment once acute renal rejection is diagnosed.

Cardiac/hepatic allograft rejection, steroid-resistant.

5 mg/day for 10–14 days with treatment beginning after determination that corticosteroids will not reverse the rejection.

NURSING CONSIDERATIONS

ADMINISTRATION/STORAGE

IV 1. Give methylprednisolone sodium succinate, 8 mg/kg IV, 1–4 hr before dose to decrease incidence of first-dose reactions. Acetaminophen and antihistamines, given together, may reduce early reactions.

2. Initiate treatment as soon as acute renal rejection is diagnosed.

3. Give the dose in less than 1 min.

4. Do not give the drug by IV infusion or with any other drug solutions.

5. If the body temperature is 37.8°C (100°F), do not initiate drug therapy.

6. Draw the solution (which is a protein) into a syringe through a 0.2- or 0.22-µm filter; discard the filter and attach a 20-gauge needle.

7. Do not add or infuse other drugs through the same IV line. If the same IV line is used for sequential infusion of different drugs, flush the line with saline before and after infusion of muromonab-CD3.

8. The appearance of a few translucent particles of protein does not affect the potency of the preparation.

9. Use ampule immediately after opening; no bacteriostatic agent in product. Discard any unused drug.

10. Decrease dose of other immunosuppressant drugs as follows during muromonab-CD3 use: prednisone, 0.5 mg/kg/day; azathioprine, 25 mg/day. Cyclosporine should be discontinued. Maintenance doses of these drugs can be resumed approximately 3 days prior to termination of muromonab-CD3.

11. Store at 2–8°C (36–46°F); do not freeze or shake.

ASSESSMENT

1. Determine any past use and assess closely for evidence of antibodies. Drug is usually only given for one course of therapy.

2. Note any sensitivity to murine derivatives.

3. Monitor CBC and T-cell assays with CD_3 antigen daily.

INTERVENTIONS

1. Anticipate pretreatment administration of an antihistamine, antipyretic, and methylprednisolone succinate

and hydrocortisone succinate post-treatment to minimize intensity of side effects.
2. Monitor I&O and weights; assess for a positive fluid balance and report rapid weight gain.
3. Obtain CXR, assess lung sounds, and report evidence of congestion.
4. Take the temperature q 4 hr; if above 37.7°C (100°F), withhold drug until the temperature drops.
5. Monitor for a decrease in urine volume and C_{CR}; these are signs of transplant rejection.
6. Administer acetaminophen for flu-like symptoms/febrile reaction.
7. Symptoms of aseptic meningitis are usually evident within 3 days characterized by fever, headache, nuchal rigidity, and photophobia.

CLIENT/FAMILY TEACHING

1. Chills, fever, SOB, and fatigue are first-dose symptoms that will diminish with therapy.
2. Report any SOB, edema, weight gain, chest pain, N&V, or infection immediately.
3. Perform frequent, careful oral care to minimize occurrence of oral inflammation.
4. Avoid vaccinia and crowds.
5. Continue to practice birth control for 12 weeks following therapy.

OUTCOMES/EVALUATE

- Reversal of kidney transplant rejection and improved organ function
- Absence of graft rejection

Mycophenolate mofetil

(**my**-koh-**FEN**-oh-layt)

PREGNANCY CATEGORY: C
CLASSIFICATION(S):
Immunosuppressant
Rx: CellCept, CellCept IV

ACTION/KINETICS

Rapidly absorbed after PO administration and hydrolyzed to the active mycophenolic acid (MPA). MPA has potent cytostatic effects on lymphocytes. Inhibits proliferative responses of T- and B-lymphocytes to both mitogenic and allospecific stimulation. MPA also suppresses antibody formation of B-lymphocytes. MPA and additional metabolites are excreted in the urine. **t½:** 17.9 hr.

USES

With cyclosporine and corticosteroids to prevent organ rejection in those receiving allogeneic renal, heart, or liver transplants. May be used in children with renal transplants. *Investigational:* Refractory uveitis. In combination with prednisolone to treat diffuse proliferative lupus nephritis.

CONTRAINDICATIONS

Hypersensitivity to mycophenolate, mycophenolic acid, or polysorbate 80 (Tween). Lactation.

SPECIAL CONCERNS

Clients receiving immunosuppressant drugs have increased susceptibility to infection and are at a higher risk of developing lymphomas and other malignancies, especially of the skin. Higher blood levels are seen in those with severe impaired renal function. Use with caution in active serious digestive system disease. Safety and efficacy have not been determined in children.

SIDE EFFECTS

Hematologic: Severe neutropenia, anemia, leukopenia, thrombocytopenia, hypochromic anemia, leukocytosis. **GI:** ***GI tract hemorrhage/perforations,*** GI tract ulceration, diarrhea, constipation, nausea, dyspepsia, vomiting, oral moniliasis, anorexia, esophagitis, flatulence, gastritis, gastroenteritis, GI moniliasis, gingivitis, gum hyperplasia, hepatitis, ileus, infection, mouth ulceration, rectal disorder. **CNS:** Tremor, insomnia, dizziness, anxiety, depression, hypertonia, paresthesia, somnolence. **GU:** UTI, hematuria, kidney tubular necrosis, urinary tract disorder, albuminuria, dysuria, hydronephrosis, impotence, pain, pyelonephritis, urinary frequency. **CV:** Hypertension, angina pectoris, atrial fibrillation, cardiovascular disorder, hypotension, palpitation, peripheral

M

vascular disorder, postural hypotension, tachycardia, thrombosis, vasodilation. **Respiratory:** Infection, dyspnea, increased cough, pharyngitis, bronchitis, pneumonia, asthma, lung disorder, lung edema, pleural effusion, rhinitis, sinusitis. **Dermatologic:** Acne, rash, alopecia, fungal dermatitis, hirsutism, pruritus, benign skin neoplasm, skin disorder, skin hypertrophy, skin ulcer, sweating. **Metabolic/Endocrine:** Peripheral edema, dehydration, hypercholesterolemia, hypophosphatemia, edema, hypokalemia, hyperkalemia, hyperglycemia, diabetes mellitus, parathyroid disorder. **Musculoskeletal:** Arthralgia, joint disorder, leg cramps, myalgia, myasthenia. **Ophthalmologic:** Amblyopia, cataract, conjunctivitis. **Body as a whole:** Pain, abdominal pain, fever, chills, headache, infection, malaise, ***sepsis,*** asthenia, chest pain, back pain. **Miscellaneous:** Increased incidence of lymphoma/lymphoproliferative disease, nonmelanoma skin carcinoma, and other malignancies. Increased incidence of opportunistic infections, including herpes simplex, CMV, herpes zoster, *Candida, Aspergillus/Mucor* invasive disease, and *Pneumocystis carinii.* Enlarged abdomen, accidental injury, cyst, facial edema, flu syndrome, ***hemorrhage,*** hernia, weight gain, pelvic pain, ecchymosis, polycythemia.

LABORATORY TEST CONSIDERATIONS

↑ Alkaline phosphatase, creatinine, gamma glutamyl transpeptidase, LDH, AST, ALT. Also, hypercalcemia, hyperlipemia, hyperuricemia, hypervolemia, hypocalcemia, hypoglycemia, hypoproteinemia, acidosis.

OD OVERDOSE MANAGEMENT

Symptoms: Nausea, vomiting, diarrhea, hematologic abnormalities, especially neutropenia. *Treatment:* Reduce dose of the drug. Removal of MPA by bile acid sequestrants (e.g., cholestyramine).

DRUG INTERACTIONS

Acyclovir / ↑ Plasma levels of both drugs due to competition for renal tubular excretion
Antacids containing aluminum/ magnesium / ↓ Absorption of mycophenolate
Cholestyramine / ↓ Absorption of mycophenolate
Cyclosporine ↓ Mycophenolic acid levels
H *Echinacea* / Do not give with mycophenolate
Ganciclovir / ↑ Plasma levels of both drugs due to competition for renal tubular excretion
Iron / ↓ Mycophenolate absorption
Levonorgestrel / Significant ↓ in levonorgestrel area under the curve
Phenytoin / ↓ Plasma protein binding of phenytoin → ↑ free phenytoin levels
Probenecid / Significant ↑ plasma levels of MPA
Salicylates / ↑ Free fraction of MPA
Theophylline / ↓ Plasma protein binding of theophylline → ↑ free theophylline levels

HOW SUPPLIED

Capsules: 250 mg; *Powder for Injection, Lyophilized:* 500 mg (as HCl); *Powder for Oral Suspension:* 200 mg/mL; *Tablets:* 500 mg

DOSAGE

• CAPSULES, IV, ORAL SUSPENSION, TABLETS

Renal transplantation.

Adults: 1 g b.i.d. (a dose of 1.5 g b.i.d. is also safe and effective).

Cardiac transplantation.

Adults: 1.5 g b.i.d.

Hepatic transplantation.

1 g b.i.d. IV or 1.5 g b.i.d. PO.

NURSING CONSIDERATIONS

ADMINISTRATION/STORAGE

1. For PO dosage forms, start therapy as soon as possible following transplantation.
2. Give on an empty stomach. In stable renal transplant clients, may be given with food if necessary.
3. The oral suspension may be given via a nasogastric tube with a minimum size of 8 French catheter.
4. Avoid doses of 1 g b.i.d. in CRF (i.e., GFR less than 25 mL/min/1.73 m^2) outside the immediate posttreatment period.
5. Mycophenolate is teratogenic; do not open or crush capsules. Avoid inhalation or direct contact with the skin

or mucous membranes; wash the area thoroughly with soap and water if contact occurs. Rinse the eyes with plain water.

6. Dispense tablets in light-resistant containers, i.e., manufacturer's original container.

7. To prepare the oral solution tap the closed bottle several times to loosen the powder. Measure 94 mL water and add ½ the total amount of water to the bottle and shake well for about 1 min. Add the remainder of the water and shake the closed bottle well for about 1 min. Remove the child-resistant cap and push the bottle adapter into neck of bottle. Close bottle with child resistant cap tightly to ensure proper seating of the bottle adapter and the child resistant status of the cap.

IV 8. Give IV over 2 or more hr by a peripheral or central vein. Do not give by rapid or IV bolus. IV not recommended for those unable to take capsules or tablets.

9. Begin 24 or less hr after transplantation and give for 14 or less days; switch to PO mycophenoloate as soon as PO medication can be tolerated.

10. Reconstitute each vial with 14 mL of D5W. Solution is slightly yellow. Discard if particulate matter or discoloration is seen. Further dilute the contents of 2 reconstituted vials into 140 mL of D5W for a 1 g dose or of 3 reconstituted vials into 210 mL of D5W for a 1.5 g dose. The final concentration of both solutions is 6 mg/mL. Use within 4 hr of reconstitution and dilution.

11. Do not mix or give IV mycophenolate via the same infusion catheter with any other IV drugs or infusion admixtures.

12. Because the drug is teratogenic in animals, use cauton in handling and preparing IV solutions. If contact occurs, wash thoroughly with soap and water; rinse eyes with plain water.

ASSESSMENT

1. Note date of transplant, other agents used and the outcome.
2. Document a negative pregnancy test 1 week prior to initiating therapy in all women of childbearing age.
3. Monitor renal and LFTs, and hematologic profiles and observe closely for severe neutropenia (day 31 to day 180) posttransplant. If ANC is less than 1.3×10^3, then drug therapy must be interrupted or decreased.

CLIENT/FAMILY TEACHING

1. Take exactly as directed on an empty stomach twice a day; taken with cyclosporine and steroids.
2. Do not remove from manufacturer's original container.
3. With increased immunosuppression the susceptibility to infection and the risk of lymphoproliferative disease and other malignancies may be increased. Report any new or unusual side effects.
4. Practice two reliable forms of contraception simultaneously before, during, and for 6 weeks following therapy.
5. Report for all scheduled lab studies to evaluate response to therapy and to identify any potential problems. Need CBC weekly during first month, twice monthly for the second and third months, and then monthly thereafter for the first year.

OUTCOMES/EVALUATE

Prevention of transplant rejection; improved organ function

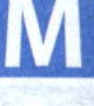

N

Nabumetone

(nah-**BYOU**-meh-tohn)

PREGNANCY CATEGORY: B
CLASSIFICATION(S):
Nonsteroidal anti-inflammatory drug
Rx: Relafen
✱Rx: Apo-Nabumetone

SEE ALSO NONSTEROIDAL ANTI-INFLAMMATORY DRUGS.

ACTION/KINETICS

Time to peak plasma levels: 2.5–4 hr. **Peak effect:** 9–12 hr. Over 99% protein-bound. **t½ of active metabolite:** 22.5–30 hr. Excreted mainly (80%) in the urine.

USES

(1) Acute and chronic treatment of osteoarthritis and rheumatoid arthritis. (2) Treat mild to moderate pain including postextraction dental pain, postsurgical episiotomy pain, and soft tissue athletic injuries.

CONTRAINDICATIONS

Lactation.

SPECIAL CONCERNS

Safety and efficacy have not been determined in children.

HOW SUPPLIED

Tablet: 500 mg, 750 mg

DOSAGE

• TABLETS

Osteoarthritis, rheumatoid arthritis.

Adults, initial: 1,000 mg as a single dose; **maintenance:** 1,500–2,000 mg/day. Doses greater than 2,000 mg/day have not been studied.

NURSING CONSIDERATIONS

SEE ALSO NURSING CONSIDERATIONS FOR NONSTEROIDAL ANTI-INFLAMMATORY DRUGS.

ADMINISTRATION/STORAGE

1. May be taken with or without food.
2. The total daily dose may be given either once or in two divided doses.
3. Use the lowest effective dose for chronic treatment.

ASSESSMENT

1. Document type, onset, and characteristics of symptoms. Rate pain level and list any other drugs used and the outcome.
2. Note any swelling, pain, inflammation, trauma, or decreased ROM.
3. Monitor CBC, liver and renal function studies with chronic therapy.

CLIENT/FAMILY TEACHING

1. Take as directed; may take with food to decrease GI upset.
2. Review side effects that require immediate reporting: persistent headaches, altered vision, rash, swelling of extremities, blood in stools.
3. Avoid tasks that require mental alertness until drug effects realized.
4. Avoid alcohol and aspirin-containing products.

OUTCOMES/EVALUATE

- Relief of pain
- Improved mobility; ↑ ROM

Nadolol

(**NAY**-doh-lohl)

PREGNANCY CATEGORY: C
CLASSIFICATION(S):
Beta-adrenergic blocking agent
Rx: Corgard
✱Rx: Alti-Nadolol, Apo-Nadol, Novo-Nadolol

SEE ALSO BETA-ADRENERGIC BLOCKING AGENTS.

ACTION/KINETICS

Manifests both beta-1- and beta-2-adrenergic blocking activity. Has no membrane stabilizing or intrinsic sympathomimetic activity. Low lipid solubility. **Peak serum concentration:** 3–4 hr. **t½:** 20–24 hr (permits once-daily dosage). **Duration:** 17–24 hr. Absorption variable, averaging 30%; steady plasma level achieved after 6–9 days of administration. Excreted unchanged by the kidney.

USES
(1) Hypertension, either alone or with other drugs (e.g., thiazide diuretic). (2) Long-term management of angina pectoris. *Investigational:* Prophylaxis of migraine, ventricular arrhythmias, aggressive behavior, essential tremor, tremors associated with lithium or parkinsonism, antipsychotic-induced akathisia, rebleeding of esophageal varices, situational anxiety, reduce intraocular pressure.

CONTRAINDICATIONS
Use in bronchial asthma or bronchospasm, including severe COPD.

SPECIAL CONCERNS
Dosage has not been established in children.

HOW SUPPLIED
Tablet: 20 mg, 40 mg, 80 mg, 120 mg, 160 mg

DOSAGE

• **TABLETS**

Hypertension.
Initial: 40 mg/day; **then,** may be increased in 40- to 80-mg increments until optimum response obtained. **Maintenance:** 40–80 mg/day although up to 240–320 mg/day may be needed.

Angina.
Initial: 40 mg/day; **then,** increase dose in 40- to 80-mg increments q 3–7 days until optimum response obtained. **Maintenance:** 40–80 mg/day, although up to 160–240 mg/day may be needed.

Aggressive behavior.
40–160 mg/day.

Antipsychotic-induced akathisia.
40–80 mg/day.

Essential tremor.
120–240 mg/day.

Lithium-induced tremors.
20–40 mg/day.

Tremors associated with parkinsonism.
80–320 mg/day.

Prophylaxis of migraine.
40–80 mg/day.

Rebleeding of esophageal varices.
40–160 mg/day.

Situational anxiety.
20 mg.

Ventricular arrhythmias.
10–640 mg/day.

Reduction of intraocular pressure.
10–20 mg b.i.d.

NOTE: For all uses decrease dose orincrease dosage intervals in clients with renal failure.

NURSING CONSIDERATIONS

SEE ALSO *NURSING CONSIDERATIONS* FOR *BETA-ADRENERGIC BLOCKING AGENTS* AND *ANTIHYPERTENSIVE AGENTS*.

ASSESSMENT
1. Note indications for therapy, medical history, sympton characteristics, and other agents trialed.
2. Document baseline VS, labs, and ECG. Reduce dose with renal dysfunction.

CLIENT/FAMILY TEACHING
1. Take only as directed; do not stop abruptly.
2. Report any rapid weight gain, increased SOB, or extremity swelling.
3. Do not perform tasks that require mental alertness until drug effects realized; may cause dizziness.
4. May cause increased sensitivity to cold; dress appropriately.

OUTCOMES/EVALUATE
- ↓ BP, ↓ HR
- ↓ Frequency/intensity of angina

Nafarelin acetate

(**NAF**-ah-rel-in)

PREGNANCY CATEGORY: X
CLASSIFICATION(S):
Gonadotropin-releasing hormone
Rx: Synarel

ACTION/KINETICS
Produced through biotechnology; differs by only one amino acid from naturally occurring GnRH. Stimulates the release of LH and FSH from the adenohypophysis. Causes estrogen and progesterone synthesis in the ovary, resulting in the maturation and subsequent release of an ovum. With repeated use of the drug, however, the pituitary becomes desensitized and no longer pro-

N

duces endogenous LH and FSH; thus endogenous estrogen is not produced, leading to a regression of endometrial tissue, cessation of menstruation, and a menopausal-like state. Broken down by the enzyme peptidase. **Peak serum levels:** 10–40 min. **t½:** 3 hr; 80% is bound to plasma proteins.

USES

(1) Endometriosis (including reduction of endometriotic lesions) in clients aged 18 or older (400 mcg/day is clinically comparable to 3.75 mg/month of Lupon Depot). (2) Central precocious puberty in children of both sexes.

CONTRAINDICATIONS

Hypersensitivity to GnRH or analogs. Abnormal vaginal bleeding of unknown origin. Pregnancy or possibility of becoming pregnant. Lactation.

SPECIAL CONCERNS

Rule out pregnancy before initiating therapy. Safety and effectiveness have not been established in children.

SIDE EFFECTS

Due to hypoestrogenic effects.

Hot flashes (common), decreased libido, vaginal dryness, headaches, emotional lability, insomnia.

Due to androgenic effects.

Acne, myalgia, reduced breast size, edema, seborrhea, weight gain, increased libido, hirsutism. **Musculoskeletal:** Decrease in vertebral trabecular bone density and total vertebral bone mass. **Miscellaneous:** Nasal irritation, depression, weight loss.

LABORATORY TEST CONSIDERATIONS

↑ Cholesterol and triglyceride levels, plasma phosphorus, eosinophils. ↓ Serum calcium, WBCs.

HOW SUPPLIED

Nasal Spray: 2 mg/mL (0.2 mg/inh)

DOSAGE

• **NASAL SPRAY**

Endometriosis.

200 mcg into one nostril in the morning and 200 mcg into the other nostril at night (400 mcg b.i.d. may be required by some women).

Central precocious puberty.

400 mcg (2 sprays) into each nostril in the morning (i.e., 4 sprays) and in the evening (total of 8 sprays/day). If adequate suppression is not achieved, 3 sprays (600 mcg) into alternating nostrils t.i.d. (i.e., a total of 9 sprays/day).

NURSING CONSIDERATIONS

ADMINISTRATION/STORAGE

1. Initiate therapy between days 2 and 4 of the menstrual cycle.
2. Use for longer than 6 months is not recommended due to the lack of safety data.
3. Store at room temperature in an upright position protected from light.

ASSESSMENT

1. Perform a complete history, noting any osteoporosis, alcohol, tobacco, or corticosteroid use; major risk factors for bone mineral loss that would preclude any repeated courses.
2. Note description of menstrual cycles and any abnormal vaginal bleeding of unknown origin; drug is contraindicated. Document abdominal/vaginal assessments and ultrasound findings.
3. Determine if pregnant; drug is teratogenic.

CLIENT/FAMILY TEACHING

1. Begin treatment between the second and fourth day of the menstrual cycle. Keep accurate records of menstrual patterns and cycles.
2. Use the spray upon arising and just before bedtime, alternating nostrils to decrease mucosal irritation.
3. Menses should cease while on therapy; report if regular menses continues.
4. Breakthrough bleeding may occur if successive doses are missed.
5. Use nonhormonal contraception; drug may cause fetal harm.
6. If a topical nasal decongestant is required during treatment, use at least 30 min after nafarelin to prevent interference with drug absorption.
7. Drug may cause hypoestrogenic and androgenic side effects; report if evident as a change in drug dosage or therapy may be indicated.

OUTCOMES/EVALUATE

• Restoration of pituitary-gonadal function in 4–8 weeks
• ↓ Number/size of endometriotic lesions

Nafcillin sodium

(naf-**SILL**-in)

PREGNANCY CATEGORY: B
CLASSIFICATION(S):
Antibiotic, penicillin
Rx: Unipen, Nallpen

SEE ALSO *ANTI-INFECTIVES* AND *PENICILLINS*.

ACTION/KINETICS
Penicillinase-resistant and acid stable. Parenteral therapy is recommended initially for severe infections. **Peak plasma levels: PO,** 7 mcg/mL after 30–60 min; **IM,** 14–20 mcg/mL after 30–60 min. **t½:** 60 min. Significantly bound to plasma proteins.

USES
Infections by penicillinase-producing staphylococci. As initial therapy if staphylococcal infection is suspected (i.e., until results of culture have been obtained).

CONTRAINDICATIONS
Use for treatment of penicillin G-susceptible staphylococcus.

ADDITIONAL SIDE EFFECTS
Sterile abscesses and thrombophlebitis occur frequently, especially in the elderly.

ADDITIONAL DRUG INTERACTIONS
When used with cyclosporine, subtherapeutic levels of cyclosporine are possible.

HOW SUPPLIED
Capsule: 250 mg; *Powder for injection:* 500 mg, 1 g, 2 g, 10 g

DOSAGE

• **IV**
Adults: 0.5–1 g q 4 hr.

• **IM**
Adults: 0.5 g q 4–6 hr. **Children and infants, less than 40 kg:** 25 mg/kg b.i.d. **Neonates:** 10 mg/kg b.i.d. Or, **for neonates weighing more than 2,000 g and less than 7 days of age:** 100 mg/kg/day in 2 divided doses; **for neonates older than 7 days:** 100 mg/kg/day in 3 divided doses; **if the weight is less than 2,000 g:** 20 mg/kg q 8 hr.

• **CAPSULES**
Mild to moderate infections.
Adults: 250–500 mg q 4–6 hr.
Severe infections.
Adults: Up to 1 g q 4–6 hr.
Pneumonia/scarlet fever.
Children: 25 mg/kg/day in four divided doses.
Staphylococcal infections.
Children: 50 mg/kg/day in four divided doses. **Neonates:** 10 mg/kg t.i.d.–q.i.d.
Streptococcal pharyngitis.
Children: 250 mg t.i.d. for 10 days.
NOTE: IV administration is not recommended for neonates or infants.

NURSING CONSIDERATIONS

SEE ALSO *NURSING CONSIDERATIONS* FOR *PENICILLINS*.

ADMINISTRATION/STORAGE

1. Reconstitute for PO use by adding powder to bottle of diluent. Replace cap tightly and shake thoroughly until all powder is in solution. Check carefully for undissolved powder at the bottom of bottle. Store in refrigerator and discard after 1 week.
2. Serum levels after PO administration are low and unpredictable.
3. Reconstitute for IM use with sterile water or NaCl injection. Shake vigorously to reconstitute.
4. Administer IM by deep intragluteal injection.
IV 5. Do not administer IV to newborn infants.
6. Reserve IV use for therapy of 24–48 hr duration due to the possibility of thrombophlebitis, especially in geriatric clients. Reduce rate of flow and report any pain, redness, or edema at IV site.
7. Reconstitute by adding required amount of sterile water. Shake vigorously. Date, time, and initial bottle. Refrigerate after reconstitution and discard unused portion after 48 hr.
8. For direct IV administration, dissolve powder in 15–30 mL of NaCl and inject over 5- to 10-min period into the tubing of flowing IV infusion. For IV drip, dissolve the required amount in

N

100–150 mL of NSS and administer over a period of 30–90 min.

ASSESSMENT

1. Note indications for therapy, symptom characteristics and culture results.
2. Monitor LFTs, renal function and CBC; assess for nafcillin induced neutropenia, especially during the third week of therapy.

CLIENT/FAMILY TEACHING

1. Take capsules 1 hr before or 2 hr after meals with a full glass of water. Report any GI distress.
2. Complete entire prescription as directed to prevent bacterial resistance.
3. Report any unusual side effects, fever, sore throat, rash, severe diarrhea, or worsening of condition.

OUTCOMES/EVALUATE

Negative culture reports with ↓ WBC, ↓ temperature and symptomatic improvement.

Naftifine hydrochloride

(**NAF**-tih-feen)

N

PREGNANCY CATEGORY: B
CLASSIFICATION(S):
Antifungal
Rx: Naftin, Naftin-MP

SEE ALSO *ANTI-INFECTIVES.*

ACTION/KINETICS

Synthetic antifungal agent with a broad spectrum of activity. Thought to inhibit squalene 2,3-epoxidase, which is responsible for synthesis of sterols. The decreased levels of sterols (especially ergosterol) and the accumulation of squalene in cells result in fungicidal activity. Although used topically, approximately 6% of the drug is absorbed. Naftifine and its metabolites are excreted via the feces and urine. **t½:** 2–3 days.

USES

To treat tinea cruris, tinea pedis, and tinea corporis caused by *Candida albicans, Epidermophyton floccosum, Microsporum canis, M. audouinii, M. gypseum, Trichophyton rubrum, T. mentagrophytes,* and *T. tonsurans.*

CONTRAINDICATIONS

Ophthalmic use.

SPECIAL CONCERNS

Discontinue nursing while using naftifine and for several days after the last application. Safety and efficacy in children have not been determined.

SIDE EFFECTS

- **TOPICAL**

Cream: Burning, stinging, dryness, itching, local irritation, erythema.

- **TOPICAL**

Gel: Burning, stinging, itching, rash, tenderness, erythema.

HOW SUPPLIED

Cream: 1%; *Gel/jelly:* 1%

DOSAGE

- **TOPICAL CREAM (1%), TOPICAL GEL (1%)**

Massage into affected area and surrounding skin once daily if using the cream and twice daily (morning and evening) if using the gel.

NURSING CONSIDERATIONS

SEE ALSO *GENERAL NURSING CONSIDERATIONS FOR ANTI-INFECTIVES.*

CLIENT/FAMILY TEACHING

1. Wash hands before and after use.
2. Avoid contact with eyes, nose, mouth, or other mucous membranes; for external use only.
3. Avoid occlusive dressings, diapers, or wrappings; do not cover area.
4. Report any excessive itching, burning or irritation.
5. Beneficial effects are usually observed within 1 week; treatment should be continued for 1–2 weeks after symptoms diminish. If no beneficial effects after 4 weeks of treatment, seek reevaluation.

OUTCOMES/EVALUATE

Negative cultures; clinical improvement

Nalbuphine hydrochloride

(**NAL**-byou-feen)

CLASSIFICATION(S):
Narcotic agonist/antagonist
Rx: Nubain

SEE ALSO *NARCOTIC ANALGESICS.*

ACTION/KINETICS
Synthetic compound resembling oxymorphone and naloxone. Potent analgesic with both narcotic agonist and antagonist actions. Analgesic potency is approximately equal to that of morphine, while its antagonistic potency is approximately one-fourth that of nalorphine. **Onset: IV,** 2–3 min; **SC or IM,** < 15 min. **Peak effect:** 30–60 min. **Duration:** 3–6 hr; **t½:** 5 hr.

USES
Moderate to severe pain. Preoperative analgesia, anesthesia adjunct, obstetric analgesia.

CONTRAINDICATIONS
Hypersensitivity to drug. Children under 18 years.

SPECIAL CONCERNS
Safe use during pregnancy (except for delivery) and lactation not established. Use with caution in presence of head injuries and asthma, MI (if client is nauseous or vomiting), biliary tract surgery (may induce spasms of sphincter of Oddi), renal insufficiency. Clients dependent on narcotics may experience withdrawal symptoms.

ADDITIONAL SIDE EFFECTS
Even though nalbuphine is an agonist-antagonist, it may cause dependence and may precipitate withdrawal symptoms in an individual physically dependent on narcotics. **CNS:** Sedation is common. Crying, feelings of unreality, and other psychologic reactions. **GI:** Cramps, dry mouth, bitter taste, dyspepsia. **Skin:** Itching, burning, urticaria, sweaty, clammy skin. **Other:** Blurred vision, difficulty with speech, urinary frequency.

DRUG INTERACTIONS
Concomitant use with CNS depressants, other narcotics, phenothiazines, may result in additive depressant effects.

HOW SUPPLIED
Injection: 10 mg/mL, 20 mg/mL

DOSAGE

- **SC, IM, IV**

Analgesia.

Adults: 10 mg/70 kg q 3–6 hr as needed (single dose should not exceed 20 mg q 3–6 hr; do not exceed a total daily dose of 160 mg).

NURSING CONSIDERATIONS

SEE ALSO NURSING CONSIDERATIONS FOR NARCOTIC ANALGESICS.

IV ADMINISTRATION/STORAGE
May be administered IV, undiluted. Administer each 10 mg or less over a 3- to 5-min period.

ASSESSMENT
1. Note any narcotic dependence; may precipitate withdrawal symptoms with narcotic addiction.
2. Document sulfite sensitivity.
3. Determine onset, location, duration, and intensity of pain. Use a pain-rating scale to assess pain.
4. Note any history of head injuries, asthma, or cardiac dysfunction.

CLIENT/FAMILY TEACHING
1. Take only as directed; do not share meds.
2. Physical dependence may result from long term use.
3. Report any symptoms of allergic reaction or withdrawal symptoms.
4. Avoid activities that require mental alertness.

OUTCOMES/EVALUATE
Desired level of pain control

Nalidixic acid

(nah-lih-**DICKS**-ick **AH**-sid)

PREGNANCY CATEGORY: B
CLASSIFICATION(S):
Urinary anti-infective
Rx: NegGram

ACTION/KINETICS
Thought to inhibit the DNA synthesis, probably by interfering with DNA polymerization. Is either bacteriostatic or bactericidal. Rapidly absorbed from the GI tract. **Peak plasma concentration:** 20–40 mcg/mL after 1–2 hr; **peak urine levels:** 150–200 mcg/mL after 3–4 hr. **t½, plasma:** 1.5 hr (increased to 21 hr in anuric clients); **t½, urine:** 6 hr. Metabolized in the liver to hydroxy-

nalidixic acid (comparable activity to nalidixic acid) and inactive compounds which are rapidly excreted. Extensively protein bound.

Sensitivity determinations are recommended before and periodically during prolonged administration of nalidixic acid. Renal and liver function tests are advisable if course of therapy exceeds 2 weeks.

USES

Acute and chronic UTIs caused by susceptible gram-negative organisms, including *Escherichia coli, Proteus, Enterobacter,* and *Klebsiella.*

CONTRAINDICATIONS

Lactation. Use in infants less than 3 months of age.

SPECIAL CONCERNS

Use with caution in prepubertal children, clients with liver disease, severely impaired kidney function, epilepsy, and severe cerebral arteriosclerosis.

SIDE EFFECTS

GI: N&V, diarrhea, abdominal pain. **CNS:** Drowsiness, headache, dizziness, weakness, vertigo, toxic psychoses, intracranial hypertension, ***seizures (rare)***. Also, increased intracranial pressure with bulging anterior fontanel, papilledema, and headache; sixth cranial nerve palsy in children and infants. **Allergic:** Photosensitivity (e.g., erythema, painful bullae on exposed skin), skin rashes, arthralgia (joint swelling and stiffness), pruritus, urticaria, angioedema, eosinophilia, anaphylaxis (rare). **Hematologic:** Leukopenia, thrombocytopenia, ***hemolytic anemia*** (especially in clients with G6PD deficiency). **Ophthalmic:** Reversible subjective visual disturbances, including overbrightness of lights, difficulty in focusing, changes in color perception, double vision, decreased visual acuity. **Other:** Metabolic acidosis, cholestatic jaundice, cholestasis, paresthesia.

LABORATORY TEST CONSIDERATIONS

False + for urinary glucose with Benedict's solution, Fehling's solution, or Clinitest Reagent tablets. Falsely elevated 17-ketosteroids.

OD OVERDOSE MANAGEMENT

Symptoms: Toxic psychoses, convulsions, increased intracranial pressure, nausea, vomiting, lethargy, metabolic acidosis. *Treatment:* Gastric lavage if the overdose is identified early. If absorption has occurred, fluid administration is increased with supportive measures. In severe cases, use of anticonvulsants may be necessary.

DRUG INTERACTIONS

Antacids, oral / ↓ Nalidixic acid effect R/T ↓ GI tract absorption
Anticoagulants, oral / ↑ Anticoagulant effect R/T ↓ plasma protein binding
Nitrofurantoin / ↓ Effect of nalidixic acid

HOW SUPPLIED

Suspension: 250 mg/5 mL; *Tablet:* 250 mg, 500 mg, 1 g

DOSAGE

• **ORAL SUSPENSION, TABLETS**

Adults: initially, 1 g q.i.d. for 1–2 weeks; **maintenance,** if necessary, 0.5 g q 6 hr. Maximum daily dose: 4 g. **Children, 3 months to 12 years, initial:** 55 mg/kg/day in four equally divided doses; **maintenance:** 33 mg/kg/day.

NURSING CONSIDERATIONS

SEE ALSO *GENERAL NURSING CONSIDERATIONS* FOR *ANTI-INFECTIVES.*

ADMINISTRATION/STORAGE

Underdosage (less than 4 g/day) may lead to emergence of bacterial resistance.

ASSESSMENT

1. Note indications for therapy, frequency and other agents trialed.
2. Obtain CBC, urine culture, liver and renal function studies; note any dysfunction.
3. Assess for adverse CNS effects (seizures, psychosis, severe headaches, ↑ ICP); withhold drug.

CLIENT/FAMILY TEACHING

1. Take 1 hr before meals, on an empty stomach. If GI upset occurs, may be taken with food. Drink at least 2–3 L/day of water. Avoid antacids for 2 hr before and after dose.
2. Do not perform tasks that require mental alertness; may cause drowsiness, confusion, blurred vision, and dizziness.
3. Avoid prolonged exposure to sunlight or ultraviolet light; wear protective clothing and sunscreen if exposed.

Photosensitivity may remain for 3 months following therapy.

OUTCOMES/EVALUATE

Negative urine cultures; symptomatic improvement (↓ dysuria, ↓ frequency)

Nalmefene hydrochloride

(**NAL**-meh-feen)

PREGNANCY CATEGORY: B
CLASSIFICATION(S):
Narcotic antagonist
Rx: Revex

SEE ALSO *NARCOTIC ANTAGONISTS*.

ACTION/KINETICS

Prevents or reverses respiratory depression, sedation, and hypotension due to opioids, including propoxyphene, nalbuphine, pentazocine, and butorphanol. Has a significantly longer duration of action than naloxone. Does not produce respiratory depression, psychotomimetic effects, or pupillary constriction (i.e., it has no intrinsic activity). Also, tolerance, physical dependence, or abuse potential have not been noted. **Onset, after IV:** 2 min. **Duration:** Up to 8 hr. **t½:** 10.8 hr. Metabolized by the liver and excreted in the urine.

USES

For complete or partial reversal of the effects of opioid drugs postoperatively. Management of known or suspected overdose of opiates.

SPECIAL CONCERNS

Will precipitate acute withdrawal symptoms in those who have some degree of tolerance and dependence on opioids. Use with caution during lactation, in high CV risk clients, or in those who have received potentially cardiotoxic drugs. Reversal of buprenorphine-induced respiratory depression may be incomplete; therefore artificial respiration may be necessary. Safety and effectiveness have not been determined in children.

SIDE EFFECTS

CV: Tachycardia, hypertension, hypotension, vasodilation, bradycardia, arrhythmia. **GI:** N&V, diarrhea, dry mouth. **CNS:** Dizziness, somnolence, depression, agitation, nervousness, tremor, confusion, withdrawal syndrome, myoclonus. **Body as a whole:** Fever, headache, chills, postoperative pain. **Miscellaneous:** Pharyngitis, pruritus, urinary retention.

LABORATORY TEST CONSIDERATIONS

↑ AST.

HOW SUPPLIED

Injection: 1 mg/mL, 100 mcg/mL

DOSAGE

• **IV**

Reversal of postoperative depression due to opiates.

Adults: Titrate in 0.25-mcg/kg incremental doses at 2–5-min intervals until the desired degree of reversal is achieved (i.e., adequate ventilation and alertness without significant pain or discomfort). If client is an increased CV risk, use an incremental dose of 0.1 mcg/kg (the drug may be diluted 1:1 with saline or sterile water). A total dose greater than 1 mcg/kg does not provide additional effects.

Management of known or suspected overdose of opiates.

Adults, initial: 0.5 mg/70 kg; **then,** 1 mg/70 kg 2–5 min later, if needed. Doses greater than 1.5 mg/70 kg do not increase the beneficial effect. If there is a reasonable suspicion of dependence on opiates, give a challenge dose of 0.1 mg/70 kg first; if there is no evidence of withdrawal in 2 min, give the recommended dose.

NURSING CONSIDERATIONS

SEE ALSO *NURSING CONSIDERATIONS* FOR *NARCOTIC ANTAGONISTS*.

ADMINISTRATION/STORAGE

1. May give SC or IM at doses of 1 mg if IV access is lost or not readily obtainable; effective in 5–15 min.

IV 2. Treatment should follow, not precede, establishment of a patent airway, ventilatory assistance, oxygen, and circulatory access.

N

3. Nalmefene is supplied in two concentrations—ampules containing 1 mL (blue label) at a concentration suitable for postoperative use (100 mcg) and ampules containing 2 mL (green label) suitable for management of overdose (1 mg/mL), i.e., **10 times as concentrated.** Follow specific guidelines, as indicated.

ASSESSMENT

1. Document type and amount of agent used and when administered/ingested.
2. Note any opioid dependence; may induce acute withdrawal S&S. Perform challenge test if opiod dependency suspected.
3. Identify high CV risk or if received cardiotoxic drugs; increases risk for cardiac complications.
4. Observe carefully for recurrent respiratory depression. Compared to naloxone (1.1 hr) the half-life of nalmefene is much longer (10.8 hr). Overdose with long-acting opiates (e.g., methadone, LAAM) may cause recurrence of respiratory depression.
5. With renal failure, if more than one dose required, administer incremental doses slowly (over 60 sec) to prevent dizziness and hypertension.
6. Client may experience N&V, fever, headaches, chills, pain, dizziness, and tachycardia.

OUTCOMES/EVALUATE

Reversal of opioid-induced drug effects; ↓ risk of renarcotization

Naloxone hydrochloride

(nal-**OX**-ohn)

PREGNANCY CATEGORY: B
CLASSIFICATION(S):
Narcotic antagonist
Rx: Narcan

SEE ALSO *NARCOTIC ANTAGONISTS.*

ACTION/KINETICS

Combines competitively with opiate receptors and blocks or reverses the action of narcotic analgesics. Since the duration of action of naloxone is shorter than that of the narcotic analgesics, the respiratory depression may return when the narcotic antagonist has worn off. **Onset: IV,** 2 min; **SC, IM:** <5 min. **Time to peak effect:** 5–15 min. **Duration:** Dependent on dose and route of administration but may be as short as 45 min. **t½:** 60–100 min. Metabolized in the liver to inactive products; eliminated through the kidneys.

USES

(1) Respiratory depression induced by natural and synthetic narcotics, including butorphanol, methadone, nalbuphine, pentazocine, and propoxyphene. Drug of choice when nature of depressant drug is not known. (2) Diagnosis of acute opiate overdosage. Not effective when respiratory depression is induced by hypnotics, sedatives, or anesthetics and other nonnarcotic CNS depressants. (3) Adjunct to increase BP in septic shock. *Investigational:* Treatment of Alzheimer's dementia, alcoholic coma, and schizophrenia.

CONTRAINDICATIONS

Sensitivity to drug. Narcotic addicts (drug may cause severe withdrawal symptoms). Use in neonates.

SPECIAL CONCERNS

Safe use during lactation and in children is not established.

SIDE EFFECTS

N&V, sweating, hypertension, tremors, sweating due to reversal of narcotic depression. If used postoperatively, excessive doses may cause ***VT and fibrillation,*** hypo- or hypertension, pulmonary edema, and ***seizures (infrequent).***

HOW SUPPLIED

Injection: 0.02 mg/mL, 0.4 mg/mL, 1 mg/mL

DOSAGE

- **IV, IM, SC**

  Narcotic overdose.

Initial: 0.4–2 mg IV; if necessary, additional IV doses may be repeated at 2- to 3-min intervals. If no response after 10 mg, reevaluate diagnosis. **Pediatric, initial:** 0.01 mg/kg IV; **then,** 0.1 mg/kg IV, if needed. The SC or IM route may be used if an IV route is not available.

To reverse postoperative narcotic depression.
Adults: IV, initial, 0.1- to 0.2-mg increments at 2- to 3-min intervals; **then,** repeat at 1- to 2-hr intervals if necessary. Supplemental IM dosage increases the duration of reversal. **Children: Initial,** 0.005–0.01 mg IV at 2- to 3-min intervals until desired response is obtained.
Reverse narcotic-induced depression in neonates.
Initial: 0.01 mg/kg IV, IM, or SC. May be repeated using adult administration guidelines.

NURSING CONSIDERATIONS

SEE ALSO *NURSING CONSIDERATIONS* FOR *NARCOTIC ANTAGONISTS*.

ADMINISTRATION/STORAGE

IV 1. May administer undiluted at a rate of 0.4 mg over 15 sec with narcotic overdosage. May reconstitute 2 mg in 500 mL of NSS or D5W to provide a 4 mcg/mL or 0.004 mg/mL concentration. Administration rate varies with client response.
2. Do not mix with preparations containing bisulfite, metabisulfite, long-chain or high molecular weight anions, or alkaline pH solutions.
3. When mixed with other solutions, use within 24 hr.

ASSESSMENT

1. Identify any evidence of narcotic addiction. Note agent and half-life.
2. Document cardiopulmonary and neurologic assessments.
3. Make appropriate referrals for those requiring substance abuse counselling.

INTERVENTIONS

1. The duration of the narcotic may exceed naloxone (the antagonist). Therefore, more than one dose may be necessary to counteract the effects of the narcotic.
2. Monitor VS at 5-min intervals, then every 30 min once stabilized.
3. Titrate to avoid interfering with pain control or readminister narcotic at a lower dosage to maintain pain control.

OUTCOMES/EVALUATE

Reversal of narcotic-induced respiratory depression

Naltrexone

(nal-**TREX**-ohn)

PREGNANCY CATEGORY: C
CLASSIFICATION(S):
Narcotic antagonist
Rx: Depade, ReVia

SEE ALSO *NARCOTIC ANTAGONISTS*.

ACTION/KINETICS
Competitively binds to opiate receptors, thereby reversing or preventing the effects of narcotics. **Peak plasma levels:** 1 hr. **Duration:** 24–72 hr. Metabolized in the liver; a major metabolite—6-beta-naltrexol—is active. **Peak serum levels, after 50 mg: naltrexone,** 8.6 ng/mL; **6-beta-naltrexol,** 99.3 ng/mL. **t½: naltrexone,** approximately 4 hr; **6-beta-naltrexol,** 13 hr. Naltrexone and its metabolites are excreted in the urine.

USES
To prevent narcotic use in former narcotic addicts. Adjunct to the psychosocial treatment for alcoholism. *Investigational:* To treat eating disorders and postconcussional syndrome not responding to other approaches.

CONTRAINDICATIONS
Those taking narcotic analgesics, dependent on narcotics, or in acute withdrawal from narcotics. Liver failure, acute hepatitis.

SPECIAL CONCERNS
Use with caution during lactation. Safety in children under 18 years of age has not been established.

SIDE EFFECTS
CNS: Headache, anxiety, nervousness, sleep disorders, dizziness, change in energy level, depression, confusion, restlessness, disorientation, hallucinations, nightmares, bad dreams, paranoia, fatigue, drowsiness. **GI:** N&V, diarrhea, constipation, anorexia, abdominal pain or cramps, flatulence, ulcers, increased appetite, weight gain or loss, increased thirst, xerostomia, hemorrhoids. **CV:** Phlebitis, edema, increased BP, changes in ECG, palpitations, epistaxis, tachycardia. **GU:** Delayed ejaculation, increased urinary frequency or

N

urinary discomfort, increased or decreased interest in sex. **Respiratory:** Cough, sore throat, nasal congestion, rhinorrhea, sneezing, excess secretions, hoarseness, SOB, heaving breathing, sinus trouble. **Dermatologic:** Rash, oily skin, itching, pruritus, acne, cold sores, alopecia, athlete's foot. **Musculoskeletal:** Joint/muscle pain, muscle twitches, tremors, pain in legs, knees, or shoulders. **Ophthalmologic:** Blurred vision, aching or strained eyes, burning eyes, light-sensitive eyes, swollen eyes. **Other:** Hepatotoxicity, tinnitus, painful or clogged ears, chills, swollen glands, inguinal pain, cold feet, "hot" spells, "pounding" head, fever, yawning, side pains.

A severe narcotic withdrawal syndrome may be precipitated if naltrexone is administered to a dependent individual. The syndrome may begin within 5 min and may last for up to 2 days.

HOW SUPPLIED

Tablet: 50 mg

DOSAGE

• TABLETS

To produce blockade of opiate actions.

Initial: 25 mg followed by an additional 25 mg in 1 hr if no withdrawal symptoms occur. **Maintenance:** 50 mg/day.

Alternate dosing schedule for blockade of opiate actions.

The weekly dose of 350 mg may be given as: (a) 50 mg/day on weekdays and 100 mg on Saturday; (b) 100 mg/48 hr; (c) 100 mg every Monday and Wednesday and 150 mg on Friday; or, (d) 150 mg q 72 hr.

Alcoholism.

50 mg once daily for up to 12 weeks. Treatment for longer than 12 weeks has not been studied.

NURSING CONSIDERATIONS

SEE ALSO *NURSING CONSIDERATIONS* FOR *NARCOTIC ANTAGONISTS.*

ADMINISTRATION/STORAGE

1. *Never* initiate therapy until determined that client is not dependent on narcotics (i.e., a naloxone challenge test should be completed).
2. Client should be opiate free for at least 7–10 days before beginning therapy.
3. When initiating therapy, begin with 25 mg and observe for 1 hr for any signs of narcotic withdrawal.
4. The blockade produced by naltrexone may be overcome by taking large doses of narcotics; such doses may be fatal.
5. Clients taking naltrexone may not respond to preparations containing narcotics for use in coughs, diarrhea, or pain.

ASSESSMENT

1. Determine if opiate addicted and when last dose was ingested; must be opiate free for 7–10 days before initiating therapy. Check urinalysis to confirm absence of opiates; note naloxone challenge test results.
2. Monitor ECG and VS. Report if respirations severely lowered or difficulty breathing evident.
3. Obtain LFTs; monitor monthly during the first 6 months of therapy.

CLIENT/FAMILY TEACHING

1. This drug blocks the effects of narcotics and opiates. It also may help to prevent alcohol consumption. Taking an opiate with this therapy may prove fatal as the amount needed to overcome the blockade is quite high.
2. May take with food or milk to diminish GI upset.
3. Headaches, restlessness, and irritability may be caused by naltrexone.
4. Report loss of appetite, unusual fatigue, yellowing of skin or sclera, or itching. Abdominal pain or difficulty with bowel function may warrant a dosage reduction.
5. Remain drug free; identify individuals, agencies, and support groups that may assist in remaining drug free.
6. Attend support groups and behavioral therapy sessions.

OUTCOMES/EVALUATE

Maintenance of narcotic-free state in detoxified addicts

Naproxen

(nah-**PROX**-en)

PREGNANCY CATEGORY: B
Rx: EC-Naprosyn, Gen-Naproxen EC, Naprosyn
♣**Rx:** Apo-Naproxen, Apo-Naproxen SR, Naxen, Novo–Naprox, Nu-Naprox, Riva-Naproxen

Naproxen sodium

(nah-**PROX**-en)

PREGNANCY CATEGORY: B
Rx: Anaprox, Anaprox DS, Naprelan
♣**Rx:** Apo-Napro-Na, Apo-Napro-Na DS, Novo–Naprox Sodium, Novo-Naprox Sodium DS, Novo-Naprox SR, Synflex, Synflex DS
OTC: Aleve
CLASSIFICATION(S):
Nonsteroidal anti-inflammatory drug

SEE ALSO *NONSTEROIDAL ANTI-INFLAMMATORY DRUGS.*

ACTION/KINETICS

Peak serum levels of naproxen: 2–4 hr; **for sodium salt:** 1–2 hr. **$t_{1/2}$ for naproxen:** 12–15 hr; **for sodium salt:** 12–13 hr. **Onset, immediate release for analgesia:** 1–2 hr. **Duration, analgesia:** Approximately 7 hr. **Onset (both immediate and delayed release):** 30 min; **duration:** 24 hr. **Onset, anti-inflammatory effects:** Up to 2 weeks; **duration:** 2–4 weeks. Over 99% plasma protein bound. Food delays the rate but not the amount of drug absorbed. 95% excreted in the urine.

USES

Rx. Mild to moderate pain. (1) Musculoskeletal and soft tissue inflammation including rheumatoid arthritis, osteoarthritis, bursitis, tendinitis, ankylosing spondylitis. (2) Primary dysmenorrhea, acute gout. (3) Juvenile rheumatoid arthritis (naproxen only). *NOTE:* The delayed-release or enteric-coated products are not recommended for initial treatment of pain because, compared to other naproxen products, absorption is delayed. *Investigational:* Antipyretic in cancer clients, sunburn, acute migraine (sodium salt only), prophylaxis of migraine, migraine due to menses, PMS (sodium salt only). Lower risk of Alzheimer's disease (long-term use). **OTC.** Relief of minor aches and pains due to the common cold, headache, toothache, muscular aches, backache, minor arthritis pain, pain due to menstrual cramps. Decrease fever.

CONTRAINDICATIONS

Simultaneous use of naproxen and naproxen sodium. Lactation. Use of delayed-release product for initial treatment of acute pain.

SPECIAL CONCERNS

Safety and effectiveness of naproxen have not been determined in children less than 2 years of age; the safety and effectiveness of naproxen sodium have not been established in children. Geriatric clients may manifest increased total plasma levels of naproxen.

LABORATORY TEST CONSIDERATIONS

Naproxen may increase urinary 17-ketosteroid values. Both forms may interfere with urinary assays for 5-HIAA.

DRUG INTERACTIONS

Alendronate / ↑ Risk of gastric ulcers
Methotrexate / Possibility of a fatal interaction
Probenecid / ↓ Plasma clearance of naproxen

HOW SUPPLIED

Naproxen: *Suspension:* 125 mg/mL; *Tablet:* 250 mg, 375 mg, 500 mg; *Tablet, Delayed Release:* 375 mg, 500 mg; **Naproxen sodium:** *Gelcap:* 220 mg; *Tablet:* 275 mg, 550 mg; *Tablet, Extended Release:* 412.5 mg, 550 mg

DOSAGE

NAPROXEN, NAPROXEN SODIUM

• **ORAL SUSPENSION, TABLETS**

Rheumatoid arthritis, osteoarthritis, ankylosing spondylitis, pain, dysmenorrhea, acute tendinitis, bursitis.

Naproxen tablets: 250–500 mg b.i.d. May increase to 1.5 g for short periods of time. **Naproxen suspension:** 250 mg (10 mL), 375 mg (15 mL), or 500 mg (20 mL) b.i.d. **Naproxen, delayed-release (EC-Naprosyn):** 375–500 mg b.i.d. **Naproxen sodium:** 275–500 mg b.i.d. May; increase to 1.65 g/day for limited periods. **Naproxen sodium, controlled release (Naprelan):** 750 mg or 1000 mg once daily, not to exceed 1500 mg/day. Do not exceed 1.25 g naproxen (1.375 g naproxen sodium) per day. If no improvement is seen within 2 weeks, consider an additional 2-week course of therapy.

Acute gout.

Naproxen, adults, initial: 750 mg; **then,** 250 mg naproxen q 8 hr until symptoms subside. **Naproxen sodium, adults, initial:** 825 mg; **then,** 275 mg q 8 hr until symptoms subside. **Naproxen sodium, controlled-release (Naprelean):** 1000–1500 mg once daily on the first day; **then,** 1000 mg once daily until symptoms subside.

Juvenile rheumatoid arthritis.

Naproxen only, 10 mg/kg/day in two divided doses. If the suspension is used, the following dosage can be used: **13 kg:** 2.5 mL b.i.d.; **25 kg:** 5 mL b.i.d.; **38 kg:** 7.5 mL b.i.d.

Mild to moderate pain, primary dyspmenorrhea,acute tendinitis, bursitis.

Naproxen, initial: 500 mg; **then,** 500 mg q 12 hr or 250 mg q 6–8 hr, not to exceed 1.25 g/day. Thereafter, do not exceed 1000 mg/day. **Naproxen sodium, initial:** 550 mg; **then,** 550 mg q 12 hr or 275 mg q 6–8 hr, not to exceed 1.375 g/day. Thereafter, do not exceed 1100 mg/day. **Naproxen sodium, controlled-release (Naprelan):** 1000 mg once daily. For a limited time, 1500 mg/day may be used. Thereafter, do not exceed 1000 mg/day.

• **TABLETS (OTC)**

Adults: 200 mg q 8–12 hr with a full glass of liquid. For some clients, 400 mg initially followed by 200 mg 12 hr later will provide better relief. Do not exceed 600 mg in a 24-hr period. Do not exceed 200 mg q 12 hr for geriatric clients. Not for use in children less than 12 years of age unless directed by a physician.

NURSING CONSIDERATIONS

SEE ALSO *NURSING CONSIDERATIONS* FOR *NONSTEROIDAL ANTI-INFLAMMATORY DRUGS.*

ADMINISTRATION/STORAGE

1. To be taken in the morning and in the evening. The doses do not have to be equal.
2. Do not give to children.
3. Naproxen suspension can be used to treat children with RA.
4. Delayed-release naproxen is not recommended for acute pain.
5. Do not use the OTC product for more than 10 days for pain or 3 days for fever unless prescribed.

ASSESSMENT

1. Note any NSAID hypersensitivity.
2. Document indications for therapy, onset and characteristics of symptoms. With pain, rate using a pain-rating scale.
3. Note any joint swelling, pain, trauma, inflammation, or decreased ROM.
4. Determine any GI bleeding or ulcers; use GI protectant if needed. Enteric coated product (EC-Naprosyn) reduces GI side effects.
5. Monitor CBC, liver and renal function studies with chronic therapy.

CLIENT/FAMILY TEACHING

1. Take with food to ↓ GI upset; in the morning and evening for optimal effects.
2. May cause dizziness or drowsiness; avoid activities that require mental alertness until effects realized.
3. Report any lack of response, worsening of symptoms, persistent abdominal pain, sore throat, fever, rash, altered vision, joint pain, edema, or dark-colored stools.
4. Avoid alcohol and all other OTC agents.

OUTCOMES/EVALUATE

- Improved joint pain and mobility
- Relief of headaches/pain
- ↓ Uterine cramping

Naratriptan hydrochloride

(**NAR**-ah-trip-tan)

PREGNANCY CATEGORY: C
CLASSIFICATION(S):
Antimigraine drug
Rx: Amerge

ACTION/KINETICS

Binds to serotonin 5-HT_{1D} and 5-HT_{1B} receptors. Activation of these receptors located on intracranial blood vessels, including those on arteriovenous anastomoses, leads to vasoconstriction and thus relief of migraine. Another possibility is that activation of these receptors on sensory nerve endings in trigeminal system causes inhibition of pro-inflammatory neuropeptide release. Well absorbed from GI tract. **Peak levels:** 2–3 hr. Unchanged drug and metabolites are primarily eliminated in urine. **t½, elimination:** 6 hr. Excretion is decreased in moderate liver or renal impairment.

USES

Acute treatment of migraine attacks in adults with or without aura.

CONTRAINDICATIONS

Use for prophylaxis of migraine or for management of hemiplegic or basilar migraine. Use in clients with ischemic cardiac, cerebrovascular, or peripheral vascular syndromes; use in uncontrolled hypertension; severe renal impairment (C_{CR} less than 15 mL/min); severe hepatic impairment; within 24 hr of treatment with another 5-HT_1 agonist, dihydroergotamine, or methysergide.

SPECIAL CONCERNS

Safety and efficacy have not been determined for use in cluster headaches or for use in children. Use with caution during lactation and with diseases that may alter the absorption, metabolism, or excretion of drugs, such as impaired renal or hepatic function.

SIDE EFFECTS

Most common side effects follow.

CNS: Paresthesia, dizziness, drowsiness, malaise, fatigue. **GI:** Nausea. **Miscellaneous:** Throat and neck symptoms, pain and pressure sensation.

Side effects that occurred in 0.1% to 1% of clients follow.

GI: Hyposalivation, vomiting, dyspeptic symptoms, diarrhea, GI discomfort and pain, gastroenteritis, constipation. **CNS:** Vertigo, tremors, cognitive function disorders, sleep disorders, disorders of equilibrium, anxiety, depression, detachment. **CV:** Palpitations, increased BP, tachyarrhythmias, syncope, abnormal ECG (PR prolongation, QTc prolongation, ST/T wave abnormalities, premature ventricular contractions, atrial flutter, or atrial fibrillation). **Musculoskeletal:** Muscle pain, arthralgia, articular rheumatism, muscle cramps and spasms, joint and muscle stiffness, tightness, and rigidity. **Dermatologic:** Sweating, skin rashes, pruritus, urticaria. **GU:** Bladder inflammation, polyuria, diuresis. **Body as a whole:** Chills, fever, descriptions of odor or taste, edema and swelling, allergies, allergic reactions, warm/cold temperature sensations, feeling strange, burning/stinging sensation. **Respiratory:** Bronchitis, cough, pneumonia. **Ophthalmic:** Photophobia, blurred vision. **ENT:** Ear, nose, and throat infections; phonophobia, sinusitis, upper respiratory inflammation, tinnitus. **Endocrine/Metabolic:** Thirst, polydipsia, dehydration, fluid retention. **Hematologic:** Increased WBCs.

OD OVERDOSE MANAGEMENT

Symptoms: Increased BP, chest pain. *Treatment:* Standard supportive treatment. Possible use of antihypertensive therapy. Monitor ECG if chest pain presents.

DRUG INTERACTIONS

Dihydroergotamine / Prolonged vasospastic reaction; effects additive
Methysergide / Prolonged vasospastic reaction; effects additive
Oral contraceptives / ↑ Mean plasma levels of naratriptan
Selective serotonin reuptake inhibitors / Possible weakness, hyperreflexia, and incoordination
Serotonin 5-HT_1 agonists / Additive effects

HOW SUPPLIED

Tablets: 1 mg, 2.5 mg

DOSAGE

• TABLETS

Migraine headaches.

Adults: Single doses of 1 mg or 2.5 mg taken with fluid. If headache returns or client has had only partial response, dose may be repeated once after 4 hr, for maximum of 5 mg in a 24-hr period. Doses of 5 mg/24 hr do not provide greater relief than 2.5 mg/24 hr.

NURSING CONSIDERATIONS

ADMINISTRATION/STORAGE

1. A dose of 2.5 mg is usually more effective than 1 mg but causes more side effects. Choice of dose is made on individual basis, weighing possible benefit of 2.5-mg dose with greater risk for side effects.
2. Safety of treating, on average, more than 4 headaches in 30-day period has not been established.
3. In clients with mild-to-moderate renal or hepatic impairment, do not exceed a dose of 2.5 mg over a 24-hr period. Consider a lower starting dose.
4. Store medication at controlled room temperature away from light.

ASSESSMENT

1. Document onset, frequency, duration, and characteristics of migraines.
2. List all drugs consumed to ensure none interact.
3. Monitor ECG, liver, and renal function studies; assess for dysfunction and dosage adjustment. In mild to moderate renal or hepatic impairment, do not exceed a dose of 2.5 mg over a 24-hr period. Consider a lower initial dose.

CLIENT/FAMILY TEACHING

1. Take exactly as directed to relieve headache. Will not reduce or prevent number of attacks experienced.
2. Review package insert and do not use with other similar headache meds.
3. May repeat once every 4 hr if headache returns or if only partial response attained. Do not exceed 5 mg/24 hr.
4. Report any unusual side effects including chest pain, SOB, or palpitations.
5. Practice reliable contraception.
6. Attempt to identify migraine triggers. Keep a headache log (identifying all factors surrounding each HA) for provider review. Continue other remedies i.e. noise reduction, reduced lighting, bed rest, that assist to control s&s.

OUTCOMES/EVALUATE

Relief of migraine headache

N

Natamycin

(nah-tah-**MY**-sin)

PREGNANCY CATEGORY: C
CLASSIFICATION(S):
Antifungal
Rx: Natacyn

SEE ALSO *ANTI-INFECTIVES.*

ACTION/KINETICS

Antifungal antibiotic derived from *Streptomyces natalensis.* Binds to the fungal cell membrane, resulting in alteration of permeability and loss of essential intracellular materials. Is fungicidal. After topical administration, therapeutic levels are reached in the corneal stroma but not in the intraocular fluid. Not absorbed systemically.

USES

For ophthalmic use only. (1) Drug of choice for *Fusarium solanae* keratitis. (2) For treatment of fungal blepharitis, conjunctivitis, and keratitis caused by susceptible organisms. (3) It is active against a variety of yeasts and filamentous fungi including *Candida, Aspergillus, Cephalosporium, Fusarium,* and *Penicillium.* Before initiating therapy, determine the susceptibility of the infectious organism to drug in smears and cultures of corneal scrapings. Effectiveness of natamycin for use as single agent in fungal endophthalmitis not established.

CONTRAINDICATIONS

Hypersensitivity to drug.

SPECIAL CONCERNS

Use with caution during lactation. Effectiveness as a single agent to treat fungal endophthalmitis has not been established. Safety and effectiveness have not been determined in children.

SIDE EFFECTS

Eye irritation, occasional allergies.

HOW SUPPLIED

Suspension: 5%

DOSAGE

• **OPHTHALMIC SUSPENSION (5%)**

Fungal keratitis.

Initially, 1 gtt in conjunctival sac q 1–2 hr; can be reduced usually, after

3–4 days to 1 gtt 6–8 times/day. Continue therapy for 14–21 days, during which dosage can be reduced gradually at 4 to 7-day intervals.

Fungal blepharitis/conjunctivitis. 1 gtt 4–6 times/day.

NURSING CONSIDERATIONS

SEE ALSO *GENERAL NURSING CONSIDERATIONS FOR ALL ANTI-INFECTIVES.*

ADMINISTRATION/STORAGE

1. Store at room temperature or in refrigerator avoiding exposure to light and excessive heat. Do not freeze.
2. Shake well before using.
3. Avoid contamination of dropper.
4. Discontinue if toxicity suspected.
5. Review therapy if no improvement noted after 7–10 days.

ASSESSMENT

Note indications for therapy, clinical presentation, and culture/scraping results.

CLIENT/FAMILY TEACHING

1. Continue as prescribed even if condition controlled. Keep all f/u appointments.
2. Report increased itching, pain, burning, visual difficulty, or stinging.
3. May experience sun and light sensitivity; wear sunglasses for several hours after administration.
4. To prevent reinfection, do not share eye makeup, washcloths, towels, or eye medications.

OUTCOMES/EVALUATE

Ophthalmic/symptomatic improvement

Nateglinide

PREGNANCY CATEGORY: C
CLASSIFICATION(S):
Antidiabetic agent, oral
Rx: Starlix

SEE ALSO *ANTIDIABETIC AGENTS, HYPOGLYCEMIC AGENTS.*

ACTION/KINETICS

Lowers blood glucoseand reduces post-mealtime glucose spikes by stimulating insulin secretion from the pancreas. Action depends on functioning beta-cells in pancreatic islets. Interacts with the ATP-sensitive potassium (K+ATP) channel on pancreatic beta cells causing depolarization of the beta cells. This opens the calcium channel-producing calcium influx and insulin secretion. Drug is highly tissue selective with a low affinity for heart and skeletal muscle. **Peak plasma levels:** 1 hr. Extent of absorption unaffected by food but there is a delay in the rate of absorption. Peak plasma levels are significantly reduced if administered 10 min prior to a liquid meal. Metabolized by the liver with most excreted through the urine. **t½, elimination:** About 1.5 hr.

USES

Type 2 diabetes in clients when hyperglycemia can not be controlled adequately by diet and exercise and who have not been treated chronically with other antidiabetic drugs. Nateglinide may be added to, but not substituted for, metformin. Do not switch clients to nateglinide when hyperglycemia is not adequately controlled with glyburide or other insulin secretagogues; do not add nateglinide to their treatment.

CONTRAINDICATIONS

Use in type I diabetes or diabetic ketoacidosis. Lactation.

SPECIAL CONCERNS

Use with caution in chronic liver disease or moderate to severe liver disease. Transient loss of glycemic control with fever, infection, trauma, surgery; insulin therapy may be required during these times. Safety and efficacy have not been determined in children.

SIDE EFFECTS

Metabolic: Hypoglycemia. **Respiratory:** URTI, bronchitis, coughing. **Miscellaneous:** Diarrhea, arthropathy, dizziness, flu symptoms, back pain, accidental trauma.

OD OVERDOSE MANAGEMENT

Symptoms: Hypoglycemia, including coma, seizure, neurological symptoms. *Treatment:* Treat severe symptoms with IV glucose.

DRUG INTERACTIONS
Beta-adrenergic blocking agents, nonselective / Possible potentiation of hypoglycemic effect
Corticosteroids / Possible reduction of hypoglycemic effect
NSAIDs / Possible potentiation of hypoglycemic effect
MAO inhibitors / Possible potentiation of hypoglycemic effect
Salicylates / Possible potentiation of hypoglycemic effect
Sympathomimetics / Possible reduction of hypoglycemic effect
Thiazides / Possible reduction of hypoglycemic effect
Thyroid products / Possible reduction of hypoglycemic effect
HOW SUPPLIED
Tablet: 60 mg, 120 mg

DOSAGE
• **TABLETS**
Type 2 diabetes mellitus.
120 mg t.i.d. before meals, with or without metformin. Use the 60 mg dose, alone or with metformin, in those who are near their HbA1c goal when treatment is initiated.

N

NURSING CONSIDERATIONS

SEE ALSO *ANTIDIABETIC AGENTS, HYPOGLYCEMIC AGENTS.*
ADMINISTRATION/STORAGE
Store at 15–30°C (59–86°F). Dispense in a tight container.
ASSESSMENT
1. Document indications for therapy, onset/type of disease, and all therapies trialed.
2. Obtain baseline labs noting any liver dysfunction; monitor throughout therapy.
3. Determine understanding of disease and refer for diabetes and nutrition education.
CLIENT/FAMILY TEACHING
1. Food delays absorption. Take 1–30 min before meals. Do not take while eating as drug will cause hypoglycemia.
2. Drug only helps to control blood sugar. Must continue diet, exercise, and lifestyle changes conducive to diabetes control.
3. Skip scheduled dose if client misses the meal, thus reducing the risk of hyopglycemia.
4. Drug is generally used initially when diet and exercise fail. May be added to metformin therapy but not in those whose DM is not adequately controlled with glyburide or other related agents.
OUTCOMES/EVALUATE
Control of blood sugar; HbA1c < 7

Nedocromil sodium

(neh-**DAH**-kroh-mill)

PREGNANCY CATEGORY: B
CLASSIFICATION(S):
Antiasthmatic drug
Rx: Alocril, Tilade

ACTION/KINETICS
Is a mast cell stabilizer. Thus, inhibits the release of various mediators, such as histamine, leukotriene C_4, and prostaglandin D_2, from a variety of cell types associated with asthma. Has no intrinsic bronchodilator, antihistamine, or glucocorticoid activity; also, systemic bioavailability is low. **t½:** 3.3 hr. About 89% bound to plasma protein; excreted unchanged. Only about 4% of the ophthalmic product is absorbed systemically.
USES
Systemic. Maintenance therapy in adults and children (age two and older) with mild to moderate bronchial asthma. **Ophthalmic.** Itching associated with allergic conjuctivitis in adults and children over 3 years old.
CONTRAINDICATIONS
Use for the reversal of acute bronchospasms, especially status asthmaticus.
SPECIAL CONCERNS
Use with caution during lactation. Safety and efficacy have not been established in children less than 12 years of age. Has not been shown to be able to substitute for the total dose of corticosteroids.
SIDE EFFECTS
• **AFTER SYSTEMIC USE.**
Respiratory: Coughing, pharyngitis, rhinitis, URTI, increased sputum, bron-

chitis, dyspnea, ***bronchospasm.*** **GI:** N&V, dyspepsia, abdominal pain, dry mouth, diarrhea. **CNS:** Dizziness, dysphonia. **Skin:** Rash, sensation of warmth. **Body as a whole:** Headache, chest pain, fatigue, arthritis. **Miscellaneous:** Viral infection, unpleasant taste.

• **AFTER OPHTHALMIC USE.**

Headache, ocular burning, irritation, stinging, unpleasant taste, nasal congestion, asthma, conjunctivitis, eye redness, photophobia, rhinitis.

LABORATORY TEST CONSIDERATIONS

↑ ALT.

HOW SUPPLIED

Metered dose inhaler: 1.75 mg/inh; *Ophthalmic solution:* 2%

DOSAGE

• **METERED DOSE INHALER**

Bronchial asthma.

Adults and children over 12 years of age: Two inhalations q.i.d. at regular intervals in order to provide 14 mg/day. If the client is under good control on q.i.d. dosing (i.e., requiring inhaled or oral beta agonist no more than twice a week or no worsening of symptoms occur with respiratory infections), a lower dose can be tried. In such instances, reduce the dose to 10.5 mg/day (i.e., used t.i.d.); then, after several weeks with good control, the dose can be reduced to 7 mg/day (i.e., used b.i.d.).

• **OPHTHALMIC SOLUTION**

Allergic conjunctivitis.

1 or 2 gtt in each eye b.i.d. Continue treatment until pollen season is over or until exposure to allergen is terminated.

NURSING CONSIDERATIONS

ADMINISTRATION/STORAGE

1. Each actuation releases 1.75 mg.
2. Must be used regularly, even during symptom-free period, in order to achieve beneficial effects.
3. Teach the proper method of use of the drug. An illustrated pamphlet is included in each pack of nedocromil.
4. Add nedocromil to existing treatment (e.g., bronchodilators). When clinical response is seen and if asthma is under good control, a gradual decrease in the concomitant medication can be tried.
5. Store metered dose inhaler between 2–30°C (36–86°F) and do not freeze.
6. Store ophthalmic solution between 2–25°C (36–77°F). Keep tightly closed and out of the reach of children.

ASSESSMENT

1. Document symptoms, noting type, onset, characteristics and triggers. List other agents trialed and the outcome.
2. Assess respiratory status thoroughly; not for use with status asthmaticus or for reversal of acute bronchospasm.
3. Monitor peak flow and vital capacity measurements (PFTs).
4. Document systemic and inhaled steroid therapy accurately. When a reduction is in progress, nedocromil cannot substitute for total steroid dose/requirements.
5. Review drug usage/time between prescriptions to ensure proper use.

CLIENT/FAMILY TEACHING

1. Review correct procedure for administration; use the step-by-step instructions provided with the drug.
2. Use ophthalmic solution as directed throughout pollen season.
3. Beneficial *preventative* effects will not be obtained if incorrectly administered by topical lung application. Drug is an inhaled anti-inflammatory that reduces lung inflammation. Continue to monitor peak flows and report loss of lung function or drop in readings.
4. Do not stop therapy during symptom-free periods; must be taken at regular intervals. Continue to use with other prescribed therapies.
5. Report any persistent headaches, unpleasant taste in mouth that interferes with nutrition, severe nausea, or chest pain.
6. Report any coughing, wheezing, or bronchospasm following use; drug should be discontinued, lungs assessed, and alternative therapy substituted.

OUTCOMES/EVALUATE

↓ Severity/frequency of asthmatic episodes ↓ eye itching

N

Nefazodone hydrochloride

(nih-**FAY**-zoh-dohn)

PREGNANCY CATEGORY: C
CLASSIFICATION(S):
Antidepressant, miscellaneous
Rx: Serzone
★**Rx:** Serzone-5HT_2

ACTION/KINETICS
Exact antidepressant mechanism not known. Inhibits neuronal uptake of serotonin and norepinephrine and antagonizes central 5-HT_2 receptors and alpha-1-adrenergic receptors (which may cause postural hypotension). Produces none to slight anticholinergic effects, moderate sedation, and slight orthostatic hypotension. **Peak plasma levels:** 1 hr. **t½:** 2–4 hr. **Time to reach steady state:** 4–5 days. Extensively metabolized by the liver with less than 1% excreted unchanged in the urine. Food delays the absorption of nefazodone and decreases the bioavailability by approximately 20%.

USES
Treatment of depression.

CONTRAINDICATIONS
Use with pimozide; in combination with an MAO inhibitor or within 14 days of discontinuing MAO inhibitor therapy. Clients hypersensitive to nefazodone or other phenylpiperazine antidepressants.

SPECIAL CONCERNS
Use with caution in clients with a recent history of MI, unstable heart disease and taking digoxin, or a history of mania. Use with caution during lactation. Safety and efficacy have not been determined in individuals below 18 years of age. There is a possibility of a suicide attempt in depression that may persist until significant remission occurs.

SIDE EFFECTS
CNS: Dizziness, insomnia, agitation, somnolence, lightheadedness, activation of mania or hypomania, confusion, memory impairment, paresthesia, abnormal dreams, decreased concentration, ataxia, incoordination, psychomotor retardation, tremor, hypertonia, decreased libido, vertigo, twitching, depersonalization, hallucinations, ***suicide thoughts/attempt,*** apathy, euphoria, hostility, abnormal gait/thinking, derealization, paranoid reaction, dysarthria, myoclonus, ***neuroleptic malignant syndrome (rare)***. **CV:** Postural hypotension, hypotension, sinus bradycardia, tachycardia, hypertension, syncope, ventricular extrasystoles, angina pectoris, ***CVA (rare)***. **GI:** Nausea, dry mouth, constipation, dyspepsia, diarrhea, increased appetite, vomiting, eructation, periodontal abscess, gingivitis, colitis, gastritis, mouth ulceration, stomatitis, esophagitis, peptic ulcer, rectal hemorrhage. **Dermatologic:** Pruritus, dry skin, acne, alopecia, urticaria, maculopapular/vesiculobullous rash, eczema. **Musculoskeletal:** Asthenia, arthralgia, arthritis, tenosynovitis, muscle stiffness, bursitis. **Respiratory:** Pharyngitis, increased cough, dyspnea, bronchitis, asthma, pneumonia, laryngitis, voice alteration, epistaxis, hiccups. **Hematologic:** Ecchymosis, anemia, leukopenia, lymphadenopathy. **Ophthalmologic:** Blurred vision, scotomata, abnormal vision, visual field defect, dry eye, eye pain, abnormal accommodation, diplopia, conjunctivitis, mydriasis, keratoconjunctivitis, photophobia, night blindness. **Body as a whole:** Headache, infection, flu syndrome, chills, fever, neck rigidity, allergic reaction, malaise, photosensitivity, facial edema, hangover effect, enlarged abdomen, hernia, pelvic pain, halitosis, cellulitis, weight loss, gout, dehydration. **GU:** Urinary frequency/retention/urgency, UTI, vaginitis, breast pain, cystitis, metrorrhagia, amenorrhea, polyuria, vaginal hemorrhage, breast enlargement, menorrhagia, urinary incontinence, abnormal ejaculation, hematuria, nocturia, kidney calculus. **Miscellaneous:** Peripheral edema, thirst, abnormal LFTs, ear pain, hyperacusis, deafness, taste loss.

LABORATORY TEST CONSIDERATIONS
↑ AST, ALT, LDH. ↓ Hematocrit. Hypercholesterolemia, hypoglycemia.

OD OVERDOSE MANAGEMENT
Symptoms: N&V, somnolence, increased incidence of severity of any of the reported side effects. *Treatment:* Symptomatic and supportive in the cases of hypotension or excessive sedation. Gastric lavage may be used.

DRUG INTERACTIONS
Alprazolam / ↑ Alprazolam plasma levels
Buspirone / ↑ Levels of both drugs → lightheadedness, somnolence, dizziness, asthenia
Carbamazepine / ↑ Carbamazepine plasma levels
Cisapride / ↑ Risk of serious cardiac arrhythmias
Digoxin / ↑ Digoxin plasma levels
HMG-CoA reductase inhibitors / ↑ Risk of rhabdomyolysis and myositis
MAO inhibitors / Serious and possibly fatal reactions including symptoms of hyperthermia, rigidity, myoclonus, autonomic instability with possible rigid fluctuations of VS, and mental status changes that may include extreme agitation progressing to delirium and coma
Pimozide / ↑ Plasma levels of pimozide resulting in QT prolongation and possible serious CV events, including death due to ventricular tachycardia of the torsades de pointes type
Propranolol / ↓ Propranolol plasma levels
Sibutramine / Serotonin syndrome, including CNS irritability, motor weakness, shivering, myoclonus, and altered consciousness
Trazodone / Serotonin syndrome, including CNS irritability, motor weakness, shivering, myoclonus, and altered consciousness
Triazolam / ↑ Triazolam plasma levels

HOW SUPPLIED
Tablet: 50 mg, 100 mg, 150 mg, 200 mg, 250 mg

DOSAGE

• **TABLETS**

Antidepressant.

Adults, initial: 200 mg/day given in two divided doses. Increase dose in increments of 100–200 mg/day at intervals of no less than 1 week. The effective dose range is 300–600 mg/day. The initial dose for elderly or debilitated clients is 100 mg/day given in two divided doses.

NURSING CONSIDERATIONS

ADMINISTRATION/STORAGE

1. May take several weeks for full beneficial effect to be observed.
2. Although long-term use has not been studied, it is usually recommended that the drug be given for a period of 6 months or longer.
3. At least 14 days should elapse between discontinuation of an MAO inhibitor and initiation of therapy with nefazodone; also, at least 7 days should elapse after stopping nefazodone and before starting an MAO inhibitor.

ASSESSMENT

1. Document indications for therapy, onset and characteristics of symptoms, and any precipitating factors/triggers.
2. List drugs currently prescribed to ensure none interact unfavorably.
3. Determine any CAD, recent MI, or conditions requiring digoxin administration.
4. Monitor CBC, ECG, liver and renal function studies.

CLIENT/FAMILY TEACHING

1. Take before meals; food may inhibit absorption.
2. Do not perform activities that require mental alertness or coordination until drug effects realized; may cause dizziness, drowsiness, confusion, incoordination, decreased concentration and response time.
3. Avoid all OTC agents, alcohol and any other CNS depressants.
4. May take several weeks (2–4) before any effects are realized; do not become discouraged.
5. Report any unusual sensations or side effects, increased depression, or suicidal thoughts/behavior.
6. Use reliable birth control.

OUTCOMES/EVALUATE

Symptomatic improvement; ↓ depression, improved sleeping and eating patterns, ↓ fatigue, and ↑ social interaction

N

Nelfinavir mesylate

(nel-**FIN**-ah-veer)

PREGNANCY CATEGORY: B
CLASSIFICATION(S):
Antiviral, protease inhibitor
Rx: Viracept

SEE ALSO *ANTIVIRAL DRUGS*.

ACTION/KINETICS
HIV-1 protease inhibitor, resulting in prevention of cleavage of gagpol polyprotein resulting in production of immature, non-infectious viruses. Activity is increased when used with didanosine, lamivudine, stavudine, zalcitabine, or zidovudine. **Peak plasma levels:** 2–4 hr. **Steady-state plasma levels:** 3–4 mcg/mL. Food increases plasma levels 2–3 fold. **t$^{1}/_{2}$, terminal:** 3.5–5 hr. Metabolites (one of which is as active as parent compound) and unchanged drug excreted mainly in feces.

USES
Treat HIV infection when antiretroviral therapy is required.

CONTRAINDICATIONS
Administration with midazolam, rifampin, or triazolam.

SPECIAL CONCERNS
Use with caution with hepatic impairment. Safety and efficacy have not been determined in children less than 2 years of age.

SIDE EFFECTS
Side effects were determined when used in combination with other antiviral drugs. **GI:** N&V, diarrhea, flatulence, abdominal pain, anorexia, dyspepsia, epigastric pain, GI bleeding, hepatitis, mouth ulcers, pancreatitis. **CNS:** Anxiety, depression, dizziness, emotional lability, hyperkinesia, insomnia, migraine, paresthesia, ***seizures,*** sleep disorder, somnolence, ***suicide ideation.*** **Hematologic:** Anemia, leukopenia, thrombocytopenia. **Respiratory:** Dyspnea, rhinitis, sinusitis, pharyngitis. **GU:** Kidney calculus, sexual dysfunction, urine abnormality. **Ophthalmic:** Eye disorder, acute iritis. **Musculoskeletal:** Arthralgia, arthritis, cramps, myalgia, myasthenia, myopathy. **Dermatologic:** Dermatitis, folliculitis, fungal dermatitis, maculopapular rash, pruritus, urticaria, sweating. **Miscellaneous:** Asthenia, dehydration, allergic reaction, back pain, fever, headache, malaise, pain, accidental injury.

LABORATORY TEST CONSIDERATIONS
↑ ALT, AST, creatine phosphokinase, alkaline phosphatase, amylase, lactic dehydrogenase, GGT. Hyperlipidemia, hyperuricemia, hypoglycemia. Abnormal LFTs.

OD OVERDOSE MANAGEMENT
Symptoms: See side effects. *Treatment:* Emesis or gastric lavage, followed by activated charcoal.

DRUG INTERACTIONS
Anticonvulsants / Possible ↓ nelfinavir plasma levels
Didanosine / ↓ Absorption of nelfinavir
Indinavir / Significant ↑ in nelfinavir levels
Methadone / ↓ Methadone plasma levels → possible withdrawal symptoms
Oral contraceptives / ↓ Drug effects; use alternative contraceptive measures
Rifabutin / ↑ Rifabutin levels; reduce rifabutin dose one-half
Rifampin / Significant ↓ in nelfinavir levels; do not coadminister

HOW SUPPLIED
Powder for Reconstitution: 50 mg/1 g; *Suspension*, 50 mg/5 mL; *Tablet, Film-Coated:* 250 mg

DOSAGE
- **POWDER, SUSPENSION, TABLETS**
  HIV.

Adults: 750 mg (i.e., 3-250 mg tablets) t.i.d. or 1250 mg b.i.d. in combination with nucleoside analogs. **Children, 2 to 13 years:** 20-30 mg/kg/dose t.i.d.

NURSING CONSIDERATIONS

SEE ALSO *NURSING CONSIDERATIONS FOR ANTIVIRAL DRUGS*.

ASSESSMENT
1. Document disease onset, characteristics, and other agents trialed.
2. List drugs prescribed/consumed to ensure none interact unfavorably.
3. Monitor CBC, CD_4 counts, viral load, liver and renal function.

N

CLIENT/FAMILY TEACHING

1. Drug is not a cure but helps to manage disease symptoms.
2. Take as prescribed with snack or light meal to enhance absorption.
3. Do not reconstitute powder with water in its original container. Mix powder with small amount of water, milk, formula, soy formula/milk or dietary supplement. Once mixed, consume entire amount for full dose. Do not mix with acidic foods or juice (e.g., orange or apple juice, apple sauce) due to their bitter taste.
4. Take drug with nucleoside analogs as prescribed.
5. Report any evidence of increased bruising/ bleeding, severe headache/ fatigue/lethargy, N&V, rash, breathing problems or changes in stool/urine color.
6. Oral contraceptives may be ineffective; use barrier contraception.
7. Drug does not prevent transmission of disease; practice safe sex.

OUTCOMES/EVALUATE

Control of HIV symptoms; ↓ viral load

Neomycin sulfate

(nee-oh-**MY**-sin)

PREGNANCY CATEGORY: D
CLASSIFICATION(S):
Antibiotic, aminoglycoside
Rx: Mycifradin Sulfate, Myciguent, Neo-fradin, Neo-Tabs

SEE ALSO *ANTI-INFECTIVES* AND *AMINOGLYCOSIDES.*

ACTION/KINETICS

Peak plasma levels: PO, 1–4 hr; **Therapeutic serum level:** 5–10 mcg/ mL. **t½:** 2–3 hr.

USES

PO: Hepatic coma, sterilization of gut prior to surgery, inhibition of ammonia-forming bacteria in GI tract in hepatic encephalopathy. Therapy of intestinal infections due to pathogenic strains of *Escherichia coli,* primarily in children. *Investigational:* Hypercholesterolemia.

Topical: Prophylaxis or treatment of infection in burns, minor cuts, wounds, and skin abrasions. As an aid to healing and for treating superficial skin infections.

ADDITIONAL CONTRAINDICATIONS

Intestinal obstruction (PO). Use of topical products in or around the eyes.

SPECIAL CONCERNS

Safe use during pregnancy has not been determined. Use with caution in clients with extensive burns, trophic ulceration, or other conditions where significant systemic absorption is possible.

SIDE EFFECTS

Chronic use of topical neomycin to inflamed skin of those with contact dermatitis and chronic dermatosis increases the chance of hypersensitivity. Ototoxicity, nephrotoxicity. Sprue-like syndrome with steatorrhea, malabsorption, and electrolyte imbalance. Skin rashes after topical or parenteral administration. Chronic use in allergic contact dermatitis and chronic dermatoses increases the risk of sensitization.

ADDITIONAL DRUG INTERACTIONS

Digoxin / ↓ Digoxin effect R/T ↓ GI tract absorption
Penicillin V / ↓ PCN effect R/T ↓ GI tract absorption
Procainamide / ↑ Muscle relaxation produced by neomycin

HOW SUPPLIED

Cream: 3.5 mg/g; *Ointment:* 3.5 mg/g; *Oral Solution:* 125 mg/5 mL; *Tablet:* 500 mg

DOSAGE

• **Oral Solution, Tablet**

Preoperatively in colorectal surgery.

1 g each of neomycin and erythromycin base for a total of three doses: the first two doses 1 hr apart the afternoon before surgery and the third dose at bedtime the night before surgery.

Hepatic coma, adjunct.

Adults, 4–12 g/day in divided doses for 5–6 days; **children:** 50–100 mg/kg/day in divided doses for 5–6 days.

N

• **TOPICAL CREAM, OINTMENT**
Neomycin alone or in combination with other antibiotics (bacitracin or gramicidin) and/or an anti-inflammatory agent (corticosteroid). Apply ointment or cream 1–3 times/day to affected area. If necessary, a bandage may be used to cover the area.

NURSING CONSIDERATIONS

SEE ALSO *NURSING CONSIDERATIONS* FOR *AMINOGLYCOSIDES*.

ASSESSMENT

1. Document indications for therapy. Note clinical presentation and symptom characteristics.
2. Describe abdominal assessment findings.
3. Assess fluid and electrolyte status and C&S.

CLIENT/FAMILY TEACHING

1. Consume 2–3 L/day of fluids.
2. Carefully follow recommended procedure to prepare the GI tract for surgery.
3. Expect slight laxative effect produced by PO neomycin. Withhold and report with S&S of intestinal obstruction.
4. Anticipate low-residue diet for preoperative disinfection and a laxative immediately preceding PO administration of neomycin sulfate.
5. When used topically, clean the affected area before applying topical ointment or solution; then apply a small amount equal to the surface area of a fingertip.

OUTCOMES/EVALUATE

- Improved level of consciousness
- Healing of skin wounds
- Bowel sterilization before surgery

Neostigmine bromide

(nee-oh-**STIG**-meen)

PREGNANCY CATEGORY: C
Rx: Prostigmin Bromide

Neostigmine methylsulfate

(nee-oh-**STIG**-meen)

PREGNANCY CATEGORY: C
Rx: Prostigmin Injection
CLASSIFICATION(S):
Cholinesterase inhibitor, indirectly-acting

ACTION/KINETICS
Acetylcholinesterase inhibitor that causes an increase in the concentration of acetylcholine at the myoneural junction, thus facilitating transmission of impulses across the myoneural junction. In myasthenia gravis, muscle strength is increased. May also act on the autonomic ganglia of the CNS. Prevents or relieves postoperative distention by increasing gastric motility and tone and prevents or relieves urinary retention by increasing the tone of the detrusor muscle of the bladder. Shorter acting than ambenonium chloride and pyridostigmine. Atropine is often given concomitantly to control side effects. **Onset: PO,** 45–75 min; **IM,** 20–30 min; **IV,** 4–8 min. **Time to peak effect, parenteral:** 20–30 min. **Duration:** All routes, 2.5–4 hr. **t½, PO:** 42–60 min; **IM:** 51–90 min; **IV:** 47–60 min. Eliminated through the urine (about 40% unchanged).

USES
(1) Diagnosis and treatment of myasthenia gravis. (2) Prophylaxis and treatment of postoperative distention or urinary retention. (3) Antidote for tubocurarine and other nondepolarizing drugs.

CONTRAINDICATIONS
Hypersensitivity, mechanical obstruction of GI or urinary tract, peritonitis, history of bromide sensitivity. Vesical neck obstruction of urinary bladder. Lactation.

SPECIAL CONCERNS
Safety and effectiveness in children have not been established. Use with caution in clients with bronchial asthma, bradycardia, vagotonia, epilepsy, hyperthyroidism, peptic ulcer, cardiac arrhythmias, or recent coronary occlusion. May cause uterine irritability and premature labor if given IV to pregnant women near term. In geriatric clients, the duration of action may be increased.

SIDE EFFECTS

GI: N&V, diarrhea, abdominal cramps, involuntary defecation, salivation, dysphagia, flatulence, increased gastric and intestinal secretions. **CV:** Bradycardia, tachycardia, hypotension, ECG changes, nodal rhythm, ***cardiac arrest,*** syncope, ***AV block,*** substernal pain, thrombophlebitis after IV use. **CNS:** Headache, ***seizures,*** malaise, weakness, dysarthria, dizziness, drowsiness, loss of consciousness. **Respiratory:** Increased oral, pharyngeal, and bronchial secretions; ***bronchospasms, skeletal muscle paralysis, laryngospasm, central respiratory paralysis, respiratory depression or arrest,*** dyspnea. **Ophthalmologic:** Miosis, double vision, lacrimation, accommodation difficulties, hyperemia of conjunctiva, visual changes. **Musculoskeletal:** Muscle fasciculations or weakness, muscle cramps or spasms, arthralgia. **Other:** Skin rashes, urinary frequency and incontinence, sweating, flushing, allergic reactions, anaphylaxis, urticaria. These effects can usually be reversed by parenteral administration of 0.6 mg of atropine sulfate, which should be readily available.

Cholinergic crisis, due to overdosage, must be distinguished from myasthenic crisis (worsening of the disease), since cholinergic crisis involves removal of drug therapy, while myasthenic crisis involves an increase in anticholinesterase therapy.

OD OVERDOSE MANAGEMENT

Symptoms: Abdominal cramps, vomiting, diarrhea, epigastric distress, excessive salivation, cold sweating, pallor, blurred vision, urinary urgency, fasciculation and ***paralysis of voluntary muscles (including the tongue),*** miosis, increased BP (may be accompanied by bradycardia), sensation of internal trembling, panic, severe anxiety. *Treatment:* Discontinue medication temporarily. Give atropine, 0.5–1 mg IV (up to 5–10 or more mg may be needed to get the HR to 80 beats/min). Supportive treatment including artificial respiration and oxygen.

DRUG INTERACTIONS

Aminoglycosides / ↑ Neuromuscular blockade
Atropine / Atropine suppresses symptoms of excess GI stimulation caused by cholinergic drugs
Corticosteroids / ↓ Effect of neostigmine
Magnesium salts / Antagonize the effects of anticholinesterases
Mecamylamine / Intense hypotensive response
Organophosphate-type insecticides/pesticides / Added systemic effects with cholinesterase inhibitors
Succinylcholine / ↑ Neuromuscular blocking effects

HOW SUPPLIED

Neostigmine bromide: *Tablet:* 15 mg. **Neostigmine methylsulfate:** *Injection:* 1:1000, 1:2000, 1:4000

DOSAGE

NEOSTIGMINE BROMIDE

• **TABLETS**

Treat myasthenia gravis.

Adults: 15 mg q 3–4 hr; adjust dose and frequency as needed. **Usual maintenance:** 150 mg/day with dosing intervals determined by client response. **Pediatric,** 2 mg/kg (60 mg/m^2) daily in six to eight divided doses.

NEOSTIGMINE METHYLSULFATE

• **IM, IV, SC**

Diagnosis of myasthenia gravis.

Adults, IM, SC: 1.5 mg given with 0.6 mg atropine; **pediatric, IM:** 0.04 mg/kg (1 mg/m^2); or, **IV:** 0.02 mg/kg (0.5 mg/m^2).

Treat myasthenia gravis.

Adults, IM, SC: 0.5 mg. **Pediatric, IM, SC:** 0.01–0.04 mg/kg q 2–3 hr.

Antidote for tubocurarine.

Adults, IV: 0.5–2 mg slowly with 0.6–1.2 mg atropine sulfate. Can repeat if necessary up to total dose of 5 mg. **Pediatric, IV:** 0.04 mg/kg with 0.02 mg/kg atropine sulfate.

Prevention of postoperative GI distention or urinary retention.

Adults, IM, SC: 0.25 mg (1 mL of the 1:4,000 solution) immediately after surgery repeated q 4–6 hr for 2–3 days.

Treatment of postoperative GI distention.
Adults, IM, SC: 0.5 mg (1 mL of the 1:2,000 solution) as required.
Treatment of urinary retention.
Adults, IM, SC: 0.5 mg (1 mL of the 1:2,000 solution). If urination does not occur within 1 hr after 0.5 mg, the client should be catheterized. After the bladder is emptied, 0.5 mg is given q 3 hr for at least five injections.

NURSING CONSIDERATIONS

ADMINISTRATION/STORAGE

1. Determine interval doses individually to achieve optimum effects.
2. If greater fatigue occurs at certain times of the day, give a larger part of the daily dose at these times.
3. Do not give if high concentrations of halothane or cyclopropane are present.

IV 4. May administer IV form undiluted at a rate of 0.5 mg/min.

ASSESSMENT

1. Note clinical presentation and indications for therapy.
2. Assess for any bromide sensitivity or to drugs in this category.
3. Identify drugs consumed to determine if any interact unfavorably.

INTERVENTIONS

1. Report symptoms of generalized cholinergic stimulation (evidence of a toxic reaction). Have atropine available as antidote.
2. Monitor VS for the first hour. If hypotension occurs, keep recumbent until BP stabilizes.
3. When used as an antidote for nondepolarizing drugs, provide ventilatory assistance.

CLIENT/FAMILY TEACHING

1. With myasthenia, maintain a written record of periods of muscle strength or weakness so that dosage can be evaluated and adjusted accordingly; space activities to avoid excessive fatigue. Therapy is lifelong.
2. Take the dose exactly as prescribed; taking it late may result in myasthenic crisis whereas taking it early may result in cholinergic crisis.
3. If difficulty with coordination or vision avoid use of heavy machinery until effects wear off.
4. If taking for myasthenia gravis, any onset of weakness 1 hr after administration usually indicates overdosage of drug. Weakness 3 hr or more after administration usually indicates underdosage and/or resistance. Report as well as any associated difficulty with respirations or increase in muscle weakness as drug tolerance can develop.
5. Wear and/or carry ID noting therapy with neostigmine and why.

OUTCOMES/EVALUATE

- ↑ Muscle strength and function, improved chewing, swallowing and breathing with myasthenia gravis
- Relief of postoperative ileus or urinary retention
- Reversal of respiratory depression R/T nondepolarizing drugs

Nesiritide

(nih-**SIR**-ih-tide)

PREGNANCY CATEGORY: C
CLASSIFICATION(S):
Vasodilator, peripheral
Rx: Natrecor

ACTION/KINETICS

Nesiritide is a human B-type natriuretic peptide (hBNP) made from *E. coli* using recombinant DNA technology. Human BNP binds to the particulate guanylate cyclase receptor in vascular smooth muscle and endothelial cells, leading to increased intracellular levels of guanosine 3'5'-cyclic monophosphate (cGMP) and smooth muscle cell relaxation. Cyclic GMP serves as a second messenger to dilate veins and arteries. In acutely decompensated CHF, the drug reduces pulmonary capillary wedge pressure and improves dyspnea. **t¹/₂, initial elimination:** About 2 min; **t¹/₂, mean terminal, elimination:** About 18 min. Human BNP is cleared from the circulation by three mechanisms: (1) Binding to cell surface clearance receptors with subsequent cellular internalization and lysosomal proteolysis; (2) Proteolytic cleavage of the peptide by endopeptidases, such as neutral endopeptidase (present on the vascular lumenal surface); and, (3) renal filtration.

USES
IV treatment of acutely decompensated CHF in those who have dyspnea at rest or with minimal activity.

CONTRAINDICATIONS
Use as primary therapy for those with cardiogenic shock or in those with a systolic BP < 90 mm Hg. Hypersensitivity to any of the product components. Use in those suspected of having, or known to have, low cardiac filling pressures. Use in those for whom vasodilating agents are not appropriate, including valvular stenosis, restrictive or obstructive cardiomyopathy, constrictive pericarditis, pericardial tamponade, or other conditions in which cardiac output is dependent on venous return.

SPECIAL CONCERNS
Use with caution during lactation. Safety and efficacy have not been determined in children.

SIDE EFFECTS
CV: Hypotension (symptomatic, asymptomatic), ventricular tachycardia, nonsustained ventricular tachycardia, ventricular extrasystoles, angina pectoris, bradycardia, tachycardia, atrial fibrillation, AV node conduction abnormalities. **CNS:** Headache, insomnia, dizziness, anxiety, confusion, paresthesia, somnolence, tremor. **GI:** N&V. **Dermatologic:** Sweating, pruritus, rash. **Respiratory:** Increased cough, hemoptysis, apnea. **Miscellaneous:** Back pain, abdominal pain, hypersensitivity reactions, catheter pain, fever, injection site reaction, leg cramps, amblyopia, anemia.

LABORATORY TEST CONSIDERATIONS
↑ Creatinine.

DRUG INTERACTIONS
↑ Symptomatic hypotension when used with ACE inhibitors.

HOW SUPPLIED
Powder for injection, lyophilized: 1.58 mg

DOSAGE

• **IV ONLY**

Acutely decompensated CHF.

IV bolus of 2 mcg/kg, followed by a continuous IV infusion of 0.01 mcg/kg/min.

NURSING CONSIDERATIONS

ADMINISTRATION/STORAGE

IV 1. Do not start nesiritide at a dose greater than the recommended dose.
2. Prime the IV tubing with an infusion of 0.25 mL before connecting to the client's vascular access port and prior to giving the bolus or starting the infusion.
3. After preparing the infusion bag, withdraw the bolus volume and give over about 60 seconds through an IV port in the tubing. Immediately following the bolus, infuse nesiritide at a flow rate of 0.1 mL/kg/hr (this will deliver an infusion dose of 0.01 mcg/kg/min).
4. To calculate the appropriate bolus volume and infusion flow rate to deliver 0.01 mcg/kg/min dose, use the following formulas: Bolus volume (mL) = 0. 33 x client weight (kg)

Infusion flow rate (mL/hr) = 0.1 x client weight (kg).

5. To prepare the infusion, use the following procedure:
• Reconstitute one 1.5 mg vial by adding 5 mL of diluent removed from a prefilled 250 mL plastic IV bag containing the diluent of choice (D5/0.9% NaCl, D5/0.45% NaCl, or D5/0.2% NaCl).
• Do not shake the vial but rock gently so that all surfaces, including the stopper, are in contact with diluent to ensure complete reconstitution. Use only a clear, essentially colorless solution.
• Withdraw the entire contents of the reconstituted vial and add to the 250 mL plastic IV bag. This will yield a solution with a nesiritide concentration of about 6 mcg/mL. Invert the IV bag several times to ensure complete mixing of the solution.
• Use the reconstituted solution within 24 hr, as there are no preservatives in the product. Inspect visually for particulate matter and discoloration prior to use.
6. If hypotension occurs during administration, reduce or discontinue the dose and begin other measures to support BP (e.g., IV fluids, changes in

N

body position). The drug may be restarted at a dose that is reduced by 30% (with no bolus given). Hypotension may be prolonged; thus, before restarting the drug, a period of observation may be needed.
7. Nesiritide is physically and chemically incompatible with injections of heparin, insulin, ethacrynate sodium, bumetamide, enalaprilat, hydralazine, and furosemide. Do not give these drugs as infusions in the same IV catheter as nesiritide.
8. Do not give injectable drugs that contain sodium metabisulfate in the same infusion line; incompatible with nesiritide. Flush the catheter between administration of nesiritide and incompatible drugs.
9. Nesiritide binds to heparin. Thus, do not give through a central line heparin-coated catheter.
10. Store at controlled room temperature between 20–25°C (68–77°F) or refrigerated at 2–8°C (36–46°F). Reconstituted vials may be left at controlled room temperature or refrigerated for 24 hr or less. Keep in carton until time of use.

N

ASSESSMENT
1. Note indications for therapy, other agents trialed, ejection fraction, and NYHA class.
2. For IV use only; avoid infusing through central line heparin-coated catheters.
3. Review list of drugs not compatible for co-administration.
4. Monitor VS; if SBP < 90 mm Hg reduce dose or stop infusion and report.
5. Administer in a closely monitored environment by trained individuals; monitor heart pressures and assess closely for arrhythmias.

OUTCOMES/EVALUATE
Improved exercise tolerance; ↓ SOB with mild exertion and at rest

Nevirapine

(neh-**VYE**-rah-peen)

PREGNANCY CATEGORY: C

CLASSIFICATION(S):
Antiviral, non-nucleoside reverse transcriptase inhibitor
Rx: Viramune

SEE ALSO *ANTIVIRAL DRUGS*.

ACTION/KINETICS
By binding tightly to reverse transcriptase, nevirapine prevents viral RNA from being converted into DNA. In combination with a nucleoside analogue, it reduces the amount of virus circulating in the body and increases CD4+ cell counts. Readily absorbed, with peak plasma levels occurring 4 hr after a 200-mg dose. Extensively metabolized in the liver. Excreted through both the urine (about 90%) and the feces (about 10%). Induces its own metabolism; following chronic use the half-life decreases from about 45 hr following a single dose to 25 to 30 hr following multiple dosing with 200 or 400 mg daily.

USES
In combination with nucleoside analogues (e.g., Zidovudine, lamivudine, didanosine, zalcitabine) or protease inhibitors (e.g., saquinavir, indinavir, nelfinavir, aritonavir) for the treatment of HIV-1 infections in adults and children 2 months or older who have experienced clinical and immunologic deterioration. Always use in combination with at least one other antiretroviral agent, as resistant viruses emerge rapidly when nevirapine is used alone.

CONTRAINDICATIONS
Lactation.

SPECIAL CONCERNS
The duration of benefit from therapy may be limited. Is not a cure for HIV infections; clients may continue to experience illnesses associated with HIV infections, including opportunistic infections. Has not been shown to reduce the risk of transmitting HIV to others through sexual contact or blood contamination. Use with caution in impaired renal or hepatic function.

SIDE EFFECTS
GI: Nausea, diarrhea, abdominal pain, ulcerative stomatitis, hepatitis, ***severe, life-threatening (sometimes fatal) he-***

patotoxicity (especially during the first 12 weeks of therapy). **CNS:** Headache, fatigue, paresthesia. **Hematologic:** Decreased hemoglobin, decreased platelets, decreased neutrophils, granulocytopenia (occurs more in children). **Miscellaneous:** ***Rash (may be severe and life-threatening),*** fever, peripheral neuropathy, myalgia.

LABORATORY TEST CONSIDERATIONS

↑ ALT, AST, GGT, total bilirubin. Abnormal LFTs.

DRUG INTERACTIONS

Ketoconazole / Significant ↓ plasma ketoconacole levels; do not use together
Methadone / ↓ Plasma methadone levels due to ↑ metabolsim; ↑ methadone dose
Oral contraceptives / ↓ OC plasma levels → ↓ effect
Protease inhibitors / ↓ Plasma levels of protease inhibitors
Rifabutin / ↓ Nevirapine trough concentrations
Rifampin / ↓ Nevirapine trough concentrations
Warfarin / Possible ↓ anticoagulant activity

HOW SUPPLIED

Suspension: 50 mg/5 mL; *Tablet:* 200 mg

DOSAGE

- **SUSPENSION, TABLETS**

HIV-1 infections.

Adults, initial: 200 mg/day for 14 days. **Maintenance:** 200 mg b.i.d. (e.g., 7:00 a.m. and 7:00 p.m.) in combination with a nucleoside analogue antiretroviral agent. **Children, 2 months–8 years:** 4 mg/kg once daily for 14 days followed by 7 mg/kg b.i.d. **Children, 8 years and older:** 4 mg/kg once daily for 14 days followed by 4 mg/kg once daily. Do not exceed a total daily dose of 400 mg for any client.

NURSING CONSIDERATIONS

SEE ALSO *NURSING CONSIDERATIONS FOR ANTIVIRAL DRUGS* AND *ANTI-INFECTIVES.*

ADMINISTRATION/STORAGE

1. Clients who interrupt nevirapine dosing for more than 7 days should restart therapy using one 200-mg tablet daily (4 mg/kg for children) for the first 14 days, followed by 200 mg b.i.d. (4 or 7 mg/kg b.i.d., according to age, for children).
2. The suspension is used for children. Shake suspension gently prior to administration.
3. Store tablets and suspension in a tightly closed bottle at 15–30°C (59–86°F).

ASSESSMENT

1. Document disease onset, symptom characteristics, other agents trialed and the outcome.
2. List drugs currently prescribed to ensure none interact unfavorably.
3. Monitor CBC, CD4 counts, viral load, liver and renal function studies. Most serious hepatic side effects occur during the first 12 weeks of therapy. Perform LFTs at least monthly during the first 12 weeks, especially at baseline and before and 2 weeks after a dose increase. Monitor liver function frequently thereafter.
4. Stop and do not resume at the first sign of liver toxicity.

CLIENT/FAMILY TEACHING

1. Drug is not a cure but helps control disease symptoms.
2. Can be taken with or without food.
3. If a dose is skipped, take the next dose as soon as possible; do not double the dose.
4. Take exactly as directed. Should be taken with another antiretroviral agent to prevent emergence of resistant viruses.
5. A rash may occur in the first few weeks of therapy; do not increase dosage until subsides. Any severe rash or rash accompanied by flu-like symptoms warrants immediate reporting.
6. Drug does not prevent transmission through sexual contact or blood contamination. Practice barrier contraception and nonhormonal form of birth control.

OUTCOMES/EVALUATE

Improved CD4 cell counts; ↓ Viral load

Niacin (Nicotinic acid)

(**NYE**-ah-sin, nih-koh-**TIN**-ick **AH**-sid)

PREGNANCY CATEGORY: C
Rx: Niacor, Niaspan
OTC: Nicotinex, Slo-Niacin

Niacinamide

(nye-ah-**SIN**-ah-myd)

PREGNANCY CATEGORY: C
Rx: Injection
OTC: Tablets
CLASSIFICATION(S):
Vitamin B complex

N

ACTION/KINETICS

Niacin (nicotinic acid) and niacinamide are water-soluble, heat-resistant vitamins prepared synthetically. Niacin (after conversion to the active niacinamide) is a component of the coenzymes nicotinamide-adenine dinucleotide and nicotinamide-adenine dinucleotide phosphate, which are essential for oxidation-reduction reactions involved in lipid metabolism, glycogenolysis, and tissue respiration. Deficiency of niacin results in pellagra, the most common symptoms of which are dermatitis, diarrhea, and dementia. In high doses niacin also produces vasodilation. Niacin, but not nicotinamide, reduces total and LDL cholesterol, triglycerides, and apolipoprotein B-100, and increases HDL cholesterol. Mechanism is unknown but may involve a decrease in esterification of hepatic triglycerides. Rapidly absorbed from the GI tract. **Peak serum levels:** 30–60 min; **t½:** 20–45 min. About 88% of a PO dose of niacin is eliminated by the kidneys unchanged or as nicotinuric acid.

USES

Niacin. (1) Prophylaxis and treatment of pellagra; niacin deficiency. (2) Adjunct therapy in adults wtih very high serum triglycerides (Types IV and V hyperlipidemia) who are at risk of pancreatitis and who do not respond adequately to diet. **Niacinamide.** Prophylaxis and treatment of pellagra. *Investigational:* Treatment of various dermatologic disorders.

CONTRAINDICATIONS

Severe hypotension, hemorrhage, arterial bleeding, liver dysfunction, active peptic ulcer. Use of the extended-release tablets and capsules in children.

SPECIAL CONCERNS

Extended-release niacin may be hepatotoxic. Use with caution in diabetics, gall bladder disease, in those who consume a large amount of alcohol, and clients with gout.

SIDE EFFECTS

GI: N&V, diarrhea, peptic ulcer activation, abdominal pain, severe hepatic toxicity. **Dermatologic:** Flushing, warm feeling, skin rash, pruritus, dry skin, itching and tingling feeling, keratosis nigricans. **Other:** Hypotension, headache, macular cystoid edema, amblyopia, rhabdomyolysis (rare). *NOTE:* Megadoses are accompanied by serious toxicity including the symptoms listed in the preceding as well as liver damage, hyperglycemia, hyperuricemia, arrhythmias, tachycardia, and dermatoses.

DRUG INTERACTIONS

Chenodiol / ↓ Effect of chenodiol
.*HMG-CoA Reductase Inhibitors* / ↑ Risk of myopathy and rhabdomyolysis
Probenecid / Niacin may ↓ uricosuric effect of probenecid
Sulfinpyrazone / Niacin ↓ uricosuric effect of sulfinpyrazone
Sympathetic blocking agents / Additive vasodilating effects → postural hypotension

HOW SUPPLIED

Niacin: *Capsule, Extended Release:* 125 mg, 250 mg, 400 mg, 500 mg; *Elixir:* 50 mg/5 mL; *Tablet:* 50 mg, 100 mg, 250 mg, 500 mg; *Tablet, Extended Release:* 250 mg, 500 mg, 750 mg, 1,000 mg. **Niacinamide:** *Tablet:* 100 mg, 500 mg

DOSAGE

NIACIN

• **EXTENDED-RELEASE CAPSULES, TABLETS, EXTENDED-RELEASE TABLETS, ELIXIR**

Pellagra.

Adults: Up to 500 mg/day; **pediatric:** Up to 300 mg/day.

Antihyperlipidemic.

Adults: 1–2 g of immediate release produce b.i.d. or t.i.d. Initiate therapy at 250 mg as a single dose after the evening meal. Frequency of dosing and total daily dose can be increased every 4–7 days until desired response reached. If adequate response not achieved after 2 months at 1.5–2 g/day, increase at 2–4 week intervals to 3 g/day (i.e., 1 g t.i.d.) Do not exceed 6 g/day. For extended release products, give 500 mg at bedtime for 1–4 weeks; then, 1,000 mg at bedtime during weeks 5–8. If resonse to 1,000 mg/day is inadequate, increase dose to 1,500 mg/day, up to a maximum of 2,000 mg/day if needed. Do not increase daily dose more than 500 mg in a 4-week period.

• **IM, IV**

Pellagra.

Adults, IM: 50–100 mg 5 or more times/day. **IV, slow:** 25–100 mg 2 or more times/day. **Pediatric, IV slow:** Up to 300 mg/day.

NIACINAMIDE

• **TABLETS**

Pellagra.

Adults: 100–500 mg/day. **Pediatric:** Up to 300 mg/day.

NURSING CONSIDERATIONS

ADMINISTRATION/STORAGE

1. Do not substitute sustained release niacin products for equivalent doses of immediate-release niacin.

IV 2. Other niacins can not be substituted for Niaspan.

3. May administer IV form diluted (to 2 mg/mL solution concentration) at a rate not exceeding 2 mg/min.

ASSESSMENT

1. Note indications for therapy. Monitor glucose, HbA1-C, LFTs, and plasma lipid levels.

2. Note any history of PUD or liver or gallbladder dysfunction.

3. Assess diet, exercise, and any lifestyle changes necessary to decrease coronary risk factors.

4. If and when used with statins monitor LFTs closely as they both utilize the same metabolic pathway.

5. When using the regular strength tablets for hyperlipidemia, start low and go slow to enhance client tolerance. With the extended release tablets, titrate up and advise to take at bedtime with an ASA to diminish side effects.

CLIENT/FAMILY TEACHING

1. Take nicotinic acid PO only with cold water (no hot beverages). Can be taken with meals if GI upset occurs.

2. May experience a warm flushing in the face and ears within 2 hr after taking. To prevent/reduce take one aspirin or a small low fat snack 1 hr prior to dosing. Alcohol may increase these effects.

3. Lie down if feeling weak and dizzy after taking niacin (until this feeling passes) and inform provider if persists.

4. Identify foods sources high in niacin (dairy products, meats, tuna, and eggs); assess consumption.

5. With diabetes, do not take niacin unless specifically ordered and then the BS levels must be closely monitored for hyperglycemia; also monitor for ketonuria and glucosuria. Antidiabetic agents may require adjustment.

6. Report any skin color changes or yellowing of the sclera.

7. Clients predisposed to gout may experience flank, joint, or stomach pains; report immediately.

8. If blurred vision or skin lesions occur, remain out of direct sunlight.

9. No unsupervised excessive vitamin ingestion; high doses may impair liver function.

10. Report as scheduled for regular labs and f/u.

OUTCOMES/EVALUATE

• ↓ Triglyceride levels

• Relief of symptoms of pellagra and niacin deficiency

Nicardipine hydrochloride

(nye-**KAR**-dih-peen)

PREGNANCY CATEGORY: C

N

CLASSIFICATION(S):
Calcium channel blocker
Rx: Cardene, Cardene SR, Cardene IV

SEE ALSO *CALCIUM CHANNEL BLOCKING AGENTS.*

ACTION/KINETICS
Moderately increases CO and significantly decreases peripheral vascular resistance. **Onset of action:** 20 min. **Maximum plasma levels:** 30–120 min. Significant first-pass metabolism. Food (especially fats) will decrease the amount of drug absorbed from the GI tract. Steady-state plasma levels are reached after 2–3 days of therapy. **Therapeutic serum levels:** 0.028–0.050 mcg/mL. **t½, at steady state:** 8.6 hr. **Maximum BP-lowering effects, immediate release:** 1–2 hr; **maximum BP-lowering effects, sustained release:** 2–6 hr. **Duration:** 8 hr. Highly bound to plasma protein (> 95%) and metabolized by the liver with excretion through both the urine and feces.

USES
Immediate release: Chronic stable angina (effort-associated angina) alone or in combination with beta-adrenergic blocking agents. Congestive heart failure. **Immediate and sustained released:** Hypertension alone or in combination with other antihypertensive drugs. **IV:** Short-term treatment of hypertension when PO therapy is not desired or possible. *Investigational:* CHF.

CONTRAINDICATIONS
Use in advanced aortic stenosis due to the effect on reducing afterload. During lactation.

SPECIAL CONCERNS
Safety and efficacy in children less than 18 years of age have not been established. Use with caution in clients with CHF, especially in combination with a beta blocker due to the possibility of a negative inotropic effect. Use with caution in clients with impaired liver function, reduced hepatic blood flow, or impaired renal function. Initial increase in frequency, duration, or severity of angina.

SIDE EFFECTS
CV: Pedal edema, flushing, increased angina, palpitations, tachycardia, other edema, abnormal ECG, hypotension, postural hypotension, syncope, ***MI, AV block,*** ventricular extrasystoles, PVD. **CNS:** Dizziness, headache, somnolence, malaise, nervousness, insomnia, abnormal dreams, vertigo, depression, confusion, amnesia, anxiety, weakness, psychoses, hallucinations, paranoia. **GI:** N&V, dyspepsia, dry mouth, constipation, sore throat. **Neuromuscular:** Asthenia, myalgia, paresthesia, hyperkinesia, arthralgia. **Miscellaneous:** Rash, dyspnea, SOB, nocturia, polyuria, allergic reactions, abnormal LFTs, hot flashes, impotence, rhinitis, sinusitis, nasal congestion, chest congestion, tinnitus, equilibrium disturbances, abnormal or blurred vision, infection, atypical chest pain.

OD OVERDOSE MANAGEMENT
Symptoms: Marked hypotension, bradycardia, palpitations, flushing, drowsiness, confusion, and slurred speech following PO overdose. Lethal overdose may cause systemic hypotension, bradycardia (following initial tachycardia), and progressive AV block.
Treatment:

- Treatment is supportive. Monitor cardiac and respiratory function.
- If client is seen soon after ingestion, emetics or gastric lavage should be considered, followed by cathartics.
- *Hypotension:* IV calcium, dopamine, isoproterenol, metaraminol, or norepinephrine. Also, provide IV fluids. Place client in Trendelenburg position.
- *Ventricular tachycardia:* IV procainamide or lidocaine; cardioversion may be necessary. Also, provide slow-drip IV fluids.
- *Bradycardia, asystole, AV block:* IV atropine sulfate (0.6–1 mg), calcium gluconate (10% solution), isoproterenol, norepinephrine; also, cardiac pacing may be indicated. Provide slow-drip IV fluids.

DRUG INTERACTIONS
Cimetidine / ↑ Bioavailability of nicardipine → ↑ plasma levels

Cyclosporine / ↑ Plasma levels of cyclosporine possibly leading to renal toxicity
Grapefruit juice / ↑ Bioavailability of nicardipine R/T ↓ liver metabolism of nicardipine in the gut wall
Ranitidine / ↑ Bioavailability of nicardipine

HOW SUPPLIED
Capsule: 20 mg, 30 mg; *Capsule, Extended Release:* 30 mg, 45 mg, 60 mg; *Injection:* 2.5 mg/mL

DOSAGE

• **CAPSULES, IMMEDIATE RELEASE**
Angina, hypertension.
Initial, usual: 20 mg t.i.d. (range: 20–40 mg t.i.d.). Wait 3 days before increasing dose to ensure steady-state plasma levels.

• **CAPSULES, EXTENDED RELEASE**
Hypertension.
Initial: 30 mg b.i.d. (range: 30–60 mg b.i.d.).
NOTE: Initial dose in renal impairment: 20 mg t.i.d. Initial dose in hepatic impairment: 20 mg b.i.d.

• **IV**
Hypertension.
Individualize dose. Initial: 5 mg/hr; the infusion rate may be increased to a maximum of 15 mg/hr (by 2.5-mg/hr increments q 15 min). For a more rapid reduction in BP, initiate at 5 mg/hr but increase the rate q 5 min in 2.5-mg/hr increments until a maximum of 15 mg/hr is reached. **Maintenance:** 3 mg/hr. The IV infusion rate to produce an average plasma level similar to a particular PO dose is as follows: 20 mg q 8 hr is equivalent to 0.5 mg/hr; 30 mg q 8 hr is equivalent to 1.2 mg/hr; and 40 mg q 8 hr is equivalent to 2.2 mg/hr.

NURSING CONSIDERATIONS

SEE ALSO *NURSING CONSIDERATIONS* FOR *CALCIUM CHANNEL BLOCKING AGENTS.*

ADMINISTRATION/STORAGE

1. When used for treating angina, may be administered safely along with sublingual nitroglycerin, prophylactic nitrates, or beta blockers.
2. When used to treat hypertension, may be administered safely along with diuretics or beta blockers.
3. During initial therapy and when dosage is increased, may experience an increase in the frequency, duration, or severity of angina.
4. If transfer to PO antihypertensives other than nicardipine is planned, initiate therapy after discontinuing infusion. If PO nicardipine is used at a dosage regimen of three times daily, give the first dose 1 hr prior to discontinuing infusion.
IV 5. Ampules must be diluted before infusion. Acceptable diluents are 5% dextrose, D5/0.45% NaCl, D5W with 40 mEq potassium, 0.45% NaCl, and 0.9% NaCl. Nicardipine is incompatible with 5% $NaHCO_3$ and RL solution.
6. The infusion concentration is 0.1 mg/mL. The diluted product is stable at room temperature for 24 hr.
7. Store ampules at room temperature; freezing does not affect the product. Protect ampules from light and elevated temperatures.

ASSESSMENT

1. Document indications for therapy. List other agents prescribed and the outcome.
2. Note CHF and if beta blockers prescribed, monitor closely.
3. Monitor ECG, liver and renal function studies; note any dysfunction.
4. Monitor VS. When the immediate-release product is used for hypertension, the maximum lowering of BP occurs 1–2 hr after dosing. Evaluate BP at trough (8 hr after dosing). When the sustained-release product is used, maximum lowering of BP occurs 2–6 hr after dosing.
5. Monitor BP frequently during and following IV infusion. Avoid too rapid or excessive decrease in BP and discontinue infusion if significant hypotension or tachycardia.

CLIENT/FAMILY TEACHING

1. Take at the same time each day.
2. Report any persistent and/or bothersome side effects such as dizziness,

N

flushing, increased angina, weight gain or edema.
3. Maintain proper intake of fluids to avoid constipation. Avoid caffeine and alcohol.
4. May experience impotence.
5. Anginal attacks may persist up to 30 min following drug ingestion due to reflex tachycardia; use nitrates as prescribed.
6. Report any change in psychologic state—depression, anxiety, sleep problems, or decreased mental acuity. Particularly important when working with elderly clients since there is a tendency to misdiagnose as senility.

OUTCOMES/EVALUATE

- Control of hypertension
- ↓ Frequency/intensity of anginal attacks
- Therapeutic drug levels (0.028–0.050 mcg/mL)

Nicotine polacrilex (Nicotine Resin Complex)

(**NIK**-oh-teen)

PREGNANCY CATEGORY: X
CLASSIFICATION(S):
Smoking deterrent
OTC: Nicorette, Nicotine Gum
✱**OTC:** Nicorette Plus

ACTION/KINETICS

Following chewing, nicotine is released from an ion exchange resin in the gum product, providing blood nicotine levels approximating those produced by smoking cigarettes. The amount of nicotine released depends on the rate and duration of chewing. **Time to peak levels:** 15–30 min. **Peak plasma levels:** 5–10 ng/mL. If the gum is swallowed, only a minimum amount of nicotine is released. **t½:** 3–4 hr. Metabolized mainly by the liver, with about 10%–20% excreted unchanged in the urine.

USES

Adjunct with behavioral modification in smokers wishing to give up the smoking habit. Is considered only as an initial aid, with the ultimate goal being abstention from all forms of nicotine. Most likely to benefit are individuals with the following characteristics: (a) smoke brands of cigarettes containing more than 0.9 mg nicotine; (b) smoke more than 15 cigarettes daily; (c) inhale cigarette smoke deeply and frequently; (d) smoke most frequently during the morning; (e) smoke the first cigarette of the day within 30 min of arising; (f) indicate cigarettes smoked in the morning are the most difficult to give up; (g) smoke even if the individual is ill and confined to bed; (h) find it necessary to smoke in places where smoking is not allowed. *NOTE:* Nicotine may be effective in improving the course of difficult-to-treat ulcerative colitis.

CONTRAINDICATIONS

Pregnancy, lactation, nonsmokers, serious arrhythmias, angina, vasospastic disease, active temporomandibular joint disease. Use in individuals less than 18 years of age.

SPECIAL CONCERNS

Safety and effectiveness in children and adolescents who smoke have not been determined. Use with caution in hypertension, PUD, oral or pharyngeal inflammation, gastritis, stomatitis, hyperthyroidism, IDDM, and pheochromocytoma.

SIDE EFFECTS

CNS: Dizziness, irritability, headache. **GI:** N&V, indigestion, GI upset, salivation, eructation. **Other:** Sore mouth or throat, hiccoughs, sore jaw muscles.

OD OVERDOSE MANAGEMENT

Symptoms: GI: N&V, diarrhea, salivation, abdominal pain. *CNS:* Headache, dizziness, confusion, weakness, fainting, ***seizures.*** *Respiratory:* Labored breathing, ***respiratory paralysis (cause of death).*** *Other:* Cold sweat, disturbed hearing and vision, hypotension, and rapid, weak pulse. *Treatment:* Syrup of ipecac if vomiting has not occurred, saline laxative, gastric lavage followed by activated charcoal (if client is unconscious), maintenance of respiration, maintenance of CV function.

DRUG INTERACTIONS
Caffeine / Possibly ↓ caffeine blood levels R/T ↑ rate of liver breakdown
Catecholamines / ↑ Catecholamine levels
Cortisol / ↑ Cortisol levels
Furosemide / Possible ↓ diuretic effect of furosemide
Imipramine / Possibly ↓ imipramine blood levels R/T ↑ rate of liver breakdown
Pentazocine / Possibly ↓ pentazocine blood levels R/T ↑ rate of liver breakdown
Theophylline / Possibly ↓ theophylline blood levels R/T ↑ rate of liver breakdown

HOW SUPPLIED
Gum: 2 mg/square, 4 mg/square

DOSAGE

• **GUM**

If the client smokes less than 25 cigarettes/day, start with the 2 mg nicotine gum. If the client smokes more than 25 cigarettes/day, start with 1 piece q 1–2 hr for weeks 1–6; then, 1 piece q 2–4 hr for weeks 7–9 and 1piece q 4–8 hr for weeks 10–12.

NURSING CONSIDERATIONS

ADMINISTRATION/STORAGE

1. All products are over-the-counter.
2. Client must stop smoking completely when beginning to use the gum.
3. Those who smoke more than 25 cigarettes/day should be started on the 4-mg dose.
4. Have client chew gum slowly until it tingles; then, park it between the cheek and gum. When the tingle is gone, have client begin chewing again until the tingle returns. Repeat the process until most of the tingle is gone (about 30 min).
5. Advise client not to eat or drink for 15 min before chewing the nicotine gum or while chewing a piece.
6. To improve chances of quitting, have client chew at least 9 pieces/day for the first 6 weeks. If there are strong and frequent cravings, use a second piece within the hour. Do not have client use continuously 1 piece after the other as hiccoughs, heartburn, nausea, and other side effects may occur.
7. Do not use more than 24 pieces/day. Stop using nicotine gum at the end of 12 weeks.
8. After gum has been chewed, place used chewing pieces in a wrapper and dispose so that children or pets can not obtain them.

ASSESSMENT

1. Document nicotine profile: type and brand (cigarettes, chewing tobacco, or cigars), amount used per day, when used, and what triggers/increases usage.
2. Note any temporomandibular joint syndrome or cardiac arrhythmia; precludes gum therapy.

CLIENT/FAMILY TEACHING

1. Must want to stop smoking and should do so immediately.
2. Avoid activities, persons, and locations that stimulate the desire to smoke (i.e drinking, bars, smokers).
3. Use gum only as directed. When client has the urge to smoke, chew one piece slowly for about 30 min. If a slight tingling becomes evident, stop chewing until sensation subsides.
4. Acidic beverages, such as coffee, juices, soft drinks, and wine, interfere with buccal absorption of nicotine; thus, avoid eating and drinking 15 min before and during chewing.
5. Gum will not stick to dentures or appliances.
6. Identify individuals and local support groups that can help with smoking cessation and provide emotional and psychologic support throughout the endeavor. Participate in a formal smoking program.

OUTCOMES/EVALUATE

Control of nicotine withdrawal symptoms with smoking cessation

Nicotine transdermal system

(NIK-oh-teen)

PREGNANCY CATEGORY: D

CLASSIFICATION(S):
Smoking deterrent
OTC: Habitrol, Nicoderm CQ, Nicotine Transdermal System, Nicotrol

ACTION/KINETICS

Nicotine transdermal system is a multilayered film that provides systemic delivery of varying amounts of nicotine over a 24-hr period after applying to the skin. Nicotine's reinforcing activity is due to stimulation of the cortex (via the locus ceruleus), producing increased alertness and cognitive performance and a "reward" effect due to an action in the limbic system. At low doses the stimulatory effects predominate, whereas at high doses the reward effects predominate. The nicotine transdermal system produces an initial (first day of use) increase in BP, an increase in HR (3%–7%), and a decrease in SV after 10 days. **Time to peak levels:** 2–12 hr. **Peak plasma levels:** 5–17 ng/mL. **t½:** 3–4 hr. Metabolized in the liver to a large number of metabolites, all of which are less active than nicotine.

USES

As an aid to stopping smoking for the relief of nicotine withdrawal symptoms. Should be used in conjunction with a comprehensive behavioral smoking cessation program.

CONTRAINDICATIONS

Hypersensitivity or allergy to nicotine or any components of the therapeutic system. Use in children and during pregnancy, labor, delivery, and lactation. Use in those with heart disease, hypertension, a recent MI, severe or worsening angina pectoris, those taking certain antidepressants or antiasthmatic drugs, or in severe renal impairment.

SPECIAL CONCERNS

Encourage pregnant smokers to try to stop smoking using educational and behavioral interventions before using the nicotine transdermal system. Use during pregnancy only if the potential benefit outweighs the potential risk of nicotine to the fetus. The use of nicotine transdermal systems for longer than 3 months has not been studied. Before use, screen clients with coronary heart disease (history of MI and/or angina pectoris), serious cardiac arrhythmias, or vasospastic diseases (e.g., Buerger's disease, Prinzmetal's variant angina) carefully. Use with caution in clients with hyperthyroidism, pheochromocytoma, IDDM (nicotine causes the release of catecholamines), in active peptic ulcers, in accelerated hypertension, and during lactation.

SIDE EFFECTS

NOTE: The incidence of side effects is complicated by the fact that clients manifest effects of nicotine withdrawal or by concurrent smoking. **Dermatologic:** Erythema, pruritus, or burning at the site of application; cutaneous hypersensitivity, sweating, rash at application site. **Body as a whole:** Allergy, back pain. **GI:** Diarrhea, dyspepsia, dry mouth, abdominal pain, constipation, N&V. **Musculoskeletal:** Arthralgia, myalgia. **CNS:** Abnormal dreams, somnolence, dizziness, impaired concentration, headache, insomnia. **CV:** Tachycardia, hypertension. **Respiratory:** Increased cough, pharyngitis, sinusitis. **GU:** Dysmenorrhea.

OD OVERDOSE MANAGEMENT

Symptoms: Pallor, cold sweat, N&V, abdominal pain, salivation, diarrhea, headache, dizziness, disturbed hearing and vision, mental confusion, weakness, tremor. Large overdoses may cause prostration, hypotension, ***respiratory failure, seizures, and death.*** *Treatment:* Remove the transdermal system immediately. The surface of the skin may be flushed with water and dried; soap should not be used as it may increase the absorption of nicotine. Diazepam or barbiturates may be used to treat seizures and atropine can be given for excessive bronchial secretions or diarrhea. Respiratory support for respiratory failure and fluid support for hypotension and CV collapse. If transdermal systems are ingested PO, activated charcoal should be given to prevent seizures. If the client is unconscious, the charcoal should be administered by a NGT. A saline cathartic or sorbitol added to the first dose of activated charcoal may hasten GI passage of the system.

Doses of activated charcoal should be repeated as long as the system remains in the GI tract as nicotine will continue to be released for many hours.

HOW SUPPLIED

Film, Extended Release, dose absorbed/24 hr: **Habitrol, Nicoderm CQ, Nicotine Transdermal System:** 21 mg/day, 14 mg/day, 7 mg/day; **Nicotrol:** 15 mg/16 hr.

DOSAGE

• TRANSDERMAL SYSTEM

HABITROL, NICOTINE TRANSDERMAL SYSTEM

21 mg/day for the first 4 weeks, 14 mg/day for the next 2 weeks, and 7 mg/day for the last 2 weeks (total course of therapy: 8–10 weeks).

NICODERM

21 mg/day for the first 6 weeks, 14 mg/day for the next 2 weeks, and 7 mg/day for the last 2 weeks (total course of therapy: 8–10 weeks). Start witih 14 mg/day for 6 weeks for those who smoke 10 or less cigarettes/day; decrease dose to 7 mg/day for the last 2 weeks.

NICOTROL

15 mg/day for 6 weeks.

NURSING CONSIDERATIONS

ADMINISTRATION/STORAGE

1. All products are over-the-counter.
2. There will be differences in the duration and length of therapy, depending on the product prescribed.
3. Apply the transdermal system promptly after its removal from the protective pouch to prevent loss of nicotine due to evaporation. Only use systems where the pouch is intact.
4. Apply system once daily to a nonhairy, clean, and dry site on the trunk or upper, outer arm. Hold for 10 seconds. Wash hands thoroughly after application. Do not wear more than 1 patch at a time. Do not cut the patch in half or in smaller pieces.
5. For Habitrol or Nicoderm, remove the used system after 24 hr and apply a new system to an alternate skin site. Do not leave the patch on for more than 24 hr as skin irritation may occur and potency is lost. Apply at the same time each day. If clients have vivid dreams or other sleep disturbances, patch may be removed at bedtime and a new patch applied in the morning.
6. For Nicotrol, apply a new system each day upon waking and remove at bedtime. If client forgets to remove the patch at bedtime, vivid dreams or other sleep disturbances may result. Do not wear patch more than 16 hr.
7. When a used system is removed, fold it over and place in the protective pouch that contained the new system. Dispose of the used system to prevent access by children or pets.
8. The goal of therapy with nicotine transdermal systems is complete abstinence. If still smoking by the fourth week of therapy, discontinue treatment.
9. Do not store Nicotrol above 30°C (86°F). Store Habitrol and Nicoderm CQ at 20–25°C (68–77°F).

ASSESSMENT

1. Document nicotine profile: type and brand (cigarettes, chewing tobacco, or cigars), amount used per day, when used, and what increases usage.
2. Determine any CAD, liver or renal dysfunction.
3. List meds currently prescribed. Cessation of smoking, with or without nicotine replacement, may alter the response to certain drugs.
4. Document any skin disorders; nicotine transdermal systems may be irritating with skin disorders such as atopic or eczematous dermatitis.

CLIENT/FAMILY TEACHING

1. Use extreme caution during application; avoid contact with active systems. If contact occurs, wash area with water only. The eyes should not be touched. These systems can be a dermal irritant and cause contact dermatitis.
2. Report any persistent skin irritations such as erythema, edema, or pruritus at the application site as well as any generalized skin reactions such as hives, urticaria, or a generalized rash; remove system.

N

3. Follow manufacturer's guidelines for proper system application. Review information sheet that comes with the product which contains instructions on how to use and dispose of the transdermal systems.
4. Stop smoking completely. If smoking continues, may experience adverse side effects due to higher nicotine levels in the body.
5. Participate in a formal smoking program. The success or failure of smoking cessation depends on the quality, intensity, and frequency of supportive care.
6. Nicotine in any form can be toxic and addictive; transdermal systems may lead to dependence. To minimize this risk, withdraw system gradually after 4–8 weeks of use.
7. Symptoms of nicotine withdrawal include craving, nervousness, restlessness, irritability, mood lability, anxiety, drowsiness, sleep disturbances, impaired concentration, increased appetite, headache, myalgia, constipation, fatigue, and weight gain; report as dosage may require adjustment.
8. Change site of application daily; do not reuse same site for 1 week.
9. With Nicotrol, remove patch at bedtime and apply upon arising.
10. Keep all products used and unused away from children and pets; sufficient nicotine is still present in used systems to cause toxicity.
11. If therapy is unsuccessful after 4 weeks, discontinue and identify reasons for failure so that a later attempt may be more successful.

OUTCOMES/EVALUATE

Smoking cessation; control of nicotine withdrawal symptoms

Nifedipine

(nye-**FED**-ih-peen)

PREGNANCY CATEGORY: C

CLASSIFICATION(S):

Calcium channel blocker

Rx: Adalat, Adalat CC, Nifedical XL, Procardia, Procardia XL

✱Rx: Adalat P.A. 10 and 20, Adalat XL, Apo-Nifed, Apo-Nifed PA, Nifedipine PA 10 and 20, Novo-Nifedin, Nu-Nifed, Nu-Nifedipine-PA

SEE ALSO *CALCIUM CHANNEL BLOCKING AGENTS.*

ACTION/KINETICS

Variable effects on AV node effective and functional refractory periods. CO is moderately increased while peripheral vascular resistance is significantly decreased. **Onset:** 20 min. **Peak plasma levels:** 30 min (up to 4 hr for extended-release). **t½:** 2–5 hr. **Therapeutic serum levels:** 0.025–0.1 mcg/mL. **Duration:** 4–8 hr (12 hr for extended-release). Low-fat meals may slow the rate but not the extent of absorption. Metabolized in the liver to inactive metabolites.

USES

(1) Vasospastic (Prinzmetal's or variant) angina. (2) Chronic stable angina without vasospasm, including angina due to increased effort (especially in clients who cannot take beta blockers or nitrates or who remain symptomatic following clinical doses of these drugs). (3) Essential hypertension (sustained-release only). *Investigational:* PO, sublingually, or chewed in hypertensive emergencies. Also prophylaxis of migraine headaches, primary pulmonary hypertension, severe pregnancy-associated hypertension, esophageal diseases, Raynaud's phenomenon, CHF, asthma, premature labor, biliary and renal colic, and cardiomyopathy. To prevent strokes and to decrease the risk of CHF in geriatric hypertensives.

CONTRAINDICATIONS

Hypersensitivity. Lactation.

SPECIAL CONCERNS

Use with caution in impaired hepatic or renal function and in elderly clients. Initial increase in frequency, duration, or severity of angina (may also be seen in clients being withdrawn from beta blockers and who begin taking nifedipine).

SIDE EFFECTS

CV: Peripheral and pulmonary edema, MI, hypotension, palpitations, syncope, CHF (especially if used with a beta blocker), decreased platelet aggregation, arrhythmias, tachycardia. Increased frequency, length, and duration of angina when beginning nifedipine therapy. **GI:** Nausea, diarrhea, constipation, flatulence, abdominal cramps, dysgeusia, vomiting, dry mouth, eructation, gastroesophageal reflux, melena. **CNS:** Dizziness, lightheadedness, giddiness, nervousness, sleep disturbances, headache, weakness, depression, migraine, psychoses, hallucinations, disturbances in equilibrium, somnolence, insomnia, abnormal dreams, malaise, anxiety. **Dermatologic:** Rash, dermatitis, urticaria, pruritus, photosensitivity, erythema multiforme, ***Stevens-Johnson syndrome.*** **Respiratory:** Dyspnea, cough, wheezing, SOB, respiratory infection, throat, nasal, or chest congestion. **Musculoskeletal:** Muscle cramps or inflammation, joint pain or stiffness, arthritis, ataxia, myoclonic dystonia, hypertonia, asthenia. **Hematologic:** Thrombocytopenia, leukopenia, purpura, anemia. **Other:** Fever, chills, sweating, blurred vision, sexual difficulties, flushing, transient blindness, hyperglycemia, hypokalemia, gingival hyperplasia, allergic hepatitis, hepatitis, tinnitus, gynecomastia, polyuria, nocturia, erythromelalgia, weight gain, epistaxis, facial and periorbital edema, hypoesthesia, gout, abnormal lacrimation, breast pain, dysuria, hematuria.

LABORATORY TEST CONSIDERATIONS

↑ Alkaline phosphatase, CPK, LDH, AST, ALT. Positive Coombs' test.

ADDITIONAL DRUG INTERACTIONS

Anticoagulants, oral / Possibility of ↑ PT

Cimetidine / ↑ Bioavailability of nifedipine

Digoxin / ↑ Effect of digoxin by ↓ excretion by kidney

Grapefruit juice / ↑ Nifedipine plasma levels R/T ↓ metabolism

Magnesium sulfate / ↑ Neuromuscular blockade and hypotension

Melatonin / Melatonin may ↓ antihypertensive effect

Quinidine / Possible ↓ quinidine effect R/T ↓ plasma levels; ↑ risk of hypotension, bradycardia, AV block, pulmonary edema, and VT

Ranitidine / ↑ Nifedipine bioavailability

Theophylline / Possible ↑ effect of theophylline

HOW SUPPLIED

Capsule: 10 mg, 20 mg; *Tablet, Extended Release:* 30 mg, 60 mg, 90 mg

DOSAGE

• CAPSULES

Individualized. Initial: 10 mg t.i.d. (range: 10–20 mg t.i.d.); **maintenance:** 10–30 mg t.i.d.–q.i.d. Clients with coronary artery spasm may respond better to 20–30 mg t.i.d.–q.i.d. Doses greater than 120 mg/day are rarely needed while doses greater than 180 mg/day are not recommended.

• EXTENDED-RELEASE TABLETS

Initial: 30 or 60 mg once daily for Procardia XL and 30 mg once daily for Adalat CC. Titrate over a 7- to 14-day period. Dosage can be increased as required and as tolerated, to a maximum of 120 mg/day for Procardia XL and 90 mg/day for Adalat CC.

Investigational, hypertensive emergencies.

10–20 mg given PO (capsule is punctured several times and then chewed).

NURSING CONSIDERATIONS

SEE ALSO *NURSING CONSIDERATIONS* FOR *CALCIUM CHANNEL BLOCKING AGENTS*.

ADMINISTRATION/STORAGE

1. Do not exceed a single dose (other than sustained-released) of 30 mg.
2. Before increasing the dose, carefully monitor BP.
3. Use only the sustained-release tablets to treat hypertension.
4. Sublingual nitroglycerin and long-acting nitrates may be used concomitantly with nifedipine.
5. Concomitant therapy with beta-adrenergic blocking agents may be used. In these cases, note any potential drug interactions.
6. Clients withdrawn from beta blockers may manifest symptoms of

increased angina which cannot be prevented by nifedipine; in fact, nifedipine may increase the severity of angina in this situation.
7. Clients with angina may be switched to the sustained-release product at the nearest equivalent total daily dose. Use doses greater than 90 mg/day with caution.
8. Protect capsules from light and moisture and store at room temperature in the original container.
9. During initial therapy and when dosage is increased, may experience an increase in the frequency, duration, or severity of angina.
10. Food may decrease the rate but not the extent of absorption; can be taken without regard to meals.

ASSESSMENT

1. Document sensitivity to CCBs.
2. Note any pulmonary edema, ECG abnormalities, or palpitations. Document cardiopulmonary assessment findings.

INTERVENTIONS

1. During titration period, note any hypotensive response and increased HR that result from peripheral vasodilation; may precipitate angina.
2. Although beta-blocking drugs may be used concomitantly with chronic stable angina, the combined effects of the drugs cannot be predicted (especially with compromised LV function or cardiac conduction abnormalities). Pronounced hypotension, heart block, and CHF may occur.
3. If therapy with a beta blocker is to be discontinued, gradually decrease dosage to prevent withdrawal syndrome.

CLIENT/FAMILY TEACHING

1. May take with or without food. Sustained-release tablets should not be chewed or divided. Grapefruit juice may caused increased serum drug levels.
2. There is no cause for concern if an empty tablet appears in the stool.
3. Maintain a fluid intake of 2–3 L/day to avoid constipation.
4. Do not use OTC agents unless approved; avoid alcohol and caffeine.
5. Report any symptoms of persistent headache, flushing, nausea, palpitations, weight gain, dizziness, or lightheadedness.
6. Perform weekly weights and note any extremity swelling. Peripheral edema may result from arterial vasodilatation precipitated by nifedipine or swelling may indicate increasing ventricular dysfunction and should be reported.
7. If also receiving beta-adrenergic blocking agents, report any evidence of hypotension, exacerbation of angina, or evidence of heart failure.
8. Once beta-blocking agents have been discontinued, report increased anginal pain.

OUTCOMES/EVALUATE

- ↓ Frequency and intensity of anginal episodes; ↓ BP
- Improved peripheral circulation
- Prevention of strokes and ↓ risk of CHF in geriatric hypertensives

Nilutamide

PREGNANCY CATEGORY: C
CLASSIFICATION(S):
Antineoplastic, hormone
Rx: Nilandron
★**Rx:** Anadron

SEE ALSO *ANTINEOPLASTIC AGENTS.*

ACTION/KINETICS

Antiandrogen with no estrogen, progesterone, mineralocorticoid, or glucocorticoid effects. Binds to the androgen receptor, thus blocking effects of testosterone and preventing the normal androgenic response. Rapidly and completely absorbed from the GI tract. Moderately bound to plasma proteins. Extensively metabolized by the liver; one of the five metabolites is active. Excreted mainly in the urine. **t½, elimination:** Approximately, 41–49 hr.

USES

In combination with surgical castration to treat metastatic prostate cancer (Stage D_2).

CONTRAINDICATIONS

Severe hepatic impairment, severe respiratory deficiency, hypersensitivity to nilutamide or any product components. Use in women.

SPECIAL CONCERNS
Interstitial pneumonitis and hepatitis may occur. Many experience a delay in adaptation to the dark ranging from a few seconds to a few minutes. Safety and efficacy have not been determined in children.

SIDE EFFECTS
CV: Hypertension, angina, ***heart failure***, syncope. **GI:** Nausea, constipation, diarrhea, dry mouth, GI disorder, ***GI hemorrhage,*** melena, hepatotoxicity, ***hepatitis*** (rare). **CNS:** Dizziness, nervousness, paresthesia. **Respiratory:** Increased cough, interstitial pneumonitis, lung disorder, rhinitis, dyspnea. **Ophthalmic:** Cataract, photophobia, impaired adaptation to dark, abnormal vision, colored vision. **Metabolic/Nutritional:** Edema, weight loss, intolerance to alcohol. **Miscellaneous:** UTI, malaise, arthritis, pruritus, hot flushes, leukopenia, aplastic anemia (rare).

LABORATORY TEST CONSIDERATIONS
↑ Haptoglobin, alkaline phosphatase, BUN, creatinine, AST, ALT. Hyperglycemia.

DRUG INTERACTIONS
Phenytoin / Possible phenytoin delayed elimination and ↑ serum t½ → toxic levels
Theophylline / Possible theophylline delayed elimination and ↑ serum t½ → toxic levels
Vitamin K antagonists / Possible vitamin K anatagonist delayed elimination and ↑ serum t½ → toxic levels

HOW SUPPLIED
Tablets: 50 mg

DOSAGE

• **TABLETS**
Metastatic prostate cancer.
300 mg (six 50-mg tablets) once daily for 30 days followed by 150 mg (three 50-mg tablets) once daily.

NURSING CONSIDERATIONS

SEE ALSO *NURSING CONSIDERATIONS* FOR *ANTINEOPLASTIC AGENTS.*

ASSESSMENT
1. Document indications for therapy, other agents/therapies trialed and outcome.
2. Monitor VS, PSA, labs, and ECG.
3. Anticipate first dosing on or the day after surgical castration.

CLIENT/FAMILY TEACHING
1. Take daily as directed, with or without food. Do not stop or interrupt dose without provider approval.
2. May experience difficulty driving at night or through tunnels (delayed dark adaptation); tinted glasses may alleviate this effect.
3. Report any increased SOB, chest pain, or unusual side effects.
4. Avoid alcohol, especially if experienced intolerance of alcohol following nilutamide use.

ADMINISTRATION/STORAGE
1. To ensure maximum beneficial effects, initiate treatment on the same day as or the day after surgical castration.
2. Protect from light and store at room temperature at 15–30°C (59–86°F).

ASSESSMENT
1. Document indications for therapy, other agents/therapies trialed and outcome.
2. Obtain CBS, LFTs, and CXR. Assess cardiopulmonary status closely; may cause interstitial pneumonitis.
3. Anticipate first dosing on or the day after surgical castration.

CLIENT/FAMILY TEACHING
1. Review guidelines concerning the dosage and dosing frequency.
2. May take with or without food.
3. Wear tinted glasses to prevent delay in adaptation to the dark. Drive cautiously through tunnels or at night.
4. Immediately report any symptoms of chest pain, cough with fever, jaundice, dark urine, fatigue or SOB.
5. Avoid alcohol, especially if experienced intolerance of alcohol following nilutamide use.

OUTCOMES/EVALUATE
Control of malignant cell proliferation

N

Nimodipine

(nye-**MOH**-dih-peen)

PREGNANCY CATEGORY: C
CLASSIFICATION(S):
Calcium channel blocker
Rx: Nimotop
✱Rx: Nimotop I.V.

SEE ALSO *CALCIUM CHANNEL BLOCKING AGENTS.*

ACTION/KINETICS
Has a greater effect on cerebral arteries than arteries elsewhere in the body (probably due to its highly lipophilic properties). Mechanism to reduce neurologic deficits following subarachnoid hemorrhage not known. **Peak plasma levels:** 1 hr. **t½:** 1–2 hr. Significantly bound (over 95%) to plasma protein. Undergoes first-pass metabolism in the liver; metabolites excreted through the urine.

USES
Improvement of neurologic deficits due to spasm following subarachnoid hemorrhage from ruptured congenital intracranial aneurysms irrespective of the post-ictus neurological condition. *Investigational:* Migraine headaches and cluster headaches.

CONTRAINDICATIONS
Lactation.

SPECIAL CONCERNS
Safety and efficacy have not been established in children. Use with caution in clients with impaired hepatic function and reduced hepatic blood flow. The half-life may be increased in geriatric clients.

SIDE EFFECTS
CV: Hypotension, peripheral edema, CHF, ECG abnormalities, tachycardia, bradycardia, palpitations, rebound vasospasm, hypertension, hematoma, ***DIC, DVT.*** **GI:** Nausea, dyspepsia, diarrhea, abdominal discomfort, cramps, ***GI hemorrhage,*** vomiting. **CNS:** Headache, depression, lightheadedness, dizziness. **Hepatic:** Abnormal LFT, hepatitis, jaundice. **Hematologic:** Thrombocytopenia, anemia, purpura, ecchymosis. **Dermatologic:** Rash, dermatitis, pruritus, urticaria. **Miscellaneous:** Dyspnea, muscle pain or cramps, acne, itching, flushing, diaphoresis, wheezing, hyponatremia.

LABORATORY TEST CONSIDERATIONS
↑ Nonfasting BS, LDH, alkaline phosphatase, ALT. ↓ Platelet count.

HOW SUPPLIED
Capsule: 30 mg

DOSAGE

• CAPSULES

Adults: 60 mg q 4 hr beginning within 96 hr after subarachnoid hemorrhage and continuing for 21 consecutive days. Reduce the dose to 30 mg q 4 hr in clients with hepatic impairment.

NURSING CONSIDERATIONS

SEE ALSO *NURSING CONSIDERATIONS FOR CALCIUM CHANNEL BLOCKING AGENTS.*

ADMINISTRATION/STORAGE
If unable to swallow capsule (e.g., unconscious or at time of surgery), make a hole in both ends of the capsule (soft gelatin) with an 18-gauge needle and withdraw the contents into a syringe. This may be administered into the NG tube and washed down with 30 mL of NSS.

ASSESSMENT
1. Obtain baseline labs; reduce dose with hepatic dysfunction.
2. Determine if pregnant.
3. Perform baseline neurologic scores and thoroughly document deficits. Note VS, I&O, and weights.
4. Initiate therapy within 96 hr of subarachnoid hemorrhage.

CLIENT/FAMILY TEACHING
1. Take the drug on time; sleep must be interrupted to give the medication q 4 hr ATC for 21 days.
2. Report any side effects such as nausea, lightheadedness, irregular heart beat, dizziness, muscle cramps, or muscle pain.
3. Report ↑ SOB, the need to take deep breaths on occasion, or wheezing.

OUTCOMES/EVALUATE
• ↓ Neurologic deficits R/T venospasm after subarachnoid hemorrhage
• Termination of migraine and cluster headaches

Nisoldipine

(**NYE**-sohl-dih-peen)

PREGNANCY CATEGORY: C
CLASSIFICATION(S):
Calcium channel blocker
Rx: Sular

ACTION/KINETICS
Inhibits the transmembrane influx of calcium into vascular smooth muscle and cardiac muscle, resulting in dilation of arterioles. Has greater potency on vascular smooth muscle than on cardiac muscle. Chronic use results in a sustained decrease in vascular resistance and small increases in SI and LV ejection fraction. Weak diuretic effect and no clinically important chronotropic effects. Well absorbed following PO use; however, absolute bioavailability is low due to presystemic metabolism in the gut wall. Foods high in fat result in a significant increase in peak plasma levels. **Maximum plasma levels:** 6–12 hr. **t½, terminal:** 7–12 hr. Almost completely bound to plasma proteins. Metabolized in the liver and excreted through the urine.

USES
Treatment of hypertension alone or in combination with other antihypertensive drugs.

CONTRAINDICATIONS
Use with grapefruit juice as it interferes with metabolism, resulting in a significant increase in plasma levels of the drug. Use in those with known hypersensitivity to dihydropyridine calcium channel blockers. Lactation.

SPECIAL CONCERNS
Geriatric clients may show a two- to threefold higher plasma concentration; use caution in dosing. Use with caution and at lower doses in those with hepatic insufficiency. Use with caution in clients with CHF or compromised ventricular function, especially in combination with a beta blocker.

SIDE EFFECTS
CV: Increased angina and/or MI in clients with CAD. Initially, excessive hypotension, especially in those taking other antihypertensive drugs. Vasodilation, palpitation, atrial fibrillation, ***CVA, MI,*** CHF, first-degree AV block, hypertension, hypotension, jugular venous distension, migraine, postural hypotension, ventricular extrasystoles, SVT, syncope, systolic ejection murmur, T-wave abnormalities on ECG, venous insufficiency. **Body as a whole:** Peripheral edema, cellulitis, chills, facial edema, fever, flu syndrome, malaise. **GI:** Anorexia, nausea, colitis, diarrhea, dry mouth, dyspepsia, dysphagia, flatulence, gastritis, ***GI hemorrhage,*** gingival hyperplasia, glossitis, hepatomegaly, increased appetite, melena, mouth ulceration. **CNS:** Headache, dizziness, abnormal dreams, abnormal thinking and confusion, amnesia, anxiety, ataxia, cerebral ischemia, decreased libido, depression, hypesthesia, hypertonia, insomnia, nervousness, paresthesia, somnolence, tremor, vertigo. **Musculoskeletal:** Arthralgia, arthritis, leg cramps, myalgia, myasthenia, myositis, tenosynovitis. **Hematologic:** Anemia, ecchymoses, leukopenia, petechiae. **Respiratory:** Pharyngitis, sinusitis, asthma, dyspnea, end-inspiratory wheeze and fine rales, epistaxis, increased cough, laryngitis, pleural effusion, rhinitis. **Dermatologic:** Acne, alopecia, dry skin, exfoliative dermatitis, fungal dermatitis, herpes simplex, herpes zoster, maculopapular rash, pruritus, pustular rash, skin discoloration, skin ulcer, sweating, urticaria. **GU:** Dysuria, hematuria, impotence, nocturia, urinary frequency, vaginal hemorrhage, vaginitis. **Metabolic:** Gout, hypokalemia, weight gain or loss. **Ophthalmic:** Abnormal vision, amblyopia, blepharitis, conjunctivitis, glaucoma, itchy eyes, keratoconjunctivitis, retinal detachment, temporary unilateral loss of vision, vitreous floater, watery eyes. **Miscellaneous:** Diabetes mellitus, thyroiditis, chest pain, ear pain, otitis media, tinnitus, taste disturbance.

LABORATORY TEST CONSIDERATIONS
↑ Serum creatine kinase, NPN, BUN, serum creatinine. Abnormal LFTs.

N

OD OVERDOSE MANAGEMENT
Symptoms: Pronounced hypotension. *Treatment:* Active CV support, including monitoring of CV and respiratory function, elevation of extremities, judicious use of calcium infusion, pressor agents, and fluids. Dialysis is not likely to be beneficial, although plasmapheresis may be helpful.

DRUG INTERACTIONS
Cimetidine / Significant ↑ plasma nislodipine levels
Ketoconazole / ↑ Plasma nislodipine levels R/T ↓ liver metabolism

HOW SUPPLIED
Extended-Release Tablets: 10 mg, 20 mg, 30 mg, 40 mg.

DOSAGE
• **TABLETS, EXTENDED-RELEASE**
Hypertension.
Dose must be adjusted to the needs of each person. **Initial:** 20 mg once daily; **then,** increase by 10 mg/week or longer intervals to reach adequate BP control. **Usual maintenance:** 20–40 mg once daily. Doses beyond 60 mg once daily are not recommended. **Initial dose, clients over 65 years and those with impaired renal function:** 10 mg once daily.

N

NURSING CONSIDERATIONS

SEE ALSO *NURSING CONSIDERATIONS* FOR *CALCIUM CHANNEL BLOCKING AGENTS.*

ADMINISTRATION/STORAGE
Closely monitor dosage adjustments in clients over age 65 and those with impaired liver/renal function.

ASSESSMENT
1. Document indications for therapy, onset of symptoms, agents trialed, and the outcome.
2. Reduce dosage in the elderly and with liver/renal dysfunction.
3. Obtain baseline ECG and note any history or evidence of CHF or compromised LV function.
4. List drugs prescribed to ensure none interact unfavorably.

CLIENT/FAMILY TEACHING
1. Swallow tablets whole; do not chew, divide, or crush.
2. Do not give tablets with grapefruit juice or a high-fat meal.
3. Headaches, peripheral edema, and dizziness may occur; use caution and report if persistent.
4. Report as scheduled for BP evaluation during titration period. Maintain record of BP and report any new or unusual side effects.

OUTCOMES/EVALUATE
↓ BP

Nitrofurantoin

(**nye**-troh-fyour-**AN**-toyn)

PREGNANCY CATEGORY: B
Rx: Furadantin
✱Rx: Apo-Nitrofurantoin, Novo-Furantoin

Nitrofurantoin macrocrystals

(**nye**-troh-fyour-**AN**-toyn)

PREGNANCY CATEGORY: B
Rx: Macrobid, Macrodantin
CLASSIFICATION(S):
Urinary anti-infective

SEE ALSO *ANTI-INFECTIVES.*

ACTION/KINETICS
Interferes with bacterial carbohydrate metabolism by inhibiting acetyl coenzyme A; also interferes with bacterial cell wall synthesis. Bacteriostatic at low concentrations and bactericidal at high concentrations. Tablets are readily absorbed from the GI tract; bioavailability is increased by food. **t½:** 20 min (60 min in anephric clients). **Urine levels:** 50–250 mcg/mL. If the C_{CR} is less than 40 mL/min, urine antibacterial levels are inadequate, with the subsequent higher blood levels increasing the possibility of toxicity. Antibacterial activity is best in an acid urine. From 30% to 50% excreted unchanged in the urine. Nitrofurantoin macrocrystals (Macrodantin) are available; this preparation maintains effectiveness while decreasing GI distress.

USES

UTIs due to susceptible strains of *Escherichia coli, Staphylococcus aureus* (not for treatment of pyelonephritis or perinephric abscesses), enterococci, and certain strains of *Enterobacter* and *Klebsiella.*

CONTRAINDICATIONS

Anuria, oliguria, and clients with impaired renal function (C_{CR} below 40 mL/min); pregnant women, especially near term; infants less than 1 month of age; and lactation.

SPECIAL CONCERNS

Use with extreme caution in anemia, diabetes, electrolyte imbalance, avitaminosis B, or a debilitating disease. Safety during lactation has not been established.

SIDE EFFECTS

Nitrofurantoin is a potentially toxic drug with many side effects. **GI:** N&V, anorexia, diarrhea, abdominal pain, parotitis, pancreatitis. **CNS:** Headache, dizziness, vertigo, drowsiness, nystagmus, confusion, depression, euphoria, psychotic reactions (rare). **Hematologic:** Leukopenia, thrombocytopenia, eosinophilia, megaloblastic anemia, ***agranulocytosis,*** granulocytopenia, ***hemolytic anemia (especially in clients with G6PD deficiency).*** **Allergic:** Drug fever, skin rashes, pruritus, urticaria, angioedema, exfoliative dermatitis, erythema multiforme ***(rarely, Stevens-Johnson syndrome), anaphylaxis,*** arthralgia, myalgia, chills, sialadenitis, asthma symptoms in susceptible clients; maculopapular, erythematous, or eczematous eruption. **Pulmonary:** Sudden onset of dyspnea, cough, chest pain, fever and chills; pulmonary infiltration with consolidation or pleural effusion on x-ray, elevated ESR, eosinophilia. **After subacute or chronic use:** dyspnea, nonproductive cough, malaise, interstitial pneumonitis. Permanent impairment of pulmonary function with chronic therapy. A lupus-like syndrome associated with pulmonary reactions. **Hepatic:** Hepatitis, cholestatic jaundice, chronic active hepatitis, hepatic necrosis (rare). **CV:** Benign intracranial hypertension, changes in ECG, collapse, cyanosis. **Miscellaneous:** Peripheral neuropathy, asthenia, alopecia, superinfections of the GU tract, muscle pain.

LABORATORY TEST CONSIDERATIONS

↑ AST, ALT, serum phosphorus. ↓ Hemoglobin.

OD OVERDOSE MANAGEMENT

Symptoms: Vomiting (most common). *Treatment:* Induce emesis. High fluid intake to promote urinary excretion. The drug is dialyzable.

DRUG INTERACTIONS

Acetazolamide / ↓ Nitrofurantoin effect R/T ↑ urine alkalinity produced by acetazolamide
Antacids, oral / ↓ Nitrofurantoin effect R/T ↓ GI tract absorption
Anticholinergic drugs / ↑ Nitrofurantoin effect R/T ↑ stomach absorption
Magnesium trisilicate / ↓ Nitrofurantoin absorption from GI tract
Nalidixic acid / ↓ Effect of nalidixic acid
Probenecid / High doses ↓ secretion of nitrofurantoin → toxicity
Sodium bicarbonate / ↓ Nitrofurantoin effect R/T ↑ urine alkalinity produced by sodium bicarbonate

HOW SUPPLIED

Nitrofurantoin: *Oral Suspension:* 25 mg/5 mL; **Nitrofurantoin Macrocrystals:** *Capsule:* 25 mg, 50 mg, 100 mg

N

DOSAGE

- **CAPSULES, ORAL SUSPENSION**

UTIs.

Adults: 50–100 mg q.i.d., not to exceed 600 mg/day. For cystitis, Macrobid is given in doses of 100 mg b.i.d. for 7 days. **Pediatric, 1 month of age and over:** 5–7 mg/kg/day in four equal doses.

Prophylaxis of UTIs.

Adults: 50–100 mg at bedtime. **Pediatric, 1 month of age and over:** 1 mg/kg/day at bedtime or in two divided doses daily.

NURSING CONSIDERATIONS

SEE ALSO *GENERAL NURSING CONSIDERATIONS* FOR *ANTI-INFECTIVES.*

ADMINISTRATION/STORAGE

1. Capsules containing crystals cause less GI intolerance.
2. Store PO medications in amber-colored bottles.
3. Continue for at least 3 days after obtaining a negative urine culture.

ASSESSMENT

1. Monitor CBC, urine C&S, liver and renal functions; also CXR and PFTs with chronic therapy.
2. Observe for acute or delayed-onset anaphylactic reaction.
3. Drug may alter certain lab results.
4. Monitor for recurrent UTI symptoms; urinary superinfections may occur.
5. Blacks and ethnic groups of Mediterranean and Near Eastern origin should be assessed for symptoms of anemia.

CLIENT/FAMILY TEACHING

1. Take with food or milk to minimize gastric irritation and enhance absorption; complete full course of therapy to prevent bacterial resistance.
2. Increase fluid intake; drink at least 2 qt/day of water. Acidic foods (prunes, cranberry juice, plums) enhance drug action whereas alkaline foods (milk products) minimize drug action.
3. Drug may turn urine a dark yellow or brown color.
4. Report any persistent or bothersome side effects. Respiratory dysfunction requires immediate intervention.
5. Immediately report any numbness and tingling of extremities or flu-like symptoms; indications for drug withdrawal because condition may worsen and become irreversible.
6. Report persistent N&V and diarrhea as these may be symptoms of a GI superinfection.

OUTCOMES/EVALUATE

- Negative urine culture results
- Resolution of infection; symptomatic improvement (↓ dysuria, ↓ frequency)

Nitroglycerin IV

(nye-troh-**GLIH**-sir-in)

PREGNANCY CATEGORY: C

CLASSIFICATION(S):
Vasodilator, coronary
Rx: Nitro-Bid IV, Nitroglycerin in 5% Dextrose, Tridil

SEE ALSO *ANTIANGINAL DRUGS, NITRATES/NITRITES.*

ACTION/KINETICS

Onset: 1–2 min; **duration:** 3–5 min (dose-dependent).

USES

(1) Hypertension associated with surgery (e.g., associated with ET intubation, skin incision, sternotomy, anesthesia, cardiac bypass, immediate postsurgical period). (2) CHF associated with acute MI. (3) Angina unresponsive to usual doses of organic nitrate or beta-adrenergic blocking agents. (4) Cardiac-load reducing agent. (5) Produce controlled hypotension during surgical procedures.

SPECIAL CONCERNS

Dosage has not been established in children.

HOW SUPPLIED

Injection: 0.5 mg/mL, 5 mg/mL; *Injection Solution:* 25 mg, 50 mg 100 mg, 200 mg

DOSAGE

- **IV INFUSION ONLY**

Initial: 5 mcg/min delivered by precise infusion pump. May be increased by 5 mcg/min q 3–5 min until response is seen. If no response seen at 20 mcg/min, dose can be increased by 10–20 mcg/min until response noted. Monitor titration continuously until client reaches desired level of response.

NURSING CONSIDERATIONS

SEE ALSO *NURSING CONSIDERATIONS* FOR *ANTIANGINAL DRUGS, NITRATES/NITRITES.*

ADMINISTRATION/STORAGE

IV 1. Dilute with D5W USP or 0.9% NaCl injection. Not for direct IV use; must first be diluted.
2. Use glass IV bottle only and administration set provided by the manufacturer; is readily adsorbed onto many plastics. Avoid adding unnecessary plastic to IV system.

3. Aspirate medication into a syringe and then inject immediately into a glass bottle (or polyolefin bottle) to minimize contact with plastic.
4. Do not administer with any other medications in the IV system.
5. Do not interrupt IV nitroglycerin for administration of a bolus of any other medication.
6. To provide correct dosage, remove 15 mL of solution from the IV tubing if concentration of solution is changed.
7. Administer infusion with infusion device (volumetric) in a closely monitored environment.

ASSESSMENT

1. Document indications and goals of therapy.
2. Assess and rate pain, noting location, onset, duration, and any precipitating factors.

INTERVENTIONS

1. Obtain written parameters for BP and pulse; monitor during therapy.
2. Monitor VS and ECG. Note any evidence of hypotension, nausea, sweating, and/or vomiting. Monitor CVP and/or PA pressure as ordered; document presence of tachycardia or bradycardia:
   - Elevate the legs to restore BP.
   - Reduce the rate of flow or administer additional IV fluids.
3. Assess for thrombophlebitis at the IV site; remove if reddened.
4. After the initial positive response to therapy, dosage increments will be smaller and made at longer intervals.
5. Sinus tachycardia may occur in client with angina receiving a maintenance dose of nitroglycerin (HR of 80 beats/min or less reduces myocardial demand).
6. Check that topical, PO, or SL doses are adjusted/held if on concomitant IV nitroglycerin.
7. Wean from IV nitroglycerin by gradually decreasing doses to avoid posttherapy or CV distress. Usually initiated when the client is receiving the peak effect from PO or topical vasodilators; monitor for hypertension and angina.
8. Administer nonnarcotic analgesic (usually acetaminophen) because headache is a common side effect of drug therapy.

CLIENT/FAMILY TEACHING

1. Drug is used to lower BP, control chest pain, and/or reduce cardiac work load.
2. Report pain and level so dose may be adjusted to control.
3. May experience headaches; report so meds to relieve may be administered.

OUTCOMES/EVALUATE

- Resolution/control of angina
- ↓ BP; ↑ activity tolerance
- Improvement in S&S of CHF (↑ output, ↓ rales, ↓ CVP)

Nitroglycerin sublingual

(nye-troh-**GLIH**-sir-in)

PREGNANCY CATEGORY: C
CLASSIFICATION(S):
Vasodilator, coronary
Rx: NitroQuick, Nitrostat, NitroTab

SEE ALSO *ANTIANGINAL DRUGS, NITRATES/NITRITES*.

ACTION/KINETICS
Sublingual. Onset: 1–3 min; **duration:** 30–60 min.

USES
Agent of choice for prophylaxis and treatment of angina pectoris.

SPECIAL CONCERNS
Dosage has not been established in children.

HOW SUPPLIED
Tablet: 0.3 mg, 0.4 mg, 0.6 mg

DOSAGE

- **SUBLINGUAL TABLETS**

Dissolve 1 tablet under the tongue or in the buccal pouch at first sign of attack; may be repeated in 5 min if necessary (no more than 3 tablets should be taken within 15 min). For prophylaxis, tablets may be taken 5–10 min prior to activities that may precipitate an attack.

N

NURSING CONSIDERATIONS

SEE ALSO *NURSING CONSIDERATIONS* FOR *ANTIANGINAL DRUGS, NITRATES/NITRITES.*

CLIENT/FAMILY TEACHING

1. Sit down and place sublingual tablets under the tongue and allow to dissolve; do not swallow until entirely dissolved. May sting when it comes in contact with the mucosa.
2. Take *before* stressful activity, i.e., exercise, sex.
3. Report immediately if pain is not controlled with prescribed dosage. Call 911 or for an ambulance as directed by provider if relief not attained.
4. Date sublingual container upon opening. Store in original container at room temperature protected from moisture. Discard unused tablets if 6 months has elapsed since the original container was opened.

OUTCOMES/EVALUATE

- Angina prophylaxis
- Termination of anginal attack

N

Nitroglycerin sustained-release capsules

(nye-troh-**GLIH**-sir-in)

PREGNANCY CATEGORY: C
Rx: Nitroglyn, Nitro-Time

Nitroglycerin sustained-release tablets

(nye-troh-**GLIH**-sir-in)

PREGNANCY CATEGORY: C
Rx: Nitrong
✱Rx: Nitrong SR
CLASSIFICATION(S):
Vasodilator, coronary

SEE ALSO *ANTIANGINAL DRUGS, NITRATES/NITRITES.*

ACTION/KINETICS
Sustained-release. Onset: 20–45 min; **duration:** 3–8 hr.

USES
To prevent anginal attacks. "Possibly effective" for the prophylaxis or treatment of anginal attacks.

SPECIAL CONCERNS
Dosage has not been established in children.

HOW SUPPLIED
Sustained-release capsules: 2.5 mg, 6.5 mg, 9 mg, 13 mg. **Sustained-release tablets:** 2.6 mg, 6.5 mg, 9 mg

DOSAGE

• SUSTAINED-RELEASE CAPSULES, TABLETS
Initial: 2.5 or 2.6 mg t.i.d. or q.i.d. Titrate upward to an effective dose until side effects limit dose. Dose may usually be increased by 2.5 or 2.6 mg b.i.d.–q.i.d. over a period of days or weeks. Doses as high as 26 mg q.i.d. have been reported.

NURSING CONSIDERATIONS

SEE ALSO *NURSING CONSIDERATIONS* FOR *ANTIANGINAL DRUGS, NITRATES/NITRITES.*

CLIENT/FAMILY TEACHING

1. Drug is used to control/prevent chest pain.
2. Do not chew or crush sustained-release tablets and capsules; not intended for sublingual use.
3. Take smallest effective dose 2–4 times/day with a glass of water. Report if tolerance/lack or response evident.

OUTCOMES/EVALUATE

Angina prophylaxis

Nitroglycerin topical ointment

(nye-troh-**GLIH**-sir-in)

PREGNANCY CATEGORY: C
CLASSIFICATION(S):
Vasodilator, coronary
Rx: Nitro-Bid, Nitrol

SEE ALSO *ANTIANGINAL DRUGS, NITRATES/NITRITES.*

ACTION/KINETICS
Onset: 30–60 min; **duration:** 2–12 hr (depending on amount used per unit of surface area).

USES
Prophylaxis and treatment of angina pectoris due to CAD.

SPECIAL CONCERNS
Dosage has not been established in children.

HOW SUPPLIED
Ointment: 2%

DOSAGE

• **TOPICAL OINTMENT (2%)**
1–2 in. (15–30 mg) q 8 hr; up to 4–5 in. (60–75 mg) q 4 hr may be necessary. One inch equals approximately 15 mg nitroglycerin. Determine optimum dosage by starting with ½ in. q 8 hr and increasing by ½ in. with each successive dose until headache occurs; then, decrease to largest dose that does not cause headache. When ending treatment, reduce both the dose and frequency of administration over 4–6 weeks to prevent sudden withdrawal reactions.

NURSING CONSIDERATIONS

SEE ALSO *NURSING CONSIDERATIONS* FOR *ANTIANGINAL DRUGS, NITRATES/NITRITES.*

CLIENT/FAMILY TEACHING

1. Squeeze ointment carefully onto dose-measuring application papers, which are packaged with the medicine. Use applicator to spread ointment or fold paper in half and rub back and forth.
2. Use the paper to spread the ointment onto a nonhairy area of skin. Application to the chest may be psychologically helpful, but may be applied to other nonhairy areas.
3. Rotate sites to prevent irritation. Keep a record of areas used to avoid unnecessary repetitive use of sites.
4. Apply ointment in a thin, even layer covering an area of skin 5–6 in. in diameter; remove last dose.
5. Date and tape the application paper over the area, or cover the area with a piece of plastic wrap-type material. A clear plastic cover causes less leakage of ointment, decreases skin irritation, increases absorption, and prevents clothing stains.
6. Once the dose is established, use the same type of covering to ensure that the same amount of drug is absorbed during each application.
7. Clean around tube opening and tightly cap tube after use.
8. To prevent systemic absorption protect skin from contact with ointment. Wash hands thoroughly after application to avoid headache.
9. Remove at bedtime or as directed to prevent tolerance or loss of drug effect. Remember to reapply upon awakening the next morning.

OUTCOMES/EVALUATE
Termination/prevention of anginal episodes

Nitroglycerin transdermal system

(nye-troh-**GLIH**-sir-in)

PREGNANCY CATEGORY: C
CLASSIFICATION(S):
Vasodilator, coronary
Rx: Deponit 0.2 mg/hr and 0.4 mg/hr; Minitran 0.1 mg/hr, 0.2 mg/hr; 0.4 mg/hr, and 0.6 mg/hr; Nitrek 0.2 mg/hr, 0.4 mg/hr; and 0.6 mg/hr; Nitrodisc 0.2 mg/hr, 0.3 mg/hr, and 0.4 mg/hr; Nitro-Dur 0.1 mg/hr, 0.2 mg/hr, 0.3 mg/hr, 0.4 mg/hr, 0.6 mg/hr, and 0.8 mg/hr; Transderm-Nitro 0.1 mg/hr, 0.2 mg/hr, 0.4 mg/hr, 0.6 mg/hr, and 0.8 mg/hr

SEE ALSO *ANTIANGINAL DRUGS, NITRATES/NITRITES.*

ACTION/KINETICS
Onset: 30–60 min; **duration:** 8–24 hr. The amount released each hour is indicated in the name.

USES
Prophylaxis of angina pectoris due to CAD. *NOTE:* There is some evidence that nitroglycerin patches stop preterm labor. Also, high-dose nitrate therapy with an ACE inhibitor may cause significant, progressive, and long-term enhancement of exercise tolerance within 2 months of initiation of nitrate therapy.

N

SPECIAL CONCERNS

Dosage has not been established in children.

HOW SUPPLIED

Film, Extended Release: 0.1 mg/hr, 0.2 mg/hr, 0.3 mg/hr, 0.4 mg/hr, 0.6 mg/hr, 0.8 mg/hr

DOSAGE

• TOPICAL PATCH

Initial: 0.2–0.4 mg/hr (initially the smallest available dose in the dosage series) applied each day to skin site free of hair and free of excessive movement (e.g., chest, upper arm). **Maintenance:** Additional systems or strengths may be added depending on the clinical response.

NURSING CONSIDERATIONS

SEE ALSO *NURSING CONSIDERATIONS* FOR *ANTIANGINAL DRUGS, NITRATES/NITRITES*.

ADMINISTRATION/STORAGE

1. Follow instructions for specific products on package insert.
2. When terminating therapy, gradually reduce the dose and frequency of application over 4–6 weeks.
3. Tolerance is a significant factor affecting efficacy if the system is used continuously for more than 12 hr/day. Thus, a dosage regimen would include a daily period where the patch is on for 12–14 hr and a period of 10–12 hr when the patch is off (i.e., while asleep).
4. Remove patch before defibrillating as patch may explode.
5. The various products differ in the mechanism for the delivery system; the most important factor is the amount of drug released per hour. A wide range of client variability will be noted. Variables in the absorption rate include skin, physical exercise, and elevated ambient temperature.

CLIENT/FAMILY TEACHING

1. Apply only as directed at the same time each day. Dry skin completely before applying to an area free of hair.
2. Remove old pad and rotate application sites each day to avoid skin irritation. Do not apply to distal extremities or to skin that is irritated, abraded, or scarred.
3. Date patch as a reminder that drug has been administered.
4. Once applied, do not disturb or open patch. Do not stop abruptly.
5. Remove at bedtime or as directed to prevent a diminished response (tolerance) to the drug. Remember to reapply a new system upon awakening the next morning.
6. Bathing or swimming should not interfere with therapy.

OUTCOMES/EVALUATE

Control/prevention of anginal episodes

Nitroglycerin translingual spray

(nye-troh-**GLIH**-sir-in)

PREGNANCY CATEGORY: C

CLASSIFICATION(S):

Vasodilator, coronary

Rx: Nitrolingual, Nitrolingual Pumpspray

SEE ALSO *ANTIANGINAL DRUGS, NITRATES/NITRITES*.

ACTION/KINETICS

Onset: 2 min; **duration:** 30–60 min.

USES

Coronary artery disease to relieve an acute attack or used prophylactically 10–15 min before beginning activities that can cause an acute anginal attack.

SPECIAL CONCERNS

Dosage has not been established in children.

HOW SUPPLIED

Aerosol Spray: 0.4 mg/metered dose; *Pumpspray:* 200 doses/bottle

DOSAGE

• SPRAY

Termination of acute attack.

One to two metered doses (400–800 mcg) on or under the tongue q 5 min as needed; no more than three metered doses should be administered within a 15-min period.

Prophylaxis.

One to two metered doses 5–10 min before beginning activities that might precipitate an acute attack.

NURSING CONSIDERATIONS

SEE ALSO *NURSING CONSIDERATIONS* FOR *ANTIANGINAL DRUGS, NITRATES/NITRITES*.

CLIENT/FAMILY TEACHING

1. Do *not* inhale the spray. Spray under or on the tongue 5-10 min before anticipated activity or when pain experienced.
2. Seek immediate medical attention if chest pain persists.
3. Have family/significant other learn CPR.

OUTCOMES/EVALUATE

Control/prevention of acute anginal episodes

Nitroprusside sodium

(nye-troh-**PRUS**-eyed)

PREGNANCY CATEGORY: C
CLASSIFICATION(S):
Antihypertensive, peripheral vasodilator
Rx: Nitropress

ACTION/KINETICS

Direct action on vascular smooth muscle, leading to peripheral vasodilation of arteries and veins. Acts on excitation-contraction coupling of vascular smooth muscle by interfering with both influx and intracellular activation of calcium. No effect on smooth muscle of the duodenum or uterus and is more active on veins than on arteries. May also improve CHF by decreasing systemic resistance, preload and afterload reduction, and improved CO. **Onset** (drug must be given by IV infusion): 0.5–1 min; **peak effect:** 1–2 min; **t1/2:** 2 min; **duration:** Up to 10 min after infusion stopped. Reacts with hemoglobin to produce cyanmethemoglobin and cyanide ion. Caution must be exercised as nitroprusside injection can result in toxic levels of cyanide. However, when used briefly or at low infusion rates, the cyanide produced reacts with thiosulfate to produce thiocyanate, which is excreted in the urine.

USES

(1) Hypertensive crisis to reduce BP immediately. (2) To produce controlled hypotension during anesthesia to reduce bleeding. (3) Acute CHF. *Investigational:* In combination with dopamine for acute MI. Left ventricular failure with coadministration of oxygen, morphine, and a loop diuretic.

CONTRAINDICATIONS

Compensatory hypertension where the primary hemodynamic lesion is aortic coarctation or AV shunting. Use to produce controlled hypotension during surgery in clients with known inadequate cerebral circulation or in moribund clients. Clients with congenital optic atrophy or tobacco amblyopia (both of which are rare). Acute CHF associated with decreased peripheral vascular resistance (e.g., high-output heart failure that may be seen in endotoxic sepsis). Lactation.

SPECIAL CONCERNS

Use with caution in hypothyroidism, liver or kidney impairment, during lactation, and in the presence of increased ICP. Geriatric clients may be more sensitive to the hypotensive effects of nitroprusside; also, a decrease in dose may be necessary in these clients due to age-related decreases in renal function.

SIDE EFFECTS

Excessive hypotension. ***Large doses may lead to cyanide toxicity.***

Following rapid BP reduction.

Dizziness, nausea, restlessness, headache, sweating, muscle twitching, palpitations, abdominal pain, apprehension, retching, retrosternal discomfort. **Other side effects:** Bradycardia, tachycardia, ECG changes, venous streaking, rash, vomiting or skin rash, methemoglobinemia, decreased platelet aggregation, flushing, hypothyroidism, ileus, irritation at injection site, hypothyroidism. **Symptoms of thiocyanate toxicity:** Blurred vision, tinnitus, confusion, hyperreflexia, seizures. **CNS symptoms (transitory):** Restlessness, agitation, increased ICP, and muscle twitching.

N

OD OVERDOSE MANAGEMENT
Symptoms: Excessive hypotension, cyanide toxicity, thiocyanate toxicity.
Treatment:
• Measure cyanide levels and blood gases to determine venous hyperoxemia or acidosis.
• To treat cyanide toxicity, discontinue nitroprusside and give sodium nitrite, 4–6 mg/kg (about 0.2 mL/kg) over 2–4 min (to convert hemoglobin into methemoglobin); follow by sodium thiosulfate, 150–200 mg/kg (about 50 mL of the 25% solution). This regimen can be given again, at half the original doses, after 2 hr.

DRUG INTERACTIONS
Concomitant use of other antihypertensives, volatile liquid anesthetics, or certain depressants ↑ nitroprusside response.

HOW SUPPLIED
Powder for injection: 50 mg/vial

DOSAGE
• **IV INFUSION ONLY**
Hypertensive crisis.
Adults: Average, 3 mcg/kg/min. **Range:** 0.3–10 mcg/kg/min. Smaller dose is required for clients receiving other antihypertensives. **Pediatric:** 1.4 mcg/kg/min adjusted slowly depending on the response.

Monitor BP and use as guide to regulate rate of administration to maintain desired antihypertensive effect. Do not exceed a rate of administration of 10 mcg/kg/min.

NURSING CONSIDERATIONS

SEE ALSO *NURSING CONSIDERATIONS* FOR *ANTIHYPERTENSIVE AGENTS*.

ADMINISTRATION/STORAGE
IV 1. Dissolve contents of the vial (50 mg) in 2–3 mL of D5W. This stock solution must be diluted further in 250–1,000 mL D5W.
2. If protected from light, reconstituted solution stable for 24 hr.
3. Discard solutions that are any color but light brown.
4. Do not add any other drug or preservative to solution.
5. Protect dilute solutions during administration by wrapping bag and tubing with opaque material such as aluminum foil or foil-lined bags; change setup every 24 hr. Explain that covering the IV bag protects the medication from light and maintains drug stability. Administer IV solution with an electronic infusion device in a monitored environment.
6. Cyanide toxicity is possible if more than 500 mcg/kg nitroprusside is given faster than 2 mcg/kg/min. To reduce this possibility, sodium thiosulfate can be co-infused with nitroprusside at rates of 5–10 times that of nitroprusside.
7. Protect drug from heat, light, and moisture. Store at 15–30°C (59–86°F).

ASSESSMENT
1. Document symptom characteristics and other therapies trialed.
2. Note any hypothyroidism or B_{12} deficiency.
3. Monitor CBC, electrolytes, ABGs, PAWP, renal and LFT's.

INTERVENTIONS
1. Monitor VS, I&O, and ECG. Monitor BP closely and titrate infusion.
2. Observe for symptoms of thiocyanate toxicity. Evaluate thiocyanate levels q 24–48 hr; levels should be less than 100 mcg thiocyanate/mL or 3 µmol cyanide/mL. Metabolic acidosis may precede cyanide toxicity.

CLIENT/FAMILY TEACHING
Drug is given in a monitored environment to rapidly lower BP and to reduce the workload of the heart. Aluminum foil or foil-lined bags are used to protect solutions during administration from light and to maintain drug stability.

OUTCOMES/EVALUATE
• ↓ BP
• Improved S&S of refractory CHF

Nizatidine
(nye-**ZAY**-tih-deen)

PREGNANCY CATEGORY: C
CLASSIFICATION(S):
Histamine H-2 receptor blocking drug
Rx: Axid
✱**Rx:** Apo-Nizatidine, Novo-Nizatidine
OTC: Axid AR

SEE ALSO *HISTAMINE H_2 ANTAGONISTS*.

ACTION/KINETICS

Decreases gastric acid secretion by blocking the effect of histamine on histamine H_2 receptors. Does not affect the P-450 and P-448 drug metabolizing enzymes.**Onset:** 30 min. **Peak plasma levels:** 0.5–3 hr after a PO dose. **Time to peak effect:** 0.5–3 hr. **Duration, nocturnal:** Up to 12 hr; **basal:** Up to 8 hr. **t½:** 1–2 hr. Approximately 60% of a PO dose is excreted unchanged in the urine. Clients with moderate to severe renal impairment manifest a significant prolongation of t½ with decreased clearance.

USES

(1) Treatment of acute duodenal ulcer and maintenance following healing of a duodenal ulcer. (2) GERD, including erosive and ulcerative esophagitis. (3) Short-term treatment of benign gastric ulcer. (4) OTC use to prevent meal-induced heartburn.

CONTRAINDICATIONS

Hypersensitivity to H_2 receptor antagonists. Cirrhosis of the liver, impaired renal or hepatic function. Lactation.

SPECIAL CONCERNS

Safety and efficacy have not been determined in children.

SIDE EFFECTS

CNS: Headache, fatigue, somnolence, insomnia, dizziness, abnormal dreams, anxiety, nervousness, confusion (rare). **GI:** N&V, diarrhea, pancreatitis, constipation, abdominal discomfort, flatulence, dyspepsia, anorexia, dry mouth. **Dermatologic:** Exfoliative dermatitis, erythroderma, pruritus, urticaria, erythema multiforme. **CV:** Asymptomatic VT; ***rarely, cardiac arrhythmias or arrest following rapid IV use.*** **Respiratory:** Rhinitis, pharyngitis, sinusitis, cough. **Body as a whole:** Asthenia, back pain, chest pain, infection, fever, myalgia. **Miscellaneous:** Impotence, loss of libido, thrombocytopenia, sweating, gynecomastia, hyperuricemia, eosinophilia, gout, and cholestatic or hepatocellular effects (resulting in increased AST, ALT, or alkaline phosphatase).

LABORATORY TEST CONSIDERATIONS

False + test for urobilinogen.

DRUG INTERACTIONS

Antacids containing Al and Mg hydroxides / ↓ Nizatidine absorption by about 10%
Aspirin, high doses / ↑ Salicylate serum levels
Simethicone / ↓ Nizatidine absorption by about 10%

HOW SUPPLIED

Capsule: 150 mg, 300 mg; *Tablet:* 75 mg

DOSAGE

Axid

• **CAPSULES**

Active duodenal ulcer.

Adults: Either 300 mg once daily at bedtime or 150 mg b.i.d. If the C_{CR} is 20–50 mL/min: 150 mg/day; if C_{CR} is less than 20 mL/min: 150 mg every other day.

Prophylaxis following healing of duodenal ulcer.

Adults: 150 mg/day at bedtime. If C_{CR} is 20–50 mL/min: 150 mg every other day; if C_{CR} is less than 20 mL/min: 150 mg every 3 days.

Treatment of benign gastric ulcer.

Adults: 150 mg b.i.d. or 300 mg at bedtime

GERD, including erosive and ulcerative esophagitis.

Adults: 150 mg b.i.d.

Axid AR

• **TABLETS**

Heartburn.

1 tablet b.i.d.

NURSING CONSIDERATIONS

SEE ALSO NURSING CONSIDERATIONS FOR HISTAMINE H_2 ANTAGONISTS.

ADMINISTRATION/STORAGE

1. Maintain treatment for active duodenal ulcer for up to 8 weeks.
2. Gastric malignancy may be present even though a clinical response to nizatidine has occurred.
3. Doses of 150 and 300 mg can be mixed with commercial juices (apple juice, *Gatorade, Ocean Spray,* and others); such preparations are stable for 48 hr when refrigerated. However, a

N

10% loss in potency is seen if mixed with *V8* or *Cran-Grape* juices.

ASSESSMENT

1. Document type, onset, location, and characteristics of symptoms.
2. Note any allergies to H_2 receptor antagonists.
3. Monitor hepatic and renal function studies; reduce dosage with renal insufficiency.
4. Note *H. pylori* results and diagnostic findings, i.e., radiographic and/or endoscopic.

CLIENT/FAMILY TEACHING

1. Take at bedtime due to potential sedative effects.
2. Use caution when performing tasks that require mental alertness until drug effects realized.
3. Continue to take as ordered even if symptoms subside.
4. Report any rashes, flaking of skin, or extreme sleepiness.
5. Avoid alcohol, caffeine, spicy foods, and aspirin-containing products.
6. Do not smoke, as this interferes with drug's effects.

OUTCOMES/EVALUATE

Improvement in ulcer pain/irritation; ↓ GERD S&S

N

—***COMBINATION DRUG***—

Norelgestromin/ Ethinyl estradiol transdermal system

(**nor**-el-**JES**-troh-min/**ETH**-ih-nill **es**-troh-**DYE**-all)

PREGNANCY CATEGORY: X
CLASSIFICATION(S):
Contraceptive Patch
Rx: Ortho Evra

SEE ALSO *ORAL CONTRACEPTIVES* SINCE CONTRADINDICATIONS, SPECIAL CONCERNS, SIDE EFFECTS, AND DRUG INTERACTIONS ARE SIMILAR.

CONTENT

Each patch contains norelgestromin, 6 mg and ethinyl estradiol, 0.75 mg with release rates of 0.15 mg norelgestromin and 0.02 mg ethinyl estradiol per day.

USES

Prevention of pregnancy. System uses a 4-week cycle.

DOSAGE

• **TRANSDERMAL PATCH**

Prevention of pregnancy.

A new patch is applied each week for 3 weeks (21 days total). Week 4 is patch-free. Apply a new patch on the same day of the week.

NURSING CONSIDERATIONS

SEE ALSO *NURSING CONSIDERATIONS* FOR *ORAL CONTRACEPTIVES*

ADMINISTRATION/STORAGE

1. Apply each new patch on the same day of the week —known as "Patch Change Day." The patch can be changed any time during the change day. Apply each new patch to a new spot on the skin to avoid irritation, although the same anatomic area can be used. Only 1 patch is worn at a time.
2. On the day after week 4 ends, a new 4-week cycle is started by applying a new patch. There should never be more than a 7 day patch-free interval between dosing cycles since the woman may not be protected from pregnancy and back-up contraceptive (e.g., condoms, spermicide, diaphragm) must be used for 7 days.
3. The client has two options for determining the day on which the patch is applied:
   • Apply the first patch during the first 24 hr of the menstrual period. If therapy starts after day 1 of the menstrual cycle, use a nonhormonal back-up contraceptive (e.g., condoms, spermicide, diaphragm) for the first 7 consecutive days of the first treatment cycle.
   • Apply the first patch on the first Sunday after the menstrual period starts. Back-up contraceptive must be used for the first week of the first cycle.
4. Apply the patch to clean, dry, intact, healthy skin on the buttock, abdomen, upper arm, or upper torso where it will not be rubbed by tight clothing. Do not place the patch on red, irritated, or cut skin or on the breasts.
5. To prevent interference with the adhesive properties of the patch, do

not apply make-up, creams, lotions, powders, or other topical products to the skin area where the patch will be placed.

6. The following guidelines are used if a patch is partially or completely detached:

• If the patch is detached for up to 24 hr, try to reapply to the same place or replace it with a new patch immediately. No back-up contraceptive is required. The "patch change day" will remain the same.

• If the patch is detached for more than 24 hr or if the woman is not sure how long the patch has been detached, stop the current contraceptive cycle. Start a new cycle by applying a new patch. Note that there is now a new "day 1" and a new "patch change day." Back-up contraceptive (e.g., condoms, spermicide, diaphragm) must be used for the first week of the new cycle.

• Do not reapply a patch if it is no longer sticky, if it has become stuck to itself or another surface, if it has other material stuck to it, or if has previously become loose or fallen off. If a patch cannot be reapplied, apply a new patch immediately. Do not use supplemental adhesives or wraps to hold the patch in place.

7. If the woman forgets to change her patch at the start of any patch cycle (week 1/day 1), apply a new patch as soon as she remembers. Note there is now a new "patch change day" and a new "day 1." Back-up contraceptive (e.g., condoms, spermicide, diaphragm) must be used for the first week of the new cycle.

Use the following guidelines if the woman forgets to change her patch in the middle of the patch cycle (week 2/day 8 or week 3/day 15):

• If the woman forgets for 1 or 2 days (up to 48 hr), apply a new patch immediately. Apply the next patch on the usual "patch change day". No back-up contraceptive is needed.

• If the women forgets for more than 2 days (over 48 hr), stop the current contraceptive cycle and start a new 4-week cycle immediately by putting on a new patch. Note there is now a new "patch change day" and a new "day 1." Back-up contraceptive must be used for 1 week.

• If the woman forgets to remove the patch at the end of the patch cycle (week 4/day 22), take off the patch as soon as she remembers. Start the next cycle on the usual "patch change day" which is the day after day 28. No back-up contraceptive is needed.

8. If the woman wishes to change her patch change day, complete the current cycle, removing the third patch on the correct day. During the patch-free week, an earlier patch change day can be selected by applying a new patch on the desired day. In no case should there be more than 7 consecutive patch-free days.

9. If the woman is switching from an oral contraceptive to the patch, apply the patch on the first day of withdrawal bleeding. If there is no withdrawal bleeding within 5 days of the last hormone-containing tablet, pregnancy must be ruled out. If therapy starts later than the first day of withdrawal bleeding, use a nonhormal contraceptive for 7 days. If more than 7 days have elapsed after taking the last active oral contraceptive tablet, there is the possibility of ovulation and conception.

10. A woman who wishes to use the patch after childbirth cannot be breastfeeding. Contraception using the patch should start no sooner than 4 weeks after childbirth. If a woman begins using the patch postpartum and has not yet had a period, consider the possibility that ovulation and conception may occur prior to the use of the patch. An additional method of contraception (e.g., condoms, spermicide, diaphragm) must be used for the first 7 days.

11. After an abortion or miscarriage that occurs during the first trimester, the patch may be started immediately. If use of the patch is not started within 5 days following a first trimester abortion, follow the instructions for a

N

woman starting a patch for the first time. In the meantime, a nonhormonal contraceptive must be used as ovulation may occur within 10 days after an abortion or miscarriage. Do not begin using the patch earlier than 4 weeks after a second trimester abortion or miscarriage.
12. Continue treatment if breakthrough bleeding or spotting occurs on days that the patch is worn. If breakthrough bleeding persists longer than a few cycles, consider a cause other than the patch.
13. If no withdrawal bleeding occurs during the patch-free week, resume treatment on the next scheduled change day. If the patch has been used correctly, the absence of withdrawal bleeding does not necessarily mean pregnancy. However, consider the possibility of pregnancy, especially if no withdrawal bleeding occurs in 2 consecutive cycles. If pregnancy is confirmed, discontinue the patch.
14. If the patch causes uncomfortable irritation, remove and apply a new patch to a different location until the next change day.
15. If the woman has not followed the prescribed schedule, consider the possibility of pregnancy at the time of the first missed period.
16. Store patches in their protective pouches. Apply immediately after removing the patch from the protective pouch. Do not store in the refrigerator or freezer.
17. Used patches still contain some active hormones. Thus, carefully fold each patch in half so that it sticks to itself before disposal.

CLIENT/FAMILY TEACHING

1. The patch is placed on the skin to provide a hormonal form of birth control.
2. A new patch is applied each week for 3 weeks (21 days total). Week 4 is patch-free. Apply a new patch on the same day of the week.
3. Apply the patch to clean, dry, intact, healthy skin on the buttock, abdomen, upper arm, or upper torso where it will not be rubbed by tight clothing. Do not place the patch on red, irritated, or cut skin or on the breasts.
4. To prevent interference witih the adhesive properties of the patch, do not apply make-up, creams, lotions, powders, or other topical products to the skin area where the patch will be placed.
5. Follow administration guidelines carefully especially if patch change day is missed, or starting after an abortion, or after childbirth, or if the patch falls off.
6. Have additional nonhormonal form of reliable birth control available in the event the patch becomes disengaged or is not tolerated.
7. Patch does not prevent the transmission of STDs, must use barrier protection.

OUTCOMES/EVALUATE

Prevention of pregnancy

Norfloxacin

(nor-**FLOX**-ah-sin)

PREGNANCY CATEGORY: C
CLASSIFICATION(S):
Antibiotic, fluoroquinolone
Rx: Chibroxin Ophthalmic Solution, Noroxin
Rx: Apo-Norflox, Noroxin Ophthalmic Solution, Novo-Norfloxacin, Riva-Norfloxacin

SEE ALSO *ANTI-INFECTIVES* AND *FLUOROQUINOLONES*.

ACTION/KINETICS

Active against gram-positive and gram-negative organisms by inhibiting bacterial DNA synthesis. Not effective against obligate anaerobes. **Peak plasma levels:** 1.4–1.6 mcg/mL after 1–2 hr following a dose of 400 mg and 2.5 mcg/mL 1–2 hr after a dose of 800 mg. **t½:** 3–4.5 hr. Food decreases the absorption of norfloxacin. Approximately 30% excreted unchanged in the urine and 30% through the feces.

USES

Systemic: (1) Uncomplicated UTIs (including cystitis) caused by *Escherichia coli, Klebsiella pneumoniae, Enterobacter cloacae, Proteus mirabilis, P. vulgaris, Pseudomonas aeruginosa, Citrobacter freundii, Staphylococcus aureus, S.*

epidermidis, Enterococcus faecalis, Enterobacter aerogenes, S. saprophyticus, and *S. agalactiae.* (2) Complicated UTIs caused by *Enterococcus faecalis, E. coli, K. pneumoniae, P. mirabilis, P. aeruginosa,* or *Serratia marcescens.* (3) Urethral gonorrhea and endocervical gonococcal infections due to penicillinase- or non-penicillinase-producing *Neisseria gonorrhoeae.* (4) Prostatitis due to *E. coli.* **Ophthalmic:** Superficial ocular infections involving the cornea or conjunctiva due to *Staphylococcus aureus, Streptococcus pneumoniae, E. coli, Haemophilus influenzae, S. epidermidis, Acinetobacter calcoaceticus, Aeromonas hydrophila, Proteum mirabilis, Pseudomonas aeruginosa, Serratia marcescens, S. warnerii.*

CONTRAINDICATIONS

Hypersensitivity to nalidixic acid, cinoxacin, or norfloxacin. Lactation, infants, and children. Ophthalmic use for dendritic keratitis, vaccinia, varicella, mycobacterial infections of the eye, fungal disease of the eye, and use with steroid combinations after uncomplicated removal of a corneal foreign body.

SPECIAL CONCERNS

Use with caution in clients with a history of seizures and in impaired renal function. Geriatric clients eliminate norfloxacin more slowly.

SIDE EFFECTS

See also *Side Effects* for *Fluoroquinolones.*

GI: N&V, diarrhea, abdominal pain or discomfort, dry/painful mouth, dyspepsia, flatulence, constipation, pseudomembranous colitis, stomatitis. **CNS:** Headache, dizziness, fatigue, malaise, drowsiness, depression, insomnia, confusion, psychoses. **Hematologic:** Decreased hematocrit, eosinophilia, leukopenia, neutropenia, either increased or decreased platelets. **Dermatologic:** Photosensitivity, rash, pruritus, exfoliative dermatitis, ***toxic epidermal necrolysis,*** erythema, erythema multiforme, ***Stevens-Johnson syndrome.*** **Other:** Paresthesia, hypersensitivity, fever, visual disturbances, hearing loss, crystalluria, cylindruria, candiduria, myoclonus (rare), hepatitis, pancreatitis, arthralgia.

Following ophthalmic use: Conjunctival hyperemia, photophobia, chemosis, bitter taste in mouth.

LABORATORY TEST CONSIDERATIONS

↑ AST, ALT, alkaline phosphatase, BUN, serum creatinine, and LDH.

ADDITIONAL DRUG INTERACTIONS

Nitrofurantoin ↓ antibacterial effect of norfloxacin.

HOW SUPPLIED

Ophthalmic solution: 0.3%; *Tablet:* 400 mg

DOSAGE

• TABLETS

Uncomplicated UTIs due to E. coli, K. pneumoniae, *or* P. mirabilis.

400 mg q 12 hr for 3 days.

Uncomplicated UTIs due to other organisms.

400 mg q 12 hr for 7–10 days.

Complicated UTIs.

400 mg q 12 hr for 10–21 days. Maximum dose for UTIs should not exceed 800 mg/day.

Uncomplicated gonorrhea.

800 mg as a single dose.

Impaired renal function, with C_{CR} equal to or less than 30 mL/min/1.73 m^2.

400 mg/day for appropriate duration for infection present.

Prostatis due to E. coli.

400 mg q 12 hr for 28 days.

• OPHTHALMIC SOLUTION

Acute infections.

Initially, 1–2 gtt to the affected eye(s) q.i.d. for 7 (or less) days. For more serious infections, the first day of therapy may be 1 or 2 gtt q 2 hr during waking hours.

NURSING CONSIDERATIONS

SEE ALSO ***NURSING CONSIDERATIONS FOR FLUOROQUINOLONES.***

ASSESSMENT

1. Document indications for therapy, location, onset and characteristics of symptoms. List other agents trialed and outcome.
2. Note any seizure disorder or impaired renal/liver function; reduce dose with impaired function.

N

3. Assess CBC and cultures.
4. Determine if pregnant.

CLIENT/FAMILY TEACHING

1. Take 1 hr before or 2 hr after meals, with a glass of water; food decreases drug absorption. Antacids should not be taken with or for 2 hr after dosing.
2. Take at evenly spaced intervals, generally every 12 hr.
3. To prevent crystalluria consume 2–3 L/day of fluids.
4. Use caution if operating equipment or driving a motor vehicle; may cause dizziness.
5. Females of childbearing age should practice reliable contraception.
6. Avoid prolonged sun exposure; wear sunglasses, protective clothing, and a sunscreen to prevent photosensitivity reactions.
7. Report any unusual or new side effects or lack of response.

OUTCOMES/EVALUATE

- Negative culture reports
- Symptomatic improvement (with UTI: ↓ dysuria, hematuria, and frequency; with ophthalmic use: ↓ itching, burning, and discharge).

N

Nortriptyline hydrochloride

(nor-**TRIP**-tih-leen)

PREGNANCY CATEGORY: C
CLASSIFICATION(S):
Antidepressant, tricyclic
Rx: Aventyl, Pamelor
***Rx:** Alti-Nortriptyline Hydrochloride, Apo-Nortriptyline, Gen-Nortriptyline, Norventyl, Novo-Nortriptyline, Nu-Nortriptyline, PMS-Nortriptyline

SEE ALSO *ANTIDEPRESSANTS, TRICYCLIC.*

ACTION/KINETICS

Manifests moderate anticholinergic and sedative effects but slight orthostatic hypotensive effects. **Effective plasma levels:** 50–150 ng/mL. **$t^1/_2$:** 18–44 hr. **Time to reach steady state:** 4–19 days.

USES

(1) Treatment of symptoms of depression. (2) Chronic, severe neurogenic pain. (3) Dermatologic disorders including chronic urticaria, angioedema, and nocturnal pruritus in atopic eczema. (4) Assist with smoking cessation (second-line therapy).

CONTRAINDICATIONS

Use in children (safety and efficacy have not been determined).

SIDE EFFECTS

See *Antidepressants, Tricyclic.*

LABORATORY TEST CONSIDERATIONS

↓ Urinary 5-HIAA.

HOW SUPPLIED

Capsule: 10 mg, 25 mg, 50 mg, 75 mg; *Solution:* 10 mg base/5 mL

DOSAGE

- **CAPSULES, ORAL SOLUTION**

Depression.

Adults: 25 mg t.i.d.–q.i.d. Dose individualized; begin at a low dosage and increase as needed. **Doses above 150 mg/day are not recommended. Adolescent and elderly clients:** 30–50 mg/day in divided doses or total daily dose may be given once/day.

Dermatologic disorders.

75 mg/day.

Smoking cessation.

5-100 mg/day for 12 weeks.

NURSING CONSIDERATIONS

SEE ALSO *NURSING CONSIDERATIONS FOR ANTIDEPRESSANTS, TRICYCLIC.*

ADMINISTRATION/STORAGE

Store at controlled room temperatures.

ASSESSMENT

Document indications for therapy, type, onset, and characteristics of symptoms. Identify any causative factors and rate pain when indicated.

CLIENT/FAMILY TEACHING

1. Take after meals and at bedtime to minimize GI upset.
2. May take several weeks before beneficial effects noted. Do not stop suddenly after long term use.
3. Take at bedtime with chronic pain conditions to minimize daytime sedation. Avoid activities that require mental alertness until drug effects realized.

4. Report any unusual or intolerable side effects. May require dosage adjustment or change in therapy.
5. Avoid alcohol, and CNS depressants.
6. May experience photosensitivity, use precautions.

OUTCOMES/EVALUATE

- Control of symptoms of depression (↓ fatigue, improved sleeping/eating patterns, effective coping)
- ↓ Nocturnal pruritus
- Relief of chronic neurogenic pain

Nystatin

(nye-**STAT**-in)

PREGNANCY CATEGORY: C (A FOR VAGINAL USE)
CLASSIFICATION(S):
Antifungal
Rx: Oral Suspension: Mycostatin, Nilstat, Nystex, **Tablets:** Mycostatin., **Topical Cream/Ointment:** Mycostatin, Nilstat, Nystex., **Topical Powder:** Mycostatin, Pedi-Dri., **Troches:** Mycostatin Pastilles., **Vaginal Tablets:** Mycostatin.
✱Rx: Topical Cream/Ointment: Nyaderm, **Topical Powder:** Candistatin

SEE ALSO *ANTI-INFECTIVES*.

ACTION/KINETICS

Derived from *Streptomyces noursei*; is both fungistatic and fungicidal against all species of *Candida*. Binds to fungal cell membranes (sterols), resulting in altered cellular permeability and leakage of potassium and other essential intracellular components. Poorly absorbed from the GI tract; unabsorbed nystatin is excreted in the feces.

USES

Candida infections of the skin, mucous membranes, GI tract, vagina, and mouth (thrush). The drug is too toxic for systemic infections although it can be given PO for intestinal moniliasis infections, as it is not absorbed from the GI tract.

CONTRAINDICATIONS

Use for systemic mycoses. Use of topical products in or around the eyes.

SPECIAL CONCERNS

Do not use occlusive dressings when treating candidiasis. Do not use lozenges in children less than 5 years of age.

SIDE EFFECTS

Nystatin has few toxic effects.
GI: Epigastric distress, N&V, diarrhea.
Other: Rarely, irritation.

HOW SUPPLIED

Cream: 100,000 U/gm; *Lozenge/troche:* 200,000 U; *Ointment:* 100,000 U/gm; *Powder:* 100,000 U/gm; *Suspension:* 100,000 U/mL; *Tablet, Oral:* 500,000 U; *Tablet, Vaginal:* 100,000 U

DOSAGE

• LOZENGE, ORAL SUSPENSION, TABLETS

Intestinal candidiasis.

Tablets, 500,000–1,000,000 units t.i.d.; continue treatment for 48 hr after cure to prevent relapse.

Oral candidiasis.

Oral Suspension, adults and children: 400,000–600,000 units q.i.d. (½ dose in each side of mouth, held as long as possible before swallowing); **infants:** 200,000 units q.i.d. (same procedure as with adults); **premature or low birth weight infants:** 100,000 units q.i.d. **Lozenge, adults and children:** 200,000–400,000 units 4–5 times/day, up to 14 days. *NOTE:* Lozenges should not be chewed or swallowed.

• VAGINAL TABLETS

100,000 units (1 tablet) inserted in vagina once each day for 2 weeks.

• TOPICAL CREAM, OINTMENT, POWDER (100,000 UNITS/G EACH)

Apply to affected areas b.i.d.–t.i.d., or as indicated, until healing is complete.

NURSING CONSIDERATIONS

SEE ALSO *GENERAL NURSING CONSIDERATIONS* FOR *ANTI-INFECTIVES*.

ADMINISTRATION/STORAGE

1. A powder for extemporaneous compounding of the oral suspension is available. To reconstitute, add ⅛ tsp

N

of the powder (about 500,000 units) to approximately ½–1 cup water and stir well. This product is administered immediately after mixing.
2. Protect drug from heat, light, moisture, and air.
3. The suspension can be stored for 7 days at room temperature or for 10 days in the refrigerator without loss of potency.
4. For *Candida* infections of the feet, the powder can be freely dusted on the feet as well as in socks and shoes.
5. The cream is generally used in *Candida* infections involving intertriginous areas; treat moist lesions with powder.
6. Refrigerate vaginal tablets.

ASSESSMENT

1. Document onset, location, and clinical presentation of symptoms. Note any precipitating factors/triggers.
2. Assess carefully and monitor recovery; severe oral candidiasis especially after XRT may include the esophagus and require systemic therapy as opposed to topical applications.

CLIENT/FAMILY TEACHING

1. Review the appropriate method and technique for administration. Use as directed for the amount of time designated to ensure desired results.
2. Do not mix oral suspension in foods because the medication will be inactivated.
3. Drop 1 mL of oral suspension in each side of mouth or apply with a swab to treat oral moniliasis. Swish around and keep in the mouth as long as possible before swallowing.
4. For pediatric use, 250,000 units of cherry flavor nystatin has been frozen in the form of popsicles.
5. Do not use mouthwash with oral candidiasis as this may alter normal flora and promote infections.
6. Vaginal tablets may be administered PO for candidiasis. These should be sucked on as a lozenge and not chewed or swallowed.
7. Insert vaginal tablets high in vagina with applicator.
8. Continue using vaginal tablets even when menstruating; treatment should be continued for 2 weeks. Avoid tampons.
9. Continue vaginal tablets in the gravid client for 3–6 weeks before term to reduce incidence of thrush in the newborn.
10. Discontinue and report if vaginal tablets cause irritation, redness, or swelling.
11. Drug may stain; sanitary pads may help protect clothing and linens.
12. Apply cream or ointment to mycotic lesions with a swab or wear gloves to avoid direct contact with hands as contact dermatitis may ensue.
13. To prevent reinfection, avoid intercourse during therapy or use condoms. Advise partner to seek treatment if symptomatic.
14. Report lack of response, worsening of symptoms or adverse side effects .

OUTCOMES/EVALUATE

- Negative culture results
- Improvement in skin and mucous membrane irritation/lesions with less discomfort and itching

O

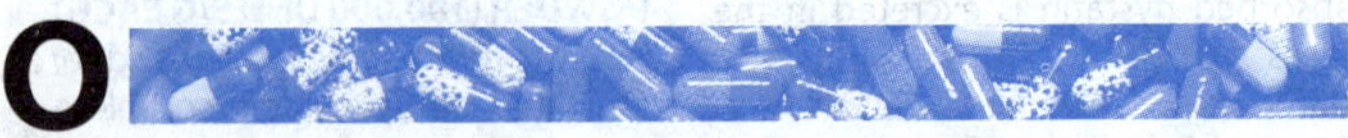

Ofloxacin

(oh-**FLOX**-ah-zeen)

PREGNANCY CATEGORY: C
CLASSIFICATION(S):
Antibiotic, fluoroquinolone

Rx: Floxin, Floxin Otic, Ocuflox
✱Rx: Apo-Oflox

SEE ALSO *ANTI-INFECTIVES*.

ACTION/KINETICS

Effective against a wide range of gram-positive and gram-negative aerobic and anaerobic bacteria. Penicillinase has no effect on the activity of ofloxacin. Widely distributed to body fluids. **Maximum serum levels:** 1–2 hr. **t½, first phase:** 5–7 hr; **second phase:** 20–25 hr. **Peak serum levels at steady state, after PO doses:** 1.5 mcg/mL after 200-mg doses, 2.4 mcg/mL after 300-mg doses, and 2.9 mcg/mL after 400-mg doses. Between 70% and 80% is excreted unchanged in the urine.

USES

Systemic: (1) Pneumonia or acute bacterial exacerbations of chronic bronchitis or community-acquired pneumonia due to *Haemophilus influenzae* or *Streptococcus pneumoniae*. Not a drug of first choice in the treatment of presumed or confirmed pneumococcal pneumonia. Not effective for syphilis. (2) Acute, uncomplicated urethral and cervical gonorrhea due to *Neisseria gonorrhoeae;* nongonococcal urethritis, and cervicitis due to *Chlamydia trachomatis.* Mixed infections of the urethra and cervix due to *N. gonorrhoeae* and *C. trachomatis.* (3) Mild to moderate skin and skin structure infections due to *Staphylococcus aureus, Streptococcus pyogenes,* or *Proteus mirabilis.* (4) Uncomplicated cystitis due to *Citrobacter diversus, Enterobacter aerogenes, E. coli, Klebsiella pneumoniae, Proteus mirabilis,* or *Pseudomonas aeruginosa.* (5) Complicated UTIs due to *Escherichia coli, K. pneumoniae, P. mirabilis, C. diversus,* or *P. aeruginosa.* (6) Prostatitis due to *E. coli.* (7) Monotherapy for PID due to *C. trachomatis* or *N. gonorrhoeae.* (8) Tuberculosis in adults.

Ophthalmic: (1) Treatment of conjunctivitis caused by *S. aureus, Staphylococcus epidermidis, S. pneumoniae, Enterobacter cloacae, H. influenzae, P. mirabilis,* and *P. aeruginosa.* (2) Corneal ulcers caused by *S. aureus, S. epidermidis, S. pneumoniae, P. aeruginosa, S. marcescens.*

Otic: (1) Otitis externa due to *S. aureus* and *P. aeruginosa* in clients one year of age and older. (2) Acute otitis media with tympanostomy tubes due to *S. aureus, S. pneumoniae, H. influenzae, Moraxella catarrhalis,* and *P. aeruginosa* (from age one to twelve). (3) Chronic suppurative otitis media due to *S. aureus, P. mirabilis,* and *P. aeruginosa* in those twelve years and older who have perforated tympanic membranes.

CONTRAINDICATIONS

Hypersensitivity to quinolone antibacterial agents. Use during lactation. Use for syphilis (ineffective). Ophthalmic use in dendritic keratitis, vaccinia, varicella, mycobacterial infections of the eye, fungal diseases of the eye, and with steroid combinations after uncomplicated removal of a corneal foreign body.

SPECIAL CONCERNS

Safety and effectiveness of the systemic forms have not been established in children, adolescents under the age of 18 years, pregnant women, and lactating women. Safety and effectiveness of the ophthalmic form have not been established in children less than 1 year of age. Use with caution in clients with known or suspected CNS disorders such as severe cerebral atherosclerosis, epilepsy, or factors that predispose to seizures.

SIDE EFFECTS

See also *Side Effects* for *Fluroquinolones*.

GI: Nausea, diarrhea, vomiting, abdominal pain or discomfort, dry or painful mouth, dyspepsia, flatulence, constipation, pseudomembranous colitis, dysgeusia, decreased appetite. **CNS:** Headache, dizziness, fatigue, malaise, somnolence, depression, insomnia, seizures, sleep disorders, nervousness, anxiety, cognitive change, dream abnormality, euphoria, hallucinations, vertigo. **CV:** Chest pain, edema, hypertension, palpitations, vasodilation. **Hypersensitivity reactions:** Dyspnea, ***anaphylaxis.*** **GU:** External genital pruritus in women, vaginitis, vaginal discharge; burning, irritation, pain, and rash of the female genitalia; glucosuria, proteinuria, hematuria, pyuria, dysmenorrhea, menorrhagia, metrorrhagia, urinary frequency or pain. **Respiratory:** Cough, rhinorrhea. **Dermatologic:** Diaphoresis, vasculitis, photosensitivity, rash, pruritus. **Hematologic:** Leukocytosis, lymphocytopenia, eosinophil-

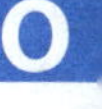

ia. **Musculoskeletal:** Asthenia, extremity pain, arthralgia, myalgia, possibility of osteochondrosis. **Miscellaneous:** Chills, malaise, syncope, hyperglycemia or hypoglycemia, whole body pain, thirst, weight loss, photophobia, trunk pain, paresthesia, visual disturbances, hypersensitivity, hearing loss, fever.

After ophthalmic use: Transient ocular burning or discomfort, stinging, redness, itching, photophobia, tearing, and dryness.

After otic use: Pruritus, application site reaction, dizziness, earache, vertigo, taste perversion, paresthesia, rash.

LABORATORY TEST CONSIDERATIONS

↑ ALT, AST.

HOW SUPPLIED

Injection: 200 mg, 400 mg; *Ophthalmic solution:* 0.3%; *Otic Solution:* 0.3%; *Tablet:* 200 mg, 300 mg, 400 mg

DOSAGE

• IV, TABLETS

Pneumonia, exacerbation of chronic bronchitis.

400 mg q 12 hr for 10 days.

Acute uncomplicated urethral or cervical gonorrhea.

One 400-mg dose. The Centers for Disease Control also recommend adding doxycycline or azithromycin.

Cervicitis/urethritis due to C. trachomatis or N. gonorrhoeae.

300 mg q 12 hr for 7 days.

Mild to moderate skin and skin structure infections.

400 mg q 12 hr for 10 days.

Uncomplicated cystitis due to E. coli *or K. pneumoniae.*

200 mg q 12 hr for 3 days.

Uncomplicated cystitis due to other organisms.

200 mg q 12 hr for 7 days.

Complicated UTIs.

200 mg q 12 hr for 10 days.

Prostatitis due to E. coli.

300 mg q 12 hr for 6 weeks.

Chlamydia.

300 mg PO b.i.d. for 7 days.

Epididymitis.

300 mg PO b.i.d. for 10 days.

PID, outpatient.

400 mg PO b.i.d. for 14 days plus metronidazole.

Tuberculosis.

Adults: 600–800 (maximum) mg/day. *NOTE:* The dose should be adjusted in clients with a C_{CR} of 50 mL/min or less. If the C_{CR} is 10–50 mL/min, the dosage interval should be q 24 hr, and if C_{CR} is less than 10 mL/min, the dose should be half the recommended dose given q 24 hr.

• OPHTHALMIC SOLUTION (0.3%)

Conjunctivitis.

Initial: 1–2 gtt in the affected eye(s) q 2–4 hr for the first 2 days; **then,** 1–2 gtt q.i.d. for seven additional days.

Bacterial corneal ulcer.

1–2 gtt q 30 min while awake. Awaken at about 4 and 6 hr after retiring and instill 1–2 gtt. **Then,** instill 1–2 gtt hourly while awake for days 3 through 7 to 9; for days 7 to 9 through treatment completion, instill 1–2 gtt q.i.d.

• OTIC SOLUTION (0.3%)

Otitis externa, acute otitis media with tympanostomy tubes.

Children, 1–12 years: 5 gtt b.i.d. for 10 days. **Children, 12 years and older:** 10 gtt b.i.d. for 10 days.

Chronic suppurative otitis media with perforated tympanic membranes.

Children,12 years and older: 10 gtt b.i.d. for 14 days.

NURSING CONSIDERATIONS

SEE ALSO *NURSING CONSIDERATIONS* FOR *FLUOROQUINOLONES* AND *ANTI-INFECTIVES*.

ADMINISTRATION/STORAGE

1. Do not take with food.
2. Store in tightly closed containers at a temperature below 30°C (86°F).
3. Do not inject the ophthalmic solution subconjunctivally and do not introduce directly into the anterior chamber of the eye.
4. Do not confuse the ophthalmic and otic dosage forms; they are not interchangeable.

IV 5. Give by IV infusion only over a period of not less than 60 min. Do not give IM, SC, IP, or intrathecally. Avoid rapid or bolus IV administration.

6. Must be diluted prior to use for a final concentration of 4 mg/mL. Can be diluted with 0.9% NaCl, D5W, D5/0.9% NaCl, 5% dextrose in lactated Ringer's,

5% sodium bicarbonate, Plasma-Lyte 56 in 5% dextrose, D5/0.45% NaCl and 0.15% KCl, sodium lactate (M/6), or water for injection.
7. The premixed bottles/flexible containers do not require further dilution as they are premixed with 5% dextrose.
8. Discard unused portions.

ASSESSMENT

1. Note any sensitivity to quinolone derivatives.
2. Document indications for therapy, type, onset, and symptom characteristics.
3. Monitor CBC, cultures, liver and renal function studies; reduce dose with altered renal function. Review other prescribed agents; probenecid may block tubular excretion.
4. Assess for any CNS disorders. Report any tremors, restlessness, confusion, and hallucinations; therapy may need to be discontinued.

CLIENT/FAMILY TEACHING

1. Do not take with food. Take PO form 1 hr before or 3 hr after meals.
2. Avoid vitamins, iron or mineral combinations, aluminum- or magnesium-based antacids 2 hr before and 2 hr after ingestion of ofloxacin.
3. Do not perform activities that require mental alertness until drug effects are realized; may cause drowsiness and lightheadedness.
4. Avoid contamination of the ophthalmic applicator tip with material from the eye or fingers.
5. Do not confuse the eye and ear dosage forms; they are not interchangeable.
6. Before using, warm ear drops by rolling the bottle in hands; instillation of cold drops may cause dizziness.
7. May experience burning, stinging, itching, or tearing after eye use; should subside.
8. Drink 2–3 L/day of fluids to assist in drug elimination.
9. Side effects include N&V and diarrhea; report if persistent.
10. Avoid direct sunlight; photosensitivity reaction may occur. If exposed, wear sunglasses, protective clothing, and sunscreen.
11. Clients with diabetes should monitor sugars closely as extreme variations may occur.

OUTCOMES/EVALUATE

Negative culture reports; symptomatic improvement

Olanzapine

(oh-**LAN**-zah-peen)

PREGNANCY CATEGORY: C
CLASSIFICATION(S):
Antipsychotic
Rx: Zyprexa, Zyprexa Zydis

ACTION/KINETICS

A thienbenzodiazepine antipsychotic believed to act by antagonizing dopamine D_{1-4} and serotonin ($5HT_2$) receptors. Also binds to muscarinic, histamine H_1, and alpha-1 adrenergic receptors, which can explain many of the side effects. Well absorbed from the GI tract. **Peak plasma levels:** 6 hr after PO dosing. Undergoes significant first-pass metabolism with about 40% metabolized before it reaches the systemic circulation. Food does not affect the rate or extent of absorption. Significantly bound to plasma proteins. Unchanged drug and metabolites are excreted through both the urine and feces.

USES

(1) Short- and long-term management (including maintenance of treatment response) of schizophrenia. (2) Short-term treatment of acute mania associated with bipolar I disorder. *Investigational:* Dementia related to Alzheimer's disease.

CONTRAINDICATIONS

Lactation.

SPECIAL CONCERNS

Use with caution in geriatric clients, as the drug may be excreted more slowly in this population. Use with caution in impaired hepatic function and in those where there is a chance of increased core body temperature (e.g., strenuous exercise, exposure to extreme heat, concomitant anticholiner-

O

gic drug administration, dehydration). Due to anticholinergic side effects, use with caution in clients with significant prostatic hypertrophy, narrow-angle glaucoma, or a history of paralytic ileus. Safety and efficacy have not been determined in children less than 18 years of age.

SIDE EFFECTS

Neuroleptic malignant syndrome: Hyperpyrexia, muscle rigidity, altered mental status, irregular pulse/BP, tachycardia, diaphoresis, cardiac dysrhythmia, rhabdomyolysis, ***acute renal failure, death.*** **GI:** Dysphagia, constipation, dry mouth, increased appetite/salivation, N&V, thirst, aphthous stomatitis, eructation, esophagitis, rectal incontinence, flatulence, gastritis, gastroenteritis, gingivitis, glossitis, hepatitis, melena, mouth ulceration, oral moniliasis, periodontal abscess, ***rectal hemorrhage,*** tongue edema. **CNS:** Tardive dyskinesia, seizures, somnolence, agitation, insomnia, nervousness, hostility, dizziness, anxiety, personality disorder, akathisia, hypertonia, tremor, amnesia, impaired articulation, euphoria, stuttering, ***suicide,*** abnormal gait, alcohol misuse, antisocial reaction, ataxia, CNS stimulation, coma, delirium, depersonalization, hypesthesia, hypotonia, incoordination, decreased libido, obsessive-compulsive symptoms, phobias, somatization, stimulant misuse, stupor, vertigo, withdrawal syndrome. **CV:** Tachycardia, orthostatic/postural hypotension, hypotension, ***CVA, hemorrhage, heart arrest,*** migraine, palpitation, vasodilation, ventricular extrasystoles. **Body as a whole:** Headache, fever, abdominal/chest pain, neck rigidity, intentional injury, flu syndrome, chills, facial edema, hangover effect, malaise, moniliasis, neck/pelvic pain, photosensitivity. **Respiratory:** Rhinitis, increased cough, pharyngitis, dyspnea, apnea, asthma, epistaxis, hemoptysis, hyperventilation, voice alteration. **GU:** PMS, hematuria, metrorrhagia, urinary incontinence, UTI, abnormal ejaculation, priapism, amenorrhea, breast pain, cystitis, decreased/increased menstruation, dysuria, female lactation, impotence, menorrhagia, polyuria, pyuria, urinary retention/frequency, impaired urination, enlarged uterine fibroids. **Hematologic:** Leukocytosis, lymphadenopathy, thrombocytopenia. **Metabolic/nutritional:** Weight gain/loss, peripheral/lower extremity edema, dehydration, hypo/hyperglycemia, hypo/hyperkalemia, hyperuricemia, hyponatremia, ketosis, water intoxication. **Musculoskeletal:** Joint/extremity pain, twitching, arthritis, back/hip pain, bursitis, leg cramps, myasthenia, rheumatoid arthritis. **Dermatologic:** Vesiculobullous rash, alopecia, contact dermatitis, dry skin, eczema, hirsutism, seborrhea, skin ulcer, urticaria. **Ophthalmic:** Amblyopia, blepharitis, corneal lesion, cataract, diplopia, dry eyes, eye hemorrhage, eye inflammation/pain, ocular muscle abnormality. **Otic:** Deafness, ear pain, tinnitus. **Miscellaneous:** DM, goiter, cyanosis, taste perversion, sleep-walking (rare).

LABORATORY TEST CONSIDERATIONS

↑ ALT, AST, GGT, alkaline phosphatase, serum prolactin, eosinophils, CPK. Hyperprolactinemia.

OD OVERDOSE MANAGEMENT

Symptoms: Drowsiness, slurred speech. Possible obtundation, seizures, dystonic reaction of the head and neck. CV symptoms, arrhythmias. *Treatment:* Establish and maintain an airway and ensure adequate oxygenation and ventilation. Gastric lavage followed by activated charcoal and a laxative can be considered, although dystonic reaction may cause aspiration with induced emesis. Begin CV monitoring immediately with continuous ECG monitoring to detect possible arrhythmias. Hypotension and circulatory collapse are treated with IV fluids or sympathomimetic agents. Do not use epinephrine, dopamine, or other sympathomimetics with beta-agonist activity, as beta stimulation may worsen hypotension.

DRUG INTERACTIONS

Antihypertensive agents / ↑ Antihypertensive effect
Carbamazepine / ↑ Olanzepine clearance R/T ↑ metabolism
CNS depressants / ↑ CNS depressant effect

Levodopa and Dopamine agonists / May antagonize the effects of levodopa and dopamine agonists
H *St. John's wort* / Possible ↓ olanzapine plasma levels R/T ↑ metabolism

HOW SUPPLIED
Tablet: 2.5 mg, 5 mg, 7.5 mg, 10 mg, 15 mg, 20 mg; *Tablets oral disintegrating:* 5 mg, 10 mg, 15 mg, 20 mg

DOSAGE

• TABLETS, TABLETS ORAL DISINTEGRATING

Schizophrenia.

Adults, initial: 5–10 mg once daily without regard to meals. Goal is 10 mg daily; increments to reach 10 mg can be in 5-mg amounts but at an interval of 1 week. Doses higher than 10 mg daily are recommended only after clinical assessment and should not be greater than 20 mg/day. The recommended initial dose is 5 mg in those who are debilitated, who have a predisposition to hypotensive reactions, who may have factors that cause a slower metabolism of olanzapine (e.g., nonsmoking female clients over 65 years of age), or who may be more sensitive to the drug. It is recommended that clients who respond to the drug be continued on it at the lowest possible dose to maintain remission with periodic evaluation to determine continued need for the drug.

Bipolar mania.

Initial:10–15 mg/day without regard to meals. Adjust dose at 5 mg increments in intervals not less than 24 hr, if needed.

Behavioral symptoms in Alzheimer's disease.

10 mg/day.

NURSING CONSIDERATIONS

ADMINISTRATION/STORAGE

Protect from light and moisture and store at a controlled room temperature of 20–25°C (68–77°F).

ASSESSMENT

1. Document onset, duration, and characteristics of symptoms; note presenting behaviors. List agents trialed and the outcome.
2. Monitor VS, ECG, CBC, liver and renal function studies. Assess carefully for dehydration especially in the elderly. Voiding before drug administration may decrease anticholinergic effects of urinary retention.

CLIENT/FAMILY TEACHING

1. To take disintegrating tablets, peel back foil on blister; do not push tablet through foil. Using dry hands, remove from foil and place entire tablet in the mouth. The tablet will disintegrate with or without liquid in about 2 min.
2. Take only as directed; do not share medications; do not exceed prescribed dosage.
3. Avoid activities or situations where overheating may occur, e.g., strenuous exercise.
4. Do not drive or perform activities that require mental alertness until drug effects realized.
5. Avoid changing positions suddenly, especially from lying to standing position R/T orthostatic effects.
6. Report any suicidal ideations, abnormal bleeding, sudden muscle pain or weakness, and irregular heart beat.
7. Avoid alcohol and any other CNS depressants or OTC agents.
8. Practice reliable birth control.
9. Report as scheduled for medication renewals, therapy sessions, and evaluation of drug effectiveness.

OUTCOMES/EVALUATE

Improved patterns of behavior with ↓ agitation, ↓ hostility, and fewer delusions.

Olopatadine hydrochloride

(oh-loh-pah-**TIH**-deen)

PREGNANCY CATEGORY: C
CLASSIFICATION(S):
Antihistamine, ophthalmic
Rx: Patanol

SEE ALSO *ANTIHISTAMINES*.

O

ACTION/KINETICS
Selective histamine H-1 receptor antagonist. Little is absorbed into the systemic circulation.
USES
Prevention of itching in allergic conjunctivitis.
CONTRAINDICATIONS
Not to be injected. Not to be instilled while the client is wearing contact lenses.
SPECIAL CONCERNS
Use with caution during lactation. Safety and efficacy have not been determined for children less than 3 years of age.
SIDE EFFECTS
Ophthalmic: Burning or stinging, dry eye, foreign body sensation, hyperemia, keratitis, lid edema, pruritus. **Nose/throat**: Pharyngitis, rhinitis, sinusitis. **Miscellaneous:** Headache, asthenia, cold syndrome, taste perversion.
HOW SUPPLIED
Solution: 0.1%

DOSAGE
- **SOLUTION (0.1%)**
  Allergic conjunctivitis.

Adults and children over 3 years of age: 1–2 drops in each affected eye b.i.d. at an interval of 6–8 hr.

NURSING CONSIDERATIONS

SEE ALSO *NURSING CONSIDERATIONS* FOR *ANTIHISTAMINES*.

ADMINISTRATION/STORAGE
Store at 4–30°C (39–86°F).
ASSESSMENT
Document indications for therapy; note onset, duration, occurrence, and characteristics of symptoms. Identify triggers.
CLIENT/FAMILY TEACHING
1. Wash hands before and after administration; do not let the dropper tip touch the eyelids or surrounding areas to prevent contamination.
2. Burning and stinging, swelling, redness, and foreign body sensation may occur; report if persistent.
3. Remove contact lens before instilling eye drops.
4. Review potential triggers and how to avoid and reduce contact to prevent increased irritation.

OUTCOMES/EVALUATE
Relief of allergic ocular manifestations.

Olsalazine sodium

(ohl-**SAL**-ah-zeen)

PREGNANCY CATEGORY: C
CLASSIFICATION(S):
Anti-inflammatory drug
Rx: Dipentum

ACTION/KINETICS
A salicylate that is converted by bacteria in the colon to 5-PAS (5-para-aminosalicylate), which exerts an anti-inflammatory effect for the treatment of ulcerative colitis. 5-PAS is slowly absorbed resulting in a high concentration of drug in the colon. The anti-inflammatory activity is likely due to inhibition of synthesis of prostaglandins in the colon. After PO use the drug is only slightly absorbed (2.4%) into systemic circulation where it has a short half-life (< 1 hr) and is more than 99% bound to plasma proteins.
USES
To maintain remission of ulcerative colitis in clients who cannot take sulfasalazine.
CONTRAINDICATIONS
Hypersensitivity to salicylates.
SPECIAL CONCERNS
Use with caution during lactation. Safety and efficacy have not been established in children. May cause worsening of symptoms of colitis.
SIDE EFFECTS
GI: Diarrhea (common), pain or cramps, nausea, dry mouth, dyspepsia, bloating, anorexia, vomiting, stomatitis. **CNS:** Headache, drowsiness, lethargy, fatigue, dizziness, vertigo. **Ophthalmic:** Dry eyes, watery eyes, blurred vision. **Miscellaneous:** Arthralgia, rash, itching, upper respiratory tract infection. *NOTE:* The following symptoms have been reported on withdrawal of therapy: diarrhea, nausea,

abdominal pain, rash, itching, headache, heartburn, insomnia, anorexia, dizziness, lightheadedness, rectal bleeding, depression.

LABORATORY TEST CONSIDERATIONS

↑ ALT, AST.

OD OVERDOSE MANAGEMENT

Symptoms: Diarrhea, decreased motor activity. *Treatment:* Treat symptoms.

HOW SUPPLIED

Capsule: 250 mg

DOSAGE

• **CAPSULES**

Adults: Total of 1 g/day in two divided doses.

NURSING CONSIDERATIONS

ASSESSMENT

1. Note any sensitivity to salicylates and/or intolerance to sulfasalazine.
2. Document indications for therapy, type, onset, and characteristics of symptoms.
3. With renal disease, monitor urinalysis, BUN, and creatinine. With chronic therapy monitor CBC and renal function studies.
4. Review radiographic/endoscopic findings.

CLIENT/FAMILY TEACHING

1. Drug should be taken with food and in evenly divided doses.
2. Report any persistent diarrhea, lethargy, fatigue, fever, or blood in the stools.

OUTCOMES/EVALUATE

Symptom remission with ulcerative colitis

Omeprazole

(oh-**MEH**-prah-zohl)

PREGNANCY CATEGORY: C

CLASSIFICATION(S):

Proton pump inhibitor

Rx: Prilosec

ACTION/KINETICS

Thought to be a gastric pump inhibitor in that it blocks the final step of acid production by inhibiting the H^+–K^+ ATPase system at the secretory surface of the gastric parietal cell. Both basal and stimulated acid secretions are inhibited. Serum gastrin levels are increased during the first 1 or 2 weeks of therapy and are maintained at such levels during the course of therapy. Because omeprazole is acid-labile, the product contains an enteric-coated granule formulation; however, absorption is rapid. **Peak plasma levels:** 0.5–3.5 hr. **Onset:** Within 1 hr. **t½:** 0.5–1 hr. **Duration:** Up to 72 hr (due to prolonged binding of the drug to the parietal H^+–K^+–ATPase enzyme). Significantly bound (95%) to plasma protein. Metabolized in the liver and inactive metabolites are excreted through the urine. Consider dosage adjustment in Asians.

USES

(1) Short-term (4 to 8-week) treatment of active duodenal ulcer, active benign gastric ulcer, erosive esophagitis (all grades), and heartburn and other symptoms associated with GERD. (2) In combination with various drugs for eradication of *Helicobacter pylori* and treatment of active duodenal ulcer. (3) Long-term maintenance therapy for healed erosive esophagitis. (4) Long-term treatment of pathologic hypersecretory conditions such as Zollinger-Ellison syndrome, multiple endocrine adenomas, and systemic mastocytosis. *Investigational:* Posterior laryngitis, enhanced efficacy of pancreatin for treating steatorrhea in cystic fibrosis.

CONTRAINDICATIONS

Lactation. Use as maintenance therapy for duodenal ulcer disease.

SPECIAL CONCERNS

Bioavailability may be increased in geriatric clients. Use with caution during lactation. Symptomatic effects with omeprazole do not preclude gastric malignancy. Safety and effectiveness have not been determined in children.

SIDE EFFECTS

CNS: Headache, dizziness. Possibly, anxiety disorders, abnormal dreams, vertigo, insomnia, nervousness, apathy, paresthesia, somnolence, depres-

O

sion, aggression, hallucinations, hemifacial dysesthesia, tremors, confusion. **GI:** Diarrhea, N&V, abdominal pain, abdominal swellling, constipation, flatulence, anorexia, fecal discoloration, esophageal candidiasis, mucosal atrophy of the tongue, dry mouth, irritable colon, gastric fundic gland polyps, gastroduodenal carcinoids. **Hepatic: *Pancreatitis.*** Overt liver disease, including hepatocellular, cholestatic, or mixed hepatitis; ***liver necrosis, hepatic failure,*** hepatic encephalopathy. **CV:** Angina, chest pain, tachycardia, bradycardia, palpitation, peripheral edema, elevated BP. **Respiratory:** URI, pharyngeal pain, bronchospasms, cough, epistaxis. **Dermatologic:** Rash, severe generalized skin reaction including ***toxic epidermal necrolysis, Stevens-Johnson syndrome;*** erythema multiforme, skin inflammation, urticaria, pruritus, alopecia, dry skin, hyperhidrosis. **GU:** UTI, acute interstitial nephritis, urinary frequency, hematuria, proteinuria, glycosuria, testicular pain, microscopic pyuria, gynecomastia. **Hematologic:** Pancytopenia, thrombocytopenia, anemia, leukocytosis, neutropenia, hemolytic anemia, ***agranulocytosis***. **Musculoskeletal:** Asthenia, back pain, myalgia, joint pain, muscle cramps, muscle weakness, leg pain. **Miscellaneous:** Rash, angioedema, fever, pain, gout, fatigue, malaise, weight gain, tinnitus, alteration in taste.

When used with clarithromycin the following *additional* side effects were noted: Tongue discoloration, rhinitis, pharyngitis, and flu syndrome.

NOTE: Data are lacking on the effect of long-term hypochlorhydria and hypergastrinemia on the risk of developing tumors.

LABORATORY TEST CONSIDERATIONS

↑ AST, ALT, gamma-glutamyl transpeptidase, alkaline phosphatase, bilirubin, serum creatinine. Glycosuria, hyponatremia, hypoglycemia.

OD OVERDOSE MANAGEMENT

Symptoms: Confusion, drowsiness, blurred vision, tachycardia, nausea, diaphoresis, flushing, headache, dry mouth. *Treatment:* Symptomatic and supportive. Omeprazole is not readily dialyzable.

DRUG INTERACTIONS

Ampicillin (esters) / Possible ↓ absorption of ampicillin esters R/T ↑ stomach pH
Clarithromycin / Possible ↑ plasma levels of both drugs
Cyanocobalamin / ↓ Cyanocobalamin absorption R/T ↑ gastric pH
Diazepam / ↑ Diazepam plasma levels R/T ↓ rate of liver metabolism
Iron salts / Possible ↓ absorption of iron salts R/T ↑ stomach pH
Ketoconazole / Possible ↓ ketoconazole absorption R/T ↑ stomach pH
Phenytoin / ↑ Plasma phenytoin levels R/T ↓ rate of liver metabolism
Sucralfate / ↓ Omeprazole absorption; take 30 min before sucralfate
Warfarin / Prolonged rate of warfarin elimination R/T ↓ rate of liver metabolism

HOW SUPPLIED

Enteric Coated Capsule: 10 mg, 20 mg, 40 mg

DOSAGE

• **CAPSULES, ENTERIC-COATED**

Active duodenal ulcer.

Adults, 20 mg/day for 4–8 weeks.

Erosive esophagitis.

Adults: 20 mg/day for 4–8 weeks. Maintenance of healing erosive esophagitis: 20 mg/day.

GERD without esophageal lesions.

20 mg/day for 4 weeks.

GERD with erosive esophgatigis.

20 mg/day for 4–8 weeks.

Treatment of H. pylori.

The following regimens may be used: (1) Clarithromycin, 500 mg b.i.d.; amoxicillin, 1 g b.i.d.; and either omeprazole, 20 mg b.i.d. or lansoprazole, 30 mg b.i.d. Each drug is given for 10 or 14 days. (2) Clarithromycin, 500 mg b.i.d.; metronidazole, 500 mg b.i.d.; and either omeprazole, 20 mg b.i.d., or lansoprazole, 30 mg b.i.d. Each drug is given for 14 days. (3) Tetracycline, 500 mg q.i.d.; metronidazole, 500 mg q.i.d., bismuth subsalicylate, 525 mg q.i.d.; and either omeprazole, 20 mg/day, or lansoprazole, 30 mg/day. Each drug is given for 14 days.

Pathologic hypersecretory conditions.

Adults, initial: 60 mg/day; then, dose individualized although doses up to

120 mg t.i.d. have been used. Daily doses greater than 80 mg should be divided.

Gastric ulcers.

Adults: 40 mg once daily for 4–8 weeks.

NURSING CONSIDERATIONS

ADMINISTRATION/STORAGE

1. Efficacy for more than 8 weeks has not been determined. However, if a client does not respond to 8 weeks of therapy, an additional 4 weeks may help. If there is a recurrence of erosive or symptomatic GERD poorly responsive to usual treatment, an additional 4 to 8 weeks of therapy may be tried.
2. Capsules should be stored in a tight container protected from light and moisture. Store between 15–30°C (59–86°F).

ASSESSMENT

1. Document indications for therapy, type, onset, triggers and characteristics of symptoms.
2. Determine if pregnant.
3. Record abdominal assessments, radiographic/endoscopic findings and *H. pylori* results.
4. Monitor CBC and LFTs; note any hepatic dysfunction.

CLIENT/FAMILY TEACHING

1. Antacids can be administered with omeprazole.
2. The capsule should be taken before eating and is to be swallowed whole; it should not be opened, chewed, or crushed.
3. Review drug associated side effects; report if diarrhea persists.
4. Report any changes in urinary elimination or pain and discomfort.
5. Avoid alcohol and OTC agents.
6. For short-term use only, drug inhibits total gastric acid secretion. Side effects of prolonged therapy and suppression of acid secretion alter bacterial colonization and lead to hypochlorhydria and hypergastrinemia which may cause an increased risk for gastric tumors.

OUTCOMES/EVALUATE

Promotion of ulcer healing; relief of pain; ↓ gastric acid production

Ondansetron hydrochloride

(on-**DAN**-sih-tron)

PREGNANCY CATEGORY: B
CLASSIFICATION(S):
Antiemetic
Rx: Zofran ODT, Zofran

ACTION/KINETICS

Cytotoxic chemotherapy is thought to release serotonin from enterochromoffin cells of the small intestine. The released serotonin may stimulate the vagal afferent nerves through the 5-HT_3 receptors, thus stimulating the vomiting reflex. Ondansetron, a 5-HT_3 antagonist, blocks this effect of serotonin. Whether the drug acts centrally and/or peripherally to antagonize the effect of serotonin is not known. **Time to peak plasma levels, after PO:** 1.7–2.1 hr. **t½, after IV use:** 3.5–4.7 hr; **after PO use:** 3.1–6.2 hr, depending on the age. A decrease in clearance and increase in half-life are observed in clients over 75 years of age, although no dosage adjustment is recommended. Clients less than 15 years of age show a shortened plasma half-life after IV use (2.4 hr). Significantly metabolized with 5% of a dose excreted unchanged in the urine.

USES

Parenteral: (1) Prevent N&V resulting from initial and repeated courses of cancer chemotherapy, including high-dose cisplatin. (2) Prophylaxis and treatment of selected cases of postoperative N&V, especially situations where there is multiple retching and long periods of N&V. **Oral:** (1) Prevention of N&V due to initial and repeated courses of cancer chemotherapy, including single-day highly emetogenic cancer chemotherapy (e.g. Cisplatin). (2) Prevention of N&V associated with radiotherapy in clients receiving either total body irradiation, single high-dose fraction, or daily fractions to the abdomen. (3) Prevention of postoperative N&V. *Investigational:* N&V due to acetamino-

O

phen poisoning, acute levodopa-induced psychosis, N&V due to prostacyclin therapy, spinal or epidural morphine-induced pruritus, social anxiety disorder, decrease in bulimic episodes in clients with bulimia nervosa. Early alcoholism to reduce intake and promote abstinence in those under age 25.

SPECIAL CONCERNS

Use with caution during lactation. Safety and effectiveness in children 3 years of age and younger are not known.

SIDE EFFECTS

GI: Diarrhea (most common), constipation, xerostomia, abdominal pain. **CNS:** Headache, dizziness, drowsiness, sedation, malaise, fatigue, anxiety, agitation, extrapyramidal syndrome, ***clonic-tonic seizures.*** **CV:** Tachycardia, chest pain, hypotension, ECG alterations, angina, bradycardia, syncope, vascular occlusive events. **Dermatologic:** Pain, redness, and burning at injection site; cold sensation, pruritus, paresthesia. **Hypersensitivity (rare):** ***Anaphylaxis, bronchospasm, shock,*** SOB, hypotension, angioedema, urticaria. **Miscellaneous:** Rash, ***bronchospasm,*** transient blurred vision, hypokalemia, weakness, fever, musculoskeletal pain, shivers, dysuria, postoperative carbon dioxide-related pain, akathisia, acute dystonic reactions, gynecologic disorder, urinary retention, wound problem.

O

LABORATORY TEST CONSIDERATIONS

↑ AST, ALT.

DRUG INTERACTIONS

Rifampin ↓ ondansetron plasma levels R/T ↑ liver metabolism.

HOW SUPPLIED

Injection: 2 mg/mL, 32 mg/50 mL; *Oral Solution:* 4 mg/5 mL; *Tablet:* 4 mg, 8 mg, 24 mg; *Tablets, Orally Disintegrating:* 4 mg (as base), 8 mg (as base)

DOSAGE

• IM, IV

Prevention of N&V due to chemotherapy.

Adults and children, 4–18 years: Three doses of 0.15 mg/kg each. For the 3-dose regimen, the first dose is infused over 15 min starting 30 min before the start of chemotherapy; the second and third doses are given 4 hr and 8 hr, respectively, after the first dose. Alternatively, a single 32-mg dose may be given over 15 min beginning 30 min before the start of chemotherapy.

N&V postoperatively.

Adults: 4 mg over 2–5 min immediately before induction of anesthesia or postoperatively as needed. **Children, 2 to 12 years weighing 40 kg or less:** 0.1 mg/kg over 2–5 min. **Children, 2 to 12 years weighing over 40 kg:** 4 mg over 2–5 min.

• TABLETS, ORAL SOLUTION, ORAL DISINTEGRATING TABLETS

In clients receiving moderately emetogenic chemotherapy agents.

Adults and children over 12 years of age: 8 mg 30 min before treatment followed by a second 8-mg dose 8 hr after the first dose; **then,** 8 mg b.i.d. for 1–2 days after chemotherapy. **Children, 4–11 years:** 4 mg t.i.d. The first dose is given 30 min before chemotherapy with subsequent doses 4 and 8 hr after the first dose. **Then,** 4 mg q 8 hr for 1–2 days after completion of chemotherapy.

In clients receiving single-day highly emetogenic cancer chemotherapy.

Adults: 24 mg once a day given 30 min before the single-day dose.

Prevention of N&V due to total body irradiation.

8 mg 1–2 hr before each fraction of radiotherapy administered each day.

Prevention of N&V in single high-dose fraction radiotherapy to the abdomen.

8 mg 1–2 hr before radiotherapy with subsequent doses 8 hr after the first dose for 1–2 days after completion of radiotherapy.

Prevention of N&V due to daily fractionated radiotherapy to the abdomen.

8 mg 1–2 hr before radiotherapy, with subsequent doses 8 hr after the first dose for each day radiotherapy is given.

Prevention of postoperative N&V.

Adults: 16 mg given as a single dose 1 hr before induction of anesthesia.

NURSING CONSIDERATIONS

SEE ALSO ***NURSING CONSIDERATIONS FOR ANTIEMETICS.***

ADMINISTRATION/STORAGE

1. With impaired hepatic function, do not exceed 8 mg PO or 8 mg IV daily infused over 15 min; 30 min prior to starting chemotherapy.
2. Tablets may be used to prepare a liquid product with cherry syrup, Syrpalta, Ora Sweet, or Ora Sweet Sugar Free. The concentration is 4 mg/5mL and is stable for 42 days at 4°C (39°F).
3. Suppositories can be made by adding pulverized tablets to a melted fatty acid base, mixing thoroughly, and pouring into suppository molds. They are stable for 30 or more days if stored in light-resistant containers under refrigeration.

IV 4. Dilute the 2-mg/mL injection in 50 mL of D5W or 0.9% NaCl injection and infuse over 15 min.

5. The diluted drug is stable at room temperature, with normal lighting, for 48 hr after dilution with 0.9% NaCl; D5W, D5/0.9% NaCl, D5/0.45% NaCl, and 3% NaCl injection.

ASSESSMENT

1. Document indications for therapy, onset and duration of symptoms, agents trialed, and outcome.
2. Monitor LFTs; adjust dosage with liver dysfunction.

CLIENT/FAMILY TEACHING

1. Drug is used to prevent N&V. It is to be given exactly as prescribed q 8 h RTC in order to ensure desired results. May be continued 1-2 day following radiation/chenotherapy to ensure prevention of N&V.
2. Report any rash, diarrhea, constipation, altered respirations (bronchospasms) or loss of response.

OUTCOMES/EVALUATE

- Prevention/control of chemotherapy-induced N&V
- Prophylaxis/relief of postoperative N&V

Oprelvekin (Interleukin 11)

(oh-**PREL**-veh-kin)

PREGNANCY CATEGORY: C

CLASSIFICATION(S):
Interleukin, human recombinant
Rx: Neumega

ACTION/KINETICS

Produced by DNA recombinant technology. Interleukin 11 is a thrombopoietic growth factor that directly stimulates proliferation of hematopoietic stem cells and megakaryocyte progenitor cells and induces megakaryocyte maturation. This results in increased platelet production. **Peak serum levels:** 3.2 hr. **t½, terminal:** 6.9 hr. Metabolized and excreted through urine.

USES

Prevention of thrombocytopenia following myelosuppressive chemotherapy in clients with nonmyeloid malignancies who are at high risk of severe thrombocytopenia.

CONTRAINDICATIONS

Use following myeloablative chemotherapy. Lactation.

SPECIAL CONCERNS

Use with caution in CHF or those who may be susceptible to developing CHF, and in those with history of heart failure who are well compensated and receiving appropriate medical therapy. Use with caution in those with history of atrial arrhythmia, in preexisting papilledema or with tumors involving CNS. Safety and efficacy have not been determined in children.

SIDE EFFECTS

Body as a whole: Edema, neutropenic fever, headache, fever, rash, conjunctival infection, asthenia, chills, pain, infection, flu-like symptoms. **GI:** N&V, mucositis, diarrhea, oral moniliasis, abdominal pain, constipation, dyspepsia. **CV:** Tachycardia, vasodilation, palpitations, syncope, atrial fibrillation or flutter, thrombocytosis, thrombotic events. **CNS:** Dizziness, insomnia, nervousness. **Respiratory:** Dyspnea, rhinitis, increased cough, pharyngitis, pleural effusion. **Miscellaneous:** Anorexia, ecchymosis, myalgia, bone pain, alopecia, mild visual blurring (transient), papilledema in children 12 years and younger.

O

In cancer clients: Also, amblyopia, dehydration, exfoliative dermatitis, eye hemorrhage, paresthesia, skin discoloration.

LABORATORY TEST CONSIDERATIONS

↓ Hemoglobin, serum albumin, transferrin, gamma globulins (all due to expansion of plasma volume).

OD OVERDOSE MANAGEMENT

Symptoms: Increased incidence of cardiovascular events if doses greater than 50 mcg/kg are given. *Treatment:* Discontinue drug and observe for signs of toxicity.

HOW SUPPLIED

Powder for injection, lyophilized: 5 mg

DOSAGE

- **SC INJECTION**

Prevent thrombocytopenia.

Adults: 50 mcg/kg once daily SC either in the abdomen, thigh, or hip. Dose of 75–100 mcg/kg in children will produce plasma levels consistent with a 50 mcg/kg dose in adults.

NURSING CONSIDERATIONS

ADMINISTRATION/STORAGE

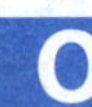

1. Initiate dosing 6 to 24 hr after completion of chemotherapy. Continue until post-nadir platelet count is 50,000 cells/mcL or more. Duration of dosing is usually 10 to 21 days; beyond 21 days is not recommended.
2. Discontinue treatment 2 or more days before starting next planned cycle of chemotherapy.
3. Reconstitute with 1 mL of sterile water for injection without preservative. Direct water at side of vial and swirl gently. Avoid excessive or vigorous shaking.
4. Reconstituted solution contains 5 mg/mL. Use within 3 hr as there is no preservative. Store vial either in refrigerator or at room temperature. Do not shake or freeze reconstituted solution.
5. Do not re-enter or reuse single-use vial. Discard unused portion.
6. Store lyophilized drug and diluent at 2–8°C (36–46°F).

ASSESSMENT

1. Document indications for therapy, onset, duration, and clinical manifestations.
2. Monitor I&O, lytes, CBC and platelet counts.
3. List chemotherapy agent and platelet nadir; initiate therapy 6-24 hr after chemotherapy completed. Stop oprelvekin at least 2 days before next round of chemotherapy.

CLIENT/FAMILY TEACHING

1. Review administration and dosage guidelines. Use as directed, SC, into abdomen, thigh, or hip; rotate sites.
2. Drug is used to prevent chemotherapy induced low platelets by stimulating bone marrow to increase platelet production.
3. Report any unusual side effects or increased bruising/bleeding.

OUTCOMES/EVALUATE

Thrombocytopenia prophylaxis; ↑ platelet production

Orlistat

(OR-lih-stat)

PREGNANCY CATEGORY: B
CLASSIFICATION(S):
Antiobesity drug
Rx: Xenical

ACTION/KINETICS

Reversible inhibitor of lipases resulting in inhibition of absorption of dietary fats. Acts in the lumen of the stomach and small intestine to form a covalent bond with the active serine residue site of gastric and pancreatic lipases. Inactivated enzymes are not available to hydrolyze dietary fat, in the form of triglycerides, into absorbable free fatty acids and monoglycerides. At therapeutic doses, it inhibits dietary fat absorption by about 30%. Effect on absorption of lipids seen as soon as 24–48 hr after dosing. Weight loss was seen within 2 weeks of starting therapy and continued for 6–12 months. Systemic absorption is not needed for activity, although a small amount is absorbed. Metabolism occurs mainly in the GI wall. Unabsorbed drug is excreted through the feces.

USES

Management of obesity, including weight loss and weight maintenance when used with a reduced calorie diet. To reduce risk for weight regain after prior weight loss. In obese clients with an initial body mass index of 30 kg/m^2 or more or 27 kg/m^2 or more in the presence of risk factors as hypertension, diabetes, dyslipidemia.

CONTRAINDICATIONS

Use in chronic malabsorption syndrome or cholestasis; known hypersensitivity to the drug. Lactation.

SPECIAL CONCERNS

Exclude organic causes of obesity (e.g., hypothyroidism) before prescribing. GI side effects may increase when taken with a high fat diet. Potential exists for misuse (e.g., in those with anorexia nervosa or bulimia). Use with caution in those with a history of hyperoxaluria or calcium oxalate nephrolithiasis. Safety and effectiveness have not been determined in children.

SIDE EFFECTS

GI: Oily spotting, flatus with discharge, fecal urgency, fatty/oily stool, oily evacuation, increased defecation, fecal incontinence, abdominal pain or discomfort, N&V, infectious diarrhea, rectal pain or discomfort, tooth disorder, gingival disorder. **CNS:** Headache, dizziness, psychiatric anxiety, depression. **Respiratory:** Influenza, URTI, lower respiratory infection, ENT symptoms. **Musculoskeletal:** Back pain, arthritis, myalgia, joint disorder. **Miscellaneous:** Fatigue, sleep disorder, rash, dry skin, menstrual irregularity, vaginitis, UTI, otitis, pedal edema.

DRUG INTERACTIONS

Beta-carotene / 30% ↓ in absorption of beta-carotene supplement

Cyclosporine / ↓ Cyclosporine blood levels due to ↓ absorption

Pravastatin / Additive lipid-lowering effects

Vitamin A / Possible malabsorption of Vitamin A

Vitamin D / Possible malabsorption of Vitamin D

Vitamin E / 60% ↓ in absorption of vitamin E acetate supplement

Vitamin K / Possible ↓ in vitamin K absorption

HOW SUPPLIED

Capsules: 120 mg

DOSAGE

- **CAPSULES**

Management of obesity.

Adults: 120 mg (1 capsule) t.i.d. with each main meal containing fat; give during or up to 1 hr after the meal. Doses greater than 120 mg t.i.d. have not been shown to produce additional benefit. Safety and effectiveness beyond 2 yr have not been determined.

NURSING CONSIDERATIONS

ASSESSMENT

1. Document indications for therapy, length of weight problem, other agents/therapies trialed and the outcome.
2. Determine any history of cholestasis, eating disorders, or malabsorption syndrome.
3. Note any thyroid dysfunction or kidney stones (drug may increase urinary oxalate).
4. List medical conditions/risk factors necessitating treatment (i.e, DM, HTN, hyperlipidemia).
5. Obtain baseline BMI, weight, VS, waist and hip circumference.
6. Assess lytes, cholesterol profile, BS, urinalysis, renal and LFTs.

CLIENT/FAMILY TEACHING

1. Drug acts by inhibiting absorption of some of the dietary fat intake.
2. Take with or within 1 hr following each main meal. If a meal is occasionally missed or contains no fat, the dose of orlistat can be omitted.
3. In order to be successful in losing weight, follow a nutritionally balanced, reduced-calorie diet containing 30% of calories from fat and perform 20 min of daily exercise. Distribute the daily intake of CHO, protein, and fat over three main meals.
4. Drug may reduce absorption of fat-soluble vitamins (A, D, E) and beta-carotene. Take supplements at least 2 hr after therapy or at bedtime.
5. Diabetics should monitor FS; improved metabolic control may require

O

a reduction of the dose of hypoglycemic agents.

6. May cause GI S&S, gas with discharge, fecal urgency/incontinence, oily or spotty discharge, abdominal pain/discomfort, diarrhea. These should subside with continued use; report any persistent side effects.

7. Report as scheduled for assessment of BP, labs, side effects, and weight.

OUTCOMES/EVALUATE

- ↓ Risk of weight gain after prior loss
- Desired weight loss and maintenance

Oseltamivir phosphate

(oh-sell-**TAM**-ih-vir)

PREGNANCY CATEGORY: C

CLASSIFICATION(S):

Antiviral

Rx: Tamiflu

ACTION/KINETICS

Hydrolyzed by hepatic esterases to the active oseltamivir carboxylate. May act by inhibiting the flu virus neuraminidase with possible alteration of virus particle aggregation and release. Drug resistance to influenza A virus is possible. Readily absorbed from the GI tract. **t½, oseltamivir carboxylate:** 6–10 hr. Over 99% is eliminated in the urine as oseltamivir carboxylate.

USES

(1) Prophylaxis of influenza in adults and adolescents 13 years and older. (2) Treatment of uncomplicated acute influenza A or B infection in clients over 1 year who have been symptomatic for 2 days or less.

SPECIAL CONCERNS

Use during lactation only if potential benefits outweigh the potential risk to the infant. Efficacy in clients who begin treatment after 40 hr of symptoms, for prophylactic use to prevent influenza, or for repeated treatment courses have not been determined. The drug is not a substitute for annual flu vaccination, which is the treatment of choice to prevent the flu. Safety and efficacy have not been determined for children less than 13 years of age.

SIDE EFFECTS

GI: N&V, diarrhea, abdominal pain. **CNS:** Dizziness, headache, insomnia, vertigo, seizure, confusion. **Miscellaneous:** Bronchitis, cough, fatigue, rash, swelling of face or tongue, arrhythmia, aggravation of diabetes. *NOTE:* For adolescents, additional side effects include otitis media, aggravated asthma, epistaxis, pneumonia, ear disorder, sinusitis, conjunctivitis.

HOW SUPPLIED

Capsules: 75 mg; *Powder for Oral Suspension:* 12 mg/mL (after reconstitution)

DOSAGE

- **CAPSULES, ORAL SUSPENSION**

Prophylaxis of influenza.

Adults and children 13 years and older: 75 mg once daily for 7 or more days. For clients with a C_{CR} between 10 and 30 mL/min, reduce dose to 75 mg every other day. Begin treatment within 2 days of exposure to flu. Safety and efficacy have been shown for use for 6 weeks or less.

Treatment of influenza.

Adults and children 13 years and older: 75 mg b.i.d. for 5 days. Begin treatment within 2 days of onset of flu symptoms.

NURSING CONSIDERATIONS

CLIENT/FAMILY TEACHING

1. Do not double up on doses. Take any missed dose as soon as remembered. If the missed dose is remembered within 2 hr of the next scheduled dose, take at the usual time and resume usual schedule.

2. Tolerability may be enhanced if taken with food. May aggravate diabetes control.

3. Initiate treatment as soon as possible at the first appearance of flu S&S.

4. Drug is used to diminish side effects and duration of illness. An annual flu shot is still required.

5. Not for use in children under age 13 ; must be provider initiated. May

cause more adverse effects in children than benefit.

OUTCOMES/EVALUATE

↓ Intensity/duration of S&S influenza A and B.

Oxacillin sodium

(ox-ah-**SILL**-in)

PREGNANCY CATEGORY: B

CLASSIFICATION(S):

Antibiotic, penicillin

Rx: Bactocill

SEE ALSO *ANTI-INFECTIVES* AND *PENICILLINS*.

ACTION/KINETICS

Penicillinase-resistant, acid-stable drug used for resistant staphylococcal infections. **Peak plasma levels: PO,** 1.6–10 mcg after 30–60 min; **IM,** 5–11 mcg/mL after 30 min. **t½:** 30 min.

USES

Infections caused by penicillinase-producing staphylococci; may be used to initiate therapy when a staphylococcal infection is suspected.

HOW SUPPLIED

Capsule: 250 mg, 500 mg; *Powder for injection:* 250 mg, 500 mg, 1 g, 2 g, 4 g, 10 g; *Powder for Oral Solution:* 250 mg/5 mL (when reconstituted)

DOSAGE

- **CAPSULES, ORAL SOLUTION**

Mild to moderate infections of the upper respiratory tract, skin, soft tissue.

Adults and children (over 20 kg): 500 mg q 4–6 hr for at least 5 days. **Children less than 20 kg:** 50 mg/kg/day in equally divided doses q 6 hr for at least 5 days.

Septicemia, deep-seated infections.

Parenteral therapy (see below) followed by PO therapy. **Adults:** 1 g q 4–6 hr; **children:** 100 mg/kg/day in equally divided doses q 4–6 hr.

- **IM, IV**

Mild to moderate infections.

Adults and children over 40 kg: 250–500 mg q 4–6 hr. **Children less than 40 kg:** 50 mg/kg/day in equally divided doses q 6 hr.

Severe infections of the lower respiratory tract or disseminated infections.

Adults and children over 40 kg: 1 g q 4–6 hr. **Children less than 40 kg:** 100 mg/kg/day in equally divided doses q 4–6 hr. **Neonates and premature infants, less than 2,000 g:** 50 mg/kg/day divided q 12 hr if less than 7 days of age and 100 mg/kg/day divided q 8 hr if more than 7 days of age. **Neonates and premature infants, more than 2,000 g:** 75 mg/kg/day divided q 8 hr if less than 7 days of age and 150 mg/kg/day divided q 6 hr if more than 7 days of age. Maximum daily dose: **Adults,** 12 g; **children,** 100–300 mg/kg.

NURSING CONSIDERATIONS

SEE ALSO *NURSING CONSIDERATIONS FOR ANTI-INFECTIVES AND PENICILLINS*.

ADMINISTRATION/STORAGE

1. Administer IM by deep intragluteal injection, rotate injection sites, and observe for pain and swelling at IM injection site.

IV 2. Reconstitution: Add NaCl or sterile water for injection in amount indicated on vial. Shake until solution is clear. For parenteral use, reconstituted solution may be kept for 3 days at room temperature or 1 week in refrigerator. Discard outdated solutions.

3. IV administration (two methods):

- For rapid, direct administration, add an equal amount of sterile water or isotonic saline to reconstituted dosage (usually 250- to 500-mg vial with 5 mL of solution) and administer over a period of 10 min.
- For IV infusion, add reconstituted solution to either dextrose, saline, or invert sugar solution for a concentration of 0.5–40 mg/mL and administer over a 6-hr period, during which time drug remains potent.
- Observe for pain, redness, and edema at IV injection site and along the course of the vein.

O

4. Do not physically mix other drugs with oxacillin.

CLIENT/FAMILY TEACHING

1. Take exactly as directed and complete entire script to prevent bacterial resistance.
2. Treatment of osteomyelitis may require several months of intensive PO therapy.
3. Report any rash, diarrhea with fever or abdominal pain, blood/mucus in stools or other adverse side effects or lack of response; return as scheduled.

OUTCOMES/EVALUATE

Improvement in S&S of infection; negative cultures

Oxaprozin

(**ox**-ah-**PROH**-zin)

PREGNANCY CATEGORY: C
CLASSIFICATION(S):
Nonsteroidal anti-inflammatory drug
Rx: Daypro

SEE ALSO *NONSTEROIDAL ANTI-INFLAMMATORY DRUGS.*

ACTION/KINETICS

Peak effect: 3–5 hr. **t½:** 42–50 hr. Over 99% plasma protein-bound. Excreted in the urine (65%) and feces (35%).

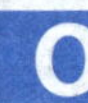

USES

Acute and chronic management of rheumatoid arthritis and osteoarthritis.

HOW SUPPLIED

Caplet: 600 mg

DOSAGE

• **TABLETS**

Rheumatoid arthritis.

Adults: 1,200 mg once daily. Lower and higher doses may be required in certain clients.

Osteoarthritis.

Adults: 1,200 mg once daily. For clients with a lower body weight or with a milder disease, 600 mg/day may be appropriate.

Maximum daily dose for either rheumatoid arthritis or osteoarthritis: 1,800 mg (or 26 mg/kg, whichever is lower) given in divided doses.

NURSING CONSIDERATIONS

SEE ALSO *NURSING CONSIDERATIONS FOR NONSTEROIDAL ANTI-INFLAMMATORY DRUGS.*

ADMINISTRATION/STORAGE

Regardless of the use, individualize and use the lowest effective dose to minimize side effects.

ASSESSMENT

1. Document type, onset, and symptom characteristics; rate pain level. List other agents used and the outcome.
2. Assess involved joint(s) and determine baseline ROM, the extent of any inflammation and functionality.
3. Monitor CBC, liver and renal function studies (q 6–12 months).

CLIENT/FAMILY TEACHING

1. Take exactly as directed with a full glass of water to enhance absorption; do not share meds. May take with food if GI upset occurs.
2. Report any evidence of unusual bruising/bleeding, blurred vision, ringing or roaring in ears (may indicate toxicity).
3. May cause dizziness or drowsiness, assess effects before driving or performing activities that require alertness.
4. Report S&S of nephrotoxicity: wt gain, edema, increased joint pain, fever, and blood in the urine.
5. May take up to one mo to note positive effects.

OUTCOMES/EVALUATE

Relief of joint pain/inflammation with improved mobility

Oxazepam

(ox-**AY**-zeh-pam)

PREGNANCY CATEGORY: D
CLASSIFICATION(S):
Antianxiety drug, benzodiazepine
Rx: Serax **C-IV**
✱Rx: Apo-Oxazepam

SEE ALSO *TRANQUILIZERS, ANTIMANIC DRUGS, AND HYPNOTICS.*

ACTION/KINETICS

Absorbed more slowly than most benzodiazepines. **Peak plasma levels:** 2–4 hr. **t½:** 5–20 hr. Broken down in the liver to inactive metabolites, which are excreted through both the urine and feces. Reputed to cause less drowsiness than chlordiazepoxide.

USES

Anxiety, tension, anxiety with depression. Adjunct in acute alcohol withdrawal.

SPECIAL CONCERNS

Dosage has not been established in children less than 12 years of age; use is not recommended in children less than 6 years of age.

ADDITIONAL SIDE EFFECTS

Paradoxical reactions characterized by sleep disorders and hyperexcitability during first weeks of therapy. Hypotension after parenteral administration.

HOW SUPPLIED

Capsule: 10 mg, 15 mg, 30 mg; *Tablet:* 15 mg

DOSAGE

• CAPSULES, TABLETS

Anxiety, mild to moderate with associated tension, irritability, or related symptoms of functional origin.

Adults: 10–15 mg t.i.d.–q.i.d.

Anxiety, tension, irritability, agitation in geriatric clients.

10 mg t.i.d.; can be increased to 15 mg t.i.d.–q.i.d.

Severe anxiety syndromes, agitation, or anxiety associated with depression.

15–30 mg t.i.d.–q.i.d.

Alcohol withdrawal.

Adults: 15–30 mg t.i.d.–q.i.d.

NURSING CONSIDERATIONS

SEE ALSO ***NURSING CONSIDERATIONS FOR TRANQUILIZERS, ANTIMANIC DRUGS, AND HYPNOTICS.***

CLIENT/FAMILY TEACHING

1. May take with milk or food to decrease GI upset. Review goals of therapy, dosage, and frequency of administration.
2. Drug may cause dizziness and drowsiness; use caution until drug effects realized.

te

OU

• ↓S

• Cont

toms

Oxcarb...

(ox-kar**BA**... een)

PREGNANCY CATEGORY: C

CLASSIFICATION(S):

Anticonvulsant, miscellaneous

Rx: Trileptal

SEE ALSO ***ANTICONVULSANTS.***

ACTION/KINETICS

Anticonvulsant mechanism not known with certainty. May block voltage-sensitive sodium channels, resulting in stabilization of hyperexcited neural membranes, inhibition of repetitive neuronal firing, and decreased propagation of synaptic impulses. These effects thought to be important in preventing seizure spread. Also, increased potassium conductance and modulation of high-voltage activated calcium channels may contribute to the anticonvulsant effects. Maximum plasma levels are higher in geriatric clients. Oxcarbazepine (active) is metabolized to the 10-monohydroxy metabolite (MHD) which is also active. MHD is further metabolized to inactive compounds. **t½, oxcarbazepine:** About 2 hr; **t½, MHD:** About 9 hr. MHD and inactive metabolites are excreted mainly in the urine.

USES

(1) Adjunctive therapy or monotherapy to treat partial seizures in adults. (2) Adjunctive therapy to treat partial seizures in children, aged 4 to 16 years of age. *Investigational:* Treat panic disorder.

CONTRAINDICATIONS

Lactation.

SPECIAL CONCERNS

About 25–30% of clients who experience hypersensitivity reactions to car-

...ence hyper-
...azepine.

...nomotor slowing, concen-...n difficulty, somnolence, fatigue, ...peech/language problems, abnormal coordination (ataxia, gait disturbances), headache, dizziness, anxiety, nystagmus, insomnia, tremor, amnesia, aggravated convulsions, emotional lability, hypoesthesia, nervousness, agitation, abnormal EEG, confusion, dysmetria, abnormal thinking, aggressive reaction, anguish, apathy, aphrasia, aura, delirum, delusion, dysphonia, dystonia, euphoria, extrapyramidal disorder, feeling "drunk," hemiplegia, hyperkinesia, hyperreflexia, hypokinesia, hyporeflexia, hypotonia, hysteria, decreased or increased libido, mania, migraine, nervousness, neuralgia, panic disorder, paralysis, paroniria, personalitiy disorder, psychosis, stupor. **GI:** N&V, abdominal pain, anorexia, dry mouth, ***rectal hemorrhage***, toothache, diarrhea, dyspepsia, constipation, gastritis, increased appetite, blood in stool, cholelithiasis, colitis, duodenal ulcer, dysphagia, enteritis, eructation, esophagitis, flatulence, gastric ulcer, gingival bleeding, gum hyperplasia, hematemesis, hemorrhoids, hiccough, biliary pain, retching, hypochondrium pain right, sialadenitis, stomatitis, ulcerative stomatitis. **CV:** Bradycardia, ***cardiac failure, cerebral hemorrhage,*** hypertension, postural hypotension, palpitations, syncope, tachycardia. **Respiratory:** Rhinitis, URTI, coughing, bronchitis, pharyngitis, epistaxis, chest infection, sinusitis, asthma, dyspnea, laryngismus, pleurisy. **GU:** UTI, frequent urination, vaginitis, dysuria, hematuria, intermenstrual bleeding, leukorrhea, menorrhagia, renal pain, urinary tract pain, polyuria, priapism, renal calculus. **Hematologic:** Leukopenia, thrombocytopenia. **Dermatologic:** Acne, hot flushes, purpura, rash, alopecia, angioedema, bruising, contact dermatitis, eczema, facial rash, flushing, folliculitis, heat rash, photosensitivity, genital pruritus, psoriasis, purpura, erythematous rash, maculopapular rash, vitiligo, erythema multiforme, ***Stevens-Johnson syndrome, toxic epidermal necrolysis***. **Musculoskeletal:** Muscle weakness, back pain, sprains, strains, involuntary muscle contractions, tetany. **Ophthalmic:** Diplopia, abnormal vision, abnormal accommodation, oculogyric crisis, ptosis, cataract, conjunctival hemorrhage, eye edema, hemianopia, mydriasis, xerophthalmia, photophobia, scotoma. **Otic:** Earache, ear infection, otitis externa, tinnitus. **Body as a whole:** Fatigue, fever, malaise, allergy, rigors, generalized edema, asthenia, weight increase or decrease, abnormal feeling, viral infection, infection. **Miscellaneous:** Thirst, precordial chest pain, leg edema, lymphadenopathy, taste perversion, systemic lupus erythematosus. Multiorgan hypersensitivity reaction with symptoms of rash, fever, lymphadenopathy, abnormal LFTs, eosinophilia, arthralgia.

LABORATORY TEST CONSIDERATIONS

↑ Gamma-GT, liver enzymes, serum transaminase. ↓ Serum sodium, T_4. Hyponatremia, hyperglycemia, hypocalcemia, hypoglcyemia, hypokalemia.

DRUG INTERACTIONS

Carbamazepine / ↓ Plasma oxcarbazepine levels R/T ↑ liver metabolism
Felodipine / ↓ Plasma felodipine levels
Lamotrigine / ↓ Lamotrigine serum levels
Oral contraceptives ↓ Plasma levels of both estrogen and progestin
Phenobarbital / ↓ Plasma oxcarbazepine levels R/T ↑ liver metabolism; ↑ plasma levels of phenobarbital
Phenytoin / ↓ Plasma oxcarbazepine levels R/T ↑ liver metabolism; ↑ plasma levels of phenytoin
Valproic acid / ↓ Plasma oxcarbazepine levels
Verapamil / ↓ Plasma oxcarbazepine levels

HOW SUPPLIED

Oral Suspension: 300 mg/5 mL; *Tablets:* 150 mg, 300 mg, 600 mg

DOSAGE

• **TABLETS, ORAL SOLUTION**

Adjunctive therapy for partial seizures in adults.

Adults: 600 mg b.i.d. If indicated, may increase by a maximum of 600 mg/

day at approximately weekly intervals. Doses greater than 2400 mg/day are not well tolerated due to CNS effects.

Conversion to monotherapy for partial seizures in adults.

Adults, initial: 600 mg b.i.d. while simultaneously reducing other anticonvulsant drug(s) over 3–6 weeks. Achieve maximum oxcarbazepine dose in 2–4 weeks. Dose may be increased by a maximum of 600 mg/day at approximatley weekly intervals to a maximum daily dose of 2400 mg.

Initiation of monotherapy for partial seizures in adults.

Adults: 600 mg b.i.d. May increase by 300 mg/day every third day to a dose of 1200 mg/day.

Adjunctive therapy for partial seizures in children.

Children, aged 4–12 years: 8–10 mg/kg, not to exceed 600 mg/day twice daily. Achieve maintenance dose over 2 weeks according to client weight as follows: **20–29 kg:** 900 mg/day; **29.1–39 kg:** 1200 mg/day; **over 39 kg:** 1800 mg/day.

NOTE: Initiate therapy at 300 mg/day in those with a C_{CR} less than 30 mL/min. May then increase slowly to achieve the desired response.

NURSING CONSIDERATIONS

SEE ALSO *NURSING CONSIDERATIONS* FOR *ANTICONVULSANTS*.

ASSESSMENT

1. Identify type, frequency and characteristics of seizures.
2. If hypersensitivity reaction to carbamezepine experienced may also have one with oxcarbazepine.
3. Monitor electrolytes, renal and LFTs.

CLIENT/FAMILY TEACHING

1. Take exactly as directed to prevent seizures.
2. May cause dizziness and drowsiness. Do not perform activities that require mental alertness until drug effects realized.
3 Avoid alcohol, may increase sedative effect.
4. Report any new or unusual side effects or seizure recurrence.
5. Practice reliable contraception.

OUTCOMES/EVALUATE

Control of seizures

Oxybutynin chloride

(ox-ee-**BYOU**-tih-nin)

PREGNANCY CATEGORY: B
CLASSIFICATION(S):
Cholinergic blocking drug
Rx: Ditropan, Ditropan XL
✱Rx: Albert Oxybutynin, Apo-Oxybutynin, Gen-Oxybutynin, Novo-Oxybutynin, Nu-Oxybutyn, Oxybutyn, PMS-Oxybutynin

ACTION/KINETICS

Causes increased vesicle capacity, decreases frequency of uninhibited contractions of the detrusor muscle, and delays initial urgency to void. Acts by exerting a direct antispasmodic effect and inhibits the muscarinic action of acetylcholine on smooth muscle. Has no effect at either the neuromuscular junction or autonomic ganglia. Has 4–10 times the antispasmodic effect of atropine but only one-fifth the anticholinergic activity. **Onset:** 30–60 min; **time to peak effect:** 3–6 hr; **duration:** 6–10 hr. Eliminated through the urine.

USES

Neurogenic bladder disease characterized by urinary retention, urinary overflow, incontinence, nocturia, urinary frequency or urgency, reflex neurogenic bladder.

CONTRAINDICATIONS

Glaucoma (angle closure), untreated narrow anterior chamber angles, GI obstruction, paralytic ileus, intestinal atony (in elderly or debilitated), megacolon, toxic megacolon complicating ulcerative colitis, severe colitis, myasthenia gravis, obstructive uropathy, unstable CV status in acute hemorrhage.

SPECIAL CONCERNS

Use with caution when increased cholinergic effect is undesirable and in the elderly. Safe use in children less

O

than 5 years of age has not been determined. Use with caution in geriatric clients; during lactation; in clients with autonomic neuropathy, renal, or hepatic disease; in clinically significant bladder outflow obstruction; and in clients with hiatal hernia with reflex esophagitis. Heat stroke and fever (due to decreased sweating) may occur if given at high environmental temperatures. Symptoms may be aggravated in hyperthyhroidism, coronary heart disease, CHF, cardiac arrhythmias, tachycardia, hypertension, hiatal hernia, and prostatic hypertrophy.

SIDE EFFECTS

Side effects due to Immediate-Release product. GI: Constipation, decreased GI motility, nausea, dry mouth. **CNS:** Dizziness, drowsiness, insomnia, hallucinations, restlessness. **CV:** Palpitations, tachycardia, vasodilation. **Dermatologic:** Decreased sweating, rash. **GU:** Urinary hesitation and retention. **Ophthalmic:** Amblyopia, cycloplegia, mydriasis, decreased lacrimation. **Miscellaneous:** Impotence, asthenia, suppressed lacatation, ***severe allergic reactions,*** drug idiosyncrasies, heat prostration when given in presence of high environmental temperatures,

Side effects due to Extended-Release product. GI: Dry mouth, constipation, nausea, dyspepsia, diarrhea, flatulence, gastroesophageal reflux. **CNS:** Somnolence, headache, dizziness, insomnia, nervousness, confusion. **CV:** Hypertension, palpitation, vasodilation. **Dermatologic:** Dry skin, rash. **GU:** Urinary hesitancy, UTI, increased post-void residual volume, urinary retention, cystitis. **Respiratory:** Upper respiratory tract infections, cough, sinusitis, rhinitis, bronchitis, dry nasal and mucous membranes, pharyngitis. **Ophthalmic:** Blurred vision, dry eyes. **Miscellaneous:** Asthenia, pain, abdominal pain, accidental injury, back pain, flu syndrome, arthritis, ***severe allergic reactions,*** drug idiosyncrasies, heat prostration when given in presence of high environmental temperatures.

OD OVERDOSE MANAGEMENT

Symptoms: Intense CNS disturbances (restlessness, psychoses), circulatory changes (flushing, hypotension) and failure, respiratory failure, paralysis, coma. *Treatment:* Stomach lavage, physostigmine (0.5–2 mg IV; repeat as necessary up to maximum of 5 mg). Supportive therapy, if necessary. Counteract excitement with sodium thiopental (2%) or chloral hydrate (100–200 mL of 2% solution) rectally. Artificial respiration may be necessary if respiratory muscles become paralyzed.

DRUG INTERACTIONS

See *Cholinergic Blocking Agents.*

HOW SUPPLIED

Syrup: 5 mg/5 mL; *Tablet, Immediate Release:* 5 mg; *Tablet, Extended-Release:* 5 mg, 10 mg, 15 mg

DOSAGE

• SYRUP, TABLETS IMMEDIATE RELEASE

Adults: 5 mg b.i.d.–t.i.d. Maximum dose: 5 mg q.i.d. **Children, over 5 years:** 5 mg b.i.d. Maximum dose: 5 mg t.i.d.

• TABLETS, EXTENDED-RELEASE

Adults, initial: 5 mg once daily. Increase, in 5- mg increments, up to a maximum of 30 mg/day.

NURSING CONSIDERATIONS

SEE ALSO *NURSING CONSIDERATIONS* FOR *CHOLINERGIC BLOCKING AGENTS.*

ADMINISTRATION/STORAGE

Dispense in tight, light-resistant containers and store at 15–30°C (59–86°F).

ASSESSMENT

1. Document type, onset, frequency, and characteristics of symptoms.
2. Assess urinary patterns: frequency, urgency, hesitation, nocturia, incontinence, distension.
3. Review conditions that may be aggravated by oxybutynin and note if present (renal, hepatic disease, hiatal hernia, reflux esophagitis).

CLIENT/FAMILY TEACHING

1. Take only as directed. Take Extended-Release tablets with or without food; swallow whole with the help of liquids (do not chew, divide, or crush).
2. Use caution driving a car or in operating dangerous machinery; drug may cause drowsiness and blurred vision.

3. Withhold medication and report if diarrhea occurs (especially with an ileostomy or colostomy); may be symptom of intestinal obstruction.
4. Consume 2–3 L/day of fluids to ensure adequate hydration and to relieve symptoms of dry mouth.
5. Vegetables, fruit, fiber, and fluids should be consumed in adequate quantities to prevent constipation.
6. Wear sunglasses, sunscreen, and protective clothing during exposure; may cause photosensitivity reaction.
7. Avoid overexposure to heat; body needs increased fluids in hot weather because sweating is drug inhibited and heat stroke may occur.
8. Report any loss of effect as dosage may require adjustment.
9. With neurogenic bladder, return as scheduled for cystometry, to evaluate response to therapy, and need for continuation of medication.

OUTCOMES/EVALUATE

- Relief of spasms and GU pain
- Normal elimination patterns
- Positive cystometry findings

—COMBINATION DRUG—

Oxycodone and acetaminophen

(ox-ee-**KOH**-dohn, ah-**SEAT**-ah-**MIN**-oh-fen)

PREGNANCY CATEGORY: C
CLASSIFICATION(S):
Analgesic
Rx: Percocet, Roxicet, Roxicet 5/500 Capsules, Roxilox, Tylox **C-II**
✱**Rx:** Endocet, Oxycocet, Percocet-Demi

SEE ALSO *ACETAMINOPHEN* AND *NARCOTIC ANALGESICS.*

CONTENT

Percocet Tablets, Roxicet Tablets: *Narcotic analgesic:* Oxycodone hydrochloride, 2.5 mg or 5 mg. *Analgesic:* Acetaminophen, 325 mg. **Roxicet Oral Solution:** Oxycodone hydrochloride, 5 mg/5 mL and Acetaminophen, 325 mg/5 mL. **Roxicet 5/500 Caplets, Roxilox Capsules, Tylox Capsules:** *Narcotic analgesic:* Oxycodone hydrochloride, 5 mg. *Analgesic:* Acetaminophen, 500 mg.

USES

Relief of moderate to moderately severe pain.

CONTRAINDICATIONS

Hypersensitivity to either oxycodone or acetaminophen.

SPECIAL CONCERNS

Can produce drug dependence and has abuse potential. The respiratory depressant effects of oxycodone can be exaggerated in clients with head injury, other intracranial lesions, or a preexisting increase in intracranial pressure. Use with caution in clients who are elderly, are debilitated, have severely impaired hepatic or renal function, are hyperthyroid, have Addison's disease, have prostatic hypertrophy, or have urethral stricture. Use for acute abdominal conditions may obscure the diagnosis or clinical course. Use with caution during lactation. Safety and efficacy in children have not been established.

SIDE EFFECTS

Commonly, dizziness, lightheadedness, N&V, and sedation; these effects are more common in ambulatory clients than nonambulatory clients. Other side effects include euphoria, dysphoria, constipation, skin rash, and pruritus. See also individual components.

DRUG INTERACTIONS

Anticholinergic drugs / Production of paralytic ileus
Antidepressants, tricyclic / ↑ Effect of either the TCAs or oxycodone
CNS depressants (including other narcotic analgesics, phenothiazines, antianxiety drugs, sedative-hypnotics, anesthetics, alcohol) / Additive CNS depression
MAO inhibitors / ↑ Effect of either the MAO inhibitor or oxycodone

HOW SUPPLIED

See Content

DOSAGE

- **ORAL SOLUTION, TABLETS**

Analgesic.
Adults: 5 mL of the oral solution q 6 hr or 1 tablet q 6 hr as needed for pain.

NURSING CONSIDERATIONS

SEE ALSO *NURSING CONSIDERATIONS FOR ACETAMINOPHEN* AND *NARCOTIC ANALGESICS*.

ASSESSMENT

1. Document indications for therapy, type, onset, and characteristics of symptoms. Use a pain-rating scale to rate pain level.
2. List other agents prescribed and the outcome.
3. Note VS, CNS assessment findings and level of consciousness.

CLIENT/FAMILY TEACHING

1. Take only as directed; may take with food to decrease GI upset. Do not share drugs, store in a safe place.
2. Drug may cause dizziness and drowsiness; do not perform activities that require mental or physical alertness and do not change positions abruptly.
3. May cause constipation, N&V, dry mouth, and physical dependence (withdrawal S&S include N&V, cramps, fever, fainting and anorexia); report.
4. Avoid alcohol and any other CNS depressants without provider approval. (*NOTE:* Oral solution contains small amounts of alcohol.)
5. Tolerance may occur; report loss of effectiveness.

OUTCOMES/EVALUATE

Pain control

Oxycodone hydrochloride

(ox-ee-**KOH**-dohn)

PREGNANCY CATEGORY: C
CLASSIFICATION(S):
Narcotic analgesic
Rx: Endocodone, M-oxy, OxyContin, OxyFAST, OxyIR, Percolone, Roxicodone, Roxicodone Intensol **C-II**
★**Rx:** Supeudol

SEE ALSO *NARCOTIC ANALGESICS*.

ACTION/KINETICS

Semisynthetic opiate causing mild sedation and little or no antitussive effect. Most effective in relieving acute pain. **Onset:** 15–30 min. **Peak effect:** 60 min. **Duration:** 4–6 hr. **t½:** 3.2 hr for immediate-release product and 4.5 hr for extended-release. Dependence liability is moderate. Oxycodone terephthalate is available but only in combination with aspirin (e.g., Percodan) or acetaminophen.

USES

Immediate release: Management of moderate to severe pain. **Controlled-release:** Management of moderate to severe pain when a continuous, around-the-clock analgesic is required for an extended period of time. To be used postoperatively if the client has received the drug prior to surgery or if the postoperative pain is expected to be moderate to severe and last for an extended period of time. Not intended for use as an "as needed" analgesic. Not for pain in the immediate postoperative period (i.e., first 12–24 hr following surgery) or if the pain is mild or not expected to persist for a long period of time. *NOTE*: The 80 mg- and 160 mg-extended-release tablets are only for use in opiate-dependent clients.

ADDITIONAL CONTRAINDICATIONS

Use in hypercarbia, paralytic ileus, children, or during labor. Clients with gastric distress, such as colitis or gastric or duodenal ulcer, and clients who have glaucoma should not receive Percodan, which also contains aspirin.

SPECIAL CONCERNS

Controlled-release tablets are as potentially addicting as morphine; chewing, snorting, or injecting can lead to death.

ADDITIONAL DRUG INTERACTIONS

Use with protease inhibitors → ↑ CNS and respiratory depression.

HOW SUPPLIED

Capsule, Immediate-Release: 5 mg; *Solution, Concentrate:* 20 mg/mL; *Solution, Oral:* 5 mg/5 mL; *Tablet:* 5 mg; *Tablet, Immediate-Release:* 15 mg, 30 mg; *Tablet, Extended Release:* 10 mg, 20 mg, 40 mg, 80 mg, 160 mg

DOSAGE

• IMMEDIATE RELEASE: CAPSULE, ORAL CONCENTRATE, ORAL SOLUTION, TABLET

Analgesia.

Adults: 10–30 mg q 4 hr (5 mg q 6 hr for OxyIR, Oxydose, or OxyFAST, as needed). Individualize dose. For those who have not been receiving opiates start with 5–15 mg q 4–6 hr. Titrate dose based on client response.

NURSING CONSIDERATIONS

SEE ALSO *NURSING CONSIDERATIONS* FOR *NARCOTIC ANALGESICS*.

ADMINISTRATION/STORAGE

1. Give clients with chronic pain around-the-clock dosing. For control of severe chronic pain, give immediate-release products on a regularly scheduled basis, q 4–6 hr at the lowest dose level that will provide adequate analgesia.
2. When converting from a fixed-ratio opiod/nonopiod regimen, determine whether or not to continue the nonopiod drug. If the nonopiod drug is to be discontinued, it may be necessary to titrate the dose of immediate-release tablets in response to the level of analgesia and side effects experienced. If the nonopiod drug is to be continued, base the oxycodone starting dose on the most recent dose of opiod as a baseline.
3. If the client has been taking opiates prior to taking immediate-release oxycodone, factor the potency of the prior opiate into the selection of the total daily dose of oxycodone.
4. Continuous evaluation of those receiving immediate-release or controlled-release oxycodone is required. Supplemental doses for breakthrough or incident pain and titration of the total daily dose may be required, especially in those with rapidly changing disease states.
5. When a client no longer requires therapy with immediate-release or controlled-release tablets, gradually discontinue over time to prevent development of withdrawal symptoms. Generally decrease therapy by 25–50% per day and monitor carefully for signs of withdrawal. If withdrawal symptoms develop, raise the dose to the previous level and titrate down more slowly.
6. For controlled-release tablets, swallow whole; do not break, chew, or crush.
7. Controlled-release tablets are intended for moderate-to-severe pain when a continuous, around-the-clock analgesic is needed for an extended period of time.
8. For controlled-release tablets, the dosing regimen must be individualized based on prior opiod and nonopiod drug treatment, as well as the general condition and medical status of the client.
9. Follow manufacturer's guidelines carefully for conversion from other opiates.
10. Controlled-release tablets, 80 and 160 mg, are for use only in opiod-tolerant clients requiring daily oxycodone equivalent dosages of 160 mg or more for the 80 mg tablets and 320 mg or more for the 160 mg (currently distribution is limited) tablet.

ASSESSMENT

Document onset, location, and duration of pain and characteristics of symptoms. Use a pain-rating scale to rate pain levels. Note other agents trialed and the outcome. Assess ability to function and perform daily activities.

CLIENT/FAMILY TEACHING

1. Take medication with food to minimize GI upset.
2. Swallow extended-release tablets whole. Ingesting broken, crushed, or chewed extended-release tablets may lead to rapid release/absorption and possibility of toxic effects.
3. Use caution; do not perform activities that require mental alertness.
4. May cause constipation, N&V, dry mouth, and physical dependence (withdrawal S&S include N&V, cramps, fever, faintning and anorexia); report.
5. Avoid alcohol in any form.
6. Do not share meds; store in a safe, protected location. Drug has a high abuse potential.
7. Tolerance may develop; report loss of effectiveness.

OUTCOMES/EVALUATE

Relief of pain

O

Oxymorphone hydrochloride

(ox-ee-**MOR**-fohn)

PREGNANCY CATEGORY: C
CLASSIFICATION(S):
Narcotic analgesic
Rx: Numorphan **C-II**

SEE ALSO *NARCOTIC ANALGESICS.*

ACTION/KINETICS

On a weight basis, is 2–10 times more potent as an analgesic than morphine, although potency depends on the route of administration. Produces mild depression of the cough reflex and significant respiratory depression and emesis. **Onset:** 5–10 min. **Peak effect:** 30–60 min. **Duration:** 3–6 hr.

USES

Moderate to severe pain. **Parenteral:** Preoperative analgesia, to support anesthesia, obstetrics, relief of anxiety in clients with dyspnea associated with pulmonary edema secondary to acute LV dysfunction.

ADDITIONAL CONTRAINDICATIONS

Use in paralytic ileus or for treatment of pulmonary edema secondary to a chemical respiratory irritant

SPECIAL CONCERNS

Safety has not been determined for use in children less than 18 years of age.

HOW SUPPLIED

Injection: 1 mg/mL, 1.5 mg/mL; *Suppository:* 5 mg

DOSAGE

• **SC, IM**

Analgesia.

Adults, initial: 1–1.5 mg q 4–6 hr; dose can be increased carefully until analgesic response obtained.

Analgesia during labor.

Adults: 0.5–1.0 mg IM.

• **IV**

Analgesia.

Adults, initial: 0.5 mg. Increase dose cautiously in nondebilitated clients until analgesia is obtained.

• **SUPPOSITORIES**

Analgesia.

Adults: 5 mg q 4–6 hr.

NOTE: For all routes of administration, use lower doses for debilitated and elderly clients and for liver disease.

NURSING CONSIDERATIONS

SEE ALSO *NURSING CONSIDERATIONS FOR NARCOTIC ANALGESICS.*

ADMINISTRATION/STORAGE

1. Store suppositories in the refrigerator.
2. Protect injections from light.
3. **IV** If the drug is to be administered IV, dilute the dosage in 5 mL of sterile water or NSS and administer over 2–3 min.

ASSESSMENT

Document indications for therapy, noting onset, location, duration and characteristics of symptoms; use a scale to rate pain to evaluate effectiveness as well as functioning level.

CLIENT/FAMILY TEACHING

1. C&DB several times each hour while awake to prevent atelectasis; incentive spirometry may be useful.
2. Drug may aggravate gallbladder conditions; report abdominal complaints.
3. Use safety precautions; drug causes drowsiness and dizziness.

OUTCOMES/EVALUATE

Relief of pain; control of anxiety

Oxytocin, parenteral

(ox-eh-**TOE**-sin)

PREGNANCY CATEGORY: X
CLASSIFICATION(S):
Oxytocic drug
Rx: Pitocin, Syntocinon

ACTION/KINETICS

Synthetic compound identical to the natural hormone isolated from the posterior pituitary. Has uterine stimulant, vasopressor, and weak antidiuretic properties. May act on uterine myofibril activity to increase the number of contracting myofibrils. Uterine sensitivity to oxytocin, as well as amplitude and duration of uterine contractions, increases gradually during gestation and just before parturition increases rapidly. Facilitates ejection of milk from the breasts by stimulating smooth muscle. **Onset, IV:** immediate; **IM,** 3–5 min; **Peak effects:** 40 min. **Steady-state plasma levels:** Reached within 40 min. **t½:** 1–6 min (decreased in late pregnancy and lactation). **Duration, IV:** 20 min after infusion is stopped; **IM:** 2–3 hr. Eliminated through the urine, liver, and functional mammary gland.

USES

Antepartum: Induction or stimulation of labor at term. To overcome true primary or secondary uterine inertia. Induction of labor with oxytocin is indicated only under certain *specific* conditions and is not usual because serious toxic effects can occur.

Oxytocin is indicated:

1. For uterine inertia.
2. For induction of labor in cases of erythroblastosis fetalis, maternal diabetes mellitus, preeclampsia, and eclampsia.
3. For induction of labor after premature rupture of membranes in last month of pregnancy when labor fails to develop spontaneously within 12 hr.
4. For routine control of postpartum hemorrhage and uterine atony.
5. To hasten uterine involution.
6. To complete inevitable abortions after the 20th week of pregnancy.
7. Intranasally for initial letdown of milk.

Investigational: Breast engorgement, oxytocin challenge test for determining antepartum fetal HR.

CONTRAINDICATIONS

Hypersensitivity to drug. Significant cephalopelvic disproportion; unfavorable fetal positions or presentations that are undeliverable without conversion prior to delivery. In obstetric emergencies where the benefit-to-risk ratio for either the mother or fetus favors surgical intervention. Fetal distress where delivery is not imminent, prolonged use in uterine inertia or severe toxemia, hypertonic or hyperactive uterine patterns, when adequate uterine activity does not achieve satisfactory progress. Induction of augmentation of labor where vaginal delivery is contraindicated, including invasive cervical cancer, cord presentation or prolapse, total placenta previa and vasa previa, active herpes genitalis. Use of oxytocin citrate in severe toxemia, CV or renal disease. Use of intranasal oxytocin during pregnancy.

Also, predisposition to thromboplastin and amniotic fluid embolism (dead fetus, abruptio placentae), history of previous traumatic deliveries, or women with four or more deliveries. Never give oxytocin IV undiluted or in high concentrations.

SIDE EFFECTS

Mother: Tetanic uterine contractions, ***anaphylaxis,*** cardiac arrhythmia, ***fatal afibrinogenemia,*** N&V, PVCs, increased blood loss, pelvic hematoma, hypertension, tachycardia, and ECG changes. Also, rarely, anxiety, dyspnea, precordial pain, edema, cyanosis or reddening of the skin, and CV spasm. Water intoxication from prolonged IV infusion, ***death due to hypertensive episodes, SAH, postpartum hemorrhage, or uterine rupture.*** Excessive dosage may cause uterine hypertonicity, spasm, tetanic contraction, or uterine rupture.

Fetus: ***Death,*** PVCs, bradycardia, tachycardia, arrhythmias, hypoxia, ***intracranial hemorrhage due to overstimulation of the uterus during labor leads to uterine tetany with marked impairment of uteroplacental blood flow.***

NOTE: Hypersensitivity reactions occur rarely. When they do, they occur most often with natural oxytocin administered IM or in concentrated IV doses and least frequently after IV infusion or diluted doses. Accidental swallowing of buccal tablets is not harmful.

OD OVERDOSE MANAGEMENT

Symptoms: ***Hyperstimulation of the uterus resulting in hypertonic or tetanic contractions. Or, a resting tone of 15–20 cm water between contractions can result in uterine rupture, cervical and vaginal lacerations, tumultuous labor, uteroplacental hypoperfusion, postpartum hemorrhage, and a variable deceleration of***

O

fetal heart rate, fetal hypoxia, hypercapnia, or death. Water intoxication with seizures can occur if large doses (40–50 mL/min) of the drug are infused for long periods of time. *Treatment:* Discontinue the drug and restrict fluid intake. Start diuresis and give a hypertonic saline solution IV. Correct electrolyte imbalance and control seizures with a barbiturate. If the client is comatose, provide special nursing care.

DRUG INTERACTIONS

Sympathomimetic amines / Severe hypertension and possible stroke

HOW SUPPLIED

Injection: 10 U/mL.

DOSAGE

- **IV INFUSION, IM**

Induction or stimulation of labor.

Dilute 10 units (1 mL) to 1,000 mL isotonic saline or 5% dextrose for IV infusion. **Initial:** 0.001–0.002 unit/min (0.1–0.2 mL/min); dose can be gradually increased at 15- to 30-min intervals by 0.001 unit/min (0.1 mL/min) to maximum of 0.02 unit/min (2 mL/min).

Reduction of postpartum bleeding.

Dilute 10–40 units (1–4 mL) to 1,000 mL with isotonic saline or 5% dextrose for IV infusion. Administer at a rate to control uterine atony, usually at a rate of 0.02–0.1 unit/min.

Incomplete or therapeutic abortion.

10 units at a rate of 0.02–0.04 unit/min by IV infusion or 10 units IM after placental delivery.

NURSING CONSIDERATIONS

ADMINISTRATION/STORAGE

IV 1. Use Y-tubing system, with one bottle containing IV solution and oxytocin, and the other containing only the IV solution. This allows for the discontinuation of the drug while maintaining the patency of the vein when it is decided to change to the drug-free infusion bottle. Give parenteral oxytocin infusions only with an electronic infusion device.

2. Oxytocin is rapidly broken down by sodium bisulfite. Have magnesium sulfate immediately available to relax the uterus in case of tetanic uterine contractions.

3. Have the provider immediately available during drug administration.

ASSESSMENT

1. Note any sensitivity to the drug.

2. Document indications for therapy, onset and characteristics of symptoms.

3. Determine fetal maturity (size), pelvic adequacy, fetal presentation/position and lack of complications prior to initiating drug therapy.

4. Provide continous observation of client checking for dilation, resting uterine tone, characteristics of uterine contractions e.g., time, duration and frequency. Record maternal/fetal HRs; intrauterine pressures.

5. Carefully review history for any contraindications prior to administering oxytocin.

For induction and stimulation of labor and/or oxytocin challenge test:

INTERVENTIONS

1. Before initiating therapy, inform client of the rationale for using oxytocic agents and reassure that the procedure is not unusual. Explain that the medication will induce contractions that may feel like menstrual cramps initially but can be very painful; analgesics should be used.

2. Remain with the client during the induction period and throughout the stimulation of labor. Titrate oxytocin to establish uterine contractions that are similar to normal labor; continuously monitor rate and strength of contractions.

3. Record VS, check I&O q 15 min.

4. Note resting uterine tone and assess contractions for frequency, duration, and strength.

5. Monitor the fetal HR and rhythm at least every 10 min. Document and immediately report any alterations.

6. Prevent uterine rupture and fetal damage by clamping off IV oxytocin, starting medication-free IV fluids, turning client on her left side to prevent fetal anoxia, providing oxygen, and reporting when the following events occur:

- If contractions occur more frequently than every 2 min and last longer than 60–90 sec with no period of uterine relaxation in between.

• If the contractions are excessively strong and/or exceed 50–65 mm Hg or stop.

• If resting uterine tone is 15–20 mm Hg or more.

• If the fetal HR indicates bradycardia, tachycardia, or irregularities of rhythm.

7. Assess for water intoxication following prolonged administration of oxytocin. Monitor I&O and serum electrolytes closely.

8. Observe for lethargy, confusion, and stupor. Note if the client has developed neuromuscular hyperexcitability with increased reflexes and muscular twitching. These symptoms should be reported immediately since convulsions and coma may occur if left untreated. Magnesium sulfate should be readily available for IV administration.

During the fourth stage of labor when oxytocin is administered for prevention or control of hemorrhage:

1. Describe the location, size, and firmness of the uterus. Report if the uterus is displaced or boggy and follow designated hospital protocol.

2. In clients with spinal anesthesia, visually inspect for any evidence of bleeding. Sensation is diminished and hemorrhage may occur insidiously.

3. Note the amount and color of the lochia. Report any bright red lochia, excessive bleeding, or the passage of clots.

4. Monitor VS until stable.

5. Closely monitor I&O. Observe for S&S of water intoxication; document and report immediately.

CLIENT/FAMILY TEACHING

Cramps will feel like strong menstrual cramps but will continue to increase in intensity. Report increased blood/fluid loss, fever, foul smelling drainage, or abdominal cramps.

OUTCOMES/EVALUATE

• Induction of labor with effective uterine contractions

• ↑ Uterine tone with ↓ postpartum bleeding

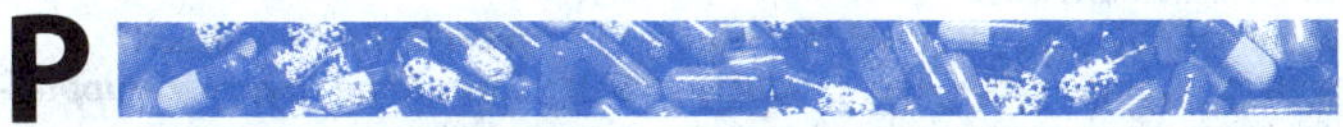

Paclitaxel

(**PACK**-lih-**tax**-el)

PREGNANCY CATEGORY: D

CLASSIFICATION(S):

Antineoplastic, miscellaneous

Rx: Onxol, Taxol

SEE ALSO *ANTINEOPLASTIC AGENTS.*

ACTION/KINETICS

Naturally occurring antineoplastic agent that promotes the assembly of microtubules from tubulin dimers and stabilizes microtubules by preventing depolymerization. The stabilization results in the inhibition of the normal dynamic reorganization of the microtubule network that is required for vital interphase and mitotic cellular functions. Also induces abnormal "bundles" of microtubules throughout the cell cycle and multiple esters of microtubules during mitosis. Following IV administration, there is a biphasic decline in plasma levels. The initial rapid decline is due to distribution to the peripheral compartment and significant elimination, whereas the second phase is due, in part, to a slow efflux of the drug from the peripheral compartment. Metabolized by the liver with small amounts of unchanged drug excreted in the urine.

USES

Onxol. (1) Advanced carconoma of the ovary as subsequent therapy. (2) Breast cancer after failure of combination chemotherapy for metastases (including use of an anthracycline unless contraindicated) or relapse within

6 months of adjuvant chemotherapy. **Taxol.** (1) Advanced carcinoma of the ovary as first-line or subsequent therapy. When used as first-line therapy, combine with cisplatin. (2) Adjuvant treatment of node-positive breast cancer given sequentially to doxorubicin-containing combination therapy. (3) Treatment of breast cancer after failure of combination chemotherapy (including use of an anthracycline unless contraindicated) for metastases or relapse within 6 months of adjuvant chemotherapy. (4) Combined with cisplatin for first-line treatment of non-small cell lung cancer in those not candidates for potentially curative surgery or radiation therapy. (5) Second-line therapy for AIDS-related Kaposi's sarcoma. *Investigational:* Alone or in combination with other chemotherapeutic drugs for advanced head and neck cancer, small-cell lung cancer, adenocarcinoma of the upper GI tract, hormone-refractory prostate cancer, non-Hodgkin's lymphoma, transitional cell carcinoma of the urothelium, pancreatic cancer, polycystic kidney disease.

CONTRAINDICATIONS

Hypersensitivity to paclitaxel, in those with a hypersensitivity to products containing polyoxymethylated castor oil (Cremophor EL), clients with solid tumors when baseline neutrophil counts are below 1,500 cells/mm^3, and those with AIDS-related Kaposi's sarcoma with baseline neutrophil counts below 1,000 cells/mm^3. Lactation.

SPECIAL CONCERNS

Use with caution in clients with moderate- to severe-impaired hepatic function. Safety and efficacy have not been determined in children.

SIDE EFFECTS

Hypersensitivity reactions: Severe symptoms, including anaphylaxis, usually occur during the first hour of therapy and occur during both the first or second course of therapy despite premedication. Severe symptoms include ***dyspnea, angioedema,*** hypotension, or generalized urticaria all of which require immediate cessation of the drug and aggressive treatment therapy. Symptoms not requiring treatment include milder dyspnea, flushing, skin reactions, hypotension, or tachycardia. **Injection site reactions:** Erythema, extravasation, tenderness, skin discoloration, swelling. Rarely, phlebitis, cellulitis, induration, skin exfoliation, necrosis, fibrosis. **Hematologic:** Neutropenia and leukopenia (common), thrombocytopenia, anemia, infections, bleeding, packed cell transfusions, platelet transfusions. **CV:** Bradycardia and hypotension (including during the infusion), hypertension, ***severe CV events (including asymptomatic VT, bigeminy, syncope, complete AV block),*** abnormal ECG (including nonspecific repolarization abnormalities, sinus tachycardia, premature beats). **Musculoskeletal:** Peripheral neuropathy (including mild paresthesia), myalgia, arthralgia. **GI:** N&V, diarrhea, mucositis, impaired liver function. **Miscellaneous:** Alopecia, fever associated with severe neutropenia; infections of the urinary tract and upper respiratory tract as well as ***sepsis due to neutropenia,*** mutagenic.

LABORATORY TEST CONSIDERATIONS

↑ Bilirubin, alkaline phosphatase, ALT, AST.

OD OVERDOSE MANAGEMENT

Symptoms: ***Bone marrow suppression,*** peripheral neurotoxicity, mucositis. Accidental inhalation may cause dyspnea, chest pain, burning eyes, sore throat, and nausea. *Treatment:* Treat symptomatically.

DRUG INTERACTIONS

Carbamazepine / ↑ Paclitaxel metabolism
Cisplatin / More profound myelosuppression when paclitaxel was given after cisplatin than when paclitaxel was given before cisplatin, due to a 1/3 decrease in paclitaxel clearance
Cyclosporine / ↓ Paclitaxel metabolism R/T inhibition of drug metabolism
Diazepam / ↓ Paclitaxel metabolism R/T inhibition of drug metabolism
Doxorubicin / ↑ Levels of doxorubicin and doxorubicinol; also, ↓ paclitaxel metabolism R/T inhibition of drug metabolism
Felodipine / ↓ Paclitaxel metabolism R/T inhibition of drug metabolism

Ketoconazole / ↓ Paclitaxel metabolism R/T inhibition of drug metabolism
Midazolam / ↓ Paclitaxel metabolism R/T inhibition of drug metabolism
Phenobarbital / ↑ Paclitaxel metabolism
Retinoic acid / ↓ Paclitaxel metabolism R/T inhibition of drug metabolism
Troleandomycin / ↓ Paclitaxel metabolism R/T inhibition of drug metabolism

HOW SUPPLIED

Injection: 6 mg/mL

DOSAGE

• **IV INFUSION**

Carcinoma of the ovary.

The following regimens may be used: (1) **Adults:** 135 mg/m² given IV over 3 hr q 3 weeks. (2) **Adults:** Paclitaxel, 135 mg/m², IV over 24 hr q 3 weeks, followed by cisplatin, 75 mg/m² in previously untreated clients (Taxol only). (3) **Adults:** Paclitaxel, 135 mg/m² or 175 mg/m², IV over 3 hr every 3 weeks in those previously receiving chedmotherapy.

Adjuvant treatment of node-positive breast cancer.

Adults: 175 mg/m² given IV over 3 hr q 3 weeks for 4 courses given sequentially to doxorubicin-containing combination therapy.

Metastatic breast cancer or relapse within 6 months of adjuvant therapy.

Adults: 175 mg/m² IV over 3 hr every 3 weeks after failure of initial chemotherapy.

Non-small cell lung carcinoma.

135 mg/m² over 24 hr followed by cisplatin, 75 mg/m², q 3 weeks.

AIDS-related Kaposi's sarcoma.

135 mg/m² given IV over 3 hr q 3 weeks or 100 mg/m² given IV over 3 hr q 2 weeks.

NURSING CONSIDERATIONS

SEE ALSO *NURSING CONSIDERATIONS* FOR *ANTINEOPLASTIC AGENTS*.

ADMINISTRATION/STORAGE

IV 1. Do not allow the undiluted concentrate to come in contact with plasticized polyvinylchloride equipment or devices used to prepare solutions for infusion.
2. Premedicate before use to prevent severe hypersensitivity reactions. Premedication may consist of oral dexamethasone, 20 mg, given 12 and 6 hr before paclitaxel; diphenhydramine (or equivalent), 50 mg IV, 30–60 min before; and cimetidine, 300 mg IV, or ranitidine, 50 mg IV, 30–60 min before paclitaxel.
3. In those with advanced HIV disease, reduce dose of dexamethasone to 10 mg PO; initiate or repeat treatment only if neutrophil count is 1,000 cells/mm³ or greater; begin concomitant hematopoietic growth factor as needed.
4. Dilute paclitaxel concentrate prior to infusion in 0.9% NSS, D5W, D5/0.9% NaCl, or D5/RL to a final concentration of 0.3–1.2 mg/mL. Diluted solutions are stable for up to 24 hr at room temperature.
5. Administer diluted solution through an in-line filter with a microporous membrane not greater than 0.22 μm.
6. The dilutions may show haziness, which is due to the formulation vehicle. No significant loss of potency has been noted following simulated delivery of the solution through IV tubing containing an in-line (0.22-μm) filter.
7. To minimize client exposure to the plasticizer DHEP which may be leached from PVC infusion bags or sets, store diluted paclitaxel solutions in bottles (glass, polypropylene) or plastic bags (polypropylene, polyolefin) and administered through polyethylene-lined administration sets.
8. Unopened vials of the concentrate are stable when stored under refrigeration, protected from light, in the original package.
9. Do not undertake repeat courses until the neutrophil count is at least 1,500 cells/mm³ and the platelet count is at least 100,000 cells/mm³. Reduce dose by 20% for subsequent courses in those who experience a neutrophil count below 500 cells/mm³ for 1 week or more or if there is se-

P

vere peripheral neuropathy during therapy.
10. Use gloves when handling the drug. If the solution comes in contact with the skin, wash the skin immediately and thoroughly with soap and water. If the drug comes in contact with mucous membranes, thoroughly flush the membranes with water.
11. *Treatment of Hypersensitivity Reactions:* Stop the infusion and treat with bronchodilators (such as albuterol or theophylline), epinephrine, antihistamines, and corticosteroids.
12. Store paclitaxel between 20–25°C (68–77°F).

ASSESSMENT

1. Document tumor location, previous therapy (include agents, dosage, and duration), especially radiation because this may enhance myelosuppressive drug effects. Determine if client has received this drug and the response.
2. Administer pretreatment medications. If symptoms of severe hypersensitivity reaction (dyspnea, hypotension, angioedema, or generalized urticaria) appear, interrupt infusion and report. Hypersensitivity reactions usually occur during the first hour and despite premedication.
3. Document any severe hypersensitivity reaction so that client is *NOT* rechallenged with paclitaxel.
4. Monitor VS, I&O, CBC, liver and renal function studies; ensure that neutrophil count is 1,500 cells/mm^3 before drug administration (with AIDS-related Kaposi's sarcoma with baseline neutrophil counts > 1,000 cells/mm^3) and that platelet count is at least 100,000 cells/mm^3. Neutrophil nadir: 11 days; platelet nadir 8–9 days.

CLIENT/FAMILY TEACHING

1. Anticipate hair loss.
2. Joint pain and discomfort may be experienced 2–3 days after therapy but should resolve in several days.
3. Report any severe N&V, fever, chills, sore throat, infection, abnormal bruising or bleeding, or CNS symptoms, especially numbness and tingling in fingers/toes.
4. Avoid alcohol, aspirin, and NSAIDs.
5. Use reliable contraception during and for 4 months following therapy.

OUTCOMES/EVALUATE

↓ Tumor size and spread

Palivizumab

(**pal**-ih-**VIZ**-you-mab)

PREGNANCY CATEGORY: C
CLASSIFICATION(S):
Monoclonal antibody
Rx: Synagis

ACTION/KINETICS

Humanized monoclonal antibody produced by recombinant DNA technology. The antibody exhibits neutralizing and fusion-inhibitory activity against respiratory syncytial virus (RSV), leading to a reduction in the quantity of RSV in the lower respiratory tract. **t½, children:** 20 days.

USES

Prevention of serious lower respiratory tract disease due to RSV in pediatric clients at high risk of RSV disease.

CONTRAINDICATIONS

Use in adults. Pediatric clients with a history of severe reaction to palivizumab or other components of the product.

SPECIAL CONCERNS

Safety and efficacy have not been determined for treatment of established RSV disease.

SIDE EFFECTS

Respiratory: URTI, rhinitis, pharyngitis, cough, wheezing, bronchiolitis, pneumonia, bronchitis, asthma, croup, dyspnea, sinusitis, apnea. **GI:** Diarrhea, vomiting, gastroenteritis, abnormal liver function, oral monilia. **Dermatologic:** Rash, fungal dermatitis, eczema, seborrhea. **Miscellaneous:** Otitis media, fever, pain, hernia, failure to thrive, nervousness, injection site reaction, conjunctivitis, viral infection, anemia, flu syndrome, allergic reactions.

LABORATORY TEST CONSIDERATIONS

↑ AST, ALT.

HOW SUPPLIED

Injection, lyophilized: 50 mg, 100 mg

DOSAGE

- **IM ONLY**

Prevention of RSV disease.

Children: 15 mg/kg per month IM (preferably in the anterolateral part of the thigh). To calculate the monthly dose: [patient weight (kg) x 15 mg/kg divided by 100 mg/mL of palivizumab]

NURSING CONSIDERATIONS

ADMINISTRATION/STORAGE

1. Give injection volumes greater than 1 mL in divided doses.
2. To prepare for administration, slowly add 1 mL of sterile water for injection to a 100 mg vial. Swirl gently for 30 seconds to avoid foaming (do not shake vial). Allow reconstituted drug to stand at room temperature for a minimum of 20 minutes until the solution clarifies.
3. Reconstituted palivizumab does not contain a preservative; administer within 6 hr of reconstitution.
4. Prior to reconstitution store between 2–8°C (35–46°F) in its original container. Do not freeze.

ASSESSMENT

1. Identify candidates for therapy i.e., premature infants at 35 weeks or less gestation without BPD and infants with BPD requiring intervention for RSV in the past 6 mo.
2. Give monthly doses throughout the RSV season. In the northern hemisphere, the RSV season usually begins in November and lasts through April (may be different in some communities).
3. Give the first dose prior to the beginning of the RSV season to ensure protection.
4. Due to the possibility of sciatic nerve damage, do not use the gluteal site routinely as the injection site. Give volumes greater than 1 mL in divided doses.
5. Follow dosing guidelines for correct dosage.

CLIENT/FAMILY TEACHING

1. Therapy consists of monthly injections based on body weight, during the RSV season. Protect child from exposure to infection while on therapy; i.e. limit visitors, providers may need to wear masks and gloves, avoid infected persons.
2. May experience URI, runny nose, sore throat, ear infections, rash or pain at injection site; report fever, other infections and difficulty breathing.

OUTCOMES/EVALUATE

RSV prophylaxis in high risk infants

Pamidronate disodium

(pah-**MIH**-droh-nayt)

PREGNANCY CATEGORY: C
CLASSIFICATION(S):
Bone growth regulator, bisphosphonate
Rx: Aredia

ACTION/KINETICS

Inhibits both normal and abnormal bone resorption without inhibiting bone formation and mineralization. Precise mechanism is not known, but the drug may inhibit dissolution of hydroxyapatite crystal or have an effect on bone reabsorbing cells. Causes decreased serum phosphate levels probably due to a decreased release of phosphate from bone and increased renal excretion as parathyroid levels return to normal. Urinary calcium/creatinine and urinary hydroxyproline/creatinine ratios decrease and usually return to normal or below normal after treatment. **t½:** Biphasic, 1.6 hr (alpha) and 27.3 hr (beta). Approximately 50% of an IV infused dose is excreted unchanged in the urine within 72 hr.

USES

(1) In conjunction with hydration to treat moderate to severe hypercalcemia of malignancy associated with breast and lung cancers and multiple myeloma (with or without bone metastases). (2) Moderate to severe Paget's disease. (3) Prevent bone loss during treatment of prostate cancer. *Investigational:* Postmenopausal osteoporosis;

P

hyperparathyroidism; prophylaxis of glucocorticoid-induced osteoporosis; reduce bone pain in clients with prostatic carcinoma; treat immobilization-induced hypercalcemia.

CONTRAINDICATIONS

Hypersensitivity to bisphosphonates.

SPECIAL CONCERNS

Use with caution during lactation. Safety and effectiveness have not been determined in children. Pamidronate has not been tested in clients who have creatinine levels greater than 5 mg/dL.

SIDE EFFECTS

Metabolic/Electrolytes: Hypocalcemia, hypokalemia, hypomagnesemia, hypophosphatemia. **Body as a whole:** Slight increase in body temperature, fluid overload, generalized pain, back pain, fatigue, fever, moniliasis. **GI:** N&V, constipation, abdominal pain, anorexia, ***GI hemorrhage,*** ulcerative stomatitis. **CNS:** Somnolence, insomnia, dizziness, headache, paresthesia, abnormal vision, slight possibility of ***seizures.*** **CV:** Hypertension, atrial fibrillation, syncope, tachycardia. **Respiratory:** Rales, rhinitis, URTI. **GU:** UTI. **Musculoskeletal:** Bone pain. **At site of administration:** Redness, swelling or induration, pain on palpation. **Miscellaneous:** Anemia, hypothyroidism, sweating.

HOW SUPPLIED

Powder for injection: 30 mg, 60 mg, 90 mg

DOSAGE

• IV INFUSION

Moderate hypercalcemia (corrected serum calcium of about 12–13.5 mg/dL) of malignancy.

Initial therapy: 60–90 mg. The 60-mg dose is given as an initial single dose over at least 4 hr; the 90-mg dose must be given as an initial single dose over 2–24 hr.

Severe hypercalcemia (corrected serum calcium greater than 13.5 mg/dL) of malignancy.

Initial therapy: 90 mg as a single initial dose given over 2–24 hr. If retreatment is necessary, use the same dose as for initial therapy; at least 7 days should elapse before retreatment.

Moderate to severe Paget's disease.

30 mg/day given as a 4-hr infusion on 3 consecutive days (total dose: 90 mg). If retreatment is necessary, the same dosage schedule is used.

Osteolytic bone lesions of multiple myeloma.

90 mg given as a 4-hr infusion every month. Those with marked Bence-Jones proteinuria and dehydration should receive adequate hydration before infusion of pamidronate.

Osteolytic bone metastases.

90 mg given as a 2-hr infusion q 3 to 4 weeks.

NURSING CONSIDERATIONS

ADMINISTRATION/STORAGE

IV 1. If hypercalcemia recurs, may retreat provided a minimum of 7 days has elapsed to allow full response to the initial dose.

2. Reconstitute drug by adding 10 mL sterile water for injection, which results in a concentration of 30, 60, or 90 mg/10 mL with a pH of 6–7.4.

3. For hypercalcemia of malignancy, dilute in 1,000 mL of sterile 0.45% or 0.9% NaCl or D5W. This solution is stable for 24 hr at room temperature.

4. For treating Paget's disease or osteolytic bone lesions of multiple myeloma, dilute the recommended dose in 500 mL of sterile 0.45% or 0.9% NaCl or D5W.

5. If reconstituted with sterile water, drug may be stored in the refrigerator for up to 24 hr at 2–8°C (36–46°F).

6. Do not mix with calcium-containing infusion solutions such as Ringer's solution.

7. Give as a single IV solution and in a separate line.

ASSESSMENT

1. Note indications for therapy, i.e., hypercalcemia of malignancy, symptomatic Paget's disease, postmenopausal osteoporosis, bone pain and presenting symptoms.

2. Document any biphosphonate hypersensitivity.

3. Note any cardiac disease.

4. Obtain baseline ECG, serum Ca, Mg, K, PO_4, CBC, and renal function studies.

INTERVENTIONS

1. Monitor VS and I&O. Ensure adequate administration of fluids to correct hypovolemia and correct any volume deficits before administering diuretics.
2. During drug administration, vigorous saline hydration should be undertaken for moderate to severe hypercalcemia to restore urine output to about 2 L/day. For less severe hypercalcemia, more conservative approaches can be taken including saline hydration with or without loop diuretics. Overhydration should be avoided, especially with CHF. Weigh daily; observe for edema.
3. Assess for seizure activity; incorporate seizure precautions.

CLIENT/FAMILY TEACHING

1. Review dietary sources of calcium (dark green vegetables, yogurt, cheese, milk, etc.) that should be avoided with hypercalcemia.
2. May experience transient mild temperature elevations for up to 48 hr following therapy.
3. Maintain adequate hydration; keep a log of I&O.
4. Report any increase in N&V, bone pain, thirst, or lethargy R/T hypercalcemia.

OUTCOMES/EVALUATE

- Desired calcium levels
- ↓ Bone pain/instability

Pancrelipase (Lipancreatin)

(pan-kree-**LY**-payz)

PREGNANCY CATEGORY: C
CLASSIFICATION(S):
Digestive enzyme
Rx: Cotazym, Cotazym-S, Ilozyme, Ku-Zyme HP, Lipram, Pancrease, Pancrease MT 4, 10, 16, 20, 25, Protilase, Ultrase MT12 or 20, Viokase, Zymase
✱**Rx:** Creon 5, 10, 20, 25, Digess 8000, Pancrease MT, Ultrase, Ultrase MT

ACTION/KINETICS

Enzyme concentrate from hog pancreas, which contains lipase, amylase, and protease, enzymes that replace or supplement naturally occurring enzymes. More active at neutral or slightly alkaline pH. Has 12 times the lipolytic activity and 4 times both the proteolytic and amylolytic activity of pancreatin. Certain products have an enteric coating that protects the enzymes from deactivation in the stomach.

USES

(1) Pancreatic deficiency diseases such as chronic pancreatitis, cystic fibrosis of the pancreas, pancreatectomy, ductal obstructions caused by cancer of the pancreas or common bile duct, steatorrhea of malabsorption syndrome or postgastrectomy or postgastrointestinal surgery. (2) Presumptive test for pancreatic function, especially in insufficiency due to chronic pancreatitis.

CONTRAINDICATIONS

Hog protein sensitivity. Acute pancreatitis, acute exacerbation of chronic pancreatic disease.

SPECIAL CONCERNS

Safety for use during lactation and in children less than 6 months of age not established. Methacrylic acid copolymer, which is found in the enteric coating of certain products, may cause fibrosing colonopathy.

SIDE EFFECTS

GI: Nausea, diarrhea, abdominal cramps following high doses. **Other:** Inhalation of the powder is irritating to the skin and mucous membranes and may result in an asthma attack. High doses cause hyperuricemia and hyperuricosuria.

OD OVERDOSE MANAGEMENT

Symptoms: Diarrhea, intestinal upset.

DRUG INTERACTIONS

Calcium carbonate / ↓ Effect of pancreatic enzymes
Iron / Response to oral iron may ↓ if given with pancreatic enzymes
Magnesium hydroxide / ↓ Effect of pancreatic enzymes

HOW SUPPLIED

Capsule; Enteric Coated capsule; Enteric Coated tablet; Powder; Tablet

P

DOSAGE

• CAPSULES; ENTERIC-COATED MICROSPHERES, MICROTABLETS, SPHERES, PELLETS; POWDER; TABLETS

Pancreatic insufficiency.

Adults and children over 12 years of age: 4,000–48,000 units of lipase with each meal and with snacks. **Children, 7–12 years:** 4,000–12,000 units of lipase with each meal and snacks; **1–6 years:** 4,000–8,000 units of lipase with each meal and 4,000 units lipase with snacks. **6–12 months:** 2,000 units lipase with each meal. Dosage has not been established in children less than 6 months of age. Severe deficiencies may require up to 64,000–88,000 units of lipase with meals (or the frequency of administration can be increased if side effects are not manifested).

Pancreatectomy or obstruction of pancreatic ducts.

Adults: 8,000–16,000 units of lipase at 2 hr intervals or as directed by a physician.

Cystic fibrosis.

Use 0.7 g of the powder with meals.

NURSING CONSIDERATIONS

ADMINISTRATION/STORAGE

1. When administering to young children, may sprinkle capsule contents on food.
2. After several weeks of use, adjust the dosage according to the therapeutic response.
3. Store unopened preparations in tight containers at a temperature not to exceed 25°C (77°F).
4. Do not crush or chew enteric-coated products (i.e., microspheres, microtablets). If unable to swallow, the capsule may be opened and shaken on a small amount of soft, cold food (e.g., applesauce, gelatin) that does not require chewing. Swallow immediately without chewing (the enzymes may irritate the mucosa). Follow with a glass of juice or water to ensure complete swallowing of the product. Enteric-coated products that come in contact with foods with a pH greater than 5.5 will dissolve.
5. Generally, 300 mg of pancrelipase is required to digest every 17 g of dietary fat.
6. Products are not bioequivalent; do not interchange without approval.

ASSESSMENT

1. Obtain a thorough history and document indications for therapy.
2. Determine any sensitivity or allergy to pork, since hog protein is the main constituent of pancrelipase.

CLIENT/FAMILY TEACHING

1. Review the appropriate dietary recommendations (usually low fat, high calorie, high protein); utilize a dietitian for dietary counseling and assistance in meal planning. It takes 300 mg of pancrelipase to digest 17 g of dietary fat.
2. Take just before or with meals and snacks and with plenty of liquids to prevent oral mucosal irritation. Do not crush or chew enteric-coated capsules; drug will deactivate in acid stomach environment-swallow whole.
3. Report any joint pain/swelling/soreness or breathing difficulty. With nausea, cramping, or diarrhea, dosage needs adjustment to control steatorrhea.

OUTCOMES/EVALUATE

- Improved digestion/nutritional status with deficiency states
- Control of diarrhea, ↓ steatorrhea

Pancuronium bromide

(pan-kyou-**ROH**-nee-um)

PREGNANCY CATEGORY: C

CLASSIFICATION(S):

Neuromuscular blocking drug

Rx: Pavulon

SEE ALSO ***NEUROMUSCULAR BLOCKING AGENTS.***

ACTION/KINETICS

Five times as potent as d-tubocurarine. Anticholinesterase agents will reverse effects. Possesses vagolytic activity although it is not likely to cause histamine release. **Onset:** Within 45 sec. **Time to peak effect:** 3–4.5 min (depending on the dose). **Duration:** 35–45 min (increased with multiple doses). **t½, elimination:** 89–161 min. Forty percent is excreted through the urine either unchanged or as metabolites; 10% is excreted through the bile. In clients with renal failure, the t½ is doubled. Significantly bound to plasma protein.

USES

Adjunct to anesthesia to produce relaxation of skeletal muscle. Facilitate ET intubation. Facilitate management of clients undergoing mechanical ventilation.

SPECIAL CONCERNS

Children up to 1 month of age may be more sensitive to the effects of pancuronium. Clients with myasthenia gravis or Eaton-Lambert syndrome may have profound effects from small doses.

ADDITIONAL SIDE EFFECTS

Respiratory: ***Apnea, respiratory insufficiency.*** **CV:** Increased HR and MAP. **Miscellaneous:** Salivation, skin rashes, ***hypersensitivity reactions (e.g., bronchospasm,*** flushing, hypotension, redness, tachycardia).

ADDITIONAL DRUG INTERACTIONS

Azathioprine / Reverses effects of pancuronium
Bacitracin / Additive muscle relaxation
Enflurane / ↑ Muscle relaxation
Isoflurane / ↑ Muscle relaxation
Metocurine / ↑ Muscle relaxation but duration is not prolonged
Quinine / ↑ Effect of pancuronium
Sodium colistimethate / ↑ Muscle relaxation
Succinylcholine / ↑ Intensity and duration of action of pancuronium
Tetracyclines / Additive muscle relaxation
Theophyllines / ↓ Effects of pancuronium; also, possible cardiac arrhythmias
Tricyclic antidepressants with halothane / Administration of pancuronium may cause severe arrhythmias
Tubocurarine / ↑ Muscle relaxation but duration is not prolonged

HOW SUPPLIED

Injection: 1 mg/mL, 2 mg/mL

DOSAGE

- **IV ONLY**

Muscle relaxation during anesthesia.
Adults and children over 1 month of age, initial: 0.04–0.1 mg/kg. Additional doses of 0.01 mg/kg may be administered as required (usually q 20–60 min). **Neonates:** Administer a test dose of 0.02 mg/kg first to determine responsiveness.

ET intubation.
0.06–0.1 mg/kg as a bolus dose. Can undertake intubation in 2 to 3 min.

NURSING CONSIDERATIONS

SEE ALSO NURSING CONSIDERATIONS FOR NEUROMUSCULAR BLOCKING AGENTS.

ADMINISTRATION/STORAGE

IV 1. Additional doses significantly increase the duration of skeletal muscle relaxation.
2. May be mixed with D5W, D5/NSS, RL, and 0.9% NSS. When mixed with any of these solutions, the drug is stable with no change in pH or potency for 2 days in glass or plastic containers.
3. Administer in a continuously monitored environment.
4. Have appropriate anticholinesterase agents available to reverse drug effects; pyridostigmine bromide, neostigmine, or edrophonium and are usually administered with atropine or glycopyrrolate.

INTERVENTIONS

1. Provide ventilatory support.
2. Monitor and record VS, ECG, and I&O. Drug can cause vagal stimulation resulting in bradycardia, hypotension, and cardiac arrhythmias.
3. A peripheral nerve stimulator may be used to evaluate neuromuscular response and recovery.
4. Consciousness is not affected by pancuronium. Explain all procedures and provide emotional support. Do not conduct any discussions that should not be overheard.
5. With short-term therapy, reassure will be able to talk and move once the drug effects are reversed.
6. Muscle fasciculations may cause soreness or injury after recovery. Ad-

P

minister prescribed nondepolarizing agent and reassure that soreness likely caused by the unsynchronized contractions of adjacent muscle fibers just before the onset of paralysis.

7. Position for comfort and so that the body is in proper alignment. Turn and perform mouth care and eye care frequently (protect eyes and instill liquid tears q 2 h as blink reflex is suppressed).

8. Assess airway at frequent intervals. Have a suction machine at the bedside.

9. Check to be certain that the ventilator alarms are set and on at all times. *Never* leave client unmonitored.

10. Determine client need and administer medications for anxiety, pain, and/or sedation regularly (valium, morphine).

OUTCOMES/EVALUATE

- Desired level of paralysis; suppression of twitch response
- Facilitation of ET intubation; tolerance of mechanical ventilation

Pantoprazole sodium

(pan-**TOH**-prah-zohl)

P

PREGNANCY CATEGORY: B
CLASSIFICATION(S):
Proton pump inhibitor
Rx: Protonix, Protonix I.V.
✱**Rx:** Panto IV, Pantoloc

ACTION/KINETICS

Proton pump inhibitor that suppresses the final step in gastric acid production by forming a covalent bond to two sites of the (H^+, $K+$)–ATPase enzyme system at the secretory surface of the gastric parietal cell. Results in inhibition of both basal and stimulated gastric acid secretion regardless of the stimulus. Duration greater than 24 hr due to binding to the ATPase. Gastrin levels increase. Absorption begins only after the tablet leaves the stomach although it occurs rapidly. Absorption is not affected by antacids, although food may delay absorption up to 2 hr or longer. Extensively metabolized in the liver through the CYP system. Excreted in both the urine (71%) and feces (18%).

USES

PO: (1) Short-term treatment (up to 8 weeks) of erosive esophagitis associated with GERD. An additional 8 weeks therapy may be indicated for those who have not healed after the initial 8 weeks of therapy. (2) Maintenance of healing of erosive esophagitis and reduction in relapse rates of day- and night-time heartburn symptoms in those with GERD. **IV:** Short-term (7–10 days) treatment of GERD (as an alternate to PO therapy in those unable to continue taking PO medication). *Investigational:* Treatment of Zollinger-Ellison syndrome.

CONTRAINDICATIONS

Hypersensitivity to any component of the formulation. Lactation.

SPECIAL CONCERNS

Safety and efficacy for children or for maintenance therapy (i.e., beyond 16 weeks) have not been established. Safety and efficacy of IV use as initial treatment for GERD not established. Use with caution in severe hepatic impairment as there may be modest drug accumulation when dosed once/day.

SIDE EFFECTS

Side effects listed are those with an incidence of 1% or more. **GI:** Diarrhea, flatulence, abdominal pain, eructation, constipation, dyspepsia, gastroenteritis, GI disorder, N&V, rectal disorder. **CNS:** Headache, insomnia, anxiety, dizziness, migraine. **Respiratory:** Bronchitis, increased cough, dyspnea, pharyngitis, rhinitis, sinusitis, URTI. **GU:** Urinary frequency, UTI. **Body as a whole:** Rash, asthenia, flu syndrome, infection, pain, arthralgia. **Miscellaneous:** Back/chest/neck pain.

LABORATORY TEST CONSIDERATIONS

↑ SGOT, creatinine. Hyperlipemia, hyperglycemia, hypercholesterolemia, hyperuricemia. Abnormal LFTs.

DRUG INTERACTIONS

Due to the prolonged effect on inhibition of gastric acid secretion, pantoprazole may interfere with absorption of drugs where gastric pH is an important factor in their bioavailability (e.g., ampicillin esters, iron salts, ketoconazole).

HOW SUPPLIED
Powder for Injection, Freeze-dried: 40 mg/vial; *Tablets, Delayed Release:* 20 mg, 40 mg

DOSAGE

• **DELAYED RELEASE TABLETS**

Erosive esophagitis.

Adults: 40 mg once daily for up to 8 weeks; an additional 8 weeks therapy may be considered.

Maintenance of healing of erosive esophagitis.

Adults: 40 mg once daily.

• **IV**

Erosive esophagitis.

Adults: 40 mg once daily for 7–10 days.

NURSING CONSIDERATIONS

ADMINISTRATION/STORAGE

IV 1. Reconstitute for IV use with 10 mL of 0.9% NaCl injection; further diliute with 100 mL of D5W, 0.9% NaCl, or lactated Ringer's injection to a final concentration of 0.4 mg/mL.
2. Give IV admixtures over about 15 min at a rate of 3 mg or less/min through a dedicated line using the in-line filter provided. The filter must be used to remove precipitates that may form when the reconstituted drug is mixed with IV solutions.
3. If use of a Y-site is preferred, the in-line filter must be positioned below the Y-site that is closest to the client.
4. Flush the IV line before and after IV pantoprazole with either D5W injection, 0.9% NaCl injection, or lactated Ringer's injection.
5. Do not give IV pantoprazole simultaneously through the same line with other IV solutions.
6. Discontinue IV therapy as soon as the client is able to resume PO therapy.
7. Store IV product at 2–8°C (36–46°F). Protect from light. Store in-line filters at room temperature.
8. Do not freeze reconstitiuted drug. Reconstituted solution may be stored at room temperature for up to 2 hr. The admixed solution may be stored for up to 12 hr at room temperature. It is not necessary to protect either the reconstituted or admixed solution from light.

ASSESSMENT

1. Note indications for therapy, onset and characteristics of symptoms. Record abdominal assessment and endoscopic findings if available.
2. Assess LFTs; may reduce dose to qod with dysfunction to prevent drug accumulations.
3. List drugs prescribed to ensure none require acidity for metabolism.

CLIENT/FAMILY TEACHING

1. Take as directed. Do not split, crush, or chew the delayed release tablets; swallow whole.
2. May take with or without food in the stomach. Antacid consumption will not affect.
3. Report any unusual side effects and keep F/U appointments to assess drug response.

OUTCOMES/EVALUATE

Reduced gastric acidity with relief of S&S erosive esophagitis

Papaverine

(pah-**PAV**-er-een)

PREGNANCY CATEGORY: C
CLASSIFICATION(S):
Vasodilator, peripheral
Rx: Pavabid Plateau Caps, Pavagen TD

ACTION/KINETICS
Direct spasmolytic effect on smooth muscle, possibly by inhibiting cyclic nucleotide phosphodiesterase, thus increasing levels of cyclic AMP. This effect is seen in the vascular system, bronchial muscle, and in the GI, biliary, and urinary tracts. Large doses produce CNS sedation and sleepiness. May also directly relax cerebral vessels as it increases cerebral blood flow and decreases cerebral vascular resistance. Depresses cardiac conduction and irritability and prolongs the myocardial refractory period. Localized in fat tissues and liver. Steady plasma concentration maintained when drug is

P

given q 6 hr. **Peak plasma levels:** 1–2 hr. **t½:** 30–120 min. Sustained-release products may be poorly and erratically absorbed. Metabolized in the liver and inactive metabolites excreted in the urine.

USES

Relief of cerebral and peripheral ischemia associated with arterial spasm and myocardial ischemia complicated by arrhythmias.

CONTRAINDICATIONS

Complete AV block.

SPECIAL CONCERNS

Safe use during lactation or for children not established. Use with extreme caution in coronary insufficiency and glaucoma.

SIDE EFFECTS

CV: Flushing of face, hypertension, increase in HR and depth of respiration. Large doses can depress AV and intraventricular conduction, causing serious arrhythmias. **GI:** Nausea, anorexia, abdominal distress, constipation or diarrhea, dry mouth and throat. **CNS:** Headache, drowsiness, sedation, vertigo. **Miscellaneous:** Sweating, malaise, pruritus, skin rashes, chronic hepatitis, hepatic hypersensitivity, jaundice, eosinophilia, altered LFTs.

LABORATORY TEST CONSIDERATIONS

↑ AST, ALT, and bilirubin.

P

OD OVERDOSE MANAGEMENT

NOTE: Both acute and chronic poisoning may result from use of papaverine. Symptoms are extensions of side effects.

Symptoms (Acute Poisoning): Nystagmus, diplopia, drowsiness, weakness, lassitude, incoordination, coma, cyanosis, ***respiratory depression.*** *Treatment (Acute Poisoning):* Delay absorption by giving tap water, milk, or activated charcoal followed by gastric lavage or induction of vomiting and then a cathartic. Maintain BP and take measures to treat respiratory depression and coma. Hemodialysis is effective.

Symptoms (Chronic Poisoning): Ataxia, blurred vision, drowsiness, anxiety, headache, GI upset, depression, urticaria, erythematous macular eruptions, blood dyscrasias, hypotension. *Treatment (Chronic Poisoning):* Discontinue medication. Monitor and treat blood dyscrasias. Provide symptomatic treatment. Treat hypotension by IV fluids, elevation of legs, and a vasopressor with inotropic effects.

DRUG INTERACTIONS

Diazoxide IV / Additive hypotension
Levodopa / ↓ Levodopa effect by blocking dopamine receptors

HOW SUPPLIED

Capsule, Extended Release: 150 mg; *Injection:* 30 mg/mL

DOSAGE

• **CAPSULES, TIMED-RELEASE**

Ischemia.

150 mg q 12 hr. May be increased to 150 mg q 8 hr or 300 mg q 12 hr in difficult cases.

NURSING CONSIDERATIONS

ASSESSMENT

1. Document indications for therapy, type, onset, duration, and characteristics of symptoms.
2. Determine any cardiac dysfunction; monitor VS, ECG, and LFTs.
3. Document mental status; assess all extremities for color, warmth, and pulses.

CLIENT/FAMILY TEACHING

1. Take with meals or milk to minimize GI upset.
2. Do not perform activities that require mental alertness until drug effects are realized; may cause dizziness or drowsiness.
3. Avoid tobacco products as nicotine may cause vasospasm.

OUTCOMES/EVALUATE

↓ Pain symptoms R/T ischemia

Paregoric (Camphorated opium tincture)

(pair-eh-**GOR**-ick)

PREGNANCY CATEGORY: C
CLASSIFICATION(S):
Antidiarrheal
Rx: C-III

SEE ALSO *NARCOTIC ANALGESICS.*

ACTION/KINETICS
The active principle of the mixture is opium (0.04% morphine). The preparation also contains benzoic acid, camphor, and anise oil. Morphine increases the muscular tone of the intestinal tract, decreases digestive secretions, and inhibits normal peristalsis. The slowed passage of the feces through the intestines promotes desiccation, which is a function of the time the feces spend in the intestine. **t½:** 2–3 hr. **Duration:** 4–5 hr.
USES
Acute diarrhea.
CONTRAINDICATIONS
See *Morphine Sulfate*. Use in clients with diarrhea caused by poisoning until toxic substance has been eliminated. Treatment of pseudomembranous colitis due to lincomycin, penicillins, and cephalosporins. Rubbing paregoric on the gums of a teething child. Use to treat neonatal opioid dependence.
SIDE EFFECTS
See *Narcotic Analgesics*.
DRUG INTERACTIONS
See *Narcotic Analgesics*.
HOW SUPPLIED
Oral Liquid: 2 mg morphine equivalent/5 mL

DOSAGE

• **LIQUID**

Adult: 5–10 mL 1–4 times/day (5 mL contains 2 mg of morphine). **Pediatric:** 0.25–0.5 mL/kg 1–4 times/day.

NURSING CONSIDERATIONS

SEE ALSO *NURSING CONSIDERATIONS* FOR *NARCOTIC ANALGESICS*.

ADMINISTRATION/STORAGE

1. Administer with water to ensure that it reaches the stomach; mixture will have a milky appearance.
2. Store in a light-resistant container.
3. Carefully distinguish between paregoric and tincture of opium. Tincture of opium contains 25 times more morphine than paregoric.
4. Paregoric preparations are subject to the Controlled Substances Act and must be charted accordingly.
5. Have naloxone available to treat any overdosage.

ASSESSMENT

1. Document onset, duration, and condition requiring paregoric, level of effectiveness, other agents prescribed and the outcome.
2. Note any hepatic dysfunction or drug dependence.

CLIENT/FAMILY TEACHING

1. Adhere to prescribed regimen.
2. Report if the diarrhea persists. Consume adequate warm clear fluids to replace loss and avoid dehydration.
3. Stop medication once diarrhea has abated. Continued use may result in constipation.

OUTCOMES/EVALUATE

Relief of diarrhea

Paricalcitol

(**pair**-ee-**KAL**-sih-tohl)

PREGNANCY CATEGORY: C
CLASSIFICATION(S):
Treatment of hyperparathyroidism
Rx: Zemplar

ACTION/KINETICS
Synthetic vitamin D analog that reduces parathyroid hormone levels in chronic renal failure with no significant changes in the incidence of hypercalcemia or hyperphosphatemia. Serum phosphorous, calcium, and calcium x phosphorous product may increase. **Peak levels:** 5 min which decrease quickly within 2 hr. **t½:** About 15 hr. Hepatobiliary excretion is most common.
USES
Prevention and treatment of secondary hyperparathyroidism associated with chronic renal failure.
CONTRAINDICATIONS
Evidence of vitamin D toxicity, hypercalemia, or hypersensitivity to any part of the product. Use of phosphate or vitamin D-related compounds concomitantly with paricalcitol.
SPECIAL CONCERNS
Use with caution during lactation or if given with digitalis compounds. Safety

P

and efficacy have not been determined in children.

SIDE EFFECTS

GI: N&V, GI bleeding, dry mouth. **CV:** Palpitation. **CNS:** Lightheadedness. **Respiratory:** Pneumonia. **Body as a whole:** Edema, chills, fever, flu, sepsis, not feeling well.

OD OVERDOSE MANAGEMENT

Symptoms: Hypercalcemia. Early symptoms include weakness, headache, somnolence, nausea, vomiting, dry mouth, constipation, muscle pain, bone pain, and metallic taste. Late symptoms include anorexia, weight loss, conjunctivitis, pancreatitis, photophobia, rhinorrhea, pruritus, hyperthermia, decreased libido, elevated BUN, hypercholesterolemia, elevated AST and ALT, ectopic calcification, hypertension, cardiac arrhythmias, somnolence, overt psychosis, death (rarely). *Treatment:* Immediately reduce or discontinue therapy. Institute a low calcium diet and withdraw calcium supplements. Mobilize client, give attention to fluid and electrolyte imbalances, assess ECG abnormalities (especially if also taking digitalis), and undertake hemodialysis or peritoneal dialysis against a calcium-free dialysate. Monitor serum calcium levels frequently until normal values are obtained.

DRUG INTERACTIONS

Digitalis toxicity is potentiated by hypercalcemia.

HOW SUPPLIED

Injection: 5 mcg/mL

DOSAGE

• **INJECTION**

Treat hyperparathyroidism associated with chronic renal failure.

Initial: 0.04–0.1 mcg/kg (2.8 to 7 mcg) as a bolus dose no more frequently than every other day at any time during dialysis. Doses as high as 0.24 mcg/kg (16.8 mcg) have been used safely. If a satisfactory response is not seen, the dose may be increased by 2 to 4 mcg at 2- to 4-week intervals. During any dosage adjustment period, monitor serum calcium and phosphorous levels more frequently. If an elevated calcium level or Ca x P product greater than 75 is noted, immediately reduce or stop the drug until parameters are normal. Then, restart at a lower dose. Doses may need to be decreased as the parathyroid levels decrease in response to therapy.

NURSING CONSIDERATIONS

ADMINISTRATION/STORAGE

Store at 25°C (77°F). Discard unused portion.

ASSESSMENT

1. Note indications for therapy.
2. Initially and with dose adjustment monitor Ca and P twice weekly and then q mo once dose established. Monitor PTH every 3 mo.

CLIENT/FAMILY TEACHING

1. Adhere to a dietary regimen of calcium supplementation and phosphorous restriction.
2. Avoid excessive use of aluminum-containing compounds.
3. Drug is used for the prevention and treatment of secondary hyperparathyroidism associated with CRF.
4. May experience nausea, vomiting, and edema; report if persistent or intolerable.

OUTCOMES/EVALUATE

↓ PTH concentrations

Paromomycin sulfate

(pair-oh-moh-**MY**-sin)

PREGNANCY CATEGORY: C
CLASSIFICATION(S):
Antibiotic, aminoglycoside
Rx: Humatin

SEE ALSO *AMINOGLYCOSIDES*.

ACTION/KINETICS

Obtained from *Streptomyces rimosus forma paromomycina.* Spectrum of activity resembles that of neomycin and kanamycin. Poorly absorbed from the GI tract and is ineffective against systemic infections when given PO.

USES

(1) Inhibition of ammonia-forming bacteria in GI tract in hepatic encephalopathy. (2) Intestinal amebiasis. (3) Preoperative suppression of intestinal flora. (4) Hepatic coma. *Investigation-*

al: Anthelmintic, to treat *Dientamoeba fragilis, Diphyllobothrium latum, Taenia saginata, T. solium, Dipylidium caninum,* and *Hymenolepis nana.*

CONTRAINDICATIONS

Intestinal obstruction.

SPECIAL CONCERNS

Use during pregnancy only if benefits outweigh risks. Use with caution in the presence of GI ulceration because of possible systemic absorption.

ADDITIONAL SIDE EFFECTS

Diarrhea or loose stools. Heartburn, emesis, and pruritus ani. Superinfections, especially by monilia.

DRUG INTERACTIONS

Paromomycin inhibits penicillin.

HOW SUPPLIED

Capsule: 250 mg

DOSAGE

• **CAPSULES**

Hepatic coma.

Adults: 4 g/day in divided doses for 5–6 days.

Intestinal amebiasis.

Adults and children: 25–35 mg/kg/day administered in three doses with meals for 5–10 days.

D. fragilis infections.

25–30 mg/kg/day in three divided doses for 1 week.

H. nana infections.

45 mg/kg/day for 5–7 days.

D. latum, T. saginata, T. solium, D. caninum infections.

Adults: 1 g/ q 15 min for a total of four doses; **pediatric:** 11 mg/kg/15 min for four doses.

NURSING CONSIDERATIONS

SEE ALSO ***NURSING CONSIDERATIONS*** FOR ***AMINOGLYCOSIDES.***

ADMINISTRATION/STORAGE

Do not administer parenterally and/or concurrently with penicillin.

CLIENT/FAMILY TEACHING

1. Take before or after meals.
2. Report any persistent diarrhea, dehydration, and general weakness.

OUTCOMES/EVALUATE

Suppression of intestinal flora

Paroxetine hydrochloride

(pah-**ROX**-eh-teen)

PREGNANCY CATEGORY: B

CLASSIFICATION(S):

Antidepressant, selective serotonin reuptake inhibitor

Rx: Paxil, Paxil CR

SEE ALSO ***SELECTIVE SEROTONIN REUPTAKE INHIBITORS.***

ACTION/KINETICS

Completely absorbed from the GI tract. **Time to peak plasma levels:** 5.2 hr. **Peak plasma levels:** 61.7 ng/mL. **t½:** 21–24 hr. **Time to reach steady state:** 7–14 days. Plasma levels are increased in impaired renal and hepatic function as well as in geriatric clients. Extensively metabolized in the liver to inactive metabolites. Approximately two-thirds of the drug is excreted through the urine and one-third is excreted in the feces.

USES

(1) Treatment of major depressive episodes. (2) Panic disorder with or without agoraphobia (as defined in DSM-IV). (3) Obsessive-compulsive disorders in clients with OCD (as defined in DSM-IV). (4) Social anxiety disorder (social phobia, as defined in DSM-IV). (5) Generalized anxiety disorder (as defined in DSM-IV). *Investigational:* Chronic headaches, diabetic neuropathy, premature ejaculation, fibromyalgia syndrome, premenstrual dysphoric disorder. With lithium for bipolar depression. Reduce incidence and severity of interferon-related depression in clients with malignant melanoma (allows completion of therapy).

ADDITIONAL CONTRAINDICATIONS

Use of alcohol. Concomitant use of thioridazine.

SPECIAL CONCERNS

Use with caution and initially at reduced dosage in elderly clients as well as in those with impaired hepatic or renal function, with a history of mania,

P

with a history of seizures, in clients with diseases or conditions that could affect metabolism or hemodynamic responses. Concurrent administration of paroxetine with lithium or digoxin should be undertaken with caution.

SIDE EFFECTS

The side effects listed were observed with a frequency up to 1 in 1,000 clients.

CNS: Headache, somnolence, insomnia, agitation, ***seizures,*** tremor, anxiety, activation of mania or hypomania, dizziness, nervousness, paresthesia, drugged feeling, myoclonus, CNS stimulation, confusion, amnesia, impaired concentration, depression, emotional lability, vertigo, abnormal thinking, akinesia, alcohol abuse, ataxia, ***convulsions, possibility of a suicide attempt,*** depersonalization, hallucinations, hyperkinesia, hypertonia, incoordination, lack of emotion, manic reaction, paranoid reaction. **GI:** Nausea, abdominal pain, diarrhea, dry mouth, vomiting, constipation, decreased appetite, flatulence, oropharynx disorder ("lump" in throat, tightness in throat), dyspepsia, increased appetite, bruxism, dysphagia, eructation, gastritis, glossitis, increased salivation, mouth ulceration, ***rectal hemorrhage,*** abnormal LFTs. **Hematologic:** Anemia, leukopenia, lymphadenopathy, purpura. **CV:** Palpitation, vasodilation, postural hypotension, hypertension, syncope, tachycardia, bradycardia, conduction abnormalities, abnormal ECG, hypotension, migraine, peripheral vascular disorder. **Dermatologic:** Sweating, rash, pruritus, acne, alopecia, dry skin, ecchymosis, eczema, furunculosis, urticaria. **Metabolic/Nutritional:** Edema, weight gain, weight loss, hyperglycemia, peripheral edema, thirst. **Respiratory:** Respiratory disorder (cold symptoms or URI), pharyngitis, yawn, increased cough, rhinitis, asthma, bronchitis, dyspnea, epistaxis, hyperventilation, pneumonia, respiratory flu, sinusitis. **GU:** Abnormal ejaculation (usually delay), erectile difficulties, sexual dysfunction, impotence, urinary frequency, urinary difficulty or hesitancy, decreased libido, anorgasmia in women, difficulty in reaching climax/orgasm in women, abortion, amenorrhea, breast pain, cystitis, dysmenorrhea, dysuria, menorrhagia, nocturia, polyuria, urethritis, urinary incontinence, urinary retention, vaginitis. **Musculoskeletal:** Asthenia, back pain, myopathy, myalgia, myasthenia, neck pain, arthralgia, arthritis. **Ophthalmologic:** Blurred vision, abnormality of accommodation, eye pain, mydriasis. **Otic:** Ear pain, otitis media, tinnitus. **Miscellaneous:** Fever, chest pain, trauma, taste perversion or loss, chills, malaise, allergic reaction, ***carcinoma,*** face edema, moniliasis, anorexia.

NOTE: Over 4- to 6-week period, there was evidence of adaptation to side effects such as nausea and dizziness but less adaptation to dry mouth, somnolence, and asthenia.

OD OVERDOSE MANAGEMENT

Symptoms: N&V, drowsiness, sinus tachycardia, dilated pupils. *Treatment:*

- Establish and maintain an airway.
- Ensure adequate oxygenation and ventilation.
- Induction of emesis, lavage, or both; following evacuation, 20–30 g activated charcoal may be given q 4–6 hr during the first 24–48 hr after ingestion.
- Take an ECG and monitor cardiac function if there is any evidence of abnormality.
- Provide supportive care with monitoring of VS.

ADDITIONAL DRUG INTERACTIONS

Antiarrhythmics, Type IC / Possible ↑ effect R/T ↓ liver breakdown
Cimetidine / ↑ Paroxetine effect R/T ↓ liver breakdown
Digoxin / Possible ↓ plasma levels
Phenobarbital / Possible ↓ Paroxetine effect R/T ↑ liver breakdown
Phenytoin / Possible ↓ Paroxetine effect R/T ↑ liver breakdown; also, ↓ phenytoin levels
Procyclidine / ↓ Procyclidine dose due to significant anticholinergic effects
Risperidone / ↑ Plasma risperidone levels R/T ↓ metabolism
H *St. John's wort* / Possible CNS depression
Theophylline / ↑ Theophylline levels
Thioridazine / ↑ Plasma levels of thioridazine → possible prolongation of QTc interval

HOW SUPPLIED

Suspension: 10 mg/5 mL; *Tablet:* 10 mg, 20 mg, 30 mg, 40 mg

DOSAGE

• **SUSPENSION, TABLETS**

Depression.

Adults, initial: 20 mg/day, usually given as a single dose in the morning. Some clients not responding to the 20-mg dose may benefit from increasing the dose in 10-mg/day increments, up to a maximum of 50 mg/day. Make dose changes at intervals of at least 1 week. **Maintenance:** Doses average about 30 mg/day.

Panic disorders.

Adults, initial: 10 mg/day usually given in the morning; **then,** increase by 10-mg increments each week until a dose of 40 mg/day is reached. Maximum daily dose: 60 mg.

Obsessive-compulsive disorders.

Adults, initial: 20 mg/kg; **then,** increase by 10-mg increments a day in intervals of at least 1 week until a dose of 40 mg/kg is reached. Maximum daily dose: 60 mg.

Social anxiety disorder.

Adults, initial: 20 mg/day, given as a single dose with or without food, usually in the morning. Dose range is 20–60 mg/day.

Generalized anxiety disorder.

Adults, initial: 20 mg/day, given as a single dose with or without food, usually in the morning. Dose range is 20–50 mg/day. Change doses in 10 mg/day increments at intervals of 1 week or more. Doses greater than 20 mg/day do not provide additional benefit.

Headaches.

10–50 mg/day.

Diabetic neuropathy.

10–60 mg/day.

Premature ejaculation in men.

20 mg/day.

NOTE: Geriatric or debilitated clients, those with severe hepatic or renal impairment, **initial:** 10 mg/day, up to a maximum of 40 mg/day for all uses.

NURSING CONSIDERATIONS

SEE ALSO *NURSING CONSIDERATIONS* FOR *SELECTIVE SEROTONIN REUPTAKE INHIBITORS.*

ADMINISTRATION/STORAGE

1. Even though beneficial effects may be seen in 1–4 weeks, continue therapy as prescribed.
2. Effectiveness is maintained for up to 1 year with daily doses averaging 30 mg.

ASSESSMENT

1. Document type, onset, and duration of symptoms, any previous treatment, and the outcome.
2. Note clinical presentation and behavioral manifestations.
3. Document any mania, altered metabolic or hemodynamic states, or seizures.
4. List drugs currently prescribed to ensure no unfavorable interactions. Do not use in combination with a MAO or within 14 days of discontinuing treatment with a MAO.
5. Monitor weight, VS, ECG, electrolytes, CBC, liver and renal function studies; note any dysfunction.
6. Closely monitor infants born to mothers who took paroxetine during pregnancy due to the possibility of a withdrawal syndrome.
7. During management of overdose, always entertain the possibility of multiple drug involvement.

CLIENT/FAMILY TEACHING

1. Take only as directed. Prescriptions may be for small quantities to ensure compliance and to discourage overdose. Allow up to 4 weeks for therapeutic effects.
2. Do not engage in tasks that require mental alertness until drug effects realized.
3. Avoid alcohol and OTC products.
4. Report excessive weight loss/gain and adjust diet/exercise to compensate.
5. Notify provider if pregnancy is suspected or planned.
6. Report any thoughts of suicide or increased suicide ideations. Advise

P

family not to leave severely depressed individuals alone; possibility of a suicide attempt is inherent in depression and may persist until significant remission is observed.

7. Participate in therapy sessions designed to assist with underlying problems. With prolonged use may require gradual titrated withdrawl.

OUTCOMES/EVALUATE

- ↓ Anxiety/depression
- Improved eating/sleeping patterns; ↑ social involvement/activity
- ↓ Panic attacks; ↓ palpitations; ↓ obsessive repetitive behaviors

Pegaspargase (PEG-L-asparaginase)

(peg-**ASS**-pair-gays)

PREGNANCY CATEGORY: C

CLASSIFICATION(S):

Antineoplastic, miscellaneous

Rx: Oncaspar

SEE ALSO *ANTINEOPLASTIC AGENTS*.

ACTION/KINETICS

Pegaspargase is a modification of the enzyme L-asparaginase. L-asparaginase, derived from *Escherichia coli*, is modified by conjugating covalently units of monomethoxypolyethylene glycol (PEG), thus forming the active PEG-L-asparaginase. Leukemic cells are not able to synthesize asparagine due to a lack of the enzyme asparaginase synthetase and are thus dependent on exogenous asparaginase for survival. Rapid depletion of asparagine, due to administration of asparaginase, kills leukemic cells. Normal cells, which can synthesize their own asparagine, are less affected.

USES

Clients with acute lymphoblastic leukemia who have developed hypersensitivity to the native forms of L-asparaginase. Used in combination with other antineoplastic drugs, including vincristine, methotrexate, cytarabine, daunorubicin, and doxorubicin. Only use pegaspargase as a single agent when therapy with multiple drugs is determined to be inappropriate for the client.

CONTRAINDICATIONS

Pancreatitis or history thereof. Significant hemorrhagic events associated with prior L-asparaginase therapy. Previous allergic reactions, such as generalized urticaria, bronchospasm, laryngeal edema, hypotension, or other side effects to pegaspargase that are not acceptable. Lactation.

SPECIAL CONCERNS

Clients taking pegaspargase are at a higher risk for bleeding problems, especially with simultaneous use of other drugs that have anticoagulant properties (e.g., aspirin, NSAIDs). Safety and efficacy have not been determined in clients from 1 to 21 years of age with known previous hypersensitivity to L-asparaginase.

SIDE EFFECTS

Most commonly hypersensitivity reactions, chemical hepatotoxicity, and coagulopathies. **Allergic reactions: *Hypersensitivity reactions*** (acute or delayed), including ***life-threatening anaphylaxis,*** may occur during therapy, especially in clients with known hypersensitivity to other forms of L-asparaginase. Also, skin rashes, erythema, edema, pain, fever, chills, urticaria, dyspnea, ***bronchospasm,*** increased ALT, N&V, malaise, arthralgia, induration, hives, tenderness, swelling, lip edema. **GI:** Pancreatitis (may be severe), abdominal pain, anorexia, diarrhea, constipation, flatulence, GI pain, indigestion, mucositis, mouth tenderness, severe colitis. **Coagulation disorders:** Decreased anticoagulant effect, ***DIC,*** decreased fibrinogen, increased thromboplastin, increased coagulation time, prolonged PTs, prolonged PTTs, ***clinical hemorrhage (may be fatal),*** decreased antithrombin III, superficial and deep venous thrombosis, sagittal sinus thrombosis, venous catheter thrombosis, atrial thrombosis, decreased platelet count, purpura, ecchymosis, easy bruisability. **Hepatic:** Jaundice, abnormal LFTs, liver fatty deposits, hepatomegaly, ascites, ***liver failure.*** **CV:** Hypotension (may be severe), tachycardia, thrombosis, chest pain, hypertension, subacute bacterial endocarditis, edema. **Hematologic:**

Hemolytic anemia, leukopenia, pancytopenia, thrombocytopenia, ***agranulocytosis,*** anemia. **CNS:** ***Convulsions, status epilepticus,*** temporal lobe seizures, headache, paresthesia, mild to severe confusion, disorientation, dizziness, emotional lability, somnolence, ***coma,*** mental status changes, Parkinson-like syndrome. **Respiratory:** Dyspnea, ***bronchospasm,*** increased cough, epistaxis, URI. **Dermatologic:** Injection site hypersensitivity, rash, petechial rash, erythema simplex, pruritus, itching, alopecia, fever blister, hand whiteness, fungal changes, nail whiteness and ridging. **GU:** Hematuria, increased urinary frequency, abnormal kidney function, severe hemorrhagic cystitis, ***renal failure,*** uric acid nephropathy. **Musculoskeletal:** Arthralgia, myalgia, bone pain, joint disorder, diffuse and local musculoskeletal pain, joint stiffness, cramps. **Miscellaneous:** Pain in the extremities, injection site reaction (including pain, swelling, or redness), night sweats, peripheral edema, increased or decreased appetite, excessive thirst, weight loss, face edema, lesional edema, ***septic shock, sepsis,*** infection, malaise, fatigue, metabolic acidosis.

LABORATORY TEST CONSIDERATIONS

↑ AST, amylase, lipase, gamma-glutamyltranspeptidase, BUN, creatinine. Bilirubinemia, hyperglycemia, hyperuricemia, hypoglycemia, hypoproteinemia, hyperammonemia, hyponatremia, hypoalbuminemia, proteinuria.

DRUG INTERACTIONS

Depletion of serum proteins by pegaspargase may ↑ the toxicity of other drugs which are protein bound. ↑ Predisposition to bleeding when used with warfarin, heparin, dipyridamole, aspirin, or NSAIDs. May ↓ the effect of methotrexate.

HOW SUPPLIED

Injection: 750 IU/mL

DOSAGE

- **IM (PREFERRED), IV**

As a component of selected multi-drug regimens.

Adults: 2,500 IU/m² q 14 days. This dose is also used if the drug is given as a sole agent. **Children with a BSA greater than 0.6 m²:** 2,500 IU/m² q 14 days. **Children with a BSA less than 0.6 m²:** 82.5 IU/kg q 14 days.

NURSING CONSIDERATIONS

SEE ALSO *NURSING CONSIDERATIONS* FOR *ANTINEOPLASTIC AGENTS.*

ADMINISTRATION/STORAGE

1. The preferred route of administration is IM due to a lower risk of hepatotoxicity, coagulopathy, and GI and renal disorders.
2. Do not give if there is any indication it has been frozen; freezing destroys pegaspargase activity.
3. When given IM, do not exceed 2 mL to a single injection site; if more than 2 mL is necessary, use multiple injection sites.
4. When remission is obtained, appropriate maintenance therapy may be instituted.
5. Do not shake; avoid excessive agitation. Do not use if cloudy, if a precipitate is present, or if it's been stored at room temperature for more than 48 hr.
6. Store at 2–8°C (36–46°F).
7. Use only one dose per vial; do not reenter the vial. Discard any unused portions.

IV 8. When used IV, administer over a 1- to 2-hr period in 100 mL of NSS or D5W, through an infusion tube of a solution that is already running.

ASSESSMENT

1. Document previous therapy and outcome. Use the National Cancer Institute Common Toxic Criteria to grade the severity of any hypersensitivity reaction.
2. Anticipate administration with other antineoplastic agents.
3. Monitor continuously for anaphylaxis during the first hour of therapy.
4. Assess for early S&S of infection due to immunosuppressive effects; or pancreatitis.
5. IM administration may decrease many of the drug-associated adverse systemic effects.
6. Monitor liver and renal function studies, uric acid, hematologic and

P

coagulation profiles. Assess PFT's and CXR; obtain CXR q 2 weeks during therapy and watch for severe pulmonary effects i.e. bronchospasm, fibrosis or infiltrates.

CLIENT/FAMILY TEACHING

1. Report any increased bruising or bleeding, any early S&S of infection.
2. Avoid agents that may increase bleeding (e.g., aspirin/NSAIDs, alcohol).
3. Report any persistent N&V, yellow skin discoloration, difficulty breathing, chest pain, rash, or severe abdominal pain immediately.
4. Report any altered mental status or evidence of seizure activity.
5. Increase fluid intake 2-3L/day to prevent urate deposits/calculi formation. Consume diet low in purines to maintain alkaline urine.
6. Drug lowers resistance to infections; avoid situations that may put one at risk (i.e., crowds, persons with infectious diseases, vaccinia).

OUTCOMES/EVALUATE

Improved hematologic parameters; remission of acute lymphoblastic leukemia

Peginterferon alfa-2b

(peg-**in**-ter-**FEER**-on)

PREGNANCY CATEGORY: C
CLASSIFICATION(S):
Immunomodulator
Rx: PEG-Intron

ACTION/KINETICS

Effect due to the interferon alfa-2b moiety which binds to specific membrane receptors on the cell surface. This initiates a complex series of intracellular effects, including suppression of cell proliferation, enhancement of phagocytic activity of macrophages, augmentation of specific cytotoxicity of lymphocytes for target cells, and inhibition of virus replication in virus-infected cells. **Maximum serum levels:** 15–44 hr; serum levels sustained for 48 hr (or less)–72 hr. **t½, elimination:** About 40 hr. About 30% excreted in the urine. Clearance is decreased by about one-half in those with impaired renal function.

USES

Monotherapy or with ribavirin to treat chronic hepatitis C in those 18 years or older not previously treated with interferon alpha and who have compensated liver disease. *Investigational:* Renal carcinoma.

CONTRAINDICATIONS

Hypersensitivity to the drug or any component of the product, autoimmune hepatitis, decompensated liver disease. Lactation.

SPECIAL CONCERNS

Serious, acute hypersensitivity reactions, although rare, may occur. When combined with ribavirin, side effects are common and severe. Use with caution in those with a creatinine clearance less than 50 mL/min, in the elderly, and in CV disease. May be development or worsening of autoimmune disorders (e.g., thyroiditis, thrombocytopenia, rheumatoid arthritis, interstitial nephritis, systemic lupus erythematosus, psoriasis). Safety and efficacy have not been determined in children less than 18 years of age, for the treatment of clients with HCV coinfected with HIV or HBV, or to treat hepatitis C in clients who have received liver or other organ transplants.

SIDE EFFECTS

CNS: Headache, depression, suicidal behavior (attempt, ideation), anxiety, emotional lability, irritability, insomnia, dizziness, relapse of drug addiction/overdose, loss of consciousness. **GI:** Nausea, anorexia, diarrhea, abdominal pain, vomiting, dyspepsia, ***fatal/nonfatal ulcerative and hemorrhagic colitis, fatal/nonfatal pancreatitis***. **Respiratory:** Pharyngitis, sinusitis, coughing, dyspnea, pulmonary infiltrates, pneumonitis, pneumonia. **Dermatologic:** Alopecia, pruritus, dry skin, increased sweating, rash, flushing, aggravated psoriasis, urticaria. **Hematologic:** Thrombocytopenia, neutropenia, autoimmune thrombocytopenia. **CV:** ***Cardiomyopathy, MI,*** hypotension, arrhythmia, TIA, supraventricular arrhythmias. **Ophthalmic:** Retinal hemorrhages, cotton wool spots, retinal artery/vein obstruction, retinal ischemia, retinal vein thrombosis. **Body as a whole:** Flu-like symptoms, musculoskeletal pain, fatigue, rigors, fever, weight decrease, abscess, lupus-like syndrome, rheumatoid arthritis, viral infection, malaise. **Hypersensitivity reaction:** Urticaria, angioedema, bronchoconstriction, ***anaphylaxis***. **At injection site:** Bruising, itchiness, irritation, pain, alopecia. **Miscellaneous:** Right upper quadrant pain, hepatomegaly, hypertonia, hypo-/hyperthyroidism, nerve palsy (facial, oculomotor), interstitial nephritis.

LABORATORY TEST CONSIDERATIONS

↑ ALT. ↓ Neutrophils, platelet counts. TSH abnormalities. Appearance of serum neutralizing antibodies.

HOW SUPPLIED

Powder for injection, lyophilized: 100 mcg/mL, 160 mcg/mL, 240 mcg/mL, 300 mcg/mL

DOSAGE

• **SC**

Chronic hepatitis C.

Initial: Based on weight. Dose is given once weekly (on the same day of each week) for 1 year. **37–45 kg:** 40 mcg (0.4 mL of the 100 mcg/mL strength); **46–56 kg:** 50 mcg (0.5 mL of the 100 mcg/mL strength); **57–72 kg:** 64 mcg (0.4 mL of the 160 mcg/mL strength); **73–88 kg:** 80 mcg (0.5 mL of the 160 mcg/mL strength); **89–106 kg:** 96 mcg (0.4 mL of the 240 mcg/mL strength); **107–136 kg:** 120 mcg (0.5 mL of the 240 mcg/mL strength); **137–160 kg:** 150 mcg (0.5 mL of the 300 mcg/mL strength).

NURSING CONSIDERATIONS

ADMINISTRATION/STORAGE

Store unreconstituted drug between 15–30°C (59–86°F). After reconstitution use immediately but may be stored for 24 hr or less between 2–8°C (36–46°F). Do not freeze.

ASSESSMENT

1. Document onset of disease, associated factors, and other agents trialed.
2. Determine renal and LFTs; assess viral load. Assess clients with impaired renal function for S&S of interferon toxicity; adjust dose accordingly.
3. Ensure adequate hydration, especially during initial stages of treatment.

CLIENT/FAMILY TEACHING

1. To minimize flu-like symptoms, administer the drug at bedtime once a week. Use antipyretics as needed.
2. It is not known if treatment will cure hepatitis C or prevent cirrhosis, liver failure, or liver cancer that may result from infection with the hepatitis C virus. It is also not known if the drug will prevent transmission of HCV infection to others.
3. Once reconstituted, may only store in the refrigerator up to 24 hr.
4. Proper disposal of needles is imperative; do not reuse needles or syringes. A puncture-resistant container will be supplied for disposal of used needles and syringes at home.
5. Drug may cause depression, flu-like symptoms, bleeding abnormalities, and autoimmune dysfunction. Report any unusual side effects to provider for evaluation.
6. Labs are required before beginning therapy and at periodic set intervals; must comply to continue on therapy.

OUTCOMES/EVALUATE

Inhibition of progression of hepatitis C; improved LFTs

P

Pemoline

(**PEM**-oh-leen)

PREGNANCY CATEGORY: B
CLASSIFICATION(S):
CNS stimulant
Rx: Cylert, Cylert Chewable, PemADD, PemADD CT, **C-IV**

ACTION/KINETICS

Believed to act by dopaminergic mechanisms. Causes a decrease in hyperactivity and a prolonged attention span in children. **Peak serum levels:** 2–4 hr. **Duration:** Up to 8 hr. **t½:** 12 hr. **Steady state:** 2–3 days; beneficial effects may not be noted for 3–4 weeks.

Approximately 50% is bound to plasma protein. Metabolized by the liver, and approximately 50% is excreted unchanged by the kidneys.

USES

Attention-deficit disorders. Due to possible life-threatening hepatic failure, not usually first-line therapy. *Investigational:* Narcolepsy, fatigue, and excessive daytime sleepiness.

CONTRAINDICATIONS

Hypersensitivity to drug. Hepatic insufficiency. Tourette's syndrome. Children under 6 years of age.

SPECIAL CONCERNS

Safe use during lactation has not been established. Use with caution in significantly impaired kidney function or in emotionally unstable clients. Chronic use in children may cause growth suppression.

SIDE EFFECTS

CNS: Insomnia (most common). Dyskinesia of the face, tongue, lips, and extremities; precipitation of Tourette's syndrome. Mild depression, headache, nystagmus, dizziness, hallucinations, irritability, drowsiness, abnormal oculomotor function (nystagmus, oculogyric crisis), ***seizures.*** Exacerbation of behavior disturbances and thought disorders in psychotic children. Possibility of psychological or physical dependence. **GI:** Transient weight loss, anorexia, gastric upset, nausea. **Miscellaneous:** Skin rash, hepatic toxicity, ***hepatic failure, aplastic anemia (rare).***

LABORATORY TEST CONSIDERATIONS

↑ AST, ALT, serum LDH.

OD OVERDOSE MANAGEMENT

Symptoms: Symptoms of CNS stimulation and sympathomimetic effects including agitation, confusion, delirium, euphoria, headache, muscle twitching, mydriasis, vomiting, hallucinations, flushing, sweating, tachycardia, hyperreflexia, tremors, ***hyperpyrexia,*** hypertension, ***seizures (may be followed by coma).*** *Treatment:* Reduce external stimuli. If symptoms are not severe, induce vomiting or undertake gastric lavage. Chlorpromazine can be used to decrease the CNS stimulation and sympathomimetic effects.

DRUG INTERACTIONS

↓ Seizure threshold when used with antiepileptic drugs.

HOW SUPPLIED

Chew Tablet: 37.5 mg; *Tablet:* 18.75 mg, 37.5 mg, 75 mg

DOSAGE

• TABLETS, CHEW TABLETS

Attention-deficit disorders.

Children, 6 years and older, initial: 37.5 mg/day as a single dose in the morning; increase at 1-week intervals by 18.75 mg until desired response is attained up to maximum of 112.5 mg/day. **Usual maintenance:** 56.25–75 mg/day.

Narcolepsy.

Adults: 50–200 mg/day in two divided doses.

NURSING CONSIDERATIONS

ADMINISTRATION/STORAGE

Interrupt treatment once or twice annually to determine whether behavioral symptoms still necessitate therapy.

ASSESSMENT

1. Document indications for therapy, type, onset, and characteristics of symptoms; describe clinical presentation.
2. Assess renal and LFTs, mental status and child for growth retardation. Assess LFTs at baseline and every 2 weeks thereafter; discontinue if clinical signs of hepatic failure occur or if ALT values increase to clinically significant levels or 2 or more times the upper limit of normal.

CLIENT/FAMILY TEACHING

1. Administer early in the morning to minimize insomnia.
2. Do not perform activities that require mental alertness until drug effects are realized.
3. Avoid excessive consumption of caffeine-containing products.
4. Advise school health department of medication regimen. Do not stop abruptly; withdraw over several weeks.
5. Measure height every month, and weigh child twice/week. Graph all measurements and bring to each visit. Report weight loss or failure to grow.
6. Continue therapy; behavioral changes take 3–4 weeks to occur.

7. Instruct when to interrupt drug administration, and to observe and record behavior without the medication, to determine whether therapy should be resumed.
8. Stress importance of bringing the child in periodically for LFTs to assess for toxicity.
9. Identify signs of overdosage, such as agitation, restlessness, hallucinations, and tachycardia; withhold drug, protect the child, and report immediately.

OUTCOMES/EVALUATE

Improved attention span; ↓ hyperactivity with ability to sit quietly and concentrate

Penbutolol sulfate

(pen-**BYOU**-toe-lohl)

PREGNANCY CATEGORY: C
CLASSIFICATION(S):
Beta-adrenergic blocking agent
Rx: Levatol

SEE ALSO *BETA-ADRENERGIC BLOCKING AGENTS.*

ACTION/KINETICS

Has both beta-1- and beta-2-receptor blocking activity. It has no membrane-stabilizing activity but does possess minimal intrinsic sympathomimetic activity. High lipid solubility. **t½:** 5 hr. 80%–98% protein bound. Metabolized in the liver and excreted through the urine.

USES

Alone or in combination with other antihypertensive drugs for mild to moderate arterial hypertension

CONTRAINDICATIONS

Bronchial asthma or bronchospasms, including severe COPD.

SPECIAL CONCERNS

Dosage has not been established in children. Geriatric clients may manifest increased or decreased sensitivity to the usual adult dose.

HOW SUPPLIED

Tablet: 20 mg

DOSAGE

• **TABLETS**

Hypertension.

Initial: 20 mg/day either alone or with other antihypertensive agents. **Maintenance:** Same as initial dose. Doses greater than 40 mg/day do not result in a greater antihypertensive effect.

NURSING CONSIDERATIONS

SEE ALSO *NURSING CONSIDERATIONS FOR ANTIHYPERTENSIVE AGENTS.*

ADMINISTRATION/STORAGE

Doses of 10 mg/day are effective but full effects are not evident for 4–6 weeks. The full effect of a 20- to 40-mg dose may not be observed for 2 weeks.

CLIENT/FAMILY TEACHING

1. May cause postural hypotension; to avoid, rise slowly from a sitting or lying position.
2. Take only as prescribed; full effects may not be realized for a month or more.
3. May cause an increased sensitivity to cold; dress appropriately.
4. Avoid alcohol. Do not stop drug suddenly, may exacerbate heart disease.

OUTCOMES/EVALUATE

↓ BP

Penciclovir

(pen-**SIGH**-kloh-veer)

PREGNANCY CATEGORY: B
CLASSIFICATION(S):
Antiviral
Rx: Denavir

SEE ALSO *ANTIVIRAL DRUGS.*

ACTION/KINETICS

Active against herpes simplex viruses (HSVs), including HSV-1 and HSV-2. In infected cells, viral thymidine kinase phosphorylates penciclovir to a monophosphate form which then is converted to penciclovir triphosphate by cellular kinases. Penciclovir triphosphate inhibits HSV polymerase competitively with deoxyguanosine triphosphate which inhibits herpes vi-

P

ral DNA synthesis and replication. Not absorbed through the skin.

USES

Treatment of recurrent herpes labialis (cold sores) in adults.

CONTRAINDICATIONS

Lactation. Application of the drug to mucous membranes.

SPECIAL CONCERNS

Use with caution if applied around the eyes due to the possibility of irritation. The effect of the drug in immunocompromised clients has not been determined. Safety and efficacy have not been determined in children.

SIDE EFFECTS

Dermatologic: Reaction at the site of application, hypesthesia, local anesthesia, erythematous rash, mild erythema. **Miscellaneous:** Headache, taste perversion.

HOW SUPPLIED

Cream: 10 mg/g.

DOSAGE

• **CREAM**

Cold sores.

Apply q 2 hr while awake for 4 days.

NURSING CONSIDERATIONS

SEE ALSO *NURSING CONSIDERATIONS* FOR *ANTIVIRAL DRUGS.*

ADMINISTRATION/STORAGE

1. Start treatment as soon as possible during the prodrome or when lesions appear.
2. Use only on the lips and face.

ASSESSMENT

Document onset, location, description, and extent of lesions. Note frequency of occurrence and any triggers or prodrome.

CLIENT/FAMILY TEACHING

1. Wash hands before and after application. Apply q 2 hr while awake for 4 days at first cold sore symptoms.
2. Avoid contact with mucous membranes and eyes; apply to lips and face only.
3. Use sunscreens and lip balms with a sunscreen when sun exposed to prevent recurrence and to diminish intersity of outbreaks.
4. Report if lesions do not improve or if a foul odor or purulent drainage appears.

OUTCOMES/EVALUATE

↓ Intensity/pain; clearing of herpes lesions

Penicillamine

(pen-ih-**SILL**-ah-meen)

PREGNANCY CATEGORY: D
CLASSIFICATION(S):
Antirheumatic
Rx: Cuprimine, Depen

ACTION/KINETICS

A chelating agent for mercury, lead, iron, and copper; forms soluble complexes, thus decreasing toxic levels of the metal (e.g., copper in Wilson's disease). Anti-inflammatory activity may be due to its ability to inhibit T-lymphocyte function and therefore decrease cell-mediated immune response. May also protect lymphocytes from hydrogen peroxide generated at the site of inflammation by inhibiting release of lysosomal enzymes and oxygen radicals. Beneficial effects may not be seen for 2 to 3 months when used for rheumatoid arthritis. In cystinuria, is able to reduce excess cystine excretion, probably by disulfide interchange between penicillamine and cystine. This results in penicillamine-cysteine disulfide, which is a complex that is more soluble than cystine and is thus readily excreted. Well absorbed from the GI tract and excreted in urine. Food decreases the absorption of penicillamine over 50%. **Peak plasma levels:** 1–3 hr. About 80% is bound to plasma albumin. **t½:** Approximately 2 hr. Metabolites are excreted through the urine.

USES

Wilson's disease, cystinuria, and rheumatoid arthritis (severe active disease unresponsive to conventional therapy). Heavy metal antagonist. *Investigational:* Primary biliary cirrhosis. Scleroderma.

CONTRAINDICATIONS

Pregnancy, lactation, penicillinase-related aplastic anemia or agranulocytosis, hypersensitivity to drug. Clients allergic to penicillin may cross-react with penicillamine. Renal insufficiency or history thereof.

SPECIAL CONCERNS

Use for juvenile rheumatoid arthritis has not been established. Clients older than 65 years may be at greater risk of developing hematologic side effects.

SIDE EFFECTS

This drug manifests a large number of potentially serious side effects. Clients should be carefully monitored.

GI: Altered taste perception (common), N&V, diarrhea, anorexia, GI pain, stomatitis, oral ulcerations, reactivation of peptic ulcer, glossitis, cheilosis, colitis, gingivostomatitis (rare). **CNS:** Tinnitus, myasthenia gravis, peripheral sensory and motor neuropathies (with or without muscle weakness), reversible optic neuritis, polyradiculopathy (rare). **Hematologic:** Thrombocytopenia, leukopenia, ***agranulocytosis, aplastic anemia,*** eosinophilia, monocytosis, red cell aplasia, thrombocytopenia, ***hemolytic anemia,*** leukocytosis, thrombocytosis. **Renal:** Proteinuria, hematuria, nephrotic syndrome, ***Goodpasture's syndrome*** (a severe and ultimately fatal glomerulonephritis). **Allergic:** Rashes (common), lupus-like syndrome, drug fever, pruritus, pemphigoid-type symptoms (e.g., bullous lesions), arthralgia, lymphadenopathy, dermatoses, urticaria, thyroiditis, hypoglycemia, migratory polyarthralgia, polymyositis, allergic alveolitis. **Respiratory:** Obliterative bronchiolitis, pulmonary fibrosis, pneumonitis, bronchial asthma, interstitial pneumonitis. **Dermatologic:** Increased skin friability, excessive skin wrinkling, development of small white papules at venipuncture and surgical sites, alopecia or falling hair, lichen planus, dermatomyositis, nail disorders, ***toxic epidermal necrolysis,*** cutaneous macular atrophy. **Hepatic:** Pancreatitis, hepatic dysfunction, intrahepatic cholestasis, toxic hepatitis (rare). **Other:** Thrombophlebitis, hyperpyrexia, polymyositis, mammary hyperplasia, renal vasculitis (may be fatal), hot flashes, lupus erythematosus–like syndrome.

LABORATORY TEST CONSIDERATIONS

↑ Serum alkaline phosphatase, LDH. Positive thymol turbidity test and cephalin flocculation test.

DRUG INTERACTIONS

Antacids / ↓ Effect of penicillamine R/T ↓ absorption from GI tract
Antimalarial drugs / ↑ Risk of blood dyscrasias and adverse renal effects
Cytotoxic drugs / ↑ Risk of blood dyscrasias and adverse renal effects
Digoxin / Penicillamine ↓ effect of digoxin
Gold therapy / ↑ Risk of blood dyscrasias and adverse renal effects
Iron salts / ↓ Effect of penicillamine R/T ↓ absorption from GI tract
Pyridoxine / ↑ Pyridoxine requirements

HOW SUPPLIED

Capsule: 125 mg, 250 mg; *Tablet, titratable:* 250 mg

DOSAGE

- **CAPSULES, TABLETS**

Rheumatoid arthritis.

Adults, individualized, initial: 125–250 mg/day. Dosage may be increased at 1- to 3-month intervals by 125- to 250-mg increments until adequate response is attained. **Maximum:** 500–750 mg/day. Up to 500 mg/day can be given as a single dose; higher dosages should be divided. **Maintenance, individualized. Range:** 500–750 mg/day. If the client is in remission for 6 or more months, a gradual stepwise decrease in dose of 125 or 250 mg/day at about 3-month intervals can be attempted.

Wilson's disease.

Dosage is usually calculated on the basis of the urinary excretion of copper. One gram of penicillamine promotes excretion of 2 mg of copper. **Adults and adolescents, usual, initial:** 250 mg q.i.d. Dosage may have to be increased to 2 g/day. A further increase does not produce additional excretion. **Pediatric, 6 months—young children:** 250 mg as a single dose given in fruit juice.

Antidote for heavy metals.

Adults: 0.5–1.5 g/day for 1–2 months; **pediatric:** 30–40 mg/kg/day (600–750 mg/m²/day) for 1–6 months.

P

Cystinuria.
Individualized and based on excretion rate of cystine (100–200 mg/day in clients with no history of stones, below 100 mg with clients with history of stones or pain). Initiate at low dosage (250 mg/day) and increase gradually to minimum effective dosage. **Adult, usual:** 2 g/day (range: 1–4 g/day); **pediatric:** 7.5 mg/kg q.i.d. If divided in fewer than four doses, give larger dose at night.

Primary biliary cirrhosis.
Adults: 600–900 mg/day.

NURSING CONSIDERATIONS

ADMINISTRATION/STORAGE

1. If unable to tolerate dosage for cystinuria, the bedtime dosage should be larger and should be continued.
2. Administer the contents of the capsule in 15–30 mL of chilled juice or pureed fruit if unable to swallow capsules or tablets.
3. When treating rheumatoid arthritis, discontinue if doses up to 1.5 g/day for 2–3 months do not produce improvement.
4. Alternative dosage forms may be prepared if needed. An elixir containing 50 mg/mL may be prepared by dissolving the contents of 48 capsules in 100 mL of water. This is then filtered, and 100 mL of cherry syrup and 30 mL of alcohol stirred in. The volume is then brought up to 240 mL with water. The preparation is shaken well and stored in the refrigerator. Suppositories (750 mg) may be prepared by melting 51 g of cocoa butter and dissolving the contents of 150 capsules in the cocoa butter; the mixture is poured into a prelubricated suppository mold and then frozen and stored in a refrigerator.

ASSESSMENT

1. Determine indications, presenting symptoms, other therapies prescribed and outcome.
2. Note if taking any medication with which penicillamine will interact unfavorably; impedes absorption of many drugs.
3. Assess hearing to detect any evidence of hearing loss.
4. Document CNS assessment and neurologic status.
5. With arthritis, assess joints for pain, stiffness, soreness, swelling, and ↓ ROM.
6. Test for pregnancy; drug can cause fetal damage.
7. White papules appearing at the site of venipuncture or at surgical sites may indicate sensitivity to penicillamine or the presence of infection.
8. If to undergo surgery, anticipate dosage reduction to 250 mg/day until wound healing is complete.
9. Monitor CBC, LFTs, and urinalysis. If WBC falls below 3,500/mm^3 or the platelet count falls below 100,000/mm^3, withhold drug and report. If counts are low for three successive lab tests, a temporary interruption of therapy is indicated.
10. A positive ANA test indicates client may develop a lupus-like syndrome in the future. The drug need not be discontinued.

CLIENT/FAMILY TEACHING

1. Give on an empty stomach 1 hr before or 2 hr after meals; wait 1 hr after ingestion of any other food, milk, or drug. With Wilson's disease take 30-60 min before meals and at bedtime.
2. Take temperature nightly during the first few months of therapy. A fever may indicate a hypersensitivity reaction.
3. Report any evidence of fever, sore throat, chills, skin rash, bruising, or bleeding; early S&S of granulocytopenia.
4. If stomatitis occurs, report immediately and stop drug. Practice regular oral hygiene such as brushing teeth with a soft toothbrush, flossing daily, and using alcohol free mouth rinses.
5. Inspect mucosal surfaces at regular intervals. Report if ulcers appear and are severe or persistent, may need to reduce drug dose as it may interfere with wound healing.
6. Penicillamine increases the body's need for pyridoxine. May be given pyridoxine (25 mg/day po).
7. A loss of taste perception or a metallic taste may develop; relates to zinc chelation and may last for 2 months or more. With N&V or diarrhea, monitor

weight and I&O. Report jaundice or other signs of hepatic dysfunction.
8. If to receive an oral iron preparation, at least 2 hr should elapse between ingestion of penicillamine and the dose of therapeutic iron. Iron decreases the cupruretic effects of penicillamine.
9. Skin tends to become friable and susceptible to injury; avoid activities that could injure skin. Elderly should avoid excessive pressure on the shoulders, elbows, knees, toes, and buttocks.
10. Report cloudy urine or urine that is smoky brown (signs of proteinuria and hematuria).
11. Practice reliable birth control; report missed menstrual period or other symptoms of pregnancy.
12. With Wilson's disease:
• Eat a diet low in copper. Exclude foods such as chocolate, nuts, shellfish, mushrooms, liver, molasses, broccoli, and copper-enriched cereals.
• Use distilled or demineralized water if drinking water contains more than 0.1 mg/L copper.
• Unless taking iron supplements, take sulfurated potash or Carbo-Resin with meals to minimize the absorption of copper.
• It may take 1–3 months for neurologic improvements to occur. Therefore, continue the therapy even if no improvements seem evident.
• Check any vitamin preparations being used to ensure that they do not contain copper.
13. If cystinuria occurs, do the following:
• Drink large amounts of fluid to prevent the formation of renal calculi. Drink 500 mL of fluid at bedtime and another pint during the night, when the urine tends to be the most concentrated and most acidic. The greater the fluid intake, the lower the required dose of penicillamine.
• Measure specific gravity and determine pH. The urine specific gravity should be maintained at less than 1.010 and the pH maintained at 7.5–8.0.
• Obtain yearly X-ray of the kidneys to detect presence of renal calculi.
• Eat a diet low in methionine, a major precursor of cystine. Exclude foods high in cystine such as rich meat, soups and broths, milk, eggs, cheeses, and peas.
• If client is pregnant or a child, diets low in methionine are also low in calcium; consider calcium supplementation.
14. With rheumatoid arthritis, continue using other therapies and meds to achieve relief from symptoms; penicillamine may take 4–6 mo to have therapeutic effect. As improvement begins, analgesic drugs and NSAIDs may be slowly tapered.

OUTCOMES/EVALUATE

• ↑ Urinary excretion of copper
• ↓ Cystine excretion and prevention of renal calculi in cystinuria
• ↓ Joint pain, swelling, inflammation, and stiffness with ↑ mobility

—COMBINATION DRUG—

Penicillin G benzathine and Procaine combined, intramuscular

(pen-ih-**SILL**-in, **BEN**-zah-theen, **PROH**-kain)

PREGNANCY CATEGORY: B
CLASSIFICATION(S):
Antibiotic, penicillin
Rx: Bicillin C-R, Bicillin C-R 900/300

SEE ALSO *ANTI-INFECTIVES* AND *PENICILLINS*.

CONTENT

The injection contains the following: *300,000 units/dose:* 150,000 units each of penicillin G benzathine and penicillin G procaine. *600,000 units/dose:* 300,000 units each of penicillin G benzathine and penicillin G procaine. *1,200,000 units/dose:* 600,000 units each of penicillin G benzathine and penicillin G procaine. *2,400,000 units/dose:* 1,200,000

P

units each of penicillin G benzathine and penicillin G procaine. *Injection, 900/300 per dose.* 900,000 units of penicillin G benzathine and 300,000 units of penicillin G procaine.

USES

Streptococcal infections (A, C, G, H, L, and M) without bacteremia, of the upper respiratory tract, skin, and soft tissues. Scarlet fever, erysipelas, pneumococcal infections, and otitis media. *Note:* For severe pneumonia, empyema, bacteremia, pericarditis, meningitis, peritonitis, and arthritis of pneumococcal etiology, use aqueous penicillin G during the acute stage.

CONTRAINDICATIONS

Use to treat syphilis, gonorrhea, yaws, bejel, and pinta. IV use.

ADDITIONAL DRUG INTERACTIONS

Aspirin, ethacrynic acid, furosemide, indomethacin, sulfonamides, or thiazide diuretics may compete with penicillin G for renal tubular secretion → prolongation of serum t½ of penicillin

HOW SUPPLIED

See Content

DOSAGE

• **IM ONLY**

Streptococcal infections.

Adults and children over 27 kg: 2,400,000 units, given at a single session using multiple injection sites or, alternatively, in divided doses on days 1 and 3; **children 13.5–27 kg:** 900,000–1,200,000 units; **infants and children under 13.5 kg:** 600,000 units.

Pneumococcal infections, except pneumococcal meningitis.

Adults: 1,200,000 units; **pediatric:** 600,000 units. Give q 2–3 days until temperature is normal for 48 hr.

NURSING CONSIDERATIONS

SEE ALSO *NURSING CONSIDERATIONS* FOR *PENICILLINS.*

ADMINISTRATION/STORAGE

1. For adults, administer by deep IM injection in the upper outer quadrant of the buttock. For infants and children, use the midlateral aspect of the thigh.
2. Rotate injection sites for repeated doses.
3. Refrigerate but protect from freezing.

ASSESSMENT

Note indications for therapy, symptom type/onset and disease confirmation. Assess cultures.

OUTCOMES/EVALUATE

Resolution of infection

Penicillin G benzathine, intramuscular

(pen-ih-**SILL**-in, **BEN**-zah-theen)

PREGNANCY CATEGORY: B

CLASSIFICATION(S):

Antibiotic, penicillin

Rx: Bicillin L-A, Permapen

✱**Rx:** Penicillin G/Penicillin V

SEE ALSO *ANTI-INFECTIVES* AND *PENICILLINS.*

ACTION/KINETICS

Penicillin G is neither penicillinase resistant nor acid stable. The product is a long-acting (repository) form of penicillin in an aqueous vehicle; it is administered as a sterile suspension. **Peak plasma levels: IM** 0.03–0.05 unit/mL.

USES

(1) URTI (mild to moderate) due to susceptible streptococci. (2) Sexually transmitted diseases, such as syphilis, yaws, bejel, and pinta. (3) Prophylaxis of rheumatic fever or chorea. (4) Follow-up prophylactic therapy for rheumatic heart disease and acute glomerulonephritis.

CONTRAINDICATIONS

IV use.

ADDITIONAL DRUG INTERACTIONS

Aspirin, ethacrynic acid, furosemide, indomethacin, sulfonamides, or thiazide diuretics may compete with penicillin G for renal tubular secretion → prolongation of serum t½ of penicillin

HOW SUPPLIED

Injection: 300,000 U/mL; 600,000 U/dose; 1,200,000 U/dose; 2,400,000 U/dose

DOSAGE

• **PARENTERAL SUSPENSION (IM ONLY)**

URTI due to Group A streptococcus.

Adults: 1,200,000 units as a single

dose; **older children:** 900,000 units as a single dose; **children under 27 kg:** 300,000–600,000 units as a single dose; **neonates:** 50,000 units/kg as a single dose.

Early syphilis (primary, secondary, or latent).

Adults: 2,400,000 units as a single dose. **Children:** 50,000 units/kg, up to the adult dose.

Gummas and cardiovascular syphilis.

Adults: 2,400,000 units q 7 days for 3 weeks. **Children:** 50,000 units/kg, up to adult dose.

Neurosyphilis.

Adults: Aqueous penicillin G, 18,000,000–24,000,000 units IV/day (3–4 million units q 4 hr) for 10–14 days followed by penicillin G benzathine, 2,400,000 units IM q week for 3 weeks. An alternative regimen is procaine penicillin G, 2,400,000 units/day plus probenecid, 500 mg PO, q.i.d., both for 10–14 days. Some recommend benzathine G penicillin, 2.4 million units following completion of this regimen.

Yaws, bejel, pinta.

1,200,000 units in a single dose.

Prophylaxis of rheumatic fever and glomerulonephritis.

Following an acute attack, 1,200,000 units once a month or 600,000 units q 2 weeks.

NURSING CONSIDERATIONS

SEE ALSO *NURSING CONSIDERATIONS* FOR *PENICILLINS*.

ADMINISTRATION/STORAGE

1. Shake multiple-dose vial vigorously before withdrawing the desired dose because medication tends to clump on standing. Check that all medication is dissolved and that no residue is present at bottom of bottle.
2. Use a 20-gauge needle and do not allow medication to remain in the syringe and needle for long periods of time before administration because the needle may become plugged and the syringe "frozen."
3. Inject slowly and steadily into muscle; *do not massage* injection site.
4. For adults, use the upper outer quadrant of the buttock; for infants and small children, the midlateral aspect of the thigh should be used. Do not administer in the gluteal region in children less than 2 years of age.
5. *Do not administer IV.* Before injection of medication, aspirate to ensure that needle is not in a vein.
6. Rotate and chart site of injections.
7. Divide between two injection sites if dose is large or available muscle mass is small.
8. Refrigerate, but do not freeze.

CLIENT/FAMILY TEACHING

1. Must return as scheduled for repository penicillin injections.
2. Obtain sexual counseling. Sexual partner should also undergo treatment.

OUTCOMES/EVALUATE

- Prophylaxis of poststreptococcal rheumatic fever
- Resolution of infection

Penicillin G (Aqueous)

(pen-ih-**SILL**-in)

PREGNANCY CATEGORY: B
CLASSIFICATION(S):
Antibiotic, penicillin
Rx: Pfizerpen

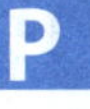

SEE ALSO *ANTI-INFECTIVES* AND *PENICILLINS*.

ACTION/KINETICS

The first choice for treatment of many infections due to low cost. Rapid onset makes it especially suitable for fulminating infections. Is neither penicillinase resistant nor acid stable. **Peak plasma levels: IM or SC,** 6–20 units/mL after 15–30 min **t½:** 30 min.

USES

Streptococci of groups A, C, G, H, L, and M are sensitive to penicillin G. High serum levels are effective against streptococci of the D group.

ADDITIONAL SIDE EFFECTS

Rapid IV administration may cause hyperkalemia and cardiac arrhythmias. Renal damage occurs rarely.

ADDITIONAL DRUG INTERACTIONS
Aspirin, ethacrynic acid, furosemide, indomethacin, sulfonamides, or thiazide diuretics may compete with penicillin G for renal tubular secretion → prolongation of serum t½ of penicillin

HOW SUPPLIED
Injection, premixed: 1 million U/vial, 2 million U/vial, 3 million U/vial; *Powder for injection:* 1 million U, 5 million U, 20 million U.

DOSAGE

• **IM CONTINUOUS, IV INFUSION**

Serious streptococcal infections (empyema, endocarditis, meningitis, pericarditis, pneumonia).
Adults: 5–24 million units/day in divided doses q 4 to 6 hr. **Pediatric:** 150,000 units/kg/day given in equal doses q 4 to 6 hr. **Infants over 7 days of age:** 75,000 units/kg/day in divided doses q 8 hr. **Infants less than 7 days of age:** 50,000 units/kg/day given in divided doses q 12 hr. For group B streptococcus, give 100,000 units/kg/day.

Meningococcal meningitis/septicemia.
Adults: 1–2 million units IM q 2 hr or 20–30 million units/day continuous IV drip for 14 days or until afebrile for 7 days. Or, 200,000–300,000 units/kg/day q 2–4 hr in divided doses for a total of 24 doses.

P

Meningitis due to susceptible strains of Pneumococcus or *Meningococcus.*
Children: 250,000 units/kg/day divided in equal doses q 4 to 6 hr for 7 to 14 days (maximum daily dose: 12–20 million units). **Infants over 7 days of age:** 200,000–300,0000 units/kg/day divided into equal doses given q 6 hr. **Infants less than 7 days of age:** 100,000–150,000 units/kg/day.

Anthrax.
Adults: A minimum of 5 million units/day (up to 12–20 million units have been used).

Clostridial infections.
Adults: 20 million units/day in divided doses q 4–6 hr used with an antitoxin.

Actinomycosis.
Adults: *Cervicofacial:* 1–6 million units/day. *Thoracic and abdominal disease:* **initial,** 10–20 million units/day divided into equal doses given q 4–6 hr IV for 6 weeks followed by penicillin V, PO, 500 mg q.i.d. for 2–3 months.

Rat-bite fever, Haverhill fever.
Adults: 12–20 million units/day q 4 to 6 hr for 3–4 weeks. **Children:** 150,000–250,000 units/kg/day in equal doses q 4 hr for 4 weeks.

Endocarditis due to Listeria.
Adults: 15–20 million units/day q 4 to 6 hr for 4 weeks.

Endocarditis due to Erysipelothrix rhusiopathiae.
Adults: 12–20 million units/day q 4 to 6 hr for 4–6 weeks.

Meningitis due to Listeria.
Adults: 15–20 million units/day q 4 to 6 hr for 2 weeks.

Pasteurella infections causing bacteremia and meningitis.
Adults: 4–6 million units/day q 4 to 6 hr for 2 weeks.

Severe fusospirochetal infections of the oropharynx, lower respiratory tract, and genital area.
Adults: 5–10 million units/day q 4 to 6 hr.

Pneumococcal infections causing empyema.
Adults: 5–24 million units/day in divided doses q 4–6 hr.

Pneumococcal infections causing meningitis.
Adults: 20–24 million units/day for 14 days.

Pneumococcal infections causing endocarditis, pericarditis, peritonitis, suppurative arthritis, osteomyelitis, mastoiditis.
Adults: 12–20 million units/day for 2–4 weeks.

Adjunct with antitoxin to prevent diphtheria.
Adults: 2–3 million units/day in divided doses q 4 to 6 hr for 10–12 days. **Children:** 150,000–250,000 units/kg/day in equal doses q 6 hr for 7–10 days.

Neurosyphilis.
Adults: 18–24 million units/day (3–4 million units q 4 hr) for 10–14 days (can be followed by benzathine penicillin G, 2.4 million units IM weekly for 3 weeks).

Disseminated gonococcal infections. **Adults:** 10 million units/day q 4 to 6 hr (for meningococcal meningitis/septicemia, give q 2 hr). **Children, less than 45 kg:** Arthritis, 100,000 units/kg/day in 4 equally divided doses for 7 to 10 days. Endocarditis: 250,000 units/kg/day in equal doses q 4 hr for 4 weeks. Meningitis: 250,000 units/kg/day in equal doses q 4 hr for 10 to 14 days. **Children, over 45 kg:** Arthritis, endocarditis, meningitis: 10 million units/day in 4 equally divided doses (duration depends on type of infection).

Syphilis (congenital, neurosyphilis) after the newborn period.
200,000–300,000 kunits/kg/day (given as 50,000 units/kg q 4–6 hr) for 10–14 days.

Symptomatic or asymptomatic congenital syphilis in infants.
Infants: 50,000 units/kg/dose IV q 12 hr the first 7 days; then, q 8 hr for a total of 10 days. **Children:** 50,000 units/kg q 4–6 hr for 10 days.

NURSING CONSIDERATIONS

SEE ALSO *NURSING CONSIDERATIONS* FOR *PENICILLINS*.

ADMINISTRATION/STORAGE

1. IM administration is preferred; discomfort is minimized by using solutions of up to 100,000 units/mL.
2. Use 1%–2% lidocaine solution as diluent for IM (if ordered) to lessen pain at injection site. Do not use procaine as diluent for aqueous penicillin.
3. Electrolyte contents: Pfizerpen contains 0.3 mEq sodium and 1.68 m Eq potassium/million units.
4. If Pencillin G is to be given by intrapleural or other local infusion and fluid is aspirated, give infusion in a volume equal to ¼ or ½ the amount of fluid aspirated. Otherwise, prepare as for the IM injection.
5. Intrathecal use must be highly individualized and used only with full consideration of possible irritating effects of penicillin when given intrathecally. The preferred route in bacterial meningitis is IV supplemented by IM.

IV 6. Use sterile water, isotonic saline, or D5W and mix with recommended volume for desired strength.
7. For intermittent IV administration (q 6 hr) reconstitute with 100 mL of dextrose or saline solution and infuse over 1 hr.
8. Loosen powder by shaking bottle before adding diluent.
9. Hold vial horizontally and rotate slowly while directing the stream of diluent against the vial wall, then shake vigorously.
10. Solutions may be stored at room temperature for 24 hr or in refrigerator for 1 week. Discard remaining solution.
11. When larger doses are needed, give by continuous IV infusion.
12. The following drugs should *not* be mixed with penicillin during IV administration: aminophylline, amphotericin B, ascorbic acid, chlorpheniramine, chlorpromazine, gentamicin, heparin, hydroxyzine, lincomycin, metaraminol, novobiocin, oxytetracycline, phenylephrine, phenytoin, polymyxin B, prochlorperazine, promazine, promethazine, sodium bicarbonate, sodium salts of barbiturates, sulfadiazine, tetracycline, tromethamine, vancomycin, vitamin B complex.

ASSESSMENT

1. Document indications for therapy, type, onset, and characteristics of symptoms.
2. Order drug by specifying sodium or potassium salt.
3. Monitor I&O. Dehydration decreases drug excretion and may raise blood level of penicillin G to dangerously high levels causing kidney damage. GI disturbances may lead to dehydration.
4. Very high doses (>20 million units) may cause seizures or platelet dysfunction, especially with impaired renal function.
5. Obtain baseline CBC, liver and renal function studies and cultures.

CLIENT/FAMILY TEACHING

1. The drug must be given by injection to clear up infection.

P

2. Report any ususual bruising, bleeding, N&V, sore mouth, diarrhea, rash, fever or difficulty breathing.

OUTCOMES/EVALUATE

- Symptomatic improvement; negative culture reports
- Resolution of infective process

Penicillin G procaine, intramuscular

(pen-ih-**SILL**-in, **PROH**-caine)

PREGNANCY CATEGORY: B
CLASSIFICATION(S):
Antibiotic, penicillin
Rx: Wycillin

SEE ALSO *ANTI-INFECTIVES* AND *PENICILLINS*.

ACTION/KINETICS

Long-acting (repository) form in aqueous or oily vehicle. Destroyed by penicillinase. Because of slow onset, a soluble penicillin is often administered concomitantly for fulminating infections.

USES

Penicillin-sensitive staphylococci, pneumococci, streptococci, and bacterial endocarditis (for *Streptococcus viridans* and *S. bovis* infections). Gonorrhea, all stages of syphilis. *Prophylaxis:* Rheumatic fever, pre- and postsurgery. Diphtheria, anthrax, fusospirochetosis (Vincent's infection), erysipeloid, rat-bite fever. *Note:* Severe pneumonia, empyema, bacteremia, pericarditis, meningitis, peritonitis, and purulent or septic arthritis due to pneumococcus are better treated with aqueous penicillin G during the acute stage.

CONTRAINDICATIONS

Use in newborns due to possible sterile abcesses and procaine toxicity.

ADDITIONAL DRUG INTERACTIONS

Aspirin, ethacrynic acid, furosemide, indomethacin, sulfonamides, or thiazide diuretics may compete with penicillin G for renal tubular secretion → prolongation of serum t½ of penicillin

HOW SUPPLIED

Injection: 600,000 U/unit dose; 1,200,000 U/unit dose; 2,400,000 U/unit dose

DOSAGE

- **IM ONLY**

Pneumococccal, streptococcal (Group A, including tonsillitis, erysipelas, scarlet fever, URTI, and skin and skin structure infections), staphylococcal infections.

Adults, usual: 600,000–1 million units/day for 10–14 days. **Children, less than 27.2 kg:** 300,000 units/day.

Bacterial endocarditis (only very sensitive S. viridans or *S. bovis* infections).

Adults: 600,000–1 million units/day.

Diphtheria carrier state.

300,000 units/day for 10 days.

Diphtheria, adjunct with antitoxin.

300,000–600,000 units/day.

Anthrax (cutaneous), erysipeloid, rate-bite fever.

600,000 to 1 million units/day.

Fusospirochetosis: Vincent's gingivitis, pharyngitis.

600,000 to 1 million units/day. Obtain necessary dental care.

Gonococcal infections.

4.8 million units divided into at least two doses at one visit and given with 1 g PO probenecid (given 30 min before the injections).

Neurosyphilis.

2.4 million units/day for 10 to 14 days (given at two sites) with probenecid 500 mg PO q.i.d.; **then,** benzathine penicillin G, 2.4 million units/week for 3 weeks. *NOTE:* For yaws, bejel, and pinta, treat the same as syphilis in corresponding stage of disease.

Congenital syphilis in infants, symptomatic and asymptomatic.

50,000 units/kg/day for 10 days.

Syphilis: primary, secondary, latent with negative spinal fluid.

Adults and children over 12 years: 600,000 units/day for 8 days (total of 4.8 million units).

Syphilis: tertiary, neurosyphilis, latent with positive spinal-fluid.

Adults: 600,000 units/day for 10 to 15 days (total of 6 to 9 million units).

NURSING CONSIDERATIONS

SEE ALSO *NURSING CONSIDERATIONS* FOR *ANTI-INFECTIVES* AND *PENICILLINS*.

ADMINISTRATION/STORAGE

1. Shake multiple-dose vial thoroughly to ensure uniform suspension be-

fore injection. If the medication is clumped at the bottom of the vial, shake until clump dissolves.
2. Use a 20-gauge needle and aspirate immediately after withdrawing medication from the vial; otherwise needle may become clogged and syringe may "freeze."
3. Administer into two sites if dose is large or available muscle mass is small.
4. Aspirate to check that the needle is not in a vein.
5. Inject slowly, deep into the muscle.
6. For IM use only. Rotate and chart injection sites. Do not massage site.

ASSESSMENT

Document indications for therapy, type, onset and characteristics of symptoms, any other treatments prescribed, and culture results.

CLIENT/FAMILY TEACHING

1. Drug can only be given IM.
2. Report a wheal or other skin reactions at injection site that may indicate reaction to procaine as well as to penicillin. Report N&V, diarrhea, mouth sores, severe pain at injection site, unusual bruising/bleeding, or difficulty breathing.
3. Obtain sexual counseling; have sexual partner also undergo treatment.
4. With a history of rheumatic fever or congenital heart disease, must remember to use antibiotic prophylaxis prior to any invasive medical/dental procedure.

OUTCOMES/EVALUATE

Resolution of infection; infection prophylaxis

Penicillin V potassium (Phenoxymethylpenicillin potassium)

(pen-ih-**SILL**-in)

PREGNANCY CATEGORY: B
CLASSIFICATION(S):
Antibiotic, penicillin

Rx: Beepen-VK, Penicillin VK, Pen-Vee K, Veetids, Veetids '250'
✤**Rx:** Apo-Pen-VK, Nadopen-V, Novo–Pen-VK, Nu-Pen-VK

SEE ALSO *ANTI-INFECTIVES* AND *PENICILLINS*.

ACTION/KINETICS

Related closely to penicillin G. Products are not penicillinase resistant but are acid stable and resist inactivation by gastric secretions. Well absorbed from the GI tract and not affected by foods. **Peak plasma levels:** Penicillin V, **PO:** 2.7 mcg/mL after 30–60 min; penicillin V potassium, **PO:** 1–9 mcg/mL after 30–60 min. **t½:** 30 min. Periodic blood counts and renal function tests are indicated during long-term usage.

USES

(1) Mild to moderate upper respiratory tract streptococcal infections, including scarlet fever and erysipelas. (2) Mild to moderate upper respiratory tract pneumococcal infections, including otitis media. (3) Mild staphylococcal infections of the skin and soft tissue. (4) Mild to moderate fusospirochetosis (Vincent's infection) of the oropharynx. (5) Prophylaxis of recurrence following rheumatic fever or chorea. *Investigational:* Prophylactically to reduce *S. pneumoniae* septicemia in children with sickle cell anemia, mild to moderate anaerobic infections, Lyme disease.

CONTRAINDICATIONS

PO penicillin V to treat severe pneumonia, empyema, bacteremia, pericarditis, meningitis, and arthritis during the acute stage. Prophylactic uses for GU instrumentation or surgery, sigmoidoscopy, or childbirth.

SPECIAL CONCERNS

More and more strains of staphylococci are resistant to penicillin V, necessitating culture and sensitivity studies.

ADDITIONAL DRUG INTERACTIONS

Contraceptives, oral / ↓ Effectiveness of oral contraceptives
Neomycin, oral / ↓ Absorption of penicillin V

P

HOW SUPPLIED
Powder for oral solution: 125 mg/5 mL, 250 mg/5 mL; *Tablet:* 250 mg, 500 mg

DOSAGE

• **ORAL SOLUTION, TABLETS**

Streptococcal infections, including scarlet fever and mild erysipelas.

Adults and children over 12 years: 125–250 mg q 6–8 hr for 10 days. **Children, usual:** 500 mg q 8 hr for pharyngitis.

Staphylococcal infections (including skin and soft tissue), fusospirochetosis of oropharynx.

Adults and children over 12 years: 250 mg q 6–8 hr.

Pneumococcal infections, including otitis media.

Adults and children over 12 years: 250 mg q 6 hr until afebrile for at least 2 days.

Prophylaxis of recurrence of rheumatic fever/chorea.

Adults and children over 12 years: 125–250 mg b.i.d., on a continuing basis.

Prophylaxis of septicemia caused by Staphylococcus pneumoniae *in children with sickle cell anemia.*

125 mg b.i.d.

Anaerobic infections.

250 mg q.i.d. See also *Penicillin G, Procaine, Aqueous, Sterile.*

Lyme disease.

250–500 mg q.i.d. for 10–20 days (for children less than 2 years of age, 50 mg/kg/day in four divided doses for 10–20 days).

NOTE: 250 mg penicillin V is equivalent to 400,000 units.

NURSING CONSIDERATIONS

SEE ALSO *NURSING CONSIDERATIONS* FOR *ANTI-INFECTIVES* AND *PENICILLINS*.

ADMINISTRATION/STORAGE

1. Twice-daily dosing of penicillin V, 500–1000 mg/day is equivalent to 3-4 times daily dosing.
2. Administer without regard to meals. Blood levels may be slightly higher when administered on an empty stomach.
3. Store reconstituted solution in the refrigerator; discard unused portion after 14 days.

ASSESSMENT
Note indications for therapy, type, onset, and characteristics of symptoms, and culture results.

CLIENT/FAMILY TEACHING

1. Clients with a history of rheumatic fever or congenital heart disease need to use and understand the importance of antibiotic prophylaxis prior to any invasive medical or dental procedure.
2. Report if throat and/or ear symptoms do not improve after 48 hr of therapy; may need to reevaluate and alter therapy.
3. With oral administration, if a reaction is going to occur, you usually see it after the second dose. Seek medical intervention immediately if respiratory distress or skin wheals appear.
4. Use an additional nonhormonal form of birth control if taking oral contraceptives because their effectiveness may be diminished.

OUTCOMES/EVALUATE

• Symptomatic improvement
• Negative lab C&S reports
• Endocardits/rheumatic fever prophylaxis

Pentamidine isethionate

(pen-**TAM**-ih-deen)

PREGNANCY CATEGORY: C
CLASSIFICATION(S):
Antibiotic, miscellaneous
Rx: NebuPent, Pentacarinate, Pentam 300

ACTION/KINETICS
Inhibits synthesis of DNA, RNA, phospholipids, and proteins, thereby interfering with cell metabolism. May interfere also with folate transformation. About one-third of the dose excreted unchanged in the urine. Plasma levels following inhalation are significantly lower than after a comparable IV dose.

USES
Parenteral: Pneumonia caused by *Pneumocystis carinii.* **Inhalation:** Prophylaxis of *P. carinii* in high-risk HIV-

infected clients defined by one or both of the following: (a) a history of one or more cases of pneumonia caused by *P. carinii* and/or (b) a peripheral CD4+ lymphocyte count less than 200/mm^3. *Investigational:* Trypanosomiasis, visceral leishmaniasis.

CONTRAINDICATIONS

Anaphylaxis to inhaled or parenteral pentamidine.

SPECIAL CONCERNS

Use with caution in clients with hepatic or kidney disease, hypertension or hypotension, hyperglycemia or hypoglycemia, hypocalcemia, leukopenia, thrombocytopenia, anemia, ventricular tachycardia, pancreatitis, Stevens-Johnson syndrome.

SIDE EFFECTS

• PARENTERAL

CV: Hypotension, ***ventricular tachycardia,*** phlebitis. **GI:** Nausea, anorexia, bad taste in mouth. **Hematologic:** Leukopenia, thrombocytopenia, anemia. **Electrolytes/glucose:** Hypoglycemia, hypocalcemia, hyperkalemia. **CNS:** Dizziness without hypotension, confusion, hallucinations. **Miscellaneous:** Acute renal failure, ***Stevens-Johnson syndrome,*** elevated serum creatinine, elevated LFTs, pain or induration at IM injection site, sterile abscess at injection site, rash, neuralgia.

• INHALATION

Most frequent include the following. **GI:** Decreased appetite, N&V, metallic taste, diarrhea, abdominal pain. **CNS:** Fatigue, dizziness, headache. **Respiratory:** SOB, cough, pharyngitis, chest pain, chest congestion, ***bronchospasm,*** pneumothorax. **Miscellaneous:** Rash, night sweats, chills, myalgia, headache, anemia, edema.

HOW SUPPLIED

Injection: 300 mg; *Powder for injection, lyophilized:* 300 mg; *Powder for inhalation,* 300 mg

DOSAGE

• IV, DEEP IM

Adults and children: 4 mg/kg/day for 14 days. Dosage should be reduced in renal disease.

• AEROSOL

Prevention of P. carinii *pneumonia.* 300 mg q 4 weeks given via the Respirgard II nebulizer.

NURSING CONSIDERATIONS

SEE ALSO *GENERAL NURSING CONSIDERATIONS* FOR *ANTI-INFECTIVES.*

ADMINISTRATION/STORAGE

1. For use in the nebulizer, reconstitute by dissolving vial contents in 6 mL sterile water for injection. Do not use saline solution because it causes the drug to precipitate. Do not mix with other meds in the nebulizer chamber.
2. Deliver the dose using the nebulizer until the chamber is empty (30–45 min). The suggested flow rate is 5–7 L/min from a 40- to 50-psi (pounds per square inch) air or oxygen source.
3. When used for nebulization, do not mix with any other drug.
4. The solution for nebulization is stable at room temperature for 48 hr if protected from light.
5. To prepare IM solution, dissolve one vial in 3 mL of sterile water for injection.

IV 6. To prepare IV solution, dissolve one vial in 3–5 mL of sterile water for injection or D5W. The drug is then further diluted in 50–250 mL of D5W. Infuse slowly over 60 min.

7. IV solutions in concentrations of 1 and 2.5 mg/mL in D5W are stable for 48 hr at room temperature.

ASSESSMENT

1. Document indications for therapy and assess extent of infection.
2. Determine history of kidney disease, hypertension, and past blood disorders. Monitor cultures, CBC, electrolytes, blood sugar, calcium, CD_4 counts, liver and renal function.
3. Note results of TB skin test.
4. Auscultate lung sounds; document CXR and respiratory assessment findings.

INTERVENTIONS

1. Observe for symptoms of hypoglycemia, hypocalcemia, and/or hyperkalemia.
2. During IV therapy monitor BP (q 15 min during therapy and q 2 hr after

P

therapy until stable); monitor VS and I&O.
3. Obtain apical pulse; auscultate for evidence of arrhythmia.
4. During administration of aerosolized pentamidine, follow precautions to protect the health care worker. Do not administer if pregnant; remove contact lenses. Administer with the Respirgard II nebulizer. Document worker exposure(s) and report any persistent or unusual symptoms, especially chronic URIs. Wear:
• Eye protection with side shields
• Disposable gowns
• Respiratory protective equipment such as an organic dust-mist respirator unless client is under hood stalls or in a ventilated booth
• Gloves
5. Follow appropriate institutional guidelines and Occupational Safety and Health Administration (OSHA) standards for administration of drug. Incorporate Universal Precautions.

CLIENT/FAMILY TEACHING
1. Parenteral drug therapy must be given every day (IV/IM). Inhalation therapy must be used once every 4 weeks. Follow appropriate guidelines for administration.
2. Report any bruising, blood in urine/stools, or unusual bleeding. Expect frequent blood tests and BP checks.
3. Avoid aspirin-containing compounds, alcohol, IM injections, or rectal thermometers.
4. Use a soft toothbrush, electric razor, and night light to prevent injury and falls.
5. Be alert for S&S of hypoglycemia (which may be severe); report.
6. Report early signs of Stevens-Johnson syndrome (characterized by high fever, severe headaches, mouth, eye, nose or penis inflammation or swelling.
7. Consume 2–3 L/day of fluids.
8. Rise from a prone position slowly and dangle legs before standing as drug may cause dizziness and low BP.
9. During inhalation, a metallic taste and GI upsets may be experienced. Eat small, frequent meals and perform regular mouth care to offset.

OUTCOMES/EVALUATE
• (Parenterally) Improvement in symptoms of PCP
• (Inhalation) PCP prophylaxis

Pentostatin (2'-deoxycoformycin; DCF)

(**PEN**-toh-**stah**-tin)

PREGNANCY CATEGORY: D
CLASSIFICATION(S):
Antineoplastic, antibiotic
Rx: Nipent

SEE ALSO *ANTINEOPLASTIC AGENTS.*

ACTION/KINETICS
Isolated from *Streptomyces antibioticus;* inhibits the enzyme ADA. Inhibition of ADA, especially in the presence of adenosine or deoxyadenosine, results in cellular toxicity (T cells, B cells) due to elevated intracellular levels of dATP; this blocks the synthesis of DNA through inhibition of ribonucleotide reductase. Also inhibits RNA synthesis and causes increased DNA damage. **t½, distribution:** 11 min; **terminal:** 5.7 hr. Approximately 90% is excreted in the urine as unchanged pentostatin or metabolites.

USES
Hairy cell leukemia in adults who are refractory to alpha-interferon; such individuals have progressive disease after a minimum of 3 months of alpha-interferon therapy or no response after a minimum of 6 months of alpha-interferon therapy.

CONTRAINDICATIONS
In combination with fludarabine phosphate. Lactation.

SPECIAL CONCERNS
Treat clients with infection only if the potential benefit outweighs the risk; infection should be treated before pentostatin therapy is initiated or resumed. Safety and effectiveness have not been determined in children.

SIDE EFFECTS
Hematologic: Leukopenia, anemia, thrombocytopenia, ecchymosis, lymphadenopathy, petechia, abnormal

erythrocytes, leukocytosis, pancytopenia, purpura, splenomegaly, eosinophilia, hematologic disorder, hemolysis, lymphoma-like reaction. **GI:** N&V, anorexia, abdominal pain, diarrhea, constipation, flatulence, stomatitis, colitis, dysphagia, dyspepsia, eructation, gastritis, ***GI hemorrhage,*** gum hemorrhage, intestinal obstruction, leukoplakia, melena, periodontal abscess, proctitis, abnormal stools, esophagitis, gingivitis, mouth disorder. **Hepatic:** Hepatitis, hepatomegaly, ***hepatic failure.*** **CNS:** Headache, anxiety, abnormal thinking, confusion, depression, dizziness, insomnia, nervousness, paresthesia, somnolence, agitation, amnesia, ataxia, abnormal dreams, depersonalization, emotional lability, hyperesthesia, hypesthesia, hypertonia, incoordination, decreased libido, neuropathy, stupor, tremor, vertigo, ***coma, seizures.*** **CV:** Arrhythmia, abnormal ECG, ***hemorrhage,*** thrombophlebitis, aortic stenosis, arterial anomaly, cardiomegaly, CHF, ***cardiac arrest,*** flushing, hypertension, ***MI,*** palpitation, varicose vein, ***shock.*** **Dermatologic:** Rash, skin disorder, eczema, dry skin, herpes simplex, herpes zoster, maculopapular rash, pruritus, seborrhea, skin discoloration, sweating, vesiculobullous rash, acne, alopecia, exfoliative dermatitis, contact dermatitis, fungal dermatitis, benign skin neoplasm, psoriasis, SC nodule, skin hypertrophy, urticaria. **GU:** GU disorder, dysuria, hematuria, fibrocystic breasts, gynecomastia, hydronephrosis, oliguria, polyuria, pyuria, toxic nephropathy, urinary frequency, urinary retention, urinary urgency, UTI, impaired urination, urolithiasis, vaginitis. **Musculoskeletal:** Myalgia, arthralgia, asthenia, facial paralysis, abnormal gait, arthritis, bone pain, osteomyelitis, neck rigidity, pathologic fracture. **Respiratory:** Cough, URI, lung disorder, bronchitis, dyspnea, epistaxis, lung edema, pneumonia, pharyngitis, rhinitis, sinusitis, asthma, atelectasis, hemoptysis, hyperventilation, hypoventilation, increased sputum, laryngitis, larynx edema, lung fibrosis, pleural effusion, pneumothorax, ***pulmonary embolus.*** **Body as a whole:** Fever, infection, fatigue, weight loss or gain, peripheral edema, pain, allergic reaction, chills, sepsis, chest pain, back pain, flu syndrome, malaise, neoplasm, abscess, enlarged abdomen, ascites, acidosis, dehydration, diabetes mellitus, gout, abnormal healing, cellulitis, facial edema, cyst, fibrosis, granuloma, hernia, hemorrhage or inflammation of the injection site, moniliasis, pelvic pain, photosensitivity, ***anaphylaxis,*** mucous membrane disorder, immune system disorder, neck pain. **Ophthalmic:** Abnormal vision, conjunctivitis, eye pain, blepharitis, cataract, diplopia, exophthalmos, lacrimation disorder, optic neuritis, retinal detachment. **Miscellaneous:** Ear pain, deafness, otitis media, parosmia, taste perversion, tinnitus.

LABORATORY TEST CONSIDERATIONS

↑ LFT, BUN, creatinine, LDH, CPK, gamma globulins. Albuminuria, glycosuria, hyponatremia, hypocholesterolemia.

OD OVERDOSE MANAGEMENT

Symptoms: ***Severe renal, hepatic, pulmonary, and CNS toxicity; death can result****.* *Treatment:* General supportive measures.

DRUG INTERACTIONS

Fludarabine / ↑ Risk of fatal pulmonary toxicity

Vidarabine / ↑ Effect of vidarabine, including side effects

HOW SUPPLIED

Powder for Injection: 10 mg

DOSAGE

- **IV BOLUS, IV INFUSION**

Alpha-interferon-refractory hairy cell leukemia.

4 mg/m² every other week.

NURSING CONSIDERATIONS

SEE ALSO *NURSING CONSIDERATIONS* FOR *ANTINEOPLASTIC AGENTS.*

ADMINISTRATION/STORAGE

IV 1. The optimum duration of treatment has not been determined; if major toxicity has not occurred, continue treatment until a complete re-

sponse has been achieved. Follow by two additional doses and then stop treatment. If, after 12 months, there is only a partial response, discontinue treatment.
2. Withhold if there is severe rash, CNS toxicity, infection, or elevated serum creatinine.
3. Temporarily withhold if the absolute neutrophil count falls below 200 cells/mm³ during treatment in a client who had an initial neutrophil count greater than 500 cells/mm³. Continue treatment when the count returns to pretreatment levels.
4. Store vials in the refrigerator at 2–8°C (36–46°F). Reconstituted vials or reconstituted vials further diluted may be stored at room temperature and ambient light for up to 8 hr.
5. To reconstitute, add 5 mL of sterile water for injection to the vial; mix thoroughly to obtain complete dissolution for a concentration of 2 mg/mL.
6. May be given by IV bolus or diluted in 25–50 mL of D5W or 0.9% NaCl injection and administered over 30 min. Dilution of the entire contents of the reconstituted vial with 25 or 50 mL provides a concentration of diluted pentostatin of 0.33 or 0.18 mg/mL, respectively. Such a dilution does not interact with polyvinylchloride infusion containers or administration sets.

P

ASSESSMENT

1. Note previous experience with alpha-interferon and response.
2. Obtain baseline hematologic parameters, renal and LFTs.
3. Question client initially and note any symptoms of infection.

CLIENT/FAMILY TEACHING

1. Report the development of rashes as these may require discontinuation of drug therapy.
2. Practice effective birth control.
3. Avoid direct sun exposure; use protection when necessary.
4. Report for scheduled lab studies to evaluate hematologic parameters. Periodic bone marrow aspirates and biopsies may be necessary (q 2-3 mo).
5. Avoid immunizations, crowds, and those with infections. Report any fever, sore throat, bruising/bleeding, or S&S of infection.

OUTCOMES/EVALUATE

Improved hematologic parameters (↑ hemoglobin, granulocyte, and platelet counts) with hairy cell leukemia

Pentoxifylline

(pen-tox-**EYE**-fih-leen)

PREGNANCY CATEGORY: C
CLASSIFICATION(S):
Drug affecting blood viscosity
Rx: Pentoxifylline Extended-Release, Trental
✱Rx: Albert Pentoxifylline, Apo-Pentoxifylline SR, Nu-Pentoxifylline-SR

ACTION/KINETICS

Drug and active metabolites decrease the viscosity of blood and improve erythrocyte flexibility. Results in increased blood flow to the microcirculation and an increase in tissue oxygen levels. Mechanism may include (1) decreased synthesis of thromboxane A_2, thus decreasing platelet aggregation, (2) increased blood fibrinolytic activity (decreasing fibrinogen levels), and (3) decreased RBC aggregation and local hyperviscosity by increasing cellular ATP. **Peak plasma levels:** 2–4 hr. Significant first-pass effect. **t½:** pentoxifylline, 0.4–0.8 hr; metabolites, 1–1.6 hr. Excreted in the urine.

USES

Intermittent claudication; not intended to replace surgery. Night cramps symptomatic of peripheral vascular disease. *Investigational:* To improve circulation in clients with cerebrovascular insufficiency, TIAs, sickle cell thalassemia, diabetic angiopathies and neuropathies, high-altitude sickness, strokes, acute and chronic hearing disorders, circulation disorders of the eye, severe recurrent aphthous stomatitis, leg ulcers, asthenozoospermia, and Raynaud's phenomenon.

CONTRAINDICATIONS

Intolerance to pentoxifylline, caffeine, theophylline, or theobromine. Recent cerebral or retinal hemorrhage.

SPECIAL CONCERNS

Use with caution in impaired renal function and during lactation. Safety and efficacy in children less than 18 years of age not established. Geriatric clients may be at greater risk for manifesting side effects.

SIDE EFFECTS

CV: Angina, chest pain, hypotension, edema. **GI:** Abdominal pain, flatus/bloating, belching, dyspepsia, salivation, bad taste in mouth, N&V, anorexia, constipation, dry mouth and thirst, cholecystitis. **CNS:** Dizziness, headache, tremor, anxiety, confusion, depression, ***seizures.*** **Ophthalmologic:** Blurred vision, conjunctivitis, scotomata. **Dermatologic:** Pruritus, rash, urticaria, brittle fingernails, angioedema. **Respiratory:** Dyspnea, laryngitis, nasal congestion, epistaxis. **Miscellaneous:** Flu-like symptoms, leukopenia, sore throat, swollen neck glands, change in weight, earache, malaise.

OD OVERDOSE MANAGEMENT

Symptoms: Agitation, fever, flushing, hypotension, nervousness, ***seizures,*** somnolence, tremors, loss of consciousness. *Treatment:* Gastric lavage followed by activated charcoal. Monitor BP and ECG. Support respiration, control seizures, and treat arrhythmias.

DRUG INTERACTIONS

Antihypertensives / Small ↓ in BP; may need to ↑ antihypertensive dose
Theophylline / ↑ Theophylline levels → ↑ risk of toxicitiy
Warfarin / Prolonged PT

HOW SUPPLIED

Tablet: 400 mg; *Tablet, Extended Release:* 400 mg

DOSAGE

• TABLETS, EXTENDED-RELEASE TABLETS

Intermittent claudication.

Adults: 400 mg t.i.d. with meals for at least 8 weeks, although beneficial effects may be seen in 2–4 weeks. If side effects occur, reduce dose to 400 mg b.i.d.

Severe idiopathic recurrent aphthous stomatitis.

400 mg t.i.d. for 1 month.

NURSING CONSIDERATIONS

ASSESSMENT

1. Note any sensitivity to caffeine, theophylline, or theobromine.
2. Document indications for therapy, type, onset, and characteristics of symptoms. List other agents trialed and any studies performed (i.e., ABIs, Dopplers) to rule out blockage.
3. Determine if pregnant.
4. Monitor CBC and renal function studies.

CLIENT/FAMILY TEACHING

1. Take with meals to minimize GI upset.
2. Report any unusual bruising/bleeding, chest pain or palpitations.
3. Continue the treatment for at least 8 weeks, even though effectiveness may not yet be apparent.
4. Do not perform activities that require mental alertness until drug effects are realized as dizziness and blurred vision may occur.
5. Avoid all nicotine-containing products; nicotine constricts blood vessels.
6. Walk every day to the point of tears past pain, rest and then resume walking. Wear cotton socks and comfortable, well-fitting shoes. Pay attention to foot care because of diminished blood flow to feet.
7. Report for F/U to evaluate drug effectiveness.

OUTCOMES/EVALUATE

↓ Pain and cramping in lower extremities during activity

Pergolide mesylate

(**PER**-go-lyd)

PREGNANCY CATEGORY: B
CLASSIFICATION(S):
Antiparkinson drug
Rx: Permax

SEE ALSO *ANTIPARKINSON AGENTS.*

ACTION/KINETICS

Potent dopamine receptor (both D_1 and D_2) agonist. May act by directly stimulating postsynaptic dopamine

P

receptors in the nigrostriatal system, thus relieving symptoms of parkinsonism. Also inhibits prolactin secretion; causes a transient rise in serum levels of growth hormone and a decrease in serum levels of LH. About 90% of the drug is bound to plasma proteins. Metabolized in the liver and excreted through the urine.

USES

Adjunct with levodopa/carbidopa in Parkinson's disease.

SPECIAL CONCERNS

Use with caution during lactation and in clients prone to cardiac dysrhythmias, preexisting dyskinesia, and preexisting states of confusion or hallucinations. Safety and efficacy have not been determined in children.

SIDE EFFECTS

The most common side effects are listed. **CV:** Postural hypotension, palpitation, vasodilation, syncope, hypotension, hypertension, ***arrhythmias, MI.*** **GI:** Nausea (common), vomiting, diarrhea, constipation, dyspepsia, anorexia, dry mouth. **CNS:** Dyskinesia (common), dizziness, dystonia, hallucinations, confusion, insomnia, somnolence, anxiety, tremor, depression, abnormal dreams, psychosis, personality disorder, extrapyramidal syndrome, akathisia, paresthesia, incoordination, akinesia, neuralgia, hypertonia, speech disorders. **Musculoskeletal:** Arthralgia, bursitis, twitching, myalgia. **Respiratory:** Rhinitis, dyspnea, hiccup, epistaxis. **Dermatologic:** Sweating, rash. **Ophthalmologic:** Abnormal vision, double vision, eye disorders. **GU:** UTI, urinary frequency, hematuria. **Whole body:** Pain in chest, abdomen, neck, or back; headache, asthenia, flu syndrome, chills, facial edema, infection. **Miscellaneous:** Taste alteration, peripheral edema, anemia, weight gain.

OD OVERDOSE MANAGEMENT

Symptoms: Include agitation, hypotension, N&V, hallucinations, involuntary movements, palpitations, tingling of arms and legs. *Treatment:* Activated charcoal (usually recommended instead of or in addition to gastric lavage or induction of vomiting). Maintain BP. An antiarrhythmic drug may be helpful. A phenothiazine or butyrophenone may help any CNS stimulation. Support ventilation.

DRUG INTERACTIONS

Butyrophenones / ↓ Pergolide effect R/T dopamine antagonist effect
Metoclopramide / ↓ Pergolide effect R/T dopamine antagonist effect
Phenothiazines / ↓ Pergolide effect R/T dopamine antagonist effect
Thioxanthines / ↓ Pergolide effect R/T dopamine antagonist effect

HOW SUPPLIED

Tablet: 0.05 mg, 0.25 mg, 1 mg

DOSAGE

• TABLETS

Parkinsonism.

Adults, initial: 0.05 mg/day for the first 2 days; **then,** increase dose gradually by 0.1 or 0.15 mg/day every third day over the next 12 days. The dosage may then be increased by 0.25 mg/day every third day until the therapeutic dosage level is reached. The mean therapeutic daily dosage is 3 mg used concurrently with levodopa/carbidopa (expressed as levodopa) at a dose of 650 mg/day. The effectiveness of doses of pergolide greater than 5 mg/day has not been evaluated.

NURSING CONSIDERATIONS

SEE ALSO *NURSING CONSIDERATIONS* FOR *ANTIPARKINSON AGENTS*.

ADMINISTRATION/STORAGE

1. Usually given in divided doses 3 times/day.
2. When determining the therapeutic dose for pergolide, the dosage of concurrent levodopa/carbidopa may be decreased cautiously.

ASSESSMENT

1. Note any sensitivity to ergot derivatives.
2. Document cardiac arrhythmias and monitor for arrhythmia inducement in at risk clients.
3. Describe tremor, rigidity, motor fluctuations and movements.
4. Assess neuro status and for evidence of dyskinesia.

CLIENT/FAMILY TEACHING

1. Pergolide is to be taken concurrently with prescribed dose of levodo-

P

pa/carbidopa. Do not exceed prescribed dosage.
2. Do not perform tasks that require mental alertness until drug effects realized; may cause drowsiness or dizziness.
3. Rise slowly from a sitting or lying position to minimize hypotensive effects. May need to curtail activities until side effects subside.
4. Report for all scheduled lab and medical appointments so that drug therapy may be evaluated and adjusted as needed.

OUTCOMES/EVALUATE

Improved levodopa/carbidopa response evidenced by ↓ muscle weakness, ↓ rigidity, ↓ salivation, and improved mobility

Perindopril erbumine

(per-**IN**-doh-pril)

PREGNANCY CATEGORY: C (FIRST TRIMESTER), D (SECOND AND THIRD TRIMESTERS)
CLASSIFICATION(S):
Antihypertensive, ACE inhibitor
Rx: Aceon
✱**Rx:** Coversyl

SEE ALSO *ANGIOTENSIN CONVERTING ENZYME (ACE) INHIBITORS.*

ACTION/KINETICS

Converted in the liver to the active perindoprilat.

USES

Treatment of essential hypertension, either alone or combined with other antihypertensive classes, especially thiazide diuretics.

CONTRAINDICATIONS

Use in those with a history of angioedema related to previous ACE inhibitor therapy.

SPECIAL CONCERNS

Safety and efficacy have not been determined in clients with a C_{CR} less than 30 mL/min. There is a higher incidence of angioedema in blacks compared to nonblacks. Use with caution during lactation. Safety and efficacy have not been determined in children.

SIDE EFFECTS

GI: Diarrhea, abdominal pain, N&V, dyspepsia, flatulence, dry mouth, dry mucous membrane, increased appetite, gastroenteritis, ***hepatic necrosis/failure***. **CNS:** Headache, dizziness, sleep disorder, paresthesia, depression, migraine, amnesia, vertigo, anxiety, psychosexual disorder. **CV:** Palpitation, abnormal ECG, ***CVA, MI,*** orthostatic symptoms, hypotension, ventricular extrasystole, vasodilation, syncope, abnormal conduction, heart murmur. **Respiratory:** Cough, sinusitis, URTI, rhinitis, pharyngitis, posterior nasal drip, bronchitis, rhinorrhea, throat disorder, dyspnea, sneezing, epistaxis, hoarseness, pulmonary fibrosis. **Body as a whole:** Asthenia, viral infection, fever, edema, rash, seasonal allergy, malaise, pain, cold/hot sensation, chills, fluid retention, angioedema, ***anaphylaxis***. **Musculoskeletal:** Back pain, upper extremity pain, lower extremity pain, chest pain, neck pain, myalgia, arthralgia, arthritis. **GU:** UTI, male sexual dysfunction, menstrual disorder, vaginitis, kidney stone, flank pain, urinary frequency, urinary retention. **Dermatologic:** Sweating, skin infection, tinea, pruritus, dry skin, erythema, fever blisters, purpura, hematoma. **Miscellaneous:** Hypertonia, ear infection, injury, tinnitus, facial edema, gout, ecchymosis.

LABORATORY TEST CONSIDERATIONS

↑ Alkaline phosphatase, uric acid, cholesterol, AST, ALT, creatinine, glucose. ↓ Potassium. Hematuria, proteinuria.

DRUG INTERACTIONS

Concomitant use of diuretics may cause an excessive ↓ BP.

HOW SUPPLIED

Tablets: 2 mg, 4 mg, 8 mg

DOSAGE

- **TABLETS**

Uncomplicated essential hypertension.

Adults, initial: 4 mg once daily (may also be given in 2 divided doses). May increase dose until BP, when meas-

P

ured just before the next dose, is controlled. **Usual maintenance:** 4–8 mg, up to a maximum of 16 mg/day. For elderly clients, give doses greater than 8 mg/day cautiously.

Use with a diuretic for essential hypertension.

If possible, discontinue the diuretic 2–3 days before beginning perindopril therapy. If BP is not controlled with perindopril, resume the diuretic. When using both drugs, use an initial dose of 2–4 mg of perindopril daily in 1 or 2 divided doses. Carefully supervise until BP has stabilized.

In clients with a C_{CR} greater than 30 mL/min, give an initial dose of 2 mg/day. Daily dose should not exceed 8 mg.

NURSING CONSIDERATIONS

SEE ALSO *NURSING CONSIDERATIONS FOR ANGIOTENSIN CONVERTING ENZYME (ACE) INHIBITORS.*

ASSESSMENT

1. Note indications for therapy, other medical conditions, previous agents trialed, and outcome.
2. Monitor electrolytes, urinalysis, renal and LFTs; reduce dose with renal dysfunction.

CLIENT/FAMILY TEACHING

1. Take as directed at the same time(s) each day.
2. May experience cough, headaches, palpitations, sinusitis and dizziness; report if persistent.
3. Do not perform activities that require mental alertness until drug effects known.
4. Practice reliable contraception.
5. Continue life style changes useful in controlling BP; i.e.; regular exercise, weight loss, low fat/salt diet, smoking cessation, reduced alcohol intake, and stress reduction.
6. Monitor BP at different times during the day and keep a log for provider review.
7. Report any unusual side effects and avoid all OTC agents esp. cold/cough remedies without provider approval.

OUTCOMES/EVALUATE

Control of HTN; ↓ BP

P

Perphenazine

(per-**FEN**-ah-zeen)

PREGNANCY CATEGORY: C
CLASSIFICATION(S):
Antipsychotic, phenothiazine
Rx: Trilafon
✱Rx: Apo-Perphenazine

SEE ALSO *ANTIPSYCHOTIC AGENTS, PHENOTHIAZINES.*

ACTION/KINETICS

Resembles chlorpromazine. High incidence of extrapyramidal effects; strong antiemetic effects; moderate anticholinergic effects; and a low incidence of orthostatic hypotension and sedation. **Onset, IM:** 10 min. **Maximum effect, IM:** 1–2 hr. **Duration, IM:** 6 hr (up to 24 hr).

USES

Psychotic disorders. IV to treat severe N&V and intractable hiccoughs.

SPECIAL CONCERNS

Use during pregnancy only if benefits clearly outweigh risks. Dosage has not been established in children less than 12 years of age. Geriatric, emaciated, or debilitated clients usually require a lower initial dose.

HOW SUPPLIED

Concentrate: 16 mg/5 mL; *Injection:* 5 mg/mL; *Tablet:* 2 mg, 4 mg, 8 mg, 16 mg

DOSAGE

- **CONCENTRATE, TABLETS**

Psychoses.

Nonhospitalized clients: 4–8 mg t.i.d. **Hospitalized clients:** 8–16 mg b.i.d.–q.i.d. Avoid doses greater than 64 mg/day.

- **IM**

Psychotic disorders.

Adults and adolescents, nonhospitalized: 5 mg q 6 hr, not to exceed 15 mg/day. **Hospitalized clients: initial,** 5–10 mg; total daily dose should not exceed 30 mg.

- **IV**

Severe N&V.

Adults: Up to 5 mg diluted to 0.5 mg/mL with 0.9% sodium chloride injection. Give in divided doses of not more than 1 mg q 1–3 hr. Can also be given as an infusion at a rate not to exceed 1 mg/min. Restrict use to hospitalized recumbent adults. Do not exceed a single dose of 5 mg.

NURSING CONSIDERATIONS

SEE ALSO *NURSING CONSIDERATIONS* FOR *ANTIPSYCHOTIC AGENTS, PHENOTHIAZINES.*

ADMINISTRATION/STORAGE

1. When rapid action is required, administer IM using 5 mg. Inject deep into the muscle, and repeat at 6-hr intervals as needed. Place client in a recumbent position and retain in that position for at least 1 hr after IM administration.
2. Protect from light and store solutions in an amber-colored container.
3. Avoid skin contact with oral solution; may cause contact dermatitis.
IV 4. For IV use dilute with NSS to a concentration of 0.5 mg/mL and administer 1 mg over at least 1 min.

ASSESSMENT

1. Document indications for therapy, describe behavioral manifestations, and note onset and characteristics of symptoms.
2. List other agents prescribed, duration of therapy, and outcome.
3. Assess for dehydration. Obtain baseline CBC, ECG, and LFTs.
4. Monitor VS closely; may cause hypotension, tachycardia, and/or bradycardia. Supervise activity until drug effects realized.
5. Observe for tardive dyskinesia and other extrapyramidal symptoms; would require a dosage reduction/discontinuation.

CLIENT/FAMILY TEACHING

1. May dilute each 5.0 mL of oral concentrate with 60 mL of water, homogenized milk, saline, carbonated orange drink, or orange, pineapple, apricot, prune, tomato, and grapefruit juice. Avoid skin contact with drug solution.
2. Do not mix with caffeinated beverges (e.g., tea, coffee, cola), grape juice, or apple juice; precipitates.
3. Avoid activities that require mental alertness, may cause drowsiness/dizziness.
4. Report any rash, fever, or urinary retention as well as tardive dyskinesia (fine tongue movements) and extrapyramidal symptoms (tremors, jerking movements) .
5. May discolor urine pinkish brown.
6. Wear protective clothes and sunscreen when exposure necessary; may discolor skin a bluish color.
7. Drug impairs body temperature regulation; dress appropriately and avoid temperature extremes.
8. Avoid alcohol/CNS depressants.

OUTCOMES/EVALUATE

- ↓ Agitation/excitability or withdrawn behaviors
- Control of severe N&V

Phenazopyridine hydrochloride (Phenylazodiamino-pyridine HCl)

(fen-**AY**-zoh-**PEER**-ih-deen)

PREGNANCY CATEGORY: B
CLASSIFICATION(S):
Urinary tract drug
Rx: Geridium, Pyridiate, Pyridium, Pyridium Plus, Urodine, Urogesic, UTI Relief
✱Rx: Phenazo
OTC: Azo-Standard, Baridium, Prodium

ACTION/KINETICS

An azo dye with local analgesic and anesthetic effects on the urinary tract. Sixty-five percent excreted unchanged or as metabolites within 24 hr.

USES

Relief of pain, urgency or frequency, and burning in chronic UTIs or irritation, including cystitis, urethritis and pyelitis, trauma, surgery, or urinary tract instrumentation. As an adjunct to antibacterial therapy. Determine the underlying cause of the irritation.

P

CONTRAINDICATIONS
Renal insufficiency. Use in children less than 12 years of age. Chronic use to treat undiagnosed pain of the urinary tract.

SIDE EFFECTS
GI: Nausea. **Hematologic:** Methemoglobinemia, ***hemolytic anemia*** (especially in clients with G6PD deficiency). **Dermatologic:** Yellowish tinge of the skin or sclerae may indicate accumulation of drug due to renal insufficiency, pruritus, rash. **Miscellaneous:** Renal and hepatic toxicity, headache, anaphylactoid reaction, staining of contact lenses.

LABORATORY TEST CONSIDERATIONS
Ehrlich's test for urine urobilinogen, phenolsulfonphthalein excretion test for kidney function, urine bilirubin, Clinistix or Tes-Tape, colorimetric laboratory test procedures (e.g., urine ketone tests, urine protein tests, urine steroid determinations).

OD OVERDOSE MANAGEMENT
Symptoms: Methemoglobinemia following massive overdoses. Hemolysis due to G6PD deficiency. *Treatment:* Methylene blue, 1–2 mg/kg IV or 100–200 mg PO of ascorbic acid to treat methemoglobinemia.

HOW SUPPLIED
Tablet: 95 mg, 97.2 mg, 100 mg, 150 mg, 200 mg

P

DOSAGE

• **TABLETS**

Adults: 200 mg t.i.d. with or after meals for not more than 2 days when used together with an antibacterial agent for UTI. **Pediatric, 6–12 years:** 4 mg/kg t.i.d. with food for 2 days.

NURSING CONSIDERATIONS

ASSESSMENT
1. Document indications for therapy, type, onset, and characteristics of symptoms.
2. Assess for any liver/renal dysfunction.

CLIENT/FAMILY TEACHING
1. Take with or after meals to prevent GI upset.
2. Use for only 2 days when taken together with an antibacterial agent for UTIs; continue antibiotic for entire prescription.
3. Consume 2–3 L/day of fluids.
4. With diabetes, check finger sticks regularly.
5. May cause staining of contact lenses.
6. Drug turns urine orange-red; may stain fabrics. Wear a sanitary napkin to avoid staining garments. A 0.25% sodium dithionate or sodium hydrosulfite solution, available from a pharmacy, will remove these stains.
7. Report any itching/yellowing of skin or lack or response.

OUTCOMES/EVALUATE
Relief of pain and discomfort with UTI

Phenobarbital
(fee-no-**BAR**-bih-tal)

PREGNANCY CATEGORY: D
Rx: Bellatal, Solfoton, **C-IV**

Phenobarbital sodium
(fee-no-**BAR**-bih-tal)

PREGNANCY CATEGORY: D
Rx: Luminal Sodium, **C-IV**
CLASSIFICATION(S):
Sedative-hypnotic, barbiturate

ACTION/KINETICS
Depressant and anticonvulsant effects may be related to its ability to increase and/or mimic the inhibitory activity of GABA on nerve synapses. Is not an analgesic; not to be given to relieve pain. Long-acting. **t½:** 53–140 hr. **Onset:** 30 to more than 60 min. **Duration:** 10–16 hr. **Anticonvulsant therapeutic serum levels:** 15–40 mcg/mL. **Time for peak effect, after IV:** up to 15 min. Distributed more slowly than other barbiturates due to lower lipid solubility. Is 50%–60% protein bound. Twenty-five percent eliminated unchanged in the urine.

USES
PO: Sedative, hypnotic (short-term), anticonvulsant (partial and generalized tonic-clonic or cortical focal sei-

zures); emergency control of acute seizure disorders such as status epilepticus, meningitis, tetanus, eclampsia, toxicity of local anesthetics. **Parenteral:** Sedative, hypnotic (short-term), preanesthetic, anticonvulsant, emergency control of acute seizure disorders.

CONTRAINDICATIONS

Hypersensitivity to barbiturates, severe trauma, pulmonary disease when dyspnea or obstruction is present, edema, uncontrolled diabetes, history of porphyria, and impaired liver function and for clients in whom they produce an excitatory response. Also, clients who have been addicted previously to sedative-hypnotics.

SPECIAL CONCERNS

Use with caution during lactation and in clients with CNS depression, hypotension, marked asthenia (characteristic of Addison's disease, hypoadrenalism, and severe myxedema), porphyria, fever, anemia, hemorrhagic shock, cardiac, hepatic or renal damage, and a history of alcoholism in suicidal clients. Geriatric clients usually manifest increased sensitivity to barbiturates, as evidenced by confusion, excitement, mental depression, and hypothermia. Reduce the dose in geriatric and debilitated clients, as well as those with impaired hepatic or renal function. When given in the presence of pain, restlessness, excitement, and delirium may result.

SIDE EFFECTS

CNS: Sleepiness, drowsiness, agitation, confusion, hyperkinesia, ataxia, CNS depression, nightmares, nervousness, psychiatric disturbances, hallucinations, insomnia, anxiety, dizziness, headache, abnormal thinking, vertigo, lethargy, hangover, excitement, appearance of being inebriated. Irritability and hyperactivity in children. **Musculoskeletal:** Localized or diffuse myalgic, neuralgic, or arthritic pain, especially in psychoneurotic clients. Pain is often most intense in the morning and is frequently located in the neck, shoulder girdle, and arms. **Respiratory:** Hypoventilation, ***apnea, respiratory depression.*** **CV:** Bradycardia, hypotension, syncope, ***circulatory collapse.*** **GI:** N&V, constipation, liver damage (especially with chronic use of phenobarbital). **Allergic:** Skin rashes, ***angioedema,*** exfoliative dermatitis (including ***Stevens-Johnson syndrome and toxic epidermal necrolysis***). Allergic reactions are most common in clients who have asthma, urticaria, angioedema, and similar conditions. Symptoms include localized swelling (especially of the lips, cheeks, or eyelids) and erythematous dermatitis).

• **AFTER IV USE**

CV: Circulatory depression, thrombophlebitis, ***peripheral vascular collapse, seizures with cardiorespiratory arrest, myocardial depression, cardiac arrhythymias.*** **Respiratory:** ***Apnea, laryngospasm, bronchospasm,*** dyspnea, rhinitis, sneezing, coughing. **CNS:** Emergence delirium, headache, anxiety, prolonged somnolence and recovery, restlessness, ***seizures.*** **GI:** N&V, abdominal pain, diarrhea, cramping. **Hypersensitivity:** ***Acute allergic reactions, including erythema, pruritus, anaphylaxis.*** **Miscellaneous:** Pain or nerve injury at injection site, salivation, hiccups, skin rashes, shivering, skeletal muscle hyperactivity, ***immune hemolytic anemia with renal failure,*** and radial nerve palsy.

• **AFTER IM USE**

Pain at injection site.

Although barbiturates can induce physical and psychologic dependence if high doses are used regularly for long periods of time, the incidence of dependence on phenobarbital is low. Withdrawal symptoms usually begin after 12–16 hr of abstinence. Manifestations of withdrawal include anxiety, weakness, N&V, muscle cramps, delirium, and even ***tonic-clonic seizures.*** Chronic use may result in headache, fever, and megaloblastic anemia.

LABORATORY TEST CONSIDERATIONS

Interference with test method: ↑ 17-Hydroxycorticosteroids. ↑ Creatinine phosphokinase, alkaline phosphatase, serum transaminase, serum testoste-

P

rone (in certain women), urinary estriol, porphobilinogen, coproporphyrin, uroporphyrin. ↓ PT in clients on coumarin. ↑ or ↓ Bilirubin. False + lupus erythematosus test.

OD OVERDOSE MANAGEMENT

Symptoms (Acute Toxicity): Characterized by cortical and ***respiratory depression; anoxia; peripheral vascular collapse;*** feeble, rapid pulse; pulmonary edema; decreased body temperature; clammy, cyanotic skin; depressed reflexes; stupor; and ***coma.*** After initial constriction the pupils become dilated. ***Death results from respiratory failure or arrest followed by cardiac arrest.*** *Symptoms (Chronic Toxicity):* Prolonged use of barbiturates at high doses may lead to physical and psychologic dependence, as well as tolerance. Symptoms of dependence are similar to those associated with chronic alcoholism, and withdrawal symptoms are equally severe. Withdrawal symptoms usually last for 5–10 days and are terminated by a long sleep. *Treatment (Acute Toxicity):*

- Maintenance of an adequate airway, oxygen intake, and carbon dioxide removal are essential.
- After PO ingestion, gastric lavage or gastric aspiration may delay absorption. Emesis should not be induced once the symptoms of overdosage are manifested, as the client may aspirate the vomitus into the lungs. Also, if the dose of barbiturate is high enough, the vomiting center in the brain may be depressed.
- Absorption following SC or IM administration of the drug may be delayed by the use of ice packs or tourniquets.
- Maintain renal function.
- Removal of the drug by peritoneal dialysis or an artificial kidney should be carried out.
- Supportive physiologic methods have proven superior to use of analeptics.

Treatment (Chronic Toxicity): Cautious withdrawal of the hospitalized addict over a 2–4-week period. A stabilizing dose of 200–300 mg of a short-acting barbiturate is administered q 6 hr. The dose is then reduced by 100 mg/day until the stabilizing dose is reduced by one-half. The client is then maintained on this dose for 2–3 days before further reduction. The same procedure is repeated when the initial stabilizing dose has been reduced by three-quarters. If a mixed spike and slow activity appear on the EEG, or if insomnia, anxiety, tremor, or weakness is observed, the dosage is maintained at a constant level or increased slightly until symptoms disappear.

DRUG INTERACTIONS

GENERAL CONSIDERATIONS

1. Phenobarbital stimulates the activity of enzymes responsible for the metabolism of a large number of other drugs by a process known as *enzyme induction.* As a result, when phenobarbital is given to clients receiving such drugs, their therapeutic effectiveness may be markedly reduced or even abolished.
2. The CNS depressant effect of the barbiturates is potentiated by many drugs. Concomitant administration may result in coma or fatal CNS depression. Barbiturate dosage should either be reduced or eliminated when other CNS drugs are given.
3. Barbiturates also potentiate the toxic effects of many other agents.

Acetaminophen / ↑ Risk of hepatotoxicity when used with large or chronic doses of barbiturates
Alcohol / Potentiation or addition of CNS depressant effects. Concomitant use may lead to drowsiness, lethargy, stupor, respiratory collapse, coma, or death
Anesthetics, general / See *Alcohol*
Anorexiants / ↓ Effect of anorexiants due to opposite activities
Antianxiety drugs / See *Alcohol*
Anticoagulants, oral / ↓ Effect of anticoagulants R/T ↓ GI tract absorption and ↑ liver breakdown
Antidepressants, tricyclic / ↓ Antidepressant effects R/T ↑ liver breakdown
Antidiabetic agents / Prolong the effects of barbiturates
Antihistamines / See *Alcohol*

Beta-adrenergic agents / ↓ Beta blockade R/T ↑ liver breakdown
Carbamazepine / ↓ Serum carbazepine levels may occur
Charcoal / ↓ Absorption of barbiturates from the GI tract
Chloramphenicol / ↑ Effect of barbiturates R/T ↓ liver breakdown and ↓ effect of chloramphenicol by ↑ liver breakdown
Clonazepam / Barbiturates may ↑ excretion of clonazepam → loss of efficacy
Clozapine / ↓ Clozapine plasma levels R/T ↑ liver metabolism
CNS depressants / See *Alcohol*
Corticosteroids / ↓ Effect of corticosteroids R/T ↑ liver breakdown
Doxorubicin / ↓ Effect of doxorubicin R/T ↑ excretion
Doxycycline / ↓ Effect of doxycycline R/T ↑ liver breakdown (effect may last up to 2 weeks after barbiturates are discontinued)
Estrogens / ↓ Effect of estrogen R/T ↑ liver breakdown
Felodipine / ↓ Plasma levels of felodipine → ↓ effect
Fenoprofen / ↓ Bioavailability of fenoprofen
Furosemide / ↑ Risk or intensity of orthostatic hypotension
Griseofulvin / ↓ Effect of griseofulvin R/T ↓ absorption from GI tract
Haloperidol / ↓ Effect of haloperidol R/T ↑ liver breakdown
H *Indian snakeroot* / Additive CNS depression
H *Kava kava* / Potentiation of CNS depression
MAO inhibitors / ↑ Effect of barbiturates R/T ↓ liver breakdown
Meperidine / CNS depressant effects may be prolonged
Methadone / ↓ Effect of methadone
Methoxyflurane / ↑ Kidney toxicity R/T ↑ liver breakdown of methoxyflurane to toxic metabolites
Metronidazole / ↓ Effect of metronidazole
Narcotic analgesics / See *Alcohol*
Oral contraceptives / ↓ Effect of contraceptives R/T ↑ liver breakdown
Phenothiazines / ↓ Effect of phenothiazines R/T ↑ liver breakdown; also see *Alcohol*
Phenytoin / Effect variable and unpredictable; monitor carefully
Procarbazine / ↑ Effect of barbiturates
Quinidine / ↓ Effect of quinidine R/T ↑ liver breakdown
Rifampin / ↓ Effect of barbiturates R/T ↑ liver breakdown
Sedative-hypnotics, nonbarbiturate / See *Alcohol*
Theophyllines / ↓ Effect of theophyllines R/T ↑ liver breakdown
Valproic acid / ↑ Effect of barbiturates R/T ↓ liver breakdown
Verapamil / ↑ Excretion of verapamil → ↓ effect
Vitamin D / Barbiturates may ↑ requirements for vitamin D R/T ↑ liver breakdown

HOW SUPPLIED

Phenobarbital: *Capsule:* 16 mg; *Elixir:* 15 mg/5mL, 20 mg/5 mL; *Tablet:* 15 mg, 16 mg, 16.2 mg, 30 mg, 60 mg, 90 mg, 100 mg. **Phenobarbital sodium:** *Injection:* 30 mg/mL, 60 mg/mL, 65 mg/mL, 130 mg/mL

DOSAGE

PHENOBARBITAL, PHENOBARBITAL SODIUM

- **CAPSULES, ELIXIR, TABLETS**

Sedation.

Adults: 30–120 mg/day in two to three divided doses. **Pediatric:** 2 mg/kg (60 mg/m^2) t.i.d.

Hypnotic.

Adults: 100–200 mg at bedtime. **Pediatric:** Dose should be determined by provider, based on age and weight.

Anticonvulsant.

Adults: 60–200 mg/day in single or divided doses. **Pediatric:** 3–6 mg/kg/day in single or divided doses.

- **IM, IV**

Sedation.

Adults: 30–120 mg/day in two to three divided doses.

Preoperative sedation.

Adults: 100–200 mg IM only, 60–90 min before surgery. **Pediatric:** 1–3 mg/kg IM or IV 60–90 min prior to surgery.

P

Hypnotic.

Adults: 100–320 mg IM or IV.

Acute convulsions.

Adults: 200–320 mg IM or IV; may be repeated in 6 hr if needed. **Pediatric:** 4–6 mg/kg/day for 7–10 days to achieve a blood level of 10–15 mcg/mL (or 15 mg/kg/day, IV or IM).

Status epilepticus.

Adults: 15–20 mg/kg IV (given over 10–15 min); may be repeated if needed. **Pediatric:** 15–20 mg/kg given over a 10- to 15-min period.

NURSING CONSIDERATIONS

ADMINISTRATION/STORAGE

1. When used for seizures, give the major fraction of the dose according to when seizures are likely to occur (i.e., on arising for daytime seizures and at bedtime when seizures occur at night).
2. When used as an anticonvulsant in infants and children, a loading dose of 15–20 mg/kg achieves blood levels of about 20 mcg/mL shortly after administration. To achieve therapeutic blood levels of 10–20 mcg/mL, higher doses per kilogram may be needed compared with adults.
3. When used IM, inject into a large muscle (e.g., gluteus maximus, vastus lateralis). Injection into or near peripheral nerves may cause permanent neurological deficit.
4. In most cases, when used for epilepsy, drug must be taken regularly to avoid seizures, even when no seizures are imminent.
5. When used for seizures, give the lowest dose possible to avoid adding to the depression that may follow seizures.

IV 6. Reserve IV use for conditions when other routes are not feasible. There is the possibility of overdose, including respiratory depression, even with slow injection of fractional doses.

7. Freshly prepare the aqueous solution for injection.
8. Some ready-dissolved solutions for injection are available; the vehicle is propylene glycol, water, and alcohol.
9. For IV administration, inject slowly at a rate of 50 mg/min.
10. Avoid extravasation as tissue damage and necrosis may result.

ASSESSMENT

1. Document indications for therapy, type, onset, and characteristics of symptoms.
2. List other agents prescribed and the outcome.
3. Assess VS, CBC, liver and renal function studies. Reduce dose with impairment and in debilitated/elderly clients.

CLIENT/FAMILY TEACHING

1. Take only as directed and do not stop abruptly. Store away from bedside and out of childs reach.
2. May initially cause drowsiness; assess effects before performing tasks that require mental alertness.
3. Phenobarbital may require an increase in vitamin D consumption; consume foods high in vitamin D. It may also contribute to a folate deficiency; may require supplemental folic acid.
4. Drug decreases the effect of oral contraceptives; practice other nonhormonal forms of birth control.
5. Avoid alcohol and OTC agents without approval.
6. Do not stop abruptly following long term use; may precipitate seizures. Tolerance may develop and require dosage adjustment.
7. Report any loss of effects, adverse effects or fever, sore throat, rash or bruising/bleeding.

OUTCOMES/EVALUATE

- Sedation; control of seizures
- Therapeutic anticonvulsant drug levels (10–40 mcg/mL)

Phensuximide

(fen-**SUCKS**-ih-myd)

CLASSIFICATION(S):

Anticonvulsant, succinimide

Rx: Milontin

SEE ALSO *ANTICONVULSANTS* AND *SUCCINIMIDES*.

ACTION/KINETICS

Less effective and less toxic than other succinimides. May color the urine pink, red, or red-brown. **t½:** 5–12 hr. **Peak effect:** 1–4 hr. Excreted through the bile and urine.

USES

Absence seizures.

SPECIAL CONCERNS

Use with caution in clients with intermittent porphyria.

ADDITIONAL SIDE EFFECTS

Kidney damage, hematuria, urinary frequency.

HOW SUPPLIED

Capsule: 500 mg

DOSAGE

• CAPSULES

Absence seizures.

Individualize dose. **Adults and children, initial:** 0.5–1 g b.i.d.–t.i.d. The total dose may vary between 1 and 3 g/day (average 1.5 g/day). May be used with other anticonvulsants in the presence of multiple types of epilepsy.

NURSING CONSIDERATIONS

SEE ALSO *NURSING CONSIDERATIONS* FOR *ANTICONVULSANTS* AND *SUCCINIMIDES*.

CLIENT/FAMILY TEACHING

1. Take exactly as directed, do not stop abruptly. May take with food or milk if GI upset.
2. May discolor urine a pink-brown. Report changes in elimination such as pain, frequency, or blood.
3. Report any adverse side effects and loss of seizure control.

OUTCOMES/EVALUATE

Control of seizures

Phentolamine mesylate

(fen-**TOLL**-ah-meen)

PREGNANCY CATEGORY: C
CLASSIFICATION(S):
Alpha-adrenergic blocking drug
Rx: Regitine

ACTION/KINETICS

Phentolamine competitively blocks both presynaptic (alpha-2) and postsynaptic (alpha-1) adrenergic receptors producing vasodilation and a decrease in peripheral resistance. The drug has little effect on BP. In CHF, phentolamine reduces afterload and pulmonary arterial pressure as well as increases CO. **Onset** (parenteral): Immediate. **Duration:** Short. Poorly absorbed from the GI tract. About 10% excreted unchanged in the urine after parenteral use.

USES

(1) Prophylaxis or treatment of hypertension in pheochromocytoma as a result of stress or manipulation prior to or during surgery. (2) Dermal necrosis and sloughing following IV use or extravasation of norepinephrine or dopamine. (3) To test for pheochromocytoma (not the method of choice). *Investigational:* Hypertensive crisis secondary to MAO inhibitor/sympathomimetic amine interactions; rebound hypertension due to withdrawal of clonidine, propranolol, or other antihypertensive drugs. In combination with papaverine as an intracavernous injection for impotence.

CONTRAINDICATIONS

CAD including angina, MI, or coronary insufficiency.

SPECIAL CONCERNS

Use during pregnancy and lactation only if benefits clearly outweigh risks. Geriatric clients may have a greater risk of developing hypothermia. Use with great caution in the presence of gastritis, ulcers, and clients with a history thereof. Defer use of cardiac glycosides until cardiac rhythm returns to normal.

SIDE EFFECTS

CV: Acute and prolonged hypotension, tachycardia, ***MI, cerebrovascular spasm, cerebrovascular occlusion,*** and arrhythmias, especially after parenteral administration. Orthostatic hypotension, flushing. **GI:** N&V, diarrhea. **Other:** Dizziness, weakness, nasal stuffiness.

OD OVERDOSE MANAGEMENT

Symptoms: ***Hypotension, shock.*** *Treatment:* Maintain BP by giving IV norepinephrine (DO NOT USE EPINEPHRINE).

P

DRUG INTERACTIONS

Ephedrine / Vasoconstrictor and hypertensive effect antagonized

Epinephrine / Vasoconstrictor and hypertensive effect antagonized

HOW SUPPLIED

Injection: 5 mg; *Powder for injection:* 5 mg

DOSAGE

• **IV, IM**

Prevent hypertension in pheochromocytoma, preoperative.

Adults, IV: 5 mg 1–2 hr before surgery; dose may be repeated if needed. **Pediatric, IV, IM:** 1 mg (or 0.1 mg/kg) 1–2 hr before surgery; dose may be repeated if needed.

Prevent or control hypertension during surgery.

Adults, IV: 5 mg. **IV infusion:** 0.5–1 mg/min. **Pediatric, IV:** 0.1 mg/kg (3 mg/m^2). May be repeated, if necessary. During surgery 5 mg for adults and 1 mg for children may be given to prevent or control symptoms of epinephrine intoxication (e.g., paroxysms of hypertension, respiratory depression, seizures, tachycardia).

Dermal necrosis/sloughing following IV or extravasation of norepinephrine.

Prevention: 10 mg/1,000 mL norepinephrine solution; *treatment:* 5–10 mg/10 mL saline injected into area of extravasation within 12 hr. **Pediatric:** 0.1–0.2 mg/kg to a maximum of 10 mg.

CHF.

Adults, IV infusion: 0.17–0.4 mg/min.

Diagnosis of pheochromocytoma.

Adults, rapid IV, initial: 2.5 mg (if response is negative, a 5-mg test should be undertaken before concluding the test is negative); **children, rapid IV:** 1 mg. **Adults, IM:** 5 mg; **children, IM:** 3 mg.

• **INTRACAVERNOSAL**

Impotence.

Adults: Papaverine, 30 mg, and 0.5–1 mg phentolamine; adjust dose according to response.

NURSING CONSIDERATIONS

ADMINISTRATION/STORAGE

IV 1. For IV administration, reconstitute 5 mg with 1 mL sterile water or 0.9% NaCl and inject over 1 min.

2. Drug may also be further diluted: 5–10 mg in 500 mL of D5W and titrated to desired response.

3. When norepinephrine or dopamine infusion infiltrates, use 5–10 mg of phentolamine in 10–15 mL of 0.9% NaCl SC at the site and within 12 hr for beneficial effects.

ASSESSMENT

Note indications for therapy and any history of CAD, gastritis, or PUD; monitor VS and ECG.

INTERVENTIONS

1. Monitor VS during parenteral administration until stabilized.

2. To avoid postural hypotension, keep supine for at least 30 min after injection. Then dangle legs over the side of the bed and rise slowly to avoid orthostatic hypotension.

3. With S&S of drug overdose, place in Trendelenburg position. Have levarterenol available to minimize hypotension. *Do not use epinephrine.*

For the diagnosis of pheochromocytoma:

1. The test should not be undertaken on normotensive clients.

2. Sedatives, analgesics, and other nonessential medication should be withheld for 24 hr (and preferably 72 hr) prior to the test.

3. When testing for pheochromocytoma, keep in a supine position, preferably in a dark, quiet room.

4. If the IV test is used, BP should be measured immediately after the injection, at 30-sec intervals for the first 3 min and at 60-sec intervals for the next 7 min. If the IM test is used, BP should be measured every 5 min for 30–45 min.

5. The test is most reliable with sustained hypertension and least reliable with paroxysmal hypertension.

6. A positive response is a drop of more than 35 mm Hg systolic and 25 mm Hg diastolic pressure. Maximal decreases in BP usually occur within 2 min after injection and return to preinjection pressure within 15–30 min. A negative response is indicated when the BP is unchanged, elevated, or reduced less than 35 mm Hg systolic and 25 mm Hg diastolic pressure.

OUTCOMES/EVALUATE

- ↓ BP
- Prevention of tissue necrosis
- Pheochromocytoma diagnosis
- Treatment of erectile dysfunction

Phenylephrine hydrochloride

(fen-ill-**EF**-rin)

PREGNANCY CATEGORY: C
CLASSIFICATION(S):
Sympathomimetic
Rx: Nasal: AH-chew D, Alconefrin, Alconefrin 12 and 25, Children's Nostril, Neo-Synephrine Solution, Nostril, Rhinall, Vicks Sinex. **Ophthalmic:** AK-Dilate, AK-Nefrin, Mydfrin 2.5%, Neo-Synephrine, Neo-Synephrine Viscous, Phenoptic, Prefrin Liquifilm, Relief. **Parenteral:** Neo-Synephrine . (Rx: Parenteral and Ophthalmic Solutions 2.5% or greater; OTC: Nasal products and ophthalmic solutions 0.12% or less)
✱Rx: Ophthalmic: Dionephrine

SEE ALSO *SYMPATHOMIMETIC DRUGS*.

ACTION/KINETICS

Stimulates alpha-adrenergic receptors, producing pronounced vasoconstriction and hence an increase in both SBP and DBP; reflex bradycardia results from increased vagal activity. Also acts on alpha receptors producing vasoconstriction in the skin, mucous membranes, and the mucosa as well as mydriasis by contracting the dilator muscle of the pupil. Resembles epinephrine, but it has more prolonged action and few cardiac effects. **IV: Onset:** immediate; **duration:** 15–20 min. **IM, SC: Onset:** 10–15 min; **duration:** 0.5–2 hr for IM and 50–60 min for SC. *Nasal decongestion (topical):* **Onset:** 15–20 min; **duration:** 30 min–4 hr. *Ophthalmic:* **Time to peak effect for mydriasis:** 15–60 min for 2.5% solution and 10–90 min for 10% solution. **Duration:** 0.5–1.5 hr for 0.12%, 3 hr for 2.5%, and 5–7 hr with 10% (when used for mydriasis). Excreted in urine.

USES

Systemic: (1) Vascular failure in shock, shock-like states, drug-induced hypotension or hypersensitivity. (2) To maintain BP during spinal and inhalation anesthesia; to prolong spinal anesthesia. As a vasoconstrictor in regional analgesia. (3) Paroxysmal SVT. **Nasal:** Nasal congestion due to allergies, sinusitis, common cold, or hay fever. **Ophthalmologic: 0.12%:** Temporary relief of redness of the eye associated with colds, hay fever, wind, dust, sun, smog, smoke, contact lens. **2.5% and 10%:** (1) Decongestant and vasoconstrictor. (2) Treatment of uveitis with posterior synechiae. (3) Open-angle glaucoma. (4) Refraction without cycloplegia, ophthalmoscopic examination, funduscopy, prior to surgery.

CONTRAINDICATIONS

Severe hypertension, VT.

SPECIAL CONCERNS

Use with extreme caution in geriatric clients, severe arteriosclerosis, bradycardia, partial heart block, myocardial disease, hyperthyroidism and during pregnancy and lactation. Systemic absorption with nasal or ophthalmic use. Use of the 2.5% or 10% ophthalmic solutions in children may cause hypertension and irregular heart beat. In geriatric clients, chronic use of the 2.5% or 10% ophthalmic solutions may cause rebound miosis and a decreased mydriatic effect.

SIDE EFFECTS

CV: Reflex bradycardia, arrhythmias (rare). **CNS:** Headache, excitability, restlessness. **Ophthalmologic:** Rebound miosis and decreased mydriatic response in geriatric clients, blurred vision.

OD OVERDOSE MANAGEMENT

Symptoms: Ventricular extrasystoles, short paroxysms of ventricular tachycardia, sensation of fullness in the head, tingling of extremities. *Treatment:* Administer an alpha-adrenergic blocking agent (e.g., phentolamine).

ADDITIONAL DRUG INTERACTIONS

Anesthetics, halogenated hydrocarbon / May sensitize myocardium → serious arrhythmias

P

Bretylium / ↑ Effect of phenylephrine → possible arrhythmias

HOW SUPPLIED

Nasal. *Solution:* 0.125%, 0.16%, 0.25%, 0.5%, 1%; *Tablet, chewable:* 10 mg. **Ophthalmic.** *Solution:* 0.12%, 2.5%, 10 %. **Parenteral.** *Injection:* 10 mg/mL

DOSAGE

• IM, IV, SC

Vasopressor, mild to moderate hypotension.

Adults: 2–5 mg (range: 1–10 mg), not to exceed an initial dose of 5 mg IM or SC repeated no more often than q 10–15 min; or, 0.2 mg (range: 0.1–0.5 mg), not to exceed an initial dose of 0.5 mg IV repeated no more often than q 10–15 min. **Pediatric:** 0.1 mg/kg (3 mg/m²) IM or SC repeated in 1–2 hr if needed.

Vasopressor, severe hypotension and shock.

Adults: 10 mg by continuous IV infusion using 250–500 mL D5W or 0.9% NaCl injection given at a rate of 0.1–0.18 mg/min initial; **then,** give at a rate of 0.04–0.06 mg/min.

Prophylaxis of hypotension during spinal anesthesia.

Adults: 2–3 mg IM or SC 3–4 min before anesthetic given; subsequent doses should not exceed the previous dose by more than 0.1–0.2 mg. No more than 0.5 mg should be given in a single dose. **Pediatric:** 0.044–0.088 mg/kg IM or SC.

Hypotensive emergencies during spinal anesthesia.

Adults, initial: 0.2 mg IV; dose can be increased by no more than 0.2 mg for each subsequent dose not to exceed 0.5 mg/dose.

Prolongation of spinal anesthesia.

2–5 mg added to the anesthetic solution increases the duration of action up to 50% without increasing side effects or complications.

Vasoconstrictor for regional anesthesia.

Add 1 mg to every 20 mL of local anesthetic solution. If more than 2 mg phenylephrine is used, pressor reactions can be expected.

Paroxysmal SVT.

Initial: 0.5 mg (maximum) given by rapid IV injection (over 20–30 seconds). Subsequent doses are determined by BP and should not exceed the previous dose by more than 0.1–0.2 mg and should never be more than 1 mg.

• NASAL SOLUTION, NASAL SPRAY

Adults and children over 12 years of age: 2–3 gtt of the 0.25% or 0.5% solution into each nostril q 3–4 hr as needed. In resistant cases, the 1% solution can be used but no more often than q 4 hr. **Children, 6–12 years of age:** 2–3 gtt of the 0.25% solution q 3–4 hr as needed. **Infants, greater than 6 months of age:** 1–2 gtt of the 0.16% solution into each nostril q 3–4 hr.

• OPHTHALMIC SOLUTION, 0.12%, 2.5%, 10%

Vasoconstriction, pupillary dilation.

1 gtt of the 2.5% or 10% solution on the upper limbus a few minutes following 1 gtt of topical anesthetic (prevents stinging and dilution of solution by lacrimation). An additional drop may be needed after 1 hr.

Uveitis.

1 gtt of the 2.5% or 10% solution with atropine. To free recently formed posterior synechiae, 1 gtt of the 2.5% or 10% solution to the upper surface of the cornea. Continue treatment the following day, if needed. In the interim, apply hot compresses for 5–10 min t.i.d. using 1 gtt of 1% or 2% atropine sulfate before and after each series of compresses.

Glaucoma.

1 gtt of 10% solution on the upper surface of the cornea as needed. Both the 2.5% and 10% solutions may be used with miotics in clients with open-angle glaucoma.

Surgery.

2.5% or 10% solution 30–60 min before surgery for wide dilation of the pupil.

Refraction.

Adults: 1 gtt of a cycloplegic (homatropine HBr, atropine sulfate, cyclopentolate, tropicamide HCl, or a combination of homatropine and cocaine HCl) in each eye followed in 5 min with 1 gtt of 2.5% phenylephrine solution and in 10 min with another drop of cycloplegic. The eyes are ready for refraction in 50–60 min. **Children:** 1 gtt of atropine sulfate, 1%, in each eye followed in 10–15 min with 1 gtt of phenylephrine solution, 2.5%, and in 5–10 min with a second drop of atropine sulfate, 1%. The eyes are ready for refraction in 1–2 hr.

Ophthalmoscopic examination.
1 gtt of 2.5% solution in each eye. The eyes are ready for examination in 15–30 min and the effect lasts for 1–3 hr.

Minor eye irritations.
1–2 gtt of the 0.12% solution in the eye(s) up to q.i.d. as needed.

NURSING CONSIDERATIONS

SEE ALSO *NURSING CONSIDERATIONS* FOR *SYMPATHOMIMETIC DRUGS.*

ADMINISTRATION/STORAGE

1. Store drug in a brown bottle and away from light.
2. Instill a drop of local anesthetic before administering the 10% ophthalmic solution.
IV 3. For IV administration, dilute each 1 mg with 9 mL of sterile water and administer over 1 min. Further dilution of 10 mg in 500 mL of dextrose, Ringer's, or saline solution may be titrated to client response.
4. When used parenterally, monitor infusion site closely to avoid extravasation. If evident, administer SC phentolamine locally to prevent tissue necrosis.
5. Prolonged exposure to air or strong light may result in oxidation and discoloration. Do not use solution if it changes color, becomes cloudy, or contains a precipitate.

ASSESSMENT

1. Document indications for therapy, type, onset, and characteristics of symptoms; note goals of therapy.
2. During IV administration monitor cardiac rhythm and BP continuously until stabilized, noting any evidence of bradycardia or arrhythmias.

CLIENT/FAMILY TEACHING

1. Ophthalmic instillations and nasal decongestants may produce systemic sympathomimetic effects; chronic excessive use may cause rebound congestion.
2. Wear sunglasses in bright light. Report if symptoms of photosensitivity and blurred vision persist after 12 hr. Blurred vision should decrease with repeated use.
3. With ophthalmic solution, report if there is no relief of symptoms within 2 days.
4. When using for nasal decongestion, blow nose before administering; report if no relief of symptoms within 3 days. Rebound nasal congestion may occur with longer therapy.

OUTCOMES/EVALUATE

- ↑ BP
- Termination of paroxysmal SVT
- Relief of nasal congestion
- ↓ Conjunctivitis/allergic S&S
- Dilatation of pupils

Phenylpropanolamine hydrochloride

(fen-ill-**proh**-pah-**NOHL**-ah-meen)

PREGNANCY CATEGORY: C
CLASSIFICATION(S):
Sympathomimetic
NOTE: The FDA has found phenylpropanolamine not generally recognized as safe and effective for use as a decongestant or an appetite suppressant in OTC products and these have been removed from the market due to the possibility of hemorrhagic stroke. Action may also be taken to remove this drug from prescription products.

SEE ALSO *STIMULANTS* AND *SYMPATHOMIMETIC DRUGS.*

ACTION/KINETICS

Thought to stimulate both alpha and beta receptors as well as to act indirectly through release of norepinephrine from storage sites. Increases in BP are due mainly to increased CO rather than to vasoconstriction; has minimal CNS effects. Acts on alpha-adrenergic receptors to produce a decongestant effect in the nasal mucosa. **Onset, de-**

P

congestant: 15–30 min; **peak plasma levels:** 1–2 hr; **duration, capsules and tablets:** 3 hr; **extended-release tablets:** 12–16 hr. **Peak plasma levels:** 100 ng. **t½:** 3–4 hr. Eighty percent to 90% excreted in the urine unchanged.

USES

Nasal congestion due to colds, hay fever, allergies.

CONTRAINDICATIONS

Arteriosclerosis, depression, glaucoma, hypertension, diabetes, kidney disease, hyperthyroidism, during or within 14 days of use of MAO inhibitors, hypersensitivity to sympathomimetics. Use as an anorexiant for children less than 12 years of age. Sustained-release forms during lactation and in children less than 12 years of age.

SPECIAL CONCERNS

Safety and efficacy during pregnancy and lactation and for children not established. Children less than 6 years of age may be at greater risk for developing psychiatric disorders when using phenylpropanolamine. Individualize the anorexiant dose for children 12–18 years of age. An association has been found between use and hemorrhagic stroke.

SIDE EFFECTS

CNS: Dizziness, headache, insomnia, restlessness, bizarre behavior. Serious effects due to abuse include: agitation, tremor, increased motor activity, hallucinations, ***seizures, stroke, and death.*** **CV:** Palpitations, ***hypertension (may be severe and lead to crisis), hemorrhagic stroke,*** tachycardia. **Miscellaneous:** Dry mouth, dysuria, renal failure, nausea, nasal dryness.

ADDITIONAL DRUG INTERACTIONS

Bromocriptine / Worsening of side effects of bromocriptine; possibility of VT and cardiac dysfunction
Caffeine / ↑ Serum caffeine levels → ↑ risk pharmacologic/toxic effects
Indomethacin / Possibility of severe hypertensive episode

HOW SUPPLIED

Capsule: 37.5 mg; *Capsule, Extended Release:* 75 mg; *Tablet:* 25 mg, 37.5 mg, 50 mg; *Tablet, Extended Release:* 75 mg

DOSAGE

• CAPSULES, TABLETS

Decongestant.

Adults: 25 mg q 4 hr or 50 mg q 6–8 hr (not to exceed 150 mg/day); **Children, 2–6 years:** 6.25 mg q 4 hr, not to exceed 37.5 mg in 24 hr; **6–12 years:** 12.5 mg q 4 hr, not to exceed 75 mg in 24 hr.

Anorexiant.

Adults: 25 mg t.i.d. 30 min before meals, not to exceed 75 mg in 24 hr.

• EXTENDED-RELEASE CAPSULES, EXTENDED-RELEASE TABLETS

Decongestant.

Adults: 75 mg q 12 hr.

Anorexiant.

Adults: 75 mg once daily in the morning.

NURSING CONSIDERATIONS

SEE ALSO *NURSING CONSIDERATIONS* FOR *STIMULANTS* AND *SYMPATHOMIMETIC DRUGS.*

CLIENT/FAMILY TEACHING

1. Continue regular exercise, reduced caloric intake, and behavioral modification programs in the overall management of obesity.
2. Men should report difficulties in voiding; they may experience drug-induced urinary retention.
3. Drug may cause dizziness and tremors.
4. Avoid any caffeine-containing products or foods.

OUTCOMES/EVALUATE

- ↓ Nasal congestion
- ↓ Appetite; weight loss

Phenytoin

(**FEN**-ih-toyn, dye-**fen**-ill-hy-**DAN**-toyn)

PREGNANCY CATEGORY: C
Rx: Dilantin Infatab, Dilantin-125
★Rx: Dilantin-30 Pediatric

Phenytoin sodium, extended

(**FEN**-ih-toyn)

PREGNANCY CATEGORY: C
Rx: Dilantin Kapseals

Phenytoin sodium, parenteral

(**FEN**-ih-toyn)

PREGNANCY CATEGORY: C
Rx: Dilantin Sodium

Phenytoin sodium prompt

(**FEN**-ih-toyn)

PREGNANCY CATEGORY: C
CLASSIFICATION(S):
Anticonvulsant, hydantoin

SEE ALSO *ANTICONVULSANTS* AND *ANTIARRHYTHMIC AGENTS*.

ACTION/KINETICS

Acts in the motor cortex of the brain to reduce the spread of electrical discharges from the rapidly firing epileptic foci in this area. This is accomplished by stabilizing hyperexcitable cells possibly by affecting sodium efflux. Also, phenytoin decreases activity of centers in the brain stem responsible for the tonic phase of grand mal seizures. Has few sedative effects.

Monitor serum levels because the serum concentrations of phenytoin increase disproportionately as the dosage is increased. Phenytoin extended is designed for once-a-day dosage. It has a slow dissolution rate—no more than 35% in 30 min, 30%–70% in 60 min, and less than 85% in 120 min. Absorption is variable following PO dosage. **Peak serum levels: PO,** 4–8 hr. Since the rate and extent of absorption depend on the particular preparation, the same product should be used for a particular client. **Peak serum levels (following IM):** 24 hr (wide variation). **Therapeutic serum levels:** 5–20 mcg/mL. **t$^1/_2$:** 8–60 hr (average: 20–30 hr). **Steady state:** 7–10 days after initiation. Biotransformed in the liver. Both inactive metabolites and unchanged drug are excreted in the urine.

As an antiarrhythmic, phenytoin increases the electrical stimulation threshold of heart muscle, although it is less effective than quinidine, procainamide, or lidocaine. **Onset:** 30–60 min. **Duration:** 24 hr or more. **t$^1/_2$:** 22–36 hr. **Therapeutic serum level:** 10–20 mcg/mL.

USES

(1) Chronic epilepsy, especially of the tonic-clonic, psychomotor type. Not effective against absence seizures and may even increase the frequency of seizures in this disorder. (2) Parenteral phenytoin is sometimes used to treat status epilepticus and to control seizures during neurosurgery.

(3) PO for certain PVCs and IV for PVCs and tachycardia. Particularly useful for arrhythmias produced by digitalis overdosage.

Investigational: Paroxysmal choreoathetosis; to treat blistering and erosions in clients with recessive dystrophic epidermolysis bullosa; episodic dyscontrol; trigeminal neuralgia; as a muscle relaxant in neuromyotonia, myotonia congenita, or myotonic muscular dystrophy; to treat cardiac symptoms in overdosage of tricyclic antidepressants. Severe preeclampsia.

CONTRAINDICATIONS

Hypersensitivity to hydantoins, exfoliative dermatitis, sinus bradycardia, second- and third-degree AV block, clients with Adams-Stokes syndrome, SA block. Lactation.

SPECIAL CONCERNS

Use with caution in acute, intermittent porphyria. Administer with extreme caution to clients with a history of asthma or other allergies, impaired renal or hepatic function, and heart disease (hypotension, severe myocardial insufficiency). Abrupt withdrawal may cause status epilepticus. Combined drug therapy is required if petit mal seizures are also present.

SIDE EFFECTS

CNS: Most commonly, drowsiness, ataxia, dysarthria, confusion, insomnia, nervousness, irritability, depression, tremor, numbness, headache, psychoses, ***increased seizures.*** Choreoathetosis following IV use. **GI:** Gingival hyperplasia, N&V, either diarrhea

P

or constipation. **Dermatologic:** Various dermatoses including a measles-like rash (common), scarlatiniform, maculopapular, and urticarial rashes. Rarely, drug-induced lupus erythematosus, ***Stevens-Johnson syndrome,*** exfoliative or purpuric dermatitis, and ***toxic epidermal necrolysis.*** Alopecia, hirsutism. Skin reactions may necessitate withdrawal of therapy. **Hematopoietic:** Leukopenia, granulocytopenia, thrombocytopenia, pancytopenia, ***agranulocytosis,*** macrocytosis, megaloblastic anemia, leukocytosis, monocytosis, eosinophilia, simple anemia, ***aplastic anemia, hemolytic anemia.*** **Hepatic:** Liver damage, toxic hepatitis, hypersensitivity reactions involving the liver including hepatocellular degeneration and ***fatal hepatocellular necrosis.*** **Ophthalmic:** Diplopia, nystagmus, conjunctivitis. **Miscellaneous:** Hyperglycemia, chest pain, edema, fever, photophobia, weight gain, ***pulmonary fibrosis,*** lymph node hyperplasia, gynecomastia, periarteritis nodosa, depression of IgA, soft tissue injury at injection site, coarsening of facial features, Peyronie's disease, enlarged lips.

Rapid parenteral administration may cause serious CV effects, including hypotension, arrhythmias, CV collapse, and heart block, as well as CNS depression.

Many clients have a partial deficiency in the ability of the liver to degrade phenytoin, and as a result, toxicity may develop after a small PO dose. Liver and kidney function tests and hematopoietic studies are indicated prior to and periodically during drug therapy.

LABORATORY TEST CONSIDERATIONS

Alters LFTs, ↑ blood glucose values, and ↓ PBI values. ↑ Gamma globulins. Phenytoin ↓ immunoglobulins A and G. False + Coombs' test.

OD OVERDOSE MANAGEMENT

Symptoms: Initially, ataxia, dysarthria, and nystagmus followed by unresponsive pupils, hypotension, and ***coma.*** Plasma levels greater than 40 mcg/mL result in significant decreases in mental capacity. *Treatment:* Treat symptoms. Hemodialysis may be effective. In children, total-exchange transfusion has been used.

DRUG INTERACTIONS

Acetaminophen / ↓ Acetaminophen effect R/T ↑ liver breakdown; hepatotoxicity may ↑
Alcohol, ethyl / ↓ Phenytoin effect in alcoholics R/T ↑ liver breakdown
Allopurinol / ↑ Phenytoin effect R/T ↓ liver breakdown
Amiodarone / ↑ Phenytoin or amiodarone effect R/T ↓ liver breakdown
Antacids / ↓ Phenytoin effect R/T ↓ GI absorption
Anticoagulants, oral / ↑ Phenytoin effect R/T ↓ liver breakdown. Also, possible ↑ anticoagulant effect R/T ↓ plasma protein binding
Antidepressants, tricyclic / ↑ Risk of epileptic seizures or ↑ phenytoin effect by ↓ plasma protein binding
Barbiturates / Phenytoin effect may be ↑, ↓, or not changed; possible ↑ effect of barbiturates
Benzodiazepines / ↑ Phenytoin effect R/T ↓ liver breakdown
Carbamazepine / ↓ Phenytoin or carbamazepine effect R/T ↑ liver breakdown
Charcoal / ↓ Phenytoin effect R/T ↓ absorption from GI tract
Chloramphenicol / ↑ Phenytoin effect R/T ↓ liver breakdown
Chlorpheniramine / ↑ Phenytoin effect
Cimetidine / ↑ Phenytoin effect R/T ↓ liver breakdown
Clonazepam / ↓ Plasma levels of clonazepam or phenytoin; ↑ risk of phenytoin toxicity
Contraceptives, oral / Estrogen-induced fluid retention may precipitate seizures; also, ↓ effect of contraceptives R/T ↑ liver breakdown
Corticosteroids / ↓ Corticosteroid effect R/T ↑ liver breakdown; also, corticosteroids may mask hypersensitivity reactions due to phenytoin
Cyclosporine / ↓ Cyclosporine effect R/T ↑ liver breakdown
Diazoxide / ↓ Phenytoin effect R/T ↑ liver breakdown
Dicumarol / ↓ Dicumarol effect R/T ↑ liver breakdown
Digitalis glycosides / ↓ Digitalis effect R/T ↑ liver breakdown

Disopyramide / ↓ Disopyramide effect R/T ↑ liver breakdown
Disulfiram / ↑ Phenytoin effect R/T ↓ liver breakdown
Dopamine / IV phenytoin → hypotension and bradycardia; also, ↓ dopamine effect
Doxycycline / ↓ Doxycycline effect R/T ↑ liver breakdown
Estrogens / See *Contraceptives, oral*
Fluconazole / ↑ Phenytoin effect R/T ↓ liver breakdown
Folic acid / ↓ Phenytoin effect
Furosemide / ↓ Furosemide effect R/T ↓ absorption
Haloperidol / ↓ Haloperidol effect R/T ↑ liver breakdown
Ibuprofen / ↑ Phenytoin effect
Isoniazid / ↑ Phenytoin effect R/T ↓ liver breakdown
Itraconazole / Possible ↓ itracoazole plasma levels
Levodopa / ↓ Levodopa effect
Levonorgestrel / ↓ Levonorgestrel effect
Lithium / ↑ Risk of lithium toxicity
Loxapine / ↓ Phenytoin effect
Mebendazole / ↓ Mebendazole effect
Meperidine / ↓ Meperidine effect R/T ↑ liver breakdown; toxic effects of meperidine may ↑ due to accumulation of active metabolite (normeperidine)
Methadone / ↓ Methadone effect R/T ↑ liver breakdown
Metronidazole / ↑ Phenytoin effect R/T ↓ liver breakdown
Metyrapone / ↓ Metyrapone effect R/T ↑ liver breakdown
Mexiletine / ↓ Mexiletine effect R/T ↑ liver breakdown
Miconazole / ↑ Phenytoin effect R/T ↓ liver breakdown
H *Milk thistle*/ Helps prevent liver damage from phenytoin
Nitrofurantoin / ↓ Phenytoin effect
Omeprazole / ↑ Phenytoin effect R/T ↓ liver breakdown
Phenothiazines / ↑ Phenytoin effect R/T ↓ liver breakdown
Primidone / Possible ↑ primidone effect
Pyridoxine / ↓ Phenytoin effect
Quetiapine / ↓ Peak and trough quetiapine levels R/T ↑ liver metabolism
Quinidine / ↓ Quinidine effect R/T ↑ liver breakdown
Rifampin / ↓ Phenytoin effect R/T ↑ liver breakdown
Salicylates / ↑ Phenytoin effect R/T ↓ plasma protein binding
Sucralfate / ↓ Phenytoin effect R/T ↓ absorption from GI tract
Sulfonamides / ↑ Phenytoin effect R/T ↓ liver breakdown
Sulfonylureas / ↓ Sulfonylurea effect
Theophylline / ↓ Effect of both drugs R/T ↑ liver breakdown
Trimethoprim / ↑ Phenytoin effect R/T ↓ liver breakdown
Valproic acid / ↑ Phenytoin effect R/T ↓ liver breakdown and ↓ plasma protein binding; phenytoin may also ↓ effect of valproic acid R/T ↑ liver breakdown

HOW SUPPLIED

Phenytoin: *Chew Tablet:* 50 mg; *Suspension:* 125 mg/5 mL; **Phenytoin sodium, extended:** *Capsule, Extended Release:* 30 mg, 100 mg; **Phenytoin sodium, parenteral:** *Injection:* 50 mg/mL; **Phenytoin sodium prompt:** *Capsule:* 100 mg

DOSAGE

• ORAL SUSPENSION, CHEWABLE TABLETS

Seizures.

Adults, initial: 100 mg (125 mg of the suspension) t.i.d.; adjust dosage at 7- to 10-day intervals until seizures are controlled; **usual, maintenance:** 300–400 mg/day, although 600 mg/day (625 mg of the suspension) may be required in some. **Pediatric, initial:** 5 mg/kg/day in two to three divided doses; **maintenance,** 4–8 mg/kg (up to maximum of 300 mg/day). Children over 6 years may require up to 300 mg/day. **Geriatric:** 3 mg/kg initially in divided doses; **then,** adjust dosage according to serum levels and response. Once dosage level has been established, the extended capsules may be used for once-a-day dosage.

• CAPSULES, EXTENDED-RELEASE CAPSULES

Seizures.

Adults, initial: 100 mg t.i.d.; adjust dose at 7- to 10-day intervals until control is achieved. An initial loading dose of 12–15 mg/kg divided into two to three doses over 6 hr followed by 100 mg t.i.d. on subsequent days may be preferred if seizures are frequent. **Pediatric:** See dose for Oral Suspension and Chewable Tablets.

Arrhythmias.

Adults: 200–400 mg/day.

• **IV**

Status epilepticus.

Adults, loading dose: 10–15 mg/kg at a rate not to exceed 50 mg/min; **then,** 100 mg PO or IV q 6–8 hr. **Pediatric, loading dose:** 15–20 mg/kg in divided doses of 5–10 mg/kg given at a rate of 1–3 mg/kg/min.

Arrhythmias.

Adults: 100 mg q 5 min up to maximum of 1 g.

• **IM**

Dose should be 50% greater than the PO dose.

Neurosurgery.

100–200 mg q 4 hr during and after surgery (during first 24 hr, administer no more than 1,000 mg; after first day, give maintenance dosage).

NURSING CONSIDERATIONS

SEE ALSO *NURSING CONSIDERATIONS* FOR *ANTICONVULSANTS* AND *ANTIARRHYTHMIC AGENTS*.

ADMINISTRATION/STORAGE

1. Full effectiveness of PO administered hydantoins is delayed and may take 6–9 days to be fully established. A similar period of time will elapse before effects disappear completely.
2. When hydantoins are substituted for or added to another anticonvulsant medication, their dosage is gradually increased, while dosage of the other drug is decreased proportionally.
3. Avoid IM, SC, or perivascular injections. Pain, inflammation, and necrosis may be caused by the highly alkaline solutions.
4. If receiving tube feedings of Isocal or Osmolite, the PO absorption of phenytoin may be decreased. Do not administer together.
5. Due to potential differences in bioavailability between PO products, do not interchange brands. Also, when switching from extended to prompt products, dosage adjustments may be required.
6. IV Use of IV infusion is not recommended, as the drug is poorly soluble and may form a precipitate. Inject slowly and directly into a large vein through a large-gauge needle or IV catheter.
7. For parenteral preparations:
   • Use only a clear solution.
   • Dilute with special diluent supplied by manufacturer.
   • Shake the vials until the solution is clear. It may take about 10 min for the drug to dissolve.
   • To hasten the process, warm the vial in warm water after adding the diluent.
   • The drug is incompatible with acid solutions.
8. *Do not* add phenytoin to an already running IV solution.
9. If IV infusion is used, a rate of 50 mg/min should not be exceeded in adults or 1–3 mg/kg/min in neonates.
10. Following IV administration, administer NSS through the same needle or IV catheter to avoid local irritation of the vein due to alkalinity of the solution. Do not use dextrose solutions.
11. For treatment of status epilepticus, inject IV slowly at a rate not to exceed 50 mg/min. May repeat the dose 30 min after the initial administration if needed.

ASSESSMENT

1. Document indications for therapy, onset and characteristics of symptoms.
2. Note history and nature of seizures, addressing location, frequency, duration, causes, and characteristics.
3. Determine if hypersensitive to hydantoins or has exfoliative dermatitis. Consider fosphenytoin in those unable to tolerate phenytoin.
4. Do not breast-feed following delivery.
5. Monitor ECG, CBC, liver, and renal function studies.

INTERVENTIONS

1. During IV administration, monitor for hypotension.
2. Monitor serum drug levels:
   • Seven to 10 days may be required to achieve recommended serum levels. Drug is highly protein bound; may

order free and bound drug levels to better assess response. Drug is metabolized much slower by the elderly; thus most may be managed with once a day dosing.

• If receiving drugs that interact with hydantoins or with impaired liver function, obtain level more frequently. Dilantin induces hepatic microsomal enzymes for drug metabolism.

3. Oral form has variable absorption; do not administer with tube feedings. Administer separately, flush, and clamp tube for 20 min to ensure absorption.

CLIENT/FAMILY TEACHING

1. May take with food to minimize GI upset. Do not take within 2–3 hr of antacid ingestion.
2. Use care when performing tasks that require mental alertness. Drug may cause drowsiness, dizziness, and blurred vision.
3. Do not substitute products or exchange brands; bioavailability of phenytoin may vary. Seizure control may be lost or toxic blood levels may develop with substitutions.
4. Prompt-release forms cannot be substituted for another unless the dosage is also adjusted.
   • If taking phenytoin extended, do not substitute chewable tablets for capsules. The strengths of the medications are not equal.
   • If taking phenytoin extended, check bottle carefully. Chewable tablets are never extended form.
   • With extended, take only a single dose daily; take only as directed and only in the brand prescribed.
5. If a dose is missed, take as soon as it is remembered. Then resume the usual schedule. Do not double up to make up for the missed dose. If the doses of drug are scheduled throughout the day, and one of the doses is missed, take the drug as soon as it is realized unless it's within 4 hr of the next dose. In that case, omit unless otherwise instructed.
6. Do not take any other agents. Hydantoins interact with many other medications and may require adjustment of the anticonvulsant dose.
7. Avoid alcohol in any form and CNS depressants.
8. With diabetes, monitor FS and report changes; may have to to adjust insulin dosage and/or diet.
9. May cause urine to appear pink, red, or brown; do not be alarmed.
10. To minimize bleeding from the gums and prevent gingival hyperplasia, practice good oral hygiene. Brush teeth with a soft toothbrush, massage the gums, and floss every day. Advise dentist of therapy.
11. Hydantoin has an androgenic effect on the hair follicle. Acne may develop; practice good skin care.
12. Report any excessive hair growth on the face and trunk and any discolorations or skin rash; may require dermatologist referral.
13. Complaints of weakness, ease of fatigue, headaches, or feeling faint may be signs of folic acid deficiency or megaloblastic anemia. Dietitian evaluation as well as hematologic evaluations may be indicated.
14. Report for lab studies as ordered, including CBC, drug levels, and renal and liver function studies.
15. Drug may alter thyroid function results. If thyroid studies are conducted, for ensured accuracy, they should be repeated 10 days after therapy has been discontinued.
16. Do not stop abruptly. Report all bothersome side effects because these may be dose-related.
17. Practice reliable birth control; drug may interfere with oral contraceptives.

OUTCOMES/EVALUATE

• Control of seizures
• Termination of ventricular arrhythmias; stable cardiac rhythm
• Therapeutic drug levels (5–20 mcg/mL)

Physostigmine salicylate

(fye-zoh-**STIG**-meen)

PREGNANCY CATEGORY: C

P

CLASSIFICATION(S):
Cholinesterase inhibitor, indirectly-acting
Rx: Antilirium

SEE ALSO *NEOSTIGMINE.*

ACTION/KINETICS
Reversible acetylcholinesterase inhibitor causing an increased concentration of acetylcholine at nerve endings; antagonizes anticholinergic drugs. Produces miosis, increased accommodation, and a decrease in intraocular pressure with decreased resistance to outflow of aqueous humor. **Onset, IV:** 3–5 min. **Duration, IV:** 1–2 hr. **$t^1/_2$:** 1–2 hr. No dosage alteration is necessary in clients with renal impairment.

USES
Overdosage due to cholinergic blocking drugs (e.g., atropine) and tricyclic antidepressant overdosage. Friedreich's and other inherited ataxias (FDA has granted orphan status for this use). *Investigational:* Treat delirium tremens (DTs) and Alzheimer's disease. May also antagonize the CNS depressant effect of diazepam.

CONTRAINDICATIONS
Acute-angle glaucoma, history of retinal detachment, ocular hypotension, asthma, epilepsy, parkinsonism, gangrene, diabetes, CV disease, GI or GU tract obstruction, spastic GI conditions, vasomotor instability, severe bradycardia or hypotension, recent MI, lactation, in those receiving choline esters or depolarizing neuromuscular blocking drugs.

SPECIAL CONCERNS
Use with caution during lactation. Reserve systemic use in children for life-threatening situations only. Benzyl alcohol, found in the parenteral product, may cause a fatal "gasping syndrome" in premature infants. The parenteral form also contains sulfites that may cause allergic reactions.

SIDE EFFECTS
Nausea, GI discomfort, diarrhea, hypotension, bronchial constriction, increased salivation. If IV administration is too rapid, bradycardia, hypersalivation, breathing difficulties, and ***seizures*** may occur.

P

OD OVERDOSE MANAGEMENT
Symptoms: Cholinergic crisis. *Treatment:* IV atropine sulfate: ***Adults:*** 0.4–0.6 mg; ***infants and children up to 12 years of age:*** 0.01 mg/kg q 2 hr as needed (maximum single dose should not exceed 0.4 mg). A short-acting barbiturate may be used for seizures not relieved by atropine.

DRUG INTERACTIONS
Anticholinesterases, systemic / Additive effects → toxicity
Succinylcholine / ↑ Risk of respiratory and CV collapse

HOW SUPPLIED
Injection: 1 mg/mL.

DOSAGE

- **IM, IV**

Anticholinergic drug overdose.
Adults, IM, IV: 0.5–2 mg at a rate of 1 mg/min; may be repeated if necessary. **Pediatric, IV:** 0.02 mg/kg IM or by slow IV injection (0.5 mg given over a period of at least 1 min). Dose may be repeated at 5–10 min if needed to a maximum of 2 mg if no toxic effects are manifested.

Postanesthesia.
0.5–1 mg given IM or by slow IV (less than 1 mg/min). May be repeated at 10- to 30-min intervals to attain desired response.

NURSING CONSIDERATIONS

SEE ALSO *NURSING CONSIDERATIONS* FOR *NEOSTIGMINE.*

ADMINISTRATION/STORAGE
IV May administer IV undiluted: 1 mg/min; 0.5 mg/min for children. Product contains benzyl alcohol and sulfites.

ASSESSMENT
1. Determine type of overdosage (drug or plant ingestion), amount and time ingested.
2. During IV administration, monitor ECG and VS; report any bradycardia, hypersalivation, respiratory difficulty, or seizure activity.

INTERVENTIONS
If possible, have client void prior to administering. If incontinence occurs, may be caused by too high a dose.

OUTCOMES/EVALUATE
Reversal of toxic CNS symptoms R/T drug overdosage or plant toxins

Phytonadione (Vitamin K_1)

(fye-toe-nah-**DYE**-ohn)

PREGNANCY CATEGORY: C
CLASSIFICATION(S):
Vitamin K derivative
Rx: Aqua-Mephyton, Mephyton

ACTION/KINETICS

Vitamin K is essential for the hepatic synthesis of factors II, VII, IX, and X, all of which are essential for blood clotting. Vitamin K deficiency causes an increase in bleeding tendency, demonstrated by ecchymoses, epistaxis, hematuria, GI bleeding, and postoperative and intracranial hemorrhage. Phytonadione is similar to natural vitamin K. GI absorption occurs only via intestinal lymphatics and requires the presence of bile salts. Vitamin K is not effective in reversing the anticoagulant effect of heparin. Frequent determinations of PT are indicated during therapy. **IM: Onset,** 1–2 hr. *Control of bleeding:* Parenteral, 3–6 hr. *Normal PT:* 12–14 hr. **PO: Onset,** 6–12 hr.

USES

Coagulation disorders due to faulty formation of factors II, VII, IX, and X when caused by Vitamin K deficiency or interference with vitamin K activity.

PO. Anticoagulant-induced PT deficiency. Hypoprothrombinemia secondary to antibacterial therapy or salicylates. Secondary to obstructive jaundice and biliary fistulas (use only if bile salts are given together with phytonadione). **Parenteral.** Anticoagulant-induced prothrombin deficiency. Hypoprothrombinemia secondary to conditions limiting absorption or synthesis of vitamin K. Drug-induced hypoprothrombinemias due to interference with vitamin K metabolism. Prophylaxis and therapy of hemorrhagic disease in newborns.

CONTRAINDICATIONS

Severe liver disease.

SPECIAL CONCERNS

Use with caution in clients with sulfite sensitivity and during lactation as phytonadione is excreted in breast milk. Safety and efficacy have not been determined in children. Benzyl alcohol, contained in some preparations, may cause toxicity in newborns. IV use may result in severe reactions, including death even with appropriate precautions. Restrict IV use to situations where other routes are not feasible and the serious risk is justified.

SIDE EFFECTS

May be transient flushing of the face, sweating, a sense of constriction of the chest, and weakness. Cramp-like pain, weak and rapid pulse, convulsive movements, chills and fever, hypotension, cyanosis, or hemoglobinuria has been reported occasionally. ***Shock and cardiac and respiratory failure*** may be observed. **Allergic:** Rash, urticaria, ***anaphylaxis.*** **After PO use:** N&V, stomach upset, headache. **After parenteral use:** Flushing, alteration of taste, sweating, hypotension, dizziness, rapid and weak pulse, dyspnea, cyanosis, delayed skin reactions. Pain, swelling, and tenderness at injection site. ***IV administration may cause severe reactions (e.g., shock, cardiac or respiratory arrest, anaphylaxis) leading to death.*** These effects may occur when receiving vitamin K for the first time. **Newborns: *Fatal kernicterus,*** hemolysis, jaundice, hyperbilirubinemia (especially in premature infants).

DRUG INTERACTIONS

Antibiotics / May inhibit vitamin K production → bleeding; give vitamin K supplements
Anticoagulants, oral / Antagonizes anticoagulant effect
Cholestyramine / ↓ Phytonadione effect R/T ↓ GI tract absorption
Colestipol / ↓ Phytonadione effect R/T ↓ GI tract absorption
Hemolytics / ↑ Potential for toxicity
Mineral oil / ↓ Phytonadione effect R/T ↓ GI tract absorption
Quinidine, Quinine / ↑ Requirement for vitamin K

P

Salicylates / High doses → ↑ vitamin K requirements
Sulfonamides / ↑ Requirements for vitamin K
Sucralfate / ↓ Phytonadione effect R/T ↓ GI tract absorption

HOW SUPPLIED

Injection, aqueous colloidal: 2 mg/mL; *Injection, aqueous dispersion:* 10 mg /mL; *Tablet:* 5 mg

DOSAGE

- **PARENTERAL, TABLETS**

Hypoprothrombinemia, anticoagulant-induced.

Adults: 2.5–10 mg (up to 25 mg). Dose may be repeated after 6–8 hr (parenteral use) or 12–48 hr (PO use) if PT has not been shortened sufficiently.

Hypoprothrombinemia due to other causes.

Adults: 2.5–25 mg (rarely up to 50 mg). Amount and route of administration depend on severity of condition and client response. Avoid PO route when condition would prevent proper absorption.

Hemorrhagic disease of the newborn.

Prophylaxis: Single IM dose of 0.5–1 mg within 1 hr after birth. May be repeated after 2–3 weeks if mother has received anticoagulant, anticonvulsant, antituberculosis treatment, or recent antibiotic therapy during pregnancy. Twelve-24 hr before delivery, 1–5 mg may be given to the mother. *Treatment:* 1 mg SC or IM. Higher doses if mother has received PO anticoagulants.

NURSING CONSIDERATIONS

ADMINISTRATION/STORAGE

1. Mix suspension (injection) only with water or D5W.
2. Mix colloidal injection with D5W, isotonic NaCl, or D5/NSS.
3. Protect vitamin K from light.
4. Store injectable emulsion or colloidal solutions in cool, 5–15°C (41–59°F), dark place.
5. Do not freeze.
6. Heparin may be used to reverse effects from overdosage.

ASSESSMENT

1. Document sensitivity to sulfites.
2. Note drugs prescribed to ensure none interact.
3. Monitor PT/PTT, liver and hematologic values.
4. Determine history or lab evidence of advanced liver disease. This results in loss of protein synthesis and is not responsive to vitamin K.

INTERVENTIONS

1. Note any frank bleeding. Test stools, urine, and GI drainage for occult blood.
2. Observe hospitalized clients with poor nutrition (receiving TPN), uremia, recent surgery, and multiple antibiotic therapy for vitamin K deficiency.
3. Administer slowly. Rapid parenteral administration can produce dyspnea, chest and back pain, and even death.
4. With decreased bile secretion, administer bile salts to ensure absorption of PO phytonadione.
5. If receiving bile acid–binding resins such as colestipol or cholestyramine, monitor PT and assess carefully for malabsorption of vitamin K.

CLIENT/FAMILY TEACHING

1. Take only as directed.
2. Dietary sources high in vitamin K include dairy products, meats, and green leafy vegetables. The dietary requirement is low since it is also synthesized by colonized bacteria in the intestine.
3. Report any evidence of unusual bruising or bleeding.
4. Use a soft toothbrush, electric razor, and a night light at night; wear shoes and avoid IM shots and flossing to prevent injury with bleeding.
5. Avoid alcohol, aspirin, and ibuprofen compounds (NSAIDs) as well as any other OTC preparations.

OUTCOMES/EVALUATE

- Prevention/control of bleeding
- Prophylaxis of hypoprothrombinemia during prolonged TPN
- Prevention of hemorrhagic disease in the newborn

Pilocarpine hydrochloride

(pie-low-**CAR**-peen)

PREGNANCY CATEGORY: C

Rx: Adsorbocarpine, Akarpine, Isopto Carpine, Pilocar, Piloptic-½ -1, -2, -3, -4, and -6, Pilopto-Carpine, Pilostat, Salagen
✱Rx: Diocarpine, Miocarpine, Pilopine HS, Scheinpharm Pilocarpine

Pilocarpine ocular therapeutic system

(pie-low-**CAR**-peen)

PREGNANCY CATEGORY: C
Rx: Ocusert Pilo-20 and -40
CLASSIFICATION(S):
Cholinergic agonist

ACTION/KINETICS

Onset: *Gel/Solution:* 10–30 min; **duration:** 4–8 hr. *Nitrate:* The ocular therapeutic system is placed in the cul-de-sac of the eye for release of pilocarpine. The drug is released from the ocular therapeutic system three times faster during the first few hours and then decreases (within 6 hr) to a rate of 20 or 40 mcg/hr for 1 week. *Ocular system:* **Onset:** 60 min. **peak effect:** 1.5–2 hr; **duration:** 7 days. When used to treat dry mouth due to radiotherapy in head and neck cancer clients, pilocarpine stimulates residual functioning salivary gland tissue to increase saliva production.

USES

HCl: (1) Chronic simple glaucoma (especially open-angle). Chronic angle-closure glaucoma, including after iridectomy. Acute angle-closure glaucoma (alone or with other miotics, epinephrine, beta-adrenergic blocking agents, carbonic anhydrase inhibitors, or hyperosmotic agents). (2) To reverse mydriasis (i.e., after cycloplegic and mydriatic drugs). (3) Pre- and postoperative intraocular tension. (4) Salagen (Pilocarpine HCl) has been approved for treatment of radiation-induced dry mouth in head and neck cancer clients, as well as in Sjogren's syndrome. **Ocular Therapeutic System:** Glaucoma alone or with other ophthalmic medications. *Investigational:* Hydrochloride used to treat xerostomia in clients with malfunctioning salivary glands.

CONTRAINDICATIONS

Inflammatory eye disease, acute-angle glaucoma, history of retinal detachment, ocular hypotension, asthma, epilepsy, parkinsonism, gangrene, diabetes, CV disease, GI or GU tract obstruction, spastic GI conditions, vasomotor instability, severe bradycardia or hypotension, recent MI, lactation, in those receiving choline esters or depolarizing neuromuscular blocking drugs.

SPECIAL CONCERNS

Use with caution in those with narrow angles (angle closure may result), in those with known or suspected cholelithiasis or biliary tract disease, and in clients with controlled asthma, chronic bronchitis, or COPD. Safety and efficacy have not been established in children.

SIDE EFFECTS

After ophthalmic use: Painful contraction of ciliary muscle, pain in eye, blurred vision, spasms of accommodation, darkened vision, failure to accommodate to darkness, twitching, headaches, painful brow.

Use of pilocarpine ocular system: Conjunctival irritation, including mild erythema with or without a slight increase in mucous secretion upon initial use.

Oral use (tablets). **Dermatologic:** Sweating, flushing, rash, pruritus. **GI:** N&V, dyspepsia, diarrhea, abdominal pain, taste perversion, anorexia, increased appetite, esophagitis, tongue disorder. **CV:** Hypertension, tachycardia, bradycardia, ECG abnormality, palpitations, syncope. **CNS:** Dizziness, asthenia, headache, tremor, anxiety, confusion, depression, abnormal dreams, hyperkinesia, hypesthesia, nervousness, paresthesias, speech disorder, twitching. **Respiratory:** Sinusitis, rhinitis, pharyngitis, epistaxis, increased sputum, stridor, yawning. **Ophthalmic:** Lacrimation, amblyopia, conjunctivitis, abnormal vision, eye pain, glaucoma. **GU:** Urinary frequency, dysuria, metrorrhagia, urinary impairment. **Body as a whole:** Chills, edema, body odor, hypo-

P

thermia, mucous membrane abnormality. **Miscellaneous:** Dysphagia, voice alteration, myalgias, seborrhea.

OD OVERDOSE MANAGEMENT

Treatment: Titrate with atropine (0.5–1 mg SC or IM) and supportive measures to maintain circulation and respiration. If there is severe cardiovascular depression or bronchoconstriction, epinephrine (0.3–1 mg SC or IV) may be used.

HOW SUPPLIED

Pilocarpine hydrochloride: *Ophthalmic gel:* 4%; *Ophthalmic Solution:* 0.25%, 0.5%, 1%, 2%, 3%, 4%, 5%, 6%, 8%, 10%; *Tablet:* 5 mg. **Pilocarpine ocular therapeutic system:** *Device:* 20 mcg/hr, 40 mcg/hr

DOSAGE

PILOCARPINE HYDROCHLORIDE

- **OPHTHALMIC GEL, 4%**

Glaucoma.

Adults and adolescents: ½-in. ribbon in the lower conjunctival sac of the affected eye(s) once daily at bedtime.

- **OPHTHALMIC SOLUTION, ¼%, ½%, 1%, 2%, 3%, 4%, 5%, 6%, 8%**

Doses listed are all for adults and adolescents.

Chronic glaucoma.

1 gtt of a 0.5%–4% solution q.i.d.

Acute angle-closure glaucoma.

1 gtt of a 1% or 2% solution q 5–10 min for three to six doses; then, 1 gtt q 1–3 hr until pressure is decreased.

Miotic, to counteract sympathomimetics.

1 gtt of a 1% solution.

Miosis, prior to surgery.

1 gtt of a 2% solution q 4–6 hr for one or two doses before surgery.

Miosis before iridectomy.

1 gtt of a 2% solution for four doses immediately before surgery.

- **TABLET**

5 mg t.i.d. Up to 10 mg t.i.d. for those not responding adequately and those who tolerate lower doses.

PILOCARPINE OCULAR SYSTEM

Insert and remove as directed on package insert or by physician. Ocusert Pilo-20 is approximately equal to the 0.5% or 1% drops, while Ocusert Pilo-40 is approximately equal to the 2% or 3% solution.

NURSING CONSIDERATIONS

ADMINISTRATION/STORAGE

1. Concentrations greater than 4% of pilocarpine HCl may be more effective in clients with dark pigmented eyes; however, the incidence of side effects increases.
2. Myopia may be observed during the first several hours of therapy with the ocular therapeutic system. Thus, insert the system at bedtime so by morning the myopia is stable.
3. For acute, narrow-angle glaucoma, give pilocarpine in the unaffected eye to prevent angle-closure glaucoma.
4. Store the solution, protected from light, at 8–30°C (46–86°F). Refrigerate the gel at 2–8°C (36–46°F) until dispensed. Do not freeze gel; discard any unused portion after 8 weeks. Refrigerate the ocular therapeutic system at 2–8°C (36–46° F).

ASSESSMENT

Clients with acute infectious conjunctivitis or keratitis should be carefully evaluated before use of the pilocarpine ocular system.

CLIENT/FAMILY TEACHING

1. Review how to insert and how to check the conjunctival sac for presence of the ocular system. Follow these general guidelines for insertion:
   - Wash hands.
   - Do not permit drug to touch any surface.
   - Rinse insert with cool water.
   - Pull down lower eyelid.
   - Place according to manufacturer's directions.
   - System may be moved under closed eyelids to upper eyelid for sleep. Use caution and report any pain as corneal abrasion or irritation may be present.
   - Insert at bedtime to diminish side effects; check for presence of ocular system at bedtime and also upon awakening each day. If retention is a problem, the system can be placed in the superior cul-de-sac. The unit can be moved from the lower to upper conjunctival cul-de-sac by gentle digital massage through the eyelid. For best retention, move the unit to the

P

upper conjunctival cul-de-sac before sleep.
• Report if eye irritation, redness, or mucus production persist with the ocular system.
2. If other glaucoma medication (i.e., drops) is used with the gel at bedtime, instill the drops at least 5 min before the gel.
3. Report for periodic eye pressure readings to evaluate drug effectiveness.
4. Use only as directed. Refrigerate gel and ocular system.

OUTCOMES/EVALUATE

• ↓ IOP; pupillary constriction
• ↑ Saliva production; relief of radiation-induced or Sjogren's syndrome dry mouth

Pimecrolimus

(**peem**-eh-**KROH**-lih-mus)

PREGNANCY CATEGORY: C
CLASSIFICATION(S):
Immunomodulator
Rx: Elidel

ACTION/KINETICS

Mechanism not known for beneficial effect in atopic dermatitis. Binds with high affinity to macrophilin-12 and inhibits calcineurin (calcium-dependent phosphatase). As a result, it inhibits T-cell activation by blocking the transcription of early cytokines. It specifically inhibits interleukin-2, interferon gamma (Th1-type), interleukin-4, and interleukin-10 (Th2-type) cytokine synthesis in human T-cells. It also prevents release of inflammatory cytokines and mediators from mast cells. Poorly absorbed systemically.

USES

Short-term and intermittent long-term therapy to treat mild to moderate atopic dermatitis in nonimmunocompromised clients over 2 years of age.

CONTRAINDICATIONS

Pimecrolimus or any ingredients in the product. Use on areas of active cutaneous viral infections. Lactation.

SPECIAL CONCERNS

May be an increased risk of varicella zoster or herpes simplex virus infections or eczema herpeticum.

SIDE EFFECTS

Dermatologic: Skin papilloma, warts, application site burning/erythema/irritation/pruritus, skin infection, impetigo, folliculitis, molluscum contagiosum, herpes simplex dermatitis, urticaria, acne. **GI:** Gastroenteritis, abdominal pain (upper), sore throat, vomiting, diarrhea, nausea, toothache, constipation, loose stools. **Respiratory:** URTI, nasopharyngitis, sinusitis, pneumonia, pharyngitis (including streptococcal), bronchitis, cough, nasal congestion, rhinorrhea, aggravated asthma, sinus congestion, rhinitis, wheezing, asthma, epistaxis, dyspnea, tonsillitis. **Musculoskeletal:** Back pain, arthralgias. **Otic:** Ear infection, otitis media, earache. **Ophthalmic:** Eye infection, conjunctivitis. **Body as a whole:** Influenza, lymphadenopathy, bacterial/staphylococcal/viral infection, herpes simplex, chickenpox, pyrexia, hypersensitivity. **Miscellaneous:** Dysmenorrhea, laceration, headache.

DRUG INTERACTIONS

Coadminister known inhibitors (e.g., calcium channel blockers, cimetidine, erythromycin, fluconazole, itraconazole, ketoconazole) of the drug metabolizing CYP3A enzyme with caution in those with widespread or erythrodermic disease.

HOW SUPPLIED

Cream: 1%

DOSAGE

• **CREAM**

Atopic dermatitis.

Apply a thin layer to the affected skin b.i.d. and rub in gently and completely.

NURSING CONSIDERATIONS

ADMINISTRATION/STORAGE

1. Use b.i.d. for as long as signs and symptoms persist. If symptoms persist for over 6 weeks, reevaluate client.
2. Store between 15–30°C (59–86°F). Do not freeze.

P

ASSESSMENT

1. Describe skin condition and area being treated, photos may be useful. List other agents trialed and outcome.
2. Note drugs currently prescribed to ensure none compete with CYP3A enzyme in those with large areas for treatment.
3. Ensure no diseases/conditions that may predispose clients to immunocompromised states.

CLIENT/FAMILY TEACHING

1. Apply as directed twice daily to affected areas. May be used on all skin surfaces, including the head, neck,and intertriginous areas.
2. For external use only. Wash hands after application unless hands are being treated.
3. Do not apply any occlusive covering or dressings. May experience mild to moderate feeling or warmth or burning sensation upon application. Report if severe or persists > 1 week.
4. Minimize or avoid exposure to natural or artificial sunlight during therapy.
5. Once lesions cleared may stop therapy. Report if no improvement after 6 weeks of therapy or if condition worsens. May resume therapy at the first evidence of recurrence.

OUTCOMES/EVALUATE

Healing/clearing of atopic dermatitis lesions

P

Pindolol

(**PIN**-doh-lohl)

PREGNANCY CATEGORY: B
CLASSIFICATION(S):
Beta-adrenergic blocking agent
Rx: Visken
✱Rx: Apo-Pindol, Gen-Pindolol, Novo–Pindol, Nu-Pindol, PMS-Pindolol

SEE ALSO *BETA-ADRENERGIC BLOCKING AGENTS.*

ACTION/KINETICS
Manifests both beta-1 and beta-2 adrenergic blocking activity. Also has significant intrinsic sympathomimetic effects and minimal membrane-stabilizing activity. Moderate lipid solubility. **$t^1/_2$:** 3–4 hr; however, geriatric clients have a variable half-life ranging from 7 to 15 hr, even with normal renal function. Metabolized by the liver, and the metabolites and unchanged (35%–40%) drug are excreted through the kidneys.

USES
Alone or in combination with other antihypertensive agents (e.g., thiazide diuretics) to treat hypertension. *Investigational:* Ventricular arrhythmias and tachycardias, antipsychotic-induced akathisia, situational anxiety.

CONTRAINDICATIONS
Bronchial asthma or bronchospasm, including severe COPD.

SPECIAL CONCERNS
Dosage has not been established in children.

LABORATORY TEST CONSIDERATIONS
↑ AST and ALT. Rarely, ↑ LDH, uric acid, alkaline phosphatase.

HOW SUPPLIED
Tablet: 5 mg, 10 mg

DOSAGE

- **TABLETS**

Hypertension.
Initial: 5 mg b.i.d. (alone or with other antihypertensive drugs). If no response in 3–4 weeks, increase by 10 mg/day q 3–4 weeks to a maximum of 60 mg/day.

Antipsychotic-induced akathisia.
5 mg/day.

NURSING CONSIDERATIONS

SEE ALSO *NURSING CONSIDERATIONS FOR BETA-ADRENERGIC BLOCKING AGENTS* AND *ANTIHYPERTENSIVE AGENTS.*

ASSESSMENT

1. Document indications for therapy, onset and characteristics of symptoms; list other agents trialed.
2. Assess diet, salt consumption, weight, exercise regimens, and lifestyle.
3. Document VS and cardiopulmonary assessments.

CLIENT/FAMILY TEACHING

1. Take as directed, do not stop abruptly. May take at bedtime to decrease orthostatic hypotension.

2. Avoid activities that require mental alertness until drug effects realized.
3. Report any difficulty breathing, fever, sore throat, rash, slow pulse, confusion, or depression.
4. Avoid alcohol and OTC cold preparations.

OUTCOMES/EVALUATE

↓ BP; ↓ anxiety

Pioglitazone hydrochloride

(**pie**-oh-**GLIT**-ah-zohn)

PREGNANCY CATEGORY: C
CLASSIFICATION(S):
Antidiabetic, oral; thiazolidinedione
Rx: Actos

SEE ALSO *ORAL HYPOGLYCEMIC AGENTS.*

ACTION/KINETICS

Depends on the presence of insulin to act. Decreases insulin resistance in the periphery and liver resulting in increased insulin-dependent glucose disposal and decreased hepatic glucose output. It is not an insulin secretagogue. Is an agonist for peroxisome proliferator-activated receptor (PPAR) gamma, which is found in adipose tissue, skeletal muscle, and liver. Activation of these receptors modulates the transcription of a number of insulin responsive genes that control glucose and lipid metabolism. Reduces fasting plasma glucose 39–65 mg/dL from placebo and HbA1c 1–1.6% from placebo. After PO, steady state serum levels are reached within 7 days. **Peak levels:** 2 hr; food slightly delays the time to peak serum levels to 3–4 hr, but does not change the extent of absorption. Extensively protein-bound (over 99%). Metabolized to both active and inactive metabolites. Unchanged drug and metabolites are excreted in the feces. **t½:** 3–7 hr (pioglitazone); 16–24 hr (total pioglitazone).

USES

Adjunct to diet and exercise in type 2 diabetes. Used either as monotherapy or in combination with a sulfonylurea, metformin, or insulin when diet and exercise plus the single drug does not adequately control blood glucose.

CONTRAINDICATIONS

In type I diabetes, diabetic ketoacidosis, active liver disease, with ALT levels that exceed 2.5 times ULN, in clients with NYHA Class II or IV cardiac status, lactation, or in pediatric clients less than 18 years of age.

SPECIAL CONCERNS

Treatment may result in resumption of ovulation in premenopausal anovulatory clients with insulin resistance. Use with caution in clients with edema. Safety and efficacy have not been determined in children.

SIDE EFFECTS

Metabolic: Hypoglycemia, aggravation of diabetes mellitus. **Respiratory:** URTI, sinusitis, pharyngitis. **Miscellaneous:** Headache, myalgia, tooth disorder, anemia, edema.

LABORATORY TEST CONSIDERATIONS

↑ ALT, creatine phosphokinase (sporadic and transient); ↓ H&H.

DRUG INTERACTIONS

Ketoconazole / Significant inhibition of pioglitazone metabolism
Oral contraceptives (containing ethinyl estradiol/norethindrone / ↓ Plasma levels of both hormones; possible loss of contraception

HOW SUPPLIED

Tablets: 15 mg, 30 mg, 45 mg

DOSAGE

• **TABLETS**

Type II diabetes as monotherapy.

Adults: 15 mg or 30 mg once daily in clients not adequately controlled with diet and exercise. Initial dose can be increased up to 45 mg once daily for those who respond inadequately.

Type II diabetes as combination therapy.

If combined with a sulfonylurea, initiate pioglitazone at 15 or 30 mg once daily. The current sulfonylurea dose can be continued unless hypoglycemia occurs; then, reduce the sulfonylurea dose. If combined with metformin, initiate pioglitazone at 15 or 30 mg once daily. The current metformin dose can be continued; it is unlikely the metformin dose will have to be adjusted due to hypoglycemia. If combined with insulin, initiate pioglitazone at 15 or 30 mg once daily. The current insulin dose can be continued unless hypoglycemia occurs or plasma glucose levels decrease to less than 100 mg/dL; then, decrease the insulin dose by 10% to 25%. Individualize further dosage adjustments based on glucose-lowering response.

Daily dose should not exceed 45 mg.

NURSING CONSIDERATIONS

SEE ALSO *NURSING CONSIDERATIONS* FOR *ANTI-DIABETIC AGENTS: HYPOGLYCEMIC AGENTS.*

ASSESSMENT

1. Note indications for therapy, onset and characteristics of disease, other agents trialed and outcome.
2. List drugs prescribed to ensure none interact.
3. Obtain CBC, HbA1c, renal and LFTs. Ensure clients undergo periodic monitoring of liver enzymes. Evaluate ALT prior to initiation of therapy, every two months for the first year of therapy, and periodically thereafter. Obtain LFTs if symptoms suggest hepatic dysfunction. Discontinue if jaundice is seen.

CLIENT/FAMILY TEACHING

1. Take once daily without regard to meals.
2. May cause edema, resumption of ovulation, and hypoglycemia.
3. Report if dark urine, abdominal pain, fatigue or unexplained N&V occur.
4. Practice reliable contraception if pregnancy is not desired.
5. Follow dietary guidelines, perform regular exercise and other life style changes consistent with controlling diabetes.
6. Monitor FS at different times during the day and maintain log for provider review.

OUTCOMES/EVALUATE

Control of NIDDM by ↓ insulin resistance; normalization of glucose and HbA1c < 7

Pipecuronium bromide

(pih-peh-kyour-**OHN**-ee-um)

PREGNANCY CATEGORY: C
CLASSIFICATION(S):
Neuromuscular blocking drug
Rx: Arduan

SEE ALSO *NEUROMUSCULAR BLOCKING AGENTS.*

ACTION/KINETICS

Competes for cholinergic receptors at the motor end plate and is antagonized by acetylcholinesterase inhibitors. Has no effect on consciousness, pain threshold, or cerebration; thus, use must be accompanied by adequate anesthesia. **Maximum time for blockade:** 5 min following single doses of 70–85 mcg/kg. **Time to recovery to 25% of control:** 30–175 min under balanced anesthesia following single doses of 70 mcg/kg. **t½, distribution:** 6.22 min (4.33 min in renal transplant clients); **t½, elimination:** 1.7 hr (4 hr in renal transplant clients). Increased plasma levels are seen in clients with impaired renal function. Metabolized in the liver; metabolites and unchanged drug eliminated in the urine.

USES

Adjunct to general anesthesia to provide relaxation of skeletal muscle during surgery. Skeletal muscle relaxation for ET intubation. Recommended for procedures lasting 90 or more minutes.

CONTRAINDICATIONS

Due to the long duration of action, do not use in myasthenia gravis or Eaton-Lambert syndrome, as low doses can lead to a profound effect. Clients undergoing cesarean section. Use of pipecuronium before succinylcholine in order to reduce side effects of succinylcholine. In those requiring prolonged mechanical ventilation in the ICU or prior to or following other nondepolarizing neuromuscular blocking agents.

SPECIAL CONCERNS

Although the drug is used in infants and children, no information is available on maintenance dosing. Also, children 1–14 years of age under balanced or halothane anesthesia may be less sensitive to the drug than adults. Use with caution in clients with impaired renal function. The drug should be administered only if there are adequate facilities for intubation, artificial respiration, oxygen therapy, and administration of an antagonist. Obesity may prolong the duration of action. Conditions resulting in an increased volume of distribution (e.g., old age, edematous states, slower circulation time in CV disease) may cause a delay in the time of onset.

SIDE EFFECTS

Neuromuscular: ***Prolongation of blockade including skeletal muscle paralysis resulting in respiratory insufficiency or apnea.*** Muscle atrophy, difficult intubation. **CV:** Hypotension, bradycardia, hypertension, CVA, thrombosis, myocardial ischemia, atrial fibrillation, ventricular extrasystole. **CNS:** Hypesthesia, CNS depression. **Respiratory:** Dyspnea, respiratory depression, laryngismus, atelectasis. **Metabolic:** Hypoglycemia, hyperkalemia, increased creatinine. **Miscellaneous:** Rash, urticaria, anuria.

OD OVERDOSE MANAGEMENT

Symptoms: ***Skeletal muscle paralysis including depressed respiration.*** *Treatment:* Artificial respiration until effects of drug have worn off. Antagonize neuromuscular blockade by administration of neostigmine, 0.04 mg/kg. Do not use edrophonium.

DRUG INTERACTIONS

Aminoglycosides / ↑ Intensity and duration of neuromuscular blockade
Bacitracin / ↑ Intensity and duration of neuromuscular blockade
Colistin/Sodium colistimethate / ↑ Intensity and duration of neuromuscular blockade
Enflurane / ↑ Duration of action of pipecuronium
Halothane / ↑ Duration of action of pipecuronium
Isoflurane / ↑ Duration of action of pipecuronium
Magnesium salts / ↑ Intensity of neuromuscular blockade when used for toxemia of pregnancy
Polymyxin B / ↑ Intensity and duration of neuromuscular blockade
Quinidine / ↑ Risk of recurrent paralysis
Tetracyclines / ↑ Intensity and duration of neuromuscular blockade

HOW SUPPLIED

Powder for injection, lyophilized: 10 mg

DOSAGE

- **IV ONLY**

Adjunct to general anesthesia.

Adults: Initial dose may be based on the C_{CR} and the ideal body weight (see information provided by manufacturer). Dose is individualized. The dose range is 50–100 mcg/kg.

ET intubation using balanced anesthesia.

70–85 mcg/kg with halothane, isoflurane, or enflurane in clients with normal renal function who are not obese; duration of muscle relaxation is 1–2 hr using this dosage range.

Use following recovery from succinylcholine.

50 mcg/kg in clients with normal renal function who are not obese; duration of muscle relaxation using this dose is 45 min. *Maintenance.* **Adults:** 10–15 mcg/kg given at 25% recovery of control T_1 will provide muscle relaxation for an average of 50 min using balanced anesthesia; lower doses should be used in clients receiving inhalation anesthetics. **Pediatric:** The duration of action in infants following a dose of 40 mcg/kg ranged from 10 to 44 min while the duration in children following a dose of 57 mcg/kg ranged from 18 to 52 min.

P

NURSING CONSIDERATIONS

SEE ALSO *NURSING CONSIDERATIONS* FOR *NEUROMUSCULAR BLOCKING AGENTS.*

ADMINISTRATION/STORAGE

IV 1. Administer only under the supervision of individuals experienced with the use of neuromuscular blocking agents.
2. Reconstitute using 0.9% NaCl, D5/NSS, D5W, RL, sterile water, and bacteriostatic water for injection.
3. If used in newborns, do not reconstitute with bacteriostatic water for injection (contains benzyl alcohol).
4. When reconstituted with bacteriostatic water for injection, store the solution at room temperature or in the refrigerator; use within 5 days.
5. When reconstituted with sterile water or other IV solutions, refrigerate and use within 24 hr.
6. Do not dilute with or administer from large volumes of IV solutions.
7. Store at 2–30°C (35–86°F) and protect from light.

ASSESSMENT

1. Document indications for therapy and anticipated duration of use.
2. Determine height and weight; note if obese; correlate drug dose for *ideal* body weight.
3. Assess for myasthenia gravis or Eaton-Lambert syndrome.
4. List drugs prescribed because many interact unfavorably.
5. Determine diarrhea presence and duration; may alter desired neuromuscular blockade.
6. Monitor ECG, VS, electrolytes, and renal function studies.

INTERVENTIONS

1. The twitch response should be used to evaluate neuromuscular blockade and recovery and to minimize overdosage potential. Use a peripheral nerve stimulator to assess the height of the twitch wave.
2. Allow more time for pipecuronium to achieve maximum effect in older clients with slowed circulation, CV diseases, and/or edematous states. *Do not* increase drug dose because this will produce a longer duration of action.
3. Monitor VS and observe postrecovery for adequate clinical evidence of antagonism:
- 5-sec head lift
- Adequate pronation
- Effective airway and ventilatory patterns

4. Monitor ECG. Drug can cause vagal stimulation resulting in bradycardia, hypotension, and cardiac arrhythmias.
5. Muscle fasciculations may cause client to be sore or injured after recovery. Reassure that the soreness is likely caused by the unsynchronized contractions of adjacent muscle fibers just before the onset of paralysis.
6. Document duration of therapy. Use drug only on a short-term basis and in a continuously monitored environment.
7. Remember client is fully conscious and aware of surroundings and conversations.
8. Drug does not affect pain or anxiety; administer analgesics and antianxiety agents as needed.
9. Prolonged use, as in an ICU setting, may lead to skeletal muscle weakness and symptoms consistent with muscle disuse atrophy. This may complicate ventilator weaning and some clients may require extensive physical therapy.

OUTCOMES/EVALUATE

- Skeletal muscle relaxation/paralysis
- Suppression of twitch response

Piperacillin sodium

(pie-**PER**-ah-sill-in)

PREGNANCY CATEGORY: B
CLASSIFICATION(S):
Antibiotic, penicillin
Rx: Pipracil

SEE ALSO *PENICILLINS.*

ACTION/KINETICS

Semisynthetic, broad-spectrum penicillin for parenteral use. It is not penicillinase resistant. Penetrates CSF in the presence of inflamed meninges. **Peak serum level:** 244 mcg/mL. **t½:** 36–72 min. Excreted unchanged in urine and bile.

USES

(1) Intra-abdominal infections (including hepatobiliary and surgical infections) due to *Escherichia coli, Pseudomonas aeruginosa, Clostridium* sp., enterococci, anaerobic cocci, *Bacteroides* sp., including *B. fragilis*. (2) URIs due to *E. coli, P. aeruginosa, Proteus* sp. (including *P. mirabilis* and enterococci), *Klebsiella* sp. (3) Urinary tract infections due to *E. coli, Klebsiella* species, *P. aeruginosa, Proteus* species, including *P. mirabilis* and enterococci. (4) Gynecologic infections (including endometritis, PID, pelvic cellulitis) due to *Bacteroides* sp. (including *B. fragilis*), anaerobic cocci, enterococci (*Streptococcus faecalis*), *Neisseria gonorrhoeae.* (5) Septicemia (including bacteremia) due to *E. coli, P. mirabilis, S. pneumoniae, P. aeruginosa, Klebsiella* sp., *Enterobacter* sp., *Serratia* sp., *Bacteroides* sp., anaerobic cocci. (6) Lower respiratory tract infections due to *E. coli, P. aeruginosa, Haemophilus influenzae, Klebsiella* sp., *Enterobacter* sp., *Serratia* sp., *Bacteroides* sp., anaerobic cocci. (7) Skin and skin structure infections due to *E. coli, Klebsiella* sp., *Serratia* sp., *Acinetobacter* sp., *Enterobacter* sp., *P. aeruginosa, P. mirabilis,* indole-positive *Proteus* sp., *Bacteroides* sp. (including *B. fragilis*), anaerobic cocci, enterococci. (8) Bone and joint infections due to *P. aeruginosa, Bacteroides* sp., enterococci, anaerobic cocci. (9) Uncomplicated gonococcal urethritis. (10) Infections due to streptococcus species, including Group A β–hemolytic streptococcus and *S. pneumoniae.* (11) Prophylaxis in surgery, including GI and biliary procedures, vaginal and abdominal hysterectomy, and cesarean section.

SPECIAL CONCERNS

Possible antibiotic resistance when used to treat *Pseudomonas aeruginosa* infections.

ADDITIONAL SIDE EFFECTS

Rarely, prolonged muscle relaxation.

LABORATORY TEST CONSIDERATIONS

Positive Coombs' test; ↑ (especially in infants) AST, ALT, LDH, bilirubin.

ADDITIONAL DRUG INTERACTIONS

Piperacillin may prolong the neuromuscular blockade of vecuronium.

HOW SUPPLIED

Powder for injection: 2g, 3g, 4g, 40g

DOSAGE

- **IM, IV**

Serious infections, including septicemia, nosocomial pneumonia, intra-abdominal infections, aerobic and anaerobic gyn infections, and skin and soft tissue infections.

Adults, IV: 3–4 g q 4–6 hr (12–18 g/day, not to exceed 24 g/day) as a 20- to 30-min infusion. Average duration is 7 to 10 days (3 to 10 days for gynecologic infections and at least 10 days for group A β–hemolytic streptococcal infections). If C_{CR} is 20–40 mL/min, give 12 g/day (4 g q 8 hr); if C_{CR} is less than 20 mL/min, give 8 g/day (4 g q 12 hr). Dosage has not been determined for children less than 12 years of age. However, use the following guidelines: **Neonates, less than 36 weeks old:** 75 mg/kg IV q 12 hr during the first week of life; **then,** q 8 hr during the second week. **Full-term:** 75 mg/kg IV q 8 hr during the first week of life; **then,** q 6 hr thereafter. **Children, other conditions:** 200–300 mg/kg/day, up to a maximum of 24 g/day divided q 4 to 6 hr.

Complicated UTIs.

Adults, IV: 8–16 g/day (125–200 mg/kg/day) in divided doses q 6–8 hr. If C_{CR} is 20–40 mL/min, give 9 g/day (3 g q 8 hr); if C_{CR} is less than 20 mL/min, give 6 g/day (3 g q 12 hr).

Uncomplicated UTIs and most community-acquired pneumonias.

Adults, IM, IV: 6–8 g/day (100–125 mg/kg/day) in divided doses q 6–12 hr. If C_{CR} is less than 20 mL/min, give 6 g/day (3 g q 12 hr).

Uncomplicated gonorrhea infections.

2 g **IM** with 1 g probenecid **PO** 30 min before injection (both given as single dose).

P

Prophylaxis in surgery.
Intra-abdominal surgery: 2 g IV just prior to anesthesia, 2 g during surgery, and 2 g q 6 hr post surgery for no more than 24 hr. *Vaginal hysterectomy:* 2 g IV just prior to anesthesia, 2 g 6 hr after initial dose, and 2 g 12 hr after first dose. *Cesarean section:* 2 g IV after cord is clamped, 2 g 4 hr after initial dose, and 2 g 8 hr after first dose. *Abdominal hysterectomy:* 2 g IV just prior to anesthesia, 2 g on return to recovery room, and 2 g after 6 hr.

For cystic fibrosis.
350–500 mg/kg/day divided q 4–6 hr.

NURSING CONSIDERATIONS

SEE ALSO *NURSING CONSIDERATIONS* FOR *PENICILLINS.*

ADMINISTRATION/STORAGE

1. For IM administration, use upper, outer quadrant of gluteus or well-developed deltoid muscle. Do not use lower or mid-third of upper arm.
2. Do not administer more than 2 g IM at any one site.

IV 3. For IV administration reconstitute each gram with at least 5 mL diluent, such as sterile or bacteriostatic water for injection, NaCl or bacteriostatic NaCl for injection, D5W, D5/ 0.9% NaCl, and lidocaine HCl 0.5% to 1% without epinephrine (only for IM use). Shake until dissolved.

P

4. Inject IV slowly over a period of 3–5 min to avoid vein irritation.
5. Administer over 20–30 min by intermittent IV infusion in at least 50 mL of dextrose or saline solutions.
6. After reconstitution, store at room temperature for 24 hr, refrigerate for 1 week, or freeze for 1 month.

ASSESSMENT

1. Document indications for therapy, onset and characteristics of symptoms.
2. Monitor cultures, electrolytes, hematologic, renal and LFTs.
3. Assess for diarrhea or other evidence of superinfection.

OUTCOMES/EVALUATE

- Infection prophylaxis
- Symptomatic improvement
- Negative C&S reports

Piperacillin sodium and Tazobactam sodium

(pie-**PER**-ah-**sill**-in, tay-zoh-**BAC**-tam)

PREGNANCY CATEGORY: B
CLASSIFICATION(S):
Antibiotic, penicillin
Rx: Zosyn
✱**Rx:** Tazocin

SEE ALSO *PENICILLINS* AND *PIPERACILLIN SODIUM.*

ACTION/KINETICS

A combination of piperacillin sodium and tazobactam sodium, a beta-lactamase inhibitor. Tazobactam inhibits beta-lactamases, thus ensuring activity of piperacillin against beta-lactamase-producing microorganisms. Thus, tazobactam broadens the antibiotic spectrum of piperacillin to those bacteria normally resistant to it. **Peak plasma levels:** Attained immediately after completion of an IV infusion. **t½, piperacillin and tazobactam:** 0.7–1.2 hr. Both drugs are eliminated through the kidney with piperacillin and tazobactam both excreted unchanged and as inactive metabolites. The t½ of both drugs is increased in clients with renal impairment and in hepatic cirrhosis (dose adjustment not required).

USES

(1) Appendicitis complicated by rupture or abscess and peritonitis caused by piperacillin-resistant, beta-lactamase-producing strains of *Escherichia coli, Bacteroides fragilis, B. ovatus, B. thetaiotaomicron,* or *B. vulgatus.* (2) Uncomplicated and complicated skin and skin structure infections (including cellulitis, cutaneous abscesses, and ischemic/diabetic foot infections) caused by piperacillin-resistant, beta-lactamase-producing strains of *Staphylococcus aureus.* (3) Postpartum endometritis or PID caused by piperacillin-resistant, beta-lactamase-producing strains of *E. coli.* (4) Community-acquired pneumonia of moderate severity caused by piperacillin-

resistant, beta-lactamase-producing strains of *Haemophilus influenzae.* (5) Moderate to severe nosocomial pneumonia caused by piperacillin-resistant, beta-lactamase-producing strains of *S. aureus.* (6) Infections caused by piperacillin-susceptible organisms for which piperacillin is effective may also be treated with this combination. The treatment of mixed infections caused by piperacillin-susceptible organisms and piperacillin-resistant, beta-lactamase-producing organisms susceptible to this combination does not require addition of another antibiotic.

CONTRAINDICATIONS

Hypersensitivity to penicillins, cephalosporins, or beta-lactamase inhibitors.

SPECIAL CONCERNS

Use with caution during lactation. Safety and efficacy have not been determined in children less than 12 years of age.

SIDE EFFECTS

See *Penicillins*. The highest incidence of side effects include the following:

GI: Diarrhea, constipation, N&V, dyspepsia, stool changes, abdominal pain. **CNS:** Headache, insomnia, fever, agitation, dizziness, anxiety. **Dermatologic:** Rash, including maculopapular, bullous, urticarial, and eczematoid; pruritus. **Hematologic:** Thrombocytopenia, eosinophilia, leukopenia, neutropenia. **Miscellaneous:** Pain, moniliasis, hypertension, chest pain, edema, rhinitis, dyspnea.

LABORATORY TEST CONSIDERATIONS

↓ H&H. Transient ↑ AST, ALT, alkaline phosphatase, and bilirubin. ↑ Serum creatinine, BUN. Prolonged PT and PTT. Positive direct Coombs' test. Proteinuria, hematuria, pyuria, abnormalities in electrolytes (↑ and ↓ sodium, potassium, calcium), hyperglycemia, ↓ total protein or albumin.

DRUG INTERACTIONS

Heparin / Possible ↑ heparin effect
Oral anticoagulants / Possible ↑ anticoagulant effect
Tobramycin / ↓ Area under the curve, renal clearance, and urinary recovery of tobramycin
Vecuronium / Prolongation of neuromuscular blockade

HOW SUPPLIED

Powder for Injection: 2 g-0.25 g, 3 g-0.375 g, 4 g-0.5 g, 36 g-4.5g (first number refers to amount of piperacillin sodium)

DOSAGE

• **IV INFUSION**

Susceptible infections.

Adults: 12 g/day piperacillin and 1.5 g/day tazobactam, given as 3.375 g (i.e., 3 g piperacillin and 0.375 g tazobactam) q 6 hr for 7–10 days. In clients with renal insufficiency, the IV dose is adjusted depending on the extent of impaired function. If C_{CR} is 20–40 mL/min, the dose is 8 g/day piperacillin and 1 g/day tazobactam in divided doses of 2.25 g q 6 hr. If the C_{CR} is less than 20 mL/min, the dose is 6 g/day piperacillin and 0.75 g/day tazobactam in divided doses of 2.25 g q 8 hr.

Moderate to severe nosocomial pneumonia due to piperacillin-resistant, beta-lactamase-producing S. aureus.

Adults: 3.375 g q 4 hr with an aminoglycoside for 7 to 14 days.

NURSING CONSIDERATIONS

SEE ALSO *NURSING CONSIDERATIONS FOR PIPERACILLIN SODIUM* AND *PENICILLINS*.

ADMINISTRATION/STORAGE

IV 1. For IV administration or by infusion, reconstitute the powder for injection with 5 mL suitable diluent/g piperacillin. IV diluents that can be used include 0.9% NaCl, sterile water for injection, dextran 6% in saline, D5W, KCl 40 mEq, bacteriostatic saline/parabens, bacteriostatic water/parabens, bacteriostatic saline/benzyl alcohol, bacteriostatic water/benzyl alcohol. *LR is not compatible.*

2. After the diluent is added, shake vial well until the powder is dissolved. May further dilute to the desired final volume with the diluent.

3. If intermittent IV infusion is used, the 5 mL diluent/g piperacillin is further diluted to a volume of at least 50

P

mL. Give the infusion over a period of 30 min. During the infusion, discontinue the primary infusion solution.
4. If concomitant therapy with aminoglycosides is indicated, give piperacillin/tazobactam and the aminoglycoside separately, as penicillin can inactivate the aminoglycoside if they are mixed.
5. Use single-dose vials immediately after reconstitution. Discard any unused drug after 24 hr if stored at room temperature or after 48 hr if stored in the refrigerator at 2–8°C (36–46°F).
6. After reconstitution, is stable in glass and plastic syringes, IV bags, and tubing. Is stable in IV bags for up to 24 hr at room temperature and up to 1 week in the refrigerator. Is stable in an ambulatory IV infusion pump for 24 hr at room temperature.

ASSESSMENT

1. Document indications for therapy, type, location, and characteristics of symptoms.
2. Determine any sensitivity to penicillins, cephalosporins, beta-lactamase inhibitors, or other allergens.
3. List drugs prescribed to ensure none interact unfavorably. Use of heparin and oral anticoagulants may require dosage adjustments.
4. Monitor electrolytes, urinalysis, hematologic and coagulation profile, liver and renal function studies. Reduce dosage with renal impairment.

OUTCOMES/EVALUATE

Resolution of infection

Pipobroman

(pip-oh-**BROH**-man)

PREGNANCY CATEGORY: D
CLASSIFICATION(S):
Antineoplastic, alkylating

SEE ALSO *ANTINEOPLASTIC AGENTS* AND *ALKYLATING AGENTS*.

ACTION/KINETICS

The mechanism, metabolism, and excretion are not known. Well absorbed from the GI tract.

USES

Polycythemia vera; chronic granulocytic leukemia in clients refractory to busulfan.

ADDITIONAL CONTRAINDICATIONS

Children under 15 years of age. Lactation. Bone marrow depression due to chemotherapy or X rays.

SPECIAL CONCERNS

Bone marrow depression may not occur for 4 or more weeks after therapy is started.

SIDE EFFECTS

Hematologic: Leukopenia, anemia, thrombocytopenia. **GI:** N&V, diarrhea, abdominal cramps. **Dermatologic:** Skin rashes.

OD OVERDOSE MANAGEMENT

Symptoms: Hematologic toxicity, especially with chronic overdosage. *Treatment:* Monitor hematologic status; if necessary, begin vigorous supportive treatment.

HOW SUPPLIED

Tablet: 25 mg

DOSAGE

• TABLETS

Polycythemia vera.

1 mg/kg/day. Up to 1.5–3 mg/kg/day may be required in clients refractory to other treatment; do not use such doses until a dose of 1 mg/kg/day has been given for at least 30 days with no improvement. When hematocrit has been reduced to 50%–55%, **maintenance dosage** of 100–200 mcg/kg is instituted.

Chronic granulocytic leukemia.

Initial: 1.5–2.5 mg/kg/day; **maintenance:** 7–175 mg/day, to be instituted when leukocyte count approaches 10,000/mm³.

NURSING CONSIDERATIONS

SEE ALSO *NURSING CONSIDERATIONS FOR ANTINEOPLASTIC AGENTS*.

ASSESSMENT

1. Document indications for therapy, other agents trialed and the outcome.
2. Obtain baseline hematologic profile and monitor closely for dosing parameters, leukopenia and thrombocytopenia. Bone marrow depression

may occur latently in therapy (after 4 weeks) (Nadir: 14–21 days).

CLIENT/FAMILY TEACHING

1. Discuss with provider and review literature for benefits/dangers of drug therapy.
2. Report evidence of infection such as fever, shaking chills, SOB, or painful urination; drug may decrease body's ability to fight infections.
3. Nausea, vomiting, or hair loss may occur with this drug.
4. Avoid aspirin-containing products and use alcohol in moderation, if at all.
5. Identify if candidate for sperm/egg harvesting; drug may cause permanent sterility in men and women.
6. Use reliable birth control; may cause birth defects.

OUTCOMES/EVALUATE

- ↓ Hematocrit (50%–55%) with polycythemia vera
- Hematologic recovery with leukemia
- Inhibition of malignant cell proliferation

Pirbuterol acetate

(peer-**BYOU**-ter-ohl)

PREGNANCY CATEGORY: C
CLASSIFICATION(S):
Sympathomimetic
Rx: Maxair Autohaler, Maxair Inhaler

SEE ALSO *SYMPATHOMIMETIC DRUGS*.

ACTION/KINETICS

Causes bronchodilation by stimulating beta-2-adrenergic receptors. Has minimal effects on beta-1 receptors. Also inhibits histamine release from mast cells, causes vasodilation, and increases ciliary motility. **Onset, inhalation:** Approximately 5 min. **Time to peak effect:** 30–60 min. **Duration:** 5 hr.

USES

Alone or with theophylline or steroids for prophylaxis and treatment of bronchospasm in asthma and other conditions with reversible bronchospasms (e.g., exercise-induced bronchospasm), including bronchitis, emphysema, bronchiectasis, obstructive pulmonary disease.

CONTRAINDICATIONS

Cardiac arrhythmias due to tachycardia; tachycardia caused by digitalis toxicity.

SPECIAL CONCERNS

Safety and efficacy have not been determined in children less than 12 years of age.

ADDITIONAL SIDE EFFECTS

CV: PVCs, hypotension. **CNS:** Hyperactivity, hyperkinesia, anxiety, confusion, depression, fatigue, syncope. **GI:** Diarrhea, dry mouth, anorexia, loss of appetite, bad taste or taste change, abdominal pain, abdominal cramps, stomatitis, glossitis. **Dermatologic:** Rash, edema, pruritus, alopecia. **Miscellaneous:** Flushing, numbness in extremities, weight gain.

HOW SUPPLIED

Autohaler or Inhaler: 0.2 mg/inh

DOSAGE

- **INHALATION AEROSOL**

Bronchodilation.

Adults and children over 12 years: 0.2–0.4 mg (1–2 inhalations) q 4–6 hr, not to exceed 12 inhalations (2.4 mg) daily.

NURSING CONSIDERATIONS

SEE ALSO *NURSING CONSIDERATIONS* FOR *SYMPATHOMIMETIC DRUGS*.

ASSESSMENT

Document indications for therapy, noting onset, duration, and characteristics of symptoms. Assess lungs and note ECG, CXR, and PFTs.

CLIENT/FAMILY TEACHING

1. Review methods, frequency, and indication for administration. Use a spacer (chamber) to enhance dispersion.
2. Report if condition or peak flows deteriorate or if inhaler is ineffective in relieving symptoms at prescribed dosage.

OUTCOMES/EVALUATE

Improved airway exchange; ↓ airway resistance

P

Piroxicam

(peer-**OX**-ih-kam)

PREGNANCY CATEGORY: C
CLASSIFICATION(S):
Nonsteroidal anti-inflammatory drug
Rx: Feldene
✱Rx: Alti-Piroxicam, Apo-Piroxicam, Gen-Piroxicam, Novo–Pirocam, Nu-Pirox

SEE ALSO *NONSTEROIDAL ANTI-INFLAMMATORY DRUGS.*

ACTION/KINETICS
May inhibit prostaglandin synthesis. Effect is comparable to that of aspirin, but with fewer GI side effects and less tinnitus. May be used with gold, corticosteroids, and antacids. **Peak plasma levels:** 1.5–2 mcg/mL after 3–5 hr (single dose). **Steady-state plasma levels** (after 7–12 days): 3–8 mcg/mL. **t½:** 50 hr. **Analgesia, onset:** 1 hr; **duration:** 2–3 days. **Anti-inflammatory activity, onset:** 7–12 days; **duration:** 2–3 weeks. 98.5% plasma-protein bound. Metabolites and unchanged drug excreted in urine and feces.

USES
Acute and chronic treatment of rheumatoid arthritis and osteoarthritis. *Investigational:* Juvenile rheumatoid arthritis, primary dysmenorrhea, sunburn.

CONTRAINDICATIONS
Safe use during pregnancy has not been determined. Use in children less than 14 years old. Lactation.

SPECIAL CONCERNS
Safety and efficacy have not been established in children. Increased plasma levels and elimination half-life may be observed in geriatric clients (especially women).

LABORATORY TEST CONSIDERATIONS
Reversible ↑ BUN.

HOW SUPPLIED
Capsule: 10 mg, 20 mg

DOSAGE

- **CAPSULES**

Rheumatoid arthritis, osteoarthritis.
Adults: 20 mg/day in one or more divided doses. Do not assess the effect of therapy for 2 weeks.

NURSING CONSIDERATIONS

SEE ALSO *NURSING CONSIDERATIONS* FOR *NONSTEROIDAL ANTI-INFLAMMATORY DRUGS.*

ADMINISTRATION/STORAGE
1. Steady-state plasma levels may not be reached for 2 weeks.
2. Clients over 70 years of age generally require one-half the usual adult dose of medication.

ASSESSMENT
1. Document indications for therapy, symptom characteristics, other agents prescribed, and the outcome. Rate pain level.
2. Assess involved joints and note ROM, erythema, swelling, pain, and warmth.

CLIENT/FAMILY TEACHING
1. Take as directed with food or milk to decrease GI upset. A stomach protectant (i.e., Cytotec) may be prescribed for those with a history of ulcer disease.
2. Take at anti-inflammatory dose to prevent further joint destruction during acute exacerbations.
3. Therapeutic effects of the medication cannot be evaluated fully for at least 2 weeks after treatment onset.
4. Aspirin decreases the effectiveness of piroxicam and may increase the occurrence of side effects. Avoid aspirin, ethanol, and OTC products.
5. Report any increased abdominal pain, abnormal bruising or bleeding, malaise, or changes in the color of the stool immediately.
6. Drug side effects may not be evident for 7–10 days.
7. Report for scheduled labs.

OUTCOMES/EVALUATE
↓ Joint pain and inflammation with improved mobility

Plicamycin (Mithramycin)

(plye-kah-**MY**-sin, mith-rah-**MY**-sin)

PREGNANCY CATEGORY: X

CLASSIFICATION(S):
Antineoplastic, antibiotic
Rx: Mithracin (Abbreviation: MTH)

SEE ALSO *ANTINEOPLASTIC AGENTS*.

ACTION/KINETICS
Antibiotic produced by *Streptomyces plicatus, S. argillaceus,* and *S. tanashiensis.* Complexes with DNA in the presence of magnesium (or other divalent cations), resulting in inhibition of cellular and enzymatic RNA synthesis. Decreases blood calcium by blocking the hypercalcemic effect of vitamin D, acting on osteoclasts, and preventing the action of parathyroid hormone. Cleared rapidly from the blood and is concentrated in the Kupffer cells of the liver, renal tubular cells, and along formed bone surfaces. Crosses the blood-brain barrier. Excreted through the urine.

USES
Malignant testicular tumors usually associated with metastases and when radiation or surgery is not an alternative. Hypercalcemia and hypercalciuria associated with advanced malignancy and not responsive to other therapy.

ADDITIONAL CONTRAINDICATIONS
Thrombocytopenia, thrombocytopathy, coagulation disorders, and increased tendency to hemorrhage. Impaired bone marrow function. Pregnancy. Lactation. Do not use for children under 15 years of age.

SPECIAL CONCERNS
Use with caution in impaired liver or kidney function.

ADDITIONAL SIDE EFFECTS
Severe thrombocytopenia, ***hemorrhagic tendencies.*** Facial flushing. Hepatic and renal toxicity. Extravasation may cause irritation or cellulitis. Electrolyte imbalance including hypocalcemia, hypokalemia, and hypophosphatemia.

LABORATORY TEST CONSIDERATIONS
↓ Serum calcium, potassium, and phosphorus. ↑ Serum BUN, creatinine, AST, ALT, alkaline phosphatase, bilirubin, isocitric dehydrogenase, ornithine carbamyltransferase, LDH. ↑ BSP retention.

OD OVERDOSE MANAGEMENT
Symptoms: Hematologic toxicity. *Treatment:* Monitor hematologic status, especially clotting factors. Also, closely monitor serum electrolytes and hepatic and renal functions.

HOW SUPPLIED
Powder for injection: 2.5 mg

DOSAGE

• IV ONLY

Testicular tumor.

Dose individualized. Usual: 25–30 (maximum) mcg/kg (given over a period of 4–6 hr) daily for 8–10 (maximum) days. Alternatively, 25–50 mcg/kg on alternate days for an average of eight doses.

Hypercalcemia, hypercalciuria.

Dose individualized: 15–25 mcg/kg (given over a period of 4–6 hr) daily for 3–4 days. Additional courses of therapy may be warranted at weekly intervals if initial course is unsuccessful.

NURSING CONSIDERATIONS

SEE ALSO *NURSING CONSIDERATIONS FOR ANTINEOPLASTIC AGENTS*.

ADMINISTRATION/STORAGE

IV 1. Store vials of medication in refrigerator at temperatures below 10°C (36°F). Discard unused portion of drug.
2. Reconstitute fresh for each day of therapy.
3. Drug is unstable in acid solution (pH 5 and below) and in reconstituted solutions (pH 7) and thus deteriorates rapidly.
4. Add 4.9 mL of sterile water to the 2.5-mg vial of plicamycin (or as recommended on the package insert) and shake to dissolve the drug. Final concentration 500 mcg/mL.
5. Add the calculated dosage of drug to the IV solution ordered (recommended 1 L of D5W) and adjust the rate of flow as ordered (recommended infusion time is 4–6 hr/L).
6. Closely check peripheral IV for extravasation. Stop IV if extravasation occurs; apply moderate heat to disperse drug and to reduce pain and tissue damage. Restart IV at another site.
7. Use only for hospitalized clients.

P

ASSESSMENT

1. Document indications for therapy and any other treatments prescribed.
2. Monitor CBC, calcium, potassium, phosphorus, hepatic and renal function studies; correct electrolytes and minerals throughout therapy.
3. Assess for evidence of abnormal bleeding such as epistaxis, hemoptysis, hematemesis, purpura, or ecchymoses. Drug may cause granyulocyte and platelet suppression. Nadir: 10–14 days; recovery: 21 days.

INTERVENTIONS

1. Administer antiemetic drugs before or during mithramycin therapy.
2. Monitor I&O. Correct dehydration; administer 2–3 L/day of fluids during therapy.
3. Rapid IV drug flow precipitates more severe GI side effects; administer slowly over 4–6 hr.
4. Calcium and phosphate may rebound after therapy; check levels.
5. Practice reliable birth control during and for several months following therapy.

OUTCOMES/EVALUATE

- ↓ Tumor size/spread
- ↓ Serum calcium levels

P

Polymyxin B sulfate, parenteral

(pol-ee-**MIX**-in)

PREGNANCY CATEGORY: C

Polymyxin B sulfate, sterile ophthalmic

(pol-ee-**MIX**-in)

PREGNANCY CATEGORY: C
CLASSIFICATION(S):
Antibiotic, polymyxin

SEE ALSO *ANTI-INFECTIVES.*

ACTION/KINETICS

Derived from the spore-forming soil bacterium *Bacillus polymyxa.* Bactericidal against most gram-negative organisms; rapidly inactivated by alkali, strong acid, and certain metal ions. Increases the permeability of the plasma cell membrane of the bacterium (i.e., similar to detergents), causing leakage of essential metabolites and ultimately inactivation. **Peak serum levels: IM,** 2 hr. **t½:** 4.3–6 hr. Longer in presence of renal impairment. Sixty percent of drug excreted in urine. Virtually unabsorbed from the GI tract except in newborn infants. Remains in plasma after parenteral administration.

USES

Systemic: (1) Acute infections of the urinary tract and meninges, septicemia caused by *Pseudomonas aeruginosa.* (2) Meningeal infections caused by *Haemophilus influenzae,* UTIs caused by *Escherichia coli,* bacteremia caused by *Enterobacter aerogenes* or *Klebsiella pneumoniae.* (3) Combined with neomycin for irrigation of the urinary bladder to prevent bacteriuria and bacteremia from indwelling catheters.

Ophthalmic: Conjunctival and corneal infections (e.g., conjunctivitis, keratitis, keratoconjunctivitis, corneal ulcers, blepharitis, blepharoconjunctivitis, acute meibomianitis, dacryocystitis) due to *E. coli, H. influenzae, H. parainfluenzae, K. pneumoniae, E. aerogenes,* and *P. aeruginosa.*

CONTRAINDICATIONS

Hypersensitivity. A potentially toxic drug to be reserved for the treatment of severe, resistant infections in hospitalized clients. Not indicated for clients with severely impaired renal function or nitrogen retention. Ophthalmic use in dendritic keratitis, vaccinia, varicella, mycobacterial infections of the eye, fungal diseases of the eye, use with steroid combinations after uncomplicated removal of a foreign body from the cornea. Ophthalmic use in deep-seated ophthalmic infections or in those likely to become systemic infections.

SPECIAL CONCERNS

Safe use during pregnancy has not been established.

SIDE EFFECTS

Nephrotoxic: Albuminuria, cylindruria, azotemia, hematuria, proteinuria, leukocyturia, electrolyte loss. **Neuro-**

logic: Dizziness, flushing of face, mental confusion, irritability, nystagmus, muscle weakness, drowsiness, paresthesias, blurred vision, slurred speech, ataxia, ***coma, seizures. Neuromuscular blockade may lead to respiratory paralysis.*** **GI:** N&V, diarrhea, abdominal cramps. **Miscellaneous:** Fever, urticaria, skin exanthemata, eosinophilia, ***anaphylaxis.*** **Following intrathecal use:** Meningeal irritation with fever, stiff neck, headache, increase in leukocytes and protein in the CSF. Nerve-root irritation may result in neuritic pain and urine retention. **Following IM use:** Irritation, severe pain. **Following IV use:** Thrombophlebitis. **Following ophthalmic use:** Burning, stinging, irritation, inflammation, angioneurotic edema, itching, urticaria, vesicular and maculopapular dermatitis.

LABORATORY TEST CONSIDERATIONS

False + or ↑ levels of urea nitrogen and creatinine. Casts and RBCs in urine.

DRUG INTERACTIONS

Aminoglycoside antibiotics / Additive nephrotoxic effects
Cephalosporins / ↑ Risk of renal toxicity
Phenothiazines / ↑ Risk of respiratory depression
Skeletal muscle relaxants (surgical) / Additive muscle relaxation

HOW SUPPLIED

Powder for injection: 500,000 U; *Powder for ophthalmic solution:* 500,000 units

DOSAGE

• **IV**

Infections.

Adults and children: 15,000–25,000 units/kg/day (maximum) in divided doses q 12 hr. **Infants,** up to 40,000 units/kg/day.

• **IM**

Not usually recommended due to pain at injection site.

Infections.

Adults and children: 25,000–30,000 units/kg/day in divided doses q 4–6 hr. **Infants,** up to 40,000 units/kg/day.

Both IV and IM doses should be reduced in renal impairment.

• **INTRATHECAL**

Meningitis.

Adults and children over 2 years: 50,000 units/day for 3–4 days; **then,** 50,000 units every other day until 2 weeks after cultures are negative; **children under 2 years,** 20,000 units/day for 3–4 days or 25,000 units once every other day; dosage of 25,000 units should be continued every other day for 2 weeks after cultures are negative.

• **OPHTHALMIC SOLUTION**

1–2 gtt 2–6 times/day, depending on the infection. Treatment may be necessary for 1–2 months or longer.

NURSING CONSIDERATIONS

SEE ALSO *GENERAL NURSING CONSIDERATIONS* FOR *ANTI-INFECTIVES.*

ADMINISTRATION/STORAGE

1. Store and dilute as directed on package insert.
2. Lessen pain on IM injection by reducing drug concentration as much as possible. It is preferable to give drug more frequently in more dilute doses. If ordered, procaine hydrochloride (2 mL of a 0.5%–1.0% solution per 5 units of dry powder) may be used for mixing the drug for IM injection.
IV 3. For IV administration, reconstitute 500,000 units with 300–500 mL of D5W and infuse over 60–90 min.
4. *Never use preparations containing procaine hydrochloride for IV or intrathecal use.*

ASSESSMENT

1. Note indications: type, onset, and characteristics of symptoms.
2. Determine kidney function and urinary output; note edema. Assess respiratory function; note any prior problems.
3. Obtain specimens for C&S.
4. Note any muscle weakness and early signs of muscle paralysis related to neuromuscular blockade. Assess for evidence of respiratory paralysis; withhold drug and report.
5. Monitor I&O; reduce dose with impaired renal function; observe for

P

nephrotoxicity, characterized by albuminuria, urinary casts, nitrogen retention, and hematuria.
6. Ambulatory or bedridden clients with neurologic disturbances require supervision.

CLIENT/FAMILY TEACHING

1. Avoid hazardous tasks until drug effects realized; may cause dizziness, vertigo, and ataxia.
2. Consume at least 2 L/day of fluids.
3. Report any neurologic disturbances, i.e., dizziness, blurred vision, irritability, circumoral and peripheral numbness and tingling, weakness, and ataxia; usually gone 24–48 hr after drug discontinued; associated with high drug levels.
4. Anticipate a prolonged regimen of topical application of solution because drug is not toxic when used in wet dressings, and provider may wish to prevent emergence of resistant strains.
5 When used in the eye(s), tilt the head back and place the medication in the conjunctival sac. Light finger pressure should be applied on the lacrimal sac for 1 min.
6. To avoid contamination, do not allow the tip of the container to touch any surface.

OUTCOMES/EVALUATE

Negative cultures; resolution of infection; symptomatic improvement

P

Poractant alfa

(poor-**ACK**-tant **AL**-fah)

CLASSIFICATION(S):
Lung surfactant
Rx: Curosurf

ACTION/KINETICS

Preterm infants may be deficient in pulmonary surfactant resulting in respiratory distress syndrome (RDS). Poractant, a porcine lung surfactant, compensates for the deficiency and restores surface activity to the lungs. It suppresses the secretion of tumor necrosis factor by resting and through lipopolysaccharide-stimulate human monocytes. Reduces mortality and pneumothoraces due to RDS.

USES

Treatment of respiratory distress syndrome (RDS) in premature infants. *Investigational:* RDS prophylaxis; adult RDS due to viral pneumonia; HIV-infected infants with *Pneumocystis carinii* pneumonia; adult RDS following near drowning.

SPECIAL CONCERNS

Transient episodes of bradycardia, decreased oxygen saturation, reflux of the drug into the endotracheal tube, hypotension, and airway obstruction have occurred during dosing. If these occur, administration must be interrupted and measures taken to alleviate. After stabilization, dosing may resume with appropriate monitoring.

SIDE EFFECTS

Transient effects: Bradycardia, hypotension, endotracheal tube blockage, oxygen desaturation. **Respiratory:** Acquired pneumonia, bronchopulmonary dysplasia, pneumothorax, pulmonary interstitial emphysema. **CV: Intracranial hemorrhage,** patent ductus arteriosus. **Miscellaneous:** ***Acquired septicemia.***

OD OVERDOSE MANAGEMENT

Symptoms: Effects on respiration, ventilation, or oxygenation. *Treatment:* Aspirate as much of the suspension as possible. Provide supportive treatment, with attention to fluid and electrolyte balance.

HOW SUPPLIED

Suspension, intratracheal: 1.5 mL (120 mg phospholipids), 3.0 mL (240 mg phospholipids)

DOSAGE

• **SUSPENSION, INTRATRACHEAL**

RDS in premature infants.

Initial: 2.5 mL/kg birth weight. Up to 2 subsequent doses of 1.25 mL/kg birth weight can be given at 12-hr intervals, if needed (i.e., infants who remain intubated and need mechanical ventilation and supplemental oxygen). **Maximum total dose:** 5 mL/kg.

NURSING CONSIDERATIONS

ADMINISTRATION/STORAGE

1. Slowly withdraw the entire contents of the vial into a 3 or 5 mL plastic

syringe through a 20 gauge or large needle. Attach the pre-cut 8-cm 5 French catheter to the syringe and fill the catheter with the poractant. Discard excess drug through the catheter so that only the total dose to be given remains in the syringe.
2. Administer through the 5 French end-hole catheter (8-cm in length) inserted into the endotracheal tube of the infant. Position the tip distally in the endotracheal tube. Do not extend the catheter tip beyond the distal tip of the endotracheal tube. The endotracheal tube may be suctioned before giving poractant. Allow the infant to stabilize before proceeding with dosing.
3. Give each dose as 2 aliquots, with each aliquot given into 1 of the 2 main bronchi by positioning the infant with either the right or left side dependent.
4. Immediately before drug administration, change the ventilator setting of the infant to a rate of 40–60 breaths/min, inspiratory time 0.5 sec, and supplemental oxygen sufficient to maintain SaO_2 at > 92%.
5. Keep the infant in a neutral position (head and body in alignment without inclination). Briefly disconnect the endotracheal tube from the ventilator. Insert the catheter, as described above, and instill the first aliquot of 1.25 mL/kg birth weight. Position the infant as described above.
6. After the first aliquot is instilled, remove the catheter from the endotracheal tube and manually ventilate the infant with 100% oxygen at a rate of 40–60 breaths/min for 1 min. When the infant is stable, reposition so that the other side is dependent and give the remaining aliquot using the same procedure.
7. After giving the second aliquot, remove the catheter without flushing. Do not suction for 1 hr after drug instillation, unless signs of significant airway obstruction occur.
8. After dosing is completed, resume usual ventilator management and clinical care.
9. Store in a refrigerator at 2–8° C (36–46° F). Unopened vials may be warmed to room temperature for 24 hr prior to use. Do not return warmed vials to the refrigerator more than once.
10. Protect from light and do not shake. Vials are for single use only. Discard any unused drug after opening the vial.

ASSESSMENT

1. Drug is administered by intratracheal means via catheter into each bronchus.
2. May suction before drug instillation but do not suction for 1 hr after instillation unless extreme airway obstruction evidenced.
3. Observe infant frequently for S&S respiratory distress, hypotension, bradycardia and oxygen desaturation. Correct acidosis, hypotension, anemia, hypoglycemia, and hypothermia before giving poractant.

OUTCOMES/EVALUATE

- Management of RDS in premature infants
- Restoration of surface activity to lungs
- ↓ Mortality in RDS

Porfimer sodium

(**POOR**-fih-mer)

PREGNANCY CATEGORY: C
CLASSIFICATION(S):
Antineoplastic, miscellaneous
Rx: Photofrin

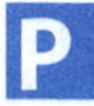

ACTION/KINETICS

A photosensitizing drug used in the photodynamic therapy (PDT) of tumors. The effects are both light and oxygen dependent. Following IV injection, porfimer is retained for a prolonged period of time in tumors, skin, and organs of the reticuloendothelial system (including liver and spleen). Drug administration is followed by illumination with 630 nm of light, which causes a photochemical (not a thermal) effect. Cellular damage is the result of propagation of radical reactions, including formation of superoxide and hydroxyl radicals. Tumor death may also occur through ischemic necrosis secondary to vascular occlusion that is likely mediated through release of thromboxane A_2. **t½, elimination:** 250 hr. **Mean plasma levels after 48 hr:** 2.6 mcg/mL. About 90% bound to serum proteins.

USES

(1) Completely obstructing esophageal cancer or those with partially obstructing esophageal cancer who cannot be treated satisfactorily with Nd:YAG laser therapy. (2) Microinvasive endobronchial non-small cell lung cancer where surgery and radiotherapy are not indicated.

CONTRAINDICATIONS

Known allergies to porphyrins. Use of PDT in existing tracheoesophageal or bronchoesophageal fistulas or tumors eroding into a major blood vessel. Lactation.

SPECIAL CONCERNS

Those treated with porfimer sodium will be photosensitive and must observe precautions to avoid exposure of the skin and eyes to direct sunlight or bright indoor lighting. Use with extreme caution in esophageal varices and where treatment-induced inflammation can obstructe the main airway. Safety and efficacy have not been determined in children.

SIDE EFFECTS

Side effects listed are those possible from porfimer PDT. Over 95% of clients experienced one or more side effects. Location of the tumor was predictive for three side effects: esophageal edema if the tumor was in the upper one-third of the esophagus, atrial fibrillation if in the middle third, and anemia if in the lower third. Clients with large tumors (greater than 10 cm) were more likely to manifest anemia. Some GI, CV, and respiratory side effects may be due to mediastinal inflammation.

GI: Constipation, N&V, abdominal pain, dysphagia, esophageal edema, esophageal tumor bleeding, hematemesis, dyspepsia, esophageal stricture, diarrhea, eructation, esophagitis, melena, esophageal perforation, gastric ulcer, ileus, jaundice, peritonitis. **Respiratory:** Pleural effusion, dyspnea, pneumonia, pharyngitis, respiratory insufficiency, coughing, tracheoesophageal fistula, bronchitis, ***bronchospasm, respiratory distress, laryngotracheal edema, pulmonary hemorrhage, respiratory failure,*** pneumonitis, pulmonary edema, stridor. **CNS:** Insomnia, anorexia, confusion, anxiety. **CV:** Atrial fibrillation, cardiac failure, tachycardia, hypertension, hypotension, angina pectoris, bradycardia, ***MI,*** sick sinus syndrome, SVT. **Body as a whole:** Fever, pain, chest pain, back pain, peripheral edema, asthenia, substernal chest pain, generalized edema, surgical complications, weight decrease, dehydration. **Ophthalmic:** Abnormal vision, diplopia, eye pain, photophobia, ocular sensitivity, photosensitivity reaction. **Miscellaneous:** Anemia (due to tumor bleeding), moniliasis, UTI, ***sepsis.***

OD OVERDOSE MANAGEMENT

Symptoms: Photosensitivity. Increased symptoms and damage to normal tissue following an overdose of light. *Treatment:* Treat photosensitivity by protecting eyes and skin from direct sunlight or bright indoor light for 30 days. Then, test clients for residual photosensitivity. Porfimer is not dialyzable.

DRUG INTERACTIONS

Allopurinol / ↓ Effect of porfimer
Beta-carotene / ↓ PDT activity
Calcium channel blockers / ↓ Effect of porfimer
Ethanol / ↓ PDT activity
Glucocorticoids / ↓ PDT activity
Griseofulvin / ↑ Photosensitivity reaction
Hypoglycemic drugs / ↑ Photosensitivity reaction
Mannitol / ↓ PDT activity
Phenothiazines / ↑ Photosensitivity reaction
Prostaglandin synthesis inhibitors / ↓ Effect of porfimer
Sulfonamides / ↑ Photosensitivity reaction
Tetracyclines / ↑ Photosensitivity reaction
Thiazide diuretics / ↑ Photosensitivity reaction

HOW SUPPLIED

Cake or Freeze-Dried Powder for Injection: 75 mg.

DOSAGE

- **IV INJECTION**

Esophageal cancer.

The first stage is IV injection of porfimer, 2 mg/kg, given over 3–5 min. Illumination with laser light (300 J/cm of tumor length at a wavelength of 630 nm) 40–50 hr later is the second stage of therapy. A second laser light application may be given 96–120 hr after the porfimer injection, which is preceded by gentle debridement of residual tumor. This regimen may be repeated 30 days after the initial therapy; up to three courses of treatment (each separated by a minimum of 30 days) may be given.

NURSING CONSIDERATIONS

ADMINISTRATION/STORAGE

IV 1. Vials of porfimer sodium are freeze-dried cake or powder for injection. Reconstitute each vial with 31.8 mL of either D5W or 0.9% NaCl injection. The final concentration is 2.5 mg/mL with a pH of 7–8. Shake well until the drug is dissolved. The reconstituted product is an opaque solution; detection of particulate matter by visual inspection is difficult.

2. Protect reconstituted drug from bright light; administer immediately.
3. Do not mix with other drugs in the same solution.
4. Avoid extravasation at injection site. If occurs, protect area from light.
5. The laser light is delivered to the tumor by cylindrical *Optiguide* fiberoptic diffusers that are passed through the operating channel of an endoscope.
6. Wipe any spills with a damp cloth. Avoid skin and eye contact due to the potential for photosensitivity reactions when exposed to light. Use of rubber gloves and eye protection is recommended.
7. Dispose of contaminated materials in a special polyethylene bag consistent with local regulations.
8. Store the unreconstituted drug at 20–25°C (68–77°F).

ASSESSMENT

1. Document indications for therapy, symptom onset, any other treatments/procedures trialed.
2. Evaluate before each course of treatment for evidence of tracheo/bronchoesophageal fistula.
3. Note size and location of the tumor to help anticipate and prepare for potential side effects. For example, if tumor is in the upper third of the esophagus, esophageal edema may develop; if in the middle third may see atrial fibrillation; and if in the lower third may see anemia. With tumors that are larger than 10 cm, anemia may occur.

CLIENT/FAMILY TEACHING

1. Review the method of therapy and stages, e.g., IV injection of drug followed in 2–4 days by illumination with laser light. This laser therapy may be repeated in another 2–4 days after residual tumor debridement and then repeated for up to three courses of therapy.
2. Avoid any exposure to sunlight or to bright lighting for 30 days as drug renders one photosensitive. Skin must be covered and protected. Sunglasses must be worn. Report any chest pain or eye sensitivity.

OUTCOMES/EVALUATE

Control of malignant cell proliferation

Potassium Salts

Potassium acetate, parenteral

PREGNANCY CATEGORY: C

Potassium acetate, Potassium bicarbonate, and Potassium citrate (Trikates)

Rx: Oral Solution: Tri-K

Potassium bicarbonate

Rx: Oral Solution: K + Care ET

Potassium bicarbonate and Citric acid

Rx: Effervescent Tablets: K+ Care ET

Potassium bicarbonate and Potassium chloride

Rx: Effervescent Tablets: Klorvess, Klor-Con/EF, K-Lyte/Cl, K-Lyte/Cl 50
✱**Rx: Effervescent Granules:** Neo-K. **Effervescent Tablets:** Potassium-Sandoz

Potassium bicarbonate and Potassium citrate

Rx: Effervescent Tablets: K-Lyte, Effer-K, Effervescent Potassium

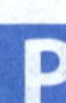

Potassium chloride

Rx: Extended-Release Capsules: K-Lease, K-Norm, Micro-K 10 Extencaps., Micro-K Extencaps **Extended-Release Tablets:** K+ 10, Kaon-Cl, Kaon-Cl-10, K-Dur 10 and 20, Klor-Con 8 and 10, Klotrix, K-Tab, Slow-K, Ten-K, **Injection:** Potassium Chloride for Injection Concentrate., **Oral Solution:** Cena-K 10% and 20%, Kaochlor 10%, Kaochlor S-F 10%, Kaon-Cl 20% Liquid, Kay Ciel, Klorvess 10% Liquid, Potasalan, Rum-K., **Powder for Oral Solution:** Gen-K, K+ Care, Kay Ciel, K-Lor, Klor-Con Powder, Klor-Con/25 Powder, K-Lyte/Cl Powder, Micro-K LS.
✱**Rx: Extended-Release Tablets:** Apo-K, Kalium Durules, K-Long, Novolente-K, Slo-Pot 600, Slow-K, **Oral Solution:** K-10, Kaochlor-10 and -20, KCl 5%

Potassium chloride, Potassium bicarbonate, and Potassium citrate

Rx: Effervescent Granules: Klorvess Effervescent Granules

Potassium gluconate

Rx: Elixir: Kaon, Kaylixir, K-G Elixir
✱**Rx: Elixir:** Potassium-Rougier, Royonate., **Tablets:** Kaon

Potassium gluconate and Potassium chloride

Rx: Oral Solution and Powder for Oral Solution: Kolyum

Potassium gluconate and Potassium citrate

Rx: Oral Solution: Twin-K
CLASSIFICATION(S):
Electrolyte

GENERAL STATEMENT

Potassium is the major cation of the body's intracellular fluid. It is essential for the maintenance of important physiologic processes, including cardiac, smooth, and skeletal muscle function, acid-base balance, gastric secretions, renal function, protein and carbohydrate metabolism. Symptoms of hypokalemia include weakness, cardiac arrhythmias, fatigue, ileus, hyporeflexia or areflexia, tetany, polydipsia, and, in severe cases, flaccid paralysis and inability to concentrate urine. Loss of potassium is usually accompanied by a loss of chloride resulting in hypochloremic metabolic alkalosis.

The usual adult daily requirement of potassium is 40–80 mg. In adults, the normal extracellular concentration of potassium ranges from 3.5 to 5 mEq/L with the intracellular levels being 150–160 mEq/L. Extracellular concentrations of up to 5.6 mEq/L are normal in children.

Both hypokalemia and hyperkalemia, if uncorrected, can be fatal; thus, potassium must always be administered cautiously.

ACTION/KINETICS

Potassium is readily and rapidly absorbed from the GI tract. Though a number of salts can be used to supply the potassium cation, potassium chloride is the agent of choice since hypochloremia frequently accompanies potassium deficiency. Dietary measures can often prevent and even correct potassium deficiencies. Potassium-rich foods include most meats (beef, chicken, ham, turkey, veal), fish, beans, broccoli, brussels sprouts, lentils, spinach, potatoes, milk, bananas, dates, prunes, raisins, avocados, watermelon, cantaloupe, apricots, and molasses.

From 80% to 90% of potassium intake is excreted by the kidney and is partially reabsorbed from the glomerular filtrate.

USES

PO: (1) Treat hypokalemia due to digitalis intoxication, diabetic acidosis, diarrhea and vomiting, familial periodic paralysis, certain cases of uremia, hyperadrenalism, starvation and debilitation, and corticosteroid or diuretic therapy. (2) Hypokalemia with or without metabolic acidosis and following surgical conditions accompanied by nitrogen loss, vomiting and diarrhea, suction drainage, and increased urinary excretion of potassium. (3) Prophylaxis of potassium depletion when dietary intake is not adequate in the following conditions: clients on digitalis and diuretics for CHF, hepatic cirrhosis with ascites, excess aldosterone with normal renal function, significant cardiac arrhythmias, potassium-losing nephropathy, and certain states accompanied by diarrhea. *Investigational:* Mild hypertension.

NOTE: Use potassium chloride when hypokalemia is associated with alkalosis; potassium bicarbonate, citrate, acetate, or gluconate should be used when hypokalemia is associated with acidosis.

IV: (1) Prophylaxis and treatment of moderate to severe potassium loss when PO therapy is not feasible. (2) Potassium acetate is used as an additive for preparing specific IV formulas when client needs cannot be met by usual nutrient or electrolyte preparations. (3) Potassium acetate is also used in the following conditions: marked loss of GI secretions due to vomiting, diarrhea, GI intubation, or fistulas; prolonged parenteral use of potassium-free fluids (e.g., dextrose or NSS); diabetic acidosis, especially during treatment with insulin and dextrose infusions; prolonged diuresis; metabolic alkalosis; hyperadrenocorticism; primary aldosteronism; overdose of adrenocortical steroids, testosterone, or corticotropin; attacks of hereditary or familial periodic paralysis; during the healing phase of burns or scalds; and cardiac arrhythmias, especially due to digitalis glycosides.

CONTRAINDICATIONS

Severe renal function impairment with azotemia or oliguria, postoperatively before urine flow has been reestablished. Crush syndrome, Addison's disease, hyperkalemia from any cause, anuria, heat cramps, acute dehydration, severe hemolytic reactions, adynamia episodica hereditaria, clients receiving potassium-sparing diuretics or aldosterone-inhibiting drugs. Solid dosage forms in clients in whom there is a reason for delay or arrest in passage of tablets through the GI tract.

SPECIAL CONCERNS

Safety during lactation and in children has not been established. Geriatric clients are at greater risk of developing hyperkalemia due to age-related changes in renal function. Administer with caution in the presence of cardiac and renal disease. Potassium loss is often accompanied by an obligatory loss of chloride resulting in hypochloremic metabolic alkalosis; thus, the underlying cause of the potassium loss should be treated.

P

SIDE EFFECTS

Hypokalemia. **CNS:** Dizziness, mental confusion. **CV:** Arrhythmias; weak, irregular pulse; hypotension, ***heart block,*** ECG abnormalities, ***cardiac arrest.*** **GI:** Abdominal distention, anorexia, N&V, **Neuromuscular:** Weakness, paresthesia of extremities, flaccid paralysis, areflexia, muscle or ***respiratory paralysis,*** weakness and heaviness of legs. **Other:** Malaise.

Hyperkalemia. **CV:** Bradycardia, then tachycardia, ***cardiac arrest.*** **GI:** N&V, diarrhea, abdominal cramps, GI bleeding or obstruction. Ulceration or perforation of the small bowel from enteric-coated potassium chloride tablets. **GU:** Oliguria, anuria. **Neuromuscular:** Weakness, tingling, paralysis. **Other:** Skin rashes, hyperkalemia.

Effects due to solution or IV technique used. Fever, infection at injection site, venous thrombosis, phlebitis extending from injection site, extravasation, venospasm, hypervolemia, hyperkalemia.

OD OVERDOSE MANAGEMENT

Symptoms: Mild (5.5–6.5 mEq/L) to moderate (6.5–8 mEq/L) hyperkalemia (may be asymptomatic except for ECG changes). ECG changes include progression in height and peak of T waves, lowering of the R wave, decreased amplitude and eventually disappearance of P waves, prolonged PR interval and QRS complex, shortening of the QT interval, ***ventricular fibrillation, death. Muscle weakness that may progress to flaccid quadriplegia and respiratory failure,*** although dangerous cardiac arrhythmias usually occur before onset of complete paralysis. *Treatment (plasma potassium levels greater than 6.5 mEq/L):* All measures must be monitored by ECG. Measures consist of actions taken to shift potassium ions from plasma into cells by:

• ***Sodium bicarbonate:*** IV infusion of 50–100 mEq over period of 5 min. May be repeated after 10–15 minutes if ECG abnormalities persist.

• ***Glucose and insulin:*** IV infusion of 3 g glucose to 1 unit regular insulin to shift potassium into cells.

• ***Calcium gluconate—or other calcium salt*** (only for clients not on digitalis or other cardiotonic glycosides): IV infusion of 0.5–1 g (5–10 mL of a 10% solution) over period of 2 min. Dosage may be repeated after 1–2 min if ECG remains abnormal. When ECG is approximately normal, the excess potassium should be removed from the body by administration of polystyrene sulfonate, hemodialysis, or peritoneal dialysis (clients with renal insufficiency), or other means.

• ***Sodium polystyrene sulfonate, hemodialysis, peritoneal dialysis:*** To remove potassium from the body.

DRUG INTERACTIONS

ACE inhibitors / May cause potassium retention → hyperkalemia

Digitalis glycosides / Cardiac arrhythmias

Potassium-sparing diuretics / Severe hyperkalemia with possibility of cardiac arrhythmias or arrest

HOW SUPPLIED

Potassium acetate, parenteral: *Injection:* 2 mEq/mL, 4 mEq/mL; **Potassium acetate**, **potassium bicarbonate**, and **potassium citrate:** *Liquid:* 45 mEq/15 mL; **Potassium bicarbonate:** *Tablet, effervescent:* 25 mEq, 650 mg; **Potassium bicarbonate** and **potassium citrate:** *Tablet, effervescent:* 25 mEq; **Potassium bicarbonate** and **potassium chloride:** *Granule for reconstitution:* 20 mEq; *Tablet, effervescent*: 25 mEq, 50 mEq; **Potassium chloride:** *Capsule, extended release:* 8 mEq, 10 mEq; *Injection:* 1.5 mEq/mL, 2 mEq/mL, 10 mEq/50 mL, 10 mEq/100 mL, 20 mEq/50 mL, 20 mEq/100 mL, 30 mEq/100 mL, 40 mEq/100 mL, 100 mEq/L, 200 mEq/L; *Liquid:* 20 mEq/15 mL, 30 mEq/15 mL, 40 mEq/15 mL; *Powder for reconstitution:* 20 mEq, 25 mEq, 200 mEq; *Tablet*: 180 mg; *Tablet, extended release:* 8 mEq, 10 mEq, 20 mEq; **Potassium gluconate:** *Elixir:* 20 mEq/15 mL; *Tablet:* 486 mg, 500 mg, 550 mg, 595 mg, 610 mg, 620 mg; *Tablet, extended release:* 595 mg; **Potassium gluconate** and **potassium citrate:** *Liquid:* 20 mEq/15 mL

DOSAGE

Highly individualized. Oral administration is preferred because the slow absorption from the GI tract prevents sudden, large increases in plasma potassium levels. Dosage is usually expressed as mEq/L of potassium. The bicarbonate, chloride, citrate, and gluconate salts are usually administered PO. The chloride, acetate, and phosphate may be administered by **slow IV** infusion.

- **IV INFUSION**

Serum K less than 2.0 mEq/L.

400 mEq/day at a rate not to exceed 40 mEq/hr. Use a maximum concentration of 80 mEq/L.

Serum K more than 2.5 mEq/L.

200 mEq/day at a rate not to exceed 20 mEq/hr. Use a maximum concentration of 40 mEq/L.

Pediatric: Up to 3 mEq potassium/kg (or 40 mEq/m^2) daily. Adjust the volume administered depending on the body size.

- **EFFERVESCENT GRANULES, EFFERVESCENT TABLETS, ELIXIR, EXTENDED-RELEASE CAPSULES, EXTENDED RELEASE GRANULES, EXTENDED-RELEASE TABLETS, ORAL SOLUTION, POWDER FOR ORAL SOLUTION, TABLETS**

Prophylaxis of hypokalemia.

16–24 mEq/day.

Potassium depletion.

40–100 mEq/day.

NOTE: Usual dietary intake of potassium is 40–250 mEq/day.

For clients with accompanying metabolic acidosis, use an alkalizing potassium salt (potassium bicarbonate, potassium citrate, potassium acetate, or potassium glucosate).

NURSING CONSIDERATIONS

ADMINISTRATION/STORAGE

1. Give PO doses 2–4 times/day. Correct hypokalemia slowly over a period of 3–7 days to minimize risk of hyperkalemia.
2. With esophageal compression, administer dilute liquid solutions of potassium rather than tablets.

IV 3. Do not administer potassium IV undiluted. Usual method is to administer by slow IV infusion in dextrose solution at a concentration of 40–80 mEq/L and at a rate not to exceed 10–20 mEq/hr.

4. Avoid "layering" of potassium by inverting container during addition of potassium solution and properly agitating the prepared IV solution. Squeezing the plastic container will not prevent KCL from settling to the bottom. Never add potassium to an IV bottle that is hanging.
5. Check site of administration frequently for pain and redness because drug is extremely irritating.
6. In critical clients, KCL may be given slow IV in a solution of saline (unless contraindicated) since dextrose may lower serum potassium levels by producing an intracellular shift.
7. Administer all concentrated potassium infusions and riders with an infusion control device.
8. Have sodium polystyrene sulfonate (Kayexalate) available for oral or rectal administration in the event of hyperkalemia.

ASSESSMENT

1. Note indications for therapy; document electrolytes and ECG.
2. Note any impaired renal function. Assess for adequate urinary flow before administering potassium. Impaired function can lead to hyperkalemia.

P

INTERVENTIONS

1. Withhold and report if abdominal pain, distention, or GI bleeding occurs.
2. Complaints of weakness, fatigue, or the presence of cardiac arrhythmias may be symptoms of hypokalemia indicating a low *intracellular* potassium level, although the level may appear to be within normal limits.
3. Monitor I&O. Withhold drug and report oliguria, anuria, or azoturia.
4. Observe for symptoms of adrenal insufficiency or extensive tissue breakdown.
5. Report complaints of weakness or heaviness of the legs, the presence of a gray pallor, cold skin, listlessness,

mental confusion, flaccid paralysis, hypotension, or cardiac arrhythmias (S&S of hyperkalemia).

6. Monitor serum potassium levels during parenteral therapy; normal level is 3.5–5.0 mEq/L.

CLIENT/FAMILY TEACHING

1. Dilute or dissolve PO liquids, effervescent tablets, or soluble powders in 3–8 oz of cold water, fruit or vegetable juice, or other suitable liquid and drink slowly. Chill to improve taste.
2. If GI upset occurs, products can be taken after meals or with food with a full glass of water.
3. Swallow enteric-coated tablets and extended-release capsules and tablets; do not chew or dissolve in the mouth.
4. Salt substitutes should not be used concomitantly with potassium preparations.
5. If receiving potassium-sparing diuretics, such as spironolactone or triamterene, do not take potassium supplements or eat foods high in potassium.
6. Identify high-potassium sources in the diet: spinach, collards, brussel sprouts, beet greens, tomato juice, celery. Once parenteral potassium is discontinued, ingest potassium-rich foods such as citrus juices, bananas, apricots, raisins, and nuts. The daily adult requirement is usually 40–80 mg. A dietitian may assist with meal planning.
7. Avoid self-prescribed enemas, and large amounts of licorice.
8. Report any adverse side effects and keep all visits for lab and exams.

OUTCOMES/EVALUATE

Correction of potassium deficiency; potassium levels within desired range

Pramipexole

(prah-mih-**PEX**-ohl)

PREGNANCY CATEGORY: C
CLASSIFICATION(S):
Antiparkinson drug
Rx: Mirapex

ACTION/KINETICS

Thought to act by stimulating dopamine (especially D_3) receptors in striatum. Rapidly absorbed. **Peak levels:** 2 hr. Food increases time for maximum levels to occur. **t½, terminal:** About 8 hr (12 hr in geriatric clients). Excreted mainly unchanged in urine. Clearance decreases with age.

USES

Idiopathic Parkinson's disease.

CONTRAINDICATIONS

Lactation.

SPECIAL CONCERNS

Possible sudden, overwhelming urge to sleep. Safety and efficacy have not been determined in children.

SIDE EFFECTS

CNS: Hallucinations (especially in elderly), dizziness, somnolence, insomnia, confusion, amnesia, hypesthesia, dystonia, akathisia, abnormal thinking, decreased libido, myoclonus. **CV:** Orthostatic hypotension. **Body as a whole:** Asthenia, general edema, malaise, fever. **GI:** Nausea, constipation, anorexia, dysphagia. **Miscellaneous:** Vision abnormalities, impotence, peripheral edema, decreased weight.

DRUG INTERACTIONS

Butyrophenones / Possible ↓ effect of pramipexole
Cimetidine / ↑ Levodopa levels and half-life
CNS Depressants / Additive CNS depression
Levodopa / ↑ Levodopa levels; also, may cause or worsen pre-existing dyskinesia
Metoclopramide / Possible ↓ effect of pramipexole
Phenothiazines / Possible ↓ effect of pramipexole
Thioxanthines / Possible ↓ effect of pramipexole

HOW SUPPLIED

Tablets: 0.125 mg, 0.25 mg, 0.5 mg, 1 mg, 1.5 mg

DOSAGE

• **TABLETS**

Parkinsonism.

Initial: Start with 0.125 mg t.i.d.; **then,** increase dose by 0.125 mg t.i.d. weekly for seven weeks (i.e., dose at week seven is 1.5 mg t.i.d.). **Maintenance:** 1.5–4.5 mg/day in equally divided doses t.i.d. with or without comcomitant levodopa (about 800 mg/day). Impaired renal function: C_{CR} over 60 mL/min: Start with 0.125 mg t.i.d., up to maximum of 1.5 mg t.i.d. C_{CR} 25–59 mL/min: Start with 0.125 mg b.i.d., up to maximum of 1.5 mg b.i.d. C_{CR} 15–24 mL/min: Start with 0.125 mg once daily, up to maximum of 1.5 mg once daily.

NURSING CONSIDERATIONS

ADMINISTRATION/STORAGE

1. Consider decrease in levodopa dose if taken with pramipexole.
2. Discontinue pramipexole over 1 week period.

ASSESSMENT

1. Document disease onset, extent of motor function, reflexes, gait, strength of grip, and amount of tremor.
2. With tremor, assess for muscle weakness, muscle rigidity, difficulty walking, or changing directions.
3. Monitor mental status, VS, ECG, liver and renal function studies.

CLIENT/FAMILY TEACHING

1. Take only as prescribed; may take with food to decrease nausea.
2. Rise slowly from sitting or lying position to prevent postural effects.
3. Do not drive or perform activities that require mental/motor alertness until stabilized on drug. May cause dizziness, fainting, blackouts, hypotension, sudden urge to sleep, and sedative effects.
4. Practice reliable contraception.
5. Report any vision problems; obtain regular eye exams.
6. May cause hallucinations; report if evident.
7. Do not stop abruptly; must do so over one week period.
8. Avoid alcohol and any other CNS depressants, may exaggerate drowsiness and dizziness.

OUTCOMES/EVALUATE

Control of Parkinsonian symptoms (e.g., improvement in motor function, reflexes, gait, strength of grip, and amount of tremor)

Pravastatin sodium

(prah-vah-**STAH**-tin)

PREGNANCY CATEGORY: X
CLASSIFICATION(S):
Antihyperlipidemic, HMG-CoA reductase inhibitor
Rx: Pravachol
✱**Rx:** Lin-Pravastatin

SEE ALSO *ANTIHYPERLIPIDEMIC, HMG-COA REDUCTASE INHIBITORS*

ACTION/KINETICS

Drug increases survival in heart transplant recipients. Rapidly absorbed from the GI tract. **Peak plasma levels:** 1–1.5 hr. Significant first-pass extraction and metabolism in the liver, which is the site of action of the drug; thus, plasma levels may not correlate well with lipid-lowering effectiveness. **t½, elimination:** 1.5–3.2 hr. Metabolized in the liver; excreted in the urine (47%) and feces (53%).

USES

(1) Adjunct to diet for reducing elevated total and LDL cholesterol and triglyceride levels in clients with primary hypercholesterolemia (type IIa and IIb) and mixed dyslipidemia when the response to a diet with restricted saturated fat and cholesterol has not been effective. Treat elevated serum triglyceride levels (Fredrickson Type IV) and primary dysbetalipoproteinemia (Fredrickson Type III). Reduction of apolipoprotein B serum levels. (2) Reduce the risk of recurrent MI in those with previous MI and normal cholesterol levels; reduce risk of undergoing myocardial revascularization procedures; reduce risk of stroke or TIA. (3) Reduce risk of MI in hypercholesterolemia without evidence of coronary heart disease; reduce risk of CV mortality with no increase in death from noncardiovascular causes. (4) Slow the progression of coronary atherosclerosis and reduce risk of acute coronary events in hypercholesterolemia with clinically evident CAD, including prior MI. *Investigational:* To lower cholesterol

P

levels in those with heterozygous familial hypercholesterolemia, familial combined hyperlipidemia, diabetic dyslipidemia in non-insulin-dependent diabetics, hypercholesterolemia secondary to nephrotic syndrome, homozygous familial hypercholesterolemia in those not completely devoid of LDL receptors but who have a decreased level of LDL receptor activity.

ADDITIONAL CONTRAINDICATIONS

To treat hypercholesterolemia due to hyperalphaproteinemia.

SPECIAL CONCERNS

Use with caution in clients with a history of liver disease or renal insufficiency.

SIDE EFFECTS

Musculoskeletal: Rhabdomyolysis with renal dysfunction secondary to myoglobinuria, myalgia, myopathy, arthralgias, localized pain, muscle cramps, leg cramps, bursitis, tenosynovitis, myasthenia, tendinous contracture, myositis. **CNS:** CNS vascular lesions characterized by ***perivascular hemorrhage,*** edema, and mononuclear cell infiltration of perivascular spaces; headache, dizziness, psychic disturbances. Dizziness, vertigo, memory loss, anxiety, insomnia, somnolence, abnormal dreams, emotional lability, incoordination, hyperkinesia, torticollis, psychic disturbances. **GI:** N&V, diarrhea, abdominal pain, cramps, constipation, flatulence, heartburn, anorexia, gastroenteritis, dry mouth, rectal hemorrhage, esophagitis, eructation, glossitis, mouth ulceration, increased appetite, stomatitis, cheilitis, duodenal ulcer, dysphagia, enteritis, melena, gum hemorrhage, stomach ulcer, tenesmus, ulcerative stomach. **CV:** Palpitation, vasodilation, syncope, migraine, postural hypotension, phlebitis, arrhythmia. **Hepatic:** Hepatitis (including chronic active hepatitis), fatty change in liver, cirrhosis, ***fulminant hepatic necrosis, hepatoma,*** pancreatitis, cholestatic jaundice, biliary pain. **GU:** Gynecomastia, erectile dysfunction, loss of libido, cystitis, hematuria, impotence, dysuria, kidney calculus, nocturia, epididymitis, fibrocystic breast, albuminuria, breast enlargement, nephritis, urinary frequency, incontinence, retention and urgency, abnormal ejaculation, vaginal or uterine hemorrhage, metrorrhagia, UTI. **Ophthalmic:** Progression of cataracts, lens opacities, ophthalmoplegia. **Hypersensitivity reaction:** Vasculitis, purpura, polymyalgia rheumatica, ***angioedema,*** lupus erythematosus–like syndrome, thrombocytopenia, ***hemolytic anemia,*** leukopenia, positive ANA, arthritis, arthralgia, urticaria, asthenia, ESR increase, fever, chills, photosensitivity, malaise, dyspnea, ***toxic epidermal necrolysis, Stevens-Johnson syndrome.*** **Dermatologic:** Alopecia, pruritus, rash, skin nodules, discoloration of skin, dryness of skin and mucous membranes, changes in hair and nails, contact dermatitis, sweating, acne, urticaria, eczema, seborrhea, skin ulcer. **Neurologic:** Dysfunction of certain cranial nerves resulting in alteration of taste, impairment of extraocular movement, and facial paresis; paresthesia, peripheral neuropathy, tremor, vertigo, memory loss peripheral nerve palsy. **Respiratory:** Common cold, rhinitis, cough. **Hematologic:** Anemia, transient asymptomatic eosinophilia, thrombocytopenia, leukopenia, ecchymosis, lymphadenopathy, petechiae. **Miscellaneous:** Cardiac chest pain, fatigue, influenza.

LABORATORY TEST CONSIDERATIONS

↑ CPK, AST, ALT, alkaline phosphatase, bilirubin. Abnormalities in thyroid function tests.

ADDITIONAL DRUG INTERACTIONS

Bile acid sequestrants / ↓ Bioavailability of pravastatin

Clofibrate / ↑ Risk of myopathy

HOW SUPPLIED

Tablet: 10 mg, 20 mg, 40 mg

DOSAGE

• **TABLETS**

Initial: 10–20 mg once daily at bedtime. **Maintenance dose:** 10–40 mg once daily at bedtime. Alternatively, an optional starting dose of 40 mg/day may be given any time of the day with or without food. Use a starting dose of 10 mg/day at bedtime in renal/hepatic dysfunction and in the elderly (maximum maintenance dose for geriatric clients is 20 mg/day).

NURSING CONSIDERATIONS

SEE ALSO *NURSING CONSIDERATIONS* FOR *ANTIHYPERLIPIDEMIC HMG-COA REDUCTASE INHIBITORS.*

ADMINISTRATION/STORAGE

1. In clients taking immunosuppressants (e.g., cyclosporine), begin pravastatin therapy at 10 mg/day at bedtime and titrate to higher doses with caution. Usual maximum dose is 20 mg/day.
2. Place on a standard cholesterol-lowering diet for 3–6 months before beginning pravastatin and continue during therapy.
3. Drug may be taken without regard to meals.
4. When given with a bile-acid binding resin (e.g., cholestyramine, colestipol), give pravastatin either 1 hr or more before or 4 or more hr after the resin.
5. The maximum effect is seen within 4 weeks during which time periodic lipid determinations should be undertaken.

ASSESSMENT

1. Determine that secondary causes for hypercholesterolemia are ruled out. Secondary causes include hypothyroidism, poorly controlled diabetes mellitus, dysproteinemias, obstructive liver disease, nephrotic syndrome, alcoholism, and other drug therapy.
2. Determine if pregnant.
3. Assess for liver disease or alcohol abuse.
4. Document all CAD risk factors. Initiate therapy during hospitalization for MI/angioplasty procedure.
5. Monitor cholesterol profile, CBC, liver and renal function studies.

INTERVENTIONS

1. Obtain LFTs prior to pravastatin therapy and 6 weeks after starting therapy; if wnl may monitor at 6-month intervals.
2. Pravastatin should be discontinued if markedly elevated CPK levels occur or myopathy is diagnosed.
3. Pravastatin should be discontinued temporarily in clients experiencing an acute or serious condition (e.g., sepsis, hypotension, major surgery, trauma, uncontrolled epilepsy, or severe metabolic, endocrine, or electrolyte disorders) predisposing to the development of renal failure secondary to rhabdomyolysis.

CLIENT/FAMILY TEACHING

1. Take as directed at bedtime.
2. Review the prescribed dietary recommendations (restricted cholesterol and saturated fats); continue diet during drug therapy.
3. Continue a regular exercise program and strive to attain recommended weight loss.
4. Report unexplained muscle pain, tenderness, or weakness, especially if accompanied by malaise or fever.
5. Practice reliable barrier contraception; report if pregnancy is suspected as drug therapy hazardous to a developing fetus.
6. Report severe GI upset, unusual bruising/bleeding, vision changes, dark urine or light colored stools.

OUTCOMES/EVALUATE

↓ Serum cholesterol and LDL levels; heart attack prophylaxis in those with atherosclerosis and hypercholesterolemia

Praziquantel

(pray-zih-**KWON**-tell)

PREGNANCY CATEGORY: B
CLASSIFICATION(S):
Anthelmintic
Rx: Biltricide

ACTION/KINETICS

Causes increased cell permeability in the helminth, resulting in a loss of intracellular calcium with massive contractions, and paralysis of musculature with breakdown of the integrity of the organism. Also causes vacuolization and disintegration of phagocytes to the parasite, resulting in death. **Maximum serum levels:** 1–3 hr. **t½:** 0.8–1.5 hr. Levels in the CSF are approximately 14%–20% of the total amount of the drug in the plasma. Significant first-pass effect. Excreted primarily in the urine.

P

USES
Schistosomal infections due to *Schistosoma japonicum, S. mansoni, S. mekongi,* and *S. hematobium.* Liver flukes (*Clonorchis sinensis, Opisthorchis viverrini*). *Investigational:* Neurocysticercosis, other tissue flukes, and intestinal cestodes. Low doses of oxamniquine and praziquantel as a single-dose treatment of schistosomiasis.

CONTRAINDICATIONS
Ocular cysticercosis. Lactation.

SPECIAL CONCERNS
Safety in children less than 4 years of age not established. When schistosomiasis or fluke infection is associated with cerebrasl cysticercosis, hospitalize client for treatment duration.

SIDE EFFECTS
GI: Nausea, abdominal discomfort. **CNS:** Malaise, headache, dizziness, drowsiness. **Miscellaneous:** Fever, urticaria (rare). *NOTE:* These side effects may also be due to the helminth infection itself.

OD OVERDOSE MANAGEMENT
Symptoms: Extension of side effects. *Treatment:* Administer a fast-acting laxative.

DRUG INTERACTIONS
H-2 Antagonists / ↑ Plasma praziquantel levels → ↑ effectiveness and side effects
Hydantoins / Possible ↓ serum praziquantel levels

HOW SUPPLIED
Tablet: 600 mg

DOSAGE
• **TABLETS**
Schistosomiasis.
Three doses of 20 mg/kg as a 1-day treatment with an interval between doses not less than 4 hr or more than 6 hr.
Chonorchiasis and opisthorchiasis.
Three doses of 25 mg/kg as a 1-day treatment with an interval between doses not less than 4 hr or more than 6 hr.

NURSING CONSIDERATIONS

ASSESSMENT
1. Document indications for therapy, onset, characteristics, duration of symptoms, and source of infestation.
2. Determine if the schistosomiasis or fluke infection is accompanied by cerebral cysticercosis; if so, hospitalize for treatment.
3. Note any liver dysfunction as reduced dosage may be indicated.
4. List drugs currently prescribed to ensure none interact unfavorably or deactivate drug (i.e., hydantoins).

CLIENT/FAMILY TEACHING
1. Swallow tablets unchewed with liquid during meals. Keeping the tablets in the mouth may cause gagging or vomiting; do not chew the tablets as their bitter taste can cause retching and vomiting.
2. Use caution while driving or performing tasks requiring alertness; may cause dizziness/drowsiness, .
3. Do not nurse baby on treatment day and for 3 days following.
4. With schistosomiasis, larvae enter through the skin and are usually acquired by swimming in cercaria-infested water found in many parts of the world esp Africa and Middle East. Schistosomal worms are usually dead 7 days following treatment.
5. Report any high fever or sustained headaches with cestode infection. May require corticosteroids for treatment of cerebral cysticerosis caused by the pork tapeworm.

OUTCOMES/EVALUATE
Eradication of parasitic infestation; negative cultures

Prazosin hydrochloride

(**PRAY**-zoh-sin)

PREGNANCY CATEGORY: C
CLASSIFICATION(S):
Antihypertensive, alpha-1-adrenergic blocking drug
Rx: Minipress
✱Rx: Alti-Prazosin, Apo-Prazo, Novo-Prazin, Nu-Prazo

SEE ALSO *ALPHA-1-ADRENERGIC BLOCKING AGENTS* AND *ANTIHYPERTENSIVE AGENTS*.

ACTION/KINETICS
Produces selective blockade of postsynaptic alpha-1-adrenergic receptors. Dilates arterioles and veins, thereby decreasing total peripheral resistance and decreasing DBP more than SBP. CO, HR, and renal blood flow are not affected. Can be used to initiate antihypertensive therapy; most effective when used with other agents (e.g., diuretics, beta-adrenergic blocking agents). **Onset:** 2 hr. Absorption not affected by food. **Maximum effect:** 2–3 hr; **duration:** 6–12 hr. **t½:** 2–3 hr. Full therapeutic effect: 4–6 weeks. Metabolized extensively; excreted primarily in feces.

USES
Mild to moderate hypertension alone or in combination with other antihypertensive drugs. *Investigational:* CHF refractory to other treatment. Raynaud's disease, BPH.

SPECIAL CONCERNS
Safe use in children has not been established. Use with caution during lactation. Geriatric clients may be more sensitive to the hypotensive and hypothermic effects; may be necessary to decrease the dose in these clients due to age-related decreases in renal function.

SIDE EFFECTS
First-dose effect: Marked hypotension and syncope 30–90 min after administration of initial dose (usually 2 or more mg), increase of dosage, or addition of other antihypertensive agent. **CNS:** Dizziness, drowsiness, headache, fatigue, paresthesias, depression, vertigo, nervousness, hallucinations. **CV:** Palpitations, syncope, tachycardia, orthostatic hypotension, aggravation of angina. **GI:** N&V, diarrhea or constipation, dry mouth, abdominal pain, pancreatitis. **GU:** Urinary frequency or incontinence, impotence, priapism. **Respiratory:** Dyspnea, nasal congestion, epistaxis. **Dermatologic:** Pruritus, rash, sweating, alopecia, lichen planus. **Miscellaneous:** Asthenia, edema, symptoms of lupus erythematosus, blurred vision, tinnitus, arthralgia, myalgia, reddening of sclera, eye pain, conjunctivitis, edema, fever.

LABORATORY TEST CONSIDERATIONS
↑ Urinary metabolites of norepinephrine, VMA.

OD OVERDOSE MANAGEMENT
Symptoms: Hypotension, ***shock.*** *Treatment:* Keep client supine to restore BP and HR. If shock is manifested, use volume expanders and vasopressors; maintain renal function.

DRUG INTERACTIONS
Antihypertensives (other) / ↑ Antihypertensive effect
Beta-adrenergic blocking agents / Enhanced acute postural hypotension after first dose of prazosin
Clonidine / ↓ Antihypertensive effect
Diuretics / ↑ Antihypertensive effect
Indomethacin / ↓ Effect of prazosin
Nifedipine / ↑ Hypotensive effect
Propranolol / Especially pronounced additive hypotensive effect
Verapamil / ↑ Hypotensive effect; ↑ sensitivity to prazosin-induced postural hypotension

HOW SUPPLIED
Capsule: 1 mg, 2 mg, 5 mg

DOSAGE
- **CAPSULES**

Hypertension.
Individualized: Initial, 1 mg b.i.d.–t.i.d.; **maintenance:** if necessary, increase gradually to 6–15 mg/day in two to three divided doses. Do not exceed 20 mg/day, although some clients have benefitted from doses of 40 mg daily. If used with diuretics or other antihypertensives, reduce dose to 1–2 mg t.i.d. **Pediatric, less than 7 years of age, initial:** 0.25 mg b.i.d.–t.i.d. adjusted according to response. **Pediatric, 7–12 years of age, initial:** 0.5 mg b.i.d.–t.i.d. adjusted according to response.

NURSING CONSIDERATIONS

SEE ALSO NURSING CONSIDERATIONS FOR ANTIHYPERTENSIVE AGENTS AND ALPHA-1-ADRENERGIC BLOCKING AGENTS.

P

ADMINISTRATION/STORAGE

Reduce the dose to 1 or 2 mg t.i.d. if a diuretic or other antihypertensive agent is added to the regimen and then retitrate client.

CLIENT/FAMILY TEACHING

1. Take the first dose at bedtime. Also, take the first dose of each increment at bedtime to reduce the incidence of syncope.
2. Do not drive or operate machinery for 24 hr after the first dose; may cause dizziness and drowsiness.
3. Food may delay absorption and minimize side effects of the drug.
4. Avoid rapid changes in body position that may precipitate weakness, dizziness, and syncope. Lie down or sit down and put head below knees to avoid fainting if a rapid heartbeat is felt.
5. Avoid dangerous situations that may lead to fainting.
6. Report any bothersome side effects because reduction in dosage may be indicated. Use sips of water and sugarless gum or candies for dry mouth effects.
7. Do not stop medication unless directed.
8. Avoid cold, cough, and allergy medications. The sympathomimetic component of such medications will interfere with the action of prazosin.
9. Comply with prescribed drug regimen; full drug effect may not be evident for 4–6 weeks.

OUTCOMES/EVALUATE

↓ BP; ↓ symptoms of refractory CHF

P

Prednisolone

(pred-**NISS**-oh-lohn)

PREGNANCY CATEGORY: C
Rx: Syrup: Prelone., **Tablets:** Delta-Cortef

Prednisolone acetate

(pred-**NISS**-oh-lohn)

PREGNANCY CATEGORY: C
Rx: Ophthalmic Suspension: Econopred, Econopred Plus, Key-Pred 25 and 50, **Parenteral:** Pred Forte Ophthalmic, Pred Mild Ophthalmic, Predalone 50, Predcor-50, Prednisolone Acetate Ophthalmic
✱Rx: Ophthalmic Suspension: Diopred, Ophtho-Tate

Prednisolone sodium phosphate

(pred-**NISS**-oh-lohn)

PREGNANCY CATEGORY: C
Rx: Ophthalmic Solution: AK-Pred Ophthalmic, **Oral Solution:** Orapred, Inflamase Forte Ophthalmic, Inflamase Mild Ophthalmic, Pediapred, **Oral Solution:** Key-Pred-SP, **Parenteral:** Hydeltrasol

Prednisolone tebutate

(pred-**NISS**-oh-lohn)

PREGNANCY CATEGORY: C
Rx: Prednisol TPA
CLASSIFICATION(S):
Glucocorticoid

SEE ALSO *CORTICOSTEROIDS*.

ACTION/KINETICS

Intermediate-acting. Is five times more potent than hydrocortisone and cortisone. Minimal side effects except for GI distress. Moderate mineralocorticoid activity. **Plasma t½:** over 200 min.

CONTRAINDICATIONS

Lactation.

SPECIAL CONCERNS

Use with particular caution in diabetes.

HOW SUPPLIED

Prednisolone: *Syrup:* 5 mg/5 mL, 15 mg/5 mL; *Tablet:* 5 mg. **Prednisolone acetate:** *Injection:* 25 mg/mL, 50 mg/mL; *Ophthalmic Suspension:* 0.12%, 0.125%, 1%. **Prednisolone sodium phosphate:** *Injection:* 20 mg/mL; *Liquid, Oral:* 5 mg/5 mL, 15 mg (base)/5 mL; *Ophthalmic Solution:* 0.125%, 1%. **Prednisolone tebutate:** *Injection:* 20 mg/mL.

DOSAGE

PREDNISOLONE

- **TABLETS, SYRUP**

Most uses.

5–60 mg/day, depending on disease being treated.

Multiple sclerosis (exacerbation).
200 mg/day for 1 week; **then,** 80 mg on alternate days for 1 month.
Pleurisy of tuberculosis.
0.75 mg/kg/day (then taper) given concurrently with antituberculosis therapy.
PREDNISOLONE ACETATE
• **IM**
4–60 mg/day. **Not for IV use.**
Multiple sclerosis (exacerbation).
See *Prednisolone.*
• **INTRALESIONAL, INTRA-ARTICULAR, SOFT TISSUE INJECTION**
4–100 mg (larger doses for large joints).
• **OPHTHALMIC SUSPENSION (0.12%, 0.125%, 1%)**
Instill 1–2 gtt into the conjunctival sac b.i.d.–q.i.d. During the first 24 to 48 hr, the frequency of dosing may be increased if necessary.
PREDNISOLONE SODIUM PHOSPHATE
• **PO SOLUTION**
Most uses.
5–60 mg/day in single or divided doses.
Adrenocortical insufficiency.
Pediatric: 0.14 mg/kg (4 mg/m^2) daily in three to four divided doses.
Other pediatric uses.
0.5–2 mg/kg (15–60 mg/m^2) daily in three to four divided doses.
• **IM, IV**
4–60 mg/day.
Multiple sclerosis (exacerbation).
See *Prednisolone.*
• **INTRALESIONAL, INTRA-ARTICULAR, SOFT TISSUE INJECTION**
2–30 mg, depending on site and severity of disease.
• **OPHTHALMIC SOLUTION (0.125%, 1%)**
1–2 gtt into the conjunctival sac q hr during the day and q 2 hr during the night; **then,** after response obtained, decrease dose to 1 gtt q 4 hr and then later 1 gtt t.i.d.–q.i.d.
PREDNISOLONE TEBUTATE
• **INTRA-ARTICULAR, INTRALESIONAL, SOFT TISSUE INJECTION**
4–30 mg, depending on site and severity of disease. Doses higher than 40 mg are not recommended.

NURSING CONSIDERATIONS

SEE ALSO *NURSING CONSIDERATIONS* FOR *CORTICOSTEROIDS.*

ADMINISTRATION/STORAGE

1. Before administering, check spelling and dose carefully; is frequently confused with prednisone.
2. Check if provider wants PO form administered with an antacid.
3. Prednisolone sodium phosphate oral solution produces a 20% higher peak plasma level than tablets.
4. Shake the suspension well before using.
IV 5. The IV form (sodium phosphate) may be administered at a rate not to exceed 10 mg/min.

ASSESSMENT

1. Document indications for therapy, onset and characteristics of symptoms. Note any previous experiences with this drug and the outcome.
2. Monitor VS, CBC, electrolytes, blood sugar, weight, and mental status.

CLIENT/FAMILY TEACHING

1. Take as directed and do not stop suddenly without provider approval as adrenal crisis may occur.
2. Report any loss of effect as dose may need adjustment.
3. Avoid exposure to infected persons and crowds.
4. Report nausea, anorexia, fatigue, joint pain, weakness, dizziness, or sob; symptoms of adrenal insufficiency.
5. With joint injections, do not overuse joint after therapy despite improvement in rom and pain.
6. Assess for weight gain and adjust diet and exercise to control.

OUTCOMES/EVALUATE

• Replacement therapy during adrenocortical hypofunction
• Symptomatic relief of allergic, immune, and inflammatory manifestations

Prednisone

(**PRED**-nih-sohn)

PREGNANCY CATEGORY: C

P

CLASSIFICATION(S):
Glucocorticoid
Rx: Oral Solution: Prednisone Intensol Concentrate. **Syrup:** Liquid Pred. **Tablets:** Deltasone, Meticorten, Orasone 1, 5, 10, 20, and 50, Panasol-S, Prednicen-M, Sterapred DS
★Rx: Tablets: Apo-Prednisone, Winpred

SEE ALSO *CORTICOSTEROIDS*.

ACTION/KINETICS
Three to five times as potent as cortisone or hydrocortisone. May cause moderate fluid retention. Metabolized in the liver to prednisolone, the active form.

SPECIAL CONCERNS
Dose must be highly individualized.

HOW SUPPLIED
Oral Solution: 5 mg/5 mL; *Syrup:* 5 mg/5 mL; *Tablet:* 1 mg, 2.5 mg, 5 mg, 10 mg, 20 mg, 50 mg

DOSAGE

- **ORAL SOLUTION, SYRUP, TABLETS**

Acute, severe conditions.

Initial: 5–60 mg/day in four equally divided doses after meals and at bedtime. Decrease gradually by 5–10 mg q 4–5 days to establish minimum maintenance dosage (5–10 mg) or discontinue altogether until symptoms recur.

Replacement.

Pediatric: 0.1–0.15 mg/kg/day.

COPD.

30–60 mg/day for 1–2 weeks; then taper.

Ophthalmopathy due to Graves' disease.

60 mg/day; **then,** taper to 20 mg/day.

Duchenne's muscular dystrophy.

0.75–1.5 mg/kg/day (used to improve strength).

NURSING CONSIDERATIONS

SEE ALSO *NURSING CONSIDERATIONS* FOR *CORTICOSTEROIDS*.

ASSESSMENT

1. Document indications for therapy, type, onset, and characteristics of symptoms. List other agents prescribed and the outcome.
2. Monitor CBC, ESR, electrolytes, blood sugar, weights, and mental status.
3. With chronic back pain, titrate dose to assess for relief; if relief attained may send for trigger point injections. Generally if pain is diffuse/severe or involves joints other than spine, trigger point injections are usually not effective. Titrate to lowest dose possible to control symptoms and to ensure adequate physical functioning level. Address benefits versus risks with client and family.
4. With COPD provide rescue doses and instruct client how and when to use i.e during acute exacerbation when sputum is clear to white and no fever. May suggest 30mg to start and decrease by 5 mg per day until down to 5 mg and continue for 5 days then off. If no relief advise to call for instructions or seek hospitalization depending on severity of symptoms.

CLIENT/FAMILY TEACHING

1. Take in the morning to prevent insomnia and with food to decrease GI upset.
2. Do not stop abruptly with long-term therapy. Take as directed and wean when indicated.
3. Report any S&S of adrenal insufficiency or loss of effectiveness.
4. Avoid alcohol and OTC agents.
5. With weight gain, adjust caloric intake and exercise to control.
6. Avoid vaccines, crowds and infected persons when on suppressive therapy.

OUTCOMES/EVALUATE
Relief of allergic, immune, and inflammatory manifestations

Primaquine phosphate

(**PRIM**-ah-kwin)

PREGNANCY CATEGORY: C
CLASSIFICATION(S):
Antimalarial, 8-aminoquinolone

ACTION/KINETICS
Mechanism of action not known, but the drug binds to and may alter the properties of DNA leading to decreased protein synthesis. Both the gametocyte and exoerythrocyte forms

are inhibited. Some gametocytes are destroyed while others cannot undergo maturation division in the gut of the mosquito. Well absorbed from GI tract. **Peak plasma levels:** 1–3 hr. Poorly distributed in body tissues. **t½ elimination:** 4 hr. Rapidly metabolized.

USES

Only for the radical cure of *Plasmodium vivax* malaria, the prophylaxis of relapse in *P. vivax* malaria, or following the termination of chloroquine phosphate suppressive therapy in areas where *P. vivax* is endemic.

CONTRAINDICATIONS

Concomitant use with quinacrine. In clients with rheumatoid arthritis or lupus erythematosus who are acutely ill or who have a tendency to develop granulocytopenia. Concomitant use with other bone marrow depressants or hemolytic drugs.

SPECIAL CONCERNS

Use during pregnancy only when benefits outweigh risks.

SIDE EFFECTS

GI: Abdominal cramps, epigastric distress, N&V. **Hematologic:** Leukopenia. Methemoglobinemia in NADH methemoglobin reductase deficient individuals. Blacks and members of certain Mediterranean ethnic groups (Sardinians, Sephardic Jews, Greeks, Iranians) manifest a high incidence of G6PD deficiency and as a result have a low tolerance for primaquine. These individuals manifest ***marked hemolytic anemia*** following primaquine administration. **Miscellaneous:** Headache, pruritus, interference with visual accommodation, ***cardiac arrhythmias,*** hypertension.

OD OVERDOSE MANAGEMENT

Symptoms: Abdominal cramps, vomiting, burning and epigastric distress, cyanosis, methemoglobinemia, anemia, moderate leukocytosis or leukopenia, CNS and CV disturbances. Granulocytopenia and ***acute hemolytic anemia*** in sensitive clients. *Treatment:* Treat symptoms.

DRUG INTERACTIONS

Bone marrow depressants, hemolytic drugs / Additive side effects

Quinacrine / ↓ Metabolic degradation of primaquine → ↑ effects. **Do not give primaquine** to clients who are receiving or have received quinacrine within the past 3 months.

HOW SUPPLIED

Tablet: 26.3 mg

DOSAGE

• TABLETS

Acute attack of vivax malaria, clients with parasitized RBCs.

15 mg (base) daily for 14 days together with chloroquine phosphate (to destroy erythrocytic parasites).

Suppression of malaria.

Adults: 26.3 mg (15 mg base) daily for 14 days or 78.9 mg once a week for 8 weeks; **children:** 0.5 mg/kg/day (0.3 mg/kg base) for 14 days.

NURSING CONSIDERATIONS

SEE ALSO *GENERAL NURSING CONSIDERATIONS* FOR *ANTI-INFECTIVES*

ADMINISTRATION/STORAGE

1. Store in tightly closed containers.
2. For suppression therapy, initiate during the last 2 weeks of or after suppressive therapy with chloroquine or a similar drug.

ASSESSMENT

1. Note any history of rheumatoid arthritis or lupus.
2. List other drugs prescribed to ensure no unfavorable interactions.
3. Determine if pregnant. Do not give during first trimester and preferably not until after delivery.
4. Obtain hematologic profile and cultures. Monitor for indications to withdraw drug: dark urine may indicate hemolysis.
5. Assess dark-skinned clients closely. Because of a possible inborn deficiency of G6PD, these clients are particularly susceptible to hemolytic anemia while on primaquine.

CLIENT/FAMILY TEACHING

1. Take immediately before or after meals or with antacids to minimize gastric irritation.
2. For suppressive therapy, take drug on same day each week.

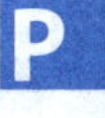

3. Monitor color of urine; report darkening or brown discoloration.
4. Must complete a full course of therapy for effective results.
5. Report GI, CNS, and CV disturbances; symptoms of overdose.

OUTCOMES/EVALUATE

Termination of acute malarial attacks; suppression of malarial symptoms

Primidone

(**PRIH**-mih-dohn)

CLASSIFICATION(S):
Anticonvulsant, miscellaneous
Rx: Mysoline
✱Rx: Apo-Primidone

ACTION/KINETICS

Closely related to the barbiturates; however, the anticonvulsant mechanism is unknown. Produces a greater sedative effect than barbiturates when used for seizure treatment. Side effects usually subside with use. **Peak plasma levels:** 3 hr. Primidone is converted in the liver to two active metabolites, phenobarbital and phenylethylmalonamide (PEMA). **Peak plasma levels (PEMA):** 7–8 hr. **t¹/₂ (primidone):** 5–15 hr; **t¹/₂ (PEMA):** 10–18 hr; **t¹/₂ (phenobarbital):** 53–140 hr. The appearance of phenobarbital in the plasma may be delayed several days after initiation of therapy. **Therapeutic plasma levels, primadone:** 5–12 mcg/mL; **phenobarbital,** 15–40 mcg/mL. Primidone and metabolites are excreted through the kidneys, although 40% of primidone is excreted unchanged.

USES

Alone or with other anticonvulsants to treat psychomotor, focal , or tonic-clonic seizures (including those refractory to barbiturate-hydantoin regimens). *Investigational:* Benign familial tremor.

CONTRAINDICATIONS

Porphyria. Hypersensitivity to phenobarbital. Lactation.

SPECIAL CONCERNS

Safe use during pregnancy has not been determined. Use during lactation may result in drowsiness in the neonate. Children and geriatric clients may react to primidone with restlessness and excitement. Abrupt withdrawal may precipitate status epilepticus.

SIDE EFFECTS

CNS: Drowsiness, ataxia, vertigo, fatigue, hyperirritability, emotional disturbances, personality disturbances with mood changes and paranoia. **GI:** N&V, anorexia, painful gums. **Hematologic:** Megaloblastic anemia, thrombocytopenia. **Ophthalmologic:** Diplopia, nystagmus. **Miscellaneous:** Impotence, morbilliform and maculopapular skin rashes. Occasionally has caused hyperexcitability, especially in children. ***Postpartum hemorrhage and hemorrhagic disease of the newborn.*** Symptoms of SLE.

DRUG INTERACTIONS

SEE ALSO *BARBITURATES.*

Acetazolamide / ↓ Effect of primidone R/T ↓ levels
Carbamazepine / ↓ Plasma levels of primidone and phenobarbital and ↑ plasma levels of carbamazepine
Hydantoins / ↑ Plasma levels of primidone, phenobarbital, and PEMA
Isoniazid / ↑ Effect of primidone R/T ↓ liver breakdown
Nicotinamide / ↑ Effect of primidone R/T ↓ rate of clearance from body
Oral contraceptives / ↓ Plasma levels of estrogens/progestins → ↓ effect
Succinimides / ↓ Plasma levels of primidone and phenobarbital

HOW SUPPLIED

Suspension: 250 mg/5 mL; *Tablet:* 50 mg, 250 mg

DOSAGE

- **ORAL SUSPENSION, TABLETS**

Seizures, in clients on no other anticonvulsant medication.

Adults and children over 8 years, initial: Days 1–3, 100–125 mg at bedtime; days 4–6, 100–125 mg b.i.d.; days 7–9, 100–125 mg t.i.d.; **maintenance:** 250 mg t.i.d.–q.i.d. (may be increased to 250 mg 5–6 times/day; not to exceed 500 mg q.i.d.). **Children under 8 years, initial:** days 1–3, 50 mg at bedtime; days 4–6, 50 mg b.i.d.; days 7–9, 100 mg b.i.d.; **maintenance:** 125 mg b.i.d.–250 mg t.i.d. (10–25 mg/kg in divided doses).

Seizures, in clients receiving other anticonvulsants.
Initial: 100–125 mg at bedtime; **then,** increase to maintenance levels as other drug is slowly withdrawn (transition should take at least 2 weeks).

Benign familial tremor.
750 mg/day.

NURSING CONSIDERATIONS

SEE ALSO *NURSING CONSIDERATIONS* FOR *ANTICONVULSANTS.*

ADMINISTRATION/STORAGE

Due to bioequivalence problems, brand interchange is not recommended unless bioavailability data are available.

ASSESSMENT

1. Document age of seizure onset, frequency of occurrence, characteristics, and cause if known.
2. List other agents prescribed and the outcome.
3. Monitor CBC, liver and renal function studies.

CLIENT/FAMILY TEACHING

1. May be taken with food if GI upset occurs.
2. Review the following conditions that should be reported:
   - Hyperexcitability in children
   - Excessive loss of hair
   - Edema of eyelids and legs
   - Visual disturbances
   - Mental status changes
   - Impotence
   - Loss of seizure control
3. Vitamin K may be prescribed during the last month of pregnancy to prevent postpartum hemorrhage in the mother and hemorrhagic disease of the newborn.
4. Do not stop abruptly as withdrawal symptoms may occur.
5. Avoid alcohol and CNS depressants. Do not perform activities that require mental alertness until drug effects realized; may cause dizziness and drowsiness.

OUTCOMES/EVALUATE

- Control of refractory seizures
- Therapeutic drug levels (5–12 mcg/mL)

Probenecid

(proh-**BEN**-ih-sid)

PREGNANCY CATEGORY: B
CLASSIFICATION(S):
Antigout drug, uricosuric
✱Rx: Benuryl

ACTION/KINETICS

A uricosuric agent that increases the excretion of uric acid by inhibiting the tubular reabsorption of uric acid; this results in a decreased serum level of uric acid. Also inhibits the renal secretion of penicillins and cephalosporins; this effect is often taken advantage of in the treatment of infections because concomitant administration of probenecid will increase plasma levels of antibiotics. **Peak plasma levels:** 2–4 hr. **Time to peak effect, uricosuric:** 0.5 hr; **for suppression of penicillin excretion:** 2 hr. **Therapeutic plasma levels for inhibition of antibiotic secretion:** 40–60 mcg/mL; **therapeutic plasma levels for uricosuric effect:** 100–200 mcg/mL. **t½:** approximately 5–8 hr. **Duration for inhibition of penicillin excretion:** 8 hr. Metabolized in the liver to active metabolites; excreted in urine (5%–10% unchanged). Excretion is increased in alkaline urine.

USES

(1) Hyperuricemia in chronic gout and gouty arthritis. (2) Adjunct in therapy with penicillins or cephalosporins to elevate and prolong plasma antibiotic levels.

CONTRAINDICATIONS

Hypersensitivity to drug, blood dyscrasias, uric acid, and kidney stones. Use for hyperuricemia in neoplastic disease or its treatment. Use in children less than 2 years of age. Concomitant use of salicylates or use with penicillin in renal impairment.

SPECIAL CONCERNS

Use with caution in renal disease, porphyria, G6PD deficiency, history of allergy to sulfa drugs, and peptic ulcer.

P

SIDE EFFECTS

CNS: Headaches, dizziness. **GI:** Anorexia, N&V, diarrhea, constipation, and abdominal discomfort. **Allergic:** Skin rash, dermatitis, pruritus, drug fever, and rarely ***anaphylaxis.*** **GU:** Nephrotic syndrome, uric acid stones with or without hematuria, urinary frequency, renal colic or costovertebral pain. **Miscellaneous:** Flushing, ***hemolytic anemia (possibly related to G6PD deficiency),*** anemia, sore gums, ***hepatic necrosis, aplastic anemia.***

Initially, the drug may increase frequency of acute gout attacks due to mobilization of uric acid.

DRUG INTERACTIONS

Acyclovir / ↓ Renal excretion of acyclovir
Allopurinol / Additive effects to ↓ uric acid serum levels
AZT / ↑ Bioavailability of AZT; possible malaise, myalgia, fever
Benzodiazepines / More rapid onset and longer duration of benzodiazepine effects
Cephalosporins / ↑ Cephalosporin effect R/T ↓ kidney excretion
Ciprofloxacin / 50% ↑ in systemic levels of ciprofloxacin
Clofibrate / ↑ Clofibric acid (active) levels → ↑ effects
Dapsone / ↑ Dapsone effects
Dyphylline / ↑ Dyphylline effect R/T ↓ kidney excretion
Methotrexate / ↑ Methotrexate effect and toxicity R/T ↓ kidney excretion
Niacin ↓ Uric acid-lowering effects of probenecid
NSAIDs / ↑ NSAID effects R/T ↓ kidney excretion
Pantothenic acid / ↑ Pantothenic acid effects
Penicillamine / ↓ Penicillamine effects
Penicillins / ↑ Pencillin effects R/T ↓ kidney excretion
Pyrazinamide / Inhibits hyperuricemia produced by pyrazinamide
Rifampin / ↑ Rifampin effects R/T ↓ kidney excretion
Salicylates / Inhibits uricosuric activity of probenecid
Sulfinpyrazone / ↑ Sulfinpyrazone effects R/T ↓ kidney excretion
Sulfonamides / ↑ Sulfonamide effects R/T ↓ plasma protein binding
Sulfonylureas, oral / ↑ Sulfonylurea effect → ↑ hypoglycemia
Thiopental / ↑ Thiopental effects

HOW SUPPLIED

Tablet: 500 mg

DOSAGE

• TABLETS

Gout.

Adults, initial: 250 mg b.i.d. for 1 week. **Maintenance:** 500 mg b.i.d. Dosage may have to be increased further (by 500 mg/day q 4 weeks to maximum of 2 g) until urate excretion is less than 700 mg in 24 hr. Colbenemid, a combination tablet containing colchicine (0.5 mg) and probenecid (500 mg), is available.

Adjunct to penicillin or cephalosporin therapy.

Adults: 500 mg q.i.d. Dosage is decreased for elderly clients with renal damage. **Pediatric, 2–14 years, initial:** 25 mg/kg (or 700 mg/m^2); **maintenance,** 10 mg/kg q.i.d. (or 300 mg/m^2 q.i.d.). **For children 50 kg or more:** give adult dosage.

Gonorrhea, uncomplicated.

Adults: 1 g (as a single dose) 30 min before 4.8 million units of penicillin G procaine aqueous; **pediatric, less than 45 kg:** 25 mg/kg (up to a maximum of 1 g) with appropriate antibiotic therapy.

Neurosyphilis.

Adults: 0.5 g q.i.d. with penicillin G procaine aqueous, 2.4 million units/day IM, both for 10–14 days.

Pelvic inflammatory disease.

Adults: 1 g (as a single dose) plus cefoxitin, 2 g IM given concurrently.

NURSING CONSIDERATIONS

ADMINISTRATION/STORAGE

1. Do not start therapy until acute gouty attack has subsided. If an acute attack is precipitated during therapy, continue the drug.
2. To prevent kidney stones, take at least 6 to 8 (8-oz) glasses of water.
3. Maintain an alkaline urine by taking sodium bicarbonate, 3–7.5 g/day, or potassium citrate, 7.5 g/day.

ASSESSMENT

1. Document indications for therapy, type, onset and characteristics of symptoms.
2. Determine any PUD, G6PD deficiency, uricemia R/T neoplastic disease, kidney stones, sulfa allergy, or blood dyscrasia.
3. Assess involved joints, noting pain, inflammation, heat, swelling, deformity, and ROM.
4. Monitor CBC, uric acid, liver and renal function studies. Note urate excretion levels and urine alkalinity as urates crystalize in acid urine.
5. Hypersensitivity reactions may occur more frequently with intermittent therapy.
6. Assess for toxic plasma antibiotic levels if excretion is inhibited by probenecid; adjust dosage.

CLIENT/FAMILY TEACHING

1. Take with food or milk to minimize gastric irritation. Report gastric intolerance so dosage may be corrected without loss of therapeutic effect.
2. Take a liberal amount of fluid (2.5–3 L/day) to prevent the formation of sodium urate stones. Avoid cranberry juice or vitamin C preparations, which acidify urine. Sodium bicarbonate may be used to maintain an alkaline urine to prevent urates from crystallizing and forming kidney stones.
3. Acute gout attacks may initially be more frequent due to mobilization of uric acid. Report any increase in the number of acute attacks at the initiation of therapy since colchicine may need to be added. Continue to take during acute attacks with colchicine unless otherwise specified.
4. Report any unexplained fever, fatigue, skin rash, persistent GI upset, flushing, increased sweating, headaches, or dizziness.
5. Do not take salicylates or use caffeine or alcohol during uricosuric therapy. Acetaminophen preparations may be used for analgesia.
6. Monitor FS closely; drug may increase hypoglycemic effects of PO antidiabetic agents.

OUTCOMES/EVALUATE

- ↓ Uric acid levels; ↓ gout attacks
- ↓ Joint pain and swelling
- Elevated/prolonged antibiotic (penicillin or cephalosporin) levels

Procainamide hydrochloride

(proh-**KAYN**-ah-myd)

PREGNANCY CATEGORY: C
CLASSIFICATION(S):
Antiarrhythmic, Class IA
Rx: Procanbid, Pronestyl-SR , Pronestyl
✱**Rx:** Apo-Procainamide, Procan SR

SEE ALSO *ANTIARRHYTHMIC AGENTS.*

ACTION/KINETICS

Produces a direct cardiac effect to prolong the refractory period of the atria and to a lesser extent the bundle of His-Purkinje system and ventricles. Large doses may cause AV block. Some anticholinergic and local anesthetic effects. **Onset: PO,** 30 min; **IV,** 1–5 min. **Time to peak effect, PO:** 90–120 min; **IM,** 15–60 min; **IV,** immediate. **Duration:** 3 hr. **t½:** 2.5–4.7 hr. **Therapeutic serum level:** 4–8 mcg/mL. **Protein binding:** 15%. From 40% to 70% excreted unchanged. Metabolized in the liver (16%–21% by slow acetylators and 24%–33% by fast acetylators) to the active N-acetylprocainamide (NAPA); has antiarrhythmic properties with a longer half-life than procainamide.

USES

Documented ventricular arrhythmias (e.g., sustained ventricular tachycardia) that may be life threatening in clients where benefits of treatment clearly outweigh risks. Antiarrhythmic drugs have not been shown to improve survival in clients with ventricular arrhythmias.

CONTRAINDICATIONS

Hypersensitivity to drug, complete AV heart block, lupus erythematosus, torsades de pointes, asymptomatic ventric-

P

ular premature contractions. Lactation.

SPECIAL CONCERNS

There is an increased risk of death in those with non-life-threatening arrhythmias. Although used in children, safety and efficacy have not been established. Use with extreme caution in clients for whom a sudden drop in BP could be detrimental, in CHF, acute ischemic heart disease, or cardiomyopathy. Also, use with caution in clients with liver or kidney dysfunction, preexisting bone marrow failure or cytopenia of any type, development of first-degree heart block while on procainamide, myasthenia gravis, and those with bronchial asthma or other respiratory disorders. May cause more hypotension in geriatric clients; also, in this population, the dose may have to be decreased due to age-related decreases in renal function.

SIDE EFFECTS

Body as a whole: Lupus erythematosus–like syndrome especially in those on maintenance therapy and who are slow acetylators. Symptoms include arthralgia, pleural or abdominal pain, arthritis, pleural effusion, pericarditis, fever, chills, myalgia, skin lesions, hematologic changes. **CV:** Following IV use: Hypotension, ***ventricular asystole or fibrillation, partial or complete heart block.*** Rarely, second-degree heart block after PO use. **GI:** N&V, diarrhea, anorexia, bitter taste, abdominal pain. **Hematologic:** Thrombocytopenia, ***agranulocytosis,*** neutropenia. ***Rarely, hemolytic anemia.*** **Dermatologic:** Urticaria, pruritus, angioneurotic edema, flushing, maculopapular rash. **CNS:** Depression, dizziness, weakness, giddiness, psychoses, hallucinations. **Other:** Granulomatous hepatitis, weakness, fever, chills.

LABORATORY TEST CONSIDERATIONS

May affect LFTs. False + ↑ in serum alkaline phosphatase. Positive ANA test. High levels of lidocaine and meprobamate may inhibit fluorescence of procainamide and NAPA.

OD OVERDOSE MANAGEMENT

Symptoms: Plasma levels of 10–15 mcg/mL are associated with toxic symptoms. Progressive widening of the QRS complex, prolonged QT or PR intervals, lowering of R and T waves, increased AV block, increased ventricular extrasystoles, ***ventricular tachycardia or fibrillation. IV overdose may result in hypotension, CNS depression, tremor, respiratory depression.*** *Treatment:*

- Induce emesis or perform gastric lavage followed by administration of activated charcoal.
- To treat hypotension, give IV fluids and/or a vasopressor (dopamine, phenylephrine, or norepinephrine).
- Infusion of 1⁄6 molar sodium lactate IV reduces the cardiotoxic effects.
- Hemodialysis (but not peritoneal dialysis) is effective in reducing serum levels.
- Renal clearance can be enhanced by acidification of the urine and with high flow rates.
- A ventricular pacing electrode can be inserted as a precaution in the event AV block develops.

DRUG INTERACTIONS

Acetazolamide / ↑ Procainamide effect R/T ↓ kidney excretion
Anticholinergic agents, atropine / Additive anticholinergic effects
Antihypertensive agents / Additive hypotensive effect
Cholinergic agents / Anticholinergic activity of procainamide antagonizes effect of cholinergic drugs
Cimetidine / ↑ Procainamide effect R/T ↑ bioavailability
Disopyramide / ↑ Risk of enhanced prolongation of conduction or depression of contractility and hypotension
Ethanol / Effect of procainamide may be altered, but because the main metabolite is active as an antiarrhythmic, specific outcome not clear
H *Henbane leaf* / ↑ Anticholinergic effects
Kanamycin / ↑ Kanamycin-induced muscle relaxation
Lidocaine / Additive cardiodepressant effects
Magnesium salts / ↑ Magnesium-induced muscle relaxation

Neomycin / ↑ Neomycin-induced muscle relaxation
Propranolol / ↑ Serum procainamide levels
Quinidine / ↑ Risk of enhanced prolongation of conduction or depression of contractility and hypotension
Ranitidine / ↑ Procainamide effect R/T ↑ bioavailability
Sodium bicarbonate / ↑ Procainamide effect R/T ↓ kidney excretion
Succinylcholine / ↑ Succinylcholine-induced muscle relaxation
Trimethoprim / ↑ Procainamide effect R/T ↑ serum levels

HOW SUPPLIED

Capsule: 250 mg, 375 mg, 500 mg; *Injection:* 100 mg/mL, 500 mg/mL; *Tablet:* 250 mg, 375 mg, 500 mg; *Tablet, extended release:* 250 mg, 500 mg, 750 mg, 1000 mg

DOSAGE

• CAPSULES, EXTENDED-RELEASE TABLETS, TABLETS

Adults, initial: 50 mg/kg/day in divided doses q 3 hr. **Usual, 40–50 kg:** 250 mg q 3 hr of standard formulation or 500 mg q 6 hr of sustained-release; **60–70 kg:** 375 mg q 3 hr of standard formulation or 750 mg q 6 hr of sustained-release; **80–90 kg:** 500 mg q 3 hr of standard formulation or 1 g q 6 hr of sustained-release; **over 100 kg:** 625 mg q 3 hr of standard formulation or 1.25 g q 6 hr of sustained-release. **Pediatric:** 15–50 mg/kg/day divided q 3–6 hr (up to a maximum of 4 g/day).

• PROCANBID EXTENDED-RELEASE TABLETS

Life-threatening arrhythmias.

500 or 1,000 mg b.i.d.

• IM

Ventricular arrhythmias.

Adults, initial: 50 mg/kg/day divided into fractional doses of 1/8–1/4 given q 3–6 hr until PO therapy is possible. **Pediatric:** 20–30 mg/kg/day divided q 4–6 hr (up to a maximum of 4 g/day).

Arrhythmias associated with surgery or anesthesia.

Adults: 100–500 mg.

• IV

Initial loading infusion: 20 mg/min (for up to 25–30 min). **Maintenance infusion:** 2–6 mg/min. **Pediatric, initial loading dose:** 3–5 mg/kg/dose over 5 min (maximum of 100 mg); **maintenance:** 20–80 mcg/kg/min continuous infusion (maximum of 2 g/day).

NURSING CONSIDERATIONS

SEE ALSO *NURSING CONSIDERATIONS* FOR *ANTIARRHYTHMIC AGENTS.*

ADMINISTRATION/STORAGE

1. Procainamide HCl extended-release is *not* interchangeable with procainamide HCl sustained-release.
2. Extended-release tablets are not recommended for use in children or for initiating treatment.
3. IM therapy may be used as an alternative to PO in clients with less threatening arrhythmias but who are nauseated or vomiting, who cannot take anything PO (e.g., preoperatively), or who have malabsorptive problems.
4. If more than three IM injections are required, assess the age, renal function, and blood levels of procainamide and NAPA; adjust dosage accordingly.
IV 5. Reserve IV use for emergency situations.
6. For IV initial therapy, dilute the drug with D5W; give a maximum of 1 g slowly to minimize side effects by one of the following methods:

• Direct injection into a vein or into tubing of an established infusion line at a rate not to exceed 50 mg/min. Dilute either the 100- or 500-mg/mL vials prior to injection to facilitate control of the dosage rate. Doses of 100 mg may be given q 5 min until arrhythmia is suppressed or until 500 mg has been given (then wait 10 or more min before resuming administration).
• Loading infusion containing 20 mg/mL (1 g diluted with 50 mL of D5W) given at a constant rate of 1 mL/min for 25–30 min to deliver 500–600 mg.

P

7. For IV maintenance infusion, dose is usually 2–6 mg/min. Administer with electronic infusion device.
8. Discard solutions that are darker than light amber or otherwise colored. Solutions that have turned slightly yellow on standing may be used. Consult pharmacist if unsure.

ASSESSMENT

1. Document indications for therapy, type, onset, and characteristics of symptoms. List other agents prescribed and the outcome.
2. Assess cardiopulmonary status and note findings. Note any sensitivity to tartrazine, pregnancy, or heart block.
3. Monitor VS, ECG, CBC, electrolytes, ANA titers, liver and renal function studies.

INTERVENTIONS

1. Place in a supine position during IV infusion and monitor BP. Discontinue if SBP falls 15 mm Hg or more during administration or if increased SA or AV block is noted.
2. Reduce dose with liver or renal dysfunction, or if client <120 lbs.
3. Assess for symptoms of SLE, manifested by polyarthralgia, arthritis, pleuritic pain, fever, myalgia, and skin lesions.

CLIENT/FAMILY TEACHING

1. Take with a full glass of water to lessen GI symptoms. Take either 1 hr before or 2 hr after meals.
2. If GI symptoms are severe and persistent may take with meals or with a snack to ensure adherence.
3. Sustained-release preparations should be swallowed whole. They should not be crushed, broken, or chewed. The wax matrix of sustained-release tablets may be evident in the stool and is considered normal.
4. Report any sore throat, fever, rash, chills, bruising, diarrhea or increased palpitations. With long term use may note loss of effectiveness.
5. Do not take any OTC drugs.

OUTCOMES/EVALUATE

- Termination of arrhythmias with restoration of stable cardiac rhythm
- Therapeutic drug levels (4–8 mcg/mL)

Procarbazine hydrochloride (PCB, MIH, N-Methylhydrazine)

(pro-**KAR**-bah-zeen)

PREGNANCY CATEGORY: D
CLASSIFICATION(S):
Antineoplastic, miscellaneous
Rx: Matulane
★**Rx:** Natulan

SEE ALSO *ANTINEOPLASTIC AGENTS.*

ACTION/KINETICS

May inhibit synthesis of protein, RNA, and DNA and inhibit transmethylation of methyl groups of methionine into t-RNA. Absences of t-RNA could result in cessation of protein synthesis and subsequently DNA and RNA synthesis. Also, hydrogen peroxide formed during auto-oxidation of the drug may attack protein sulfhydryl groups found in residual protein that is tightly bound to DNA. Rapidly absorbed from GI tract. Drug equilibrates between plasma and CSF (peak CSF levels occur within 30–90 min and peak plasma levels occur within 60 min). **t½, after IV:** 10 min. Metabolized in the liver and kidneys to cytotoxic products. About 70% eliminated in urine, mostly as metabolites, after 24 hr.

USES

As an adjunct in the treatment of Hodgkin's disease (stage III and stage IV) as part of MOPP (nitrogen mustard, vincristine, procarbazine, prednisone) or ChIVPP (chlorambucil, vinblastine, procarbazine, prednisone) therapies. *Investigational:* Non-Hodgkin's lymphomas, malignant melanoma, primary brain tumors, lung cancer, multiple myeloma, polycythemia vera.

CONTRAINDICATIONS

Inadequate bone marrow reserve as shown by bone marrow aspiration (i.e., in clients with leukopenia, thrombocytopenia, or anemia). Lactation. Hypersensitivity to drug.

SPECIAL CONCERNS

Use with caution in impaired kidney or liver function. Due to the possibility of tremors, convulsions, and coma, close monitoring is necessary when used in children.

SIDE EFFECTS

GI: N&V, anorexia, stomatitis, dry mouth, dysphagia, abdominal pain, hematemesis, melena, diarrhea, constipation. **CNS:** Paresthesias, neuropathies, headache, dizziness, depression, apprehension, nervousness, insomnia, nightmares, hallucinations, falling, weakness, fatigue, lethargy, drowsiness, unsteadiness, ataxia, foot drop, decreased reflexes, tremors, confusion, ***coma, convulsions.*** **CV:** Hypotension, tachycardia, syncope. **Respiratory:** Pleural effusion, pneumonitis, cough. **Hematologic:** Leukopenia, anemia, thrombocytopenia, pancytopenia, eosinophilia, ***hemolytic anemia,*** petechiae, purpura, epistaxis, hemoptysis. **GU:** Hematuria, urinary frequency, nocturia. **Dermatologic:** Dermatitis, pruritus, rash, urticaria, herpes, hyperpigmentation, flushing, alopecia. **Ophthalmic:** Retinal hemorrhage, nystagmus, photophobia, diplopia, inability to focus, papilledema. **Hepatic:** Jaundice, hepatic dysfunction. **Miscellaneous:** Gynecomastia in prepubertal and early pubertal boys, pain, myalgia and arthralgia, pyrexia, diaphoresis, chills, intercurrent infections, edema, hoarseness, generalized allergic reactions, hearing loss, slurred speech, second nonlymphoid malignancies (including acute myelocytic leukemia, malignant myelosclerosis) and azoospermia in those treated with procarbazine combined with other chemotherapy or radiation.

OD OVERDOSE MANAGEMENT

Symptoms: N&V, diarrhea, enteritis, hypotension, tremors, seizures, coma, hematologic and hepatic toxicity. *Treatment:* Induce vomiting or undertake gastric lavage. IV fluids. Perform frequent blood counts and LFTs.

DRUG INTERACTIONS

Alcohol / Antabuse-like reaction
Antihistamines / Additive CNS depression
Antihypertensive drugs / Additive CNS depression
Barbiturates / Additive CNS depression
Chemotherapy / Depressed bone marrow activity
Digoxin / ↓ Digoxin plasma levels
Guanethidine / Excitation and hypertension
Hypoglycemic agents, oral / ↑ Hypoglycemic effect
Insulin / ↑ Hypoglycemic effect
Levodopa / Flushing and hypertension within 1 hr of administration
MAO inhibitors / Possibility of hypertensive crisis
Methyldopa / Excitation and hypertension
Narcotics / Significant CNS depression → possible deep coma/death
Phenothiazines / Additive CNS depression; also, possible hypertensive crisis
Sympathomimetics, indirectly acting / Possibility of hypertensive crisis
Tricyclic antidepressants / Possible toxic and fatal reactions, including excitability, fluctuations in BP, seizures, and coma
Tyramine-containing foods / Possibility of hypertensive crisis

HOW SUPPLIED

Capsule: 50 mg

DOSAGE

• CAPSULES

When used alone.

Adults: 2–4 mg/kg/day for first week; **then,** 4–6 mg/kg/day until leukocyte count falls below 4,000/mm³ or platelet count falls below 100,000/mm³. If toxic symptoms appear, discontinue drug and resume treatment at rate of 1–2 mg/kg/day; **maintenance:** 1–2 mg/kg/day. **Children, highly individualized:** 50 mg/m²/day for first week; then 100 mg/m² (to nearest 50 mg) until maximum response obtained or until leukopenia or thrombocytopenia occurs. When maximum response is reached, maintain the dose at 50 mg/m²/day.

P

When used in combination with other antineoplastic drugs (e.g., MOPP or ChlVPP therapies).
100 mg/m² for 14 days.

NURSING CONSIDERATIONS

SEE ALSO *NURSING CONSIDERATIONS* FOR *ANTINEOPLASTIC AGENTS*.

ASSESSMENT

1. Document indications for therapy and other agents/treatments prescribed.
2. Document cardiopulmonary and neurologic assessments.
3. Monitor CBC, uric acid, liver and renal function studies. May cause granulocyte and platelet suppression. Nadir: 14 days; recovery: 21–28 days.

CLIENT/FAMILY TEACHING

1. Consult provider before taking any other medication because procarbazine has MAO inhibitory activity. Avoid sympathomimetic drugs and foods with a high tyramine content (yeasts, yogurt, caffeine, chocolate, aged cheese, liver, smoked or pickled fish, fermented sausage, etc.) during and for 2 weeks after completing therapy; may precipitate a hypertensive crisis.
2. Do not drive or perform tasks that require mental alertness until drug effects are realized.
3. Consume adequate fluids (2–3 L/day) to prevent dehydration.
4. Drug increases effect of insulin and oral hypoglycemic agents; report symptoms as medication adjustment may be necessary.
5. Avoid exposure to sun or to ultraviolet rays because a photosensitive skin reaction may occur. Wear sunscreen, sunglasses, and protective clothing if exposure is necessary.
6. Avoid alcohol; a disulfiram-type reaction may occur.
7. Practice reliable contraception.
8. Report fever, rash, chills, SOB, abnormal bruising/bleeding, persistent constipation (especially if diet, increased fluids, and bulk are ineffective); laxatives may be needed.

OUTCOMES/EVALUATE

Suppression of malignant cell proliferation

P

Prochlorperazine

(proh-klor-**PAIR**-ah-zeen)

PREGNANCY CATEGORY: C
Rx: Compazine, Compro Suppositories
✱Rx: Stemetil Suppositories

Prochlorperazine edisylate

(proh-klor-**PAIR**-ah-zeen)

Rx: Compazine

Prochlorperazine maleate

(proh-klor-**PAIR**-ah-zeen)

Rx: Compazine
✱Rx: Nu-Prochlor, Stemetil
CLASSIFICATION(S):
Antipsychotic, phenothiazine

SEE ALSO *ANTIPSYCHOTIC AGENTS, PHENOTHIAZINES*.

ACTION/KINETICS

Prochlorperazine causes a high incidence of extrapyramidal and antiemetic effects, moderate sedative effects, and a low incidence of anticholinergic effects and orthostatic hypotension.

USES

Psychotic disorders. Short-term treatment of generalized nonpsychotic anxiety (not drug of choice). Postoperative N&V, radiation sickness, vomiting due to toxins. Severe N&V. *Investigational:* Acute headache.

CONTRAINDICATIONS

Use in clients who weigh less than 44 kg or who are under 2 years of age.

SPECIAL CONCERNS

Safe use during pregnancy has not been established. Geriatric, emaciated, and debilitated clients usually require a lower initial dose.

HOW SUPPLIED

Prochlorperazine: *Injection:* 5 mg/mL; *Suppository:* 2.5 mg, 5 mg, 25 mg; **Prochlorperazine Edisylate:** *Injection:* 5 mg/mL; *Syrup:* 5 mg/5 mL; **Prochlorperazine maleate:** *Capsule, extended release:* 10 mg, 15 mg, 30 mg; *Tablet:* 5 mg, 10 mg, 25 mg

DOSAGE

• EDISYLATE SYRUP, MALEATE EXTENDED-RELEASE CAPSULES, TABLETS

Psychotic disorders.

Adults and adolescents: 5 or 10 mg t.i.d. or q.i.d. for mild conditions. For severe conditions, for hospitalized, or adequately supervised clients: 10 mg t.i.d. or q.i.d. Dose can be increased gradually q 2–3 days as needed and tolerated. For extended-release capsules, up to 100–150 mg/day can be given. **Pediatric, 2–12 years:** 2.5 mg b.i.d.–t.i.d. Do not give more than 10 mg on the first day.

N&V.

Adults and adolescents: 5–10 mg t.i.d.–q.i.d. (up to 40 mg/day). For extended-release capsules, the dose is 15–30 mg once daily in the morning (or 10 mg q 12 hr, up to 40 mg/day). **Pediatric, 18–39 kg:** 2.5 mg (base) t.i.d. (or 5 mg b.i.d.), not to exceed 15 mg/day; **14–17 kg:** 2.5 mg (base) b.i.d.–t.i.d., not to exceed 10 mg/day; **9–13 kg:** 2.5 mg (base) 1–2 times/day, not to exceed 7.5 mg/day. The total daily dose for children should not exceed 10 mg the first day; on subsequent days, the total daily dose should not exceed 20 mg for children 2–5 years of age or 25 mg for children 6–12 years of age.

Anxiety.

Adults and adolescents: 5 mg t.i.d.–q.i.d. on arising. Or, 15 mg sustained release on arising or 10 mg sustained release q 12 hr. Do not give more than 20 mg/day for more than 12 weeks.

• IM, EDISYLATE INJECTION

Psychotic disorders, for immediate control of severely disturbed clients.

Adults and adolescents, initial: 10–20 mg; dose can be repeated q 2–4 hr as needed (usually up to three or four doses). If prolonged therapy is needed: 10–20 mg q 4–6 hr. **Children, less than 12 years of age:** 0.03 mg/kg by deep IM injection. After control is achieved (usually after 1 injection), switch to PO at same dosage level or higher.

N&V.

Adults and adolescents: 5–10 mg; repeat the dose q 3–4 hr as needed. **Pediatric, 2–12 years:** 0.132 mg/kg.

N&V during surgery.

Adults and adolescents: 5–10 mg (base) given as a slow injection or infusion 15–30 min before induction of anesthesia; to control symptoms during or after surgery the dose can be repeated once. The rate of infusion should not exceed 5 mg/mL/min.

• RECTAL SUPPOSITORIES

Pediatric, 2–12 years: 2.5 mg b.i.d.–t.i.d. with no more than 10 mg given on the first day. No more than 20 mg/day for children 2–5 years of age and 25 mg/day for children 6–12 years of age.

NURSING CONSIDERATIONS

SEE ALSO *NURSING CONSIDERATIONS* FOR *ANTIPSYCHOTIC AGENTS, PHENOTHIAZINES*.

ADMINISTRATION/STORAGE

1. Store all forms of the drug in tight-closing amber-colored bottles; store suppositories below 37°C (98.6°F).
2. Due to local irritation, do not give SC.
3. Do not mix with other agents in a syringe.
4. Do not dilute with any material containing the preservative parabens.
5. When given IM to children for N&V, the duration of action may be 12 hr.
6. Parenteral prescribing limits are 20 mg/day for children 2–5 years of age and 25 mg/day for children 6–12 years of age.

ASSESSMENT

1. Document indications for therapy, onset and characteristics of symptoms.
2. Assess mental status and note behavioral manifestations.
3. Monitor CBC, LFTs, and ECG.

INTERVENTIONS

1. Monitor I&O and VS.

P

2. Auscultate bowel sounds and assess function.
3. Incorporate safety precautions during the treatment of an overdose. If taking spansules, continue treatment until all signs of overdosage are no longer evident. Saline laxatives may be used to hasten the evacuation of pellets that have not yet released their medication.

CLIENT/FAMILY TEACHING

1. Do not exceed the prescribed dose of drug. Avoid skin contact with the solution. Do not crush or chew sustained release tablets.
2. Add desired dosage of concentrate to 60 mL of beverage (e.g., tomato or fruit juice, milk, soup) or semisolid food just before administration to disguise the taste.
3. Withhold drug and report if child shows signs of restlessness and excitement. Report symptoms of extrapyramidal effects and tardive dyskinesia (tremor, involuntary twitching).
4. Do not drive or operate machinery until drug effects are realized; drowsiness or dizziness may occur.
5. Consume adequate fluids to prevent dehydration and use precautions against heatstroke in hot weather. Urine may be pink to reddish-brown.
6. Use protection when in the sun to prevent photosensitivity reaction.
7. Rise and change positions slowly to prevent orthostatic effects.
8. Report adverse side effects, fever, sore throat, rashes, tremors, dark urine, pale stools, impaired vision, or lack of response.

OUTCOMES/EVALUATE

- Control of N&V
- Reduction in agitation, excitability, or withdrawn behaviors

Progesterone gel

(pro-**JES**-ter-ohn)

CLASSIFICATION(S):
Progesterone
Rx: Crinone 4%, Crinone 8%

SEE ALSO PROGESTERONE AND PROGESTINS.

ACTION/KINETICS

t½, absorption: 25–50 hr. **t½, elimination:** 5–20 min. Extensively bound to plasma proteins. Metabolized in liver; excreted through urine and feces.

USES

Progesterone supplementation or replacement as part of assisted reproductive technology treatment for infertile women with progesterone deficiency. Secondary amenorrhea.

CONTRAINDICATIONS

Undiagnosed vaginal bleeding, liver disease or dysfunction, known or suspected malignancy of breast or genital organs, missed abortion, active thrombophlebitis or thromboembolic disease (or history of such). Concurrent use with other local intravaginal therapy.

SPECIAL CONCERNS

Safety and efficacy have not been determined in children.

SIDE EFFECTS

See Progesterone and Progestins.

HOW SUPPLIED

Vaginal gel: 45 mg/1.125 g (Crinone 4%), 90 mg/1.125 g (Crinone 8%)

DOSAGE

- **VAGINAL GEL: CRINONE 8%**

Assisted reproductive technology.

90 mg once daily for women who require progesterone supplementation. Administer 90 mg b.i.d. in women with partial or complete ovarian failure who require progesterone replacement. If pregnancy occurs, treatment may be continued until placental autonomy has been achieved (up to 10–12 weeks).

- **VAGINAL GEL: CRINONE 4%**

Secondary amenorrhea.

45 mg every other day up to total of 6 doses. For women who fail to respond, Crinone 8% (90 mg) may be given every other day up to total of 6 doses.

NURSING CONSIDERATIONS

SEE ALSO *NURSING CONSIDERATIONS FOR PROGESTERONE AND PROGESTINS.*

ADMINISTRATION/STORAGE

1. Dosage increase from 4% gel can only be accomplished by using 8%

gel. Increasing volume of gel does not increase amount absorbed.

2. If other local intravaginal therapy is to be used, wait at least 6-hr before or after Crinone administration.

3. Store at controlled room temperature below 25°C (77°F).

ASSESSMENT

1. Document indications for therapy, with physical and GYN findings.

2. Assess for liver disease, breast or genital malignancy, undiagnosed vaginal bleeding, or history of thromboembolic disease; precludes drug therapy.

CLIENT/FAMILY TEACHING

1. Review product information sheet on how to use product; use only as directed.

2. Do not use with other intravaginal products; if concurrent therapy prescribed, wait for 6 hr.

3. May experience breast enlargement, constipation, headaches, sleepiness, and perineal pain.

4. Report any overt symptoms or depression.

OUTCOMES/EVALUATE

Progesterone replacement/supplementation

Promethazine hydrochloride

(proh-**METH**-ah-zeen)

PREGNANCY CATEGORY: C
CLASSIFICATION(S):
Antihistamine, first generation, phenothiezine
Rx: Suppositories: Phenergan, **Syrup:** Phenergan Fortis, Phenergan Plain, **Tablets:** Phenergan, **Parenteral:** Anergan 50 Phenergan

SEE ALSO *ANTIHISTAMINES* AND *ANTIEMETICS*.

ACTION/KINETICS

Antiemetic effects are likely due to inhibition of the CTZ. Effective in vertigo by its central anticholinergic effect which inhibits the vestibular apparatus and the integrative vomiting center as well as the CTZ. May cause severe drowsiness. **Onset, PO, IM, PR:** 20 min; **IV:** 3–5 min. **Duration, antihistaminic:** 6–12 hr; **sedative:** 2–8 hr. Slowly eliminated through urine and feces.

USES

(1) PO and PR for prophylaxis and treatment of motion sickness. (2) Prophylaxis of N&V due to anesthesia or surgery (also postoperatively). (3) Pre- or postoperative sedative, obstetric sedative. (4) Hypersensitivity reactions, including perennial and seasonal allergic rhinitis, vasomotor rhinitis, allergic conjunctivitis, urticaria, angioedema, allergic reactions to blood or plasma, dermographism. (5) Adjunct in the treatment of anaphylaxis or anaphylactoid reactions. (6) Adjunct to analgesics for postoperative pain. (7) IV with meperidine or other narcotics in special surgical procedures as bronchoscopy, ophthalmic surgery, or in poor-risk clients.

CONTRAINDICATIONS

Lactation. Comatose clients, CNS depression due to drugs, previous phenothiazine idiosyncrasy, acutely ill or dehydrated children (due to greater susceptibility to dystonias). Children up to 2 years of age. SC or intra-arterial use due to tissue necrosis and gangrene.

SPECIAL CONCERNS

Safe use during pregnancy has not been established. Use in children may cause paradoxical hyperexcitability and nightmares. Geriatric clients are more likely to experience confusion, dizziness, hypotension, and sedation.

ADDITIONAL SIDE EFFECTS

Leukopenia and ***agranulocytosis (especially if used with cytotoxic agents)***.

HOW SUPPLIED

Injection: 25 mg/mL, 50 mg/mL (IM only); *Suppository:* 12.5 mg, 25 mg, 50 mg; *Syrup:* 6.25 mg/5 mL, 25 mg/5 mL; *Tablet:* 12.5 mg, 25 mg, 50 mg

DOSAGE

• **SUPPOSITORIES, SYRUP, TABLETS**
Hypersensitivity reactions.
Adults: 12.5 mg q.i.d. before meals and at bedtime (or 25 mg at bedtime if

P

needed). **Pediatric over 2 years:** 0.125 mg/kg (3.75 mg/m^2) q 4–6 hr; 0.5 mg/kg (15 mg/m^2) at bedtime if needed; or, 6.25–12. mg t.i.d. (or 25 mg at bedtime if needed).

Antiemetic.

Adults: 25 mg (usual); 12.5–25 mg q 4–6 hr as needed. **Pediatric, over 2 years:** 0.25–0.5 mg/kg (7.5–15 mg/m^2) q 4–6 hr as needed (or 12.5–25 mg q 4–6 hr).

Sedation.

Adults: 25–50 mg at bedtime; **pediatric, over 2 years:** 0.5–1 mg/kg (15–30 mg/m^2) or 12.5–25 mg at bedtime.

Motion sickness.

Adults: 25 mg b.i.d. **Pediatric, over 2 years:** 12.5–25 mg b.i.d.

Analgesia adjunct.

Adults: 50 mg with an equal amount of meperidine and an appropriate dose of an atropine-like agent. **Pediatric, over 2 years:** 1.2 mg/kg with an equal amount of meperidine and an atropine-like agent.

• **IM, IV**

Hypersensitivity reactions.

Adults: 25 mg repeated in 2 hr if needed; **pediatric, 2–12 years:** 12.5 mg or less, not to exceed half the adult dose. Resume PO therapy as soon as possible.

P

Antiemetic.

Adults: 12.5–25 mg q 4 hr if needed. If used postoperatively, reduce doses of concomitant hypnotics, analgesics, or barbiturates. **Pediatric, 2–12 years:** Do not exceed half the adult dose. Do not use when the cause of vomiting is unknown.

Sedation.

Adults: 25–50 mg at bedtime. May be combined with hypnotics for pre- and postoperative sedation. **Pediatric, 2–12 years:** Do not exceed half the adult dose.

Sedation during labor.

Adults: 50 mg during early stages of labor, not to exceed 100 mg/24 hr.

Analgesia adjunct.

Adults: 25–50 mg in combination with reduced doses of analgesics and hypnotics; give atropine-like drugs as needed. **Pediatric, 2–12 years:** 1.2 mg/kg in combination with an equal dose of analgesic or barbiturate and an appropriate dose of an atropine-like drug.

NURSING CONSIDERATIONS

SEE ALSO *NURSING CONSIDERATIONS FOR ANTIHISTAMINES* AND *ANTIEMETICS*.

ADMINISTRATION/STORAGE

Decrease dosage in dehydrated clients or those with oliguria.

ASSESSMENT

Document indications for therapy, onset and characteristics of symptoms. Note age; older clients may manifest more adverse side effects.

CLIENT/FAMILY TEACHING

1. Take only as directed and do not exceed dose, as arrhythmias may occur. May take with food or milk to decrease GI upset.
2. When used to prevent motion sickness, take 30–60 min before travel. On successive travel days, take on rising and again before the evening meal.
3. Avoid activities requiring mental alertness until drug effects realized.
4. Do not consume alcohol or any OTC agents.
5. Drug may alter skin testing; stop 72 hr before testing.
6. Consume adequate fluids to prevent dehydration; use caution in hot weather to prevent heat stroke.
7. Avoid prolonged sun exposure, may cause photosensitivity reaction. Wear sunscreen and protection if exposed.

OUTCOMES/EVALUATE

• Prevention of vertigo
• Control of N&V
• Promotion of sleep
• Control of allergic manifestations

Propafenone hydrochloride

(proh-pah-**FEN**-ohn)

PREGNANCY CATEGORY: C
CLASSIFICATION(S):
Antiarrhythmic, Class IC
Rx: Rythmol

ACTION/KINETICS

Manifests local anesthetic effects and a direct stabilizing action on the myocardium. Reduces upstroke velocity (Phase O) of the monophasic action potential, reduces the fast inward current carried by sodium ions in the Purkinje fibers, increases diastolic excitability threshold, and prolongs the effective refractory period. Also, spontaneous activity is decreased. Slows AV conduction and causes first-degree heart block. Has slight beta-adrenergic blocking activity. **Peak plasma levels:** 3.5 hr. **Therapeutic plasma levels:** 0.5–3 mcg/mL. Significant first-pass effect. Most metabolize rapidly (**t½**: 2–10 hr) to two active metabolites: 5-hydroxypropafenone and N-depropylpropafenone. However, approximately 10% (as well as those taking quinidine) metabolize the drug more slowly (**t½:** 10–32 hr). Because the 5-hydroxy metabolite is not formed in slow metabolizers and because steady-state levels are reached after 4–5 days in all clients, the recommended dosing regimen is the same for all clients.

USES

Documented life-threatening ventricular arrhythmias, such as sustained ventricular tachycardia where the benefits outweigh the risks. Paroxysmal atrial fibrillation or flutter and paroxysmal supraventricular tachycardia associated with disabling symptoms. Do not use in less severe ventricular arrhythmias even if the client is symptomatic. Antiarrhythmic drugs have not been shown to improve survival in clients with ventricular arrhythmias. *Investigational:* Arrhythmias associated with Wolff-Parkinson-White syndrome.

CONTRAINDICATIONS

Uncontrolled CHF, cardiogenic shock, sick sinus node syndrome or AV block in the absence of an artificial pacemaker, bradycardia, marked hypotension, bronchospastic disorders, electrolyte disorders, hypersensitivity to the drug. MI more than 6 days but less than 2 years previously. Lactation.

SPECIAL CONCERNS

There is an increased risk of death in those with non-life-threatening arrhythmias. Use with caution during labor and delivery. Safety and effectiveness have not been determined in children. Use with caution in clients with impaired hepatic or renal function. Geriatric clients may require lower dosage.

SIDE EFFECTS

CV: *New or worsened arrhythmias.* First-degree AV block, intraventricular conduction delay, palpitations, PVCs, proarrhythmia, bradycardia, atrial fibrillation, angina, syncope, CHF, ***ventricular tachycardia, second-degree AV block,*** increased QRS duration, chest pain, hypotension, bundle branch block. Less commonly, atrial flutter, AV dissociation, flushing, hot flashes, sick sinus syndrome, sinus pause or arrest, SVT, ***cardiac arrest.*** **CNS:** Dizziness, headache, anxiety, drowsiness, fatigue, loss of balance, ataxia, insomnia. Less commonly, abnormal speech, abnormal dreams, abnormal vision, confusion, depression, memory loss, ***apnea,*** psychosis/mania, vertigo, ***seizures, coma,*** numbness, paresthesias. **GI:** Unusual taste, constipation, nausea and/or vomiting, dry mouth, anorexia, flatulence, abdominal pain, cramps, diarrhea, dyspepsia. Less commonly, gastroenteritis and liver abnormalities (cholestasis, hepatitis, elevated enzymes, hepatitis). **Hematologic: *Agranulocytosis,*** increased bleeding time, anemia, granulocytopenia, bruising, leukopenia, purpura, anemia, thrombocytopenia. **Miscellaneous:** Blurred vision, dyspnea, weakness, rash, edema, tremors, diaphoresis, joint pain, possible decrease in spermatogenesis. Less commonly, tinnitus, unusual smell sensation, alopecia, eye irritation, hyponatremia, inappropriate ADH secretion, impotence, increased glucose, kidney failure, lupus erythematosus, muscle cramps or weakness, nephrotic syndrome, pain, pruritus.

LABORATORY TEST CONSIDERATIONS

↑ ANA titers.

P

OD OVERDOSE MANAGEMENT

Symptoms: Bradycardia, hypotension, IA and intraventricular conduction disturbances, somnolence. ***Rarely, high-grade ventricular arrhythmias and seizures.*** *Treatment:* To control BP and cardiac rhythm, defibrillation and infusion of dopamine or isoproterenol. If seizures occur, diazepam, IV, can be given. External cardiac massage and mechanical respiratory assistance may be required.

DRUG INTERACTIONS

Beta-adrenergic blockers / ↑ Plasma levels of beta blockers metabolized by the liver
Cimetidine / ↓ Propafenone plasma levels
Cyclosporine / ↑ Blood trough levels; ↓ renal function
Digoxin / ↑ Plasma levels → ↓ digoxin dose
Local anesthetics / May ↑ risk of CNS side effects
Mexiletine / ↓ Metabolic clearance of mexiletine in extensive metabolizers → no differences between extensive and poor metabolizers
Quinidine / ↑ Propafenone serum levels in rapid metabolizers → possible ↑ effect
Rifampin / ↓ Propafenone effect R/T ↑ clearance
Warfarin / May ↑ warfarin plasma levels; ↓ warfarin dose

HOW SUPPLIED

Tablet: 150 mg, 225 mg, 300 mg

DOSAGE

• TABLETS

Adults, initial: 150 mg q 8 hr; dose may be increased at a minimum of q 3–4 days to 225 mg q 8 hr and, if necessary, to 300 mg q 8 hr.

NURSING CONSIDERATIONS

SEE ALSO *NURSING CONSIDERATIONS FOR ANTIARRHYTHMIC AGENTS.*

ADMINISTRATION/STORAGE

1. Always initiate therapy in a hospital setting.
2. The effectiveness and safety of doses exceeding 900 mg/day have not been determined.
3. There is no evidence that the use of propafenone affects the survival or incidence of sudden death with recent MI or SVT.

ASSESSMENT

1. Assess ECG and baseline arrhythmias; note any cardiac problems.
2. Monitor CBC, electrolytes, liver and renal function studies. Determine any renal or hepatic disease.
3. Report any significant widening of the QRS complex or any evidence of second- or third-degree AV block.
4. May induce new or more severe arrhythmias; titrate dose based on client response and tolerance.
5. Increase dose more gradually in elderly clients as well as those with previous myocardial damage.
6. Evaluate hematologic studies for anemia, agranulocytosis, leukopenia, thrombocytopenia, or altered prothrombin and coagulation times.

CLIENT/FAMILY TEACHING

1. Drink adequate quantities of fluid (2–3 L/day) and add bulk to the diet to avoid constipation.
2. May experience unusual taste in the mouth; report if interferes with eating and nutritional status.
3. Report any increased or unusual bruising/bleeding or S&S of hepatic dysfunction such as yellow sclera, dark-yellow urine, or yellow skin.
4. Report any urinary tract problems or decreased urinary output.
5. Record BP and pulse readings.

OUTCOMES/EVALUATE

• Termination of life-threatening VT; restoration of stable rhythm
• Therapeutic drug levels (0.5–3 mcg/mL)

Propantheline bromide

(proh-**PAN**-thih-leen)

PREGNANCY CATEGORY: C
CLASSIFICATION(S):
Cholinergic blocking drug, quaternary ammonium compound
Rx: Pro-Banthine
✱Rx: Propanthel

SEE ALSO *CHOLINERGIC BLOCKING AGENTS.*

ACTION/KINETICS
Duration: 6 hr. Metabolized in the liver and excreted through the urine.
USES
Adjunct in peptic ulcer therapy. Spastic and inflammatory disease of GI and urinary tracts. Control of salivation and enuresis. Duodenography. Second-line therapy for urinary incontinence.
SPECIAL CONCERNS
Safety and effectiveness for use in children with peptic ulcer have not been established.
ADDITIONAL DRUG INTERACTIONS
Propantheline, due to slowing of GI motility, ↑ absorption of metformin
HOW SUPPLIED
Tablet: 7.5 mg, 15 mg

DOSAGE
• **TABLETS**
GI problems.
Adults: 15 mg 30 min before meals and 30 mg at bedtime. Reduce dose to 7.5 mg t.i.d. for mild symptoms, geriatric clients, or clients of small stature. **Pediatric:** 0.375 mg/kg (10 mg/m²) q.i.d. with dose being adjusted as needed.
Urinary incontinence.
Adults: 7.5–30 mg 3–5 times/day; in some, doses as high as 15–60 mg q.i.d. may be needed.

NURSING CONSIDERATIONS

SEE ALSO *NURSING CONSIDERATIONS* FOR *CHOLINERGIC BLOCKING AGENTS.*

ASSESSMENT
1. Document indications for therapy, type, onset, and characteristics of symptoms.
2. With ulcer disease or persistent GI complaints, assess for *H. pylori*. Review UGI/endoscopic findings.
3. A liquid diet is recommended during initiation of therapy with edematous duodenal ulcer.
CLIENT/FAMILY TEACHING
1. May cause drowsiness or dizziness. Do not drive or operate equipment until drug effects realized. Avoid alcohol.
2. May impair visual acuity; dark glasses may be necessary. Report if symptoms are persistent.
3. Increase dietary intake of fluids and fiber to minimize the constipating effects of drug therapy.
4. Report any symptoms of urinary retention and persistent constipation as well as rash, sob, irregular heart beat etc.
OUTCOMES/EVALUATE
• Relief of GI pain R/T PUD
• Control of urinary incontinence

Propoxyphene hydrochloride

(proh-**POX**-ih-feen)

PREGNANCY CATEGORY: C
Rx: Darvon, **C-IV**
★**Rx:** 642 Tablets

Propoxyphene napsylate

(proh-**POX**-ih-feen)

PREGNANCY CATEGORY: C
Rx: Darvon-N , **C-IV**
CLASSIFICATION(S):
Narcotic analgesic

ACTION/KINETICS
Resembles narcotics with respect to its mechanism and analgesic effect; it is one-half to one-third as potent as codeine. Is devoid of antitussive, anti-inflammatory, or antipyretic activity. When taken in excessive doses for long periods, psychologic dependence and occasionally physical dependence and tolerance will be manifested. **Peak plasma levels:** *hydrochloride:* 2–2.5 hr; *napsylate:* 3–4 hr. **Analgesic onset:** 30–60 min. **Peak analgesic effect:** 2–2.5 hr. **Duration:** 4–6 hr. **Therapeutic serum levels:** 0.05–0.12 mcg/mL. **t½, propoxyphene:** 6–12 hr; **norpropoxyphene:** 30–36 hr. Extensive first-pass effect; metabolites are excreted in the urine.

USES
Relief of mild to moderate pain. *Investigational:* Suppress the withdrawal syndrome from narcotics (napsylate).
CONTRAINDICATIONS
Hypersensitivity to drug. Use in children or in those who are suicidal or addiction-prone.
SPECIAL CONCERNS
Safe use during pregnancy has not been established. Use with caution during lactation and in those taking tranquilizers, antidepressants, and who use excess alcohol.
SIDE EFFECTS
GI: N&V, constipation, abdominal pain. **CNS:** Sedation, dizziness, lightheadedness, headache, weakness, euphoria, dysphoria. **Other:** Skin rashes, visual disturbances. Propoxyphene can produce psychologic dependence, as well as physical dependence and tolerance.
OD OVERDOSE MANAGEMENT
Symptoms: Stupor, respiratory depression, ***apnea,*** hypotension, pulmonary edema, ***circulatory collapse, cardiac arrhythmias,*** conduction abnormalities, ***coma, seizures,*** respiratory-metabolic acidosis. *Treatment:* Maintain an adequate airway, artificial respiration, and naloxone, 0.4–2 mg IV (repeat at 2- to 3-min intervals) to combat respiratory depression. Gastric lavage or administration of activated charcoal may be helpful. Correct acidosis and electrolyte imbalance. Acidosis due to lactic acid may require IV sodium bicarbonate.
DRUG INTERACTIONS
Alcohol, antianxiety drugs, antipsychotic agents, narcotics, sedative-hypnotics / Concomitant use → drowsiness, lethargy, stupor, respiratory depression, and coma
Carbamazepine / ↑ Carbamazepine effects R/T ↓ liver breakdown
Charcoal / ↓ Propoxyphene absorption from GI tract
CNS depressants / Additive CNS depression
Orphenadrine / Concomitant use → confusion, anxiety, and tremors
Phenobarbital / ↑ Phenobarbital effects R/T ↓ liver breakdown
Protease inhibitors / Do not use together
Skeletal muscle relaxants / Additive respiratory depression
Warfarin / ↑ Warfarin hypoprothrombinemic effects
HOW SUPPLIED
Hydrochloride: *Capsule:* 65 mg; **Napsylate:** *Tablet:* 100 mg

DOSAGE

- **CAPSULES (HYDROCHLORIDE)**
  Analgesia.

Adults: 65 mg q 4 hr, not to exceed 390 mg/day.

- **TABLETS (NAPSYLATE)**
  Analgesia.

Adults: 100 mg q 4 hr, not to exceed 600 mg/day. Reduce the dose of propoxyphene in renal or hepatic impairment.

NURSING CONSIDERATIONS

SEE ALSO *NURSING CONSIDERATIONS* FOR *NARCOTIC ANALGESICS*.

ASSESSMENT
1. Document indications for therapy; note onset, duration, and characteristics of pain. Use a pain-rating scale to assess pain. Note other agents prescribed and outcome.
2. Assess for opiate or alcohol dependency.
3. Monitor liver and renal function studies; reduce dose with dysfunction.
4. Determine if smoker; smoking reduces drug effect by increasing metabolism.
5. Use with caution in the elderly and review drug profile to ensure other prescribed agents do not cause additive CNS effects.

CLIENT/FAMILY TEACHING
1. Take only as directed. Do not share meds or take for conditions other than prescribed. Store out of childs reach.
2. May take with food/milk to decrease GI upset.
3. Avoid activities that require mental alertness; may cause dizziness/drowsiness.
4. Report lack of response, any unusual side effects, or loss of effective-

ness. Tolerance may develop over time.

5. Do not smoke (induces liver enzymes that rapidly metabolize propoxyphene), consume alcohol, or any OTC agents.

OUTCOMES/EVALUATE

Relief of pain

Propranolol hydrochloride

(proh-**PRAN**-oh-lohl)

PREGNANCY CATEGORY: C

CLASSIFICATION(S):

Beta-adrenergic blocking agent

Rx: Inderal, Inderal LA, Propranolol Intensol

✱**Rx:** Apo-Propranolol, Nu-Propranolol

SEE ALSO *BETA-ADRENERGIC BLOCKING AGENTS.*

ACTION/KINETICS

Manifests both beta-1- and beta-2-adrenergic blocking activity. Antiarrhythmic action is due to both beta-adrenergic receptor blockade and a direct membrane-stabilizing action on the cardiac cell. Has no intrinsic sympathomimetic activity and has high lipid solubility. **Onset, PO:** 30 min; **IV:** immediate. **Maximum effect:** 1–1.5 hr. **Duration:** 3–5 hr. **t½:** 2–3 hr (8–11 hr for long-acting). **Therapeutic serum level, antiarrhythmic:** 0.05–0.1 mcg/mL. Completely metabolized by liver and excreted in urine. Although food increases bioavailability, absorption may be decreased.

USES

(1) Hypertension, alone or in combination with other antihypertensive agents. (2) Angina pectoris when caused by coronary atherosclerosis. (3) Hypertrophic subaortic stenosis (especially to treat exercise or other stress-induced angina, palpitations, and syncope). (4) Treat MI. (5) Adjunctive treatment of pheochromocytoma after primary therapy with an alpha-adrenergic blocker. (6) Prophylaxis of migraine. (7) Essential tremor (familial or hereditary). (8) Cardiac arrhythmias, including supraventricular, ventricular, tachyarrhythmias of digitalis intoxication and resistant tachyarrhythamias due to excessive catecholamines during anesthesia.

Investigational: Schizophrenia, tremors due to parkinsonism, aggressive behavior, antipsychotic-induced akathisia, rebleeding due to esophageal varices, situational anxiety, acute panic attacks, gastric bleeding in portal hypertension, vaginal contraceptive, anxiety, alcohol withdrawal syndrome, winter depression.

CONTRAINDICATIONS

Bronchial asthma, bronchospasms including severe COPD.

SPECIAL CONCERNS

It is dangerous to use propranolol for pheochromocytoma unless an alpha-adrenergic blocking agent is already in use.

ADDITIONAL SIDE EFFECTS

Psoriasis-like eruptions, skin necrosis, SLE (rare).

LABORATORY TEST CONSIDERATIONS

↑ Blood urea, serum transaminase, alkaline phosphatase, LDH. Interference with glaucoma screening test.

ADDITIONAL DRUG INTERACTIONS

Gabapentin / Possible paroxysmal dystonic movements in the hands

Haloperidol / Severe hypotension

Hydralazine / ↑ Effect of both agents

Methimazole / May ↑ propranolol effects

Phenobarbital / ↓ Propranolol effect R/T ↑ liver breakdown

Propylthiouracil / May ↑ propranolol effects

Rifampin / ↓ propranolol effect R/T ↑ liver breakdown

Smoking / ↓ Serum levels and ↑ clearance of propranolol

HOW SUPPLIED

Capsule, sustained release: 60 mg, 80 mg, 120 mg, 160 mg; *Oral Solution Concentrate:* 80 mg/mL; *Injection:* 1 mg/mL; *Solution, oral:* 4 mg/mL, 8 mg/mL; *Tablet:* 10 mg, 20 mg, 40 mg, 60 mg, 80 mg, 90 mg

P

DOSAGE

• TABLETS, SUSTAINED-RELEASE CAPSULES, ORAL SOLUTION, ORAL SOLUTION CONCENTRATE

Hypertension.

Initial: 40 mg b.i.d. or 80 mg of sustained-release/day; **then,** increase dose to maintenance level of 120–240 mg/day given in two to three divided doses or 120–160 mg of sustained-release medication once daily. Do not exceed 640 mg/day. **Pediatric, initial:** 0.5 mg/kg b.i.d.; dose may be increased at 3- to 5-day intervals to a maximum of 1 mg/kg b.i.d. Calculate the dosage range by weight and not by body surface area.

Angina.

Initial: 80–320 mg b.i.d., t.i.d., or q.i.d.; or, 80 mg of sustained-release once daily; **then,** increase dose gradually to maintenance level of 160 mg/day of sustained-release capsule. Do not exceed 320 mg/day.

Arrhythmias.

10–30 mg t.i.d.–q.i.d. given after meals and at bedtime.

Hypertrophic subaortic stenosis.

20–40 mg t.i.d.–q.i.d. before meals and at bedtime or 80–160 mg of sustained-release medication given once daily.

MI prophylaxis.

180–240 mg/day given in three to four divided doses. Do not exceed 240 mg/day.

Pheochromocytoma, preoperatively.

60 mg/day for 3 days before surgery, given concomitantly with an alpha-adrenergic blocking agent.

Pheochromocytoma, inoperable tumors.

30 mg/day in divided doses.

Migraine.

Initial: 80 mg sustained-release medication given once daily; **then,** increase dose gradually to maintenance of 160–240 mg/day in divided doses. If a satisfactory response has not been observed after 4–6 weeks, discontinue the drug and withdraw gradually.

Essential tremor.

Initial: 40 mg b.i.d.; **then,** 120 mg/day up to a maximum of 320 mg/day.

Aggressive behavior.

80–300 mg/day.

Antipsychotic-induced akathisia.

20–80 mg/day.

Tremors associated with Parkinson's disease.

160 mg/day.

Rebleeding from esophageal varices.

20–180 mg b.i.d.

Schizophrenia.

300–5,000 mg/day.

Acute panic symptoms.

40–320 mg/day.

Anxiety.

80–320 mg/day.

Intermittent explosive disorder.

50–1,600 mg/day.

Nonvariceal gastric bleeding in portal hypertension.

24–480 mg/day.

• IV

Life-threatening arrhythmias or those occurring under anesthesia.

1–3 mg not to exceed 1 mg/min; a second dose may be given after 2 min, with subsequent doses q 4 hr. Begin PO therapy as soon as possible. Although use in pediatrics is not recommended, investigational doses of 0.01–0.1 mg/kg/dose, up to a maximum of 1 mg/dose (by slow push), have been used for arrhythmias.

NURSING CONSIDERATIONS

SEE ALSO *NURSING CONSIDERATIONS* FOR *BETA-ADRENERGIC BLOCKING AGENTS* AND *ANTIHYPERTENSIVE AGENTS*.

ADMINISTRATION/STORAGE

1. Do not administer for a minimum of 2 weeks of MAO drug use.

IV 2. Reserve IV use for life-threatening arrhythmias or those occurring during anesthesia.

3. If signs of serious myocardial depression occur, slowly infuse isoproterenol (Isuprel) IV.

4. For IV use, dilute 1 mg in 10 mL of D5W and administer IV over at least 1 min. May be further reconstituted in 50 mL of dextrose or saline solution and infused IVPB over 10–15 min.

5. After IV administration, have emergency drugs and equipment available

to combat hypotension or circulatory collapse.

ASSESSMENT

1. Document indications for therapy, type, onset, characteristics of symptoms, and other agents prescribed.
2. Note ECG, VS, and cardiopulmonary assessment. Assess for pulmonary disease, bronchospasms, or depression.
3. Report rash, fever, and/or purpura; S&S of hypersensitivity reaction.
4. Monitor VS, I&O. Observe for S&S of CHF (e.g., SOB, rales, edema, and weight gain).

CLIENT/FAMILY TEACHING

1. May cause drowsiness; assess drug response before performing activities that require mental alertness.
2. Do not smoke; smoking decreases serum levels and interferes with drug clearance.
3. May mask symptoms of hypoglycemia; monitor FS carefully.
4. Check BP and HR weekly; report any significant changes.
5. Do not stop abruptly; may precipitate hypertension, myocardial ischemia, or cardiac arrhythmias.
6. Dress appropriately; may cause increased sensitivity to cold.
7. Avoid alcohol and any OTC agents containing alpha-adrenergic stimulants or sympathomimetics.
8. Report any persistent side effects, e.g., skin rashes, abnormal bleeding, unusual crying, or feelings of depression.

OUTCOMES/EVALUATE

- ↓ BP, ↓ HR
- ↓ Angina; prophylaxis of myocardial reinfarction
- Migraine prophylaxis
- Control of tachyarrhythmias
- Desired behavioral changes
- Therapeutic drug levels as an antiarrhythmic (0.05–0.1 mcg/mL)

Propylthiouracil

(proh-pill-thigh-oh-**YOUR**-ah-sill)

PREGNANCY CATEGORY: D

CLASSIFICATION(S):
Antithyroid drug
✦Rx: Propyl-Thyracil

ACTION/KINETICS

Inhibits (partially or completely) the production of thyroid hormones by the thyroid gland by preventing the incorporation of iodide into tyrosine and coupling of iodotyrosines. Does not affect release or activity of preformed hormone; thus, it may take several weeks for the therapeutic effect to become established. May be preferred for treatment of thyroid storm, as it inhibits peripheral conversion of thyroxine to triiodothyronine. Rapidly absorbed from the GI tract. **Duration:** 2–3 hr. **t½:** 1–2 hr. **Onset:** 10–20 days. **Time to peak effect:** 2–10 weeks. Eighty percent is protein bound. Metabolized by the liver and excreted through the kidneys.

USES

Hyperthyroidism; prior to surgery or radiotherapy. Adjunct in treatment of thyrotoxicosis or thyroid storm. To reduce mortality due to alcoholic liver disease.

CONTRAINDICATIONS

Lactation—may cause hypothyroidism in infant.

SPECIAL CONCERNS

Incidence of vasculitis is increased. Use with caution in the presence of CV disease. Monitor PT due to possible hypoprothrombinemia and bleeding.

SIDE EFFECTS

Hematologic: ***Agranulocytosis,*** thrombocytopenia, granulocytopenia, hypoprothrombinemia, ***aplastic anemia,*** leukopenia. **GI:** N&V, taste loss, epigastric pain, sialadenopathy. **CNS:** Headache, paresthesia, drowsiness, vertigo, depression, CNS stimulation. **Dermatologic:** Skin rash, urticaria, alopecia, skin pigmentation, pruritus, exfoliative dermatitis, erythema nodosum. **Miscellaneous:** Jaundice, arthralgia, myalgia, neuritis, edema, lymphadenopathy, vasculitis, lupus-like syndrome, drug fever, periarteritis, hepatitis, nephritis, interstitial

P

pneumonitis, insulin autoimmune syndrome resulting in hypoglycemic coma.

OD OVERDOSE MANAGEMENT

Symptoms: N&V, headache, fever, pruritus, epigastric distress, arthralgia, pancytopenia, ***agranulocytosis*** (most serious). Rarely, exfoliative dermatitis, hepatitis, neuropathies, CNS stimulation or depression. *Treatment:* Maintain a patent airway and support ventilation and perfusion. Very carefully monitor and maintain VS, blood gases, and serum electrolytes. Monitor bone marrow function.

DRUG INTERACTIONS

Propylthiouracil may produce hypoprothrombinemia, adding to the effect of anticoagulants.

HOW SUPPLIED

Tablet: 50 mg

DOSAGE

• TABLETS

Hyperthyroidism.

Adults, initial: 300 mg/day (up to 900 mg/day may be required in some clients with severe hyperthyroidism) given as one to four divided doses; **maintenance, usual:** 100–150 mg/day. **Pediatric, 6–10 years, initial:** 50–150 mg/day in one to four divided doses; **over 10 years, initial:** 150–300 mg/day in one to four divided doses. Maintenance for all pediatric use is based on response. **Alternative dose for children, initial:** 5–7 mg/kg/day (150–200 mg/m²/day) in divided doses q 8 hr; **maintenance:** ⅓–⅔ the initial dose when the client is euthyroid.

Thyrotoxic crisis.

Adults: 200–400 mg q 4 hr during the first day as an adjunct to other treatments.

Neonatal thyrotoxicosis.

10 mg/kg daily in divided doses.

P

NURSING CONSIDERATIONS

ASSESSMENT

1. Document onset of illness, symptoms experienced, physical presentation, and any underlying cause.
2. Determine if pregnant.
3. Monitor VS, I&O, and weights; PT, CBC, ECG, and thyroid function studies.
4. Assess thyroid gland noting any enlargement, pain, asymmetry, nodules, or bruits.
5. Check children every 6 months for appropriate growth and development; plot on a graph.

CLIENT/FAMILY TEACHING

1. It takes 6–12 weeks for the drug to produce full effect. Take regularly and exactly as directed q 8 hr around the clock. Hyperthyroidism may recur if not taken properly. Regularly record heart rate and weight.
2. Report symptoms of hyperthyroidism or thyrotoxicosis (palpitations, increased HR, nervousness, sleeplessness, sweating, diarrhea, weight loss, fever).
3. Report symptoms of hypothyroidism (weak, listless, tired, headache, dry skin, cold intolerance, constipation) as dosage may require adjustment.
4. Report any sore throat, enlargement of the cervical lymph nodes, GI disturbances, fever, skin rashes, itching, or jaundice; may require either a dosage reduction or withdrawal of the drug.
5. May alter taste perception; increase use of herbs and nonsodium seasonings.
6. Report symptoms of iodism (cold symptoms, skin lesions, stomatitis, GI upset, metallic taste)
7. Identify dietary sources of iodine (iodized salt, shellfish, turnips, cabbage, kale) that may need to be omitted from the diet.
8. Report unusual bleeding, alopecia, nausea, loss of taste, or epigastric pain.
9. When drug is taken for 1 year, more than half the clients achieve a permanent remission. Those who relapse are usually treated with radioiodine.
10. Carry ID listing medical problems and currently prescribed meds.
11. Avoid all OTC agents without approval. Report as scheduled for evaluation and labs.

OUTCOMES/EVALUATE

• Normal metabolism; control of S&S (↑ weight, ↓ sweating, ↓ HR)

• Suppression of thyroid hormones (↓ T_3, T_4); thyroid function studies within desired range (euthyroid)

Protamine sulfate

(**PROH**-tah-meen)

PREGNANCY CATEGORY: C
CLASSIFICATION(S):
Heparin antagonist

ACTION/KINETICS
A strong basic polypeptide that complexes with strongly acidic heparin to form an inactive stable salt. The complex has no anticoagulant activity. Heparin is neutralized within 5 min after IV protamine. **Duration:** 2 hr (but depends on body temperature). The t½ of protamine is shorter than heparin; thus, repeated doses may be required. Upon metabolism, the complex may liberate heparin (heparin rebound).
USES
Only for treatment of heparin overdose.
CONTRAINDICATIONS
Previous intolerance to protamine. Use to treat spontaneous hemorrhage, postpartum hemorrhage, menorrhagia, or uterine bleeding. Administration of over 50 mg over a short period.
SPECIAL CONCERNS
Use with caution during lactation. Safety and efficacy have not been determined in children. Rapid administration may cause severe hypotension and anaphylaxis.
SIDE EFFECTS
CV: Sudden fall in BP, bradycardia, transitory flushing, warm feeling, ***acute pulmonary hypertension, circulatory collapse (possibly irreversible) with myocardial failure*** and decreased CO. Pulmonary edema in clients on cardiopulmonary bypass undergoing CV surgery. *Anaphylaxis:* Severe respiratory distress, capillary leak, and noncardiogenic pulmonary edema. **GI:** N&V. **CNS:** Lassitude. **Other:** Dyspnea, back pain in conscious clients undergoing cardiac catheterization, hypersensitivity reactions.
OD OVERDOSE MANAGEMENT
Symptoms: Bleeding. Rapid administration may cause dyspnea, bradycardia, flushing, warm feeling, severe hypotension, hypertension. In assessing overdose, there may be the possibility of multiple drug overdoses leading to drug interactions and unusual pharmacokinetics. *Treatment:* Replace blood loss with blood transfusions or fresh frozen plasma. Fluids, epinephrine, dobutamine, or dopamine to treat hypotension.
HOW SUPPLIED
Injection: 10 mg/mL

DOSAGE
• **SLOW IV**
Give no more than 50 mg of protamine sulfate in any 10-min period. One mg of protamine sulfate can neutralize about 90 USP units of heparin derived from lung tissue or about 115 USP units of heparin derived from intestinal mucosa. *NOTE:* The dose of protamine sulfate depends on the amount of time that has elapsed since IV heparin administration. For example, if 30 min has elapsed, one-half the usual dose of protamine sulfate may be sufficient because heparin is cleared rapidly from the circulation.

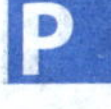

NURSING CONSIDERATIONS
ADMINISTRATION/STORAGE
IV 1. Incompatible with several penicillins and with cephalosporins.
2. To minimize side effects, give slowly over 10 min. May also be diluted in 50 mL of D5W or saline solution and administered at a rate of 50 mg over 10–15 min. Do not store diluted solutions.
3. Refrigerate at 2–8°C (36–46°F).
ASSESSMENT
1. Determine amount, time of overdose and source to ensure appropriate antidote dosing.
2. Request type and crossmatch; assess need for fresh frozen plasma or whole blood.

3. Coagulation studies should be performed 5–15 min after protamine has been administered; repeat in 2–8 hr to assess for heparin rebound (increased bleeding, lowered BP, and/or shock).
4. Monitor VS, I&O; assess for sudden fall in BP, bradycardia, dyspnea, transitory flushing, or sensations of warmth.

OUTCOMES/EVALUATE

Stable H&H; control of heparin-induced hemorrhage

Pseudoephedrine hydrochloride

(soo-doh-eh-**FED**-rin)

PREGNANCY CATEGORY: B
Rx: Children's Silfedrine, Dynafed Pseudo, Mini-Thin Pseudo, Pediatric Nasal Decongestant, Sudafed 12 Hour Caplets, Sudex, Triaminic AM Decongestant Formula
OTC: Allermed, Cenafed, Children's Congestion Relief, Congestion Relief, Decofed Syrup, DeFed-60, Dorcol Children's Decongestant Liquid, Efidac/24, Genaphed, Halofed, PediaCare Infants' Oral Decongestant Drops, Pseudo, Pseudo-Gest, Seudotabs, Sinustop Pro, Sudafed
✱OTC: Balminil Decongestant Syrup, Contac Cold 12 Hour Relief Non Drowsy, Eltor 120, PMS-Pseudoephedrine, Triaminic Oral Pediatric Drops

P

Pseudoephedrine sulfate

(soo-doh-eh-**FED**-rin)

PREGNANCY CATEGORY: B
OTC: Afrin Extended-Release Tablets, Drixoral Non-Drowsy Formula
✱OTC: Drixoral Day, Drixoral N.D.
CLASSIFICATION(S):
Sympathomimetic

SEE ALSO *SYMPATHOMIMETIC DRUGS.*

ACTION/KINETICS

Produces direct stimulation of both alpha-(pronounced) and beta-adrenergic receptors, as well as indirect stimulation through release of norepinephrine from storage sites. Results in decongestant effect on the nasal mucosa. Systemic administration eliminates possible damage to the nasal mucosa. **Onset:** 15–30 min. **Time to peak effect:** 30–60 min. **Duration:** 3–4 hr. **Extended-release: duration,** 8–12 hr. Urinary excretion slowed by alkalinization, causing reabsorption of drug.

USES

Nasal congestion associated with sinus conditions, otitis, allergies. Relief of eustachian tube congestion.

ADDITIONAL CONTRAINDICATIONS

Lactation. Use of sustained-release products in children less than 12 years of age.

SPECIAL CONCERNS

Use with caution in newborn and premature infants due to a higher risk of side effects. Geriatric clients may be more prone to age-related prostatic hypertrophy.

HOW SUPPLIED

Pseudoephedrine hydrochloride: *Capsule:* 60 mg; *Drops:* 7.5 mg/0.8 mL; *Liquid:* 15 mg/5 mL, 30 mg/5 mL; *Tablet:* 30 mg, 60 mg; *Tablet, extended release:* 120 mg, 240 mg. **Pseudoephedrine sulfate:** *Tablet, extended release* 120 mg

DOSAGE

HYDROCHLORIDE

• **CAPSULES, LIQUID, DROPS, TABLETS**

Decongestant.

Adults: 60 mg q 4–6 hr, not to exceed 240 mg in 24 hr. **Pediatric, 6–12 years:** 30 mg using the drops or liquid or syrup q 4–6 hr, not to exceed 120 mg in 24 hr; **2–6 years:** 15 mg using the drops or liquid q 4–6 hr, not to exceed 60 mg in 24 hr. Individualize the dose for children less than 2 years of age.

SULFATE

• **EXTENDED-RELEASE TABLETS**

Decongestant.

Adults and children over 12 years: 120 mg q 12 hr. Use is not recommended for children less than 12 years of age.

NURSING CONSIDERATIONS

SEE ALSO *NURSING CONSIDERATIONS* FOR *SYMPATHOMIMETIC DRUGS.*

ASSESSMENT

Note indications for therapy, onset, and characteristics of symptoms. Assess lung/heart sounds and note any allergy history.

CLIENT/FAMILY TEACHING

1. Avoid taking near bedtime; stimulation may produce insomnia.
2. With hypertension, report headaches, dizziness, or increased BP. Any extreme restlessness or sensitivity reactions should be reported.
3. Take exactly as directed. Do not crush or chew extended-release products. Continuous use or excessive dosing may cause rebound congestion.
4. Avoid OTC meds; may also contain ephedrine or other sympathomimetic amines and intensify drug action.
5. Report if symptoms do not improve after 3–5 days or worsen. Identify triggers and practice avoidance esp with seasonal allergies.

OUTCOMES/EVALUATE

Relief of nasal, sinus, or eustachian tube congestion

Psyllium hydrophilic muciloid

(**SILL**-ee-um hi-droh-**FILL**-ik)

CLASSIFICATION(S):

Laxative, bulk-forming

OTC: Alramucil, Fiberall Natural Flavor, Fiberall Orange Flavor, Fiberall Wafers, Genfiber, Hydrocil Instant, Konsyl, Konsyl-D, Konsyl-Orange, Maalox Daily Fiber Therapy, Maalox Daily Fiber Therapy Sugar Free, Metamucil, Metamucil Lemon-Lime Flavor, Metamucil Orange Flavor, Metamucil Sugar Free, Metamucil Sugar Free Orange Flavor, Modane Bulk, Mylanta Natural Fiber Supplement, Natural Fiber Laxative, Natural Fiber Laxative Sugar Free, Natural Vegetable, Perdiem Fiber, Reguloid Natural, Reguloid Orange, Reguloid Sugar Free Regular, Restore, Restore Sugar Free, Serutan, Syllact, V-Lax

✱**OTC:** Novo-Mucilax

SEE ALSO *LAXATIVES.*

ACTION/KINETICS

Obtained from the fruit of various species of plantago. The powder forms a gelatinous mass with water, which adds bulk to the stools and stimulates peristalsis. Also has a demulcent effect on an inflamed intestinal mucosa. Products may also contain dextrose, sodium bicarbonate, monobasic potassium phosphate, citric acid, and benzyl benzoate. Laxative effects usually occur in 12–24 hr. The full effect may take 2–3 days. Dependence may occur.

USES

(1) Prophylaxis of constipation in clients who should not strain during defecation. (2) Short-term treatment of constipation; useful in geriatric clients with diminished colonic motor response and during pregnancy and postpartum to reestablish normal bowel function. (3) To soften feces during fecal impaction.

CONTRAINDICATIONS

Severe abdominal pain or intestinal obstruction.

SIDE EFFECTS

Obstruction of the esophagus, stomach, small intestine, and rectum.

DRUG INTERACTIONS

Do not use concomitantly with salicylates, nitrofurantoin, or cardiac glycosides (e.g., digitalis).

HOW SUPPLIED

Effervescent Powder; Granule; Powder; Wafer

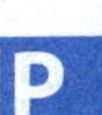

DOSAGE

Dose depends on the product. General information on adult dosage follows.

- **GRANULES, POWDER**

Adults: 1–2 teaspoons 1–3 times/day spread on food or with a glass of water.

- **EFFERVESCENT POWDER**

Adults: 1 packet in water 1–3 times/day.

- **WAFERS**

Adults: 2 wafers followed by a glass of water 1–3 times/day.

NURSING CONSIDERATIONS

SEE ALSO *NURSING CONSIDERATIONS* FOR *LAXATIVES.*

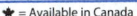

CLIENT/FAMILY TEACHING

1. Mix powder with plenty of liquid just prior to administering; otherwise, the mixture may become thick and difficult to drink.
2. The powder may be noxious and irritating when removing from the packets or canister. Open in a well-ventilated area and avoid inhaling particulate matter.
3. Take exactly as directed. Report lack of response or intolerable side effects.

OUTCOMES/EVALUATE

Prophylaxis/relief of constipation

Pyrantel pamoate

(pie-**RAN**-tell)

PREGNANCY CATEGORY: C
CLASSIFICATION(S):
Anthelmintic
OTC: Antiminth, Pin-Rid, Pin-X, Reese's Pinworm
★**Rx:** Combantrin

ACTION/KINETICS

Has neuromuscular blocking effect which paralyzes the helminth, allowing it to be expelled through the feces. Also inhibits cholinesterases. Poorly absorbed from GI tract. **Peak plasma levels:** 0.05–0.13 mcg/mL after 1–3 hr. Partially metabolized in liver. Fifty percent is excreted unchanged in feces and less than 15% excreted unchanged in urine.

USES

Pinworm (enterobiasis) and roundworm (ascariasis) infestations. Multiple helminth infections, as it is also effective against roundworm and hookworm.

CONTRAINDICATIONS

Pregnancy. Hepatic disease.

SPECIAL CONCERNS

Use with caution in presence of liver dysfunction. Safe use in children less than 2 years of age has not been established.

SIDE EFFECTS

GI (most frequent): Anorexia, N&V, abdominal cramps, diarrhea. **Hepatic:** Transient elevation of AST. **CNS:** Headache, dizziness, drowsiness, insomnia. **Miscellaneous:** Skin rashes.

DRUG INTERACTIONS

Use with piperazine for ascariasis results in antagonism of the effect of both drugs.

HOW SUPPLIED

Capsule, soft gel: 180 mg (as pamoate); *Liquid:* 50 mg (as pamoate)/mL; *Suspension, oral:* 50 mg (as pamoate)/mL

DOSAGE

• LIQUID, ORAL SUSPENSION, CAPSULES, SOFT GEL

Adults and children: One dose of 11 mg/kg (maximum). **Maximum total dose:** 1.0 g.

NURSING CONSIDERATIONS

ASSESSMENT

Note indications for therapy, symptom characteristics, and stool culture results. Identify close contacts.

CLIENT/FAMILY TEACHING

1. May be taken without regard to food intake. May take with milk or fruit juices.
2. May cause dizziness or drowsiness; do not engage in activities that require mental alertness.
3. Purging is not required. Report rash, severe headaches/GI upset, joint pain, or prolonged dizziness.
4. When treating pinworms, review client/family precautions R/T transmission.
   - strict handwashing and hygiene measures
   - launder undergarments, bed linens, sleep clothes in hot water daily
   - disinfect toilet facilities daily and bathroom floors
   - wet mop bedroom floors to prevent egg spread
   - do not share towels or wash clothes
   - treat all family members

OUTCOMES/EVALUATE

Resolution of infection; negative stool and perianal swabs

Pyridostigmine bromide

(peer-id-oh-**STIG**-meen)

PREGNANCY CATEGORY: C
CLASSIFICATION(S):
Cholinesterase inhibitor, indirectly-acting
Rx: Mestinon, Regonol
✱**Rx:** Mestinon-SR

FOR ALL INFORMATION, SEE ALSO *NEOSTIGMINE*.

ACTION/KINETICS

Has a slower onset, longer duration of action, and fewer side effects than neostigmine. **Onset, PO:** 30–45 min for syrup and tablets and 30–60 min for extended-release tablets; **IM:** 15 min; **IV:** 2–5 min. **Duration, PO:** 3–6 hr for syrup and tablets and 6–12 hr for extended-release tablets; **IM, IV:** 2–4 hr. Poorly absorbed from the GI tract; excreted in urine up to 72 hr after administration.

USES

Myasthenia gravis. Antidote for nondepolarizing muscle relaxants (e.g., tubocurarine).

ADDITIONAL CONTRAINDICATIONS

Sensitivity to bromides.

SPECIAL CONCERNS

Safe use during pregnancy and during lactation has not been established. May cause uterine irritability and premature labor if given IV to pregnant women near term. Duration of action may be increased in the elderly.

ADDITIONAL SIDE EFFECTS

Skin rash. Thrombophlebitis after IV use.

OD OVERDOSE MANAGEMENT

Symptoms: Abdominal cramps, vomiting, diarrhea, epigastric distress, excessive salivation, cold sweating, pallor, blurred vision, urinary urgency, fasciculation and ***paralysis of voluntary muscles*** (including the tongue), miosis, increased BP (may be accompanied by bradycardia), sensation of internal trembling, panic, severe anxiety. *Treatment:* Discontinue medication temporarily. Give atropine, 0.5–1 mg IV (up to 5–10 mg or more may be needed to get HR to 80 beats/min). Supportive treatment including artificial respiration and oxygen.

HOW SUPPLIED

Injection: 5 mg/mL; *Syrup:* 60 mg/5 mL; *Tablet:* 60 mg; *Tablet, extended release:* 180 mg

DOSAGE

- **SYRUP, TABLETS**

Myasthenia gravis.

Adults: 60–120 mg q 3–4 hr with dosage adjusted to client response. **Maintenance:** 600 mg/day (range: 60 mg–1.5 g). **Pediatric:** 7 mg/kg (200 mg/m^2) daily in five to six divided doses.

- **SUSTAINED-RELEASE TABLETS**

Myasthenia gravis.

Adults: 180–540 mg 1–2 times/day with at least 6 hr between doses. Sustained-release tablets not recommended for use in children.

- **IM, IV**

Myasthenia gravis.

Adults, IM, IV: 2 mg (about 1/30 the adult dose) q 2–3 hr.

Neonates of myasthenic mothers.

IM: 0.05–0.15 mg/kg q 4–6 hr.

Antidote for nondepolarizing drugs.

Adults, IV: 10–20 mg with 0.6–1.2 mg atropine sulfate given IV.

NURSING CONSIDERATIONS

SEE ALSO *NURSING CONSIDERATIONS* FOR *NEOSTIGMINE*.

ADMINISTRATION/STORAGE

1. During dosage adjustment, administer in a closely monitored environment.

IV 2. Parenteral dosage is 1/30 of the PO dose. May give undiluted at a rate of 0.5 mg IV over 1 min for myasthenia and at a rate of 5 mg IV over 1 min (with atropine) for reversal of nondepolarizing drug effects.

ASSESSMENT

1. Monitor VS and observe for toxic reactions demonstrated by generalized cholinergic stimulation.

P

2. Assess for muscular weakness; may signal impending myasthenic crisis and cholinergic overdose.
3. Determine the best individualized administration schedule according to client's routines and life-style.

CLIENT/FAMILY TEACHING

1. Myasthenia is an autoimmune disease with an unclear etiology. Medications correct acetycholine and cholinesterase imbalance at myoneural junction, which facilitates muscle contraction.
2. Do not crush and do not take extended-release tablets more often than q 6 hr; may be taken with conventional tablets, if prescribed.
3. With rest, muscle weakness and fatigue are temporarily resolved.
4. Rest and report symptoms of toxic reaction and myasthenic crisis.
5. Take medication as prescribed, since too early administration may result in cholinergic crisis whereas too late administration may result in myasthenic crisis.
6. Drug resistance may develop; close medical supervision and prompt reporting of all side effects is paramount.
7. Identify local support groups that may assist to understand and cope with this disorder.

P

OUTCOMES/EVALUATE

• Improvement in muscle strength/function
• Reversal of nondepolarizing drugs

Pyridoxine hydrochloride (Vitamin B_6)

(peer-ih-**DOX**-een)

PREGNANCY CATEGORY: A (C FOR DOSES THAT EXCEED THE RDA)
CLASSIFICATION(S):
Vitamin B complex
OTC: Aminoxin, Nestrex (Rx: Injection, OTC: Tablets)

ACTION/KINETICS

A water-soluble, heat-resistant vitamin that is destroyed by light. Acts as a coenzyme in the metabolism of protein, carbohydrates, and fat. As the amount of protein increases in the diet, the pyridoxine requirement increases. However, pyridoxine deficiency alone is rare. **t½:** 2–3 weeks. Metabolized in the liver and excreted through the urine.

USES

Pyridoxine deficiency including poor diet, drug-induced (e.g., oral contraceptives, isoniazid), and inborn errors of metabolism. *Investigational:* Hydrazine poisoning, PMS, high urine oxalate levels, N&V due to pregnancy, carpal tunnel syndrome, tardive dyskinesia due to antipsychotic drugs.

SPECIAL CONCERNS

Safety and effectiveness have not been established in children for doses that exceed the RDA.

SIDE EFFECTS

CNS: Unstable gait; decreased sensation to touch, temperature, and vibration; paresthesia, sleepiness; numbness of feet; awkwardness of hands; perioral numbness, photoallergic reaction, ataxia. *NOTE:* Abuse and dependence have been noted in adults administered 200 mg/day.

OD OVERDOSE MANAGEMENT

Symptoms: Ataxia, severe sensory neuropathy. *Treatment:* Discontinue pyridoxine; allow up to 6 months for CNS sensation to return.

DRUG INTERACTIONS

Chloramphenicol / ↑ Pyridoxine requirements
Contraceptives, oral / ↑ Pyridoxine requirements
Cycloserine / ↑ Pyridoxine requirements
Ethionamide / ↑ Pyridoxine requirements
Hydralazine / ↑ Pyridoxine requirements
Immunosuppressants / ↑ Pyridoxine requirements
Isoniazid / ↑ Pyridoxine requirements
Levodopa / Doses exceeding 5 mg/day pyridoxine antagonize the therapeutic effect of levodopa
Penicillamine / ↑ Pyridoxine requirements

Phenobarbital / ↓ Serum phenobarbital levels
Phenytoin / ↓ Serum phenytoin levels

HOW SUPPLIED

Enteric coated tablet: 20 mg; *Injection:* 100 mg/mL; *Tablet:* 25 mg, 50 mg, 100 mg, 250 mg, 500 mg; *Tablet, extended release:* 200 mg

DOSAGE

• ENTERIC-COATED TABLETS, TABLETS

RDAs.

The RDAs are as follows: **Adult males:** 1.7–2 mg. **Adult females:** 1.4–1.6 mg.

Dietary supplement.

Adults: 10–20 mg/day for 2 weeks; **then,** 2–5 mg/day as part of a multivitamin preparation for several weeks. **Pediatric,** 2.5–10 mg/day for 3 weeks; **then,** 2–5 mg/day as part of a multivitamin preparation for several weeks.

Isoniazid-induced deficiency.

Adults, prophylaxis: 6–100 mg/day for isoniazid. **Adults, treatment:** 50–200 mg/day for 3 weeks followed by 25–100 mg/day to prevent relapse. **Adults, alcoholism:** 50 mg/day for 2–4 weeks; if anemia responds, continue pyridoxine indefinitely.

PMS.

40–500 mg/day.

High urine oxalate levels.

25–300 mg/day.

Carpal tunnel syndrome.

100–200 mg/day for 12 or more weeks.

Tardive dyskinesia due to antipsychotic drugs.

100 mg/day for 4 weeks.

• IM, IV

Isoniazid-induced deficiency.

Adults: 50–200 mg/day for 3 weeks followed by 25–100 mg/day as needed.

Cycloserine poisoning.

Adults: 300 mg/day.

Isoniazid poisoning.

Adults: 1 g for each gram of isoniazid taken.

NURSING CONSIDERATIONS

ADMINISTRATION/STORAGE

1. If receiving levodopa, avoid preparations of vitamins containing B_6 as this decreases the availability of levodopa to the brain.

IV 2. May be administered by direct IV or placed in infusion solutions.

ASSESSMENT

1. Document characteristics of symptoms, and nutritional status. Identify reasons for drug therapy, e.g., to prevent toxicity (peripheral neuropathy) with long term isoniazid or contraceptive therapy, to replace vitamin B_6 with inborn errors of metabolism or with poor nutrition.

2. Take a complete dietary/drug history. Report cycloserine, isoniazid, or oral contraceptive use as these increase pyridoxine requirements.

CLIENT/FAMILY TEACHING

1. Foods high in vitamin B_6 include potatoes, lima beans, broccoli, bananas, chicken breast, liver, yeast, wheat germ, whole-grain cereals. Well-balanced diets are the best source of vitamins.

2. If prescribed levodopa, avoid vitamin supplements containing vitamin B_6. More than 5 mg of the vitamin antagonizes levodopa effect. At the same time, concomitant carbidopa administration will prevent effects of vitamin B_6 on levodopa.

3. If taking phenobarbital and/or phenytoin, obtain serum drug levels routinely, as pyridoxine alters serum concentrations.

4. Pyridoxine may inhibit lactation. Protein rich diet increases pyridoxine needs. Usual RDA for adults 2.2 mg; in pregnancy/lactation 2.6 mg.

5. Do not take OTC vitamin preparations without provider approval.

OUTCOMES/EVALUATE

• Relief of symptoms of pyridoxine deficiency

• Prophylaxis of drug-induced deficiency; ↓ toxic drug side effects

P

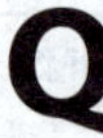

Quetiapine fumarate

(kweh-**TYE**-ah-peen)

PREGNANCY CATEGORY: C
CLASSIFICATION(S):
Antipsychotic
Rx: Seroquel

ACTION/KINETICS

Mechanism unknown but may act as an antagonist at dopamine D_2 and serotonin $5HT_2$ receptors. Side effects may be due to antagonism of other receptors (e.g., histamine H_1, dopamine D_1, adrenergic alpha-1 and alpha-2, serotonin $5HT_{1A}$). Rapidly absorbed. **Peak plasma levels:** 1.5 hr. Metabolized by liver and excreted through urine and feces. **t½, terminal:** About 6 hr.

USES

Treatment of schizophrenia.

CONTRAINDICATIONS

Lactation.

SPECIAL CONCERNS

Use with caution in liver disease, in those at risk for aspiration pneumonia, and in those with history of seizures or conditions that lower seizure threshold (e.g., Alzheimer's). Safety and efficacy have not been determined in children.

SIDE EFFECTS

Side effects with incidence of 1% or more are listed. **Body as a whole:** Asthenia, rash, fever, weight gain, back pain, flu syndrome. **CNS:** Headache, somnolence, dizziness, hypertonia, dysarthria. **GI:** Constipation, dry mouth, dyspepsia, anorexia, abdominal pain. **CV:** Orthostatic hypotension, syncope, tachycardia, palpitation. **Respiratory:** Pharyngitis, rhinitis, increased cough, dyspnea. **Miscellaneous:** Peripheral edema, hyperprolactinemia, sweating, leukopenia, ear pain. *NOTE:* ***Neuroleptic malignant syndrome*** and ***seizures,*** although rare, may occur.

LABORATORY TEST CONSIDERATIONS

↑ ALT during initial therapy, AST, total cholesterol, triglycerides.

OD OVERDOSE MANAGEMENT

Symptoms: Drowsiness, sedation, tachycardia, hypotension, dystonic reaction of the head and neck, seizures, obtundation. *Treatment:* Cardiovascular monitoring for arrhythmias. If antiarrhythmic therapy is used, disopyramide, procainamide, and quinidine increase risk of prolongation of QT. Treat hypotension and circulatory shock with IV fluids or sympathomimetic drugs (do not use epinephrine or dopamine as they may worsen hypotension). Use anticholinergic drugs to treat severe extrapyramidal symptoms.

DRUG INTERACTIONS

Barbiturates / ↓ Quetiapine effect R/T ↑ liver breakdown
Carbamazepine / ↓ Quetiapine effect R/T ↑ liver breakdown
Dopamine agonists / Quetiapine antagonizes effect
Glucocorticoids / ↓ Quetiapine effect R/T ↑ liver breakdown
Levodopa / Quetiapine antagonizes effect
Phenytoin / ↓ Quetiapine effect R/T ↑ liver breakdown
Rifampin / ↓ Quetiapine effect R/T ↑ liver breakdown
Thioridazine / ↑ Quetiapine clearance

HOW SUPPLIED

Tablets: 25 mg, 100 mg, 200 mg, 300 mg

DOSAGE

• TABLETS

Psychoses.

Initial: 25 mg b.i.d., with increases of 25 to 50 mg b.i.d. or t.i.d. on second and third day, as tolerated. Target dose range, by fourth day, is 300 to 400 mg daily. Further dosage adjustments can occur at intervals of two or more days. The antipsychotic dose range is 150 to 750 mg/day.

NURSING CONSIDERATIONS

ADMINISTRATION/STORAGE

1. Effectiveness for more than 6 weeks has not been evaluated. Evalu-

ate long-term usefulness periodically. Continue therapy at lowest dose to maintain remission.
2. Slower rate of dose titration and lower target dose is considered for elderly, in hepatic impairment, debilitated clients, and in those predisposed to hypotension.
3. Titration is not required when restarting clients who have had an interval of less than one week off quetiapine. Initial titration schedule is followed if clients have been off drug for more than one week.

ASSESSMENT

1. Document clinical presentation and behavioral manifestations.
2. Note any predisposition to hypotensive reactions if debilitated or if hepatic impairment present.
3. Document ophthalmic exam initially, and at 6 mo intervals, to assess for cataract formation.
4. Assess for S&S of Alzheimers disease, or history of seizures or cardiovascular disease; note VS, ECG, and LFTs.

CLIENT/FAMILY TEACHING

1. May take with or without food.
2. Total daily dose is divided and given two or three times a day.
3. Do not perform activities that require mental alertness until after titration period and until drug effects realized; may impair judgement and motor skills, and cause sleepiness. Change positions slowly to prevent postural effects.
4. Avoid alcohol and any OTC agents without approval.
5. Use reliable contraception; report if pregnancy suspected. Do not breastfeed.
6. Report any evidence of extrapyramidal symptoms; tardive dyskinesia (involuntary movements).
7. Avoid situations where overheating or dehydration may occur.
8. Long-term usefulness must be evaluated periodically while on lowest dose to maintain remission.

OUTCOMES/EVALUATE

Control of S&S of psychotic disorders

Quinapril hydrochloride

(**KWIN**-ah-prill)

PREGNANCY CATEGORY: D
CLASSIFICATION(S):
Antihypertensive, ACE inhibitor
Rx: Accupril

SEE ALSO *ANGIOTENSIN-CONVERTING ENZYME INHIBITORS.*

ACTION/KINETICS

Onset: 1 hr. **Time to peak serum levels:** 1 hr. **Peak decrease in BP:** 2–6 hr. Metabolized to quinaprilat, the active metabolite. **t½, quinaprilat:** 2–3 hr. **Duration:** 18–24 hr. Significantly bound to plasma proteins. Food reduces absorption. Metabolized with approximately 60% excreted through the urine and 37% excreted in the feces. Also appears to improve endothelial function, an early marker of coronary atherosclerosis.

USES

(1) Alone or in combination with a thiazide diuretic for the treatment of hypertension. (2) Adjunct with a diuretic or digitalis to treat CHF in those not responding adequately to diuretics or digitalis.

SPECIAL CONCERNS

Use with caution during lactation. Safety and effectiveness have not been determined in children. Geriatric clients may be more sensitive to the effects of quinapril and manifest higher peak quinaprilat blood levels.

SIDE EFFECTS

CV: Vasodilation, tachycardia, ***heart failure,*** palpitations, chest pain, hypotension, ***MI, CVA, hypertensive crisis,*** angina pectoris, orthostatic hypotension, ***cardiac rhythm disturbances, cardiogenic shock***. **GI:** Dry mouth or throat, constipation, diarrhea, N&V, abdominal pain, hepatitis, pancreatitis, ***GI hemorrhage.*** **CNS:** Somnolence, vertigo, insomnia, sleep disturbances, paresthesias, nervousness, depression, headache, dizziness, fatigue. **Hematologic:** ***Agranulocyto-***

Q

sis, bone marrow depression, thrombocytopenia. **Dermatologic: *Angioedema of the lips, tongue, glottis, and larynx;*** sweating, pruritus, exfoliative dermatitis, photosensitivity, dermatopolymyositis, flushing, rash. **Body as a whole:** Malaise, edema, back pain. **GU:** Oliguria and/or progressive azotemia and rarely ***acute renal failure and/or death in severe heart failure.*** Impotence. Worsening renal failure. **Respiratory:** Pharyngitis, cough, asthma, bronchospasm, dyspnea. **Musculoskeletal:** Myalgia, arthralgia. **Miscellaneous:** Oligohydramnios in fetuses exposed to the drug in utero. Abnormal liver function tests, syncope, hyperkalemia, amblyopia, syncope, viral infection.

OD OVERDOSE MANAGEMENT

Symptoms: Commonly, hypotension. *Treatment:* IV infusion of normal saline to restore blood pressure.

DRUG INTERACTIONS

Potassium-containing salt substitutes / ↑ Risk of hyperkalemia
Potassium-sparing diuretics / ↑ Risk of hyperkalemia
Potassium supplements / ↑ Risk of hyperkalemia
Tetracyclines / ↓ Absorption R/T high Mg^{++} content of quinapril tablets

HOW SUPPLIED

Tablet: 5 mg, 10 mg, 20 mg, 40 mg

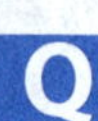

DOSAGE

• TABLETS

Hypertension, client not on diuretics.

Initial: 10 or 20 mg once daily; **then,** adjust dosage based on BP response at peak (2–6 hr) and trough (predose) blood levels. The dose should be adjusted at 2-week intervals. **Maintenance:** 20, 40, or 80 mg daily as a single dose or in two equally divided doses. With impaired renal function, the initial dose should be 10 mg if the C_{CR} is greater than 60 mL/min, 5 mg if the C_{CR} is between 30 and 60 mL/min, and 2.5 mg if the C_{CR} is between 10 and 30 mL/min. If the initial dose is well tolerated, the drug may be given the following day as a b.i.d. regimen.

CHF.

Initial: 5 mg b.i.d. If this dose is well tolerated, titrate clients at weekly intervals until an effective dose, usually 20–40 mg daily in two equally divided doses, is attained. Undesirable hypotension, orthostasis, or azotemia may prevent this dosage level from being reached.

NURSING CONSIDERATIONS

SEE ALSO *ANGIOTENSIN-CONVERTING ENZYME INHIBITORS* AND *ANTIHYPERTENSIVE AGENTS.*

ADMINISTRATION/STORAGE

1. If taking a diuretic, discontinue the diuretic 2–3 days prior to beginning quinapril. If the BP is not controlled, reinstitute the diuretic. If the diuretic cannot be discontinued, the initial dose should be 1.25 mg.
2. If the antihypertensive effect decreases at the end of the dosing interval with once-daily therapy, consider either twice-daily administration or increasing the dose.
3. The antihypertensive effect may not be observed for 1–2 weeks.

ASSESSMENT

1. Observe infants exposed to quinapril in utero for the development of hypotension, oliguria, and hyperkalemia.
2. If angioedema occurs, stop drug, assess airway, and observe until swelling resolved. Antihistamines may help relieve symptoms.
3. Monitor VS, I&O, weights, electrolytes, CBC, and renal function studies. Agranulocytosis and bone marrow depression seen more often with renal impairment, especially if collagen vascular disease (e.g., SLE, scleroderma) present.
4. Clients with unilateral or bilateral renal artery stenosis may manifest increased BUN and serum creatinine if given quinapril. Assess renal function closely the first few weeks of therapy.

CLIENT/FAMILY TEACHING

1. Take as directed; food/antacids reduces absorption so take 1-2hr before.
2. Avoid activities that require mental alertness until drug effects realized.
3. Report any unusual bruising/bleeding, fever, sore throat, or persistent side effects.
4. Any increased SOB, palpitations,

swelling, or persistent nonproductive cough should be evaluated.

5. Keep a log of BP readings for provider review.

OUTCOMES/EVALUATE

↓ BP

Quinidine gluconate

(**KWIN**-ih-deen)

PREGNANCY CATEGORY: C
Rx: Quinaglute Dura-Tabs, Quinalan

Quinidine polygalacturonate

(**KWIN**-ih-deen)

PREGNANCY CATEGORY: C
Rx: Cardioquin

Quinidine sulfate

(**KWIN**-ih-deen)

PREGNANCY CATEGORY: C
Rx: Quinidex Extentabs, Quinora
✱**Rx:** Apo-Quinidine
CLASSIFICATION(S):
Antiarrhythmic, Class IA

SEE ALSO *ANTIARRHYTHMIC AGENTS*.

ACTION/KINETICS

Reduces the excitability of the heart and depresses conduction velocity and contractility. Prolongs the refractory period and increases conduction time. It also decreases CO and possesses anticholinergic, antimalarial, antipyretic, and oxytocic properties. **PO: Onset:** 0.5–3 hr. **Maximum effects, after IM:** 30–90 min. **t½:** 6–7 hr. **Time to peak levels, PO:** 3–5 hr for gluconate salt, 1–1.5 hr for sulfate salt, and 6 hr for polygalacturonate salt; **IM:** 1 hr. **Therapeutic serum levels:** 2–6 mcg/mL. **Protein binding:** 60%–80%. **Duration:** 6–8 hr for tablets/capsules and 12 hr for extended-release tablets. Metabolized by liver. Urine pH affects rate of urinary excretion (10%–50% excreted unchanged).

USES

(1) Premature atrial, AV junctional, and ventricular contractions. (2) Treatment and control of atrial flutter, established atrial fibrillation, paroxysmal atrial tachycardia, paroxysmal AV junctional rhythm, paroxysmal and chronic atrial fibrillation, paroxysmal ventricular tachycardia not associated with complete heart block. (3) Maintenance therapy after electrical conversion of atrial flutter or fibrillation. The parenteral route is indicated when PO therapy is not feasible or immediate effects are required. *Investigational:* Gluconate salt for life-threatening *Plasmodium falciparum* malaria.

CONTRAINDICATIONS

Hypersensitivity to drug or other cinchona drugs. Myasthenia gravis, history of thrombocytopenic purpura associated with quinidine use, digitalis intoxication evidenced by arrhythmias or AV conduction disorders. Also, complete heart block, left bundle branch block, or other intraventricular conduction defects manifested by marked QRS widening or bizarre complexes. Complete AV block with an AV nodal or idioventricular pacemaker, aberrant ectopic impulses and abnormal rhythms due to escape mechanisms. History of drug-induced torsades de pointes or long QT syndrome.

SPECIAL CONCERNS

Safety in children and during lactation has not been established. Use with extreme caution in clients in whom a sudden change in BP might be detrimental or in those suffering from extensive myocardial damage, subacute endocarditis, bradycardia, coronary occlusion, disturbances in impulse conduction, chronic valvular disease, considerable cardiac enlargement, frank CHF, and renal or hepatic disease. Use with caution in acute infections, hyperthyroidism, muscular weakness, respiratory distress, and bronchial asthma. The dose in geriatric clients may have to be reduced due to age-related changes in renal function.

SIDE EFFECTS

CV: Widening of QRS complex, hypotension, ***cardiac asystole,*** ectopic ventricular beats, ***ventricular tachycardia or fibrillation, torsades de pointes,*** paradoxical tachycardia, ***arterial embolism,*** ventricular extrasystoles (one or more every 6 beats), prolonged QT interval, ***complete AV block, ventricular flutter.*** **GI:** N&V, abdominal pain, anorexia, diarrhea, urge to defecate as well as urinate, esophagitis (rare). **CNS:** Syncope, headache, confusion, excitement, vertigo, apprehension, delirium, dementia, ataxia, depression. **Dermatologic:** Rash, urticaria, exfoliative dermatitis, photosensitivity, flushing with intense pruritus, eczema, psoriasis, pigmentation abnormalities. **Allergic:** Acute asthma, angioneurotic edema, ***respiratory arrest,*** dyspnea, fever, ***vascular collapse,*** purpura, vasculitis, hepatic dysfunction (including granulomatous hepatitis), ***hepatic toxicity.*** **Hematologic:** Hypoprothrombinemia, ***acute hemolytic anemia,*** thrombocytopenic purpura, ***agranulocytosis,*** thrombocytopenia, leukocytosis, neutropenia, shift to left in WBC differential. **Ophthalmologic:** Blurred vision, mydriasis, alterations in color perception, decreased field of vision, double vision, photophobia, optic neuritis, night blindness, scotomata. **Other:** Liver toxicity including hepatitis, lupus nephritis, tinnitus, decreased hearing acuity, arthritis, myalgia, increase in serum skeletal muscle CPK, lupus erythematosus.

LABORATORY TEST CONSIDERATIONS

False + or ↑ PSP, 17-ketosteroids, PT.

OD OVERDOSE MANAGEMENT

Symptoms: CNS: Lethargy, confusion, ***coma, seizures, respiratory depression or arrest,*** headache, paresthesia, vertigo. CNS symptoms may be seen after onset of CV toxicity. *GI:* Vomiting, diarrhea, abdominal pain, hypokalemia, nausea. *CV:* Sinus tachycardia, ***ventricular tachycardia or fibrillation, torsades de pointes, depressed automaticity and conduction*** (including bundle branch block, sinus bradycardia, SA block, prolongation of QRS and QTc, sinus arrest, AV block, ST depression, T inversion), syncope, ***heart failure.*** Hypotension due to decreased conduction and CO and vasodilation. *Miscellaneous:* Cinchonism, visual and auditory disturbances, hypokalemia, tinnitus, acidosis. *Treatment:*

- Perform gastric lavage, induce vomiting, and administer activated charcoal if ingestion is recent.
- Monitor ECG, blood gases, serum electrolytes, and BP.
- Institute cardiac pacing, if necessary.
- Acidify the urine.
- Use artificial respiration and other supportive measures.
- Infusions of 1/6 molar sodium lactate IV may decrease the cardiotoxic effects.
- Treat hypotension with metaraminol or norepinephrine after fluid volume replacement.
- Use phenytoin or lidocaine to treat tachydysrhythmias.
- Hemodialysis is effective but not often required.

DRUG INTERACTIONS

Acetazolamide, Antacids / ↑ Quinidine effect R/T ↓ renal excretion
Amiodarone / ↑ Quinidine levels with possible fatal cardiac dysrhythmias
Anticholinergic agents, Atropine / Additive effect on blockade of vagus nerve action
Anticoagulants, oral / Additive hypoprothrombinemia with possible hemorrhage
Barbiturates / ↓ Quinidine effect R/T ↑ liver breakdown
H *Belladonna leaf/root* / Increased anticholinergic effect
Cholinergic agents / Quinidine antagonizes effect of cholinergic drugs
Cimetidine / ↑ Quinidine effect R/T ↓ liver breakdown
Digoxin / ↑ Symptoms of digoxin toxicity
Disopyramide / Either ↑ disopyramide levels or ↓ quinidine levels
Guanethidine / Additive hypotensive effect
H *Henbane leaf* / ↑ Anticholinergic effects
Itraconazole / ↑ Risk of tinnitus and ↓ hearing

H *Lily-of-the-valley* / ↑ Effect and side effects of quinidine
Methyldopa / Additive hypotensive effect
Metoprolol / ↑ Metoprolol effect in fast metabolizers
Neuromuscular blocking agents / ↑ Respiratory depression
Nifedipine / ↓ Quinidine effect
H *Pheasant's eye herb* / ↑ Effect and side effects of quinidine
Phenobarbital, Phenytoin / ↓ Quinidine effect R/T ↑ rate of liver metabolism
Potassium / ↑ Quinidine effect
Procainamide / ↑ Procainamide effects with possible toxicity
Propafenone / ↑ Serum propafenone levels in rapid metabolizers
Propranolol / ↑ Propranolol effect in fast metabolizers
Rifampin / ↓ Quinidine effect R/T ↑ liver breakdown
H *Scopolia root* / ↑ Quinidine effect
Skeletal muscle relaxants / ↑ Skeletal muscle relaxation
Sodium bicarbonate / ↑ Quinidine effect R/T ↓ renal excretion
H *Squill* / ↑ Effect and side effects of quinidine
Sucralfate / ↓ Serum quinidine levels → ↓ effect
Thiazide diuretics / ↑ Quinidine effect R/T ↓ renal excretion
Tricyclic antidepressants / ↑ TCA effect R/T ↓ clearance
Verapamil / ↓ Verapamil clearance → ↑ hypotension, bradycardia, AV block, VT, and pulmonary edema

HOW SUPPLIED

Quinidine gluconate: *Injection:* 80 mg/mL; *Tablet, extended release:* 324 mg. **Quinidine polygalacturonate:** *Tablet:* 275 mg. **Quinidine sulfate:** *Tablet:* 200 mg, 300 mg; *Tablet, extended release:* 300 mg

DOSAGE

• QUINIDINE POLYGALACTURONATE TABLETS, QUINIDINE SULFATE TABLETS

Premature atrial and ventricular contractions.

Adults: 200–300 mg t.i.d.–q.i.d.

Paroxysmal SVTs.

Adults: 400–600 mg q 2–3 hr until the paroxysm is terminated.

Conversion of atrial flutter.

Adults: 200 mg q 2–3 hr for five to eight doses; daily doses can be increased until rhythm is restored or toxic effects occur.

Conversion of atrial flutter, maintenance therapy.

Adults: 200–300 mg t.i.d.–q.i.d. Large doses or more frequent administration may be required in some clients.

• QUINIDINE GLUCONATE EXTENDED-RELEASE TABLETS, QUINIDINE SULFATE EXTENDED-RELEASE TABLETS

All uses.

Adults: 300–600 mg q 8–12 hr.

• QUINIDINE GLUCONATE INJECTION (IM OR IV)

Acute tachycardia.

Adults, initial: 600 mg IM; **then,** 400 mg IM repeated as often as q 2 hr.

Arrhythmias.

Adults: 330 mg IM or less IV (as much as 500–750 mg may be required).

P. falciparum malaria.

Two regimens may be used. (1) *Loading dose:* 15 mg/kg in 250 mL NSS given over 4 hr; **then,** 24 hr after beginning the loading dose, institute 7.5 mg/kg infused over 4 hr and given q 8 hr for 7 days or until PO therapy can be started. (2) *Loading dose:* 10 mg/kg in 250 mL NSS infused over 1–2 hr followed immediately by 0.02 mg/kg/min for up to 72 hr or until parasitemia decreases to less than 1% or PO therapy can be started.

NURSING CONSIDERATIONS

SEE ALSO *NURSING CONSIDERATIONS* FOR *ANTIARRHYTHMIC AGENTS*.

ADMINISTRATION/STORAGE

1. A preliminary test dose may be given. **Adults:** 200 mg quinidine sulfate or quinidine gluconate administered PO or IM. **Children:** Test dose of 2 mg/kg of quinidine sulfate.
2. The extended-release forms are not interchangeable.
IV 3. Prepare IV solution by diluting 10 mL of quinidine gluconate injec-

Q

tion (800 mg) with 50 mL of D5W; give at a rate of 1 mL/min.

4. Use only colorless clear solution for injection. Light may cause quinidine to crystallize, which turns solution brownish.

ASSESSMENT

1. Note any allergic reactions to antiarrhythmic drugs or tartrazine, which is found in some formulations. Perform a test dose; observe for hypersensitivity reactions and check for intolerance.
2. Document indications for therapy, onset, and symptom characteristics.
3. Obtain CXR; monitor electrolytes, CBC, liver and renal function studies.
4. Assess VS and ECG; note heart and lung sounds.

INTERVENTIONS

1. Report any increased AV block, cardiac irritability, or rhythm suppression during IV administration.
2. Monitor I&O, VS; observe for hypotension. Drug induces urinary alkalization.
3. Report any neurologic deficits/sensory impairment (i.e., numbness, confusion, pyschosis, depression, or involuntary movements).
4. Report any persistent diarrhea. Among the elderly, there is a higher risk of toxicity, reduced CO, and unpredictable effects from drug.
5. Clients with long-standing atrial fibrillation or CHF with atrial fibrillation run a risk of embolization from mural thrombi when converting to sinus rhythm.

CLIENT/FAMILY TEACHING

1. Take with food to minimize GI effects.
2. Avoid activities that require mental alertness until drug effects realized; may cause dizziness or blurred vision.
3. Add fruit and grain to diet. A high intake of fruits and vegetables (alkaline-ash foods) may prolong drug half-life.
4. Report any of the following symptoms:
   - Severe skin rash, hives or itching
   - Severe headache
   - Unexplained fever
   - Ringing in the ears, buzzing, or hearing loss
   - Unusual bruising or bleeding
   - Blurred vision
   - Irregular heart beat, palpitations, or faintness
   - Continued diarrhea
5. Wear dark glasses if photophobic.
6. Report for labs, ECG, PFTs, and eye exams.

OUTCOMES/EVALUATE

- Restoration of stable rhythm
- Therapeutic drug levels (2–6 mcg/mL)

Quinine sulfate

(**KWYE**-nine)

PREGNANCY CATEGORY: X
CLASSIFICATION(S):
Antimalarial
✱**Rx:** Quinine-Odan

ACTION/KINETICS

Natural alkaloid having antimalarial, antipyretic, analgesic, and oxytocic properties. Use in treating malaria is important due to emergence of resistant forms of vivax and falciparum; no resistant forms of the parasite have been found for quinine. Antimalarial mechanism not known precisely; quinine does affect DNA replication and may raise intracellular pH. Eradicates the erythrocytic stages of plasmodia. Increases the refractory period of skeletal muscle, decreases the excitability of the motor end-plate region, and affects the distribution of calcium within the muscle fiber, thus making it useful for nocturnal leg cramps. Is oxytocic and may cause congenital malformations. Rapidly and completely absorbed from the upper small intestine; widely distributed in body tissues. **Peak plasma levels:** 1–3 hr; **plasma levels following chronic use:** 7 mcg/mL. **t½:** 4–5 hr. Highly bound to protein (70%–85%); about 5% excreted unchanged in urine. Small amounts found in saliva, bile, feces, and gastric juice. Acidifying the urine increases the rate of excretion.

Pharmacokinetics of quinine are affected by malaria, with a decrease in volume of distribution and systemic clearance. Protein binding, which is normally 70% to 85%, increases to more than 90% in clients with cerebral malaria, in pregnancy, and in children.

USES

(1) Alone or in combination with pyrimethamine and a sulfonamide or a tetracycline for chloroquine-resistant forms of *Plasmodium falciparum.* (2) As alternative therapy for chloroquine-sensitive stains of *P. falciparum, P. malariae, P. ovale,* and *P. vivax.* Mefloquine and clindamycin may also be used with quinine, depending on where the malaria was acquired. *Investigational:* Prevention and treatment of nocturnal recumbency leg cramps.

CONTRAINDICATIONS

Use with tinnitus, G6PD deficiency, optic neuritis, history of blackwater fever, and thrombocytopenia purpura associated with previous use of quinine. Pregnancy.

SPECIAL CONCERNS

Use with caution in clients with cardiac arrhythmias and during lactation. Hemolysis, with a potential for hemolytic anemia, may occur in clients with G6PD deficiency.

SIDE EFFECTS

Use of quinine may result in a syndrome referred to as *cinchonism.* Mild cinchonism is characterized by tinnitus, headache, nausea, slight visual disturbances. Larger doses, however, may cause severe CNS, CV, GI, or dermatologic effects. **Allergic:** Flushing, cutaneous rashes (papular, scarlatinal, urticarial), fever, facial edema, pruritus, dyspnea, tinnitus, sweating, asthmatic symptoms, visual impairment, gastric upset. **GI:** N&V, epigastric pain, hepatitis. **Ophthalmologic:** Blurred vision with scotomata, photophobia, diplopia, night blindness, decreased visual fields, impaired color vision and perception, amblyopia, mydriasis, optic atrophy. **CNS:** Headache, confusion, restlessness, vertigo, syncope, fever, apprehension, excitement, delirium, hypothermia, dizziness, ***convulsions.*** **Otic:** Tinnitus, deafness. **Hematologic:** Acute hemolysis, hemolytic anemia, thrombocytopenic purpura, agranulocytosis, hypoprothrombinemia. **CV:** Symptoms of angina, ventricular tachycardia, conduction disturbances, vasculitis. **Miscellaneous:** Sweating, hypoglycemia, lichenoid photosensitivity.

OD OVERDOSE MANAGEMENT

Symptoms: Dizziness, intestinal cramping, skin rash, tinnitus. With higher doses, symptoms include apprehension, confusion, fever, headache, vomiting, and seizures. *Treatment:*

- Induce vomiting or undertake gastric lavage.
- Maintain BP and renal function.
- If necessary, provide artificial respiration.
- Sedatives, oxygen, and other supportive measures may be required.
- Give IV fluids to maintain fluid and electrolyte balance.
- Treat angioedema or asthma with epinephrine, corticosteroids, and antihistamines.
- Urinary acidification will hasten excretion; however, in the presence of hemoglobinuria, acidification of the urine will increase renal blockade.

DRUG INTERACTIONS

Acetazolamide / ↑ Blood levels with potential for quinine toxicity R/T ↓ rate of elimination
Aluminum-containing antacids / ↓ Or delayed quinine absorption
Anticoagulants, oral / Additive hypoprothrombinemia R/T ↓ synthesis of vitamin K–dependent clotting factors
Cimetidine / ↑ Quinine effect R/T ↓ rate of excretion
Digoxin / ↑ Digoxin serum levels
Heparin / ↓ Heparin effect
Mefloquine / ↑ Risk of ECG abnormalities or cardiac arrest; also, ↑ risk of convulsions. **Do not** use together; delay mefloquine administration at least 12 hr after the last dose of quinine.
Neuromuscular blocking agents (depolarizing and nondepolarizing) / ↑ Respiratory depression and apnea
Rifabutin, Rifampin / ↑ Hepatic clearance of quinine; can persist for several days following discontinuation of the rifampin

Q

Sodium bicarbonate / ↑ Quinine blood levels with potential for quinine toxicity R/T ↓ elimination rate
Succinylcholine / ↓ Succinylcholine metabolism rate due to ↓ plasma cholinesterase activity

HOW SUPPLIED
Capsule: 200 mg, 260 mg, 325 mg; *Tablet:* 260 mg

DOSAGE

- **CAPSULES, TABLETS**

Chloroquine-resistant malaria.

Adults: 650 mg q 8 hr for at least 3 days (7 days in Southeast Asia) along with pyrimethamine, 25 mg b.i.d. for the first 3 days and sulfadiazine, 2 g/day for the first 5 days. There are two alternative regimens: (1) quinine, 650 mg q 8 hr for at least 3 days (7 days in Southeast Asia) along with a tetracycline, 250 mg q 6 hr for 10 days or (2) quinine, 650 mg q 8 hr for 3 days with sulfadoxine, 1.5 g and pyrimethamine, 75 mg as a single dose.

Chloroquine-sensitive malaria.

Adults: 600 mg q 8 hr for 5–7 days. **Pediatric:** 10 mg/kg q 8 hr for 5–7 days.

Nocturnal leg cramps.

Adults: 260–300 mg at bedtime.

NURSING CONSIDERATIONS

SEE ALSO *GENERAL NURSING CONSIDERATIONS FOR ALL ANTI-INFECTIVES.*

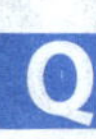

ADMINISTRATION/STORAGE

1. Dispense in a light-resistant and child-resistant container; store at controlled room temperatures of 15–30°C (59–86°F).
IV 2. The parenteral form is available from the Centers for Disease Control if client unable to take PO.

ASSESSMENT

1. Document indications for therapy, onset and symptom duration, dates of travel, and other agents trialed.
2. Note any history or evidence of cardiac arrhythmias or disease.
3. Assess leg cramps to determine that they only occur at night when recumbent.
4. Obtain baseline CBC and eye exam; monitor status.

CLIENT/FAMILY TEACHING

1. Do not take with antacids. Take with food or after meals to minimize GI irritation. Stop smoking.
2. Do not drive a car or operate machinery until drug effects realized; may cause dizziness or blurred vision.
3. Use sunglasses to protect from photophobia.
4. Avoid tonic water and OTC agents esp cold remedies. If also taking cimetidine or digoxin, may require dosage adjustment; report side effects.
5. Females should use non-hormonal contraception; drug may harm fetus.
6. Report new ringing in the ears, blurring of vision, and headache, which may be followed by digestive disturbances, impairment of hearing and sight, confusion, and delirium. May indicate intolerance or overdosage and requires immediate medical intervention.

OUTCOMES/EVALUATE

- Termination of acute malarial attack/control of malaria symptoms
- Relief of nocturnal leg cramps

Quinupristin/ Dalfopristin

(**kwin**-oo-**PRIS**-tin/**DAL**-foh-**pris**-tin)

PREGNANCY CATEGORY: B
CLASSIFICATION(S):
Antibiotic, streptogramin
Rx: Synercid

ACTION/KINETICS

A sterile, lyophilized product of two semisynthetic pristinamycin derivatives — quinupristin (30 parts) and dalfopristin (70 parts). The two act synergistically so the microbiologic activity is greater than each individually. Metabolites of the two are also active. The drugs act at the bacterial ribosome: dalfopristin inhibits the early phase of protein synthesis while quinupristin inhibits the late phase of protein synthesis. Vancomycin-resistant infections may also be resistant to this product. **t½, quinupristin and**

metabolites: 3.07 hr; **t½, dalfopristin and metabolites:** 1.04 hr. Both can interfere with the metabolism of other drugs that are associated with QTc prolongation; however, they do not themselves induce QTc prolongation. Excreted through the feces (about 75% for both drugs) and urine (about 17% for both drugs).

USES

(1) Treatment of serious or life-threatening infections associated with vancomycin-resistant *Enterococcus faecium* bacteremia. (2) Complicated skin and skin structure infections caused by *Staphylococcus aureus* (methicillin-sensitive) or *Streptococcus pyogenes*.

CONTRAINDICATIONS

Hypersensitivity to quinupristin/dalfopristin or prior hypersensitivity to other streptogramins. Use with drugs metabolized by the cytochrome P450 3A4 enzyme system that may prolong the QTc interval.

SPECIAL CONCERNS

Use with caution during lactation. Although sometimes used for emergencies in children, safety and efficacy have not been determined in clients less than 16 years of age.

SIDE EFFECTS

At infusion site: Inflammation, pain, edema, infusion site reaction. **GI:** Pseudomembranous colitis (mild to life-threatening), N&V, diarrhea, constipation, dyspepsia, oral moniliasis, pancreatitis, stomatitis. **CNS:** Headache, anxiety, confusion, dizziness, hypertonia, insomnia, leg cramps, paresthesia. **CV:** Thrombophlebitis, palpitation, phlebitis, vasodilation. **Dermatologic:** Rash, pruritus, maculopapular rash, sweating, urticaria. **Musculoskeletal:** Arthralgia, myalgia, myasthenia. **GU:** Hematuria, vaginitis. **Respiratory:** Dyspnea, pleural effusion. **Miscellaneous:** Pain, abdominal pain, worsening of underlying illness, allergic reaction, chest pain, fever, infection, superinfection.

LABORATORY TEST CONSIDERATIONS

↑ AST, ALT, bilirubin, conjugated bilirubin, LDH, alkaline phosphatase, gamma-GT, CPK, creatinine, BUN, hematocrit. ↓ Hemoglobin. ↑ or ↓ Blood glucose, bicarbonates, CO_2, sodium, potassium, platelets. Hyperbilrubinemia.

DRUG INTERACTIONS

Quinupristin/dalfopristin may cause increased plasma levels of drugs primarily metabolized by the cytochrome P450 3A4 enzyme system. These drugs include: Carbamazepine, cisapride, cyclosporine, delavirdine, diazepam, diltiazem, disopyramide, docetaxel, HMG-CoA reductase inhibitors, indinavir, lidocaine, methylprednisolone, midazolam, nevirapine, nifedipine, paclitaxel, quinidine, ritonavir, tacrolimus, verapamil, vinca alkaloids.

HOW SUPPLIED

Injection, lyophilized: 500 mg (150 mg quinupristin and 350 mg dalfopristin)/10 mL

DOSAGE

• **IV INFUSION**

Vancomycin-resistant Enterococcus faecium *infections.*

7.5 mg/kg q 8 hr. Base treatment duration on the site and severity of the infection.

Complicated skin and skin structure infections.

7.5 mg/kg q 12 hr for 7 days.

NURSING CONSIDERATIONS

ADMINISTRATION/STORAGE

IV 1. Give by IV infusion in D5W over a 60-min period.

2. Central venous access may be used to decrease venous irritation.

3. An infusion pump/device may be used to control infusion rate.

4. Prepare and give as follows:

• Reconstitute the single dose vial by slowly adding 5 mL D5W or sterile water for injection under strict aseptic conditions (e.g., laminar flow hood).

• To ensure dissolution, gently swirl the vial by manual rotation without shaking (to limit foam formation).

• Allow the solution to sit for a few minutes until all the foam has disappeared. Solution should be clear. Concentration is 100 mg/mL. Further dilution is required before administration; dilute within 30 min of reconstitution.

• According to the client's weight, add the reconstituted solution to 250 mL of D5W (about 2 mg/mL). An infusion volume of 100 mL may be used for central line infusions.
• If moderate-to-severe venous irritation occurs following peripheral administration, consider increasing the infusion volume to 500 or 750 mL, changing the infusion site, or by peripherally inserting a central venous catheter.
5. **Do not dilute/flush** with saline solution because the drugs are incompatible.
6. Do not mix with or physically add these drugs to other drugs except for the following: aztreonam (20 mg/mL), ciprofloxacin (1 mg/mL), fluconazole (2 mg/mL), haloperidol (0.2 mg/mL), metoclopramide (5 mg/mL), and potassium chloride (40 mEq/L).
7. With intermittent infusion of these drugs and other drugs through a common IV line, flush the line before and after administration with D5W.
8. Before reconstitution, refrigerate vials at 2–8° C (36–46° F).
9. Prior to infusion, the diluted solution is stable for 5 hr at room temperature or 54 hr if refrigerated. Do not freeze the solution.

ASSESSMENT

1. Note indications for therapy, characteristics of infection, and culture and sensitivity results.
2. If these drugs are used with drugs that are cytochrome P450 3A4 substrates (see drug interactions) and possess a narrow therapeutic index, monitor carefully.
3. If client develops diarrhea, test for *C. difficile* colitis.
4. Isolate client and take special precautions to identify source and to prevent spread of organism.

OUTCOMES/EVALUATE

Resolution of VRE infection

R

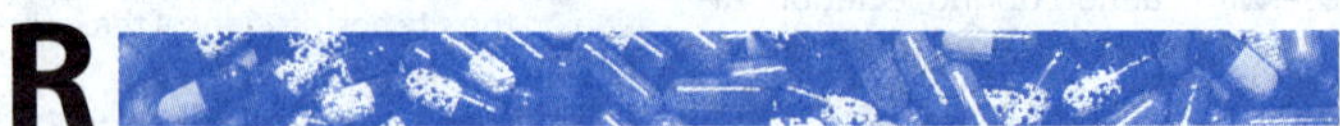

Rabeprazole sodium

(rah-**BEP**-rah-zohl)

PREGNANCY CATEGORY: B
CLASSIFICATION(S):
Proton pump inhibitor
Rx: Aciphex

R

ACTION/KINETICS

Suppresses gastric secretion by inhibiting gastric H^+,K^+ATPase at the secretory surface of parietal cells, i.e., is a gastric proton-pump inhibitor. Blocks the final step of gastric acid secretion. **Peak plasma levels:** 2–5 hr. **t½, plasma:** 1–2 hr. **Duration:** Over 24 hr. Over 96% plasma protein-bound. Extensively metabolized in the liver by P450 3A and 2C19. Excreted mainly in the urine.

USES

(1) Short-term (4–8 weeks) treatment in the healing and symptomatic relief of erosive or ulcerative gastroesophageal reflux disease (GERD). (2) Maintenance of healing and reduction in relapse rates of heartburn symptoms in clients with erosive or ulcerative GERD. (3) Short-term (up to 4 weeks) treatment in healing and symptomatic relief of duodenal ulcers. (4) Long-term treatment of pathological hypersecretory symptoms, including Zollinger-Ellison syndrome.

CONTRAINDICATIONS

Known sensitivity to rabeprazole or substituted benzimidazoles. Lactation.

SPECIAL CONCERNS

Safety and efficacy have not been determined in children. Greater sensitivity in some geriatric clients is possible. Symptomatic response to therapy does not preclude presence of gastric malignancy. Use with caution in severe hepatic impairment.

SIDE EFFECTS

GI: Diarrhea, N&V, abdominal pain, dyspepsia, flatulence, constipation, dry mouth, eructation, gastroenteritis,

rectal hemorrhage, melena, anorexia, cholelithiasis, mouth ulceration, stomatitis, dysphagia, gingivitis, cholecystitis, increased appetite, abnormal stools, colitis, esophagitis, glossitis, pancreatitis, proctitis. **CNS:** Insomnia, anxiety, dizziness, depression, nervousness, somnolence, hypertonia, neuralgia, vertigo, **convulsions**, abnormal dreams, decreased libido, neuropathy, paresthesia, tremor, coma, disorientation, delirium. **CV:** Hypertension, **MI**, abnormal EEG, migraine, syncope, angina pectoris, bundle branch block, palpitation, sinus bradycardia, tachycardia. **Musculoskeletal:** Myalgia, arthritis, leg cramps, bone pain, arthrosis, bursitis, neck rigidity, **rhabdomyolysis. Respiratory:** Dyspnea, asthma, epistaxis, laryngitis, hiccough, hyperventilation, interstitial pneumonia. **Dermatologic:** Rash, pruritus, sweating, urticaria, alopecia, jaundice, bullous and other skin eruptions. **GU:** Cystitis, urinary frequency, dysmenorrhea, dysuria, kidney calculus, metorrhagia, polyuria. **Endocrine:** Hyper/hypothyroidism. **Hematologic:** Anemia, ecchymosis, lymphadenopathy, hypochromic anemia, agranulocytosis, hemolytic anemia, leukopenia, pancytopenia, thrombocytopenia. **Metabolic:** Peripheral edema, edema, weight gain/loss, gout, dehydration. **Body as a whole:** Asthenia, fever, allergic reaction, chills, malaise, substernal chest pain, photosensitivity reaction, **sudden death**. **Ophthalmic:** Cataract, amblyopia, glaucoma, dry eyes, abnormal vision. **Otic:** Tinnitus, otitis media.

LABORATORY TEST CONSIDERATIONS

↑ Creatine phosphatase, AST, ALT, TSH, PSA. Abnormal platelets, erythrocytes, LFTs, urine, WBCs. Albuminuria, hypercholesterolemia, hyperglycemia, hyperlipemia, hypokalemia, hyponatremia, leukocytosis, leukorrhea, hyperammonemia.

DRUG INTERACTIONS

Digoxin / ↑ Plama levels of digoxin R/T changes in gastric pH

Ketoconazole / ↓ Plasma levels of ketoconazole R/T changes in gastric pH

HOW SUPPLIED

Tablet, Delayed-Release: 20 mg

DOSAGE

• **TABLET, DELAYED-RELEASE**

Healing of erosive or ulcerative GERD.

Adults: 20 mg once daily for 4–8 weeks. An additional 8 weeks of therapy may be considered for those who have not healed.

Maintenance of healing of erosive or ulcerative GERD.

Adults: 20 mg once daily.

Healing of duodenal ulcers.

Adults: 20 mg once daily after the morning meal for up to 4 weeks. A few clients may require additional time to heal.

Treatment of pathological hypersecretory conditions.

Adults, initial: 60 mg once a day. Adjust dosage to individual client needs (doses up to 100 mg/day and 60 mg b.i.d. have been used). Continue as long as clinically needed.

NURSING CONSIDERATIONS

ADMINISTRATION/STORAGE

1. No dosage adjustment is needed in elderly clients, those with renal disease, or in mild to moderate hepatic impairment.
2. Protect tablets from moisture.

ASSESSMENT

1. Document indications for therapy, onset, and characteristics of symptoms.
2. List drugs currently prescribed to ensure none interact.
3. Review UGI/endoscopy findings and H. Pylori results.

CLIENT/FAMILY TEACHING

1. Take as directed. Swallow tablets whole; do not crush, chew, or split tablets.
2. Report any unusual bleeding, acid reflux, abdominal pain, severe lightheadedness/diarrhea, rash, or lack of effectiveness.
3. Avoid alcohol, NSAIDs, and salicylates; may increase GI upset.
4. Do not perform activities that require mental alertness until drug effects realized.

R

OUTCOMES/EVALUATE

- ↓ Intraesophageal acid exposure
- Healing of duodenal ulcers; symptomatic improvement

Raloxifene hydrochloride

(ral-**OX**-ih-feen)

PREGNANCY CATEGORY: X
CLASSIFICATION(S):
Estrogen receptor modulator
Rx: Evista

ACTION/KINETICS
Selective estrogen receptor modulator that reduces bone resorption and decreases overall bone turnover. Considered an estrogen antagonist that acts by combining with estrogen receptors. Has not been associated with endometrial proliferation, breast enlargement, breast pain, or increased risk of breast cancer. Also decreases total and LDL cholesterol levels. Absorbed rapidly after PO; significant first-pass effect. **t½:** 32.5 hr (multiple doses). Excreted primarily in feces with small amounts excreted in urine.

USES
Prevention and treatment of osteoporosis in postmenopausal women. Not effective in reducing hot flashes or flushes associated with estrogen deficiency. *Investigational:* Reduce risk of breast cancer in postmenopausal women.

CONTRAINDICATIONS
In women who are or who might become pregnant , active or history of venous thromboembolic events (e.g., DVT, pulmonary embolism, retinal vein thrombosis). Use in premenopausal women, during lactation, or in pediatric clients. Concurrent use with systemic estrogen or hormone replacement therapy.

SPECIAL CONCERNS
Use with caution with highly protein-bound drugs, including clofibrate, diazepam, diazoxide, ibuprofen, indomethacin, and naproxen. Effect on bone mass density beyond 2 years of treatment is not known.

SIDE EFFECTS
CV: Hot flashes, migraine, venous thromboembolic events (e.g., pulmonary embolism, DVT), syncope, migraine. **Body as a whole:** Infection, flu syndrome, headache, chest pain, fever, weight gain, peripheral edema, infection. **CNS:** Depression, insomnia, vertigo, neuralgia, hypesthesia. **GI:** N&V, dyspepsia, diarrhea, flatulence, GI disorder, gastroenteritis, abdominal pain. **GU:** Vaginitis, UTI, cystitis, leukorrhea, endometrial disorder, uterine disorder, vaginal hemorrhage, urinary tract disorder, breast pain. **Respiratory:** Sinusitis, rhinitis, pharyngitis, bronchitis, increased cough, pneumonia, laryngitis. **Musculoskeletal:** Arthralgia, myalgia, leg cramps, arthritis, tendon disorder. **Dermatologic:** Rash, sweating. **Miscellaneous:** Conjunctivitis, hot flashes

LABORATORY TEST CONSIDERATIONS
↑ Apolipoprotein A1, steroid-binding globulin, thyroxine-binding globulin, corticosteroid-binding globulin. ↓ Total cholesterol, LDL cholesterol, fibrinogen, apolipoprotien B, lipoprotein.

DRUG INTERACTIONS
Cholestryamine / ↓ Raloxifene absorption
Diazepam / Use with caution R/T both drugs highly protein bound
Diazoxide / Use with caution R/T both drugs highly protein bound
Lidocaine / Use with caution R/T both drugs highly protein bound
Warfarin / ↓ PT

HOW SUPPLIED
Tablets: 60 mg

DOSAGE

- **TABLETS**

Prevention and treatment of osteoporosis in postmenopausal women.
Adults: 60 mg once daily.

NURSING CONSIDERATIONS

ADMINISTRATION/STORAGE

1. May be taken without regard for meals.
2. Take supplemental calcium and vitamin D if daily dietary intake is inadequate.

ASSESSMENT

1. Document indications for therapy; note bone density and onset of menopause.
2. Assess for history or evidence of CHF, active cancer or blood clots in legs, lungs or eyes.
3. Monitor LFTs; assess for any dysfunction.

CLIENT/FAMILY TEACHING

1. Take exactly as directed once daily with or without food; if dietary calcium and vitamin D intake is inadequate, consume supplemental.
2. Drug is used by women after menopause to prevent bones from becoming weak and thin.
3. Avoid prolonged immobilization and movement restrictions as with travel due to increased risk of venous thromboembolic events. Stop 3 days prior to and during prolonged immobilization as with surgery or prolonged bedrest.
4. Drug is not effective in reducing hot flashes or flushes associated with low estrogen as it does not stimulate breast or uterus.
5. Regular weight bearing exercises as well as tobacco and alcohol cessation/modification should be practiced.
6. Report any pain in calves or swelling in legs, fever, insomnia, acute migraines, emotional distress, sudden chest pain, SOB, or coughing up blood, as well as any vision changes.

OUTCOMES/EVALUATE

Postmenopausal osteoporosis prophylaxis; increased bone mineral density

Ramipril

(**RAM**-ih-prill)

PREGNANCY CATEGORY: D
CLASSIFICATION(S):
Antihypertensive, ACE inhibitor
Rx: Altace

SEE ALSO ***ANGIOTENSIN-CONVERTING ENZYME INHIBITORS.***

ACTION/KINETICS

Onset: 1–2 hr. **Time to peak serum levels:** 1 hr (1–2 hr for ramiprilat, the active metabolite). **Peak effect:** 3–6 hr. Ramiprilat has approximately six times the ACE inhibitory activity than ramipril. **t½:** 1–2 hr (13–17 hr for ramiprilat); prolonged in impaired renal function. **Duration:** 24 hr. Metabolized in the liver with 60% excreted through the urine and 40% in the feces. Food decreases the rate, but not the extent, of absorption of ramipril.

USES

(1) Alone or in combination with other antihypertensive agents (especially thiazide diuretics) for the treatment of hypertension. (2) Treatment of CHF following MI to decrease risk of CV death and decrease the risk of failure-related hospitalization and progression to severe or resistant heart failure. (3) Reduce risk of stroke, MI, and death from CV causes in clients over 55 years with a history of CAD, stroke, peripheral vascular disease, or with diabetes and one other risk factor (e.g., elevated cholesterol, cigarette smoking).

CONTRAINDICATIONS

Lactation.

SPECIAL CONCERNS

Geriatric clients may manifest higher peak blood levels of ramiprilat. May cause hyperkalemia, especially when used with salt substitutes.

SIDE EFFECTS

CV: Hypotension, chest pain, palpitations, angina pectoris, orthostatic hypotension, ***MI, CVA, arrhythmias.*** **GI:** N&V, abdominal pain, diarrhea, dysgeusia, anorexia, constipation, dry mouth, dyspepsia, enzyme changes suggesting pancreatitis, dysphagia, gastroenteritis, increased salivation. **CNS:** Headache, dizziness, fatigue, insomnia, sleep disturbances, somnolence, depression, nervousness, malaise, vertigo, anxiety, amnesia, ***convulsions,*** tremor. **Respiratory:** Cough, dyspnea, URI, asthma, ***bronchospasm.*** **Hematologic:** Leukopenia, anemia, eosinophilia. Rarely, decreases in hemoglobin or hematocrit. **Dermato-**

R

logic: Diaphoresis, photosensitivity, pruritus, rash, dermatitis, purpura, alopecia, erythema multiforme, urticaria. **Body as a whole:** Paresthesias, angioedema, asthenia, syncope, fever, muscle cramps, myalgia, arthralgia, arthritis, neuralgia, neuropathy, influenza, edema. **Miscellaneous:** Impotence, tinnitus, hearing loss, vision disturbances, epistaxis, weight gain, proteinuria, angioneurotic edema, edema, flu syndrome.

LABORATORY TEST CONSIDERATIONS

↓ H&H.

HOW SUPPLIED

Capsule: 1.25 mg, 2.5 mg, 5 mg, 10 mg

DOSAGE

• CAPSULES

Hypertension.

Initial: 2.5 mg once daily in clients not taking a diuretic; **maintenance:** 2.5–20 mg/day as a single dose or two equally divided doses. *Clients taking diuretics or who have a C_{CR} less than 40 mL/min/1.73 m^2:* initially 1.25 mg/day; dose may then be increased to a maximum of 5 mg/day.

CHF following MI.

Initial: 2.5 mg b.i.d. Clients intolerant of this dose may be started on 1.25 mg b.i.d. The target maintenance dose is 5 mg b.i.d.

Reduce risk of MI, stroke, death in clients 55 and over with risk factors.

Initial: 2.5 mg/day for 1 week followed by 5 mg/day for the next 3 weeks. **Maintenance:** 10 mg/day. If the client is hypertensive or post-MI, the dose can be divided.

NURSING CONSIDERATIONS

SEE ALSO *NURSING CONSIDERATIONS* FOR *ANGIOTENSIN-CONVERTING ENZYME INHIBITORS,* AND *ANTIHYPERTENSIVE AGENTS.*

ADMINISTRATION/STORAGE

1. If the antihypertensive effect decreases at the end of the dosing interval with once-daily dosing, consider either twice-daily administration or an increase in dose.
2. If taking a diuretic, discontinue the diuretic 2–3 days prior to beginning ramipril. If BP is not controlled, reinstitute the diuretic. If the diuretic cannot be discontinued, consider an initial dose of ramipril of 1.25 mg.

ASSESSMENT

Note indications for therapy, other agents trialed and the outcome. Assess liver and renal fuction to ensure no abnormality.

CLIENT/FAMILY TEACHING

1. For ease in swallowing, may mix contents of the capsule with water, apple juice, or apple sauce.
2. Use caution; drug may cause dizziness and postural effects with sudden changes in position.
3. Report any persistent, dry, nonproductive cough, increased SOB, edema, or unusual bruising/bleeding.
4. Do not take any OTC agents without approval.
5. Record BP at different times of day/night for provider review.

OUTCOMES/EVALUATE

- ↓ BP
- Renal protection with DM

Ranitidine bismuth citrate

(rah-**NIH**-tih-deen **BIS**-muth)

PREGNANCY CATEGORY: C, WHEN USED WITH CLARITHROMYCIN

CLASSIFICATION(S):

Treatment of *Helicobacter pylori*

Rx: Tritec

★**Rx:** Pylorid

SEE ALSO *HISTAMINE H_2 ANTAGONISTS* AND *RANITIDINE. NOTE:* SINCE CLARITHROMYCIN IS USED WITH RANITIDINE BISMUTH CITRATE, INFORMATION ON CLARITHROMYCIN MUST ALSO BE CONSULTED.

ACTION/KINETICS

A complex of ranitidine and bismuth citrate which is freely soluble in water; solubility decreases as pH is decreased. The complex is more soluble than either ranitidine or bismuth citrate given separately. Is believed the greater solubility of the complex facilitates penetration of the drug into the mucous layer that protects the epithelial cells in the GI mucosa. **Peak**

levels of ranitidine from complex: 0.5–5 hr. **t½, elimination, ranitidine from ranitidine bismuth citrate:** 2.8–3.1 hr. Ranitidine is eliminated through the kidneys. **t½, terminal, bismuth:** 11–28 days. Bismuth is excreted primarily in the feces.

USES

In combination with clarithromycin for treatment of active duodenal ulcers associated with *Helicobacter pylori* infections. *NOTE:* Ranitidine bismuth citrate should not be prescribed alone for the treatment of active duodenal ulcer.

CONTRAINDICATIONS

Hypersensitivity to the complex or any of its ingredients. Hangover. Use in those with a history of acute porphyria or in those with a C_{CR} less than 25 mL/min.

SPECIAL CONCERNS

Use with caution during lactation. Safety and efficacy of ranitidine bismuth citrate plus clarithromycin in pediatric clients have not been determined.

SIDE EFFECTS

See also side effects for *Ranitidine*.

GI: N&V, diarrhea, constipation, abdominal discomfort, gastric pain. **CNS:** Headache, dizziness, sleep disorder, tremors (rare). *Hypersensitivity:* Rash, anaphylaxis (rare). **Miscellaneous:** Pruritus, gynecologic problems, taste disturbance, chest symptoms, transient changes in liver enzymes.

LABORATORY TEST CONSIDERATIONS

False + test for urine protein using Multistix. ↑ ALT, AST.

DRUG INTERACTIONS

Antacids / Possible ↓ plasma levels of ranitidine and bismuth

Clarithromycin / ↑ Plasma levels of ranitidine and bismuth

HOW SUPPLIED

Tablet: 400 mg

DOSAGE

• TABLETS

Eradication of H. pylori *infection.*

Ranitidine bismuth citrate: 400 mg b.i.d. for 4 weeks. *Clarithromycin:* 500 mg t.i.d. for the first 2 weeks of therapy and either metronidazole, 500 mg b.i.d., amoxicillin, 1 g b.i.d., or tetracycline, 500 mg b.i.d. for the first 2 weeks of therapy.

NURSING CONSIDERATIONS

SEE ALSO NURSING CONSIDERATIONS FOR HISTAMINE H_2 ANTAGONISTS AND RANITIDINE.

ADMINISTRATION/STORAGE

Protect drug from light and store at 2–30°C (36–86°F).

ASSESSMENT

1. Document indications for therapy, onset, and characteristics of symptoms; list other agents trialed and the outcome.
2. Check serum *H. pylori* or UGI/endoscopic confirmation of disease.
3. Obtain baseline CBC, liver and renal function studies.
4. Determine any experience with these agents. Not for use with acute porphyria, a hangover, or C_{CR} < 25 mL/min.

CLIENT/FAMILY TEACHING

1. Take exactly as directed; do not skip doses or try and double up on missed doses. Take missed dose when remembered.
2. The cause for the ulcer is the bacteria *H. pylori;* drug helps kill bacteria. Must be taken with clarithromycin in order to be effective .
3. Bismuth may cause a temporary and harmless darkening (black) of the tongue or stool; do not be alarmed or confuse with melena.
4. Both ranitidine bismuth citrate and clarithromycin can be taken with or without food.
5. May experience diarrhea, headache, nausea, vomiting, and itchy skin; report if persistent and use only acetaminophen for headaches.
6. Use sugarless candies or rinse mouth frequently to diminish bad taste.
7. Do not smoke; smoking slows ulcer healing and may cause a recurrence.
8. Avoid any other medications (prescription or OTC) without approval.

OUTCOMES/EVALUATE

Healing of ulcer; ↓ abdominal pain and discomfort

R

Ranitidine hydrochloride

(rah-**NIH**-tih-deen)

PREGNANCY CATEGORY: B
CLASSIFICATION(S):
Histamine H-2 receptor blocking drug
Rx: Zantac EFFERdose, Zantac GEL-dose Capsules, Zantac
✽Rx: Alti-Ranitidine HCl, Apo-Ranitidine, Gen-Ranitidine, Novo-Ranitidine, Nu-Ranit, Scheinpharm Ranitidine
OTC: Zantac 75

SEE ALSO *HISTAMINE H₂ ANTAGONISTS.*

ACTION/KINETICS

Competitively inhibits gastric acid secretion by blocking the effect of histamine on histamine H_2 receptors. Both daytime and nocturnal basal gastric acid secretion, as well as food- and pentagastrin-stimulated gastric acid are inhibited. Weak inhibitor of cytochrome P-450 (drug-metabolizing enzymes); thus, drug interactions involving inhibition of hepatic metabolism are not expected to occur. Food increases the bioavailability. **Peak effect: PO,** 1–3 hr; **IM, IV,** 15 min. **t½:** 2.5–3 hr. **Duration, nocturnal:** 13 hr; **basal:** 4 hr. **Serum level to inhibit 50% stimulated gastric acid secretion:** 36–94 ng/mL. From 30% to 35% of a PO dose and from 68% to 79% of an IV dose excreted unchanged in urine.

USES

(1) Short-term (4–8 weeks) and maintenance treatment of duodenal ulcer. (2) Pathologic hypersecretory conditions such as Zollinger-Ellison syndrome and systemic mastocytosis. (3) Short-term treatment of active, benign gastric ulcers. (4) Maintenance of healing of gastric ulcers. (5) GERD, including erosive esophagitis. (6) Maintenance of healing of erosive esophagitis. *Investigational:* Prophylaxis of pulmonary aspiration of acid during anesthesia, prevent gastric damage from NSAIDs, prevent stress ulcers, prevent acute UGI bleeding, as part of multidrug regimen to eradicate Helicobacter pylori.

CONTRAINDICATIONS

Cirrhosis of the liver, impaired renal or hepatic function.

SPECIAL CONCERNS

Use with caution during lactation and in clients with decreased hepatic or renal function. Safety and efficacy not established in children.

SIDE EFFECTS

GI: Constipation, N&V, diarrhea, abdominal pain, pancreatitis (rare). **CNS:** Headache, dizziness, malaise, insomnia, vertigo, confusion, anxiety, agitation, depression, fatigue, somnolence, hallucinations. **CV:** Bradycardia or tachycardia, premature ventricular beats following rapid IV use (especially in clients predisposed to cardiac rhythm disturbances), ***cardiac arrest***. **Hematologic:** Thrombocytopenia, granulocytopenia, leukopenia, pancytopenia (sometimes with marrow hypoplasia), ***agranulocytosis, autoimmune hemolytic or aplastic anemia.*** **Hepatic:** Hepatotoxicity, jaundice, hepatitis, increase in ALT. **Dermatologic:** Erythema multiforme, rash, alopecia. **Allergic: *Bronchospasm, anaphylaxis,*** angioneurotic edema (rare), rashes, fever, eosinophilia. **Other:** Arthralgia, gynecomastia, impotence, loss of libido, blurred vision, pain at injection site, local burning or itching following IV use.

LABORATORY TEST CONSIDERATIONS

False + test for urine protein using Multistix.

DRUG INTERACTIONS

Antacids / May ↓ ranitidine absorption
Cyanocobalamin / ↓ Cyanocobalamin absorption R/T ↑ gastric pH
Diazepam / ↓ Diazepam effects R/T ↓ GI tract absorption
Glipizide / ↑ Glipizide effects
Procainamide / ↓ Procainamide excretion → possible ↑ effect
Theophylline / Possible ↑ theophylline pharmacologic and toxicologic effects
Warfarin / May ↑ warfarin hypoprothrombinemic effects

HOW SUPPLIED

Capsule: 150 mg, 300 mg; *Granule effervescent:* 150 mg; *Injection:* 0.5 mg/mL, 25 mg/mL; *Syrup:* 15 mg/mL; *Tablet:*

R

75 mg, 150 mg, 300 mg; *Tablet, effervescent:* 150 mg

DOSAGE

• **CAPSULES, EFFERVESCENT TABLETS AND GRANULES, SYRUP, TABLETS**

Duodenal ulcer, short-term.

Adults: 150 mg b.i.d. or 300 mg at bedtime to heal ulcer, although 100 mg b.i.d. will inhibit acid secretion and may be as effective as the higher dose. **Maintenance:** 150 mg at bedtime.

Pathologic hypersecretory conditions.

Adults: 150 mg b.i.d. (up to 6 g/day has been used in severe cases).

Benign gastric ulcer.

Adults: 150 mg b.i.d. for active ulcer. **Maintenance:** 150 mg at bedtime

Gastroesophageal reflux disease.

Adults: 150 mg b.i.d.

Erosive esophagitis.

Adults: 150 mg q.i.d.

Maintenenace of healing of erosive esophagitis.

Adults: 150 mg b.i.d.

• **IM, IV**

Treatment and maintenance for duodenal ulcer, hypersecretory conditions, gastroesophageal reflux.

Adults, IM: 50 mg q 6–8 hr. **Intermittent IV injection or infusion:** 50 mg q 6–8 hr, not to exceed 400 mg/day. **Continuous IV infusion:** 6.25 mg/hr.

Zollinger-Ellison clients.

Continuous IV infusion: Dilute ranitidine in D5W to a concentration no greater than 2.5 mg/mL with an initial infusion rate of 1 mg/kg/hr. If after 4 hr the client shows a gastric acid output of greater than 10 mEq/hr or if symptoms appear, increase the dose by 0.5-mg/kg/hr increments and measure the acid output. Doses up to 2.5 mg/kg/hr may be necessary.

NURSING CONSIDERATIONS

SEE ALSO *NURSING CONSIDERATIONS* FOR *HISTAMINE H_2 ANTAGONISTS.*

ADMINISTRATION/STORAGE

1. If the C_{CR} is less than 50 mL/min, give 150 mg PO q 24 hr or 50 mg parenterally q 18–24 hr.
2. Give antacids concomitantly for gastric pain although they may interfere with ranitidine absorption.
3. Dissolve Efferdose tablets and granules in 6–8 oz of water before taking.
4. About one-half of clients may heal completely within 2 weeks; thus, endoscopy may show no need for further treatment.
5. No dilution is required for IM use.
6. Store the syrup between 4–25°C (39–77°F).

IV 7. For IV injection, dilute 50 mg in 0.9% NaCl injection to a total volume of 20 mL. Give diluted solution over 5 min or more. For intermittent IV infusion, dilute 50 mg in 100 mL D5W; give over 15–20 min.

8. The premixed injection does not require dilution; give only by slow IV drip over 15–20 min. Do not introduce additives into the solution. If used with a primary IV fluid system, discontinue the primary solution during drug infusion.
9. For continuous IV infusion, add ranitidine injection to D5W
10. The drug is stable for 48 hr at room temperature when mixed with 0.9% NaCl, 5% or 10% dextrose injection, RL, or 5% $NaHCO_3$ injection.

ASSESSMENT

1. Document indications for therapy, onset and duration of symptoms, other agents used and anticipated treatment period.
2. Assess stomach pain, noting characteristics, frequency of occurrence and things that alter it.
3. Obtain CBC; assess for infections.
4. Note *H. pylori*, UGI, or endoscopy findings.
5. Assess for renal or liver disease.
6. Determine if pregnant.
7. Skin tests using allergens may elicit false negative results; stop drug 24–72 hr prior to testing.

CLIENT/FAMILY TEACHING

1. Take as directed with or immediately following meals. Wait 1 hr before taking an antacid.
2. Do not drive or operate machinery until drug effects are realized; dizziness or drowsiness may occur.

R

3. Avoid alcohol, aspirin-containing products, and beverages that contain caffeine (tea, cola, coffee); these increase stomach acid.
4. Avoid things that may aggravate symptoms, i.e., ETOH, aspirin, NSAIDs, caffeine, and black pepper.
5. Do not smoke; interferes with healing and drug's effectiveness.
6. Report any evidence of diarrhea and maintain adequate hydration.
7. Report any confusion or disorientation.
8. Symptoms of breast tenderness will usually disappear after several weeks; report if persistent and evaluate need to stop drug.
9. Report as scheduled to determine extent of healing and expected length of therapy.

OUTCOMES/EVALUATE
- ↓ Gastric acid production
- ↓ Abdominal pain/discomfort
- Endoscopic/radiographic evidence of duodenal ulcer healing

Remifentanil hydrochloride

(rem-ih-**FEN**-tah-nil)

PREGNANCY CATEGORY: C
CLASSIFICATION(S):
Narcotic analgesic
Rx: Ultiva, **C-II**

R

SEE ALSO *NARCOTIC ANALGESICS*.

ACTION/KINETICS
Narcotic analgesic that binds with mu-opioid receptors. Depresses respiration in a dose-dependent manner and causes muscle rigidity. Rapidly metabolized by nonspecific blood and tissue esterases; not metabolized appreciably by the liver or lung. **Onset:** 1 min. **Peak effect:** 1 min. **t½, elimination:** 3–10 min. **Recovery:** Within 5–10 min.

USES
(1) As an analgesic during the induction and maintenance of general anesthesia for inpatient and outpatient procedures and for continuation as an analgesic in the immediate postoperative period. (2) Analgesic component of monitored anesthesia care. (3) Maintenance of general anesthesia in pediatric clients, aged 1–12 years.

CONTRAINDICATIONS
Epidural or intrathecal use due to the presence of glycine in the formulation. Hypersensitivity to fentanyl analogues. Use as the sole agent in general anesthesia because LOC cannot be ensured and due to a high incidence of apnea, muscle rigidity, and tachycardia.

SPECIAL CONCERNS
Use with caution in obese clients and during lactation. Respiratory depression and other narcotic effects may be seen in newborns whose mothers are given remifentanil shortly before delivery. Geriatric clients are twice as sensitive as younger clients to the effects of the drug. Not studied in children less than 2 years of age. Possible intraoperative awareness in clients less than 55 years old when given with propofol infusion rates of 75 or less mcg/kg/min.

SIDE EFFECTS
GI: N&V, constipation, abdominal discomfort, xerostomia, gastroesophageal reflux, dysphagia, diarrhea, heartburn, ileus. **CNS:** Shivering, fever, dizziness, headache, agitation, chills, warm sensation, anxiety, involuntary movement, prolonged emergence from anesthesia, tremors, disorientation, dysphoria, nightmares, hallucinations, paresthesia, nystagmus, twitch, sleep disorder, seizures, amnesia. **CV:** Hypo/hypertension, brady/tachycardia, atrial and ventricular arrhythmias, heart block, ECG change consistent with myocardial ischemia, syncope. **Musculoskeletal:** Muscle rigidity/stiffness, musculoskeletal chest pain, delayed recovery from neuromuscular block. **Respiratory:** Respiratory depression, apnea, hypoxia, cough, dyspnea, bronchospasm, laryngospasm, rhonchi, stridor, nasal congestion, pharyngitis, pleural effusion, hiccoughs, pulmonary edema, rales, bronchitis, rhinorrhea. **Dermatologic:** Pruritus, rash, urticaria, erythema, sweating, flushing, pain at IV site. **GU:** Urine retention/incontinence, oli-

guria, dysuria. **Hematologic:** Anemia, lymphopenia, leukocytosis, thrombocytopenia. **Metabolic:** Abnormal liver function, hyperglycemia, electrolyte disorders. **Miscellaneous:** Decreased body temperature, ***anaphylactic reaction,*** visual disturbances, postoperative pain.

LABORATORY TEST CONSIDERATIONS

↑ CPK-MB levels.

OD OVERDOSE MANAGEMENT

Symptoms: Apnea, chest-wall rigidity, seizures, hypoxemia, hypotension, bradycardia. *Treatment:* Discontinue administration, maintain a patent airway, initiate assisted or controlled ventilation with oxygen, and maintain adequate CV function. A neuromuscular blocking agent or a mu-opiate receptor antagonist may be used to treat muscle rigidity. IV fluids, vasopressors, and other supportive measures are indicated to treat hypotension. Bradycardia or hypotension may also be treated with atropine or glycopyrrolate. IV naloxone is used to treat respiratory depression or muscle rigidity. Reversal of the opioid effects may lead to acute pain and sympathetic hyperactivity.

DRUG INTERACTIONS

Remifentanil is synergistic with other anesthetics. Doses of thiopental, propofol, isoflurane, and midazolam have been reduced by up to 75% with the coadministration of remifentanil.

HOW SUPPLIED

Powder for injection, lyophilized: 1 mg/mL (after reconstitution)

DOSAGE

- **CONTINUOUS IV INFUSION ONLY**

Induction of anesthesia through intubation.

0.5–1 mcg/kg/min given with a hypnotic or volatile agent. If endotracheal intubation is to occur less than 8 min after the start of the infusion of remifentanil, the initial dose of 1 mcg/kg may be given over 30 to 60 sec.

Maintenance of nitrous oxide (66%) anesthesia.

The dose of remifentanil is 0.4 mcg/kg/min (range of 0.1–2 mcg/kg/min). A supplemental IV bolus dose of 1 mcg/kg may be given.

Maintenance of isoflurance (0.4 to 1.5 MAC) or propofol (100–200 mcg/kg/min) anesthesia.

The dose of remifentanil is 0.25 mcg/kg/min (range of 0.05–2 mcg/kg/min). A supplemental IV bolus dose of 1 mcg/kg may be given.

Continuation as an analgesic into the immediate postoperative period.

0.1 mcg/kg/min (range of 0.025–0.2 mcg/kg/min). The infusion rate may be adjusted every 5 min in 0.025-mcg/kg/min increments to balance the client's level of analgesia and respiratory rate.

Analgesic component of monitored anesthesia care.

Single IV dose: 1 mcg/kg administered over 30 to 60 sec and given 90 sec before the local anesthetic. If remifentanil is given with midazolam (2 mg), the dose is 0.5 mcg/kg. **Continuous IV infusion:** 0.1 mcg/kg beginning 5 min before the local anesthetic. After the local anesthetic, the dose of remifentanil is 0.05 mcg/kg/min (range 0.025–0.2 mcg/kg/min) at 5-min intervals in order to balance the level of analgesia and respiratory rate. If remifentanil is given with midazolam (2 mg), the dose is 0.025 mcg/kg/min (range 0.025–0.2 mcg/kg/min).

NURSING CONSIDERATIONS

SEE ALSO *NURSING CONSIDERATIONS* FOR *NARCOTIC ANALGESICS*.

ADMINISTRATION/STORAGE

IV 1. Individualize choice of anesthetic and need for preanesthetic drugs.

2. Decrease starting dose by 50% in clients over age 65. Cautiously titrate to desired effect.

3. Use the adult dose for pediatric clients 2 years of age and older.

4. In obese clients (i.e., greater than 30% over ideal body weight [IBW]) base the starting dose on IBW.

5. Give continuous infusions only by an infusion device. Have the injection site close to the venous cannula.

6. Due to the rapid onset and short duration, administration during anes-

thesia can be titrated upward in 25% to 100% increments or downward in 25% to 50% decrements every 2 to 5 min to attain the desired opiate effect. With light anesthesia or transient periods of intense surgical stress, supplemental bolus doses of 1 mcg/kg may be given q 2–5 min.
7. Administer under close anesthesia supervision into the immediate postoperative period. Infusion rates greater than 0.2 mcg/kg/min are associated with respiratory depression. Manage respiratory depression by decreasing the rate of infusion by 50% or discontinue the infusion temporariliy.
8. When infusion is discontinued, clear the IV tubing to prevent inadvertant administration at a later time.
9. Due to its short duration, no opioid activity will be present within 5–10 min of discontinuation.
10. Stable for 24 hr at room temperature after reconstitution and further dilute to concentrations of 20–250 mcg/mL. Dilute with sterile water for injection, D5W, D5/0.9% NaCl, 0.9% NaCl, or 0.45% NaCl injection.
11. Compatible with propofal when coadministered into a running IV administration set.
12. Store at 2–25°C (36–77°F).

ASSESSMENT

1. Document indications and expected duration of therapy.
2. Determine if pain is acute or chronic in nature; describe distinguishing characteristics and use a pain-rating scale to rate pain level.
3. Monitor liver and renal function studies.
4. Observe for progressive respiratory depression.

CLIENT/FAMILY TEACHING

1. Call for assistance. Do not perform activites that require mental alertness for 24 hr; drug causes dizziness, drowsiness, and impaired physical and mental performance.
2. Avoid alcohol and any other CNS depressants for 24 hr after procedure.
3. Change positions slowly to prevent postural effects.

OUTCOMES/EVALUATE

Pain control and analgesia

R

Repaglinide

(re-**PAY**-glin-eyed)

PREGNANCY CATEGORY: C
CLASSIFICATION(S):
Antidiabetic, oral; meglitinide
Rx: Prandin
✱Rx: GlucoNorm

SEE ALSO *ANTIDIABETIC AGENTS, HYPOGLYCEMIC AGENTS.*

ACTION/KINETICS

Lowers blood glucose by stimulating release of insulin from pancreas. Action depends on functioning beta cells in pancreatic islets. Drug closes ATP-dependent potassium channels in beta-cell membrane due to binding at sites. Blockade of potassium channel depolarizes beta cell which leads to opening of calcium channels. This causes calcium influx which induces insulin secretion. Rapidly and completely absorbed from GI tract. **Peak plasma levels:** 1 hr. Completely metabolized in liver with most excreted in feces.

USES

(1) Adjunct to diet and exercise in type 2 diabetes mellitus where hyperglycemia can not be controlled by diet and exercise alone. (2) In combination with metformin to lower blood glucose where hyperglycemia can not be controlled by exercise, diet, or either agent alone.

CONTRAINDICATIONS

Lactation. Diabetic ketoacidosis, with or without coma. Type 1 diabetes.

SPECIAL CONCERNS

Use with caution in impaired hepatic function. Oral hypoglycemics are associated with increased CV mortality compared with diet alone or diet plus insulin. Safety and efficacy have not been determined in children.

SIDE EFFECTS

CV: Chest pain, angina, ischemia. **GI:** Nausea, diarrhea, constipation, vomiting, dyspepsia. **Respiratory:** URI, sinusitis, rhinitis, bronchitis. **Musculoskeletal:** Arthralgia, back pain. **Miscellaneous:** Hypoglycemia, headache, paresthesia, chest pain, UTI, tooth disorder, allergy.

OD OVERDOSE MANAGEMENT
Symptoms: Hypoglycemia. *Treatment:* Oral glucose. Also adjust drug dosage or meal patterns.

DRUG INTERACTIONS
See *Antidiabetic Agents, Hypoglycemic Agents.*
Clarithromycin / Possible ↑ peak plasma levels and t½ of repaglinide
Rifampin / ↓ Plasma levels and effects of repaglinide R/T ↑ liver metabolism

HOW SUPPLIED
Tablets: 0.5 mg, 1 mg, 2 mg

DOSAGE

- **TABLETS**

Type 2 diabetes mellitus.
Individualize dosage. **Initial:** In those not previously treated or whose HbA1-C is less than 8%, give 0.5 mg. For those previously treated or whose HbA1-C is 8% or more, give 1 or 2 mg before each meal. **Dose range:** 0.5–4 mg taken with meals. **Maximum daily dose:** 16 mg.

NURSING CONSIDERATIONS

SEE ALSO *NURSING CONSIDERATIONS* FOR *ANTIDIABETIC AGENTS, HYPOGLYCEMIC AGENTS.*

ADMINISTRATION/STORAGE

1. May be dosed after meals 2, 3, or 4 times daily, depending on client's meal patterns.
2. Usually taken within 15 min of meal but time may vary from immediately preceding meal to as long as 30 min before meal.
3. In renal impairment, initial dose adjustments not required. Make subsequent increases in dose carefully in impaired renal function or in renal failure requiring hemodialysis.
4. When used to replace another oral hypoglycemic, may be started the day after last dose of other drug. Observe carefully for hypoglycemia as drug effects may overlap. When transferring from a longer acting sulfonylurea (e.g., chlorpropamide), monitor for up to 1 week or longer.
5. If combined with metformin, starting dose and dose adjustments are the same as if repaglinide was used alone.

ASSESSMENT

1. Document onset, duration, and characteristics of disease; note other agents/methods trialed and outcome.
2. Monitor VS, HbA1-C, and LFTs.

CLIENT/FAMILY TEACHING

1. Take as prescribed with meals for glucose control.
2. Continue regular exercise, diabetic diet, and lifestyle modifications to control BS and prevent organ damage.
3. Record FS for provider review; report any unusual side effects or lack of response.
4. Report fever, sore throat, unusual bruising/bleeding, severe abdominal pain, or lack of effectiveness. Attend diabetic education classes and dietary instruction.

OUTCOMES/EVALUATE
HbA1-C within desired range; control of BS

Respiratory Syncytial Virus Immune Globulin Intravenous (RSV-IGIV) (Human)

PREGNANCY CATEGORY: C
CLASSIFICATION(S):
Immunosuppressant
Rx: RespiGam

ACTION/KINETICS
Is an IgG containing neutralizing antibody to RSV. The immunoglobulin is obtained and purified from pooled adult human plasma that has been selected for high titers of neutralizing antibody against RSV. Each milliliter contains 50 mg of immunoglobulin, primarily IgG with trace amounts of IgA and IgM.

USES
Prevention of serious lower respiratory tract infection caused by RSV in children less than 24 months old with bronchopulmonary dysplasia or a history of premature birth (less than 35 weeks gestation). *Investigational:* In place of IGIV during the RSV season in

R

immunocompromised children who get IGIV monthly.

CONTRAINDICATIONS

History of a severe prior reaction associated with administration of RSV-IGIV or other human immunoglobulin products. Clients with selective IgA deficiency who have the potential for developing antibodies to IgA and which could cause anaphylaxis or allergic reactions to blood products that contain IgA.

SPECIAL CONCERNS

Safety and efficacy have not been determined in children with congenital heart disease. Give close attention to the infusion rate as side effects may be related to the rate of administration. Since RSV-IGIV is made from human plasma, there is the possibility for transmission of blood-borne pathogenic organisms, although the risk is considered to be low due to screening of donors and viral inactivation and removal steps in the manufacturing process.

SIDE EFFECTS

Infusion of RSV-IGIV may cause fluid overload, especially in children with bronchopulmonary dysplasia. Aseptic meningitis syndrome has been reported within several hours to 2 days following RSV-IGIV treatment. Symptoms include severe headache, drowsiness, fever, photophobia, painful eye movements, muscle rigidity, nausea, and vomiting. The CSF shows pleocytosis, predominately granulocytic, as well as elevated protein levels.

Allergic: Hypotension, ***anaphylaxis, angioneurotic edema,*** respiratory distress. **CNS:** Fever, pyrexia, sleepiness. **Respiratory:** Respiratory distress, wheezing, rales, tachypnea, cough. **GI:** Vomiting, diarrhea, gagging, gastroenteritis. **CV:** Tachycardia, increased pulse rate, hypertension, hypotension, heart murmur. **Dermatologic:** Rash, pallor, cyanosis, eczema, cold and clammy skin. **Miscellaneous:** Hypoxia, hypoxemia, inflammation at injection site, edema, rhinorrhea, conjunctival hemorrhage.

Reactions similar to other immunoglobulins may occur as follows. **Body as a whole:** Dizziness, flushing, ***immediate allergic, anaphylactic, or hypersensitivity reactions.*** **CV:** Blood pressure changes, palpitations, chest tightness. **Miscellaneous:** Anxiety, dyspnea, abdominal cramps, pruritus, myalgia, arthralgia.

OD OVERDOSE MANAGEMENT

Symptoms: Symptoms due to fluid volume overload. *Treatment:* Administration of diuretics and modification of the infusion rate.

DRUG INTERACTIONS

Antibodies found in immunoglobulin products may interfere with the immune response to live virus vaccines, including those for mumps, rubella, and measles. Also, the antibody response to diphtheria, tetanus, pertussis, and *Haemophilus influenzae b* may be lower in RSV-IGIV recipients.

HOW SUPPLIED

Injection: 50 +/- 10 mg immunoglobulin/mL

DOSAGE

- **IV INJECTION**

Prevention of RSV infections.

1.5 mL/kg/hr for 15 min. If the clinical condition of the client allows, the rate can be increased to 3.6 mL/kg/hr for the remainder of the infusion. *Do not exceed these rates of infusion.* **Maximum dose/monthly infusion:** 750 mg/kg.

NURSING CONSIDERATIONS

ADMINISTRATION/STORAGE

IV 1. Enter the single-use vial only once. Initiate infusion within 6 hr and complete within 12 hr of removal from the vial.

2. Do not use if the solution is turbid.

3. Give separately from other drugs or medications.

4. Give through an IV line (preferably a separate line) using a constant infusion pump. Administration may be "piggy-backed" into an existing line if that line contains one of the following dextrose solutions (with or without NaCl): 2.5%, 5%, 10%, or 20% dextrose in water. If a preexisting line must be used, do not dilute RSV-IGIV more than 1:2 with one of the above solutions. Do not predilute RSV-IGIV before infusion.

5. Although use of filters is not necessary, an in-line filter with a pore size greater than 15 µm may be used.
6. Store the injection at 2–8°C (36–46°F). Do not freeze or shake (to prevent foaming).

ASSESSMENT

1. Document indications for therapy, any previous experiences with this drug and the outcome.
2. Note any IgA deficiency.
3. Assess VS, I&O, and cardiopulmonary status prior to infusion, before each rate increase, and thereafter at 30-min intervals until 30 min following infusion completion. Observe for fluid overload (increased HR, increased respiratory rate, rales, retractions), especially in infants with bronchopulmonary dysplasia. A loop diuretic (e.g., furosemide or bumetanide) should be available for management of fluid overload.

CLIENT/FAMILY TEACHING

1. The first dose of RSV-IGIV should be given prior to the beginning of the RSV season and monthly throughout the RSV season (in the Northern Hemisphere, from Nov– April) to maintain protection.
2. Drug is derived from human plasma; review potential risks related to blood-borne pathogenic agents.
3. Report any severe headaches, painful eye movements, drowsiness, fever, N&V, or muscle rigidity (symptoms of aseptic meningitis); must be evaluated to rule out other causes of meningitis.
4. If virus vaccines are given during or within 10 months after RSV-IGIV infusion, reimmunization is recommended.

OUTCOMES/EVALUATE

RSV prophylaxis; ↓ severity of RSV illness

Reteplase recombinant

(**REE**-teh-place)

PREGNANCY CATEGORY: C

CLASSIFICATION(S):
Thrombolytic, tissue plasminogen activator
Rx: Retavase

ACTION/KINETICS

Plasminogen activator that catalyzes the cleavage of endogenous plasminogen to generate plasmin. Plasmin, in turn, degrades the matrix of the thrombus, causing a thrombolytic effect. **t½:** 13 to 16 min. Cleared primarily by the liver and kidney.

USES

In adults for the management of acute MI for improvement of ventricular function, reduction of the incidence of CHF, and reduction of mortality.

CONTRAINDICATIONS

Active internal bleeding; history of CVA; recent intracranial or intraspinal surgery or trauma; intracranial neoplasm, arteriovenous malformation, or aneurysm; known bleeding diathesis; severe uncontrolled hypertension.

SPECIAL CONCERNS

Use with caution during lactation. Safety and efficacy have not been determined in children.

SIDE EFFECTS

Bleeding disorders: From internal bleeding sites, including intracranial, retroperitoneal, GI, GU, or respiratory. ***Hemorrhage may occur.*** From superficial bleeding sites, including venous cutdowns, arterial punctures, sites of recent surgery.
CV: ***Cholesterol embolism,*** coronary thrombolysis resulting in arrhythmias associated with perfusion (no different from those seen in the ordinary course of acute MI), cardiogenic shock, sinus bradycardia, accelerated idioventricular rhythm, ventricular premature depolarizations, SVT, ventricular tachycardia, ***ventricular fibrillation,*** AV block, pulmonary edema, ***heart failure, cardiac arrest, recurrent ischemia, myocardial rupture, cardiac tamponade, venous thrombosis or embolism, electromechanical dissociation, mitral regurgitation, pericardial effusion, pericarditis***. **Hypersensitivity:** Serious allergic reactions. *NOTE:*

R

Many of the CV side effects listed are frequent sequelae of MI and may or may not be attributable to reteplase recombinant.

LABORATORY TEST CONSIDERATIONS

↓ Plasminogen, fibrinogen. Degradation of fibrinogen in blood samples removed for analysis.

DRUG INTERACTIONS

Use with abciximab, aspirin, dipyridamole, heparin, or vitamin K antagonists may increase the risk of bleeding.

HOW SUPPLIED

Powder for Injection, lyophilized: 10.8 IU (18.8 mg)

DOSAGE

• **IV ONLY**

Acute MI.

Adults: 10 + 10 unit double-bolus. Each bolus is given over 2 min, with the second bolus given 30 min after initiation of the first bolus injection.

NURSING CONSIDERATIONS

SEE ALSO *NURSING CONSIDERATIONS* FOR *ALTEPLASE*.

ADMINISTRATION/STORAGE

IV 1. Initiate treatment as soon as possible after symptom onset.

2. Have available antiarrhythmic therapy for bradycardia and/or ventricular irritability.

3. Give each bolus by IV line in which no other medication is being simultaneously infused/injected. Do not add any other medication to the reteplase solution.

4. Reconstitution is performed using the diluent, syringe, needle, and dispensing pin provided with the drug as follows:

• Remove the flip-cap from one vial of sterile water (preservative free), and, with the syringe provided, withdraw 10 mL of the sterile water.

• Open the package containing the dispensing pin. Remove the needle from the syringe and discard. Remove the protective cap from the spike end of the dispensing pin and connect the syringe to the dispensing pin. Remove the protective flip-cap from one vial of reteplase.

• Remove the protective cap from the spike end of the dispensing pin, and insert the spike into the vial of reteplase. Transfer the 10 mL of sterile water through the dispensing pin into the vial.

• With the dispensing pin and syringe still attached to the vial, gently swirl the vial to dissolve the reteplase. *Do not* **shake.**

• Withdraw the 10 mL of reconstituted reteplase back into the syringe (a small amount will remain due to overfill).

• Detach the syringe from the dispensing pin, and attach the sterile 20-gauge needle provided. The solution is ready to administer.

5. Since reteplase contains no antibacterial preservatives, reconstitute just prior to use. When reconstituted as directed, the solution may be used within 4 hr when stored at 2–30°C (36–86°F).

6. Keep the kit sealed until use and store at 2–25°C (36–77°F).

ASSESSMENT

1. Document indications for therapy, noting onset, pain level, and characteristics of chest pain.

2. List drugs currently prescribed to ensure none interact unfavorably.

3. Note evidence of CVA, internal bleeding, trauma, neurosurgery, or bleeding disorders.

4. Obtain CBC, type and cross, coagulation times, cardiac panel, and liver and renal function studies.

5. Note cardiopulmonary assessments and ECG.

INTERVENTIONS

1. During administration, continuously monitor cardiac rhythm. Have medications available for management of arrhythmias.

2. Record VS every 15 min during infusion and for 2 hr following.

3. Administer first dose over 2 min and the second dose 30 min later if no serious bleeding is observed. In the event of any uncontrolled bleeding, terminate the heparin infusion and withhold the second dose.

4. Observe all puncture sites and areas for evidence of bleeding. Arterial sticks require 30 min of manual pressure

R

followed by application of a pressure dressing.
5. Assess for reperfusion reactions such as:
• Arrhythmias usually of short duration, which may include bradycardia or ventricular tachycardia
• Reduction of chest pain
• Return of elevated ST segment and smaller Q waves
6. Maintain bedrest and observe for S&S of abnormal bleeding (hematuria, hematemesis, melena, CVA, cardiac tamponade).

CLIENT/FAMILY TEACHING

1. Review goals of therapy and inherent risks of drug therapy during acute coronary artery occlusion.
2. To be effective, therapy should be instituted as soon as possible after symptom onset.
3. Encourage family members to learn CPR.

OUTCOMES/EVALUATE

Improved ventricular function; ↓ incidence of CHF, and ↓ mortality with AMI

Rh_o (D) Immune Globulin (Rh_o[D] IGIM)

Rh_o (D) Immune Globulin IV (RH_o [D] IGIV)

(roh (dee) im-**MYOUN GLOH**-byou-lin)

PREGNANCY CATEGORY: C
Rx: Rh_o [D] IGIM: BayRho-D Full Dose, RhoGAM; **Rh_o (D) IGIV:** WinRho SDF
CLASSIFICATION(S):
Immunosuppressant

ACTION/KINETICS

Sterile, freeze-dried gamma globulin (IgG) fraction containing antibodies to Rh_o (D) derived from human plasma. The manufacturing process is effective in inactivating lipid-enveloped viruses, including hepatitis B and C and HIV. Contains approximately 2 mcg IgA/1,500 international units (300 mcg). It suppresses the immune response of nonsensitized Rh_o (D) antigen-negative individuals following Rh_o (D) antigen-positive red blood cell exposure. Mechanism for ITP may be due to formation of anti-Rh_o(D) (anti-D) coated RBC complexes resulting in Fc receptor blockade; this spares antibody-coated platelets. Suppression of Rh isoimmunization decreases the possibility of hemolytic disease in an Rh_o (D) antigen-positive fetus in present and future pregnancies. For Rh_o(D) IGIV, **Peak levels, after IV:** 2 hr; **after IM:** 5–10 days. **t½, after IV:** 24 days; **after IM:** 30 days.

USES

BayRho-D Full Dose, RhoGAM. (1) Prevention of Rh hemolytic disease of the newborn (given to mother 72 hr after birth of a Rh_o(D)-positive infant. (2) Prevent isoimmunization in Rh_o(D)-negative persons who have been transfused with Rh_o(D)-positive RBCs or blood components containing RBCs. *Investigational:* Immune thrombocytopenia purpura in Rh_o(D) antigen-positive children.

WinRho SDF.(1) Suppression of Rh isoimmunization in non-sensitized Rh_o (D) antigen-negative women within 72 hr after spontaneous or induced abortions, amniocentesis, chorionic vilus sampling, ruptured tubal pregnancy, abdominal trauma, transplacental hemorrhage, or in the normal course of pregnancy unless the blood type of the fetus or father is known to be Rh_o (D) antigen-negative. (2) Suppression of Rh isoimmunization in Rh_o (D) antigen-negative female children and female adults in their childbearing years transfused with Rh_o (D) antigen-positive RBCs or blood components containing Rh_o (D) antigen-positive RBCs. (3) Treatment of non-splenectomized Rh_o (D) antigen-positive children with chronic or acute immune thrombocytopenic purpura (ITP), adults with chronic ITP, or children and adults with ITP secon-

R

dary to HIV infection in clinical situations requiring an increase in platelet count to prevent excessive hemorrhage.

CONTRAINDICATIONS

History of anaphylactic or severe systemic reaction to human globulin (i.e., due to the presence of trace amounts of IgA). Administration to Rh_o (D) antigen-negative or splenectomized individuals, as efficacy has not been shown. Use in Rh_o (D) antigen-negative clients who are Rh immunized (Rh antibody-positive), as evidenced by standard manual Rh antibody screening tests. Use in infants. IV use of Rh_o(D) IGIM.

SPECIAL CONCERNS

Use with extreme caution in those with a hemoglobin level less than 8 g/dL due to the possibility of increasing the severity of anemia. There is a risk of transmitting infectious agents since products are made from human plasma.

SIDE EFFECTS

When used for Rh isoimmunization suppression. Side effects are infrequent but include discomfort and slight swelling at the injection site and a slight elevation in temperature. There is the possibility of ***anaphylaxis.***

When used for ITP. Most commonly, headaches, chills, and fever. Decreased hemoglobin.

Immune thrombocytopenic clients positive for Rh_o antigen D-(positive) may show symptoms of intravascular hemolysis, clinically compromising anemia, and renal insufficiency.

HOW SUPPLIED

BayRho-D Full Dose. *Solution for Injection:* 15%–18% protein. **RhoGAM.** *Solution for Injection:* 5% +/- 1% gamma globuin. **WinRho SDF.** *Powder for injection, lyophilized:* 600 IU (120 mcg); 1,500 IU (300 mcg); 5,000 IU (1,000 mcg)

DOSAGE

• BAYRHO-D FULL DOSE, RHOGAM. IM ONLY.

Postpartum prophylaxis.

Give 1 vial or syringe (300 mcg) preferably within 72 hr of delivery. Dosage requirements vary with full-term deliveries depending on magnitude of fetomaternal hemorrhage. One 300 mcg dose provides sufficient antibody to prevent Rh sensitization if the RBC volume that has entered the circulation is 15 mL or less. If more than 15 mL is suspected or if the dose calculation results in a fraction, give the next higher whole number of vials or syringes.

Antenatal prophylaxis.

One-300 mcg vial or syringe given at about 28 weeks gestation. Must be followed by another 300 mcg dose, preferably within 72 hr after delivery if infant is Rh positive.

Following threatened abortion at any stage of gestation with continuation of pregnancy.

Give 300 mcg. If more than 15 mL RBCs is suspected due to fetomaternal hemorrhage, give a dose as described under postpartum prophylaxis.

Following miscarriage, abortion, or termination of ectopic pregnancy at or beyond 13 weeks' gestation.

Give 300 mcg. If more than 15 mL RBCs is suspected due to fetomaternal hemorrhage, give a dose as described under postpartum prophylaxis.

Transfusion.

After calculating the volume of Rh_o(D)-positive red cells given to an Rh_o(D)-negative recipient, divide by 15 to determine the number of vials or syringes of Rh_o(D) IGIM to give. If the dose calculated results in a fraction, give the next higher whole number of vials or syringes. Give as soon as possible after the incompatible transfusion, but within 72 hr.

• WINRHO SDF. IM, IV.

Suppression of Rh isoimmunization.

1,500 IU (300 mcg) at 28 weeks gestation. If given early in the pregnancy, administer at 12-week intervals in order to maintain an adequate level of passively acquired anti-Rh (antibodies). Give 600 IU (120 mcg) to the mother as soon as possible after delivery of a confirmed Rh_o (D) antigen-positive baby and within 72 hr after delivery. If the Rh status of the baby is not known at 72 hr, give the drug to the mother. If more than 72 hr have elapsed, do not withhold the drug but give as soon as possible up to 28 days after delivery.

Postpartum, if newborn is Rh positive.
600 IU (120 mcg).

Abortion, amniocentesis, or any other manipulation after 34 weeks gestation.
600 IU (120 mcg).

Threatened abortion at any time, amniocentesis and chorionic villus sampling before 34 weeks gestation.
1500 IU (300 mcg) immediately. Repeat dose q 12 weeks during pregnancy.

Incompatible blood transfusions or massive fetal hemorrhage.
IV: 3,000 IU (600 mcg) q 8 hr until the total dose is given. **IM:** 6,000 IU (1,200 mcg) q 12 hr until the total dose is given.

• **IV ONLY**

ITP.
Initial: 250 IU (50 mcg)/kg (125–200 IU/kg if the hemoglobin level is less than 10 g/dL). Give the initial dose as a single dose or two divided doses on separate days. If subsequent therapy is required, give 125–300 IU (25–60 mcg)/kg by IV only. If response to initial dose resulted in a satisfactory increase in platelets, maintenance therapy is 125–300 IU/kg (25–60 mcg/kg). If client did not respond to initial dose, give a subsequent dose based on hemoglobin. If hemoglobin is > 10 g/dL, redose between 250–300 IU/kg (50–60 mcg/kg); if hemoglobin is 8–10 g/dL, redose between 125–200 IU/kg (25–40 mcg/kg); if hemoglobin is < 8 g/dL, use with caution.

NURSING CONSIDERATIONS

ADMINISTRATION/STORAGE

1. Never inject Rh_o(D) IGIM IV or give to a neonate.
2. Administer Rh_o(D) IGIM preferably in the anterolateral aspects of the upper thigh and the deltoid muscle of the upper arm. Do not use the gluteal area routinely due to possible injury to the sciatic nerve. If used, only the upper, outer quadrant should be used.
3. When using a single vial or syringe of Rh_o(D) IGIM, give the entire amount. If using multiple vials or syringes, calculate the total number of vials or syringes needed. The total voloume can be given in divided doses at different sites at 1 time or the total dose may be divided and given at intervals, provided the total dose is given within 72 hr of the fetomaternal hemorrhage or transfusion.
4. Use the following administration procedure for a syringe containing Rh_o(D) IGIM:
• Remove the prefilled syringe from the package. Lift by the barrel, not the plunger.
• Twist the plunger rod clockwise until the threads are seated.
• With the rubber needle shield secured on the syringe tip, push the plunger rod forward a few millimeters to break any friction seal between the rubber stopper and the glass syringe barrel.
• Remove the needle shield and expel air bubbles.
• Proceed with puncture with the needle.
• Aspirate prior to injection to ensure needle is not in an artery or vein.
• Inject the drug. Withdraw the needle and destroy it.
5. For IM use of Rh_o(D) IGIV, reconstitute the 600 IU and the 1,500 IU product aseptically with 1.25 mL of 0.9% NaCl injection and the 5,000 IU product with 8.5 mL 0.9% NaCl injection, using the same method as for IV use. Administer into the deltoid muscle of the upper arm or the anterolateral aspects of the upper thigh. Do not use the gluteal region routinely due to the risk of sciatic nerve injury; if used, give only in the upper, outer quadrant.
6. Reduce dose (125–200 IU/kg) of Rh_o(D) IGIV if hemoglobin level is less than 10 g/dL, to reduce the risk of increasing the severity of anemia.

This information is for Rh_o(D) IGIV:

IV 7. The drug must be given IV for treating ITP, as the SC or IM routes are not effective.
8. For IV use, reconstitute the 600 IU and the 1,500 IU products aseptically with 2.5 mL of 0.9% NaCl injection and the 5,000 IU product with 8.5 mL of

R

0.9% NaCl injection. Introduce the diluent slowly onto the inside wall of the vial and wet the pellet by gentle swirling until dissolved. Do not shake. Administer into a suitable vein over 3 to 5 min.

9. Use only 0.9% NaCl injection to reconstitute the product.

10. Store unreconstituted drug vials at 2–8°C (35–46°F). If reconstituted drug not used immediately, may be stored at room temperature for up to 4 hr. Discard any unused portion. Do not freeze either unreconstituted or reconstituted product.

ASSESSMENT

1. Document indications and condition requiring therapy.

2. Determine Rh factor to ensure client is not antibody positive. Obtain blood sample for type and cross from mother and the neonate's cord. The neonate should be Rh_o(D) positive and the mother must be Rh_o(D) negative and (D^u) negative. A large fetomaternal hemorrhage late in pregnancy or following delivery may cause a weak mixed field positive (D^u) test result. Assess for a large fetomaternal hemorrhage and adjust the dose of Rh_o (D) immune globulin accordingly. Give drug if there is any doubt about the blood type of the mother.

3. Reduce dose if hemoglobin is < 10 or there is evidence of a large fetomaternal hemorrhage.

4. When used to treat ITP, monitor clinical response by assessing platelet counts, red cell counts, hemoglobin, and reticulocyte levels.

5. Monitor Rh_o clients for signs and symptoms if intravascular hemolysis, clinically compromising anemia, and renal insufficiency.

CLIENT/FAMILY TEACHING

When an Rh-negative mother carries an Rh-positive fetus, the fetal RBCs cross the placenta and enter the mother's circulation, evoking maternal antibody production against the Rh factor. When these antibodies cross to the fetal circulation, they destroy fetal RBCs, hence the need for monitoring and administration with all subsequent pregnancies. The medication prevents sensitization of an Rh-negative mother by an Rh-positive fetus, ultimately preventing hemolytic disease of the newborn.

OUTCOMES/EVALUATE

- Suppression of Rh isoimmunization
- Prevention of hemolytic disease of the newborn
- ↑ Platelets

Ribavirin

(rye-bah-**VYE**-rin)

PREGNANCY CATEGORY: X
CLASSIFICATION(S):
Antiviral
Rx: Virazole

SEE ALSO *ANTIVIRAL DRUGS*.

ACTION/KINETICS

Has antiviral activity against respiratory syncytial virus (RSV), influenza virus, and HSV. Precise mechanism not known; may act as a competitive inhibitor of cellular enzymes that act on guanosine and xanthosine. Ribavirin is distributed to the plasma, respiratory tract, and RBCs and is rapidly taken up by cells. **t½ from plasma:** 9.5 hr; **from RBCs:** 40 days. Eliminated through both the urine and feces.

USES

Hospitalized pediatric clients (including infants) with severe lower respiratory tract infections (viral pneumonia including bronchiolitis) due to RSV. Underlying conditions, such as prematurity or cardiopulmonary disease, may increase the severity of the RSV infection. Ribavirin is intended to be used along with standard treatment (including fluid management) for such clients with severe lower respiratory tract infections. *Investigational:* Ribavirin aerosol has been used against influenza A and B. Oral ribavirin has been used against herpes genitalis, acute and chronic hepatitis, measles, and Lassa fever.

CONTRAINDICATIONS

Use in adults. Infants requiring artificial respiration (the drug may precipitate in the equipment and interfere with appropriate ventilation of the client). Children with mild RSV lower respiratory tract infections who require a shorter hospital stay than required for a full course of ribavirin therapy. Pregnancy or women who may become pregnant during drug therapy (the drug may cause fetal harm and is known to be teratogenic). Lactation.

SPECIAL CONCERNS

Deterioration of respiratory function in infants with COPD or asthma.

SIDE EFFECTS

Pulmonary: Worsening of respiratory status, pneumothorax, apnea, bacterial pneumonia, dependence on ventilator, ***bronchospasm,*** pulmonary edema, hypoventilation, cyanosis, dyspnea, atelectasis. **CV:** Hypotension, ***cardiac arrest,*** manifestations of digitalis toxicity, bradycardia, bigeminy, tachycardia. **Hematologic:** Anemia (with IV or PO ribavirin), reticulocytosis. **Other:** Conjunctivitis and rash (with the aerosol).

NOTE: The following symptoms have been noted in health care workers: headache, conjunctivitis, rhinitis, nausea, rash, dizziness, pharyngitis, lacrimation, bronchospasm, chest pain. Also, damage to contact lenses after prolonged close exposure to the aerosolized product.

HOW SUPPLIED

Lyophilized powder for aerosol reconstitution: 6 g/100 mL vial

DOSAGE

• AEROSOL ONLY, TO AN INFANT OXYGEN HOOD USING THE SMALL PARTICLE AEROSOL GENERATOR-2 (SPAG-2)

The concentration administered is 20 mg/mL and the average aerosol concentration for a 12-hr period is 190 mcg/L of air. Treatment is continued for 12–18 hr a day for 3 (minimum)–7 days (maximum). See *Administration/ Storage.*

NURSING CONSIDERATIONS

ADMINISTRATION/STORAGE

1. Treatment is most effective if initiated within the first 3 days of the RSV, which causes lower respiratory tract infections.
2. Administer ribavirin aerosol using only the SPAG-2 aerosol generator.
3. Do *not* institute therapy in clients requiring artificial respiration.
4. Do not give any other aerosolized medications if using ribavirin aerosol.
5. Reconstitute with a minimum of 75 mL sterile water (USP) for injection or inhalation in the original 100-mL vial. Shake well and transfer the solution to the SPAG-2 reservoir utilizing a sterilized 500-mL wide-mouth Erlenmeyer flask and further dilute to a final volume of 300 mL with sterile water. Use water that has no antimicrobial agent or other substance added.
6. Replace solutions in the SPAG-2 reservoir daily. Also, if the liquid level is low, discard before new drug solution is added.
7. The dose and administration schedule for infants who require mechanical ventilation are the same as for those who do not.
8. For nonmechanically ventilated infants, the aerosol is delivered to an infant oxygen hood from the SPAG-2 aerosol generator. If a hood cannot be used, the aerosol is given by face mask or oxygen tent. However, due to the larger size of a tent, the delivery dynamics may be altered.
9. Store reconstituted solutions at room temperature up to 24 hr.
10. Women of childbearing age are not to administer the drug. *Post* this advisement so they do not come in contact with the drug.

INTERVENTIONS

1. Health care workers administering drug should use goggles and respirator to protect mucous membranes; remove contact lens, and monitor exposure times. Review drug related side effects.
2. It is essential that constant monitoring be undertaken for both the fluid and respiratory status of the client. Fo ventilator assisted clients be sure to drain tubing often to prevent obstruction and impaired ventilation.
3. Assess frequently for evidence of respiratory distress; stop therapy and report if distress occurs. Do not leave

R

child unattended and unstimulated in the tent for long periods.
4. Monitor and record VS and I&O.
5. Anticipate limited use in infants and adults with COPD or asthma.
6. With prolonged therapy assess for anemia; monitor VS and CBC values.

OUTCOMES/EVALUATE

Improved airway exchange; resolution of RSV pneumonia

—COMBINATION DRUG—

Ribavirin and Interferon alfa-2b recombinant

(**rye**-bah-**VYE**-rin/inter-**FEER**-on)

PREGNANCY CATEGORY: X
CLASSIFICATION(S):
Treatment for chronic hepatitis C
Rx: Rebetron

SEE ALSO *RIBAVIRIN* AND *INTERFERON ALFA-2B RECOMBINANT*. NOTE: REBETRON IS A COMBINATION PACKAGE CONTAINING RIBAVIRIN AND INTERFERON ALFA-2B RECOMBINANT. THUS, THE INFORMATION FOR EACH DRUG IS TO BE CONSULTED.

ACTION/KINETICS

The mechanism of action of the combination in inhibiting the hepatitis C virus is not known.

USES

Treatment of chronic hepatitis C in clients with compensated liver disease who either have relapsed following alpha interferon therapy or have previously been untreated with alpha-interferon therapy.

R

CONTRAINDICATIONS

Pregnancy, in those who may become pregnant, and in male partners of women who are pregnant. Lactation. Hypersensitivity, or history thereof, to alpha interferons and/or ribavirin. Use in clients with autoimmune hepatitis.

SPECIAL CONCERNS

Use with extreme caution in those with pre-existing psychiatric disorders who report a history of severe depression. Use with caution if C_{CR} is less than 50 mL/min or in pre-existing cardiac disease. Safety and efficacy have not been determined in children less than 18 years of age.

SIDE EFFECTS

See individual drugs; selected treatment-emergent side effects follow.
Hematologic: Anemia. **GI:** N&V, anorexia, dyspepsia. **CNS:** Depression, suicidal behavior, dizziness, insomnia, irritability, emotional lability, impaired concentration, nervousness. **Respiratory:** Dyspnea, pulmonary infiltrates, pneumonitis, pneumonia, sinusitis. **Musculoskeletal:** Myalgia, arthralgia, musculoskeletal pain. **Dermatologic:** Alopecia, rash, pruritus. **Body as a whole:** Headache, fatigue, rigors, fever, flu-like symptoms, asthenia, chest pain. **Miscellaneous:** Taste perversion, injection site inflammation or reaction.

LABORATORY TEST CONSIDERATIONS

↑ Bilirubin, uric acid. ↓ Hemoglobin, neutrophils.

DRUG INTERACTIONS

See individual drugs.

HOW SUPPLIED

Combination packages containing ribavirin (Rebetol) capsules, 200 mg, and interferon alfa-2b recombinant (Introl A) injectable, 3 million IU

DOSAGE

- **CAPSULES (REBETOL), SC (INTRON A)**
  Chronic hepatitis C.

Adults, 75 kg or less: Rebetol: 2 x 200 mg capsules in the a.m. and 3 x 200 mg capsules in the p.m. Intron A: 3 million I.U. 3 times weekly SC. **Adults, more than 75 kg:** Rebetol: 3 x 200 mg capsules in the a.m. and 3 x 200 mg capsules in the p.m. Intron A: 3 million I.U. three times a week SC. Reduce the dose of Rebetol by 600 mg daily and Intron A by 1.5 million I.U. three times a week if the hemoglobin is less than 10 g/dL.

NURSING CONSIDERATIONS

SEE ALSO *NURSING CONSIDERATIONS* FOR *RIBAVIRIN* AND *INTERFERON ALFA-2B RECOMBINANT*.

ADMINISTRATION/STORAGE

1. Continue the drug combination for six months (24 weeks). The safety and efficacy of the combination have not been established beyond 6 months of therapy.

2. Rebetol may be given without regard to food.
3. At provider discretion, the client may self-administer Intron A.
4. Refrigerate capsules and injection between 2–8°C (36–46°F).

ASSESSMENT

1. Detemine disease onset/diagnosis, liver function, previous therapies trialed and when if relapsed with alpha interferon therapy.
2. Note any psychiatric history or cardiac disease.
3. Initially obtain a negative pregnancy test and then monthly during therapy and for 6 mo following therapy. Providers should report any pregnancy during or for 6 mo following therapy at 1-800-727-7064.
4. Monitor CBC, renal and LFTs, chemistries and TSH per protocol.
5. Obtain eye exam prior to therapy with diabetes and HTN.

CLIENT/FAMILY TEACHING

1. Take exactly as directed. The package contains the Rebetol capsules and also the injectable Introl A for SC administration.
2. May experience flu like symptoms which should diminish with continued therapy. Take injections at bedtime to help minimize.
3. Men and women must use two forms of reliable birth control during and for 6 mo following therapy; causes severe fetal damage.
4. Report any unusual behaviors, depression, or suicide ideations immediately.
5. Visual problems or decreased acuity should be evaluated by an eye doctor.

OUTCOMES/EVALUATE

Treatment of chronic hepatitis C; ↓ viral load

Rifabutin

(**rif**-ah-**BYOU**-tin)

PREGNANCY CATEGORY: B
CLASSIFICATION(S):
Antitubercular drug
Rx: Mycobutin

ACTION/KINETICS

Inhibits DNA-dependent RNA polymerase in susceptible strains of *Escherichia coli* and *Bacillus subtilis.* Rapidly absorbed from the GI tract. **Peak plasma levels after a single dose:** 3.3 hr. **Mean terminal t½:** 45 hr. About 85% is bound to plasma proteins. High-fat meals slow the rate, but not the extent, of absorption. About 30% of a dose is excreted in the feces and 53% in the urine, primarily as metabolites. The 25-O-desacetyl metabolite is equal in activity to rifabutin.

USES

Prevention of disseminated *Mycobacterium avium* complex (MAC) disease in clients with advanced HIV infection. *Investigational:* Eradicate *H. pylori* as part of a triple-therapy (amoxicillin, pantoprazole, rifabutin), 10-day regimen.

CONTRAINDICATIONS

Hypersensitivity to rifabutin or other rifamycins (e.g., rifampin). Use in active tuberculosis. Lactation.

SPECIAL CONCERNS

Safety and efficacy have not been determined in children, although the drug has been used in HIV-positive children.

SIDE EFFECTS

GI: Anorexia, abdominal pain, diarrhea, dyspepsia, eructation, flatulence, N&V, taste perversion. **Respiratory:** Chest pain, chest pressure or pain with dyspnea. **CNS:** Insomnia, ***seizures,*** paresthesia, aphasia, confusion. **Musculoskeletal:** Asthenia, myalgia, arthralgia, myositis. **Body as a whole:** Fever, headache, generalized pain, flu-like syndrome. **Dermatologic:** Rash, skin discoloration. **Hematologic:** Neutropenia, leukopenia, anemia, eosinophilia, thrombocytopenia. **Miscellaneous:** Discolored urine, nonspecific T wave changes on ECG, hepatitis, hemolysis, uveitis.

LABORATORY TEST CONSIDERATIONS

↑ AST, ALT, alkaline phosphatase.

OD **OVERDOSE MANAGEMENT**

Symptoms: Worsening of side effects. *Treatment:* Gastric lavage followed by

R

instillation into the stomach of an activated charcoal slurry.

DRUG INTERACTIONS

Although less potent than rifampin, rifabutin induces liver enzymes and may be expected to have similar interactions as does rifampin.

Amprenavir / ↓ Rifabutin clearance; ↓ rifabutin dose by 50%

AZT / ↓ AZT steady-state plasma levels after repeated rifabutin dosing

Oral contraceptives / May ↓ OC effectiveness

HOW SUPPLIED

Capsule: 150 mg

DOSAGE

• CAPSULES

Prophylaxis of MAC disease in clients with advanced HIV infection.

Adults: 300 mg/day.

NURSING CONSIDERATIONS

SEE ALSO GENERAL NURSING CONSIDERATIONS FOR ANTI-INFECTIVES.

ASSESSMENT

1. Document indications for therapy, noting type, onset, and characteristics of symptoms.
2. Monitor CBC for neutropenia.
3. Ensure that CXR, PPD, and sputum AFB cultures have been performed to rule out active tuberculosis. Clients who develop active tuberculosis during therapy must be covered with appropriate antituberculosis medications.

CLIENT/FAMILY TEACHING

1. Take as directed and do not interupt therapy. If N&V or other GI upset occurs, may take doses of 150 mg b.i.d. with food.
2. Urine, feces, saliva, sputum, perspiration, tears, skin, and mucous membranes may be colored brown-orange. Soft contact lenses may be permanently stained.
3. Report any S&S of muscle or eye pain, irritation, or inflammation as well as any persistent vomiting or abnormal bruising/bleeding.
4. Avoid crowds and those with infections.
5. Practice nonhormonal form of birth control.

OUTCOMES/EVALUATE

Prevention of disseminated *Mycobacterium avium* complex (MAC) with advanced HIV

Rifampin

(rih-**FAM**-pin)

PREGNANCY CATEGORY: C

CLASSIFICATION(S):

Antitubercular drug

Rx: Rimactane, Rifadin

★Rx: Rofact

ACTION/KINETICS

Semisynthetic antibiotic derived from *Streptomyces mediterranei.* Suppresses RNA synthesis by binding to the beta subunit of DNA-dependent RNA polymerase. This prevents attachment of the enzyme to DNA and blockade of RNA transcription. Both bacteriostatic and bactericidal; most active against rapidly replicating organisms. Well absorbed from the GI tract; widely distributed in body tissues. **Peak plasma concentration:** 4–32 mcg/mL after 2–4 hr. **t½:** 1.5–5 hr (higher in clients with hepatic impairment). In normal clients t½ decreases with usage. Metabolized in liver; 60% is excreted in feces.

USES

(1) All types of tuberculosis. Must be used in conjunction with at least one other tuberculostatic drug (such as isoniazid, ethambutol, pyrazinamide) but is the drug of choice for retreatment. (2) Treatment of asymptomatic meningococcal carriers to eliminate *Neisseria meningitidis. Investigational:* Used in combination for infections due to *Staphylococcus aureus* and *S. epidermidis* (endocarditis, osteomyelitis, prostatitis); Legionnaire's disease; in combination with dapsone for leprosy; prophylaxis of meningitis due to *Haemophilus influenzae* and gram-negative bacteremia in infants.

CONTRAINDICATIONS

Hypersensitivity; not recommended for intermittent therapy.

SPECIAL CONCERNS
Safe use during lactation has not been established. Safety and effectiveness not determined in children less than 5 years of age. Use with extreme caution in clients with hepatic dysfunction. Use with caution, if at all, with pyrazinamide to treat latent tuberculosis in those not infected with human immunodeficeincy virus.

SIDE EFFECTS
GI: N&V, diarrhea, anorexia, gas, pseudomembranous colitis, pancreatitis, sore mouth and tongue, cramps, heartburn, flatulence. **CNS:** Headache, drowsiness, fatigue, ataxia, dizziness, confusion, generalized numbness, fever, difficulty in concentrating. **Hepatic:** Jaundice, hepatitis, ***severe/fatal liver injury when used with pyrazinamide***. Increases in AST, ALT, bilirubin, alkaline phosphatase. **Hematologic:** Thrombocytopenia, eosinophilia, hemolysis, leukopenia, ***hemolytic anemia.*** **Allergic:** Flu-like symptoms, dyspnea, wheezing, SOB, purpura, pruritus, urticaria, skin rashes, sore mouth and tongue, conjunctivitis. **Renal:** Hematuria, hemoglobinuria, renal insufficiency, acute renal failure. **Miscellaneous:** Visual disturbances, muscle weakness or pain, arthralgia, decreased BP, osteomalacia, menstrual disturbances, edema of face and extremities, adrenocortical insufficiency, increases in BUN and serum uric acid. *NOTE:* Body fluids and feces may be red-orange.

LABORATORY TEST CONSIDERATIONS
↑ AST, ALT, alkaline phosphatase, BUN, bilirubin, uric acid, BSP retention values. False + Coombs' test.

OD OVERDOSE MANAGEMENT
Symptoms: Shortly after ingestion, N&V, and lethargy will occur. Followed by severe hepatic involvement (liver enlargement with tenderness, increased direct and total bilirubin, change in hepatic enzymes) with unconsciousness. Also, brownish red or orange discoloration of urine, saliva, tears, sweat, skin, and feces. *Treatment:* Gastric lavage followed by activated charcoal slurry introduced into the stomach. Antiemetics to control N&V. Forced diuresis to enhance excretion. If hepatic function is seriously impaired, bile drainage may be required. Extracorporeal hemodialysis may be necessary.

DRUG INTERACTIONS
Acetaminophen / ↓ Acetaminophen effects R/T ↑ liver breakdown
Aminophylline / ↓ Aminophylline effects R/T ↑ liver breakdown
Amiodarone / ↓ Amiodarone serum levels R/T ↑ liver breakdown
Aminosalicylic acid / ↓ Rifampin effect; give 2 agents 8–12 hr apart
Amprenavir / Significant ↑ Amprenavir clearance; do not use together
Anticoagulants, oral / ↓ Anticoagulant effects R/T ↑ liver breakdown
Antidiabetics, oral / ↓ Antidiabetic effects R/T ↑ liver breakdown
Barbiturates / ↓ Barbiturate effects R/T ↑ liver breakdown
Benzodiazepines / ↓ Benzodiazepine effects R/T ↑ liver breakdown
Beta-adrenergic blocking agents / ↓ Beta-blocking effects R/T ↑ liver breakdown
Buspirone / ↓ Buspiron effect R/T ↑ liver metabolism
Chloramphenicol / ↓ Chloramphenicol effects R/T ↑ liver breakdown
Clofibrate / ↓ Clofibrate effects R/T ↑ liver breakdown
Contraceptives, oral / ↓ OC effects R/T ↑ liver breakdown
Corticosteroids / ↓ Corticosteroid effects R/T ↑ liver breakdown
Cyclosporine / ↓ Cyclosporine effects R/T ↑ liver breakdown
Delaviridine / ↓ Delaviridine effect R/T ↑ liver metabolism
Digoxin / ↓ Digoxin serum levels
Disopyramide / ↓ Disopyramide effects R/T ↑ liver breakdown
Doxycycline / ↓ Doxycycline serum level and half-life possibly ↓ effect
Enalapril / ↓ Enalapril effect
Estrogens / ↓ Estrogen effects R/T ↑ liver breakdown
Fluconazole / Rifampin ↑ fluconazole metabolism
Fluoroquinolones / Possible ↑ fluoroquinolone liver metabolism

R

Haloperidol / ↓ Halothane plasma levels and effect
Halothane / ↑ Risk of hepatotoxicity and hepatic encephalopathy
Hydantoins / ↓ Hydantoin effects R/T ↑ liver breakdown
Isoniazid / ↑ Risk of hepatotoxicity
Ketoconazole / Rifampin ↑ ketoconazole metabolism; ketoconazole ↓ rifampin absorption → ↓ effect of both drugs
Lamotrigine / ↓ Lamotrigine area under the curve and half-life due to ↑ liver metabolism
Losartan / Rifampin may ↑ losartan liver metabolism
Macrolide antibiotics (e.g., clarithromycin) / Possible ↑ clarithromycin liver metabolism and ↓ rifamycin liver metabolism
Methadone / ↓ Methadone effects R/T ↑ liver breakdown
Mexiletine / ↓ Mexiletine effects R/T ↑ liver breakdown
Morphine / ↓ Morphine analgesia
Nifedipine / ↓ Nifedipine effects
Ondansetron / ↓ Ondansetron plasma levels R/T ↑ liver breakdown
Propafenone / ↓ Propafenone serum levels R/T ↑ liver breakdown
Protease inhibitors (e.g., indinavir, nelfinavir, ritonavir) / Possible ↓ liver metabolism of both drugs
Pyrazinamide / Possible severe hepatitis
Quinine / ↑ Quinine liver metabolism
Quinidine / ↓ Quinidine effects R/T ↑ liver breakdown
Repaglinide / ↓ Repaglinide plasma levels and effects R/T ↑ liver metabolism
Sertraline / ↓ Sertraline effect R/T ↑ liver metabolism
Sulfapyridine / ↓ Sulfapyridine plasma levels
Sulfones / ↓ Sulfone effects R/T ↑ liver breakdown
Tacrolimus / ↓ Tacrolimus immunosuppressant effects
Terbenafine / ↓ Effect R/T ↑ liver metabolism
Theophylline / ↓ Theophylline effects R/T ↑ liver breakdown
Thyroid hormones / TSH levels may ↑ → hypothyroidism
Tocainide / ↓ Tocainide effects R/T ↑ liver breakdown
Tricyclic antidepressants / ↓ TCA levels R/T ↑ liver metabolism
Verapamil / ↓ Verapamil effects R/T ↑ liver breakdown
Zidovudine / ↓ Zidovudine effect R/T ↑ liver metabolism
Zolpidem / ↓ Zolpidem plasma levels and effect

HOW SUPPLIED

Capsule: 150 mg, 300 mg; *Powder for injection:* 600 mg

DOSAGE

• CAPSULES, IV

Pulmonary tuberculosis.

Adults: 10 mg/kg in a single daily dose, not to exceed 600 mg/day; **children over 5 years:** 10–20 mg/kg/day, not to exceed 600 mg/day.

Meningococcal carriers.

Adults: 600 mg q 12 hr for 2 days; **children, over 1 month:** 10–20 mg/kg q 12 hr for four doses, not to exceed 600 mg/day.

NURSING CONSIDERATIONS

SEE ALSO *GENERAL NURSING CONSIDERATIONS FOR ANTI-INFECTIVES.*

ADMINISTRATION/STORAGE

1. Administer capsules once daily 1 hr before or 2 hr after meals to ensure maximum absorption.
2. A PO suspension (10 mg/mL) may be prepared as follows: The contents of either four 300-mg rifampin capsules or eight 150-mg capsules are emptied into a 4-oz amber glass bottle. Add 20 mL of simple syrup; shake vigorously; then add 100 mL of simple syrup and shake again. The suspension is stable for 4 weeks when stored at room temperature or in the refrigerator.
3. Check to be sure that there is a desiccant in the bottle containing capsules of rifampin because these are relatively moisture sensitive.
4. If administered concomitantly with PAS, give drugs 8–12 hr apart because the acid interferes with the absorption of rifampin.
5. When used for tuberculosis, continue therapy for 6–9 months.

IV 6. IV use is restricted for initial treatment and retreatment of tuberculosis when the drug can not be taken PO.

7. Reconstitute 600-mg vial using 10 mL of sterile water for injection; swirl gently to dissolve. The resultant solution contains 60 mg/mL rifampin; stable at room temperature for 24 hr.

8. Add the volume of reconstituted solution needed to 500 mL of D5W and infuse over 3 hr, or may be added to 100 mL D5W and infused over 30 min. Sterile saline may be used when dextrose is contraindicated; however, the stability of rifampin is slightly less.

9. Use diluted solution within 4 hr or drug may precipitate from solution.

10. Injectable solution appears dark reddish brown.

ASSESSMENT

1. Note indications for therapy, type, onset, and characteristics of symptoms.
2. List any previous therapy.
3. Monitor CBC, cultures, liver and renal function studies; note any dysfunction.
4. Document any GI disturbances or auditory nerve impairment.
5. Obtain baseline CXR; auscultate and document lung sounds and characteristics of sputum. Note PPD skin test results.

CLIENT/FAMILY TEACHING

1. Take drug on an empty stomach 1 hr before or 2 hr after meals; report if GI upset occurs.
2. Must take daily for months to effectively treat tuberculosis. Do not stop or skip doses of medication or relapse may occur.
3. Avoid alcohol; increases risk of liver toxicity.
4. Headache, drowsiness, confusion, fever, and muscle and joint aches may occur during the first few weeks of therapy; report if symptoms persist or increase in intensity.
5. Rifampin may impart a red-orange color to urine, feces, saliva, sputum, and tears; may *permanently* discolor contact lenses.
6. Practice alternative birth control since oral contraceptives not effective; drug has teratogenic properties.

OUTCOMES/EVALUATE

- Adjunct in treating tuberculosis
- Prophylaxis of meningitis due to *H. influenzae* and gram-negative bacteremia in infants

Rifapentine

(rih-fah-**PEN**-teen)

PREGNANCY CATEGORY: C
CLASSIFICATION(S):
Antitubercular drug
Rx: Priftin

ACTION/KINETICS

Similar activity to rifampin. Inhibits DNA-dependent RNA polymerase in susceptible strains of *Mycobacterium tuberculosis*, but not in mammalian cells. Is bactericidal against both intracellular and extracellular organisms. Food increases amount absorbed. **Maximum levels:** 5–6 hr. **Steady state conditions:** 10 days after 600 mg/day. Metabolized to the active 25-desacetyl rifapentine. Both the parent drug and active metabolite are significantly bound to plasma proteins. **t½:** 13.2 hr for parent drug, 13.4 hr for active metabolite. Excreted in the feces (70%) and the urine (17%).

USES

Treatment of pulmonary tuberculosis. Must be used with at least one other antituberculosis drug.

CONTRAINDICATIONS

Hypersensitivity to other rifamycins (e.g., rifampin or rifabutin). Lactation.

SPECIAL CONCERNS

Experience is limited in HIV-infected clients. Organisms resistant to other rifamycins are likely to be resistant to rifapentine. Use with caution in clients with abnormal liver tests or liver disease. Safety and efficacy have not been determined in children less than 12 years of age.

SIDE EFFECTS

Side effects listed occurred in 1% or more of clients and were seen when rifapentine was used in combination with other antituberculosis drugs

R

(e.g., isoniazid, pyrazinamide, ethambutol).
GI: N&V, anorexia, dyspepsia, diarrhea, hemoptysis. **CNS:** Headache, dizziness. **GU:** Pyuria, proteinuria, hematuria, urinary casts. **Dermatologic:** Rash, acne, maculopapular rash. **Hematologic:** Neutropenia, lymphopenia, anemia, leukopenia, thrombocytosis. **Miscellaneous:** Hyperuricemia (probably due to pyrizinamide), hypertension, pruritus, arthralgia, pain, red coloration of body tissues and fluids.

LABORATORY TEST CONSIDERATIONS

↑ ALT, AST. Inhibition of standard microbiological assays for serum folate and vitamin B_{12}.

DRUG INTERACTIONS

Cytochrome P450 / Rifapentine is an inducer of certain cytochromes P450 → reduced activity of a number of drugs (See *Rifampin)*. Dosage adjustment may be required
Indinavir / Three-fold ↑ in clearance of indinavir.

HOW SUPPLIED

Tablets: 150 mg

DOSAGE

• **TABLETS**

Tuberculosis, intensive phase.
600 mg (four 150 mg tablets) twice weekly with an interval of 72 hr or more between doses; continue for 2 months.

Tuberculosis, continuation phase
Continue rifapentine therapy once weekly for 4 months in combination with isoniazid or another antituberculosis drug. If the client is still sputum-smear- or culture-positive, if resistant organisms are present, or if the client is HIV-positive, follow ATS/CDC treatment guidelines.

NURSING CONSIDERATIONS

ADMINISTRATION/STORAGE

Give rifapentine in combination as part of a regimen that includes other antituberculosis drugs, especially on days when rifapentine is not given.

ASSESSMENT

1. Determine onset, duration, and characteristics of disease.
2. Obtain chemistries, CBC, and LFTs; assess sputum culture. Monitor LFTs every two to four weeks during therapy.
3. List other drugs prescribed to ensure none interact.
4. Give concomitant pyridoxine in the malnourished, those predisposed to neuropathy (e.g., alcoholics, diabetics), and in adolescents.

CLIENT/FAMILY TEACHING

1. Take exactly as directed. May take with food if stomach upset, nausea, or vomiting occurs.
2. Vitamin B_6 is prescribed for clients who are malnourished or predisposed to neuropathy, and in adolescents.
3. May stain body fluids/tissues (tears, urine, saliva, sweat, skin, feces, tongue) a red-orange color.
4. Drug is administered less frequently and in conjunction with other antitubercular agents. During the two-month intensive phase, drug is taken every three days. Following this phase, rifapentine is given once a week for four months in combinations with isoniazid or other agent for susceptible organisms called the continuation phase for TB. A more frequent dosing pattern is used in HIV infected clients. Adherence to prescribed regimen is of utmost importance.
5. Report any N&V, fever, darkened urine, pain or swelling of the joints, or yellow discolorations of the skin and eyes.
6. Avoid crowds and persons with infections.
7. Practice non-hormonal method of contraception.

OUTCOMES/EVALUATE

• Treatment of pulmonary TB
• Prevention of disseminated *Mycobacterium avium* complex disease with HIV infection

Riluzole

(**RIL**-you-zohl)

PREGNANCY CATEGORY: C
CLASSIFICATION(S):
Drug for amyotropic lateral sclerosis
Rx: Rilutek

ACTION/KINETICS

Mechanism not known. Possible effects include (a) inhibition of glutamate release, (b) inactivation of voltage-dependent sodium channels, and (c) interference with intracellular events that follow transmitter binding at excitatory amino acid receptors. Well absorbed following PO use; high-fat meals decrease absorption. **t½, elimination, after repeated doses:** 12 hr. About 96% is bound to plasma proteins. Extensively metabolized, mainly in the liver, and excreted in the urine.

USES

Treatment of clients with ALS; the drug extends both survival and time to tracheostomy.

CONTRAINDICATIONS

Lactation.

SPECIAL CONCERNS

Use with caution in hepatic and renal impairment due to decreased excretion and higher plasma levels. Use with caution in the elderly, as age-related changes in renal and hepatic function may cause a decreased clearance. Clearance of riluzole in Japanese clients is 50% lower compared with Caucasians; clearance may also be lower in women. Safety and efficacy have not been determined in children.

SIDE EFFECTS

Side effects listed occurred at a frequency of 0.1% or more.

GI: N&V, diarrhea, anorexia, abdominal pain, dyspepsia, flatulence, dry mouth, stomatitis, tooth disorder, oral moniliasis, dysphagia, constipation, increased appetite, intestinal obstruction, fecal impaction, ***GI hemorrhage,*** GI ulceration, gastritis, fecal incontinence, jaundice, hepatitis, glossitis, gum hemorrhage, pancreatitis, tenesmus, esophageal stenosis. **Body as a whole:** Asthenia, malaise, weight loss or gain, peripheral edema, flu syndrome, hostility, abscess, ***sepsis,*** photosensitivity reaction, cellulitis, facial edema, hernia, peritonitis, reaction at injection site, chills, ***attempted suicide,*** enlarged abdomen, neoplasm. **CNS:** Dizziness (more common in women), vertigo, somnolence, circumoral paresthesia, headache, aggravation reaction, hypertonia, depression, insomnia, agitation, tremor, hallucination, personality disorders, abnormal thinking, coma, paranoid reaction, manic reaction, ataxia, extrapyramidal syndrome, hypokinesis, emotional lability, delusions, apathy, hypesthesia, incoordination, confusion, ***convulsion,*** amnesia, increased libido, stupor subdural hematoma, abnormal gait, delirium, depersonalization, facial paralysis, hemiplegia, decreased libido. **CV:** Hypertension, tachycardia, phlebitis, palpitation, postural hypotension, ***heart arrest, heart failure,*** syncope, hypotension, migraine, PVD, angina pectoris, ***MI,*** ventricular extrasystoles, ***cerebral hemorrhage,*** atrial fibrillation, BBB, CHF, pericarditis, lower extremity embolus, ***myocardial ischemia, shock.*** **Hematologic:** Neutropenia, anemia, leukocytosis, leukopenia, ecchymosis. **Respiratory:** Decreased lung function, pneumonia, rhinitis, increased cough, sinusitis, apnea, bronchitis, dyspnea, respiratory disorder, increased sputum, hiccup, pleural disorder, asthma, epistaxis, hemoptysis, yawn, hyperventilation, lung edema, hypoventilation, ***lung carcinoma,*** hypoxia, laryngitis, pleural effusion, pneumothorax, respiratory moniliasis, stridor. **Musculoskeletal:** Arthralgia, back pain, leg cramps, dysarthria, myoclonus, arthrosis, myasthenia, ***bone neoplasm.*** **GU:** Urinary retention/urgency/incontinence, urine abnormality, kidney calculus, hematuria, impotence, ***prostate carcinoma,*** kidney pain, metrorrhagia, priapism. **Dermatologic:** Pruritus, eczema, alopecia, exfoliative dermatitis, skin ulceration, urticaria, psoriasis, seborrhea, skin disorder, fungal dermatitis. **Metabolic:** Gout, respiratory acidosis, edema, thirst, hypokalemia, hyponatremia. **Miscellaneous:** Accidental or intentional injury, ***death,*** diabetes mellitus, thyroid neoplasia, amblyopia, ophthalmitis.

R

LABORATORY TEST CONSIDERATIONS
↑ GGT, alkaline phosphatase, gamma globulins. Abnormal LFTs, + direct Coombs' test.

DRUG INTERACTIONS
Amitriptyline / ↓ Elimination of riluzole → higher plasma levels
Caffeine / ↓ Elimination of riluzole → higher plasma levels
Charcoal-broiled foods / ↑ Elimination of riluzole → lower plasma levels
Omeprazole / ↑ Elimination of riluzole → lower plasma levels
Quinolones / ↓ Elimination of riluzole → higher plasma levels
Rifampin / ↑ Elimination of riluzole → lower plasma levels
Smoking (cigarettes) / ↑ Elimination of riluzole → lower plasma levels
Theophyllines / ↓ Elimination of riluzole → higher plasma levels

HOW SUPPLIED
Tablets: 50 mg.

DOSAGE
- **TABLETS**

Treatment of ALS.

50 mg q 12 hr. Higher daily doses will not increase the beneficial effect but will increase the incidence of side effects.

NURSING CONSIDERATIONS

ADMINISTRATION/STORAGE
Protect from bright light.

ASSESSMENT
1. Document symptom onset, characteristics, presentation, ethnic background, and familial associations.
2. Assess renal and LFTs. Elevations of several liver functions, especially bilirubin, should preclude drug use.
3. Monitor LFTs. SGPT levels should be measured q month during the first 3 months of therapy, q 3 months for the remainder of the first year, and then periodically.

CLIENT/FAMILY TEACHING
1. Take 1 hr before or 2 hr after meals to maintain drug bioavailability.
2. Take as prescribed at the same time each day. Do not double up if dose is missed or forgotten, take the next tablet as originally planned.
3. Report any febrile illnesses.
4. Drug may cause dizziness, drowsiness, or vertigo. Do not perform activities that require mental alertness until drug effects realized.
5. Severe dry mouth symptoms may require use of salagen.
6. Do not smoke. Avoid alcohol; may potentiate liver toxicity.

OUTCOMES/EVALUATE
Extension of survival or time to tracheostomy with ALS

Rimantadine hydrochloride

(rih-**MAN**-tih-deen)

PREGNANCY CATEGORY: C
CLASSIFICATION(S):
Antiviral
Rx: Flumadine

SEE ALSO *ANTIVIRAL DRUGS* AND *AMANTADINE HYDROCHLORIDE*.

ACTION/KINETICS
May act early in the viral replication cycle, possibly by inhibiting the uncoating of the virus. A virus protein specified by the virion M_2 gene may play an important role in the inhibition of the influenza A virus by rimantadine. Has little or no activity against influenza B virus. Plasma trough levels following 100 mg b.i.d. for 10 days range from 118 to 468 ng/mL; however, levels are higher in clients over the age of 70 years. Metabolized in the liver, and both unchanged drug (25%) and metabolites excreted through the urine.

USES
Adults: Prophylaxis and treatment of illness caused by strains of influenza A virus. **Children:** Prophylaxis against influenza A virus.

CONTRAINDICATIONS
Hypersensitivity to amantadine, rimantadine, or other drugs in the adamantine class. Lactation.

SPECIAL CONCERNS
Use with caution in clients with renal or hepatic insufficiency. An increased incidence of seizures is possible in clients with a history of epilepsy who have received amantadine. Influenza

A virus strains resistant to rimantadine can emerge during treatment and be transmitted, causing symptoms of influenza. Safety and efficacy of rimantadine in the treatment of symptomatic influenza infections in children have not been established. Safety and efficacy for prophylaxis of infections have not been determined in children less than 1 year of age. The incidence of side effects in geriatric clients is higher than in other clients.

SIDE EFFECTS

GI and CNS side effects are the most common.

GI: N&V, anorexia, dry mouth, abdominal pain, diarrhea, dyspepsia, constipation, dysphagia, stomatitis. **CNS:** Insomnia, dizziness, headache, nervousness, fatigue, asthenia, impairment of concentration, ataxia, somnolence, agitation, depression, gait abnormality, euphoria, hyperkinesia, tremor, hallucinations, confusion, ***convulsions,*** agitation, diaphoresis, hypesthesia. **Respiratory:** Dyspnea, ***bronchospasm,*** cough. **CV:** Pallor, palpitation, hypertension, ***cerebrovascular disorder, cardiac failure,*** pedal edema, heart block, tachycardia, syncope. **Miscellaneous:** Tinnitus, taste loss or change, parosmia, eye pain, rash, nonpuerperal lactation, increased lacrimation, increased frequency of micturition, fever, rigors.

OD OVERDOSE MANAGEMENT

Symptoms: Extensions of side effects including the possibility of agitation, hallucinations, ***cardiac arrhythmias, and death.*** *Treatment:* Supportive therapy. IV physostigmine at doses of 1–2 mg IV in adults and 0.5 mg in children, not to exceed 2 mg/hr, has been reported to be beneficial in treating overdose for amantadine (a related drug).

DRUG INTERACTIONS

Acetaminophen / ↓ Peak concentration and area under the curve for rimantadine

Aspirin / ↓ Peak plasma levels and area under the curve for rimantadine

Cimetidine / ↓ Clearance of rimantadine

HOW SUPPLIED

Syrup: 50 mg/5 mL; *Tablet:* 100 mg

DOSAGE

• **SYRUP, TABLETS**

Prophylaxis.

Adults and children over 10 years of age: 100 mg b.i.d. In clients with severe hepatic dysfunction (C_{CR} < 10 mL/min) and in elderly nursing home clients, reduce the dose to 100 mg/day. **Children, less than 10 years of age:** 5 mg/kg once daily, not to exceed a total dose of 150 mg/day.

Treatment.

Adults: 100 mg b.i.d. In clients with severe hepatic dysfunction and in elderly nursing home clients, reduce the dose to 100 mg/day.

NURSING CONSIDERATIONS

SEE ALSO *NURSING CONSIDERATIONS* FOR *AMANTADINE HYDROCHLORIDE*.

ADMINISTRATION/STORAGE

For treatment of influenza A virus infections, initiate therapy as soon as possible, preferably within 48 hr after onset of S&S. Continue treatment for approximately 7 days from the initial onset of symptoms.

ASSESSMENT

1. Document indications for therapy, noting onset and duration of symptoms or exposure.
2. Determine when immunized.
3. List other drugs prescribed to ensure none interact unfavorably.
4. Assess liver and renal function studies to determine any dysfunction; reduce dosage with severe hepatic dysfunction and with elderly nursing home clients.
5. Note any epilepsy; assess for loss of seizure control.

CLIENT/FAMILY TEACHING

1. Take only as directed; do not share meds.
2. Initiate as soon as symptoms appear and continue for 7 days.
3. Drug may cause dizziness; avoid activities that require mental alertness until drug effects realized.

R

4. Early annual vaccination is the method of choice for influenza prophylaxis. The 2- to 4-week time frame required to develop an antibody response can be managed with rimantadine.

OUTCOMES/EVALUATE

Prevention/ ↓ severity of influenza A virus

Risedronate sodium

(rih-**SEH**-droh-nayt)

PREGNANCY CATEGORY: C
CLASSIFICATION(S):
Bone growth regulator, bisphosphonate
Rx: Actonel

ACTION/KINETICS

Inhibits osteoclasts, thus leading to decreased bone resorption. Rapidly absorbed; food decreases absorption. **t½, initial:** 1.5 hr; **terminal:** 220 hr. Excreted unchanged in the urine.

USES

(1) Treatment of Paget's disease in those who (a) have a serum alkaline phosphatase level at least two times the upper limit of normal, (b) are symptomatic, or (c) are at risk for future complications from the disease. (2) Prophylaxis and treatment of postmenopausal osteoporosis and glucocorticoid-induced osteroporosis. *Investigational:* Reduce the chance of spine fractures in clients on long-term steroid therapy.

CONTRAINDICATIONS

Use in those with C_{CR} less than 30 mL/min. Hypocalcemia. Lactation.

SPECIAL CONCERNS

May cause upper GI disorders, including dysphagia, esophagitis, esophageal ulcer, or gastric ulcer. Use with caution in those with a history of UGI disorders. Safety and efficacy have not been determined in children.

SIDE EFFECTS

GI: Diarrhea, abdominal pain, nausea, constipation, belching, colitis. **CNS:** Headache, dizziness. **Body as a whole:** Flu syndrome, chest pain, asthenia, neoplasm. **Musculoskeletal:** Arthralgia, bone pain, leg cramps, myasthenia. **Respiratory:** Sinusitis, bronchitis. **Ophthalmic:** Amblyopia, dry eye. **Miscellaneous:** Peripheral edema, skin rash, tinnitus.

OD OVERDOSE MANAGEMENT

Symptoms: Hypocalemia. *Treatment:* Gastric lavage to remove unabsorbed drug. Milk or antacids to bind risedronate. IV calcium.

DRUG INTERACTIONS

Antacids, calcium-containing / ↓ Absorption of risedronate
Bone imaging agents / Risedronate interferes with these agents
Calcium / ↓ Absorption of risedronate
NSAIDs / Possible additive GI side effects

HOW SUPPLIED

Tablets: 5 mg, 30 mg

DOSAGE

- **TABLETS**

Treat Paget's disease.

Adults: 30 mg once daily for 2 months.

Prevention and treatment of postmenopausal or corticosteroid-induced osteoporosis.

5 mg daily.

NURSING CONSIDERATIONS

ADMINISTRATION/STORAGE

1. Before starting therapy, treat hypocalcemia and other disturbances of bone and mineral metabolism.
2. Following 2 mo post-treatment observation for Paget's disease, retreatment may be considered if serum alkaline phosphatase is not normal. The dose and duration of therapy is the same as for initial treatment.

ASSESSMENT

1. Note onset and characteristics of disease; list other agents trialed. Assess for GI disease/dysfunction.
2. Obtain chemistries, alkaline phosphatase, Ca, liver and renal function studies; avoid if $C_{CR} < 30$ mL/min.
3. Assess nutritional status and vitamin D and calcium intake.

CLIENT/FAMILY TEACHING

1. Take sitting or standing with a full glass of water at least 30 min before the first food or drink of the day.
2. To facilitate delivery to the stom-

ach and minimize GI side effects, take in an upright position with 6 to 8 oz of water. Avoid lying down for 30 min after taking the drug.
3. Therapy is once daily for 2 mo.
4. If dietary intake inadequate, consume supplemental calcium and vitamin D. Antacids and calcium may interfere with drug; take at different times during the day with food.
5. May experience nausea, diarrhea, bone pain, headache, and rash. Report so appropriate analgesics and skin care may be prescribed.
6. Report any swallowing difficulty, throat/ abdominal pain, muscle spasms, or dark colored urine.

OUTCOMES/EVALUATE

Remission of Paget's disease with ↓ bone resorption, ↓ pain and ↓ alkaline phosphatase levels

Risperidone

(ris-**PAIR**-ih-dohn)

PREGNANCY CATEGORY: C
CLASSIFICATION(S):
Antipsychotic
Rx: Risperdal

ACTION/KINETICS

Mechanism may be due to a combination of antagonism of dopamine (D_2) and serotonin (5-HT_2) receptors. Also has high affinity for the alpha-1, alpha-2, and histamine-1 receptors. Metabolized significantly in the liver to the active metabolite 9-hydroxyrisperidone, which has equal receptor-binding activity as risperidone. Thus, the effect is likely due to both the parent compound and the metabolite. Food does not affect either the rate or extent of absorption. The ability to convert risperidone to 9-hydroxyrisperidone is subject to genetic variation. A low percentage of Asians have the ability to metabolize the drug. **Peak plasma levels, risperidone:** 1 hr; **peak plasma levels, 9-hydroxyrisperidone:** 3 hr for extensive metabolizers and 17 hr for poor metabolizers. **t½, risperidone and 9-methylrisperidone:** 3 and 21 hr, respectively, for extensive metabolizers and 20 and 30 hr, respectively, for poor metabolizers. Clearance is decreased in geriatric clients and in clients with hepatic and renal impairment.

USES

Treatment of psychotic disorders. *Investigational:* Bipolar disorder. Management of dementia-related psychotic symptoms.

CONTRAINDICATIONS

Lactation.

SPECIAL CONCERNS

Use with caution in clients with known CV disease (including history of MI or ischemia, heart failure, conduction abnormalities), cerebrovascular disease, and conditions that predispose the client to hypotension (e.g., dehydration, hypovolemia, use of antihypertensive drugs). Use with caution in clients who will be exposed to extreme heat or when taken with other CNS drugs or alcohol. Greater risk of orthostatic hypotension, aspiration pneumonia, and toxic effects in geriatric clients with impaired renal function. The effectiveness of risperidone for more than 6–8 weeks has not been studied. Safety and effectiveness have not been established for children.

SIDE EFFECTS

Neuroleptic malignant syndrome: Hyperpyrexia, muscle rigidity, altered mental status, autonomic instability (i.e., irregular pulse or BP, tachycardia, diaphoresis, cardiac dysrhythmia), elevated CPK, rhabdomyolysis, ***ARF, death.***
CNS: Tardive dyskinesia (especially in geriatric clients), somnolence, insomnia, agitation, anxiety, aggressive reaction, extrapyramidal symptoms, headache, dizziness, ↑ dream activity, ↓ sexual desire, nervousness, impaired concentration, depression, apathy, catatonia, euphoria, ↑ libido, amnesia, ↑ duration of sleep, dysarthria, vertigo, stupor, paresthesia, confusion. **GI:** Constipation, nausea, dyspepsia, vom-

R

iting, abdominal pain, ↑ or ↓ salivation, toothache, ***anorexia***, flatulence, diarrhea, ↑ appetite, stomatitis, melena, dysphagia, hemorrhoids, gastritis. **CV:** Prolongation of the QT interval that might lead to ***torsades de pointes,***. Orthostatic hypotension, tachycardia, palpitation, hyper/hypotension, ***AV block, MI.*** **Respiratory:** Rhinitis, coughing, URI, sinusitis, pharyngitis, dyspnea. **Body as a whole:** Arthralgia, back/chest pain, fever, fatigue, rigors, malaise, edema, flu-like symptoms, ↑ or ↓ in weight. **Hematologic:** Purpura, anemia, hypochromic anemia. **GU:** Polyuria, polydipsia, urinary incontinence, hematuria, dysuria, menorrhagia, orgastic dysfunction, dry vagina, erectile dysfunction, nonpuerperal lactation, amenorrhea, female breast pain, leukorrhea, mastitis, dysmenorrhea, female perineal pain, intermenstrual bleeding, ***vaginal hemorrhage,*** failure to ejaculate. **Dermatologic:** Rash, dry skin, seborrhea, ↑ pigmentation, ↑ or ↓ sweating, acne, alopecia, hyperkeratosis, pruritus, skin exfoliation. **Ophthalmic:** Abnormal vision/accommodation, xerophthalmia. **Miscellaneous:** ↑ prolactin, photosensitivity, diabetes mellitus, thirst, myalgia, epistaxis.

LABORATORY TEST CONSIDERATIONS

↑ CPK, serum prolactin, AST, ALT. Hyponatremia.

OD OVERDOSE MANAGEMENT

Symptoms: Exaggeration of known effects, especially drowsiness, sedation, tachycardia, hypotension, and extrapyramidal symptoms. *Treatment:* Establish and secure airway, and ensure adequate oxygenation and ventilation. Follow gastric lavage with activated charcoal and a laxative. Monitor CV system, including continuous ECG readings. Provide general supportive measures. Treat hypotension and circulatory collapse with IV fluids or sympathomimetic drugs; however, do not use epinephrine and dopamine, as beta stimulation may worsen hypotension due to risperidone-induced alpha blockade. Anticholinergic drugs can be given for severe extrapyramidal symptoms.

DRUG INTERACTIONS

Carbamazepine / ↑ Risperidone clearance following chronic use of carbamazepine
Clozapine / ↓ Risperidone clearance following chronic use of clozapine
Levodopa / Risperidone antagonizes the effects of levodopa and dopamine agonists
Paroxetine / Significant ↑ in risperidone plasma levels R/T ↓ liver metabolism

HOW SUPPLIED

Oral Solution: 1 mg/mL; *Tablet:* 0.25 mg, 0.5 mg, 1 mg, 2 mg, 3 mg, 4 mg

DOSAGE

• ORAL SOLUTION, TABLETS

Antipsychotic.

Adults, initial: 1 mg b.i.d. Once daily dosing can also be used. Can be increased by 1 mg b.i.d. on the second and third days, as tolerated, to reach a dose of 3 mg b.i.d. by the third day. Further increases in dose should occur at intervals of about 1 week. **Maximal effect:** 4–8 mg/day. Doses greater than 6 mg/day were not shown to be more effective and were associated with greater incidence of side effects. Safety of doses greater than 16 mg/day have not been studied. **Maintenance:** Use lowest dose that will maintain remission. The initial dose is 0.5 mg b.i.d. for clients who are elderly or debilitated, those with severe renal or hepatic impairment, and those predisposed to hypotension or in whom hypotension would pose a risk. Dosage increases in these clients should be in increments of 0.5 mg b.i.d. Dosage increases above 1.5 mg b.i.d. should occur at intervals of about 1 week.

NURSING CONSIDERATIONS

SEE ALSO *NURSING CONSIDERATIONS* FOR *ANTIPSYCHOTIC DRUGS.*

ADMINISTRATION/STORAGE

1. Use a lower starting dose in geriatric clients and those with impaired renal or hepatic function. The PO solution may ease administration to geriatric clients and those in an acute-care setting.
2. When restarting clients who have had an interval of risperidone, follow the initial 3-day dose titration schedule.

3. If switching from other antipsychotic drugs to risperidone, immediate discontinuation of the previous antipsychotic drug is recommended when starting risperidone therapy. When switching from a depot antipsychotic injection, initiate risperidone in place of the next scheduled shot.

ASSESSMENT

1. Document indications for therapy; note onset and duration as well as presenting behavioral manifestations and mental status.
2. Perform appropriate baseline assessments. Electrolyte imbalance, bradycardia, and concomitant administration with drugs that prolong the QT interval may increase the risk of torsades de pointes.
3. Reduce dose with severe liver, cardiac, or renal dysfunction and monitor closely.
4. Note any history of drug dependency.
5. Observe for altered mental status, muscle rigidity, dyskinetic movements, or overt changes in VS.
6. The antiemetic effect of risperidone may mask the S&S of overdose with certain drugs or conditions such as intestinal obstruction, Reye's syndrome, and brain tumor.

CLIENT/FAMILY TEACHING

1. Take only as directed; do not share meds or stop abruptly.
2. Drug may impair judgment, motor skills, and thinking and cause blurred vision; determine drug effects before engaging in activities that require mental alertness.
3. Rise slowly from a lying to a sitting position, dangle legs before standing; may cause orthostatic hypotension.
4. May alter temperature regulation; avoid exposure to extreme heat.
5. Wear protective clothing, sunscreen, hat, and sunglasses when sun exposure is necessary; may cause a photosensitivity reaction.
6. Report abnormal bruising/bleeding, yellow skin discoloration, or adverse side effects.
7. Practice birth control. Report if pregnancy is suspected or desired.
8. Avoid alcohol and any other OTC agents or CNS depressants.
9. Risperidone elevates serum prolactin levels. Explore the potential relationship of prolactin and human breast cancer development; report evidence/history of breast cancer.
10. Any suicide ideations or bizarre behavior should be reported immediately. Due to the possibility of suicide attempts with schizophrenia, close supervision of high-risk clients is necessary and prescriptions will be written for the smallest quantity of tablets. Close F/U is required.

OUTCOMES/EVALUATE

Improved behavior patterns with ↓ agitation, ↓ hyperactivity, and reality orientation

Ritodrine hydrochloride

(**RYE**-toe-dreen)

PREGNANCY CATEGORY: B
CLASSIFICATION(S):
Uterine relaxant
Rx: Ritodrine HCl in 5% Dextrose, Yutopar

ACTION/KINETICS

Stimulates beta-2 receptors of smooth muscle of the uterus, which results in inhibition of uterine contractility. May also directly inhibit the actin-myosin interaction. Beta-adrenergic blocking agents inhibit the drug. Increased blood levels of insulin, glucose, and free fatty acids and decreased levels of potassium have been observed during IV infusion. **Onset, IV:** 5 min. **Peak plasma concentration, IV:** After a 9-mg infusion over 60 min, 32–50 ng/mL; **PO:** after a dose of 10 mg, 5–15 ng/mL. **Time to peak serum levels:** 20–60 min. **t½, after IV:** 15–17 hr. Ninety percent of drug excreted within 24 hr through the urine.

USES

Management of preterm labor in selected clients after week 20 of gestation. When indicated, initiate therapy as

R

early as possible after diagnosis. However, decision to use ritodrine should include determination of fetal maturity.

CONTRAINDICATIONS

Before week 20 of pregnancy and when continuation of pregnancy is hazardous to mother (e.g., eclampsia, severe preeclampsia, intrauterine fetal death, antepartum hemorrhage, pulmonary hypertension, chorioamnionitis, and maternal hyperthyroidism, cardiac disease or uncontrolled diabetes mellitus). Also, medical conditions (e.g., uncontrolled hypertension, pheochromocytoma, bronchial asthma, hypovolemia, cardiac arrhythmias due to tachycardia or digitalis toxicity) that would be aggravated by beta-adrenergic agonists. Use in diabetics.

SPECIAL CONCERNS

Maternal pulmonary edema has been noted in women treated with ritodrine. The use in advanced labor (i.e., greater than 4 cm cervical dilation or effacement greater than 80%) has not been established.

SIDE EFFECTS

All effects are related to the stimulation of beta receptors by the drug. **CV:** Increase in maternal and fetal HR, increase in maternal systolic and marked decrease in diastolic BP (widening of pulse pressure), persistent tachycardia (may indicate pulmonary edema), palpitations, ***arrhythmias including VT,*** chest pain or tightness, angina, heart murmur, ***myocardial ischemia.*** Sinus bradycardia following drug withdrawal. **GI:** N&V, bloating, ileus, epigastric distress, diarrhea or constipation. **CNS:** Headache, migraine headache, tremors, malaise, nervousness, jitteriness, restlessness, anxiety, emotional changes, drowsiness, weakness. **Metabolic:** Transient increases in insulin and blood glucose, increases in cyclic AMP and free fatty acids, decrease in potassium, glycosuria, lactic acidosis. **Respiratory:** Dyspnea, ***maternal pulmonary edema,*** hyperventilation. **Hematologic:** Leukopenia or agranulocytosis after 2–3 weeks of IV therapy (leukocyte count returned to normal after cessation of drug). **Other:** Erythema, ***anaphylactic shock,*** rash, intrauterine growth retardation, hemolytic icterus, sweating, chills, impaired liver function. *NOTE:* Neonatal effects are infrequent but may include hypoglycemia and ileus; also, hypocalcemia and hypotension in neonates whose mothers were treated with other betamimetic drugs.

LABORATORY TEST CONSIDERATIONS

↑ Plasma glucose and insulin; ↓ plasma potassium.

OD OVERDOSE MANAGEMENT

Symptoms: Excessive beta-adrenergic stimulation, including tachycardia (in both the mother and fetus), palpitations, ***cardiac arrhythmias,*** hypotension, dyspnea, tremor, dyspnea, nervousness, N&V. *Treatment:* Supportive measures. A beta-adrenergic blocking agent can be used as an antidote. The drug is dialyzable.

DRUG INTERACTIONS

Anesthetics, general / Additive hypotension or cardiac arrhythmias
Atropine / ↑ Systemic hypertension
Beta-adrenergic blocking agents / Inhibition of the effect of ritodrine
Corticosteroids / ↑ Risk of pulmonary edema
Diazoxide / Additive hypotension or cardiac arrhythmias
Magnesium sulfate / Additive hypotension or cardiac arrhythmias
Meperidine / Additive hypotension or cardiac arrhythmias
Sympathomimetics / Additive or potentiated effects of sympathomimetics

HOW SUPPLIED

Injection: 0.3 mg/mL, 10 mg/mL, 15 mg/mL

DOSAGE

- **IV**

Preterm labor.

Initial: 0.05 mg/min (10 gtt/min using microdrip chamber); **then,** depending on response, increase by 0.05 mg/min (10 microdrops/min) q 10 min until desired response occurs. **Effective dose range:** 0.15–0.35 mg/min (30–70 gtt/min). Continue infusion antepartum for a minimum of 12 hr after contractions cease.

NURSING CONSIDERATIONS

ADMINISTRATION/STORAGE

IV 1. Reconstitute with dextrose solution (150 mg in 500 mL). Final dilution will contain 0.3 mg/mL ritodrine. Avoid solutions containing NaCl; increases risk of pulmonary edema.
2. To minimize hypotension, administer while in the left lateral position.
3. Use a Y set-up, infusion pump, and microdrip tubing (60 microdrops/mL) for drug administration.
4. Do not use discolored solutions or those containing precipitate. Use diluted solution within 48 hr.
5. If other drugs must be given by the IV route, the use of piggyback or another IV site allows continued independent control of the infusion rate of ritodrine.

ASSESSMENT

1. Note characteristics, onset, and duration of contractions.
2. Assess for preeclampsia, hypertension, or diabetes.
3. Ensure that ultrasound and amniocentesis have been performed to establish fetal maturity. Determine gestational age prior to initiating drug therapy; should not be used before week 20.

INTERVENTIONS

1. Avoid concomitant administration of beta-adrenergic blocking drugs; these inhibit action of ritodrine.
2. Place in left lateral recumbent position to increase renal blood flow and to decrease hypotension. Assess response to IV therapy by evaluating strength and frequency of uterine contractions and by monitoring fetal HR; report fetal HR changes.
3. Monitor and record VS.
• Maintain BP by positioning in a left lateral position and evaluating level of hydration.
• Report any increase in SBP, decrease in DBP, and tachycardia.
4. Monitor I&O; auscultate lung sounds to assess fluid status.
5. Prevent circulatory overload. Closely monitor IV flow rate and infused volume.
6. Assess for any respiratory dysfunction (i.e., rales, dyspnea, frothy sputum) that may precede pulmonary edema, especially when also receiving corticosteroids.
7. Assess for S&S of electrolyte imbalance (hypokalemia), hyperglycemia, and acidosis with diabetes and monitor.
8. Assess postpartum client who has received both ritodrine and general anesthetic for potentiation of hypotensive effects.
9. Neonates of mothers who have received ritodrine should be assessed for hyper- or hypoglycemia, hypocalcemia, hypotension, and ileus. Have emergency medication and equipment to support neonate.

CLIENT/FAMILY TEACHING

1. Medication is administered to stop labor and requires close medical supervision for appropriate dosage.
2. Report any chest pain/tightness, palpitations, dizziness, weakness, tremors, or difficulty breathing.
3. Once infusion has been completed, ambulation may be resumed in 3–4 days if symptoms do not recur.
4. If contractions resume, membranes rupture, or spotting and/or bleeding occur, lie down immediately and notify provider.

OUTCOMES/EVALUATE

Inhibition of uterine contractions; suppression of labor

Ritonavir

(rih-**TOH**-nah-veer)

PREGNANCY CATEGORY: B
CLASSIFICATION(S):
Antiviral, protease inhibitor
Rx: Norvir
✱**Rx:** Norvir Sec.

SEE ALSO *ANITIVIRAL DRUGS.*

ACTION/KINETICS

A peptidomimetic inhibitor of both the HIV-1 and HIV-2 proteases. Inhibition of HIV protease results in the enzyme incapable of processing the "gag-pool" polyprotein precursor that leads to production of noninfectious immature HIV particles. **Peak concentrations after 600 mg of the solu-**

tion: 2 hr after fasting and 4 hr after nonfasting. **t½:** 3–5 hr. Metabolized by the cytochrome P450 system. Metabolites and unchanged drug are excreted through both the feces and urine.

USES

Alone or in combination with nucleoside analogues (ddC or AZT) for the treatment of HIV infection. Use of ritonavir may result in a reduction in both mortality and AIDS-defining clinical events. Clinical benefit has not been determined for periods longer than 6 months.

SPECIAL CONCERNS

Not considered a cure for HIV infection; clients may continue to manifest illnesses associated with advanced HIV infection, including opportunistic infections. Also, therapy with ritonavir has not been shown to decrease the risk of transmitting HIV to others through sexual contact or blood contamination. Use with caution in those with impaired hepatic function and during lactation. Hemophiliacs treated with protease inhibitors may manifest spontaneous bleeding episodes. Safety and efficacy have not been determined in children less than 12 years of age.

SIDE EFFECTS

Side effects listed are those with a frequency of 2% or greater.

GI: N&V, diarrhea, taste perversion, anorexia, flatulence, constipation, abdominal pain, dyspepsia, local throat irritation. *Neurologic:* Circumoral/peripheral paresthesia, dizziness, insomnia, paresthesia, somnolence, abnormal thinking. **Body as a whole:** Asthenia, headache, malaise, fever. **Dermatologic:** Sweating, rash. **Miscellaneous:** Vasodilation, hyperlipidemia, myalgia, pharyngitis.

LABORATORY TEST CONSIDERATIONS

↑ Triglycerides, AST, ALT, GGT, CPK, uric acid.

OD OVERDOSE MANAGEMENT

Symptoms: Extension of side effects. *Treatment:* General supportive measures, including monitoring of VS and observing the clinical status. Elimination of unabsorbed drug may be assisted by emesis or gastric lavage, with attention given to maintaining a patent airway. Activated charcoal may also help in removing any unabsorbed drug. Dialysis is not likely to be of benefit in removing the drug from the body.

DRUG INTERACTIONS

(1) Ritonavir is expected to produce large increases in the plasma levels of a number of drugs, including amiodarone, bepridil, bupropion, cisapride, clozapine, encainide, flecainide, meperidine, piroxicam, propafenone, propoxyphene, quinidine, rifabutin, tefenadine, and warfarin. This may lead to an increased risk of arrhythmias, hematologic complications, seizures, or other serious adverse effects.

(2) Ritonavir may produce a decrease in the plasma levels of the following drugs: atovaquone, clofibrate, daunorubicin, diphenoxylate, metoclopramide, and sedative/hypnotics.

(3) Coadministration of ritonavir with the following drugs may cause extreme sedation and respiratory depression and thus should not be combined: alprazolam, clorazepate, diazepam, estazolam, flurazepam, midazolam, triazolam, and zolpidem. *Clarithromycin* / ↑ Clarithromycin levels; reduce dose*Desipramine* / Significant ↑ despiramine levels; reduce dose*Ethinyl estradiol* / ↓ Ethyinyl estradiol levels; use alternative contraceptive*Fentanyl* / ↑ Risk of fentanyl-induced respiratory depression due to ↓ liver metabolism*Propulsid* / ↑ Risk of serious cardiac arrhythmias*Saquinavir* / Significant ↑ in saquinavir blood levels*Theophylline* / ↓ Theophylline levels*Warfarin* / ↓ Warfarin anticoagulant effect

HOW SUPPLIED

Capsules: 100 mg; *Oral Solution:* 80 mg/mL.

DOSAGE

• **CAPSULES, ORAL SOLUTION**

Treatment of HIV infection.

600 mg b.i.d. If nausea is experienced upon initiation of therapy, dose escalation may be tried as follows: 300 mg b.i.d. for 1 day, 400 mg b.i.d. for 2 days, 500 mg b.i.d. for 1 day, and then 600 mg b.i.d. thereafter.

NURSING CONSIDERATIONS

SEE ALSO *NURSING CONSIDERATIONS* FOR *ANTIVIRAL DRUGS.*

ADMINISTRATION/STORAGE

1. Clients prescribed combination regimens with nucleoside analogues may improve GI tolerance by starting therapy with ritonavir alone and then adding the nucleoside before completing 2 weeks of ritonavir monotherapy.
2. Until dispensed, store capsules and solution in refrigerator at 2–8°C (36–46°F) and protect from light. Capsule and solution refrigeration is recommended after dispensing; however, this is not necessary if solution is stored in the original container, used within 30 days, and kept below 25°C (77°F).

ASSESSMENT

1. Document symptom onset, serum confirmation of diagnosis, and other agents trialed with the outcome.
2. Monitor CBC, T-lymphocytes (CD_4), viral load, and LFTs. Document impaired liver function; drug hepatically metabolized via P450 system.
3. List other agents prescribed to ensure none interact unfavorably.

CLIENT/FAMILY TEACHING

1. Take with food, if possible. Taste may be improved by mixing with chocolate milk, Ensure, or Advera within 1 hr of dosing.
2. Take each day as prescribed. Do not alter dosage or discontinue without approval. If a dose is missed, the next dose should be taken as soon as possible; if a dose is skipped, do not double the next dose.
3. Use reliable birth control and barrier protection; drug does not reduce the risk of transmitting disease through sexual contact or blood contamination.
4. Drug is not a cure for HIV; illnesses associated with advanced HIV infection may still occur, including opportunistic infections.

OUTCOMES/EVALUATE

Inhibition of disease progression and death with HIV infection

Rituximab

(rih-**TUK**-sih-mab)

PREGNANCY CATEGORY: C
CLASSIFICATION(S):
Antineoplastic, monoclonal antibody
Rx: Rituxan

SEE ALSO ANTINEOPLASTIC AGENTS.

ACTION/KINETICS

Genetically engineered chimeric murine/human monoclonal antibody which binds specifically to CD20 antigen found on surface of normal and malignant B lymphocytes causing cell lysis. Cell lysis may result due to complement-dependent cytotoxicity and antibody-dependent cellular cytotoxicity. CD20 regulates early steps in activation process for cell cycle initiation and differentiation and possibly functions as calcium ion channel. Causes significant decreases in both IgM and IgG serum levels from months 5 to 11. **Mean serum t½:** 59.8 hr after first infusion and 174 hr after 4th infusion.

USES

Treat relapsed or refractory low-grade or follicular, CD20 positive, B-cell non-Hodgkin's lymphoma.

CONTRAINDICATIONS

Use in known Type I hypersensitivity or anaphylactic reactions to murine proteins or any component of product. Lactation.

SPECIAL CONCERNS

Use with caution in preexisting cardiac conditions, including arrhythmias and angina. Infusion-related symptoms may occur from 30 to 120 min at beginning of first infusion and with less frequency with subsequent infusions. Use is associated with severe infusion and hypersensitivity reactions. Safety of immunization with any vaccine, especially live viral vaccines, has not been studied. Safety and efficacy have not been determined in children.

SIDE EFFECTS

Infusion-related events: Fever, chills, and rigors are most common. Also,

R

nausea, urticaria, fatigue, headache, pruritus, bronchospasm, hypotension, angioedema, dyspnea, rhinitis, vomiting, flushing, pain at disease sites, hypoxia, pulmonary infiltrates, ***acute respiratory distress syndrome, MI, ventricular fibrillation, cardiogenic shock***. ***Retreatment events:*** Asthenia, throat irritation, flushing, tachycardia, anorexia, leukopenia, thrombocytopenia, anemia, peripheral edema, dizziness, depression, respiratory symptoms, night sweats, pruritus.

General side effects. **CV:** Arrhythmias, including VT and SVTs; trigeminy, angina, hypo/hypertension, tachycardia, postural hypotension, bradycardia. **Hematologic:** Thrombocytopenia (up to 30 days following last dose), severe anemia, neutropenia, leukopenia, lymphopenia, coagulation disorder. **Body as a whole:** Asthenia, pain, fever, infection, chills, malaise. **GI:** Abdominal pain, N&V, diarrhea, dyspepsia, taste perversion. **CNS:** Headache, paresthesia, anxiety, agitation, insomnia, hypesthesia, nervousness. **Respiratory:** ***Bronchospasm,*** increased cough, rhinitis, dyspnea, bronchiolitis obliterans, hypoxia, asthma, sinusitis, respiratory disorder, bronchitis. **Musculoskeletal:** Myalgia, arthralgia. **Dermatologic:** Pruritus, rash, urticaria, flushing, night sweats, ***mucocutaneous skin reactions (rare)***. **Miscellaneous:** Angioedema, lacrimation disorder, chest/back/tumor pain, peripheral edema, throat irritation, anorexia, abdominal enlargement, conjunctivitis, pain at injection site, hypertonia, ***tumor lysis syndrome with acute renal failure requiring dialysis***.

LABORATORY TEST CONSIDERATIONS

↑ LDH. Hyperglycemia, hypocalcemia.

HOW SUPPLIED

Injection: 10 mg/mL

DOSAGE

• **IV INFUSION**

Non-Hodgkin's lymphoma.

375 mg/m^2 as IV infusion once a week for 4 or 8 doses. Progressive disease may be retreated at the same dose, once weekly for 4 doses. *Do not administer as IV push or bolus.*

R

NURSING CONSIDERATIONS

SEE ALSO *NURSING CONSIDERATIONS FOR ANTINEOPLASTIC AGENTS.*

ADMINISTRATION/STORAGE

IV 1. To prepare for administration, withdraw necessary amount of rituximab and dilute to final concentration of 1 to 4 mg/mL into infusion bag containing either 0.9% NaCl or D5/W. Discard any unused portion left in vial.

2. Solutions for infusion are stable at 2–8°C (36–46°F) for 24 hr and at room temperature for additional 12 hr.

3. Due to the potential of hypersensitivity reactions, consider premedication with acetaminophen and diphenhydramine. Hypersensitivity reactions may respond to changes in the infusion rate. Also, institute supportive care (IV fluids, vasopressors, oxygen, bronchodilators, diphenhydramine, acetaminophen).

4. Due to the possibility of transient hypotension during infusion, consider withholding antihypertensive medication 12 hr prior to rituximab.

5. For first infusion, give at initial rate of 50 mg/hr. If hypersensitivity or infusion-related events do not occur, escalate infusion rate in 50 mg/hr increments every 30 min to maximum of 400 mg/hr. If hypersensitivity or infusion-related events occur, temporarily slow or interrupt infusion; infusion can continue at one-half previous rate until symptoms improve. Subsequent infusions can be given at initial rate of 100 mg/hr, and increased by 100 mg/hr increments at 30 min intervals to maximum of 400 mg/hr (as long as tolerated).

6. Do not mix or dilute with other drugs.

7. Protect vials from direct sunlight.

ASSESSMENT

1. Note any cardiac disease and assess for arrhythmias.

2. Therapy usually consists of once weekly infusions for four doses.

3. Infusion related reaction consisting of fever and chills/rigors may occur with first infusion.

4. Interrupt infusion if severe reaction occurs; may resume infusion at 50% initial rate once symptoms resolved.

CLIENT/FAMILY TEACHING
Practice reliable contacteption during and for up to 12 mo following therapy. Report any adverse reactions.
OUTCOMES/EVALUATE
Control of malignant cell proliferation

Rivastigmine tartrate

(rih-vah-**STIG**-meen)

PREGNANCY CATEGORY: B
CLASSIFICATION(S):
Treatment of Alzheimer's disease
Rx: Exelon

ACTION/KINETICS
Probably acts by enhancing cholinergic function by increasing levels of acetylcholine through reversible inhibition of acetylcholinesterase. There is no evidence that the drug alters the course of the underlying disease. Is rapidly and completely absorbed. Is 40% bound to plasma proteins. Is rapidly and extensively metabolized by cholinesterase-mediated hydrolysis. **t½, elimination:** About 1.5 hr. Excreted mainly in the urine.
USES
Treat mild to moderate dementia of the Alzheimer's type. *Investigational:* Treat behavioral effects in Lewy-body dementia.
CONTRAINDICATIONS
Hypersensitivity to rivastigmine or other carbamate derivatives.
SPECIAL CONCERNS
Use with caution during lactation; it is not known if rivastigmine is excreted in breast milk. Use with caution in clients with a history of asthma or obstructive pulmonary disease. Drugs that increase cholinergic activity may have vagotonic effects on the heart, cause urinary obstruction, and may cause seizures.
SIDE EFFECTS
Side effects listed are those with a frequency of 1% or greater. Significant GI side effects may occur.
GI: N&V, diarrhea, anorexia, weight loss, abdominal pain, peptic ulcers, GI bleeding, dyspepsia, constipation, flatulence, eructation, fecal incontinence, gastritis. **CNS:** Dizziness, headache, insomnia, confusion, depression, anxiety, somnolence, hallucination, tremor, aggressive reaction, abnormal gait, ataxia, paresthesia, agitation, nervousness, delusion, ***convulsions,*** paranoid reaction, confusion. **CV:** Hypotension, postural hypotension, hypertension, ***cardiac failure, MI,*** atrial fibrillation, bradycardia, palpitation, angina pectoris. **Body as a whole:** Accidental trauma, fatigue, asthenia, malaise, increased sweating, flu-like symptoms, syncope, dehydration, fever, edema, allergy, hot flushes, general infection. **Dermatologic:** Rashes, including maculopapular, eczema, bullous, exfoliative, psoriaform, erythematous. **GU:** UTI, urinary obstruction, hematuria, urinary incontinence. **Musculoskeletal:** Arthritis, leg cramps, myalgia, back pain, arthralgia, bone fracture. **Respiratory:** Rhinitis, epistaxis, upper respiratory tract infections, coughing, pharyngitis, bronchitis. **Miscellaneous:** Anemia, hypokalemia, tinnitus, cataract, rigors, chest pain, peripheral edema.
OD OVERDOSE MANAGEMENT
Symptoms: Cholinergic crisis, including symptoms of severe nausea, vomiting, salivation, sweating, bradycardia, hypotension, respiratory depression, collapse, seizures. Increasing muscle weakness with possible death if respiratory muscles are involved. *Treatment:* General supportive measures. Treat severe nausea and vomiting with antiemetics.
DRUG INTERACTIONS
Anticholinergics / Rivastigmine interferes with anticholinergic activitiy
Bethanechol / Synergistic effect
Nicotine / ↑ PO clearance of rivastigmine by 23%
Succinylcholine / Exaggeration of succinylcholine-induced muscle relaxation during anesthesia
HOW SUPPLIED
Capsule: 1.5 mg, 3 mg, 4.5 mg, 6 mg; *Solution, oral:* 2 mg/mL (all concentrations as the base)

R

DOSAGE

- **CAPSULES, ORAL SOLUTION**

Dementia due to Alzheimer's disease. **Initial:** 1.5 mg b.i.d. If the dose is well tolerated after a minimum of 2 weeks, may increase dose to 3 mg b.i.d. Attempt subsequent increases to 4.5 mg and 6 mg b.i.d. only after a minimum of 2 weeks at the previous dose.

NURSING CONSIDERATIONS

ADMINISTRATION/STORAGE

1. If side effects develop during treatment, discontinue treatment for several doses; restart at the lowest daily dose (to prevent severe vomiting) and titrate back to the maintenance dose.
2. The capsules and oral solution may be interchanged at equal doses.
3. Store the oral solution below 25°C (77°F) in an upright position. Protect from freezing.

ASSESSMENT

1. Document onset/duration of symptoms, other agents trialed, and the outcome.
2. Describe clinical presentation and functioning level.
3. Note any history of asthma, seizures, BPH, or COPD.
4. Obtain ECG, serum electrolytes, CBC, and u/a and bs.

CLIENT/FAMILY TEACHING

1. Take with food in divided doses in the morning and evening.
2. If using the oral solution, remove the oral dosing syringe provided and withdraw the correct amount of drug from the container. Each dose of rivastigmine may be swallowed directly from the syringe or first mixed with a small glass of water, cold fruit juice, or soda. When mixed with fruit juice or soda, the mixture is stable for 4 hr or less.
3. Drug may cause a high incidence of N&V; monitor weight and report if loss evident so therapy can be reassessed.
4. Stop drug and report any evidence of seizures, urinary obstruction, dizziness, and low heart rate.
5. Drug dosage may be gradually increased by provider if drug is tolerated and desired effects not evident. Report lack of response or intolerance.

OUTCOMES/EVALUATE

Improved cognitive functioning with Alzheimer's

Rizatriptan benzoate

(rise-ah-**TRIP**-tan)

PREGNANCY CATEGORY: C
CLASSIFICATION(S):
Antimigraine drug
Rx: Maxalt, Maxalt-MLT
✱Rx: Maxalt RPD

ACTION/KINETICS

Binds to 5-$HT_{IB/ID}$ receptors, resulting in cranial vessel vasocontriction, inhibition of neuropeptide release, and reduced transmission in trigeminal pain pathways. Completely absorbed after PO use; rate of absorption of Maxalt-MLT is somewhat slower. **Peak plasma levels, Maxalt:** 1–1.5 hr; **Maxalt-MLT:** 1.6–2.5 hr. Food has no effect on bioavailability, but will delay time to reach peak levels by an hr. **t½:** 2–3 hr. Metabolized by MAO-A; most is excreted through the urine. Is a significant first-pass effect.

USES

Acute treatment of migraine attacks in adults with or without aura.

CONTRAINDICATIONS

Use in children less than 18 years of age, as prophylactic therapy of migraine, or use in the management of hemiplegic or basilar migraine. Use in those with ischemic heart disease or vasospastic coronary artery disease, uncontrolled hypertension, within 24 hr of treatment with another 5-HT_1 agonist or an ergotamine-containing or ergot-type medication (e.g., dihydroergotamine, methysergide). Use concurrently with MAO inhibitors or use of rizatriptan within 2 weeks of discontinuing a MAO inhibitor. Strongly recommended the drug not be given in unrecognized coronary artery disease (CAD) predicted by the presence of risk factors, including hypertension, hypercholesterolemia, smoking, obesity, diabetes, strong family history of CAD, female with surgical or physiological menopause, or males over 40, unless a CV evaluation reveals the client is free from CAD or ischemic myocardial disease.

SPECIAL CONCERNS

Safety and efficacy have not been determined for use in cluster headache or in children. Use with caution during lactation, with diseases that may alter the absorption, metabolism, or excretion of drugs; in dialysis clients, and in moderate hepatic insufficiency. Maxalt-MLT tablets contain phenylalanine; may be of concern to phenylketonurics. Serious cardiac events may occur within a few hours after giving Maxalt.

SIDE EFFECTS

CV: ***Acute MI, coronary artery vasospasm, life-threatening disturbances in cardiac rhythm (VT, ventricular fibrillation), death, cerebral hemorrhage, subarachnoid hemorrhage, stroke, hypertensive crisis.*** Also, transient myocardial ischemia, peripheral vascular ischemia, colonic ischemia with abdominal pain and bloody diarrhea, palpitation, tachycardia, cold extremities, hypertension, arrhythmia, bradycardia. **GI:** Nausea, dry mouth, abdominal distention, vomiting, dyspepsia, thirst, acid regurgitation, dysphagia, constipation, flatulence, tongue edema. **CNS:** Somnolence, headache, dizziness, paresthesias, hypesthesia, decreased mental acuity, euphoria, tremor, nervousness, vertigo, insomnia, anxiety, depression, disorientation, ataxia, dysarthria, confusion, dream abnormality, abnormal gait, irritability, impaired memory, agitation, hyperesthesia. **Pain and pressure sensations:** Chest tightness/pressure and/or heaviness; pain/tightness/pressure in the precordium, neck, throat, jaw; regional pain, tightness, pressure, or heaviness; or unspecified pain. **Musculoskeletal:** Muscle weakness, stiffness, myalgia, muscle cramps, musculoskeletal pain, arthralgia, muscle spasm. **Respiratory:** Dyspnea, pharyngitis, nasal irritation, nasal congestion, dry throat, URI, yawning, dry nose, epistaxis, sinus disorder. **GU:** Urinary frequency, polyuria, menstrual disorder. **Dermatologic:** Flushing, sweating, pruritus, rash, urticaria. **Body as a whole:** Asthenia, fatigue, chills, heat sensitivity, hangover effect, warm/cold sensations, dehydration, hot flashes. **Ophthalmic:** Blurred vision, dry eyes, burning eye, eye pain, eye irritation, tearing. **Miscellaneous:** Facial edema, tinnitus, ear pain.

DRUG INTERACTIONS

Dihydroergotamine / Additive vasospastic reactions; do not use within 24 hr of each other

MAO Inhibitors / ↑ Rizatriptan plasma levels; do not use together

Methysergide / Additive vasospastic reactions; do not use within 24 hr of each other

Propranolol / ↑ Rizatriptan plasma levels

HOW SUPPLIED

Orally Disintegrating Tablets: 5 mg, 10 mg; *Tablets:* 5 mg, 10 mg.

DOSAGE

• ORAL DISINTEGRATING TABLETS, TABLETS

Acute treatment of migraine.

Adults: Single dose of 5 mg or 10 mg of Maxalt or Maxalt-MLT. Doses should be separated by at least 2 hr, with no more than 30 mg taken in any 24-hr period.

NURSING CONSIDERATIONS

ADMINISTRATION/STORAGE

1. In clients receiving propranolol, use the 5-mg dose of Maxalt, up to a maximum of 3 doses in any 24-hr period.
2. Store Maxalt and Maxalt-MLT tablets at room temperature.

ASSESSMENT

1. Note characteristics of migraines, when diagnosed, other agents trialed and the outcome.
2. Determine any evidence of heart disease, uncontrolled HTN, DM, or allergies. Assess risk factors for CAD. Clients over age 40 should be carefully screened for CAD.
3. List all meds consumed to ensure none interact. Reduce dose if prescribed propranolol.

R

CLIENT/FAMILY TEACHING

1. For Maxalt-MLT, do not remove the blister from the outer pouch until just before dosing. Peel open the blister (do not push through the blister) with dry hands and place the orally-disintegrating tablet on the tongue. It will dissolve and be swallowed in the saliva; fluids are not needed which eases administration.
2. May cause dizziness, drowsiness, or pressure sensation in the upper chest; do not operate equipment or drive until effects realized.
3. Do not take within 24 hr of any other prescription drug used to treat headaches or depression.
4. Review patient information sheet provided for side effects; report if persistent or intolerable.
5. If headache returns or only a partial response is attained, may repeat dose after waiting at least 2 hr. Do not exceed 30 mg in a 24-hr period.
6. Use alternative birth control and measures to prevent photosensitivity, use sun screen and protective clothing as well as sun screen.
7. Inform phenylketonuric clilents that each 5 mg of the oral disintegrating tablets contain 1.05 mg phenylalanine.

OUTCOMES/EVALUATE

Relief of migraine headache

R

Rocuronium bromide

(**roh**-kyou-**ROH**-nee-um)

PREGNANCY CATEGORY: B
CLASSIFICATION(S):
Neuromuscular blocking drug
Rx: Zemuron

SEE ALSO *NEUROMUSCULAR BLOCKING AGENTS.*

ACTION/KINETICS

A nondepolarizing neuromuscular blocking agent that acts by competing with acetylcholine for receptors at the motor end-plate. Causes histamine release in a small number of clients. Use must be accompanied by adequate anesthesia or sedation, as the drug has no effect on consciousness, pain threshold, or cerebration. Depending on the dose, it has a rapid to intermediate onset and an intermediate duration of action. **t½, rapid distribution phase:** 1–2 min; **t½, slower distribution phase:** 14–18 min. Metabolized by the liver.

USES

(1) As an adjunct to general anesthesia to facilitate rapid sequence and routine tracheal intubation. (2) To cause relaxation of skeletal muscle during surgery or mechanical ventilation.

SPECIAL CONCERNS

Use with caution in clients with pulmonary hypertension, valvular heart disease, or significant hepatic disease. Burn clients may develop resistance to nondepolarizing neuromuscular blocking agents. Elderly clients may exhibit a slightly prolonged medical clinical duration of action. Use in children less than 3 months of age has not been studied.

SIDE EFFECTS

CV: Arrhythmias, abnormal ECG, transient hypotension and hypertension, tachycardia. **GI:** N&V. **Respiratory:** Symptoms of asthma, including ***bronchospasm,*** wheezing, rhonchi; hiccup. **Dermatologic:** Rash, edema at injection site, pruritus.

OD OVERDOSE MANAGEMENT

Symptoms: Neuromuscular blockade longer than needed for anesthesia and surgery. *Treatment:* Careful monitoring of client. Artificial respiration may be required.

HOW SUPPLIED

Injection: 10 mg/ml

DOSAGE

- **IV ONLY**

Rapid sequence intubation.

0.6–1.2 mg/kg in appropriately premedicated and adequately anesthetized clients will result in good intubating conditions in less than 2 min.

Tracheal intubation.

Initial, regardless of anesthetic technique: 0.6 mg/kg. Maximum blockade is noted in less than 3 min with a mean duration of 31 min. However, a dose of 0.45 mg/kg may also be used with maximum blockade in less than 4 min with a mean duration of 22 min. Initial doses of 0.6 mg/kg in children under halothane anesthesia produce good intubating conditions within 1 min with a mean duration of 41 min in children 3 months to 1 year and 27 min in children 1–2 years of age. Maintenance doses in children of 0.075–0.125 mg/kg, given upon return of T_1 of 25% of control provide muscle relaxation for 7–10 min.

Maintenance doses.

0.1, 0.15, and 0.2 mg/kg, given at 25% recovery of control T_1 (defined as three twitches of train-of-four), provide a median of 12, 17, and 24 min of duration under opioid/nitrous oxide/oxygen anesthesia. Do not administer the dose until recovery of neuromuscular function is evident.

Continuous infusion.

Initial: 0.01–0.02 mg/kg/min only after early evidence of spontaneous recovery from an intubating dose. Upon reaching the desired level of neuromuscular blockade, the infusion must be individualized for each client; adjust the rate based on the twitch response (monitored with the use of a peripheral nerve stimulator) of the client. **Maintenance, usual:** 0.004–0.016 mg/kg/min.

NURSING CONSIDERATIONS

SEE ALSO *NURSING CONSIDERATIONS* FOR *NEUROMUSCULAR BLOCKING AGENTS.*

ADMINISTRATION/STORAGE

IV 1. Inhalation anesthetics (especially enflurane or isoflurane) may enhance the effects of rocuronium. When inhalation anesthetics are used, it may be necessary to reduce the rate of infusion by 30%–50% 45–60 min after the intubating dose.

2. Prepare solutions for infusion by mixing with D5W or RL solution. Drug is also compatible with 0.9% NaCl solution, sterile water for injection, and D5/NSS. Use solution within 24 hr after mixing; discard any unused solutions.

3. Spontaneous recovery occurs at about the same rate in children 3 mo–12 mo as in adults, but is more rapid in children 1–12 years old.

4. Do not mix rocuronium, which has an acid pH, with alkaline solutions (e.g., barbiturates) in the same syringe or give at the same time during infusion through the same needle.

5. Store at 2–8°C (36–46°F); do not freeze.

ASSESSMENT

1. Obtain ECG, liver and renal function studies.

2. In the critically ill, intubate prior to rocuronium administration.

3. Use a peripheral nerve stimulator to assess neuromuscular function and to confirm recovery from neuromuscular blockade.

4. Medicate for pain and anxiety as drug does not affect and client unable to convey.

INTERVENTIONS

1. Provide ventilatory support.

2. Monitor and record VS, ECG, and I&O. Drug can cause vagal stimulation resulting in bradycardia, hypotension, and cardiac arrhythmias.

3. A peripheral nerve stimulator may be used to evaluate neuromuscular response and recovery.

4. Consciousness is not affected by drug. Explain all procedures and provide emotional support. Do not conduct any discussions that should not be overheard.

5. With short-term therapy, reassure will be able to talk and move once the drug effects are reversed.

6. Muscle fasciculations may cause soreness or injury after recovery. Administer prescribed nondepolarizing agent and reassure that soreness likely caused by the unsynchronized contractions of adjacent muscle fibers just before the onset of paralysis.

7. Position for comfort and so that the body is in proper alignment. Turn and perform mouth care and eye care frequently (protect eyes and instill liquid tears q 2 h as blink reflex is suppressed).

8. Assess airway at frequent intervals. Have a suction machine at the bedside.

R

9. Check to be certain that the ventilator alarms are set and on at all times. *Never* leave client unmonitored.
10. Determine client need and administer medications for anxiety, pain, and/or sedation regularly (valium, morphine).

OUTCOMES/EVALUATE

• Desired level of skeletal muscle relaxation/paralysis
• Control of breathing during mechanical ventilation

Rofecoxib

(**roh**-feh-**KOX**-ib)

PREGNANCY CATEGORY: C
CLASSIFICATION(S):
Nonsteroidal anti-inflammatory drug, COX-2 inhibitor
Rx: Vioxx

SEE ALSO *NONSTEROIDAL ANTI-INFLAMMATORY DRUGS.*

ACTION/KINETICS
NSAID that acts by inhibiting prostaglandin synthesis via inhibition of cyclooxygenase-2 (COX-2). **Peak levels:** 2–3 hr. The tablets and oral suspension are bioequivalent. Bound to plasma protein (87%). Metabolized in the liver and excreted in the urine (72%) and feces (14%, including unchanged drug). **t½:** 17 hr.

USES
Relieve signs and symptoms of osteoarthritis, acute pain in adults, and treatment of dysmenorrhea.

CONTRAINDICATIONS
Advanced renal disease. Use in clients who manifested asthma, urticaria, or allergic-type reactions after taking aspirin or other NSAIDs. Use in late pregnancy due to premature closure of the ductus arteriosus. Lactation.

SPECIAL CONCERNS
Use with extreme caution in those with a prior history of ulcer disease or GI bleeding. Use with caution in fluid retention, hypertension, or heart failure. Most fatal GI events are in elderly or debilitated clients. Users may be at risk for CV side effects. Safety and efficacy have not been determined in children less than 18 years of age. Use caution not to confuse Vioxx (rofecoxib) with Zyvox (linezolid).

SIDE EFFECTS
Side effects listed occurred in at least 2% of clients.
GI: Diarrhea, nausea, constipation, heartburn, epigastric discomfort, dyspepsia, abdominal pain. **CNS:** Headache. **Respiratory:** Bronchitis, URTI. **CV:** Hypertension. **GU:** UTI. **Body as a whole:** Lower extremity edema, asthenia, fatigue, dizziness, flu-like disease, fever. **Miscellaneous:** Back pain, sinusitis, post-dental extraction alveolitis.

LABORATORY TEST CONSIDERATIONS
↑ ALT, AST.

DRUG INTERACTIONS
ACE inhibitors / ↓ ACE inhibitor effect
Antacids (Mg-Al containing, Calcium carbonate) / ↓ Absorption of rofecoxib
Aspirin / ↑ Risk of GI ulceration and other complications
Furosemide / ↓ Natriuertic effect of furosemide
Lithium / ↑ Risk of lithium toxicity
Methotrexate / ↑ Risk of methotrexate toxicity
Rifampin / ↓ Plasma levels of rifampin R/T ↑ liver metabolism
Thiazide diurtetics / ↓ Natriuretic effect of thiazides
Warfarin / ↑ PT with possible bleeding

HOW SUPPLIED
Oral Suspension: 12.5 mg/5 mL, 25 mg/5 mL; *Tablets:* 12.5 mg, 25 mg, 50 mg

DOSAGE

• **ORAL SUSPENSION, TABLETS**

Osteoarthritis.

Adults, initial: 12.5 mg once daily, up to a maximum of 25 mg once daily.

Acute pain, primary dysmenorrhea.

Adults, initial: 50 mg once daily; **then,** 50 mg once daily as needed.

NURSING CONSIDERATIONS

SEE ALSO *NURSING CONSIDERATIONS FOR NONSTEROIDAL ANTI-INFLAMMATORY DRUGS.*

R

ADMINISTRATION/STORAGE

1. Can be given without regard to meals.
2. Seek the lowest dose for each client.
3. Use for more than 5 days for pain has not been studied.
4. Store the tablets and oral suspension between 15–30°C (59–86°F).

ASSESSMENT

1. Note indications for therapy, onset and characteristics of disease, ROM, deformity/loss of function, instability, pain level, other agents trialed and the outcome.
2. Determine any GI bleed or ulcer history, aspirin or other NSAID-induced asthma/sensitivity, urticaria, or allergic-type reactions.
3. Assess for liver/renal dysfunction; monitor lytes, renal and LFTs.

CLIENT/FAMILY TEACHING

1. Take as directed at the same time each day, with food, a full glass of water, or after meals if GI upset occurs.
2. Report any GI discomfort as drug may cause GI bleeding, ulcerations or perforation.
3. Do not take aspirin, alcohol, or other NSAIDS while taking rofecoxib.
4. Report weight gain, swelling of ankles, chest pain, SOB, black tarry stools, stomach pain, unexplained lethargy, itching, jaundice, flu-like symptoms, skin rash, or lack of response.

OUTCOMES/EVALUATE

Relief of joint pain/inflammation with improved mobility

Ropinirole hydrochloride

(roh-**PIN**-ih-roll)

PREGNANCY CATEGORY: C
CLASSIFICATION(S):
Antiparkinson drug
Rx: Requip

SEE ALSO *ANTIPARKINSON AGENTS.*

ACTION/KINETICS

Mechanism is not known but believed to involve stimulation of postsynaptic D_2 dopamine receptors in caudate-putamen in brain. Causes decreases in both systolic and diastolic BP at doses above 0.25 mg. Rapidly absorbed. **Peak plasma levels:** 1–2 hr. Food reduces maximum concentration. **t½, elimination:** 6 hr. First pass effect; extensively metabolized in liver.

USES

Treat signs and symptoms of idiopathic Parkinson's disease, both as initial therapy and adjunctive therapy with levodopa.

CONTRAINDICATIONS

Lactation.

SPECIAL CONCERNS

Safety and efficacy have not been determined in children.

SIDE EFFECTS

CNS: Hallucinations, cause and/or exacerbate pre-existing dyskinesia. **CV:** Syncope (sometimes with bradycardia), postural hypotension.

OD OVERDOSE MANAGEMENT

Symptoms: Agitation, increased dyskinesia, grogginess, sedation, orthostatic hypotension, chest pain, confusion, N&V. *Treatment:* General suppportive measures. Maintain vital signs. Gastric lavage.

DRUG INTERACTIONS

Ciprofloxacin / Significant ↑ in ropinirole plasma levels
Estrogens / ↓ Oral clearance of ropinirole

HOW SUPPLIED

Tablets: 0.25 mg, 0.5 mg, 1 mg, 2 mg, 4 mg, 5 mg

DOSAGE

• **TABLETS**

Parkinson's disease.

Week 1: 0.25 mg t.i.d. **Week 2:** 0.5 mg t.i.d. **Week 3:** 0.75 mg t.i.d. **Week 4:** 1 mg t.i.d. After week 4, daily dose, if necessary, may be increased by 1.5 mg/day on weekly basis up to dose of 9 mg/day. This may be followed by increase of up to 3 mg/day weekly to total dose of 24 mg/day.

R

NURSING CONSIDERATIONS

SEE ALSO *NURSING CONSIDERATIONS* FOR *ANTIPARKINSON AGENTS*.

ADMINISTRATION/STORAGE

1. If taken with l-dopa, decrease dose of l-dopa gradually, as tolerated.
2. When discontinued, do so gradually over 7-day period. Reduce frequency of administration to twice daily for 4 days. For remaining 3 days, reduce frequency to once daily prior to complete withdrawal.

ASSESSMENT

1. Document disease onset, extent of motor function, reflexes, gait, strength of grip, and amount of tremor.
2. With tremor, note extent, muscle weakness, muscle rigidity, difficulty walking or changing direction.
3. Monitor VS, ECG.

CLIENT/FAMILY TEACHING

1. May be taken with or without food.
2. May cause dizziness and syncope, use caution; report if persists.
3. Avoid tasks that require mental alertness until drug effects realized.
4. Report any loss of effect or evidence of dyskinesia.
5. Do not stop abruptly. Drug must be gradually withdrawn over seven day period.
6. Report as scheduled for periodic lab tests, CXR, eye and medical evaluations.

OUTCOMES/EVALUATE

Control of tremor

R

Rosiglitazone maleate

(**roh**-sih-**GLIH**-tah-zohn)

PREGNANCY CATEGORY: C
CLASSIFICATION(S):
Antidiabetic, oral; thiazolidinedione
Rx: Avandia

SEE ALSO *ANTIDIABETIC AGENTS: HYPOGLYCEMIC AGENTS*.

ACTION/KINETICS

Improves blood glucose levels by improving insulin sensitivity in type II diabetes insulin resistance. Active only in the presence of insulin. A highly selective and potent agonist for the peroxisome proliferator-activated receptor (PPAR)-gamma which is found in adipose tissue, skeletal muscle, and liver. Activation of these receptors regulates the transcription of insulin-responsive genes involved in the control of glucose production, transport, and use. The genes also participate in regulation of fatty acid metabolism. Fasting blood glucose decreases from 31–64 mg/dL from placebo and HbA1c decreases from 0.8–1.5% from placebo. **Peak plasma levels:** 1 hr (over 99% bioavailable). Food decreases the rate of absorption but not the total amount absorbed. Approximately 99.8% bound to plasma proteins. **t½, distribution:** 3–4 hr. Extensively metabolized in the liver and excreted in the urine and feces.

USES

(1) As an adjunct to diet and exercise to improve glycemic control in type II diabetes. (2) In combination with a sulfonylurea or metformin in clients with type II diabetes when diet and exercise and either single agent does not achieve adequate control. (3) In combination with insulin to treat type II diabetes.

CONTRAINDICATIONS

Type I diabetes, diabetic ketoacidosis, active liver disease, if serum ALT levels are 2.5 times ULN, in clients with NYHA Class III and IV cardiac status (unless the expected benefit outweighs the potential risk), and during lactation.

SPECIAL CONCERNS

Treatment may result in resumption of ovulation in premenopausal anovulatory clients with insulin resistance. Use with caution in clients with edema. Safety and efficacy have not been determined in clients less than 18 years of age.

SIDE EFFECTS

CV: ***Cardiac failure,*** cardiac effects. **Respiratory:** URTI, sinusitis. **Metabolic:** Hyperglycemia, hypoglycemia. **Miscellaneous:** Injury, headache, back ache, fatigue, diarrhea, anemia, edema, hepatitis, hepatic enzyme elevations.

LABORATORY TEST CONSIDERATIONS

↑ ALT. ↓ H&H. Changes in serum lipids. Hyperbilirubinemia.

HOW SUPPLIED

Tablets: 2 mg, 4 mg, 8 mg

DOSAGE

• **TABLETS**

Type II diabetes, monotherapy.

Adults, initial: 4 mg once daily or in divided doses b.i.d. If the response is inadequate after 8–12 weeks, the dose can be increased to 8 mg as a single dose once daily or in divided doses b.i.d. A dose of 4 mg b.i.d. resulted in the greatest decrease in fasting blood glucose and HbA1c.

Type II diabetes, combination therapy with sulfonylurea or metformin.

Adults, initial: 4 mg once daily or in divided doses b.i.d. If the response is inadequate after 12 weeks, the dose can be increased to 8 mg (maximum daily dose) as a single dose once daily or in divided doses b.i.d.

NURSING CONSIDERATIONS

SEE ALSO *NURSING CONSIDERATIONS FOR ANTIDIABETIC AGENTS: HYPOGLYCEMIC AGENTS.*

ASSESSMENT

1. Note disease onset, other agents trialed, dietary/exercise adherance.
2. Note any history of CAD and NYHA class.
3. List agents prescribed to ensure none interact.
4. Monitor liver enzymes following initiation of therapy, every 2 months during the first year of use, and periodically thereafter. If ALT levels increase to 3X ULN at any time, recheck liver enzymes as soon as possible. If ALT levels remain greater than 3X ULN, discontinue therapy.
5. Monitor fasting blood glucose and HbA1c levels.

CLIENT/FAMILY TEACHING

1. Take once or twice daily as prescribed with meals. If dose missed may be taken at next meal.
2. May cause edema, resumption of ovulation, and hypoglycemia.
3. Report if dark urine, abdominal pain fatigue, or unexplained N&V occur. Also report any fever, sore throat, unusual bleeding/bruising, rash, or hypoglycemic reactions.
4. Practice reliable barrier contraception if using hormonal contraception and pregnancy is not desired.
5. Follow dietary guidelines, perform regular exercise and other life style changes consistent with controlling diabetes.
6. Monitor FS at different times during the day and maintain log for provider review.
7. Must report as scheduled for regular monitoring of renal and LFTs and bs.

OUTCOMES/EVALUATE

Control of NIDDM by ↓ insulin resistance; HbA1c < 7

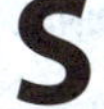
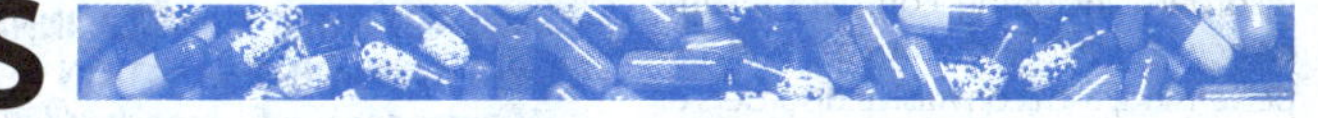

S

Salmeterol xinafoate

(sal-**MET**-er-ole)

PREGNANCY CATEGORY: C

CLASSIFICATION(S):

Sympathomimetic

Rx: Serevent, Serevent Diskus

SEE ALSO *SYMPATHOMIMETIC DRUGS.*

ACTION/KINETICS

Selective for beta-2 adrenergic receptors, located in the bronchi and heart. Acts by stimulating intracellular adenyl cyclase, the enzyme that converts ATP to cyclic AMP. Increased AMP levels cause relaxation of bronchial smooth muscle and inhibition of release of mediators of immediate hypersensitivity, especially from mast cells. **Onset:** Within 20 min. **Duration:**

12 hr. Significantly bound to plasma proteins. Cleared by hepatic metabolism.

USES

(1) Long-term maintenance treatment of asthma or bronchospasm in clients 12 years and older (4 years and older for inhalation powder) associated with reversible obstructive airway disease. Includes those with symptoms of nocturnal asthma who require regular treatment with inhaled, short-acting β_2–agonists. Not for use in asthmatics who can be managed by occasional use of a short-acting β_2–agonist. May be used with or without concurrent inhaled or systemic steroid therapy. (2) Prevention of exercise-induced bronchospasms in clients 12 years and older (4 years and older for inhalation powder). (3) Chronic treatment of bronchospasms associated with COPD, including emphysema and chronic bronchitis.

CONTRAINDICATIONS

Use in clients who can be controlled by short-acting, inhaled beta-2 agonists. Use to treat acute symptoms of asthma or in those who have worsening or deteriorating asthma. Lactation.

SPECIAL CONCERNS

Not a substitute for PO or inhaled corticosteroids. The safety and efficacy of using salmeterol with a spacer or other devices has not been studied adequately. Use with caution in impaired hepatic function; with cardiovascular disorders, including coronary insufficiency, cardiac arrhythmias, and hypertension; with convulsive disorders or thyrotoxicosis; and in clients who respond unusually to sympathomimetic amines. Because of the potential of the drug interfering with uterine contractility, use of salmeterol during labor should be restricted to those in whom benefits clearly outweigh risks. Safety and efficacy have not been determined in children less than 12 years of age.

SIDE EFFECTS

Respiratory: Paradoxical bronchospasms, upper or lower respiratory tract infection, nasopharyngitis, disease of nasal cavity/sinus, cough, pharyngitis, allergic rhinitis, laryngitis, tracheitis, bronchitis. **Allergic:** ***Immediate hypersensitivity reactions,*** including urticaria, rash, and ***bronchospasm.*** **CV:** Palpitations, chest pain, increased BP, tachycardia. **CNS:** Headache, sinus headache, tremors, nervousness, malaise, fatigue, dizziness, giddiness. **GI:** Stomachache. **Musculoskeletal:** Joint pain, back pain, muscle cramps, muscle contractions, myalgia, myositis, muscle soreness. **Miscellaneous:** Flu, dental pain, rash, skin eruption, dysmenorrhea.

LABORATORY TEST CONSIDERATIONS

↓ Serum potassium.

OD OVERDOSE MANAGEMENT

Symptoms: Tachycardia, arrhythmia, tremors, headache, muscle cramps, hypokalemia, hyperglycemia. *Treatment:* Supportive therapy. Consider judicious use of a beta-adrenergic blocking agent, although these drugs can cause bronchospasms. Cardiac monitoring is necessary. Dialysis is not an appropriate treatment of overdosage.

DRUG INTERACTIONS

Diuretics / Worsening of diuretic-induced ECG changes and hypokalemia
MAO Inhibitors / ↑ Salmeterol effect
Tricyclic antidepressants / ↑ Salmeterol effect

HOW SUPPLIED

Metered dose inhaler (Aerosol): 25 mcg base/inh; *Powder for Inhalation:* 50 mcg/inh

DOSAGE

• METERED DOSE AEROSOL INHALER, POWDER FOR INHALATION

Maintenance of bronchodilation, prevention of symptoms of asthma, including nocturnal asthma.

Adults and children over 12 years of age: Two inhalations (42 mcg) using the aerosol b.i.d. (morning and evening, approximately 12 hr apart). **Children 4 years and over:** 1 inhalation (50 mcg) using the inhalation powder b.i.d. (morning and evening, approximately 12 hr apart).

Prevention of exercise-induced bronchospasms.

Adults and children over 12 years of age: Two inhalations (42 mcg) of the aerosol or 1 inhalation (50 mcg) of the inhalation powder at least 30–60 min before exercise. Additional doses should not be used for 12 hr.

Maintenance treatment of asthma or bronchospasm associated with COPD. **Adults and children over 12 years of age:** Two inhalations (42 mcg) of the aerosol b.i.d. in the morning and evening (about 12 hr apart).

NOTE: Even though the metered dose inhaler and the inhalation powder are used for the same conditions, they are not interchangeable.

NURSING CONSIDERATIONS

SEE ALSO *NURSING CONSIDERATIONS* FOR *SYMPATHOMIMETIC DRUGS*.

ADMINISTRATION/STORAGE

1. Ensure doses spaced q 12 hr.
2. The safety of more than 8 inhalations per day of short-acting beta-2 agonists with salmeterol has not been established.
3. If a previously effective dose fails to provide the usual response, contact provider immediately.
4. If using salmeterol twice daily, do not use additional doses to prevent exercise-induced bronchospasms.
5. Use only with the actuator provided. Do not use the actuator with other aerosol medications.
6. Store the aerosol from 15–30°C (59– 86°F). Store the canister nozzle end down; protect from freezing temperatures, direct sunlight.
7. Store the inhalation powder from 20–25°C (68–77°F) in a dry place away from direct heat or sunlight.
8. Do not spray in the eyes.
9. Shake canister well before using at room temperature; therapeutic effect may diminish if cold.
10. For the inhalation of powder (Diskus), a built-in dose counter shows the number of doses remaining.

ASSESSMENT

1. Document onset, duration, and characteristics of symptoms; note agents trialed and outcome.
2. Determine any cardiac or liver dysfunction, thyrotoxicosis, hypertension, or seizure disorders.
3. Document PFTs and lung sounds.
4. Monitor VS, liver enzymes, PFTs (ABGs, PEFR, and FEV).

CLIENT/FAMILY TEACHING

1. Review proper use (with actuator) and obtain instruction. Record peak flows and identify critical zones.
2. Use only as prescribed and do not exceed prescribed dosage and administration frequency (drug effects last 12 hr).
3. Do not use this drug during an acute asthma attack.
4. Review procedure for use of the short-acting beta-2 agonist prescribed to treat symptoms of asthma that occur between the salmeterol dosing schedule. Increased utilization warrants medical evaluation (e.g., when used more than 4 times/day or more than one canister of 200 inhalations/8 weeks).
5. May experience palpitations, chest pain, headaches, tremors, and nervousness as side effects.
6. Report immediately if chest pain, fast pounding irregular heart beat, hives, increased wheezing, or difficulty breathing occurs.
7. Take 30–60 min before activity to prevent acute bronchospasms.
8. Salmeterol does not replace inhaled or systemic steroids; do not stop prescribed steroid therapy abruptly without approval.
9. Identify appropriate support groups that may assist client to cope and live a normal life with asthma.
10. Stop smoking; avoid smokey environments and any other triggers that may aggravate breathing condition.

OUTCOMES/EVALUATE

- Prevention and control of asthmatic symptoms (e.g., decreased wheezing, dyspnea, orthopnea, and cough)
- Prevention of exercise-induced bronchospasms

Saquinavir mesylate

(sah-**KWIN**-ah-veer)

PREGNANCY CATEGORY: B

S

CLASSIFICATION(S):
Antiviral, protease inhibitor
Rx: Fortovase, Invirase

SEE ALSO *ANTIVIRAL DRUGS*.

ACTION/KINETICS

HIV protease cleaves viral polyprotein precursors to form functional proteins in HIV-infected cells. Cleavage of viral polyprotein precursors is required for maturation of the infectious virus. Saquinavir inhibits the activity of HIV protease and prevents the cleavage of viral polyproteins. Has a low bioavailability after PO use, probably due to incomplete absorption and first-pass metabolism. A high-fat meal or high-calorie meal increases the amount of drug absorbed. Over 98% bound to plasma protein. About 87% metabolized in the liver by the cytochrome P450 system. Both metabolites and unchanged drug are excreted mainly through the feces. It is believed the bioavailability of Fortovase is greater than Invirase.

USES

Combined with antiretroviral drugs for treatment of HIV infection in selected clients.

CONTRAINDICATIONS

Lactation. Use with cisapride, ergot derivatives, midazolam, triazolam.

SPECIAL CONCERNS

Photoallergy or phototoxicity may occur; take protective measures against exposure to ultraviolet or sunlight until tolerance is assessed. Use with caution in those with hepatic insufficiency and in the elderly. Hemophiliacs treated with protease inhibitors for HIV infections may manifest spontaneous bleeding episodes. Safety and efficacy have not been determined in HIV-infected children or adolescents less than 16 years of age.

SIDE EFFECTS

Side effects listed are for saquinavir combined with either Zidovudine or ddC.

GI: Diarrhea, abdominal discomfort, nausea, dyspepsia, abdominal pain, ulceration of buccal mucosa, cheilitis, constipation, dysphagia, eructation, blood-stained or discolored feces, gastralgia, gastritis, GI inflammation, gingivitis, glossitis, ***rectal hemorrhage,*** hemorrhoids, hepatomegaly, hepatosplenomegaly, melena, pain, painful defecation, pancreatitis, parotid disorder, pelvic salivary glands disorder, stomatitis, tooth disorder, vomiting, frequent bowel movements, dry mouth, alteration in taste. **CNS:** Headache, paresthesia, numbness of extremity, dizziness, peripheral neuropathy, ataxia, confusion, ***convulsions,*** dysarthria, dysesthesia, hyperesthesia, hyperreflexia, hyporeflexia, face numbness, facial pain, paresis, poliomyelitis, progressive multifocal leukoencephalopathy, spasms, tremor, agitation, amnesia, anxiety, depression, excessive dreaming, euphoria, hallucinations, insomnia, reduced intellectual ability, irritability, lethargy, libido disorder, overdose effect, psychic disorder, somnolence, speech disorder. **Musculoskeletal:** Musculoskeletal pain, myalgia, arthralgia, arthritis, back pain, muscle cramps, musculoskeletal disorder, stiffness, tissue changes, trauma. **Body as a whole:** Allergic reaction, chest pain, edema, fever, intoxication, external parasites, retrosternal pain, shivering, wasting syndrome, weight decrease, abscess, angina tonsillaris, candidiasis, hepatitis, herpes simplex, herpes zoster, infections (bacterial, mycotic, staphylococcal), influenza, lymphadenopathy, tumor. **CV:** Cyanosis, heart murmur, heart valve disorder, hypertension, hypotension, syncope, distended vein, HR disorder. **Metabolic:** Dehydration, hyperglycemia, weight decrease, worsening of existing diabetes mellitus. **Hematologic:** Anemia, microhemorrhages, pancytopenia, splenomegaly, thrombocytopenia. **Respiratory:** Bronchitis, cough, dyspnea, epistaxis, hemoptysis, laryngitis, pharyngitis, pneumonia, respiratory disorder rhinitis, sinusitis, URTI. **GU:** Enlarged prostate, vaginal discharge, micturition disorder, UTI. **Dermatologic:** Acne, dermatitis, seborrheic dermatitis, eczema, erythema, folliculitis, furunculosis, hair changes, hot flushes, photosensitivity reaction, changes in skin pigment, maculopapular rash, skin disorder, skin nodules,

S

skin ulceration, increased sweating, urticaria, verruca, xeroderma. **Ophthalmic:** Dry eye syndrome, xerophthalmia, blepharitis, eye irritation, visual disturbance. **Otic:** Earache, ear pressure, decreased hearing, otitis, tinnitus.

LABORATORY TEST CONSIDERATIONS

↑ CPK, serum amylase, AST, ALT, total bilirubin. ↓ Neutrophils. Abnormal phosphorus.

DRUG INTERACTIONS

Carbamazepine / ↓ Saquinavir blood levels
Cisapride / Possibility of serious or life-threatening cardiac arrhythmias or prolonged sedation
Clarithromycin / ↑ Blood levels of both drugs
Cyclosporine / Significant ↑ blood levels
Delaviridine / Significant ↑ in saquinavir plasma AUC using Invirase
Dexamethasone / ↓ Saquinavir blood levels
Ergot derivatives / Possibility of serious or life-threatening cardiac arrhythmias or prolonged sedation
Grapefruit juice / ↑ Bioavailabilitiy and blood levels of saquinavir
HMG-CoA reductase inhibitors / Do not use with saquinavir; both are metbolized by the same pathway
Indinavir / Significant ↑ in AUC of saquinavir using Fortovase
Ketoconazole / ↑ Saquinavir blood levels
Midazolam / Possibility of serious or life-threatening cardiac arrhythmias or prolonged sedation; ↑ Plasma levels of midazolam
Nelfinavir / ↑ Plasma levels of both drugs
Nevirapine / ↓ Saquinavir blood levels
Phenobarbital / ↓ Saquinavir blood levels
Phenytoin / ↓ Saquinavir blood levels
Rifampin / ↓ Saquinavir blood levels
Ritonavir / ↑ Saquinavir blood levels
Sildenafil / ↑ Plasma levels of both drugs
Triazolam / Possibility of serious or life-threatening cardiac arrhythmias or prolonged sedation

HOW SUPPLIED

Capsules: 200 mg (Invirase). *Capsules, Soft Gelatin:* 200 mg (Fortovase)

DOSAGE

• **FORTOVASE CAPSULES**

HIV infections in combination with nucleoside analogs.

Six 200-mg capsules (i.e., 1,200 mg) taken t.i.d. within 2 hr of a meal.

• **INVIRASE CAPSULES**

HIV infections in combination with a nucleoside analog.

Three 200-mg t.i.d. capsules taken within 2 hr of a full meal.

NURSING CONSIDERATIONS

SEE ALSO *NURSING CONSIDERATIONS FOR ANTIVIRAL DRUGS.*

ADMINISTRATION/STORAGE

1. Fortovase soft gelatin capsules and Invirase capsules are *not* bioequivalent and are not to be used interchangeably.
2. Take within 2 hr of a full meal. If taken without food, blood levels may not be sufficiently high to exert an antiviral effect.
3. Doses less than 200 mg t.i.d. are not recommended; lower doses have not shown antiviral activity.
4. Fortovase is the recommended product. Invirase can be used if combined with antiretroviral drugs that significantly inhibit saquinavir's metabolism.
5. Do not reduce the dose when Fortovase is used with nucleoside analogs as this will cause greater than dose-proportional decreases in saquinavir plasma levels.
6. Refrigerate Fortovase from 2–8°C (36–46°F) in tightly closed bottles. Once brought to room temperature, use within 3 months. Store Inverase from 15–30°C (59–86°F) in tightly closed bottles.

ASSESSMENT

1. Document onset, duration, and characteristics of symptoms.
2. Monitor CBC, T-lymphocytes/viral load, renal and LFTs.
3. List drugs currently prescribed; drug is metabolized hepatically via cytochrome P450 system.

S

4. If serious or severe toxicity occurs, interrupt therapy until cause is determined or toxicity resolves. Monitor for opportunistic infections and treat appropiately.

CLIENT/FAMILY TEACHING

1. Take only as prescribed and within 2 hr of a full meal, as blood levels markedly reduced when taken without food.
2. Drug is not a cure for HIV infections. It does not prevent the occurrence or decrease the frequency of opportunistic infections associated with HIV.
3. Avoid sun exposure; take protective measures against UV or sunlight until tolerance assessed.
4. Continue to use barrier contraception and safe sex; drug does not inhibit disease transmission.
5. Long-term drug effects are still unknown; report side effects.

OUTCOMES/EVALUATE

Control of progression of HIV infections

Sargramostim

(sar-**GRAM**-oh-stim)

PREGNANCY CATEGORY: C
CLASSIFICATION(S):
Granulocyte colony-stimulating factor, human
Rx: Leukine
✱Rx: GM-CSF

S

ACTION/KINETICS

A granulocyte-macrophage colony-stimulating factor (rhu GM-CSF) produced by recombinant DNA technology in a yeast expression system. GM-CSF stimulates the proliferation and differentiation of hematopoietic progenitor cells. It stimulates partially committed progenitor cells to divide and differentiate in the granulocyte-macrophage pathways. Division, maturation, and activation are induced through GM-CSF binding to specific receptors located on the surface of target cells. Also activates mature granulocytes and macrophages. Increases the cytotoxicity of monocytes toward certain neoplastic cell lines as well as activates polymorphonuclear neutrophils, thus inhibiting the growth of tumor cells. Sargramostim differs from the naturally occurring GM-CSF by one amino acid and by a different carbohydrate moiety. **Peak levels:** 2–3 hr, depending on the dose. **t½, initial:** 12–17 min; **t½, terminal:** 1.6–2.6 hr, depending on the dose. Neutralizing antibodies have been detected in a small number of clients.

USES

(1) Increased myeloid recovery in clients with non-Hodgkin's lymphoma, ALL, and Hodgkin's disease undergoing autologous bone marrow transplantation. (2) Bone marrow transplantation failure or engraftment delay. (3) To shorten recovery time to neutrophil recovery and to decrease the incidence of severe and life-threatening infections in older adult clients with AML. (4) To mobilize hematopoietic progenitor cells into peripheral blood collection by leukapheresis. (5) For acceleration of myeloid recovery in allogenic bone marrow transplantation from human lymphocyte antigen-matched related donors. *Investigational:* To increase WBC counts in clients with myelodysplastic syndrome and in AIDS clients taking AZT; to correct neutropenia in clients with aplastic anemia; to decrease the nadir of leukopenia secondary to myelosuppressive chemotherapy and to decrease myelosuppression in preleukemic clients; and to decrease organ system damage following transplantation, especially in the liver and kidney.

CONTRAINDICATIONS

More than 10% leukemic myeloid blasts in the bone marrow or peripheral blood. Known hypersensitivity to GM-CSF, yeast-derived products, or any component of the product. Simultaneous use with cytotoxic chemotherapy or radiotherapy or use within 24 hr preceding or following chemotherapy or radiotherapy.

SPECIAL CONCERNS

Use with caution in clients with preexisting cardiac disease and hypoxia and during lactation. Safety and effectiveness have not been determined in children although it appears the drug is no more toxic in children than in adults. May aggravate fluid retention in clients with preexisting peripheral edema, or pleural or pericardial effusion. Insufficient data on effectiveness of sargramostim in increasing myeloid recovery after peripheral blood stem cell transplantation. It is possible that sargramostim can act as a growth factor for any tumor type, especially myeloid malignancies; thus, use with caution in any malignancy with myeloid characteristics.

SIDE EFFECTS

First-dose effects (rare): Respiratory distress, hypoxia, flushing, hypotension, syncope, tachycardia.

CV: Hypertension, ***hemorrhage,*** edema, hypotension, peripheral edema, cardiac event, tachycardia, pericardial effusion, pleural effusion, capillary leak syndrome. **GI:** N&V, diarrhea, abdominal pain, GI disorder, stomatitis, dyspepsia, anorexia, hematemesis, dysphagia, ***GI hemorrhage,*** constipation, abdominal distension, liver damage. **CNS:** Neuroclinical, neuromotor, neuropsychiatric, and neurosensory side effects. Paresthesia, headache, CNS disorder, insomnia, anxiety. **Respiratory:** Pulmonary event, pharyngitis, lung disorder, epistaxis, dyspnea, rhinitis. **Hematologic:** Blood dyscrasias, thrombocytopenia, leukopenia, petechia, agranulocytosis, coagulation disorders. **Musculoskeletal:** Bone pain, arthralgia, asthenia. **Dermatologic:** Rash, alopecia, pruritus. **GU:** Urinary tract disorder, hematuria, abnormal kidney function. **Miscellaneous:** Fever, infection, malaise, weight loss, chills, pain, chest pain, allergy, ***sepsis,*** eye hemorrhage, back pain, weight gain, sweating.

LABORATORY TEST CONSIDERATIONS

↑ Glucose, BUN, cholesterol, bilirubin, serum creatinine, ALT, alkaline phosphatase. ↓ Albumin, calcium.

OD OVERDOSE MANAGEMENT

Symptoms: Dyspnea, malaise, nausea, fever, rash, sinus tachycardia, chills, headache. *Treatment:* Discontinue therapy. Monitor for increases in WBCs and for respiratory symptoms.

DRUG INTERACTIONS

Drugs such as corticosteroids and lithium may ↑ the myeloproliferative effects of sargramostim. The effect of sargramostim may be limited in those who have received alkylating agents, anthracycline antibiotics, or antimetabolites.

HOW SUPPLIED

Injection: 500 mcg/mL; *Powder for injection, lyophilized:* 250 mcg, 500 mcg

DOSAGE

- **IV INFUSION, SC**

Myeloid reconstitution after autologous or allogenic bone marrow transplantation.

250 mcg/m²/day for 21 days as a 2-hr infusion beginning 2–4 hr after the autologous bone marrow infusion and greater than 24 hr after the last dose of chemotherapy and 12 hr after the last dose of radiotherapy. Do not give drug until the postmarrow infusion absolute neutrophil count is less than 500 cells/mm³.

Bone marrow transplantation failure or engraftment delay.

250 mcg/m²/day for 14 days as a 2-hr IV infusion. If engraftment has not occurred, therapy may be repeated after 7 days off therapy. A third course of 250 mcg/m²/day may be undertaken after another 7 days off therapy. However, if no response occurs after three courses, it is unlikely the drug will be beneficial.

Neutrophil recovery following chemotherapy in acute myelogenous leukemia.

250 mcg/m²/day given over a 4-hr period staring at about day 11 or 4 days following completion of induction chemotherapy. Use if the day 10 bone marrow is hypoplastic with less than 5% blasts. If a second cycle of therapy is needed, give about 4 days after the completion of chemotherapy if the bone marrow is hypoplastic with less than 5% blasts. Continue therapy until an absolute neutrophil count greater than 1,500/mm³ is noted for 3 consec-

S

utive days or a maximum of 42 days. If a severe adverse reaction occurs, decrease the dose by 50% or discontinue temporarily until the drug reaction is reduced.

Mobilization of peripheral blood progenitor cells (PBPCs).
250 mcg/m²/day IV over 24 hr or SC once daily. Use this dose throughout the PBPC collection period. If the WBC count is greater than 50,000 cells/mm³, reduce the dose by 50%. If sufficient numbers of progenitor cells are not collected, use other mobilization therapy.

Postperipheral blood progenitor cell transplantation.
250 mcg/m²/day IV over 24 hr or SC once daily beginning immediately after infusion of progenitor cells and continuing until an absolute neutrophil count greater than 1,500 is reached for 3 consecutive days.

NURSING CONSIDERATIONS

ADMINISTRATION/STORAGE

IV 1. Give daily dosage as a 2-hr IV infusion beginning 2–4 hr after the autologous bone marrow infusion. Ensure at least 24 hr have elapsed after last dose of chemotherapy and 12 hr elapsed since the last dose of XRT.
2. Reduce dose or discontinue if severe adverse reactions occur; may resume once reactions abate.
3. Reconstitute lyophilized powder with 1 mL of sterile water for injection without preservatives. Direct sterile water at the side of the vial, followed by a gentle swirling of the contents to avoid foaming. Avoid excessive or vigorous agitation.
4. Reconstituted solutions are clear, colorless, and isotonic with a pH of 7.4.
5. Do not reenter or reuse the vial; discard unused portion.
6. Dilute with 0.9% NaCl injection for IV infusion. If the final concentration is less than 10 mcg/mL, add human albumin at a final concentration of 0.1% to the saline before adding sargramostim, to prevent adsorption to the drug delivery system.
7. Contains no preservatives; thus, give as soon as possible, but within 6 hr, following reconstitution or dilution for IV infusion. Store the sterile powder, reconstituted solution, and dilution solution in the refrigerator at 2–8°C (36–46°F). Do not freeze or shake solutions or use beyond the expiration date on the vial.
8. Use an in-line membrane filter for IV infusion. Do not add other drugs to sargramostim infusion.

ASSESSMENT

1. Determine any sensitivity to yeast-derived products. Note any cardiac disease, hypoxia, peripheral edema, pleural or pericardial effusion, or myeloid-type malignancy.
2. Monitor CBC (ANC and platelets twice weekly during therapy), liver and renal function studies.
3. Document any therapy with drugs or radiation. Drug should *not* be administered 24 hr before or after cytotoxic chemotherapy or within 12 hr preceding or following radiation therapy. Give within 2—4 h of bone marrow infusion.

INTERVENTIONS

1. Monitor I&O, VS, and weight; assess for fluid retention or edema.
2. Monitor for respiratory symptoms during or immediately following infusion, especially with preexisting lung disease. Reduce rate of infusion by one-half if dyspnea occurs.
3. Monitor hematologic response with a CBC twice weekly. If the ANC exceeds 20,000/mm³ or the platelet count exceeds 500,000/mm³ or a severe reaction occurs, stop therapy and reduce the dose by one-half. Excessive blood counts have returned to normal levels within 3–7 days following termination of therapy.
4. Renal and hepatic function should be monitored every 2 weeks with hepatic or renal dysfunction.
5. Drug effectiveness may be limited in clients who, before autologous bone marrow transplantation, received extensive radiotherapy in the chest or abdomen to treat the primary disease; effectiveness is also limited in clients who have received multiple myelotoxic agents such as antimetabolites, alkylating agents, or anthracycline antibiotics.

OUTCOMES/EVALUATE

- Inhibition of tumor cell growth
- Improved hematologic parameters; neutrophil recovery
- Mobilization of peripheral blood progenitor cells

Scopolamine hydrobromide

(scoh-**POLL**-ah-meen)

PREGNANCY CATEGORY: C
Rx: Hyoscine Hydrobromide, Isopto Hyoscine Ophthalmic, Scopace
✱**Rx:** Buscopan

Scopolamine transdermal therapeutic system

(scoh-**POLL**-ah-meen)

PREGNANCY CATEGORY: C
Rx: Transderm-Scop
✱**Rx:** Transderm-V
CLASSIFICATION(S):
Cholinergic blocking drug, antiemetic

SEE ALSO *CHOLINERGIC BLOCKING AGENTS.*

ACTION/KINETICS

Anticholinergic with CNS depressant effects; produces amnesia when given with morphine or meperidine. Inhibits excessive motility and hypertonus of the GI tract. In the presence of pain, delirium may be produced. Causes pupillary dilation and paralyzes the muscle required to accommodate for close vision (cycloplegia). This enables the physician to examine the inner structure of the eye, including the retina, as well as to examine refractive errors of the lens without automatic accommodation by the client. Tolerance may develop if scopolamine is used alone. When used for refraction: **peak for mydriasis,** 20–30 min; **peak for cycloplegia,** 30–60 min; **duration:** 24 hr (residual cycloplegia and mydriasis may last for 3–7 days). Recovery time can be reduced by using 1–2 gtt pilocarpine (1% or 2%). To reduce absorption, apply pressure over the nasolacrimal sac for 2–3 min.

The transdermal therapeutic system contains 1.5 mg scopolamine, which is slowly released from a mineral oil–polyisobutylene matrix. Approximately 0.5 mg is released from the system per day.

USES

Ophthalmic: (1) For cycloplegia and mydriasis in diagnostic procedures. (2) Preoperatively and postoperatively in the treatment of iridocyclitis. (3) Dilate the pupil in treatment of uveitis or posterior synechiae. *Investigational:* Prophylaxis of synechiae, treatment of iridocyclitis. **Parenteral:** (1) Antiemetic, antivertigo. (2) Preanesthetic sedation and obstetric amnesia. (3) Antiarrhythmic during anesthesia and surgery. **Oral:** Prevention of motion sickness. Excessive motility and hypertonus of the GI tract. **Transdermal:** (1) Antiemetic, antivertigo. (2) Prevention of motion sickness.

ADDITIONAL CONTRAINDICATIONS

Use of the transdermal system in children or lactating women. Ophthalmic use in glaucoma or infants less than 3 months of age. Use for prophylaxis of excess secretions in children less than 4 months of age.

SPECIAL CONCERNS

Use with caution in children, infants, geriatric clients, diabetes, hypo- or hyperthyroidism, narrow anterior chamber angle.

ADDITIONAL SIDE EFFECTS

Disorientation, delirium, increased HR, decreased respiratory rate. **Ophthalmologic:** Blurred vision, stinging, increased intraocular pressure. Long-term use may cause irritation, photophobia, conjunctivitis, hyperemia, or edema. **Transdermal:** Dry mouth, drowsiness, blurred vision, dilation of pupils.

HOW SUPPLIED

Scopolamine hydrobromide: *Injection:* 0.3 mg/mL, 0.4 mg/mL, 0.86 mg/mL, 1 mg/mL; *Ophthalmic Solution:* 0.25%; *Tablet, soluble:* 0.4 mg. **Scopolamine transdermal therapeutic sys-**

S

tem: *Film, extended release:* 0.33 mg/24 hr, 0.5 mg/24 hr

DOSAGE

• **OPHTHALMIC SOLUTION**

Cycloplegia/mydriasis.

Adults: 1–2 gtt of the 0.25% solution in the conjunctiva 1 hr prior to refraction; **children:** 1 gtt of the 0.25% solution b.i.d. for 2 days prior to refraction.

Uveitis.

Adults and children: 1 gtt of the 0.25% solution in the conjunctiva 1–4 times/day, depending on the severity of the condition.

Treatment of posterior synechiae.

Adults and children: 1 gtt of the 0.25% solution q min for 5 min. (1 gtt of either a 2.5% or 10% solution of phenylephrine instilled q min for 3 min will enhance the effect of scopolamine.)

Postoperative mydriasis.

Adults: 1 gtt of the 0.25% solution once daily. For dark brown irides, administration 2 or 3 times/day may be required.

Pre- or Postoperative iridocyclitis.

Adults and children: 1 gtt of the 0.25% solution 1–4 times/day as required. Individualize the pediatric dose based on age, weight, and severity of the inflammation.

• **INJECTION (IM, IV, SC)**

Anticholinergic, antiemetic.

Adults: 0.3–0.6 mg (single dose). **Pediatric:** 0.006 mg/kg (0.2 mg/m^2) as a single dose.

Prophylaxis of excessive salivation and respiratory tract secretions in anesthesia.

Adults: 0.2–0.6 mg 30–60 min before induction of anesthesia. **Pediatric (given IM): 8–12 years:** 0.3 mg; **3–8 years:** 0.2 mg; **7 months–3 years:** 0.15 mg; **4–7 months:** 0.1 mg. Not recommended for children less than 4 months of age.

Adjunct to anesthesia, sedative-hypnotic.

Adults: 0.6 mg t.i.d–q.i.d.

Adjunct to anesthesia, amnesia.

Adults: 0.32–0.65 mg.

• **TABLETS**

Prevent motion sickness.

0.4–0.8 mg. Excessive GI tract motility and hypertonus.

• **TRANSDERMAL SYSTEM**

Antiemetic, antivertigo.

Adults: 1 transdermal system placed on the postauricular skin to deliver either 1 mg or 0.33 mg over 3 days (apply at least 4 hr before antiemetic effect is required). The Canadian product should be applied about 12 hr before the antiemetic effect is desired.

NURSING CONSIDERATIONS

SEE ALSO *NURSING CONSIDERATIONS* FOR *CHOLINERGIC BLOCKING AGENTS*.

ADMINISTRATION/STORAGE

1. Give drops into the conjunctival sac followed by digital pressure for 2–3 min after instillation.
2. Do not give alone for pain because it may cause delirium; use an analgesic or sedative as needed.
3. Protect solution from light.

ASSESSMENT

1. Document indications for therapy, onset and characteristics of symptoms.
2. With eyedrops, check for angle-closure glaucoma; may precipitate an acute glaucoma crisis.
3. Some clients may experience toxic delirium with therapeutic doses. Observe closely and have physostigmine available to reverse effects.
4. Note any conditions that may preclude therapy.

CLIENT/FAMILY TEACHING

1. Use exactly as directed. Take oral agents 30 min before meals. Do not share meds. Store safely.
2. Do not drive a car or operate dangerous machinery until drug effects realized; may cause drowsiness, confusion, disorientation, and, when used in the eye, blurred vision and dilated pupils.
3. Wear dark glasses if photosensitivity occurs and report if eye pain occurs. May temporarily impair vision.
4. Wait 5 min before instilling other eye drops.
5. With the transdermal system:
   - Wash hands before and after application
   - Apply at least 4 hr before desired effect

• Apply to a clean, nonhairy site, behind the ear
• Use pressure to apply the patch to ensure contact with the skin
• Replace with a new system if patch becomes dislodged
• System is water-proof so bathing and swimming are permitted
• System effects last for 3 days
• NOT for use in children

6. Report any extrapyramidal symptoms, urinary retention, and constipation. Increase fluids and bulk to prevent constipation and ensure adequate hydration. Avoid hot temperatures; may be heat intolerant.
7. Use gum, sugarless candies, and frequent mouth rinses to alleviate symptoms of dry mouth.
8. Avoid alcohol and any other CNS depressants.

OUTCOMES/EVALUATE

• Control of vomiting
• Preoperative sedation; postoperative amnesia
• Desired mydriasis
• Prevention of motion sickness

Sertraline hydrochloride

(**SIR**-trah-leen)

PREGNANCY CATEGORY: C
CLASSIFICATION(S):
Antidepressant, selective serotonin reuptake inhibitor
Rx: Zoloft
✱**Rx:** Apo-Sertraline, Novo-Sertraline

SEE ALSO *SELECTIVE SEROTONIN REUPTAKE INHIBITORS.*

ACTION/KINETICS

Steady-state plasma levels are usually reached after 1 week of once daily dosing but is increased to 2–3 weeks in older clients. **Time to peak plasma levels:** 4.5–8.4 hr. **Peak plasma levels:** 20–55 ng/mL. **Time to reach steady state:** 7 days. **Terminal elimination t½:** 1–4 days (including active metabolite). Washout period is 7 days. Food decreases the time to reach peak plasma levels. Undergoes significant first-pass metabolism; significant (98%) binding to serum proteins. Excreted through the urine (40–45%) and feces (40–45%). Metabolized to N-desmethylsertraline, which has minimal antidepressant activity.

USES

(1) Treatment of depression with reduced psychomotor agitation, anxiety, and insomnia. (2) Obsessive-compulsive disorders in adults and children as defined in DSM-IV. (3) Treatment of panic disorder, with or without agoraphobia, as defined in DSM-IV. (4) Treatment of posttraumatic stress disorder (over a 28-week period) in men and women. *Investigational:* Social phobia, premenstrual dysphoric disorder.

SPECIAL CONCERNS

Use with caution in hepatic or renal dysfunction, and with seizure disorders. Plasma clearance may be lower in elderly clients. The possibility of a suicide attempt is possible in depression and may persist until significant remission occurs.

SIDE EFFECTS

A large number of side effects is possible; listed are those side effects with a frequency of 0.1% or greater.
GI: Nausea and diarrhea (common), dry mouth, constipation, dyspepsia, vomiting, flatulence, anorexia, abdominal pain, thirst, increased salivation/appetite, gastroenteritis, teeth-grinding, dysphagia, eructation, taste perversion/change. **CV:** Palpitations, hot flushes, edema, hyper/hypotension, peripheral ischemia, postural hypotension or dizziness, syncope, tachycardia. **CNS:** Headache (common), insomnia (common), somnolence, agitation, nervousness, activation of mania/hypomania, seizures, anxiety, dizziness, tremor, fatigue, impaired concentration, yawning, paresthesia, hypoesthesia, twitching, hypertonia, confusion, ataxia or abnormal coordination/gait, hyperesthesia, hyper/hypokinesia, abnormal dreams, aggressive reaction, amnesia, apathy, delusion, depersonalization, depression, aggravated depression, emotional lability,

S

euphoria, hallucinations, neurosis, paranoid reaction, ***suicide ideation or attempt,*** abnormal thinking, migraine, nystagmus, vertigo. **Dermatologic:** Rash, acne, excessive sweating, alopecia, pruritus, cold/clammy skin, facial edema, erythematous rash, maculopapular rash, dry skin. **Musculoskeletal:** Myalgia, arthralgia, arthrosis, dystonia, muscle cramps/weakness. **GU:** Urinary frequency/incontinence, UTI, micturition/menstrual disorders, dysmenorrhea, dysuria, painful menstruation, intermenstrual bleeding, sexual dysfunction and decreased libido, noc-turia, polyuria, dysuria. **Respiratory:** Rhinitis, pharyngitis, bronchospasm, coughing, dyspnea, epistaxis. **Ophthalmologic:** Blurred/abnormal vision, abnormal accommodation, conjunctivitis, diplopia, eye pain, xerophthalmia. **Otic:** Tinnitus, earache. **Body as a whole:** Asthenia, fever, chest/back pain, chills, weight loss/gain, generalized edema, malaise, flushing, hot flashes, rigors, lymphadenopathy, purpura.

LABORATORY TEST CONSIDERATIONS

↑ AST or ALT, total cholesterol, triglycerides. ↓ Serum uric acid. Altered platelet function. Hyponatremia.

OD OVERDOSE MANAGEMENT

Symptoms: Intensification of side effects. *Treatment:*

- Establish and maintain an airway, ensuring adequate oxygenation and ventilation.
- Activated charcoal, with or without sorbitol, may be as or more effective than emesis or lavage.
- Cardiac and VS should be monitored.
- Provide general supportive measures and symptomatic treatment.
- Since sertraline has a large volume of distribution, it is unlikely that dialysis, forced diuresis, hemoperfusion, or exchange transfusion will be beneficial.

ADDITIONAL DRUG INTERACTIONS

Because sertraline is highly bound to plasma proteins, its use with other drugs that are also highly protein bound may lead to displacement, resulting in higher plasma levels of the drug and possibly increased side effects.

Alcohol / Concurrent use is not recommended in depressed clients
Benzodiazepines / ↓ Clearance of benzodiazepines metabolized by hepatic oxidation
Carbamazepine / Possible ↓ sertraline effect due to ↑ liver metabolism
Cimetidine / ↑ Half-life and blood levels of sertraline
Clozapine / ↑ Serum clozapine levels
Diazepam / ↑ Plasma levels of desmethyldiazepam (significance not known)
Erythromycin / Possiblity of "Serotonin Syndrome"
Hydantoins / Possible ↑ hydantoin levels
Rifampin / Possible ↓ sertraline serum levels

HOW SUPPLIED

Liquid Concentrate: 20 mg/mL; *Tablet:* 25 mg, 50 mg, 100 mg

DOSAGE

• LIQUID CONCENTRATE, TABLETS

Depression.

Adults, initial: 50 mg once daily either in the morning or evening. Clients not responding to a 50-mg dose may benefit from doses up to a maximum of 200 mg/day.

Obsessive-compulsive disorder.

Adults: 50 mg once daily either in the morning or evening; up to 200 mg/day may be required in some. **Children, 6 to 12 years:** 25 mg once a day; **adolescents, 13 to 17 years:** 50 mg once a day. Those not responding may require doses up to a maximum of 200 mg/day.

Panic attacks.

Adults, initial: 25 mg/day for the first week; **then,** increase the dose to 50 mg once daily.

Posttraumatic stress syndrome.

25 mg once daily. After 1 week, increase dose to 50 mg once daily.

NOTE: Lower the dose or space dose frequency in those with hepatic or renal impairment.

NURSING CONSIDERATIONS

SEE ALSO *NURSING CONSIDERATIONS* FOR *SELECTIVE SEROTONIN REUPTAKE INHIBITORS*.

ADMINISTRATION/STORAGE

1. Clients responding during an initial 8-week treatment period will likely benefit during an additional 8-week treatment period. The effectiveness of sertraline has not been evaluated for more than 16 weeks, although it is generally recognized that acute periods of depression require several months or longer of sustained drug therapy. Shown to be effective up to 52 weeks for depression.
2. Do not increase dosage at intervals of less than 1 week.
3. Beneficial effects may not be observed for 2–4 weeks after starting.
4. Use for more than 12 weeks for panic attacks has not been studied.

ASSESSMENT

1. Document indications for therapy, type, onset, and symptom characteristics.
2. List other drugs trialed and the outcome.
3. Note any seizure disorder.
4. Assess life-style, i.e., recent loss (death of loved one), stress, job change/loss, alcohol/drug use, or other factors that may contribute to depression.
5. Monitor ECG, renal and LFTs.

CLIENT/FAMILY TEACHING

1. Take only as directed, do not share meds, store safely, and remain under close medical supervision.
2. Prior to use of the oral concentrate, dilute with 4 oz of water, ginger ale, lemon/lime soda, lemonade, or orange juice only. Take immediately after mixing; do not mix in advance.
3. Do not perform activities that require mental and physical alertness until drug effects are realized.
4. Review side effects, noting those that require immediate medical attention.
5. Loss of appetite, persistent nausea, and diarrhea with excessive weight loss should be reported.
6. Report any suicidal thoughts or aggression. Attend counseling and maintain contact with provider so drug utilization can be assessed, as the risk of suicide is tantamount in a depressive phase.
7. Avoid OTC agents, alcohol, and any other CNS depressants.
8. Use reliable contraception; report if pregnancy suspected.

OUTCOMES/EVALUATE

- Improved eating/sleeping pattern
- ↓ Levels of agitation and anxiety
- Relief of symptoms of depression

Sevelamer hydrochloride

(seh-**VEL**-ah-mer)

PREGNANCY CATEGORY: C
CLASSIFICATION(S):
Urinary tract drug
Rx: Renagel

ACTION/KINETICS

A polymeric phosphate binder that decreases intestinal phosphate absorption. A decrease in serum phosphate decreases ectopic calcification and osteitis fibrosa. Also lowers LDL and total serum cholesterol. Is not absorbed into the systemic circulation.

USES

To reduce serum phosphorous in ESRD in clients on hemodialysis.

CONTRAINDICATIONS

Hypophosphatemia, bowel obstruction.

SPECIAL CONCERNS

No well controlled studies in lactating mothers. Use with caution in dysphagia, swallowing disorders, severe GI motility disorders, or major GI tract surgery. Safety and efficacy have not been determined in children.

SIDE EFFECTS

GI: Diarrhea, dyspepsia, vomiting. **CV:** Hypotension or hypertension, thrombosis. **Body as a whole:** Infection, pain, headache. **Respiratory:** Increased cough.

DRUG INTERACTIONS

Sevelamer may bind antiarrhythmic or anticonvulsant drugs → ↓ absorption.

HOW SUPPLIED

Capsule: 403 mg

S

DOSAGE

• **CAPSULES**

Hyperphosphatemia in ESRD

Adults, initial: 2–4 capsules with each meal, based on the following serum phosphorus levels: **Greater than 6 but less than 7.5 mg/dL:** 2 capsules t.i.d.; **7.5 mg/dL or more but less than 9 mg/dL:** 3 capsules t.i.d.; **9 mg/dL or more:** 4 capsules t.i.d. Adjust dosage to lower serum phosphorus to 6 mg/dL or less. Increase or decrease the dose by 1 capsule/meal as needed.

NURSING CONSIDERATIONS

ASSESSMENT

1. Note disease onset, dietary compliance, other agents trialed, and time on hemodialysis.
2. Assess for low P levels and bowel obstruction; determine any dysphagia, swallowing or severe GI motility disorders, or major GI surgery.
3. Monitor serum P, Ca, Cl, and bicarbonate levels.

CLIENT/FAMILY TEACHING

1. Take with meals and adhere to prescribed diet for ESRD.
2. Space doses of concomitant drugs by 1 or more hr before or 3 hr after sevelamer.
3. Swallow whole. Do not chew capsules or take apart because the capsule contents expand in water.
4. Dosage is prescribed/adjusted according to serum phosphorus levels.
5. May experience diarrhea, vomiting, GI upset, headaches, and pain; report if persistent.

S

OUTCOMES/EVALUATE

↓ Serum phosphorus to 6 mg/dL or less

Sibutramine hydrochloride monohydrate

(sih-**BYOU**-trah-meen)

PREGNANCY CATEGORY: C
CLASSIFICATION(S):
Antiobesity drug
Rx: Meridia , **C-IV**

ACTION/KINETICS

Main effect is likely due to primary and secondary amine metabolites of sibutramine. Inhibits reuptake of norepinephrine (NE) and serotonin (5HT), resulting in enhanced NE and 5HT activity and reduced food intake. Significant improvement in serum uric acid. Rapidly absorbed from GI tract. Extensive first-pass metabolism in liver. **Peak plasma levels of active metabolites:** 3–4 hr. **t½, sibutramine:** 1.1 hr; **t½, active metabolites:** 14–16 hr. Excreted in urine and feces.

USES

Management of obesity, including weight loss and maintenance of weight loss. Recommended for obese clients with initial body mass index of 30 kg/m^2 or more or 27 kg/m^2 in presence of hypertension, diabetes, or dyslipidemia. Use in conjunction with reduced calorie diet. Safety and efficacy have not been determined for more than 2 years.

CONTRAINDICATIONS

Lactation. Use in clients receiving MAO inhibitors, who have anorexia nervosa, those taking centrally-acting appetite suppressant drugs, those with history of coronary artery disease, CHF, arrhythmias, or stroke. Use in severe renal impairment or hepatic dysfunction. Use with serotonergic drugs, such as fluoxetine, fluvoxamine, paroxetine, sertraline, venlafaxine, sumatriptan, and dihydroergotamine; also, use with dextromethorphan, meperidine, pentazocine, fentanyl, lithium, or tryptophan.

SPECIAL CONCERNS

Use with caution in geriatric clients. Safety and efficacy have not been determined in children less than 16 years of age. Use with caution in narrow angle glaucoma, history of seizures, or with drugs that may raise BP (e.g., phenylpropanolamine, ephedrine, pseudoephedrine). Exclude organic causes (e.g., untreated hypothyroidism) before use.

SIDE EFFECTS

Body as a whole: Headache, back pain, flu syndrome, injury/accident, asthenia, chest pain, neck pain, allergic reaction. **GI:** Dry mouth, anorexia, abdominal pain, constipation, N&V, rectal disorder, increased appetite, dyspepsia, gastritis, diarrhea, flatulence, gastroenteritis, tooth disorder. **CNS:** Insomnia, dizziness, paresthesia, nervousness, anxiety, depression, somnolence, CNS stimulation, emotional lability, agitation, hypertonia, abnormal thinking, seizures. **CV:** Increased blood pressure and pulse, tachycardia, vasodilation, migraine, palpitation. **Dermatologic:** Sweating, rash, herpes simplex, acne, pruritus, ecchymosis. **Musculoskeletal:** Arthralgia, myalgia, tenosynovitis, joint disorder, arthritis. **Respiratory:** Rhinitis, pharyngitis, sinusitis, increase cough, laryngitis, bronchitis, dyspnea. **GU:** Dysmenorrhea, UTI, vaginal monilia, metrorrhagia, menstrual disorder. **Otic:** Ear disorder, ear pain. **Miscellaneous:** Thirst, generalized edema, taste perversion, fever, amblyopia, leg cramps.

DRUG INTERACTIONS

Alcohol / Do not use excess alcohol if taking sibutramine
Dextromethorphan / Possible life-threatening serotonin syndrome
Dihydroergotamine / Possible life-threatening serotonin syndrome
Ephedrine / ↑ BP and HR
Fentanyl / Possible life-threatening serotonin syndrome
Isocarboxazid / Possible life-threatening serotonin syndrome
Lithium / Additive serotonergic effects
Meperidine / Possible life-threatening serotonin syndrome
Pentazocine / Possible life-threatening serotonin sydnrome
Phenelzine / Possible life-threatening serotonin syndrome
Pseudoephedrine / ↑ BP and HR
Selective serotonin reuptake inhibitors / Possible life-threatening serotonin syndrome
Selegiline / Possible life-threatening serotonin syndrome
Sumatriptan / Possible life-threatening serotonin syndrome
L-Tryptophan / Possible life-threatening serotonin syndrome
Tranylcypromine / Possible life-threatening serotonin syndrome
Zolmitriptan / Possible life-threatening serotonin syndrome

HOW SUPPLIED

Capsules: 5 mg, 10 mg, 15 mg

DOSAGE

- **CAPSULES**

Obesity.

Adults, initial: 10 mg once daily (usually in morning) with or without food. Use the 5 mg dose for those who do not tolerate 10 mg. If there is inadequate weight loss, dose may be titrated after 4 weeks to total of 15 mg once daily. Do not exceed 15 mg daily.

NURSING CONSIDERATIONS

ADMINISTRATION/STORAGE

1. May take with or without food.
2. Re-evaluate therapy if client has not lost at least 4 pounds in first 4 weeks of treatment.
3. Allow at least 2 weeks to elapse between discontinuation of a MAO inhibitor and initiation of sibutramine and between discontinuation of sibutramine and initiation of a MAO inhibitor.
4. Store at controlled room temperature. Protect from heat and moisture and dispense in tight, light-resistant container.

ASSESSMENT

1. Document indications for therapy, length of weight problem, other agents/therapies trialed and outcome.
2. Assess for anorexia nervosa and MAO use.
3. Obtain weight and calculate BMI.
4. Monitor ECG, VS and labs; assess for increased BP or increased HR.

CLIENT/FAMILY TEACHING

1. Take only as directed with or without food. Do not exceed prescribed dosage.
2. Continue regular exercise, weight counselling, and low calorie diet during therapy.
3. Review package insert before starting therapy and review with each refill.
4. Report any signs of allergic reaction including rash or hives.

S

5. Pactice reliable non-hormonal form of birth control; may harm fetus.
6. Avoid alcohol and OTC agents and report all prescribed meds to prevent interactions.
7. Report regularly for F/U visits and lab work; record BP and pulse for provider review.

OUTCOMES/EVALUATE

Desired weight loss

Sildenafil citrate

(sill-**DEN**-ah-fill)

PREGNANCY CATEGORY: B
CLASSIFICATION(S):
Drug for erectile dysfunction
Rx: Viagra

ACTION/KINETICS

Nitric oxide activates the enzyme guanylate cyclase, which causes increased levels of guanosine monophosphate (cGMP) and subsequently smooth muscle relaxation in the corpus cavernosum and allowing inflow of blood. Sildenafil enhances effect of nitric oxide by inhibiting phosphodiesterase type 5 which is responsible for degradation of cGMP in the corpus cavernosum. When sexual stimulation causes local release of nitric oxide, inhibition of phosphodiesterse type 5 by sildenafil causes increased levels of cGMP in the corpus cavernosum and thus smooth muscle relaxation and inflow of blood resulting in an erection. Drug has no effect in absence of sexual stimulation. Rapidly absorbed after PO use. Absorption is decreased when taken with high fat meal. Metabolized in liver where it is converted to active metabolite (N-desmethyl sildenafil). **$t^{1/2}$, sildenafil and metabolite:** 4 hr. Excreted mainly in feces (80%) with about 13% excreted in urine. Reduced clearance is seen in geriatric clients.

USES

Treatment of erectile dysfunction. Has no effect in the absence of sexual stimulation.

CONTRAINDICATIONS

Concomitant use with organic nitrates in any form or with other treatments for erectile dysfunction. Use in men for whom sexual activity is not advisable due to underlying cardiovascular status. Use in newborns, children, or women.

SPECIAL CONCERNS

Use with caution in clients with anatomical deformation of penis, in those with predisposition to priapism (e.g., sickle cell anemia, multiple myeloma, leukemia), in bleeding disorders or active peptic ulceration, and in those with genetic disorders of retinal phosphodiesterases. Drug is potentially hazardous in those with acute coronary ischemia but not on nitrates; have CHF, borderline low BP, or borderline low volume status; are on complicated antihypertensive therapy with several drugs; are taking erythromycin or cimetidine; or have impaired hepatic or renal function.

SIDE EFFECTS

CNS: Headache, dizziness, ataxia, hypertonia, neuralgia, neuropathy, paresthesia, tremor, vertigo, depression, insomnia, somnolence, abnormal dreams, decreased reflexes, hypesthesia, seizures, anxiety. **GI:** Dyspepsia, diarrhea, vomiting, glossitis, colitis, dysphagia, gastritis, gastroenteritis, esophagitis, stomatitis, dry mouth, rectal hemorrhage, gingivitis. **CV:** Hypertension, TIA, ***MI, sudden cardiac death, ventricular arrhythmia, CVA*** especially with preexisting CV risk factors. Also, angina pectoris, AV block, migraine, syncope, tachycardia, palpitation, hypotension, postural hypotension, myocardial ischemia, cerebral thrombosis, ***cardiac arrest, heart failure, cardiomyopathy*** , abnormal ECG. **Dermatologic:** Flushing, rash, urticaria, herpes simplex, pruritus, sweating, skin ulcer, contact dermatitis, exfoliative dermatitis. **GU:** UTI, cystitis, nocturia, urinary frequency, urinary incontinence, abnormal ejaculation, genital edema and anorgasmia, prolonged erection, priaprism, hematuria, breast enlargment. **Ophthalmic:** Mild and transient predominantly color tinge to vision, increased sensitivity to light, blurred vision, mydriasis, conjunctivitis, photophobia, eye pain, eye hemorrhage, cataract, dry eyes, diplo-

S

pia, temporary vision loss, ocular redness or bloodshot appearance, ocular burning, ocular swelling/pressure, increased intraocular pressure, retinal vascular disease or bleeding, vitreous detachment/traction, paramacular edema. **Otic:** tinnitus, deafness, ear pain. **Respiratory:** Nasal congestion, respiratory tract infection, asthma, dyspnea, laryngitis, pharyngitis, sinusitis, bronchitis, increased sputum, increased cough. **Musculoskeletal:** Arthritis, arthrosis, myalgia, tendon rupture, tenosynovitis, bone pain, myasthenia, synovitis. **Miscellaneous:** Back pain, flu syndrome, face edema, shock, asthenia, pain, chills, accidental fall/injury, abdominal pain, allergic reaction, chest pain. *NOTE:* Death has occurred in some clients following use of the drug.

LABORATORY TEST CONSIDERATIONS

Abnormal LFTs.

OD OVERDOSE MANAGEMENT

Symptoms: Extension of side effects. *Treatment:* Standard supportive measures.

DRUG INTERACTIONS

Amlodipine / Additional ↓ in BP
Cimetidine / ↑ Sildenafil plasma levels
Erythromycin / Significant ↑ sildenafil plasma levels
Itraconazole / ↑ Sildenafil plasma levels
Ketoconazole / ↑ Sildenafil plasma levels
Mibefradil / ↑ Sildenafil plasma levels
Nitrites / Potentiation of vasodilatory effects → significant and potential fatal ↓ BP; do not use together
Rifampin / ↓ Sildenafil plasma levels

HOW SUPPLIED

Tablets: 25 mg, 50 mg, 100 mg

DOSAGE

• **TABLETS**

Treat erectile dysfunction.

For most clients, 50 mg no more than once daily, as needed, about 1 hr before sexual activity. Take anywhere from 0.5 hr to 4 hr before sexual activity. Depending on tolerance and effectiveness, dose may be increased to maximum of 100 mg or decreased to 25 mg. Consider a starting dose of 25 mg in those with hepatic or renal impairment, in geriatric clients, or if taken with erythromycin, itraconzole, or ketoconazole.

NURSING CONSIDERATIONS

ASSESSMENT

1. Note onset and cause of erectile dysfunction, i.e., organic, psychogenic, or combined.
2. Assess cardiovascular status and obtain ECG. Clients using nitrates should not use this drug or should be nitrate free for 24 hr prior to use.
3. List drugs prescribed as some may potentiate drug effects.
4. Assess for any retinal or bleeding disorders or active ulcers.
5. Note any conditions that may predispose client to priapism, i.e., multiple myelomas, sickle cell anemia, or leukemia.
6. Assess for any anatomical deformation of penis (Peyronie's disease, angulation, or cavernosal fibrosis).

CLIENT/FAMILY TEACHING

1. Take only as directed on an empty stomach 1 hr prior to act; high fat meal may slow absorption.
2. May experience headache, flushing, upset stomach, stuffy nose, or abnormal vision; report any unusual, persistant or bothersome effects.
3. Do not use any other agent for erections with this therapy. Effects may be evident the day after therapy; assess before taking additional drug.
4. Report all meds currently prescribed to ensure none alter effects.
5. Practice safe sex; drug does not prevent disease transmission.
6. Plan some form of sexual stimulation after ingestion to ensure desired erection obtained.
7. Do not share meds or prescriptions due to potential for adverse interactions and effects. *Never* use this drug if currently taking nitates in any form.

OUTCOMES/EVALUATE

Acquisition and maintenance of penile erection

Simvastatin

(**sim**-vah-**STAH**-tin)

PREGNANCY CATEGORY: X
CLASSIFICATION(S):
Antihyperlipidemic, HMG-CoA reductase inhibitor
Rx: Zocor

SEE ALSO *ANTIHYPERLIPIDEMIC AGENTS, HMG-COA REDUCTASE INHIBITORS.*

ACTION/KINETICS

Does not reduce basal plasma cortisol or testosterone levels or impair renal reserve. **Peak therapeutic response:** 4–6 weeks. Approximately 85% absorbed; significant first-pass effect with less than 5% of a PO dose reaching the general circulation. Ninety-four to 98% plasma protein bound. **t½:** 3 hr. Metabolites excreted in the feces (60%) and urine (13%).

USES

(1) Adjunct to diet to reduce elevated total and LDL cholesterol, apoprotein B, and triglyceride levels in hypercholesterolemia and mixed dyslipidemia (types IIa and IIb) when the response to diet and other approaches has been inadequate. (2) To increase HDL cholesterol in primary hypercholesterolemia and mixed dyslipidemias. (3) Treatment of isolated hypertriglyceridemia (Frederickson IV) and hyperlipoproteinemia (type III). (4) In coronary heart disease and hypercholesterolemia to reduce risk of total mortality by reducing coronary death; to reduce the risk of non-fatal MI; to reduce the risk for undergoing myocardial revascularization procedures; to reduce the risk of stroke or TIAs. *Investigational:* Heterozygous familial hypercholesterolemia, familial combined hyperlipidemia, diabetic dyslipidemia in non-insulin-dependent diabetes, hyperlipidemia secondary to the nephrotic syndrome, and homozygous familial hypercholesterolemia in clients with defective LDL receptors.

SPECIAL CONCERNS

Use with caution in clients who have a history of liver disease/consume large quantities of alcohol or with drugs that affect steroid levels or activity. Higher plasma levels may be observed in clients with hepatic and severe renal insufficiency. Safety and efficacy have not been determined in children less than 18 years of age.

SIDE EFFECTS

Musculoskeletal: Rhabdomyolysis with renal dysfunction secondary to myoglobinuria, myopathy, arthralgias. **GI:** N&V, diarrhea, abdominal pain, constipation, flatulence, dyspepsia, pancreatitis, anorexia, stomatitis. **Hepatic:** Hepatitis (including chronic active hepatitis), cholestatic jaundice, cirrhosis, fatty change in liver, ***fulminant hepatic necrosis, hepatoma.*** **Neurologic:** Dysfunction of certain cranial nerves resulting in alteration of taste, impairment of extraocular movement, and facial paresis. Paresthesia, peripheral neuropathy, peripheral nerve palsy. **CNS:** Headache, tremor, vertigo, memory loss, anxiety, insomnia, depression. *Hypersensitivity Reactions:* Although rare, the following symptoms have been noted. ***Angioedema, anaphylaxis,*** lupus erythematous–like syndrome, vasculitis, purpura, thrombocytopenia, leukopenia, ***hemolytic anemia,*** polymyalgia rheumatica, positive ANA, ESR increase, arthritis, arthralgia, asthenia, urticaria, photosensitivity, chills, fever, flushing, malaise, dyspnea, ***toxic epidermal necrolysis, erythema multiforme (including Stevens-Johnson syndrome).*** **GU:** Gynecomastia, loss of libido, erectile dysfunction. **Ophthalmologic:** Lens opacities, ophthalmoplegia. **Hematologic:** Transient asymptomatic eosinophilia, anemia, thrombocytopenia, leukopenia. **Miscellaneous:** URI, asthenia, alopecia, edema.

LABORATORY TEST CONSIDERATIONS

↑ CPK, AST, ALT.

ADDITIONAL DRUG INTERACTIONS

Chronic use of grapefruit juice ↑ simvastatin plasma levels due to ↓ liver metabolism

HOW SUPPLIED

Tablet: 5 mg, 10 mg, 20 mg, 40 mg, 80 mg

DOSAGE

• **TABLETS**

Hyperlipidemia.

Adults, initially: 20 mg once daily in the evening; **maintenance:** 5–80 mg/day as a single dose in the evening. Consider a starting dose of 5 mg/day for clients on immunosuppressives (e.g., cyclosporine), those with LDL less than 190 mg/dL, or in those with severe renal insufficiency. Consider a starting dose of 10 mg/day for clients with LDL greater than 190 mg/dL. Consider a starting dose of 40 mg as an alternative for those who require a reduction of more than 45% in their LDL cholesterol (most often those with CAD). For geriatric clients, the starting dose should be 5 mg/day with maximum LDL reductions seen with 20 mg or less daily. Do not exceed 10 mg/day if used in combination with fibrates or niacin.

Homozygous familial hypercholesterolemia.

Adults: 40 mg/day in the evening or 80 mg/day in 3 divided doses of 20 mg, 20 mg, and an evening dose of 40 mg. Use as an adjunct to other lipid-lowering treatments.

NURSING CONSIDERATIONS

SEE ALSO *NURSING CONSIDERATIONS FOR ANTIHYPERLIPIDEMIC AGENTS, HMG-COA REDUCTASE INHIBITORS.*

ADMINISTRATION/STORAGE

1. Place client on a standard cholesterol-lowering diet for 3–6 months before starting simvastatin. Continue the diet during drug therapy.
2. May give without regard to meals.
3. Dosage may be adjusted at intervals of at least 4 weeks.

ASSESSMENT

1. Monitor CBC, cholesterol profile, liver and renal function studies. Schedule LFTs at the beginning of therapy and semiannually for the first year of therapy. Special attention should be paid to elevated serum transaminase levels.
2. List all medications prescribed to ensure none interact unfavorably.
3. Assess level of adherence to weight reduction, exercise, and cholesterol-lowering diet.
4. Note any alcohol abuse.

CLIENT/FAMILY TEACHING

1. A low-cholesterol diet must be followed during drug therapy. Consult dietitian for assistance in meal planning and food preparation. Do not take with grapefruit juice. May enjoy grapefruit juice at other times during the day.
2. Report any S&S of infections, unexplained muscle pain, tenderness/weakness (especially if accompanied by fever or malaise), surgery, trauma, or metabolic disorders. Report as scheduled for LFTs.
3. Review importance of following a low-cholesterol diet, regular exercise, low alcohol consumption, and not smoking in the overall plan to reduce serum cholesterol levels and inhibit progression of CAD.
4. Not for use during pregnancy; use barrier contraception.
5. May experience sun sensitivity; take precautions to avoid/potect self.

OUTCOMES/EVALUATE

↓ Serum triglycerides and LDL cholesterol levels

Sirolimus

(sir-oh-**LIH**-mus)

PREGNANCY CATEGORY: C
CLASSIFICATION(S):
Immunosuppressant
Rx: Rapamune

S

ACTION/KINETICS

Inhibits both T-lymphocyte activation and proliferation that occurs in response to antigenic and interleukin IL-2, IL-4, and IL-15 stimulation. Also inhibits antibody production. Rapidly absorbed after PO use. **Peak levels:** About 1 hr in healthy clients and about 2 hr in renal transplant clients. Extensively bound to plasma proteins. The majority of the drug is sequestered in erythrocytes resulting in much higher blood levels compared with plasma levels. Extensively metabolized by cytochrome P450 IIIA4 and P-glycoprotein in the liver and gut wall. Over 90% is excreted in the feces. Adjust dosage for mild-to-moderate hepatic impairment. **t½, terminal, after multiple dosing in renal transplant clients:** About 62 hr.

USES

Use with corticosteroids and cyclosporine to prevent organ rejection in renal transplants. *Investigational:* Treatment of psoriasis.

CONTRAINDICATIONS

Hypersensitivity to sirolimus, its derivatives, or any component of the drug product. Lactation.

SPECIAL CONCERNS

Use with caution in those with impaired renal function or when using with drugs that impair renal function (e.g., aminoglycosides, amphotericin B). Safety and efficacy have not been determined in combination with other immunosuppressant drugs or in pediatric clients less than 13 years of age. Increased susceptibility to infection and possible development of lymphoma due to immunosuppression.

SIDE EFFECTS

GI: Diarrhea, nausea, constipation, vomiting, dyspepsia, anorexia, dysphagia, eructation, esophagitis, flatulence, gastritis, gastroenteritis, gingivitis, gum hyperplasia, ileus, mouth ulceration, oral moniliasis, stomatitis. **CNS:** Tremor, insomnia, anxiety, confusion, depression, dizziness, emotional lability, hypertonia, hypesthesia, hypotonia, insomnia, neuropathy, paresthesia, somnolence. **CV:** Hypertension, atrial fibrillation, CHF, hemorrhage, hypervolemia, hypotension, palpitation, peripheral vascular disorder, postural hypotension, syncope, tachycardia, thrombophlebitis, thrombosis, vasodilation. **Dermatologic:** Acne, rash, fungal dermatitis, hirsutism, pruritus, skin hypertrophy, skin ulcer, sweating. **Respiratory:** Dyspnea, URTI, pharyngitis, asthma, atelectasis, bronchitis, increased cough, epistaxis, hypoxia, lung edema, pleural effusion, pneumonia, rhinitis, sinusitis. **Hematologic:** Anemia, thrombocytopenia, leukopenia, leukocytosis, lymphadenopathy, polycythemia, thrombotic thrombocytopenic purpura (hemolytic uremic syndrome). **GU:** UTI, bladder pain, dysuria, hematuria, hydronephrosis, impotence, kidney pain, kidney tubular necrosis, nocturia, oliguria, pyuria, scrotal edema, testis disorder, toxic nephrotoxicity, increased urinary frequency, urinary incontinence, urinary retention. **Musculoskeletal:** Arthralgia, arthrosis, bone necrosis, leg cramps, myalgia, osteoporosis, tetany. **Endocrine:** Cushing's syndrome, diabetes mellitus, glycosuria. **Ophthalmic:** Abnormal vision, cataract, conjunctivitis. **Otic:** Deafness, ear pain, otitis media, tinnitus. **Miscellaneous:** Abdominal pain, asthenia, back pain, chest pain, fever, headache, pain, arthralgia, ecchymosis, dehydration, abnormal healing, weight loss, enlarged abdomen, abscess, ascites, cellulitis, chills, facial edema, flu syndrome, generalized edema, hernia, infection, lymphocele, malaise, pelvic pain, peritonitis, sepsis, increased susceptibility to infection and possible development of lymphoma.

LABORATORY TEST CONSIDERATIONS

↑ Alkaline phosphatase, BUN, creatine phosphokinase, lactic dehydrogenase, ALT, AST, serum cholesterol, triglycerides. Abnormal LFTs. Acidosis, hypercalcemia, hyperglycemia, hyperphosphatemia, hypocalcemia, hypoglycemia, hypomagnesemia, hyponatremia.

DRUG INTERACTIONS

Bromocriptine / ↑ Sirolimus blood levels R/T ↓ metabolism
Carbamazepine / ↓ Sirolimus blood levels R/T ↑ metabolism
Cimetidine / ↑ Sirolimus blood levels R/T ↓ metabolism
Cisapride / ↑ Sirolimus blood levels R/T ↓ metabolism
Clarithromycin / ↑ Sirolimus blood levels R/T ↓ metabolism
Clotrimazole / ↑ Sirolimus blood levels R/T ↓ metabolism
Cyclosporine / ↑ Sirolimus plasma levels
Danazol / ↑ Sirolimus blood levels R/T ↓ metabolism
Diltiazem / ↑ Sirolimus plasma levels

Erythromycin / ↑ Sirolimus blood levels R/T ↓ metabolism
Fluconazole / ↑ Sirolimus blood levels R/T ↓ metabolism
HIV-protease inhibitors / ↑ Sirolimus blood levels R/T ↓ metabolism
Itraconazole / ↑ Sirolimus blood levels R/T ↓ metabolism
Ketoconazole Significant ↑ sirolimus plasma levels; do not use together
Metoclopramide / ↑ Sirolimus blood levels R/T ↓ metabolism
Nicardipine / ↑ Sirolimus blood levels R/T ↓ metabolism
Phenobarbital / ↓ Sirolimus blood levels R/T ↑ metabolism
Phenytoin / ↓ Sirolimus blood levels R/T ↑ metabolism
Rifabutin / ↓ Sirolimus blood levels R/T ↑ metabolism
Rifampin / ↓ Sirolimus plasma levels R/T ↑ metabolism
Rifapentine/ ↓ Sirolimus blood levels R/T ↑ metabolism
Troleandomycin / ↑ Sirolimus blood levels R/T ↓ metabolism
Vaccines / Vaccines may be less effective
Verapamil / ↑ Sirolimus blood levels R/T ↓ metabolism

HOW SUPPLIED

Oral Solution: 1 mg/mL

DOSAGE

• ORAL SOLUTION

Prophylaxis of rejection following kidney transplantation.

Loading dose, initial: 2 mg; **maintenance dose:** 2 mg/day. Or, **Loading dose, initial:** 15 mg; **maintenance:** 5 mg/day. **Clients, 13 years and older weighing <40 kg:** Adjust the initial dose based on body surface area to 1 mg/m²/day. The loading dose should be 3 mg/m². Reduce the maintenance dose by about 33% in clients with impaired hepatic function; it is not necessary to reduce the initial loading dose.

NURSING CONSIDERATIONS

ADMINISTRATION/STORAGE

1. Use sirolimus with cyclosporine and corticosteroids. Give sirolimus 4 hr after cyclosporine.
2. Give the initial dose of sirolimus as soon as possible after transplantation.
3. To reduce dosing errors, read the label carefully. The strength of the liquid is 1 mg/mL but it is avalable in 1 mL, 2 mL, and 5 mL quantities. Thus a 2 mL vial contains 2 mg of the drug.
4. Take consistently with or without food. Grapefruit juice reduces CYP3A4-mediated metabolism; do not give sirolimus with grapefruit juice.
5. After dilution, use the product immediately. Discard the syringe after 1 use.
6. Protect the oral solution bottles and pouches from light. Refrigerate at 2–8° C (36–46° F). The oral solution is stable for 24 months under these storage conditions. Use the contents within 1 month once the bottle has been opened. If necessary, both the pouches and bottles may be stored at room temperature (25°C; 77°F) for no more than 24 hr. If the oral solution in bottles develops a slight haze when refrigerated, allow to stand at room temperature and shake gently until the haze disappears. Haze does not affect the quality of the product.

ASSESSMENT

1. Note date of transplant and for what reasons required.
2. Monitor blood sirolimus levels in pediatric clients, in those with impaired hepatic function, during concurrent administration of strong CYP3A4 inhibitors and inducers, and if cyclosporine is markedly reduced or discontinued.
3. Assess VS, ensure BP well controlled.
4. Monitor CBC, renal and LFTs as well as cyclosporine and sirolimus drug levels.

CLIENT/FAMILY TEACHING

1. Take sirolimus as prescribed with cyclosporine and corticosteroids. Take sirolimus 4 hr after cyclosporine.
2. Initial dose of sirolimus will be given as soon as possible after transplantation.
3. Review drug insert for client taking drug carefully.

S

4. Take consistently with or without food. Grapefruit juice reduces metabolism; do not give sirolimus with grapefruit juice. May enjoy juice at another time during the day.
5. Use the amber oral dose syringe to withdraw the correct amount of the oral solution. Empty from the syringe into a glass or plastic container holding 2 or more ounces of water or orange juice. Do not use any other liquids for dilution. Discard the syringe after 1 use.
6. Stir vigorously and drink at once. Refill the container with an additional volume (minimum of 4 ounces) of water or orange juice. Stir vigorously and drink at once.
7. When using the pouch, squeeze the entire contents of the pouch into a glass or plastic container containing 2 or more ounces of only water or orange juice. Stir vigorously and drink at once. Refill the container with an additional volume (minimum of 4 ounces) of water or orange juice; stir vigorously and drink at once.
8. Protect the oral solution bottles and pouches from light; refrigerate. After dilution, use the product immediately.
9. If the oral solution in bottles develops a slight haze when refrigerated, allow to stand at room temperature and shake gently until the haze disappears. Haze does not affect the quality of the product.
10. May also be prescribed antibiotics for one year to prevent *P.carinii* and CMV prophylaxis for 3 mo post transplant.
11. Females must use reliable contraception before, during and for 12 weeks after therapy has been discontinued.
12. While receiving immunosuppressive drugs, one may be more susceptible to infections and possibly lymphoma. Avoid crowds, infected persons and report any unusual side effects or symptoms of illness. Keep regularly scheduled visits at transplant center.

OUTCOMES/EVALUATE

• Prophylaxis of renal transplant rejection
• Therapeutic serum drug levels

Sodium bicarbonate

(**SO**-dee-um bye-**KAR**-bon-ayt)

PREGNANCY CATEGORY: C
CLASSIFICATION(S):
Alkalinizing agent, Antacid, Electrolyte
Rx: Neut
OTC: Arm and Hammer Pure Baking Soda, Bell/ans, Citrocarbonate, Soda Mint

ACTION/KINETICS

The antacid action is due to neutralization of hydrochloric acid by forming sodium chloride and carbon dioxide (1 g of sodium bicarbonate neutralizes 12 mEq of acid). Provides temporary relief of peptic ulcer pain and of discomfort associated with indigestion. Although widely used by the public, sodium bicarbonate is rarely prescribed as an antacid because of its high sodium content, short duration of action, and ability to cause alkalosis (sometimes desired). Is also a systemic and urinary alkalinizer by increasing plasma and urinary bicarbonate, respectively.

USES

(1) Treatment of hyperacidity, severe diarrhea (where there is loss of bicarbonate). (2) Alkalization of the urine to treat drug toxicity (e.g., due to barbiturates, salicylates, methanol). (3) Treatment of acute mild to moderate metabolic acidosis due to shock, severe dehydration, anoxia, uncontrolled diabetes, renal disease, cardiac arrest, extracorporeal circulation of blood, severe primary lactic acidosis. (4) Prophylaxis of renal calculi in gout. (5) During sulfonamide therapy to prevent renal calculi and nephrotoxicity. (6) Neutralizing additive solution to decrease chemical phlebitis and client discomfort due to vein irritation at or near the site of infusion of IV acid solutions. *Investigational:* Sickle cell anemia.

CONTRAINDICATIONS

Chloride loss due to vomiting or from continuous GI suction. With diuretics known to produce a hypochloremic alkalosis. Metabolic and respiratory alkalosis. Hypocalcemia in which alkalosis may cause tetany. Hypertension, convulsions, CHF, and other situations where administration of sodium can be dangerous. As a systemic alkalinizer when used as a neutralizing additive solution. As an antidote for strong mineral acids because carbon dioxide is formed, which may cause discomfort and even perforation.

SPECIAL CONCERNS

Use with caution in impaired renal function, toxemia of pregnancy, with oliguria or anuria, during lactation, in edema, CHF, liver cirrhosis, with low-salt diets, and in geriatric or postoperative clients with renal or CV insufficiency with or without CHF.

SIDE EFFECTS

GI: Acid rebound, gastric distention. **Milk-alkali syndrome:** Hypercalcemia, metabolic alkalosis (dizziness, cramps, thirst, anorexia, N&V, hyperexcitability, tetany, diminished breathing, ***seizures***), renal dysfunction. **Miscellaneous:** Systemic alkalosis after prolonged use. **Following rapid infusion:** Hypernatremia, alkalosis, hyperirritability, tetany, fluid or solute overload. Extravasation following IV use may manifest ulceration, sloughing, cellulitis, or tissue necrosis at the site of injection.

OD OVERDOSE MANAGEMENT

Symptoms: Severe alkalosis that may be accompanied by tetany or hyperirritability. *Treatment:* Discontinue sodium bicarbonate. Reverse symptoms of alkalosis by rebreathing expired air from a paper bag or using a rebreathing mask. Use an IV infusion of ammonium chloride solution, 2.14%, to control severe cases. Treat hypokalemia by IV sodium chloride or potassium chloride. Calcium gluconate will control tetany.

DRUG INTERACTIONS

Amphetamines / ↑ Amphetamine effect by ↑ renal tubular reabsorption
Antidepressants, tricyclic / ↑ TCA effect by ↑ renal tubular reabsorption
Benzodiazepines / ↓ Benzodiaepine effect R/T ↑ urine alkalinity
Chlorpropamide / ↑ Chlorpropamide excretion rate R/T urine alkalinization
Ephedrine / ↑ Ephedrine effect by ↑ renal tubular reabsorption
Erythromycin / ↑ Erythromycin effect in urine R/T ↑ urine alkalinity
Flecainide / ↑ Flecainide effect R/T ↑ urine alkalinity
Iron products / ↓ Iron effects R/T ↑ urine alkalinity
Ketoconazole / ↓ Ketoconazole effect R/T ↑ urine alkalinity
Lithium carbonate / Excretion of lithium proportional to amount of sodium ingested. If client on sodium-free diet, may develop lithium toxicity R/T ↓ lithium excreted
Mecamylamine / ↓ Mecamylamine excretion R/T alkalinization of the urine
Methenamine compounds / ↓ Methenamine effect R/T ↑ urine alkalinity
Methotrexate / ↑ Renal methotrexate excretion R/T alkalinization of the urine
Nitrofurantoin / ↓ Nitrofurantoin effect R/T ↑ urine alkalinity
Procainamide / ↑ Procainamide effect R/T ↓ kidney excretion
Pseudoephedrine / ↑ Pseudoephedrine effect R/T ↑ tubular reabsorption
Quinidine / ↑ Quinidine effect by ↑ renal tubular reabsorption
Salicylates / ↑ Rate of salicylate excretion R/T alkalinization of the urine
Sulfonylureas / ↓ Sulfonylurea effect R/T ↑ urine alkalinity
Sympathomimetics / ↓ Sympathomimetic renal excretion R/T alkalinization of the urine
Tetracyclines / ↓ Tetracycline effect R/T ↑ kidney excretion

HOW SUPPLIED

Injection: 4%, 4.2%, 5%, 7.5%, 8.4%; *Powder*; *Tablet:* 325 mg, 520 mg, 650 mg

DOSAGE

- **EFFERVESCENT POWDER**
  Antacid.

Adults: 3.9–10 g in a glass of cold water after meals. **Geriatric and pediatric, 6–12 years:** 1.9–3.9 g after meals.

S

• **ORAL POWDER**

Antacid.

Adults: ½ teaspoon in a glass of water q 2 hr; adjust dosage as required.

Urinary alkalinizer.

Adults: 1 teaspoon in a glass of water q 4 hr; adjust dosage as required. Dosage not established for this form for children.

• **TABLETS**

Antacid.

Adults: 0.325–2 g 1–4 times/day; pediatric, 6–12 years: 520 mg; may be repeated once after 30 min.

Urinary alkalinizer.

Adults, initial: 4 g; **then,** 1–2 g q 4 hr. **Pediatric:** 23–230 mg/kg/day; adjust dosage as needed.

• **IV**

Cardiac arrest.

Adults: 200–300 mEq given rapidly as a 7.5% or 8.4% solution. In emergencies, 300–500 mL of a 5% solution given as rapidly as possible without overalkalinizing the client. **Infants, less than 2 years of age, initial:** 1–2 mEq/kg/min given over 1–2 min; **then,** 1 mEq/kg q 10 min of arrest. Do not exceed 8 mEq/kg/day.

Severe metabolic acidosis.

90–180 mEq/L (about 7.5–15 g) at a rate of 1–1.5 L during the first hour. Adjust to needs of client.

Less severe metabolic acidosis.

Add to other IV fluids. **Adults and older children:** 2–5 mEq/kg given over a 4- to 8-hr period.

Neutralizing additive solution.

One vial of neutralizing additive solution added to 1 L of commonly used parenteral solutions, including dextrose, NaCl, and Ringer's.

S

NURSING CONSIDERATIONS

ADMINISTRATION/STORAGE

IV 1. Hypertonic solutions must be administered by trained personnel. Avoid extravasation as tissue irritation or cellulitis may result.

2. Determine IV dose by arterial blood pH, pCO_2, and base deficit; may be given IV push in arrest situation or diluted in dextrose or saline solution and given over 4–8 hr.

3. Administer isotonic solutions slowly; too-rapid administration may result in death due to cellular acidity. Check rate of flow frequently.

4. If only the 7.5% or 8.4% solution is available, dilute 1:1 with D5W when used in infants for cardiac arrest.

5. Do not exceed a rate of administration of 8 mEq/kg/day in infants with cardiac arrest to guard against hypernatremia, induction of intracranial hemorrhage, and decreasing CSF pressure.

6. In the event of severe alkalosis or tetany, have available a parenteral solution of calcium gluconate and 2.14% ammonium chloride .

7. Do not add to calcium-containing solutions, except where compatibility has been established.

8. Norepinephrine and dobutamine are incompatible with $NaHCO_3$.

ASSESSMENT

1. Note indications for therapy and any history of renal impairment or CHF.

2. Assess for edema, which may indicate inability to utilize $NaHCO_3$. May try potassium bicarbonate (sodium content is 27%).

3. If on low continuous or intermittent NG suctioning or vomiting, assess for evidence of excessive chloride loss.

4. Record I&O. Observe for dry skin and mucous membranes, polydipsia, polyuria, and air hunger; may indicate a reversal of metabolic acidosis.

5. With acidosis, assess for the relief of dyspnea and hyperpnea.

6. If prescribed to counteract metabolic acidosis, monitor electrolytes and ABGs (pH, pCO_2, and HCO_3). Test urine periodically with nitrazine paper to determine if becoming alkaline.

CLIENT/FAMILY TEACHING

1. Chew tablets thoroughly and take only as prescribed. Follow with a full glass of water.

2. If routinely taking excessive PO preparations of sodium bicarbonate to relieve gastric distress, a rebound reaction may occur, resulting either in an increased acid secretion or systemic alkalosis. Persistent symptoms of gastric distress require medical intervention.

3. Continuous, routine ingestion of sodium bicarbonate may cause for-

mation of phosphate crystals in the kidney and fluid retention.

4. Consuming sodium bicarbonate with milk or calcium may result in a milk-alkali syndrome. Report immediately if anorexia, N&V, or mental confusion occurs.

5. Avoid OTC preparations that contain sodium bicarbonate, such as Alka-Seltzer or Fizrin.

OUTCOMES/EVALUATE

- Reversal of metabolic acidosis
- ↑ Urinary and serum pH
- ↓ Gastric discomfort

Sodium chloride

(**SO**-dee-um **KLOR**-eyed)

PREGNANCY CATEGORY: C
CLASSIFICATION(S):
Electrolyte
Rx: Parenteral: Concentrated Sodium Chloride Injection (14.6%, 23.4%), Sodium Chloride IV Infusions (0.45%, 0.9%, 3%, 5%), Sodium Chloride Diluent (0.9%), Sodium Chloride Injection for Admixtures (50, 100, 625 mEq/vial)
OTC: Ophthalmic: Adsorbonac Ophthalmic, AK-NaCl, Hypersal 5%, Muro-128 Ophthalmic, Muroptic-5 **Tablets:** Slo-Salt **Topical:** Ayr Saline, HuMIST Saline Nasal, NaSal Saline Nasal, Ocean Mist, Salinex Nasal Mist.

ACTION/KINETICS

Sodium is the major cation of the body's extracellular fluid. It plays a crucial role in maintaining the fluid and electrolyte balance. Excess retention of sodium results in overhydration (edema, hypervolemia), which is often treated with diuretics. Abnormally low levels of sodium result in dehydration. Normally, the plasma contains 136–145 mEq sodium/L and 98–106 mEq chloride/L. The average daily requirement of salt is approximately 5 g.

USES

PO: Prophylaxis of heat prostration or muscle cramps, chloride deficiency due to diuresis or salt restriction, prevention or treatment of extracellular volume depletion.

Parenteral:

0.9% (Isotonic) NaCl. To restore sodium and chloride losses; to dilute or dissolve drugs for IV, IM, or SC use; flushing of IV catheters; extracellular fluid replacement; priming solution for hemodialysis; initiate and terminate blood transfusions so RBCs will not hemolyze; metabolic alkalosis when there is fluid loss and mild sodium depletion.

0.45% (Hypotonic) NaCl. Fluid replacement when fluid loss exceeds depletion of electrolytes; hyperosmolar diabetes when dextrose should not be used (need for large volume of fluid but without excess sodium ions).

3% or 5% (Hypertonic) NaCl. Hyponatremia and hypochloremia due to electrolyte losses; to dilute body water significantly following excessive fluid intake; emergency treatment of severe salt depletion.

Concentrated NaCl. Additive in parenteral therapy for clients with special needs for sodium intake.

Bacteriostatic NaCl. Used only to dilute or dissolve drugs for IM, IV, or SC injection.

Topical: Relief of inflamed, dry, or crusted nasal membranes; irrigating solution. **Ophthalmic:** Use hypertonic solutions to decrease corneal edema due to bullous keratitis; as an aid to facilitate ophthalmoscopic examination in gonioscopy, biomicroscopy, and funduscopy.

CONTRAINDICATIONS

Congestive heart failure, severely impaired renal function, hypernatremia, fluid retention. Use of the 3% or 5% solutions in elevated, normal, or only slightly depressed levels of plasma sodium and chloride. Use of bacteriostatic NaCl injection in newborns.

SPECIAL CONCERNS

Use with caution in CV, cirrhotic, or renal disease; in presence of hyperproteinemia, hypervolemia, urinary tract obstruction, and CHF; in those with concurrent edema and sodium retention and in clients receiving cortico-

S

steroids or corticotropin; and during lactation. Use with caution in geriatric or postoperative clients with renal or CV insufficiency with or without CHF.

SIDE EFFECTS

Hypernatremia.

Excessive NaCl may lead to hypopotassemia and acidosis. Fluid and solute overload leading to dilution of serum electrolyte levels, CHF, overhydration, ***acute pulmonary edema*** (especially in clients with CV disease or in those receiving corticosteroids or other drugs that cause sodium retention). Too rapid administration may cause local pain and venous irritation.

Postoperative intolerance of NaCl. Cellular dehydration, weakness, asthenia, disorientation, anorexia, nausea, oliguria, increased BUN levels, distention, deep respiration.

Symptoms due to solution or administration technique. Fever, abscess, tissue necrosis, infection at injection site, venous thrombosis or phlebitis extending from injection site, local tenderness, extravasation, hypervolemia.

Inadvertent administration of concentrated NaCl (i.e., without dilution) will cause sudden hypernatremia with the possibility of CV shock, extensive hemolysis, CNS problems, necrosis of the cortex of the kidneys, local tissue necrosis (if given extravascularly).

OD OVERDOSE MANAGEMENT

Symptoms: Irritation of GI mucosa, N&V, abdominal cramps, diarrhea, edema. Hypernatremia symptoms include: irritability, restlessness, ***weakness, seizures,*** coma, tachycardia, hypertension, fluid accumulation, ***pulmonary edema, respiratory arrest.*** *Treatment:* Supportive measures, including gastric lavage, induction of vomiting, provide adequate airway and ventilation, maintain vascular volume and tissue perfusion. Magnesium sulfate given as a cathartic.

HOW SUPPLIED

Dressing; Injection: 0.45%, 0.9%, 2.5%, 3%, 5%, 14.6%, 23.4%; *Inhalation solution:* 0.45%, 0.9%, 3%, 10%; *Irrigation solution:* 0.45%, 0.9%; *Nasal solution:* 0.4%, 0.75%; *Ophthalmic ointment:* 5%; *Ophthalmic solution:* 0.44%, 2%, 5%; *Powder for reconstitution*; *Tablet, Slow Release:* 600 mg

DOSAGE

• TABLETS (INCLUDING EXTENDED-RELEASE AND ENTERIC-COATED)

Heat cramps/dehydration.

0.5–1 g with 8 oz water up to 10 times/day; total daily dose should not exceed 4.8 g.

• IV

Individualized. Daily requirements of sodium and chloride can be met by administering 1 L of 0.9% NaCl.

To calculate sodium deficit. Amount of sodium to be given to raise serum sodium to the desired level:

Total body water (TBW): sodium deficit (mEq) = TBW × (desired plasma Na – observed plasma Na).

• OPHTHALMIC SOLUTION 2% OR 5%

1–2 gtt in eye q 3–4 hr.

• OPHTHALMIC OINTMENT 5%

A small amount (approximately ¼ in.) to the inside of the affected eye(s) (i.e., by pulling down the lower eyelid) q 3–4 hr.

NURSING CONSIDERATIONS

ADMINISTRATION/STORAGE

IV 1. Give hypertonic injections of NaCl slowly through a small-bore needle placed well within the lumen of a large vein (to minimize irritation). Avoid infiltration.

2. Concentrated NaCl injection must be diluted before use.

3. Flush IV catheters before and after the medications are given using 0.9% NaCl for injection.

4. Incompatibilities may occur when mixing NaCl injection with other additives; inspect the final product for cloudiness or a precipitate immediately after mixing, before administration, and periodically during administration. Do not store these mixtures.

ASSESSMENT

1. Note indications for therapy; monitor electrolytes, ECG, liver and renal function studies.

2. Observe for S&S of hypernatremia: flushed skin, elevated temperature, rough dry tongue, and edema. Symp-

S

toms of hyponatremia may include N&V, muscle cramps, dry mucous membranes, increased HR, and headaches.

3. Monitor VS and I&O. Assess urine specific gravity and serum sodium levels. Report if urine specific gravity is above 1.020 and serum sodium level is above 146 mEq/L.

4. Note level of consciousness; assess heart and lung sounds.

5. When administering IV the 0.45% NaCl is hypotonic, the 0.9% NaCl is isotonic, and the 3% and 5% NaCl solutions are hypertonic.

OUTCOMES/EVALUATE

- Prophylaxis of heat prostration during exposure to high temperatures or during increased activity
- Prevention of chloride deficiency R/T excessive diuresis or salt restriction or excessive sweating

Sodium ferric gluconate complex

PREGNANCY CATEGORY: B
CLASSIFICATION(S):
Antianemic, iron
Rx: Ferrlecit

ACTION/KINETICS

A stable macromolecular complex used to replete total body iron content. Iron requirements increase from erythropoietin therapy, blood loss, decreased dietary intake or absorption, surgery, malignancy, and iron sequestration due to inflammation.

USES

Iron deficiency in clients undergoing chronic hemodialysis who are receiving supplemental erythropoetin therapy.

CONTRAINDICATIONS

Hypersensitivity to sodium ferric gluconate complex. Any anemia not associated with iron deficiency. Use in neonates; product contains benzyl alcohol.

SPECIAL CONCERNS

Use with caution in the elderly and during lactation. Safety and efficacy have not been determined in children.

SIDE EFFECTS

Due to rapid IV administration of iron. Hypotension, flushing, lightheadedness, malaise, fatigue, weakness, severe pain in the chest, back, flanks, or groin. **Hypersensitivity: CV collapse, cardiac arrest, bronchospasm, oral or pharyngeal edema,** dyspnea, angioedema, urticaria, pruritus, pain and muscle spasm of the chest or back.
GI: N&V, diarrhea, rectal disorder, dyspepsia, eructation, flatulence, melena. **CNS:** Cramps, dizziness, leg cramps, paresthesias, agitation, insomnia, somnolence. **CV:** Hypotension, hypertension, syncope, tachycardia, bradycardia, angina pectoris, MI, pulmonary edema. **Hematologic:** Abnormal erythrocytes, anemia, lymphadenopathy. **Respiratory:** Dyspnea, coughing, URTI, rhinitis, pneumonia. **Musculoskeletal:** Myalgia, arthralgia. **Metabolic:** Generalized edema, leg edema, edema, hypervolemia. **Dermatologic:** Pruritus, increased sweating, rash. **Ophthalmic:** Conjunctivitis, abnormal vision. **Body as a whole:** Pain, asthenia, headache, fatigue, fever, malaise, infection, rigors, chills, flu-like syndrome, **sepsis, carcinoma. Miscellaneous:** Injection site reaction, chest pain, abdominal pain, back pain, arm pain, UTI.

LABORATORY TEST CONSIDERATIONS

Hyperkalemia, hypoglycemia, hypokalemia.

OD OVERDOSE MANAGEMENT

Symptoms: Abdominal pain, diarrhea, vomiting, pallor, cyanosis, lassitude, drowsiness, hyperventilation due to acidosis, CV collapse. *Treatment:* Treat symptoms. Product is not dialyzable.

HOW SUPPLIED

Injection: 12.5 mg/mL of elemental iron

DOSAGE

- **INJECTION**

Iron deficiency in chronic hemodialysis with erythropoetin therapy.

Therapeutic dose for iron deficiency: 10 mL (125 mg elemental iron) diluted in 100 mL of 0.9% NaCl injection

S

given over 1 hr. Do not exceed an infusion rate of 12.5 mg/min. Most will require a minimum cumulative dose of 1 g elemental iron, given over 8 sessions, at sequential dialysis treatments.

NURSING CONSIDERATIONS

ADMINISTRATION/STORAGE

IV 1. Clients may continue to require iron therapy at the lowest dose required to maintain target levels of hemoglobin, hematocrit, and lab parameters of iron storage within acceptable limits.
2. Can be infused during the dialysis session itself.
3. Do not mix with other medications or add to parenteral nutrition solutions for IV infusion.
4. Store at 20–25°C (68–77°F).
5. Use immediately after diluting with saline.

ASSESSMENT

1. Note indications for therapy, onset, characteristics and etiology of deficiency and other agents trialed.
2. Ensure that test dose has been performed before initiating therapy (25 mg in 50 mL NSS over 60 min).
3. List drugs prescribed.
4. Monitor VS, CBC, iron panel, renal and LFTs.

CLIENT/FAMILY TEACHING

1. Drug is used to replace low iron stores. The drug erythropoetin does not work to improve red blood cells effectively if the iron level is too low.
2. May be given during dialysis to prevent additional sticks.
3. Report any unusual or persistant side effects.

OUTCOMES/EVALUATE

- Restoration of serum iron levels
- Improvement in exercise tolerance and level of fatigue
- Improvement in skin pallor, color of nail beds, Hb and iron levels

Sodium polystyrene sulfonate

(**SO**-dee-um pol-ee-**STY**-reen **SUL**-fon-ayt)

PREGNANCY CATEGORY: C

CLASSIFICATION(S):
Potassium-removing resin
Rx: Kayexalate, SPS
★Rx: PMS Sodium Polystyrene Sulfonate

ACTION/KINETICS

Resin that exchanges sodium ions for potassium ions primarily in the large intestine. Thus, excess amounts of potassium (as well as calcium and magnesium) may be removed. Therapy is governed by daily monitoring of serum potassium levels. Discontinue therapy when serum potassium levels have reached 4–5 mEq/L. Monitor for serum calcium and magnesium levels.
Onset, PO: 2–12 hr.

USES

Hyperkalemia.

SPECIAL CONCERNS

Use with caution in geriatric clients because they are more likely to develop fecal impaction. Use with caution in clients sensitive to sodium overload (e.g., in CV disease) or for those receiving digitalis preparations because the action of these agents is potentiated by hypokalemia. Effective decreases in potassium may take several hours to accomplish; other treatment (e.g., IV calcium or sodium bicarbonate or glucose and insulin) may be considered in states of severe hyperkalemia (e.g., burns, renal failure).

SIDE EFFECTS

GI: N&V, constipation, anorexia, gastric irritation, diarrhea (rarely). Fecal impaction in geriatric clients. **Electrolyte:** Sodium retention, hypokalemia, hypocalcemia, hypomagnesemia. **Other:** Overhydration, ***pulmonary edema.***

DRUG INTERACTIONS

Aluminum hydroxide / ↑ Risk of intestinal obstruction; ↓ effect of resin to exchange potassium
Calcium- or magnesium-containing antacids or laxatives / ↑ Risk of metabolic alkalosis; ↓ effect of resin to exchange potassium

HOW SUPPLIED

Powder for reconstitution: About 100 mg/g; *Suspension:* 15 g/60 mL

DOSAGE

• POWDER FOR SUSPENSION, SUSPENSION

Hyperkalemia.

Adults: 15 g resin suspended in 20–100 mL water or syrup (to increase palatability) 1–4 times/day. Up to 40 g/day has been used. **Pediatric:** To calculate dose, use an exchange ratio of 1 mEq potassium/g resin (usually, 1 g/kg dose).

• ENEMA

Hyperkalemia.

Adults: 30–50 g suspended in 100 mL sorbitol or 20% dextrose in water q 6 hr.

NURSING CONSIDERATIONS

ADMINISTRATION/STORAGE

1. Designate on orders the grams of powder and the percent sorbitol and volume to be used or the amount of premixed suspension; specify frequency and route of administration.
2. Avoid inhaling the powder for suspension when admixing.

ASSESSMENT

1. Document serum potassium levels. Attempt to identify cause for increased levels. Also monitor renal function studies and levels of sodium, magnesium, and calcium.
2. Determine any history of CV disease and/or if taking any digitalis preparations.
3. Assess clients on sodium restrictions closely; drug contains 100 mg Na/g.

CLIENT/FAMILY TEACHING

1. The use of Ca- or Mg-containing antacids during PO administration of sodium polystyrene may cause metabolic alkalosis; use cautiously.
2. Take exactly as prescribed; report as scheduled for F/U.
3. Report any increase in urinary output or constipation or lack of response.
4. To treat or to prevent constipation, 10–20 mL of 70% sorbitol may be given PO q 2 hr (or as necessary) to produce 1–2 watery stools each day.
5. For PO administration, give the resin suspended in water or sorbitol syrup (3–4 mL/g resin). If necessary, the resin can be administered through a NGT, either as an aqueous suspension, mixed with dextrose, or as a peanut or olive oil emulsion.
6. Rectal administration:
   • First, administer a cleansing enema.
   • To administer medication, insert a large-size rubber tube (e.g., 28 French) into the rectum for a distance of 20 cm until it is well into the sigmoid colon and tape in place.
   • Suspend resin in appropriate vehicle (see *Dosage;* 30-50 g suspended in 100 mL sorbitol or 20% dextrose in water)at body temperature. Administer by gravity while stirring suspension.
   • Flush remaining suspension in the container with 50–100 mL fluid, clamp the tube, and leave in place.
   • Elevate hips or assume a knee-chest position for a short time if there is back leakage.
   • Keep the enema in the colon as long as possible (3–4 hr).
   • Resin is removed by colonic irrigation with 2 quarts of a *non-sodium*-containing solution warmed to body temperature. Returns are drained constantly through a Y tube.
7. With enemas, retain solution for several hours to ensure effectiveness.
8. Retention enemas are not as effective as oral administration.
9. Use freshly prepared solutions within 24 hr. Do not heat resin.
10. Oral suspension products contain sorbitol and sodium.

OUTCOMES/EVALUATE

↓ Serum K+ levels (4.0–5.5 mEq/L)

Somatrem

(**SO**-mah-trem)

PREGNANCY CATEGORY: C
Rx: Protropin

Somatropin

(so-mah-**TROH**-pin)

PREGNANCY CATEGORY: C, SEROSTIM IS B
Rx: Genotropin, Humatrope, Norditropin, Nutropin, Nutropin AQ, Nutropin Depot, Saizen, Serostim
CLASSIFICATION(S):
Growth hormone

ACTION/KINETICS

Both somatrem and somatropin are derived from recombinant DNA technology. Somatrem contains the same sequence of amino acids (191) as human growth hormone derived from the pituitary gland plus one additional amino acid (methionine). Somatropin has the identical sequence of amino acids as does human growth hormone of pituitary origin. These agents stimulate linear growth by increasing somatomedin-C serum levels, which, in turn, increases the incorporation of sulfate into proteoglycans, thereby stimulating skeletal growth. They also increase the number and size of muscle cells, increase synthesis of collagen, increase protein synthesis, and increase internal organ size. Serum insulin levels increase (indicative of insulin resistance), and there is acute mobilization of lipid. **Peak plasma levels, somatotropin:** 7.5 hr after SC. **t½, somatotropin:** 3.8 hr after SC and 4.9 hr after IM.

USES

Somatrem. Long-term treatment of growth failure in children due to lack of adequate endogenous growth hormone secretion. **Somatropin.** (1) Except for Serostim to stimulate linear growth of children who suffer from lack of adequate levels of endogenous growth hormone. (2) Long-term replacement therapy in adults with growth hormone deficiency of either childhood or adult-onset (use Genotropin, Humatrope, Nutropin, Nutropin AQ). (3) Treat growth failure associated with chronic renal insufficiency up to the time of renal transplantation (use Nutropin or Nutropin AQ only). (4) Treat growth failure in children with Prader-Willi syndrome (use Genotropin only). (5) Long-term treatment of short stature associated with Turner's syndrome (use Humatrope, Nutropin, and Nutropin AQ only). (6) Treatment of AIDS wasting or cachexia (use Serostim only). *Investigational:* Short children due to intrauterine growth retardation.

CONTRAINDICATIONS

In clients in whom epiphyses have closed. Active intracranial lesions, sensitivity to benzyl alcohol (somatrem); sensitivity to m-cresol or glycerin (diluent in Humatrope). Use of Genotropin to treat acute catabolism in critically ill clients. *NOTE:* Hypothyroidism (which may be induced by the drug) decreases the response to somatrem.

SPECIAL CONCERNS

Use with caution during lactation. Concomitant use of glucocorticoids may decrease the response to growth hormone.

SIDE EFFECTS

Development of persistent antibodies to growth hormone (30%–40% taking somatrem and 2% taking somatropin). Development of insulin resistance; hypothyroidism. Sodium retention and mild edema (especially in adults). Slipped capital femoral epiphysis or avascular necrosis of the femoral head in children with advanced renal osteodystrophy. Intracranial hypertension manifested by papilledema, visual changes, headache, N&V. **In adults:** Hyperglycemia, glucosuria; mild, transient edema; headache, weakness, muscle pain. **In children:** Injection site pain, leukemia.

Nutropin AQ: CTS, increased growth of preexisting nevi, gynecomastia, peripheral edema (rare), pancreatitis (rare). *Somatropin:* In adults, headache, localized muscle pain, weakness, mild hyperglycemia, glucosuria, mild transient edema during early treatment.

OD OVERDOSE MANAGEMENT

Symptons: In acute overdose, hypoglycemia followed by hyperglycemia. Long-term overdose can result in S&S of acromegaly or gigantism.

DRUG INTERACTIONS

Glucocorticoids inhibit the effect of somatrem on growth.

HOW SUPPLIED

Somatrem: *Protropin (Powder for injection lyophilized:* 5 mg, 10 mg. **Somatropin:** *Genotropin (Powder for injection, lyophilized):* 1.5 mg/vial, 5.8 mg/vial, 13.8 mg/vial; *Genotropin Miniquick (Powder for injection, lyophilized):* 0.2 mg/vial, 0.4 mg/vial, 0.6 mg/vial, 0.8 mg/vial, 1 mg/vial, 1.2 mg/vial, 1.4 mg/vial, 1.6 mg/vial, 1.8

mg/vial, 2 mg/vial; *Humatrope (Powder for injection, lyophilized):* 5 mg, 6 mg, 12 mg, 24 mg; *Norditropin (Injection):* 5 mg/1.5 mL, 10 mg/1.5 mL, 15 mg/1.5 mL; *Norditropin (Powder for injection, lyophilized):* 4 mg/vial, 8 mg/vial; *Nutropin (Powder for injection, lyophilized):* 5 mg, 10 mg; *Nutropin AQ (Injection):* 10 mg; *Nutropin Depot (Powder for injection):* 13.5 mg, 18 mg, 22.5 mg; *Saizen (Powder for injection, lyophilized):* 5 mg; *Serostim (Powder for injection, lyophilized):* 4 mg, 5 mg, 6 mg

DOSAGE

SOMATREM (PROTROPIN)

• **IM, SC**

Individualized. Usual: Up to 0.1 mg/kg (0.26 IU/kg) 3 times/week, not to exceed a weekly dosage of 0.30 mg/kg (about 0.90 IU/kg). The incidence of side effects increases if the dose is greater than 0.1 mg/kg.

SOMATROPIN (GENOTROPIN)

• **SC**

Adult growth hormone deficiency.

Initial: No more than 0.04 mg/kg/week. May increase dose at 4– 8–week intervals according to client response, up to a maximum of 0.08 mg/kg/week.

Pediatric growth hormone deficiency.

0.16–0.24 mg/kg/week.

Pediatric Prader-Willi syndrome.

0.24 mg/kg/week.

SOMATROPIN (HUMATROPE)

• **IM, SC**

Most uses.

Adults: Individualized. Initial: 0.006 mg/kg/day (0.018 IU/kg/day) or less SC. May be increased, depending on need, to a maximum of 0.0125 mg/kg/day (0.0375 IU/kg/day). **Pediatric:** 0.18 mg/kg/week (0.54 IU/kg/week) SC or IM divided into equal doses given either on 3 alternate days or 6 times a week. Maximum weekly replacement dose is 0.3 mg/kg (0.9 IU/kg). Divide into equal doses and given on 3 alternate days, six days a week, or daily.

Turner syndrome.

Up to 3.75 mg/kg/week (1.125 IU/kg/week) SC. Divide into equal doses given daily or on 3 alternate days.

SOMATRIPIN (NORDITROPIN)

• **IM, SC**

0.024–0.034 mg/kg 6 to 7 times a week.

SOMATROPIN (NUTROPIN, NUTROPIN AQ)

• **SC**

Growth hormone deficiency.

Adults, initial: 0.006 mg/kg or less/day in clients less than 35 years of age, up to a maximum of 0.025 mg/kg/day in those less 35 years of age and a maximum of 0.0125 mg/kig/day in those over 35 years of age. Lower doses may be needed in older or overweight clients. **Children:** Up to 0.3 mg/kg/week divided into daily SC injections.

Chronic renal insufficiency.

Up to 0.35 mg/kg/week divided into daily SC injections. May continue therapy up to renal transplantation.

Turner syndrome.

0.375 mg/kg/week or less divided into equal doses 3–7 times/week SC.

SOMATROPIN (NUTROPIN DEPOT)

• **SC**

1.5 mg/kg SC on the same day each month. Those more than 15 mg require more than 1 injection/dose. For twice-monthly injections, give 0.75 mg/kg SC twice each month on the same days of each month (e.g., days 1 and 15). Clients over 30 kg require more than 1 injection/dose.

SOMATROPIN (SAIZEN)

• **IM, SC**

0.06 mg/kg (about 0.18 IU/kg) 3 times weekly. Discontinue when epiphyses fuse.

SOMATROPIN (SEROSTIM)

• **SC**

Weight > 55 kg: 6 mg daily; **45–55 kg:** 5 mg daily; **35–45 kg:** 4 mg daily; **less than 35 kg:** 0.1 mg/kg. Give daily dose at bedtime.

NURSING CONSIDERATIONS

ADMINISTRATION/STORAGE

1. Somatrem should be prescribed only by a physician experienced in the

S

diagnosis and treatment of pituitary disorders.

2. Due to the development of insulin resistance, evaluate for possible glucose intolerance.

3. Reconstitue somatrem (Protropin – powder for injection, lyophilized) *only* with bacteriostatic water for injection (benzyl alcohol preserved).

4. If used in newborns, reconstitute somatrem with water for injection because benzyl alcohol can be toxic to newborns.

5. Inject only reconstituted somatrem solution that is clear and without particulate matter.

6. Be sure needle used for injection is at least 1 in. or longer so that the injection reaches muscle layer.

7. Use reconstituted somatrem within 7 days; do not freeze.

8. The following information is applicable to *Genotropin*:

• Divide the weekly dose into 6 or 7 SC injections and give in the thigh, buttocks, or abdomen. Rotate site of injections daily to help prevent lipoatrophy.

• Genotropin is supplied in a two-chamber cartridge with the drug in the front chamber and the diluent in the rear chamber. Use a reconstitution device to co-mix the drug and diluent following the directions on the package. Gently tip the cartridge upside down a few times until complete dissolution occurs. Do not shake.

• The 1.5-mg cartridge may be refrigerated for 24 hr or less because it contains no preservative. Use once and discard any remaining solution. The 5.8- and 13.8-mg cartridges contain a preservative and may be stored under refrigeration for up to 14 days.

9. The following information is applicable to *Humatrope:*

• Reconstitute by adding 1.5–5 mL of the diluent supplied for each 5-mg vial. Do not reconstitute with the diluent for Humatrope provided with Humatrope vials. Do not shake the vial. Do not give the reconstituted solution if it is cloudy or contains particulate material. Use a small enough syringe to ensure accuracy when the solution is withdrawn from the vial.

• Vials are stable for 14 days or less after reconstitution with diluent for Humatrope or bacteriostatic water for injection when stored in a refrigerator.

• After reconstitution with sterile water, use only one dose/Humatrope vial and discard the unused portion.

• If the solution is not used immediately, refrigerate at 2–8°C (36–46°F) and used within 24 hr.

• After reconstitution, cartridges of Humatrope are stable for up to 28 days when reconstituted with diluent for Humatrope and stored in a refrigerator. Avoid freezing.

10. The following information is applicable to *Norditropin:*

• Give in the thighs and vary injection site on the thigh on a rotating basis.

• When using the cartridges, use the corresponding color-coded Nor NNN Nordipen injection pen. The 5 mg/1.5 mL cartridge uses the orange pen, the 10 mg/1.5 mL cartridge uses the blue pen, and the 15 mg/1.5 mL cartridge uses the green pen.

• Reconstitute each 4 or 8 mg vial with the 2 mL diluent.

• Before and after reconstitution, refrigerate. Do not freeze. Use reconstituted vials within 14 days after dissolution.

• Avoid direct light.

11. The following information is applicable to *Nutropin, Nutropin AQ:*

• To reconstitute Nutropin, add 1–5 mL bacteriostatic water for injection (benzyl alcohol preserved) per each 5 mg vial and 1–10 mL per each 10 mg vial.

• Before reconstitution, refrigerate Nutropin. Reconstituted vials are stable for up to 14 days when refrigerated. Avoid freezing.

• For Nutropin AQ, vials are stable for 28 days after initial use when stored in the refrigerator. Avoid freezing.

12. The following information is applicable to *Nutropin Depot:*

• To reconstitute use only the diluent provided in the kit and give with the needles supplied.

• The suspension is viscous and thus withdrawal of the entire vial contents is not possible. Thus, vials are overfilled.

• Using the diluent volumes recommended results in a final concentraion of 19 mg/mL somatropin in each vial size.
• To reconstitute, inject the diluent into the vial against the vial wall. Swirl the vial vigorously for up to 2 min to disperse the powder. Mixing is complete when the suspension appears uniform, thick, and milky and all the powder is fully dispersed.
• Do not store the vial after reconstitution or the suspension may settle.
• Withdraw the required dose. Use only 1 vial for each injection. Replace the needle with a new needle from the kit and give the dose immediately to avoid the suspension settling in the syringe. Give the dose at a continuous rate over not more than 5 sec.
• Discard unused vial contents as the product contains no preservative.
13. The following information is applicable to *Saizen:*
• Reconstitute with 1–2 mL bacteriostatic water for injection.
• Before reconstitution store at room temperature. Reconstituted solutions are stable for up to 14 days when refrigerated. Avoid freezing.
14. The following information is applicable to *Serosim:*
• Reconstitute each vial with 1 mL sterile water for injection.
• Before reconstitution, store at room temperature. Use within 24 hr after reconstitution with diluent. Refrigerate reconstituted solutoin.

ASSESSMENT

1. Note indications for therapy, age of client, and any other therapy trialed.
2. Determine that X-ray evidence of bone growth (wrists, hands) has been conducted. Record height and weight monthly. Generally a growth increase of 2 cm/year should be attained in order for treatment to be continued.
3. If growth slow in absence of rising antibody titers, hypopituitarism should be ruled out; untreated hypothyroidism or excessive glucocorticoid replacement can impair growth.
4. Monitor blood sugar and thyroid function studies; assess for diabetes or hypothyroidism. With diabetes, assess for hyperglycemia and acidosis.
5. Note any limps or knee/hip pain because a slipped capital epiphysis may occur.

CLIENT/FAMILY TEACHING

1. Keep and review drug literature with guidelines for administration, drug preparation, and storage, after instructed by provider. Drug is given IM or SC three times per week.
2. Keep a growth record and report as scheduled for F/U.
3. Report any adverse effects or any limps or knee or hip pain. May experience sudden growth spurts with increased appetite.
4. The cost per year is based on client's weight and typically runs $10,000–$30,000.

OUTCOMES/EVALUATE

Desired skeletal growth; (growth hormone replacement with deficiency)

Sotalol hydrochloride

(**SOH**-tah-lol)

PREGNANCY CATEGORY: B
CLASSIFICATION(S):
Beta-adrenergic blocking agent
Rx: Betapace, Betapace AF
✱Rx: Alti-Sotalol, Apo-Sotalol, Gen-Sotalol, Novo-Sotalol, Nu-Sotalol, PMS-Sotalol, Rho-Sotalol, Rylosol, Sotacor

SEE ALSO ***BETA-ADRENERGIC BLOCKING AGENTS.***

ACTION/KINETICS

Blocks both beta-1- and beta-2-adrenergic receptors; has no membrane-stabilizing activity or intrinsic sympathomimetic activity. Has both Group II and Group III antiarrhythmic properties (dose dependent). Significantly increases the refractory period of the atria, His-Purkinje fibers, and ventricles. Also prolongs the QTc and JT intervals. **t½:** 12 hr. Not metabolized; excreted unchanged in the urine.

USES

(1) Treatment of documented ventricular arrhythmias such as life-threaten-

ing sustained VT. (2) Betapace AF is used for maintenance of normal sinus rhythm in those with symptomatic atrial fibrillation/atrial flutter who are in sinus rhythm; since Betapace AF can cause lifie-threatening ventricular arrhythmias, reserve use for those who are highly symptomatic. *Do not substitute Betapace for Betapace AF.*

CONTRAINDICATIONS

Use in asymptomatic PVCs or supraventricular arrhythmias due to the proarrhythmic effects of sotalol. Congenital or acquired long QT syndromes. Use in clients with hypokalemia or hypomagnesemia until the imbalance is corrected, as these conditions aggravate the degree of QT prolongation and increase the risk for torsades de pointes.

SPECIAL CONCERNS

Clients with sustained ventricular tachycardia and a history of CHF appear to be at the highest risk for serious proarrhythmia. Dose, presence of sustained ventricular tachycardia, females, excessive prolongation of the QTc interval, and history of cardiomegaly or CHF are risk factors for torsades de pointes. Use with caution in clients with chronic bronchitis or emphysema and in asthma if an IV agent is required. Use with extreme caution in clients with sick sinus syndrome associated with symptomatic arrhythmias due to the increased risk of sinus bradycardia, sinus pauses, or sinus arrest. Reduce dosage in impaired renal function. Safety and efficacy in children have not been established. Do *not* interchange Betapace and Betapace AF due to significant differences in dosage and safety, although clients can be transferred to Betapace AF from Betapace.

ADDITIONAL SIDE EFFECTS

CV: ***New or worsened ventricular arrhythmias, including sustained VT or ventricular fibrillation that might be fatal. Torsades de pointes.***

HOW SUPPLIED

Betapace Tablets: 80 mg, 120 mg, 160 mg, 240 mg; **Betapace AF Tablets**: 80 mg, 120 mg,160 mg

DOSAGE

• BETAPACE TABLETS

Ventricular arrhythmias.

Adults, initial: 80 mg b.i.d. The dose may be increased to 240 or 320 mg/day after appropriate evaluation. **Usual:** 160–320 mg/day given in two or three divided doses. Clients with life-threatening refractory ventricular arrhythmias may require doses ranging from 480 to 640 mg/day (due to potential proarrhythmias, use these doses only if the potential benefit outweighs the increased risk of side effects). Use the following doses in clients with impaired renal function: 80 mg b.i.d. if C_{CR} is greater than 60 mL/min, 80 mg once daily if the C_{CR} is between 30 and 59 mL/min, and 80 mg every 36–48 hr if the C_{CR} is between 10 and 29 mL/min. Individualize dose if the C_{CR} is < 10 mL/min.

• BETAPACE AF TABLETS

Maintenance of normal sinus rhythm in those with symptomatic atrial fibrillation/atrial flutter who are in sinus rhythm.

Dose individualized according to calculated creatinine clearance. Initial: 80 mg. **Maintenance:** 80 mg b.i.d. if C_{CR} is greater than 60 mL/min and 80 mg once daily if the C_{CR} is between 40 and 60 mL/min. Do not use in clients with a C_{CR} less than 40 mL/min. Can be titrated upward to 120 mg during initial hospitalization or after discharge on 80 mg in the event of recurrence, by rehospitalization and repating the same steps used during initiation of therapy. An increase in dose to 160 mg b.i.d. or q.d. can be considered if the 120 mg dose does not reduce the frequency of early relapse of AFIB/AFL and is tolerated without excessive QT interval prolongation. Doses higher than 160 mg b.i.d. are associated with an increased incidence of torsade de pointes.

NURSING CONSIDERATIONS

SEE ALSO *NURSING CONSIDERATIONS* FOR *BETA-ADRENERGIC BLOCKING AGENTS.*

ADMINISTRATION/STORAGE

1. Adjust dosage gradually, allowing 2–3 days between increments in dos-

age. This allows steady-state plasma levels to be reached and QT intervals to be monitored.
2. Undertake dosage initiation and increases in a hospital with facilities for cardiac rhythm monitoring. Dosage must be individualized only after appropriate clinical assessment.
3. Proarrhythmias can occur during initiation of therapy and with each dosage increment.
4. In clients with impaired renal function, alter the dosing interval as follows: if C_{CR} is 30–60 mL/min, the dosing interval is 24 hr; if C_{CR} is 10–30 mL/min, the dosing interval should be 36–48 hr. If C_{CR} is less than 10 mL/min, dose must be individualized. Undertake dosage adjustments in clients with impaired renal function only after five to six doses at the intervals described.
5. Before initiating sotalol, withdraw previous antiarrhythmic therapy with careful monitoring for a minimum of 2–3 plasma half-lives if condition permits.
6. Do not initiate sotalol after amiodarone is discontinued until the QT interval is normalized.

Initiation and Maintenance of Betapace AF Therapy

1. Determine the QT interval prior to initiation of therapy using an average of 5 beats. If the baseline QT is greater than 450 msec (JT equal to or greater than 330 msec if QRS over 100 msec), do not use Betapace AF.
2. Calculate the creatinine clearance.
3. Initiate the correct dose of Betapace AF, depending on the creatinine clearance (see Dosage).
4. Begin continuous ECG monitoring with QT interval measurements 2–4 hr after each dose.
5. If the 80 mg dose is tolerated and the QT interval remains less than 500 msec after at least 3 days (after 5 or 6 doses if client is receiving once daily dosing), the client can be discharged. Alternatively, during hospitalization, the dose can be increased to 120 mg b.i.d. if the 80 mg dose does not reduce the frequency and relapses of AFIB/AFL. Once again, the client is followed for 3 days on this dose (or 5 or 6 doses if receiving once daily dosing).
6. If the 120 mg dose b.i.d. or q.d. does not reduce the frequency of early relapses of AFIB/AFL and is tolerated without excessive QT interval prolongation (520 msec or longer), Betapace AF can be increased to 160 mg b.i.d. or q.d., provided appropriate monitoring is undertaken.
7. Re-evaluate renal function and QT regularly if medically warranted. If QT is 520 msec or greater (JT 430 msec or greater if QRS is over 100 msec), reduce the dose of Betapace AF and monitor carefully until QT returns to less than 520 msec.
8. If the QT interval is 520 msec or greater while on the lowest maintenance dose (80 mg), discontinue the drug.
9. If renal function decreases, reduce the daily dose in half and administer the drug once daily.
10. If a dose is missed, the next dose should not be doubled. The next dose should be taken at the usual time.
11. Before starting Betapace AF, withdraw previous antiarrhythmic therapy, with careful monitoring, for a minimum of 2 or 3 plasma half-lives if the clinical condition permits.
12. Do not initiate Betapace AF after amiodarone until the QT interval is normalized.

ASSESSMENT

1. Perform a thorough nursing history; note any cardiomegaly or CHF.
2. Obtain ECG and document QT interval; note symptoms associated with arrhythmia.
3. Client should be in a closely monitored environment with VS and ECG monitored during initiation and adjustment of sotalol.
4. Monitor VS, I&O, electrolytes, Mg^{+} level, renal and LFTs.

CLIENT/FAMILY TEACHING

1. Take on an empty stomach as food decreases absorption.
2. Take exactly as directed and do not stop abruptly; drug controls symptoms but does not cure condition.

S

3. Avoid activites that require mental alertness until drug effects realized; may cause dizziness/drowsiness.
4. Report increased chest pain/SOB, night cough, swelling of feet and ankles, increased fatigue, low heart rate, or unsteady gait.
5. Avoid alcohol and OTC agents.
6. Continue dietary and exercise guidelines as prescribed and healthy life-style changes.

OUTCOMES/EVALUATE

Control/conversion of life-threatening arrhythmias to stable cardiac rhythm

Sparfloxacin

(spar-**FLOX**-ah-sin)

PREGNANCY CATEGORY: C
CLASSIFICATION(S):
Antibiotic, fluoroquinolone
Rx: Zagam

SEE ALSO *FLUOROQUINOLONES*.

ACTION/KINETICS

Well absorbed. **Peak serum levels:** 4–5 hr. 50% excreted in the urine.

USES

(1) Community acquired pneumonia due to *Chlamydia pneumoniae, Haemophilus influenzae, Haemophilus parainfluenzae, Moraxella catarrhalis, Mycoplasma pneumoniae,* or *Streptococcus pneumoniae.* (2) Acute bacterial exacerbations of chronic bronchitis caused by *C. pneumoniae, Enterobacter cloacae, H. influenzae, H. parainfluenzae, Klebsiella pneumoniae, M. catarrhalis, Staphylococcus aureus,* or *S. pneumoniae.* (3) Treatment of tuberculosis.

SPECIAL CONCERNS

Safety and efficacy have not been determined in children less than 18 years of age.

HOW SUPPLIED

Tablets: 200 mg.

DOSAGE

• **TABLETS**

Community-acquired pneumonia, acute bacterial exacerbations of chronic bronchitis.

Adults over 18 years of age: Two - 200 mg tablets taken on the first day as a loading dose. Then, one - 200 mg tablet q 24 hr for a total of 10 days of therapy (i.e., a total of 11 tablets). For clients with a C_{CR} less than 50 mL/min, the loading dose is two - 200 mg tablets taken on the first day. Then, one - 200 mg tablet q 48 hr for a total of 9 days (i.e., a total of 6 tablets).

Treatment of tuberculosis.

200 mg (maximum)/day.

NURSING CONSIDERATIONS

SEE ALSO *NURSING CONSIDERATIONS FOR FLUOROQUINOLONES*.

ASSESSMENT

1. Document onset, location, duration, and characteristics of symptoms.
2. Monitor CBC, cultures, and renal function studies; reduce dose with impaired renal function.

CLIENT/FAMILY TEACHING

1. Take exactly as directed (4 hr before or 2 hr after antacids, dairy products, or zinc products); may be taken with or without food. Consume at least 2L fluid/day.
2. Do not perform activities that require mental alertness until drug effects realized.
3. Avoid prolonged sun exposue, may experience photosensitivity reaction.
4. Complete entire prescription and do not skip or double up on doses unless directed.
5. Report any unusual side effects or lack of response after 72 hr.

OUTCOMES/EVALUATE

• Symptomatic improvement
• Resolution of infection

Spectinomycin hydrochloride

(speck-tin-oh-**MY**-sin)

PREGNANCY CATEGORY: B
CLASSIFICATION(S):
Antibiotic, miscellaneous
Rx: Trobicin

SEE ALSO *ANTI-INFECTIVES*.

ACTION/KINETICS

Produced by *Streptomyces spectabilis.* It inhibits bacterial protein synthesis by binding to ribosomes (30S subunit), thereby interfering with transmission of genetic information crucial to life of microorganism. Mainly bacteriostatic. Only given IM. **Peak plasma concentration:** 100 mcg/mL (2-g dose) after 1 hr and 160 mcg/mL (4-g dose) after 2 hr. **t½:** 1.2–2.8 hr. Not significantly bound to protein. Excreted in urine.

USES

(1) Acute gonorrheal proctitis and urethritis in males and acute gonorrheal cervicitis and proctitis in females due to susceptible strains of *Neisseria gonorrhoeae.* (2) For pharyngeal infections, use only in those intolerant to cephalosporins or quinolones. It is ineffective against pharyngeal infections and against syphilis; is a poor drug to choose when mixed infections are present.

CONTRAINDICATIONS

Sensitivity to drug.

SPECIAL CONCERNS

Safe use during pregnancy, in infants, and in children has not been established. Benzyl alcohol in the product may cause a fatal gasping syndrome in infants.

SIDE EFFECTS

A single dose of spectinomycin has caused soreness at the site of injection, urticaria, dizziness, nausea, chills, fever, and insomnia. Multiple doses have caused a decrease in H&H and C_{CR} and an increase in alkaline phosphatase, BUN, and ALT. In single or multiple doses, decrease in urine output.

HOW SUPPLIED

Powder for injection: 400 mg/mL (when reconstituted)

DOSAGE

• **IM ONLY**

Gonorrheal urethritis in males, proctitis, and cervicitis.

2 g. In geographic areas where antibiotic resistance is known to be prevalent, give 4 g divided between two gluteal injection sites.

Alternative regimen for urethral, endocervical, or rectal gonococcal infections in clients who cannot take ceftriaxone.

Adults and children weighing more than 45 kg: Spectinomycin, 2 g, as a single dose followed by doxycycline. **Children weighing less than 45 kg:** 40 mg/kg given IM once.

Gonococcal infections in pregnancy where client is allergic to beta-lactams.

2 g followed by erythromycin.

Disseminated gonococcal infection where client is allergic to beta-lactams.

2 g q 12 hr.

NURSING CONSIDERATIONS

SEE ALSO *GENERAL NURSING CONSIDERATIONS FOR ALL ANTI-INFECTIVES.*

ADMINISTRATION/STORAGE

1. Powder is stable for 3 years.
2. Contains benzyl alcohol; may cause fatal gasping syndrome in infants.
3. Use reconstituted solution within 24 hr.
4. Inject deeply into the upper, outer quadrant of the gluteus muscle.
5. Injections may be divided between two sites for clients requiring 4 g. Rotate and document injection sites.

CLIENT/FAMILY TEACHING

1. Return for serologic tests monthly for 3 mo if syphilis suspected; with gonorrhea, report for repeat serologic test 3 mo after treatment.
2. Obtain counseling and encourage treatment of sexual partners.
3. Abstain from intercourse until infection is resolved; follow safe sex practices to prevent reinfections.

OUTCOMES/EVALUATE

• Negative serology/cultures for gonorrhea

• Symptomatic improvement with gonorrheal urethritis, cervicitis, and/or proctitis

Spironolactone

(speer-oh-no-**LAK**-tohn)

PREGNANCY CATEGORY: D

CLASSIFICATION(S):

Diuretic, potassium-sparing

Rx: Aldactone

✱**Rx:** Novo-Spiroton

SEE ALSO *DIURETICS, THIAZIDES.*

S

ACTION/KINETICS

Mild diuretic that acts on the distal tubule to inhibit sodium exchange for potassium, resulting in increased secretion of sodium and water and conservation of potassium. An aldosterone antagonist. Manifests a slight antihypertensive effect. Interferes with synthesis of testosterone and may increase formation of estradiol from testosterone, thus leading to endocrine abnormalities. **Onset:** Urine output increases over 1–2 days. **Peak:** 2–3 days. **Duration:** 2–3 days, and declines thereafter. Metabolized to an active metabolite (canrenone). **t½:** 13–24 hr for canrenone. Canrenone is excreted through the urine (primary) and the bile. Almost completely bound to plasma protein.

USES

(1) Primary hyperaldosteronism, including diagnosis, short-term preoperative treatment, long-term maintenance therapy for those who are poor surgical risks and those with bilateral micronodular or macronodular adrenal hyperplasia. (2) To treat edema when other approaches are inadequate or ineffective (e.g., CHF, cirrhosis of the liver, nephrotic syndrome). (3) Essential hypertension (usually in combination with other drugs). (4) Prophylaxis of hypokalemia in clients taking digitalis. *Investigational:* Hirsutism, treat symptoms of PMS, with testolactone to treat familial male precocious puberty (short-term treatment), acne vulgaris. In severe heart failure with recommended therapies to reduce mortaility.

S

CONTRAINDICATIONS

Acute renal insufficiency, progressive renal failure, hyperkalemia, and anuria. Clients receiving potassium supplements, amiloride, or triamterene.

SPECIAL CONCERNS

Use during pregnancy only if benefits clearly outweigh risks. Use with caution in impaired renal function. Geriatric clients may be more sensitive to the usual adult dose.

SIDE EFFECTS

Electrolyte: Hyperkalemia, hyponatremia (characterized by lethargy, dry mouth, thirst, tiredness). **GI:** Diarrhea, cramps, ulcers, gastritis, gastric bleeding, vomiting. **CNS:** Drowsiness, ataxia, lethargy, mental confusion, headache. **Endocrine:** Gynecomastia, menstrual irregularities, impotence, bleeding in postmenopausal women, deepening of voice, hirsutism. **Dermatologic:** Maculopapular or erythematous cutaneous eruptions, urticaria. **Miscellaneous:** Drug fever, breast carcinoma, gynecomastia, hyperchloremic metabolic acidosis in hepatic cirrhosis (decompensated), ***agranulocytosis.*** *NOTE:* Spironolactone has been shown to be tumorigenic in chronic rodent studies.

LABORATORY TEST CONSIDERATIONS

Interference with radioimmunoassay for digoxin. False + plasma cortisol (as determined by fluorometric assay of Mattingly).

DRUG INTERACTIONS

ACE inhibitors / Significant hyperkalemia
Anesthetics, general / Additive hypotension
Anticoagulants, oral / Inhibited by spironolactone
Antihypertensives / ↑ Hypotensive effect of both agents; ↓ dosage, especially of ganglionic blockers, by one-half
Captopril / ↑ Risk of significant hyperkalemia
Digoxin / ↑ Half-life of digoxin → ↓ clearance. Spironolactone may ↓ inotropic effect of digoxin. Spironolactone both ↑ and ↓ elimination t½ of digitoxin
Diuretics, others / Often given together due to potassium-sparing effect of spironolactone. Possible severe hyponatremia; monitor closely
Lithium / ↑ Risk of lithium toxicity R/T ↓ renal clearance
Norepinephrine / ↓ NE effect
Potassium salts / Hyperkalemia R/T spironolactone conserving potassium excessively. Rarely used together
Salicylates / Large doses may ↓ spironolactone effects
Triamterene / Possible hazardous hyperkalemia

HOW SUPPLIED

Tablet: 25 mg, 50 mg, 100 mg

DOSAGE

• **TABLETS**

Edema.

Adults, initial: 100 mg/day (range: 25–200 mg/day) in two to four divided doses for at least 5 days; **maintenance:** 75–400 mg/day in two to four divided doses. **Pediatric:** 3.3 mg/kg/day as a single dose or as two to four divided doses.

Antihypertensive.

Adults, initial: 50–100 mg/day as a single dose or as two to four divided doses—give for at least 2 weeks; **maintenance:** adjust to individual response. **Pediatric:** 1–2 mg/kg in a single dose or in two to four divided doses.

Hypokalemia.

Adults: 25–100 mg/day as a single dose or two to four divided doses.

Diagnosis of primary hyperaldosteronism.

Adults: 400 mg/day for either 4 days (short-test) or 3–4 weeks (long-test).

Hyperaldosteronism, prior to surgery.

Adults: 100–400 mg/day in two to four doses prior to surgery.

Hyperaldosteronism, chronic-therapy.

Use lowest possible dose.

Hirsutism.

50–200 mg/day.

Symptoms of PMS.

25 mg q.i.d. beginning on day 14 of the menstrual cycle.

Familial male precocious puberty, short-term.

Spironolactone, 2 mg/kg/day, and testolactone, 20–40 mg/kg/day, for at least 6 months.

Acne vulgaris.

100 mg/day.

Reduce mortality in severe CHF.

25–50 mg/day with other therapies (e.g., ACE inhibitor, loop diuretic).

NURSING CONSIDERATIONS

SEE ALSO *NURSING CONSIDERATIONS* FOR *DIURETICS, THIAZIDES.*

ADMINISTRATION/STORAGE

1. When used as the sole drug to treat edema, maintain the initial dose for at least 5 days. After that, adjustments may be made. If the dosage is not effective, a second diuretic may be added, especially one that acts in the proximal tubules.
2. When administered to small children, tablets may be crushed and given as suspension in cherry syrup.
3. Food may increase the absorption of spironolactone.
4. Protect the drug from light.

ASSESSMENT

1. Document indications for therapy, other agents prescribed, and the outcome.
2. With cardiac disease, be alert for irregularities R/T hypokalemia.
3. Monitor ABGs, ECG, CBC, blood sugar, uric acid, serum electrolytes, and liver and renal function studies. Record VS, I&O, and weights.
4. If client develops dysuria, urinary frequency, or renal spasm, obtain a urinalysis and urine culture.
5. Assess for drug tolerance characterized by edema and reduced urine output.

CLIENT/FAMILY TEACHING

1. Take as directed with a snack or meals to minimize GI upset. Report if nausea, bloating, anorexia, vomiting, or diarrhea persist.
2. Record BP for provider review.
3. Avoid foods or salt substitutes high in potassium; drug is potassium-sparing.
4. Record weight twice a week. Report any evidence of edema or weight gain/loss of more than 5 lb (2.2 kg) weekly.
5. Do not drive/operate dangerous machinery until drug effects realized; may cause drowsiness or unsteady gait.
6. Drug may cause gynecomastia and diminished libido by reducing testosterone levels.
7. Report if deep, rapid respirations, headaches, or mental slowing occurs; may indicate hyperchloremic metabolic acidosis.
8. Drug is metabolized in the liver. Report jaundice, tremors, or mental confusion; may develop hepatic encephalopathy with liver disease.

S

9. With CAD, drug is used to reduce mortality in those with CHF.

OUTCOMES/EVALUATE

- Enhanced diuresis with ↓ edema
- ↓ BP
- Antagonism of high levels of aldosterone
- Prevention of hypokalemia
- Reduced mortality in CAD with CHF

Stavudine

(**STAH**-vyou-deen)

PREGNANCY CATEGORY: C
CLASSIFICATION(S):
Antiviral, nucleoside reverse transcriptase inhibitor
Rx: Zerit

SEE ALSO *ANTIVIRAL AGENTS.*

ACTION/KINETICS
Inhibits replication of HIV due to phosphorylation by cellular kinases to stavudine triphosphate, which has antiviral activity. The mechanism for the antiviral activity includes inhibition of HIV reverse transcriptase by competing with the natural substrate deoxythymidine triphosphate and by causing DNA chain termination, thereby inhibiting viral DNA synthesis. Rapidly absorbed. **Peak plasma levels:** 1 hr or less. **t½, terminal:** Approximately 1.4 hr after PO use in adults and 0.96 hr in children. About 40% of the drug is eliminated through the kidney.

USES
(1) Treatment of adults with advanced HIV infection who cannot tolerate approved therapies or who have experienced significant clinical or immunologic deterioration while receiving such therapies (or for whom such therapies are contraindicated). (2) With didanosine, as well as either a protease inhibitor or nonnucleoside analog, as first-line therapy for HIV-1 infections.

CONTRAINDICATIONS
Lactation.

SPECIAL CONCERNS
The effect of stavudine on the clinical progression of HIV infection, such as incidence of opportunistic infections or survival, has not been determined. Increased risk of fatal lactic acidosis in pregnant women taking stavudine with didanosine; use together in this population only if benefits outweigh risks.

SIDE EFFECTS
Neurologic: Peripheral neuropathy (common), including numbness, tingling, or pain in feet or hands. **CNS:** Insomnia, anxiety, depression, nervousness, dizziness, confusion, migraine, somnolence, tremor, neuralgia, dementia. **GI:** Diarrhea, N&V, anorexia, dyspepsia, constipation, ulcerative stomatitis, aphthous stomatitis, ***pancreatitis, lactic acidosis and severe hepatomegaly with steatosis, hepatic failure.*** **Body as a whole:** Headache, chills, fever, asthenia, abdominal pain, back pain, malaise, weight loss, allergic reactions, flu syndrome, lymphadenopathy, pelvic pain, myalgia, ***neoplasms, death.*** **CV:** Chest pain, vasodilation, hypertension, peripheral vascular disorder, syncope. **Hematologic:** Anemia, leukopenia, thrombocytopenia. **GU:** Dysuria, genital pain, dysmenorrhea, vaginitis, urinary frequency, hematuria, impotence, urogenital neoplasm. **Respiratory:** Dyspnea, pneumonia, asthma. **Dermatologic:** Rash, sweating, pruritus, maculopapular rash, benign skin neoplasm, urticaria, exfoliative dermatitis. **Ophthalmic:** Conjunctivitis, abnormal vision.

LABORATORY TEST CONSIDERATIONS
↑ AST, ALT, amylase, bilirubin, GGT, lipase.

DRUG INTERACTIONS
Zidovudine may competitively inhibit intracellular phosphorylation of stavudine; do not use together.

HOW SUPPLIED
Capsule: 15 mg, 20 mg, 30 mg, 40 mg; *Powder for Oral Solution:* 1 mg/mL

DOSAGE

- **CAPSULES, ORAL SOLUTION**
  Advanced HIV infections.

Adults, initial: 40 mg b.i.d. for clients weighing 60 or more kg and 30 mg b.i.d. for clients weighing less than 60 kg. **Children:** 1 mg/kg/dose if weight is less than 30 kg; more than 30 kg, use adult dose. In clients developing peripheral neuropathy, the following dosage schedule may be used if symptoms of neuropathy resolve completely: 20 mg b.i.d. for clients weighing 60 or more kg and 15 mg b.i.d. for clients weighing less than 60 kg.

The following dosage schedule is recommended for clients with impaired renal function: (a) C_{CR} greater than 50 mL/min: 40 mg q 12 hr for clients weighing 60 or more kg and 30 mg q 12 hr for clients weighing less than 60 kg; (b) C_{CR} 26–50 mL/min: 20 mg q 12 hr for clients weighing 60 or more kg and 15 mg q 12 hr for clients weighing less than 60 kg; (c) C_{CR} 10–25 mL/min: 20 mg q 24 hr for clients weighing 60 or more kg and 15 mg q 24 hr for clients weighing less than 60 kg. Insufficient data are available to recommend doses for a C_{CR} less than 10 mL/min. For clients undergoing dialysis: 20 mg q 24 hr for clients weighing 60 or more kg and 15 mg q 24 hr for clients weighing less than 60 kg. Give after dialysis is completed and at the same time of day on nondialysis days.

NURSING CONSIDERATIONS

SEE *NURSING CONSIDERATIONS* FOR *ANTIVIRAL AGENTS.*

ADMINISTRATION/STORAGE

1. To reconstitute the powder for oral solution, add 202 mL purified water to the container. Shake vigorously until powder is completely dissolved. This produces 200 mL of deliverable drug at a concentration of 1 mg/mL. The solution may be slightly hazy.
2. The interval between PO doses is 12 hr.

ASSESSMENT

1. Document onset of symptoms, other agents prescribed, and date confirmed; note date of intolerance.
2. Obtain baseline CBC, CD_4 counts/viral load, PT/PTT, liver and renal function studies. Reduce dose with impaired renal function.

CLIENT/FAMILY TEACHING

1. May be taken without regard to meals.
2. Take exactly as prescribed q 12h RTC, do not exceed prescribed dose, and do not share medications.
3. Shake container with oral solution vigorously before measuring each dose. Store, tightly closed, in the refrigerator. Discard any unused portion after 30 days.
4. Drug is not a cure, but alleviates/manages the symptoms of HIV infections. May continue to acquire illnesses associated with AIDS or ARC, including opportunistic infections; must remain under close medical supervision.
5. The risk of transmission of HIV to others through blood or sexual contact is not reduced with drug therapy. Review the criteria and precautions for safe sex and do not share needles.
6. Insomnia and GI upset usually resolve after 3–4 weeks of therapy.
7. Report any S&S of infection (i.e., sore throat, swollen glands, fever).
8. Report symptoms of peripheral neuropathy characterized by numbness and tingling or pain in the hands and/or feet and discontinue drug if evident. Symptoms may temporarily worsen following cessation of drug therapy but, once resolved, drug may be reintroduced at a lower dose.
9. Report for all scheduled lab studies and follow-up visits to assess response to therapy and to identify any adverse drug effects.
10. Identify local support groups that may assist client/family to understand and cope with this disease.

OUTCOMES/EVALUATE

Clinical/immunologic improvement with AIDS and ARC

S

Streptokinase

(strep-toe-**KYE**-nayz)

PREGNANCY CATEGORY: C
CLASSIFICATION(S):
Thrombolytic enzyme
Rx: Streptase
✱**Rx:** Kabikinase

ACTION/KINETICS

Most clients have a natural resistance to streptokinase that must be overcome with the loading dose before the drug becomes effective. Streptokinase acts with plasminogen to produce an "activator complex," which enhances the conversion of plasminogen to plasmin. Plasmin then breaks down fibrinogen, fibrin clots, and other plasma proteins, promoting the dissolution (lysis) of the insoluble fibrin trapped in intravascular emboli and thrombi. Also, inhibitors of streptokinase, such as alpha-2-macroglobulin, are rapidly inactivated by streptokinase. **Onset:** rapid; **duration:** 12 hr. **t½, activator complex:** 23 min.

USES

DVT; arterial thrombosis and embolism; acute evolving transmural MI; pulmonary embolism. Also, clearing of occluded arteriovenous and IV cannulae.

CONTRAINDICATIONS

Any condition presenting a risk of hemorrhage, such as recent surgery or biopsies, delivery within 10 days, ulcerative disease. Arterial emboli originating from the left side of the heart. Also, hepatic or renal insufficiency, tuberculosis, recent cerebral embolism, thrombosis, hemorrhage, SBE, rheumatic valvular disease, thrombocytopenia. Streptokinase resistance in excess of 1 million IU. Use to restore patency to IV catheters.

SPECIAL CONCERNS

S

The use of streptokinase in septic thrombophlebitis may be hazardous. History of significant allergic response. Safety in children has not been established. Geriatric clients have an increased risk of bleeding during therapy. Serious reactions, including hypotension, hypersensitivity, apnea, and bleeding have been associated with using streptokinase for restoring catheter patency.

SIDE EFFECTS

CV: Superficial bleeding, ***severe internal bleeding.*** **Allergic:** Nausea, headache, breathing difficulties, ***bronchospasm, angioneurotic edema,*** urticaria, flushing, musculoskeletal pain, vasculitis, interstitial nephritis, periorbital swelling. **Other:** Fever, possible development of Guillain-Barre syndrome, development of antistreptokinase antibody (i.e., streptokinase may be ineffective if administered between 5 days and 6 months following prior use of streptokinase or following streptococcal infections).

LABORATORY TEST CONSIDERATIONS

↓ Fibrinogen, plasminogen. ↑ Thrombin time, PT, and activated PTT.

DRUG INTERACTIONS

The following drugs increase the chance of bleeding when given concomitantly with streptokinase: anticoagulants, aspirin, heparin, indomethacin, and phenylbutazone.

HOW SUPPLIED

Powder for injection: 250,000 IU, 750,000 IU, 1.5 million IU

DOSAGE

• **IV INFUSION**

DVT, pulmonary embolism, arterial thrombosis or embolism.

Loading dose: 250,000 IU over 30 min (use the 1,500,000 IU vial diluted to 90 mL); **maintenance:** 100,000 IU/hr for 24–72 hr for arterial thrombosis or embolism, 72 hr for deep vein thrombosis, and 24 hr (72 hr if deep vein thrombosis is suspected) for pulmonary embolism.

Acute evolving transmural MI.

1,500,000 IU within 60 min (use the 1,500,000 IU vial diluted to a total of 45 mL).

Arteriovenous cannula occlusion.

Before using, try to clear cannula using heparinized saline solution (syringe technique). If adequate flow does not occur, slowly instill 250,000 IU in 2-mL IV solution into each occluded limb of cannula and clamp off; **then,** after 2 hr aspirate cannula limbs, flush with saline, and reconnect cannula.

• **INTRACORONARY INFUSION**

Acute evolving transmural MI.

20,000 IU by bolus; **then,** 2,000 IU/min for 60 min (total dose of 140,000 IU). Use the 250,000 IU vial diluted to 125 mL.

NURSING CONSIDERATIONS

SEE ALSO *NURSING CONSIDERATIONS* FOR *ALTEPLASE, RECOMBINANT.*

ADMINISTRATION/STORAGE

IV 1. NaCl injection USP or D5W is the preferred diluent for IV use.
2. For AV cannulae, dilute 250,000 units with 2 mL of NaCl injection or D5W.
3. Reconstitute gently, as directed, without shaking vial.
4. Use within 24 hr of reconstitution.
5. Use an electronic infusion device to administer streptokinase and do not add any other medications to the line. Note any redness and/or pain at the site of infusion; may need to further dilute to prevent phlebitis.
6. Have emergency drugs and equipment available. Have corticosteroids and aminocaproic acid available for excessive bleeding.
7. Do not add other medication to streptokinase.

ASSESSMENT

1. Document indications for therapy, type, onset, and characteristics of symptoms.
2. Note any history of tuberculosis, SBE, ulcerative disease, recent surgery, or streptococcal infection.
3. Assess for bleeding tendency, heart disease, and/or allergic drug reactions.
4. Identify other drugs taking such as aspirin or NSAIDs that could increase bleeding times.
5. Clients with high allergy potential or high streptokinase antibody titer may benefit by skin testing prior to administering therapy. Drug may not be effective if administered within 5 days to 6 months of a strep infection or previous use.
6. Obtain baseline lab studies; ensure that bleeding studies, type and crossmatch, and streptokinase resistance have been completed before initiation of therapy.

INTERVENTIONS

1. Observe in a continously monitored environment; document rhythm strips and VS.
2. Check access sites for evidence of bleeding. Test stools, urine, and emesis for occult blood.
3. During IV therapy, arterial sticks require 30 min of manual pressure followed by application of a pressure dressing. To prevent bruising, avoid unnecessary handling of client.
4. If IM injections necessary, apply pressure after withdrawing the needle to prevent hematoma and bleeding from the puncture site. Observe injection sites and postoperative wounds for bleeding during therapy
5. If excessive bleeding develops from an invasive procedure, discontinue therapy and call for packed RBCs and plasma expanders *other than dextran.*
6. To prevent new thrombus formation, or rethrombosis, IV heparin and oral anticoagulants are used when therapy is concluded.
7. Note allergic reactions, ranging from anaphylaxis to moderate and mild reactions. These usually can be controlled with antihistamines and corticosteroids.
8. Fever reaction may be treated with acetaminophen.
9. Following recanalization of an occluded coronary artery, clients may develop reperfusion reactions; these may include:
- Reperfusion arrhythmias (accelerated idioventricular rhythm, sinus bradycardia) usually of short duration.
- Reduction of chest pain
- Return of elevated ST segment to near baseline levels

CLIENT/FAMILY TEACHING

1. Review inherent benefits and risks of drug therapy.
2. To be effective, the therapy should be instituted within 4–6 hr of onset of symptoms of acute MI.
3. Report any symptoms or side effects immediately.
4. Encourage family members or significant other to learn CPR.

OUTCOMES/EVALUATE

- Lysis of emboli/thrombi with restoration of normal blood flow
- ↓ Myocardial infarct size; improved ventricular function
- Catheter patency in previously occluded AV or IV cannulae

S

Streptozocin

(strep-toe-**ZOH**-sin)

PREGNANCY CATEGORY: C
CLASSIFICATION(S):
Antineoplastic, alkylating
Rx: Zanosar

SEE ALSO *ANTINEOPLASTIC AGENTS* AND *ALKYLATING AGENTS*.

ACTION/KINETICS
Cell-cycle nonspecific although it does inhibit progression out of the G_2 phase of cell division. Forms methylcarbonium ions that alkylate or bind with intracellular substances such as nucleic acids. Also cytotoxic by virtue of cross-linking of DNA strands resulting in inhibition of DNA synthesis. May cause hyperglycemia. Does not penetrate the blood-brain barrier well, although within 2 hr after administration, metabolites do and produce levels similar to those in plasma. **t½, unchanged drug, initial:** 35 min. **t½, metabolites, initial:** 6 min; **intermediate:** 3.5 hr; **terminal:** 40 hr. Unchanged drug and metabolites excreted in urine.

USES
Metastatic islet cell pancreatic carcinomas (functional and nonfunctional) in clients with symptomatic or progressive metastases. *Investigational:* Malignant carcinoid tumors.

CONTRAINDICATIONS
Lactation.

SPECIAL CONCERNS
Dosage has not been determined for children.

ADDITIONAL SIDE EFFECTS
Renal toxicity (up to two-thirds of clients) manifested by anuria, azotemia, glycosuria, hypophosphatemia, and renal tubular acidosis. ***Toxicity is dose-related and cumulative and may be fatal.*** Glucose intolerance (reversible) or insulin shock with hypoglycemia, depression.

HOW SUPPLIED
Powder for injection: 1 g (100 mg/mL)

DOSAGE

• **IV**

Daily schedule: 500 mg/m² for 5 consecutive days q 6 weeks (until maximum benefit is achieved or toxicity occurs). Do not increase dose. *Weekly schedule:* **Initial:** 1,000 mg/m²/week for 2 weeks; **then,** if no response or no toxicity, dose can be increased, not to exceed a single dose of 1,500 mg/m². Expect a response in 17–35 days.

NURSING CONSIDERATIONS

SEE ALSO *NURSING CONSIDERATIONS* FOR *ANTINEOPLASTIC AGENTS*.

ADMINISTRATION/STORAGE
IV 1. Reconstitute with 9.5 mL dextrose or 0.9% NaCl injection. Reconstituted solution is pale gold in color and contains 100 mg/mL streptozocin. This may be further diluted. Administer slowly over 1–2 hr.
2. Total storage time for reconstituted drug is 12 hr, as there are no preservatives present. The ampule is not multiple dose.
3. Observe caution (wear gloves) in handling the drug.
4. Drug is a vesicant. Infiltration may result in tissue ulceration and necrosis.

ASSESSMENT
1. Document indications for therapy, characteristics of symptoms, and other agents trialed.
2. Premedicate with antiemetic; may cause severe N&V.
3. Monitor I&O, lab studies, and weight. Consume 3 L/day of fluids to reduce the risk of renal damage; if urine output decreases streptozocin can cause anuria.
4. Monitor blood sugar, CBC, uric acid, liver and renal function studies. Drug may cause lymphocyte and platelet suppression. Nadir: 10 days; recovery: 14–17 days.

OUTCOMES/EVALUATE
↓ Tumor size and spread; suppression of malignant cell proliferation

Succinylcholine chloride

(suck-sin-ill-**KOH**-leen)

PREGNANCY CATEGORY: C

CLASSIFICATION(S):
Neuromuscular blocking drug, depolarizing
Rx: Anectine, Anectine Flo-Pack, Quelicin

SEE ALSO *NEUROMUSCULAR BLOCKING AGENTS.*

ACTION/KINETICS
Initially excites skeletal muscle by combining with cholinergic receptors preferentially to acetylcholine. Subsequently, it prevents the muscle from contracting by prolonging the time during which the receptors at the neuromuscular junction cannot respond to acetylcholine. The order of paralysis is levator muscles of the eyelid, mastication muscles, limb muscles, abdominal muscles, glottis muscles, the intercostals, the diaphragm, and all other skeletal muscles. Prolonged use may change from a depolarizing neuromuscular block (phase I block) to a block that resembles a nondepolarizing block (phase II block). This may be associated with prolonged respiratory depression and apnea. No effect on pain threshold, cerebration, or consciousness; use with sufficient anesthesia. Effects are not blocked by anticholinesterase drugs and may even be enhanced by them. May cause a change in myocardial rhythm due to vagal stimulation due to surgical procedures (especially in children) and from potassium-mediated alterations in electrical conductivity (enhanced by cyclopropane and halogenated anesthetics). **IV: onset,** 30–60 sec; **duration:** 4–6 min; **recovery:** 8–10 min. **IM: Onset,** 2–3 min; **duration:** 10–30 min. Metabolized by plasma pseudocholinesterase to succinylmonocholine, which is a nondepolarizing muscle relaxant, and then to succinic acid and choline. About 10% excreted unchanged in the urine.

USES
Adjunct to general anesthesia to facilitate ET intubation and to induce relaxation of skeletal muscle during surgery or mechanical ventilation. *Investigational:* Reduce intensity of electrically induced seizures or seizures due to drugs.

CONTRAINDICATIONS
Use in genetically determined disorders of plasma pseudocholinesterase. Personal or family history of malignant hyperthermia. Myopathies associated with elevated CPK values. Acute narrow-angle glaucoma or penetrating eye injuries. Use of IV infusion in children due to the risk of malignant hyperpyrexia.

SPECIAL CONCERNS
Use with caution during lactation. Pediatric clients may be especially prone to myoglobinemia, myoglobinuria, and cardiac effects. Use with caution in clients with severe liver disease, severe anemia, malnutrition, impaired cholinesterase activity, fractures. Also, use with caution in CV, pulmonary, renal, or metabolic diseases. Use with great caution in those with severe burns, electrolyte imbalance, hyperkalemia, those receiving quinidine, and those who are digitalized or recovering from severe trauma, as serious cardiac arrhythmias or cardiac arrest may result. Clients with myasthenia gravis may show resistance to succinylcholine. Those with fractures or muscle spasms may manifest additional trauma due to succinylcholine-induced muscle fasciculations.

SIDE EFFECTS
Skeletal muscle: May cause ***severe, persistent respiratory depression or apnea.*** Muscle fasciculations, postoperative muscle pain. **CV:** Bradycardia or tachycardia, hypertension, hypotension, ***arrhythmias, cardiac arrest.*** **Respiratory:** ***Apnea, respiratory depression.*** **Other:** Fever, salivation, hyperkalemia, postoperative muscle pain, ***anaphylaxis,*** myoglobinemia, myoglobinuria, skin rashes, increased intraocular pressure, muscle fasciculation, myalgia, jaw rigidity, perioperative dreams in children, rhabdomyolysis with possible myoglobinuric acute renal failure. Repeated doses may cause tachyphylaxis. ***Malignant hyperthermia:*** Muscle rigidity (especially

S

of the jaw), tachycardia, tachypnea unresponsive to increased depth of anesthesia, increased oxygen requirement and carbon dioxide production, increased body temperature, metabolic acidosis.

OD OVERDOSE MANAGEMENT

Symptoms: Skeletal muscle weakness, decreased respiratory reserve, low tidal volume, apnea. *Treatment:* Maintain a patent airway and respiratory support until normal respiration is ensured.

DRUG INTERACTIONS

Aminoglycoside antibiotics / Additive skeletal muscle blockade
Amphotericin B / ↑ Succinylcholine effect R/T induced electrolyte imbalance
Antibiotics, nonpenicillin / Additive skeletal muscle blockade
Beta-adrenergic blocking agents / Additive skeletal muscle blockade
Chloroquine / Additive skeletal muscle blockade
Cimetidine / Inhibits pseudocholinesterase
Clindamycin / Additive skeletal muscle blockade
Cyclophosphamide / ↑ Succinylcholine effect by ↓ breakdown by plasma pseudocholinesterase
Cyclopropane / ↑ Risk of bradycardia, arrhythmias, sinus arrest, apnea, and malignant hyperthermia
Diazepam / ↓ Succinycholine effect
Digitalis glycosides / ↑ Risk of cardiac arrhythmias, including VF
Echothiophate iodide / ↑ Succinylcholine effect by ↓ breakdown by plasma pseudocholinesterase
Furosemide / ↑ Skeletal muscle blockade
Halothane / ↑ Risk of bradycardia, arrhythmias, sinus arrest, apnea, and malignant hyperthermia
Isoflurane / Additive skeletal muscle blockade
Lidocaine / Additive skeletal muscle blockade
Lincomycin / Additive skeletal muscle blockade
Lithium carbonate / ↑ Skeletal muscle blockade
Magnesium salts / Additive skeletal muscle blockade
Narcotics / ↑ Risk of bradycardia and sinus arrest
Nitrous oxide / ↑ Risk of bradycardia, arrhythmias, sinus arrest, apnea, and malignant hyperthermia
Oxytocin / ↑ Succinylcholine effect
Phenelzine / ↑ Succinylcholine effect
Phenothiazines / ↑ Succinylcholine effect
Polymyxin / Additive skeletal muscle blockade
Procainamide / ↑ Succinylcholine effect
Procaine / ↑ Succinylcholine effect by inhibiting plasma pseudocholinesterase
Promazine / ↑ Succinylcholine effect
Quinidine / Additive skeletal muscle blockade
Quinine / Additive skeletal muscle blockade
Tacrine / ↑ Succinylcholine effect
Thiazide diuretics / ↑ Succinylcholine effect due to induced electrolyte imbalance
Thiotepa / ↑ Succinylcholine effect by ↓ breakdown by plasma pseudocholinesterase
Trimethaphan / ↑ Succinylcholine effect by inhibiting plasma pseudocholinesterase

HOW SUPPLIED

Injection: 20 mg/mL, 50 mg/mL, 100 mg/mL; *Powder for infusion:* 500 mg, 1 g

DOSAGE

• IM, IV

Short or prolonged surgical procedures.

Adults, IV, initial: 0.3–1.1 mg/kg (average: 0.6 mg/kg); **then,** repeated doses can be given based on client response. **Adults, IM:** 3–4 mg/kg, not to exceed a total dose of 150 mg.

• IV INFUSION (PREFERRED)

Prolonged surgical procedures.

Adults: Average rate ranges from 2.5 to 4.3 mg/min. Most commonly used are 0.1%–0.2% solutions in 5% dextrose, sodium chloride injection, or other diluent given at a rate of 0.5–10 mg/min depending on client response and degree of relaxation desired, for up to 1 hr.

• **INTERMITTENT IV**

Prolonged muscle relaxation.

Initial: 0.3–1.1 mg/kg; **then,** 0.04–0.07 mg/kg at appropriate intervals to maintain required level of relaxation.

• **IM, IV**

Electroshock therapy.

Adults, IV: 10–30 mg given 1 min prior to the shock (individualize dosage). **IM:** Up to 2.5 mg/kg, not to exceed a total dose of 150 mg.

ET intubation.

Pediatric, IV: 1–2 mg/kg; if necessary, dose can be repeated. **IM:** 3–4 mg/kg, not to exceed a total dose of 150 mg.

NURSING CONSIDERATIONS

SEE ALSO *NURSING CONSIDERATIONS* FOR *NEUROMUSCULAR BLOCKING AGENTS.*

ADMINISTRATION/STORAGE

IV 1. Give an initial test dose of 0.1 mg/kg to assess sensitivity and recovery time.

2. Do not mix with anesthetic.

3. For IV infusion, use 1 or 2 mg/mL solution of drug in D5W, 0.9% NaCl, or other suitable IV solution; not compatible with alkaline solutions.

4. To reduce salivation, premedicate with atropine or scopolamine.

5. Have neostigmine or pyridostigmine available to reverse neuromuscular blockade.

6. Refrigerate drug at 2–8°C (36–46°F). Multidose vials stable for 14 days or less at room temperature without significant loss of potency.

ASSESSMENT

1. List agents currently prescribed to ensure that none interact unfavorably. Note if the client is taking digitalis products or quinidine. These clients are sensitive to the release of intracellular potassium.

2. Obtain baseline ECG, lytes, liver and renal function studies. Those with low plasma pseudocholinesterase levels are sensitive to the effects of succinylcholine and require lower doses.

3. Document any evidence/history of MS, malignant hyperthermia, CPK myopathy, acute glaucoma, or eye injury; drug generally contraindicated.

4. Use a peripheral nerve stimulator to assess neuromuscular function and to confirm recovery from neuromuscular blockade.

5. Medicate for pain and anxiety as drug does not affect and client unable to convey. Reassure that they will regain function once therapy completed.

INTERVENTIONS

1. A peripheral nerve stimulator should be used to assess neuromuscular response and recovery. The order of paralysis is levator muscles of the eyelid, mastication muscles, limb muscles, abdominal muscles, glottis muscles, the intercostals, the diaphragm, and all other skeletal muscles. This is reversed with recovery.

2. Monitor VS and ECG; can cause vagal stimulation resulting in bradycardia, hypotension, and cardiac arrhythmias, especially in children.

3. Observe for excessive, transient increase in intraocular pressure.

4. Muscle fasciculations may cause the client to be sore and injured after recovery. Administer prescribed nondepolarizing agent (i.e., tubocurarine) and reassure that the soreness is likely caused by unsynchronized contractions of adjacent muscle fibers just before onset of paralysis.

5. Monitor for evidence of malignant hyperthermia, unresponsive tachycardia, jaw spasm, or lack of laryngeal relaxation.

6. Drug should be used only on a short-term basis and in a continuously monitored environment. Prolonged use may change from a depolarizing neuromuscular block (phase I block) to a block that resembles a nondepolarizing block (phase II block) which may be associated with prolonged respiratory depression and apnea.

7. Client fully conscious and aware of surroundings/conversations.

8. Drug does not affect pain or anxiety; administer analgesics and antianxiety agents as indicated.

9. When used for seizures, ensure that serum level of anticonvulsant agent is therapeutic. Succinylcholine does not cross the blood-brain barrier

and will only suppress peripheral manifestations of seizures, not the central process.

OUTCOMES/EVALUATE

- Muscle relaxation/paralysis
- Suppression of the twitch response
- Facilitation of ET intubation; control of breathing during mechanical ventilation

Sucralfate

(sue-**KRAL**-fayt)

PREGNANCY CATEGORY: B
CLASSIFICATION(S):
Antiulcer drug
Rx: Carafate
★Rx: Apo-Sucralfate, Novo-Sucralate, Nu-Sucralfate, PMS-Sucralfate, Sulcrate, Sulcrate Suspension Plus

ACTION/KINETICS

Thought to form an ulcer-adherent complex with albumin and fibrinogen at the site of the ulcer, protecting it from further damage by gastric acid. May also form a viscous, adhesive barrier on the surface of the gastric mucosa and duodenum. It adsorbs pepsin, thus inhibiting its activity. May be used in conjunction with antacids. Approximately 90% excreted in the feces. **Duration:** 5 hr.

USES

(1) Short-term treatment (up to 8 weeks) of active duodenal ulcers. (2) Maintenance for duodenal ulcer at decreased dosage after healing of acute ulcers. *Investigational:* Hasten healing of gastric ulcers, chronic treatment of gastric ulcers. Treatment of reflux and peptic esophagitis. Treatment of aspirin- and NSAID-induced GI symptoms; prevention of stress ulcers and GI bleeding in critically ill clients. The suspension has been used to treat oral and esophageal ulcers due to chemotherapy, radiation, or sclerotherapy.

NOTE: Even though healing of ulcers may result, the frequency or severity of subsequent attacks is not altered.

SPECIAL CONCERNS

Safety for use in children and during lactation has not been fully established. A successful course resulting in healing of ulcers will not alter posthealing frequency or severity of duodenal ulceration.

SIDE EFFECTS

GI: Constipation (most common); also, N&V, diarrhea, indigestion, flatulence, dry mouth, gastric discomfort. **Hypersensitivity:** Urticaria, ***angioedema, respiratory difficulty,*** rhinitis. **Miscellaneous:** Back pain, dizziness, sleepiness, vertigo, rash, pruritus, facial swelling, ***laryngospasm.***

DRUG INTERACTIONS

Antacids containing aluminum / ↑ Total body burden of aluminum
Anticoagulants / ↓ Warfarin hypoprothrombinemic effect
Cimetidine / ↓ Cimetidine absorption R/T binding to sucralfate
Ciprofloxacin / ↓ Ciprofloxacin absorption R/T binding to sucralfate
Digoxin / ↓ Digoxin absorption R/T binding to sucralfate
Ketoconazole / ↓ Ketoconaozle bioavailability
Levothyroxine / ↓ Therapeutic effect of levothyroxine due to ↓ GI absorption
Norfloxacin / ↓ Norfloxacin absorption R/T binding to sucralfate
Phenytoin / ↓ Phenytoin absorption R/T binding to sucralfate
Quinidine / ↓ Quinidine levels → ↓ effect
Ranitidine / ↓ Ranitidine absorption R/T binding to sucralfate
Tetracycline / ↓ Tetracycline absorption R/T binding to sucralfate
Theophylline / ↓ Theophylline absorption R/T binding to sucralfate

HOW SUPPLIED

Suspension: 1 g/10 mL; *Tablet:* 1 g

DOSAGE

- **SUSPENSION, TABLETS**

Adults: usual: 1 g q.i.d. (10 mL of the suspension) 1 hr before meals and at bedtime (it may also be taken 2 hr after meals). Take for 4–8 weeks unless X-ray films or endoscopy have indicated significant healing. **Maintenance (tablets only):** 1 g b.i.d.

NURSING CONSIDERATIONS

ASSESSMENT

1. Document indications for therapy, noting onset and characteristics of symptoms.
2. List other agents prescribed and the outcome.
3. Reconstitute tablets prior to administering through the NGT. When placed in a cup with a small amount of water and left for 10–15 min, the tablets will dissolve completely.
4. Assess and monitor gastric pH; maintain pH above 5.
5. Monitor CBC and serum phosphate levels. Drug binds phosphate and may lead to hypophosphatemia.

CLIENT/FAMILY TEACHING

1. Take on an empty stomach 1 hr before or 2 hr after meals. If antacids are used, take 30 min before or after.
2. Do not crush or chew tablets.
3. Take exactly as prescribed. It binds to proteins at the site of the lesions to create a protective barrier that prevents diffusion of hydrogen ions at a normal gastric pH.
4. May cause constipation; increase fluids and bulk and regular exercise.
5. Avoid smoking, alcohol, and caffeine to prevent a recurrence of ulcers. Even though healing of ulcers may result, the frequency or severity of subsequent attacks is not altered.
6. Report as scheduled for follow-up, upper GI, endoscopy, and labs.

OUTCOMES/EVALUATE

- ↓ Abdominal pain/discomfort
- Prophylaxis of GI bleeding
- Healing of duodenal ulcers

Sufentanil

(soo-**FEN**-tah-nil)

PREGNANCY CATEGORY: C
CLASSIFICATION(S):
Narcotic analgesic
Rx: Sufenta

SEE ALSO *NARCOTIC ANALGESICS.*

ACTION/KINETICS
Onset, IV: 1.3–3 min. **Anesthetic blood concentration:** 8–30 mcg/kg. **t½:** 2.5 hr. Allows appropriate oxygenation of the heart and brain during prolonged surgical procedures. May be used in children.

USES
(1) Narcotic analgesic used as an adjunct to maintain balanced general anesthesia. (2) To induce and maintain general anesthesia (with 100% oxygen), especially in neurosurgery or CV surgery.

ADDITIONAL CONTRAINDICATIONS
Use during labor.

SPECIAL CONCERNS
Decrease dose in the obese, elderly, or debilitated client.

ADDITIONAL SIDE EFFECTS
Erythema, chills, intraoperative muscle movement, bradycardia, skeletal muscle rigidity. ***Extended postoperative respiratory depression.***

ADDITIONAL DRUG INTERACTIONS
Beta adrenergic blockers / ↑ Risk of bradycardia and hypotension during induction
Calcium channel blockers / ↑ Risk of bradycardia and hypotension during induction
Nitrous oxide / CV depression

HOW SUPPLIED
Injection: 50 mcg/mL

DOSAGE

- **IV**

Analgesia.

Adults, individualized, usual initial: 1–2 mcg/kg with oxygen and nitrous oxide; **maintenance:** 10–25 mcg as required.

For complicated surgery.

Adults: 2–8 mcg/kg with oxygen and nitrous oxide; **maintenance:** 10–50 mcg.

To induce and maintain general anesthesia.

Adults: 8–30 mcg/kg with 100% oxygen and a muscle relaxant; **maintenance:** 0.5–10 mcg/kg for surgical stress (e.g., incision, sternotomy, cardiopulmonary bypass). Base maintenance infusion rate on induction dose

S

to total dose for the procedure does not exceed 30 mcg/kg.

Induction and maintenance of general anesthesia in children less than 12 years of age undergoing CV surgery.
Initial: 10–25 mcg/kg with 100% oxygen; **maintenance:** 25–50 mcg supplemental doses, as needed

Epidural use in labor and delivery.
10–15 mcg with 10 mL bupivacaine, 0.125% with or without epinephrine. Can repeat doses twice (i.e., total of 3 doses) at 1 hr or greater intervals until delivery.

NURSING CONSIDERATIONS

SEE ALSO *NURSING CONSIDERATIONS* FOR *NARCOTIC ANALGESICS*.

ADMINISTRATION/STORAGE

1. Limit epidural or intrathecal administration of preservative free drug to the lumbar area.

IV 2. Reduce the dose in the debilitated or elderly client.

3. Calculate the dose based on ideal body weight.

CLIENT/FAMILY TEACHING

1. Avoid activities that require mental alertness for at least 24 hr following procedure; dizziness and drowsiness may occur.
2. Call for assistance with ambulation and transfers.
3. Avoid alcohol and any other CNS depressants for 24 hr following procedure.

OUTCOMES/EVALUATE

Desired level of analgesia

S

Sulfacetamide sodium

(sul-fah-**SEAT**-ah-myd)

CLASSIFICATION(S):
Sulfonamide, topical
Rx: AK-Sulf, Bleph-10, Cetamide, Isopto-Cetamide, Ocusulf-10, Sebizon, Sodium Sulamyd, Storz Sulf, Sulf-10, Sulster
✱Rx: Diosulf

SEE ALSO *SULFONAMIDES*.

USES

(1) Topically for conjunctivitis, corneal ulcer, and other superficial ocular infections. (2) As an adjunct to systemic sulfonamides to treat trachoma.

CONTRAINDICATIONS

In infants less than 2 months of age. Use in the presence of epithelial herpes simplex keratitis, vaccinia, varicella, and other viral diseases of the cornea and conjunctiva. Mycobacterial or fungal infections of the ocular structures. After uncomplicated removal of a corneal foreign body.

SPECIAL CONCERNS

Safe use during pregnancy and lactation or in children less than 12 years of age has not been established. Use with caution in clients with dry eye syndrome. Ophthalmic ointments may retard corneal wound healing.

SIDE EFFECTS

When used topically: Itching, local irritation, periorbital edema, burning and transient stinging, headache, bacterial or fungal corneal ulcers. *NOTE:* Sulfonamides may cause serious systemic side effects, including severe hypersensitivity reactions. Symptoms include fever, skin rash, GI disturbances, bone marrow depression, ***Stevens-Johnson syndrome, toxic epidermal necrolysis,*** exfoliative dermatitis, photosensitivity. Fatalities have occurred.

DRUG INTERACTIONS

Preparations containing silver are incompatible.

HOW SUPPLIED

Lotion: 10%; *Ophthalmic Ointment:* 10%; *Ophthalmic Solution:* 1%, 10%, 15%, 30%

DOSAGE

• **OPHTHALMIC SOLUTION, 1%, 10%, 15%, 20%**

Conjunctivitis or other superficial ocular infections.
1–2 gtt in the conjunctival sac q 1–4 hr. Doses may be tapered by increasing the time interval between doses as the condition improves.

Trachoma.
2 gtt q 2 hr with concomitant systemic sulfonamide therapy.

• **OPHTHALMIC OINTMENT (10%)**

Apply approximately 1/4 in. into the lower conjunctival sac 3–4 times/day and at bedtime. Alternatively, 0.5–1 in. is placed in the conjunctival sac at bedtime along with use of drops during the day.

For cutaneous infections.

Apply locally (10%) to affected area b.i.d.–q.i.d.

• **LOTION**

Seborrheic dermatitis.

Apply 1–2 times/day (for mild cases, apply overnight).

Cutaneous bacterial infections.

Apply b.i.d.–q.i.d. until infection clears.

NURSING CONSIDERATIONS

SEE ALSO *GENERAL NURSING CONSIDERATIONS* FOR *ANTI-INFECTIVES* AND FOR *SULFONAMIDES*.

ADMINISTRATION/STORAGE

Solutions will darken in color if left standing for long periods; discard these products.

ASSESSMENT

1. Document indications for therapy, onset, duration, and characteristics of symptoms.
2. List other agents prescribed and the outcome.
3. Note any allergy to sulfa drugs.

CLIENT/FAMILY TEACHING

1. Use only as directed. Wash hands before and after instillation.
2. Ophthalmic products may cause sensitivity to bright light; wear sunglasses to minimize.
3. Report any purulent eye drainage as this inactivates sulfacetamide.
4. If prescribed additional eye drops, wait 5 min after sulfacetamide instillation.
5. Do not wear contact lenses until infection is resolved.
6. Discard any cloudy or dark solutions. Do not let dropper/tip touch any part of eye so as to prevent contamination of bottle/tube contents.

OUTCOMES/EVALUATE

Resolution of inflammation/infection

Sulfadiazine

(sul-fah-**DYE**-ah-zeen)

PREGNANCY CATEGORY: C
CLASSIFICATION(S):
Antibiotic, sulfonamide

SEE ALSO *SULFONAMIDES*.

ACTION/KINETICS

Short-acting; often combined with other anti-infectives.

USES

(1) UTIs caused by *Escherichia coli, Klebsiella, Enterobacter, Staphylococcus aureus, Proteus mirabilis,* and *Proteus vulgaris.* (2) Chancroid. (3) Inclusion conjunctivitis. (4) Adjunct to treat chloroquine-resistant strains of *Plasmodium falciparum.* (5) Meningitis caused by *Haemophilus influenzae,* meningococcal meningitis for sulfonamide-sensitive group A strains. (6) Nocardiosis. (7) With penicillin to treat acute otitis media caused by *H. influenzae.* (8) Rheumatic fever prophylaxis. (9) Adjunct with pyrimethamine for toxoplasmosis in selected immunocompromised clients (e.g., those with AIDS, neoplastic disease, or congenital immune compromise). (10) Trachoma.

CONTRAINDICATIONS

Use in infants less than 2 months of age unless combined with pyrimethamine to treat congenital toxoplasmosis.

SPECIAL CONCERNS

Safe use during pregnancy has not been established.

HOW SUPPLIED

Tablet: 500 mg

DOSAGE

• **TABLETS**

General use.

Adults, loading dose: 2–4 g; **maintenance:** 2–4 g/day in 3 to 6 divided doses; **infants over 2 months, loading dose:** 75 mg/kg/day (2 g/m^2); **maintenance:** 150 mg/kg/day (4 g/m^2/day) in 4 to 6 divided doses, not to exceed 6 g/day.

Rheumatic fever prophylaxis.

Under 30 kg: 0.5 g/day; **over 30 kg:** 1 g/day.

S

As adjunct with pyrimethamine in congenital toxoplasmosis.
Infants less than 2 months: 25 mg/kg q.i.d. for 3 to 4 weeks. **Children greater than 2 months:** 25–50 mg/kg q.i.d. for 3 to 4 weeks.

NURSING CONSIDERATIONS

SEE ALSO *GENERAL NURSING CONSIDERATIONS* FOR *ANTI-INFECTIVES* AND *SULFONAMIDES*.

ASSESSMENT

Document indications for therapy, onset, duration, and characteristics of symptoms. Obtain appropriate labs/cultures.

CLIENT/FAMILY TEACHING

1. Take as directed with a full glass of water to prevent dehydration and crystalluria. Do not share meds; complete entire prescription.
2. Avoid prolonged sun exposure and use protection; may cause photosensitivity reaction.
3. No OTC meds esp Aspirin or Vitamin C without provider approval.
4. Report any unusual bruising/bleeding, rash, fever, sore throat, or lack of effectiveness.

OUTCOMES/EVALUATE

- Negative culture reports
- Prophylaxis during invasive procedures

Sulfamethoxazole

(sul-fah-meth-**OX**-ah-zohl)

S

PREGNANCY CATEGORY: C
CLASSIFICATION(S):
Antibiotic, sulfonamide
Rx: Gantanol

SEE ALSO *SULFONAMIDES*.

ACTION/KINETICS

t½: 8.6 hr.

USES

(1) UTIs caused by *Escherichia coli, Klebsiella, Enterobacter, Staphylococcus aureus, Proteus mirabilis,* and *Proteus vulgaris.* (2) Chancroid. (3) Inclusion conjunctivitis. (4) Adjunct to treat chloroquine-resistant strains of *Plasmodium falciparum.* (5) Meningococcal meningitis for sulfonamide-sensitive group A strains. (6) Nocardiosis. (7) With penicillin to treat acute otitis media caused by *H. influenzae.* (8) Adjunct with pyrimethamine for toxoplasmosis in selected immunocompromised clients (e.g., those with AIDS, neoplastic disease, or congenital immune compromise). (9) Trachoma.

SPECIAL CONCERNS

May be an increased risk of severe side effects in elderly clients.

HOW SUPPLIED

Tablet: 500 mg

DOSAGE

- **TABLETS**

Mild to moderate infections.
Adults, initially: 2 g; **then,** 1 g in morning and evening.
Severe infections.
Adults, initially: 2 g; **then,** 1 g t.i.d. **Infants over 2 months, initial:** 50–60 mg/kg; **then,** 25–30 mg/kg in morning and evening, not to exceed 75 mg/kg/day. Alternative dosing: 50–60 mg/kg/day divided q 12 hr, not to exceed 3 g/24 hr.

NURSING CONSIDERATIONS

SEE ALSO *GENERAL NURSING CONSIDERATIONS* FOR *ANTI-INFECTIVES* AND *SULFONAMIDES*.

ASSESSMENT

Document indications for therapy, onset, duration, and characteristics of symptoms. Obtain appropriate labs/cultures.

CLIENT/FAMILY TEACHING

1. Take only as directed and complete entire prescription. Consume plenty of fluids to prevent dehydration and crystalluria.
2. May cause dizziness; assess response prior to any activity requiring mental alertness.
3. Use sunglasses, sunscreens, and protective clothing during sun exposure as a photosensitivity reaction may occur.

OUTCOMES/EVALUATE

Resolution of infection; symptomatic improvement

Sulfasalazine

(sul-fah-**SAL**-ah-zeen)

PREGNANCY CATEGORY: B
CLASSIFICATION(S):

Antibiotic, sulfonamide

Rx: Azulfidine, Azulfidine EN-Tabs

✱**Rx:** Alti-Sulfasalazine, S.A.S., Salazopyrin, Salazopyrin-EN Tabs

SEE ALSO *SULFONAMIDES*.

ACTION/KINETICS

About one-third of the dose of sulfasalazine is absorbed from the small intestine while two-thirds passes to the colon, where it is split to 5-aminosalicylic acid and sulfapyridine. The drug does not affect the microflora.

USES

(1) Ulcerative colitis. (2) Azulfidine EN-tabs are also used to treat rheumatoid arthritis in adults and children over 6 years of age (with juvenile arthritis involving 5 or more diseased joints) who do not respond well to NSAIDs. *Investigational:* Ankylosing spondylitis, collagenous colitis, Crohn's disease, psoriasis, juvenile chronic arthritis, psoriatic arthritis.

ADDITIONAL CONTRAINDICATIONS

Children below 2 years. In persons with marked sulfonamide, salicylate, or related drug hypersensitivity. Intestinal or urinary obstruction.

SPECIAL CONCERNS

Use with caution during lactation.

SIDE EFFECTS

Most common include anorexia, headache, N&V, gastric distress, reversible oligospermia. Less frequently, pruritus, urticaria, fever, Heinz body anemia, hemolytic anemia, cyanosis.

DRUG INTERACTIONS

Digoxin / ↓ Digoxin absorption
Folic acid / ↓ Folic acid absorption
Sulfonylureas / Sulfasalazine may impair sulfonylurea metabolism

HOW SUPPLIED

Enteric Coated Tablet: 500 mg; *Tablet:* 500 mg

DOSAGE

• ENTERIC-COATED TABLETS, TABLETS

Ulcerative colitis.

Adults, initial: 3–4 g/day in divided doses (1–2 g/day may decrease side effects); **maintenance:** 500 mg q.i.d. **Pediatric, over 2 years of age, initial:** 40–60 mg/kg/day in 3 to 6 equally divided doses; **maintenance:** 30 mg/kg/day in 4 divided doses.

For desensitization to sulfasalazine.

Reinstitute at level of 50–250 mg/day; **then,** give double dose q 4–7 days until desired therapeutic level reached. Do not attempt in those with a history of agranulocytosis or who have experienced anaphylaxis previously with sulfasalazine.

Adult rhematoid arthritis.

To reduce GI intolerance, **initial:** 0.5 g in the evening for the first week, increased to 0.5 g in the morning and evening the second week, 0.5 g in the morning and 1 g in the evening the third week; then, beginning week 4, 1 g in the morning and evening.

Juvenile rheumatoid arthritis, polyarticular course.

Children, 6 years and older: 30–50 mg/kg daily in 2 evenly divided doses (maximum 2 g/day). To reduce GI intolerance, begin with a quarter to a third of the planned maintenance dose and increase weekly until reaching the maintenance dose at 1 month.

Collagenous colitis.

2–3 g/day.

Psoriasis.

3–4 g/day.

Psoriatic arthritis.

2 g/day.

NURSING CONSIDERATIONS

SEE ALSO *GENERAL NURSING CONSIDERATIONS* FOR *ANTI-INFECTIVES* AND *SULFONAMIDES*.

ASSESSMENT

1. Note indications for therapy, including onset, location, duration, and characteristics of symptoms.

2. Document frequency, quantity, and consistency of stool production; assess abdominal pain.
3. Note joint deformity, pain, ROM, inflammation, and swelling with rheumatoid arthritis.
4. Monitor CBC, renal function studies, and urinalysis; with colitis, send stool for analysis.

CLIENT/FAMILY TEACHING

1. Take with/after meals to reduce GI upset.
2. Take exactly as ordered at the same time each day; or if intermittent therapy (2 weeks on, 2 weeks off).
3. Drug may discolor urine or skin a yellow-orange color.
4. Take at least 2–3 L/day of water to decrease incidence of dehydration and crystalluria/stone formation.
5. Avoid prolonged exposure to sunlight; may increase sensitivity. Wear protective clothing, sunglasses, and sunscreen.
6. Report any unusual bruising/bleeding, rash, fever, sore throat or lack of effect.

OUTCOMES/EVALUATE

- ↓ Frequency of loose stools; ↓ abdominal pain; ↓ colon inflammation
- Relief of pain from joint deformity, swelling, and inflammation

Sulfinpyrazone

(sul-fin-**PEER**-ah-zohn)

S

CLASSIFICATION(S):
Antigout drug, uricosuric
Rx: Anturane
✱**Rx:** Apo-Sulfinpyrazone, Nu-Sulfinpyrazone

ACTION/KINETICS

Inhibits tubular reabsorption of uric acid, thereby increasing its excretion. Also exhibits antithrombotic and platelet inhibitory actions. **Peak plasma levels:** 1–2 hr. **Therapeutic plasma levels:** Up to 160 mcg/mL following 800 mg/day for uricosuria. **Duration:** 4–6 hr (up to 10 hr in some). **t½:** 3–8 hr. Metabolized by the liver. Approximately 45% of the drug is excreted unchanged by the kidney, and a small amount is excreted in the feces.

USES

Chronic and intermittent gouty arthritis. Not effective during acute attacks of gout and may even increase the frequency of acute episodes during the initiation of therapy. However, do not discontinue during acute attacks. Concomitant administration of colchicine during initiation of therapy is recommended. *Investigational:* To decrease sudden death during first year after MI.

CONTRAINDICATIONS

Active peptic ulcer or symptoms of GI inflammation or ulceration. Blood dyscrasias. Sensitivity to phenylbutazone or other pyrazoles. Use to control hyperuricemia secondary to treatment of malignancies.

SPECIAL CONCERNS

Use with caution in pregnant women. Dosage has not been established in children. Use with extreme caution in clients with impaired renal function and in those with a history of peptic ulcers.

SIDE EFFECTS

GI: N&V, abdominal discomfort. May reactivate peptic ulcer. **Hematologic:** Leukopenia, ***agranulocytosis,*** anemia, thrombocytopenia, ***aplastic anemia.*** **Miscellaneous:** Skin rash (which usually disappears with usage), ***bronchoconstriction in aspirin-induced asthma.*** Acute attacks of gout may become more frequent during initial therapy. Give concomitantly with colchicine at this time.

OD OVERDOSE MANAGEMENT

Symptoms: N&V, diarrhea, epigastric pain, labored respiration, ataxia, seizures, coma. *Treatment:* Supportive measures.

DRUG INTERACTIONS

Acetaminophen / ↓ Effect of acetaminophen; ↑ risk of hepatotoxicity;
Anticoagulants / ↑ Anticoagulant effect R/T ↓ plasma protein binding
Niacin / ↓ Uricosuric effect of sulfinpyrazone
Salicylates / Inhibit uricosuric effect of sulfinpyrazone
Theophylline / ↓ Theophylline effect R/T to ↑ plasma clearance

Tolbutamide / ↑ Risk of hypoglycemia
Verapamil / ↓ Verapamil effect R/T ↑ plasma clearance

HOW SUPPLIED

Capsule: 200 mg; *Tablet:* 100 mg

DOSAGE

• **CAPSULES, TABLETS**

Gout.

Adults, initial: 200–400 mg/day in two divided doses with meals or milk. Clients who are transferred from other uricosuric agents can receive full dose at once. **Maintenance:** 100–400 mg b.i.d. Maintain full dosage without interruption even during acute attacks of gout.

Following MI.

Adults: 300 mg q.i.d. or 400 mg b.i.d.

NURSING CONSIDERATIONS

ASSESSMENT

1. Assess joint(s) for pain, deformity, ROM, and inflammation.
2. Monitor CBC and uric acid levels.

CLIENT/FAMILY TEACHING

1. If GI upset occurs, take with food, milk, or antacids. May still reactivate peptic ulcer.
2. Consume at least ten to twelve 8-oz glasses of fluid daily to prevent the formation of uric acid stones. Avoid cranberry juice or vitamin C preparations, as these acidify urine; acidification may cause formation of uric acid stones.
3. Sodium bicarbonate may be ordered to alkalinize the urine to prevent urates from crystallizing in acid urine and forming kidney stones.
4. Avoid alcohol and aspirin; may interfere with drug effectiveness.
5. During *acute* attacks of gout, concomitant administration of colchicine is indicated.

OUTCOMES/EVALUATE

• ↓ Pain/stiffness in joints; ↑ ROM
• ↓ Frequency/intensity gout attacks
• ↓ Serum uric acid levels

Sulfisoxazole

(sul-fih-**SOX**-ah-zohl)

PREGNANCY CATEGORY: C

Sulfisoxazole diolamine

(sul-fih-**SOX**-ah-zohl)

PREGNANCY CATEGORY: C
CLASSIFICATION(S):
Antibiotic, sulfonamide

SEE ALSO *SULFONAMIDES*.

ACTION/KINETICS

t½: 5.9 hr.

USES

(1) UTIs caused by *Escherichia coli, Klebsiella, Enterobacter, Staphylococcus aureus, Proteus mirabilis, and Proteus vulgaris.* (2) Chancroid. (3) Inclusion conjunctivitis. (4) Adjunct to treat chloroquine-resistant strains of *Plasmodium falciparum.* (5) Meningitis caused by *Haemophilus influenzae,* meningococcal meningitis for sulfonamide-sensitive group A strains. (6) Nocardiosis. (7) With penicillin to treat acute otitis media caused by *H. influenzae.* (8) Adjunct with pyrimethamine for toxoplasmosis in selected immunocompromised clients (e.g., those with AIDS, neoplastic disease, or congenital immune compromise). (9) Ophthalmically as an adjunct with systemic sulfonamides to treat trachoma.

ADDITIONAL CONTRAINDICATIONS

Use in infants less than 2 months of age except as adjunct with pyrimethamine to treat congenital toxoplasmosis. Use in the presence of epithelial herpes simplex keratitis, vaccinia, varicella, and other viral diseases of the cornea and conjunctiva. Mycobacterial or fungal infections of the ocular structures. After uncomplicated removal of a corneal foreign body.

SPECIAL CONCERNS

Safety and efficacy of the ophthalmic products have not been established in children. Use with caution in clients with severe dry eye.

ADDITIONAL SIDE EFFECTS

Following ophthalmic use: Blurred vision, itching, local irritation, epithelial keratitis, reactive hyperemia, conjunc-

S

tival edema, burning, headache or browache, transient stinging.

ADDITIONAL DRUG INTERACTIONS

Sulfisoxazole may ↑ effects of thiopental due to ↓ plasma protein binding.

HOW SUPPLIED

Sulfisoxazole: *Tablet:* 500 mg. **Sulfisoxazole diolamine:** *Ophthalmic Solution:* 4%

DOSAGE

• **TABLETS**

Adults, loading dose: 2–4 g; **maintenance:** 4–8 g/day in 4 to 6 divided doses, depending on severity of the infection. **Infants over 2 months, initial:** 75 mg/kg/day; **maintenance:** 150 mg/kg/day (4 g/m^2/day) in 4 to 6 divided doses, not to exceed 6 g/day.

• **OPHTHALMIC SOLUTION (4%)**

Conjunctivitis or corneal ulcer.

1–2 gtt into conjunctival sac q 1–4 hr, depending on the severity of the infection. Dose may be tapered by increasing the time interval between doses as the condition improves.

Trachoma.

2 gtt q 2 hr with concomitant systemic therapy.

NURSING CONSIDERATIONS

SEE ALSO *GENERAL NURSING CONSIDERATIONS* FOR *ANTI-INFECTIVES* AND *SULFONAMIDES*.

ADMINISTRATION/STORAGE

Solutions will darken in color if left standing for long periods; discard these products.

ASSESSMENT

1. Document type, onset, and characteristics of symptoms. List other agents trialed and the outcome.
2. Monitor CBC and cultures.

CLIENT/FAMILY TEACHING

1. Take tablets on an empty stomach and consume plenty of fluids to prevent dehydration and crystalluria.
2. May cause sensitivity to bright light; wear sunglasses and avoid exposures to minimize.
3. With ophthalmic use, report if no improvement after 7–8 days, if the condition worsens, or if pain, increased redness, itching, or swelling of the eye occurs.
4. Avoid OTC agents esp ASA and vitamin C. Report any unusual bruising/bleeding, rash, fever, sore throat or lack of response.

OUTCOMES/EVALUATE

Negative cultures; symptomatic improvement

Sulindac

(sul-**IN**-dak)

CLASSIFICATION(S):

Nonsteroidal anti-inflammatory drug

Rx: Clinoril

✱**Rx:** Apo-Sulin, Novo-Sundac, Nu-Sulindac

SEE ALSO *NONSTEROIDAL ANTI-INFLAMMATORY DRUGS*.

ACTION/KINETICS

Biotransformed in the liver to a sulfide, the active metabolite. **Peak plasma levels of sulfide:** after fasting, 2 hr; after food, 3–4 hr. **Onset, anti-inflammatory effect:** within 1 week; **duration, anti-inflammatory effect:** 1–2 weeks. **t½,** of sulindac: 7.8 hr; of metabolite: 16.4 hr. Over 93% plasma protein-bound. Excreted in both urine (50%) and feces (25%).

USES

Acute and chronic treatment of rheumatoid arthritis, osteoarthritis, ankylosing spondylitis, acute gouty arthritis; acute, painful shoulder; tendinitis, bursitis. *Investigational:* Juvenile rheumatoid arthritis, sunburn.

CONTRAINDICATIONS

Use with active GI lesions or a history of recurrent GI lesions.

SPECIAL CONCERNS

Safety and efficacy have not been established for children. Safe use during pregnancy has not been established. Use with caution during lactation.

ADDITIONAL SIDE EFFECTS

Hypersensitivity, pancreatitis, GI pain (common), maculopapular rash. Stupor, ***coma,*** hypotension, and diminished urine output.

ADDITIONAL DRUG INTERACTIONS

Sulindac ↑ effect of warfarin due to ↓ plasma protein binding.

HOW SUPPLIED

Tablet: 150 mg, 200 mg

DOSAGE

• **TABLETS**

Osteoarthritis, rheumatoid arthritis, ankylosing spondylitis.

Adults: 150 mg b.i.d.

Acute painful shoulder, acute gouty arthritis.

Adults: 200 mg b.i.d. for 7–14 days.

Antigout.

Adults: 200 mg b.i.d. for 7 days.

NURSING CONSIDERATIONS

SEE ALSO *NURSING CONSIDERATIONS FOR NONSTEROIDAL ANTI-INFLAMMATORY DRUGS.*

ADMINISTRATION/STORAGE

For acute conditions, reduce dosage when satisfactory response is attained.

ASSESSMENT

1. Document type, onset, and characteristics of symptoms.
2. Determine baseline ROM; describe location, inflammation, and swelling; rate pain level and note functional class of arthritis.
3. Monitor CBC, liver and renal function studies; reduce dosage with renal dysfunction.

CLIENT/FAMILY TEACHING

1. Take with food to decrease GI upset and consume plenty of water. A stomach protectant (i.e., misoprostol) may be prescribed with a history of ulcer disease.
2. Do not take aspirin because plasma levels of sulindac will be reduced. Avoid alcohol.
3. Report any incidence of unexplained bleeding such as oozing of blood from the gums, nosebleeds, or excessive bruising.
4. Drug may cause dizziness; assess response prior to any activity requiring mental alertness.
5. When used for arthritis, a favorable response usually occurs within 1 week; report lack of response.

OUTCOMES/EVALUATE

↓ Joint pain and inflammation with ↑ mobility

Sumatriptan succinate

(**soo**-mah-**TRIP**-tan)

PREGNANCY CATEGORY: C

CLASSIFICATION(S):

Antimigraine drug

Rx: Imitrex

ACTION/KINETICS

Selective agonist for a vascular 5-HT_1 receptor subtype (probably 5-HT_{1D}) located on cranial arteries, on the basilar artery, and the vasculature of the dura mater. Activates the 5-HT_1 receptor, causing vasoconstriction and therefore relief of migraine. Transient increases in BP may be observed. No significant activity at 5-HT_2 or 5-HT_3 receptor subtypes; alpha-1-, alpha-2-, or beta-adrenergic receptors; dopamine-1 or dopamine-2 receptors; muscarinic receptors; or benzodiazepine receptors. **Time to peak effect after SC:** 12 min after a 6-mg SC dose. **t½ distribution, after SC:** 15 min; **terminal t½:** 115 min. Approximately 22% of a SC dose is excreted in the urine as unchanged drug and 38% as metabolites. Rapidly absorbed after PO administration, although bioavailability is low due to incomplete absorption and a first-pass effect (bioavailability may be significantly increased in those with impaired liver function). **PO, elimination t½:** About 2.5 hr. About 60% of a PO dose is excreted through the urine and 40% in the feces.

USES

(1) Treatment of acute migraine attacks with or without aura. Photophobia, phonophobia, N&V associated with migraine attacks are also relieved. Intended to relieve migraine, but not to prevent or reduce the number of attacks experienced. (2) Acute treatment of cluster headaches (injection only). *Investigational:* Relieve persistent headaches in head and neck cancer clients despite standard drug therapy.

S

CONTRAINDICATIONS

Hypersensitivity to sumatriptan. IV use due to the possibility of coronary vasospasm. SC use in clients with ischemic heart disease, history of MI, documented silent ischemia, Prinzmetal's angina, or uncontrolled hypertension. Concomitant use with ergotamine-containing products or MAO inhibitor therapy (or within 2 weeks of discontinuing an MAO inhibitor). Use in clients with hemiplegic or basilar migraine. Use in women who are pregnant, think they may be pregnant, or are trying to get pregnant.

SPECIAL CONCERNS

Use with caution during lactation, in clients with impaired hepatic or renal function, and in clients with heart conditions. Clients with risk factors for CAD (e.g., men over 40, smokers, postmenopausal women, hypertension, obesity, diabetes, hypercholesterolemia, family history of heart disease) should be screened before initiating treatment. Safety and efficacy have not been determined for use in children.

SIDE EFFECTS

Side effects listed are for either SC or PO use of the drug.

CV: Coronary vasospasm in clients with a history of CAD. ***Serious and/or life-threatening arrhythmias, including atrial fibrillation, ventricular fibrillation, ventricular tachycardia, MI, marked ischemic ST elevations,*** chest and arm discomfort representing angina pectoris. Flushing, hypertension, hypotension, bradycardia, tachycardia, palpitations, pulsating sensations, ECG changes (including nonspecific ST- or T-wave changes, prolongation of PR or QTc intervals, sinus arrhythmia, nonsustained ventricular premature beats, isolated junctional ectopic beats, atrial ectopic beats, and delayed activation of the right ventricle), syncope, pallor, abnormal pulse, vasodilatation, atherosclerosis, bradycardia, cerebral ischemia, CV lesion, heart block, peripheral cyanosis, thrombosis, transient myocardial ischemia, vasodilation, Raynaud's syndrome. **At injection site:** Pain, redness. **Atypical sensations:** Sensation of warmth, cold, tingling, or paresthesia. Localized or generalized feeling of pressure, burning, numbness, and tightness. Feeling of heaviness, feeling strange, tight feeling in head. **CNS:** Fatigue, dizziness, drowsiness, vertigo, sedation, headache, anxiety, malaise, confusion, euphoria, agitation, relaxation, chills, tremor, shivering, prickling or stinging sensations, phonophobia, depression, euphoria, facial pain, heat sensitivity, incoordination, monoplegia, sleep disturbances, shivering. **EENT:** Throat discomfort, discomfort in nasal cavity or sinuses. Vision alterations, eye irritation, photophobia, lacrimation, otalgia, feeling of fullness in ear, disorders of sclera, mydriasis. **GI:** Abdominal discomfort, dysphagia, discomfort of mouth and tongue, gastroesophageal reflux, diarrhea, peptic ulcer, retching, flatulence, eructation, gallstones, taste disturbances, GI bleeding, hematemesis, melena. **Respiratory:** Dyspnea, diseases of the lower respiratory tract, hiccoughs, influenza, asthma. **Dermatologic:** Erythema, pruritus, skin rashes, skin eruptions, skin tenderness, dry or scaly skin, tightness or wrinkling of skin. **GU:** Dysuria, dysmenorrhea, urinary frequency, renal calculus, breast tenderness, increased urination, intermenstrual bleeding, nipple discharge, abortion, hematuria. **Musculoskeletal:** Weakness, neck pain or stiffness, myalgia, muscle cramps, joint disturbances (pain, stiffness, swelling, ache), muscle stiffness, need to flex calf muscles, backache, muscle tiredness, swelling of the extremities, tetany. **Endocrine:** Elevated TSH levels, galactorrhea, hyperglycemia, hypoglycemia, hypothyroidism, weight gain or loss. **Miscellaneous:** Chest, jaw, or neck tightness. Sweating, thirst, polydipsia, chills, fever, dehydration.

LABORATORY TEST CONSIDERATIONS

Disturbance of LFTs.

OD OVERDOSE MANAGEMENT

Symptoms: Tremor, ***convulsions,*** inactivity erythema of extremities, reduced respiratory rate, cyanosis, ataxia, mydriasis, injection site reactions (desquamation, hair loss, scab formation), paralysis. *Treatment:* Continuous monitoring of client for at least 10 hr and especially when signs and symptoms persist.

DRUG INTERACTIONS

Ergot drugs / Prolonged vasospastic reactions
Monoamine oxidase A inhibitors / ↑ t½ of sumatriptan
Selective Serotonin Reuptake Inhibitors (SSRIs) / Rarely, weakness, hyperreflexia, and incoordination

HOW SUPPLIED

Injection: 12 mg/mL; *Nasal spray:* 5 mg, 20 mg; *Tablet:* 25 mg, 50 mg, 100 mg

DOSAGE

• **SC**

Migraine headaches.

Adults: 6 mg. A second injection may be given if symptoms of migraine come back but no more than two injections (6 mg each) should be taken in a 24-hr period and at least 1 hr should elapse between doses.

• **TABLETS**

Adults: A single dose of 25 mg, 50 mg, or 100 mg with fluids as soon as symptoms of migraine appear. Doses of 50 mg or 100 mg may provide a greater effect than 25 mg. A second dose may be taken if symptoms return but not sooner than 2 hr following the first dose. **Maximum recommended dose:** 100 mg, with no more than 200 mg taken in a 24-hr period.

• **NASAL SPRAY**

A single dose of 5, 10, or 20 mg given in one nostril. The 20 mg dose increases the risk of side effects, although it is more effective. The 10-mg dose may be given as a single 5-mg dose in each nostril. If the headache returns, repeat the dose once after 2 hr, not to exceed a total daily dose of 40 mg. The safety of treating an average of more than 4 headaches in a 30-day period has not been studied.

NURSING CONSIDERATIONS

ADMINISTRATION/STORAGE

1. No increased beneficial effect has been found with the administration of a second 6-mg dose SC in clients not responding to the first injection.
2. If side effects are dose limiting, a dose lower than 6 mg SC may be given; in such cases, use the single-dose 6 mg vial. An autoinjection device can be used to deliver the drug.
3. Consideration should be given to administering the first dose of sumatriptan in the provider's office due to the possibility (although rare) of coronary events.
4. Is equally effective at whatever stage of the attack given; advisable to take as soon as possible after the onset of a migraine attack.
5. Store away from heat (no higher than 30°C; 86°F) and light.

ASSESSMENT

1. Document headache characteristics, including onset, frequency, type, and duration of symptoms. Rate pain levels.
2. Determine any cardiac problems or ischemic CV disease.
3. Review neurologic exam and CT/MRI results. A clear diagnosis of migraine should be made; the drug should not be given for headaches due to other neurologic events.
4. Assess ECG, liver, and renal function studies. Monitor VS; expect transient increases in BP.
5. Parenteral form for SC use only. IV use may cause coronary vasospasm.

CLIENT/FAMILY TEACHING

1. Review appropriate method for administration. With SC form, administer first dose in office to assess response.
2. Printed instructions concerning how to load the autoinjector, administer the medication, and remove the syringe, are enclosed and provided by the manufacturer.
3. The injection is given just below the skin as soon as migraine symptoms appear or any time during the attack. A second injection may be administered 1 hr later if migraine symptoms return; do *not* exceed two injections in 24 hr. Report lack of response or loss of effectiveness.
4. Practice safe handling, storage, and disposal of syringes.

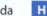

S

5. Pain and tenderness may be evident at injection site for up to an hour after administration.
6. For tablets, take a single dose with fluids as soon as symptoms appear; a second dose may be taken if symptoms return, but no sooner than 2 hr after the first dose. If there is no response to the first tablet, do not take a second tablet without consulting the provider.
7. Check expiration date before use and discard all outdated drugs.
8. Report if chest, jaw, throat, and neck pain occur after injection; this should be medically evaluated before using more Imitrex.
9. Severe chest pain or tightness, wheezing, palpitations, facial swelling, or rashes/hives should be immediately reported.
10. Symptoms of flushing, tingling, heat and heaviness, as well as dizziness or drowsiness may occur and should be reported before taking more sumatriptan.
11. Practice barrier contraception and do not use Imitrex if pregnancy is suspected.

OUTCOMES/EVALUATE

Reversal of acute migraine attack; relief of symptoms

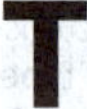

Tacrine hydrochloride (THA, Tetrahydro-aminoacridine)

(**TAH**-krin)

PREGNANCY CATEGORY: C
CLASSIFICATION(S):
Treatment of Alzheimer's disease
Rx: Cognex

ACTION/KINETICS

During early stages of Alzheimer's disease, cholinergic neuronal pathways that project from the basal forebrain to the cerebral cortex and hippocampus may be affected. Symptoms of dementia may be due to a deficiency of acetylcholine. As a reversible CNS cholinesterase inhibitor, tacrine elevates acetylcholine levels in the cerebral cortex. There is no evidence tacrine alters progression of dementia. Rapidly absorbed after PO administration. **Maximal plasma levels:** 1–2 hr. Food will affect the bioavailability of tacrine. Extensively metabolized in the liver. Undergoes first-pass metabolism; can be overcome by increasing the dose. **Elimination t½:** 2–4 hr. The average plasma levels are about 50% higher in females. Also, the mean tacrine levels in smokers are about one-third the levels of nonsmokers.

USES

Treatment of mild to moderate dementia of the Alzheimer's type.

CONTRAINDICATIONS

Hypersensitivity to tacrine or acridine derivatives. Use in clients previously treated with tacrine who developed jaundice (elevated total bilirubin > 3 mg/dL).

SPECIAL CONCERNS

May cause bradycardia—important in sick sinus syndrome. Use with caution in clients at risk for developing ulcers as the drug increases gastric acid secretion. Use with caution in clients with a history of abnormal liver function as indicated by abnormalities in serum ALT, AST, bilirubin, and GGT levels. Use with caution in clients with a history of asthma. There may be worsening of cognitive function following abrupt discontinuation of the drug. Safety and efficacy have not been determined in children with dementing illness.

SIDE EFFECTS

Hepatic: Increased transaminase levels (most common reason for stopping the drug during treatment). **GI:** N&V, diarrhea, dyspepsia, anorexia, abdominal pain, flatulence, constipation, glossitis, gingivitis, dry mouth/throat, stomatitis, increased salivation, dysphagia, esophagitis, gastritis, gastroenteritis, ***GI hemorrhage,*** stomach ulcer, hiatal hernia, hemorrhoids, bloody stools, diverticulitis, fecal impaction/incontinence, ***rectal hemorrhage,*** cholelithiasis, cholecystitis, increased appetite. **Musculoskeletal:** Myalgia, fracture, arthralgia, arthritis, hypertonia, osteoporosis, tendinitis, bursitis, gout, myopathy. **CNS:** ***Precipitation of seizures*** (may also be due to Alzheimer's), dizziness, confusion, ataxia, insomnia, somnolence, tremor, agitation, depression, abnormal thinking, anxiety, hallucinations, hostility, migraine, ***convulsions,*** vertigo, syncope, hyperkinesia, paresthesia, abnormal dreams, dysarthria, aphasia, amnesia, twitching, hypesthesia, delirium, paralysis, bradykinesia, movement disorders, cogwheel rigidity, paresis, neuritis, hemiplegia, Parkinson's disease, neuropathy, extrapyramidal syndrome, decreased/absent reflexes, tardive dyskinesia, dysesthesia, dystonia, encephalitis, ***coma,*** apraxia, oculogyric crisis, akathisia, oral facial dyskinesia, Bell's palsy, nervousness, apathy, increased libido, paranoia, neurosis, ***suicidal episodes,*** psychosis, hysteria. **Respiratory:** Rhinitis, URI, coughing, pharyngitis, sinusitis, bronchitis, pneumonia, dyspnea, epistaxis, chest congestion, asthma, hyperventilation, lower respiratory infection, hemoptysis, lung edema, ***lung cancer, acute epiglottitis.*** **CV:** Hypo/hypertension, ***heart failure, MI, CVA,*** angina pectoris, TIA, phlebitis, venous insufficiency, AAA, atrial fibrillation/flutter, palpitation, tachycardia, bradycardia, ***pulmonary embolus, heart arrest,*** PAC's, ***AV block,*** BBB. **Dermatologic:** Rash, facial/skin flushing, increased sweating, acne, alopecia, dermatitis, eczema, dry skin, herpes zoster, psoriasis, cellulitis, cyst, furunculosis, herpes simplex, hyperkeratosis, basal/squamous cell carcinoma, skin cancer, desquamation, seborrhea, skin ulcer/necrosis, ***melanoma.*** **GU:** Bladder outflow obstruction, urinary frequency/incontinence, UTI, hematuria, renal stone, kidney infection, glycosuria, dysuria, polyuria, nocturia, pyuria, cystitis, urinary retention/urgency, ***vaginal hemorrhage,*** genital pruritus, breast pain, urinary obstruction, impotence, ***prostate cancer, bladder/renal tumor, renal failure, breast/ovarian carcinoma,*** epididymitis. **Body as a whole:** Headache, fatigue, chest/back pain, weight increase/decrease, asthenia, chill, fever, malaise, peripheral/facial edema, dehydration, cachexia, lipoma, heat exhaustion, sepsis, ***cholinergic crisis, death.*** **Hematologic:** Anemia, lymphadenopathy, leukopenia, thrombocytopenia, hemolysis, pancytopenia. **Ophthalmologic:** Conjunctivitis, cataract, dry eyes, eye pain, visual field defect, diplopia, amblyopia, glaucoma, hordeolum, vision loss, ptosis, blepharitis. **Otic:** Deafness, earache, tinnitus, inner ear disturbance/infection, otitis media, labyrinthitis. **Miscellaneous:** Purpura, hypercholesterolemia, diabetes mellitus, hypo/hyperthyroid, unusual taste.

OD OVERDOSE MANAGEMENT

Symptoms: Cholinergic crisis characterized by severe N&V, sweating, bradycardia, salivation, hypotension, ***collapse, seizures, and increased muscle weakness (may paralyze respiratory muscles leading to death).*** *Treatment:* General supportive measures. IV atropine sulfate, titrated to effect, may be given in an initial dose of 1–2 mg IV with subsequent doses based on the response.

DRUG INTERACTIONS

Anticholinergic drugs / Tacrine interferes with action of these drugs
Bethanechol / Synergistic effects
Cholinesterase inhibitors / Synergistic effects
Cimetidine / ↑ Maximum tacrine levels
Succinylcholine / ↑ Muscle relaxation

Theophylline / ↑ Plasma theophylline levels; ↓ dose recommended.

HOW SUPPLIED

Capsule: 10 mg, 20 mg, 30 mg, 40 mg

DOSAGE

• **CAPSULES**

Alzheimer's disease.

Initial: 10 mg q.i.d. for at least 6 weeks; **then,** after 6 weeks, increase the dose to 20 mg q.i.d., providing there are no significant transaminase elevations and the client tolerates the treatment. Based on the degree of tolerance, the dose may be titrated, at 6-week intervals, to 30 or 40 mg q.i.d.

If transaminase elevations occur, modify the dose as follows:

• If transaminase levels are less than or equal to 2 × ULN, continue treatment according to recommended titration and monitoring schedule.

• If transaminse levels are greater than 2 but equal to or less than 3 × ULN, treatment is continued according to recommended titraiton but levels are monitored weekly until they return to normal levels.

• If transaminase levels are more than 3 but equal to or less than 5 × ULN, the daily dose is reduced by 40 mg/day. Monitor ALT/SGPT levels weekly. Dose titration is resumed and every other week monitoring is undertaken when levels return to within normal limits.

• If transaminase levels are greater than 5 × ULN, stop treatment. Monitor closely for signs and symptoms associated with hepatitis; monitor levels until they are within normal limits.

Clients who are required to stop treatment due to elevated transaminase levels may be rechallenged once levels return to within normal range. Weekly monitoring of serum ALT/SGPT levels should be undertaken after rechallenging occurs. If rechallenged, the initial dose is 10 mg t.i.d. with levels monitored weekly. After 6 weeks on this dose, the client may begin dose titration if transaminase levels are acceptable.

NURSING CONSIDERATIONS

ADMINISTRATION/STORAGE

1. Take drug between meals, if possible. If GI upset occurs, may take with meals; however, the plasma level will be decreased by 30%–40%.
2. Do not increase the initial dose for 6 weeks as there is the potential for delayed onset of transaminase elevations.
3. See increased use of Aricept due to improved side effect profile and ease of dosing.

ASSESSMENT

1. Assess mental status. Document onset/duration of symptoms and if this is a first drug trial or rechallenge. If rechallenge, check serum bilirubin and SGPT from previous treatment.
2. Note any ECG evidence of sick sinus syndrome, AV block, or any ulcer disease, asthma, or liver disease.
3. List drugs currently prescribed to ensure none interact unfavorably. Drug is a cholinesterase inhibitor; notify anesthesia before procedures.
4. Monitor ECG, hematologic, liver, and renal profiles. Serum transaminase levels (ALT/SGPT) should be monitored weekly for the first 18 weeks and then every 3 months unless dose is increased or the transaminase levels are mildly elevated; follow guidelines under *Dosage*.
5. Monitor VS; may cause bradycardia.
6. Observe and record response carefully; drug is titrated according to client tolerance.

CLIENT/FAMILY TEACHING

1. Take between meals unless GI upset is experienced. With meals, the plasma drug level will be decreased by 30–40%.
2. Take at regularly spaced intervals. Do not increase for the first 6 weeks until response and tolerance assessed. Report for labs as scheduled.
3. Clinical manifestations of mild to moderate dementia in Alzheimer's disease are thought to be related to a deficiency of acetylcholine. Tacrine is thought to act to elevate acetylcholine concentrations in the cerebral cortex. Drug does not cure disease but helps to slow its progress.
4. Report any new symptoms or any increase in existing symptoms. Keep all lab and provider appointments.

5. Smoking may interfere with serum drug levels.
6. During initiation of therapy, N&V and diarrhea may be evident; report if persistent or bothersome. Delayed-onset side effects that should be reported include rashes and yellow skin/stool discolorations.
7. Do not stop abruptly. Abrupt withdrawal may cause a decline in cognitive function and also contribute to behavioral disturbances.
8. Identify appropriate resources and support groups that may assist the family and caregivers in understanding and coping with this disorder.

OUTCOMES/EVALUATE

Improved level of cognitive functioning with Alzheimer's disease

Tacrolimus (FK506)

(tah-**KROH**-lih-mus)

PREGNANCY CATEGORY: C
CLASSIFICATION(S):
Immunosuppressant
Rx: Protopic, Prograf

ACTION/KINETICS

Produced by *Streptomyces tsukubaensis*. Mechanism of action for either systemic or topical use is not known but it inhibits T-lymphocyte activation by first binding to FKBP-12 (an intracellular protein). A complex of tacrolimus-FKBP-12, calcium, calmodulin, and calcineurin is formed leading to inhibition of phosphatase activity of calcineurin. This effect prevents dephosphorylation and translocation of nuclear factor of activated T-cells (NF-AT) which is a nuclear component thought to initiate gene transcription to form lymphokines. Tacrolimus also inhibits transcription for genes that encode factors involved in the early states of T-cell activation. Absorption from the GI tract is variable. **t½, terminal elimination:** 11.7 hr in liver transplant clients and 21.2 hr in healthy volunteers. Food decreases both the absorption and bioavailability of tacrolimus. Significantly bound to proteins and erythrocytes; extensively metabolized by the liver and excreted through the urine.

USES

Systemic: Prophylaxis of organ rejection in allogeneic liver transplants and kidney transplants; usually used with corticosteroids. **Topical:** Short-term and intermittent long-term therapy to treat moderate to severe atopic dermatitis in adults and children unable to take traditional agents or who do not respond to conventional therapy. *Investigational:* Transplants of bone marrow, heart, pancreas, pancreatic island cells, and small bowel. Treatment of autoimmune disease and severe recalcitrant psoriasis.

CONTRAINDICATIONS

Hypersensitivity to tacrolimus or HCO-60 polyoxyl 60 hydrogenated castor oil (vehicle used for the injection). Lactation. Concomitant use with cyclosporine.

SPECIAL CONCERNS

Increased risk of developing lymphomas and other malignancies (especially of the skin). Safety and efficacy of the ointment to treat infected atopic dermatitis have not been studied.

SIDE EFFECTS

After Systemic Use. CNS: Headache, tremor, insomnia, paresthesia, ***seizures, coma,*** delirium, abnormal dreams, anxiety, agitation, confusion, depression, dizziness, emotional lability, hallucinations, hypertonia, incoordination, myoclonus nervousness, psychosis, somnolence, abnormal thinking. *Neurotoxicity:* Changes in motor/sensory function, and mental status; tremor, headache.

GI: Diarrhea, nausea, constipation, abnormal LFT, anorexia, vomiting, dyspepsia, dysphasia, flatulence, ***GI hemorrhage/perforation,*** ileus, increased appetite, oral moniliasis. **Hepatic:** Hepatitis, cholangitis, cholestatic jaundice, jaundice, liver damage. **CV:** Hypertension, chest pain, abnormal ECG, ***hemorrhage,*** hypotension, tachycardia. **Hematologic:** Anemia, thrombocytopenia, leukocytosis, coagulation

T

disorder, ecchymosis, hypochromic anemia, leukopenia, decreased prothrombin. **GU:** Abnormal kidney function, nephrotoxicity, UTI, oliguria, hematuria, ***kidney failure.*** **Metabolic:** Hyper/hypokalemia, hyperglycemia, hypomagnesemia, acidosis, alkalosis, hyperlipemia, hyperphosphatemia, hyperuricemia, hypocalcemia, hypophosphatemia, hyponatremia, hypoproteinemia, bilirubinemia, diabetes mellitus. **Respiratory:** Pleural effusion, atelectasis, dyspnea, asthma, bronchitis, increased cough, pulmonary edema, pharyngitis, pneumonia, lung/respiratory disorder, rhinitis, sinusitis, alteration in voice. **Musculoskeletal:** Arthralgia, leg cramps, myalgia, myasthenia, osteoporosis, generalized spasm. **Dermatologic:** Pruritus, rash, alopecia, herpes simplex, sweating, skin disorder. **Miscellaneous:** Hypersensitivity reactions (including ***anaphylaxis***), increased incidence of malignancies, lymphoma, pain, fever, asthenia, ascites, peripheral edema, back/abdominal pain, enlarged abdomen, abscess, chills, hernia, photosensitivity, peritonitis, abnormal healing/vision, amblyopia, tinnitus.

• **AFTER TOPICAL USE.**

Dermatologic: Phototoxicity, skin burning, pruritus, skin erythema, skin infection, herpes simplex, eczema herpeticum, pustular rash, folliculitis, urticaria, maculopapular rash, fungal dermatitis, acne, sunburn, skin disorder, vesiculobullous rash, skin tingling, dry skin, benign skin neoplasm, contact dermatitis, eczema, exfoliative dermatitis. **GI:** N&V, diarrhea, abdominal pain, gastroenteritis, dyspepsia. **Respiratory:** Increased cough, asthma, pharyngitis, rhinitis, sinusitis, bronchitis, pneumonia. **CNS:** Head-ache, insomnia. **Miscellaneous:** Flu-like symptoms, allergic reaction, fever, infection, accidental injury, otitis media, alcohol intolerance, conjunctivitis, pain, lymphadenopathy, facial edema, hyperesthesia, back pain, peripheral edema, varicella zoster/herpes zoster, asthenia, dysmenorrhea, periodontal abscess, myalgia, cyst.

LABORATORY TEST CONSIDERATIONS

↑ Alkaline phosphatase, AST, ALT.

T

DRUG INTERACTIONS

Aminoglycosides / Additive or synergistic impairment of renal function
Amphotericin B / Additive or synergistic impairment of renal function
Antifungal drugs / ↑ Tacrolimus blood levels
Bromocriptine / ↑ Tacrolimus blood levels
Calcium channel blocking drugs / ↑ Tacrolimus blood levels
Carbamazepine / ↓ Tacrolimus blood levels
Chloramphenicol / ↑ Tacrolimus blood levels
Cimetidine / ↑ Tacrolimus blood levels
Cisplatin / Additive or synergistic impairment of renal function
Clarithromycin / ↑ Tacrolimus blood levels
Cyclosporine / Additive or synergistic nephrotoxicity; also, ↑ tacrolimus blood levels
Danazol / ↑ Tacrolimus blood levels
Diltiazem / ↑ Tacrolimus blood levels
H *Echinacea* / Do not give with tacrolimus
Erythromycin / ↑ Tacrolimus blood levels
Itraconazole / ↑ Tacrolimus levels
Methylprednisolone / ↑ Tacrolimus blood levels
Metoclopramide / ↑ Tacrolimus blood levels
Nefazodone / Possible tacrolimus toxicity
Nelfinavir / ↑ Tacrolimus levels probably due to ↓ liver metabolism
Phenobarbital / ↓ Tacrolimus blood levels
Phenytoin / ↓ Tacrolimus blood levels
Rifamycin / ↓ Tacrolimus blood levels
Vaccines / ↓ Effectiveness of vaccines

HOW SUPPLIED

Capsule: 1 mg, 5 mg; *Injection:* 5 mg/ml; *Ointment:* 0.03%, 0.1%

DOSAGE

• **IV INFUSION ONLY**

Immunosuppression.

Initial: 0.05–0.1 mg/kg/day as a continuous IV infusion. Early in the period following transplantation, concomitant adrenal corticosteroid use is recommended.

• **CAPSULES**

Immunosuppression.

Initial: 0.15–0.3 mg/kg/day administered in two divided doses q 12 hr. **Maintenance:** Titrate dose based on clinical assessment of rejection and tolerability. Lower doses may suffice for maintenance therapy.

• **OINTMENT**

Atopic dermatitis.

Adults: Apply a thin layer of either the 0.03% or 0.1% ointment to the affected skin areas b.i.d. **Children:** Apply a thin layer of only the 0.03% ointment to the affected skin areas b.i.d. Continue treatment for 1 week after clearing of signs and symptoms.

NURSING CONSIDERATIONS

ADMINISTRATION/STORAGE

IV 1. IV therapy may be started if unable to take capsules.

2. For both IV and PO administration, give doses for adult clients at the lower end of the dosage range and initiate doses for pediatric clients at the higher end of the dosage range (i.e., 0.1 mg/kg/day for IV use and 0.3 mg/kg/day for PO use).

3. Give the initial dose no sooner than 6 hr after implantation.

4. Prior to use dilute with either 0.9% NaCl or D5W to a concentration between 0.004 and 0.02 mg/mL.

5. Continue IV therapy only until client can be switched to PO therapy (usually within 2–3 days). Give the first PO dose 8–12 hr after discontinuing the IV infusion.

6. With renal or hepatic impairment administer at the lowest level of the dosage range.

7. Do not use tacrolimus and cyclosporine simultaneously; discontinue either agent at least 24 hr before initiating the other.

8. Store the diluted solution for infusion in glass or polyethylene containers and discard after 24 hr. Do not use PVC containers for storage due to decreased stability and the possiblity of extraction of phthalates.

ASSESSMENT

1. Injection contains castor oil derivatives; note any sensitivity.

2. Monitor serum electrolytes, CBC, uric acid, blood sugar, liver and renal function studies.

3. Determine time of transplantation; monitor in facilities equipped and staffed with adequate lab and supportive medical resources.

4. Monitor VS, labs, and I&O. Anticipate higher dosages in children to maintain trough levels and reduced dosage with impaired renal function.

5. During IV administration, observe continuously for the first 30 min and at frequent intervals until infusion completed; interrupt infusion if S&S of anaphylaxis occur.

6. Monitor tacrolimus levels; helpful in clinical evaluation of rejection and toxicity.

CLIENT/FAMILY TEACHING

1. Review the risk of therapy associated with neoplasia (lymphomas and other malignancies).

2. Must follow the written guidelines for medication therapy explicitly. Call with questions or if problems arise. The drug must be taken throughout one's lifetime to prevent transplant rejection.

3. Because this drug is so important to transplant clients in preventing rejection, a written list of all possible side effects and how to identify which side effects need to be reported will be provided.

4. Perform daily weights and I&O. Take BP and keep a log of these values for provider review. Report any persistent diarrhea, N&V and other adverse effects.

5. Report as scheduled to specialist/transplant center for assessment and labs to evaluate drug effectiveness, since dosage is based on clinical assessments of rejection and tolerability.

6. Avoid crowds, infections, and those with infections. Report any S&S of infection or if injury occurs.

7. Rub in the ointment gently and completely.

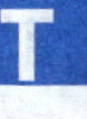

OUTCOMES/EVALUATE

- Prophylaxis of organ rejection
- Immune suppression
- Median trough blood concentrations of 9.8–19.4 ng/mL

Tamoxifen

(tah-**MOX**-ih-fen)

PREGNANCY CATEGORY: D
CLASSIFICATION(S):
Antiestrogen
Rx: Nolvadex
✱**Rx:** Apo-Tamox, Gen-Tamoxifen, Nolvadex-D, Novo–Tamoxifen, PMS-Tamoxifen, Tamofen

SEE ALSO *ANTINEOPLASTIC AGENTS*.

ACTION/KINETICS

Antiestrogen believed to compete with estrogen for estrogen-binding sites in target tissue (breast); also blocks uptake of estradiol. **Steady-state plasma levels (after 10 mg b.i.d. for 3 months):** 120 ng/mL for tamoxifen and 336 ng/mL for N-desmethyl tamoxifen. **Steady-state levels, tamoxifen:** About 4 weeks; **for N-desmethyltamoxifen:** About 8 weeks (**t½ for metabolite:** about 14 days). Metabolized to the equally active N-desmethyltamoxifen. Tamoxifen and metabolites are excreted mainly through the feces. Objective response may be delayed 4–10 weeks with bone metastases.

USES

(1) Adjuvant treatment of axillary node-negative or node-positive breast cancer in women following total or segmental mastectomy, axillary dissection, and breast irradiation. (2) Metastatic breast cancer in premenopausal women as an alternative to oophorectomy or ovarian irradiation (especially in women with estrogen-positive tumors). (3) Reduce risk of invasive breast cancer following breast surgery and radiation in women with ductal carcinoma in situ. (4) Advanced metastatic breast cancer in men. (5) To reduce the incidence of breast cancer in high-risk women, taking into account age, previous breast biopsies, age at first live birth, number of first-degree relatives with breast cancer, age at first menstrual period, and a history of lobular carcinoma in situ. *Investigational:* Mastalgia, gynecomastia (to treat pain and size), pancreatic carcinoma, advanced or recurrent endometrial and hepatocellular carcinoma.

CONTRAINDICATIONS

Lactation. Concomitant coumarin anticoagulant therapy or women with a history of deep vein thrombosis or pulmonary embolus.

SPECIAL CONCERNS

Use with caution in clients with leukopenia or thrombocytopenia. Women should not become pregnant while taking tamoxifen. Although the risk of breast cancer is significantly lowered, this benefit must be weighed against an increased risk of endometrial cancer, pulmonary embolism, and DVT. Safety and efficacy have not been determined in children.

SIDE EFFECTS

GI: N&V, distaste for food, anorexia, diarrhea, abdominal cramps. **CV:** Peripheral edema, flushing, superficial phlebitis, DVT, ***pulmonary embolism, thromboembolic disorders (especially when tamoxifen is combined with other cytotoxic agents).*** **CNS:** Depression, dizziness, lightheadedness, headache, fatigue. **Hepatic:** Rarely, fatty liver, cholestasis, hepatitis, ***hepatic necrosis.*** **GU:** Hot flashes, vaginal bleeding and discharge, menstrual irregularities, amenorrhea, altered menses, oligomenorrhea, vaginal dryness, pruritus vulvae, ovarian cysts, hyperplasia of the uterus, polyps, uterine carcinoma. **Ophthalmic:** Corneal changes, cataracts, decrease in color vision perception, retinal vein thrombosis, retinopathy. **Hematologic:** Leukopenia, thrombocytopenia. **Other:** Skin rash, skin changes, hypercalcemia, musculoskeletal pain, hyperlipidemias, weight gain or loss, increased bone and tumor pain, hair thinning or partial loss, fluid retention, coughing. In men, may be loss of libido and impotence, after discontinuing therapy.

LABORATORY TEST CONSIDERATIONS

↑ Serum calcium (transient), thyroid-binding globulin in postmenopausal women, BUN, AST, alkaline phosphatase, bilirubin, creatinine.

DRUG INTERACTIONS

Anticoagulants / ↑ Hypoprothrombinemic effect

Bromocriptine / ↑ Serum levels of tamoxifen and N-desmethyl tamoxifen

Cytotoxic drugs / ↑ Risk of thromboembolic events

HOW SUPPLIED

Tablet: 10 mg, 20 mg

DOSAGE

• TABLETS

Breast cancer.

10–20 mg b.i.d. (morning and evening) or 20 mg daily. Doses of 10 mg b.i.d.–t.i.d. for 2 years and 10 mg b.i.d. for 5 or more years have been used. There is no evidence that doses greater than 20 mg daily are more effective.

Reduction in incidence of breast cancer in high-risk women.

20 mg/day for 5 years.

Mastalgia.

10 mg/day for 4 months.

Ductal carcinoma in situ.

20 mg daily for 5 years.

NURSING CONSIDERATIONS

SEE ALSO *NURSING CONSIDERATIONS* FOR *ANTINEOPLASTIC AGENTS*.

ADMINISTRATION/STORAGE

Initiate tamoxifen during menses in sexually active women of child-bearing age. In those with menstrual irregularities, a negative B-hCG just before starting therapy is sufficient.

ASSESSMENT

1. Document onset, duration, and characteristics of symptoms, surgery and biopsy results. Note any other therapies received.
2. Assess hematologic profile and monitor. Drug may cause granulocyte suppression. Nadir: 14 days; recovery: 21 days.
3. The effect of the steroid and osteolytic metastases may result in hypercalcemia. Report symptoms of hypercalcemia (insomnia, lethargy, anorexia, N&V, coma, and vascular collapse).
4. With increased pain, administer adequate analgesics.

CLIENT/FAMILY TEACHING

1. Review side effects that should be reported; a reduction in dosage or discontinuation may be indicated.
2. Increased bone and lumbar pain or local disease flares should subside; take analgesics as needed.
3. Consume 2–3 L/day of fluids to minimize hypercalcemia.
4. Exercise to reduce calcium levels, improve circulation, and prevent thrombophlebitis. (Perform ROM exercises if bedridden.)
5. Record weights weekly; report excessive weight gain or evidence of peripheral edema.
6. May experience "hot flashes"; stay in cool environment.
7. Wear protective clothing, sunscreens, and sunglasses to prevent photosensitivity reactions.
8. Practice safe, nonhormonal methods of contraception during and for 1 mo following therapy.
9. Report decreased visual acuity, may be irreversible. Have regular eye exams, especially if higher than usual dosage.
10. Obtain regular GYN exams; report menstrual irregularities, abnormal vaginal bleeding, change in discharge, or pelvic pain/pressure.
11. Although the risk of breast cancer is significantly lowered, there is also an increased risk of endometrial cancer, pulmonary embolism, and DVT.

OUTCOMES/EVALUATE

- Suppression of tumor growth and malignant cell proliferation
- Relief of breast pain
- Prophylaxis of breast cancer in high-risk women

Tamsulosin hydrochloride

(tam-**SOO**-loh-sin)

PREGNANCY CATEGORY: B

CLASSIFICATION(S):

Alpha-adrenergic blocking drug

Rx: Flomax

ACTION/KINETICS

Blockade of alpha-1 receptors (probably $alpha_{1A)}$ in prostate results in relaxation of smooth muscles in bladder neck and prostate; thus, urine flow rate is improved and there is a decrease in symptoms of BPH. Food interferes with the rate of absorption. **t½, elimination:** 5–7 hr. Significantly bound to plasma proteins. Extensively metabolized in liver; excreted through urine and feces.

USES

Treatment of signs and symptoms of BPH. Rule out prostatic carcinoma before using tamsulosin.

CONTRAINDICATIONS

Use to treat hypertension, with other alpha-adrenergic blocking agents, or in women or children.

SPECIAL CONCERNS

Use with caution with concurrent administration of warfarin.

SIDE EFFECTS

Body as a whole: Headache, infection, asthenia, back pain, chest pain. **CV:** Postural hypotension, syncope. **GI:** Diarrhea, nausea, tooth disorder. **CNS:** Dizziness, vertigo, somnolence, insomnia, decreased libido. **Respiratory:** Rhinitis, pharyngitis, increased cough, sinusitis. **GU:** Abnormal ejaculation. **Miscellaneous:** Amblyopia.

OD OVERDOSE MANAGEMENT

Symptoms: Hypotension. *Treatment:* Keep client in supine position to restore BP and normalize HR. If this is inadequate, consider IV fluids. Vasopressors may also be used; monitor renal function.

DRUG INTERACTIONS

Cimetidine causes significant ↓ in clearance of tamsulosin.

HOW SUPPLIED

Capsules: 0.4 mg

DOSAGE

• **CAPSULES**

Benign prostatic hypertrophy.

Adult males: 0.4 mg daily given about 30 min after same meal each day. If, after 2 to 4 weeks, clients have not responded, dose can be increased to 0.8 mg daily.

NURSING CONSIDERATIONS

ADMINISTRATION/STORAGE

1. If dose is discontinued or interrupted for several days after either the 0.4 mg or 0.8 mg dose, start therapy again with 0.4 mg dose.
2. Store at 20–25°C (68–77°F).

ASSESSMENT

1. Document indications for therapy, onset, and characteristics of symptoms. Note BPH score.
2. List drugs prescribed to ensure none interact; especially cimetidine and coumadin.
3. Note PSA levels and results of digital rectal exam.

CLIENT/FAMILY TEACHING

1. Take as directed, do not chew, crush, or open capsule. Report any loss of effectiveness or increase in nighttime voiding.
2. Do not perform activities that require mental/physical alertness until drug effects realized; may cause dizziness and syncope.

OUTCOMES/EVALUATE

Improvement in BPH symptoms; decreased nocturia

Tazarotene

(taz-**AR**-oh-teen)

PREGNANCY CATEGORY: X
CLASSIFICATION(S):
Antipsoriasis drug
Rx: Tazorac

ACTION/KINETICS

A retinoid prodrug converted by deesterification to active cognate carboxylic acid of tazarotene. Mechanism not known. Little systemic absorption. **t½, after topical use:** About 18 hr. Parent drug and metabolite are further metabolized and excreted through urine and feces.

USES

Stable plaque psoriasis. Mild to moderate facial acne vulgaris.

CONTRAINDICATIONS
Pregnancy. Use on eczematous skin. Use of cosmetics or skin medications that have strong drying effect.

SPECIAL CONCERNS
Use with caution during lactation. Safety and efficacy have not been determined in children less than 12 years of age. Psoriasis may worsen from month 4 to 12 compared with first 3 months of therapy. Use with caution with drugs that cause photosensitivity.

SIDE EFFECTS
Dermatologic: Pruritus, photosensitivity, burning/stinging, erythema, worsening of psoriasis, skin pain, irritation, rash, desquamation, contact dermatitis, skin inflammation, fissuring, bleeding, dry skin, localized edema, skin discoloration.

OD OVERDOSE MANAGEMENT
Symptoms: Marked redness, peeling, discomfort. *Treatment:* Decrease or discontinue dose.

DRUG INTERACTIONS
↑ Risk of photosensitivity when used with fluoroquinolones, phenothiazines, sulfonamides, tetracyclines, thiazides.

HOW SUPPLIED
Cream: 0.05%, 0.1%; *Gel:* 0.05%, 0.1%

DOSAGE

• **CREAM, GEL**

Acne vulgaris, Psoriasis.

After skin is dry following cleaning, apply thin film (2 mg/cm^2) on lesions once daily in evening. Cover entire affected area. For psoriasis, do not apply to more than 20% of body surface area.

NURSING CONSIDERATIONS

ADMINISTRATION/STORAGE
Avoid application to unaffected skin due to increased susceptibility to irritation.

ASSESSMENT
1. Document condition requiring treatment; may photograph to assess response.
2. Determine if pregnant and begin therapy during menstrual cycle.

CLIENT/FAMILY TEACHING
1. Cleanse face gently, pat dry, apply a thin film in evening only where lesions are present.
2. Apply once daily as directed. Avoid contact with eyes and mouth; rinse thoroughly if contact occurs.
3. Report excessive itching, redness, burning, or peeling of skin. Stop therapy until skin integrity restored.
4. Avoid weather extremes such as wind or cold; may increase irritation.
5. Practice reliable contraception; drug causes fetal damage.
6. May experience photosensitivity reaction; use sunscreens and protective clothing if exposed.

OUTCOMES/EVALUATE
Clearing of psoriasis placques/acne lesions

Telmisartan

(**tell**-mih-**SAR**-tan)

PREGNANCY CATEGORY: C (FIRST TRIMESTER), D (SECOND AND THIRD TRIMESTERS)
CLASSIFICATION(S):
Antihypertensive, angiotensin II receptor blocker
Rx: Micardis

SEE ALSO *ANGIOTENSIN II RECEPTOR ANTAGONISTS* AND *ANTIHYPERTENSIVES.*

ACTION/KINETICS
Over 99.5% bound to plasma protein. Control of BP in blacks is less than in whites. **t½, terminal:** About 24 hr. Excreted mainly in the feces by way of the bile.

USES
Treat hypertension alone or in combination with other antihypertensives.

SPECIAL CONCERNS
Use with caution in impaired hepatic function or in biliary obstructive disorders.

SIDE EFFECTS
GI: Diarrhea, dyspepsia, heartburn, N&V, abdominal pain. **CNS:** Dizziness, headache, fatigue, anxiety, nervousness. **Musculoskeletal:** Pain, includ-

T

ing back and neck pain; myalgia. **Respiratory:** URI, sinusitis, cough, pharyngitis, influenza. **Miscellaneous:** Chest pain, UTI, peripheral edema, hypertension.

LABORATORY TEST CONSIDERATIONS

↑ Creatinine (in small number of clients). ↓ Hemoglobin.

OD OVERDOSE MANAGEMENT

Symptoms: Hypotension, dizziness, tachycardia or bradycardia. *Treatment:* Supportive for hypotension.

DRUG INTERACTIONS

↑ Digoxin peak plasma and trough levels.

HOW SUPPLIED

Tablets: 40 mg, 80 mg

DOSAGE

- **TABLETS**

  Antihypertensive.

Adults, initial: 40 mg/day. **Maintenance:** 20–80 mg/day. If additional BP reduction is desired beyond that achieved with 80 mg/day, add a diuretic.

NURSING CONSIDERATIONS

ADMINISTRATION/STORAGE

May be taken with or without food.

ASSESSMENT

1. Note onset and duration of disease, other agents trialed and the outcome.
2. Symptomatic hypotension may occur in clients who are volume- or salt-depleted. Correct prior to using telmisartan, use a lower starting dose and monitor closely.
3. With renal dialysis may develop orthostatic hypotension; monitor BP closely.
4. Monitor ECG, renal, LFTs and VS. With hepatic or renal dysfunction, use cautiously.

CLIENT/FAMILY TEACHING

1. Take as directed at the same time daily with or without food.
2. Regular exercise, low-salt diet, and life-style changes (i.e., no smoking, low alcohol, low-fat diet, low stress, adequate rest) contribute to enhanced BP control.
3. Use effective contraception; report pregnancy as drug during second and third trimesters associated with fetal injury and morbidity.

OUTCOMES/EVALUATE

BP control

Temazepam

(teh-**MAZ**-eh-pam)

PREGNANCY CATEGORY: X

CLASSIFICATION(S):

Sedative-hypnotic, benzodiazepine

Rx: Restoril , **C-IV**

✱Rx: Apo-Temazepam, Gen-Temazepam, Novo-Temazepam, Nu-Temazepam, PMS-Temazepam

SEE ALSO *TRANQUILIZERS, ANTIMANIC DRUGS, AND HYPNOTICS.*

ACTION/KINETICS

Benzodiazepine derivative. Disturbed nocturnal sleep may occur the first one or two nights following discontinuance of the drug. Prolonged administration is not recommended because physical dependence and tolerance may develop. See also *Flurazepam.* **Peak blood levels:** 2–4 hr. **t½, initial:** 0.4–0.6 hr; **final:** 10 hr. **Steady-state plasma levels:** 382 ng/mL (2.5 hr after 30-mg dose). Accumulation of the drug is minimal following multiple dosage. Significantly bound (98%) to plasma protein. Metabolized in the liver to inactive metabolites.

USES

Insomnia in clients unable to fall asleep, with frequent awakenings during the night and/or early morning awakenings.

CONTRAINDICATIONS

Pregnancy.

SPECIAL CONCERNS

Use with caution in severely depressed clients. Use during lactation may cause sedation and feeding problems in the infant. Geriatric clients may be more sensitive to the effects of temazepam.

SIDE EFFECTS

CNS: Drowsiness (after daytime use) and dizziness are common. Lethargy, confusion, euphoria, weakness, ataxia, lack of concentration, hallucinations. In some clients, paradoxical excitement (less than 0.5%), including stimulation and hyperactivity, occurs. **GI:** Anorexia, diarrhea. **Other:** Tremors, horizontal nystagmus, falling, palpitations. Rarely, blood dyscrasias.

HOW SUPPLIED

Capsule: 7.5 mg, 15 mg, 30 mg

DOSAGE

• CAPSULES

Adults, usual: 15–30 mg at bedtime. **In elderly or debilitated clients, initial:** 15 mg; **then,** adjust dosage to response.

NURSING CONSIDERATIONS

SEE ALSO *NURSING CONSIDERATIONS* FOR *TRANQUILIZERS, ANTIMANIC DRUGS, AND HYPNOTICS*.

ASSESSMENT

1. Note indications for therapy, onset, duration and characteristics of symptoms.
2. Assess sleep patterns; identify factors/triggers contributing to insomnia.

CLIENT/FAMILY TEACHING

1. Take only as directed and do not increase dose.
2. May cause daytime drowsiness. Avoid activities that require mental alertness until drug effects realized.
3. Avoid alcohol and CNS depressants; may increase CNS depression.
4. Avoid tobacco; decreases drug's effect.
5. Review nonpharmacologic methods of sleep induction.
6. Practice reliable birth control; may cause fetal harm.
7. For short-term use only. Long-term use can cause dependence and withdrawal symptoms. After more than 3 weeks of continuous use may experience rebound insomnia.

OUTCOMES/EVALUATE

Improved sleeping patterns; ↓ awakenings

Temozolomide

(tem-oh-**ZOHL**-oh-myd)

PREGNANCY CATEGORY: D

CLASSIFICATION(S):

Antineoplastic, miscellaneous

Rx: Temodar

✱Rx: Temodal

ACTION/KINETICS

Temozolomide is a prodrug that is hydrolyzed, nonenzymatically, at physiologic pH to the reactive 3-methyl-(triazen-1-yl)imidazole-4-carboxamide (MTIC). MTIC methylates specific guanine-rich areas of DNA that initiate transcription, leading to cytotoxicity and antiproliferative effects. Rapidly and completely absorbed after PO use. **Peak plasma levels:** 1 hr. Food reduces the rate and extent of absorption. Metabolized by hydrolysis. Excreted mainly in the urine. **t½:** 1.8 hr.

USES

Treat adults with refractory anaplastic astrocytoma, i.e., those at first relapse whose disease has progressed on a drug regimen containing a nitrosourea and procarbazine.

CONTRAINDICATIONS

Hypersensitivity to dacarbazine (DTIC) because it is also metabolized to MTIC. Lactation.

SPECIAL CONCERNS

Use with caution in the elderly and in those with severe renal or hepatic impairment. Safety and efficacy have not been determined in pediatric clients.

SIDE EFFECTS

Most common: N&V, headache, fatigue. *Myelosuppression:* Thrombocytopenia, neutropenia.

CNS: Convulsions, hemiparesis, dizziness, abnormal coordination, amnesia, insomnia, paresthesia, somnolence, paresis, ataxia, anxiety, dysphasia, depression, abnormal gait, confusion. **GI:** N&V, constipation, diarrhea, abdominal pain, anorexia. **Dermatologic:** Rash, pruritus. **Respiratory:** URTI, pharyngitis, sinusitis, coughing. **GU:** Urinary incontinence, UTI, increased frequency of micturition. **Ophthalmic:** Diplopia, blurred vision, visual deficit, vision changes, vision troubles. **Body as a whole:** Fatigue, asthenia, fever, viral infection, weight increase, myalgia. **Miscellaneous:** Headache, pe-

T

ripheral edema, back pain, adrenal hypercorticism, female breast pain.

OD OVERDOSE MANAGEMENT

Symptoms: Neutropenia, thrombocytopenia. *Treatment:* Hematologic evaluation. Supportive measures, as necessary.

DRUG INTERACTIONS

Valproic acid ↓ PO clearance of temozolomide.

HOW SUPPLIED

Capsules: 5 mg, 20 mg, 100 mg, 250 mg

DOSAGE

• **CAPSULES**

Anaplastic astrocytoma.

Adults, initial: 150 mg/m^2 once daily for 5 consecutive days per 28-day treatment cycle. If both the nadir and day of dosing (day 29, day 1 of next cycle) ANC are equal to or greater than 1.5 x 10^9 (1500/mcL), the dose may be increased to 200 mg/m^2 for 5 consecutive days per 28-day treatment cycle.

During treatment, obtain a CBC on day 22 (21 days after the first dose) or within 48 hr of that day, and weekly until the ANC is greater than 1.5 x 10^9/L (1500/mcL) and the platelet count exceeds 100 x 10^9 (100,000/mcL). Do not start the next cycle until the ANC and platelet count exceed these levels. If the ANC falls to less than 1 x 10^9/L (1000/mcL) or the platelet count is less than 50 x 10^9/L (50,000/mcL) during any cycle, reduce the next cycle by 50 mg/m^2, but not less than 100 mg/m^2 (the lowest recommended dose).

T

NURSING CONSIDERATIONS

ADMINISTRATION/STORAGE

1. Therapy can be continued until disease progression; the optimum duration is not known.
2. Consult the package insert for dosage calculations based on body surface area and suggested capsule combinations to achieve the required daily dose.
3. Follow institutional procedures for proper handling and disposal of antineoplastic agents.

ASSESSMENT

1. Note disease onset, previous drug regimen and date of relapse.
2. Determine BSA–daily dosage dependent on calculations; see package insert. Temozolomide capsule combinations based on daily dose/BSA.
3. Obtain CBC 21 days after first dose and weekly until recovery (ANC > 1.5 x 10^9/L).
4. If ANC < 1 x 10^9/L or platelet count < 50 x 10^9/L during any cycle reduce dose as directed under dosage. Nadir 21-40 days for platelets and 1-44 days for neutrophils.

CLIENT/FAMILY TEACHING

1. To reduce N&V, take on an empty stomach, preferably at bedtime.
2. May experience nausea, vomiting, fatigue, and headaches. Antiemetic therapy may be given before or after temozolomide administration.
3. Do not open or chew capsules; swallow whole with a glass of water.
4. If capsules are accidentally opened or damaged, take serious precautions to avoid inhalation or contact with the skin or mucous membranes.
5. Store away from children and pets.

OUTCOMES/EVALUATE

Treatment of refractory anaplastic astrocytoma

Tenecteplase

(teh-**NECK**-teh-plays)

PREGNANCY CATEGORY: C

CLASSIFICATION(S):

Thrombolytic, tissue plasminogen activator

Rx: TNKase

ACTION/KINETICS

A tissue plasminogen activator produced by recombinant DNA. It binds to fibrin and converts plasminogen to plasmin. In the presence of fibrin, tenecteplase conversion of plasminogen to plasmin is increased relative to conversion in the absence of fibrin. Following the drug there are decreases in circulating fibrinogen. **$t^1/_2$, initial disposition:** 20–24 min; **terminal dis-**

position: 90–130 min. Metabolized in the liver.

USES

Reduce mortality due to acute myocardial infarction.

CONTRAINDICATIONS

Active internal bleeding, history of CVA, within 2 months of intracranial or intraspinal surgery or trauma, intracranial neoplasm, arteriovenous malformation or aneurysm, known bleeding diathesis, severe uncontrolled hypertension. IM use.

SPECIAL CONCERNS

There is the possibility of cholesterol embolization and arrhythmias associated with reperfusion. Use with caution in the elderly, weighing the benefits versus risks, including bleeding. Use with caution during lactation. Safety and efficacy have not been determined in children.

SIDE EFFECTS

Bleeding.

Most common side effect. Major bleeding includes hematoma, GI tract, urinary tract, puncture site (including cardiac catheterization site), retroperitoneal, respiratory tract. Minor bleeding includes hematoma, urinary tract, puncture site (including cardiac catheterization site), pharyngeal, GI tract, and epistaxis.

CV: Cardiogenic shock, arrrhythmias, AV block, ***heart failure, cardiac arrest,*** recurrent myocardial ischemia, ***myocardial reinfarction, myocardial rupture, cardiac tamponade,*** pericarditis, pericardial effusion, mitral regurgitation, thrombosis, embolism, electromechanical dissociation. **Miscellaneous:** Pulmonary edema, N&V, hypotension, fever, ***serious allergic or anaphylactic reactions.***

LABORATORY TEST CONSIDERATIONS

Results of coagulation tests or measures of fibrinolytic activity may be unreliable; specific precautions must be taken to prevent in vitro artifacts. Degradation of fibrinogen in blood samples removed for analysis is possible.

DRUG INTERACTIONS

Heparin, vitamin K antagonists, aspirin, dipyridamole, and GP IIb/IIIa inhibitors may increase the risk of bleeding if given prior to, during, or after tenecteplase therapy.

HOW SUPPLIED

Powder for injection, lyophilized: 50 mg

DOSAGE

• **IV**

AMI.

Dose is based on client weight, but not to exceed 50 mg. Given as a single bolus dose over 5 sec. **Less than 60 kg:** 30 mg (6 mL); **60 kg–less than 70 kg:** 35 mg (7 mL); **70 kg– less than 80 kg:** 40 mg (8 mL); **80 kg– less than 90 kg:** 45 mg (9 mL); **90 kg and over:** 50 mg (10 mL).

NURSING CONSIDERATIONS

ADMINISTRATION/STORAGE

IV 1. Initiate treatment as soon as possible after the onset of symptoms of MI.

2. Reconstitute and administer as follows:

• Aseptically withdraw 10 mL sterile water for injection from that supplied. Use the red hub cannula syringe filling device. Do not discard the shield assembly. Do *not* use bacteriostatic water for injection.

• Inject the entire contents of the syringe (10 mL) into the tenecteplase vial. Direct the stream into the powder. Slight foaming may occur; any large bubbles will dissipate if allowed to stand undisturbed for several minutes.

• Swirl contents gently until completely dissolved. Do not shake. The reconstituted product is colorless to pale yellow and is transparent with a concentration of 5 mg/mL and pH of about 7.3.

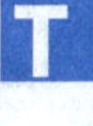

• Determine the appropriate dose of tenecteplase and withdraw the correct volume (in mL) from the reconstituted vial with the syringe. Discard any unused portion.

• With the correct dose in the syringe, stand the shield vertically on a flat surface with the green side down and passivley recap the red hub cannula.

• Remove the entire shield assembly, including the red hub cannula by twisting counter clockwise. The shield assembly also contains the clear-ended blunt plastic cannula; retain for split septum IV access.

• Administer as a single IV bolus over 5 sec.

3. Tenecteplase contains no preservatives; thus, reconstitute immediately before use.

4. If given in an IV line with dextrose, precipitation may occur. Flush dextrose-containing lines with a saline-containing solution prior to and following single bolus administration of tenecteplase.

5. Store lyophilized tenecteplase at controlled temperatures not to exceed 30°C (86°F) or under refrigeration at 2–8°C (36–46°F).

6. If reconstituted drug is not used immediately, refrigerate the tenecteplase vial at 2–8°C (36–46°F) and use within 8 hr.

ASSESSMENT

1. Note indications for therapy identifying symptom onset and site of infarct.

2. Do not use with active internal bleeding, history of CVA, recent: intracranial bleed, spinal surgery, trauma or neoplasm; AV malformation, aneurysm, or uncontrolled HTN.

3. Obtain baseline weight, CBC, bleeding times, type and crossmatch.

4. Assess for reperfusion arrhythmias after therapy which may include accelerated idioventricular rhythm, sinus bradycardia of short duration, and return of elevated ST segment to near baseline.

CLIENT/FAMILY TEACHING

1. Review inherent benefits and risks of drug therapy.

2. To be effective, the therapy should be instituted as soon as possible after symptom onset of AMI.

3. Report any adverse effects or side effects immediately.

4. Encourage family members or significant other to learn CPR.

OUTCOMES/EVALUATE

↓ Mortality with AMI; resolution on MI

Teniposide (VM-26)

(teh-**NIP**-ah-side)

PREGNANCY CATEGORY: D

CLASSIFICATION(S):

Antineoplastic, miscellaneous

Rx: Vumon

SEE ALSO *ANTINEOPLASTIC AGENTS.*

ACTION/KINETICS

Derivative of podophyllotoxin that acts in the late S or early G_2 phase of the cell cycle, preventing cells from entering mitosis. Inhibits type II topoisomerase activity resulting in both single- and double-stranded breaks in DNA and DNA:protein cross-links. Active against sublines of certain murine leukemias that have developed resistance to amsacrine, cisplatin, daunorubicin, doxorubicin, mitoxantrone, or vincristine. **Terminal t½:** 5 hr. Significantly bound to plasma proteins (over 99%). Metabolized in the liver and excreted mainly through the urine (4%–12% unchanged) with small amounts excreted in the feces.

USES

In combination with other antineoplastic agents for induction therapy in clients with refractory childhood acute lymphoblastic leukemia (ALL). Has also been used for relapsed ALL.

CONTRAINDICATIONS

Hypersensitivity to teniposide, etoposide, or the polyoxylethylated castor oil present in teniposide products. Lactation.

SPECIAL CONCERNS

Clients with both Down syndrome and leukemia may be especially sensitive to myelosuppressive chemotherapy; thus, reduce initial dosing. A life-threatening anaphylactic reaction may occur with the first dose (incidence appears to be greater in clients with brain tumors and neuroblastoma). Use with caution in clients with impaired hepatic function. Contains benzyl alcohol associated with a fatal "gasping" syndrome in premature infants.

SIDE EFFECTS

Hematologic: *Severe myelosuppression,* leukopenia, neutropenia, thrombocytopenia, anemia. *Hypersensitivity reactions:* ***Anaphylaxis*** manifested by chills, fever, ***bronchospasm,*** dyspnea, facial flushing, hypertension or hypotension, tachycardia. **CV:** Hypotension. **GI:** Mucositis, N&V, diarrhea. **Dermatologic:** Alopecia (reversible), rash, hepatic dysfunction or toxicity, peripheral neurotoxicity, infection, bleeding, renal dysfunction, metabolic abnormalities.

OD OVERDOSE MANAGEMENT

Symptoms: Myelosuppression, hypotension, anaphylaxis. *Treatment (Anaphylaxis or Overdose):*

- Treat anaphylaxis promptly with antihistamines, corticosteroids, epinephrine, IV fluids, and other supportive measures. If a client who manifested a hypersensitivity reaction must be retreated, undertake pretreatment with corticosteroids and antihistamines; carefully observe client during and after the infusion.
- If hypotension occurs, stop the infusion and give fluids. Undertake other supportive therapy as needed.
- Myelosuppression may be treated with supportive care including blood products and antibiotics.

DRUG INTERACTIONS

Antiemetic drugs / Acute CNS depression and hypotension in clients receiving high doses of teniposide and who were pretreated with antiemetics

Methotrexate / ↑ Plasma clearance of methotrexate

Sodium salicylate / ↑ Teniposide effect R/T displacement from plasma protein binding sites

Sulfamethizole / ↑ Teniposide effect R/T displacement from plasma protein binding sites

Tolbutamide / ↑ Teniposide effect R/T displacement from plasma protein binding sites

HOW SUPPLIED

Injection: 10 mg/mL

DOSAGE

- **IV INFUSION**

Regimen 1 for childhood ALL clients failing induction therapy with cytarabine.

Teniposide, 165 mg/m², and cytarabine, 300 mg/m² IV twice weekly for eight to nine doses.

Regimen 2 for childhood ALL refractory to vincristine/prednisone-containing regimens.

Teniposide, 250 mg/m², and vincristine, 1.5 mg/m², IV weekly for 4–8 weeks, and prednisone, 40 mg/m² orally for 28 days.

Note: Dosage adjustment may be needed for clients with significant renal or hepatic dysfunction.

NURSING CONSIDERATIONS

SEE ALSO *NURSING CONSIDERATIONS* FOR *ANTINEOPLASTIC AGENTS* AND *ETOPOSIDE*.

ADMINISTRATION/STORAGE

IV 1. Give over 30–60 min or longer; do not give by rapid IV infusion, as hypotension may occur.

2. The IV catheter or needle must be in the proper position and functional prior to infusion. Improper administration may cause extravasation resulting in local tissue necrosis or thrombophlebitis. Also, occlusion of central venous access devices has occurred during 24-hr infusion at concentrations of 0.1–0.2 mg/mL.

3. Dilute with either D5W or 0.9% NaCl injection to give a final concentration of 0.1, 0.2, 0.4, or 1 mg/mL.

4. Contact of undiluted teniposide with plastic equipment/devices used to prepare IV infusions may result in softening, cracking, and possible drug leakage. To prevent extraction of plasticizer DEHP, prepare and give solutions in non-DEHP-containing LVP containers such as glass or polyolefin plastic bags or containers. Do not use PVC containers.

5. Lipid administration sets or low DEHP-containing nitroglycerin sets will keep exposure to DEHP at low levels and can be used. Diluted solutions are chemically/physically compatible with the recommended IV administration sets and LVP containers for up to 24 hr at ambient room temperature and lighting conditions.

6. Use caution in handling and preparing the solution as skin reactions may occur with accidental exposure and drug is cytotoxic. Use of gloves is

recommended; if the solution comes in contact with the skin, wash immediately with soap and water. If the drug comes in contact with mucous membranes, flush thoroughly with water.
7. Heparin solution can cause precipitation of teniposide, flush administration apparatus thoroughly with D5W or 0.9% NaCl injection before and after administration.
8. Unopened ampules are stable until the date indicated if stored at 2–8°C (36–46°F) in the original package (protected from light).
9. Give solutions containing 1 mg/mL within 4 hr of preparation to reduce the potential for precipitation. Refrigeration of solutions is not recommended.
10. Precipitation of teniposide may occur at the recommended concentrations, especially if the diluted solution is agitated more than recommended during preparation. Also, minimize storage time prior to administration; take care to avoid contact of the diluted solution with other drugs or fluids.
11. Not for use in premature infants; contains benzyl alcohol.

ASSESSMENT

1. Note any sensitivity to product derivatives, especially polyoxylethylated castor oil. Product also contains benzyl alcohol.
2. Premedicate with antiemetics; observe for enhanced CNS effects.
3. Reduce dose with Down syndrome, liver or renal dysfunction.
4. If symptoms of anaphylaxis occur (chills, fever, tachycardia, chest pain, dyspnea, or altered BP), interrupt infusion and report.
5. Monitor hematologic profile, uric acid, liver and renal function studies. May cause granulocyte and platelet suppression. Withhold if platelet count < 50,000/mm^3 or ANC < 500/mm^3 do not resume treatment until hematologic recovery is evident. Nadir: 14 days; recovery: 21 days.

CLIENT/FAMILY TEACHING

1. Drug is a "possible carcinogen"; review risk of developing secondary acute nonlymphocytic leukemia with intensive therapy schedules (1–2 times/week during remission).
2. Report promptly if fever, chills, rapid heartbeat, or difficulty in breathing occurs.
3. N&V and hair loss are frequent drug side effects.
4. Drug will cause fetal harm; use reliable contraceptive measures during treatment.

OUTCOMES/EVALUATE

Remission with relapsed or refractory ALL

Tenofovir disoproxil fumarate

(teh-**NOFF**-oh-veer)

PREGNANCY CATEGORY: B
CLASSIFICATION(S):
Antiviral, nucleoside reverse transcriptase inhibitor
Rx: Viread

ACTION/KINETICS

Tenofovir disoproxil inhibits the activity of HIV reverse transcriptase by competing with the natural substrate deoxyadenosine 5′-triphosphate and, after incorporation into DNA, by DNA chain termination. **Maximum serum levels:** About 1 hr. High fat meals increase the PO bioavailability. Excreted by a combination of glomerular filtration and active tubular secretion. Impairment of renal or hepatic function affects the pharmacokinetics.

USES

In combination with other antiretroviral drugs to treat HIV-1 infection that is expected to be susceptible to tenofovir based on lab testing or treatment history.

CONTRAINDICATIONS

Use in those with renal insufficiency (C_{CR} <60 mL/min). Lactation.

SPECIAL CONCERNS

Lactic acidosis and severe hepatomegaly with steatosis (may be fatal), especially in women. Obesity and prolonged nucleoside administration may be risk factors. Use with caution in clients with known risk factors for liver disease and in the elderly.

SIDE EFFECTS
GI: N&V, diarrhea, flatulence, abdominal pain. **Miscellaneous:** ***Lactic acidosis, severe hepatomegaly with steatosis,*** asthenia, headache, anorexia.
LABORATORY TEST CONSIDERATIONS
↑ AST, ALT, creatine kinase, triglycerides, serum amylase, urine/serum glucose. ↓ Neutrophils.
DRUG INTERACTIONS
Acyclovir / ↑ Serum levels of tenofovir R/T competition for tubular secretion
Cidofovir / ↑ Serum levels of tenofovir R/T competition for tubular secretion
Didanosine / ↑ Maximum concentration and AUC of didanosine
Ganciclovir / ↑ Serum levels of tenofovir R/T competition for tubular secretion
Valacyclovir / ↑ Serum levels of tenofovir R/T competition for tubular secretion
Valganciclovir / ↑ Serum levels of tenofovir R/T competition for tubular secretion
HOW SUPPLIED
Tablet: 300 mg (equivalent to 245 mg tenofovir disoproxil)

DOSAGE
• **TABLETS**
HIV-1 infection.
300 mg once daily taken PO with a meal.

NURSING CONSIDERATIONS
ASSESSMENT
1. Identify indications for therapy, disease onset, and other therapies trialed.
2. Assess for evidence of liver disease and acidosis. Monitor CBC, renal and LFTs, and viral loads.

CLIENT/FAMILY TEACHING
1. When taken with didanosine, take the tenofovir 2 hr before or 1 hr after didanosine administration.
2. Take once a day as prescribed with a meal.
3. May experience changes in body fat, N&V, diarrhea, and gas; report if intolerable.
4. Report any yellowing of skin or eyes, abdominal pain, muscle aches/pains and stop drug therapy.
5. Keep all F/U visits for labs and clinical evaluation

OUTCOMES/EVALUATE
Control of progression of tenofovir susceptible HIV infection

Terazosin
(ter-**AY**-zoh-sin)

PREGNANCY CATEGORY: C
CLASSIFICATION(S):
Antihypertensive, alpha-1-adrenergic blocking drug
Rx: Hytrin
✤**Rx:** Alti-Terazosin, Apo-Terazosin, Novo-Terazosin, Nu-Terazosin

ACTION/KINETICS
Blocks postsynaptic alpha-1-adrenergic receptors, leading to a dilation of both arterioles and veins, and ultimately, a reduction in BP. Both standing and supine BPs are lowered with no reflex tachycardia. Also relaxes smooth muscle of the prostate and bladder neck. Usefulness in BPH is due to alpha-1 receptor blockade, which relaxes the smooth muscle of the prostate and bladder neck and relieves pressure on the urethra. Bioavailability is not affected by food. **Onset:** 15 min. **Peak plasma levels:** 1–2 hr. **$t_{1/2}$:** 9–12 hr. **Duration:** 24 hr. Excreted unchanged and as inactive metabolites in both the urine and feces.
USES
(1) Alone or in combination with diuretics or beta-adrenergic blocking agents to treat hypertension. (2) Treat symptoms of benign prostatic hyperplasia.
SPECIAL CONCERNS
Use with caution during lactation. Safety and efficacy have not been determined in children. Geriatric clients may be more sensitive to the hypotensive and hypothermic effects of terazosin.
SIDE EFFECTS
First-dose effect: Marked postural hypotension and syncope.

CV: Palpitations, tachycardia, postural hypotension, syncope, ***arrhythmias,*** chest pain, vasodilation. **CNS:** Dizziness, headache, somnolence, drowsiness, nervousness, paresthesia, depression, anxiety, insomnia, vertigo. **Respiratory:** Nasal congestion, dyspnea, sinusitis, epistaxis, bronchitis, ***bronchospasm,*** cold or flu symptoms, increased cough, pharyngitis, rhinitis. **GI:** Nausea, constipation, diarrhea, dyspepsia, dry mouth, vomiting, flatulence, abdominal discomfort or pain. **Musculoskeletal:** Asthenia, arthritis, arthralgia, myalgia, joint disorders, back pain, pain in extremities, neck and shoulder pain, muscle cramps. **Miscellaneous:** Peripheral edema, weight gain, blurred vision, impotence, chest pain, fever, gout, pruritus, rash, sweating, urinary frequency, UTI, tinnitus, conjunctivitis, abnormal vision, edema, facial edema.

LABORATORY TEST CONSIDERATIONS

↓ H&H, WBCs, albumin.

OD OVERDOSE MANAGEMENT

Symptoms: Hypotension, drowsiness, shock. *Treatment:* Restore BP and HR. Client should be kept supine; vasopressors may be indicated. Volume expanders can be used to treat shock.

DRUG INTERACTIONS

When used with finasteride → ↑ finasteride plasma levels.

HOW SUPPLIED

Capsule: 1 mg, 2 mg, 5 mg, 10 mg

DOSAGE

• **CAPSULES**

Hypertension.

Individualized, initial: 1 mg at bedtime (this dose is not to be exceeded); **then,** increase dose slowly to obtain desired response. **Range:** 1–5 mg/day; doses as high as 20 mg may be required in some clients. Doses greater than 20 mg daily do not provide further BP control.

Benign prostatic hyperplasia.

Initial: 1 mg/day; dose should be increased to 2 mg, 5 mg, and then 10 mg once daily to improve symptoms and/or urinary flow rates. Doses greater than 20 mg daily have not been studied.

T

NURSING CONSIDERATIONS

SEE ALSO *NURSING CONSIDERATIONS* FOR *ANTIHYPERTENSIVE AGENTS.*

ADMINISTRATION/STORAGE

1. The initial dosing regimen must be carefully observed to minimize severe hypotension.
2. Monitor BP 2–3 hr after dosing and at end of dosing interval to ensure BP control maintained.
3. Consider an increase in dose or b.i.d. dosing if BP control is not maintained at 24-hr interval.
4. To prevent dizziness or fainting due to a drop in BP, take the initial dose at bedtime; the daily dose can be given in the morning.
5. If terazosin must be discontinued for more than a few days, reinstitute the initial dosing regimen if restarted.
6. Due to additive effects, use caution when combined with other antihypertensive agents.
7. When treating BPH, a minimum of 4–6 weeks of 10 mg/day may be needed to determine if a beneficial effect has occurred.

ASSESSMENT

1. Document onset, duration, and characteristics of symptoms.
2. Assess prostate gland, PSA level, and BPH score.
3. A gradual increase in dose, i.e., 1 mg/day for 7 days, then 2 mg/day for 7 days, then 3 mg/day for 7 days, then 4 mg/day for 7 days, and then 5 mg /day, may assist to diminish adverse effects and enhance compliance, especially in the elderly.

CLIENT/FAMILY TEACHING

1. Take initial dose at bedtime to minimize side effects. Do not stop abruptly. Use caution when performing activities that require mental alertness until drug effects realized.
2. Do not drive or undertake hazardous tasks for 12 hr after the first dose and after increasing dose or reinstituting therapy.
3. Avoid symptoms of orthostatic hypotension by rising slowly from a sitting or lying position and waiting until symptoms subside.

4. Record weight 2 times/week; report persistent side effects or excessive weight gain or ankle edema.
5. Report if night time urinary frequency increases.

OUTCOMES/EVALUATE

- Control of BP
- Improvement in BPH symptoms

Terbinafine hydrochloride

(ter-**BIN**-ah-feen)

PREGNANCY CATEGORY: B
CLASSIFICATION(S):
Antifungal
Rx: Lamisil DermGel, 1%
✱Rx: PMS-Terbinafine
OTC: Lamisil, Lamisil AT

ACTION/KINETICS

Inhibits squalene epoxidase, a key enzyme in the sterol biosynthesis in fungi. Results in ergosterol deficiency and a corresponding accumulation of squalene leading to fungal cell death. Approximately 75% of cutaneously absorbed drug is excreted in the urine, mostly as metabolites. Well absorbed following PO administration, with first-pass metabolism being about 40%. **Peak plasma levels:** 1 mcg/mL within 2 hr. Food enhances absorption. Over 99% bound to plasma proteins. Slowly excreted from adipose tissue and skin. Extensively metabolized, with about 70% of the dose eliminated in the urine. Renal or hepatic disease decreases clearance from the body.

USES

Topical use: (1) Interdigital tinea pedis (athlete's foot), tinea cruris (jock itch), or tinea corporis (ringworm) due to *Epidermophyton floccosum, Trichophyton mentagrophytes,* or *T. rubrum.* (2) Plantar tinea pedis. (3) Tinea versicolor due to *Malassezia furfur. Investigational:* Cutaneous candidiasis and tinea versicolor. **Oral use:** Onychomycosis of the toenail or fingernail due to dermatophytes.

CONTRAINDICATIONS

Ophthalmic or intravaginal use. PO use in chronic or active liver disease or renal impairment (C_{CR} less than 50 mL/min). Lactation.

SPECIAL CONCERNS

Safety and efficacy have not been determined in children less than 12 years of age.

SIDE EFFECTS

Following topical use:
Dermatologic: Irritation, burning, itching, dryness.

Following oral use. GI: Diarrhea, dyspepsia, abdominal pain, nausea, flatulence, vomiting, rarely taste loss. **Dermatologic:** Rash, pruritus, urticaria, ***Stevens-Johnson syndrome, toxic epidermal necrolysis***. **Body as a whole:** Malaise, fatigue, arthralgia, myalgia. **Other:** Headache, taste or visual disturbances (changes in the ocular lens or retina), hair loss. Rarely, symptomatic idiosyncratic hepatobiliary dysfunction (including cholestatic hepatitis), ***hepatic failure,*** severe neutropenia, thrombocytopenia, allergic reactions (including ***anaphylaxis***).

LABORATORY TEST CONSIDERATIONS

Liver enzyme abnormalities that are two or more times the upper limit of the normal range. ↓ Absolute neutrophil counts.

DRUG INTERACTIONS

Caffeine / ↑ Clearance of IV caffeine
Cimetidine / Terbinafine clearance is ↓ by one-third
Cyclosporine / ↑ Cyclosporine clearance
Dextromethorphan / ↑ Dextromethorphan plasma levels due to ↓ liver metabolism
Rifampin / ↑ Terbinafine clearance (100%)
Warfarin / Altered PT

HOW SUPPLIED

Cream: 1%; *Gel:* 1%; *Spray:* 1%; *Tablet:* 250 mg

DOSAGE

- **CREAM, GEL**
  Interdigital tinea pedis.
  Apply to cover the affected and immediately surrounding areas b.i.d. for 1 week. The cream is otc.

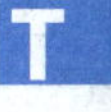

Tinea cruris or tinea corporis.
Apply to cover the affected and immediately surrounding areas 1–2 times/day for 1 week.

• **SPRAY**

Tinea pedis, Tinea versicolor.
Spray b.i.d. for one week.

Tinea corporis, Tinea cruris.
Spray once daily for one week.

• **TABLETS**

Onychomycosis.
Fingernail(s): 250 mg/day for 6 weeks. *Toenail(s):* 250 mg/day for 12 weeks. Alternatively, intermittent dosing may be used: 500 mg daily for 1 week each month (use 2 months for fingernails and 4 months for toenails). The optimal clinical effect is observed several months after mycologic cure and cessation of treatment due to slow period for outgrowth of healthy nails.

NURSING CONSIDERATIONS

ADMINISTRATION/STORAGE

1. Avoid contact of the cream with eyes, nose, mouth, or other mucous membranes.
2. Avoid occlusive dressings.
3. For topical use, many clients treated for 1–2 weeks continue to improve during the 2–4 weeks after drug therapy has been completed. Do not consider clients therapeutic failures until they have been observed for a period of 2–4 weeks off therapy.
4. Store the cream between 5–30°C (41–86°F). Protect tablets from light and store below 25°C (77°F).

ASSESSMENT

1. Describe clinical presentation and note location, onset, duration, and characteristics of symptoms.
2. If presentation unclear, document infected tissue scrapings to confirm diagnosis.
3. Note any liver or renal dysfunction.

CLIENT/FAMILY TEACHING

1. Cream for topical dermatologic use only; review application method.
2. Wash hands before and after topical application. Use a clean towel and washcloth; avoid sharing.
3. Avoid contact of cream with mouth, nose, eyes, and other mucous membranes; do not cover treated areas with occlusive dressing.
4. Take tablets with food to ensure maximal absorption.
5. Report symptoms of increased irritation or possible sensitization such as redness, itching, burning, blistering, swelling, or oozing.
6. Use for prescribed time; do not skip or double up on doses.
7. Continued improvement in skin condition and/or mycotic nails may be noted for 2–4 weeks after therapy.

OUTCOMES/EVALUATE

• Improvement in dermatologic condition
• Clearing/healing of mycotic nail beds

Terbutaline sulfate

(ter-**BYOU**-tah-leen)

PREGNANCY CATEGORY: B
CLASSIFICATION(S):
Sympathomimetic, direct-acting
Rx: Brethaire, Brethine, Bricanyl

SEE ALSO *SYMPATHOMIMETIC DRUGS.*

ACTION/KINETICS

Specific beta-2 receptor stimulant, resulting in bronchodilation and relaxation of peripheral vasculature. Minimum beta-1 activity. Action resembles that of isoproterenol. **PO: Onset:** 30 min; **maximum effect:** 2–3 hr; **duration:** 4–8 hr. **SC: Onset,** 5–15 min; **maximum effect:** 30 min–1 hr; **duration:** 1.5–4 hr. **Inhalation: Onset,** 5–30 min; **time to peak effect:** 1–2 hr; **duration:** 3–6 hr.

USES

(1) Bronchodilator in asthma, bronchitis, emphysema, bronchiectasis, pulmonary obstructive disease, and other conditions associated with reversible bronchospasms. (2) Relief of reversible bronchospasms in clients age six and up who suffer from obstructive airway diseases.

CONTRAINDICATIONS

Lactation. Use for preterm labor.

SPECIAL CONCERNS

Large IV doses may aggravate preexisting diabetes and ketoacidosis. Safe use in children less than 12 years of age not established.

ADDITIONAL SIDE EFFECTS

CV: PVCs, ECG changes (e.g., atrial premature beats, AV block, sinus pause, ST-T wave depression, T-wave inversion, sinus bradycardia, atrial escape beat with aberrant conduction), tachycardia. **Respiratory:** Wheezing. **Miscellaneous:** Hypersensitivity reactions (including vasculitis), flushing, sweating, bad taste or taste change, muscle cramps, CNS stimulation, pain at injection site.

LABORATORY TEST CONSIDERATIONS

↑ Liver enzymes.

HOW SUPPLIED

Metered dose inhaler: 0.2 mg/inh; *Injection:* 1 mg/mL; *Tablet:* 2.5 mg, 5 mg

DOSAGE

- **TABLETS**

  Bronchodilation.

Adults and children over 15 years: 5 mg t.i.d. q 6 hr during waking hours, not to exceed 15 mg q 24 hr. If disturbing side effects are observed, dose can be reduced to 2.5 mg t.i.d. without loss of beneficial effects. Anticipate use of other therapeutic measures if client fails to respond after second dose. **Children 12–15 years:** 2.5 mg t.i.d., not to exceed 7.5 mg q 24 hr.

- **SC**

  Bronchodilation.

Adults: 0.25 mg into the lateral deltoid area. May be repeated 1 time after 15–30 min if no significant clinical improvement is noted. If client does not respond to the second dose, undertake other measures. Do not exceed a dose of 0.5 mg over 4 hr.

- **METERED DOSE INHALER**

  Bronchodilation.

Adults and children over 12 years: 0.2–0.5 mg (1–2 inhalations) q 4–6 hr. Inhalations should be separated by 60-sec intervals. Dosage may be repeated q 4–6 hr.

NURSING CONSIDERATIONS

SEE ALSO *NURSING CONSIDERATIONS* FOR *SYMPATHOMIMETIC DRUGS*.

ASSESSMENT

1. Document type, onset, duration, and characteristics of symptoms.
2. Auscultate and document lung assessments and PFTs. Observe respiratory client for evidence of drug tolerance and rebound bronchospasm.
3. Determine onset, frequency, and duration of contractions and fetal HR with preterm labor.
4. Observe mother for headache, tremor, anxiety, palpitations, symptoms of pulmonary edema, and tachycardia. Assess fetus for distress; report increased contractions. Monitor both for symptoms of hypoglycemia and mother for hypokalemia.

CLIENT/FAMILY TEACHING

1. Take oral medication with meals to minimize GI upset.
2. Report any persistent or bothersome side effects. Do not increase dose or frequency if symptoms are not relieved. Report so dose can be reevaluated.
3. Increase fluid intake to help liquefy secretions.
4. With preterm labor, notify provider immediately if labor resumes or unusual side effects are noted.

OUTCOMES/EVALUATE

- Improved airway exchange
- Inhibition of premature labor

Terconazole nitrate

(ter-**KON**-ah-zohl)

PREGNANCY CATEGORY: C

CLASSIFICATION(S):

Antifungal

Rx: Terazol 3, Terazol 7

✱**Rx:** Terazol

ACTION/KINETICS

May exert its antifungal activity by disrupting cell membrane permeability leading to loss of essential intracellular materials. Also inhibits synthesis of triglycerides and phospholipids as well as inhibiting oxidative and peroxidative enzyme activity. When used for *Candida,* terconazole inhibits transformation of blastospores into the invasive mycelial form.

USES

Vulvovaginitis caused by *Candida.* Ineffective in infections due to *Trichomonas* or *Haemophilus vaginalis.*

SPECIAL CONCERNS

During lactation, consider discontinuing nursing or the drug. Safety and efficacy have not been established in children.

SIDE EFFECTS

GU: Vulvovaginal burning, irritation, or itching; dysmenorrhea, pain of the female genitalia. **Miscellaneous:** Headache (most common), body pain, photosensitivity, abdominal pain, chills, fever.

HOW SUPPLIED

Vaginal cream: 0.4%, 0.8%; *Vaginal suppository:* 80 mg

DOSAGE

• **VAGINAL CREAM (0.4%, 0.8%)**

One applicator full (5 g) intravaginally, once daily at bedtime for 7 consecutive days for the 0.4% cream and for 3 consecutive days for the 0.8% cream.

• **VAGINAL SUPPOSITORY**

One 80-mg suppository once daily at bedtime for 3 consecutive days.

NURSING CONSIDERATIONS

ASSESSMENT

1. Obtain a thorough nursing history because recurrent candidiasis may be caused by oral contraceptives, antibiotics, or diabetes whereas intractable candidiasis may be the result of undetected diabetes mellitus or reinfection.
2. Prior to a second course of therapy, the diagnosis should be confirmed to rule out other pathogens associated with vulvovaginitis.

CLIENT/FAMILY TEACHING

1. Review the appropriate method for administration and cleansing (the cream should be inserted high into the vagina). Sitz baths and vaginal douches may also be used.
2. Discontinue use and report if any burning, irritation, or pain occurs.
3. May stain clothes; use sanitary napkins during therapy and change frequently because damp sanitary napkins may harbor infecting organisms.
4. To avoid reinfection, refrain from sexual intercourse. Advise partner to use a condom as med may also irritate partner; use care as drug may interact with diaphragm and latex condoms.
5. Use for prescribed time frame even if symptoms subside.
6. Effect not affected by menses. Thus, continue to use during menses to ensure a full course of therapy.

OUTCOMES/EVALUATE

Resolution of fungal infections; symptomatic improvement

Testolactone

(tes-toe-**LACK**-tohn)

PREGNANCY CATEGORY: C
CLASSIFICATION(S):
Antineoplastic, hormone
Rx: Teslac, **C-III**

SEE ALSO *ANTINEOPLASTIC AGENTS.*

ACTION/KINETICS

Synthetic steroid related to testosterone. May act to reduce synthesis of estrone from adrenal androstenedione by inhibiting steroid aromatase activity. Well absorbed from the GI tract. Metabolized in the liver and unchanged drug and metabolites are excreted through the urine. Does not cause virilization.

USES

Palliative treatment of advanced disseminated breast cancer in postmenopausal women or in premenopausal ovariectomized clients. Is effective in only 15% of clients.

CONTRAINDICATIONS

Breast cancer in men. Lactation. Premenopausal women with intact ovaries.

SPECIAL CONCERNS

Safety and efficacy have not been determined in children.

ADDITIONAL SIDE EFFECTS

GI: N&V, glossitis, anorexia. **CNS:** Numbness or tingling of fingers, toes, face. **Miscellaneous:** Inflammation and irritation at injection site; increased BP. Hypercalcemia. Maculopapular erythema, alopecia, aches and edema of the extremities, nail growth disturbances. See also *Testosterone*.

LABORATORY TEST CONSIDERATIONS

↑ Plasma calcium, urinary excretion of creatine (24 hr) and 17-ketosteroids. ↓ Estradiol levels using radioimmunoassays.

DRUG INTERACTIONS

Testolactone may ↑ effect of oral anticoagulants.

HOW SUPPLIED

Tablet: 50 mg

DOSAGE

• **TABLETS**

250 mg q.i.d. Continue therapy for 3 months unless there is active progression of the disease.

NURSING CONSIDERATIONS

SEE ALSO *NURSING CONSIDERATIONS FOR ANTINEOPLASTIC AGENTS* AND *TESTOSTERONE*.

ASSESSMENT

Document indications for therapy, noting onset, location, and duration of symptoms and other agents or therapies trialed.

INTERVENTIONS

1. Reduce dose of anticoagulants with concomitant therapy and monitor INR.
2. The effect of the steroid and osteolytic metastases may result in hypercalcemia. Assess for symptoms of hypercalcemia (insomnia, lethargy, anorexia, N&V). Encourage high fluid intake (2–3 L/day) to minimize hypercalcemia. Assess need for diuretics if edema persists.
3. Monitor BP and report any significant increases >20 mm Hg DBP.
4. Perform ROM exercises on bedridden clients and encourage others to exercise to reduce calcium levels, improve circulation, and prevent thrombophlebitis.

CLIENT/FAMILY TEACHING

1. Drug is usually given for a minimum of 3 mo. After 6-12 weeks may assess for desired clinical response:
   • decrease in size of tumor
   • nonosseous lesion reduction by 50%
2. Report all adverse side effects; keep regularly scheduled followup appointments.

OUTCOMES/EVALUATE

↓ Tumor size and spread

Testosterone

(tess-**TOSS**-ter-ohn)

PREGNANCY CATEGORY: X
Rx: Gel: AndroGel 1%., **Pellets:** Testopel., **C-III**

Testosterone cypionate (in oil)

(tess-**TOSS**-ter-ohn)

PREGNANCY CATEGORY: X
Rx: Depo-Testosterone, **C-III**
✱**Rx:** Depo-Testosterone Cypionate

Testosterone enanthate (in oil)

(tess-**TOSS**-ter-ohn)

PREGNANCY CATEGORY: X
Rx: Delatestryl, **C-III**

Testosterone transdermal system

(tess-**TOSS**-ter-ohn)

PREGNANCY CATEGORY: X
Rx: Androderm, Testoderm, Testoderm TTS, Testoderm with Adhesive, **C-III**

CLASSIFICATION(S):
Androgen, naturally-occurring

ACTION/KINETICS

Testosterone, the primary male androgen, is produced naturally by the Leydig cells of the testes. In many tissues, the action of testosterone is due to the active metabolite, dihydrotestosterone, which binds to cytosol receptors. The steroid-receptor complex is transported to the nucleus where it initiates transcription and other cellular changes. Exogenous testosterone administration results in inhibition of endogenous testosterone release due to negative feedback of pituitary LH. Large doses of exogenous testosterone may suppress spermatogenesis through feedback inhibition of pituitary FSH. Oral testosterone is metabolized in the gut and 44% is cleared by the liver in the first pass. Thus, the parenteral, transdermal, and gel forms are use. Testosterone esters (cypionate or enanthate) are slowly absorbed after IM use. Testosterone in plasma is about 98% protein bound. The $t^1/_2$ of testosterone varies over a wide range (10–100 min). **$t^1/_2$, testosterone cypionate after IM:** 8 days. Following use of Testoderm on the scrotal skin: **Maximum serum levels:** 2–4 hr with return to baseline in about 2 hr after system is removed. Serum levels reach a plateau in 3–4 weeks. Will not produce sufficient serum levels if applied to nongenital skin. Following use of Androderm to nonscrotal skin, there is continual absorption over 24 hr. Ninety percent is excreted through the urine as metabolites and 6% is excreted through the feces.

USES

Parenteral: (1) Congenital or acquired primary hypogonadism. (2) Congenital or acquired hypogonadotropic hypogonadism. (3) Delayed puberty (use testosterone enanthate only). (4) Metastatic mammary cancer in females (uses testosterone enanthate only) who are 1–5 years postmenopausal. *Investigational:* Male contraceptive (testosterone enanthate). **Gel:** (1) Congenital or acquired primary hypogonadism. (2) Congenital or acquired hypogonadotropic hypogonadism. **Pellets:** (1) Congenital or acquired primary hypogonadism. (2) Congenital or acquired hypogonadotropic hypogonadism. (3) Stimulation of puberty in carefully selected males with clearly delayed puberty. **Transdermal products:** (1) Acquired or congenital primary hypogonadism. (2) Acquired or congenital secondary hypogonadotropic hypogonadism.

CONTRAINDICATIONS

Serious renal, hepatic, or cardiac disease due to edema formation. Prostatic or breast (males) carcinoma. Use in pregnancy (masculinization of female fetus) and lactation. Discontinue if hypercalcemia occurs.

SPECIAL CONCERNS

Prolonged use of high doses associated with development of potentially life-threatening peliosis hepatits, hepatic neoplasms, cholestatic hepatitis, jaundice, and hepatocellular carcinoma. Use with caution in young males who have not completed their growth (because of premature epiphyseal closure). Androgens may also cause virilization in females or precocious sexual development in males. Geriatric clients may manifest an increased risk of prostatic hypertrophy or prostatic carcinoma. Androgen therapy occasionally seems to accelerate metastatic breast carcinoma in women. Use of the gel has not been evaluated in women. Use with caution in children.

SIDE EFFECTS

Hepatic: Liver toxicity is the most serious side effect. Jaundice, cholestasis, alterations in BSP retention, AST, and ALT. Rarely, ***hepatic necrosis, hepatocellular neoplasms,*** peliosis hepatis, acute intermittent porphyria in clients with this disease. **GI:** N&V, diarrhea, anorexia, symptoms of peptic ulcer. **CNS:** Headache, anxiety, increased or decreased libido, insomnia, excitation, paresthesias, sleep apnea syndrome, ***CNS hemorrhage,*** chills, choreiform movements, habituation, confusion (toxic doses). **GU:** Testicular atrophy with inhibition of testicular function (e.g., oligospermia), impotence, epididymitis, irritable bladder, prepubertal phallic enlargement, gynecomastia, hypercalcemia in breast cancer. **Electrolyte:** Retention of sodium, chloride, calcium, potassium, phosphates. Edema, with or without CHF. **Miscellaneous:** Acne, flushing, suppression of clotting factors (II, V, VII, X), polycythemia, leukopenia, rashes, dermatitis, ***anaphylaxis (rare),*** muscle cramps, hypercholesterolemia, male-pattern baldness, acne, seborrhea, hirsutism. Hypercalcemia, especially in immobilized clients or those with metastatic breast carcinoma. Virilization in women.

In females, menstrual irregularities (including amenorrhea), virilization, clitoral enlargement, hirsutism, increased libido, baldness (male pattern), virilization of external genitalia of female fetus.

In males, decreased ejaculatory volume, oligospermia (high doses), gynecomastia, increased frequency and duration of penile erections.

In children, disturbances of growth, premature closure of epiphyses, precocious sexual development.

Inflammation and pain at site of IM or SC injection.

NOTE: Side effects of the cypionate and enanthate products are not readily reversible due to the long duration of action of these dosage forms.

The patch may cause itching, irritation, erythema, or discomfort of the scrotum (Testoderm) or on skin areas where applied (Androderm). Potentially, small amounts of testosterone may be transferred to a sex partner.

LABORATORY TEST CONSIDERATIONS

Altered thyroid function tests, including ↓ levels of throxine-binding globulin causing decreased total T_4 serum levels and ↑ resin uptake of T3 and T4. False + or ↑ BSP, alkaline phosphatase, bilirubin, cholesterol, and acid phosphatase (in women). Alteration of glucose tolerance tests.

DRUG INTERACTIONS

Anticoagulants, oral / ↑ Anticoagulant effect

Antidiabetic agents / Additive hypoglycemia

Barbiturates / ↓ Androgenic effect R/T ↑ breakdown by liver

Corticosteroids, ACTH / ↑ Chance of edema

Insulin / In diabetics, ↓ blood glucose → ↓ insulin requirements

Propranolol / ↑ Propranolol clearance if used with testosterone cypionate

H *Saw palmetto* / Antiandrogenic effect may ↓ testosterone activitiy

HOW SUPPLIED

Testosterone cypionate: *Injection:* 100 mg/mL, 200 mg/mL. **Testosterone enanthate:** *Injection:* 200 mg/mL. **Testosterone Gel:** *Gel:*1%; **Testosterone pellets:** *Pellets:* 75 mg; **Testosterone transdermal system:** *Film, extended release:* 2.5 mg/24 hr, 4 mg/24 hr, 5 mg/24 hr, 6 mg/24 hr

DOSAGE

• TESTOSTERONE ENANTHATE AND CYPIONATE. IM ONLY

Male hypogonadism, replacement therapy.

50–400 mg q 2–4 weeks.

Delayed puberty, males.

50–200 mg q 2–4 weeks for no more than 4–6 months.

Palliation of inoperable breast cancer in women (testosterone enanthate only).

200–400 mg q 2–4 weeks. Monitor closely as androgen therapy may accelerate the disease.

• GEL

Primary hypogonadism, Hypogonadotropic hypogonadism.

Apply 5 g (50 mg testosterone) once daily (preferable in the morning) to clean, dry, intact skin of the shoulders, upper arms, and/or abdomen.

• PELLETS

Replacement therapy.

150–450 mg SC q 3–6 months.

Delayed puberty.

Often a lower dose range is used than for replacement and for a limited time duration (e.g., 4–6 months). The number of pellets to be implanted for all uses depends on the minimum daily requirement of testosterone determined by a gradual reduction of the amount given parenterally. The usual ratio is to implant two-75 mg pellets for each 25 mg testosterone propionate required weekly. About ⅓ of the material is absorbed during the first month, ¼ the second month, and ⅙ the third month.

• TRANSDERMAL SYSTEM

Replacement therapy (congenital or acquired primary hypogonadism, congenital or acquired hypogonadotropic hypogonadism).

Testoderm and Testoderm with Adhesive: One 6-mg patch applied daily on clean, dry scrotal skin that has been dry-shaved to remove hair. Clients with a smaller scrotum can use a 4-mg patch. Are designed to be applied to scrotal skin only. The patch should be worn for 22–24 hr/day for 6–8 weeks. *Testoderm TTS:* One 5-mg patch applied to the arm, back, or upper buttocks at the same time each day. Do not apply to the scrotum. The patch can be removed and reapplied if the client wants to swim, bathe, or vigorously exercise. *Androderm:* **Initial dose, usual:** One 5-mg system or two 2.5-mg systems applied nightly for 24 hr providing a total dose of 5 mg/day. The systems are applied to a clean, dry area of the skin on the back, abdomen, upper arms, or thighs. Do not apply to the scrotum. *Note:* For the nonvirilized client, dosing may be started with one 2.5 mg system applied nightly.

NURSING CONSIDERATIONS

ADMINISTRATION/STORAGE

1. The following information is applicable to testosterone cypionate and/or testosterone enanthate:
   - Do not use testosterone enanthate interchangeable with testosterone cypionate due to differences in duration of action.
   - Redissolve crystals of testosterone enanthate or cypionate by warming and shaking the vial.
   - If needle or syringe is wet, the product may become cloudy; this does not affect potency.
   - Warm the unopened vial in warm water to decrease the viscosity of the oil. Vigorously rotate vial to resuspend drug in the oil. A film may appear on the sides of the vial. When no more suspended particles are observed on the bottom or sides of the vial, the drug has been suspended appropriately. Administer deep into the muscle; give slowly.
   - Continue therapy for at least 2 months for satisfactory response and 5 months for objective response.
   - When used for delayed puberty, consider the chronological and skeletal ages when determining initial and subsequent doses. Use is for a limited time (e.g., 4–6 mo).
2. The following information is applicable to testosterone gel:
   - When using the gel, squeeze the entire contents of the packet onto the palm of the hand and apply immediately to the application site. Allow the site to dry for a few minutes prior to dressing. Wash hands with soap and water after application. Do not apply gel to the genitals.
   - After applying the gel, wait 5–6 hr or more after before showering or swimming.
   - Measure serum testosterone levels 14 days after beginning therapy with the gel. If the desired serum testosterone levels are below the normal range or if the desired effect has not been reached, the dose may be increased from 5 to 7.5 g and from 7.5 to 10 g.
   - Testosterone from the gel will be transferred from males to female partners. Washing the area of contact on the other person as soon as possible with soap and water will remove residual testosterone from the skin surface.
3. Store testosterone pellets in a cool place.
4. The following information is applicable to *Testoderm* and *Testoderm with Adhesive* transdermal systems:
   - Dry-shave scrotal hair for optimal skin contact. Do not use chemical depilatories.
   - If the system comes off after it has been worn for more than 12 hr and it cannot be reapplied, the client may wait until it is time for the next routine application to apply a new system.
   - To determine serum total testosterone, draw blood 2–4 hr after system application after 3–4 weeks of daily system use.
   - if clients have not achieved desired results by the end of 6–8 weeks, consider another form of testosterone replacement therapy.
   - Prior to sexual activity, remove the Testoderm patch from the scrotum and wash the scrotal area to remove residue.
5. The following information is applicable to *Testoderm TTS* transdermal system:

• The area selected for application should not be oily, damaged, or irritated. Press the system firmly in place with the palm of the hand for about 10 seconds. Make sure there is good contact around the edges.
• If the system falls off, the same system may be reapplied. If the system comes off after it has been worm for more than 12 hr and it cannot be reapplied, apply a new system at the next regular application time.
• Serum testosterone levels may be measured 2–4 hr after application of the system. If the levels are too low, dose may be increased to 2 systems.
6. The following information is applicable to *Androderm* transdermal system:
• Do not apply the Androderm patch to bony areas such as the shoulders or hips; it is *not* to be applied to the scrotum.
• Sites of application should be rotated, with an interval of 7 days between applications to the same site. Areas should not be oily, damaged, or irritated.
• The system does not have to be removed during sexual intercourse or while taking a shower or bath.
• Apply Androderm immediately after opening the pouch and removing protective liner. Press the system firmly in place, making sure there is good contact with the skin, especially around the edges of the patch.
7. For all transdermal products, do not use damaged patches. Excessive heat or pressure can cause drug reservoir to burst. Discard systems safely to prevent accidental application or ingestion by children, pets, or others.
8. Due to variability in analytical values among various diagnostic labs, have testosterone levels analyzed at the some lab so results can be compared more easily.

ASSESSMENT

1. Document indications for therapy, type, onset, and characteristics of symptoms.
2. Assess for any cardiac, renal, or hepatic dysfunction. Document neurologic status, BP, respirations, heart sounds, and GU function.
3. Note hair distribution and skin texture.
4. Check prescribed medications for any drugs that may interact unfavorably (i.e., anticoagulants, hypoglycemic agents, and mineralocorticoids).
5. Determine if pregnant.
6. Monitor CBC, serum glucose, calcium, electrolytes, cholesterol, liver and renal function studies. Treatment with aplastic anemia has resulted in several cases of hepatocellular carcinoma.

INTERVENTIONS

1. Monitor for signs of mental depression such as insomnia, lack of interest in personal appearance, and withdrawal from social contacts.
2. Monitor weight, BP, pulse, and serum electrolytes. Auscultate lung sounds and note any JVD. Report edema, as sodium retention and edema can be easily treated with diuretics.
3. Assess for relaxation of the skeletal muscles and pain deep in the bones. The discomfort in the bones is caused by a honeycombing; often caused by increased calcium levels.
4. Flank pain may be caused by kidney stones from excessively high serum calcium levels. Administer large amounts of fluids to prevent renal calculi. If hypercalcemia is the result of metastases, initiate other appropriate therapy.
5. Observe for jaundice, malaise, complaints of RUQ pain, pruritus, or a change in the color/consistency of stools. Document LFTs.
6. Observe for easy bruising, bleeding, S&S sore throat or fever. Obtain CBC to rule out polycythemia and leukopenia.
7. With a child, monitor closely for growth retardation and development of precocious puberty. Use with caution as the effect on the CNS in developing children is still being explored.
• Review therapy with parents; often intermittent to allow for periods of normal bone growth.

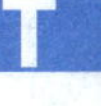

• Regular X rays to monitor bone maturation and effects on epiphyseal centers; obtain q 6 mo.
• Record height/weight regularly.
8. If female, report the signs of virilization, such as deepening of the voice, hirsuitism, acne, menstrual irregularity, and clitoral enlargement. Usually only evident with doses exceeding 200–300 mg/month.
9. Increased libido in females may be early sign of drug toxicity.
10. Report if acne is severe; may be necessary to change dose.
11. May alter serum lipid levels enhancing susceptibility to arteriosclerotic heart disease in women; monitor cholesterol panel periodically.

CLIENT/FAMILY TEACHING

1. Review method for administration/application, dosage, frequency of administration, site preparation, and time of application for the transdermal patch.
2. Report any unusual incidents of bleeding/bruising. Androgens suppress clotting factors (II, V, VII, and X); polycythemia and leukopenia may occur.
3. If drug received via pellets, sloughing can occur; report.
4. In older males, urinary obstruction may occur as a result of BPH.
5. Parents of children receiving testosterone should record weight twice a week and height every 2–3 mo. X rays will be performed periodically on prepubertal children to assess effect on bone growth.
6. Women with metastatic breast cancer need lab tests of serum and urine calcium levels, alkaline phosphatase, and serum cholesterol. If the serum cholesterol level is high, the dosage of drug may need to be changed. Follow a low-cholesterol diet and see dietitian for further assistance with diet.
7. Facial hair and acne in females are reversible once drug withdrawn.
8. Drug may cause irregularities in the menstrual cycle; in postmenopausal women may cause withdrawal bleeding.
9. Use reliable birth control during and for several weeks after therapy withdrawn. Report if pregnancy suspected; increased risk of fetal abnormalities with this drug.
10. Males should report gynecomastia or priapism; may necessitate drug withdrawal (at least temporarily).
11. Report any tingling of the fingers and toes or loss of appetite.
12. Follow a diet high in calories, proteins, vitamins, minerals, and other nutrients. Restrict sodium to reduce edema.
13. With diabetes, hypoglycemia may occur. Report extreme variations as diet and/or dose of antidiabetic agents may require modification.
14. Review potential for drug abuse. High doses of androgens for enhancement of athletic performance can result in serious irreversible side effects/permanent physical damage.

OUTCOMES/EVALUATE

• Replacement therapy with control of S&S of androgen deficiency
• Male contraceptive agent
• Suppression of breast tumor size and spread

Tetracycline hydrochloride

(teh-trah-**SYE**-kleen)

PREGNANCY CATEGORY: D
CLASSIFICATION(S):
Antibiotic, tetracycline
Rx: Achromycin Ointment, Actisite Periodontal Fiber, Nor-Tet, Panmycin, Robicaps, Sumycin 250 and 500, Sumycin Syrup, Tetracap, Tetracyn, Tetralan Syrup, Topicycline Topical Solution
★Rx: Apo-Tetra, Novo-Tetra, Nu-Tetra

SEE ALSO *TETRACYCLINES*.

ACTION/KINETICS

t½: 7–11 hr. From 40% to 70% excreted unchanged in urine; 65% bound to serum proteins. Always express dose as the hydrochloride salt.

ADDITIONAL USES

PO: (1) As part of combination therapy to eradicate *H. pylori* infections. (2) Used with gentamicin for *Vibrio vulnif-*

icus infections such as wound infections after trauma or ingestion of contaminated seafood. (3) As a mouthwash (use suspension) to treat nonspecific mouth ulcerations, aphthous ulcers, and canker sores. (4) Drug of choice for stage I Lyme disease. **Pleural:** Instilled through a chest tube as a pleural schlerosing agent in malignant pleural effusions. **Ophthalmic:** (1) Superficial ophthalmic infections due to *Staphylococcus aureus, Streptococcus, Streptococcus pneumoniae, Escherichia coli, Neisseria,* and *Bacteroides.* Prophylaxis of *Neisseria gonorrhoeae* in newborns. (2) With oral therapy for treatment of *Chlamydia trachomatis.* **Topical:** (1) Acne vulgaris. (2) Prophylaxis or treatment of infection following skin abrasions, minor cuts, wounds, or burns. **Tetracycline fiber:** Adult periodontitis. *Investigational:* Pleural sclerosing agent in malignant pleural effusions (administered by chest tube); in combination with gentamicin for *Vibrio vulnificus* infections due to wound infection after trauma or by eating contaminated seafood.

CONTRAINDICATIONS

Use of the topical ointment in or around the eyes. Ophthalmic products to treat fungal diseases of the eye, dendritic keratitis, vaccinia, varicella, mycobacterial eye infections, or following removal of a corneal foreign body.

SPECIAL CONCERNS

Use tetracycline fiber with caution in clients with a history of oral candidiasis. Use of the fiber in chronic abscesses has not been evaluated. Safety and efficacy of the fiber have not been determined in children.

ADDITIONAL SIDE EFFECTS

Temporary blurring of vision or stinging following administration. Dermatitis and photosensitivity following ophthalmic use. **Use of the tetracycline fiber:** Oral candidiasis, glossitis, staining of the tongue, severe gingival hyperplasia, minor throat irritation, pain following placement in an abscessed area, throbbing pain, hypersensitivity reactions.

HOW SUPPLIED

Tetracycline: *Syrup:* 125 mg/5 mL; **Tetracycline hydrochloride:** *Capsule:* 100 mg, 250 mg, 500 mg; *Fiber:* 12.7 mg/23 cm; *Ointment:* 3%; *Tablet:* 250 mg, 500 mg; *Topical Solution:* 2.2 mg/mL

DOSAGE

- **CAPSULES, SYRUP, TABLETS**

Mild to moderate infections.

Adults, usual: 500 mg b.i.d. or 250 mg q.i.d.

Severe infections.

Adult: 500 mg q.i.d. **Children over 8 years:** 25–50 mg/kg/day in four equal doses.

Eradication of H. pylori.

The following regimens may be used: (1) Tetracycline, 500 mg q.i.d. for 2 weeks, plus metronidazoloe, 250 mg q.i.d. for 2 weeks, plus bismsuth subsalicylate, 525 mg q.i.d. for 2 weeks, plus a H2 receptor antagonist for 28 days. (2) Clarithromycin, 500 mg b.i.d. for 2 weeks, plus ranitidine bismuth citrate, 400 mg b.i.d. for 4 weeks, plus either metronidazole, 500 mg b.i.d., or amoxicillin, 1 g b.i.d., or tetracycline, 500 mg b.i.d. for 2 weeks. (3) Tetracycline, 500 mg q.i.d. for 2 weeks, plus metronidazole, 500 mg t.i.d. for 2 weeks, plus bismuth subsalicylate, 525 mg q.i.d. for 2 weeks, plus either lansoprazole, 30 mg once daily or omeprazole, 20 mg once daily, for 2 weeks.

Lyme disease.

250 mg/day for 10 days.

Brucellosis.

500 mg q.i.d. for 3 weeks with 1 g streptomycin IM b.i.d. for first week and once daily the second week.

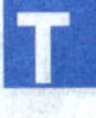

Syphilis.

Total of 30–40 g over 10–15 days.

Gonorrhea.

Initially, 1.5 g; **then,** 500 mg q 6 hr until 9 g has been given.

Gonorrhea sensitive to penicillin.

Initially, 1.5 g; **then,** 500 mg q 6 hr for 4 days (total: 9 g).

NOTE: The CDC have established treatment schedules for STDs.

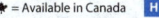

GU or rectal Chlamydia trachomatis infections.
500 mg q.i.d. for minimum of 7 days.

Severe acne.
Initially, 1 g/day; **then,** 125–500 mg/day (long-term).

• **TOPICAL**

Acne.
Apply topical solution to affected areas in the morning and at night, making sure that skin is completely wet after each application.

Infections.
Apply OTC ointment (3%) to affected areas 1–4 times/day. A sterile bandage may be used.

• **MOUTHWASH**

Mouth ulcerations, aphthous ulcers, canker sores.
5–10 mL of 125 mg/mL strength t.i.d. for 5–7 days.

• **TETRACYCLINE FIBER**

Adult periodontitis.
Place the fiber into the periodontal pocket until the pocket is filled (amount of fiber will vary with pocket depth and contour) ensuring that the fiber is in contact with the base of the pocket. Retain the fiber in place for 10 days, after which it is to be removed. Replace fibers lost before 7 days. The effectiveness of subsequent therapy with the fiber has not been assessed.

NURSING CONSIDERATIONS

SEE ALSO *NURSING CONSIDERATIONS* FOR *TETRACYCLINES* AND *ANTI-INFECTIVES.*

ADMINISTRATION/STORAGE

The tetracycline fiber product consists of a monofilament of ethylene/vinyl acetate copolymer evenly dispersed with tetracycline. The fiber provides for continuous release of tetracycline for 10 days; releases about 2 mcg/cm/hr of tetracycline.

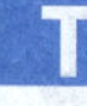

ASSESSMENT

1. Document indications for therapy, type, onset, duration, and characteristics of symptoms.
2. Monitor cultures, CBC, liver and renal function studies.

CLIENT/FAMILY TEACHING

1. Take PO form 1 hr before or 2 hr after meals with a full glass of water. Avoid dairy products, antacids, or iron preparations for 2-3 hr of ingestion.
2. May cause photosensitivity reaction; avoid exposure to sunlight and wear protective clothing and sunscreen when exposed.
3. Transient blurring of vision or stinging may occur when instilled into the eye.
4. Ointment may stain clothing.
5. Drug may cause increased yellow-brown discoloration and softening of teeth and bones. *Not* advised for children under 8 years of age.
6. Use additional nonhormonal form of contraceptive to prevent pregnancy.
7. Check expiration date; degraded drug is very nephrotoxic and may cause kidney damage.
8. With oral application for gum disease, review proper care of site(s), foods to avoid, and proper cleaning while avoiding floss or pics for the entire length of therapy. Symptoms that require immediate reporting include pain, abnormal discharge, fever, swelling, expulsion of fiber; return as scheduled for removal and follow-up.
9. Avoid actions that may dislodge the fiber; i.e., chewing hard, crusty, or sticky foods; brushing or flossing near any treated areas; engaging in hygienic practices that might dislodge the fiber; probing the treated area with tongue or fingers.
10. The fiber releases tetracycline continously for 10 days (2mcg/cm/hr). Contact dentist if the fiber is dislodged or falls out before the next scheduled visit or if pain or swelling occurs.

OUTCOMES/EVALUATE

• Resolution of infection; symptomatic improvement
• ↓ Acne lesions

Thalidomide

(thah-**LID**-ah-myd)

PREGNANCY CATEGORY: X
CLASSIFICATION(S):
Immunomodulator
Rx: Thalomid

ACTION/KINETICS

Immunomodulatory drug; mechanism of action not known. Drug may suppress excessive tumor necrosis factor–alpha (TNF–α) production and down–modulation of selected cell surface adhesion molecules involved in leukocyte migration. **Peak plasma levels:** 2.9–5.7 hr. High fat meals increase the time to peak plasma levels to about 6 hr. **t½:** 5–7 hr. Metabolized in the plasma and excreted in the urine.

USES

(1) Acute treatment of moderate to severe erythema nodosum leprosum (ENL). (2) Maintenance therapy for prevention and suppression of the cutaneous symptoms of erythema nodosum leprosum recurrence. *Investigational:* Treatment of recurrent and metastatic squamous cell carcinoma of the head and neck. Refractory Crohn's disease. Lupus erythematosus.

CONTRAINDICATIONS

Never to be used in pregnancy or in those who could become pregnant while taking the drug (even a single 50 mg dose can cause severe birth defects). Use in males unless the client meets several conditions (see package insert). Use as monotherapy for ENL in the presence of moderate to severe neuritis. Lactation.

SPECIAL CONCERNS

Due to possible birth defects, thalidomide is marketed only under a special restricted distribution program called the "System for Thalidomide Education and Prescribing Safety (STEPS). Under this program only prescribers and pharmacists registered with the program are allowed to prescribe and dispense the drug. Safety and efficacy have not been determined in children less than 12 years of age.

SIDE EFFECTS

Note: Only the most common side effects are listed. ***Human teratogenicity.*** **GI:** Constipation, diarrhea, nausea, oral moniliasis, tooth pain, abdominal pain. **CNS:** Drowsiness, somnolence, dizziness, tremor, vertigo, headache. **Neurologic:** Peripheral neuropathy. **CV:** Orthostatic hypotension, bradycardia. **Respiratory:** Pharyngitis, rhinitis, sinusitis. **Hematologic:** Neutropenia. *Hypersensitivity:* Erythematous macular rash, fever, tachycardia, hypotension. **Dermatologic:** Photosensitivity, rash, dermatitis, fungal nail disorder, pruritus. **Musculoskeletal:** Back pain, neck pain, neck rigidity. **Miscellaneous:** HIV viral load increase, impotence, peripheral edema, accidental injury, asthenia, chills, facial edema, malaise, pain.

DRUG INTERACTIONS

Alcohol / Enhanced sedative effects
Barbiturates / Enhanced sedative effects
Chlorpromazine / Enhanced sedative effects
Reserpine / Enhanced sedative effects

HOW SUPPLIED

Capsules: 50 mg

DOSAGE

• **CAPSULES**

Cutaneous ENL, initial therapy.

Adults, initial: 100–300 mg once daily with water, preferably at bedtime and at least 1 hr after the evening meal. Clients weighing less then 50 kg should be started at the low end of the dose range. In those with severe cutaneous ENL or who have required higher doses previously, dosing may be started at doses up to 400 mg once daily at bedtime or in divided doses with water 1 hr after meals. Continue initial dosing until signs and symptoms of active reaction have been eliminated (usually at least 2 weeks). Following this, taper clients off medication in 50 mg decrements q 2 to 4 weeks.

Maintenance therapy for prevention and suppression of ENL recurrence.

Maintain on the minimum dose (see initial therapy) necessary to control the reaction. Attempt tapering of medication q 3 to 6 months, in decrements of 50 mg q 2 to 4 weeks.

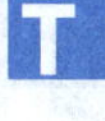

NURSING CONSIDERATIONS

ADMINISTRATION/STORAGE

1. The product is supplied only to pharmacists registered with the STEPS program. The drug is dispensed in no

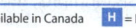

more than a 1–month supply and only on presentation of a new prescription written within the previous 14 days and client signature.
2. Specific informed consent and compliance with the mandatory client registry and survey are required of all male and female clients prior to dispensing the drug. The drug must not be repackaged.

ASSESSMENT

1. Document indications for therapy. With leprosy, note characteristics including number of painful skin nodules and any systemic manifestations (fever, neuritis, malaise). With multiple myeoloma note protein levels and steroid failures. List other agents trialed and outcome.
2. Obtain negative pregnancy test. Drug is teratogenic; only one dose taken during pregnancy can cause severe birth defects. Pregnancy tests will be performed weekly during the first month of therapy and then monthly thereafter with regular menses and every two weeks with irregular menses.
3. Drug will only be dispensed under a restricted distribution program (STEPS) requiring written consent. With relapsed MM client must still sign consent and agree to required monitoring.
4. If HIV-seropositive, monitor viral load the first and third month of treatment and then every 3 mo.

CLIENT/FAMILY TEACHING

1. Take as prescribed at least one hr after evening meal or at bedtime unless otherwise directed.
2. May cause dizziness/drowsiness; avoid activities that require mental acuity.
3. Avoid alcohol and CNS depressants.
4. Women of child bearing age must practice two methods of reliable birth control or abstain continously from heterosexual sexual intercourse. Males must always wear a latex condom when engaging in sexual intercourse with women of childbearing age, despite successful vasectomy.
5. Report any numbness, tingling, pain, or burning in the hands or feet. Peripheral neuropathy may occur and may be irreversible.
6. During therapy do not donate blood or sperm.
7. Drug is continued until S&S of active reaction subsides (approx. 2 weeks). The dosage may then be tapered by provider every 2-4 weeks.
8. Drug will be dispensed in a one month supply only and upon presentation of a valid prescription written within past 14 days.
9. Drug therapy requires informed consent and compliance with the mandatory patient registry and survey prior to dispensing and clinical monitoring during therapy.

OUTCOMES/EVALUATE

Suppression of cutaneous manifestations with ENL; inhibition of malignant cell proliferation

Theophylline

(thee-**OFF**-ih-lin)

PREGNANCY CATEGORY: C
CLASSIFICATION(S):

Antiasthmatic, xanthine derivative
Rx: Immediate-release Capsules, Tablets: Bronkodyl, Elixophyllin, Quibron-T Dividose, Slo-Phyllin, Theolair. **Liquid Products:** Accurbron, Aquaphyllin, Asmalix, Elixomin, Elixophyllin, Lanophyllin, Slo-Phyllin, Theoclear-80, Theolair, Theophylline Oral, Theostat-80. **Timed-release Capsules:** Slo-Bid Gyrocaps, Slo-Phyllin Gyrocaps, Theo-24, Theobid Duracaps, Theoclear L.A.-130, Theoclear L.A.-260, Theospan-SR, Theovent. **Timed-release Tablets:** Quibron-T/SR Dividose, Respid, Sustaire, Theochron, Theo-Dur, Theolair-SR, Theophyline SR, Theophylline Extended-Release, Theo-Sav, Theo-X, T-Phyl, Uni-Dur, Uniphyl.
✱**Rx:** Apo-Theo LA, Novo-Theophyl SR, Quibron-T/SR, Theochron-SR, Theolair, Theolixir

ACTION/KINETICS

Theophylline stimulates the CNS, directly relaxes the smooth muscles of the bronchi and pulmonary blood vessels (relieve bronchospasms), produces diuresis, inhibits uterine contractions, stimulates gastric acid secretion, and increases the rate and force of contraction of the heart. Directly relaxes the bronchiolar smooth muscle (relieves bronchospasm) and pulmonary blood vessels. Although the exact mechanism is not known, theophyllines may alter the calcium levels of smooth muscle, blocking adenosine receptors, inhibiting the effect of prostaglandins on smooth muscle, and inhibiting the release of slow-reacting substance of anaphylaxis and histamine. Well absorbed from uncoated plain tablets and PO liquids. **Time to peak serum levels, oral solution:** 1 hr; **uncoated tablets:** 2 hr; **chewable tablets:** 1–1.5 hr; **enteric-coated tablets:** 5 hr; **extended-release capsules and tablets:** 4–7 hr. **Therapeutic plasma levels:** 10–20 mcg/mL. **t½:** 3–15 hr in nonsmoking adults, 4–5 hr in adult heavy smokers, 1–9 hr in children, and 20–30 hr for premature neonates. An increased t½ may be seen in individuals with CHF, alcoholism, liver dysfunction, or respiratory infections. Because of great variations in the rate of absorption (due to dosage form, food, dose level) as well as its extremely narrow therapeutic range, theophylline therapy is best monitored by determination of the serum levels. In healthy adults, about 60% is bound to plasma protein whereas in neonates 36% is bound to plasma protein. Eighty-five percent to 90% metabolized in the liver and various metabolites, including the active 3-methylxanthine. Theophylline is metabolized partially to caffeine in the neonate. The premature neonate excretes 50% unchanged theophylline and may accumulate the caffeine metabolite. Excretion is through the kidneys (about 10% unchanged in adults).

USES

(1) Prophylaxis and treatment of bronchial asthma. (2) Reversible bronchospasms associated with chronic bronchitis, emphysema, and COPD. **Oral liquid**: Neonatal apnea as a respiratory stimulant. **Theophylline and dextrose injection**: Respiratory stimulant in neonatal apnea and Cheyne-Stokes respiration.

CONTRAINDICATIONS

Hypersensitivity to any xanthine, peptic ulcer, seizure disorders (unless on medication), hypotension, CAD, angina pectoris.

SPECIAL CONCERNS

Use during lactation may result in irritability, insomnia, and fretfulness in the infant. Use with caution in premature infants due to the possible accumulation of caffeine. Xanthines are not usually tolerated by small children because of excessive CNS stimulation. Geriatric clients may manifest an increased risk of toxicity. Use with caution in the presence of gastritis, alcoholism, acute cardiac diseases, hypoxemia, severe renal and hepatic disease, severe hypertension, severe myocardial damage, hyperthyroidism, glaucoma.

SIDE EFFECTS

Side effects are uncommon at serum theophylline levels less than 20 mcg/mL. At levels greater than 20 mcg/mL, 75% of individuals experience side effects including N&V, diarrhea, irritability, insomnia, and headache. At levels of 35 mcg/mL or greater, individuals may manifest ***cardiac arrhythmias,*** hypotension, tachycardia, hyperglycemia, ***seizures, brain damage, or death.***
GI: N&V, diarrhea, anorexia, epigastric pain, hematemesis, dyspepsia, rectal irritation (following use of suppositories), rectal bleeding, gastroesophageal reflux during sleep or while recumbent (theophylline). **CNS:** Headache, insomnia, irritability, fever, dizziness, lightheadedness, vertigo, reflex hyperexcitability, ***seizures,*** depression, speech abnormalities, alternating periods of mutism and hyperactivity, ***brain damage, death.*** **CV:** Hypotension, ***life-threatening ventricular arrhythmias,*** palpitations, tachycardia, ***peripheral vascular collapse,*** extrasystoles. **Renal:** Proteinuria, excretion of erythrocytes and renal tubular cells, dehydration due to diuresis,

urinary retention (men with prostatic hypertrophy). **Other:** Tachypnea, ***respiratory arrest,*** fever, flushing, hyperglycemia, antidiuretic hormone syndrome, leukocytosis, rash, alopecia.

LABORATORY TEST CONSIDERATIONS

↑ Plasma free fatty acids, bilirubin, urinary catecholamines, ESR. Interference with uric acid tests and tests for furosemide and probenecid.

OD OVERDOSE MANAGEMENT

Symptoms: Agitation, headache, nervousness, insomnia, tachycardia, extrasystoles, anorexia, N&V, fasciculations, tachypnea, ***tonic-clonic seizures.*** The first signs of toxicity may be seizures or ventricular arrhythmias. Toxicity is usually associated with parenteral administration but can be observed after PO administration, especially in children. *Treatment:*

- Have ipecac syrup, gastric lavage equipment, and cathartics available to treat overdose if the client is conscious and not having seizures. Otherwise a mechanical ventilator, oxygen, diazepam, and IV fluids may be necessary for the treatment of overdosage.
- For postseizure coma, maintain an airway and oxygenate the client. To remove the drug, perform only gastric lavage and give the cathartic and activated charcoal by a large-bore gastric lavage tube. Charcoal hemoperfusion may be necessary.
- Treat atrial arrhythmias with verapamil and treat ventricular arrhythmias with lidocaine or procainamide.
- Use IV fluids to treat acid-base imbalance, hypotension, and dehydration. Hypotension may also be treated with vasopressors.
- To treat hyperpyrexia, use a tepid water sponge bath or a hypothermic blanket.
- Treat apnea with artificial respiration.
- Monitor serum levels of theophylline until they fall below 20 mcg/mL as secondary rises of theophylline may occur, especially with sustained-release products.

DRUG INTERACTIONS

Allopurinol / ↑ Theophylline levels
Aminoglutethimide / ↓ Theophylline levels
Barbiturates / ↓ Theophylline levels
Benzodiazepines / Sedative effect may be antagonized by theophylline
Beta-adrenergic agonists / Additive effects
Beta-adrenergic blocking agents / ↑ Theophylline levels
Calcium channel blocking drugs / ↑ Theophylline levels
Carbamazepine / Either ↑ or ↓ theophylline levels
Charcoal / ↓ Theophylline levels R/T ↑ metabolism
Cimetidine / ↑ Theophylline levels
Ciprofloxacin / ↑ Theophylline plasma; ↑ possibility of side effects
Corticosteroids / ↑ Theophylline levels
Digitalis / ↑ Digitalis toxicity
Disulfiram / ↑ Theophylline levels
Ephedrine and other sympathomimetics / ↑ Theophylline levels
Erythromycin / ↑ Theophylline effect R/T ↓ liver metabolism
Ethacrynic acid / Either ↑ or ↓ theophylline levels
Furosemide / Either ↑ or ↓ theophylline levels
Halothane / ↑ Risk of cardiac arrhythmias
Interferon / ↑ Theophylline levels
Isoniazid / Either ↑ or ↓ theophylline levels
Ketamine / Seizures of the extensor-type
Ketoconazole / ↓ Theophylline levels
Lithium / ↓ Lithium effect R/T ↑ rate of excretion
Loop diuretics / ↓ Theophylline levels
Mexiletine / ↑ Theophylline levels
Muscle relaxants, nondepolarizing / ↓ Muscle relaxation
Oral contraceptives / ↑ Theophylline effect R/T ↓ liver metabolism
Phenytoin / ↓ Theophylline levels
Propofol / ↓ Sedative effect of propofol
Quinolones / ↑ Theophylline levels
Reserpine / ↑ Risk of tachycardia
Rifampin / ↓ Theophylline levels
H *St. John's wort* / Possible ↓ theophylline plasma levels R/T ↑ metabolism
Sulfinpyrazone / ↓ Theophylline levels
Sympathomimetics / ↓ Theophylline levels

T

Tetracyclines / ↑ Risk of theophylline toxicity
Thiabendazole / ↑ Theophylline levels
Thyroid hormones / ↓ Theophylline levels in hypothyroid clients
Tobacco smoking / ↓ Theophylline effect R/T ↑ liver metabolism
Troleandomycin / ↑ Theophylline effect R/T ↓ liver metabolism
Verapamil / ↑ Theophylline effect
Zafirlukast / Possible ↑ theophylline levels

ADDITIONAL DRUG INTERACTIONS

Possible ↑ Serum theophylline levels when used with zafirlukast.

HOW SUPPLIED

Capsule: 100 mg, 200 mg; *Capsule, extended release:* 50 mg, 75 mg, 100 mg, 125 mg, 130 mg, 200 mg, 250 mg, 260 mg, 300 mg; *Elixir:* 80 mg/15 mL; *Solution:* 80 mg/15 mL; *Syrup:* 80 mg/15 mL, 150 mg/15 mL; *Tablet:* 100 mg, 125 mg, 200 mg, 250 mg, 300 mg; *Tablet, extended release:* 100 mg, 200 mg, 250 mg, 300 mg, 400 mg, 450 mg, 500 mg, 600 mg

DOSAGE

• CAPSULES, ELIXIR, ORAL SOLUTION, SYRUP, TABLETS

Bronchodilator, acute attacks, in clients not currently on theophylline therapy.

Adults and children over 1 year of age, loading dose: 5 mg/kg. **Maintenance, Adults, nonsmoking:** 3 mg/kg q 8 hr; **Older clients, those with cor pulmonale:** 2 mg/kg q 8 hr. **Clients with CHF:** 1–2 mg/kg q 12 hr; **Children, 9–16 years of age and young adult smokers:** 3 mg/kg q 6 hr; **Children, 1–9 years of age:** 4 mg/kg q 6 hr.

Infants, 6–52 weeks, initial maintenance dose: Calculate as follows: [(0.2 x age in weeks) + 5] x kg = 24 hr dose in mg. For infants up to 26 weeks, divide into q 8 hr dosing; for infants 26–52 weeks, divide into q 6 hr dosing.

Bronchodilator, acute attacks, in clients currently receiving theophylline.

Adults and children up to 16 years of age: If possible, a serum theophylline level should be obtained first. Then, base loading dose on the premise that each 0.5 mg theophylline/kg lean body weight will result in a 0.5–1.6-mcg/mL increase in serum theophylline levels. If immediate therapy is needed and a serum level cannot be obtained, a single dose of the equivalent of 2.5 mg/kg of anhydrous theophylline in a rapidly absorbed form can be given.

Chronic therapy, based on anhydrous theophylline.

Adults and children, initial: 16 mg/kg/24 hr, up to a maximum of 400 mg/day in three to four divided doses at 6–8-hr intervals; **then,** dose can be increased in 25% increments at 2–3 day intervals up to a maximum, as follows: **Adults and children over 16 years of age:** 13 mg/kg, not to exceed 900 mg/day; **12–16 years:** 18 mg/kg/day; **9–12 years:** 20 mg/kg/day; **1–9 years:** 24 mg/kg/day.

• EXTENDED RELEASE CAPSULES AND TABLETS

Bronchodilator, chronic therapy, based on equivalent of anhydrous theophylline.

Adults, initial: 6–8 mg/kg up to a maximum of 400 mg/day in three to four divided doses at 6–8-hr intervals; **then,** dose may be increased, if needed and tolerated, by increments of 25% at 2–3 day intervals up to a maximum of 13 mg/kg/day or 900 mg/day, whichever is less, without measuring serum theophylline. **Pediatric, over 12 years of age, initial:** 4 mg/kg q 8–12 hr; **then,** dose may be increased by 2–3 mg/kg/day at 3-day intervals up to the following maximum doses (without measuring serum levels): **16 years and older:** 13 mg/kg/day or 900 mg/day, whichever is less; **12–16 years:** 18 mg/kg/day.

• ELIXIR, ORAL SOLUTION, SYRUP

Neonatal apnea.

Loading dose: Using the equivalent of anhydrous theophylline administered by NGT, 5 mg/kg; **maintenance:** 2 mg/kg/day in two to three divided doses given by NGT.

• IV

Bronchodilator, acute attacks.

See above doses using PO products.

NURSING CONSIDERATIONS

ADMINISTRATION/STORAGE

1. Individualize dosage to maintain serum levels of 10–20 mcg/mL.
2. Calculate dosage based on lean body weight (theophylline does not distribute to body fat). Once stabilized on a dosage, serum levels tend to remain constant.
3. Review list of agents with which theophylline derivatives interact.
4. Monitor serum theophylline levels in chronic therapy, especially if the maximum maintenance doses are used or exceeded.
5. The extended-release tablets or capsules are not recommended for children less than 6 years of age. Dosage for once-a-day products has not been established in children less than 12 years of age.
6. Serum levels may vary significantly following brand interchange.
7. When converting from an immediate release to a sustained release product, keep the total daily dose the same; only the dosing interval is adjusted.

IV 8. Wait to initiate PO therapy for at least 4–6 hr after switching from IV therapy.

9. Dilute drugs and maintain proper infusion rates to minimize problems of overdosage.

ASSESSMENT

1. Assess for any hypersensitivity to xanthine compounds. Note any experience with this class of drugs.
2. Document indications for therapy, type, onset, and characteristics of symptoms.
3. Note any history of hypotension, CAD, angina, PUD, or seizure disorders; avoid drug or use very cautiously in these conditions.
4. Assess for cigarette/marijuana use; induces hepatic metabolism of drug and may require increase in dosage from 50% to 100%.
5. Assess diet habits which can influence the excretion of theophylline. A high-protein and/or low-carbohydrate diet will cause an increased drug excretion. A low-protein and/or high-carbohydrate diet will decrease excretion of drug.
6. Assess lung fields closely. Note characteristics of sputum and cough; assess CXR, ABGs, and PFTs.
7. Obtain the serum sample at the time of peak absorption (1–2 hr after administration for immediate release and 5–9 hr after the morning dose or sustained release products). The client must not have missed doses during the previous 48 hr and the dosing intervals must have been reasonably typical during this time.

INTERVENTIONS

1. Observe for S&S of toxicity such as nausea, anorexia, insomnia, irritability, hyperexcitability, or cardiac arrhythmias; monitor serum levels.
2. Observe small children for excessive CNS stimulation; children often are unable to report side effects.

CLIENT/FAMILY TEACHING

1. To avoid epigastric pain, take with a snack or with meals. Avoid or minimize consumption of charbroiled foods (e.g., burgers).
2. Take ATC and only as prescribed; more is *not* better. Report nausea, vomiting, GI pain, or restlessness.
3. Do not crush or break slow-release forms of the drug.
4. Do not smoke; may aggravate underlying medical conditions as well as interfere with drug absorption. Attend smoking cessation program.
5. Protect from acute exacerbations of illness by avoiding crowds, dressing warmly in cold weather, obtaining the pneumonia vaccine and seasonal flu shot, covering mouth and nose so cold air is not directly inhaled, staying in air conditioning during excessively hot and humid weather, maintaining proper diet and nutrition, exercising daily, and consuming adequate fluids.
6. Report S&S of infections, adverse drug effects, difficulty breathing, and significant peak flow readings.
7. Caffeine- and xanthine-containing beverages and foods (chocolate, coffee, colas) and daily intake of charbroiled foods should be avoided; tend to increase drug side effects.
8. When secretions become thick and tacky, increase intake of fluids, avoiding

milk/milk products. This thins secretions and assists in their removal.
9. Do not take any OTC cough, cold, or breathing preparations without provider approval.
10. Learn to pace activity and avoid overexertion at all times.
11. Hold medication and report any side effects or CNS depression in children and infants.
12. Identify local support groups that may assist in understanding and coping with chronic respiratory dysfunction.

OUTCOMES/EVALUATE

• Knowledge/understanding of disease management; compliance with prescribed regimen
• Improved airway exchange and breathing patterns; ↓ wheezing
• Therapeutic drug levels (10–20 mcg/mL)
• Stimulation of respirations in the neonate

Thiabendazole

(thigh-ah-**BEN**-dah-zohl)

PREGNANCY CATEGORY: C
CLASSIFICATION(S):
Anthelmintic
Rx: Mintezol

ACTION/KINETICS

Interferes with the enzyme fumarate reductase, which is specific to several helminths. Readily absorbed from the GI tract. **Peak plasma levels:** 1–2 hr. **t½:** 0.9–2 hr. Most excreted within 24 hr, mainly through the urine.

USES

(1) Primarily for threadworm infections, cutaneous larva migrans, visceral larva migrans when these infections occur alone or if pinworm is also present. (2) Use in the following infections only if specific therapy is not available or cannot be used or if a second drug is desirable: hookworm, whipworm, large roundworm. (3) To reduce symptoms of trichinosis during the invasive phase.

CONTRAINDICATIONS

Lactation. Use in mixed infections with ascaris as it may cause worms to migrate.

SPECIAL CONCERNS

Safety and efficacy not established in children less than 13.6 kg. Use with caution in clients with hepatic disease or impaired hepatic function.

SIDE EFFECTS

GI: N&V, anorexia, diarrhea, epigastric distress. **CNS:** Dizziness, drowsiness, headache, irritability, weariness, giddiness, numbness, psychic disturbances, collapse, ***seizures.*** **Allergic:** Pruritus, ***angioedema,*** flushing of face, chills, fever, skin rashes, ***Stevens-Johnson syndrome, anaphylaxis,*** lymphadenopathy, conjunctival injection, erythema multiforme. **Hepatic:** Jaundice, cholestasis, parenchymal liver damage. **GU:** Crystalluria, hematuria, enuresis, foul odor of urine. **Ophthalmic:** Blurred vision, abnormal sensation in the eyes, yellow appearance of objects, drying of mucous membranes. **Miscellaneous:** Tinnitus, hypotension, hyperglycemia, transient leukopenia, perianal rash, appearance of live *Ascaris* in nose and mouth.

LABORATORY TEST CONSIDERATIONS

Rarely, ↑ AST and cephalin flocculation.

OD OVERDOSE MANAGEMENT

Symptoms: Psychic changes, transient vision changes. *Treatment:* Induce vomiting or perform gastric lavage. Treat symptoms.

DRUG INTERACTIONS

↑ Serum levels of xanthines to potentially toxic levels due to ↓ breakdown by liver.

HOW SUPPLIED

Chew Tablet: 500 mg; *Suspension:* 500 mg/5 mL

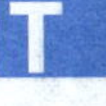

DOSAGE

• ORAL SUSPENSION, CHEWABLE TABLETS

Over 68 kg: 1.5 g/dose; **less than 68 kg:** 22 mg/kg/dose.

NURSING CONSIDERATIONS

ADMINISTRATION/STORAGE

1. Take with food to reduce stomach upset.

2. Chew chewable tablets before swallowing.
3. Cleansing enemas are not required after drug therapy.
4. For strongyloidiasis, cutaneous larva migrans, hookworm, whipworm, or roundworm: two doses daily are given for 2 days. For trichinelliasis, give two doses daily for 2–4 days. For visceral larva migrans, give two doses/day for 7 successive days.

ASSESSMENT

1. Document indications for therapy, onset/duration, and characteristics of symptoms. Determine how and when acquired. Culture for ova and parasites.
2. List agents currently prescribed to ensure none interact.

CLIENT/FAMILY TEACHING

1. Administer with food or after meals to decrease stomach upset; chew tablets thoroughly.
2. Report any CNS disturbances, including muscular weakness and loss of mental alertness.
3. Do not operate hazardous machinery; drug may cause dizziness and drowsiness.
4. May notice a urine odor 24 hr following ingestion; this is normal.
5. Report any evidence of rash, fever, or itching immediately.
6. With pinworms, treat all household members. Practice strict handwashing and hygiene measures, launder all bedlinens, underwear and sleep attire daily in hot water, disinfect toilets daily and bathroom and bedroom floors should be wet mopped; do not share towels and washclothes.

OUTCOMES/EVALUATE

- Negative consecutive stool cultures
- Eradication of infestation

T

Thiamine hydrochloride (Vitamin B_1)

(**THIGH**-ah-min)

PREGNANCY CATEGORY: A (PARENTERAL USE; C IF DOSES > RDA USED)

CLASSIFICATION(S):
Vitamin B complex
Rx: Injection, OTC: Tablets

ACTION/KINETICS

Water-soluble vitamin, stable in acid solution. Decomposed in neutral or acid solutions. Required for the synthesis of thiamine pyrophosphate, a coenzyme required in carbohydrate metabolism. The maximum amount absorbed PO is 8–15 mg/day although absorption may be increased by giving in divided doses with food.

USES

(1) Prophylaxis and treatment of thiamine deficiency states and associated neurologic and CV symptoms. (2) Prophylaxis and treatment of beriberi. (3) Alcoholic neuritis, neuritis of pellagra, and neuritis of pregnancy. (4) To correct anorexia due to thiamine insufficiency. *Investigational:* Treatment of subacute necrotizing encephalomyelopathy, maple syrup urine disease, pyruvate carboxylase deficiency, hyperalaninemia.

SPECIAL CONCERNS

Use with caution during lactation.

SIDE EFFECTS

Serious hypersensitivity reactions, including anaphylaxis; thus, intradermal testing is recommended if sensitivity is suspected. **Dermatologic:** Pruritus, urticaria, sweating, feeling of warmth. **CNS:** Weakness, restlessness. **Other:** Nausea, tightness in throat, ***angioneurotic edema,*** cyanosis, ***hemorrhage into the GI tract, pulmonary edema, CV collapse. Death has been reported.*** **Following IM use:** Induration, tenderness.

DRUG INTERACTIONS

Thiamine is unstable in neutral or alkaline solutions; do not use with substances that yield alkaline solutions, such as citrates, barbiturates, carbonates, or erythromycin lactobionate IV.

HOW SUPPLIED

Enteric Coated Tablet: 20 mg; *Injection:* 100 mg/mL; *Tablet:* 50 mg, 100 mg, 250 mg, 500 mg

DOSAGE

• **TABLETS, ENTERIC-COATED TABLETS**

Mild beriberi or maintenance following severe beriberi.

Adults: 5–10 mg/day (as part of a multivitamin product); **infants:** 10 mg/day.

Treatment of deficiency.

Adults: 5–10 mg/day; **pediatric:** 10–50 mg/day.

Alcohol-induced deficiency.

Adults: 40 mg/day.

Dietary supplement.

Adults: 1–2 mg/day; **pediatric:** 0.3–0.5 mg/day for infants and 0.5 mg/day for children.

Genetic enzyme deficiency disease.

10–20 mg/day (up to 4 g/day has been used in some clients).

• **SLOW IV, IV**

Thiamine deficiency.

Doses as high as 100 mg/L of fluid as rapidly as possible until deficiency is corrected.

Wet beriberi with myocardial failure.

Adults: 10–30 mg t.i.d.

Infantile beriberi.

25 mg if collapse occurs.

Wernicke-Korsakoff syndrome.

Initial: 100 mg IV; **then,** 50–100 mg IM until client is consuming a regular, balanced diet.

Marginal thiamine status in those receiving dextrose.

100 mg in each of the first few liters of IV fluid to avoid precipitating heart failure.

• **IM**

Beriberi.

10–20 mg t.i.d. for 2 weeks. Give a PO multivitamin product containing 5–10 mg/day thiamine for 1 month to cause body saturation.

Neuritis of pregnancy.

5–10 mg/day if vomiting is severe enough to preclude PO therapy.

Recommended dietary allowance.

Adult males: 1.2–1.5 mg; **adult females:** 1.1 mg.

NURSING CONSIDERATIONS

ADMINISTRATION/STORAGE

IV 1. May administer direct IV undiluted over at least 5 min or may be reconstituted in dextrose or saline solution and administered with daily solution therapy.

2. Drug may enhance the effects of neuromuscular blocking agents. Have epinephrine available to treat for anaphylactic shock if large dose of thiamine ordered.

ASSESSMENT

1. Document type, onset, and characteristics of symptoms.

2. List other agents prescribed to ensure none interact.

3. Note neurologic assessment and clinical presentation.

CLIENT/FAMILY TEACHING

Review dietary sources high in thiamine (enriched and whole grain cereals, meats, especially pork, and fresh vegetables); consult dietitian for assistance in meal plan/preparation. Eat well balanced meals regularly and avoid alcohol.

OUTCOMES/EVALUATE

- Prophylaxis of deficiency
- Prevention/reduction of neuritis symptoms

Thioguanine (6-TG)

(thigh-oh-**GWON**-een)

PREGNANCY CATEGORY: D

CLASSIFICATION(S):

Antineoplastic, antimetabolite

Rx: 6-Thioguanine, TG

✱**Rx:** Lanvis

SEE ALSO *ANTINEOPLASTIC AGENTS.*

ACTION/KINETICS

Purine antagonist that is cell-cycle specific for the S phase of cell division. Converted to 6-thioguanylic acid, which in turn interferes with the synthesis of guanine nucleotides by competing with hypoxanthine and xanthine for the enzyme phosphoribosyltransferase (HGPRTase). Ultimately the synthesis of RNA and DNA is inhibited. Resistance to the drug may result from increased breakdown of 6-thioguanylic acid or loss of HGPRTase activity. Partially absorbed (30%) from GI tract. **t½:** 80 min. Detoxified by liver and excreted in the urine. More effective in children than in adults. Cross-resistance with mercaptopurine. Perform platelet counts weekly; discontinue drug if abnormally large fall in blood count is noted, indicating severe bone marrow depression.

USES

(1) Acute and nonlymphocytic leukemias (usually in combination with other drugs such as cyclophosphamide, cytarabine, prednisone, vincristine). (2) Chronic myelogenous leukemia (not first-line therapy).

CONTRAINDICATIONS

Resistance to mercaptopurine or thioguanine. Lactation.

ADDITIONAL SIDE EFFECTS

Loss of vibration sense, unsteadiness of gait. ***Hepatotoxicity,*** myelosuppression (common), hyperuricemia. Adults tend to show a more rapid fall in WBC count than children.

LABORATORY TEST CONSIDERATIONS

↑ Uric acid in blood and urine.

OD OVERDOSE MANAGEMENT

Symptoms: N&V, hypertension, malaise, and diaphoresis may be seen immediately, which may be followed by myelosuppression and azotemia. ***Severe hematologic toxicity.*** *Treatment:* Induce vomiting if client is seen immediately after an acute overdosage. Treat symptoms. Hematologic toxicity may be treated by platelet transfusions (for bleeding) and granulocyte transfusions. Antibiotics are indicated for sepsis.

HOW SUPPLIED

Tablet: 40 mg

DOSAGE

• **TABLETS**

Individualized and determined by hematopoietic response.

Adults and pediatric, initial: 2 mg/kg/day (or 75–100 mg/m²) given at one time. From 2 to 4 weeks may elapse before beneficial results become apparent. Compute dose to nearest multiple of 20 mg. If no response, dosage may be increased to 3 mg/kg/day. **Usual maintenance dose (even during remissions):** 2–3 mg/kg/day (or 100 mg/m²). Dosage of thioguanine does not have to be decreased during administration of allopurinol (to inhibit uric acid production).

NURSING CONSIDERATIONS

SEE ALSO *NURSING CONSIDERATIONS FOR ANTINEOPLASTIC AGENTS.*

ASSESSMENT

1. Note indications for therapy, onset, duration, and characteristics of symptoms; list other agents trialed and the outcome.
2. Identify those experiencing loss of vibration sense and with unsteady gaits; (may be unable to rely on canes) may require assistance.
3. Expect hyperuricemia after tumor lysis, which may be reduced with administration of allopurinol, by preventing purine breakdown and excessive uric acid formation.
4. Monitor CBC, uric acid, liver and renal function studies. Obtain CBC weekly and LFTs monthly during course of therapy; may cause granulocyte and platelet suppression. Nadir: 10 days; recovery: 21 days.

CLIENT/FAMILY TEACHING

1. Take on an empty stomach for best results.
2. Increase fluid intake (2–3 L/day) to minimize hyperuricemia and hyperuricosuria.
3. Withhold drug and report if jaundice, decreased urine output, diarrhea, S&S of anemia (fatigue, dyspnea), or extremity swelling occurs.
4. Any sore throat, fever, or flu-like symptoms as well as increased bruising and bleeding tendencies require immediate reporting.
5. Avoid crowds, vaccinia, and persons with infectious diseases.
6. Practice reliable contraception.

OUTCOMES/EVALUATE

• Suppression of malignant cell proliferation

• Hematologic evidence of leukemia remission

Thioridazine hydrochloride

(thigh-oh-**RID**-ah-zeen)

PREGNANCY CATEGORY: C

CLASSIFICATION(S):
Antipsychotic, phenothiazine
Rx: Mellaril, Mellaril-S, Thioridazine HCl Intensol Oral
★**Rx:** Apo-Thioridazine

SEE ALSO *ANTIPSYCHOTIC AGENTS, PHENOTHIAZINES.*

ACTION/KINETICS
High incidence of hypotension; moderate incidence of sedative and anticholinergic effects and weak antiemetic and extrapyramidal effects. May be used in clients intolerant of other phenothiazines. **Peak plasma levels** (after PO administration): 1–4 hr. May impair its own absorption at higher doses due to the strong anticholinergic effects. **t½:** 10 hr. Metabolized in the liver to both active and inactive metabolites.

USES
Management of psychotic disorders in those who do not show an adequate response to treatment with other antipsychotics, either due to ineffectiveness or inability to reach an acceptable dose due to intolerable side effects.

CONTRAINDICATIONS
Use with fluvoxamine, fluoxetine, paroxetine, pindolol, propranolol, any drug that inhibits the cytochrome P450 2D6 isozyme, and with any drug that prolongs the QTc interval. In those with reduced levels of cytochrome P450 2D6 isozyme, those with congenital long QT syndrome, and those with a history of cardiac arrhythmias.

SPECIAL CONCERNS
Safe use during pregnancy has not been established. Dosage has not been established in children less than 2 years of age. Geriatric, emaciated, or debilitated clients usually require a lower initial dose.

ADDITIONAL SIDE EFFECTS
Dose-related prolongation of QTc interval with increased likelihood of ***torsade de pointes and sudden death.*** More likely to cause pigmentary retinopathy than other phenothiazines.

OD OVERDOSE MANAGEMENT
Treatment: Immediate CV monitoring, including continuous ECG to detect arrhythmias. Avoid drugs (e.g., disopyramide, procainamide, quinidine) that produce additive QT-prolongation.

ADDITIONAL DRUG INTERACTIONS
Fluvoxamine / ↑ Thioridazine blood levels → prolongation of QTc interval
Fluoxetine / ↑ Thioridazine blood levels → prolongation of QTc interval
Paroxetine / ↑ Thioridazine blood levels → prolongation of QTc interval
Pindolol / ↑ Thioridazine blood levels → prolongation of QTc interval
Propranolol / ↑ Thioridazine blood levels → prolongation of QTc interval

HOW SUPPLIED
Oral Concentrate: 30 mg/mL, 100 mg/mL; *Oral Suspension:* 25 mg/5 mL, 100 mg/5 mL; *Tablet:* 10 mg, 15 mg, 25 mg, 50 mg, 100 mg, 150 mg, 200 mg

DOSAGE

• ORAL SUSPENSION, ORAL SOLUTION, TABLETS

Psychotic disorders.

Adults, initial: 50–100 mg t.i.d. Increase gradually to a maximum of 800 mg/day, if needed to control symptoms. Then, reduce gradually to the minimum maintainence dose. Dose range: 200–800 mg/day divided into two to four doses.

Psychoneurotic symptoms.

Initial: 25 mg t.i.d. Dose range: 10 mg b.i.d.–q.i.d. in milder cases to 50 mg t.i.d. or q.i.d. Dose range: 20–200 mg/day.

Behavioral disorders in children.

Ages 2 to 12: 0.5 mg/kg/day to a maximum of 3 mg/kg/day. For moderate disorders, initially use 10 mg b.i.d.–t.i.d. For hospitalized, severely disturbed or psychotic children: 25 mg b.i.d.–t.i.d.

NURSING CONSIDERATIONS

SEE ALSO *NURSING CONSIDERATIONS* FOR *ANTIPSYCHOTIC AGENTS, PHENOTHIAZINES.*

ADMINISTRATION/STORAGE
Dilute each dose of concentrate just before administration with distilled

water, acidified tap water, or suitable juices. Preparation and storage of bulk dilutions are not recommended.

ASSESSMENT

1. Document mental status; assess behavioral manifestations. Note behaviors requiring treatment and presence/type of hallucinations if evident.
2. Determine baseline ECG and serum K levels before starting therapy. Prior to therapy, be sure clients have a QTc interval less than 450 msec and normal values for ECG and serum K. Monitor ECG, CBC, liver and renal function studies.

CLIENT/FAMILY TEACHING

1. Take only as directed; do not stop abruptly, as withdrawal may activate N&V, gastritis, dizziness, tachycardia, headache, and insomnia.
2. Avoid skin contact with solutions; may cause dermatitis.
3. Do not perform activities that require mental alertness, drug may cause drowsiness.
4. Wear protective clothing and sunscreens to prevent a photosensitivity reaction.
5. May cause retinal deposits viewed as a "browning of vision."
6. May impair temperature regulation; avoid temperature extremes, consume adequate fluids, and dress appropriately.
7. Doses exceeding 300 mg/day may cause reversible T-wave abnormalities on ECG. Doses above 800 mg/day have been associated with retinal deposits and cardiac toxicity.

OUTCOMES/EVALUATE

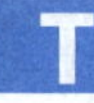

- ↓ Agitation, combativeness or explosive hyperexcitable behaviors and improved coping mechanisms
- ↓ Anxiety levels; ↓ depression; ↓ sleep disturbances

Thiotepa (Thio)

(thigh-oh-**TEP**-ah)

PREGNANCY CATEGORY: D
CLASSIFICATION(S):
Antineoplastic, alkylating
Rx: Thioplex

SEE ALSO *ANTINEOPLASTIC AGENTS* AND *ALKYLATING AGENTS*.

ACTION/KINETICS

Cell-cycle nonspecific; thought to act by causing the release of ethylenimmonium ions that bind or alkylate various intracellular substances such as nucleic acids. Is cytotoxic by virtue of cross-linking of DNA and RNA strands as well as by inhibition of protein synthesis. Rapidly cleared from the plasma following IV use. **t½, elimination:** About 2.3 hr. May be significantly absorbed through the bladder mucosa. Approximately 85% excreted through the urine, mainly as metabolites.

USES

(1) Adenocarcinoma of the breast or ovary. (2) To control intracavitary effusions secondary to diffuse or localized neoplastic disease of various serosal cavities. (3) Superficial papillary carcinoma of the urinary bladder. (4) Lymphosarcoma and Hodgkin's disease, although other treatments are used more often.

CONTRAINDICATIONS

Lactation. Pregnancy. Renal, hepatic, or bone marrow damage. Acute leukemia. Use with other alkylating agents due to increased toxicity.

SPECIAL CONCERNS

Is both carcinogenic and mutagenic. Use with caution in renal and hepatic dysfunction. Safety and efficacy have not been determined in children.

SIDE EFFECTS

GI: N&V, abdominal pain, anorexia. **CNS:** Dizziness, headache, blurred vision, fatigue, weakness, febrile reaction. **Dermatologic:** Contact dermatitis, alopecia, pain at injection site, dermatitis, skin depigmentation following topical use. **GU:** Dysuria, urinary retention, chemical or hemorrhagic cystitis following intravesical use, amenorrhea, interference with spermatogenesis. *Hypersensitivity:* Rash, urticaria, wheezing, ***laryngeal edema, asthma, anaphylactic shock.*** **Miscellaneous:** Conjunctivitis, discharge from a SC lesion due to tumor tissue breakdown. Significant toxicity to the hematopoietic system.

OD OVERDOSE MANAGEMENT

Symptoms: ***Hematopoietic toxicity.*** *Treatment:* Transfusions of whole blood, platelets, or leukocytes have been used.

DRUG INTERACTIONS
Alkylating agents / Combination with other alkylating agents ↑ toxicity
Pancuronium / Prolonged muscle paralysis and respiratory depression
Succinylcholine / Risk of ↑ apnea

HOW SUPPLIED
Powder for injection, lyophilized: 15 mg

DOSAGE

• **IV (MAY BE RAPID)**

0.3–0.4 mg/kg at 1- to 4-week intervals by rapid administration or 0.2 mg/kg for 4–5 days q 2–4 weeks.

• **INTRATUMOR OR INTRACAVITARY ADMINISTRATION**

0.6–0.8 mg/kg q 1–4 weeks; through the same tubing used to remove fluid from the cavity.

• **INTRAVESICAL ADMINISTRATION (BLADDER CANCER)**

After dehydrating client with papillary carcinoma of the bladder for 8–12 hr, instill 60 mg thiotepa in 30–60 mL of sterile water for injection in the bladder using a catheter. Retain, if possible, for 2 hr. If it is not possible to retain 60 mL, give the dose in a volume of 30 mL. Reposition client q 15 min for maximum contact area. This dose is given once a week for 4 weeks.

NURSING CONSIDERATIONS

SEE ALSO *NURSING CONSIDERATIONS* FOR *ANTINEOPLASTIC AGENTS*.

ADMINISTRATION/STORAGE

IV 1. Reconstitute with sterile water (usually 1.5 mL to give a concentration of 5 mg/0.5 mL). The reconstituted solution can then be mixed with NaCl, dextrose, dextrose and NaCl, Ringer's, or RL injection (i.e., if a large volume is needed for intracavitary use, IV drip, or perfusion).
2. Minimize pain on injection and retard rate of absorption by simultaneous administration of local anesthetics. Drug may be mixed with procaine HCl 2% or epinephrine HCl 1:1,000, or both, as ordered.
3. Store vials in the refrigerator. Reconstituted solutions may be stored for 5 days in the refrigerator without substantial loss of potency.
4. Since thiotepa is not a vesicant, it may be injected quickly and directly into the vein with the desired volume of sterile water. Usual amount of diluent is 1.5 mL.
5. Do not use NSS as a diluent.
6. Discard solutions grossly opaque or with precipitate.
7. When used for bladder carcinoma, a second or third course of treatment may be undertaken, although bone marrow depression may be increased.

ASSESSMENT

1. Document indications for therapy, onset/type of symptoms, any other agents trialed and any previous therapy with this agent.
2. Note cystoscopy findings with bladder lesions and all biopsy results.
3. Monitor CBC, uric acid, liver and renal function studies. Drug causes platelet and granulocyte suppression. Nadir: 21 days; recovery: 40–50 days.

INTERVENTIONS

1. Encourage clients who receive drug as bladder instillations to retain fluid for 2 hr. They should be NPO for 6 hr to ensure drug retention. Observe for hematuria and dysuria.
2. With bladder instillation, reposition q 15 min to ensure maximum bladder area contact.
3. Advise to practice contraception; drug is carcinogenic and mutagenic.

OUTCOMES/EVALUATE

Control of tumor size and malignant cell proliferation

Tiagabine hydrochloride

(tye-**AG**-ah-been)

PREGNANCY CATEGORY: C
CLASSIFICATION(S):
Anticonvulsant, miscellaneous
Rx: Gabatril

SEE ALSO *ANTICONVULSANTS*.

ACTION/KINETICS
Mechanism not known but activity of GABA, an inhibitory neurotransmitter, may be enhanced. Drug may block

T

uptake of GABA into presynaptic neurons allowing more GABA to bind to post-synaptic cells. This prevents propagation of neural impulses that contribute to seizures due to GABA-ergic action. **Peak plasma levels:** About 45 min when fasting. High fat meals decrease rate but not extent of absorption. Metabolized in liver; excreted in urine and feces. **t½, elimination:** 7–9 hr. Diurnal effect occurs with levels being lower in evening compared with morning.

USES

Adjunctive therapy for partial seizures.

CONTRAINDICATIONS

Lactation.

SPECIAL CONCERNS

Safety and efficacy have not been determined in children less than 12 years old.

SIDE EFFECTS

CNS: Dizziness, asthenia, somnolence, nervousness, tremor, insomnia, difficulty with concentration or attention, ataxia, confusion, speech disorder, difficulty with memory, paresthesia, depression, emotional lability, abnormal gait, hostility, nystagmus, problems with language, agitation. **GI:** N&V, diarrhea, increased appetite, mouth ulceration. **Respiratory:** Pharyngitis, increased cough. **Dermatologic:** Rash, pruritus. **Miscellaneous:** Abdominal pain, unspecified pain, vasodilation, myasthenia.

OD OVERDOSE MANAGEMENT

Symptoms: Somnolence, impaired consciousness, agitation, confusion, speech difficulties, hostility, depression, weakness, myoclonus. *Treatment:* Emesis or gastric lavage, maintain an airway. General supportive treatment.

DRUG INTERACTIONS

Carbamazepine / ↑ Clearance due to ↑ metabolism

Phenobarbital / ↑ Clearance due to ↑ metabolism

Phenytoin / ↑ Clearance due to ↑ metabolism

Valproate / ↑ Clearance due to ↑ metabolism

HOW SUPPLIED

Tablets: 2 mg, 4 mg, 12 mg, 16 mg, 20 mg

DOSAGE

• TABLETS

Partial seizures.

Adults and children over 18 years, initial: 4 mg once daily. Total daily dose may be increased by 4 to 8 mg at weekly intervals until clinical effect is observed or daily dose is 56 mg/day. **Children, 12 to 18 years, initial:** 4 mg once daily. Total daily dose may be increased by 4 mg at beginning of week 2. Thereafter, dose may be increased by 4 to 8 mg at weekly intervals until clinical effect is seen or dose is 32 mg/day. For all ages, give total daily dose in 2 to 4 divided doses.

NURSING CONSIDERATIONS

SEE ALSO *NURSING CONSIDERATIONS* FOR *ANTICONVULSANTS*.

ADMINISTRATION/STORAGE

1. It is not necessary to modify dose of concomitant anticonvulsant drugs, unless clinically indicated.
2. Dose must be titrated in those taking enzyme-inducing anticonvulsant drugs; consult package insert.

ASSESSMENT

1. Document indications for therapy, characteristics of seizures, other agents trialed and outcome.
2. Monitor LFTs; decrease dosage or dosing intervals with dysfunction.

CLIENT/FAMILY TEACHING

1. Take with food as directed.
2. Do not perform activities requiring mental alertness until drug effects realized; may cause dizziness, sleepiness, or confusion.
3. Report any increased frequency or loss of seizure control, rash, weakness, or visual disturbances.
4. Do not stop abruptly; may trigger seizures.
5. Practice reliable contraception; do not breast feed.

OUTCOMES/EVALUATE

Control of seizures

Ticarcillin disodium

(tie-kar-**SILL**-in)

PREGNANCY CATEGORY: B

CLASSIFICATION(S):
Antibiotic, penicillin
Rx: Ticar

SEE ALSO *ANTI-INFECTIVES* AND *PENICILLINS.*

ACTION/KINETICS
A parenteral, semisynthetic antibiotic with an antibacterial spectrum of resembling that of carbenicillin. **Peak plasma levels: IM,** 25–35 mcg/mL after 1 hr; **IV,** 15 min. **t½:** 70 min. Elimination complete after 6 hr.

USES
Primarily suitable for treatment of gram-negative organisms but also effective for mixed infections. (1) Bacterial septicemia, skin and soft tissue infections, acute and chronic respiratory tract infections caused by susceptible strains of *Pseudomonas aeruginosa, Proteus, Escherichia coli,* and other gram-negative organisms. Combined therapy with gentamicin or tobramycin is sometimes indicated for treatment of *Pseudomonas* infections. (2) GU tract infections (complicated and uncomplicated) caused by the above organisms and by *Enterobacter* and *Streptococcus faecalis.* (3) Anaerobic bacteria causing empyema, anaerobic pneumonitis, lung abscess, bacterial septicemia, peritonitis, intra-abdominal abscess, skin and soft tissue infections, salpingitis, endometritis, pelvic inflammatory disease, pelvic abscess. Ticarcillin may be used in infections in which protective mechanisms are impaired such as during use of oncolytic or immunosuppressive drugs or in clients with acute leukemia.

ADDITIONAL CONTRAINDICATIONS
Pregnancy.

SPECIAL CONCERNS
Use with caution in presence of impaired renal function and for clients on restricted salt diets.

ADDITIONAL SIDE EFFECTS
Neurotoxicity and neuromuscular excitability, especially in clients with impaired renal function.

LABORATORY TEST CONSIDERATIONS
↑ Alkaline phosphatase, AST, ALT.

ADDITIONAL DRUG INTERACTIONS
Effect of carbenicillin may be enhanced when used in combination with gentamicin or tobramycin for *Pseudomonas* infections.

HOW SUPPLIED
Powder for injection: 1 g, 3 g, 6 g, 20 g, 30 g

DOSAGE

• IV INFUSION, DIRECT IV, IM

Bacterial septicemia, intra-abdominal infections, skin and soft tissue infections, infections of the female genital system and pelvis, respiratory tract infections.

Adults: 200–300 mg/kg/day by IV infusion in divided doses q 4 or 6 hr (3 g q 4 hr or 4 g q 6 hr), depending on the weight and severity of the infection. **Pediatric, less than 40 kg:** 200–300 mg/kg/day by IV infusion q 4 or 6 hr (daily dose should not exceed the adult dose).

UTIs, uncomplicated.

Adults: 1 g IM or direct IV q 6 hr. **Pediatric, less than 40 kg:** 50–100 mg/kg/day IM or direct IV in divided doses q 6 or 8 hr.

UTIs, complicated.

Adults: 150–200 mg/kg/day by IV infusion in divided doses q 4 or 6 hr (usual dose is 3 g q.i.d. for a 70-kg client).

Neonates with sepsis due to Pseudomonas, Proteus, *or E. coli.*

Less than 7 days of age and less than 2 kg, 75 mg/kg q 12 hr; **more than 7 days of age and less than 2 kg,** 75 mg/kg q 8 hr; **less than 7 days of age and more than 2 kg,** 75 mg/kg q 8 hr; **more than 7 days of age and more than 2 kg,** 100 mg/kg q 8 hr. Can be given IM or by IV infusion over 10–20 min.

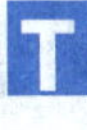

Clients with renal insufficiency should receive a loading dose of 3 g **IV,** and subsequent doses, as follows by C_{CR}. C_{CR} over 60 mL/min: 3 g IV q 4 hr; C_{CR} from 30–60 mL/min: 2 g IV q 4 hr; C_{CR} from 10–30 mL/min: 2 g IV q 8 hr; C_{CR}, less than 10 mL/min: 2 g IV q 12 hr or 1 g IM q 6 hr; C_{CR}, less than 10 mL/min with hepatic dysfunction: 2 g IV q 24 hr or 1 g IM q 12 hr. Clients on peritoneal dialysis: 3 g IV q 12 hr; clients on hemodialysis: 2 g IV q 12 hr and 3 g after each dialysis.

NURSING CONSIDERATIONS

SEE ALSO NURSING CONSIDERATIONS FOR PENICILLINS.

ADMINISTRATION/STORAGE

1. Clients seriously ill should receive higher doses such as in serious urinary tract and systemic infections.
2. For IM use, reconstitute each gram with 2 mL sterile water for injection, NaCl injection, or 1% lidocaine HCl (without epinephrine) to prevent pain and induration. Use the reconstituted solution quickly; inject well into a large muscle.
3. Do not administer more than 2 g of the drug in each IM site.
4. Give the adult dose to children weighing over 40 kg.
5. Do not mix ticarcillin together with amikacin, gentamicin, or tobramycin due to the gradual inactivation of these aminoglycosides.
6. Discard unused reconstituted solutions after 24 hr when stored at room temperature and after 72 hr when refrigerated.

IV 7. For IV use, reconstitute each gram with 4 mL of the desired solution. Administer slowly to prevent vein irritation and phlebitis. A dilution of 1 g/20 mL (or more) will decrease the chance of vein irritation.

8. For an IV infusion, use 50 or 100 mL *ADD-Vantage* container of either D5W or NaCl injection and give by intermittent infusion over 30–120 min in equally divided doses.

ASSESSMENT

1. Document type, onset, and characteristics of symptoms.
2. Monitor bleeding times, cultures, liver and renal function studies. Reduce dosage with liver or renal dysfunction.
3. With high doses, monitor for signs of electrolyte imbalance (especially Na and K levels).
4. Note sodium content of drug (usually 4.75 mEq Na/g) and calculate accordingly if Na restricted.

CLIENT/FAMILY TEACHING

1. Report any symptoms of bleeding abnormalities, such as petechiae, ecchymosis, or frank bleeding.
2. Edema, weight gain, or respiratory distress may be precipitated by drug's large sodium content.
3. Review drug side effects that should be reported if evident.

OUTCOMES/EVALUATE

- Negative cultures
- Symptomatic improvement

—COMBINATION DRUG—

Ticarcillin disodium and Clavulanate potassium

(tie-kar-**SILL**-in, klav-you-**LAN**-ate poe-**TASS**-ee-um)

PREGNANCY CATEGORY: B
CLASSIFICATION(S):
Antibiotic, penicillin
Rx: Timentin

SEE ALSO TICARCILLIN DISODIUM AND PENICILLINS.

CONTENT
Each vial of the Powder for Injection and the Solution contains: ticarcillin disodium, 3.1 g, and clavulanate potassium, 0.1 g.

ACTION/KINETICS
Contains clavulanic acid, which protects the breakdown of ticarcillin by beta-lactamase enzymes, thus ensuring appropriate blood levels of ticarcillin.

USES
(1) Septicemia, including bacteremia, due to β–lactamase producing strains of *Klebsiella* sp., *Staphylococcus aureus*, and *Pseudomonas aeruginosa* (and other *Pseudomonas* species). (2) Lower respiratory tract infections due to β–lactamase producing strains of *S. aureus, Haemophilus influenzae,* and *Klebsiella* sp. (3) Bone and joint infections due to β–lactamase producing strains of *S. aureus.* (4) Skin and skin structure infections due to β–lactamase producing strains of *S. aureus,*

Klebsiella sp., and *E. coli.* (5) UTIs (complicated and uncomplicated) due to β–lactamase producing strains of *E. coli, Klebsiella* sp., *P. aeruginosa* (and other *Pseudomonas* species), *Citrobacter* sp., *Enterobacter cloacae, Serratia marcescens,* and *S. aureus.* (6) Endometritis due to β–lactamase producing strains of *B. melaninogenicus, Enterobacter* sp. (including *E. cloacae), E. coli, Klebsiella pneumoniae, S. aureus,* and *Staphylococcus epidermidis.* (7) Peritonitis due to β–lactamase producing strains of *E. coli, K. pneumoniae,* and *Bacteroides fragilis* group.

HOW SUPPLIED

See Content

DOSAGE

- **IV INFUSION**

Systemic and UTIs.

Adults more than 60 kg: 3.1 g (containing 0.1 g clavulanic acid) q 4–6 hr for 10–14 days. **Adults less than 60 kg:** 200–300 mg ticarcillin/kg/day in divided doses q 4–6 hr for 10–14 days.

Gynecologic infections.

Adults more than 60 kg, moderate infections: 200 mg/kg/day in divided doses q 6 hr; **severe infections:** 300 mg/kg/day in divided doses q 4 hr.

In renal insufficiency.

Initially, loading dose of 3.1 g ticarcillin and 0.1 g clavulanic acid; **then,** dose based on C_{CR} as follows. C_{CR} over 60 mL/min: 3.1 g q 4 hr; C_{CR} from 30–60 mL/min: 2 g q 4 hr; C_{CR} from 10–30 mL/min: 2 g q 8 hr; C_{CR}, less than 10 mL/min: 2 g q 12 hr; C_{CR}, less than 10 mL/min with hepatic dysfunction: 2 g q 24 hr. Clients on peritoneal dialysis: 3.1 g q 12 hr; clients on hemodialysis: 2 g q 12 hr and 3.1 g after each dialysis.

NURSING CONSIDERATIONS

SEE ALSO *NURSING CONSIDERATIONS* FOR *PENICILLINS* AND *TICARCILLIN DISODIUM*.

ADMINISTRATION/STORAGE

1. To attain the appropriate dilution for 3.1 g ticarcillin and 0.1 g clavulanic acid, dilute with 13 mL of either NaCl or sterile water for injection. Further dilutions can be undertaken with D5W, RL injection, or NaCl.
2. Administer over a 30-min period, either through a Y-type IV infusion or by direct infusion.
3. This product is incompatible with sodium bicarbonate.
4. Dilutions with NaCl or RL injection may be stored at room temperature for 24 hr or refrigerated for 7 days. Dilutions with D5W are stable at room temperature for 12 hr or for 3 days if refrigerated.
5. If used with another anti-infective agent (e.g., an aminoglycoside), give each drug separately.

ASSESSMENT

1. Document type, onset, and characteristics of symptoms.
2. Monitor bleeding times, cultures, liver and renal function studies. Reduce dosage with liver or renal dysfunction.

OUTCOMES/EVALUATE

Resolution of infection; symptomatic improvement

Ticlopidine hydrochloride

(tie-**KLOH**-pih-deen)

PREGNANCY CATEGORY: B
CLASSIFICATION(S):
Antiplatelet drug
Rx: Ticlid
★**Rx:** Alti-Ticlopidine, Gen-Ticlopidine, Nu-Ticlopidine, Apo-Ticlopidine

ACTION/KINETICS

Irreversibly inhibits ADP-induced platelet-fibrinogen binding and subsequent platelet-platelet interactions. This results in inhibition of both platelet aggregation and release of platelet granule constituents as well as prolongation of bleeding time. **Peak plasma levels:** 2 hr. **Maximum platelet inhibition:** 8–11 days after 250 mg b.i.d. **Steady-state plasma levels:** 14–21 days. **$t^{1/2}$, elimination:** 4–5 days. After discontinuing therapy, bleeding time and other platelet function tests return to normal within 14 days. Rapidly absorbed; bioavailability is increased

T

by food. Highly bound (98%) to plasma proteins. Extensively metabolized by the liver with approximately 60% excreted through the kidneys; 23% is excreted in the feces (with one-third excreted unchanged). Clearance of the drug decreases with age.

USES

(1) With aspirin to decrease the incidence of subacute stent thrombosis in clients undergoing successful coronary stent implantation. (2) To reduce the risk of fatal or nonfatal thrombotic stroke in clients who have manifested precursors of stroke or who have had a completed thrombotic stroke. Due to the risk of neutropenia or agranulocytosis, this use should be reserved for clients who are intolerant to aspirin therapy or who have failed aspirin therapy. *Investigational:* Chronic arterial occlusion, coronary artery bypass grafts, intermittent claudication, open heart surgery, primary glomerulonephritis, subarachnoid hemorrhage, sickle cell disease, uremic clients with AV shunts or fistulas.

CONTRAINDICATIONS

Use in the presence of neutropenia and thrombocytopenia, hemostatic disorder, or active pathologic bleeding such as bleeding peptic ulcer or intracranial bleeding. Severe liver impairment. Lactation.

SPECIAL CONCERNS

Use with caution in clients with ulcers (i.e., where there is a propensity for bleeding). Consider reduced dosage in impaired renal function. Geriatric clients may be more sensitive to the effects of the drug. Severe hematological side effects (including thrombotic thrombocytopenic purpura) may occur within a few days of the start of ticlopidine therapy. Safety and effectiveness have not been established in children less than 18 years of age.

SIDE EFFECTS

Hematologic: ***Neutropenia, agranulocytosis, thrombotic thrombocytopenia purpura,*** thrombocytopenia, pancytopenia, immune thrombocytopenia, ***hemolytic anemia with reticulocytosis.*** **GI:** Diarrhea, N&V, GI pain, dyspepsia, flatulence, anorexia, GI fullness, peptic ulcer. **Hepatic:** Hepatitis, cholestatic jaundice, hepatocellular jauncide, ***hepatic necrosis.*** *Bleeding complications:* Ecchymosis, hematuria, epistaxis, conjunctival hemorrhage, ***GI bleeding,*** perioperative bleeding, posttraumatic bleeding, ***intracerebral bleeding (rare).*** **Dermatologic:** Maculopapular or urticarial rash, pruritus, urticaria. Rarely, erythema multiforme, exfoliative dermatitis, ***Stevens-Johnson syndrome.*** **CNS:** Dizziness, headache. **Neuromuscular:** Asthenia, SLE, peripheral neuropathy, arthropathy, myositis. **Miscellaneous:** Tinnitus, pain, allergic pneumonitis, vasculitis, nephrotic syndrome, renal failure, angioedema, hyponatremia, serum sickness.

LABORATORY TEST CONSIDERATIONS

↑ Alkaline phosphatase, ALT, AST, serum cholesterol, and triglycerides. Abnormal LFTs.

DRUG INTERACTIONS

Antacids / ↓ Ticlopidine plasma levels
Aspirin / ↑ Effect of aspirin on collagen-induced platelet aggregation
Carbamazepine / ↑ Carbazepine plasma levels → toxicity
Cimetidine / ↓ Ticlopidine clearance R/T ↓ liver metabolism
Digoxin / Slight ↓ in digoxin plasma levels
H *Evening primrose oil* / Potential for ↑ antiplatelet effect
H *Feverfew* / Potential for ↑ antiplatelet effect
H *Garlic* / Potential for ↑ antiplatelet effect
H *Ginger* / Potential for ↑ antiplatelet effect
H *Ginkgo biloba* / Potential for ↑ antiplatelet effect
H *Ginseng* / Potential for ↑ antiplatelet effect
H *Grapeseed extract* / Potential for ↑ antiplatelet effect
Phenytoin / ↑ Phenytoin plasma levels → somnolence and lethargy
Theophylline / ↑ Theophylline plasma levels R/T ↓ clearance

HOW SUPPLIED

Tablet: 250 mg

DOSAGE

• **TABLETS**

Reduce risk of thrombotic stroke, Adjunct with aspirin to reduce subacute stent thrombosis.

250 mg b.i.d.

NURSING CONSIDERATIONS

ADMINISTRATION/STORAGE

1. To increase bioavailability and decrease GI discomfort, take with food or just after eating.
2. If switched from an anticoagulant or fibrinolytic drug to ticlopidine, discontinue the former drug before initiation of ticlopidine therapy.
3. IV methylprednisolone (20 mg) may normalize prolonged bleeding times, usually within 2 hr.

ASSESSMENT

1. Note any liver disease, bleeding disorders, or ulcer disease.
2. Ascertain aspirin intolerance.
3. See increased use of plavix due to less side effect profile and once daily dosing advantage.
4. Determine baseline hematologic profile (e.g., CBC, PT, PTT, INR), liver and renal function studies.
5. Monitor blood biweekly to screen for possibly fatal thrombotic thrombocytopenic purpura.

CLIENT/FAMILY TEACHING

1. Take with food or after meals to minimize GI upset.
2. It may take longer than usual to stop bleeding; report unusual bleeding as severe hematological side effects may occur.
3. Brush teeth with a soft-bristle tooth brush, use an electric razor for shaving, wear shoes when ambulating, use caution and avoid injury, as bleeding times may be prolonged.
4. During the first 3 months of therapy, neutropenia can occur, resulting in an increased risk of infection. Come for scheduled blood tests and report any symptoms of infection (e.g., fever, chills, sore throat).
5. Any severe or persistent diarrhea, SC bleeding, skin rashes, or evidence of cholestasis (e.g., yellow skin or sclera, dark urine, light-colored stools) should be reported.

OUTCOMES/EVALUATE

Prevention of a complete or recurrent cerebral thrombotic event

Tiludronate disodium

(tye-**LOO**-droh-nayt)

PREGNANCY CATEGORY: C
CLASSIFICATION(S):
Bone growth regulator, biphosphonate
Rx: Skelid

ACTION/KINETICS
Inhibits activity of osteoclasts and decreases bone turnover. Does not interfere with bone mineralization. Poorly absorbed from GI tract when fasting and in presence of food. **Peak serum levels:** 2 hr. Not metabolized; excreted in urine. **t½:** About 150 hr.

USES
Treatment of Paget's disease where level of serum alkaline phosphatase is at least twice upper limit of normal, in those who are symptomatic, or who are at risk for future complications of disease.

CONTRAINDICATIONS
Not recommended for those with C_{CR} less than 30 mL/min.

SPECIAL CONCERNS
Use with caution during lactation and in those with dysphagia, symptomatic esophageal disease, gastritis, duodenitis, or ulcers. Safety and efficacy have not been determined in children.

SIDE EFFECTS
GI: Diarrhea, N&V, dyspepsia, flatulence, tooth disorder, abdominal pain, constipation, dry mouth, gastritis. **Body as whole:** Pain, back pain, accidental injury, flu-like symptoms, chest pain, asthenia, syncope, fatigue, flushing. **CNS:** Headache, dizziness, paresthesia, vertigo, anorexia, somnolence, anxiety, nervousness, insomnia. **CV:** Dependent edema, peripheral edema, hypertension, syncope. **Musculoskeletal:** Arthralgia, arthrosis, pathological fracture, involuntary muscle contractions. **Respiratory:** Rhinitis, sinusitis, URTI, coughing, pharyngitis, bronchitis. **Dermatologic:** Rash, skin disorder, pruritus, increased sweating, Stevens-Johnson

type syndrome (rare). **Ophthalmic:** Cataract, conjunctivitis, glaucoma. **Miscellaneous:** Hyperparathyroidism, vitamin D deficiency, UTI, infection.

OD OVERDOSE MANAGEMENT

Symptoms: Hypocalcemia. *Treatment:* Supportive.

DRUG INTERACTIONS

Antacids, aluminum- or magnesium-containing / Antacids, taken 1 hr before, ↓ tiludronate bioavailability
Aspirin / Aspirin, taken 2 hr after, ↓ tiludronate bioavailability by 50%
Calcium / ↓ Tiludronate bioavailability when taken at same time
Indomethacin / ↑ Tiludronate bioavailability by 2- to 4-fold

HOW SUPPLIED

Tablets: 240 mg (equivalent to 200 mg tiludronic acid)

DOSAGE

• **TABLETS**

Paget's disease.

Adults: Single 400 mg dose/day taken with 6 to 8 oz of plain water for period of only 3 months.

NURSING CONSIDERATIONS

ADMINISTRATION/STORAGE

Allow an interval of 3 months to assess response.

CLIENT/FAMILY TEACHING

1. Take with 6 to 8 oz of plain water. Do not take within 2 hr of food. Beverages other than water, food, and some medications reduce absorption of tiludronate.
2. Do not take aspirin, indomethacin, or calcium or mineral supplements within 2 hr of taking drug.
3. Do not remove tablets from foil strips until they are to be used.
4. May experience nausea, diarrhea, and GI upset; report if severe.
5. Report any rashes, itching, hives, severe stomach pains, bloody or black tarry stools.
6. Consume diet high in calcium and vitamin D.

OUTCOMES/EVALUATE

Inhibition of Paget's disease progression

T

Timolol maleate

(**TIE**-moh-lohl)

PREGNANCY CATEGORY: C
CLASSIFICATION(S):

Beta-adrenergic blocking agent
Rx: Betimol, Blocadren, Timoptic, Timoptic-XE
★**Rx:** Apo-Timol, Apo-Timop, Gen-Timolol, Novo-Timol, Nu-Timolol, PMS-Timolol, Rhoxal-timolol, Tim-AK

SEE ALSO *BETA-ADRENERGIC BLOCKING AGENTS*.

ACTION/KINETICS

Exerts both beta-1- and beta-2-adrenergic blocking activity. Has minimal sympathomimetic effects, direct myocardial depressant effects, or local anesthetic action. Does not cause pupillary constriction or night blindness. The mechanism of the protective effect in MI is not known. **Peak plasma levels:** 1–2 hr. **t½:** 4 hr. Metabolized in the liver. Metabolites and unchanged drug excreted through the kidney.Also reduces both elevated and normal IOP, whether or not glaucoma is present; thought to act by reducing aqueous humor formation and/or by slightly increasing outflow of aqueous humor. Does not affect pupil size or visual acuity. For use in eye: **Onset:** 30 min. **Maximum effect:** 1–2 hr. **Duration:** 24 hr.

USES

Tablets: (1) Hypertension (alone or in combination with other antihypertensives such as thiazide diuretics). (2) Reduce CV mortality and risk of reinfarction in clinically stable MI survivors. (3) Prophylaxis of migraine. *Investigational:* Ventricular arrhythmias and tachycardias, essential tremors.

Ophthalmic solution (Betimol, Timoptic): Lower IOP in chronic open-angle glaucoma, selected cases of secondary glaucoma, ocular hypertension, aphakic (no lens) clients with glaucoma. **Gel-Forming Solution (Timoptic-XE):** Reduce elevated IOP in open-angle glaucoma or ocular hypertension.

CONTRAINDICATIONS
Hypersensitivity to drug. Bronchial asthma or bronchospasm including severe COPD.

SPECIAL CONCERNS
Use ophthalmic preparation with caution in clients for whom systemic beta-adrenergic blocking agents are contraindicated. Safe use in children not established.

SIDE EFFECTS
Systemic following use of tablets: See *Beta-Adrenergic Blocking Agents.*

Following use of ophthalmic product: Few. Occasionally, ocular irritation, local hypersensitivity reactions, slight decrease in resting HR.

LABORATORY TEST CONSIDERATIONS
↑ BUN, serum potassium, and uric acid. ↓ H&H.

DRUG INTERACTIONS
When used ophthalmically, possible potentiation with systemically administered beta-adrenergic blocking agents.

HOW SUPPLIED
Gel forming solution: 0.25%, 0.5%; *Ophthalmic solution:* 0.25%, 0.5%; *Tablet:* 5 mg, 10 mg, 20 mg

DOSAGE

- **TABLETS**

Hypertension.

Initial: 10 mg b.i.d. alone or with a diuretic; **maintenance:** 20–40 mg/day (up to 60 mg/day in two doses may be required), depending on BP and HR. If dosage increase is necessary, wait 7 days.

MI prophylaxis in clients who have survived the acute phase.

10 mg b.i.d.

Migraine prophylaxis.

Initially: 10 mg b.i.d. **Maintenance:** 20 mg/day given as a single dose; total daily dose may be increased to 30 mg in divided doses or decreased to 10 mg, depending on the response and client tolerance. If a satisfactory response for migraine prophylaxis is not obtained within 6–8 weeks using the maximum daily dose, discontinue the drug.

Essential tremor.

10 mg/day.

- **OPHTHALMIC SOLUTION (BETIMOL OR TIMOPTIC, EACH 0.25% OR 0.5%)**

Glaucoma.

1 gtt of 0.25%–0.50% solution in each eye b.i.d. If the decrease in intraocular pressure is maintained, reduce dose to 1 gtt once a day.

- **OPHTHALMIC GEL-FORMING SOLUTION (TIMOPTIC-XE 0.25% OR 0.5%)**

Glaucoma.

1 gtt once daily.

NURSING CONSIDERATIONS

SEE ALSO *NURSING CONSIDERATIONS* FOR *BETA-ADRENERGIC BLOCKING AGENTS* AND *ANTIHYPERTENSIVE AGENTS.*

ADMINISTRATION/STORAGE

1. When transferring from another antiglaucoma agent, continue old medication on day 1 of timolol therapy (1 gtt of 0.25% solution). Then, discontinue former therapy. Initiate with 0.25% solution. Increase to 0.50% solution if response is insufficient. Further dosage increases are ineffective.
2. When transferring from several antiglaucoma agents, individualize the dose. If one of the agents is a beta-adrenergic blocking agent, discontinue it before starting timolol. Dosage adjustments should involve one drug at a time at 1-week intervals. Continue the antiglaucoma drugs with the addition of timolol, 1 gtt of 0.25% solution b.i.d. (if response is inadequate, 1 gtt of 0.5% solution may be used b.i.d.). The following day, discontinue one of the other antiglaucoma agents while continuing the remaining agents or discontinue based on client response.
3. Before using the gel, invert the closed container and shake once before each use.
4. Administer other ophthalmics at least 10 min before the gel.
5. The ocular hypotensive effect has been maintained when switching clients from timolol solution given b.i.d. to the gel once daily.

T

ASSESSMENT

1. Document indications for therapy, onset, duration, and characteristics of symptoms.
2. Monitor renal and LFTs.

CLIENT/FAMILY TEACHING

1. Review procedure for ophthalmic administration.
• Apply finger lightly to lacrimal sac for 1 min following administration.
• Regular intraocular measurements by an ophthalmologist are required because ocular hypertension may recur without any overt S&S.
2. When tablets used for long-term prophylaxis against MI, do not interrupt therapy; abrupt withdrawal may precipitate reinfarction.
3. Report any evidence of rash, dizziness, heart palpitations, SOB, edema, or depression.
4. Do not perform tasks such as driving or operating machinery until drug effects are realized; may cause dizziness.
5. May cause increased sensitivity to cold; dress appropriately.
6. With diabetes, monitor FS as drug may mask S&S of hypoglycemia.
7. Continue life-style modifications (i.e., weight reduction, regular exercise, reduced intake of sodium and alcohol, and no smoking) in the overall goal of BP control.

OUTCOMES/EVALUATE

• ↓ BP
• Myocardial reinfarction prophylaxis
• Migraine prophylaxis
• ↓ Intraocular pressures

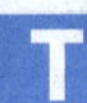

Tinzaparin sodium

(tin-**ZAH**-pah-rin)

PREGNANCY CATEGORY: B
CLASSIFICATION(S):
Anticoagulant, low molecular weight heparin
Rx: Innohep

SEE ALSO *HEPARIN, LOW MOLECULAR WEIGHT*

ACTION/KINETICS

Maximum plasma levels: 4–5 hr. **Maximum plasma levels:** 0.25–0.87 IU/mL within 4 to 5 hrs. after a single SC dose of 4,500 IU. Metabolized in the liver. **t½:** 3–4 hr. Excreted mainly in the urine. Clearance was reduced in impaired renal function.

USES

Treat acute symptomatic deep vein thrombosis (DVT) with or without pulmonary embolism when given with warfarin sodium.

ADDITIONAL CONTRAINDICATIONS

Use in those with a history of heparin-induced thrombocytopenia (HIT). Sensitivity to heparin, sulfites, benzyl alcohol, or pork products. Mixing with other injections or infusions.

SPECIAL CONCERNS

See also *Heparins, Low Molecular Weight.* Use with caution in pregnancy and only if clearly needed since benzyl alcohol in the product may cross the placenta and cause a fatal "gasping syndrome" in premature neonates. Use with caution during lactation. Safety and efficacy have not been determined in children.

SIDE EFFECTS

CV: Bleeding, ***hemorrhage,*** hypo/hypertension, tachycardia, angina pectoris, deep/deep leg thrombophlebitis, peripheral ischemia, hemoptysis, ocular hemorrhage, rectal bleeding. **Hematologic:** Thrombocytopenia, anemia, agranulocytosis, pancytopenia. **GI:** N&V, abdominal pain, diarrhea, constipation, flatulence, GI disorder, dyspepsia, cholestatic hepatitis. **CNS:** Headache, dizziness, insomnia, confusion. **GU:** Priapism, UTI, hematuria, urinary retention, dysuria. **Respiratory:** ***Pulmonary embolism,*** dyspnea, epistaxis, pneumonia, respiratory disorder. **Dermatologic:** Rash, erythematous rash, pruritus, bullous eruption, skin disorder, epidermal necrolysis, ischemic necrosis, urticaria. **At injection site:** Mild local irritation, pain, hematoma, ecchymosis, necrosis, abscess. *Hypersensitivity:* ***Anaphylaxis,*** angioedema. **Body as a whole:** Fever, impaired healing, infection. **Miscellaneous:** Back/chest pain, pain, rash, neonatal hypotonia.

ADDITIONAL DRUG INTERACTIONS

Anticoagulants, oral / ↑ Risk of bleeding

Dextran / ↑ Risk of bleeding
Thrombolytics / ↑ Risk of bleeding

HOW SUPPLIED

Injection: 20,000 anti-Factor Xa IU/mL

DOSAGE

• **SC**

Deep vein thrombosis.

175 anti-Xa IU/kg once daily for 6 days or until client is adequately anticoagulated with warfarin (INR at least 2.0 for two consecutive days). Initiate warfarin when appropriate (usually 1–3 days after tinzaparin initiation).

NURSING CONSIDERATIONS

SEE ALSO *NURSING CONSIDERATIONS FOR HEPARIN, LOW MOLECULAR WEIGHT*

ADMINISTRATION/STORAGE

1. To assure withdrawal of the correct volume, use an appropriately calibrated syringe.
2. Inspect visually before administration to ensure there is no particulate matter or discoloration of the vial contents.
3. Have client lying down or sitting and give by deep SC injection only. Alternate sites between the left and right anterolateral and left and right posterolateral abdominal wall. Vary the injection site daily.
4. Introduce the whole length of the needle into a skin fold held between the thumb and forefinger. Hold the skin fold throughout the injection.
5. To minimize bruising, do not rub the injection site after completion of the injection.
6. Store between 15–30°C (59–86°F).

ASSESSMENT

1. Assess for any active major bleeding, HIT, or any hypersensitivity to heparin sulfite, benzyl alcohol or pork products.
2. Use cautiously with history of recent GI ulcerations, diabetic retinopathy, hemorrhage, uncontrolled HTN, or bleeding diathesis.
3. Confirm PE by segmental lung scan defect and/or DVT by US. Start SC tinzaparin treatment x 6 days; add coumadin on day 2 and titrate to an INR of 2-3.
4. Weigh client; calculate dose for client weight (kg x 0.00875 mL/Kg = voulme in mL to be administered sc).
5. Monitor PT, INR, platelet count, CBC, renal function and FOB. May have to adjust for renal dysfunction.

CLIENT/FAMILY TEACHING

1. Review indications for therapy, self administration techniques, and importance of site rotation.
2. To minimize bruising do not rub site after administering and avoid OTC agents such as NSAIDS or aspirin.
3. Use caution to prevent injury; soft bristle tooth bush, electric razor to prevent bleeding.
4. Report any unusual bruising, bleeding, chest pain, acute SOB, itching, rash, or swelling. Keep f/u to evaluate blood tests.

OUTCOMES/EVALUATE

• Anticoagulation and prevention of complications due to clot formation
• Resolution of DVT

Tioconazole

(tie-oh-**KON**-ah-zohl)

PREGNANCY CATEGORY: C
CLASSIFICATION(S):
Antifungal
★Rx: Gynecure, Trosyd AF, Trosyd J
OTC: Monistat 1, Vagistat-1

ACTION/KINETICS

Antifungal activity thought to be due to alteration of the permeability of the cell membrane of the fungus, causing leakage of essential intracellular compounds. The systemic absorption of the drug in nonpregnant clients is negligible.

USES

Vulvovaginal candidiasis, including moniliasis and vaginal yeast infections.

CONTRAINDICATIONS

Use of a vaginal applicator during pregnancy may be contraindicated.

SPECIAL CONCERNS

Safety and effectiveness have not been determined during lactation or in children.

SIDE EFFECTS
GU: Burning, itching, irritation, vulvar edema and swelling, discharge, vaginal pain, dysuria, dyspareunia, nocturia, desquamation, dryness of vaginal secretions.

HOW SUPPLIED
Ointment: 6.5%

DOSAGE

- **VAGINAL OINTMENT, 6.5%**

Single dose of about 4.6 g (one applicator full) intravaginally at bedtime.

NURSING CONSIDERATIONS

ASSESSMENT

Obtain a thorough nursing history and carefully evaluate symptoms and sources of infection.

CLIENT/FAMILY TEACHING

1. Review appropriate method for administration (the cream should be inserted high into the vagina). Administer just prior to bedtime.
2. Report if burning, irritation, or pain occurs.
3. May stain clothes; use sanitary napkins during therapy.
4. To avoid reinfection, refrain from sexual intercourse. The ointment base may interact with rubber and latex; avoid condoms or diaphragms for 3 days following treatment.
5. Effectiveness is not altered by menstruation.
6. Symptomatic improvement is usually seen within 3 days and complete relief within 7 days.

OUTCOMES/EVALUATE

Resolution of fungal infection; symptomatic improvement

T

Tirofiban hydrochloride

(**ty**-roh-**FYE**-ban)

PREGNANCY CATEGORY: B
CLASSIFICATION(S):
Antiplatelet drug
Rx: Aggrastat

ACTION/KINETICS
Non–peptide antagonist of the platelet glycoprotein (GP) IIb/IIIa receptor, which is the major platelet surface receptor involved in platelet aggregation. Activation of the receptor leads to binding of fibrinogen and von Willebrand's factor to platelets, and thus aggregation. Tirofiban is a reversible antagonist of fibrinogen binding to the GP IIb/IIIa receptor, thus inhibiting platelet aggregation. **t½:** About 2 hr. Cleared from the plasma mainly unchanged by renal excretion (65%) and feces (25%). Plasma clearance is lower in clients over 65 years of age and is significantly decreased in those with a C_{CR} less than 30 mL/min.

USES
In combination with heparin for acute coronary syndrome (ACS), including those being treated medically and those undergoing PTCA or atherectomy.

CONTRAINDICATIONS
Active internal bleeding or history of diathesis within the previous 30 days; history of intracranial hemorrhage, intracranial neoplasm, AV malformation, or aneurysm; history of thrombocytopenia following prior use of tirofiban; history of stroke within 30 days or any history of hemorrhagic stroke; major surgical procedure or severe physical trauma within the last month; history, findings, or symptoms suggestive of aortic dissection; severe hypertension (systolic BP greater than 180 mm Hg or diastolic BP greater than 110 mm Hg); concomitant use of another parenteral GP IIb/IIIa inhibitor; acute pericarditis.

SPECIAL CONCERNS
Use with caution in clients with a platelet count less than 150,000/mm^3 in hemorrhagic retinopathy, with other drugs that affect hemostasis (e.g., warfarin). Safety and efficacy in children less than 18 years of age have not been established. Safety when used in combination with thrombolytic drugs has not been determined.

SIDE EFFECTS
Most common is bleeding, including intracranial bleeding, retroperitoneal bleeding, major GI and GU bleeding. Female and elderly clients have a higher incidence of bleeding than male or younger clients.

Miscellaneous: Nausea, fever, headache, bradycardia, coronary artery dissection, dizziness, edema or swelling, leg pain, pelvic pain, vasovagal reaction, sweating.

LABORATORY TEST CONSIDERATIONS

↓ H&H, platelets. ↑ Urine and fecal occult blood.

OD OVERDOSE MANAGEMENT

Symptoms: Bleeding, including minor mucocutaneous bleeding events and minor bleeding at the site of cardiac catheterization. *Treatment:* Assess clinical condition. Adjust or cease infusion, as appropriate. Can be removed by hemodialysis.

DRUG INTERACTIONS

Aspirin / ↑ Bleeding
H *Evening primrose oil* / Potential for ↑ antiplatelet effect
H *Feverfew* / Potential for ↑ antiplatelet effect
H *Garlic* / Potential for ↑ antiplatelet effect
H *Ginger* / Potential for ↑ antiplatelet effect
H *Ginkgo biloba* / Potential for ↑ antiplatelet effect
H *Ginseng* / Potential for ↑ antiplatelet effect
H *Grapeseed extract* / Potential for ↑ antiplatelet effect
Heparin / ↑ Bleeding
Levothyroxine / ↑ Tirofiban clearance
Omeprazole / ↑ Tirofiban clearance

HOW SUPPLIED

Injection: 50 mcg/mL; *Injection, Concentrate:* 250 mcg/mL

DOSAGE

• **IV**

Acute coronary syndrome.

Initial: 0.4 mcg/kg/min for 30 min; **then,** 0.1 mcg/kg/min. Use half the usual rate in those with severe renal impairment. Consult package insert for the guide to dosage adjustment by weight of the client.

NURSING CONSIDERATIONS

ADMINISTRATION/STORAGE

IV 1. May be given in the same IV line as heparin, dopamine, lidocaine, potassium chloride, and famotidine. Do not give in the same IV line as diazepam.

2. Tirofiban injection (250 mcg/mL) must be diluted to the same strength as tirofiban injection premixed (50 mcg/mL). One of three methods can be used to achieve a final concentration of 50 mcg/mL (mix well prior to use):

- Withdraw and discard 100 mL from a 500 mL bag of either sterile 0.9% NaCl or D5W; replace this volume with 100 mL of tirofiban injection (i.e., from two 50 mL vials).
- Withdraw and discard 50 mL from a 250 mL bag of either sterile 0.9% NaCl or D5W and replace this volume with 50 mL of tirofiban injection (i.e., from two-25 mL vials or one-50 mL vial).
- Add the contents of a 25 mL vial to a 100 mL bag of sterile 0.9% NaCl or D5W.

3. Tirofiban injection premix comes in 500 mL *Intravia* containers with 0.9% NaCl and tirofiban, 50 mcg/mL. To open the *Intravia* container, remove the dust cover. The plastic may be opaque due to moisture absorption during sterilization; the opacity will decrease gradually. Check for leaks by firmly squeezing the inner bag. Sterility may be suspected if leaks are found; discard the solution. Do not use unless the solution is clear and the seal is intact.

4. Do not add other drugs or remove tirofiban from the bag without a syringe.

5. Do not use plastic containers in series connections as an air embolism can result by drawing air from the first container if it is empty.

6. Store at 25°C (77°F); do not freeze and protect from light.

7. Discard any unused solution 24 hr after start of the infusion.

ASSESSMENT

1. Note indications for therapy, onset, and characteristics of symptoms.

2. Determine any history of intracranial hemorrhage or neoplasm, AV malformation, or aneurysm.

3. Monitor VS, H&H, platelets, PTT initially and 6 hr after loading infusions of tirofiban and heparin and daily; moni-

tor renal function studies and reduce dosage with dysfunction (C_{CR} < 30 mL/min).

CLIENT/FAMILY TEACHING

1. Drug is used IV with heparin to reduce death and symptoms associated with heart vessel blockage.
2. May experience bleeding so all sites will be carefully assessed and blood work evaluated frequently.
3. Encourage family to learn CPR.

OUTCOMES/EVALUATE

Inhibition of platelet aggregation with ↓ refractory ischemia, MI, and death

Tizanidine hydrochloride

(tye-**ZAN**-ih-deen)

PREGNANCY CATEGORY: C
CLASSIFICATION(S):
Skeletal muscle relaxant, centrally-acting
Rx: Zanaflex

SEE ALSO ***SKELETAL MUSCLE RELAXANTS, CENTRALLY ACTING.***

ACTION/KINETICS

Acts on central α-2 adrenergic receptors; reduces spasticity by increasing presynaptic inhibition of motor neurons possibly by reducing release of excitatory amino acids. Greatest effects are on polysynaptic pathways. Also may reduce postsynaptic excitatory transmitter activity, decrease the firing rate of noradrenergic locus ceruleas neurons, and inhibit synaptic transmission of nociceptive stimuli in the spinal pathways. **Peak effect:** 1–2 hr. **Duration:** 3–6 hr. Extensive first pass metabolism. **t½:** About 2.5 hr. Excreted in urine and feces. Elderly clear drug more slowly.

USES

Acute and intermittent management of muscle spasticity.

CONTRAINDICATIONS

Use with α-2-adrenergic agonists.

SPECIAL CONCERNS

Use with caution in renal impairment, in elderly and during laction. Use with extreme caution in hepatic insufficiency. Safety and efficacy have not been determined in children.

SIDE EFFECTS

Note: Side effects listed are those with a frequency of 0.1% or greater.
CV: Hypotension, vasodilation, postural hypotension, syncope, migraine, arrhythmia. **GI:** Hepatotoxicity, dry mouth, constipation, pharyngitis, vomiting, abdominal pain, diarrhea, dyspepsia, dysphagia, cholelithiasis, fecal impaction, flatulence, ***GI hemorrhage*** hepatitis, melena. **CNS:** Dizziness, dyskinesia, nervousness, somnolence, sedation, hallucinations, psychotic-like symptoms, depression, anxiety, paresthesia, tremor, emotional lability, seizures, paralysis, abnormal thinking, vertigo, abnormal dreams, agitation, depersonalization, euphoria, stupor, dysautonomia, neuralgia. **GU:** Urinary frequency, UTI, urinary urgency, cystitis, menorrhagia, pyelonephritis, urinary retention, kidney calculus, enlarged uterine fibroids, vaginal moniliasis, vaginitis. **Hematologic:** Ecchymosis, anemia, leukopenia, leukocytosis. **Musculoskeletal:** Myasthenia, back pain, pathological fracture, arthralgia, arthritis, bursitis. **Respiratory:** Sinusitis, pneumonia, bronchitis, rhinitis. **Dermatologic:** Rash, sweating, skin ulcer, pruritus, dry skin, acne, alopecia, urticaria. **Body as a whole:** Flu syndrome, weight loss, infection, ***sepsis, cellulitis, death,*** allergic reaction, moniliasis, malaise, asthenia, fever, abscess, edema. **Ophthalmic:** Glaucoma, amblyopia, conjunctivitis, eye pain, optic neuritis, retinal hemorrhage, visual field defect. **Otic:** Ear pain, tinnitus, deafness, otitis media. **Miscellaneous:** Speech disorder.

LABORATORY TEST CONSIDERATIONS

↑ ALT. Abnormal LFTs. Hypercholesterolemia, hyperlipemia, hypothyroidism, adrenal cortical insufficiency, hyperglycemia, hypokalemia, hyponatremia, hypoproteinemia.

DRUG INTERACTIONS

Alcohol / ↑ Tizanidine side effects; additive CNS depressant effects
Alpha-2-adrenergic agonists / Additive hypotension

Oral contraceptives / ↓ Tizanidine clearance

HOW SUPPLIED

Tablets: 2 mg, 4 mg

DOSAGE

• **TABLETS**

Muscle spasticity.

Initial: 4 mg; **then,** increase dose gradually in 2 to 4 mg steps to optimum effect. Dose can be repeated at 6–8-hr intervals, to maximum of 3 doses/24 hr, not to exceed 36 mg/day. There is no experience with repeated, single, daytime doses greater than 12 mg or total daily doses of 36 mg or more.

NURSING CONSIDERATIONS

SEE ALSO *NURSING CONSIDERATIONS* FOR *SKELETAL MUSCLE RELAXANTS, CENTRALLY ACTING.*

ASSESSMENT

Note indications for therapy, onset and characteristics of symptoms. Monitor ROM, pain level, erythema, swelling, VS, liver, and renal function studies.

CLIENT/FAMILY TEACHING

1. Do not perform activities that require mental alertness; drug causes sedation.
2. Report if hallucinations or delusions experienced.
3. May cause orthostatic hypotension; avoid sudden changes in position.
4. Avoid alcohol and any other CNS depressants.
5. Report loss of effect, ↓ ROM, or worsening of symptoms.

OUTCOMES/EVALUATE

↓ Spasticity; ↑ muscle relaxation

Tobramycin sulfate

(toe-brah-**MY**-sin)

PREGNANCY CATEGORY: D (B FOR OPHTHALMIC USE)
CLASSIFICATION(S):
Antibiotic, aminoglycoside

Rx: Inhalation: TOBI. **Ophthalmic:** AKTob Ophthalmic Solution, Defy Ophthalmic Solution, Tobrex Ophthalmic Ointment, Tobrex Ophthalmic Solution,. **Parenteral:** Nebcin, Nebcin Pediatric

✱Rx: PMS-Tobramycin, Tomycine

SEE ALSO *AMINOGLYCOSIDES.*

ACTION/KINETICS

Similar to gentamicin and can be used concurrently with carbenicillin. **Therapeutic serum levels: IM,** 4–8 mcg/mL. **t½:** 2–2.5 hr. **Toxic serum levels:** > 12 mcg/mL (peak) and > 2 mcg/mL (trough).

USES

Systemic: (1) Complicated and recurrent UTIs due to *Pseudomonas aeruginosa, Proteus, Escherichia coli, Klebsiella, Enterobacter, Serratia, Staphylococcus aureus, Citrobacter,* and *Providencia.* (2) Lower respiratory tract infections due to *P. aeruginosa, Klebsiella, Enterobacter, E. coli, Serratia,* and *S. aureus* (penicillinase– and non–penicillinase producing). (3) Intra-abdominal infections (including peritonitis) due to *E. coli, Klebsiella,* and *Enterobacter.* (4) Septicemia in neonates, children, and adults due to *P. aeruginosa, E. coli,* and *Klebsiella.* (5) Skin, bone, and skin structure infections due to *P. aeruginosa, Proteus, E. coli, Klebsiella, Enterobacter,* and *S. aureus.* (6) Serious CNS infections, including meningitis. Can be used with penicillins or cephalosporins in serious infections when results of susceptibility testing are not yet known.

Ophthalmic: Treat superficial ocular infections due to Staphylococcus, *S. aureus, Streptococcus, S. pneumoniae,* beta-hemolytic streptococci, *Corynebacterium, E. coli, Haemophilus aegyptius, H. ducreyi, H. influenzae, H. parainfluenzae, Klebsiella pneumoniae, Neisseria, N. gonorrhoeae, Proteus, Acinetobacter calcoaceticus, Enterobacter, Enterobacter aerogenes, Serratia marcescens, Moraxella, Pseudomonas aeruginosa,* and *Vibrio.*

Inhalation: Management of lung infections *(P. aeruginosa)* in cystic fibrosis clients.

CONTRAINDICATIONS
Ophthalmically to treat dendritic keratitis, vaccinia, varicella, fungal or mycobacterial eye infections, after removal of a corneal foreign body. Lactation.

SPECIAL CONCERNS
Use with caution in premature infants and neonates. Ophthalmic ointment may retard corneal epithelial healing.

ADDITIONAL SIDE EFFECTS
Ophthalmic use: Transient irritation, burning, stinging, itching, inflammation, angioneurotic edema, urticaria, vesicular and maculopapular dermatitis.

OD OVERDOSE MANAGEMENT
Symptoms (Ophthalmic Use): Edema, lid itching, punctate keratitis, erythema, lacrimation.

ADDITIONAL DRUG INTERACTIONS
Carbenicillin or ticarcillin: ↑ Tobramycin effect when used for *Pseudomonas* infections.

HOW SUPPLIED
Inhalation Solution: 60 mg/mL; *Injection:* 10 mg/mL, 40 mg/mL; *Powder for injection:*1.2 g; *Ophthalmic Ointment:* 0.3%; *Ophthalmic Solution:* 0.3%

DOSAGE

• **IM, IV**

Non-life-threatening serious infections.

Adults: 3 mg/kg/day in three equally divided doses q 8 hr.

Life-threatening infections.

Up to 5 mg/kg/day in three or four equal doses. **Pediatric:** Either 2–2.5 mg/kg q 8 hr or 1.5–1.9 mg/kg q 6 hr; **neonates 1 week of age or less:** up to 4 mg/kg/day in two equal doses q 12 hr.

Impaired renal function.

Initially: 1 mg/kg; **then,** maintenance dose calculated according to information supplied by manufacturer.

• **OPHTHALMIC OINTMENT (0.3%)**

Acute infections.

0.5-in. ribbon q 3–4 hr until improvement is noted.

Mild to moderate infections.

0.5-in. ribbon b.i.d.–t.i.d.

• **OPHTHALMIC SOLUTION (0.3%)**

Acute infections.

Initial: 1–2 gtt q 15–30 min until improvement noted; **then,** reduce dosage gradually.

Moderate infections.

1–2 gtt 2–6 times/day.

• **INHALATION SOLUTION**

Pseudomonas aeruginosa in cystic fibrosis.

Dose using a nebulizer b.i.d. for 10–15 min in cycles of 28 days on and then 28 days off. See package insert for detailed instructions for administration.

NURSING CONSIDERATIONS

SEE ALSO NURSING CONSIDERATIONS FOR AMINOGLYCOSIDES.

ADMINISTRATION/STORAGE

1. Use the inhalation solution as close as possible to q 12 hr, but not less than q 6 hr.
2. Do not mix TOBI with dornase alfa in the nebulizer.
3. IV Prepare IV solution by diluting drug with 50–100 mL of dextrose or saline solution; infuse over 30–60 min.
4. Use proportionately less diluent for children than for adults.
5. Do not mix with other drugs for parenteral administration.
6. Discard solution of drug containing up to 1 mg/mL after 24 hr at room temperature.
7. Store drug at room temperature no longer than 2 years.

CLIENT/FAMILY TEACHING

1. Drink plenty of fluids (2–3 L/day) during parenteral drug therapy.
2. With eye infections, avoid wearing contact lenses until infection is cleared and provider approves.
3. With inhalation therapy the time frame is usually a month of therapy and then a month off. Follow guidelines for proper equipment cleaning and care.
4. Report if symptoms do not improve or if they worsen after several days of therapy.

OUTCOMES/EVALUATE

• Negative cultures; resolution of infection

• Therapeutic drug levels (peak: 4–10 mcg/mL; trough: 1–2 mcg/mL)

T

Tocainide hydrochloride

(toe-**KAY**-nyd)

PREGNANCY CATEGORY: C
CLASSIFICATION(S):
Antiarrhythmic, Class IB
Rx: Tonocard

SEE ALSO *ANTIARRHYTHMIC AGENTS.*

ACTION/KINETICS

Similar to lidocaine. Decreases the excitability of cells in the myocardium by decreasing sodium and potassium conductance. Increases pulmonary and aortic arterial pressure and slightly increases peripheral resistance. Effective in both digitalized and nondigitalized clients. **Peak plasma levels:** 0.5–2 hr. **t½:** 11–15 hr. **Therapeutic serum levels:** 4–10 mcg/mL. **Duration:** 8 hr. Approximately 10% is bound to plasma protein. From 28% to 55% is excreted unchanged in the urine. Alkalinization decreases the excretion of the drug although acidification does not produce any changes in excretion.

USES

Life-threatening ventricular arrhythmias, including ventricular tachycardia. Has not been shown to improve survival in clients with ventricular arrhythmias. *Investigational:* Myotonic dystrophy, trigeminal neuralgia.

CONTRAINDICATIONS

Allergy to amide-type local anesthetics, second- or third-degree AV block in the absence of artificial ventricular pacemaker. Lactation.

SPECIAL CONCERNS

Increased risk of death when used in those with non-life-threatening cardiac arrhythmias. Safety and efficacy have not been established in children. Use with caution in clients with impaired renal or hepatic function (dose may have to be decreased). Geriatric clients may have an increased risk of dizziness and hypotension; the dose may have to be reduced in these clients due to age-related impaired renal function.

SIDE EFFECTS

CV: ***Increased arrhythmias,*** increased ventricular rate (when given for atrial flutter or fibrillation), CHF, tachycardia, hypotension, ***conduction disturbances,*** bradycardia, chest pain, LV failure, palpitations. **CNS:** Dizziness, vertigo, headache, tremors, confusion, disorientation, hallucinations, ataxia, paresthesias, numbness, nervousness, altered mood, anxiety, incoordination, walking disturbances. **GI:** N&V, anorexia, diarrhea. **Respiratory:** ***Pulmonary fibrosis, fibrosing alveolitis,*** interstitial pneumonitis, ***pulmonary edema,*** pneumonia. **Hematologic:** Leukopenia, ***agranulocytosis,*** hypoplastic anemia, ***aplastic anemia,*** bone marrow depression, neutropenia, ***thrombocytopenia and sequelae as septicemia and septic shock.*** **Musculoskeletal:** Arthritis, arthralgia, myalgia. **Dermatologic:** Rash, skin lesion, diaphoresis. **Other:** Blurred vision, visual disturbances, nystagmus, tinnitus, hearing loss, lupus-like syndrome.

LABORATORY TEST CONSIDERATIONS

Abnormal LFTs (esp. in early therapy). ↑ ANA.

OD OVERDOSE MANAGEMENT

Symptoms: Initially are CNS symptoms including tremor (see above). GI symptoms may follow (see above). *Treatment:* Gastric lavage and activated charcoal may be useful. In the event of respiratory depression or arrest or seizures, maintain airway and provide artificial ventilation. An IV anticonvulsant (e.g., diazepam, thiopental, thiamylal, pentobarbital, secobarbital) may be required if seizures are persistent.

DRUG INTERACTIONS

Cimetidine / ↓ Tocainide bioavailability
Metoprolol / Additive effects on wedge pressure and cardiac index
Rifampin / ↓ Tocainide bioavailability

HOW SUPPLIED

Tablet: 400 mg, 600 mg

DOSAGE

• **TABLETS**

Antiarrhythmic.

Adults, individualized, initial: 400 mg q 8 hr, up to a maximum of 2,400 mg/day; **maintenance:** 1,200–1,800 mg/day in divided doses. Total daily dose of 1,200 mg may be adequate in clients with liver or kidney disease.

Myotonic dystrophy.

800–1,200 mg/day.

Trigeminal neuralgia.

20 mg/kg/day in three divided doses.

NURSING CONSIDERATIONS

SEE ALSO *NURSING CONSIDERATIONS* FOR *ANTIARRHYTHMIC AGENTS.*

ASSESSMENT

1. Document indications for therapy, type, onset, and characteristics of symptoms.
2. Monitor ECG, CBC, electrolytes, liver and renal function studies; correct potassium deficits.
3. Document cardiac and pulmonary assessment findings.

CLIENT/FAMILY TEACHING

1. Take in the morning with food to minimize GI upset.
2. Do not drive or operate machinery until drug effects are realized; may cause drowsiness or dizziness.
3. Report any abnormal bruising, bleeding, fever, sore throat, or chills (S&S of blood dyscrasia).
4. Avoid alcohol during therapy.
5. Pulmonary symptoms such as wheezing, coughing, or dyspnea should be reported immediately; may indicate pulmonary fibrosis.

OUTCOMES/EVALUATE

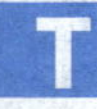

• Control of lethal ventricular arrhythmias
• ↓ Muscle spasm and pain
• Therapeutic drug levels (4–10 mcg/mL)

Tolazamide

(toll-**AZ**-ah-myd)

PREGNANCY CATEGORY: C

CLASSIFICATION(S):

Antidiabetic, oral; first generation sulfonylurea

Rx: Tolinase

SEE ALSO *ANTIDIABETIC AGENTS: HYPOGLYCEMIC AGENTS.*

ACTION/KINETICS

Effective in some with a history of coma or ketoacidosis; may be effective in clients who do not respond well to other oral antidiabetics. Use with insulin is not recommended for maintenance. Absorbed more slowly than other sulfonylureas. **Onset:** 4–6 hr. **t½:** 7 hr. **Time to peak levels:** 3–4 hr. **Duration:** 12–24 hr. Metabolized in liver to metabolites with minor hypoglycemic activity. Excreted through the kidneys.

ADDITIONAL CONTRAINDICATIONS

Renal glycosuria.

ADDITIONAL DRUG INTERACTIONS

Concomitant use of alcohol and tolazamide may → photosensitivity.

HOW SUPPLIED

Tablet: 100 mg, 250 mg, 500 mg

DOSAGE

• **TABLETS**

Diabetes.

Adults, initial: 100 mg/day if fasting blood sugar is less than 200 mg/100 mL, or 250 mg/day if fasting blood sugar is greater than 200 mg/100 mL. Adjust dose to response, not to exceed 1 g/day; adjust dosage in increments of 100–250 mg at weekly intervals based on client response. If more than 500 mg/day is required, give in two divided doses, usually before the morning and evening meals. **Maintenance, average:** 250–500 mg/day. **Elderly, malnourished, underweight clients or those not eating properly:** 100 mg once daily with breakfast, adjusting dose by increments of 50 mg/day each week. Doses greater than 1 g/day will probably not improve control.

NURSING CONSIDERATIONS

SEE ALSO *NURSING CONSIDERATIONS* FOR *ANTIDIABETIC AGENTS: HYPOGLYCEMIC AGENTS.*

ADMINISTRATION/STORAGE

Use the following guidelines when transferring type 2 diabetics on insulin to tolazamide monotherapy:

- If the insulin dose is less than 20 units, initially give tolazamide, 100 mg/day. Insulin may be discontinued abruptly.
- If the insulin dose is 20–40 units, initially give tolazamide, 250 mg/day. Insulin may be discontinued abruptly.
- If the insulin dose is more than 40 units, initially give tolazamide, 250 mg/day. Reduce insulin dose by 50%; further reduce as response occurs. Consider hospitalization.

CLIENT/FAMILY TEACHING

1. Take in the am with or before meals; do not take if vomiting or unable to eat.
2. Monitor fingersticks and maintain a record (different times on different days) for provider review.
3. Avoid alcohol as a disulfiram-like reaction may occur.
4. Use caution; may cause dizziness.
5. Use nonhormonal contraception.
6. Wear protective clothing and a sunscreen to prevent a photosensitivity reaction.
7. Continue diet, exercise, and weight loss in the overall management of diabetes.

OUTCOMES/EVALUATE

Serum glucose/HbA1 C levels within desired range

Tolbutamide

(toll-**BYOU**-tah-myd)

PREGNANCY CATEGORY: C
Rx: Orinase
Rx: Apo-Tolbutamide

Tolbutamide sodium

(toll-**BYOU**-tah-myd)

PREGNANCY CATEGORY: C
Rx: Orinase Diagnostic
CLASSIFICATION(S):
Antidiabetic, oral; first generation sulfonylurea

SEE ALSO *ANTIDIABETIC AGENTS: HYPOGLYCEMIC AGENTS.*

ACTION/KINETICS

Onset: 1 hr. **t½:** 4.5–6.5 hr. **Time to peak levels:** 3–4 hr. **Duration:** 6–12 hr. Changed in liver to inactive metabolites. Excreted through the kidneys.

ADDITIONAL USES

Most useful for clients with poor general physical status who should receive a short-acting compound.

Tolbutamide sodium is used to diagnose pancreatic islet cell tumors. It causes blood glucose, in the presence of a tumor, to drop quickly after IV administration and remain low for 3 hr.

ADDITIONAL SIDE EFFECTS

Melena (dark, bloody stools) in some clients with a history of peptic ulcer. Relapse or secondary failure may occur a few months after therapy has been started. May cause hyponatremia and a mild goiter.

ADDITIONAL DRUG INTERACTIONS

Alcohol / Photosensitivity reactions
Fluvoxamine / ↓ Tolbutamide clearance
Sulfinpyrazone / ↑ Effect of tolbutamide due to ↓ breakdown by liver

HOW SUPPLIED

Tolbutamide: *Tablet:* 500 mg; **Tolbutamide sodium:** *Powder for injection:* 1 g/vial

DOSAGE

- **TABLETS**

Diabetes mellitus.

Adults, initial: 1–2 g/day. Adjust dosage depending on response, up to 3 g/day. **Usual maintenance:** 0.25–3 g/day. A daily dose greater than 2 g is seldom required.

NURSING CONSIDERATIONS

SEE ALSO *NURSING CONSIDERATIONS* FOR *ANTIDIABETIC AGENTS: HYPOGLYCEMIC AGENTS.*

ADMINISTRATION/STORAGE

1. Transfer from other oral antidiabetic drugs to tolbutamide conservatively. When transferring from chlorpropamide, take special care the first 2 weeks due to the long duration of action of chlorpropamide.

T

2. Use the following guidelines when transferring type 2 diabetics on insulin to tolbutamide monotherapy:
• If the insulin dose is less than 20 units, initially give tolbutamide, 1–2 g/day. Insulin may be discontinued abruptly.
• If the insulin dose is 20–40 units, initially give tolbutamide, 1–2 g/day. Reduce insulin by 30–50%; further reduce based on response.
• If the insulin dose is more than 40 units, initially give tolbutamide, 1–2 g/day. Reduce insulin dose by 20%; further reduce as response occurs. Consider hospitalization.

CLIENT/FAMILY TEACHING

1. Take 30 min before meals for best results. May take as a single dose before breakfast or as divided doses before the morning and evening meals. Divided doses may improve GI tolerance.
2. Maintain log of fingersticks for provider review.
3. Drug may cause dizziness, use caution.
4. Avoid alcohol and any OTC meds without approval.
5. May cause a photosensitivity reaction; wear protective clothing and sunscreen when exposed.
6. Use a nonhormonal form of birth control.
7. Continue diet, exercise, and weight loss in the overall management of diabetes.

OUTCOMES/EVALUATE

• Serum glucose/HbA1-C levels within desired range
• Pancreatic islet cell tumor presence

T

Tolcapone

(**TOHL**-kah-pohn)

PREGNANCY CATEGORY: C
CLASSIFICATION(S):
Antiparkinson drug
Rx: Tasmar

ACTION/KINETICS

Reversible inhibitor of catechol-O-methyltransferase (COMT), resulting in an increase in plasma levodopa. When given with levodopa/carbidopa, plasma levels of levodopa are more sustained, allowing for more constant dopaminergic stimulation of the brain. May also increase side effects of levodopa. Rapidly absorbed from the GI tract; **peak levels:** 2 hr. Food given within 1 hr before or 2 hr after PO use decreases bioavailability by 10%–20%. Over 99.9% bound to plasma protein. **t½, elimination:** 2–3 hr. Almost completely metabolized in the liver; excreted in the urine (60%) and feces (40%).

USES

Adjunct to levodopa and carbidopa for the treatment of idiopathic Parkinson's disease. Reserved for clients taking levodopa-carbidopa who have symptom fluctuations and are not responding to or candidates for other therapies.

CONTRAINDICATIONS

Use with a nonselective MAO inhibitor. In clients with liver disease, history of nontraumatic rhabdomyolysis or hyperpyrexia, confusion possibly related to the drug, and in those withdrawn from tolocapone due to hepatocellular injury.

SPECIAL CONCERNS

Use with caution in severe renal or hepatic impairment and during lactation.

SIDE EFFECTS

GI: N&V, anorexia, diarrhea, constipation, xerostomia, abdominal pain, dyspepsia, flatulence, ***acute fulminant liver failure***. **CNS:** Hallucinations, dyskinesias, sleep disorder, dystonia, excessive dreaming, somnolence, confusion, dizziness, headache, syncope, loss of balance, hyperkinesia, paresthesia, hypokinesia, agitation, irritability, mental deficiency, hyperactivity, panic reaction, euphoria, hypertonia. **CV:** Orthostatic hypotension, chest pain, hypotension, chest discomfort. **Respiratory:** URTI, dyspnea, sinus congestion. **Musculoskeletal:** Muscle cramps, stiffness, arthritis, neck pain. **GU:** Hematuria, UTIs, urine discoloration, micturition disorder, uterine tumor. **Dermatologic:** Increased sweating, dermal bleeding, skin tumor, alopecia. **Ophthalmic:**

Cataract, eye inflammation. **Body as a whole:** Falling, fatigue, influenza, burning, malaise, fever, rhabdomyolysis.

NOTE: Clients over 75 years of age may develop more hallucinations but less dystonia. Females may develop somnolence more frequently than males.

LABORATORY TEST CONSIDERATIONS

↑AST, ALT.

OD OVERDOSE MANAGEMENT

Symptoms: Nausea, vomiting, dizziness, possibility of respiratory difficulties. *Treatment:* Hospitalization is advised. Give supportive care.

HOW SUPPLIED

Tablets: 100 mg, 200 mg

DOSAGE

- **TABLETS**

Adjunct for Parkinsonism.

Initial: 100 t.i.d. with or without food. Use 200 mg t.i.d. only if anticiapted benefit is justified. Do not increase the dose to 200 mg t.i.d. in those with moderate to severe liver cirrhosis.

NURSING CONSIDERATIONS

ADMINISTRATION/STORAGE

1. Even though 200 mg t.i.d. is reasonably well tolerated, the prescriber may start with 100 mg t.i.d. due to the potential for increased dopaminergic side effects and the possibility of adjustment of the concomitant levodopa/carbidopa dose.
2. A suggested dosing regimen is to give the first dose of tolcapone of the day with the first dose of levodopa/carbidopa; subsequent doses of tolcapone can be given 6 to 12 hr later.
3. Reductions in the daily dose of levodopa may be required.
4. Tolcapone can be used with either the immediate or sustained–release formulations of levodopa/carbidopa.

ASSESSMENT

1. Document indications for therapy, characteristics/duration of symptoms, and other agents trialed.
2. List drugs currently prescribed to ensure none interact unfavorably.
3. May cause severe hepatotoxicity. Do not use with clinical evidence of liver disease or if ALT or AST 2x ULN. When used, monitor LFTs q 2 weeks for the first year of therapy, then q 4 weeks for the next six months and then q 8 weeks for the remainer of use. Stop drug with any evidence of liver dysfunction.

CLIENT/FAMILY TEACHING

1. Take as directed with your levodopa/carbidopa. Drug increases the action of levodopa by decreasing its metabolism in the peripheral tissues. If taken without levodopa there is no treatment benefit.
2. Do not drive or perform activities requiring mental alertness until drug effects realized; may cause sedation.
3. Stop drug and report any evidence of liver dysfunction: fatigue, loss of appetite, yellow skin discoloration, or clay colored stools.
4. Rise slowly from a sitting or lying position to prevent orthostatic effects.
5. May experience nausea initially and an increase in involuntary repetitive movements; these should subside. Six weeks into therapy may experience diarrhea; report if persistent or severe.
6. May discolor urine bright yellow.
7. Practice reliable birth control; do not nurse.
8. Report any unusual symptoms or side effects; labs will be required frequently during the first year of therapy to protect from liver toxicity.

OUTCOMES/EVALUATE

Control of S&S Parkinson's disease

Tolmetin sodium

(**TOLL**-met-in)

PREGNANCY CATEGORY: C
CLASSIFICATION(S):

Nonsteroidal anti-inflammatory drug

Rx: Tolectin 200, Tolectin 600, Tolectin DS

✱**Rx:** Novo-Tolmetin, Tolectin

SEE ALSO *NONSTEROIDAL ANTI-INFLAMMATORY DRUGS.*

ACTION/KINETICS
Peak plasma levels: 30–60 min. **t½:** 2–7 hr. **Therapeutic plasma levels:** 40 mcg/mL. Over 93% plasma-protein bound. **Onset, anti-inflammatory effect:** within 1 week; **duration, anti-inflammatory effect:** 1–2 weeks. Inactivated in liver and excreted in urine.

USES
Acute and chronic treatment of rheumatoid arthritis and osteoarthritis. Juvenile rheumatoid arthritis. *Investigational:* Sunburn.

SPECIAL CONCERNS
Use with caution during lactation. Dosage has not been determined in children less than 2 years of age.

LABORATORY TEST CONSIDERATIONS
Tolmetin metabolites give a false + test for proteinuria using sulfosalicylic acid.

HOW SUPPLIED
Capsule: 400 mg; *Tablet:* 200 mg, 600 mg

DOSAGE

- **CAPSULES, TABLETS**

Rheumatoid arthritis, osteoarthritis.

Adults: 400 mg t.i.d. (one dose on arising and one at bedtime); adjust dosage according to client response. **Maintenance:** *rheumatoid arthritis,* 600–1,800 mg/day in three to four divided doses; *osteoarthritis,* 600–1,600 mg/day in three to four divided doses. Doses larger than 1,800 mg/day for rheumatoid arthritis and osteoarthritis are not recommended.

Juvenile rheumatoid arthritis.

2 years and older, initial: 20 mg/kg/day in three to four divided doses to start; **then,** 15–30 mg/kg/day. Doses higher than 30 mg/kg/day are not recommended. Beneficial effects may not be observed for several days to a week.

NURSING CONSIDERATIONS

SEE ALSO *NURSING CONSIDERATIONS* FOR *NONSTEROIDAL ANTI-INFLAMMATORY DRUGS.*

ASSESSMENT

1. Document indications for therapy; note joint pain and pain level, deformity, swelling, inflammation, and ROM.
2. Monitor CBC and renal function studies.

CLIENT/FAMILY TEACHING

1. Doses should be spaced so that one dose is taken in the morning on arising, one during the day, and one at bedtime. The dosage is based on the treatment condtition and varies according to indications. Take as directed.
2. May administer with meals, milk, a full glass of water, or antacids if gastric irritation occurs. Never administer with sodium bicarbonate. The elderly are particularly susceptible to gastric irritation and should take with milk, meals, an antacid or stomach protectant if prescribed.
3. Assess response; drug may cause drowsiness or dizziness.
4. Report any unusual bruising or bleeding, weight gain, edema, fever, blood in urine or increased joint pain.
5. It may take several weeks before effects are evident.
6. Avoid alcohol and any OTC meds without approval.
7. Report for labs to evaluate renal function and hematologic parameters.

OUTCOMES/EVALUATE
↓Joint pain and inflammation; ↑mobility

Tolnaftate

(toll-**NAF**-tayt)

CLASSIFICATION(S):
Antifungal

OTC: Absorbine Athlete's Foot Cream, Absorbine Footcare, Aftate for Athlete's Foot, Aftate for Jock Itch, Genaspor, Quinsana Plus, Tinactin, Tinactin for Jock Itch, Ting
✱OTC: Pitrex, ZeaSorb AF

SEE ALSO *ANTI-INFECTIVES.*

ACTION/KINETICS
Exact mechanism not known; is thought to stunt mycelial growth causing a fungicidal effect.

T

USES

(1) Tinea pedis, tinea cruris, tinea corporis, and tinea versicolor. (2) Fungal infections of moist skin areas.

CONTRAINDICATIONS

Scalp and nail infections. Avoid getting into eyes. Use in children less than 2 years of age.

SIDE EFFECTS

Mild skin irritation.

HOW SUPPLIED

Cream: 1%; *Gel:* 1%; *Powder:* 1%; Spray *Powder:* 1%; *Solution:* 1%; *Spray Liquid:* 1%

DOSAGE

• **TOPICAL: CREAM, GEL, POWDER, SPARY POWDER, SOLUTION, SPRAY LIQUID**

Apply b.i.d. for 2–3 weeks although treatment for 4–6 weeks may be necessary in some instances.

NURSING CONSIDERATIONS

SEE ALSO *GENERAL NURSING CONSIDERATIONS* FOR *ALL ANTI-INFECTIVES*.

ASSESSMENT

1. Inspect source of infection; document presentation because the choice of vehicle is important for effective therapy.

• Powders are used in mild conditions as adjunctive therapy.

• For primary therapy and prophylaxis, creams, liquids, or ointments are used, especially if the area is moist.

• Liquids and solutions are used if the area is hairy.

2. Assess cultures; use concomitant therapy if bacterial or *Candida* infections are also present.

CLIENT/FAMILY TEACHING

1. Skin should be thoroughly cleaned and dried before applying.

2. Use care; do not rub medication into or near the eye.

3. Report any bothersome side effects; local relief of symptoms should be evident within the first 24–48 hr. Report if no improvement noted within 10 days.

4. Continue to use as directed, despite improvement of symptoms. Takes 2–6 weeks to clear infection.

OUTCOMES/EVALUATE

• Symptomatic relief; skin healing

• Eradication of fungal infection

Tolterodine tartrate

(tohl-**TER**-oh-deen)

PREGNANCY CATEGORY: C

CLASSIFICATION(S):

Urinary tract drug

Rx: Detrol, Detrol LA

ACTION/KINETICS

Acts as a competitive muscarinic receptor antagonist in the bladder to cause increased bladder control. Metabolized by first pass effect in the liver to the active 5–hydroxymethyl derivative, which has similar activity as tolterodine. Rapidly absorbed with peak serum levels within 1–2 hr. Food increases bioavialability. Highly bound to plasma proteins. Excreted in the urine.

USES

Treat overactive bladder with symptoms of urinary frequency, urgency, or urge incontinence.

CONTRAINDICATIONS

Urinary retention, gastric retention, uncontrolled narrow–angle glaucoma, lactation.

SPECIAL CONCERNS

Use with caution in renal impairment, in bladder outflow obstruction, in GI obstructive disorders (e.g., pyloric stenosis), and in those being treated for narrow–angle glaucoma. Doses greater than 1 mg b.i.d. not to be given to those with significantly decreased hepatic function. Safety and efficacy have not been determined in children.

SIDE EFFECTS

GI: Dry mouth (common), dyspepsia, constipation, abdominal pain, N&V, diarrhea, flatulence. **CNS:** Headache, vertigo, dizziness, somnolence, paresthesia, nervousness. **Respiratory:** URI, bronchitis, coughing, pharyngitis, rhinitis, sinusitis. **Dermatologic:** Rash, erythema, dry skin, pruritus. **GU:** UTI, dysuria, micturition frequency, urinary retention. **Ophthalmic:** Abnormalities with vision, including accommodation. **Musculoskeletal:** Arthralgia, back pain, chest pain. **Miscellaneous:** Fatigue, flu–like symptoms, infection, hypertension, weight gain, fall, fungal infection.

OD OVERDOSE MANAGEMENT

Symptoms: Significant anticholinergic symptoms. *Treatment:* Symptomatic. Monitor ECG.

DRUG INTERACTIONS

Clarithromycin / ↑ Tolterodine plasma levels R/T ↓ liver metabolism; do not give tolterodine >1 mg b.i.d.
Cyclosporine / ↑ Tolterodine plasma levels R/T ↓ liver metabolism; do not give tolterodine >1 mg b.i.d.
Erythromycin / ↑ Tolterodine plasma levels R/T ↓ liver metabolism; do not give tolterodine >1 mg b.i.d.
Fluoxetine / ↓ Tolterodine metabolism in EM1, EM2, and poor metabolizers
Itraconazole / ↑ Tolterodine plasma levels R/T ↓ liver metabolism; do not give tolterodine >1 mg b.i.d.
Ketoconazole / ↑ Tolterodine plasma levels R/T ↓ liver metabolism; do not give tolterodine >1 mg b.i.d.
Miconazole / ↑ Tolterodine plasma levels R/T ↓ liver metabolism; do not give tolterodine >1 mg b.i.d.
Vinblastine / ↑ Tolterodine plasma levels R/T ↓ liver metabolism; do not give tolterodine >1 mg b.i.d.
Warfarin / Prolonged INR values → possible bleeding

HOW SUPPLIED

Capsules, Extended Release: 2 mg, 4 mg; *Tablets:* 1 mg, 2 mg

T

DOSAGE

• **TABLETS, IMMEDIATE RELEASE**

Treat overactive bladder.

Initial: 2 mg b.i.d. Dose may be lowered to 1 mg b.i.d. based on individual response and side effects. Adjust dose to 1 mg b.i.d. in those with significantly reduced hepatic funtion or who are currently taking drugs that are inhibitors of cytochrome P450 3A4 (see *Drug Interactions*).

• **CAPSULES, EXTENDED RELEASE**

Treat overactive bladder.

4 mg once daily taken with liquids and swallowed whole. May lower dose to 2 mg daily based on response and tolerability. For those with significantly decreased hepatic or renal function or who are taking drugs that are inhibitors of cytochrome P450 3A4, the recommended dose is 2 mg daily.

NURSING CONSIDERATIONS

ASSESSMENT

1. Note indications for therapy, onset, duration, and characteristics of incontinence and symptoms.
2. List drugs currently prescribed to ensure none interact or alter dosage.
3. Determine any evidence of urinary retention or gastric retention; GI obstructive disorders or glaucoma.
4. Monitor renal and LFTs; decrease dose with hepatic dysfunction.

CLIENT/FAMILY TEACHING

1. Take as directed with or without food.
2. Drug is used to help reduce the frequency and urgency associated with urination. It is not for stress incontinence or UTI but is for treatment of an overactive bladder.
3. May experience dizziness/drowsiness and headache; use caution and report if persistent.
4. There is a user support number. Call 1-800-896-8596 to enroll and to receive free information/updates and 24-hr hotline access.

OUTCOMES/EVALUATE

↑ Bladder control with ↓ urinary frequency, urgency, or urge incontinence

Topiramate

(toh-**PYRE**-ah-mayt)

PREGNANCY CATEGORY: C
CLASSIFICATION(S):
Anticonvulsant, miscellaneous
Rx: Topamax

SEE ALSO *ANTICONVULSANTS*.

ACTION/KINETICS

Precise mechanism not known. The following effects may contribute to the anticonvulsant activity. (1) Action potentials seen repetitively by sustained depolarization of neurons are blocked in a time-dependent manner, suggesting an effect to block sodium channels. (2) Increases the frequency at which GABA activates $GABA_A$ receptors, thus enhancing the ability of GABA to cause a flux of chloride ions into neurons (i.e., enhanced effect of the inhibitory transmitter, $GABA_A$). (3) Antagonizes the ability of kainate to activate the kainate/AMPA subtype of excitatory amino acid aspartate, thus reducing the excitatory effect. Rapidly absorbed; **peak plasma levels:** About 2 hr. **t½, elimination:** 21 hr. Steady state is reached in about 4 days in those with normal renal function. Excreted mostly unchanged in the urine.

USES

(1) Adjunct treatment for partial onset seizures in adults and children, 2–16 years. (2) Adjunct treatment for primary generalized tonic-clonic seizures in adults and children, 2–16 years old. (3) Adjunct treatment of seizures associated with Lennox-Gastaut syndrome in clients 2 years of age and older.

CONTRAINDICATIONS

Lactation.

SPECIAL CONCERNS

Use with caution in impaired hepatic and renal function. Safety and efficacy have not been determined in children less than 2 years old.

SIDE EFFECTS

Note: Side effects with an incidence of 0.1% or greater are listed.

CNS: Psychomotor slowing, including difficulty with concentration and speech or language problems. Somnolence, fatigue, dizziness, ataxia, nystagmus, paresthesia, nervousness, difficulty with memory, tremor, confusion, depression, abnormal coordination, agitation, mood problems, aggressive reaction, hypoesthesia, apathy, emotional lability, depersonalization, hypokinesia, vertlgo, stupor, ***clonic/tonic seizures,*** hyperkinesia, hypertonia, insomnia, personality disorder, impotence, hallucinations, euphoria, psychosis, decreased libido, ***suicide attempt,*** hyporeflexia, neuropathy, migraine, apraxia, hyperesthesia, dyskinesia, hyperreflexia, dysphonia, scotoma, dystonia, coma, encephalopathy, upper motor neuron lesion, paranoid reaction, delusion, paranoia, delirium, abnormal dreaming, neuroses. **GI:** Nausea, dyspepsia, anorexia, abdominal pain, constipation, dry mouth, gingivitis, halitosis, diarrhea, vomiting, fecal incontinence, flatulence, gastroenteritis, gum hyperplasia, hemorrhoids, increased appetite, tooth caries, stomatitis, dysphagia, melena, gastritis, increased saliva, hiccough, gastroesophageal reflux, tongue edema, esophagitis, gall bladder disorder, gingival bleeding. **CV:** Palpitation, hypertension, hypotension, postural hypotension, AV block, bradycardia, bundle branch block, angina pectoris, vasodilation. **Body as a whole:** Asthenia, back pain, chest pain, flu-like symptoms, leg pain, hot flashes, body odor, edema, rigors, fever, malaise, syncope, enlarged abdomen. **Respiratory:** URI, pharyngitis, sinusitis, dyspnea, coughing, bronchitis, asthma, ***bronchospasm, pulmonary embolism.*** **Dermatologic:** Acne, alopecia, dermatitis, nail disorder, folliculitis, dry skin, urticaria, skin discoloration, eczema, photosensitivity reaction, erythematous rash, seborrhea, decreased sweating, abnormal hair texture, facial edema. **GU:** Breast pain, renal stone formation, dysmenorrhea, menstrual disorder, hematuria, intermenstrual bleeding, leukorrhea, menorrhagia, vaginitis, amenorrhea, UTI, micturition frequency, urinary incontinence, dysuria, renal calculus, ejaculation disorder, breast discharge, urinary retention, renal pain, nocturia, albuminuria, polyuria, oliguria, kidney stones. **Musculoskeletal:** Arthralgia, muscle weakness, arthrosis, osteoporosis, myalgia, leg cramps. **Metabolic:** Increased weight, decreased weight, dehydration, xeropthalmia. **Hematologic:** Anemia, leukopenia, lymphadenopathy, eosinophilia, lymphopenia, granulocytopenia, lymphocytosis, thrombocytothemia, purpura, thrombocyto-

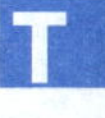

penia. **Dermatologic:** Rash, pruritus, increased sweating, flushing. **Ophthalmic:** Diplopia, abnormal vision, eye pain, conjunctivitis, abnormal accommodation, photophobia, abnormal lacrimation, strabismus, color blindness, acute myopia, mydriasis, ptosis, visual field defect, secondary angle closure glaucoma. **Miscellaneous:** Decreased hearing, epistaxis, taste perversion, tinnitus, taste loss, parosmia, goiter, basal cell carcinoma.

LABORATORY TEST CONSIDERATIONS

↑ AST, ALT, alkaline phosphatase, creatinine. Hypokalemia, hypocalcemia, hyperlipemia, acidosis, hyperglycemia, hyperchloremia.

OD OVERDOSE MANAGEMENT

Symptoms: See side effects. *Treatment:* Gastric lavage or induction of emesis if ingestion is recent. Supportive treatment. Hemodialysis.

DRUG INTERACTIONS

Alcohol / CNS depression and cognitive and neuropsychiatric side effects
Carbamazepine / ↓ Topiramate plasma levels
Carbonic anhydrase inhibitors / ↑ Risk of renal stone formation
CNS depressants / CNS depression and cognitive and neuropsychiatric side effects
Digoxin / ↓ Serum digoxin AUC; clinical relevance not established
Oral contraceptives / ↓ Effect of oral contraceptives
Phenytoin / ↓ Topiramate plasma levels and ↑ phenytoin plasma levels
Valproic acid / ↓ Plasma levels of both topiramate and valproic acid

HOW SUPPLIED

Sprinkle Capsule: 15 mg, 25 mg; *Tablets:* 25 mg, 100 mg, 200 mg.

DOSAGE

• **SPRINKLE CAPSULE, TABLETS**
All uses.

Adults, 17 years and older, initial: 25–50 mg/day; **then,** titrate in increments of 25 to 50 mg/week until an effective daily dose is reached. Doses greater than 400 mg/day have not been shown to improve the response. If C_{CR} < 70 mL/1.73 m², use one half of the usual adult dose. **Children, 2–16 years:** 5–9 mg/kg/day in two divided doses. Begin titration at 25 mg or less (based on a range of 1–3 mg/kg/day) nightly for the first week. Then, increase dose at 1- or 2-week intervals by increments of 1–3 mg/kg/day (given in 2 divided doses) to reach optimal clinical response.

NURSING CONSIDERATIONS

SEE ALSO *NURSING CONSIDERATIONS* FOR *ANTICONVULSANTS.*

ASSESSMENT

1. Document age at onset, type, and characteristics of seizures.
2. Monitor CBC, liver and renal function studies; reduce dose with renal dysfunction.
3. List drugs currently prescribed to ensure none interact or lose effectiveness; MAO inhibitors may promote kidney stones.
4. Document baseline psychomotor and mental status; assess for psychomotor slowing, speech or expression problems, difficulty concentrating, fatigue, or sleepiness.
5. Evaluate for acute myopia or secondary angle closure glaucoma. Immediately discontinue drug if symptoms present.

CLIENT/FAMILY TEACHING

1. Take exactly as prescribed. Due to the bitter taste of the drug, do not break tablets. Can be taken without regard for meals.
2. For sprinkle capsules, either swallow whole or carefully open capsule and spinkle the entire contents on a small amount (teaspoon) of soft food. Swallow the drug/food mixture immediately. Do not chew and do not store for future use.
3. Distinguish if drug affects motor or mental capacity before driving or performing activities that require mental alertness; may cause dizziness, confusion, drowsiness, and altered concentration.
4. Increase fluid intake to decrease substance concentration as drug may precipitate renal stone formation by increasing urinary pH and reducing urinary citrate excretion.

5. Use reliable, nonhormonal form of birth control; drug may compromise efficacy of PO contraceptives.
6. Do not stop drug abruptly due to risk of increased seizure frequency.
7. Review list of side effects, noting those that require attention.

OUTCOMES/EVALUATE
Adjunctive therapy in the control of partial onset seizures.

Topotecan hydrochloride

(toh-poh-**TEE**-kan)

PREGNANCY CATEGORY: D
CLASSIFICATION(S):
Antineoplastic, hormone
Rx: Hycamtin

SEE ALSO *ANTINEOPLASTIC AGENTS.*

ACTION/KINETICS
An inhibitor of topoisomerase I. Topoisomerase I relieves torsional strain in DNA by causing reversible single-strand breaks. Topotecan binds to the topoisomerase I-DNA complex and prevents religation of single-strand breaks. Cytotoxicity thought to be caused by double-strand DNA damage produced during DNA synthesis when replication enzymes interact with the ternary complex formed by topotecan, topoisomerase I, and DNA. Hydrolyzed to the active lactone form of the drug. About 30% of the drug is excreted in the urine. **t½, terminal:** 2 to 3 hr.

USES
(1) Metastatic cancer of the ovary after failure of initial or subsequent chemotherapy. (2) Small cell lung cancer sensitive disease after failure of first-line chemotherapy.

CONTRAINDICATIONS
Pregnancy, lactation. Severe bone marrow depression, including those with baseline neutrophil counts less than 1,500 cells/mm^3.

SPECIAL CONCERNS
Safety and efficacy have not been determined in children.

SIDE EFFECTS
Hematologic: Bone marrow suppression, including neutropenia, thrombocytopenia, anemia, sepsis or fever/infection with grade 4 neutropenia, platelet or RBC infusions. **GI:** N&V, abdominal pain, constipation, diarrhea, intestinal obstruction, stomatitis. **CNS:** Asthenia, headache, pain, paresthesias. **Musculoskeletal:** Arthralgia, myalgia. **Body as a whole:** Anorexia, fatigue, malaise, fever, pain. **Respiratory:** Dyspnea, coughing. **Dermatologic:** Total alopecia, rash, servere dermatitis, severe pruritus. **Miscellaneous:** Chest pain, allergic reactions, ***anaphylaxis, angioedema.***

LABORATORY TEST CONSIDERATIONS
↑ AST, ALT, bilirubin.

DRUG INTERACTIONS
Cisplatin / More severe myelosuppression
Filgrastim / Prolonged duration of neutropenia

HOW SUPPLIED
Powder for injection: 4 mg

DOSAGE

• IV INFUSION

Metastatic ovarian cancer, small cell lung cancer.

Adults: 1.5 mg/m^2 by IV infusion over 30 min daily for 5 consecutive days, starting on day 1 of a 21-day course of therapy. A minimum of four courses is recommended. If severe neutropenia occurs, reduce the dose by 0.25 mg/m^2 for subsequent courses. Also, for severe neutropenia, filgrastim may be given following the subsequent course and before dosage reduction starting from day 6 of the course (i.e., 24 hr after completion of topotecan administration).

Reduce the dose to 0.75 mg/m^2 for clients with a C_{CR} of 20–39 mL/min. No dosage reduction is required if the C_{CR} is 40–60 mL/min.

NURSING CONSIDERATIONS

SEE ALSO *NURSING CONSIDERATIONS FOR ANTINEOPLASTIC AGENTS.*

T

ADMINISTRATION/STORAGE

IV 1. To begin therapy, clients must have a baseline neutrophil count greater than 1,500 cells/mm³, a platelet count greater than 100,000 cells/mm³, and a hemoglobin level of 9 mg/dL or higher. Do not retreat until neutrophils are greater than 1,000 cells/mm³, platelets are greater than 100,000 cells/mm³, and hemoglobin levels are 9 mg/dL or greater.
2. Reconstitute the 4-mg topotecan vial with 4 mL of sterile water for injection. This may then be further diluted either with 0.9% NaCl or D5W and administered over 30 min.
3. Reconstituted vials diluted for infusion are stable at controlled room temperature and ambient lighting conditions for 24 hr.
4. Store vials in their original carton, protected from light, at controlled room temperature of 20–25°C (68–77°F).

ASSESSMENT

1. Document indications for therapy, other agents/therapies trialed, and when administered.
2. Monitor CBC and renal function studies; reduce dose with C_{CR} of 20–39 mL/m² . Ensure baseline neutrophil count above 1,500 cells/mm³ and platelet count at 100,000/mm³. Do not readminister until neutrophils are above 1,000, platelets are 100,000 cells/mm³, and hemoglobin levels are at least 9 mg/dL. Drug causes neutropenia and anemia. Nadir: 15 days.

OUTCOMES/EVALUATE

Control of malignant cell proliferation in metastatic cancer

T

Toremifene citrate

(**TOR**-em-ih-feen)

PREGNANCY CATEGORY: D
CLASSIFICATION(S):
Antineoplastic, hormone
Rx: Fareston

SEE ALSO *ANTINEOPLASTIC AGENTS.*

ACTION/KINETICS

Antiestrogen that binds to estrogen receptors and may cause estrogenic, antiestrogenic, or both effects, depending on duration of treatment, gender, and endpoint/target organ selected. Antitumor effect is likely due to antiestrogenic effect, i.e., competes for estrogen at receptor and blocks growth-stimulating effects of estrogen in tumor. Well absorbed from GI tract. **Peak plasma levels:** 3 hr. **t½, distribution:** About 4 hr. **t½, elimination:** About 5 days. Extensively metabolized in liver and mainly excreted in feces.

USES

Metastatic breast cancer in postmenopausal women with positive estrogen-receptor (ER) or ER unknown tumors.

CONTRAINDICATIONS

Use with history of thromboembolic disease or in pediatric clients.

SPECIAL CONCERNS

Hypercalcemia and tumor flare in some breast cancer clients with bone metastases during first weeks of treatment. Use with caution during lactation.

SIDE EFFECTS

CV: *Cardiac failure, MI, pulmonary embolism, CVA,* TIA. **GI:** Constipation, nausea. **Hematologic:** Leukopenia, thrombocytopenia. **Dermatologic:** Skin discoloration, dermatitis, alopecia, pruritus. **Ophthalmic:** Cataracts, dry eyes, abnormal visual fields, corneal keratopathy, glaucoma, reversible corneal opacity. **CNS:** Tremor, vertigo, depression. **Miscellaneous:** Dyspnea, paresis, anorexia, asthenia, jaundice, rigors, vaginal bleeding.

LABORATORY TEST CONSIDERATIONS

↑ AST, alkaline phosphatase, bilirubin. Hypercalcemia.

OD OVERDOSE MANAGEMENT

Symptoms: Vertigo, headache, dizziness. Possibly, hot flashes, vaginal bleeding, vertigo, dizziness, ataxia, nausea. *Treatment:* General supportive measures.

DRUG INTERACTIONS

Carbamazepine / ↓ Toremifene blood levels R/T ↑ liver breakdown
Clonazepam / ↓ Toremifene blood levels R/T ↑ liver breakdown
Erythromycin / Inhibition of toremifene breakdown

Ketoconazole / Inhibition of toremifene breakdown
Macrolide antibiotics / Inhibition of toremifene breakdown
Phenobarbital / ↓ Toremifene blood levels R/T ↑ liver breakdown
Phenytoin / ↓ Toremifene blood levels R/T ↑ liver breakdown
Warfarin / ↑ PT

HOW SUPPLIED

Tablets: 60 mg

DOSAGE

• **TABLETS**

Metastatic breast cancer.

Adults: 60 mg once daily. Continue until disease progression is observed.

NURSING CONSIDERATIONS

SEE ALSO *NURSING CONSIDERATIONS FOR ANTINEOPLASTIC AGENTS.*

ASSESSMENT

1. Document indications for therapy, characteristics of symptoms, other agents trialed and outcome.
2. Note any history or evidence of thromboembolic disorders.
3. Monitor CBC, calcium, and LFTs.

CLIENT/FAMILY TEACHING

1. Take once daily as directed.
2. Report any unusual vaginal bleeding.
3. May experience "tumor flare," syndrome of diffuse musculoskeletal pain and erythema with increased size of tumor lesions that regress later; if accompanied by hypercalcemia must stop drug.
4. Use reliable barrier birth control as drug may induce ovulation.

OUTCOMES/EVALUATE

Control of malignant cell proliferation

Torsemide

(**TOR**-seh-myd)

PREGNANCY CATEGORY: B

CLASSIFICATION(S):

Diuretic, loop

Rx: Demadex

SEE ALSO *DIURETICS, LOOP.*

ACTION/KINETICS

Onset, IV: Within 10 min; **PO:** within 60 min. **Peak effect, IV:** Within 60 min; **PO:** 60–120 min. **Duration:** 6–8 hr. **t½:** 210 min. Metabolized by the liver and excreted through the urine. Food delays the time to peak effect by about 30 min, but the overall bioavailability and the diuretic activity are not affected.

USES

Congestive heart failure, acute or chronic renal failure, hepatic cirrhosis, hypertension.

CONTRAINDICATIONS

Lactation.

SPECIAL CONCERNS

Clients sensitive to sulfonamides may show allergic reactions to torsemide. Safety and efficacy in children have not been determined.

SIDE EFFECTS

CNS: Headache, dizziness, asthenia, insomnia, nervousness, syncope. **GI:** Diarrhea, constipation, nausea, dyspepsia, edema, ***GI hemorrhage,*** rectal bleeding. **CV:** ECG abnormality, chest pain, atrial fibrillation, hypotension, ***ventricular tachycardia,*** shunt thrombosis. **Respiratory:** Rhinitis, increase in cough. **Musculoskeletal:** Arthralgia, myalgia. **Miscellaneous:** Sore throat, excessive urination, rash.

LABORATORY TEST CONSIDERATIONS

Hyperglycemia, hyperuricemia, hypokalemia, hypovolemia.

HOW SUPPLIED

Injection: 10 mg/mL; *Tablet:* 5 mg, 10 mg, 20 mg, 100 mg

DOSAGE

• **TABLETS, IV**

Congestive heart failure.

Adults, initial: 10 or 20 mg once daily.

Chronic renal failure.

Adults, initial: 20 mg once daily.

Hepatic cirrhosis.

Adults, initial: 5 or 10 mg once daily given with an aldosterone antagonist or a potassium-sparing diuretic.

Hypertension.

Adults, initial: 5 mg once daily. If this dose does not lead to an adequate decrease in BP within 4–6 weeks, the

T

dose may be increased to 10 mg once daily. If the 10-mg dose is not adequate, an additional antihypertensive agent is added to the treatment regimen.

NURSING CONSIDERATIONS

SEE ALSO *NURSING CONSIDERATIONS* FOR *DIURETICS, LOOP.*

ADMINISTRATION/STORAGE

1. If the response is inadequate for the initial dose used for CHF, chronic renal failure, or hepatic cirrhosis, the dose can be doubled until the desired diuretic response is obtained. Doses greater than 200 mg for CHF or chronic renal failure and greater than 40 mg for hepatic cirrhosis have not been adequately studied.
2. May be given without regard for meals.
3. It is not necessary to adjust the dose for geriatric clients.
IV 4. Give the IV dose slowly over a period of 2 min or as a continuous infusion.
5. Oral and IV doses are therapeutically equivalent; may switch to and from the IV form with no change in dose.

ASSESSMENT

1. Document indications for therapy, type and onset of symptoms. List agents trialed and the outcome.
2. Note any sensitivity to sulfonamides.
3. Monitor VS, weight, I&O, blood sugar, uric acid, and potassium; drug may increase blood sugar and uric acid levels.
4. Document pulmonary, renal, and CV assessments.

CLIENT/FAMILY TEACHING

1. Take only as directed. May take with food to decrease GI upset.
2. With hypertension, keep a BP log for provider review.
3. Report immediately any chest pain, increased SOB, or sudden weight gain with edema.
4. Drug may cause dizziness, lightheadedness, and fatigue; use caution.
5. Rise slowly from a sitting or lying position to minimize orthostatic drug effects.
6. May experience blurred vision, yellowing of vision, or sensitivity to sunlight. Report any unusual, persistent symptoms or lack of response.

OUTCOMES/EVALUATE

- ↓ Edema; ↑ diuresis; ↓ BP
- Reduction of interdialysis weight gain and promotion of Na, Cl, and water excretion

Tramadol hydrochloride

(**TRAM**-ah-dol)

PREGNANCY CATEGORY: C
CLASSIFICATION(S):
Analgesic, centrally-acting
Rx: Ultram

ACTION/KINETICS

A centrally acting analgesic not related chemically to opiates. Precise mechanism is not known. It may bind to mu-opioid receptors and inhibit reuptake of norepinephrine and serotonin. The analgesic effect is only partially antagonized by the antagonist naloxone. Causes significantly less respiratory depression than morphine. In contrast to morphine, tramadol does not cause release of histamine. Produces dependence of the mu-opioid type (i.e., like codeine or dextropropoxyphene); however, there is little evidence of abuse. Tolerance occurs but is relatively mild; the withdrawal syndrome is not as severe with other opiates. Rapidly absorbed after PO administration. Food does not affect the rate or extent of absorption. **Onset:** 1 hr. **Peak effect:** 2–3 hr. **Peak plasma levels:** 2 hr. **t½, plasma:** Approximately 7 hr after multiple doses. Extensively metabolized by one of the P-450 isoenzymes. Excreted in the urine, with about 30% excreted unchanged and 60% as metabolites. The M-metabolite is active.

USES

Management of moderate to moderately severe pain.

CONTRAINDICATIONS
Hypersensitivity to tramadol. In acute intoxication with alcohol, hypnotics, centrally acting analgesics, opiates, or psychotropic drugs. Use in clients with past or present addiction or opiate dependence or in those with a prior history of allergy to codeine or opiates. Use for obstetric preoperative medication or for postdelivery analgesia in nursing mothers. Use in children less than 16 years of age, as safety and efficacy have not been determined.

SPECIAL CONCERNS
Use with great caution in those taking MAO inhibitors, as tramadol inhibits norepinephrine and serotonin uptake. Dosage reduction is recommended with impaired hepatic or renal function and in clients over 75 years of age. Use with caution in increased intracranial pressure or head injury, in epilepsy, or in clients with an increased risk for seizures, including head trauma, metabolic disorders, alcohol or drug withdrawal, and CNS infections. Tramadol may complicate the assessment of acute abdominal conditions. Has abuse potential for some clients.

SIDE EFFECTS
CNS: Dizziness, vertigo, headache, somnolence, CNS stimulation, anxiety, confusion, incoordination, euphoria, nervousness, sleep disorders, ***seizures,*** paresthesia, cognitive dysfunction, hallucinations, tremor, amnesia, concentration difficulty, abnormal gait, migraine, development of drug dependence, increased risk of seizures. **GI:** Nausea, constipation, vomiting, dyspepsia, dry mouth, diarrhea, abdominal pain, anorexia, flatulence, GI bleeding, hepatitis, stomatitis, dysgeusia. **CV:** Vasodilation, syncope, orthostatic hyper/hypotension, tachycardia, abnormal ECG, myocardial ischemia, palpitations. **Dermatologic:** Pruritus, sweating, rash, urticaria, vesicles. **Body as a whole:** Asthenia, malaise, allergic reaction, accidental injury, weight loss, ***suicidal tendency.*** **GU:** Urinary retention/frequency, menopausal symptoms, dysuria, menstrual disorder. **Miscellaneous:** ***Anaphylaxis,*** visual disturbances, cataracts, deafness, tinnitus, hypertonia, dyspnea.

LABORATORY TEST CONSIDERATIONS
↑ Creatinine, liver enzymes. ↓ Hemoglobin. Proteinuria.

OD OVERDOSE MANAGEMENT
Symptoms: Extension of side effects, especially ***respiratory depression and seizures.*** *Treatment:* Naloxone will reverse some, but not all, of the symptoms of overdose. General supportive treatment, with special attention to maintenance of adequate respiration. Diazepam or barbiturates may help if seizures occur. Hemodialysis is not helpful.

DRUG INTERACTIONS
Alcohol / ↑ Respiratory depression
Anesthetics, general / ↑ Respiratory depression
Carbamazepine / ↓ Tramadol effect R/T ↑ metabolism
CNS depressants / Additive CNS depression
MAO Inhibitors / ↑ Risk of seizures
Naloxone / ↑ Risk of seizures if naloxone used for tramadol overdose.
Quinidine / ↑ Levels of tramadol and ↓ levels of M1 R/T inhibition of metabolism
Warfarin ↑ PT and INR

HOW SUPPLIED
Tablet: 50 mg

DOSAGE

• **TABLETS**

Management of pain.

Adults: 50–100 mg q 4–6 hr, as needed, but not to exceed 400 mg/day. For moderate pain, 50 mg, initially, may be adequate, and for severe pain, 100 mg, initially, is often more effective. For moderate chronic pain not requiring rapid analgesic onset, use 25 mg/day to improve tolerability; titrate in 25 mg increments, as separate doses, q 3 days to 100 mg/day. Can then be titrated by 50 mg q 3 days to 200 mg/day, not to exceed 400 mg/day. For clients over 75 years of age, the recommended dose is no more than 300 mg/day in divided doses. In im-

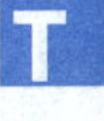

paired renal function with a C_{CR} less than 30 mL/min, the dosing interval should be increased to 12 hr, with a maximum daily dose of 200 mg. The recommended dose for clients with cirrhosis is 50 mg q 12 hr.

NURSING CONSIDERATIONS

SEE ALSO *NURSING CONSIDERATIONS* FOR *NARCOTIC ANALGESICS*.

ASSESSMENT

1. Document indications for therapy, location, onset, and characteristics of symptoms. Use a pain-rating scale to rate pain.
2. Assess for history of drug addiction, allergy to opiates or codeine, or seizures; drug may increase the risk of convulsions.
3. Monitor liver and renal function studies; reduce dose with dysfunction and if over 75 years old.

CLIENT/FAMILY TEACHING

1. Take only as directed. May be taken without regard to meals. Do not exceed single or daily doses of tramadol; do not share meds, store safely out of reach of child.
2. Do not perform activities that require mental alertness; drug may impair mental or physical performance.
3. Review list of side effects (nausea, dizziness, constipation, somnolence, pruritus, and constipation) that one may experience; report if persistent or intolerable.
4. May mask abdominal pathology and obscure intracranial pathology due to miosis. Carry ID of drugs currently prescribed.

OUTCOMES/EVALUATE

Pain control

T

Trandolapril

(tran-**DOHL**-ah-pril)

PREGNANCY CATEGORY: C (FIRST TRIMESTER); D (SECOND AND THIRD TRIMESTERS)

CLASSIFICATION(S):

Antihypertensive, ACE inhibitor

Rx: Mavik

SEE ALSO *ANGIOTENSIN CONVERTING ENZYME (ACE) INHIBITORS*.

ACTION/KINETICS

Rapidly absorbed; food slows rate, but not amount absorbed. **Onset:** 2–4 hr. **Peak plasma levels, trandolapril:** 30–60 min; **trandolaprilat:** 4–10 hr. **t½, trandolapril:** About 5 hr; **t½, trandoprilat:** About 10 hr. **Peak effect:** 4–10 hr. Metabolized in liver to active trandolaprilat. **Duration:** 24 hr. About ⅓ trandolaprilat is excreted in urine and ⅔ in feces.

USES

(1) Hypertension, alone or in combination with other antihypertensives such as hydrochlorothiazide. (2) To treat heart failure after MI or ventricular dysfunction after MI.

CONTRAINDICATIONS

In those with history of angioedema with ACE inhibitors.

SPECIAL CONCERNS

Safety and efficacy have not been determined in children.

SIDE EFFECTS

See also *ACE Inhibitors*. **Hypersensitivity: *Angioedema*. CNS:** Dizziness, headache, fatigue, insomnia, paresthesias, drowsiness, vertigo, anxiety. **GI:** Diarrhea, dyspepsia, gastritis, abdominal pain, vomiting, constipation, pancreatitis. **CV:** Hypotension, bradycardia, chest pain, ***cardiogenic shock*** , intermittent claudication, stroke. **Respiratory:** Cough, dyspnea, URTI, epistaxis, throat inflammation. **Hepatic: *Hepatic failure,*** including cholestatic jaundice, ***fulminant hepatic necrosis, death.*** **Dermatologic:** Photosensitivity, pruritus, rash. **GU:** UTI, impotence, decreased libido. **Miscellaneous:** Neutropenia, syncope, myalgia, asthenia, muscle cramps, hypocalemia, intermittent claudication, edema, extremity pain, gout.

LABORATORY TEST CONSIDERATIONS

Hyperkalemia, hypocalcemia. ↑ Serum uric acid, BUN, creatinine.

DRUG INTERACTIONS

Diuretics / Excessive hypotensive effects
Diuretics, potassium-sparing: ↑ Risk of hyperkalemia
Lithium / ↑ Risk of lithium toxicity

HOW SUPPLIED
Tablet: 1 mg, 2 mg, 4 mg.

DOSAGE

• **TABLETS**

Hypertension.

Initial: 1 mg once daily in nonblack clients (2 mg once daily in black clients) for those not receiving a diuretic. Adjust dosage according to response; usually, adjustments are made at intervals of 1 week. **Maintenance, usual:** 4 mg once daily (twice daily dosing may be needed in some). If BP is still not adequately controlled, diuretic may be added.

Heart failure post–MI/Left ventricular dysfunction post–MI.

Initial: 1 mg/day. Then, increase the dose, as tolerated, to a target dose of 4 mg/day. If 4 mg is not tolerated, continue with the highest tolerated dose.

If C_{CR} is less than 30 mL/min or if there is hepatic cirrhosis, initial dose is 0.5 mg daily.

NURSING CONSIDERATIONS

SEE ALSO *NURSING CONSIDERATIONS* FOR *ANGIOTENSIN CONVERTING ENZYME (ACE) INHIBITORS.*

ADMINISTRATION/STORAGE

If client is on diuretic, discontinue 2 to 3 days prior to beginning therapy with trandolapril to reduce likelihood of hypotension. If diuretic can not be discontinued, use initial dose of trandolapril of 0.5 mg. Titrate subsequent dosage.

ASSESSMENT

1. Note indications for therapy, disease onset, other agents trialed and outcome.
2. Monitor liver and renal function studies; reduce dosage with impairment.

CLIENT/FAMILY TEACHING

1. Take only as directed.
2. May experience cough, dizziness, and diarrhea; report if persistent.
3. Practice reliable contraception, stop drug and report if pregnancy suspected.
4. Continue lifestyle changes i.e., regular exercise, smoking/alcohol cessation, low fat, low salt diet in overall goal of BP control.

OUTCOMES/EVALUATE

• ↓ BP
• Control of heart failure/ventricular dysfunction after MI

Trastuzumab

(traz-**TOO**-zah-mab)

PREGNANCY CATEGORY: B
CLASSIFICATION(S):
Antineoplastic, miscellaneous
Rx: Herceptin

SEE ALSO *ANTINEOPLASTIC AGENTS.*

ACTION/KINETICS
A recombinant DNA-derived humanized monoclonal antibody that selectively binds with high affinity to the extracellular domain of the human epidermal growth factor receptor 2 protein (HER2). Results in inhibition of the proliferation of human tumor cells that overexpress HER2 and mediates antibody-dependent cellular cytotoxicity. The HER2 protein is overexpressed in 25% to 30% of primary breast cancers. **t½, following loading dose of 4 mg/kg and weekly dose of 2 mg/kg:** Average of 5.8 days. Mean serum trough levels of trastuzumab, when given with paclitaxel, were elevated 1.5 fold compared to use in combination with anthracycline plus cyclophosphamide.

USES
First-line treatment of metastatic breast cancer with tumor overexpressing the HER2 protein either alone or in combination with paclitaxel in those who have not received chemotherapy for their metastatic disease. Use only in those whose tumors have HER2 protein overexpression.

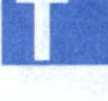

CONTRAINDICATIONS
Lactation and for six months after the last trastuzumab dose.

SPECIAL CONCERNS
Use with extreme caution in those with preexisting cardiac dysfunction.

Probability of cardiac dysfunction is highest in those receiving trastuzumab with an anthracycline; advanced age may also increase the incidence of cardiac dysfunction. Adult respiratory distress syndrome, anaphylaxis, and death within 24 hr have been noted after the first dose, during infusion, or within 12 hrs after the first infusion. Use with caution during pregnancy and in those with sensitivity to Chinese hamster ovary proteins. Increased risk for severe pulmonary side effects in those with symptomatic intrinsic pulmonary disease (e.g., asthma, COPD) or those with extensive tumor involvement of the lungs. Safety and efficacy have not been determined in children.

SIDE EFFECTS

CV: Tachycardia, ***vascular thrombosis,*** pericardial effusion, ***heart arrest, hemorrhage, shock, arrhythmia,*** hypotension, syncope. Cardiomyopathy, including ventricular dysfunction and CHF. Cardiac dysfunction, including dyspnea, increased cough, paroxysmal nocturnal dyspnea, peripheral edema, S_3 gallop, reduced ejection fraction. **GI:** Diarrhea, anorexia, N&V, ***hepatic failure,*** gastroenteritis, hematemesis, ileus, intestinal obstruction, colitis, esophageal ulcer, stomatitis, pancreatitis, hepatitis. **CNS:** Dizziness, insomnia, paresthesia, peripheral neuritis, depression, neuropathy, convulsion, ataxia, confusion, manic reaction. **Respiratory:** Increased cough, dyspnea, pharyngitis, rhinitis, sinusitis, apnea, pneumothorax, asthma, hypoxia, laryngitis, pulmonary infiltrates, pleural effusions, noncardiogenic pulmonary edema, pulmonary insufficiency, pneumonitis, pulmonary fibrosis, ***acute respiratory distresss syndrome***. **Dermatologic:** Rash, acne, herpes simplex/zoster, skin ulceration. **Hematologic:** Anemia, leukopenia, pancytopenia, acute leukemia, coagulation disorder, lymphangitis. **Musculoskeletal:** Arthralgia, bone pain/necrosis, pathological fractures, myopathy. **GU:** Hydronephrosis, kidney failure, cervical cancer, hematuria, hemorrhagic cystitis, pyelonephritis. **Metabolic:** Peripheral edema, edema, hypoglycemia, growth retardation, weight loss. **First-infusion-associated symptoms:** Chills, fever, N&V, pain, rigors, headache, dizziness, dyspnea, hypotension, rash, asthenia. **Miscellaneous:** Increased incidence of infections, especially of the URT; abdominal/back pain, accidental injury, allergic reaction, asthenia, chills, fever, flu syndrome, headache, pain, UTI, cellulitis, ***anaphylactoid reaction, extreme respiratory distress,*** ascites, hydrocephalus, radiation injury, deafness, amblyopia, hypothyroidism.

LABORATORY TEST CONSIDERATIONS

Hypercalcemia, hypomagnesemia, hyponatremia.

DRUG INTERACTIONS

Hypoprothrombinemia and ↑ risk of bleeding when usedwith warfarin.

HOW SUPPLIED

Powder, lyophilized: 440 mg

DOSAGE

• **IV**

Metastatic breast cancer.

Initial: 4 mg/kg infused over 90 min; **maintenance:** 2 mg/kg weekly, infused over 30 min if initial dose was tolerated.

NURSING CONSIDERATIONS

SEE ALSO *NURSING CONSIDERATIONS* FOR *ANTINEOPLASTIC AGENTS.*

ADMINISTRATION/STORAGE

IV 1. Do not give as an IV push or bolus.

2. Follow carefully the specific guidelines for reconstitution of trastuzumab, including use of the proper diluent, correct amount of diluent, and proper administration.

3. Reconstitute with 20 mL bacteriostatic water for injection, 1.1% benzyl alcohol, as supplied. Resulting solution contains 21 mg/mL.

4. For those with sensitivity to benzyl alcohol, reconstitute with sterile water for injection rather than bacteriostatic water for injection. Do not mix with dextrose solutions.

5. After reconstitution, immediately label the vial in the area marked "Do not

use after" with the date 28 days from the reconstitution date.
6. Determine the dose needed based on a loading or maintenance dose. Calculate the volume needed from the reconstituted vial; withdraw this amount and add it to an infusion bag containing 250 mL of 0.9% NaCl. Gently invert the bag to mix the solution. The reconstituted preparation is a colorless to pale yellow transparent solution.
7. May give in outpatient setting.
8. Do not mix or dilute with other drugs.
9. Prior to reconstitution, vials are stable at 2–8°C (36–46°F). When reconstituted with bacteriostatic water for injection, as supplied, is stable for 28 days when stored at 2–8°C and may be preserved for multiple use. If reconstituted with unpreserved sterile water for injection, use immediately and discard any unused portion. Do not freeze reconstituted drug.
10. Trastuzumab diluted in polyvinylchloride or polyethylene bags containing 0.9% NaCl for injection may be stored at 2–8°C (36–46°F) or at room temperature for 24 hr or less. Since this solution contains no effective preservative, refrigeration is recommended.

ASSESSMENT

1. Document breast cancer onset/diagnosis, other therapies trialed, and the outcome. Determine if first-line therapy or second-or third-line therapy for tumors overexpressing the HER2 protein.
2. During infusion assess for fever, chills, and other infusion-associated symptoms (see *Side Effects*).
2. Assess cardiac function. Obtain ECG, echocardiogram and/or MUGA to evaluate left ventricular function prior to and during therapy.

CLIENT/FAMILY TEACHING

1. Drug is used in combination regimens to treat metastatic disease. It is administered as an IV infusion once a week. May be given in an outpatient setting.
2. Tylenol may help with flu-like symptoms after infusion; may also experience diarrhea, anemia, and infections during therapy; report.
3. Report any S&S of ventricular dysfunction and congestive heart failure: SOB, cough, swelling of extremities, immediately. Drug may cause cardiac toxicity.

OUTCOMES/EVALUATE

Inhibition of malignant cells that overexpress HER2 protein

Travoprost

(**TRAH**-voh-prahst)

PREGNANCY CATEGORY: C
CLASSIFICATION(S):
Antiglaucoma drug
Rx: Travatan

ACTION/KINETICS

A synthetic prostaglandin $F_{2\alpha}$ analog. Believed to act by increasing uveoscleral aqueous humor outflow. **Onset:** About 2 hr. **Maximum effect:** After 12 hr. Is absorbed through the cornea.

USES

Decrease intraocular pressure in open-angle glaucoma or ocular hypertension.

CONTRAINDICATIONS

Hypersensitivity to travoprost, benzalkonium chloride, or other ingredients in the product. Use during pregnancy or by women attempting to become pregnant.

SPECIAL CONCERNS

Has not been evaluated for treatment of angle closure, inflammatory, or neovascular glaucoma. May cause increased brown pigmentation of the iris, darkening of the eyelid, and increased pigmentation and growth of eyelashes, changes may be permanent. Use with caution in active intraocular inflammation (e.g., iritis, uveitis), in aphakic or pseudophakic clients with a torn posterior lens capsule, in those with known risk factors for macular edema, and during lactation. Contamination of the product may cause bacterial keratitis. Safety and ef-

T

ficacy have not been determined in children.

SIDE EFFECTS

Ophthalmic: Ocular hyperemia, decreased visual acuity, eye discomfort, foreign body sensation, pain, pruritus, abnormal vision, blepharitis, blurred vision, cataract, cells, conjunctivitis, dry eye, eye disorder, flare, iris discoloration, keratitis, lid margin crusting, photophobia, subjunctival hemorrhage, tearing, bacterial keratitis. **CV:** Angina pectoris, bradycardia, hypertension, hypotension. **GI:** Dyspepsia, GI disorder. **CNS:** Anxiety, depression, headache. **Body as a whole:** Accidental injury, infection, pain, arthritis. **GU:** Urinary incontinence, UTI, prostate disorder. **Respiratory:** Bronchitis, sinusitis. **Miscellaneous:** Back pain, chest pain, cold syndrome, hypercholesterolemia.

HOW SUPPLIED

Solution, Ophthalmic: 0.004%

DOSAGE

- **SOLUTION, OPHTHALMIC**

  Elevated IOP.

1 gtt in the affected eye(s) once daily in the evening.

NURSING CONSIDERATIONS

ADMINISTRATION/STORAGE

Store between 2–25°C (36–77°F). Discard the container within 6 weeks of removing it from the sealed pouch.

ASSESSMENT

1. Note indications for therapy, other agents trialed, and pressure readings. Used with open angle glaucoma or ocular hypertension.
2. Assess eye for inflammation, exudate, pain, level of vision, and note iris color.
3. May alter BP, breathing and elimination patterns.

CLIENT/FAMILY TEACHING

1. Use once daily as directed, more frequent use may decrease the IOP-lowering effect.
2. Do not let tip of dropper touch any part of eye or surrounding tissue. Rinse well if contact suspected and do not share eye dropper.
3. May be used together with other topical ophthalmic drug products to lower IOP. If more than 1 eye drop is used, administer them at least 5 min apart.
4. Do not administer while wearing contact lenses. Remove contact lenses prior to instillation, lenses may be reinserted 15 min after drug administration.
5. May cause irreversible pigmentation changes to iris (brown color) and skin around the eye and lid. May also cause increased eyelash growth which may be of more concern if only one eye is being treated.
6. Report any unusual or intolerable side effects. Keep all F/U appointments to evaluate response to treatment. Do not drive or perform hazardous functions until vision clears.

OUTCOMES/EVALUATE

↓ IOP

Trazodone hydrochloride

(**TRAYZ**-oh-dohn)

PREGNANCY CATEGORY: C
CLASSIFICATION(S):
Antidepressant, miscellaneous
Rx: Desyrel, Desyrel Dividose
✱Rx: Alti-Trazodone, Alti-Trazodone Dividose, Apo-Trazodone, Apo-Trazodone D, Novo-Trazodone, Nu-Trazodone, Nu-Trazodone-D, PMS-Trazodone, Trazorel

ACTION/KINETICS

A novel antidepressant that does not inhibit MAO and is also devoid of amphetamine-like effects. Response usually occurs after 2 weeks (75% of clients), with the remainder responding after 2–4 weeks. May inhibit serotonin uptake by brain cells, therefore increasing serotonin concentrations in the synapse. May also cause changes in binding of serotonin to receptors. Causes moderate sedative and orthostatic hypotensive effects and slight anticholinergic effects. **Peak plasma levels:** 1 hr (empty stomach) or 2 hr (when taken with food). **$t^1/_2$, initial:** 3–6 hr; **final:** 5–9 hr. **Effective plasma levels:** 800–1,600 ng/mL. **Time to reach**

steady state: 3–7 days. Three-fourths of those with a therapeutic effect respond by the end of the second week of therapy. Metabolized in liver and excreted through both the urine and feces.

USES

Depression with or without accompanying anxiety. *Investigational:* In combination with tryptophan for treating aggressive behavior. Panic disorder or agoraphobia with panic attacks. Treatment of cocaine withdrawal. In combination with a selective serotonin reuptake inhibitor to treat insomnia. Alcoholism.

CONTRAINDICATIONS

During the initial recovery period following MI. Concurrently with electroshock therapy.

SPECIAL CONCERNS

Use with caution during lactation. Safety and efficacy in children less than 18 years of age have not been established. Geriatric clients are more prone to the sedative and hypotensive effects.

SIDE EFFECTS

General: Dermatitis, edema, blurred vision, constipation, dry mouth, nasal congestion, skeletal muscle aches and pains. **CV:** Hypertension or hypotension, syncope, palpitations, tachycardia, SOB, chest pain. **GI:** Diarrhea, N&V, bad taste in mouth, flatulence. **GU:** Delayed urine flow, priapism, hematuria, increased urinary frequency. **CNS:** Nightmares, confusion, anger, excitement, decreased ability to concentrate, dizziness, disorientation, drowsiness, lightheadedness, fatigue, insomnia, nervousness, impaired memory. Rarely, hallucinations, impaired speech, hypomania. **Other:** Incoordination, tremors, paresthesias, decreased libido, appetite disturbances, red eyes, sweating or clamminess, tinnitus, weight gain or loss, anemia, hypersalivation. Rarely, akathisia, muscle twitching, increased libido, impotence, retrograde ejaculation, early menses, missed periods.

OD OVERDOSE MANAGEMENT

Symptoms: CNS depresssion, including ***respiratory arrest, seizures,*** ECG changes, hypotension, priapism as well as an increase in the incidence and severity of side effects noted above (vomiting and drowsiness are the most common). *Treatment:* Treat symptoms (especially hypotension and sedation). Gastric lavage and forced diuresis to remove the drug from the body.

DRUG INTERACTIONS

Alcohol / ↑ Depressant effects
Antihypertensives / Additive hypotension
Barbiturates / ↑ Depressant effects
Carbamazepine / ↓ Plasma levels of trazodone and its active metabolite
Clonidine / ↓ Clonidine effects
CNS depressants / ↑ CNS depression
Digoxin / ↑ Serum digoxin levels
MAO inhibitors / Initiate therapy cautiously if used together
Phenothiazines / ↑ Trazodone serum levels
Phenytoin / ↑ Serum phenytoin levels
Selective serotonin reuptake inhibitors / "Serotonin syndrome," including irritability, shivering, myoclonus, increased muscle tone, and altered consciousness
Warfarin / Either ↑ or ↓ PT

HOW SUPPLIED

Tablet: 50 mg, 100 mg, 150 mg, 300 mg

DOSAGE

• TABLETS

Treat depression.

Adults and adolescents, initial: 150 mg/day in divided doses; **then,** increase by 50 mg/day every 3–4 days to maximum of 400 mg/day in divided doses (outpatients). Inpatients may require up to, but not exceeding, 600 mg/day in divided doses. **Maintenance:** Use lowest effective dose. **Geriatric clients:** 75 mg/day in divided doses; dose can then be increased, as needed and tolerated, at 3- to 4-day intervals.

Treat aggressive behavior.

Trazodone, 50 mg b.i.d., with tryptophan, 500 mg b.i.d. Dosage adjustments may be required to reach a

T

therapeutic response or if side effects develop.

Panic disorder or agoraphobia with panic attacks.

300 mg/day.

Insomnia.

25–75 mg, often with a selective serotonin reuptake inhibitor.

Alcoholism.

50–100 mg/day.

NURSING CONSIDERATIONS

ADMINISTRATION/STORAGE

1. Initiate dose at the lowest possible level; increase gradually.
2. Beneficial effects may be observed within 1 week with optimal effects seen within 2 weeks.

ASSESSMENT

1. Document indications for therapy, onset of symptoms, and any associated factors.
2. Note any history of recent MI.
3. Monitor ECG, CBC, liver and renal function studies.

CLIENT/FAMILY TEACHING

1. Take with food to enhance absorption and minimize dizziness and/or lightheadedness. Take major portion of dose at bedtime to reduce daytime side effects.
2. Use caution when driving or when performing other hazardous tasks; may cause drowsiness/dizziness.
3. Avoid alcohol and CNS depressants.
4. Report any persistent/bothersome side effects.
5. Use sugarless gum or candies and frequent mouth rinses to diminish dry mouth effects.
6. Inform surgeon if elective surgery is planned to minimize interaction with anesthetic agent.
7. Encourage family to share responsibility for drug therapy to optimize treatment, prevent overdosage, and observe for any suicidal cues. Clients taking antidepressants and emerging from deepest phases of depression are more prone to suicide.
8. May take 2–4 weeks for full drug effects to be realized.

OUTCOMES/EVALUATE

- ↓ Depression (e.g., improved sleeping/eating patterns, ↓ fatigue, and ↑ social interactions)
- Control of overwhelming anxiety/panic symptoms
- ↓ Insomnia

Tretinoin (Retinoic acid, Vitamin A acid)

(**TRET**-ih-noyn)

PREGNANCY CATEGORY: C (TOPICAL PRODUCTS), D (ORAL PRODUCTS)
CLASSIFICATION(S):
Retinoid
Rx: Avita, Renova, Retin-A, Retin-A Micro, Vesanoid
✱**Rx:** Rejuva-A

ACTION/KINETICS

Topical tretinoin is believed to decrease microcomedone formation by decreasing the cohesiveness of follicular epithelial cells. Also believed to increase mitotic activity and increase turnover of follicular epithelial cells as well as decrease keratin synthesis. Some systemic absorption occurs (approximately 5% is recovered in the urine).

The mechanism of action for PO use in acute promyelocytic leukemia (APL) is not known. Absorption is enhanced when the drug is taken with food. **Time to peak levels:** 1–2 hr. Is over 95% bound to plasma proteins (mainly to albumin). **Terminal elimination t½:** 0.5–2 hr in APL clients. Metabolized by the liver, with about two-thirds excreted in the urine and one-third in the feces.

USES

Dermatologic: *Avita, Retin-A:* Acne vulgaris. *Retin-A* and *Renova:* As an adjunct to comprehensive skin care and sun avoidance to treat fine wrinkles, mottled hyperpigmentation, and roughness of facial skin caused by age and the sun. For those individuals who do not achieve palliation using comprehensive skin care and sun avoidance programs alone. *Investiga-*

tional (*Retin-A*): (1) Treat various forms of skin cancer. (2) Dermatologic conditions including lamellar ichthyosis, mollusca contagiosa, verrucae plantaris, verrucae planae juveniles, ichthyosis vulgaris, bullous congenital ichthyosiform, and pityriasis rubra pilaris. (3) To enhance the percutaneous absorption of topical minoxidil.

Oral: To induce remission in APL. After induction therapy with tretinoin, clients should be given a standard consolidation or maintenance chemotherapy regimen for APL, unless contraindicated.

CONTRAINDICATIONS

Eczema, sunburn. Use if inherently sensitive to sunlight or if taking other drugs that increase sensitivity to sunlight. Use of Renova if client is also taking drugs known to be photosensitizers (e.g., fluoroquinolones, phenothiazines, sulfonamides, tetracyclines, thiazides). Those allergic to parabens (preservative in the gelatin capsules). Use of PO form during lactation. Use around the eyes, mouth, angles of the nose, and mucous membranes.

SPECIAL CONCERNS

Use with caution during lactation. Safety and effectiveness have not been determined in children. Excessive sunlight and weather extremes (e.g., wind and cold) may be irritating. Use Avita and Renova with caution with concomitant topical medications, medicated or abrasive soaps, shampoos, cleansers, cosmetics with a strong drying effect, permanent wave solutions, electrolysis, hair depilatories or waxes, and products with high concentrations of alcohol, astringents, spices, or lime. Safety and efficacy of Renova have not been determined in children less than 18 years of age, in individuals over the age of 50 years, or in individuals with moderately or heavily pigmented skin. Use of the PO form has resulted in retonic acid-APL syndrome, especially during the first month of treatment. The safety and efficacy of oral tretinoin at doses less than 45 mg/m^2/day have not been evaluated in children.

SIDE EFFECTS

Following topical use.

Dermatologic: Red, edematous, crusted, or blistered skin; hyperpigmentation or hypopigmentation, increased susceptibility to sunlight, erythema, peeling, stinging, pruritus, burning, dryness. Excessive application will cause redness, peeling, or discomfort with no increase in results.

Following oral use.

Retinoic acid-APL syndrome: Fever, dyspnea, weight gain, radiographic pulmonary infiltrate, pleural or pericardial effusions. Occasional impaired myocardial contractility and episodic hypotension; possibility of concomitant leukocytosis. ***Progressive hypoxemia with possible fatal outcome.*** Respiratory symptoms, including upper respiratory tract disorders, respiratory insufficiency, pneumonia, rales, expiratory wheezing, lower respiratory tract disorders, bronchial asthma, ***pulmonary or larynx edema,*** unspecified pulmonary disease. *Pseudotumor cerebri (especially in children):* Papilledema, headache, N&V, visual disturbances. *Typical retinoid toxicity (similar to ingestion of high doses of vitamin A):* Headache, fever, dryness of skin and mucous membranes, bone pain, N&V, rash, mucositis, pruritus, increased sweating, visual disturbances, ocular disorders, alopecia, skin changes, changed visual acuity, bone inflammation, visual field defects. **Body as a whole:** Malaise, shivering, ***hemorrhage, DIC,*** infections, peripheral edema, pain, chest discomfort, edema, weight increase, anorexia, weight decrease, myalgia, flank pain, cellulitis, facial edema, fluid imbalance, pallor, lymph disorders, acidosis, hypothermia, ascites. **GI:** ***GI hemorrhage,*** abdominal pain, various GI disorders, diarrhea, constipation, dyspepsia, abdominal distension, hepatosplenomegaly, hepatitis, ulcer, unspecified liver disorders. **CV:** Arrhythmias, flushing, hypotension, hypertension, phlebitis, ***cardiac failure, cardiac arrest, stroke,*** MI, enlarged heart, heart murmur, ischemia, myo-

carditis, pericarditis, pulmonary hypertension, secondary cardiomyopathy. **CNS:** Dizziness, paresthesias, anxiety, insomnia, depression, confusion, ***cerebral hemorrhage, intracranial hypertension,*** agitation, hallucinations, abnormal gait, agnosia, aphasia, asterixis, cerebellar edema, cerebellar disorders, ***convulsions, coma,*** CNS depression, dysarthria, encephalopathy, facial paralysis, hemiplegia, hyporeflexia, hypotaxia, no light reflex, neurologic reaction, spinal cord disorder, tremor, leg weakness, unconsciousness, dementia, forgetfulness, somnolence, slow speech. **GU:** Renal insufficiency, dysuria, acute renal failure, micturition frequency, renal tubular necrosis, enlarged prostate. **Otic:** Earache, feeling of fullness in the ears, hearing loss, unspecified auricular disorders, irreversible hearing loss. **Other:** Erythema nodosum, basophilia, hyperhistaminemia, Sweet's syndrome, organomegaly, hypercalcemia, pancreatitis, myositis.

LABORATORY TEST CONSIDERATIONS

Elevated LFTs following use of PO product.

DRUG INTERACTIONS

1. Concomitant use of topical tretinoin products with sulfur, resorcinol, benzoyl peroxide, or salicylic acid may cause significant skin irritation.
2. Do not use topical tretinoin products with fluoroquinolones, phenothiazines, sulfonamides, tetracycles, and thiazides (all known photosensitizers) due to the possibility of increased phototoxicity.

HOW SUPPLIED

Cream: 0.02%, 0.025%, 0.05%, 0.1%; *Gel:* 0.01%, 0.025%, 0.1%; *Liquid:* 0.05%; *Capsules:* 10 mg

DOSAGE

• **CREAM, GEL, OR LIQUID**

Acne vulgaris.

Apply lightly over the affected areas once daily at bedtime. Beneficial effects many not be seen for 2–6 weeks.

• **CREAM, 0.025%, 0.05%, 0.1%**

Palliation for skin conditions.

Apply once daily at bedtime, using only enough to lightly cover the entire affected area. Up to 6 months of therapy may be needed before effects are seen.

• **CAPSULES**

APL.

Adults: 45 mg/m²/day given as two evenly divided doses. Given until complete remission is obtained. Discontinue 30 days after achieving complete remission or after 90 days of treatment, whichever comes first.

NURSING CONSIDERATIONS

ADMINISTRATION/STORAGE

1. Apply the liquid carefully with the fingertip, cotton swab, or gauze pad only to affected areas.
2. Excessive amounts of the gel will cause a "pilling" effect which minimizes the likelihood of overapplication.
3. Wash hands thoroughly immediately after applying tretinoin.
4. Before applying Renova, wash the face gently with a mild soap and pat the skin dry, waiting 20–30 min before applying. When applied, take care to avoid contact with eyes, ears, nostrils, and mouth.
5. Do not freeze Renova cream.
6. Treatment with Renova for more than 24 weeks does not appear to increase improvement. The results of continued irritation of the skin for more than 48 weeks are not known.

ASSESSMENT

1. Note indications for therapy, type, onset, and characteristics of symptoms.
2. With acne, thoroughly describe pretreatment skin condition; obtain photographs to compare with results of therapy.
3. Determine if pregnant.
4. Monitor hematologic, liver, and renal function studies.

CLIENT/FAMILY TEACHING

Topical:

1. Keep away from normal skin, mucous membranes, eyes, ears, mouth, nostrils, and nose angles.
2. Wash with mild soap and warm water and pat skin dry. Wait 20–30 min before applying tretinoin. Do not wash face for 1 hr or more after applying tretinoin.

3. On application there will be a transitory feeling of warmth and stinging.
4. Wash hands thoroughly before and after applying tretinoin.
5. Expect dryness and peeling of skin from the affected areas.
6. May be more sensitive to wind and cold. Do not apply to wind or sunburned skin or to open wounds.
7. Avoid alcohol-containing preparations such as shaving lotions and creams, perfumes, cosmetics with drying effects, skin cleansers, and medicated soaps.
8. Initially, lesions may worsen, caused by the effect of the drug on deep lesions that had been previously undetected. Report if lesions become severe; discontinue drug until skin integrity restored.
9. Improvement should be evident in 6 weeks but therapy should be continued for at least 3 months.
10. Practice reliable birth control.
11. Avoid excessive exposure to sunlamps and to the sun. If exposed, use a sunscreen and protective clothing over affected areas.

Oral:

1. Drug will be administered until complete remission is obtained. It will be stopped 30 days after remission or after 90 days of therapy, whichever comes first. This does not replace standard maintenance chemotherapy for APL.
2. Take with food to enhance absorption. Follow a low fat diet and exercise regularly to reduce drug induced elevated triglyceride levels.
3. Take exactly as prescribed; do not exceed or skip doses.
4. Review list of potential drug side effects, noting those that require immediate reporting. Avoid pregnancy.
5. Do not donate blood while on this therapy as it may cause harm.

OUTCOMES/EVALUATE

- ↓ Size/number of acne eruptions
- Clearing of skin condition; symptomatic improvement
- Remission with APL

Triamcinolone

(try-am-**SIN**-oh-lohn)

PREGNANCY CATEGORY: C
Rx: Dental Paste: Kenalog in Orabase, Oracort, Oralone. **Tablets:** Aristocort, Atolone, Kenacort

Triamcinolone acetonide

(try-am-**SIN**-oh-lohn)

PREGNANCY CATEGORY: C
Rx: Inhalation Aerosol: Azmacort, **Parenteral:** Kenaject-40. **Topical Aerosol:** Kenalog. **Topical Cream:** Aristocort. **Topical Lotion:** Kenalog. **Topical Ointment:** Aristocort, Aristocort A, Aristocort A, Delta-Tritex, Flutex, Kenac, Kenalog, Kenalog-10 and -40, Kenalog-H, Kenonel, Nasacort, Nasacort AQ, Tac-3 and -40, Triacet, Triam-A, Triamonide 40, Triaderm, Triderm, Tri-Kort, Trilog, Tri-Nasal
✱**Rx: Dental Paste:** Oracort.

Triamcinolone diacetate

(try-am-**SIN**-oh-lohn)

PREGNANCY CATEGORY: C
Rx: Aristocort Intralesional. **Parenteral:** Amcort, Aristocort Forte, Clinacort, Triam-Forte, Trilone, Tristoject. **Syrup:** Kenacort Syrup
✱**Rx: Parenteral:** Aristocort Parenteral. **Syrup:** Aristocort Syrup

Triamcinolone hexacetonide

(try-am-**SIN**-oh-lohn)

PREGNANCY CATEGORY: C
Rx: Aristospan Intra-Articular, Aristospan Intralesional
CLASSIFICATION(S):
Glucocorticoid

SEE ALSO *CORTICOSTEROIDS*.

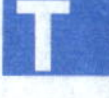

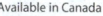

ACTION/KINETICS

More potent than prednisone. Intermediate-acting. Has no mineralocorticoid activity. **Onset:** Several hours. **Duration:** One or more weeks. **$t^{1/2}$:** Over 200 min.

ADDITIONAL USES

(1) Pulmonary emphysema accompanied by bronchospasm or bronchial edema. (2) Diffuse interstitial pulmonary fibrosis. (3) With diuretics to treat refractory CHF or cirrhosis of the liver with ascites. (4) Multiple sclerosis. (5) Inflammation following dental procedures. **Triamcinolone acetonide:** (1) PO inhalation is used for maintenance treatment of asthma. (2) Nasally for seasonal and perennial allergic rhinitis in adults and children 6 years and older. **Triamcinolone hexacetonide:** Restricted to intra-articular or intralesional treatment of rheumatoid arthritis and osteoarthritis.

SPECIAL CONCERNS

Use during pregnancy only if benefits clearly outweigh risks. Use with special caution with decreased renal function or renal disease. Dose must be highly individualized.

ADDITIONAL SIDE EFFECTS

Intra-articular, intrasynovial, or intrabursal administration may cause transient flushing, dizziness, local depigmentation, and rarely, local irritation. Exacerbation of symptoms has also been reported. A marked increase in swelling and pain and further restricted joint movement may indicate septic arthritis. Intradermal injection may cause local vesicular ulceration and persistent scarring. ***Syncope and anaphylactoid reactions*** have been reported with triamcinolone regardless of route of administration.

HOW SUPPLIED

Triamcinolone: *Tablet:* 1 mg, 2 mg, 4 mg, 8 mg. **Triamcinolone acetonide:** *Metered dose inhaler (nasal):* 50 mcg/inh, 55 mcg/inh; *Metered dose inhaler (oral)* 100 mcg/inh; *Cream:* 0.025%, 0.1%, 0.5%; *Injection, Suspension:* 3 mg/mL, 10 mg/mL, 40 mg/mL; *Lotion:* 0.025%, 0.1%; *Ointment:* 0.025%, 0.05%, 0.1%, 0.5%; *Paste:* 0.1%; *Topical Spray:* 0.147 mg/g. **Triamcinolone diacetate:** *Injection:* 25 mg/mL, 40 mg/mL; *Syrup:* 4 mg/5mL; **Triamcinolone hexacetonide:** *Injection:* 5 mg/mL, 20 mg/mL.

DOSAGE

TRIAMCINOLONE

• **TABLETS**

Adrenocortical insufficiency (with mineralocorticoid therapy).

4–12 mg/day.

Acute leukemias (children).

1–2 mg/kg.

Acute leukemia or lymphoma (adults).

16–40 mg/day (up to 100 mg/day may be necessary for leukemia).

Edema.

16–20 mg (up to 48 mg may be required until diuresis occurs).

Tuberculosis meningitis.

32–48 mg/day.

Rheumatic disease, dermatologic disorders, bronchial asthma.

8–16 mg/day.

SLE.

20–32 mg/day.

Allergies.

8–12 mg/day.

Hematologic disorders.

16–60 mg/day.

Ophthalmologic diseases.

12–40 mg daily.

Respiratory diseases.

16–48 mg/day.

TRIAMCINOLONE ACETONIDE

• **IM ONLY (NOT FOR IV USE)**

2.5–60 mg/day, depending on the disease and its severity.

• **INTRA-ARTICULAR, INTRABURSAL, TENDON SHEATHS**

2.5–5 mg for smaller joints and 5–15 mg for larger joints, although up to 40 mg has been used.

• **INTRADERMAL**

1 mg/injection site (use 3 mg/mL or 10 mg/mL suspension only).

• **TOPICAL: 0.025%, 0.1%, 0.5% OINTMENT OR CREAM; 0.025%, 0.1% LOTION; 0.1% PASTE; AEROSOL (TO DELIVER 0.2 MG)**

Apply sparingly to affected area b.i.d.–q.i.d. and rub in lightly.

• **METERED DOSE INHALER (AZMACORT)**

Adults, usual: 2 inhalations (200 mcg) t.i.d.–q.i.d. or 4 inhalations (400 mcg) b.i.d., not to exceed 1,600 mcg/day. High initial doses (1,200–1,600 mcg/day) may be needed in some clients with severe asthma. **Pediatric, 6–12 years:** 1–2 inhalations (100–200 mcg) t.i.d.–q.i.d. or 2–4 inhalations b.i.d., not to exceed 1,200 mcg/day. Use in children less than 6 years of age has not been determined.

• **INTRANASAL SPRAY (NASACORT, NASACORT AQ)**

Seasonal and perennial allergic rhinitis.

Adults and children over 6 years of age: 2 sprays (110 mcg) into each nostril once a day (i.e., for a total dose of 220 mcg/day). In adults, the dose may be increased to 440 mcg/day given either once daily or q.i.d. (1 spray/nostril). If using Nasacort AQ in children, start with 110 mcg/day given as 1 spray in each nostril/day; maximum dose is 220 mcg/day as 2 sprays/nostril once daily.

TRIAMCINOLONE DIACETATE

• **IM ONLY**

40 mg/week.

• **INTRA-ARTICULAR, INTRASYNOVIAL**

5–40 mg.

• **INTRALESIONAL, SUBLESIONAL**

5–48 mg (no more than 12.5 mg/injection site and 25 mg/lesion).

TRIAMCINOLONE HEXACETONIDE

Not for IV use.

• **INTRA-ARTICULAR**

2–6 mg for small joints and 10–20 mg for large joints.

• **INTRALESIONAL/SUBLESIONAL**

Up to 0.5 mg/sq. in. of affected area.

NURSING CONSIDERATIONS

SEE ALSO *NURSING CONSIDERATIONS* FOR *CORTICOSTEROIDS*.

ADMINISTRATION/STORAGE

1. Initially, use the aerosol concomitantly with a systemic steroid. After 1 week, initiate a gradual withdrawal of systemic steroid. Make the next reduction after 1–2 weeks, depending on the response. If symptoms of insufficiency occur, the dose of systemic steroid can be increased temporarily. Also, the dose of systemic steroid may need to be increased in times of stress or a severe asthmatic attack.
2. Do not use the acetonide products if they clump due to exposure to freezing temperatures.
3. A single IM dose of the diacetate provides control from 4–7 days up to 3–4 weeks.
4. Triamcinolone acetonide nasal spray for allergic rhinitis may be effective as soon as 12 hr after initiation of therapy. Reevaluate if improvement is not seen within 2–3 weeks.
5. For best results, store the canister at room temperature and shake well before use.
6. Nasacort AQ is viscous at rest but a liquid when shaken. This allows the drug to stay in the nasal airways at the site of inflammation for up to 2 hr.

ASSESSMENT

1. Document indications for therapy; note type, onset, and characteristics of symptoms.
2. Assess area/condition requiring treatment and describe findings.
3. Monitor blood sugar, CBC, electrolytes, and renal function.

CLIENT/FAMILY TEACHING

1. Take at the same time each day.
2. Ingest a liberal amount of protein; with regular use may experience gradual weight loss, associated with anorexia, muscle wasting, and weakness. See dietitian for assistance in meal plans/preparation.
3. Lie down if feeling faint; report if syncopal episodes persist and interfere with daily activities.
4. Report any evidence of abnormal bruising, bleeding, weight gain, edema, or dyspnea.
5. Drug may suppress reactions to skin allergy testing.
6. With topical therapy, apply to clean, slightly moist skin. Report if area does not improve with therapy or if symptoms worsen.
7. With nasal spray or inhaler, review appropriate method of administration and proper care and storage of equipment. Always rinse mouth and equipment after use.
8. Report immediately any new onset of depression as well as aggravation of existing depressive symptoms.

T

OUTCOMES/EVALUATE

- ↓ Immune and inflammatory responses in autoimmune disorders and allergic reactions
- Improved airway exchange
- Restoration of skin integrity
- Relief of pain/inflammation; improved joint mobility

Triamterene

(try-**AM**-ter-een)

PREGNANCY CATEGORY: B
CLASSIFICATION(S):
Diuretic, potassium-sparing
Rx: Dyrenium

SEE ALSO *DIURETICS*.

ACTION/KINETICS

Acts directly on the distal tubule to promote the excretion of sodium—which is exchanged for potassium or hydrogen ions—bicarbonate, chloride, and fluid. It increases urinary pH and is a weak folic acid antagonist. **Onset:** 2–4 hr. **Peak effect:** 6–8 hr. **Duration:** 7–9 hr. **t½:** 3 hr. From one-half to two-thirds of the drug is bound to plasma protein. Metabolized to hydroxytriamterene sulfate, which is also active. About 20% is excreted unchanged through the urine.

USES

Edema due to CHF, hepatic cirrhosis, nephrotic syndrome, steroid therapy, secondary hyperaldosteronism, and idiopathic edema. May be used alone or with other diuretics. *Investigational:* Prophylaxis and treatment of hypokalemia, adjunct in the treatment of hypertension.

CONTRAINDICATIONS

Hypersensitivity to drug, severe or progressive renal insufficiency, severe hepatic disease, anuria, hyperkalemia, hyperuricemia, gout, history of nephrolithiasis. Lactation.

SPECIAL CONCERNS

Safety and efficacy have not been determined in children.

SIDE EFFECTS

Electrolyte: Hyperkalemia, electrolyte imbalance. **GI:** Nausea, vomiting (may also be indicative of electrolyte imbalance), diarrhea, dry mouth. **CNS:** Dizziness, drowsiness, fatigue, weakness, headache. **Hematologic:** Megaloblastic anemia, thrombocytopenia. **Renal:** Azotemia, interstitial nephritis. **Miscellaneous:** ***Anaphylaxis,*** photosensitivity, hypokalemia, jaundice, muscle cramps, rash.

LABORATORY TEST CONSIDERATIONS

Triamterene may impart blue fluorescence to urine, interfering with fluorometric assays (e.g., lactic dehydrogenase, quinidine). ↑ BUN, creatinine. ↑ Serum uric acid in clients predisposed to gouty arthritis.

OD OVERDOSE MANAGEMENT

Symptoms: Electrolyte imbalance, especially hyperkalemia. Also, nausea, vomiting, other GI disturbances, weakness, hypotension, reversible acute renal failure. *Treatment:* Immediately induce vomiting or perform gastric lavage. Evaluate electrolyte levels and fluid balance and treat if necessary. Dialysis may be beneficial.

DRUG INTERACTIONS

Amantadine / ↑ Toxic amantadine effects R/T ↓ renal excretion
Angiotensin-converting enzyme inhibitors / Significant hyperkalemia
Antihypertensives / Potentiated by triamterene
Captopril / ↑ Risk of significant hyperkalemia
Cimetidine / ↑ Bioavailability and ↓ clearance of triamterene
Digitalis / Inhibited by triamterene
Indomethacin / ↑ Risk of nephrotoxicity and acute renal failure
Lithium / ↑ Chance of toxicity R/T ↓ renal clearance
Potassium salts / Additive hyperkalemia
Spironolactone / Additive hyperkalemia

HOW SUPPLIED

Capsule: 50 mg, 100 mg

DOSAGE

- **Capsules.**
  Diuretic.

Adults, initial: 100 mg b.i.d. after meals; **maximum daily dose:** 300 mg.

NURSING CONSIDERATIONS

SEE ALSO *NURSING CONSIDERATIONS* FOR *DIURETICS*.

ADMINISTRATION/STORAGE

1. Minimize nausea by giving the drug after meals.
2. Dosage is usually reduced by one-half when another diuretic is added to the regimen.

ASSESSMENT

1. Document indications for therapy; list agents prescribed to ensure none interact.
2. Assess for alcoholism; megaloblastic anemia may occur because triamterene is a weak antagonist of folic acid.
3. Monitor ECG, CBC, uric acid, electrolytes, and renal function.

CLIENT/FAMILY TEACHING

1. Take in the am with food to minimize GI upset/nausea.
2. Report any sore throat, rash, or fever (S&S of blood dyscrasia) or lack of effectiveness.
3. Persistent headaches, drowsiness, vomiting, restlessness, mental wandering, lethargy, and foul breath may be signs of uremia; report.
4. Drug may cause dizziness.
5. Avoid alcohol and OTC agents. Also avoid potassium supplements, salt substitutes that contain potassium, and foods high in potassium; drug is potassium-sparing.
6. Urine may appear pale fluorescent blue.
7. Avoid direct sunlight for prolonged periods; may cause a photosensitivity reaction. Use sunscreens, sunglasses, hat, and long sleeves and pants when exposed.

OUTCOMES/EVALUATE

↓ Edema; ↑ diuresis; ↓ BP

Triazolam

(try-**AYZ**-oh-lam)

PREGNANCY CATEGORY: X
CLASSIFICATION(S):
Sedative-hypnotic, benzodiazepine
Rx: Halcion , **C-IV**
🍁**Rx:** Apo-Triazo, Gen-Triazolam

SEE ALSO *TRANQUILIZERS, ANTIMANIC DRUGS, AND HYPNOTICS*.

ACTION/KINETICS

Decreases sleep latency, increases the duration of sleep, and decreases the number of awakenings. **Time to peak plasma levels:** 0.5–2 hr. **t½:** 1.5–5.5 hr. Metabolized in liver; inactive metabolites excreted in the urine.

USES

Insomnia (short-term management, not to exceed 1 month). May be beneficial in preventing or treating transient insomnia from a sudden change in sleep schedule.

CONTRAINDICATIONS

Use concomitantly with itraconazole, ketoconazole, nefaxodone. Lactation (may cause sedation and feeding problems in infants).

SPECIAL CONCERNS

Safety and efficacy in children under 18 years of age not established. Geriatric clients may be more sensitive to the effects of triazolam.

SIDE EFFECTS

CNS: Rebound insomnia, anterograde amnesia, headache, ataxia, decreased coordination, "traveler's" amnesia. Psychologic and physical dependence. **GI:** N&V.

DRUG INTERACTIONS

↑ Triazolam effect when used with azole antifungals, clarithromycin, erythromycin, grapefruit juice, protease inhibitors, and selective serotonin reuptake inhibitors R/T ↓ liver metabolism.

HOW SUPPLIED

Tablet: 0.125 mg, 0.25 mg

DOSAGE

• **TABLETS**

Adults, initial: 0.25–0.5 mg before bedtime. **Geriatric or debilitated clients, initial:** 0.125 mg; **then,** depending on response, 0.125–0.25 mg before bedtime.

NURSING CONSIDERATIONS

SEE ALSO *NURSING CONSIDERATIONS* FOR *TRANQUILIZERS, ANTIMANIC DRUGS, AND HYPNOTICS*.

T

ASSESSMENT

1. Document indications for therapy, onset, duration, and characteristics of symptoms.
2. Assess mental status and note behavioral manifestations.
3. Monitor CBC and LFTs.
4. Evaluate sleep patterns; determine underlying cause of insomnia so that source may be removed. With simple insomnia, try nonpharmacologic interventions to induce sleep, such as soft music, guided imagery, or progressive muscle relaxation.
5. Initiate safety precautions (i.e., side rails, supervised ambulation, frequent observations), especially with elderly and confused clients.
6. Assess for tolerance and for psychologic and physical dependence. Monitor closely for CNS toxic effects especially during prolonged therapy (longer than 2 weeks).

CLIENT/FAMILY TEACHING

1. Take only as directed. Store away from bedside.
2. Avoid alcohol and CNS depressants.
3. Use caution when driving or operating machinery until daytime sedative effects evaluated.
4. Drug is for short-term use only; may cause physical and psychologic dependence. Try warm baths/milk, and other methods to induce sleep, such as white noise simulator, soft music, guided imagery, or progressive muscle relaxation, rather than become dependent on drugs for insomnia.
5. Report unusual side effects including hallucinations, nightmares, depression, or periods of confusion.

OUTCOMES/EVALUATE

Improved sleeping patterns; insomnia relief

Trifluoperazine

(try-**flew**-oh-**PER**-ah-zeen)

PREGNANCY CATEGORY: C
CLASSIFICATION(S):
Antipsychotic, phenothiazine

Rx: Stelazine
★**Rx:** Apo-Trifluoperazine

SEE ALSO *ANTIPSYCHOTIC AGENTS, PHENOTHIAZINES.*

ACTION/KINETICS

Causes a high incidence of extrapyramidal symptoms and antiemetic effects and a low incidence of sedation, orthostatic hypotension, and anticholinergic side effects. **Maximum therapeutic effect:** Usually 2–3 weeks after initiation of therapy.

USES

(1) To manage psychotic disorders. Suitable for clients with apathy or withdrawal. (2) Short-term treatment of nonpsychotic anxiety (not the drug of choice).

SPECIAL CONCERNS

Use during pregnancy only when benefits clearly outweigh risks. Dosage has not been established in children less than 6 years of age. Geriatric, emaciated, or debilitated clients usually require a lower initial dose.

HOW SUPPLIED

Injection: 2 mg/mL; *Oral Concentrate:* 10 mg/mL; *Tablet:* 1 mg, 2 mg, 5 mg, 10 mg

DOSAGE

• **ORAL CONCENTRATE, TABLETS**

Psychotic disorders.

Adults and adolescents, initial: 2–5 mg (base) b.i.d.; **maintenance:** 15–20 mg/day in two or three divided doses. **Pediatric, 6–12 years:** 1 mg (base) 1–2 times/day; adjust dose as required and tolerated.

Anxiety.

Adults and adolescents: 1–2 mg b.i.d, not to exceed 6 mg/day. Not to be given for this purpose longer than 12 weeks.

• **IM**

Pyschoses.

Adults: 1–2 mg q 4–6 hr, not to exceed 10 mg/day. Switch to PO therapy as soon as possible. **Pediatric:** *Severe symptoms only:* 1 mg 1–2 times/day.

NURSING CONSIDERATIONS

SEE ALSO *NURSING CONSIDERATIONS* FOR *ANTIPSYCHOTIC AGENTS, PHENOTHIAZINES.*

ADMINISTRATION/STORAGE

1. Dilute concentrate just before administration with 60 mL of juice (tomato or fruit), carbonated drinks, water, milk, orange or simple syrup, coffee, tea, or semisolid foods (e.g., applesauce, pudding, soup).
2. Protect liquid forms from light.
3. Discard strongly colored solutions.
4. Avoid skin contact with liquid form to prevent contact dermatitis.
5. To prevent cumulative effects, allow at least 4 hr between injections.

ASSESSMENT

1. Document indications for therapy, onset of symptoms, and behavioral manifestations.
2. Note other agents prescribed and the outcome.
3. Assess/note mental status findings.
4. Monitor CBC, ECG, and LFTs.

CLIENT/FAMILY TEACHING

1. Take exactly as prescribed; prevent skin contact with solution.
2. Avoid activities that require mental alertness until drug effects realized.
3. Consume plenty of fluids to prevent dehydration; use caution in hot weather to prevent heatstroke.
4. Use sunscreen and protective clothing when out and avoid prolonged sun exposure.
5. Report any unusual side effects or lack/loss of response.

OUTCOMES/EVALUATE

- Reduction in paranoid, excitable, or withdrawn behaviors
- ↓ Levels of anxiety, tension, and agitation

Trifluridine

(try-**FLUR**-ih-deen)

PREGNANCY CATEGORY: C
CLASSIFICATION(S):
Antiviral
Rx: Viroptic

SEE ALSO *ANTI-INFECTIVES* AND *ANTIVIRAL DRUGS.*

ACTION/KINETICS

Closely resembles thymidine; inhibits thymidylic phosphorylase and specific DNA polymerases necessary for incorporation of thymidine into viral DNA. Trifluridine, instead of thymidine, is incorporated into viral DNA, resulting in faulty DNA and the ability to infect or reproduce in tissue. Also incorporated into mammalian DNA. Has activity against herpes simplex virus types 1 and 2 and vaccinia virus. **t½:** 12–18 min.

USES

(1) Primary keratoconjunctivitis and recurrent epithelial keratitis caused by HSV types 1 and 2. (2) Epithelial keratitis resistant to idoxuridine or if ocular toxicity or hypersensitivity to idoxuridine has occurred. (3) Infections resistant to vidarabine.

CONTRAINDICATIONS

Hypersensitivity or chemical intolerance to drug.

SPECIAL CONCERNS

Safe use during pregnancy not established. Use with caution during lactation.

SIDE EFFECTS

Ophthalmic: Mild, transient burning or stinging when instilled. Palpebral edema, superficial punctate keratopathy, epithelial keratopathy, hypersensitivity reaction, stomal edema, irritation, eratitis sicca, hyperemia, increased IOP.

HOW SUPPLIED

Ophthalmic Solution: 1%

DOSAGE

- **SOLUTION, 1%**

1 gtt solution q 2 hr onto cornea, up to maximum of 9 gtt/day in each eye during acute stage (presence of corneal ulcer). Following reepithelialization, decrease dosage to 1 gtt/4 hr (or minimum of 5 gtt/day in each eye) for 7 days. Do not use for more than 21 days.

NURSING CONSIDERATIONS

SEE ALSO *GENERAL NURSING CONSIDERATIONS* FOR *ANTI-INFECTIVES* AND *ANTIVIRAL DRUGS.*

ADMINISTRATION/STORAGE

1. May be used concomitantly in the eye with antibiotics (chloramphenicol, bacitracin, polymyxin B sulfate, erythromycin, neomycin, gentamicin, tetracycline, sulfacetamide sodium), corticosteroids, anticholinergics, epinephrine HCl, and NaCl.
2. Drug is heat-sensitive. Store in refrigerator at 2–8°C (36–46°F).

CLIENT/FAMILY TEACHING

1. Instill drop onto cornea. Apply finger pressure lightly to inside corner of eye for 1 min after instillation.
2. A mild, transient burning sensation may occur on instillation.
3. Report any new or bothersome side effects but do not stop medication without specific instructions as herpetic keratitis may recur. Have regular eye exams.
4. Improvement usually occurs within 7 days and healing takes place within 14 days. Thereafter, 7 more days of therapy are necessary to prevent recurrence. Report if no improvement noted within 7 days.
5. Do not administer for more than 21 days because toxicity may occur (discard remaining drug after 21 days).
6. Store drug in refrigerator.

OUTCOMES/EVALUATE

- Resolution of infection
- Reepithelialization of herpetic eye lesions

Trihexyphenidyl hydrochloride

(try-hex-ee-**FEN**-ih-dill)

PREGNANCY CATEGORY: C
CLASSIFICATION(S):
Antiparkinson drug
Rx: Artane, Artane Sequels, Trihexy-2 and -5
✱**Rx:** Apo-Trihex

SEE ALSO *CHOLINERGIC BLOCKING AGENTS* AND *ANTIPARKINSON DRUGS*.

ACTION/KINETICS

Synthetic anticholinergic, which relieves rigidity but has little effect on tremors. Causes a direct antispasmodic effect on smooth muscle. High incidence of side effects. Small doses cause CNS depression, whereas larger doses may result in CNS excitation. **Onset, PO:** 60 min. **Duration, PO:** 6–12 hr.

USES

(1) Adjunct in the treatment of all types of parkinsonism (arteriosclerotic, idiopathic, drug- or chemical-induced, postencephalitic). As an adjunct to levodopa/carbidopa. (2) Drug-induced extrapyramidal symptoms. Sustained-release medication is for maintenance dosage only.

ADDITIONAL CONTRAINDICATIONS

Arteriosclerosis and hypersensitivity to drug.

ADDITIONAL SIDE EFFECTS

Serious CNS stimulation (restlessness, insomnia, delirium, agitation) and psychotic manifestations.

ADDITIONAL DRUG INTERACTIONS

↑ Effectiveness with levodopa; do not use together for psychoses.

HOW SUPPLIED

Capsules, sustained-release: 5 mg; *Elixir:* 2 mg/5 mL; *Tablet:* 2 mg, 5 mg

DOSAGE

- **ELIXIR, SUSTAINED-RELEASE CAPSULES, TABLETS**

Parkinsonism.

Initial (day 1): 1–2 mg; **then,** increase by 2 mg q 3–5 days until daily dose is 6–10 mg given in divided doses. Some clients may require 12–15 mg/day (especially those with postencephalitic parkinsonism).

Adjunct with levodopa.

Adults: 3–6 mg/day in divided doses.

Drug-induced extrapyramidal reactions.

Initial: 1 mg/day; **then,** increase as needed to total daily dose of 5–15 mg.

NURSING CONSIDERATIONS

SEE ALSO *NURSING CONSIDERATIONS FOR CHOLINERGIC BLOCKING AGENTS* AND *ANTIPARKINSON DRUGS*.

ASSESSMENT

Assess for and note extent of involuntary movements, drooling, pill rolling, and muscle spasms/rigidity. Note mental status.

CLIENT/FAMILY TEACHING

1. Take with or after meals to minimize GI upset.
2. May cause dizziness or drowsiness and othostatic effects.
3. Increase fluids and bulk in diet to prevent constipation.
4. May impair perspiration; avoid overheating and hot weather exposures. Report urinary retention.
5. This drug has a high incidence of side effects; report as early detection and intervention are imperative.
6. Report any evidence of extrapyramidal symptoms or increase in restlessness, insomnia, agitation, or psychotic manifestations; dosage may need adjusting.

OUTCOMES/EVALUATE

- Control of S&S of parkinsonism
- Prevention of drug-induced extrapyramidal symptoms

Trimethobenzamide hydrochloride

(try-meth-oh-**BENZ**-ah-myd)

PREGNANCY CATEGORY: C
CLASSIFICATION(S):
Antiemetic
Rx: Pediatric Triban, Tebamide, T-Gen, Ticon, Tigan, Trimazide

SEE ALSO *ANTIEMETICS.*

ACTION/KINETICS

Related to the antihistamines but with weak antihistaminic properties. Less effective than the phenothiazines but has fewer side effects. Not suitable as sole agent for severe emesis. Can be used PR. Appears to control vomiting by depressing the CTZ in the medulla. **Onset: PO and IM,** 10–40 min. **Duration:** 3–4 hr after PO and 2–3 hr after IM. 30%–50% of drug excreted unchanged in urine in 48–72 hr.

USES

Control of nausea and vomiting.

CONTRAINDICATIONS

Hypersensitivity to drug, benzocaine, or similar local anesthetics. Use of suppositories premature infants or neonates; IM use in children.

SPECIAL CONCERNS

Use during pregnancy only if benefits outweigh risks. Use with caution during lactation.

SIDE EFFECTS

CNS: Depression of mood, disorientation, headache, drowsiness, dizziness, ***seizures, coma,*** Parkinson-like symptoms. **Other:** Hypersensitivity reactions, hypotension, blood dyscrasias, jaundice, muscle cramps, opisthotonos, blurred vision, diarrhea, allergic skin reactions. **After IM injection:** Pain, burning, stinging, redness at injection site.

DRUG INTERACTIONS

Avoid use with atropine-like drugs and CNS depressants, including alcohol.

HOW SUPPLIED

Capsule: 100 mg, 250 mg; *Injection:* 100 mg/mL; *Solution:* 50 mg/5 mL; *Suppository:* 100 mg, 200 mg

DOSAGE

- **CAPSULES, SOLUTION**

Adults: 250 mg t.i.d.–q.i.d.; **pediatric, 13.6–40.9 kg:** 100–200 mg t.i.d.–q.i.d.

- **SUPPOSITORIES**

Adults: 200 mg t.i.d.–q.i.d.; **pediatric, under 13.6 kg:** 100 mg t.i.d.–q.i.d.; **13.6–40.9 kg:** 100–200 mg t.i.d.–q.i.d.

- **IM**

Adults only: 200 mg t.i.d.–q.i.d. *IM route not to be used in children.*

NURSING CONSIDERATIONS

SEE ALSO *NURSING CONSIDERATIONS FOR ANTIEMETICS.*

ADMINISTRATION/STORAGE

1. Inject drug IM deeply into the upper, outer quadrant of the gluteus muscle. To minimize local reaction, use care to avoid escape of fluid from the needle.
2. Do not administer suppositories to clients allergic to benzocaine or similar anesthetics.

ASSESSMENT

1. Identify cause for N&V.

2. Document any sensitivity to benzocaine. Assess for any skin reaction (first sign of drug hypersensitivity).
3. Note any local reaction to the suppositories.

CLIENT/FAMILY TEACHING

1. Use only as directed; report any adverse drug effects. Store out of reach of child.
2. Do not drive or operate machinery until drug effects are realized; may cause drowsiness and dizziness.
3. Avoid alcohol and any other CNS depressants.

OUTCOMES/EVALUATE

Prevention/control of N&V

—COMBINATION DRUG—

Trimethoprim and Sulfamethoxazole

(try-**METH**-oh-prim, sul-fah-meh-**THOX**-ah-zohl)

PREGNANCY CATEGORY: C
CLASSIFICATION(S):
Antibiotic, combination
Rx: Bactrim, Bactrim DS, Bactrim Pediatric, Cotrim, Cotrim D.S., Cotrim Pediatric, Septra, Septra DS, Sulfatrim, Bactrim IV, Septra IV
✱Rx: Apo-Sulfatrim, Novo-Trimel, Novo-Trimel D.S., Nu-Cotrimix, Septra Injection

SEE ALSO *SULFONAMIDES*.

CONTENT

These products contain the antibacterial agents sulfamethoxazole and trimethoprim. See also *Sulfamethoxazole.*

Oral Suspension: Sulfamethoxazole, 200 mg and trimethoprim, 40 mg/5 mL.

Tablets: Sulfamethoxazole, 400 mg and trimethoprim, 80 mg/tablet.

Double Strength (DS) Tablets: Sulfamethoxazole, 800 mg and trimethoprim, 160 mg/tablet.

Concentrate for injection: Sulfamethoxazole, 80 mg and trimethoprim, 16 mg/mL.

USES

PO, Parenteral: (1) UTIs due to *Escherichia coli, Klebsiella, Enterobacter, Pseudomonas mirabilis* and *vulgaris,* and *Morganella morganii.* (2) Enteritis due to *Shigella flexneri* or *S. sonnei. Pneumocystis carinii* pneumonitis in children and adults. **PO:** (1) Acute otitis media in children due to *Haemophilus influenzae* or *Streptococcus pneumoniae.* (2) Traveler's diarrhea in adults due to *E. coli.* (3) Prophylaxis of *P. carinii* pneumonia in immunocompromised clients (including those with AIDS). (4) Acute exacerbations of chronic bronchitis in adults due to *H. influenzae* or *S. pneumoniae. Investigational:* Cholera, salmonella, nocardiosis, prophylaxis of recurrent UTIs in women, prophylaxis of neutropenic clients with *P. carinii* infections or leukemia clients to decrease incidence of gram-negative rod bacteremia. Treatment of acute and chronic prostatitis. Decrease chance of urinary and blood bacterial infections in renal transplant clients.

ADDITIONAL CONTRAINDICATIONS

Infants under 2 months of age. During pregnancy at term. Megaloblastic anemia due to folate deficiency. Lactation.

SPECIAL CONCERNS

Use with caution in impaired liver or kidney function and in clients with possible folate deficiency. AIDS clients may not tolerate or respond to this product.

LABORATORY TEST CONSIDERATIONS

Jaffe alkaline picrate reaction overestimation of creatinine by 10%.

ADDITIONAL DRUG INTERACTIONS

Alcohol / Possible disulfiram-like reaction
Cyclosporine / ↓ Cyclosporine effect; ↑ risk of nephrotoxicity
Dapsone / ↑ Effect of both dapsone and trimethoprim
Methotrexate / ↑ Risk of toxicity R/T displacement from plasma protein binding sites
Phenytoin / ↑ Effect R/T ↓ hepatic clearance
Sulfonylureas / ↑ Hypoglycemic effect
Thiazide diuretics / ↑ Risk of thrombocytopenia with purpura in geriatric clients
Warfarin / ↑ PT
Zidovudine / ↑ AZT serum levels R/T ↓ renal clearance

HOW SUPPLIED
See Content

DOSAGE

• ORAL SUSPENSION, DOUBLE-STRENGTH TABLETS, TABLETS

UTIs, shigellosis, bronchitis, acute otitis media.

Adults: 1 DS tablet, 2 tablets, or 4 teaspoonfuls of suspension q 12 hr for 10–14 days. **Pediatric:** Total daily dose of 8 mg/kg trimethoprim and 40 mg/kg sulfamethoxazole divided equally and given q 12 hr for 10–14 days. (*NOTE:* For shigellosis, give adult or pediatric dose for 5 days.) For clients with impaired renal function the following dosage is recommended: C_{CR} of 15–30 mL/min: one-half the usual regimen and for C_{CR} less than 15 mL/min: use is not recommended.

Chancroid.

1 DS tablet b.i.d. for at least 7 days (alternate therapy: 4 DS tablets in a single dose).

Pharyngeal gonococcal infection due to penicillinase-producing Neisseria gonorrhoeae.

720 mg trimethoprim and 3,600 mg sulfamethoxazole once daily for 5 days.

Prophylaxis of P. carinii pneumonia.

Adults: 160 mg trimethoprim and 800 mg sulfamethoxazole q 24 hr. **Children:** 150 mg/m² of trimethoprim and 750 mg/m² sulfamethoxazole daily in equally divided doses b.i.d. on three consecutive days per week. Do not exceed a total daily dose of 320 mg trimethoprim and 1,600 mg sulamethoxazole.

Treatment of P. carinii *pneumonia.*

Adults and children: Total daily dose of 15–20 mg/kg trimethoprim and 100 mg/kg sulfamethoxazole divided equally and given q 6 hr for 14–21 days.

Prophylaxis of P. carinii *pneumonia* in immunocompromised clients.

1 DS tablet daily.

Traveler's diarrhea.

Adults, 1 DS tablet q 12 hr for 5 days.

Prostatitis, acute bacterial.

1 DS tablet b.i.d. until client is afebrile for 48 hr; treatment may be required for up to 30 days.

Prostatitis, chronic bacterial.

1 DS tablet b.i.d. for 4–6 weeks.

• IV

UTIs, shigellosis, acute otitis media.

Adults and children: 8–10 mg/kg/day (based on trimethoprim) in two to four divided doses q 6, 8, or 12 hr for up to 14 days for severe UTIs or 5 days for shigellosis.

Treatment of P. carinii *pneumonia*

Adults and children: 15–20 mg/kg/day (based on trimethoprim) in 3–4 divided doses q 6–8 hr for up to 14 days.

NURSING CONSIDERATIONS

SEE ALSO *GENERAL NURSING CONSIDERATIONS FOR ALL ANTI-INFECTIVES* AND FOR *SULFONAMIDES*.

ADMINISTRATION/STORAGE

IV 1. Administer IV infusion over a 60–90 min period.

2. Each 5-mL vial must be diluted to 125 mL with D5W and used within 6 hr. If the amount of fluid should be restricted, each 5 mL can be diluted up to 75 mL with D5W and used within 2 hr. Do not refrigerate the diluted solution.

3. Do not mix the IV infusion with any other drugs or solutions.

4. If the diluted IV infusion is cloudy or precipitates after mixing, discard and prepare a new solution.

ASSESSMENT

1. Document indications for therapy, onset, duration, and characteristics of symptoms.

2. Monitor cultures, CBC, liver and renal function studies; reduce dose with renal dysfunction.

3. Assess for megaloblastic anemia; drug inhibits ability to produce folinic acid. Simultaneous administration of folinic acid (6–8 mg/day) may prevent antifolate drug effects.

4. Document if infected with AIDS virus; may be intolerant to product.

CLIENT/FAMILY TEACHING

1. Take only as directed. Complete entire prescription and do not share.

T

2. Report any symptoms of drug fever, vasculitis, N&V, rash, joint pain/swelling or CNS disturbances.
3. Consume 2.5–3 L of fluids/day.

OUTCOMES/EVALUATE

- Resolution of infection
- *P. carinii* pneumonia prophylaxis

Trimipramine maleate

(try-**MIP**-rah-meen)

PREGNANCY CATEGORY: C
CLASSIFICATION(S):
Antidepressant, tricyclic
Rx: Surmontil
✱Rx: Apo-Trimip, Novo-Tripramine, Nu-Trimipramine, Rhotrimine

SEE ALSO *ANTIDEPRESSANTS, TRICYCLIC.*

ACTION/KINETICS
Causes moderate anticholinergic and orthostatic hypotensive effects and significant sedative effects. **Effective plasma levels:** 180 ng/mL. **Time to reach steady state:** 2–6 days. **t½:** 7–30 hr.

USES
Treatment of symptoms of depression. PUD. May be more effective in endogenous depression than in other types of depression.

CONTRAINDICATIONS
Use in children less than 12 years of age.

HOW SUPPLIED
Capsule: 25 mg, 50 mg, 100 mg

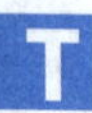

DOSAGE

- **CAPSULES**

Antidepressant.

Adults, outpatients, initial: 75 mg/day in divided doses up to 150 mg/day, but not to exceed 200 mg/day; **maintenance:** 50–150 mg/day. Total dose can be given at bedtime. **Adults, hospitalized, initial:** 100 mg/day in divided doses up to 200 mg/day. If no improvement in 2–3 weeks, increase to 250–300 mg/day. **Adolescent/geriatric clients, initial:** 50 mg/day up to 100 mg/day. Not recommended for children.

NURSING CONSIDERATIONS

SEE ALSO *NURSING CONSIDERATIONS FOR ANTIDEPRESSANTS, TRICYCLIC.*

ADMINISTRATION/STORAGE
To minimize relapse, continue maintenance therapy for about 3 months.

ASSESSMENT
Document indications for therapy, onset, duration, and characteristics of symptoms. Note any predisposing factors/events.

CLIENT/FAMILY TEACHING

1. Take as prescribed. Do not stop suddenly after long-term use.
2. Avoid activities that require mental alertness, may cause dizziness and drowsiness.
3. Use protection and avoid prolonged sun exposure.
4. Avoid alcohol and any other CNS depressants.
5. Report any unusual side effects. Desired effects may take 2-3 weeks.

OUTCOMES/EVALUATE

- ↓ Depressive symptoms
- Control of symptoms of PUD

Tripelennamine hydrochloride

(try-pell-**EN**-ah-meen)

CLASSIFICATION(S):
Antihistamine, first generation, ethylenediamine
Rx: PBZ, PBZ-SR

SEE ALSO *ANTIHISTAMINES.*

ACTION/KINETICS
GI effects more pronounced than other antihistamines. Moderate sedative effects and low to no anticholinergic activity. **Duration:** 4–6 hr.

CONTRAINDICATIONS
Use in neonates.

SPECIAL CONCERNS
Safe use during pregnancy has not been established. Geriatric clients may be more sensitive to the usual adult dose.

SIDE EFFECTS
Low incidence. Moderate sedation, mild GI distress, paradoxical excitation, hyperirritability.

HOW SUPPLIED
Tablet: 25 mg, 50 mg; *Tablet, Extended Release:* 100 mg

DOSAGE

• **TABLETS**

Adults, usual: 25–50 mg q 4–6 hr; as little as 25 mg or as high as 600 mg may be given to control symptoms. **Pediatric:** 5 mg/kg/day or 150 mg/m^2/day divided into 4–6 doses, not to exceed 300 mg/day.

• **EXTENDED-RELEASE TABLETS**

Adults: 100 mg q 8–12 hr as needed, up to a maximum of 600 mg/day. Do not use sustained-release form in children.

NURSING CONSIDERATIONS

SEE ALSO *NURSING CONSIDERATIONS* FOR *ANTIHISTAMINES*.

CLIENT/FAMILY TEACHING

1. May take with food if GI upset. Swallow extended-release tablets whole; never crush or chew.
2. Avoid alcohol; excessive sedation may occur.
3. Use caution, may cause dizziness or drowsiness.
4. Report any unusual or persistant side effects or lack of response.

OUTCOMES/EVALUATE
↓ Allergic manifestations

Triptorelin pamoate

(**TRIP**-toh-rel-in)

PREGNANCY CATEGORY: X
CLASSIFICATION(S):
Antineoplastic, gonadotropin-releasing hormone analog
Rx: Trelstar Depot, Trelstar LA

ACTION/KINETICS
A synthetic decapeptide agonist analog of luteinizing hormone releasing hormone (LHRH or GnRH). Potent inhibitor of gonadotropic secretion when given continuously. Initially, there is a transient surge in circulating LH, FSH, estradiol, and testosterone. However, after 2–4 weeks, a sustained decrease in LH and FSH secretion and marked reduction of testicular and ovarian steroidogenesis occurs. In men, levels of serum testosterone fall to those seen in surgically castrated men. Thus, tissues and functions that depend on testosterone for maintenance become quiescent. These effects are reversible upon discontinuing therapy. IM injection of the depot formulation achieves plasma levels over a 1 month period. Metabolism is unknown but probably involves hepatic microsomal enzymes. Eliminated by the liver and kidneys. Is distributed and eliminated by a 3-compartment model; **t½'s:** About 6 min, 45 min, and 3 hr.

USES
Palliative treatment of advanced prostate cancer when orchiectomy or estrogen therapy are either not indicated or unacceptable.

CONTRAINDICATIONS
Hypersensitivity to triptorelin, other components of the product, other LHRH agonists, or LHRH. Lactation.

SPECIAL CONCERNS
Initially, due to transient increase in serum testosterone levels, there may be worsening signs and symptoms of prostate cancer during the first few weeks of treatment.

SIDE EFFECTS
Worsening of signs/symptoms of prostate cancer: Bone pain, neuropathy, hematuria, urethral or bladder outlet obstruction, spinal cord compression with weakness or paralysis of lower extremities. **GI:** Vomiting, diarrhea. **CNS:** Headache, insomnia, dizziness, emotional lability. **GU:** Impotence, urinary retention, UTI. **Miscellaneous:** Hypertension, hot flushes, skeletal pain, injection site pain, pain, leg pain, fatigue, anemia, pruritus.

LABORATORY TEST CONSIDERATIONS
Suppression of the pituitary-gonadal axis may cause misleading results of diagnostic tests.

DRUG INTERACTIONS
Do not give hyperprolactinemic drugs together with triptorelin since hyperprolactinemia reduces the number of pituitary GnRH receptors.
HOW SUPPLIED
Microgranules for injection, lyophilized: 3.75 mg triptorelin peptide base

DOSAGE

- **IM ONLY**

Advanced prostate cancer

3.75 mg monthly as a single IM injection. *Note:* Trelstar LA delivers triptorelin continuously over a 3-month period.

NURSING CONSIDERATIONS

ADMINISTRATION/STORAGE

1. Alter the IM injection site periodically.
2. Prepare as follows:
• Withdraw 2 mL sterile water for injection using a syringe with a sterile 20-gauge needle. Do not use other diluents. Inject into the drug vial.
• Shake well to disperse particles thoroughly and to obtain a uniform suspension. The suspension will appear milky.
• Withdraw contents of the vial into the syringe and inject the reconstituted suspension immediately.
3. Store from 15–30°C (59–86°F).
4. Discard if not used immediately after reconstitution.

ASSESSMENT

1. Document symptom onset, PSA levels, biopsy and staging results, and other therapies trialed with the outcome.
2. Obtain and monitor PSA, renal and LFTs, and testosterone levels.

CLIENT/FAMILY TEACHING

1. Drug therapy consists of monthly IM injections. Must continue to prevent progression of disease.
2. Hot flashes may occur with drug therapy.
3. May initially experience worsening of symptoms and/or onset of new symptoms such as bone pain, blood in the urine, urethral or bladder outlet obstruction, neuropathy symptoms during the first few weeks of therapy. Immediately report any weakness, numbness, respiratory difficulty or impaired urination.
4. Identify local support groups that assist in coping with illness.

OUTCOMES/EVALUATE

↓ Prostate tumor size and spread

Tromethamine

(troh-**METH**-ah-meen)

PREGNANCY CATEGORY: C
CLASSIFICATION(S):
Alkalinizing agent
Rx: Tham

ACTION/KINETICS
Actively binds hydrogen ions, thereby decreasing and correcting acidosis. It promotes the excretion of acids, carbon dioxide, and electrolytes and is thought to be able to neutralize some intracellular acid. It acts as an osmotic diuretic, increasing urine flow. Seventy-five percent of the drug is eliminated within 8 hr, the remainder within 3 days.
USES
Prevention and correction of systemic acidosis, especially that accompanying cardiac bypass surgery, correction of acidity of acid citrate dextrose (ACD) blood in cardiac bypass surgery, and cardiac arrest.
CONTRAINDICATIONS
Uremia and anuria.
SPECIAL CONCERNS
Use with caution in newborns and infants and in clients with renal disorders.
SIDE EFFECTS
Respiratory: Respiratory depression, especially in those with chronic hypoventilation or getting drugs that depress respiration. **Other:** Fever, hypervolemia, transient decrease of blood glucose. **At injection site:** Extravasation may cause inflammation, vascular spasms, and tissue damage (e.g., chemical phlebitis, thrombosis, necrosis, sloughing). **In newborn:** ***Hemor-***

rhagic liver necrosis when given by umbilical vein.

OD OVERDOSE MANAGEMENT

Symptoms: Alkalosis, overhydration, hypoglycemia (severe and prolonged), solute overload. *Treatment:* Discontinue the infusion and treat symptoms.

HOW SUPPLIED

Injection: 3.6 g/100 mL

DOSAGE

Minimum amount to correct acid-base imbalance. The amount of tromethamine can be estimated using the buffer base deficit of the extracellular fluid: mL of 0.3 M tromethamine solution required = body weight (kg) × base deficit (mEq/L) × 1.1

• **SLOW IV INFUSION**

Acidosis in cardiac bypass surgery.

Adults: 500 mL (150 mEq or 18 g) as a single dose. Severe cases may require 1,000 mL. Do not exceed 500 mg/kg in a period less than 1 hr.

• **INJECTION INTO VENTRICULAR CAVITY OR LARGE PERIPHERAL VEIN**

Acidosis in cardiac arrest (given at the same time as other standard procedures are being applied).

If chest is open. Adults: 62–185 mL (2–6 g) into the ventricular cavity (not into the cardiac muscle). **If chest closed. Adults:** 111–333 mL (3.6–10.8 g) into a large peripheral vein.

• **ADDITION TO PUMP OXYGENATOR ACID CITRATE DEXTROSE BLOOD**

For acidity in ACD blood.

15–77 mL (0.5–2.5 g) added to each 500 mL of ACD blood. Usually 62 mL (2 g) added to 500 mL of ACD blood is adequate.

NURSING CONSIDERATIONS

ADMINISTRATION/STORAGE

IV 1. Analyze blood pH, pCO_2, HCO_3, glucose, and electrolytes before, during, and after administration.
2. Concentration of solution administered *must not* exceed 0.3 M.
3. Prepare a 0.3-M solution of tromethamine by adding 1,000 mL of sterile water for injection to 36 g of lyophilized tromethamine.
4. Infuse slowly into the largest antecubital vein through a large needle or indwelling catheter and elevate limb.
5. For treatment of cardiac arrest, the drug may be injected into the ventricular cavity if the chest is open. If the chest is not open, the drug may be injected into a large peripheral vein.
6. Do not administer longer than 1 day unless acute life-threatening situation exists.
7. Discontinue administration *immediately,* if extravasation occurs:
• Administer 1% procaine hydrochloride with hyaluronidase to reduce venospasm and to dilute the drug in the tissues.
• Phentolamine mesylate (Regitine) has been used for local infiltrates for adrenergic blocking properties.
• If necessary, a nerve block of the autonomic fibers may be done.

ASSESSMENT

1. Note any history of urinary or bladder problems.
2. Determine if pregnant.
3. Obtain and analyze baseline pH, pCO_2, bicarbonate, glucose, electrolytes, liver and renal function studies.

INTERVENTIONS

1. Observe for respiratory depression; have mechanical ventilatory equipment available.
2. Document and report any complaints of weakness, presence of moist pale skin, tremors, and a full bounding pulse (symptoms of hypoglycemia, which can occur after rapid- or high-dose administration).
3. Record I&O. Assess for nausea, diarrhea, tachycardia, oliguria, weakness, numbness, or tingling sensations (S&S of hyperkalemia).
4. Observe closely for extravasation; drug is extremely irritating to veins.

OUTCOMES/EVALUATE

• Neutralization of ACD blood in pump oxygenator
• Correction of systemic acidosis; serum pH within desired range

Trovalfloxacin mesylate injection

(**TROH**-vah-**FLOX**-ah-sin)

PREGNANCY CATEGORY: C
Rx: Trovan

Alatrofloxacin mesylate injection

(al-**AY**-troh-**flox**-ah-sin)

PREGNANCY CATEGORY: C
Rx: Trovan I.V.
CLASSIFICATION(S):
Antibiotic, fluoroquinolone

SEE ALSO *FLUOROQUINOLINES*.

ACTION/KINETICS
After IV use, alatrofloxacin is rapidly converted to trovafloxacin. Trovafloxacin is rapidly absorbed from GI tract. **t½, trovafloxacin:** 10.5–12.2 hr, depending on dose and after multiple doses. **t½, alatrofloxacin:** 11.7–12.7 hr, depending on dose and after multiple doses. About 50% excreted unchanged in urine and feces; remainder is metabolized by liver.

USES
IV, PO: (1) Nosocomial pneumonia caused by *Escherichia coli, Pseudomonas aeruginosa, Haemophilus influenzae,* or *Staphylococcus aureus.* For *P. aeruginosa* may need to combine with an aminoglycoside or aztreonam. (2) Community acquired pneumonia caused by *Streptococcus pneumoniae, H. influenzae, Klebsiella pneumoniae, S. aureus, Mycoplasma pneumoniae, Moraxella catarrhalis, Legionella pneumophila,* or *Chlamydia pneumoniae.* (3) Complicated intra-abdominal infections, including post-surgical infections caused by *E. coli, Bacteroides fragilis,* viridans group streptococci, *P. aeruginosa, K. pneumoniae, Peptostreptococcus* species, or *Prevotella* species. (4) Gynecologic or pelvic infections, including endomyometritis, parametritis, septic abortion, and post-partum infections caused by *E. coli, B. fragilis,* viridans group streptococci, *Enterococcus faecalis, Streptococcus agalactiae, Peptostreptococcus* species, *Prevotella* species, or *Gardnerella vaginalis.* (5) Complicated skin and skin structure infections, including diabetic foot infections due to *S. aureus, S. agalactiae, P. aeruginosa, E. faecalis, E.coli, or Proteus mirabilis.*

Note: Due to the risk of liver toxicity, it is recommended that trovafloxacin/alatrofloxacin be used only as follows: (1) clients who have 1 or more of several specified infections that are life- or limb-threatening; (2) therapy is started in inpatient health care facilities; or, (3) the benefit clearly outweight the risk. Therapy is not indicated for more than 14 days and is to be discontinued if the client shows signs of liver dysfunction.

CONTRAINDICATIONS
Use in those with history of hypersensitivity to trovafloxacin, alatrofloxacin, or quinolone antimicrobial agents. Use when safer, alternative antimicrobial drugs will be effective.

SPECIAL CONCERNS
Safety and efficacy in children less than 18 years of age, in pregnant women, and during lactation have not been studied. Serious liver injury, leading to liver transplantation or death, may occur especially if used for over 2 weeks. Reserve use for clients with serious, life-, or limb-threatening infections where initial treatment is in a hospital or long-term nursing facility and the provider believes the benefits outweigh the potential risks.

SIDE EFFECTS
Side effects listed occur at rate of 1% or greater.**GI:** N&V, diarrhea, abdominal pain. **CNS:** Dizziness, headache, lightheadedness. **Dermatologic:** Pruritus, rash. **Miscellaneous:** Vaginitis, reaction at injection site, eosinophila.

LABORATORY TEST CONSIDERATIONS
↑ Platelets, ALT, AST, alkaline phosphatase, BUN, creatinine. ↓ Hemoglobin, hematocrit, protein, albumin, sodium, bicarbonate. ↑ or ↓ WBCs.

DRUG INTERACTIONS
Aluminum hydroxide / ↓ Plasma levels of trovafloxacin

Ferrous sulfate / ↓ Plasma levels of trovafloxacin
Magnesium hydroxide / ↓ Plasma levels of trovafloxacin
Morphine / ↓ Plasma levels of trovafloxacin
Omeprazole / ↓ Plasma levels of trovafloxacin
Sucralfate / ↓ Plasma levels of trovafloxacin
Warfarin / ↑ INR

HOW SUPPLIED

Tablets (Trovafloxacin mesylate): 100 mg, 200 mg; *Injection (Alatrofloxacin mesylate):* 5 mg/mL

DOSAGE

• **IV, TABLETS**

Nosocomial pneumonia.

300 mg IV followed by 200 mg/day PO for 10–14 days. If due to *P. aeruginosa*, combination therapy with either aminoglycoside or aztreonam may be indicated.

Community acquired pneumonia.

200 mg PO or 200 mg IV followed by 200 mg PO/day for 7–14 days.

Complicated intra-abdominal infections, including post-surgical infections.

300 mg IV followed by 200 mg /day PO for 7–14 days.

Gynecologic and pelvic infections.

300 mg IV followed by 200 mg PO/day for 7–14 days.

Skin and skin structure infections, complicated, including diabetic foot infections.

200 mg PO or 200 mg IV, followed by 200 mg/day PO for 10–14 days.

NURSING CONSIDERATIONS

SEE ALSO *NURSING CONSIDERATIONS* FOR *FLUOROQUINOLINES*.

ADMINISTRATION/STORAGE

1. Doses are given once q 24 hr for no more than 2 weeks.
2. Tablets can be given without regard to food.
3. Give PO doses at least 2 hr before or 2 hr after antacids containing Mg or Al, sucralfate, citric acid buffered with sodium citrate, or ferrous sulfate.
4. Give IV morphine at least 2 hr after PO trovafloxacin in fasting state and at least 4 hr after PO trovafloxacin is taken with food.
5. No dosage adjustment is necessary when switching from IV or PO dosing. Switching is at discretion of provider.
6. Reduce dose in mild to moderate cirrhosis. If dose in normal hepatic function is 300 mg IV, give 200 mg IV in chronic hepatic disease. If dose in normal hepatic function is 200 mg IV or PO, give 100 mg IV or PO in chronic hepatic disease. If dose is 100 mg PO in normal hepatic function, do not decrease PO dose in chronic hepatic disease.

IV 7. Alatrofloxacin mesylate injection is given only by IV infusion. It is not for IM, SC, intrathecal, or intraperitoneal use.

8 When 300 mg IV is indicated, decrease to 200 mg as soon as clinically indicated.

9. Give IV by direct infusion or through Y-type IV infusion set over period of 60 min.

10. Alatrofloxacin I.V. single use vials, containing 5 mg/mL must be further diluted with appropriate solution before IV administration.

11. Compatible IV solutions include D5W, 0.45% NaCl injection, D5/0.45% NaCl, D5/0.2% NaCl, and D5/LR.

12. There is no preservative or bacteriostatic in alatrofloxacin IV; discard any unused portion.

13. Do not add any additives or other medications to single use vials or through same IV line.

14. If the same IV line is used for sequential infusion of different drugs, flush the line before and after infusion of alatrofloxacin with a solution compatible with any other drugs to be given in same line.

15. Diluted concentrations of 0.5 to 2 mg/mL (as trovafloxacin) are stable for up to 7 days when refrigerated or up to 3 days at room temperature if stored in glass bottles or plastic (PVC type) IV containers.

16. Store alatrofloxacin vials, prior to dilution, at 15–30°C (59–86°F). Protect from light and do not freeze.

ASSESSMENT

Document indications for therapy noting onset, duration, culture results, and characteristics of symptoms. Evaluate ID consult as drug is not for indiscriminate use and has potential severe side effect profile.

CLIENT/FAMILY TEACHING

1. May take without regard to meal. Avoid antacids, vitamins, or minerals with iron, or sucralfate 2 hr before or 2 hr after dose. Increase fluid intake during therapy.
2. May cause dizziness and lightheadedness; avoid activities requiring mental/physical alertness until response evaluated.
3. Stop drug and report any pain, inflammation, rash, or tendon rupture.
4. If skin rash, hives, or other skin reactions occur, or difficulty swallowing or breathing occurs, report immediately; may be hypersensitivity reaction.
5. Avoid excessive sunlight or UV exposure; stop drug and report if phototoxicity reaction occurs.
6. Report if symptoms do not improve or worsen after 3-4 days of therapy.

OUTCOMES/EVALUATE

Resolution of infection

Tubocurarine chloride

(too-boh-kyour-**AR**-een)

PREGNANCY CATEGORY: C
CLASSIFICATION(S):
Neuromuscular blocking drug

T

SEE ALSO ***NEUROMUSCULAR BLOCKING AGENTS.***

ACTION/KINETICS

Cumulative effects may occur. Most likely of the nondepolarizing drugs to cause histamine release. Narrow margin between therapeutic dose and toxic dose. **Onset, IV:** 1 min; **IM:** 15–25 min. **Time to peak effect, IV:** 2–5 min. **Duration, IV:** 20–90 min. **t½:** 1–3 hr. About 43% excreted unchanged in urine.

USES

(1) Muscle relaxant during surgery or setting of fractures and dislocations. (2) Spasticity caused by injury to or disease of CNS. (3) Treat seizures electrically induced or induced by drugs. (4) Diagnosis of myasthenia gravis.

ADDITIONAL CONTRAINDICATIONS

Clients in whom release of histamine is hazardous.

SPECIAL CONCERNS

Use with caution during pregnancy and lactation and in children. If repeated doses are used before delivery, the newborn may manifest decreased skeletal muscle activity. Children up to 1 month of age may be more sensitive to the effects of tubocurarine. Use with extreme caution in clients with renal dysfunction, liver disease, or obstructive states.

ADDITIONAL SIDE EFFECTS

Allergic reactions. Excessive secretion and circulatory collapse.

OD OVERDOSE MANAGEMENT

Treatment: Overdosage chiefly treated by artificial respiration, although neostigmine, atropine, and edrophonium chloride should also be on hand.

ADDITIONAL DRUG INTERACTIONS

Acetylcholine / Antagonizes effect of tubocurarine
Anticholinesterases / Antagonizes effect of tubocurarine
Calcium salts / ↑ Tubocurarine effect
Diazepam / ↑ Risk of malignant hyperthermia
Potassium / Antagonizes effect of tubocurarine
Propranolol / ↑ Tubocurarine effect
Quinine / ↑ Tubocurarine effect
Succinylcholine chloride / ↑ Relaxant effect of both drugs

HOW SUPPLIED

Injection: 3 mg (20 units)/mL

DOSAGE

• **IV, IM**

Adjunct to surgical anesthesia.

Adults, IM, IV, initial: 6–9 mg (40–60 units); **then,** 3–4.5 mg (20–30 units) in 3–5 min if needed. Supplemental doses of 3 mg (20 units) can be given for prolonged procedures. Dosage can be calculated on the basis of 1.1

units/kg. **Pediatric, up to 4 weeks of age, IV, initial:** 0.3 mg/kg; **then,** give subsequent doses in increments of 1/5–1/6 the initial dose. **Infants and children, IV:** 0.6 mg/kg.

Electroshock therapy.

Adults, IV: 0.165 mg/kg (1.1 units/kg) given over 30–90 sec. It is recommended that the initial dose be 3 mg less than the calculated total dose.

Diagnosis of myasthenia gravis.

Adults, IV: 0.004–0.033 mg/kg. A test dose should be given within 2–3 min with IV neostigmine, 1.5 mg, to minimize prolonged respiratory paralysis.

NURSING CONSIDERATIONS

SEE ALSO *NURSING CONSIDERATIONS* FOR *NEUROMUSCULAR BLOCKING AGENTS*.

ADMINISTRATION/STORAGE

IV 1. Give IV as a sustained injection over 1–1.5 min. May also be given IM.
2. Give in incremental doses until relaxation is reached.
3. Decrease the initial dose if the inhalation anesthetic used enhances the action of curariform drugs or with compromised renal function.
4. Review the drugs with which tubocurarine interacts.
5. Tubocurarine is incompatible with alkaline solutions and may form a precipitate when mixed with them (e.g., methohexital sodium or thiopental sodium).
6. Have neostigmine methylsulfate available as an antidote.

ASSESSMENT

1. Document indications for therapy, onset, duration, and characteristics of symptoms.
2. Utilize a peripheral nerve stimulator to assess neuromuscular response and recovery.
3. Document length of time receiving the drug. It should be used only on a short-term basis and in a continuously monitored environment.
4. Remember that client may be fully conscious and aware of surroundings and conversations.
5. Drug does not affect pain or anxiety; administer analgesics and antianxiety agents as needed.
6. Monitor VS, ECG, and lab studies. Drug can cause vagal stimulation resulting in bradycardia, hypotension, and cardiac arrhythmias.

OUTCOMES/EVALUATE

- Skeletal muscle relaxation
- Control of drug or electrically induced seizures
- Diagnosis of myasthenia gravis

U 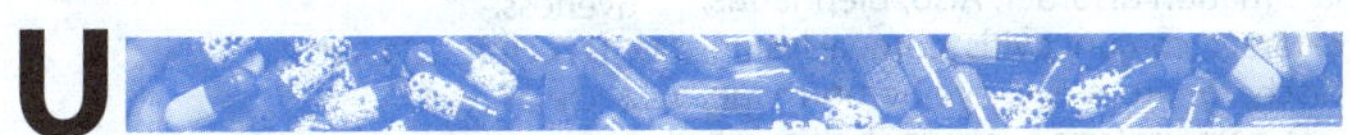

Unoprostone isopropyl ophthalmic solution

(you-noh-**PROST**-ohn)

PREGNANCY CATEGORY: C
CLASSIFICATION(S):
Antiglaucoma drug
Rx: Rescula

ACTION/KINETICS

Reduces elevated IOP by increasing outflow of aqueous humor. Exact mechanism unknown. Drug does not affect CV or pulmonary function. Absorbed through the cornea and conjunctival epithelium where it is hydrolyzed by esterases to unoprostone free acid. Little systemic absorption. However, what is absorbed is rapidly eliminated in the urine — **t½:** 14 min.

USES

Lower IOP in open-angle glaucoma or ocular hypertension in those who are intolerant of other intraocular pressure lowering drugs or who have not achieved the target IOP after multiple measurements over time to another

IOP lowering drug. Drug has not been evaluated to treat angle closure, inflammatory, or neovascular glaucoma.

CONTRAINDICATIONS

Hypersensitivity to unoprostone isopropyl, benzalkonium chloride, or any other components of the product. Use while wearing contact lenses.

SPECIAL CONCERNS

May increase the amount of brown pigment in the iris, which may be permanent. Change in iris color occurs slowly and may not be noticed for months to several years. Use with caution in clients with active intraocular inflammation (uveitis), in renal or hepatic impairment, and during lactation. The benzalkonium chloride in the product may be adsorbed by contact lenses. Safety and efficacy have not been determined in pediatric clients.

SIDE EFFECTS

Ophthalmic: Bacterial keratitis due to inadvertent contamination by clients with concurrent corneal disease or a disruption of the ocular epithelial surface. Burning/stinging, including upon drug instillation; dry eyes, itching, increased length of eyelashes, injection, increased amount of brown pigment, abnormal vision, eyelid disorder, foreign body sensation, lacrimation disorder. Also, blepharitis, cataract, conjunctivitis, corneal lesion, discharge from eye, eye hemorrhage, eye pain, irritation, photophobia, vitreous disorder, elevated IOP, color blindness, corneal deposits, corneal edema, corneal opacity, diplopia, hyperpigmentation of the eyelid, increased number of eyelashes, iritis, optic atrophy, ptosis, retinal hemorrhage, visual field defect. **Nonocular side effects:** Accidental injury, allergic reaction, back pain, bronchitis, increased cough, diabetes mellitus, dizziness, headache, hypertension, insomnia, pharyngitis, pain, rhinitis, sinusitis.

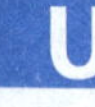

HOW SUPPLIED

Ophthalmic solution: 0.15%

DOSAGE

• OPHTHALMIC DROPS

Reduce IOP.

1 gtt in affected eye(s) b.i.d.

NURSING CONSIDERATIONS

ADMINISTRATION/STORAGE

Store between 2–25°C (36–77°F).

CLIENT/FAMILY TEACHING

1. Drops are used to reduce pressure in the eye with open-angle glaucoma or ocular hypertension in those intolerant of or unresponsive to other agents. Lack of treatment may lead to loss of vision.
2. Avoid allowing the tip of the dispensing container to contact the eye or surrounding structures so that the tip does not become contaminated.
3. May be used with other topical ophthalmic drugs to lower IOP. If using more than one topical ophthalmic drug, wait at least 5 min between use.
4. Remove contact lenses prior to instilling the drug. Lenses may be reinserted 15 min after drug therapy.
5. Drops may gradually change eye color by increasing the amount of brown pigment in the iris; this may not be reversible.
6. Report any eyelid retractions, irritation, pain, discharge, or redness immediately. F/U with eye provider to check IOP and to evaluate drug effectiveness.

OUTCOMES/EVALUATE

↓ IOP

Urokinase

(your-oh-**KYE**-nayz)

PREGNANCY CATEGORY: B

CLASSIFICATION(S):

Thrombolytic enzyme

Rx: Abbokinase, Abbokinase Open-Cath

ACTION/KINETICS

Urokinase converts plasminogen to plasmin; plasmin then breaks down fibrin clots, fibrinogen, and other plasma proteins. A decrease in plasma fibrinogen and plasminogen and increased circulating FDP may persist for 12–24 hr. **Onset:** rapid; **duration:** 12 hr. t½: < 20 min, although effect on coagulation disappears after a few hours.

USES

Acute pulmonary thromboembolism. To clear IV catheters that are blocked by fibrin or clotted blood. Coronary artery thrombosis. *Investigational:* Acute arterial thromboembolism, acute arterial thrombosis, to clear arteriovenous cannula.

CONTRAINDICATIONS

Active internal bleeding, history of CVA, within 2 months of intracranial or intraspinal surgery or trauma, recent cardiopulmonary resuscitation, intracranial neoplasm, arteriovenous malformation or aneurysm, known bleeding diathesis, severe uncontrolled arterial hypertension. Any condition presenting a risk of hemorrhage, such as recent surgery or biopsies, delivery within 10 days, pregnancy, ulcerative disease. Also hepatic or renal insufficiency, tuberculosis, recent cerebral embolism, thrombosis, hemorrhage, SBE, rheumatic valvular disease, thrombocytopenia.

SPECIAL CONCERNS

Use in septic thrombophlebitis may be hazardous. Produced from cultures of human source materials; thus, there is the potential to transmit infectious agents, although procedures are used to reduce such risk. Use with caution during lactation. Safe use in children has not been established.

SIDE EFFECTS

CV: Superficial bleeding, ***severe internal bleeding,*** transient hypotension or hypertension, tachycardia. **Allergic:** Rarely, skin rashes, ***bronchospasm.*** **Other:** Fever, chills, rigors, N&V, dyspnea, cyanosis, back pain, hypoxemia, acidosis.

DRUG INTERACTIONS

Anticoagulants, aspirin, heparin, and indomethacin ↑ the risk of bleeding when given with urokinase.

HOW SUPPLIED

Powder for injection, lyophilized: 250,000 IU; *Powder for catheter clearance, lyophilized*

DOSAGE

- **IV INFUSION ONLY**

Pulmonary embolism.

Loading dose: 4,400 IU/kg mixed with either 0.9% NaCl or D5W given at a rate of 90 mL/hr over 10 min; **maintenance:** 4,400 IU/kg/hr given at a rate of 15 mL/hr for 12 hr. At the end of therapy, treat with continuous IV heparin to prevent thrombosis recurrence. Do not begin heparin therapy without a loading dose until TT has decreased to less than twice the normal control value (about 3–4 hr after completing infusion).

Coronary artery thrombi.

Initial bolus: Heparin, as a bolus of 2,500–10,000 units **IV; then,** begin infusion of urokinase at a rate of 6,000 IU/min (4 mL/min) for up to 2 hr (average total dose of urokinase may be 500,000 IU). Urokinase should be administered until the artery is opened maximally (15–30 min after initial opening although it has been given for up to 2 hr).

Clear IV catheter.

Instill into the catheter 1–1.8 mL of a solution containing 5,000 IU/mL.

NURSING CONSIDERATIONS

SEE ALSO *NURSING CONSIDERATIONS* FOR *STREPTOKINASE* AND *ALTEPLASE, RECOMBINANT.*

ADMINISTRATION/STORAGE

1. If catheters are occluded by substances other than fibrin clots, urokinase is ineffective.
2. Avoid excessive pressure when injected into the catheter as force could rupture or expel the clot into the circulation.

IV 3. Reconstitute only with sterile water for injection without preservatives. Do not use bacteriostatic water.
4. To reconstitute, roll and tilt the vial but do not shake. Reconstitute immediately before using.

5. Dilute reconstituted urokinase before IV administration in 0.9% NSS or D5W.
6. At the end of therapy for pulmonary embolism, ensure that the total dose is given by using the following flush procedure: Give a solution of 0.9% NaCl or D5W via the pump approximately equal to the volume of the tubing in the infusion set. Flush the admixture from the entire length of the infusion set at a rate of 15 mL/hr.
7. Discard any unused portion.
8. Type and cross and have blood for transfusion available. Aminocaproic acid may be employed with severe bleeding or hemorrhage.
9. Store the powder for injection at 2–8°C (35–47°F). Store the powder for catheter clearance below 25°C (77°F) and avoid freezing.

ASSESSMENT

1. Note indications for therapy, type, onset, and symptom characteristics.
2. Monitor ECG, CBC, PT, PTT, liver and renal function studies.
3. Assess for conditions that may preclude drug therapy (recent surgery, cerebral embolism, thrombosis, hermorrhage, SBE, thrombocytopenia, pregnancy, TB).
4. Have additional IV access and Heparin drip ready for therapy.

CLIENT/FAMILY TEACHING

1. Review benefits and risks of drug therapy. Drug is used to break up clots with pulmonary embolism or from coronary arteries that are obstructed.
2. For best results, the therapy should be instituted within 4–6 hr of onset of S&S of MI and within one week of other thrombic event.
3. Report any adverse side effects immediately.
4. Encourage family members or significant other to learn CPR.

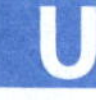

OUTCOMES/EVALUATE

• Lysis of thrombi with restoration of blood flow and prevention of tissue infarction
• Restoration of catheter/cannula patency

Ursodiol

(ur-so-**DYE**-ohl)

PREGNANCY CATEGORY: B
CLASSIFICATION(S):
Gallstone solubilizing drug
Rx: Actigall
✱Rx: Urso

ACTION/KINETICS

Naturally occurring bile acid that inhibits the hepatic synthesis and secretion of cholesterol; it also inhibits intestinal absorption of cholesterol. Acts to solubilize cholesterol in micelles and to cause dispersion of cholesterol as liquid crystals in aqueous media. Undergoes a significant first-pass effect where it is conjugated with either glycine or taurine and then secreted into hepatic bile ducts.

USES

(1) Dissolution of gallstones in clients with radiolucent, noncalcified gallstones (<20 mm) in whom elective surgery would be risky (i.e., systemic disease, advanced age, idiosyncratic reactions to general anesthesia) or in those who refuse surgery. (2) Prevent gallstones in obese clients undergoing rapid weight loss. (3) Primary biliary cirrhosis (Urso).

CONTRAINDICATIONS

Clients with calcified cholesterol stones, radiopaque stones, or radiolucent bile pigment stones. Acute cholecystitis, cholangitis, biliary obstruction, gallstone pancreatitis, biliary-gastrointestinal fistula, allergy to bile acids, chronic liver disease. Provide appropriate specifc treatment in those with variceal bleeding, hepatic encephalopathy, ascites, or in need of an urgent liver transplant.

SPECIAL CONCERNS

Use with caution during lactation. Safety and efficacy have not been determined in children. Safety for use beyond 24 months is not known.

SIDE EFFECTS

GI: N&V, dyspepsia, metallic taste, abdominal pain, biliary pain, cholecystitis, constipation, stomatitis, flatulence, diarrhea. *Skin:* Pruritus, rash, dry skin, urticaria. **CNS:** Headache, fatigue, anxiety, depression, sleep disorders. **Other:** Sweating, thinning of hair, back pain, arthralgia, myalgia, rhinitis, cough.

OD OVERDOSE MANAGEMENT

Symptoms: Diarrhea. *Treatment:* Treat with supportive measures.

DRUG INTERACTIONS

Antacids, aluminum-containing / ↓ Ursodiol effect R/T ↓ GI tract absorption
Cholestyramine / ↓ Ursodiol effect R/T ↓ GI tract absorption
Clofibrate / ↓ Ursodiol effect R/T ↑ hepatic cholesterol secretion
Colestipol / ↓ Ursodiol effect R/T ↓ GI tract absorption
Contraceptives, oral / ↓ Ursodiol effect R/T ↑ hepatic cholesterol secretion
Estrogens / ↓ Ursodiol effect R/T ↑ hepatic cholesterol secretion

HOW SUPPLIED

Capsule: 300 mg

DOSAGE

• **CAPSULES (ACTIGALL)**

Gallstones.

Adults: 8–10 mg/kg/day in two or three divided doses, usually with meals.

Prevent gallstones in rapid weight loss in obesity.

Adults: 300 mg b.i.d. during period of weight loss.

• **TABLETS (URSO)**

Primary biliary cirrhosis.

Adults: 13–15 mg/kg/day given in 4 divided doses with food.

NURSING CONSIDERATIONS

ADMINISTRATION/STORAGE

1. If partial stone dissolution is not observed within 12 months, the drug will probably not be effective.
2. For the first year of therapy, perform gallbladder ultrasound every 6 mo to determine response.

ASSESSMENT

1. Document indications for therapy, expected duration, and any conditions that may preclude therapy.
2. Drug is not indicated for calcified cholesterol, radiopaque, or radiolucent bile pigment stones.
3. Obtain ultrasound of gallbladder and LFTs; monitor q 6 mo.
4. Determine if pregnant.

CLIENT/FAMILY TEACHING

1. Avoid taking antacids unless prescribed. Many antacids have an aluminum base, which adsorbs the drug.
2. Ursodiol therapy may take up to 24 months; drug will need to be taken 2–3 times/day for stones.
3. Stones may recur after the dissolution of the current stones.
4. With primary biliary cirrhosis, take tablets in 4 divided doses with food.
5. Report any persistent N&V, abdominal pain, diarrhea, presence of a metallic taste in the mouth, headaches, itching, rash, or altered bowel function.
6. Any new-onset headache, anxiety, depression, and sleep disorders should be reported.
7. Practice reliable birth control to avoid pregnancy. The use of estrogens and oral contraceptives may decrease effectiveness of the drug; use alternative birth control.
8. Report for follow-up visits, labs, and ultrasonography to evaluate the drug effectiveness.
9. Ursodiol therapy will be continued for 1–3 months following stone dissolution and then reconfirmed with ultrasound.

OUTCOMES/EVALUATE

• Radiographic evidence of a reduction or complete dissolution of radiolucent, noncalcified gallstones.
• Reversal of intracellular accumulation of toxic bile acids

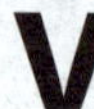

Valacyclovir hydrochloride

(**val**-ah-**SIGH**-kloh-veer)

PREGNANCY CATEGORY: B
CLASSIFICATION(S):
Antiviral
Rx: Valtrex

SEE ALSO *ANTIVIRAL DRUGS*.

ACTION/KINETICS
Rapidly converted to acyclovir, which has inhibitory activity against herpes simplex virus types 1 (HSV-1) and 2 (HSV-2) and varicella-zoster virus. Acts by inhibiting replication of viral DNA by competitive inhibition of viral DNA polymerase, incorporation and termination of the growing viral DNA chain, and inactivation of the viral DNA polymerase. Rapidly absorbed after PO administration and is rapidly and nearly completely converted to acyclovir and l-valine by first-pass intestinal or hepatic metabolism. **Time to peak levels:** Approximately 1.5 hr. **Peak plasma levels:** Less than 0.5 mcg/mL of valacyclovir at all doses. **t½, acyclovir:** 2.5–3.3 hr. Approximately 50% is excreted through the urine.

USES
(1) Treatment of recurrent episodes of genital herpes in immunocompetent adults. (2) Treatment of herpes zoster in immunocompetent adults. (3) Suppression of genital herpes in adults who have experienced previous outbreaks.

CONTRAINDICATIONS
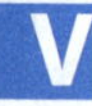
Hypersensitivity or intolerance to acyclovir or valacyclovir. Use in immunocompromised individuals. Lactation.

SPECIAL CONCERNS
Use with caution in renal impairment or in those taking potentially nephrotoxic drugs. Dosage reduction may be necessary in geriatric clients depending on the renal status. Safety and efficacy have not been determined in children.

SIDE EFFECTS
GI: N&V, diarrhea, constipation, abdominal pain, anorexia. **CNS:** Headache, dizziness. **Miscellaneous:** Asthenia, precipitation of acyclovir in renal tubules resulting in acute renal failure and anuria.

OD OVERDOSE MANAGEMENT
Symptoms: Precipitation of acyclovir in renal tubules if the solubility (2.5 mg/mL) is exceeded in the intratubular fluid. *Treatment:* Hemodialysis until renal function is restored. About 33% of acyclovir in the body is removed during a 4-hr hemodialysis session.

DRUG INTERACTIONS
Administration of cimetidine and/or probenecid decreased the rate, but not the extent, of conversion of valacyclovir to acyclovir. Also, the renal clearance of acyclovir was decreased.

HOW SUPPLIED
Tablet: 500 mg, 1 g

DOSAGE

• **TABLETS**

Herpes zoster (shingles).

Adults: 1 g t.i.d. for 7 days. *Dosage with renal impairment:* C_{CR}, 30–49 mL/min: 1 g q 12 hr; C_{CR}, 10–29 mL/min: 1 g q 24 hr; and, C_{CR}, less than 10 mL/min: 500 mg q 24 hr.

Recurrent genital herpes.

Adults: 500 mg b.i.d. for 3 days. *Dosage with renal impairment:* C_{CR}, 30–49 mL/min: 500 mg q 12 hr; C_{CR}, 10–29 mL/min: 500 mg q 24 hr; and, C_{CR}, less than 10 mL/min: 500 mg q 24 hr.

Suppression of genital herpes.

Adults: 1 g once daily (500 mg once daily for those who have 9 or fewer recurrences per year).

NURSING CONSIDERATIONS

SEE ALSO *NURSING CONSIDERATIONS* FOR *ANTIVIRAL DRUGS*.

ADMINISTRATION/STORAGE

Begin therapy as soon as possible after herpes zoster has been diagnosed. The drug is most effective when started within 48 hr after the onset of rash.

For recurrent genital herpes, initiate at the first S&S of a flare.

ASSESSMENT

1. Document indications for therapy and onset. With herpes zoster, note dermatone(s) location and characteristics of lesions. Drug is most effective if initiated within 48 hr of rash or within 72 hr of symptoms.
2. With recurrent genital herpes, note extent of lesions; initiate at first S&S of outbreak.
3. Monitor CBC and renal function studies; reduce dose if C_{CR} below 50 mL/min.

CLIENT/FAMILY TEACHING

1. Take exactly as prescribed; do not share meds or skip or double up on doses. Complete entire course of therapy.
2. May take without regard to meals; food may decrease GI upset.
3. Vesicles usually become red or pustular after 4 or 5 days and by the 7th to 10th day dry up and crust over. The acute phase is completed by approximately 3 weeks, when the scabs slough from the skin.
4. Immunocompromised clients usually experience a more severe case and the disease course usually doubles.
5. During the acute stage, cover the area and avoid contact with immunocompromised individuals, pregnant women, or anyone else that has not had the chicken pox virus.
6. Report any persistent pain once lesions have healed (postherpetic neuralgia) or if there is ocular involvement or any other unusual symptoms or behaviors.
7. Report pain and headaches so appropriate analgesics can be prescribed.
8. With genital herpes, abstain from sexual contact during acute outbreaks to prevent infecting partner; use condoms during all other times.

OUTCOMES/EVALUATE

- ↓ Duration/progression of herpes zoster outbreak with reduced healing time; symptomatic relief
- ↓ Pain, ↓ duration, and ↓ intensity with genital herpes outbreak

Valdecoxib

(**val**-dih-**KOX**-ib)

CLASSIFICATION(S):
Nonsteroidal anti-inflammatory drug, COX-2 inhibitor
Rx: Bextra

ACTION/KINETICS

Acts to inhibit prostaglandin synthesis by inhibiting cyclooxygenase-2 (COX-2). Has anti-inflammatory, analgesic, and antipyretic effects. **Maximum plasma levels:** 3 hr. Time to peak plasma levels delayed 1–2 hr by food. About 98% bound to plasma proteins. Undergoes extensive liver metabolism. Excreted mainly in the urine. **t½, terminal:** 8–11 hr.

USES

(1) Relief of signs and symptoms of osteoarthritis and adult rheumatoid arthritis. (2) Treatment of primary dysmenorrhea.

CONTRAINDICATIONS

Use in those with severe hepatic impairment (Child-Pugh Class C); in advanced kidney disease; in those who have experienced asthma, urticaria, or allergic-type reactions after taking aspirin or NSAIDs; or, in late pregnancy (may cause premature closing of the ductus arteriosus). Lactation.

SPECIAL CONCERNS

Use with caution in clients with mild to moderate hepatic impairment, hypertension, heart failure, and fluid retention. Safety and efficacy have not been determined in children less than 18 years of age. Use with extreme caution in those with a history of ulcer disease or GI bleeding (especially the elderly).

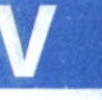

SIDE EFFECTS

GI: Serious GI toxicity, including bleeding, ulceration, and ***perforation of the stomach, small intestine, or large intestine.*** Also, dyspepsia, diarrhea, abdominal pain, flatulence, N&V, abnormal stools, constipation, diverticulosis, dry mouth, duodenal ulcer, duodenitis, eructation, esophagitis, fecal incontinence, gastritis, gastroenteritis, gastroesophageal reflux, hematemesis, hemorrhoids (including bleeding), hiatal hernia, melena, stomatitis, increased stool frequency, tenesmus, tooth disorder, halitosis, abnormal hepatic function, hepatitis. **Hematologic:** Anemia, thrombocytopenia. **CV:** Edema, fluid retention, hypertension, aneurysm, angina pectoris, arrhythmia, cardiomyopathy, CHF, CAD, heart murmur, hypotension, bradycardia, palpitation, tachycardia, intermittent claudication, varicose vein. **CNS:** Dizziness, headache, cerebrovascular disorder, hypertonia, hypoesthesia, migraine, neuralgia, neuropathy, paresthesia, tremor, twitching, vertigo, anorexia, anxiety, increased appetite, confusion, depression, insomnia, nervousness, morbid dreaming, somnolence. **Musculoskeletal:** Myalgia, arthralgia, accidental fracture, neck stiffness, osteoporosis, synovitis, tendonitis. **Respiratory:** Epistaxis, abnormal breath sounds, bronchitis, bronchospasm, coughing, dyspnea, emphysema, laryngitis, pneumonia, pharyngitis, pleurisy, rhinitis. **Dermatologic:** Acne, alopecia, dermatitis (including fungal), photosensitivity, eczema, allergic reaction, pruritus, erythematous rash, maculopapular rash, psoriaform rash, dry skin, skin hypertrophy, skin ulceration, increased sweating, urticaria. **GU:** Albuminuria, cystitis, dysuria, hematuria, increased micturition, pyuria, urinary incontinence, UTI, amenorrhea, dysmenorrhea, leukorrhea, mastitis, menstrual disorder, menorrhagia, menstrual bleeding, vaginal hemorrhage, impotence, prostatic disorder. **Body as a whole:** Allergic reaction, aggravated allergies, asthenia, chest pain, chills, generalized edema, facial edema, fatigue, fever, hot flashes, malaise, pain, peripheral pain, ecchymosis, hematoma, herpes simplex/zoster, fungal infection, soft tissue/viral infection, moniliasis (including genital), increased or decreased weight. **Ophthalmic:** Periorbital swelling, blurred vision, cataract, conjunctival hemorrhage, conjunctivitis, eye pain, keratitis, abnormal vision, xerophthalmia. **Otic:** Ear abnormality, earache, tinnitus, otitis media. **Miscellaneous:** Goiter, taste perversion, increased thirst, gout, diabetes mellitus.

LABORATORY TEST CONSIDERATIONS

↑ ALT, AST, alkaline phosphatase, BUN, CPK, creatinine, LDH. Glycosuria, hypercholesterolemia, hyperglycemia, hyperkalemia or hypokalemia, hyperlipemia, hyperuricemia, hypocalcemia.

OD OVERDOSE MANAGEMENT

Symptoms: N&V, lethargy, drowsiness, epigastric pain, GI bleeding. Rarely, hypertension, acute renal failure, respiratory depression, coma, anaphylactoid reaction. *Treatment:* Symptomatic and supportive care.

DRUG INTERACTIONS

ACE Inhibitors / ↓ Antihypertensive effect of ACE inhibitors
Aspirin / ↑ Risk of GI ulceration and complications
Dextromethorphan / Significant ↑ in plasma dextromethorphan levels
Fluconazole / Significant ↑ in valdecoxib plasma levels
Furosemide / ↓ Diuretic effect
Ketoconazole / Significant ↑ in valdecoxib plasma levels
Lithium / ↑ Plasma lithium levels R/T significant ↓ lithium clearance
Thiazide diuretics / ↓ Diuretic effect
Warfarin / Significant ↑ in plasma exposures of R-warfarin and S-warfarin

HOW SUPPLIED

Tablets: 10 mg, 20 mg

DOSAGE

• TABLETS

Osteoarthritis, Rheumatoid arthritis.
10 mg once daily.

Primary dysmenorrhea.
20 mg b.i.d., as needed.

NURSING CONSIDERATIONS

SEE ALSO *NURSING CONSIDERATIONS* FOR *NSAIDS*

ASSESSMENT

1. Document indications for therapy, onset and characteristics of disease, ROM, deformity/loss of function, level of

pain, other agents trialed and the outcome.
2. Determine any GI bleed or ulcer history, sulfonamide allergy, aspirin or other NSAID-induced asthma, urticaria, or allergic-type reactions.
3. List drugs prescribed to ensure none interact.
4. Assess hydration level. Use caution when initiating treatment in those with significant dehydration; rehydrate first.
5. Assess for liver/renal dysfunction; monitor lytes, renal and LFTs.

CLIENT/FAMILY TEACHING

1. Seek the lowest dose for each client. Take exactly as directed and generally at the same time each day.
2. Report any unusual or persistent side effects including dyspepsia, abdominal pain, dizziness, and changes in stool or skin color.
3. Avoid therapy during pregnancy.
4. Report weight gain, swelling of ankles, chest pain, SOB, or lack of response.

OUTCOMES/EVALUATE

Relief of joint pain and inflammation with improved mobility

Valganciclovir hydrochloride

(**val**-gan-**SIGH**-kloh-veer)

PREGNANCY CATEGORY: C
CLASSIFICATION(S):
Antiviral
Rx: Valcyte

SEE ALSO *ANTIVIRAL DRUGS.*

ACTION/KINETICS

Is a prodrug and is metabolized to ganciclovir by intestinal and hepatic esterases. In CMV-infected cells, ganciclovir is first phosphorylated to ganciclovir monophosphate and then further phosphorylated to ganciclovir triphosphate. The triphosphate inhibits viral DNA synthesis. Resistant viruses to ganciclovir occur after prolonged treatment with valganciclovir. Well absorbed from the GI tract. No other metabolites than ganciclovir have been identified. Excreted by the kidney. **t½, terminal:** About 4 hr.

USES

Treatment of cytomegalovirus (CMV) retinitis in AIDS clients.

CONTRAINDICATIONS

Hypersensitivity to ganciclovir or valganciclovir. Use if the absolute neutrophil count is < 500 cells/mm^3, the platelet count is < 25,000/mm^3, or the hemoglobin is < 8 g/dL. Lactation.

SPECIAL CONCERNS

Use with caution in pre-existing cytopenias or in those who have received or are receiving myelosuppressive drugs or irradiation. Safety and efficacy have not been determined in children.

SIDE EFFECTS

See also *Ganciclovir.*
Hematologic: Granulocytopenia, anemia, thrombocytopenia, severe leukopenia, neutropenia, pancytopenia, bone marrow depression, ***aplastic anemia.*** **GI:** Diarrhea, N&V, abdominal pain. **CNS:** Headache, insomnia, paresthesia, convulsions, psychosis, hallucinations, confusion, agitation. **Miscellaneous:** Peripheral neuropathy, local and systemic infections and sepsis, ***potential life-threatening bleeding due to thrombocytopenia,*** hypersensitivity.

LABORATORY TEST CONSIDERATIONS

↑ Serum creatinine.

DRUG INTERACTIONS

Since valganciclovir is rapidly metabolized to ganciclovir, any drug interactions will be those for ganciclovir. Thus, see *Ganciclovir.*

HOW SUPPLIED

Tablet: 450 mg

DOSAGE

- **TABLETS**

CMV retinitis.
Induction: 900 mg (2-450 mg tablets) b.i.d. for 21 days with food. **Maintenance:** Following induction or in those with inactive CMV retinitis, give 900 mg (2-450 mg tablets) once daily with food. Adjust the dose as follows in those with renal impairment: If C_{CR} is

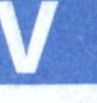

40 to 59 mL/min, give 450 mg b.i.d. for the induction dose and 450 mg once daily for the maintenance dose, If C_{CR} is 25 to 39 mL/min, give 450 mg once daily for the induction dose and 450 mg q 2 days for the maintenance dose, If C_{CR} is 10 to 24 mL/min, give 450 mg q 2 days for the induction dose and 450 mg twice weekly for the maintenance dose.

NURSING CONSIDERATIONS

SEE ALSO *NURSING CONSIDERATIONS* FOR *ANTIVIRAL DRUGS* AND *GANCICLOVIR*.

ADMINISTRATION/STORAGE

1. Valganciclovir tablets cannot be substituted for ganciclovir tablets on a one-to-one basis.
2. Use caution in handling valganciclovir tablets. Do not break or crush tablets. The drug is a potential teratogen and carcinogen, thus, use caution in handling broken tablets. Avoid direct contact of broken or crushed tablets with the skin or mucous membranes. If contact occurs, wash thoroughly with soap and water, rinse eyes thoroughly with plain water.
3. Cytopenia may occur at any time during treatment and may increase with continued dosing. Cell counts usually begin to recover within 3 to 7 days after stopping the drug.

ASSESSMENT

1. Note indications for therapy, characteristics of symptoms, other agents trialed, and the outcome.
2. Determine CMV retinitis by indirect ophthalmoscopy.
3. Assess orientation and mentation levels.
4. Review history and assess carefully for pre-existing cytopenias or if have received or are receiving myelosuppressive drugs or irradiation.
5. Monitor CBC, hold and report if ANC is < 500 cells/mm³, the platelet count is < 25,000/mm3, or the hemoglobin is < 8 g/dL. Anticipate reduced dose with renal dysfunction, see dosing guidelines.

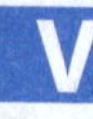

CLIENT/FAMILY TEACHING

1. Take with food to maximize bioavailability.
2. Follow directions carefully for induction and then maintenance dosing. Valganciclovir cannot be substituted for ganciclovir on a mg to mg basis.
3. If others must handle the tablets, do so with caution. Do not break/crush or handle broken tablets and if contact with skin or mucous membranes occurs, wash thoroughly with soapy water and rinse eyes well with plain water. Drug is a potential teratogen and carcinogen.
4. Do not perform activities requiring mental alertness until drug effects realized, may cause dizziness, seizures, ataxia, and confusion.
5. Report any abnormal bruising or bleeding, drug impairs clotting.
6. Drug is not a cure, it controls symptoms and progression of disease.
7. Women/men of childbearing/reproductive potential should practice reliable contraception during and for 90 days following therapy.
8. Report to eye doctor q 4-6 weeks as scheduled for evaluation/F/U.

OUTCOMES/EVALUATE

↓ Progression of CMV retinitis

Valproic acid

(val-**PROH**-ick)

PREGNANCY CATEGORY: D
Rx: Depacon, Depakene
✱Rx: Alti-Valproic, Apo-Valproic, Epiject I.V., Gen-Valproic, Novo-Valproic, Nu-Valproic, PMS-Valproic Acid, PMS-Valproic Acid E.C., Rhoxal-valproic, Rhoxal-valproic EC

Divalproex sodium

(die-val-**PROH**-ex)

PREGNANCY CATEGORY: D
Rx: Depakote, Depakote ER
✱Rx: Apo-Divalproex, Epival, Novo-Divalproex, Nu-Divalproex
CLASSIFICATION(S):
Anticonvulsant, miscellaneous

SEE ALSO *ANTICONVULSANTS*.

ACTION/KINETICS
The following information also applies to divalproex sodium (Depakote, Epival ✱). The precise anticonvulsant action is unknown; may increase brain levels of the neurotransmitter GABA. Other possibilities include acting on postsynaptic receptor sites to mimic or enhance the inhibitory effect of GABA, inhibiting an enzyme that catabolizes GABA, affecting the potassium channel, or directly affecting membrane stability. Absorption is more rapid with the syrup (sodium salt) than capsules. **Peak levels, with syrup:** 15 min–2 hr. Equivalent PO doses of divalproex sodium and valproic acid deliver equivalent amounts of valproate ion to the system. **Peak serum levels, capsules and syrup:** 1–4 hr (delayed if the drug is taken with food); **peak serum levels, enteric-coated tablet (divalproex sodium):** 3–4 hr. **t½:** 9–16 hr, with the lower time usually seen in clients taking other anticonvulsant drugs (e.g., primidone, phenytoin, phenobarbital, carbamazepine). **t½, children less than 10 days:** 10–67 hr; **t½, children over 2 months:** 7–13 hr. **t½, cirrhosis or acute hepatitis:** Up to 18 hr. **Therapeutic serum levels:** 50–100 mcg/mL. Approximately 90% bound to plasma protein. Metabolized in the liver and inactive metabolites are excreted in the urine; small amounts of valproic acid are excreted in the feces.

USES
(1) Alone or in combination with other anticonvulsants for treatment of simple and complex absence seizures (petit mal). (2) As an adjunct in multiple seizure patterns that include absence seizures. (3) Alone or as adjunct to treat complex partial seizures that occur either in isolation or in association with other types of seizures. (4) Divalproex sodium delayed release used for the acute treatment of manic episodes in bipolar disorder and for prophylaxis of migraine headaches. *Investigational:* Alone or in combination to treat atypical absence, myoclonic, and grand mal seizures. May be useful to treat intractable status epilepticus that has not responded to other therapies (used with phenytoin and phenobarbital). Subchronically to treat minor incontinence after ileoanal anastomosis. Management of anxiety disorders or panic attacks.

CONTRAINDICATIONS
Liver disease or dysfunction.

SPECIAL CONCERNS
Use with caution during lactation. Use with caution in children 2 years of age or less as they are at greater risk for developing fatal hepatotoxicity. Life-threatening/fatal pancreatitis reported in children and adults. Use lower doses in geriatric clients because they may have increased free, unbound valproic acid levels in the serum. Safety and efficacy of divalproex sodium have not been determined for treating acute mania in children less than 18 years of age or for treating migraine in children less than 16 years of age.

SIDE EFFECTS
GI: (most frequent): N&V, indigestion. Also, abdominal cramps, abdominal pain, dyspepsia, taste perversion, diarrhea, constipation, anorexia with weight loss or increased appetite with weight gain, fecal incontinence, flatulence, gastroenteritis, glossitis, periodontal abscess, dry mouth, stomatitis, tooth disorder. **CNS:** Sedation, asthenia, somnolence, ataxia, emotional lability, abnormal thinking, amnesia, euphoria, nervousness, paresthesia, insomnia, depression, tremor, hallucinations, ataxia, headache, asterixis, dysarthria, abnormal dreams, abnormal gait, agitation, catatonic reaction, confusion, hypertonia, hyperkinesia, tardive dyskinesia, dizziness, confusion, hypesthesia, vertigo, incoordination, parkinsonism, reversible cerebral atrophy, dementia. Rarely, coma (alone or in with phenobarbital), encephalopathy with fever. **CV:** Hypertension, hypotension, palpitations, postural hypotension, tachycardia, vascular anomaly, vasodilation. **Ophthalmologic:** Nystagmus, amblyopia, diplopia, "spots before eyes." **Hematologic:** Thrombocytopenia, relative

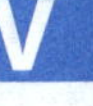

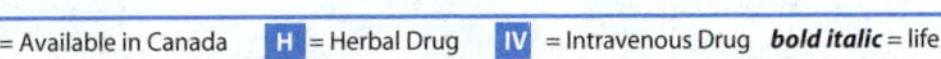

lymphocytosis, macrocytosis, hypofibrinogenemia, myelodysplastic-type syndrome, leukopenia, eosinophilia, anemia, bone marrow supression, pancytopenia, aplastic anemia, acute intermittent porphyria, bruising, hematoma formation, epistaxis, frank hemorrhage. **Dermatologic:** Transient alopecia, petechiae, erythema multiforme, ecchymosis, skin rashes. photosensitivity, pruritus, discoid lupus erythematosus, dry skin, furunculosis, maculopapular rash, seborrhea, ***Stevens-Johnson syndrome, toxic epidermal necrolysis (rare)***. **Hepatic:** ***Hepatotoxicity, pancreatitis.*** Also, minor increases in AST, ALT, LDH, serum bilirubin, and serum alkaline phosphatase values. **Endocrine:** Breast enlargement, galactorrhea, swelling of parotid gland, abnormal thyroid function tests. **GU:** Dysuria, urinary incontinence, cystitis, menstural irregularities, secondary amenorrhea, dysmenorrhea, metrorrhagia, vaginal bleeding. **Musculoskeletal:** Arthralgia, arthrosis, leg cramps, twitching, myalgia. **Otic:** Hearing loss, ear pain, otitis media, tinnitus. **Miscellaneous:** Weakness, asthenia, hyperammonemia, hyperglycinemia, hypocarnitinemia, edema of arms and legs, weakness, inappropriate ADH secretion, Fanconi's syndrome (rare and seen mostly in children), lupus erythematosus, fever, enuresis, hearing loss, fever, chest pain, infection.

LABORATORY TEST CONSIDERATIONS

False + for ketonuria. Altered thyroid function tests.

OD OVERDOSE MANAGEMENT

Symptoms: Motor restlessness, asterixis, visual hallucinations, somnolence, heart block, ***deep coma.*** *Treatment:* Perform gastric lavage if client is seen early enough (valproic acid is absorbed rapidly). Undertake general supportive measures making sure urinary output is maintained. Naloxone has been used to reverse the CNS depression (however, it could also reverse the anticonvulsant effect). Hemodialysis and hemoperfusion have been used with success.

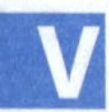

DRUG INTERACTIONS

Alcohol / ↑ Incidence of CNS depression

Carbamazepine / Variable changes in carbamazepine levels with possible loss of seizure control

Charcoal / ↓ Valproic acid absorption from the GI tract

Chlorpromazine / ↓ Clearance and ↑ t½ of valproic acid → ↑ pharmacologic effects

Cholestyramine / ↓ Valproic acid serum levels with possible loss of seizure control

Cimetidine / ↓ Clearance and ↑ t½ of valproic acid → ↑ pharmacologic effects

Clonazepam / ↑ Chance of absence seizures (petit mal) and ↑ toxicity

CNS depressants / ↑ Incidence of CNS depression

Diazepam / ↑ Diazepam effect R/T ↓ plasma binding and ↓ metabolism

Erythromycin / ↑ Serum valproic acid levels → valproic acid toxicitiy

Ethosuximide / ↑ Ethosuximide effect R/T ↓ metabolism

Felbamate / ↑ Mean peak valproic acid levels

Lamotrigine / ↓ Valproic acid serum levels and ↑ lamotrigine serum levels; reduce dose of lamotrigine

Phenobarbital / ↑ Phenobarbital effect R/T ↓ liver breakdown

Phenytoin / ↑ Phenytoin effect R/T ↓ liver breakdown or ↓ effect of valproic acid R/T ↑ metabolism

Salicylates (aspirin) / ↑ Effect of valproic acid R/T ↓ plasma protein binding and ↓ metabolism

Tricyclic antidepressants / ↑ TCA plasma levels and side effects

Warfarin sodium / ↑ Effect of valproic acid R/T ↓ plasma protein binding. Also, additive anticoagulant effect

Zidovudine / ↓ Clearance in HIV-seropositive clients

HOW SUPPLIED

Valproic acid: *Capsule:* 250 mg; *Injection (as sodium valproate):* 100 mg/mL; *Syrup (as sodium valproate):* 250 mg/5 mL; **Divalproex sodium:** *Capsule, Sprinkle:* 125 mg; *Tablet, Delayed-Release:* 125 mg, 250 mg, 500 mg

DOSAGE

• **CAPSULES, SYRUP, ENTERIC-COATED CAPSULES AND TABLETS (DIVALPROEX)**

Complex partial seizures.

Adults and children 10 years and older: 10–15 mg/kg/day. Increase by 5–10 mg/kg/week until seizures are controlled or side effects occur, up to a maximum of 60 mg/kg/day. If the total daily dose exceeds 250 mg, divide the dose. Dosage of concomitant anticonvulsant drugs can usually be reduced by about 25% every 2 weeks. Divalproex sodium may be added to the regimen at a dose of 10–15 mg/kg/day; the dose may be increased by 5–10 mg/kg/week to achieve the optimal response (usually less than 60 mg/kg/day).

Simple and complex absence seizures.

Initial: 15 mg/kg/day, increasing at 1-week intervals by 5–10 mg/kg/day until seizures are controlled or side effects occur.

Acute manic episodes in bipolar disorder (use divalproex sodium).

Initial: 250 mg t.i.d.; **then,** increase dose q 2–3 days until a trough serum level of 50 mcg/mL is reached. The maximum dose is 60 mg/kg/day.

Prophylaxis of migraine (use divalproex sodium).

250 mg/day b.i.d., although some may require up to 1,000 mg daily.

• **IV**

Epilepsy.

Give as a 60 min infusion at 20 mg or less/min with the same frequency as PO products.

• **RECTAL**

Intractable status epilepticus that has not responded to other treatment.

Adults: 200–1,200 mg q 6 hr rectally with phenytoin and phenobarbital. **Children:** 15–20 mg/kg.

NURSING CONSIDERATIONS

SEE ALSO *NURSING CONSIDERATIONS* FOR *ANTICONVULSANTS*.

ADMINISTRATION/STORAGE

1. Divide daily dosage if it exceeds 250 mg/day.
2. Do not confuse Depkote ER, an extended release divalproex sodium, with Depakote delayed release. The two forms are not substitutable. Depakote still requires dosing q 8–12 hr whereas Depakote ER is given once daily.
3. To minimize GI irritation, initiate at a lower dose, give with food, or use delayed-release (Depakote).
4. To minimize CNS depression, give at bedtime.
5. To avoid local irritation, swallow valproic acid capsules whole. However, capsules can either be swallowed whole or the contents sprinkled on teaspoonful of a soft food (e.g., applesauce, pudding) and swallowed immediately without chewing.
6. Do not administer valproic acid syrup to clients whose *sodium* intake must be restricted. Consult provider if a sodium-restricted client is unable to swallow capsules.
7. In clients taking valproic acid, conversion to divalproex sodium can be undertaken at the same total daily dose and dosing schedule.
8. Reduce the starting dose in geriatric clients, depending on the response. Younger children will require larger maintenance doses, especially if they are receiving enzyme-inducing drugs.

IV 9. Rapid IV infusion has been associated with an increase in side effects.

10. IV use for more than 14 days has not been studied. Switch to PO valproate products as soon as feasible.

ASSESSMENT

1. Note indications for therapy, type, onset, and symptom duration.
2. Document characteristics of seizure activity, including onset and prodrome if evident.
3. Identify type, frequency, and duration of behaviors that warrant therapy; list other agents prescribed and the outcome.
4. Monitor LFTs due to increased potential for hepatoxicity.

CLIENT/FAMILY TEACHING

1. Take with or after meals to minimize GI upset and at bedtime to minimize sedative effects. Do not chew

tablets or capsules, swallow whole to prevent irritation of mouth and throat.
2. Take only as directed and do not stop suddenly; seizures may occur with seizure disorder.
3. Do not drive or perform activities that require mental alertness until drug effects realized and seizure control verified.
4. Report any unexplained fever, sore throat, skin rash, yellow skin discoloration, or unusual bruising/bleeding.
5. With diabetes, drug may cause a false positive urine test for ketones. Report symptoms of ketoacidosis (dry mouth, thirst, dry flushed skin).
6. Report any loss of seizure control.
7. Avoid alcohol and any other CNS depressants or OTC products without approval.
8. Report for periodic CBC, serum glucose/acetone, and LFTs.
9. Practice reliable contraception.

OUTCOMES/EVALUATE

• Control of seizures
• Migraine headache prophylaxis
• Control of manic episodes
• Therapeutic drug levels (50–100 mcg/mL)

Valrubicin

(val-**ROO**-bih-sin)

PREGNANCY CATEGORY: C
CLASSIFICATION(S):
Antineoplastic, antibiotic
Rx: Valstar

SEE ALSO *ANTINEOPLASTIC AGENTS.*

ACTION/KINETICS

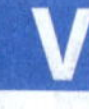

Related to doxorubicin. Inhibits incorporation of nucleosides into nucleic acids, causes extensive chromosome damage, and arrests cell cycle G_2. Although minimal metabolism occurs when instilled into the bladder, valrubicin metabolites interfere with normal DNA breaking-resealing action of DNA topoisomerase II. It penetrates the bladder wall. Almost completely excreted by voiding the instillate.

USES

Intravesical therapy of BCG-refractory carcinoma in situ of the urinary bladder.

CONTRAINDICATIONS

Hypersensitivity to anthracyclines or Cremophor EL. Concurrent UTIs, small bladder capacity (i.e., unable to hold 75 mL instillation). Use in those with a perforated bladder or when the integrity of the bladder mucosa has been compromised. IM or IV use. Lactation.

SPECIAL CONCERNS

Use with caution in severe irritable bladder symptoms. Safety and efficacy have not been determined in children.

SIDE EFFECTS

GU: Local bladder symptoms, urinary frequency/urgency/incontinence/ retention, dysuria, urinary bladder spasm, hematuria, bladder pain, urinary cystitis, nocturia, local burning symptoms, urethral pain, pelvic pain, UTI, poor urine flow, urethritis. **GI:** Abdominal pain, N&V, diarrhea, flatulence, taste loss. **Metabolic:** Hyperglycemia, peripheral edema. **CNS:** Headache, dizziness. **Dermatologic:** Rash, pruritus, local skin irritation. **Body as a whole:** Asthenia, malaise, fever, myalgia. **Miscellaneous:** Back/chest pain, anemia, vasodilation, pneumonia, tenesmus.

LABORATORY TEST CONSIDERATIONS

↑ NPN.

HOW SUPPLIED

Solution for intravesical instillation: 40 mg/mL

DOSAGE

• **SOLUTION FOR INTRAVESICAL USE**

Bladder cancer.

Adults: 800 mg once a week for 6 weeks.

NURSING CONSIDERATIONS

SEE ALSO *NURSING CONSIDERATIONS FOR ANTINEOPLASTIC AGENTS.*

ADMINISTRATION/STORAGE

1. Use aseptic techniques during administration to avoid introducing contaminants into the GU tract or traumatizing the urinary mucosa.

2. Delay use for 2 or more weeks after transurethral resection or fulguration.
3. Insert a urethral catheter under aseptic conditions, drain the bladder, and instill 75 mL valrubicin (diluted) slowly via gravity flow for several minutes. Withdraw the catheter. Have client retain the drug for 2 hr before voiding.
4. Maintain adequate hydration following treatment.
5. Cremophor EL, which contains the valrubicin, may leach a hepatotoxic plasticizer from PVC bags and IV tubing. Thus, prepare and store the drug in glass, polypropylene, or polyolefin containers and tubing.
6. Do not mix with other drugs.
7. For each instillation, warm four - 5 mL vials to room temperature slowly (do not heat). Withdraw 20 mL from the 4 vials and dilute with 55 mL 0.9% NaCl injection.
8. Valrubicin solution is clear red.
9. Valrubicin diluted in 0.9% NaCl is stable for 12 hr at temperatures up to 25°C (77°F).
10. At temperatures less than 4°C (30°F), Cremophor EL may form a waxy precipitate. If this occurs, warm the vial in the hand until the solution is clear. If particulate matter is still seen, do not use.
11. Store unopened vials at 2–8°C (36–46°F). Do not freeze or heat vials.

ASSESSMENT

Document diagnosis or BCG failure; ensure client is unable to undergo, or not a candidate for cystectomy.

CLIENT/FAMILY TEACHING

1. Drug induces complete response in only about 1 in 5 clients. Delaying cystectomy could lead to metastatic bladder cancer.
2. Drug is administered into the bladder by a catheter once a week for 6 weeks. Retain the drug in the bladder for 2 hr and then void.
3. For the first 24–48 hr following instillation, red-tinged urine is typical.
4. Consume adequate fluids during therapy.
5. Men are to refrain from sexual intercourse during therapy.
6. Evaluation for recurrence of bladder cancer should be done every 3 mo with a biopsy, cystoscopy, and urine cytology.

OUTCOMES/EVALUATE

Control of bladder cancer

Valsartan

(val-**SAR**-tan)

PREGNANCY CATEGORY: C (1ST TRIMESTER), D (2ND AND 3RD TRIMESTERS)

CLASSIFICATION(S):

Antihypertensive, angiotensin II receptor blocker

Rx: Diovan

SEE ALSO ***ANGIOTENSIN II RECEPTOR ANTAGONISTS*** AND ***ANTIHYPERTENSIVES***.

ACTION/KINETICS

Reduces both BP and left ventricular hypertrophy. Food decreases absorption. **Peak plasma levels:** 2–4 hr. Highly bound to plasma proteins. **t½, terminal:** 11–15 hr. Eliminated mostly unchanged in feces (80%) and urine (about 20%).

USES

Alone or in combination to treat hypertension. *Investigational:* Heart failure.

SIDE EFFECTS

CNS: Headache, dizziness, fatigue, anxiety, insomnia, paresthesia, somnolence. **GI:** Abdominal pain, diarrhea, nausea, constipation, dry mouth, dyspepsia, flatulence. **Respiratory:** URI, cough, rhinitis, sinusitis, pharyngitis, dyspnea. **Body as a whole:** Viral infection, edema, asthenia, allergic reaction. **Musculoskeletal:** Arthralgia, back pain, muscle cramps, myalgia. **Dermatologic:** Pruritus, rash. **Miscellaneous:** Palpitations, vertigo, neutropenia, impotence.

LABORATORY TEST CONSIDERATIONS

↓ H&H. ↑ Serum potassium, liver enzymes, serum bilirubin.

HOW SUPPLIED

Capsules: 80 mg, 160 mg; *Tablets:* 320 mg

DOSAGE

- **CAPSULES, TABLETS**

Hypertension.

Adults, initial: 80 mg once daily as monotherapy in clients who are not volume depleted. **Dose range:** 80–320 mg once daily. If additional antihypertensive effect is needed, dose may be increased to 160 mg or 320 mg once daily or diuretic may be added (has greater effect than valsartan dose increases beyond 80 mg).

NURSING CONSIDERATIONS

ADMINISTRATION/STORAGE

1. Give on an empty stomach.
2. Antihypertensive effect is usually seen within 2 weeks with maximum reduction after 4 weeks.

ASSESSMENT

1. Note disease onset, characteristics of symptoms, other agents trialed and the outcome.
2. Obtain liver and renal function studies; note dysfunction.

CLIENT/FAMILY TEACHING

1. May take with or without food and with other prescribed antihypertensive agents.
2. Change positions slowly and avoid dehydration to prevent postural effects and dizziness.
3. Practice reliable contraception; report if pregnancy suspected as drug may cause fetal death.
4. Continue low fat, low sodium diet, regular exercise, weight loss, smoking and alcohol cessation, and stress reduction in goal of BP control.
5. May experience headaches, coughing, diarrhea, nausea, and joint aches; report if persistent.

OUTCOMES/EVALUATE

↓ BP

Vancomycin hydrochloride

(van-koh-**MY**-sin)

PREGNANCY CATEGORY: C (B FOR CAPSULES ONLY)

CLASSIFICATION(S):

Antibiotic, miscellaneous

Rx: Vancocin, Vancoled

SEE ALSO *ANTI-INFECTIVES.*

ACTION/KINETICS

Appears to bind to bacterial cell wall, arresting its synthesis and lysing the cytoplasmic membrane by a mechanism that is different from that of penicillins and cephalosporins. May also change the permeability of the cytoplasmic membranes of bacteria, thus inhibiting RNA synthesis. Bactericidal for most organisms and bacteriostatic for enterococci. Poorly absorbed from the GI tract. Diffuses in pleural, pericardial, ascitic, and synovial fluids after parenteral administration. **Peak plasma levels, IV:** 33 mcg/mL 5 min after 0.5-g dosage. **t½, after PO:** 4–8 hr for adults and 2–3 hr for children; **t½, after IV:** 4–11 hr for adults and ranging from 2–3 hr in children to 6–10 hr for newborns. The half-life is increased markedly in the presence of renal impairment (240 hr has been noted). Primarily excreted in urine unchanged. Auditory and renal function tests are indicated before and during therapy.

USES

PO: (1) Antibiotic-induced pseudomembranous colitis due to *Clostridium difficile.* (2) Staphylococcal enterocolitis. (3) Severe or progressive antibiotic-induced diarrhea caused by *C. difficile* that is not responsive to the causative antibiotic being discontinued; also for debilitated clients.

IV: (1) Severe staphylococcal infections in clients who have not responded to penicillins or cephalosporins, who cannot receive these drugs, or who have resistant infections. Infections include lower respiratory tract infections, bone infections, endocarditis, septicemia, and skin and skin structure infections. (2) Alone or in combination with aminoglycosides to treat endocarditis caused by *Streptococcus viridans* or *S. bovis.* Must combine with an aminoglycoside to treat endocarditis due to Streptococcus faecalis. (3) Used with rifampin, an aminoglycoside (or both) to treat early onset prosthetic valve endocarditis caused by *Staphylococcus epidermidis* or other diphtheroids. (4) Prophylaxis of bacterial endocarditis in pencillin-allergic clients who have congenital heart disease or rheumatic or other acquired or valvular heart disease if such clients are undergoing dental or surgical procedures of the upper respiratory tract. (5) The parenteral dosage form may be given PO to treat pseudomembranous colitis or staphylococcal enterocolitis due to *C. difficile*.

CONTRAINDICATIONS

Hypersensitivity. Minor infections. Lactation.

SPECIAL CONCERNS

Use with extreme caution in the presence of impaired renal function or previous hearing loss. Geriatric clients are at a greater risk of developing ototoxicity.

SIDE EFFECTS

Ototoxicity (may lead to deafness; deafness may progress after drug is discontinued), nephrotoxicity (may lead to uremia).

Red-neck syndrome. Sudden and profound drop in BP with or without a maculopapular rash over the face, neck, upper chest, and extremities. **CV:** Exaggerated hypotension (due to rapid bolus administration), including ***shock and possibly cardiac arrest.*** **GU:** Renal failure (rare), interstitial nephritis (rare). **Respiratory:** Wheezing, dyspnea. **Dermatologic:** Urticaria, pruritus, macular rashes, exfoliative dermatitis, ***Stevens-Johnson syndrome, toxic epidermal necrolysis,*** vasculitis. **Allergic:** Drug fever, hypersensitivity, ***anaphylaxis.*** **At injection site:** Tissue irritation, including pain, tenderness, necrosis, thrombophlebitis. **Miscellaneous:** Nausea, chills, tinnitus, eosinophilia, neutropenia (reversible), pseudomembranous colitis.

DRUG INTERACTIONS

Aminoglycosides / ↑ Risk of nephrotoxicity

Anesthetics / ↑ Risk of erythema and histamine-like flushing in children

Muscle relaxants, nondepolarizing / ↑ Neuromuscular blockade

Nephrotoxic/Neurotoxic drugs / Carefully monitor with concurrent or sequential systemic or topical use

HOW SUPPLIED

Capsule: 125 mg, 250 mg; *Powder for injection:* 500 mg, 1 g, 5 g, 10 g; *Powder for oral solution:* 1 g, 10 g

DOSAGE

• CAPSULES, ORAL SOLUTION

Adults: 0.5–2 g/day in three to four divided doses for 7–10 days. Alternatively, 125 mg t.i.d.–q.i.d. for *C. difficile* may be as effective as the 500-mg dosage. **Children:** 40 mg/kg/day in three to four divided doses for 7–10 days, not to exceed 2 g/day. **Neonates:** 10 mg/kg/day in divided doses.

• IV

Severe staphylococcal infections.

Adults: 500 mg q 6 hr or 1 g q 12 hr. **Children:** 10 mg/kg/6 hr. **Infants and neonates, initial:** 15 mg/kg for one dose; **then,** 10 mg/kg q 12 hr for neonates in the first week of life and q 8 hr thereafter up to 1 month of age.

Prophylaxis of bacterial endocarditis in dental, oral, or upper respiratory tract procedures in penicillin-allergic clients.

Adults: 1 g vancomycin over 1 hr plus 1.5 mg/kg gentamicin (IV or IM), not to exceed 80 mg, 1 hr before the procedure. May repeat once, 8 hr after the initial dose. **Children:** 20 mg/kg vancomycin plus 2 mg/kg gentamicin (IV or IM), not to exceed 80 mg, 1 hr before the procedure. May repeat once, 8 hr after the initial dose.

NURSING CONSIDERATIONS

SEE ALSO *GENERAL NURSING CONSIDERATIONS* FOR *ANTI-INFECTIVES*.

ADMINISTRATION/STORAGE

1. Reduce dosage in renal disease; see package insert for procedure.
2. The PO solution is prepared by adding 115 mL distilled water to the 10-g container. The appropriate dose of PO solution may be mixed with 1 oz of

water or flavored syrup to improve the taste. The diluted drug may also be given by NGT.
3. The parenteral form may be administered PO by diluting the 1-g vial with 20 mL distilled or deionized water (each 5 mL contains about 250 mg vancomycin).
IV 4. For IV use, dilute each 500-mg vial with 10 mL of sterile water. This may be further diluted in 200 mL of dextrose or saline solution and infused over 60 min.
5. Intermittent infusion is the preferred route, but continuous IV drip may be used.
6. Avoid rapid IV administration because this may result in hypotension, nausea, warmth, and generalized tingling. Administer over 1 hr in at least 200 mL of NSS or D5W.
7. Avoid extravasation during injections; may cause tissue necrosis.
8. Reduce risk of thrombophlebitis by rotating injection sites or adding additional diluent.
9. Aqueous solution is stable for 2 weeks.
10. Once rubber stopper is punctured, ampule should be refrigerated to maintain stability.

ASSESSMENT

1. Document indications for therapy, type, onset, and characteristics of symptoms.
2. Assess renal and auditory functions (including 8th CN function).
3. Monitor CBC, cultures, and renal function studies; reduce dose with renal dysfunction.

INTERVENTIONS

1. Record weight, VS, and I&O; ensure adequate hydration.
2. Report any adverse drug effects, such as:

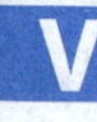

• Ototoxicity, demonstrated by tinnitus, progressive hearing loss, dizziness, and/or nystagmus; may occur latently
• Nephrotoxicity, demonstrated by albuminuria, hematuria, anuria, casts, edema, and uremia

3. During IV administration ensure that peak and trough drug levels are performed at the prescribed dosing interval, usually 30 min prior to scheduled IV dose (trough) and 1 hr following IV dose (peak) to accurately assess serum levels.

OUTCOMES/EVALUATE

• Negative cultures
• Relief of S&S R/T infection
• Serum levels within therapeutic range (trough 1–5 mcg/mL; peak 20–50 mcg/mL)

Vasopressin

(vay-so-**PRESS**-in)

PREGNANCY CATEGORY: C
CLASSIFICATION(S):
Pituitary hormone
Rx: Pitressin Synthetic
★Rx: Pressyn

ACTION/KINETICS

Released from the anterior pituitary gland; regulates water conservation by promoting reabsorption of water by increasing the permeability of the collecting ducts in the kidney. Depending on the concentration, the hormone acts on both V_1 and V_2 receptors. Also causes vasoconstriction (pressor effect) of the splanchnic and portal vessels (and to a lesser extent of peripheral, cerebral, pulmonary, and coronary vessels). Also increases the smooth muscular activity of the bladder, GI tract, and uterus. **IM, SC: Onset,** variable; **duration,** 2–8 hr. **t½:** 10–20 min. **Effective plasma levels:** 4.5–6 microunits.

USES

(1) Neurogenic (central) diabetes insipidus (ineffective when diabetes insipidus is of renal origin—nephrogenic diabetes insipidus). (2) Relief of postoperative abdominal distention. (3) To dispel gas shadows in abdominal roentgenography. *Investigational:* Bleeding esophageal varices, treat refractory septic shock (low doses), treat ventricular fibrillation/pulseless ventricular tachycardia cardiac arrest.

CONTRAINDICATIONS

Vascular disease, especially when involving coronary arteries; angina pectoris. Chronic nephritis until reasonable blood nitrogen levels are attained. Never give the tannate IV.

SPECIAL CONCERNS

Pediatric and geriatric clients have an increased risk of hyponatremia and water intoxication. Use caution during lactation and in the presence of asthma, epilepsy, migraine, CAD, and CHF.

SIDE EFFECTS

GI: N&V, increased intestinal activity (e.g., belching, cramps, urge to defecate), abdominal cramps, flatus. **CV:** Circumoral pallor, arrhythmias, decreased cardiac output, ***cardiac arrest,*** angina, myocardial ischemia, peripheral vasoconstriction, gangrene. **CNS:** Tremor, vertigo, "pounding" in head. **Dermatologic:** Sweating, urticaria, skin blanching, cutaneous gangrene. **Miscellaneous:** Tremor, ***allergic reactions, bronchoconstriction, anaphylaxis,*** water intoxication (drowsiness, headache, ***coma, convulsions.***

• **IV**

Use of vasopressin may result in severe vasoconstriction; local tissue necrosis if extravasation occurs. IM use of tannate may cause pain and sterile abscesses at site of injection.

OD OVERDOSE MANAGEMENT

Symptoms: Water intoxication. *Treatment:* Withdraw vasopressin until polyuria occurs. If water intoxication is serious, administration of mannitol (i.e., an osmotic diuretic), hypertonic dextrose, or urea alone (or with furosemide) is indicated.

DRUG INTERACTIONS

Alcohol / May decrease antidiuretic effect of vasopressin
Carbamazepine / May potentiate antidiuretic effect of vasopressin
Chlorpropamide / May potentiate antidiuretic effect of vasopressin
Clofibrate / May potentiate antidiuretic effect of vasopressin
Demeclocycline / May decrease antidiuretic effect of vasopressin
Fludrocortisone / May potentiate antidiuretic effect of vasopressin
Ganglionic blocking drugs / May ↑ significantly sensitivity to pressor effects of vasopressin
Heparin / May decrease antidiuretic effect of vasopressin
Lithium / May decrease antidiuretic effect of vasopressin
Norepinephrine/ May decrease antidiuretic effect of vasopressin
Tricyclic antidepressants / May potentiate antidiuretic effect of vasopressin

HOW SUPPLIED

Injection: 20 pressor units/mL.

DOSAGE

• **IM, SC**

Diabetes insipidus.

Adults: 5–10 U b.i.d.–t.i.d.; **pediatric:** 2.5–10 U t.i.d.–q.i.d.

Abdominal distention.

Adults, initial: 5 U IM; **then,** 10 U IM q 3–4 hr; **pediatric:** individualize the dose (usual: 2.5–5 U).

Abdominal roentgenography.

IM, SC: 2 injections of 10 U each 2 hr and ½ hr before X rays are taken.

Esophageal varices.

Initial: 0.2 U/min IV or selective IA; **then,** 0.4 U/min if bleeding continues. The maximum recommended dose is 0.9 U/min.

• **INTRANASAL (USING INJECTION SOLUTION)**

Diabetes insipidus.

Individualize the dose using the injection solution on cotton pledgets, by nasal spray, or by dropper.

NURSING CONSIDERATIONS

ADMINISTRATION/STORAGE

Administration of 1–2 glasses of water prior to use for diabetes insipidus will reduce side effects such as nausea, cramps, and skin blanching.

ASSESSMENT

1. Document indications for therapy, type, onset, and characteristics of symptoms.
2. Note any history of vascular disease, especially involving the coronary arteries (e.g., hypertension, CHF, CAD).
3. Document any asthma, seizures, or migraine headaches.

INTERVENTIONS

1. Check skin turgor, mucous membranes, and presence of thirst to assess for dehydration.

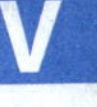

2. Monitor BP and I&O; report any excessive BP elevation or lack of response characterized by a ↓ BP.
3. Record weight daily and assess for edema; report rapid gains.
4. Perform urine specific gravity and report if < 1.005 or > than 1.030. Determine urine osmolarity.
5. With abdominal distention, assess and document presence/characteristics of bowel sounds and passage of flatus/stool. A rectal tube may facilitate expulsion of gas.

CLIENT/FAMILY TEACHING

1. Review appropriate method for administration/instillation.
2. Avoid alcohol and OTC agents without approval.

OUTCOMES/EVALUATE

- Prevention of dehydration: ↓ urinary frequency, ↑ urine osmolarity
- Control of intra-arterial bleeding
- ↓ Abdominal distention/discomfort; elimination of intestinal gas

Vecuronium bromide

(vh-kyour-**OH**-nee-um)

PREGNANCY CATEGORY: C
CLASSIFICATION(S):
Neuromuscular blocking drug, depolarizing
Rx: Norcuron

SEE ALSO *NEUROMUSCULAR BLOCKING AGENTS*.

ACTION/KINETICS

Less likely than other agents to cause histamine release. Effects can be antagonized by anticholinesterase drugs. **Onset:** 2.5–3 min; **peak effect:** 3–5 min; **duration:** 25–40 min using balanced anesthesia. About one-third more potent than pancuronium, but its duration of action is shorter at initial equipotent doses. No cumulative effects noted after repeated administration. **t½, elimination:** 65–75 min; a shortened half-life (35–40 min) has been noted in late pregnancy. Metabolized in liver and excreted through the kidney and bile. Is bound to plasma protein. Recovery may be doubled in clients with cirrhosis or cholestasis; renal failure does not affect recovery time.

USES

(1) To induce skeletal muscle relaxation during surgery or mechanical ventilation. (2) To facilitate ET intubation. (3) As an adjunct to general anesthesia. *Investigational:* To treat electrically induced seizures or seizures induced by drugs.

ADDITIONAL CONTRAINDICATIONS

Use in neonates, obesity. Sensitivity to bromides.

SPECIAL CONCERNS

Those from 7 weeks to 1 year of age are more sensitive to the effects of vecuronium leading to a recovery time up to 1½ times that for adults. The dose for children aged 1–10 years of age must be individualized and may, in fact, require a somewhat higher initial dose and a slightly more frequent supplemental dosing schedule than adults. Those with myasthenia gravis or Eaton-Lambert syndrome may experience profound effects with small doses of vecuronium. Cardiovascular disease, old age, and edematous states result in increased volume of distribution and thus a delay in onset time—the dose should *not* be increased.

ADDITIONAL SIDE EFFECTS

Moderate to severe skeletal muscle weakness, which may require artificial respiration. ***Malignant hyperthermia.***

ADDITIONAL DRUG INTERACTIONS

Bacitracin / High IV or IP bacitracin doses → ↑ muscle relaxation
Sodium colistimethate / High IV or IP sodium colistimethate doses → ↑ muscle relaxation
Tetracyclines / High IV or IP tetracycline doses → ↑ muscle relaxation
Succinylcholine ↑ Vecuronium effect

HOW SUPPLIED

Powder for injection: 10 mg, 20 mg

DOSAGE

- **IV ONLY**

Intubation.

Adults and children over 10 years of age. 0.08–0.1 mg/kg.

For use after succinylcholine-assisted ET intubation.

0.04–0.06 mg/kg for inhalation anesthesia and 0.05–0.06 mg/kg using balanced anesthesia. (*NOTE:* For halothane anesthesia, doses of 0.15–0.28 mg/kg may be given without adverse effects.)

For use during anesthesia with enflurane or isoflurane after steady state established.

0.06–0.085 mg/kg (about 15% less than the usual initial dose).

Supplemental use.

IV only: 0.01–0.015 mg/kg given 25–40 min following the initial dose; **then,** given q 12–15 min as needed. **IV infusion:** Initiated after recovery from effects of initial IV dose of 0.08–0.1 mg/kg has started. **Initial:** 0.001 mcg (1 mg)/kg; **then** adjust according to client response and requirements. Average infusion rate: 0.0008–0.0012 mg/kg/min (0.8–1.2 mcg/kg/min). After steady-state enflurane, isoflurane, and possibly halothane anesthesia has been established: reduce IV infusion by 25%–60%.

NURSING CONSIDERATIONS

SEE ALSO *NURSING CONSIDERATIONS* FOR *NEUROMUSCULAR BLOCKING AGENTS.*

ADMINISTRATION/STORAGE

IV 1. Dosage must be individualized and depends on prior or concomitant use of anesthetics or succinylcholine.

2. May be mixed with saline, D5W alone or with saline, RL solution, and sterile water for injection.

3. Refrigerate after reconstitution. Use within 8 hr of reconstitution.

4. Have neostigmine, pyridostigmine, or edrophonium available to reverse vecuronium; atropine helps counteract muscarinic effects.

ASSESSMENT

1. Document indications for therapy and anticipated time frame for use.

2. Monitor ECG, VS, CBC, electrolytes, liver and renal function studies.

3. Use a nerve stimulator to determine neuromuscular blockade. Anticholinesterase will reverse neuromuscular blockade.

INTERVENTIONS

1. May use peripheral nerve stimulator to assess neuromuscular response/recovery.

2. Monitor VS and ECG. Can cause vagal stimulation resulting in bradycardia, hypotension, and cardiac arrhythmias.

3. Muscle fasciculations may cause soreness or injury after recovery. Give prescribed nondepolarizing agent and reassure that soreness is likely caused by unsynchronized contractions of adjacent muscle fibers just before onset of paralysis.

4. Monitor closely for any evidence of malignant hyperthermia, unresponsive tachycardia, jaw spasm, or lack of laryngeal relaxation. Stop infusion and report; temperature elevations are late S&S.

5. Drug should only be used on a short-term basis and in a continuously monitored environment.

6. Client is fully conscious and aware of surroundings and conversations. Drug does not affect pain or anxiety; give analgesics and antianxiety agents.

7. Prolonged use, as in an ICU setting, may lead to skeletal muscle weakness and symptoms consistent with muscle disuse atrophy. This may complicate ventilator weaning; some may require extensive physical therapy.

OUTCOMES/EVALUATE

- Skeletal muscle relaxation
- Facilitation of intubation; tolerance of mechanical ventilation

Venlafaxine hydrochloride

(ven-lah-**FAX**-een)

PREGNANCY CATEGORY: C
CLASSIFICATION(S):
Antidepressant, miscellaneous
Rx: Effexor, Effexor XR

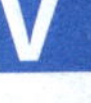

ACTION/KINETICS

Not related chemically to any of the currently available antidepressants. A potent inhibitor of the uptake of neuronal serotonin and norepinephrine in the CNS and a weak inhibitor of the uptake of dopamine. Has no anticholinergic, sedative, or orthostatic hypotensive effects. The major metabolite—O-desmethylvenlafaxine (ODV)—is active. The drug and metabolite are eliminated through the kidneys. **t½, venlafaxine:** 5 hr; **t½, ODV:** 11 hr. **Time to reach steady state:** 3–4 days. The half-life of the drug and metabolite are increased in clients with impaired liver or renal function. Food has no effect on the absorption of venlafaxine.

USES

(1) Treatment of depression. (2) Prevention of major depressive disorder relapse. (3) Chronic treatment of generalized anxiety disorder (extended-release product). *Investigational:* Treat hot flashes in women who survive breast cancer.

CONTRAINDICATIONS

Use with a MAO inhibitor or within 14 days of discontinuation of a MAO inhibitor. Use of alcohol. Lactation.

SPECIAL CONCERNS

Use with caution with impaired hepatic or renal function, in clients with a history of mania, and in those with diseases or conditions that could affect the hemodynamic responses or metabolism. Although it is possible for a geriatric client to be more sensitive, dosage adjustment is not necessary. Use for more than 4–6 weeks has not been evaluated. Safety and efficacy of the immediate release product have not been determined in children less than 18 years of age.

SIDE EFFECTS

Side effects with an incidence of 0.1% or greater are listed.

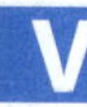

CNS: Anxiety, nervousness, insomnia, mania, hypomania, ***seizures, suicide attempts,*** dizziness, somnolence, tremors, abnormal dreams, hypertonia, paresthesia, decreased libido, agitation, confusion, abnormal thinking, depersonalization, depression, twitching, migraine, emotional lability, trismus, vertigo, apathy, ataxia, circumoral paresthesia, CNS stimulation, euphoria, hallucinations, hostility, hyperesthesia, hyperkinesia, hypertonia, hypotonia, incoordination, increased libido, myoclonus, neuralgia, neuropathy, paranoid reaction, psychosis, psychotic depression, sleep disturbance, abnormal speech, stupor, torticollis. **CV:** Sustained increase in BP (hypertension), vasodilation, tachycardia, postural hypotension, angina pectoris, extrasystoles, hypotension, peripheral vascular disorder, syncope, thrombophlebitis, peripheral edema. **GI:** Anorexia, N&V, dry mouth, constipation, diarrhea, dyspepsia, flatulence, dysphagia, eructation, colitis, edema of tongue, esophagitis, gastroenteritis, gastritis, glossitis, gingivitis, hemorrhoids, ***rectal hemorrhage,*** melena, stomatitis, stomach ulcer, mouth ulceration. **Body as a whole:** Headache, asthenia, infection, chills, chest pain, trauma, yawn, weight loss, accidental injury, malaise, neck pain, enlarged abdomen, allergic reaction, cyst, facial edema, generalized edema, hangover effect, hernia, intentional injury, neck rigidity, moniliasis, substernal chest pain, pelvic pain, photosensitivity reaction. **Respiratory:** Bronchitis, dyspnea, asthma, chest congestion, epistaxis, hyperventilation, laryngismus, laryngitis, pneumonia, voice alteration. **Dermatologic:** Acne, alopecia, brittle nails, contact dermatitis, dry skin, herpes simplex, herpes zoster, maculopapular rash, urticaria. **Hematologic:** Ecchymosis, anemia, leukocytosis, leukopenia, lymphadenopathy, lymphocytosis, thrombocytopenia, thrombocythemia, abnormal WBCs. **Endocrine:** Hypothyroidism, hyperthyroidism, goiter. **Musculoskeletal:** Arthritis, arthrosis, bone pain, bone spurs, bursitis, joint disorder, myasthenia, tenosynovitis. **Ophthalmic:** Blurred vision, mydriasis, abnormal accommodation, abnormal vision, cataract, conjunctivitis, corneal lesion, diplopia, dry eyes, exophthalmos, eye pain, photophobia, subconjunctival hemorrhage, visual field defect. **GU:** Urinary retention, abnormal ejaculation, impotence, urinary frequency, impaired urination, disturbed orgasm, menstrual disorder, anorgasmia, dysuria, hematuria, metrorrhagia, vaginitis, amenorrhea, kidney calculus, cystitis, leukorrhea, menorrhagia, nocturia, bladder pain, breast pain, kidney pain, polyuria, prostatitis, pyelonephritis, pyuria, urinary incontinence, urinary urgency, enlarged uterine fibroids, ***uterine hemorrhage, vaginal hemorrhage,*** vaginal moniliasis. **Miscellaneous:** Sweating, tinnitus, taste perversion, thirst, diabetes mellitus, alcohol intolerance, gout, hypoglycemic reaction, hemochromatosis, ear pain, otitis media.

Withdrawal syndrome.

Anxiety, agitation, tremors, vertigo, headache, nausea, tachycardia, tinnitus, akathisia.

LABORATORY TEST CONSIDERATIONS

↑ Alkaline phosphatase, creatinine, AST, ALT. Glycosuria, hyperglycemia, hyperlipemia, bilirubinemia, hyperuricemia, hypercholesterolemia, hypoglycemia, hypokalemia, hyperkalemia, hyperphosphatemia, hyponatremia, hypophosphatemia, hypoproteinemia, uremia, albuminuria.

OD OVERDOSE MANAGEMENT

Symptoms: Extensions of side effects, especially somnolence. Other symptoms include prolongation of QTc, mild sinus tachycardia, and ***seizures.*** *Treatment:* General supportive measures; treat symptoms. Ensure an adequate airway, oxygenation, and ventilation. Monitor cardiac rhythm and VS. Activated charcoal, induction of emesis, or gastric lavage may be helpful.

DRUG INTERACTIONS

Cimetidine / ↓ First-pass metabolism of venlafaxine
Haloperidol / ↑ Serum levels
MAO inhibitors / Serious and possibly fatal reaction, including hyperthermia, rigidity, myoclonus, autonomic instability with rapid changes in VS, extreme agitation, coma
H *St. John's wort* / ↑ Sedation/hypnosis
Trazodone / Possible "serotonin syndrome," including shivering, irritability, myoclonus, increased muscle tone, and altered consciousness

HOW SUPPLIED

Capsule, Extended-Release: 37.5 mg, 75 mg, 150 mg; *Tablet:* 25 mg, 37.5 mg, 50 mg, 75 mg, 100 mg

DOSAGE

- **TABLETS**

Depression.

Adults, initial: 75 mg/day given in two or three divided doses. Depending on the response, the dose can be increased to 150–225 mg/day in divided doses. Make dosage increments up to 75 mg/day at intervals of 4 or more days. Severely depressed clients may require 375 mg/day in divided doses. **Maintenance:** Sufficient studies have not been undertaken to determine length of treatment.

- **CAPSULES, EXTENDED-RELEASE**

Depression.

Adults, initial: 75 mg once daily. Dose can be increased by up to 75 mg no more often than every 4 days, to a maximum of 225 mg/day.

Generalized anxiety disorder.

Usual: 75–225 mg/day. To avoid overstimulation, some may need to start with 37.5 mg/day. Take on a daily basis not on an as-needed basis.

NURSING CONSIDERATIONS

ADMINISTRATION/STORAGE

1. Take with food.
2. If switching from the immediate-release to extended-release, use the dosage form at the nearest equivalent dose. Individual dosage adjustments may be needed.
3. Reduce the dose by 50% with moderate hepatic impairment and by 25% with mild to moderate renal impairment.
4. When discontinuing venlafaxine, taper the dose over a 2– 4–week period to minimize the risk of withdrawal syndrome.
5. At least 14 days should elapse between discontinuation of a MAO inhibitor and initiation of venlafaxine therapy; at least 7 days should elapse after stopping venlafaxine before starting a MAO inhibitor.

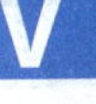

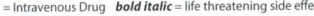

6. Take the extended-release form in the morning.

ASSESSMENT

1. Document indications for therapy, onset, duration and characteristics of symptoms.
2. List other agents prescribed to ensure none interact unfavorably.
3. Monitor CBC, serum lipid levels, renal and LFTs; reduce dose with hepatic or renal impairment.
4. Due to possible sustained hypertension, monitor HR and BP.

CLIENT/FAMILY TEACHING

1. Take only as directed; *do not* stop abruptly may cause withdrawal syndrome.
2. Do not perform activities that require mental alertness until drug effects realized; may cause dizziness or drowsiness.
3. Report any rash, hives, or other allergic manifestations immediately.
4. Drug may impair appetite and induce weight loss; report if excessive.
5. May experience anxiety, palpitations, headaches, and constipation; report if persistent or intolerable.
6. Avoid alcohol and any unprescribed or OTC preparations.
7. Use birth control. Notify provider if pregnant or intends to become pregnant while taking drug.
8. Any suicide ideations or abnormal behaviors should be reported. Due to the possibility of suicide, high-risk clients should be observed closely during initial therapy. Prescriptions should be written for the smallest quantity to reduce the risk of overdose. Have family supervise medication administration with severely depressed clients.

OUTCOMES/EVALUATE

Improvement in symptoms of depression

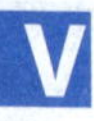

Verapamil

(ver-**AP**-ah-mil)

PREGNANCY CATEGORY: C
CLASSIFICATION(S):
Calcium channel blocker

Rx: Calan, Calan SR, Isoptin, Isoptin SR, Verelan, Verelan PM
★Rx: Alti-Verapamil, Apo-Verap, Chronovera, Gen-Verapamil, Gen-Verapamil SR, Isoptin I.V., Novo-Veramil, Novo-Veramil SR, Nu-Verap

SEE ALSO *CALCIUM CHANNEL BLOCKING AGENTS.*

ACTION/KINETICS

Slows AV conduction and prolongs effective refractory period. IV doses may slightly increase LV filling pressure. Moderately decreases myocardial contractility and peripheral vascular resistance. Worsening of heart failure may result if verapamil is given to clients with moderate to severe cardiac dysfunction. **Onset: PO,** 30 min; **IV,** 3–5 min. **Time to peak plasma levels (PO):** 1–2 hr (5–7 hr for extended-release). **t½, PO:** 4.5–12 hr with repetitive dosing; **IV, initial:** 4 min; **final:** 2–5 hr. **Therapeutic serum levels:** 0.08–0.3 mcg/mL. **Duration, PO:** 8–10 hr (24 hr for extended-release); **IV:** 10–20 min for hemodynamic effect and 2 hr for antiarrhythmic effect. Metabolized to norverapamil, which possesses 20% of the activity of verapamil.

NOTE: Covera HS is designed to deliver verapamil in concert with the 24-hr circadian variations in BP. Verelan PM allows for bedtime dosing and incorporates a 4- to 5-hr delay in drug delivery so there are maximum plasma levels in the morning.

USES

PO: (1) Angina pectoris due to coronary artery spasm (Prinzmetal's variant), chronic stable angina including angina due to increased effort, unstable angina (preinfarction, crescendo). (2) With digitalis to control rapid ventricular rate at rest and during stress in chronic atrial flutter or atrial fibrillation. (3) Prophylaxis of repetitive paroxysmal supraventricular tachycardia. (4) Essential hypertension. (5) Sustained-release tablets are used to treat essential hypertension (Step I therapy). (6) Prophylaxis of migraine headaches. (7) Cardiomyopathy. **IV:** (1) Supraventricular tachyarrhythmias. (2) Atrial flutter or fibrillation. *Investigational:* Manic depression (alternate therapy), exercise-induced asthma, recumbent nocturnal leg cramps, hypertrophic, cluster headaches.

CONTRAINDICATIONS

Severe hypotension, second- or third-degree AV block, cardiogenic shock, severe CHF, sick sinus syndrome (unless client has artificial pacemaker), severe LV dysfunction. Cardiogenic shock and severe CHF unless secondary to SVT that can be treated with verapamil. Lactation. Use of verapamil, IV, with beta-adrenergic blocking agents (as both depress myocardial contractility and AV conduction). Ventricular tachycardia.

SPECIAL CONCERNS

Infants less than 6 months of age may not respond to verapamil. Use with caution in hypertrophic cardiomyopathy, impaired hepatic and renal function, and in the elderly.

SIDE EFFECTS

CV: CHF, bradycardia, ***AV block, asystole,*** premature ventricular contractions and tachycardia (after IV use), peripheral and pulmonary edema, hypotension, syncope, palpitations, AV dissociation, ***MI, CVA.*** **GI:** Nausea, constipation, abdominal discomfort or cramps, dyspepsia, diarrhea, dry mouth. **CNS:** Dizziness, headache, sleep disturbances, depression, amnesia, paranoia, psychoses, hallucinations, jitteriness, confusion, drowsiness, vertigo. IV verapamil may increase intracranial pressure in clients with supratentorial tumors at the time of induction of anesthesia. **Dermatologic:** Rash, dermatitis, alopecia, urticaria, pruritus, erythema multiforme, ***Stevens-Johnson syndrome.*** **Respiratory:** Nasal or chest congestion, dyspnea, SOB, wheezing. **Musculoskeletal:** Paresthesia, asthenia, muscle cramps or inflammation, decreased neuromuscular transmission in Duchenne's muscular dystrophy. **Other:** Blurred vision, equilibrium disturbances, sexual difficulties, spotty menstruation, sweating, rotary nystagmus, flushing, gingival hyperplasia, polyuria, nocturia, gynecomastia, claudication, hyperkeratosis, purpura, petechiae, bruising, hematomas, tachyphylaxis.

LABORATORY TEST CONSIDERATIONS

↑ Alkaline phosphatase, transaminase.

OD OVERDOSE MANAGEMENT

Symptoms: Extension of side effects. *Treatment:* Beta-adrenergics, IV calcium, vasopressors, pacing, and resuscitation.

ADDITIONAL DRUG INTERACTIONS

Antihypertensive agents / Additive hypotensive effects
Barbiturates / ↓ Verapamil bioavailability
Calcium salts / ↓ Verapamil effect
Carbamazepine / ↑ Carbamazepine effect R/T ↓ liver breakdown
Cimetidine / ↑ Verapamil bioavailability
Clarithromycin / Possible severe hypotension and bradycardia
Cyclosporine / ↑ Cyclosporine plasma levels → possible renal toxicity
Digoxin / ↑ Risk of digoxin toxicity R/T ↑ plasma levels
Disopyramide / Additive depressant effects on myocardial contractility and AV conduction
Etomidate / Anesthetic effect may be ↑ with prolonged respiratory depression and apnea
Grapefruit juice / ↑ Verapamil plasma levels R/T ↓ liver metabolism
Lithium / ↓ Lithium levels; lithium toxicity also observed
Muscle relaxants, nondepolarizing / ↑ Neuromuscular blockade R/T verapamil effect on calcium channels
Prazosin / Acute hypotensive effect
Quinidine / Possibility of bradycardia, hypotension, AV block, VT, and pulmonary edema
Ranitidine / ↑ Verapamil bioavailability
Rifampin / ↓ Verapamil effect
Sulfinpyrazone / ↑ Verapamil clearance
Theophyllines / ↑ Theophylline effect
Vitamin D / ↓ Verapamil effect
Warfarin / Possible ↑ effect of either drug R/T ↓ plasma protein binding

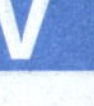

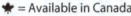

NOTE: Since verapamil is significantly bound to plasma proteins, interaction with other drugs bound to plasma proteins may occur.

HOW SUPPLIED

Capsule, sustained release: 100 mg, 120 mg, 180 mg, 200 mg, 240 mg, 300 mg; *Injection:* 2.5 mg/mL; *Tablet:* 40 mg, 80 mg, 120 mg; *Tablet, sustained release:* 120 mg, 180 mg, 240 mg

DOSAGE

• TABLETS

Angina at rest and chronic stable angina.

Individualized. Adults, initial: 80–120 mg t.i.d. (40 mg t.i.d. if client is sensitive to verapamil); **then,** increase dose to total of 240–480 mg/day. Covera HS is given once daily at bedtime in doses of either 180 or 240 mg.

Arrhythmias.

Dosage range in digitalized clients with chronic atrial fibrillation: 240–320 mg/day in divided doses t.i.d.–q.i.d. For prophylaxis of nondigitalized clients: 240–480 mg/day in divided doses t.i.d.–q.i.d. Maximum effects are seen within 48 hr.

Essential hypertension.

Initial, when used alone: 80 mg t.i.d. Doses up to 360 mg daily may be used. Effects are seen in the first week of therapy. In the elderly or in people of small stature, initial dose should be 40 mg t.i.d.

Prophylaxis of migraine headache.

40–80 mg t.i.d. or q.i.d.

• EXTENDED-RELEASE CAPSULES AND TABLETS

Essential hypertension.

Initial: 240 mg/day in the a.m (120 mg/day in the elderly or people of small stature). If response is inadequate, increase dose to 240 mg in the a.m. and 120 mg in the evening and then 240 mg q 12 hr. Covera HS is given once daily at bedtime in doses of either 180 or 240 mg. The dose of Verelan PM is 200 mg once daily at bedtime.

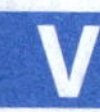

• IV, SLOW

Supraventricular tachyarrhythmias.

Adults, initial: 5–10 mg (0.075–0.15 mg/kg) given over 2 min (over 3 min in older clients); **then,** 10 mg (0.15 mg/kg) 30 min later if response is not adequate. **Infants, up to 1 year:** 0.1–0.2 mg/kg (0.75–2 mg) given as an IV bolus over 2 min; **1–15 years:** 0.1–0.3 mg/kg (2–5 mg, not to exceed 5 mg total dose) over 2 min. If response to initial dose is inadequate, it may be repeated after 30 min, but not more than a total of 10 mg should be given to clients from 1 to 15 years of age.

NURSING CONSIDERATIONS

SEE ALSO NURSING CONSIDERATIONS FOR CALCIUM CHANNEL BLOCKING AGENTS.

ADMINISTRATION/STORAGE

1. The SR tablets (120 mg) may be useful for small stature and elderly clients who require less medication.
2. Take the SR tablets with food.
3. Verelan pellet filled capsules may be carefully opened and the contents sprinkled on a spoonful of applesauce. Swallow the applesauce immediately without chewing and follow with a glass of cool water to ensure complete swallowing of the pellets. Subdividing the contents of a capsule is not recommended.

IV 4. Before administration, inspect ampules for particulate matter or discoloration.
5. Administer IV dosage under continuous ECG monitoring with resuscitation equipment readily available.
6. Give as a slow IV bolus (5–10 mg) over 2 min (3 min to elderly clients) to minimize toxic effects.
7. Store ampules at 15–30°C (59–86°F) and protect from light.
8. Do not give verapamil in an infusion line containing 0.45% NaCl with $NaHCO_3$ because a crystalline precipitate will form.
9. Do not give verapamil by IV push in the same line used for nafcillin infusion because a milky white precipitate will form.
10. Do not mix with albumin, amphotericin B, hydralazine, trimethoprim/sulfamethoxazole, or diluted with sodium lactate in PVC bags.

11. Verapamil will precipitate in any solution with a pH greater than 6.
12. Always individualize dose in the elderly because the pharmacologic effects are more pronounced and more prolonged.

ASSESSMENT

1. Document indications for therapy, onset and duration of symptoms. List agents trialed and outcome.
2. Review list of prescribed medications to ensure none interact.
3. Monitor ECG, CBC, liver and renal function studies; reduce dose with hepatic or renal impairment.

INTERVENTIONS

1. Monitor VS; assess for bradycardia and hypotension, symptoms that may indicate overdosage. Verapamil may lower BP to dangerously low levels if BP already low.
2. *Do not* administer concurrently with IV beta-adrenergic blocking agents.
3. Unless treating verapamil overdosage, withhold any med that may elevate calcium levels.
4. Clients receiving concurrent digoxin therapy should be assessed for symptoms of toxicity and have digoxin levels checked periodically.
5. If disopyramide is to be used, do not administer for at least 48 hr before to 24 hr after verapamil dose.
6. Administer extended-release tablets with food to minimize fluctuations in serum levels.

CLIENT/FAMILY TEACHING

1. Take SR capsule in the am with food; do not cut, crush, or chew, swallow capsules whole.
2. Drug may cause dizziness and orthostatic effects; use caution.
3. Keep a log of BP and pulse for provider review.
4. Avoid alcohol, CNS depressants, and any OTC preparations without approval.
5. Continue life-style modifications (low-fat and low-salt diet, decreased caloric and alcohol consumption, no smoking, and regular exercise) in the overall goal of BP control.
6. Increase bulk and fiber in diet to prevent constipation. With higher doses constipation occurs more frequently. Report if bothersome or pronounced, as psyllium may be prescribed or, if severe, drug therapy may be changed.

OUTCOMES/EVALUATE

- ↓ Frequency/severity of anginal attacks
- Control of BP
- Restoration of stable rhythm
- Therapeutic drug levels (0.08–0.3 mcg/mL)

Verteporfin

(ver-teh-**POR**-fin)

PREGNANCY CATEGORY: C
CLASSIFICATION(S):
Ophthalmic phototherapy
Rx: Visudyne

ACTION/KINETICS

A light-activated drug that is transported in the plasma, mainly by lipoproteins. Once activated by light in the presence of oxygen, highly reactive, short-lived singlet oxygen and reactive oxygen radicals are activated. Light activation causes local damage to neovascular endothelium, resulting in vessel occluson. Damaged endothelium releases procoagulant and vasoactive fctors through leukotriene and eicosanoids (e.g., thromboxane) pathways, resulting in platelet aggregation, fibrin clot formation, and vasoconstriction. The drug appears to accumulate preferentially in neovasculature, including choroidal neovasculature. The drug may also accumulate in the retina causing collateral damage to retinal structures, including retinal pigmented epithelium and outer nuclear layer of the retina. **t½:** 5–6 hr. Metabolized to a small extent by liver and plasma esterases. Excreted through the feces.

USES

Treatment of predominantly classic subfoveal choroidal neovascularization due to age-related macular degeneration, pathologic myopia, or presumed ocular histoplasmosis. *Investigational:* Psoriasis, psoriatic arthritis, rheumatoid arthritis.

CONTRAINDICATIONS

Use with porphyria or hypersensitivity to any component of the product.

SPECIAL CONCERNS

Use with caution during lactation and in those with moderate-to-severe hepatic impairment. A reduced effect may be seen with increasing age.

SIDE EFFECTS

Ophthalmic: Severe vision decrease (equivalent of 4 or more lines) within 7 days after treatment. Blepharitis, blurred vision, decreased visual acuity, visual field defects, cataracts, conjunctivitis/conjunctival injection, diplopia, dry eyes, ocular itching, severe vision loss with or without subconjunctival, subretinal, or vitreous hemorrhage. **At site of infusion:** Injection site reactions, including extravasation and rashes. **CNS:** Hypesthesia, sleep disorder, headaches, vertigo. **CV:** Atrial fibrillation, hypertension, peripheral vascular disorder, varicose veins. **GI:** Constipation, GI cancers, nausea. **Hematologic:** Anemia, decreased or increased WBC count. **Musculoskeletal:** Arthralgia, arthrosis, myasthenia. **Respiratory:** Pharyngitis, pneumonia, cough. **Miscellaneous:** Photosensitivity reactions, decreased hearing, lacrimation disorder, asthenia, back pain (primarily during infusion), eczema, fever, flu syndrome, prostatic disorder.

LABORATORY TEST CONSIDERATIONS

↑ Creatinine. Albuminuria. Elevated LFTs.

OD OVERDOSE MANAGEMENT

Symptoms: Overdose of drug or light in the treated eye may cause nonperfusion of normal retinal vessels with possible severe decreased vision that could be permanent. Prolongation of the time during which there is photosensitivity to bright light. *Treatment:* Extend photosensitivity precautions for a time proportional to the overdose.

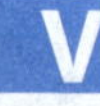

DRUG INTERACTIONS

Calcium channel blockers, polymyxin B, or radiation might increase the rate of verteporfin uptake by vascular endothelium.

HOW SUPPLIED

Lyophilized cake: 15 mg (reconstituted to 2 mg/mL)

DOSAGE

• **IV**

AMD.

Treatment consists of two steps—drug (first step) and light (second step). **Step 1:** verteporfin, 6 mg/m^2. **Step 2:** Initiate 689 nm wavelength laser light delivery 15 min after the start of the 10-min drug infusion with verteporfin.

NURSING CONSIDERATIONS

ADMINISTRATION/STORAGE

IV 1. Reconstitute each vial of verteporfin with 7 mL sterile water for injection to provide 7.5 mL containing 2 mg/mL. Reconstituted drug is an opaque dark-green solution. Protect reconstituted drug from light and use within 4 hr.

2. Withdraw the volume of reconstituted drug to achieve the desired dose of 6 mg/m^2 and dilute with D5W to a total infusion volume of 30 mL.

3. The full infusion volume is given IV over 10 min at a rate of 3 mL/min, using an appropriate syringe pump and inline filter.

4. Take care to prevent extravasation at the injection site. If extravasation occurs, protect the site from light.

5. Photoactivation of verteporfin is controlled by the total light dose delivered. The recommended light dose is 50 J/cm^2 of neovascular lesion administration at an intensity of 600 mW/cm^2. The dose is given over 83 sec.

6. Clinical trials only allowed treatment of 1 eye/client. In those who have lesions in both eyes, evaluate the potential benefits versus risks of treating both eyes concurrently. If the client has already received previous verteporfin therapy in 1 eye with acceptable safety, both eyes can be treated together after a single admin-

istration of drug. Treat the more aggressive lesion first at 15 min after the start of infusion. Immediately after completing the laser treatment of the first eye, adjust the settings for the second eye (with the same light dose and intensity as the first eye) starting 20 min or less from the start of infusion.
7. In clients who present for the first time with eligible lesions in both eyes without previous verteporfin therapy, treat only the most aggressive lesion at the first course. One week after the first course, if no significant safety issues are noted, the second eye can be treated using the same treatment regimen after a second verteporfin infusion. About 3 months later, evaluate both eyes and concurrent treatment following a new verteporfin infusion can be started if both lesions still show evidence of leakage.
8. Wipe up spills with a damp cloth. Avoid skin and eye contact because of possible photosensitivity reactions upon exposure to light. Use rubber gloves and eye protection.
9. Store verteporfin between 20–25°C (68–77°F).

CLIENT/FAMILY TEACHING

1. Advise that AMD is a progressive disease with no known cure. This therapy consists of a two step process involving IV administration of the drug followed by light therapy from a laser about 15 min after the start of the infusion.
2. Report any pain or swelling at injection site as extravasation should be avoided.
3. Avoid skin exposure to direct sunlight or bright indoor light for at least 5 days after therapy.
4. Wear protective clothing and dark glasses if it is necessary to go out in daytime. UV sunscreens are not protective due to the skin deposition of drug.
5. May expose skin to low indoor light to help inactivate drug in skin through the process of photobleaching. Avoid complete darkness.
6. Report if there are any adverse reactions or deterioration in baseline vision levels.

OUTCOMES/EVALUATE

Improved vision in those with impairment R/T AMD

Vidarabine

(vye-**DAIR**-ah-been)

PREGNANCY CATEGORY: C
CLASSIFICATION(S):
Antiviral
Rx: Vira-A

SEE ALSO *ANTIVIRAL AGENTS* AND *ANTI-INFECTIVES*.

ACTION/KINETICS

Phosphorylated in the cell to arabinosyl adenosine monophosphate (ara-AMP) or the triphosphate (ara-ATP). These compounds cause inhibition of viral DNA polymerase, inhibition of virus-induced ribonucleotide reductase. The drug may also incorporate into the viral DNA molecule leading to chain termination. Due to low solubility, systemic absorption is not expected to occur after ophthalmic use. Trace amounts seen in the aqueous humor only if there is a corneal epithelial defect.

USES

(1) Acute keratoconjunctivitis and recurrent epithelial keratitis caused by HSV types 1 and 2. (2) Superficial keratitis caused by HSV that is resistant to idoxuridine or when toxic or hypersensitivity reactions have resulted from idoxuridine. It is more effective than idoxuridine for deep recurrent infections.

CONTRAINDICATIONS

Hypersensitivity to drug. Concomitant use of corticosteroids usually contraindicated. Use in presence of sterile trophic ulcers.

SIDE EFFECTS

Photophobia, lacrimation, conjunctival infection, foreign body sensation, temporal visual haze, burning, irritation, superficial punctate keratitis, pain, punctal occlusion, sensitivity to bright light.

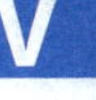

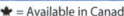

LABORATORY TEST CONSIDERATIONS
↑ Bilirubin, AST.

HOW SUPPLIED
Ophthalmic ointment: 3%

DOSAGE

• **OPHTHALMIC OINTMENT, 3%**

1/2 in. applied to lower conjunctival sac 5 times/day at 3-hr intervals. Continue therapy for 7 days after complete reepithelialization but at reduced dosage (e.g., b.i.d.). If there are no signs of improvement after 7 days or if complete reepithelialization has not occurred within 21 days, consider other therapy.

NURSING CONSIDERATIONS

SEE ALSO *GENERAL NURSING CONSIDERATIONS* FOR *ANTI-INFECTIVES*.

ADMINISTRATION/STORAGE

1. To be effective, initiate as soon as possible, but no later than 72 hr after the appearance of vesicular lesions.
2. Topical corticosteroids or antibiotics may be used concomitantly with vidarabine, but benefits and risks must be assessed.
3. Wait 10 min before use of an additional topical ointment.
4. Ophthalmic use may result in sensitivity to bright light that can be minimized by wearing sunglasses.

ASSESSMENT

Document indications for therapy, onset, duration and clinical presentation. Must initiate within 72 hr of lesion appearance to be effective.

CLIENT/FAMILY TEACHING

1. Take only as directed and do not share medications. Drug must be initiated within 72 hr of appearance of vesicular lesions to be effective.
2. Wash hands before and after applying ointment. If other agents prescribed, wait 10 min before use.
3. Ophthalmic ointment will cause a temporary haze after instillation. Avoid hazardous activities until vision clears.
4. Report any new, persistent, or bothersome side effects.
5. Wear sunglasses outside and avoid bright lights; may cause photophobic reactions.
6. Do not wear contact lenses until eye infection clears.
7. Remain under close ophthalmic supervision while receiving therapy for eye problem.

OUTCOMES/EVALUATE

• Healing of skin lesions
• Reepithelialization of herpetic eye lesions; healing in 1–3 weeks

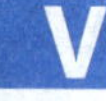

Vinblastine sulfate (VLB)

(vin-**BLAS**-teen)

PREGNANCY CATEGORY: D
CLASSIFICATION(S):
Antineoplastic, Vinca alkaloid
Rx: Velban

SEE ALSO *ANTINEOPLASTIC AGENTS*.

ACTION/KINETICS

Believed to interfere with metabolic pathways of amino acids leading from glutamic acid to the citric acid cycle and urea. Also affects cell energy production needed for mitosis (affects growing cells in metaphase) and interferes with nucleic acid synthesis. Rapidly cleared from plasma but poor penetration to the brain. About 75% bound to serum proteins. Almost completely metabolized in the liver after IV administration. **t1/2, triphasic:** initial, 3.7 min; intermediate, 1.6 hr; final, 24.8 hr. Metabolites are excreted in the bile with smaller amounts in the urine. No cross-resistance with vincristine.

USES

Palliative treatment of generalized Hodgkin's disease (stages III and IV, Ann Arbor modification of Rye staging system); lymphocytic lymphoma (nodular and diffuse, poorly and well differentiated); histiocytic lymphoma; advanced stages of mycosis fungoides; advanced testicular carcinoma; Kaposi's sarcoma; Letterer-Siwe disease (histiocytosis X).

Less effective for palliative treatment of choriocarcinoma resistant to other chemotherapy; breast cancer unresponsive to endocrine surgery and hormonal therapy.

Usually given in combination therapy. However, it has been used as a single agent to treat Hodgkin's disease and advanced testicular germinal-cell cancers (although combination therapy is more effective).

CONTRAINDICATIONS

Leukopenia, significant granulocytopenia (unless it is due to the disease being treated). Bacterial infections. Lactation.

SPECIAL CONCERNS

The drug is fatal if given intrathecally.

ADDITIONAL SIDE EFFECTS

Toxicity is dose-related and more pronounced in clients over age 65 or in those suffering from cachexia (profound general ill health) or skin ulceration. **GI:** Ileus, rectal bleeding, ***hemorrhagic enterocolitis,*** vesiculation of the mouth, ***bleeding from a former ulcer.*** *Dermatologic:* Total epilation, skin vesiculation. *Respiratory:* Acute SOB, ***severe bronchospasm.*** *Neurologic:* Paresthesias, neuritis, mental depression, loss of deep tendon reflexes, ***seizures.*** Extravasation may result in phlebitis and cellulitis with sloughing.

OD OVERDOSE MANAGEMENT

Symptoms: Exaggeration of side effects (see the above). Neurotoxicity. *Treatment:*

- If ingestion is discovered early enough, oral activated charcoal slurry should be given followed by a cathartic.
- Treat side effects due to inappropriate secretion of ADH.
- Prevent ileus (e.g., enemas, cathartic).
- Administer an anticonvulsant (e.g., phenobarbital), if necessary.
- Monitor the CV system.
- Monitor blood counts daily to determine risk of infection and whether blood transfusions are necessary.

DRUG INTERACTIONS

Bleomycin sulfate and cisplatin / Combination of bleomycin, cisplatin, and vinblastine may produce signs of Raynaud's disease in clients with testicular cancer

Erythromycin / Severe myalgia, neutropenia, and constipation

Glutamic acid / Inhibits effect of vinblastine

Mitomycin C / Severe bronchospasm with SOB

Phenytoin / ↓ Effect of phenytoin due to ↓ plasma levels

Tryptophan / Inhibits effect of vinblastine

HOW SUPPLIED

Injection: 1 mg/mL; *Powder for injection:* 10 mg

DOSAGE

• **IV**

Individualized, using WBC count as guide. Administered once every 7 days. **Adults, initial:** 3.7 mg/m^2; **then,** after 7 days, graded doses of 5.5, 7.4, 9.25, and 11.1 mg/m^2 at intervals of 7 days (maximum dose should not exceed 18.5 mg/m^2). **Children, initial:** 2.5 mg/m^2; **then,** after 7 days, graded doses of 3.75, 5.0, 6.25, and 7.5 mg/m^2 at intervals of 7 days (maximum dose should not exceed 12.5 mg/m^2). **Maintenance** doses are calculated based on WBC count—at least 4,000/mm^3.

NURSING CONSIDERATIONS

SEE ALSO *NURSING CONSIDERATIONS* FOR *ANTINEOPLASTIC AGENTS.*

ADMINISTRATION/STORAGE

IV 1. Reconstitute under a laminar flow hood; add 10 mL of bacteriostatic NaCl, which is preserved with either benzyl alcohol or phenol for a final concentration of 1 mg/mL.

2. Do not reconstitute with solutions that raise or lower the pH from between 3.5 and 5.5.

3. Inject into tubing of flowing IV infusion or directly into vein and administer over 1 min. May be further diluted in 50–100 mL of NSS and infused over 15–30 min.

4. Assess peripheral IV site for patency to prevent extravasation, local irritation and pain. If extravasation occurs, move infusion to another vein. Treat affected area with hyaluronidase in-

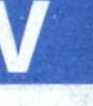

jection and application of moderate heat to decrease local reaction.
5. After reconstitution and removal of a portion from the vial, the remainder may be stored in the refrigerator for 30 days. Unopened vials should be refrigerated at temperatures of 2–8°C (36–46°F).
6. If drug gets into the eye, immediately wash eye thoroughly with water to prevent irritation and ulceration.

ASSESSMENT

1. Take a thorough drug history; note indications for therapy.
2. Document any neuropathies.
3. Monitor uric acid, renal function, and hematologic profiles. Drug may cause granulocyte and platelet suppression. Nadir: 10 days; recovery: 21 days.
4. Do not increase the dose after WBC count is reduced to about 3000 cells/mm^3. When the dose causes such a degree of leukopenia, give a dose one increment smaller at weekly intervals for maintenance. Even though 7 days has elapsed, do not give the next dose until the WBC has returned to at least 4000 cells/mm^3.

INTERVENTIONS

1. Administer antiemetic for N&V.
2. Monitor I&O. Encourage fluid intake of 2–3 L/day.
3. Observe for cyanosis and pallor of extremities and S&S of Raynaud's disease if also receiving bleomycin.
4. Check for manifestations of neurotoxicity and report if evident; dosage may need to be adjusted. Monitor neurologic toxicity by checking reflexes and strength of hand grip.
5. Observe for symptoms of gout. May empirically add allopurinol to decrease uric acid levels.

CLIENT/FAMILY TEACHING

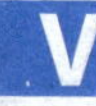

1. Report any signs of infection, fever, sore throat, unusual bruising, or bleeding.
2. Practice barrier contraception.
3. Avoid vaccinations and exposure to persons with infectious diseases.
4. To prevent constipation, eat a high-fiber diet, increase intake of fluids, remain active, and take stool softeners as prescribed.
5. Wear protective clothing, sunglasses, and a sunscreen if exposure to sunlight is necessary.
6. Partial hair loss may occur; plan for cosmetic replacement.
7. Report any S&S of neurotoxicity: paresthesias, difficulty walking, and diminished reflexes; indication to discontinue drug therapy.

OUTCOMES/EVALUATE

Control/regression of malignant process

Vincristine sulfate (VCR, LCR)

(vin-**KRIS**-teen)

PREGNANCY CATEGORY: D
CLASSIFICATION(S):
Antineoplastic, Vinca alkaloid
Rx: Oncovin, Vincasar PFS

SEE ALSO *ANTINEOPLASTIC AGENTS.*

ACTION/KINETICS

Inhibits mitosis at metaphase. The antineoplastic effect is due to interference with intracellular tubulin function by binding to microtubule and spindle proteins in the S phase. After IV use, drug is distributed within 15–30 min to tissues. Poorly penetrates blood-brain barrier. **t½, triphasic:** initial, 5 min; intermediate, 2.3 hr; final, 85 hr. Approximately 80% is excreted in the feces and up to 20% in the urine. No cross-resistance with vinblastine.

USES

(1) Frequently used in combination therapy. (2) ALL in children. Hodgkin's and non-Hodgkin's lymphomas (lymphocytic, mixed-cell, histiocytic, undifferentiated, nodular, and diffuse). (3) Wilms' tumor, neuroblastoma, lymphosarcoma, rhabdomyosarcoma, reticulum cell sarcoma. *Investigational:* ITP; cancer of the breast, ovary, cervix, lung, colorectal area; malignant melanoma, osteosarcoma, multiple myeloma, ovarian germ cell tumors, mycosis fungoides, CLL, CML, Kaposi's sarcoma.

CONTRAINDICATIONS
Use in demyelinating Charcot-Marie-Tooth syndrome or during radiation therapy. Lactation.

SPECIAL CONCERNS
Geriatric clients are more susceptible to the neurotoxic effects. Intrathecal use may cause death.

ADDITIONAL SIDE EFFECTS
Neurologic: Paresthesias, depression of DTRs, foot drop, ***seizures,*** difficulties in gait. **GI:** ***Intestinal necrosis or perforation.*** Constipation, paralytic ileus. **Renal:** Inappropriate ADH secretion (polyuria or dysuria). Acute uric acid nephropathy. **Ophthalmic:** Blindness, ptosis, diplopia, photophobia. **Miscellaneous:** CNS leukemia, leukopenia or complicating infection, ***bronchospasm,*** SOB. Less bone marrow depression than vinblastine. Significant tissue irritation if leakage occurs during IV use.

OD OVERDOSE MANAGEMENT
Symptoms: Exaggeration of side effects. *Treatment:*

- Treat side effects due to inappropriate secretion of ADH.
- Use an anticonvulsant (e.g., phenobarbital), if necessary.
- Prevent ileus by use of enemas, cathartics, or decompression of the GI tract.
- Monitor the CV system.
- Monitor blood counts daily to determine risk of infection and whether blood transfusions are necessary.
- Folinic acid, 100 mg IV q 3 hr for 24 hr and then q 6 hr for a minimum of 48 hr, may help with treating the symptoms of overdose.

DRUG INTERACTIONS
L-Asparaginase / ↓ Vincristine renal clearance; give vincristine 12–14 hr before asparaginase
Digoxin / ↓ Digoxin plasma levels
Calcium channel blocking drugs / ↑ Accumulation of vincristine in cells
Digoxin / ↓ Effect of digoxin
Glutamic acid / Inhibits effect of vincristine
Itraconazole / ↑ Risk of neurotoxicity R/T ↓ vincristine metabolism
Methotrexate / Possible hypotension
Mitomycin C / Severe bronchospasm and acute SOB
Phenytoin / ↓ Phenytoin effect R/T ↓ plasma levels

HOW SUPPLIED
Injection: 1 mg/mL

DOSAGE

- **IV ONLY (DIRECT, INFUSION)**

Individualized with extreme care as overdose can be fatal.

Adults, usual, initial: 0.4–1.4 mg/m^2 (or 0.01–0.03 mg/kg) 1 time/week; **children:** 1.5–2 mg/m^2 1 time/week. **Children less than 10 kg or with body surface area less than 1 m^2:** 0.05 mg/kg 1 time/week.

For hepatic insufficiency.
If serum bilirubin is 1.5–3, administer 50% of the dose; if serum bilirubin is more than 3.1 or AST is more than 180, omit the dose.

NURSING CONSIDERATIONS

SEE ALSO *NURSING CONSIDERATIONS* FOR *ANTINEOPLASTICS* AND *VINBLASTINE.*

ADMINISTRATION/STORAGE
IV 1. Dissolve powder in sterile water or isotonic saline injection to a concentration ranging from 0.01 to 1 mg/mL.
2. Do not mix with anything other than NSS or glucose in water.
3. Do not mix with any solution that alters the pH outside the range of 3.5–5.5.
4. Inject either directly into a vein or into the tubing of a flowing IV infusion over a period of 1 min.
5. If extravasation occurs, move to another vein. Treat affected area with hyaluronidase injection (150 U/mL in 1 mL NaCl) and apply moderate heat to decrease local reaction.
6. Protect from light exposure.
7. Store in refrigerator. Dry powder is stable for 6 mo. Solutions are stable for 2 weeks under refrigeration.

ASSESSMENT
1. Note indications for therapy. Document neurologic assessment; monitor for early S&S of neurologic and neuromuscular side effects (e.g., sensory im-

pairment and paresthesias) before neuritic pain and motor difficulties are apparent because neuromuscular manifestations are irreversible.
2. Monitor CBC, uric acid, liver and renal function studies. May cause granulocyte suppression. Nadir: 10 days; recovery: 21 days.

INTERVENTIONS

1. Premedicate and regularly administer antiemetic to control N&V.
2. Record I&O, weights, and assessment of nutritional status.
3. Observe for S&S of gout. May add allopurinol empirically to decrease uric acid levels.
4. Use laxatives and enemas to treat high colon impaction.
5. Absence of bowel sounds are indicative of paralytic ileus; temporarily discontinue drug.

CLIENT/FAMILY TEACHING

1. Prevent constipation by increased intake of fluids (2–3 L/day), regular exercise, a high-fiber diet, and stool softeners as needed.
2. Report any S&S of neurotoxicity: paresthesias, difficulty walking, and diminished reflexes.
3. Avoid vaccinations and persons with infectious diseases.
4. Practice reliable birth control during and for 2 mo following therapy.
5. Report any increased dyspnea, cough, or fatigue.
6. Avoid alcohol and OTC agents.

OUTCOMES/EVALUATE

Inhibition of malignant cell proliferation

Vinorelbine tartrate

(vin-**OR**-el-been)

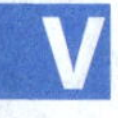

PREGNANCY CATEGORY: D
CLASSIFICATION(S):
Antineoplastic, Vinca alkaloid
Rx: Navelbine

ACTION/KINETICS

Semisynthetic vinca alkaloid thought to act by inhibiting mitosis at metaphase through the drug's interaction with tubulin. Other possible actions may include interference with (a) amino acid, cyclic AMP, and glutathione metabolism, (b) calmodulin-dependent calcium transport ATPase activity, (c) cellular respiration, and (d) nucleic acid and lipid biosynthesis. Following IV use, plasma levels decay in a triphasic manner. The initial rapid decline is due to distribution of the drug to peripheral compartments. The prolonged terminal phase is due to a slow efflux of the drug from peripheral compartments. **Terminal phase t½:** Averages 27.7–43.6 hr. Metabolized by the liver and excreted through the urine and feces.

USES

Alone or in combination with cisplatin for first-line treatment of ambulatory clients with unresectable, advanced non-small-cell lung cancer. In clients with Stage IV non-small-cell lung cancer, can be used as a single agent or with cisplatin. In stage II non-small-cell lung cancer, vinorelbine is not indicated for use with cisplatin. *Investigational:* Breast cancer, cisplatin-resistant ovarian carcinoma, and Hodgkin's disease.

CONTRAINDICATIONS

Clients with pretreatment granulocyte counts less than 1,000 cells/mm^3. Lactation.

SPECIAL CONCERNS

For IV use only; intrathecal use of other vinca alkaloids has been fatal. Use with caution in clients with severe hepatic injury or impairment. Use with extreme caution in clients whose bone marrow reserve may have been compromised by chemotherapy or prior to irradiation; also, in those whose bone marrow function is recovering from the effects of previous chemotherapy. Older clients may be more sensitive to the effects of the drug. Safety and efficacy have not been determined in children.

SIDE EFFECTS

Hematologic: Granulocytopenia (may require hospitalization), leukopenia, thrombocytopenia, anemia. **GI:** N&V, constipation (may be severe), diarrhea, paralytic ileus, anorexia, stomatitis, intestinal obstruction, necrosis, perforation, dysphagia, mucositis. **CNS:** Mild to severe peripheral neuropathy including paresthesia and hypesthesia, loss of DTRs. Headache. **CV:** Chest pain, especially in those with a history of CV disease or tumor within the chest; phlebitis, hypertension, hypotension, vasodilation, tachycardia, pulmonary edema. **Respiratory:** SOB (may be severe), dyspnea, interstitial pulmonary changes, pneumonia. **Dermatologic: At injection site:** vein discoloration, chemical phlebitis along the vein proximal to the site of injection, localized rash and urticaria, blister formation, skin sloughing. Erythema. **Miscellaneous:** Alopecia, asthenia, fatigue, jaw pain, myalgia, arthralgia, rash, hemorrhagic cystitis, SIADH secretion, vestibular and auditory deficits (especially when used with cisplatin). Also, flushing, musculoskeletal aches and pains, back pain, abdominal pain, pain in tumor-containing tissue, radiation recall events (e.g., dermatitis, esophagitis). Systemic allergic reactions, including pruritus, urticaria, angioedema, ***anaphylaxis.***

LABORATORY TEST CONSIDERATIONS

↑ Total bilirubin, AST. Transient elevations of liver enzymes.

OD OVERDOSE MANAGEMENT

Symptoms: Bone marrow suppression, peripheral neurotoxicity. *Treatment:* There is no known antidote for vinorelbine. For overdosage, begin general supportive measures together with appropriate blood transfusions and antibiotics, as necessary.

DRUG INTERACTIONS

Cisplatin / ↑ Incidence of granulocytopenia

Mitomycin / Acute pulmonary reactions

Paclitaxel / Possible neuropathy when used together or sequentially

HOW SUPPLIED

Injection: 10 mg/mL

DOSAGE

- **IV ONLY**

Non-small-cell lung cancer.

Granulocytes (1,500 or more cells/mm³) on the day of treatment: 30 mg/m² weekly given over 6–10 min into the side port of a free-flowing IV closest to the IV bag followed by flushing with at least 75–125 mL of the solution used to dilute the product. May also be given, at the same dose level, with cisplatin, 120 mg/m² on days 1 and 29 and then q 6 weeks. **Granulocytes (1,000–1,499 cells/mm³) on the day of treatment:** 15 mg/m² weekly given over 6–10 min as described previously.

Breast cancer, Hodgkin's disease.

30 mg/m²/week.

NURSING CONSIDERATIONS

SEE ALSO *NURSING CONSIDERATIONS* FOR *ANTINEOPLASTIC AGENTS.*

ADMINISTRATION/STORAGE

IV 1. During therapy, if clients have manifested fever or sepsis while granulocytopenic or had two consecutive weekly doses held due to granulocytopenia, give subsequent doses of vinorelbine as follows: 22.5 mg/m² for granulocytes equal to or > 1,500 cells/mm³ or 11.25 mg/m² for granulocytes from 1,000 to 1,499 cells/mm³.

2. Ensure granulocyte counts are equal to or > 1,000 cells/mm³ prior to giving vinorelbine. Base dosage on granulocyte counts on the day of drug treatment.

3. If hyperbilirubinemia develops during treatment, adjust the dose of vinorelbine as follows: 30 mg/m² for a total bilirubin of 2 or less mg/dL, 15 mg/m² for a total bilirubin of 2.1–3 mg/dL, and 7.5 mg/m² for a total bilirubin > 3 mg/dL.

4. Before any drug is given, properly position the needle or catheter, as leakage into surrounding tissue may cause considerable irritation, local tissue necrosis, or thrombophlebitis. If extravasation occurs, stop the injection immediately and give the remaining dose in another vein. Use institutional guidelines to treat extravasation.

5. Due to the toxicity of vinorelbine, wear gloves and use caution in handling/preparing the solution. If it

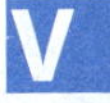

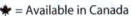

and water. If the eye is affected, flush with water immediately.

6. Must be diluted in either a syringe or IV bag. If an IV bag is used, dilute the dose to a concentration between 0.5 and 2 mg/mL using one of the following solutions: D5W, 0.45% or 0.9% NaCl, D5/0.45% NaCl, Ringer's or RL injection. When dilution in a syringe is used, dilute the dose to a concentration between 1.5 and 3 mg/mL with D5W or 0.9% NaCl.

7. Diluted vinorelbine solutions may be used for up to 24 hr under normal room light when stored in polypropylene syringes or PVC bags at 5–30°C (41–96°F). Unopened vials are stable until the expiration date indicated if stored under refrigeration at 2–8°C (36–46°F). Protect unopened vials from light and do not freeze. Do not use if particulate matter present.

ASSESSMENT

1. Document indications for therapy, other agents and therapies prescribed and when administered.

2. Monitor CBC, uric acid, liver, and renal function studies. Reduce dose with impaired liver and hematologic function. Do not administer if granulocyte counts are not at least 1,000 cells/mm^3. Granulocyte nadir 7–10 days; recovery 7–14 days thereafter.

CLIENT/FAMILY TEACHING

1. Report any fever or chills immediately; drug-induced granulocytopenia makes client much more susceptible to infections.

2. Avoid crowds, persons with infectious diseases, and vaccinations during therapy.

3. Practice reliable contraception during and for several months after therapy.

4. Rinse mouth frequently and brush teeth often to prevent stomatitis; use unwaxed floss.

5. Report any S&S of neurotoxicity: paresthesias, difficulty walking, and diminished reflexes.

OUTCOMES/EVALUATE

Control of malignant cell proliferation.

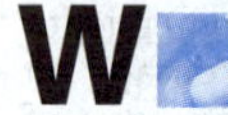

Warfarin sodium

(**WAR**-far-in)

PREGNANCY CATEGORY: X
CLASSIFICATION(S):
Anticoagulant, Coumarin derivative
Rx: Coumadin
✱**Rx:** Warfilone

ACTION/KINETICS

Interferes with synthesis of vitamin K–dependent clotting factors resulting in depletion of clotting factors II, VII, IX, and X. Has no direct effect on an established thrombus although therapy may prevent further extension of a formed clot as well as secondary thromboembolic problems. Well absorbed from the GI tract although food affects the rate (but not the extent) of absorption. Suitable for parenteral administration. **Peak activity:** 1.5–3 days; **duration:** 2–5 days. **t½:** 1–2.5 days. Highly bound to plasma proteins. Metabolized in the liver and inactive metabolites are excreted through the urine and feces.

USES

(1) Prophylaxis and treatment of venous thrombosis and its extension. (2) Prophylaxis and treatment of atrial fibrillation with embolization. (3) Prophylaxis and treatment of pulmonary embolism. Prophylaxis and treatment of thromboembolic complications associated with atrial fibrillation. *Investigational:* Adjunct to treat small cell carcinoma of the lung with chemotherapy and radiation. Prophylaxis of recurrent transient ischemic attacks and to reduce the risk of re-

current MI. In combination with aspirin to reduce risk of a second MI.

CONTRAINDICATIONS

Lactation. IM use. Use of a large loading dose (30 mg) is not recommended due to increased risk of hemorrhage and lack of more rapid protection.

SPECIAL CONCERNS

Geriatric clients may be more sensitive. Anticoagulant use in the following clients leads to increased risk: trauma, infection, renal insufficiency, sprue, vitamin K deficiency, severe to moderate hypertension, polycythemia vera, severe allergic disorders, vasculitis, indwelling catheters, severe diabetes, anaphylactic disorders, surgery or trauma resulting in large exposed raw surfaces. Use with caution in impaired hepatic and renal function. Safety and efficacy have not been determined in children less than 18 years of age. Careful monitoring and dosage regulation are required during dentistry and surgery.

SIDE EFFECTS

CV: ***Hemorrhage*** is the main side effect and may occur from any tissue or organ. Symptoms of hemorrhage include headache, paralysis; pain in the joints, abdomen, or chest; difficulty in breathing or swallowing; SOB, unexplained swelling or shock. **GI:** N&V, diarrhea, sore mouth, mouth ulcers, anorexia, abdominal cramping, paralytic ileus, intestinal obstruction (due to intramural or submucosal hemorrhage). **Hepatic:** Hepatotoxicity, cholestatic jaundice. **Dermatologic:** Dermatitis, exfoliative dermatitis, urticaria, alopecia, necrosis or gangrene of the skin and other tissues (due to protein C deficiency). **Miscellaneous:** Pyrexia, red-orange urine, priapism, leukopenia, systemic cholesterol microembolization ("purple toes" syndrome), hypersensitivity reactions, compressive neuropathy secondary to hemorrhage adjacent to a nerve (rare).

LABORATORY TEST CONSIDERATIONS

False ↓ levels of serum theophylline determined by Schack and Waxler UV method (warfarin and dicumarol). Metabolites of indanedione derivatives may color alkaline urine red; color disappears upon acidification.

OD OVERDOSE MANAGEMENT

Symptoms: Early symptoms include melena, petechiae, microscopic hematuria, oozing from superficial injuries (e.g., nicks from shaving, excessive bruising, bleeding from gums after teeth brushing), excessive menstrual bleeding. *Treatment:* Discontinue therapy. Administer oral or parenteral phytonadione (e.g., 2.5–10 mg PO or 5–25 mg parenterally). In emergency situations, 200–250 mL fresh frozen plasma or commercial factor IX complex. Fresh whole blood may be needed in clients unresponsive to phytonadione.

DRUG INTERACTIONS

Warfarin is responsible for more adverse drug interactions than any other group. Clients on anticoagulant therapy must be monitored carefully each time a drug is added or withdrawn. Monitoring usually involves determination of PT or INR. In general, a lengthened PT or INR means potentiation of the anticoagulant. Since potentiation may mean hemorrhages, a lengthened PT or INR warrants **reduction of the dosage of the anticoagulant.** However, the anticoagulant dosage must again be increased when the second drug is discontinued. A shortened PT or INR means inhibition of the anticoagulant and may require an increase in dosage.

Acetaminophen / ↑ Anticoagulant effect

Alcohol, ethyl / Chronic use ↓ warfarin effect

Aminoglutethimide / ↓ Warfarin effect R/T ↑ liver breakdown

Aminoglycoside antibiotics / ↑ Warfarin effect R/T interference with vitamin K

Amiodarone / ↑ Warfarin effect R/T ↓ liver breakdown

Androgens / ↑ Warfarin effect

Ascorbic acid / ↓ Warfarin effect by unknown mechanism

Barbiturates / ↓ Warfarin effect R/T ↑ liver breakdown

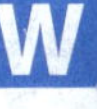

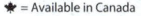

Beta-adrenergic blockers / ↑ Warfarin effect
H *Bromelain* / ↑ Tendency for bleeding
Capecitabine / ↑ Risk of bleeding and altered coagulation
Carbamazepine / ↓ Warfarin effect R/T ↑ liver breakdown
Celecoxib / ↑ PT
Cephalosporins / ↑ Warfarin effect R/T effects on platelet function
Chloral hydrate / ↑ Warfarin effect R/T ↓ plasma protein binding
Chloramphenicol / ↑ Warfarin effect R/T ↓ liver breakdown
Cholestyramine / ↓ Anticoagulant effect R/T binding and ↓ absorption from GI tract
Cimetidine / ↑ Anticoagulant effect R/T ↓ liver breakdown
H *Cinchona bark* / ↑ Anticoagulant effect
Clarithromycin / ↑ Warfarin effect R/T ↓ liver metabolism
Clofibrate / ↑ Anticoagulant effect
Contraceptives, oral / ↓ Anticoagulant effect R/T ↑ activity of certain clotting factors (VII and X); rarely, the opposite effect of ↑ risk of thromboembolism
Contrast media containing iodine / ↑ Warfarin effect by ↑ PT
Corticosteroids / ↑ Warfarin effect; also ↑ risk of GI bleeding R/T steroids ulcerogenic effect
Cyclophosphamide / ↑ Anticoagulant effect
Dextrothyroxine / ↑ Warfarin effect
Dicloxacillin / ↓ Warfarin effect
Diflunisal / ↑ Anticoagulant effect and ↑ risk of bleeding R/T effect on platelet function and GI irritation
Disulfiram / ↑ Warfarin effect
H *Dong quai* / Potential for ↑ anticoagulant effects
Erythromycin / ↑ Warfarin effect R/T ↓ liver metabolism
Estrogens / ↓ Anticoagulant response by ↑ activity of certain clotting factors; rarely, the opposite effect of ↑ risk of thromboembolism
Etretinate / ↓ Warfarin effect R/T ↑ liver breakdown
H *Evening primrose oil* / Potential to ↓ platelet aggregation
H *Feverfew* / Potential to ↓ platelet aggregation
Fluconazole / ↑ Warfarin effect
H *Garlic* / Potential to ↓ platelet aggregation
Gemfibrozil / ↑ Warfarin effect
H *Ginger* / Potential to ↓ platelet aggregation
H *Ginkgo biloba* / Potential to ↓ platelet aggregation
H *Ginseng, panax* / Potential to ↓ platelet aggregation
Glucagon / ↑ Warfarin effect
Glutethimide / ↓ Warfarin effect R/T ↑ liver breakdown
H *Grapeseed extract* / Potential to ↓ platelet aggregation
Griseofulvin / ↓ Warfarin effect
Hydantoins / ↑ Warfarin effect; also, ↑ hydantoin serum levels
Hypoglycemics, oral / ↑ Warfarin effect R/T ↓ plasma protein binding; also, ↑ effect of sulfonylureas
Ifosfamide / ↑ Warfarin effect R/T ↓ liver breakdown and displacement from protein binding sites
Indomethacin / ↑ Warfarin effect R/T effect on platelet function; also, indomethacin is ulcerogenic → GI hemorrhage
Isoniazid / ↑ Warfarin effect
Itraconazole / Anticoagulant effect is enhanced
Ketoconazole / ↑ Warfarin effect
Loop diuretics / ↑ Warfarin effect by displacement from protein binding sites
Lovastatin / ↑ Warfarin effect R/T ↓ liver breakdown
Metronidazole / ↑ Warfarin effect R/T ↓ liver breakdown
Miconazole / ↑ Bleeding or bruising
Mineral oil / ↑ Hypoprothrombinemia by ↓ absorption of vitamin K from GI tract; also mineral oil may ↓ absorption of warfarin from GI tract
Moricizine / ↑ Warfarin effect
Nafcillin / ↓ Warfarin effect
Nalidixic acid / ↑ Warfarin effect R/T displacement from protein binding sites
Nevirapine / Possible ↓ anticoagulant effect
Nonsteroidal anti-inflammatory agents / ↑ Warfarin effect; ↑ risk of bleeding R/T effects on platelet function and GI irritation

Omeprazole / ↑ Warfarin effect R/T ↓ liver breakdown
Penicillins / ↑ Warfarin effect → ↑ risk of bleeding R/T effects on platelet function
Propafenone / ↑ Warfarin effect R/T ↓ liver breakdown
Propoxyphene / ↑ Warfarin effect
Quinidine, quinine / ↑ Warfarin effect R/T ↓ liver breakdown
Quinolones / ↑ Warfarin effect
Rifampin / ↓ Anticoagulant effect R/T ↑ liver breakdown
Ritonavir / Possible ↓ anticoagulant effect
H *St. John's wort* / Possible ↓ warfarin plasma levels R/T ↑ metabolism
Salicylates / ↑ Warfarin effect and ↑ risk of bleeding R/T effect on platelet function and GI irritation
Spironolactone / ↓ Warfarin effect R/T hemoconcentration of clotting factors due to diuresis
Streptokinase / ↑ Warfarin effect
Sucralfate / ↓ Warfarin effect
Sulfamethoxazole and Trimethoprim / ↑ Warfarin effect R/T ↓ liver breakdown
Sulfinpyrazone / ↑ Anticoagulant effect R/T ↓ liver breakdown and inhibition of platelet aggregation
Sulfonamides / ↑ Sulfonamide effects
Sulindac / ↑ Warfarin effect
Tamoxifen / ↑ Warfarin effect
Tetracyclines / ↑ Warfarin effect R/T interference with vitamin K
Thiazide diuretics / ↓ Warfarin effect R/T hemoconcentration of clotting factors due to diuresis
Thioamines / ↑ Warfarin effect
Thiopurines / ↓ Warfarin effect R/T ↑ synthesis or activation of prothrombin
Thyroid hormones / ↑ Anticoagulant effect with ↑ risk of bleeding
Tolterodine / Prolonged INR values
Trazodone / ↓ Warfarin effect
Trastuzumab / Increased risk of bleeding
Troglitazone / Possible ↑ warfarin effect R/T ↓ liver breakdown or displacement from plasma proteins
Urokinase / ↑ Warfarin effect
Vitamin A / Possible ↑ anticoagulant if using large doses of Vitamin A
Vitamin C / Slightly prolonged PT
Vitamin E / ↑ Warfarin effect R/T interference with vitamin K
Vitamin K / ↓ Warfarin effect

HOW SUPPLIED

Powder for injection, lyophilized: 2 mg; *Tablet:* 1 mg, 2 mg, 2.5 mg, 3 mg, 4 mg, 5 mg, 6 mg, 7.5 mg, 10 mg

DOSAGE

• **TABLETS, IV**

Induction.

Adults, initial: 5–10 mg/day for 2–4 days; **then,** adjust dose based on prothrombin or INR determinations. A lower dose should be used in geriatric or debilitated clients or clients with increased sensitivity. Dosage has not been established for children.

Maintenance.

Adults: 2–10 mg/day, based on prothrombin or INR.

Prevent blood clots with prosthetic heart valve replacement.

2–5 mg daily.

NURSING CONSIDERATIONS

ADMINISTRATION/STORAGE

1. Frequent monitoring of PT/INR is recommended during the first week of therapy, or during adjustment periods, and monthly thereafter.
2. Do not change brands; there may be differences in bioavailability.
3. To transfer from heparin therapy, give heparin and warfarin together from the first day (as there is a delayed onset of oral anticoagulant effects). Alternatively, warfarin may be started on the third to sixth day of heparin therapy.
4. Levels of anticoagulation that are recommended for specific indications by the American College of Chest Physicians and the National Heart, Lung, and Blood Institute should be followed.
5. Protect from light; store at controlled room temperature. Dispense in a tight, light-resistant container.

IV 6. Give IV as slow bolus over 1–2 min into peripheral vein.

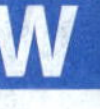

7. Reconstitute for IV use by adding 2.7 mL sterile water for injection. Inspect for particulate matter and discoloration.
8. After reconstitution, injection is stable for 4 hr at room temperature. There is no preservative; take care to assure sterility of prepared solution.
9. Do not use the vial for multiple use; discard unused solution.

ASSESSMENT

1. Note indications for therapy, timeframe (i.e., DVT (initial) 6 mo; recurrent/multiple and heart valve replacement — lifetime), and desired PT/INR range.
2. List drugs currently prescribed to ensure that none interacts unfavorably by increasing or decreasing PT as a result of competition for protein binding at receptor sites.
3. Note any bleeding tendencies. Review PMH for conditions that may preclude therapy: PUD, chronic GI tract ulcerations, alcoholic, severe renal or liver dysfunction, endocardial infections.
4. Determine if pregnant. May cause fetal malformations and neonatal hemorrhage.
5. Monitor ECG, CBC, PT/PTT, INR, renal and LFTs.
6. Adjust oral anticoagulant weekly, esp. if receiving one of the many drugs known to interact or compete.
7. Have available vitamin K, FFP, or factor IX concentrate for warfarin overdoses.

INTERVENTIONS

1. Request written parameters noting the desired range for PT or INR, once anticoagulated (orally). It usually takes 36–48 hr for drug to reach steady state; therefore allow time to equilibrate. The INR is the PT ratio (test/control) obtained from human brain thromboplastin and is universally considered most accurate to calculate dosage.
2. Drug inhibits production of factors II, VII, IX, and X; onset in response is delayed because of degradation of clotting factors that have already been synthesized.
3. Question about bleeding (gums, urine, stools, vomit, bruises). If urine discolored, determine cause, i.e., from drug therapy or hematuria. Indanedione-type anticoagulants turn alkaline urine a red-orange color; acidify urine or test for occult blood.
4. Sudden lumbar pain may indicate retroperitoneal hemorrhage.
5. GI dysfunction may indicate intestinal hemorrhage. Test for blood in urine and feces; check H&H to assess for abnormal bleeding.
6. Observe for "purple toes" syndrome related to inhibition of protein C and S.

CLIENT/FAMILY TEACHING

1. Take oral warfarin as prescribed and at the same time each day; must be compliant with therapy.
2. This drug does not dissolve clots but decreases the clotting ability of the blood and helps to prevent the formation of harmful blood clots in the blood vessels and heart valves.
3. Avoid activities and contact sports that may cause injury or cuts and bruises. Use a soft toothbrush, electric razor to shave, wear shoes and use a night light to avoid falls at night.
4. Report immediately any unusual bruising or bleeding, dark brown or blood-tinged body secretions, injury or trauma, dizziness, abdominal pain or swelling, back pain, severe headaches, and joint swelling and pain.
5. May carry vitamin K for emergency use. (The usual dosage is 5–20 mg, to be used in the event of excessive bleeding.)
6. Avoid foods high in vitamin K: asparagus, broccoli, cabbage, brussels sprouts, spinach, turnips, milk, and cheese, or consume in limited quantities as these may alter INR.
7. Use reliable birth control.
8. Menstruation may be prolonged and flow slightly increased. Report if excessive and unusual.
9. Skin eruptions may develop as an allergic reaction; report.
10. Do not change brands of drug; may alter response.
11. Avoid OTC drugs. Check prior to taking any OTC drugs that have anticoagulant-type effects such as salicylates, NSAIDS, steroids, vitamin K,

mineral preparations from health food stores, vitamins, or alcohol.
12. Wear identification and alert all providers of anticoagulant therapy.
13. Avoid smoking as this increases dose requirements.
14. Identify social/economic situations that may alter compliance; identify reliable resources.
15. Report as scheduled for labs to evaluate effectiveness of therapy and need for dosage changes.
16. The elderly are more prone to developing bleeding complications.
17. Unusual hair loss and itching are common with the elderly; advise to report if intolerable or skin break down occurs.
18. Many elderly use multiple pharmacies and shop for value; stress that they know what they are taking and why and to carry the name and dosage of ALL drugs prescribed. Remind not to skip a dose as it only works for 24 hr and must be readministered in order to be effective.

OUTCOMES/EVALUATE

- PT within desired range (1.5–2 times the control)
- INR within desired range (2.0–3.0 with standard therapy; 2.5–4.0 with high-dose therapy)
- ↓ Risk of thromboembolism with prosthetic heart valves
- Resolution/prophylaxis of DVT

Z

Zafirlukast

(zah-**FIR**-loo-kast)

PREGNANCY CATEGORY: B
CLASSIFICATION(S):
Antiasthmatic drug
Rx: Accolate

ACTION/KINETICS

A selective and competitive antagonist of leukotriene receptors D_4 and E_4, which are components of slow-reacting substance of anaphylaxis. It is believed that cysteinyl leukotriene occupation of receptors causes asthma, including airway edema, smooth muscle constriction, and altered cellular activity assoĉiated with the inflammatory process. Zafirlukast inhibits bronchoconstriction caused by sulfur dioxide and cold air in clients with asthma. It also attenuates the early- and late-phase reaction in asthmatics caused by inhalation of antigens such as grass, cat dander, ragweed, and mixed antigens. Rapidly absorbed after PO use; bioavailabilty may be decreased when taken with food. **Peak plasma levels:** 3 hr. **t½, terminal:** About 10 hr. Over 99% bound to plasma proteins. Extensively metabolized in the liver, with about 90% excreted in the feces and 10% in the urine. Inhibits certain cytochrome P450 isoenzymes.

USES

Prophylaxis and chronic treatment of asthma in adults and children 5 years of age and older.

CONTRAINDICATIONS

Use to terminate an acute asthma attack, including status asthmaticus. Lactation.

SPECIAL CONCERNS

The clearance is reduced in clients 65 years of age and older. Safety and efficacy have not been determined in children less than 12 years of age.

SIDE EFFECTS

GI: N&V, diarrhea, abdominal pain, dyspepsia.
CNS: Headache, dizziness. **Hepatic:** Hepatic dysfunction, especially in women and girls. Rarely, symptomatic hepatitis and hyperbilirubinemia. **Hypersensitivity reactions:** Urticaria, angioedema, rashes (with and without blistering). **Miscellaneous:** Infec-

tion (especially in the elderly), generalized pain, asthenia, accidental injury, myalgia, arthralgia, fever, back pain, systemic eosinophilia with vasculitis consistent with Churg-Strauss syndrome.

LABORATORY TEST CONSIDERATIONS
↑ ALT.

DRUG INTERACTIONS
Aspirin / ↑ Zafirlukast plasma levels
Erythromycin / ↓ Zafirlukast plasma levels
Theophylline / ↓ Zafirlukast plasma levels; possible ↑ theophylline serum levels
Warfarin / Significant ↑ PT

HOW SUPPLIED
Tablet: 10 mg, 20 mg

DOSAGE

• **TABLETS**
Asthma.
Adults and children aged 12 and older: 20 mg b.i.d. **Children, 7–11 years:** 10 mg (use minitablet) b.i.d., even during symptom-free periods.

NURSING CONSIDERATIONS

ADMINISTRATION/STORAGE

Protect from light and moisture; store at controlled room temperatures of 20–25°C (68–77°F).

ASSESSMENT

1. Document indications for therapy, onset, duration, and characteristics of symptoms. List other agents trialed with the outcome.
2. If liver dysfunction is suspected, discontinue therapy and perform LFTs immediately. If LFTs are consistent with hepatic dysfunction, do not resume therapy.
3. Note cardiopulmonary assessment findings.
4. Monitor labs and PFTs.

CLIENT/FAMILY TEACHING

1. Take 1 hr before or 2 hr after meals to prevent loss of bioavailability.
2. Take drug regularly during symptom-free periods. Do not increase or decrease dose without approval.
3. Drug is not appropriate for acute episodes of asthma. Continue all other antiasthma medications as prescribed.
4. Review peak flow meter use and set targets for intervention or additional therapy.
5. Avoid triggers, i.e., dust, chemicals, cigarette smoke, pollutants, pets, and perfumes.
6. Practice reliable birth control; do not breast feed during therapy.

OUTCOMES/EVALUATE

Inhibition of bronchoconstriction; improved breathing patterns

Zalcitabine (Dideoxycytidine, ddC)

(zal-**SIGH**-tah-been)

PREGNANCY CATEGORY: C
CLASSIFICATION(S):
Antiviral, nucleoside reverse transcriptase inhibitor
Rx: Hivid

SEE ALSO *ANTIVIRAL DRUGS,* AND *ANTI-INFECTIVE DRUGS.*

ACTION/KINETICS
Converted in cells to the active metabolite, dideoxycytidine 5′-triphosphate (ddCTP), by cellular enzymes. ddCTP serves as an alternative substrate to deoxycytidine triphosphate for HIV-reverse transcriptase, thereby inhibiting the in vitro replication of HIV-1 and inhibiting viral DNA synthesis. The incorporation of ddCTP into the growing DNA chain leads to premature chain termination. ddCTP serves as a competitive inhibitor of the natural substrate for deoxycytidine triphosphate for the active site of the viral reverse transcriptase, which further inhibits viral DNA synthesis. Food reduces the rate of absorption. Does not appear to undergo significant metabolism by the liver. **Elimination t½:** 1–3 hr. Approximately 70% of a PO dose is excreted through the kidneys and 10% in the feces. Prolonged elimination (t½ up to 8.5 hr) is observed in clients with impaired renal function.

Z

USES

In combination with antiretroviral drugs to treat HIV infection.

CONTRAINDICATIONS

Hypersensitivity. Use in moderate or severe peripheral neuropathy or with drugs that have the potential to cause peripheral neuropathy (see *Drug Interactions)*. Concomitant use with didanosine. Lactation.

SPECIAL CONCERNS

Use with extreme caution in clients with low CD_4 cell counts (< $50/mm^3$). Use with caution in clients with a history of pancreatitis or known risk factors for the development of pancreatitis. Clients with a C_{CR} less than 55 mL/min may be at a greater risk for toxicity due to decreased clearance. Clients may continue to develop opportunistic infections and other complications of HIV infection. Safety and efficacy have not been determined in HIV-infected children less than 13 years of age.

SIDE EFFECTS

The incidence of certain side effects is dependent on the duration of use and the dose of the drug.

Neurologic: Peripheral neuropathy (may be severe) characterized by numbness and burning dysesthesia involving the distal extremities; this may be followed by sharp shooting pains or severe continuous burning pain if the drug is not withdrawn. The neuropathy may progress to severe pain requiring narcotic analgesics and may be irreversible. **GI:** ***Fatal pancreatitis*** when given alone or with AZT. Esophageal ulcers, oral/esophageal ulcers, nausea, dysphagia, anorexia, abdominal pain, vomiting, constipation, ulcerative stomatitis, aphthous stomatitis, diarrhea, dry mouth, dyspepsia, glossitis, ***rectal hemorrhage,*** hemorrhoids, enlarged abdomen, gum disorders, flatulence, anorexia, tongue ulceration, dysphagia, eructation, gastritis, ***GI hemorrhage,*** left quadrant pain, salivary gland enlargement, esophageal pain, esophagitis, rectal ulcers, melena, painful swallowing, mouth lesion, acute pharyngitis, abdominal bloating or cramps, anal/rectal pain, colitis, dental abscess, epigastric pain, gagging with pills, gingivitis, heartburn, ***hemorrhagic pancreatitis,*** increased salivation, odynophagia, painful sore gums, rectal mass, sore tongue, sore throat, tongue disorder, toothache, unformed/loose stools. **Dermatologic:** Rash (including erythematous, maculopapular, follicular), pruritus, night sweats, dermatitis, skin lesions, acne, alopecia, bullous eruptions, increased sweating, urticaria, hot flashes, lip blister or lesions, carbuncle/furuncle, cellulitis, dry skin, dry rash desquamation, exfoliative dermatitis, finger inflammation, impetigo, infection, itchy rash, moniliasis, mucocutaneous/skin disorder, nail disorder, photosensitivity, skin fissure, skin ulcer. **CNS:** Headache, dizziness, seizures, ataxia, abnormal coordination, Bell's palsy, dysphonia, hyperkinesia, hypokinesia, migraine, neuralgia, neuritis, stupor, aphasia, decreased neurologic function, disequilibrium, facial nerve palsy, focal motor seizures, memory loss, paralysis, speech disorder, ***status epilepticus,*** tremor, vertigo, hypertonia, hand tremor, twitching, confusion, impaired concentration, insomnia, agitation, depersonalization, hallucinations, emotional lability, nervousness, anxiety, depression, euphoria, manic reaction, dementia, amnesia, somnolence, abnormal thinking, crying, loss of memory, decreased concentration, acute psychotic disorder, acute stress reaction, decreased motivation, decreased sexual desire, mood swings, paranoid states, ***suicide attempt***. **Respiratory:** Coughing, dyspnea, respiratory distress, rales/rhonchi, nasal discharge, flu-like symptoms, cyanosis, acute nasopharyngitis, chest congestion, dry nasal mucosa, hemoptysis, sinus congestion, sinus pain, sinusitis, wheezing. **Musculoskeletal:** Myalgia, arthralgia, arthritis, arthropathy, cold extremities, leg cramps, myositis, joint pain or inflammation, weakness in leg muscle, generalized muscle weakness, back pain, backache, bone aches and pains, bursitis, pain in extremities,

Z

joint swelling, muscle disorder, muscle stiffness, muscle cramps, arthrosis, myopathy, neck pain, rib pain, stiff neck. **Hepatic:** Exacerbation of hepatic dysfunction, especially in those with preexisting liver disease or with a history of alcohol abuse. Abnormal hepatic function, hepatitis, jaundice, hepatocellular damage, severe hepatomegaly with steatosis, cholecystitis. **CV: *Cardiomyopathy,*** CHF, abnormal cardiac movement arrhythmia, atrial fibrillation, ***cardiac failure,*** cardiac dysrhythmias, heart racing, hypertension, palpitations, ***subarachnoid hemorrhage,*** syncope, tachycardia, ventricular ectopy, epistaxis. **Hematologic:** Anemia, leukopenia, thrombocytopenia, alteration of absolute neutrophil count, granulocytosis, eosinophilia, neutropenia, hemoglobinemia, neutrophilia, platelet alteration, purpura, thrombus, unspecified hematologic toxicity, alteration of WBCs. **Hypersensitivity:** Urticaria, ***anaphylaxis*** (rare). **Endocrine:** Diabetes mellitus, gout, hot flushes, hypoglycemia, hyperglycemia, hypocalcemia, hypophosphatemia, hypernatremia, hyponatremia, hypomagnesemia, hyperkalemia, hypokalemia, hyperlipidemia, polydipsia. **GU:** Dysuria, toxic nephropathy, polyuria, renal calculi, ***acute renal failure,*** hyperuricemia, increased frequency of micturition, abnormal renal function, renal cyst, albuminuria, bladder pain, genital lesion/ulcer, nocturia, painful/sore penis, penile edema, testicular swelling, urinary retention, vaginal itch/ulcer/pain, vaginal/cervix disorder. **Ophthalmologic:** Abnormal vision, burning or itching eyes, xerophthalmia, eye pain or abnormality, blurred or decreased vision, eye inflammation/irritation, eye redness/hemorrhage, increased tears, mucopurulent conjunctivitis, photophobia, dry eyes, unequal sized pupils, yellow sclera. **Otic:** Ear pain/blockage, fluid in ears, hearing loss, tinnitus. **Body as a whole:** Fatigue, fever, rigors, chest pain or tightness, weight decrease, pain, malaise, asthenia, generalized edema, general debilitation, chills, difficulty moving, facial pain or swelling, flank pain, flushing, pelvic/groin pain. **Miscellaneous:** Lymphadenopathy, taste perversion, decreased taste, parosmia, lactic acidosis.

LABORATORY TEST CONSIDERATIONS

↑ ALT, AST, alkaline phosphatase, CPK, amylase, nonprotein nitrogen. Abnormal gamma-glutamyl transferase, GGT, LDH, lactate dehydrogenase, triglycerides, lipase. Bilirubinemia. ↓ Hematocrit.

DRUG INTERACTIONS

1. The following drugs have the potential to cause peripheral neuropathy. **Concomitant use is not recommended.** Drugs include: chloramphenicol, cisplatin, dapsone, didanosine, disulfiram, ethionamide, glutethimide, gold, hydralazine, iodoquinol, isoniazid, metronidazole, nitrofurantoin, phenytoin, ribavirin, vincristine.
2. Drugs such as amphotericin, foscarnet, and aminoglycosides may increase the risk of peripheral neuropathy by interfering with the renal clearance of zalcitabine, thus increasing plasma levels.

Antacids (Mg/Al-containing) / ↓ Zalcitabine absorption
Cimetidine / ↓ Zalcitabine elimination by ↓ renal tubular secretion
Pentamidine / ↑ Risk of fulminant pancreatitis
Probenecid / ↓ Zalcitabine elimination by ↓ renal tubular secretion

HOW SUPPLIED

Tablet: 0.375 mg, 0.75 mg

DOSAGE

• TABLETS

In combination with antiretroviral drugs (e.g., AZT) in advanced HIV infection.

Adults: 0.75 mg q 8 hr given at the same time with 200 mg AZT q 8 hr for a total daily dose of 2.25 mg zalcitabine and 600 mg AZT.

NURSING CONSIDERATIONS

ADMINISTRATION/STORAGE

1. Greater effect noted when new antiretroviral drugs are started at the same time as zalcitabine.

2. If C_{CR} is 10–40 mL/min, reduce dose to 0.75 mg/12 hr; if C_{CR} <10 mL/min, reduce dose to 0.75 mg/24 hr.
3. Dosage reduction not required for weights down to 30 kg.

ASSESSMENT

1. Clients with a history of pancreatitis or elevated serum amylase should be followed closely while on zalcitabine therapy.
2. Baseline serum amylase and triglyceride levels should be performed in clients with a history of pancreatitis, increased amylase, those on parenteral nutrition, or those with a history of drug abuse.
3. Frequent monitoring of hematologic indices is recommended to detect serious anemia or granulocytopenia. In clients manifesting hematologic toxicity, decreases in hemoglobin may occur as early as 2–4 weeks after beginning therapy, whereas granulocytopenia may be seen after 6–8 weeks of therapy.
4. Monitor CBC, CD_4 counts/viral loads, liver and renal function studies.
5. Assess for symptoms of peripheral neuropathy: pain, numbness, and tingling. If symptoms evident, the drug may be reintroduced at 50% of the initial dose (i.e., 0.375 mg/8 hr) once all symptoms related to the peripheral neuropathy have improved to mild. Permanently discontinue the drug if severe discomfort due to peripheral neuropathy progresses for 1 week or longer.

CLIENT/FAMILY TEACHING

1. Take with or without food (with concurrently prescribed AZT, if appropriate) every 8 hr.
2. May continue to develop opportunistic infections and other complications of HIV infection; remain under close medical supervision.
3. Use reliable contraceptive and practice safe sex.
4. Drug is not a cure, but helps to alleviate and manage the symptoms of HIV infections.
5. Discontinue and report if symptoms of peripheral neuropathy occur, especially if they are bilateral and progress for more than 72 hr. Symptoms include numbness, tingling, or burning sensation especially in the feet or tips of the toes. Peripheral neuropathy may continue to worsen despite interruption of therapy. If symptoms improve, then drug may be reintroduced at a lower dose.
6. Schedule retinal exams q 6 mo to assess for retinal depigmentation.
7. Identify local support groups that may assist client/family to understand and cope with this disease.

OUTCOMES/EVALUATE

Improved CD_4 cell counts, ↓ viral load, ↓ incidence of opportunistic infection, and improved survival rates in clients with advanced HIV infections

Zaleplon

(**ZAL**-leh-plon)

PREGNANCY CATEGORY: C
CLASSIFICATION(S):
Sedative-hypnotic, nonbenzodiazepine
Rx: Sonata , **C-IV**
✱**Rx:** Starnoc

ACTION/KINETICS

Nonbenzodiazepine hypnotic. However, it interacts with the GABA-benzodiazepine receptor complex. It binds selectively to the brain omega-1 receptor located on the alpha subunit of $GABA_A$ receptor complex and potentiates t-butyl-bicyclophosphorothionate (TBPS) binding. Although it decreases the time to sleep, it does not increase total sleep time or decrease the number of awakenings. Decreased hangover effect. Rapidly and almost completely absorbed. **Peak plasma levels:** 1 hr. Undergoes significant first-pass metabolism. A high-fat or heavy meal prolongs absorption. Extensively metabolized to inactive metabolites which are excreted in the urine (70%) and feces (17%). **t½:** About 1 hr.

USES

Treatment of insomnia for up to 5 weeks.

CONTRAINDICATIONS

Use with alcohol, severe hepatic impairment, or during lactation.

SPECIAL CONCERNS

Use with caution in diseases or conditions that could affect metabolism or hemodynamic responses, in clients with compromised respiratory function, or in clients showing signs or symptoms of depression. Abuse potential is similar to benzodiazepine and benzodiazepine-like hypnotics. The products contain tartrazine (FD&C yellow #5) which may cause an allergic-type reaction, especially in those with aspirin hypersensitivity. May cause amnesia and dependence.

SIDE EFFECTS

Listed are side effects with an incidence of 0.1% or greater.

CNS: Dizziness, amnesia, somnolence, anxiety, paresthesia, depersonalization, hypesthesia, tremor, hallucinations, vertigo, depression, hypertonia, nervousness, abnormal thinking/concentration, abnormal gait, agitation, apathy, ataxia, circumoral paresthesia, confusion, emotional lability, euphoria, hyperesthesia, hyperkinesia, hypotonia, incoordination, insomnia, decreased libido, neuralgia, nystagmus. **GI:** Nausea, dyspepsia, anorexia, colitis, constipation, dry mouth, eructation, esophagitis, flatulence, gastritis, gastroenteritis, gingivitis, glossitis, increased appetite, melena, mouth ulceration, rectal hemorrhage, stomatitis. **CV:** Migraine, angina pectoris, bundle branch block, hypertension, hypotension, palpitation, syncope, tachycardia, vasodilation, ventricular extrasystoles. **Dermatologic:** Pruritus, rash, acne, alopecia, contact dermatitis, dry skin, eczema, maculopapular rash, skin hypertrophy, sweating, urticaria, vesiculobullous rash. **GU:** Bladder pain, breast pain, cystitis, decreased urine stream, dysuria, hematuria, impotence, kidney calculus, kidney pain, menorrhagia, metorrhagia, urinary frequency, urinary incontinence, urinary urgency, vaginitis, dysmenorrhea. **Respiratory:** Bronchitis, asthma, dyspnea, laryngitis, pneumonia, snoring, voice alteration. **Musculoskeletal:** Arthritis, arthrosis, bursitis, joint disorder (swelling, stiffness, pain), myasthenia, tenosynovitis. **Hematologic:** Anemia, ecchymosis, lymphadenopathy. **Metabolic:** Edema, gout, hypercholesterolemia, thirst, weight gain. **Ophthalmic:** Eye pain, abnormal vision, conjunctivitis, diplopia, dry eyes, photophobia, watery eyes. **Otic:** Ear pain, hyperacusis, tinnitus. **Body as a whole:** Headache, asthenia, myalgia, fever, malaise, chills, generalized edema. **Miscellaneous:** Abdominal pain, photosensitivity, peripheral edema, epistaxis, back pain, chest pain, substernal chest pain, face edema, hangover effect, neck rigidity, parosmia.

DRUG INTERACTIONS

Cimetidine / Significantly ↑ zaleplon serum levels

CNS depressants (anticonvulsants, antihistamines, ethanol) / Additive CNS depression

Rifampin / Significantly ↓ zaleplon serum levels

HOW SUPPLIED

Capsules: 5 mg, 10 mg

DOSAGE

- **CAPSULES**

Insomnia.

Adults, nonelderly: 10 mg for no more than 7–10 days. Consider 20 mg for the occasional client who does not benefit from the lower dose. Do not exceed a dose of 20 mg. **Mild to moderate hepatic impairment, elderly clients, or low-weight individuals:** 5 mg, not to exceed 10 mg.

NURSING CONSIDERATIONS

ASSESSMENT

1. Note characteristics of insomnia and assess for contributing factors.
2. Assess for depression, respiratory dysfunction, alcohol or drug dependence. Drug may cause dependence and amnesia.
3. Contains tartrazine (FD&C yellow #5); note any aspirin hypersensitivity.

4. Note drugs prescribed to ensure none interact; with cimetidine initially reduce zaleplon dose to 5 mg and assess response.
5. Monitor renal and LFTs; reduce dose with liver dysfunction.

CLIENT/FAMILY TEACHING

1. Due to its rapid onset, ingest immediately prior to going to bed or after the client has gone to bed and experienced difficulty falling asleep.
2. Taking zaleplon with or immediately after a heavy, high-fat meal causes slower absorption leading to a reduced effect on sleep latency.
3. Do not engage in activities requiring mental alertness after ingesting drug and during the next day until drug effects realized.
4. Avoid alcohol and CNS depressants.
5. May experience amnesia. Obtain at least 4 hr sleep after ingestion and before activity.
6. If also taking cimetidine, take an initial lowered dose of 5 mg of zaleplon.
7. May experience withdrawal symptoms or worsening of insomnia with abrupt drug discontinuation especially with daily use for an extended period of time.
8. If behaviorial changes or unusual thinking occur involving aggressiveness, confusion, loss of personal identity, agitation, hallucinations, increased depression or suicide ideations, report.
9. Store out of the reach of children.
10. Identify triggers (caffeine, day time naps) and alternative methods to induce sleep i.e soft music, warm milk, white noise simulator etc.

OUTCOMES/EVALUATE

Relief of insomnia

Zanamivir

(zah-**NAM**-ih-vir)

PREGNANCY CATEGORY: C
CLASSIFICATION(S):
Antiviral
Rx: Relenza

ACTION/KINETICS

Selectively inhibits influenza virus neuraminidase. The enzyme allows virus release from infected cells, prevents virus aggregation, and possibly decreases virus inactivation by respiratory mucus. Zanamivir may alter virus particle aggregation and release. There is the possibility of emergence of resistance. Does not prevent complications from bacterial infections. About 4%–17% is absorbed systemically. **Peak serum levels:** 17–142 ng/mL within 1–2 hr after a 10-mg dose. Readily excreted as unchanged drug in the urine. **t½:** 2.5–5.1 hr after PO inhalation.

USES

Treatment of uncomplicated acute illness due to influenza virus A and B (limited) in adults and children 7 years and older who have been symptomatic for 2 or less days. *Note:* There is no evidence that zanamivir is effective in any illness caused by agents other than influenza virus A and B.

CONTRAINDICATIONS

Use in asthma or COPD.

SPECIAL CONCERNS

Use with caution during lactation. It is possible the elderly may be more sensitive to effects of the drug. Safety and efficacy have not been determined in children less than 7 years of age, in clients with underlying chronic pulmonary disease, for prophylactic use to prevent influenza (clients should still take annual flu vaccinations), or in those with high-risk underlying medical conditions (e.g., respiratory disease).

SIDE EFFECTS

GI: Diarrhea, N&V. **Respiratory:** Nasal S&S, bronchitis, bronchospasm, dyspnea, cough, sinusitis, infections of the ENT. **Miscellaneous:** Dizziness, arrhythmias, headache, seizures, syncope, malaise, fatigue, fever, abdominal pain, myalgia, arthralgia, urticaria, allergic reactions (including oropharyngeal edema and serious skin rashes), serious bacterial infections with flu-like symptoms or as complications of flu.

LABORATORY TEST CONSIDERATIONS
↑ Liver enzymes, CPK. Lymphopenia, neutropenia.

HOW SUPPLIED
Powder for Inhalation, Blisters: 5 mg

DOSAGE

- **POWDER FOR ORAL INHALATION**
  Influenza treatment.

Adults and children over 7 years: 2 inhalations (one 5-mg blister per inhalation for a total dose of 10 mg) b.i.d. for 5 days. Two doses are taken on the first day of treatment whenever possible, provided there is 2 or more hr between doses. On subsequent days, doses are taken about 12 hr apart (i.e., morning and evening) at about the same time each day. Safety and efficacy of repeated treatment courses have not been studied.

NURSING CONSIDERATIONS

ADMINISTRATION/STORAGE
Store at 25°C (77°F).

ASSESSMENT
Document indications for therapy, onset and characteristics of symptoms, and any other medical conditions; note drug allergies.

CLIENT/FAMILY TEACHING
1. To be given by oral inhalation only, using the Diskhaler provided. Review/demonstrate use of the delivery system.
2. Do not puncture any Relenza Rotadisk blister until taking a dose using the Diskhaler.
3. Continue complete treatment (5 days) despite feeling better. Take oral inhalations twice a day 12 hr apart at approximately the same time each day.
4. If client is to use an inhaled bronchodilator at the same time as zanamivir, use the bronchodilator before taking zanamivir.
5. Safety and efficacy of repeated treatment courses have not been evaluated.
6. Does not reduce the risk of transmisstion of flu to others.
7. Vaccination is still the primary means to prevent and control influenza.
8. Clients with asthma or COPD may experience bronchospasm with zanamivir; have a fast-acting inhaled bronchodilator available, stop zanamivir and contact provider immediately if worsening of respiratory symptoms experienced.

OUTCOMES/EVALUATE
Relief of influenza S&S

Zidovudine (Azidothymidine, AZT)

(zye-**DOH**-vyou-deen, ah-**zee**-doh-**THIGH**-mih-deen)

PREGNANCY CATEGORY: C
CLASSIFICATION(S):
Antiviral, nucleoside reverse transcriptase inhibitor
Rx: Retrovir
🍁**Rx:** Apo-Zidovudine, Novo-AZT

SEE ALSO *ANTIVIRAL DRUGS* AND *ANTI-INFECTIVE DRUGS*.

ACTION/KINETICS
The active form of the drug is Zidovudine triphosphate, which is derived from Zidovudine by cellular enzymes. Zidovudine triphosphate competes with thymidine triphosphate (the natural substrate) for incorporation into growing chains of viral DNA by retroviral reverse transcriptase. Once incorporated, Zidovudine triphosphate causes premature termination of the growth of the DNA chain. Delays appearance of AIDS symptoms. Low concentrations of Zidovudine also inhibit the activity of *Shigella, Klebsiella, Salmonella, Enterobacter, Escherichia coli,* and *Citrobacter,* although resistance develops rapidly. Rapidly absorbed from the GI tract and is distributed to both plasma and CSF. **Peak serum levels:** 0.1–1.5 hr. **t½:** approximately 1 hr. Metabolized rapidly by the liver and excreted through the urine.

USES

PO: (1) Initial treatment of HIV-infected adults who have a CD_4 cell count of 500/mm³ or less. Superior to either didanosine or zalcitabine monotherapy for initial treatment of HIV-infected clients who have not had previous antiretroviral therapy. (2) To prevent HIV transmission from pregnant women to their fetuses. (3) For HIV-infected children over 3 months of age who have HIV-related symptoms or are asymptomatic with abnormal laboratory values indicating significant immunosuppression. (4) In combination with zalcitabine in selected clients with advanced HIV disease (CD_4 cell count of 300 cells/mm³ or less).

IV: Selected adults with symptomatic HIV infections who have a history of confirmed *Pneumocystis carinii* pneumonia or an absolute CD_4 (T_4 helper/inducer) lymphocyte count of less than 200 cells/mm3 in the peripheral blood prior to therapy.

CONTRAINDICATIONS

Allergy to Zidovudine or its components. Lactation.

SPECIAL CONCERNS

Use with caution in clients who have a hemoglobin level of less than 9.5 g/dL or a granulocyte count less than 1,000/mm³. Zidovudine is not a cure for HIV; thus, clients may continue to acquire opportunistic infections and other illnesses associated with ARC or HIV. Zidovudine has not been shown to reduce the risk of HIV transmission to others through sexual contact or blood contamination.

SIDE EFFECTS

Adults.

Hematologic: Anemia (severe), granulocytopenia. **Body as a whole:** Headache, asthenia, fever, diaphoresis, malaise, body odor, chills, edema of the lip, flu-like syndrome, hyperalgesia, abdominal/chest/back pain, lymphadenopathy. **GI:** Nausea, GI pain, diarrhea, anorexia, vomiting, dyspepsia, constipation, dysphagia, edema of the tongue, eructation, flatulence, bleeding gums, mouth ulcers, ***rectal hemorrhage.*** **CNS:** Somnolence, dizziness, paresthesia, insomnia, anxiety, confusion, emotional lability, depression, nervousness, vertigo, loss of mental acuity. **CV:** Vasodilation, syncope, vasculitis (rare). **Musculoskeletal:** Myalgia, myopathy, myositis, arthralgia, tremor, twitch, muscle spasm. **Respiratory:** Dyspnea, cough, epistaxis, rhinitis, pharyngitis, sinusitis, hoarseness. **Dermatologic:** Rash, pruritus, urticaria, acne, pigmentation changes of the skin and nails. **GU:** Dysuria, polyuria, urinary hesitancy or frequency. **Other:** Amblyopia, hearing loss, photophobia, ***severe hepatomegaly with steatosis,*** lactic acidosis, change in taste perception, hepatitis, pancreatitis, hypersensitivity reactions, including ***anaphylaxis,*** hyperbilirubinemia (rare), ***seizures***.

Children.

The following side effects have been observed in children, although any of the side effects reported for adults can also occur in children. **Body as a whole:** Granulocytopenia, anemia, fever, headache, phlebitis, bacteremia. **GI:** N&V, abdominal pain, diarrhea, weight loss. **CNS:** Decreased reflexes, nervousness, irritability, insomnia, ***seizures.*** **CV:** Abnormalities in ECG, left ventricular dilation, CHF, generalized edema, ***cardiomyopathy,*** S_3 gallop. **GU:** Hematuria, viral cystitis

OD OVERDOSE MANAGEMENT

Symptoms: N&V. Transient hematologic changes. Headache, dizziness, drowsiness, confusion, lethargy. *Treatment:* Treat symptoms. Hemodialysis will enhance the excretion of the primary metabolite of Zidovudine.

DRUG INTERACTIONS

Acetaminophen / ↑ Risk of granulocytopenia
Adriamycin / ↑ Risk of cytotoxicity, nephrotoxicity, or hematologic toxicity
Dapsone / ↑ Risk of cytotoxicity, nephrotoxicity, or hematologic toxicity
Flucytosine / ↑ Risk of cytotoxicity, nephrotoxicity, or hematologic toxicity
Fluconazole / ↑ Zidovudine Levels

Z

Ganciclovir / ↑ Risk of hematologic toxicity
Interferon alfa / ↑ Risk of hematologic toxicity
Interferon beta-1b / ↑ Zidovudine serum levels
Phenytoin / Levels of phenytoin may ↑, ↓, or remain unchanged; also, ↓ Zidovudine excretion
Probenecid / ↓ Biotransformation or renal excretion of Zidovudine → flu-like symptoms, including myalgia, malaise or fever, and maculopapular rash
Rifampin / ↓ Zidovudine levels
Trimethoprim / ↑ Zidovudine serum levels
Vinblastine / ↑ Risk of cytotoxicity, nephrotoxicity, or hematologic toxicity
Vincristine / ↑ Risk of cytotoxicity, nephrotoxicity, or hematologic toxicity

HOW SUPPLIED

Capsule: 100 mg; *Injection:* 10 mg/mL; *Syrup:* 50 mg/5 mL; *Tablet:* 300 mg

DOSAGE

• CAPSULES, SYRUP, TABLETS

Symptomatic HIV infections.

Adults: 100 mg (one 100-mg capsule or 10 mL syrup) q 4 hr around the clock (i.e., total of 600 mg daily).

Asymptomatic HIV infections.

Adults: 100 mg q 4 hr while awake (500 mg/day); **Pediatric, 3 months–12 years, initial:** 180 mg/m^2 q 6 hr (720 mg/m^2/day, not to exceed 200 mg q 6 hr).

Prevent transmission of HIV from mothers to their fetuses (after week 14 of pregnancy).

Maternal dosing: 100 mg 5 times a day until the start of labor. During labor and delivery, Zidovudine IV at 2 mg/kg over 1 hr followed by continuous IV infusion of 1 mg/kg/hr until clamping of the umbilical cord. **Infant dosing:** 2 mg/kg PO q 6 hr beginning within 12 hr after birth and continuing through 6 weeks of age. Infants unable to take the drug PO may be given Zidovudine IV at 1.5 mg/kg, infused over 30 min q 6 hr.

In combination with zalcitabine.

Zidovudine, 200 mg, with zalcitabine, 0.75 mg, q 8 hr.

• IV

1–2 mg/kg infused over 1 hr. The IV dose is given q 4 hr around the clock only until PO therapy can be instituted. Dosage adjustment may be necessary due to hematologic toxicity.

NURSING CONSIDERATIONS

SEE ALSO *GENERAL NURSING CONSIDERATIONS* FOR *ALL ANTI-INFECTIVES.*

ADMINISTRATION/STORAGE

1. Protect capsules and syrup from light.

IV 2. Do not mix with blood products or protein solutions.

3. Remove dose from 20-mL vial and dilute in 5% dextrose injection to a concentration not to exceed 4 mg/mL. Administer calculated dose IV at a constant rate over 1 hr.

4. After dilution, the solution is stable at room temperature for 24 hr and if refrigerated (2–8°C, 36–46°F) for 48 hr. To ensure safety from microbial contamination, give within 8 hr if stored at room temperature and 24 hr if refrigerated.

ASSESSMENT

1. Document indications for therapy, onset, other therapies trialed and baseline CD_4 counts and viral load.

2. Initially monitor CBC at least q 2 weeks. If anemia or granulocytopenia severe, the dose must be adjusted or discontinued. Epoetin alfa recombinant may be administered with iron to stimulate RBC production. A blood transfusion may also be required.

3. Safety and effectiveness of chronic Zidovudine therapy are not known, especially in those with a less advanced form of disease.

4. When used to prevent maternal-fetal transmission of HIV, Zidovudine should be initiated in pregnant women between 14 and 24 weeks of gestation; also, IV Zidovudine should be given during labor up until the cord is clamped, and newborn infants should receive Zidovudine syrup. Mothers may not breast feed.

CLIENT/FAMILY TEACHING

1. Take with or without food q 4 hr ATC as ordered; sleep must be interrupted to take medication.
2. Report for all labs, especially CBC, because drug causes anemia, and additional medications or blood transfusions may be necessary.
3. Report early S&S of anemia, e.g.; SOB, weakness, lightheadedness, palpitations, and increased fatigue.
4. Consume 2–3 L/day fluids to ensure adequate hydration. Maintain a record of weights and I&O.
5. Report any S&S of superinfections (e.g., furry tongue, mouth lesions, vaginal/rectal itching, rash).
6. Avoid acetaminophen and any other unprescribed drugs that may exacerbate the toxicity of Zidovudine.
7. Drug is not a cure but helps to alleviate and manage symptoms of HIV infections. May continue to develop opportunistic infections and other complications due to AIDS or ARC.
8. Do not share and do not exceed the prescribed dose of Zidovudine.
9. The risk of transmission of HIV to others through blood or sexual contact is not reduced in individuals on Zidovudine therapy. Practice safe sex and do not share needles.
10. With pregnancy, Zidovudine therapy should start after the 14-week gestation period to help prevent the transmission from mother to infant. Once delivered, do not nurse infant.
11. Identify local support groups that may assist one to understand/cope with this disease.

OUTCOMES/EVALUATE

- Control of symptoms of HIV, AIDS, or ARC
- ↑ CD_4 counts; ↓ viral load
- ↓ Maternal fetal HIV transmission

Zileuton

(zye-**LOO**-ton)

PREGNANCY CATEGORY: C

CLASSIFICATION(S):
Antiasthmatic, leukotriene receptor antagonist
Rx: Zyflo

ACTION/KINETICS
Specific inhibitor of 5-lipoxygenase; thus, inhibits the formation of leukotrienes. Leukotrienes are substances that induce various biological effects including aggregation of neutrophils and monocytes, leukocyte adhesion, increase of neutrophil and eosinophil migration, increased capillary permeability, and contraction of smooth muscle. These effects of leukotrienes contribute to edema, secretion of mucus, inflammation, and bronchoconstriction in asthmatic clients. By inhibiting leukotriene formation, zileuton reduces bronchoconstriction due to cold air challenge in asthmatics. Rapidly absorbed from the GI tract; **peak plasma levels:** 1.7 hr. Metabolized in liver and mainly excreted through the urine. **t½:** 2.5 hr.

USES
Prophylaxis and chronic treatment of asthma in adults and children over 12 years of age.

CONTRAINDICATIONS
Active liver disease or transaminase elevations greater than or equal to three times the upper limit of normal. Hypersenstivity. Treatment of bronchoconstriction in acute asthma attacks, including status asthmaticus. Lactation.

SPECIAL CONCERNS
Use with caution in clients who ingest large quantities of alcohol or who have a past history of liver disease. Safety and efficacy have not been determined in children less than 12 years of age.

SIDE EFFECTS
GI: Dyspepsia, N&V constipation, flatulence. **CNS:** Headache, dizziness, insomnia, malaise, nervousness, somnolence. **Body as a whole:** Unspecified pain, abdominal pain, chest pain, asthenia, accidental injury, fever. **Musculoskeletal:** Myalgia, arthralgia, neck pain/rigidity. **GU:** UTI, vaginitis.

Z

Miscellaneous: Conjunctivitis, hypertonia, lymphadenopathy, pruritus.

LABORATORY TEST CONSIDERATIONS

↑ LFTs. Low WBC count.

DRUG INTERACTIONS

Propranolol / ↑ Propranolol effect
Theophylline / Doubling of serum theophylline levels → ↑ effect
Warfarin / ↑ PT

HOW SUPPLIED

Tablets: 600 mg.

DOSAGE

• **TABLETS**

Symptomatic treatment of asthma.

Adults and children over 12 years of age: 600 mg q.i.d.

NURSING CONSIDERATIONS

ADMINISTRATION/STORAGE

Do not decrease dose or stop taking any other antiasthmatics when taking zileuton.

ASSESSMENT

1. Document onset, characteristics, and severity of disease. Note triggers; list currently prescribed therapy.
2. Monitor CBC, PFTs, and LFTs.
3. Screen for excessive alcohol use and any evidence of liver disease.

CLIENT/FAMILY TEACHING

1. Take regularly as directed (may take with meals and at bedtime) and continue other antiasthmatic medications as prescribed.
2. Drug will not reverse bronchospasm during acute asthma attack; use bronchodilators and seek medical attention if symptoms are severe or peak flow readings indicate need.
3. Drug inhibits formation of those substances that cause bronchoconstrictive symptoms in asthmatics.
4. Use peak flow meter readings to monitor airway effectiveness, to increase medications, and to seek immediate medical attention.
5. Use caution, may cause dizziness.
6. Report immediately if experiencing RUQ pain, lethargy, itching, jaundice, fatigue, or flu-like symptoms (S&S of liver toxicity).
7. Report for CBC, regularly scheduled LFTs and evaluation of pulmonary status. Bring record of peak flow readings.
8. Review triggers (i.e., smoke, cold air, and exercise) that may cause increased hyperresponsiveness which can last up to a week. If more than the usual or maximum number of inhalations of short-acting bronchodilator treatment in a 24-hr period are required, notify provider.

OUTCOMES/EVALUATE

Asthma prophylaxis; ↑ airway exchange.

Ziprasidone hydrochloride

(zigh-**PRAYZ**-oh-dohn)

PREGNANCY CATEGORY: C

CLASSIFICATION(S):

Antipsychotic

Rx: Geodon

ACTION/KINETICS

Mechanism unknown but thought to be due to a combination of dopamine (D_2) and serotonin (5-HT_2) receptor antagonism. Well absorbed; **peak plasma levels:** 6–8 hr. Absorption increased up to 2-fold in the presence of food. Greater than 99% plasma protein bound. Extensively metabolized in the liver with about 20% excreted in the urine and 66% eliminated in the feces. **t½, terminal:** 7 hr.

USES

Treatment of schizophrenia. Due to the possibility of causing prolongation of the QT/QTc interval, other drugs should be considered first.

CONTRAINDICATIONS

Do not use with other drugs that prolong the QT interval, including dofetilide, moxifloxacin, quinidine, pimozide, sotalol, sparfloxacin, or thioridazine. Do not use in clients with a known history of QT prolongation, with recent acute MI, with uncompensated heart failure, or cardiac arrhythmia. Lactation.

SPECIAL CONCERNS

Ziprasidone has a greater capacity to prolong the QT/QTc interval compared with other antipsychotic drugs. Prolongation of the QTc interval is associated in some other drugs with causing torsade de pointes-type arrhythmia, which is a potentially fatal ventricular tachycardia. It is not known whether ziprasidone will cause torsade de pointes or increase the rate of sudden death. Use of antipsychotic drugs may cause tardive dyskinesia and/or neuroleptic malignant syndrome. Use with caution in those with a history of MI, ischemic heart disease, heart failure, or conduction abnormalities; in cerebrovascular disease; in conditions that predispose to hypotension; or in those with a history of seizures or conditions that potentially lower the seizure threshold (e.g., Alzheimer's). Safety and efficacy have not been established in children.

SIDE EFFECTS

Mainly listed are side effects with an incidence of 1% or more.

GI: Nausea, constipation, dyspepsia, diarrhea, dry mouth, anorexia. **CNS:**Seizures, somnolence, suicide attempts, akathisia, dizziness, extrapyramidal syndrome, dystonia, hypertonia. **CV:** Orthostatic hypotension, tachycardia. **Respiratory:** Cold symptoms, URTI, rhinitis, increased cough. **Dermatologic:** Rash, urticaria, fungal dermatitis. **Body as a whole:** Asthenia, accidental injury. **Miscellaneous:** Myalgia, abnormal vision.

LABORATORY TEST CONSIDERATIONS

↑ Prolactin.

OD OVERDOSE MANAGEMENT

Symptoms: Hypotension, circulatory collapse, severe extrapyramidal symptoms. *Treatment:* Establish and maintain an airway and ensure adequate oxygenation and ventilation. Establish IV access. Undertake gastric lavage if necessary and consider activated charcoal with a laxative. Monitor CV status, including continuous electrocardiographic monitoring to detect possible arrhythmias. Treat hypotension and circulatory collapse with IV fluids (do not use epinephrine or dopamine). Give anticholinergic drugs to treat severe extrapyramidal symptoms.

DRUG INTERACTIONS

Antihypertensive drugs / Additive hypotension with certain antihypertensive drugs

Carbamazepine / ↓ ziprasidone plasma levels due to ↑ liver metabolism

Centrally-acting drugs / Use caution due to CNS effects of ziprasidone

Dopamine agonists / Antagonism of agonist effect

Ketoconazole / ↑ ziprasidone plasma levels due to inhibition of metabolism

Levodopa / Antagonism of levodopa effects

HOW SUPPLIED

Capsules: 20 mg, 40 mg, 60 mg, 80 mg

DOSAGE

- **CAPSULES**

Schizophrenia.

Initial: 20 mg b.i.d. with food. Adjust dose based on individual clinical status, up to 80 mg b.i.d. If needed, adjust dose at intervals of 2 or more days, as steady state is reached in 1–3 days. **Maintenance:** Efficacy is maintained for 52 weeks or less at a dose of 20–80 mg b.i.d. Periodically assess to determine need for continued treatment.

NURSING CONSIDERATIONS

ASSESSMENT

1. Determine onset of disease, symptom characteristics, presenting behaviors, and other agents trialed.
2. Note any history of CAD, abnormal QT interval, arrhythmias, CVA, Alzheimer's disease or seizures.
3. List drugs currently prescribed to ensure none interact unfavorably.
4. Monitor CBC, U/A, LFTs, electrolytes, and Mg levels. Those being considered for ziprasidone therapy who are at risk for significant electrolyte disturbances, especially hypokalemia, should have baseline serum K and Mg levels. Hypokalemia and/or hypomagnesemia may increase the risk of QT prolongation and arrhythmias.

CLIENT/FAMILY TEACHING

1. Take as directed, twice a day with food. Do not stop suddenly; drug

Z

should be withdrawn slowly to prevent adverse side effects.
2. Report any changes in behavior, loss of control, increased tremor or evidence of seizures.
3. Avoid activities that require mental alertness until drug effects realized.
4. Change positions slowly to prevent postural effects. Avoid hot baths/showers, hot tubs as low BP may occur. Do not perform strenuous activites in warm weather, may have heat stroke.
5. Drug may alter electrolyte levels. Report as scheduled for periodic labs.
6. Continue regular psychotherapy sessions.
7. Avoid OTC drugs and ETOH. Report any unusual side effects or lack of response.

OUTCOMES/EVALUATE

Improved patterns of behavior with less agitation, less hyperactivity, and reality orientation

Zoledronic acid for injection

(**ZOH**-leh-**dron**-ick **AS**-id)

PREGNANCY CATEGORY: C
CLASSIFICATION(S):
Bone growth regulator, bisphosphonate
Rx: Zometa

ACTION/KINETICS

Hyperactivity of osteoclasts causes excessive bone resorption in hypercalcemia of malignancy. Such hypercalcemia causes polyuria and GI disturbances with progressive dehydration and decreased glomerular filtration rate. Reducing excessive bone resorption and maintaining adequate fluid intake are essential to managing hypercalcemia of malignancy. Zoledronic acid acts to inhibit bone resorption perhaps by inhibiting osteoclastic activity and inducing osteoclast apoptosis. Zoledronic acid also blocks the osteoclastic resorption of mineralized bone and cartilage by binding to bone. It inhibits the increased osteoclastic activity and skeletal calcium release induced by various stimulatory factors released by tumors. **t½:** 0.23 hr, 1.75 hr, and 167 hr for the distribution, elimination, and terminal elimination, respectively. Is primarily excreted through the urine unchanged.

USES

Treatment of hypercalcemia of malignancy.

CONTRAINDICATIONS

Hypersensitivity to zoledronic acid or other bisphosphonates.

SPECIAL CONCERNS

Use with caution in aspirin-sensitive asthma. Safety and efficacy have not been determined in treating hypercalcemia associated with hyperparathyroidism or other non-tumor-related diseases. Use with caution during lactation and in the elderly. Safety and efficacy have not been determined in children.

SIDE EFFECTS

GU: Renal toxicity, including deterioration of renal function and potential renal failure, UTI. **GI:** N&V, constipation, diarrhea, abdominal pain, anorexia, dysphagia. **CNS:** Insomnia, anxiety, confusion, agitation, headache, somnolence. **CV:** Hypotension. **Body as a whole:** Fever, progression of cancer, flu-like syndrome (fever, chills, bone pain, arthralgias, myalgias), rash, pruritus, chest pain, non-specific infection, dehydration, asthenia, leg edema, mucositis, metastases. **Hematologic:** Anemia, granulocytopenia, thrombocytopenia, pancytopenia. **Respiratory:** Dyspnea, coughing, pleural effusion. **Musculoskeletal:** Skeletal pain, arthralgia. **Infusion site reaction:** Redness, swelling. **Miscellaneous:** Moniliasis.

LABORATORY TEST CONSIDERATIONS

↑ Creatinine. Hypocalcemia, hypophosphatemia, hypomagnesemia.

DRUG INTERACTIONS

Aminoglycosides / Possible additive effect to lower serum calcium levels for prolonged periods
Diuretics, loop / ↑ Risk of hypocalcemia

HOW SUPPLIED
Injection: 4 mg/vial

DOSAGE

- **IV ONLY**

Hypercalcemia of malignancy.

Maximum recommended dose: 4 mg infused over no less than 15 min. Consider retreatment if serum calcium does not return to normal or remain normal after initial treatment. Allow 7 days to elapse before retreatment.

NURSING CONSIDERATIONS

ADMINISTRATION/STORAGE

IV 1. Do not use diuretic therapy until hypovolemia is corrected.
2. Due to the risk of significant deterioration of renal function, do not exceed single doses of 4 mg of zoledronic acid with the duration of infusion no less than 15 minutes.
3. Use the following criteria in those who experience a decrease in renal function after zoledronic acid:
- If the serum creatinine was normal prior to zoledronic acid and there is an increase of 0.5 mg/dL within 2 weeks of the next dose, withhold zoledronic acid until serum creatinine is at least within 10% of the baseline value.
- If the serum creatinine is abnormal prior to zoledronic acid and there is an increase of 1.0 mg/dL within 2 weeks of the next dose, withhold zoledronic acid until serum creatinine is at least within 10% of the baseline value.

4. Reconstitute by adding 5 mL sterile water for injection to each vial. The resulting solution allows for withdrawal of 4 mg zoledronic acid. Completely dissolve before withdrawing solution.
5. The maximum 4-mg dose must be further diluted in100 mL sterile 0.9% NaCl or D5W. Give as a single IV infusion over no less than 15 min.
6. Refrigerate if not used immediately after reconstitution. The total time between reconstitution, dilution, storage, and end of administration must not exceed 24 hr.
7. Do not mix with calcium-containing solutions, such as lactated Ringer's. Administer in a line separate from all other drugs.

ASSESSMENT

1. Note indications for therapy, source of malignancy, serum Ca levels, and other agents/methods trialed.
2. Initiate vigorous NSS hydration to ensure UO is 2L/day during treatment.
3. Avoid diuretics until client is adequately hydrated.
4. Ensure albumin corrected calcium level: (Cca, mg/dL= Ca + 0.8).
5. Monitor CBC, Ca, PO_4, Mg, and renal function. Assess for renal failure and deficiency states, replacement needed.

CLIENT/FAMILY TEACHING

This drug is administered IV to reduce high calcium levels which result from tumors that cause increased bone activity and skeletal calcium release.

OUTCOMES/EVALUATE

↓ Serum calcium levels in malignancy, Inhibition of bone resorption

Zolmitriptan

(zohl-mih-**TRIP**-tin)

PREGNANCY CATEGORY: C
CLASSIFICATION(S):
Antimigraine drug
Rx: Zomig, Zomig ZMT

ACTION/KINETICS
Binds to serotonin 5-$HT_{1B/1D}$ receptors on intracranial blood vessels and in sensory nerves of trigeminal system. This results in cranial vessel constriction and inhibition of pro-inflammatory neuropeptide release. Well absorbed after PO use. Orally disintegrating tablets may have a faster onset. **Peak plasma levels:** 2 hr. **t½, elimination:** 3 hr (for zolmitriptan and active metabolite). Excreted in feces and urine.

USES
Treatment of acute migraine in adults with or without aura. Use only when there is clear diagnosis of migraine.

Z

CONTRAINDICATIONS

Prophylaxis of migraine or management of hemiplegic or basilar migraine. Use in angina pectoris, history of MI, documented or silent ischemia, ischemic heart disease, coronary artery vasospasm (including Prinzmetal's variant angina), other significant underlying CV disease. Also use in uncontrolled hypertension, within 24 hr of treatment with another serotonin HT_1 agonist or an ergotamine-containing or ergot-type drug (e.g., dihydroergotamine, methysergide). Concurrent use with MAO inhibitor or within 2 weeks of discontinuing MAO inhibitor.

SPECIAL CONCERNS

Use with caution in liver disease and during lactation. A significant increase in BP may occur in those with moderate-to-severe hepatic impairment. Safety and efficacy have not been determined for cluster headache. Safety for treating >3 headaches in a 30-day period has not been determined.

SIDE EFFECTS

GI: Dry mouth, dyspepsia, dysphagia, nausea, increased appetite, tongue edema, esophagitis, gastroenteritis, abnormal liver function, thirst. **CV:** Palpitations, arrhythmias, hypertension, syncope. **Atypical sensations:** Hypesthesia, paresthesia, warm/cold sensation. **CNS:** Dizziness, somnolence, vertigo, agitation, anxiety, depression, emotional lability, insomnia. **Pain pressure sensations:** Chest pain, tightness, pressure and/or heaviness. Pain, tightness, or heaviness in the neck, throat, or jaw. Heaviness, pressure, tightness other than in the chest or neck. **Musculoskeletal:** Myalgia, myasthenia, back pain, leg cramps, tenosynovitis. **Respiratory:** Bronchitis, ***bronchospasm,*** epistaxis, hiccup, laryngitis, yawn. **Dermatologic:** Sweating, pruritus, rash, urticaria, ecchymosis, photosensitivity. **GU:** Hematuria, cystitis, polyuria, urinary frequency or urgency. **Body as a whole:** Asthenia, allergic reaction, chills, facial edema, edema, fever, malaise. **Miscellaneous:** Dry eye, eye pain, hyperacusis, ear pain, parosmia, tinnitus.

DRUG INTERACTIONS

Cimetidine / t½ of zolmitriptan is doubled
Ergot-containing drugs / Prolonged vasospastic reactions
MAO Inhibitors / ↑ Zolmitriptan levels
Oral contraceptives / ↑ Zolmitriptan plasma levels
Selective serotonin reuptake inhibitors / Rarely, weakness, hyperreflexia, and incoordination

HOW SUPPLIED

Tablets: 2.5 mg, 5 mg; *Tablets, Orally Disintegrating:* 2.5 mg, 5 mg

DOSAGE

• TABLETS

Migraine headaches.

Adults, initial: 2.5 mg or lower (break tablet in half). Dose of 5 mg may be required. If headache returns, repeat dose after 2 hr, not to exceed 10 mg in 24-hr period.

• TABLETS, ORALLY DISINTEGRATING

Migraine headaches.

Single dose of 2.5 mg. If headache returns, repeat dose after 2 hr, not to exceed 10 mg in 24-hr period.

NURSING CONSIDERATIONS

ADMINISTRATION/STORAGE

1. Use doses less than 2.5 mg in those with liver disease. Doses less than 2.5 mg may be obtained by manually breaking 2.5 mg tablet in half.
2. Safety of treating more than 3 headaches in 30 day period has not been established.

ASSESSMENT

1. Document frequency, duration, and characteristics of migraines. Note neurologist headache evaluation/diagnosis.
2. Assess neurologic status; noting LOC, N&V, vision changes/blurring, tingling in extremities and if precedes headache.
3. Note any evidence/history or CAD as this precludes therapy.
4. List drugs prescribed to ensure none interact.
5. Determine if pregnant.
6. Monitor VS, ECG, liver, and renal function studies; reduce dose with dysfunction and monitor BP.

CLIENT/FAMILY TEACHING

1. Take exactly as directed; strictly for migraine headaches. Do not exceed dosage or dosing intervals of 2 hr apart and total of 10 mg/24 hr.
2. If using the orally disintegrating tablet, remove from the blister just prior to dosing. Place on the tongue where it will dissolve and be swallowed with saliva. Taking a liquid is not necessary. Do not break the orally disintegrating tablet.
3. Report if chest pain, SOB, chest tightness, or wheezing persists.
4. Do not perform activities that require mental alertness until drug effects realized.
5. Practice reliable contraception; report if pregnancy suspected.
6. Report any loss of effect, unusual, or adverse side effects.
7. Attempt to identify triggers.

OUTCOMES/EVALUATE

Relief of migraine headache

Zolpidem tartrate

(**ZOL**-pih-dem)

PREGNANCY CATEGORY: B
CLASSIFICATION(S):

Sedative-hypnotic, nonbenzodiazepine

Rx: Ambien , **C-IV**

ACTION/KINETICS

May act by subunit modulation of the GABA receptor chloride channel macromolecular complex resulting in sedative, anticonvulsant, anxiolytic, and myorelaxant properties. Although unrelated chemically to the benzodiazepines or barbiturates, it interacts with a GABA-benzodiazepine receptor complex and shares some of the pharmacologic effects of the benzodiazepines. Specifically, it binds the omega-1 receptor preferentially. No evidence of residual next-day effects or rebound insomnia at usual doses; little evidence for memory impairment. Sleep time spent in stage 3 to 4 (deep sleep) was comparable to placebo with only inconsistent, minor changes in REM sleep at recommended doses. Rapidly absorbed from the GI tract. **t½:** About 2.5 hr (increased in geriatric clients and those with impaired hepatic function). Bound significantly (92.5%) to plasma proteins. Food decreases the bioavailability of zolpidem. Metabolized in the liver; inactive metabolites are excreted primarily through the urine.

USES

Short-term treatment of insomnia.

CONTRAINDICATIONS

Lactation.

SPECIAL CONCERNS

Use with caution and at reduced dosage in clients with impaired hepatic function, in compromised respiratory function, in those with impaired renal function, and in clients with S&S of depression. Impaired motor or cognitive performance after repeated use or unusual sensitivity to hypnotic drugs may be noted in geriatric or debilitated clients. Closely observe individuals with a history of dependence on or abuse of drugs or alcohol. Safety and efficacy have not been determined in children less than 18 years of age.

SIDE EFFECTS

Symptoms of withdrawal: Although there is no clear evidence of a withdrawal syndrome, the following symptoms were noted with zolpidem following placebo substitution: fatigue, nausea, flushing, lightheadedness, uncontrolled crying, emesis, stomach cramps, panic attack, nervousness, abdominal discomfort.

The most common side effects following use for up to 10 nights included drowsiness, dizziness, and diarrhea. The side effects listed in the following are for an incidence of 1% or greater. **CNS:** Headache, drowsiness, dizziness, lethargy, drugged feeling, lightheadedness, depression, abnormal dreams, amnesia, anxiety, nervousness, sleep disorder, ataxia, confusion, euphoria, insomnia, vertigo. **GI:** Nausea, diarrhea, dyspepsia, abdominal pain, constipation, anorexia, vomiting. **Musculoskeletal:** Myalgia, ar-

Z

thralgia. **Respiratory:** URI, sinusitis, pharyngitis, rhinitis. **Body as a whole:** Allergy, back pain, flu-like symptoms, chest pain, fatigue. **Ophthalmologic:** Diplopia, abnormal vision. **Miscellaneous:** Rash, UTI, palpitations, dry mouth, infection.

LABORATORY TEST CONSIDERATIONS

↑ ALT, AST, BUN. Hyperglycemia, hypercholesterolemia, hyperlipidemia, abnormal hepatic function.

OD OVERDOSE MANAGEMENT

Symptoms: Symptoms ranging from somnolence to light coma. Rarely, CV and respiratory compromise. *Treatment:* Gastric lavage if appropriate. General symptomatic and supportive measures. IV fluids as needed. Flumazenil may be effective in reversing CNS depression. Monitor hypotension and CNS depression and treat appropriately. Sedative drugs should not be used, even if excitation occurs. Zolpidem is not dialyzable.

DRUG INTERACTIONS

CNS depressants/ Additive CNS depression

Ketoconazole / ↑ Plasma ketoconazole levels

HOW SUPPLIED

Tablet: 5 mg, 10 mg

DOSAGE

- **TABLETS**

Hypnotic.

Adults, individualized, usual: 10 mg just before bedtime. In hepatic insufficiency, use an initial dose of 5 mg.

NURSING CONSIDERATIONS

ADMINISTRATION/STORAGE

1. Limit therapy to 7–10 days. Reevaluate if the drug is required for more than 2–3 weeks.
2. Do not prescribe in quantities exceeding a 1-month supply.
3. Do not exceed 10 mg daily.

ASSESSMENT

1. Note indications for therapy, onset, and symptom characteristics.
2. Determine any respiratory dysfunction (sleep apnea).
3. Note any drug or alcohol dependence; assess for symptoms of depression. Monitor CBC, LFTs.
5. Review sleep patterns (trouble falling/staying asleep, early am awakenings) and life-style. Identify underlying cause(s) of insomnia (i.e., napping during the daytime, lack of exercise, ↑ stress, depression).

CLIENT/FAMILY TEACHING

1. Take only as directed, on an empty stomach at bedtime.
2. Do not perform any activities that require mental or physical alertness. Evaluate response the following day to ensure that no residual depressant effects are evident.
3. Avoid alcohol and any unprescribed or OTC drugs.
4. Drug is only for short-term use; keep a log and identify factors that may be contributing to insomnia.
5. Review alternative methods for inducing sleep such as relaxation techniques, daily exercise, soft music, no daytime napping, guided imagery, white noise or special effects simulator.
6. Those with depression are at a higher risk for suicide or intentional overdose. Advise family that these clients warrant closer observation and limited prescriptions and to report any evidence of suicidal thoughts or aggressive behavior.
7. Keep out of reach of children and store in a safe place; drug has a high potential for abuse.

OUTCOMES/EVALUATE

Relief of insomnia

Zonisamide

(zoh-**NISS**-ah-myd)

PREGNANCY CATEGORY: C

CLASSIFICATION(S):

Anticonvulsant, miscellaneous

Rx: Zonegran

ACTION/KINETICS

Precise mechanism unknown. May block sodum channels and reduce voltage-dependent, transient inward currents (T-type Ca^{2+} currents), thus stabilizing neuronal membranes and suppressing neuronal hypersynchronization. May bind to the GABA/

Z

benzodiazepine receptor ionophore complex. **Peak plasma levels:** 2–5 mcg/mL in 2–6 hr. Food delays time to maximum levels but does not affect bioavailability. Extensively binds to erythrocytes and is about 40% plasma protein-bound. **t½, elimination:** About 63 hr from plasma and about 105 hr from erythrocytes. Excreted primarily in the urine as unchanged drug and the glucuronide metabolite.

USES

Adjunctive therapy to treat partial seizures in adults with epilepsy.

CONTRAINDICATIONS

Hypersensitivity to sulfonamides or zonisamide. Lactation.

SPECIAL CONCERNS

Hypersensitivity reactions are possible (zonisamide is a sulfonamide). Safety and efficacy have not been determined in pediatric clients.

SIDE EFFECTS

Side effects listed are those with an incidence of 0.1% or more. **Hypersensitivity:** ***Stevens-Johnson syndrome, toxic epidermal necrolysis, fulminant hepatic necrosis, agranulocytosis, aplastic anemia.***

CNS: Somnolence, dizziness, headache, agitation, irritability, tiredness, ataxia, confusion, depression, difficulty concentrating, difficulty with memory, insomnia, mental slowing, nystagmus, paresthesia, schizophrenia/schizophrenic behavior, tremor, convulsion, ***status epilepticus,*** abnormal gait, hyperesthesia, incoordination, hypertonia, twitching, abnormal dreams, vertigo, decreased libido, neuropathy, hyperkinesia, movement disorder, disarthria, hypotonia, peripheral neuritis, increased reflexes. **GI:** Anorexia, nausea, abdominal pain, diarrhea, dry mouth, taste perversion, dyspepsia, constipation, vomiting, flatulence, gingivitis, gum hyperplasia, gastritis, gastroenteritis, stomatitis, cholelithiasis, glossitis, melena, rectal hemorrhage, ulcerative stomatitis, gastro-duodenal ulcer, dysphagia, gum hemorrhage. **CV:** Palpitation, tachycardia, vascular insufficiency, ***CVA,*** hypertension, hypotension, thrombophlebitis, syncope, bradycardia. **Respiratory:** Pharyngitis, increased cough, dyspnea, rhinitis. **Musculoskeletal:** Leg cramps, myalgia, myasthenia, arthralgia, arthritis. **Dermatologic:** Pruritus, maculopapular rash, acne, alopecia, dry skin, sweating, eczema, ecchymosis, urticaria, hirsutism, pustular rash, vesiculobullous rash. **GU:** Urinary frequency, dysuria, urinary incontinence, hematuria, kidney stones, impotency, urinary retention, urinary urgency, amenorrhea, polyuria, nocturia. **Hematologic:** Leukopenia, anemia, immunodeficiency lymphadenopathy. **Metabolic:** Peripheral edema, weight gain, edema, thirst, dehydration. **Ophthalmic:** Diplopia, amblyopia, conjunctivitis, visual field defect, glaucoma, photophobia, iritis. **Miscellaneous:** Difficulties in verbal expression, speech abnormalities, flu syndrome, weight loss, tinnitus, parosmia, deafness, accidental injury, asthenia, chest pain, flank pain, malaise, allergic reaction, facial edema, neck rigidity, ***unexplained death.***

LABORATORY TEST CONSIDERATIONS

↑ Serum creatinine, BUN, serum alkaline phosphatase.

DRUG INTERACTIONS

Carbamazepine / ↓ Zonisamide t½ due to ↑ liver metabolism

Phenobarbital / ↓ Zonisamide t½ R/T ↑ liver metabolism

Phenytoin / ↓ Zonisamide t½ R/T ↑ liver metabolism

HOW SUPPLIED

Capsule: 100 mg

DOSAGE

• CAPSULES

Partial seizures.

Adults and those over 16 years of age: Individualize **Initial:** 100 mg/day. May increase to 200 mg/day after 2 weeks. Additional increases to 300 and 400 mg/day may be made in 2 weeks or longer to achieve steady state. Administer dosage once or twice daily except for the 100–mg dose

Z

NURSING CONSIDERATIONS

ASSESSMENT

1. Document type, onset, and characteristics of seizures; note other agents trialed and the outcome.
2. Note any sulfonamide allergy.
3. Monitor CBC, renal, and LFTs.
4. List other drugs prescribed to ensure none interact.

CLIENT/FAMILY TEACHING

1. Take capsules once or twice a day as directed. May take with or without food but should swallow capsules whole.
2. May cause drowsiness; do not perfom tasks that require alertness until drug effects realized and able to determine if drug affects performance.
3. Increase fluid intake to reduce kidney stone risk. Report increased back or abdominal pain or any blood in urine.
4. Stop drug and report immediately if a rash occurs or seizures worsen.
5. Report any new onset fever, sore throat, easy bruising, oral ulcers, or lack of sweating with fever.
6. Practice reliable birth control. Report if pregnancy suspected/anticipated or if breast feeding as drug should be avoided.
7. Abrupt withdrawal may precipitate increased seizure frequency or status epilepticus. Gradually reduce dose.

OUTCOMES/EVALUATE

Control of seizures

appendix 1

Drug Preview

Information for the following drugs was received subsequent to the submission of the manuscript for PDR-2003. This appendix may contain limited information for these drugs; a more complete profile will be included in next year's edition of this book.

-----COMBINATION DRUG-----

Etonogestrel/Ethinyl estradiol vaginal ring

PREGNANCY CATEGORY: X
CLASSIFICATION:
Contraceptive
Rx: NuvaRing

SEE ALSO *ESTROGENS* AND *ORAL CONTRACEPTIVES: ESTROGEN-PROGESTERONE COMBINATIONS*

CONTENT

In each ring: 11.7 mg etonogestrel and 2.7 mg ethinyl estradiol

ACTION/KINETICS

The product is a nonbiodegradable, flexible, transparent, colorless to almost colorless contraceptive vaginal ring containing a progestin (etonogestrel) and an estrogen (ethinyl estradiol). In the vagina, each ring releases an average of 0.12 mg/day of etonogestrel and 0.015 mg/day of ethinyl estradiol over a 3-week period of use. The primary action is inhibition of ovulation although changes in the cervical mucus (decrease sperm motility) and the endometrium (reduce possibility of implantation) add to the contraceptive effectiveness. Both hormones are rapidly absorbed into the systemic circulation and are metabolized by the liver cytochrome P450 3A4 isoenzyme. Both hormones are excreted in the urine, bile, and feces.

USES

Prevention of pregnancy.

CONTRAINDICATIONS

See *Estrogens* and *Oral Contraceptives: Estrogen-Progesterone Combinations.*

SPECIAL CONCERNS

See *Estrogens* and *Oral Contraceptives: Estrogen-Progesterone Combinations.*

SIDE EFFECTS

See also *Estrogens* and *Oral Contraceptives: Estrogen-Progesterone Combinations*

Most common: Vaginitis, headache, URTI, leukorrhea, sinusitis, weight gain, nausea. **Device-related events:** Foreign body sensation, coital problems, device expulsion, vaginal discomfort, vaginitis, leukorrhea, headache, emotional lability, weight gain. **Serious:** ***Thrombophlebitis, venous thrombosis with or without embolism, arterial thromboembolism, pulmonary embolism, MI, cerebral hemorrhage, cerebral thrombosis, hepatic adenomas,*** hypertension, gall bladder disease, benign liver tumors, mesenteric thrombosis, retinal thrombosis. **GI:** Cholestatic jaundice, abdominal cramps, bloating, N&V. **GU:** Amenorrhea, breakthrough bleeding, breast tenderness/enlargement/secretion, change in cervical erosion and secretion, change in menstrual flow, decrease in lactation when given immediately postpartum, spotting, temporary infertility after discontinuing treatment, vaginal candidiasis. **Miscellaneous:** Increase or decrease in weight, steepening of corneal curvature, edema, intolerance to contact lenses, Melasma, mental depression, migraine, allergic rash, decreased tolerance to carbohydrates.

DRUG INTERACTIONS

See *Estrogens* and *Oral Contraceptives: Estrogen-Progesterone Combinations.*

HOW SUPPLIED

See *Content*

DOSAGE

• **VAGINAL RING**

Prevention of pregnancy.

One vaginal ring inserted by the woman in the vagina. Ring remains in place for 3 weeks and is removed for a 1-week break A new ring is inserted 1 week after the last ring was removed on the same day of the week as it was inserted on the previous cycle.

NURSING CONSIDERATIONS

SEE ALSO *ESTROGENS* AND *ORAL CONTRACEPTIVES: ESTROGEN-PROGESTERONE COMBINATIONS.*

ADMINISTRATION/STORAGE

1. Withdrawal bleeding usually starts on day 2 to 3 after removal but may not have finished before the next ring is inserted. However, the new ring must be inserted 1 week after the previous one was removed in order to maintain contraceptive efficacy.
2. The woman can select the insertion position that is most comfortable to her (e.g., standing with one leg up, squatting, or lying down). Compress the ring and insert into the vagina. The exact position of the ring inside the vagina is not critical for activity.
3. Remove the vaginal ring after three weeks in place by hooking the index finger under the forward rim or by grasping the rim between the index and middle finger and pulling it out. Place the used ring in the foil pouch and discard in a waste receptacle out of the reach of children and pets. Do not flush in the toilet.
4. It is possible that ovulation and conception may occur before the first use of the vaginal ring. During the first cycle, an additional method of contraception should be used until after the first 7 days of ring use.
5. If no preceding hormonal contraceptive was used in the past month, count the first day of menses as day 1 and insert the vaginal ring on or prior to day 5 of the cycle, even if menses has not finished.
6. If switching from a combination oral contraceptive to the vaginal ring, insert the vaginal ring anytime within 7 days after the last combination oral contraceptive tablet and no later than the day that a new cycle of tablets would have started. No backup method of contraception is required.
7. If switching from a progestin-only method, insert the first vaginal ring as follows:

• Any day of the month when switching from a progestin-only tablet; do not skip any days between the last tablet and the first day of vaginal ring use.

• On the same day as the contraceptive implant removal.

• On the same day as removal of a progestin-containing IUD.

• On the day when the next contraceptive injection would be due.

In all of these situations, advise use of an additional method of contraception for the first 7 days after insertion of the ring.

8. The client may start using the vaginal ring within the first 5 days following a complete first trimester abortion. No additional method of contraception is required. If the vaginal ring is not inserted within 5 days, see Number 5 above.
9. Following delivery or a second-trimester abortion, insert the vaginal ring 4 weeks postpartum in women not breast feeding. Woman who are breast feeding should not use the vaginal ring until the child is weaned. Initiate use of the vaginal ring 4 weeks after a second-trimester abortion. However, there is an increased risk of thromboembolic disease. If a woman begins using the vaginal ring postpartum and has not yet had a period, it is possible that ovulation and conception has occurred prior to the insertion of the vaginal ring.
10. If there has been inadvertent removal, expulsion, or prolonged ring-free intervals during the 3-week use period, rinse the ring with cool to lukewarm (not hot) water and reinsert as soon as possible, at the latest within 3 hours. Contraceptive effectiveness is reduced if the ring has been out of the vagina for more than 3 hours. Thus, use an additional form of contraception until the ring has been

used continuously for 7 days. Consider the possibility of pregnancy if the ring-free interval has been extended beyond 1 week.

11. If the vaginal ring has been left in place for up to 1 extra week, remove it and insert a new ring after a 1-week ring-free interval. Rule out pregnancy if the vaginal ring has been left in place for more than 4 weeks.

12. If the client has not adhered to the prescribed regimen, consider the possibility of pregnancy at the time of the first missed period. Discontinue the use of the vaginal ring if pregnancy is confirmed. Rule out pregnancy if the client has adhered to the regimen and misses 2 consecutive periods.

13. Once dispensed to the user, the vaginal rings can be stored for up to 4 months at 15 - 30°C (59 - 86°F). Avoid storing in direct sunlight. When dispensed to the user, place an expiration date on the label. The date should not be more than 4 months from the date of dispensing or the expiration date, whichever comes first.

Pegfilgrastim

PREGNANCY CATEGORY: C
CLASSIFICATION:
Hematopoietic agent
Rx: Neulasta

ACTION/KINETICS

A colony stimulating factor that binds to specific cell surface receptors of hematopoietic cells resulting in proliferation, differentiation, commitment, and end cell function activation. Has same mechanism of action as filgrastim but has decreased renal clearance and prolonged activity compared with filgrastim. Clients with higher body weights experienced higher systemic exposure after receiving a dose normalized for body weight. **t½:** 15 - 80 hr after SC.

USES

Decrease incidence of infection, as demonstrated by febrile neutropenia, in clients with nonmyeloid malignancies who are receiving myelosuppressive anticancer drugs associated with a significant incidence of febrile neutropenia.

CONTRAINDICATIONS

Known hypersensitivity to *Escherichia coli*-derived proteins, pegfilgrastim, filgrastim, or any component of the product. Use of the 6 mg fixed-dose single-use syringe formulation in infants, children, and smaller adolescents weighing less than 45 kg. Use between 14 days before and 24 hr after cytotoxic chemotherapy due to the potential for an increase in sensitivity of rapidly dividing myeloid cells to cytotoxic chemotherapy.

SPECIAL CONCERNS

The possibility that pegfilgrastim can act as a growth factor for any tumor type cannot be excluded. Use with caution during lactation. Safety and efficacy have not been established in children.

SIDE EFFECTS

Most side effects appear to be due to the underlying malignancy or cytotoxic chemotherapy. **GI:** Nausea, diarrhea, vomiting, constipation, anorexia, taste perversion, dyspepsia, abdominal pain, stomatitis, mucositis. **CNS:** Headache, insomnia, dizziness. **Allergic:** ***Anaphylaxis,*** skin rash, urticaria. **Body as a whole:** Fatigue, alopecia, fever, skeletal pain, myalgia, arthralgia, generalized weakness, peripheral edema. **Hematologic:** Granulocytopenia, leukocytosis, neutropenic fever. **Miscellaneous:** Medullary bone pain (most common), hypoxia, splenic rupture (rare), ***adult respiratory distress syndrome,*** sickle cell crisis in those with sickle cell disease.

LABORATORY TEST INTERFERENCES

↑ LDH, alkaline phosphatase, uric acid (all are reversible).

DRUG INTERACTIONS

Lithium may potentiate the release of neutrophils; if used together with pegfilgrastim, monitor neutrophil counts more frequently.

HOW SUPPLIED

Single-dose syringe: Preservative-free solution containing 6 mg (0.6 mL) of pegfilgrastim (10 mg/mL)

DOSAGE

• **SC**

Myelosuppressive chemotherapy.

Single 6 mg dose given once per chemotherapy cycle.

NURSING CONSIDERATIONS

ADMINISTRATION/STORAGE

1. Visually inspect for discoloration and particulate matter before administration. Do not give if discoloration/particulate matter is noted.
2. Refrigerate at 2 - 8°C (36 - 46°F) and keep syringes in their carton to protect from light until use.
3. Avoid shaking. May be allowed to reach room temperature for a maximum of 48 hr before use, but protect from light. Discard any drug left at room temperature for more than 48 hr.
4. Avoid freezing. If accidentally frozen, allow to thaw in the refrigerator before administration. Discard if frozen a second time.

CLIENT/FAMILY TEACHING

1. Inform of the signs and symptoms of allergic drug reactions and advise of the appropriate actions to take.
2. Counsel on the importance of compliance and the need for regular monitoring of blood counts.
3. A client or caregiver may give the medication at home if provided with appropriate instruction on the proper use of the drug. Caution against the reuse of syringes, needles, or drug product and thoroughly instruct on the proper disposal techniques. Make available a puncture-resistant container for disposal of used needles and syringes.

appendix 2

Controlled Substances in the United States and Canada

Controlled Substances Act—United States

The U.S. Federal Controlled Substances Act of 1970 placed drugs controlled by the Act into five categories or schedules based on their potential to cause psychologic and/or physical dependence as well as on their potential for abuse. The schedules are defined as follows:

Schedule I [C-I]: Includes substances for which there is a high abuse potential and no current approved medical use (e.g., heroin, marijuana, LSD, other hallucinogens, certain opiates and opium derivatives).

Schedule II [C-II]: Includes drugs that have a high ability to produce physical or psychologic dependence and for which there is a current approved or acceptable medical use (e.g. narcotics, amphetamines)

Schedule III [C-III]: Includes drugs for which there is less potential for abuse than drugs in Schedule II and for which there is a current approved medical use and moderate dependence liability. Certain drugs in this category are preparations containing limited quantities of codeine and nonbarbituate sedatives. Anabolic steroids are classified in Schedule III.

Schedule IV [C-IV]: Includes drugs for which there is less abuse potential than for Schedule III, for which there is a current approved medical use, and that have limited dependence liability.

Schedule V [C-V]: Drugs in this category consist mainly of preparations containing limited amounts of certain narcotic drugs for use as antitussives and antidiarrheals. Federal law provides that limited quantities of these drugs (e.g., codeine) may be bought without a prescription by an individual at least 18 years of age if allowed under state statutes. The product must be purchased from a pharmacist, who must keep appropriate records. However, state laws vary, and in many states such products require a prescription.

NOTE: Generally prescriptions for Schedule II (high abuse potential) drugs cannot be transmitted over the phone and they cannot be refilled. Prescriptions for Schedule III, IV, and V drugs may be refilled up to five times within 6 months. Schedule II drugs are not necessarily "stronger" than drugs in Schedules III, IV, or V; Schedule II drugs are classified as such due to their high abuse potential.

Controlled Substances—Canada

In Canada, narcotics are governed by the Narcotics Control regulations and are designated by the letter N. Drugs that are considered subject to abuse, have an approved medical use, and are not narcotics are designated by the letter C.

	Drug Schedule	
Drug	*United States*	*Canada*
Alfentanil	II	N
Alprazolam	IV	*
Amobarbital sodium	II	C
Amphetamine sulfate	II	Not available
Aprobarbital	III	*
Benzphetamine HCl	III	Not available
Buprenorphine HCl	V	*
Butabarbital sodium	III	C
Butorphanol tartrate	IV	C
Chloral hydrate	IV	*
Chlordiazepoxide	IV	*
Clonazepam	IV	*
Clorazepate dipotassium	IV	*
Codeine	II	N
Dexmethylphenidate HCl	II	Not available
Dextroamphetamine sulfate	II	C
Diazepam	IV	*
Diethylpropion HCl	IV	C
Estazolam	IV	*
Ethchlorvynol	IV	*
Fentanyl	II	N
Fluoxymesterone	III	*
Flurazepam HCl	IV	*
Glutethimide	II	*
Halazepam	IV	Not available
Hydrocodone	Not available alone (usually C-III in combination drugs)	N
Hydromorphone HCl	II	N
Levomethadyl acetate HCl	II	Not available
Levorphanol tartrate	II	N
Lorazepam	IV	*
Meperidine HCl	II	N
Mephobarbital	IV	C
Meprobamate	IV	*
Methadone HCl	II	N
Methamphetamine HCl	II	Not available
Methylphenidate HCl	II	C
Methyltestosterone	III	*
Midazolam	IV	*
Morphine sulfate	II	N
Nalbuphine	*	C
Nandrolone decanote	III	*
Opium	II	N
Oxandrolone	III	*
Oxazepam	IV	*
Oxycodone HCl	II	N

Oxymetholone	III	*
Oxymorphone HCl	II	N
Paraldehyde	IV	*
Paregoric	III	N
Pemoline	IV	*
Pentazocine	IV	N
Pentobarbital sodium		
PO	II	C
Rectal	III	C
Phendimetrazine tartrate	III	Not available
Phenobarbital	IV	C
Phentermine HCl	IV	C
Propoxyphene	IV	N
Quazepam	IV	Not available
Remifentanil HCl	II	-
Secobarbital sodium	II	C
Sibutramine HCl	IV	
Stanozolol	III	*
Sufentanil citrate	II	N
Temazepam	IV	*
Testosterone (all forms)	III	*
Triazolam	IV	*
Zaleplon	IV	-
Zolpidem tartrate	IV	*

*Not controlled

appendix 3

Pregnancy Categories: FDA Assigned

The U.S. Food and Drug Administration's use-in-pregnancy rating system weighs the degree to which available information has ruled out risk to the fetus against the drug's potential benefit to the patient. The ratings, and their interpretation, are as follows:

Category	Interpetation
A	**CONTROLLED STUDIES SHOW NO RISK.** Adequate, well-controlled studies in pregnant women have failed to demonstrate a risk to the fetus in any trimester of pregnancy.
B	**NO EVIDENCE OF RISK IN HUMANS.** Either animal studies show risk but human findings do not, or if no adequate human studies have been done, animal findings are negative.
C	**RISK CANNOT BE RULED OUT.** Human studies are lacking, and animal studies are either positive for fetal risk or lacking. However, potential benefits may justify the potential risks.
D	**POSITIVE EVIDENCE OF RISK.** Investigational or post-marketing data show risk to the fetus. However, potential benefits may outweigh the potential risks. If needed in a life-threatening situation or serious disease, the drug may be acceptable if safer drugs cannot be used or are ineffective.
X	**CONTRAINDICATED IN PREGNANCY.** Studies in animals or humans, or investigational or post-marketing reports, have demonstrated positive evidence of fetal abnormalities or risk which clearly outweighs any possible benefit to the patient.

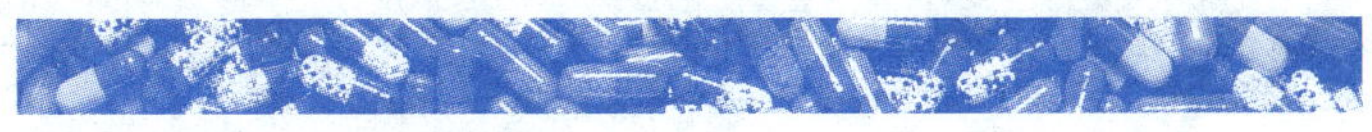

appendix 4

Nomogram for Estimating Body Surface Area

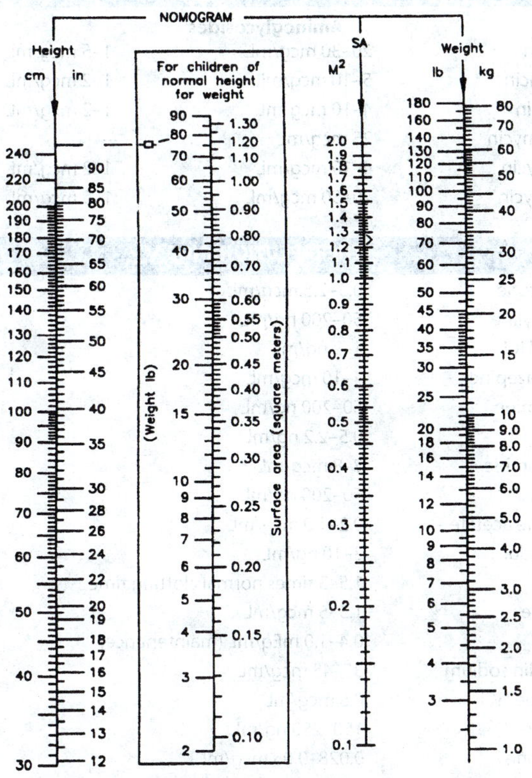

Directions for use: (1) Determine client height. (2) Determine client weight. (3) Draw a straight line to connect the height and weight. Where the line intersects on the surface area line is the derived body surface area (M^2).

Reprinted with permission from Behrman, R. E., Kliegman, R., and Arvin, A. M., eds. *Nelson Textbook of Pediatrics,* 15th ed. (Philadelphia: W. B. Saunders Company, 1996).

appendix 5

Commonly Accepted Therapeutic Drug Levels

DRUG	PEAK	TROUGH
	Aminoglycosides	
Amikacin	20–30 mcg/mL	1–5 mcg/mL
Gentamicin	5–10 mcg/mL	1–2 mcg/mL
Netilmicin	4–10 mcg/mL	1–2 mcg/mL
Streptomycin	25 mcg/mL	–
Tobramycin	4–10 mcg/mL	1–2 mcg/mL
Vancomycin	20–50 mcg/mL	1–5 mcg/mL

DRUG	THERAPEUTIC RANGE
Amiodarone	0.5–2.5 mcg/mL
Amitriptyline	50–200 ng/mL
Bepridil HCl	1–2 ng/mL
Carbamazepine	4–10 mcg/mL
Desipramine	50–200 ng/mL
Digoxin	0.5–2.2 ng/mL
Disopyramide	2–8 mcg/mL
Doxepin	50–200 ng/mL
Flecainide acetate	0.2–1.0 mcg/mL
Haloperidol	3–10 ng/mL
Heparin	1.5–3 times normal clotting time
Lidocaine	1.5–5 mcg/mL
Lithium	0.4–1.0 mEq/mL (maintenance)
Mezlocillin sodium	35–45 mcg/mL
Mexiletine HCl	0.5 mcg/mL
Milrinone	150–250 ng/mL
Nicardipine	0.028–0.05 mcg/mL
Nifedipine	0.025–0.1 mcg/mL
Phenobarbital	15–40 mcg/mL (as anticonvulsant)
Phenytoin	10–20 mcg/mL
Primidone	5–12 mcg/mL
Procainamide	4–8 mcg/mL

DRUG	THERAPEUTIC RANGE
Propafenone	0.5–3 mcg/mL
Propranolol	50–200 ng/mL
Quinidine	2–6 mcg/mL
Salicylic acid	150–300 mcg/mL (as anti-inflammatory)
Theophylline	10–20 mcg/mL (desired 7-12 mcg/mL)
Tocainide HCl	4–10 mcg/mL
Valproic acid	50–100 mcg/mL
Verapamil	0.08–0.3 mcg/mL

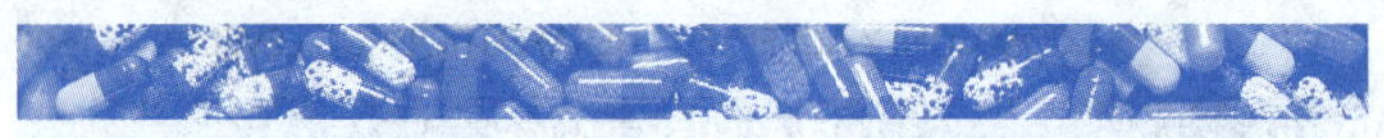

appendix 6

Tables of Weights and Measures

Weights	Exact Equivalents	Approximate Equivalents
1 ounce (oz)	28.35 g	30 g
1 pound (lb)	453.6 g	454 g
1 gram (g)	0.0353 oz	0.035 oz
1 kilogram (kg)	2.205 lb	2.2 lb
Fluid Measures		
1 teaspoon (t)		5 mL
1 tablespoon (T)	3 tsp	15 mL (1/2 fl oz)
1 fluid ounce (fl oz)	29.57 mL	30 mL
1 pint (16 fl oz)	473.0 mL	473 mL
1 quart (32 fl oz)	946 mL	945 mL
1 gallon (128 fl oz)	3.785 L	3.8 L
1 milliliter (mL)	0.0352 fl oz (Imperial)	0.0345 fl oz
1 liter (L)	2.11 pt	2 pt
Lengths		
1 inch (in)	2.54 cm	2.5 cm
1 foot (ft)	30.48 cm	30.0 cm
1 yard (yd)	0.914 m	0.9 m
1 centimeter (cm)	0.3937 in	
1 meter (m)	39.4 in	

Approximate Conversions to Metric Measures

To Convert	To	Multiply By
Inches	Centimeters	2.54
Feet	Centimeters	30.48
Grains	Grams	0.065
Ounces	Grams	28.35
Pounds	Kilograms	0.45
Teaspoons, Medical	Milliliters	5.0
Tablespoons	Milliliters	15.0
Fluid ounces	Milliliters	29.57
Cups	Liters	0.24
Pints	Liters	0.47
Quarts	Liters	0.95
Gallons	Liters	3.8

Approximate Conversions to Metric Measures

To Convert	To	Multiply By
Millimeters	Inches	0.039
Centimeters	Inches	0.39
Grams	Grains	15.432
Kilograms	Pounds	2.2
Milliliters	Fluid ounces	0.034
Liters	Pints	2.1
Liters	Quarts	1.06
Liters	Gallons	0.26
Deg. Fahrenheit	Deg. Celsius	5/9 (after subtracting 32)
Deg. Celsius	Deg. Fahrenheit	9/5 (then add 32)

appendix 7
Elements of a Prescription

To safely communicate the exact elements desired on a prescription, the following items should be addressed:

A. The prescriber: Name, address, phone number, and associated practice/speciality

B. The client: Name, age, address and Social Security number

C. The prescription itself: Name of the medication (generic or trade); quantity to be dispensed (e.g., tablets or capsules, 1 vial, 1 tube, volume of liquid); the strength of the medication (e.g., 125-mg tablets, 250 mg/5 mL, 80 mg/1 mL, 10%); and directions for use (e.g., 1 tablet po t.i.d.; 2 gtt to each eye q.i.d.; 1 teaspoonful po q 8 hr for 10 days; apply a thin film to lesions b.i.d. for 14 days)

D. Other elements: Date prescription is written, signature of the provider, number of refills; provider number: state license number and Drug Enforcement Agency (DEA) number (when applicable); and brand-product-only indication (when applicable)

A typical prescription as follows:

A. **Julia Bryan, MSN, RN, CPNP**
Pediatric Associates
1611 Kirkwood Highway
Wilmington, DE 19805
302-645-8261

Date: July 10, 2002

B. For: Kathryn Woods, Age 8
27 East Parkway
Lewes, DE 19958
123-555-1234

C. Rx Amoxicillin susp. 250 mg/5 mL
Disp. 150 mL
Sig: 1 teaspoon PO q 8 hr x 10 days

D. Refills: 0
Provider signature
Provider/State license number

Interpretation of prescription: The above prescription is written by Pediatric Nurse Practitioner Julia Bryan for Kathryn Woods and is for amoxicillin suspension. The concentration desired is 250 mg/5 mL. The directions for taking the medication are 1 teaspoon (i.e., 5 mL) by mouth every 8 hr for 10 days. The prescriber wants 150 mL dispensed and there are no refills allowed.

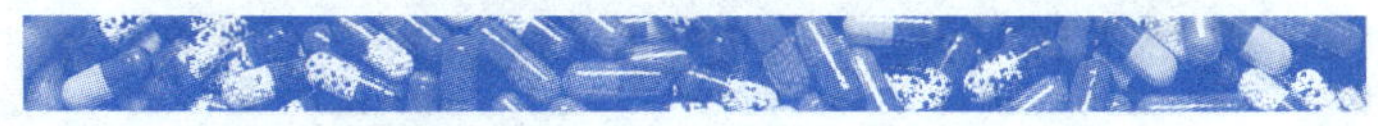

appendix 8

Easy Formulas for IV Rate Calculation

In order to calculate the continuous drip rate for an IV infusion, the following information is necessary:

a. amount of solution to be infused
b. time for infusion to be administered
c. *drop factor (found in the tubing package)

$$\frac{\text{Total volume to be infused}}{\text{Total hours for infusion}} \times \frac{\text{*drop factor}}{\text{60 min/hr}} = \text{gtt/min}$$

*If drop factor is:

- 60 gtt/min, then use 1 in the formula
- 10 gtt/min, then use 1/6 in the formula
- 15 gtt/min, then use 1/4 in the formula
- 20 gtt/min, then use 1/3 in the formula

This gives you $\frac{\text{gtt}}{\text{min}}$.

Example: Infuse 1,000 cc over 8 hr using tubing with a drop factor of 10 gtt/min.

$$\frac{\text{1,000 cc}}{\text{8 hr}} \times \frac{1}{6} = 20.8 \text{ or } 21 \ \frac{\text{gtt}}{\text{min}}$$

Complete equation is:

$$\frac{\text{1,000 cc}}{\text{8 hr}} \times \frac{\text{10 gtt/min}}{\text{60 min/1 hr}} = \frac{\text{1,000 cc}}{\text{8 hr}} \times \frac{\text{10 gtt}}{\text{cc}} \times \frac{\text{1hr}}{\text{60 min}} = 21 \ \frac{\text{gtt}}{\text{min}}$$

To get $\frac{\text{cc}}{\text{hr}}$ invert drop factor and multiply by $\frac{\text{gtt}}{\text{min}}$, or:

$$\frac{6}{1} \times 21 \ \frac{\text{gtt}}{\text{min}} = 126 \ \frac{\text{cc}}{\text{hr}}$$

When administering intermittent infusions, as with antibiotic therapy, use the following formula:

$$\text{Total volume to be infused} \div \frac{\text{minutes to administer}}{\text{60 min/hr}} = \frac{\text{mL}}{\text{hr}}$$

Example: Administer 3 g Zosyn in 100 cc of D5W over 45 min

$$100 \div \frac{45}{60} \text{ (invert to multiply)}$$

or

$$100 \times \frac{60}{45} = 133.3 \text{ or } 134 \ \frac{\text{mL}}{\text{hr}}$$

appendix 9

Adult IVPB Medication Administration Guidelines and Riders

Adult IVPB Medication Guidelines

Medication	*Solutions(s)*	*Amount*	*Infuse Over*
Amikin (Amikacin)	D5W; NSS	250–500 mg/100 mL	30–60 min
Amphotericin B (Fungizone)	D5W	50 mg/500 mL	6 hr
Ampicillin (Polycillin-N)	NSS	1 g/50 mL	15–30 min
Ancef (Cefazolin Na)	D5W; NSS	1 g/50 mL	40 min
Azactam (Aztreonam)	D5W; NSS	1 g/50 mL	20–30 min
Bactrim (Septra/Co-Trimoxazole)	D5W	Premixed, usually 5 mL/125 mL	60–90 min
Cefotan (Cefotetan disodium)	D5W; NSS	1–2 g/75 mL	30 min
Cipro (Ciprofloxacin)	D5W; NSS	400 mg/200 mL	60 min
Claforan (Cefotaxime)	D5W; NSS	1 g/50 mL	30 min
Cleocin (Clindamycin)	D5W; NSS	300–900 mg/100 mL	20–40 min
Decadron (Dexamethasone)	D5W; NSS	40 mg/50 mL	15–30 min
Doxycycline (Vibramycin)	D5W; NSS	100 mg/100 mL	1–2 hr
Erythromycin (Erythrocin)	NSS, RL	500 mg/100 mL	30–60 min
Famotidine (Pepcid)	D5W; NSS	20 mg/50–100 mL	15–30 min
Flagyl (Metronidazole)	Prepackaged	—	60 min
Foscavir (Foscarnet)	D5W	60–90 mg/kg q 8 hr	2 hr
Fortaz (Ceftazidime)	D5W; NSS	1–2 g/100 mL	30 min
Gentamycin (Garamycin)	D5W; NSS	80 mg/50 mL	30–60 min
Nafcillin (Nafcin)	D5W; NSS	1 g/50–100 mL	30–60 min
Penicillin G	D5W; NSS	5,000,000 U/100 mL	40 min
Primaxin (Imipenem-Cilastatin Na)	D5W; NSS	500 mg/100 mL	20–30 min
Rocephin (Ceftriaxone Na)	D5W; NSS	1–2 g/100 mL	30 min
Solumedrol (Methylprednisolone)	D5W; NSS	10–250 mg/50 mL	20 min

Tagamet (Cimetidine)	D5W; NSS	300 mg/50 mL	15–20 min
Tetracycline (Achromycin IV)	D5W; NSS	250–500 mg/100 mL	60 min
Tobramycin (Nebcin)	D5W; NSS	80 mg/100 mL	30 min
Vancomycin (Vancocin)	D5W; NSS	1 g/200 mL	60 min
Zantac (Ranitidine HCl)	D5W; NSS	50 mg/100 mL	15–20 min

Riders

When ordered for nonemergent IV infusion, the following guidelines may be used for administration:

- Calcium gluconate: 1 ampule Ca gluconate in 100 mL D5W given over 1 hr (each ampule contains approximately 940 mg Ca)

- Magnesium sulfate: 1 g in 100 mL D5W given over 1 hr

- Potassium chloride: 40 mEq in 150 mL D5W given over 4 hr or 60 mEq in 250 mL D5W given over 6 hr. With KCl, a good rule of thumb is not to infuse more than 10 mEq/hr.

- Potassium phosphate: 15 mM phosphate (contains 22 mEq K) in 100 mL D5W given over 2–3 hr

appendix 10
Therapeutic Classification of Wounds and Dressings

Wounds heal best in a moist environment; thus moisture-retentive or occlusive dressings should be used. With a moist wound environment, granulation tissue formation and collagen synthesis are improved, cell migration and epithelial resurfacing occur faster, and crusts, scabs, and eschars do not form. A careful wound assessment should be performed to determine the wound stage and any other factors contributing to the skin breakdown, such as infection, lack of nutrition, or necrotic tissues. Wounds are staged by determining which tissue layers are involved. Products that enhance wound care management continue to proliferate. A list of the categories of wound care products with their composition and purpose is included.

A careful wound assessment should be performed to determine the ulcer stage and any other factors contributing to the skin breakdown, such as infection or necrotic tissues. Wounds are staged by determining which tissue layers are involved:

WOUND STAGING

Stage I: Erythema of intact skin; nonblanchable. A stage I pressure ulcer is an observable pressure-related alteration of intact skin. Indicators include changes in one or more of the following: skin temperature (warmth/coolness), tissue consistency (firm/boggy), or sensation (pain/itching). The ulcer appears as a specific area of persistent redness in lightly pigmented skin; with darker skin tones, the ulcer may appear with red, blue, or purple hues.

Stage II: Partial-thickness skin loss involving epidermis and/or dermis; appears as a shallow crater, blister, or abrasion. Includes partial or complete skin tear. A stage II pressure ulcer involves the epidermis, dermis, or both. It is a superficial wound and may present as an abrasion, blister, or shallow crater.

Stage III: Full-thickness skin loss of subcutaneous tissue involving damage or necrosis that may extend down to the fascia; appears as a deep crater. A stage III pressure ulcer involves subcutaneous tissue that may extend down to, but not through, underlying fascia. May present as a deep crater with or without undermining of tissue.

Stage IV: Full-thickness skin loss with extensive necrosis, destruction, or damage to muscle, bone, or supporting structures; may also see sinus tracts or undermining with this stage. A stage IV pressure ulcer involves muscle, bone, or supporting structures. Sinus tract undermining may be present.

Unstageable: An unstageable pressure ulcer is not assessable due to eschar or slough that covers the wound, prohibiting complete assessment.

WOUND MANAGEMENT BY STAGE

Stage I: Wounds

Cover/protect skin: Skin protectant (cream or ointment), skin sealant, transparent film, thin hydrocolloid, thin foam, heel and elbow protectors

Cleanse intact skin: Skin cleanser

Moisturize intact skin: Skin protectant (cream or ointment)

Stage II: Wounds

Protect intact skin: Skin protectant, skin sealant, skin cleanser, transparent film, thin hydrocolloid, heel and elbow protectors

Cleanse wound: Wound cleanser

Manage wound exudate—Scant or minimal drainage: Transparent film, thin hydrocolloid, thin foam, absorptive gauze

—Moderate drainage: Hydrocolloid, foam, calcium alginate, collagen, absorptive gauze

—Heavy drainage: Calcium alginate, foam, absorptive gauze, dressing combinations, wound beads, pastes or powders

Stage III: Wounds

Protect intact skin: Skin protectant, skin sealant, skin cleanser, transparent film, thin hydrocolloid, heel and elbow protectors

Cleanse wound: Wound cleanser

Manage wound exudate—Scant or minimal drainage: Transparent film, thin hydrocolloid, thin foam, absorptive gauze

—Moderate drainage: Hydrocolloid, foam, calcium alginate, collagen, absorptive gauze, dressing combinations

—Heavy drainage: Calcium alginate, foam, absorptive gauze, dressing combinations, wound beads, pastes or powders

Debride wound—Dry: Transparent film, hydrogel, moist saline gauze, hydrating impregnated gauze

—Moist/wet: Hydrocolloid, foam, calcium alginate, absorptive gauze

—Heel ulcers may be left undebrided with pressure relief provided; dressings may be used alone or in combination with mechanical and sharp debridement

Hydrate wound: Hydrogel, hydrating impregnated gauze, moist saline gauze

Manage wound odor: Wound cleanser, odor absorbent dressing, room deodorizer, more frequent dressing changes, antimicrobial topical agent

Fill in dead space: Calcium alginate, hydrating or absorptive gauze, moist saline gauze, foam cavity dressing, wound beads, pastes or powders, collagen

Stage IV: Wounds

Protect intact skin: Skin protectant, skin sealant, skin cleanser, transparent film, thin hydrocolloid, skin barrier, heel and elbow protectors

Cleanse wound: Wound cleanser

Manage wound exudate—Scant or minimal drainage: transparent film, thin hydrocolloid/foam, absorptive gauze

—Moderate drainage: Hydrocolloid, foam, calcium alginate, collagen, absorptive gauze

—Heavy drainage: Calcium alginate, foam, absorptive gauze, dressing combinations, wounds beads, pastes or powders

Debride, hydrate, manage wound odor, fill in dead space: As identified under stage III wounds

Unstageable Wounds

Protect intact skin: Skin protectant, skin sealant, skin cleanser, transparent film, thin hydrocolloid, heel and elbow protectors

Debride wound—Dry: Transparent film, hydrogel, moist saline gauze, hydrating impregnating gauze

—Moist/wet: Hydrocolloid, foam, calcium alginate, absorptive gauze

Manage wound odor: Wound cleanser, odor absorbent dressing, room deodorizer, more frequent dressing changes

ADJUNCTIVE THERAPIES IN WOUND CARE

Compression: Elastic stockings or bandages applied to the lower extremities. Promotes venous blood return, prevents blood pooling, decreases edema.

Electrical stimulation: Electrical current applied to stimulate tissue regeneration. Increases oxygen and nutrient transport to tissues, reduces edema and pain, increases fibroblastosis and collagen development, improves scar tissue elasticity.

Hydrotherapy: Partial to full-body immersion in which injected air produces water turbulence and agitation. Promotes debridement (thermal/non-thermal), cleans the wound, induces circulatory and neurologic effects.

Hyperbaric oxygen: In a chamber at >1 atmosphere of pressure (14.7 psi), the patient breathes 100% oxygen. By increasing tissue oxygenation, wound healing is fostered by supporting bacterial destruction by WBCs, allowing fibroblasts to proliferate and build collagen, and developing new epithelial tissue.

Negative pressure therapy (vacuum-assisted wound closure): Uses continuous or intermittent vacuum over a wound, using negative pressure up to 125 mm. Do not use over open bowel. With stage III and IV wounds, protect tendons, bone, or graft sites with Adaptic.

Nutritional support: High-calorie, high-protein, moderate-fat diet that contains enough non-nitrogen calories to prevent the body from using amino acids for energy; vitamin or mineral deficiencies must be corrected. 2L/day fluid intake recommended. Decreases susceptibility of soft tissue breakdown.

Support surface: Available as cushions (for chairs and wheelchairs), mattress overlays, and beds (air-fluidized or air suspension); requires turning/repositioning schedule. Provides skeleton stability, distributes body weight over a larger area and reduces tissue pressure, controls shear forces on the skin.

Topical growth factors: Biologically developed product applied directly to the wound; effects depend on target cell of the specific product. Increase wound healing by increasing wound strength, controlling collagen deposition, increasing cellular content.

Ultrasound: High-frequency sound waves transmitted through water or sonic gel to the wound. Increases collagen elasticity, decreases muscle and joint stiffness. Diminishes pain, decreases muscle spasms, increases oxygen transport, decreases hyperemia, accelerates wound recovery, decreases edema.

WOUND CARE PRODUCT INGREDIENTS

Alginates

Form: Sheets, ropes

Composition/purpose: Calcium alginate (water-insoluble salt or alginic acid) creates fibers that gel on contact with a solution containing sodium. Sodium alginate causes gelling. The greater the amount of sodium alginate, the more the alginate gels.

Collagen

Form: Powder, sheets, pastes

Composition: Type I bovine collagen/Type I avian collagen

Purpose: Absorbs wound fluid and provides a biocompatible matrix for granulation tissue

Foams

Form: Sheets of various thicknesses, with or without adhesive coatings that may have film coatings on one side

Composition: Polyurethane

Purpose: Creates the open/closed cell foam structure that is the body of the foam and used as a transparent film coating on one side of the foam, rendering it waterproof.

Hydrocolloids

Form: Sheets of various thicknesses, inherently adhesive

Composition/purpose: Polyisobutylene provides adhesive qualities. Pectin, gelatin, carboxymethylcellulose provide absorptive capacity and gelling-pectin may be fibrinolytic. Polyurethane is a backing film.

Hydrofibers

Form: Sheets, strips

Composition: Carboxymethyl cellulose

Purpose: Absorbs wound fluid

Hydrogels, Amorphous

Form: Viscous liquids

Composition/purpose: Starch-based polymers, polyvinylpyrrolidone, carboxymethylcellulose, and sodium create a viscous mixture with water. Water creates a viscous mixture with the polymer component. Alginate, collagen, peptides, aloe vera are minor additives that enhance absorbency or performance. Propylene glycol and paraben preserve.

Hydrogels, Sheet

Form: Sheets with or without adhesive borders

Composition/purpose: Polyethylene oxide, polyvinylpyrrolidone creates a microscopic, three-dimensional cross-linked structure that binds water. Water binds into the polymer matrix to form the gel. Glycerin retards evaporation of water from the matrix. Propylene glycol preserves and moistens. Paraben strengthens the gel sheet with its internal netting or “scrim” structure. Acrylic is used as an adhesive that attaches to the skin.

Pastes, powders

Composition: Xanthan gum, guar gum

Purpose: Absorbs wound fluid

Superabsorbent Particles

Purpose: Enhance absorbent capacity

Composition/purpose: Activated charcoal cloth or paper absorbs odor molecules and binds certain bacteria to control odors. Acrylics, polyurethanes used as an adhesive that attaches to the skin.

Transparent Films

Form: Flexible sheets coated on one side with adhesive

Composition: Composed of polyurethanes, copolymer mixtures

Purpose: Transpire moisture vapor and gases but not liquids. Acrylics and vinyl ethers are used as an adhesive that attaches to the skin.

The goal in topical wound management is to keep the wound moist, clean, and free from physical trauma. In stage I, stage II, stage III, and stage IV pressure ulcers, the goal of care is to restore skin integrity and to avoid infection. Using the most effective dressings and therapies and implementing appropriate wound care procedures help achieve this goal. There are over 2,000 wound care products on the market. Use the wound characteristics to stage the wound and identify the appropriate product to use. In many cases one product can achieve more than one therapeutic goal, e.g., moist dressing can support wound healing and also debride. Always consult someone experienced or trained in wound assessment and management to evaluate your client, reassess the wound at regular intervals, and to make recommendations and changes based on the clinical presentation.

REFERENCES

Hess, C. T. (1999). *Clinical guide to wound care* (3rd ed.). Philadelphia: Springhouse.

Hollister Incorporated. (2001). *Wound and skin care guide.*

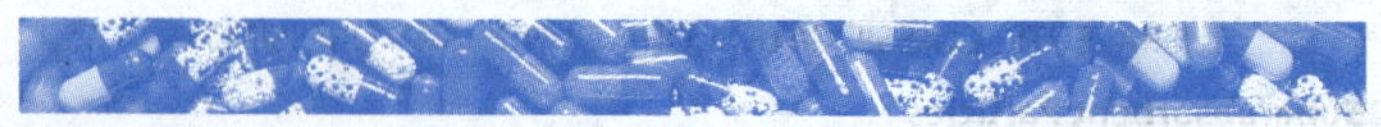

appendix 11

Medication Errors: The Importance of Reporting

There has been a lot of attention in the media to the loss of unnecessary life due to medication errors, many of which were preventable. It has been estimated that adverse drug reactions to prescriptions and over-the-counter medications kill at least 100,000 Americans and seriously injure an additional 2.1 million each year.

Some of the more common types of errors are:

- Drugs with similar sounding names
- Inappropriate abbreviations
- Poor handwriting; misplaced decimals and zeroes
- Confusion of metric and other dosing units
- Environmental factors such as noise, distractions, lighting
- Lack of complete patient data on allergies, medical conditions, and so forth

The National Coordinating Council for Medication Error Reporting and Prevention (http://www.nccmerp.org) defines a medication error as "any preventable event that may cause or lead to inappropriate medication use or patient harm while the medication is in the control of the health care professional, patient, or consumer. Such events may be related to professional practice, health care products, procedures, and systems including prescribing; order communication; product labeling; packaging; and nomenclature; compounding; dispensing; distribution; administration; education; monitoring; and use." (Copyright 1998-2002 NCC MERP. All rights reserved.)

The FDA maintains a site for medication errors: http://www.fda.gov/cder/MedErrors.

The FDA began monitoring reports of medication errors in 1992. They reviewed reports that were sent to the FDA from the United States Pharmacopeia (USP) and the Institute for Safe Medication Practices (ISMP). The Med Watch reports were also reviewed. The Division of Medication Errors and Technical Support includes a medication error prevention program. This is staffed with pharmacists and support personnel so they can review the medication error reports sent to the USP-ISMP Medication Errors Reporting Program (MERP) and Med Watch. Since many medical errors are related to medication errors, it is felt that if they share the knowledge gained, then this information may lead to improved patient safety.

The FDA maintains other searchable safety databases related to medical devices, biologic products, recalls, drug shortages, vaccine safety and dietary supplements to name a few. All reports are voluntary and without penalty. Forms are easily downloaded for completion or can be completed on line.

All medication error reports should be filed with the MERP. Observed errors may be reported confidentially.

1-800-23-ERROR
http://www.usp.org

The website alerts the health care professional about the need for practice changes and alerts industry and regulatory professionals about pharmaceutical labeling, packaging, and nomenclature that may foster error by their design. When you report errors, you are asked for your recommendations. Links are also maintained to the ISMP, USP, and FDA (for adverse drug reports). They also maintain international reporting links.

FDA's Medwatch Online Reporting Form
http://www.fda.gov/medwatch/index.html
1-800-FDA-1088

Voluntarily report medications errors and fill out Form 3500, which you can download from the site and mail or fax back or you can report the error by phone.

American Society of Consultant Pharmacists
http://www.ascp.com/medreporting

Center for Drug Error Reporting (FDA)
http://www.fda.gov/cder

This site has highlights of new drugs, new safety information, drugs recently approved, and generic and OTC products.

appendix 12

Commonly Used Combination Drugs

NOTE: Please consult individual drugs for more extensive information.

NOTE: Table entries are alphabetized by generic name.

Accuretic (quinapril hydrochloride and hydrochlorothiazide)
Advair Diskus (fluticasone and salmeterol)
Aggrenox (aspirin and dipyridamole)
Aldactazide (spironolactone and hydrochlorothiazide)
Aldoril (methyldopa and hydrochlorothiazide)
Arthrotec (diclofenac sodium and misoprostol)
Atacand HCT (candesartan cilexetil and hydrochlorothiazide)
Axocet (butalbital and acetaminophen)
Brontex (codeine phosphate and guaifenesin)
Claritin-D (loratidine and pseudoephedrine)
Combivent (ipratropium bromide and albuterol sulfate)
Cosopt (dorzolamide hydrochloride and timolol maleate)
Darvocet-N50, Darvocet N-100 (acetaminophen and propoxyphene napsylate)
Darvon Compound 65 (aspirin, caffeine and propoxyphene hydrochloride)
Donnatal (atropine sulfate, hyoscyamine sulfate, scopolamine hydrobromide, and phenobarbital)
Dyazide, Maxzide, Maxide-25 MG, Apo-Triazide, Novo-Triamzide, Nu-Triazide, Protriazide (triamterene and hydrochlorothiazide)
Equagesic (aspirin and meprobamate)
Fiorinal (aspirin, butalbital and caffeine)
Fiorinal with codeine (aspirin, butalbital, caffeine, and codeine phosphate)
Glucovance (glyburide and metformin hydrochloride)
Hycodan (hydrocodone bitartrate and homatropine methylbromide)
Hyzaar (losartan potassium and hydrochlorothiazide)
Inderide, Inderide LA (propranolol hydrochloride and hydrochlorothiazide)
Kaletra (lopinavir and ritonavir)
Librax (chlordiazepoxide and clidinium bromide)
Lotrel (amlodipine and benazepril hydrochloride)
Lotrisone (clotrimazole and betamethasone propionate)
Malarone (atovaquone and proguanil hydrochloride)
Micardis HCT (telmisarten and hydrochlorothiazide)
Moduretic (amiloride and hydrochlorothiazide)
Pediazole (erythromycin ethylsuccinate and sulfisoxazole)
Prinzide, Zestoretic (lisinopril and hydrochlorothiazide)
Rifamate, Rimactane/INH (rifampin and isoniazid)
Rifater (rifampin, isoniazid and pyrazinamide)
Talwin NX (pentazocine hydrochloride and naloxone hydrochloride)
Triavil (amitriptyline hydrochloride and perphenazine)
Trizivir (abacavir sulfate, lamivudine, zidovudine)

Tylenol with codeine (acetaminophen and codeine phosphate)
Ultracet (tramadol hydrochloride, acetaminophen)
Vaseretic (enalapril maleate and hydrochlorothiazide)
Vicoprofen (hydrocodone bitartrate and ibuprofen)
Ziac (bisoprolol fumarate and hydrochlorothiazide)
Zyrtec-D 12 Hour (cetirizine, pseudoephedrine)

Generic Name (Content)	Trade Name	Use	Dose
Abacavir sulfate (300 mg), Lamivudine (150 mg), Zidovudine (300 mg)	Trizivir	Alone or with other antiretroviral drugs to treat HIV-1 infections.	**Adults and adolescents, 40 kg or more:** 1 tablet b.i.d. (Not for use in those weighing less than 40 kg or if creatinine clearance is 50 mL/min or less due to it being a fixed-dose tablet).
Acetaminophen (300 mg/tablet or 120 mg/5mL), Codeine phosphate (15 mg–No. 2, 30 mg–No. 3, 60 mg–No. 4 tablets and 12 mg/5mL elixir).	Tylenol with Codeine (Rx, C-III: Tablets, C-V: Elixir).	Mild to moderate pain.	**Tablets. Adults, individualized, usual:** 1–2 No. 2 or No. 3 Tablets q 2–4 hr as needed for pain. Or, 1-No. 4 Tablet q 4 hr as needed. Maximum 24-hr dose: 360 mg codeine phosphate and 4,000 mg acetaminophen. **Elixir. Adults, individualized, usual:** 15 mL q 4 hr as needed; **pediatric, 7–12 years:** 10 mL t.i.d.–q.i.d.; **3–6 years:** 5 mL t.i.d.–q.i.d. Use cautiously with liver dysfunction.
Acetaminophen (325 or 650 mg), Propoxyphene napsylate (50 or 100 mg)	Darvocet-N 50, Darvocet-N 100 (Rx, C-IV)	Mild to moderate pain (may be used if fever is present)	2-Darvocet-N 50 tablets or 1-Darvocet-100 tablet q 4 hr, not to exceed 600 mg propoxyphene napsylate/day. Reduce dose in impaired renal/hepatic function.

Generic Name (Content)	Trade Name	Use	Dose
Amiloride (5 mg), Hydrochlorothiazide (50mg)	Moduretic (Rx)	Hypertension or CIIF, especially when hypokalemia occurs. May be used with other anti-hypertensives.	**Initial:** 1 tablet/day; **then**, can increase to 2 tablets/day.
Amitriptyline HCl (10, 25, or 50 mg),Perphenazine (2 or 4 mg)	Triavil 2-10, 2-25, 4-10, 4-25, 4-50 (Rx)	Depression with moderate to severe anxiety and/or agitation (including those with chronic physical disease). Schizophrenia with symptoms of depression.	**Initial:** 1 Triavil 2-25 or 4-25 tablet t.i.d.–q.i.d. or 1 Triavil tablet 4-50 b.i.d. (for schizophrenia, use 2 Triavil 4-50 t.i.d. with a fourth dose at bedtime if needed). **Maintenance:** 1 Triavil 2-25 or 4-25 b.i.d.–q.i.d. or 1 Triavil 4-50 b.i.d.
Amlodipine (2.5 or 5 mg), Benazepril HCl (10 or 20 mg)	Lotrel 2.5/10, 5/10, or 5/20 (Rx)	Hypertension if control not achieved with either drug alone.	One 2.5/10, 5/10, or 5/20 capsule daily. For the small, elderly, frail, or hepatically impaired, initial amlodipine dose is 2.5 mg.
Aspirin (325 mg), Butalbital (50 mg), Caffeine (40 mg)	Fiorinal (Rx, C-III)	Tension headaches.	1–2 tablets or capsules q 4 hr, not to exceed 6 tablets or capsules/day.

Generic Name (Content)	Trade Name	Use	Dose
Aspirin (325 mg), Butalbital (50 mg), Caffeine (40 mg), Codeine phosphate (7.5 mg, 15 mg, or 30 mg)	Fiorinal with Codeine (Rx, C-III)	Analgesic for all types of pain.	**Initial:** 1–2 capsules; **then,** dose may be repeated, if necessary, up to maximum of 6 capsules/day.
Aspirin (389 mg), Caffeine (32.4 mg), Propoxyphene HCl (65 mg)	Darvon Compound 65 (Rx, C-IV)	Mild to moderate pain, with or without fever.	1-Capsule q 4 hr, not to exceed 390 mg propoxyphene HCl/day. Decrease total daily dose in impaired renal/hepatic function.
Aspirin (25 mg), Dipyridamole (200 mg)	Aggrenox (Rx)	Reduce risk of stroke in clients who have had transient ischemia of the brain or completed ischemic stroke due to thrombosis.	One capsule b.i.d., in the morning and evening. Swallow capsules whole without chewing.
Aspirin (325 mg), Meprobamate (200 mg)	Equagesic (Rx, C-IV)	Short-term treatment of pain due to musculoskeletal disease accompanied by anxiety and tension.	**Adults:** 1–2 tablets t.i.d.–q.i.d.

Generic Name (Content)	Trade Name	Use	Dose
Atovaquone (250 mg/tablet or 62.5 mg/pediatric tablet), Proguanil hydrochloride (100 mg/tablet or 25 mg/pediatric tablet)	Malarone	Prophylaxis of *Plasmodium falciparum* malaria including areas where chloroquine resistence seen. Treatment of acute, uncomplicated *P. falciparum*, even in areas where resistance to other drugs seen.	*Prophylaxis.* **Adults:** 1 adult tablet/day. **Children, 11-20 kg:** 1 pediatric tablet/day; **21-30 kg:** 2 pediatric tablets/day as a single dose; **31-40 kg:** 3 pediatric tablets/day as a single dose; **>40 kg:** 1 adult strength tablet/day. *Treatment.* **Adults:** 4 adult strength tablets/day as a single dose/day for 3 consecutive days. **Children, 11-20 kg:** 1 adult strength tablet/day for 3 consecutive days; **21-30 kg:** 2 adult strength tablets/day for 3 consecutive days; **31-40 kg:** 3 adult strength tablets/day for 3 consecutive days; **>40 kg:** Use adult dose. Take daily dose at same time each day with food or a milky drink.
Atropine sulfate (0.0194 mg), Hyoscyamine sulfate (0.1037 mg), Scopolamine HBr (0.0065 mg), Phenobarbital (16.2 mg) in each tablet, capsule, or 5 mL elixir	Donnatal (Rx)	Adjunct to treat irritable colon, spastic colon, mucous colitis, acute enterocolitis.	**Adults, usual:** 1–2 tablets or capsules t.i.d.–q.i.d. or 1-Extentab q 12 hr, or 5–10 mL elixir t.i.d.–q.i.d. **Pediatric:** Use elixir as follows: **4.5–9.0 kg:** 0.5 mL q 4 hr or 0.75 mL q 6 hr. **9.1–13.5 kg:** 1.0 mL q 4 hr or 1.5 mL q 6 hr; **13.6–22.6 kg:** 1.5 mL q 4 hr or 2.0 mL q 6 hr; **22.7–33.9 kg:** 2.5 mL q 4 hr or 3.75 mL q 6 hr; **34.0–45.3 kg:** 3.75 mL q 4 hr or 5 mL q 6 hr; **45.4 kg:** 5 mL q 4 hr or 7.5 mL q 6 hr.

Generic Name (Content)	Trade Name	Use	Dose
Bisoprolol fumarate (2.5, 5, or 10 mg), Hydrochlorothiazide (6.25 mg)	Ziac (Rx)	Mild to moderate hypertension (first-line therapy).	1 2.5/6.25 mg tablet once daily; dose may be increased q 14 days to a maximum of 2 10/6.25 tablets once daily.
Butalbital (50 mg), Acetaminophen (650 mg)	Axocet (Rx)	Tension headaches.	1 Capsule q 4 hr, not to exceed 6 capsules/day.
Candesartan cilexetil (16 mg or 32 mg), Hydrochlorothiazide (12.5 mg)	Atacand HCT 16-12.5 or Atacand HCT 32-12.5 (Rx)	Hypertension (not for initial treatment)	**Initial:** 1 tablet of Atacand HCT 16-12.5. Depending on response, can increase to Atacand 32-12.5
Cetirizine, Pseudoephedrine	Zyrtec-D 12 Hour	Relief of nasal and nonnasal symptoms associated with seasonal or perennial allergic rhinitis in adults and children over 12 years of age.	**Adults and children over 12 years:** q tablet b.i.d. given with or without food. Give 1 tablet once/day if creatinine clearance is between 11 and 31 mL/min, client is on hemodialysis, or if hepatically impaired.
Chlordiazepoxide (5 mg), Clidinium Br (2.5 mg)	Librax (Rx)	Adjunct in the treatment of irritable colon, spastic colon, mucous colitis, and acute enterocolitis.	**Adults, individualized, usual:** 1–2 capsules t.i.d.–q.i.d before meals and at bedtime.
Clotrimazole (10 mg) and Betamethasone dipropionate (0.64 mg) per gram of cream	Lotrisone	Symptomatic inflammatory tinea pedis, tinea cruris, and tinea corporis due to *Epidermophyton, rubrum, Trichophyton metagrophytes,* or *T. rubrum*	Gently massage cream or lotion into the affected skin areas b.i.d. in the morning and evening.

Generic Name (Content)	Trade Name	Use	Dose
Codeine phosphate (10 mg/tablet or 20 mL), Guaifenesin (300 mg/tablet or 20 mL)	Brontex (Rx, C-III)	Relief of cough due to cold or inhaled irritants. Loosen mucus and thin bronchial secretions.	**Adults and children over 12 years:** 1 Tablet or 20 mL q 4 hr. **Children, 6–12 years:** 10 mL q 4 hr.
Diclofenac sodium (50 or 75 mg), Misoprostol (200 mcg)	Arthrotec 50, Arthrotec 75 (Rx)	Osteoarthritis or rheumatoid arthritis in those at high risk of developing NSAID-induced gastric and duodenal ulcers.	*Osteoarthritis:* 1-Arthrotec 50 tablet with food t.i.d. If intolerance occurs, give Arthrotec 50 or Arthrotec 75 b.i.d., although this dose is less effective in preventing ulcers. *Rheumatoid arthritis:* 1-Arthrotec 50 tablet with food t.i.d. or q.i.d. If intolerance occurs, give Arthrotec 50 or Arthrotec 75 b.i.d., atlhough this dose is less effective in preventing ulcers.
Dorzolamide HCl (2%), Timolol maleate (0.5%)	Cosopt (Rx)	Reduce elevated IOP in open-angle glaucoma or ocular hypertension in those inadequately controlled with beta blockers.	**Adults:** 1 gtt in the affected eye(s) b.i.d.
Enalapril maleate (5 mg or 10 mg), Hydrochlorothiazide (12.5 or 25 mg)	Vaseretic (Rx)	Hypertenstion	**Adults:** 1-2 tablets once daily.

Generic Name (Content)	Trade Name	Use	Dose
Erythromycin ethylsuccinate (200 mg) and Sulfisoxazole (600 mg) in 5 mL of oral suspension.	Pediazole (Rx)	Acute otitis media in children due to *Haemophilus influenzae.*	**Usual:** Equivalent of 50 mg/kg/day of erythromycin and 150 mg/kg/day of sulfisoxazole, up to a maximum of 6 g/day. **Over 45 kg:** 10 mL q 6 hr; **24 kg:** 7.5 mL q 6 hr; **16 kg:** 5 mL q 6 hr; **8 kg:** 2.5 mL q 6 hr; **less than 8 kg:** calculate dose according to body weight.
Fluticasone (100 mcg), Salmetcrol (50 mcg)	Advair Diskus (Rx)	Maintenance treatment of asthma in clients 12 years and older.	One inhalation b.i.d. (morning and evening) approximately 12 hr apart.
Glyburide (1.25 mg, 2.5 mg, or 5 mg), Metformin hydrochloride (250 mg or 500 mg)	Glucovance (Rx)	Initial therapy, as an adjunct to diet and exercise, to treat type 2 diabetics whose hyperglycemia can not be treated by diet and exercise alone.	Individualize. **Initial:** 1.25 mg/250 mg once or twice daily with meals. **Use in previously treated clients (second-line therapy):** 2.5 mg/500 mg or 5 mg/500 mg b.i.d. with meals. Do not exceed 20 mg glyburide and 2000 mg metformin/day.
Hydrocodone bitartrate (5 mg), Homatropine methylbromide (1.5 mg) in each tablet or 5 mL	Hycodan (Rx, C-III)	Relief of symptoms of cough.	**Adults and children over 12 years:** 1 Tablet or 5 mL q 4–6 hr, not to exceed 6 tablets or 30 mL in 24 hr. **Children, 6–12 years:** ½ Tablet or 2.5 mL q 4–6 hr, as needed, not to exceed 3 tablets or 15 mL in 24 hr.

Generic Name (Content)	Trade Name	Use	Dose
Hydrocodone bitartrate (7.5 mg), Ibuprofen (200 mg)	Vicoprofen (Rx, C-III)	Short-term (less than 10 days) treatment of pain.	**Adults:** 1 tablet q 4 - 6 hr, as needed, not to exceed 5 tablets in a 24-hr period. Adjust dose/frequency of dosing to client needs.
Ipratropium bromide (18 mcg) and Albuterol sulfate (103 mcg) in each actuation of metered dose inhaler.	Combivent (Rx)	Treatment of COPD in those who are on regular aerosol bronchodilator therapy and who require a second bronchodilator.	2 Inhalations q 6 hr, not to exceed 12 inhalations/24 hr.
Lisinopril (20 mg), Hydrochlorothiazide (12.5 mg or 25 mg)	Prinzide 12.5 and 25, Zestoretic 20–12.5 and 20–25 (Rx)	Hypertension in clients where combination therapy is appropriate. Not for initial therapy.	**Individualized, usual:** 1 or 2 tablets daily of one of the products.
Lopinavir (133.3 mg/capsule, 80 mg/mL solution), Ritonavir (33.3 mg/capsule, 20 mg/mL solution)	Kaletra (Rx)	With other antiretroviral drugs to treat HIV infections.	3 Capsules or 5 mL b.i.d. with food.
Loratidine (5 mg), Pseudoephedrine (120 mg)	Claritin-D (Rx)	Relieve symptoms of seasonal allergic rhinitis, including asthma.	**Adults and children over 12 years:** 1 Tablet q 12 hr on an empty stomach. Give 1 tablet/day in those with a GFR less than 30 mL/min.

Generic Name (Content)	Trade Name	Use	Dose
Loratidine (10 mg), Pseudoephedrine (240 mg)	Claritin-D 24 Hour Extented Release (Rx)	Relieve symptoms of seasonal allergic rhinitis, including asthma.	**Adults:** 1 Tablet daily.
Losartan potassium (50 mg), Hydrochlorothiazide (12.5 mg)	Hyzaar (Rx)	Hypertension (not for initial treatment). Use when losartan alone is not effective or hydrochlorothiazide (25 mg) alone causes hypokalemia.	**Adults:** 1 Tablet daily. If BP not controlled after 3 weeks, can increase dose to a maximum of 2 tablets/day.
Methyldopa (250 or 500 mg), Hydrochlorothiazide (15, 25, 30, or 50 mg)	Aldoril 15, 25, D30, and D50 (Rx)	Hypertension (not for initial treatment).	**Adults:** 1 Tablet b.i.d.–t.i.d. for the first 48 hr; **then,** increase dose, depending on response, in intervals of not less than 2 days to a maximum daily dose of 3 g methyldopa and 100–200 mg hydrochlorothiazide.
Pentazocine HCl (50 mg), Naloxone HCl (0.5 mg)	Talwin NX (Rx, C-IV)	Moderate to severe pain.	**Adults:** 1 Tablet q 3–4 hr, up to 2 tablets q 3–4 hr. Daily dose should not exceed 600 mg pentazocine.

Generic Name (Content)	Trade Name	Use	Dose
Propranolol HCl (40, 80, 120, or 160 mg), Hydrochlorothiazide (25 or 50 mg)	Inderide 40/25, Inderide 80/25, Inderide LA 80/50, Inderide LA 120/50, Inderide LA 160/50 (Rx)	Hypertension (not for initial therapy).	*Inderide Tablets:* 1–2 tablets b.i.d., up to 320 mg propranolol/day. *Inderide LA Capsules:* 1 capsule per day.
Quinapril hydrochloride (10 mg or 20 mg), Hydrochlorothiazide (12.5 mg or 25 mg)	Accuretic (Rx)	Hypertension (not for initial treatment).	One 10/12.5 or 20/12.5 tablet/day if BP not controlled by quinapril alone. Also for those whose BP adequately controlled by 25 mg hydrochlorothiazide but have significant potassium loss. Those adequately treated with 20 mg quinapril and 25 mg hydrochlorothiazide may switch to 20/25 dosage form.
Rifampin (300 mg), Isoniazid (150 mg)	Rifamate, Rimactane/INH Dual Pack (Rx)	Pulmonary tuberculosis following completion of initial therapy. In malnourished clients, adolescents, or those predisposed to neuropathy, also treat with pyridoxine.	Two capsules once daily.

Generic Name (Content)	Trade Name	Use	Dose
Rifampin (120 mg), Isoniazid (50 mg), Pyrazinamide (300 mg)	Rifater (Rx)	nitial phase of the short-course (2 months) treatment of pulmonary tuberculosis. If resistance is high, add streptomycin or ethambutol. In malnourished clients, adolescents, or those predisposed to neuropathy, also treat with pyridoxine. Follow the 2-month course of treatment with Rifamate.	**Weight less than 44 kg:** 4 tablets/day given at the same time; **45–54 kg:** 5 tablets/day given at the same time; **Over 55 kg:** 6 tablets/day given at the same time.
Spironolactone (25 or 50 mg), Hydrochlorothiazide (25 or 50 mg)	Aldactazide 25 and 50 (Rx)	CHF, essential hypertension, nephrotic syndrome. Edema and/or ascites in cirrhosis of the liver.	*Edema.* **Adults, usual:** 100 mg of each drug daily (range 25–200 mg) given as single or divided doses. **Children, usual:** Equivalent to 1.65–3.3 mg/kg spironolactone. *Essential hypertension.* **Adults, usual:** 50–100 mg of each drug daily in single or divided doses.

Generic Name (Content)	Trade Name	Use	Dose
Telmisartin (40 or 80 mg), Hydrochlorothiazide (12.5 mg)	Micardis HCT	Hypertension (second-line treatment).	**Initial:** 40 mg of telmisartin once/day (range: 20–80 mg). Effective dose of hydrochlorothiazide is 12.5–50 mg once daily. Not for use in those with severe hepatic impairment.
Tramadol hydrochloride (37.5 mg), Acetaminophen (325 mg)	Ultracet	Short-term (5 days or less) management of acute pain.	Two tablets q 4–6 hr as needed for pain relief, up to a maximum of 8 tablets per day.
Triamterene (37.5 or 75 mg for capsules or tablets), Hydrochlorothiazide (25 mg for capsules, 25 or 50 mg for tablets)	Apo-Triazide, Dyazide, Maxzide, Maxide-25 MG, Novo-Triamzide, Nu-Triazide, Pro-Triazide (Rx)	Hypertension or edema in clients who manifest hypokalemia on hydrochlorothiazide alone. Not first line of therapy except in those in whom hypokalemia should be avoided	Triamterene/Hydrochlorothiazide: **37.5 mg/25 mg:** 1 or 2 capsules/tablets daily; **50 mg/25 mg:** 1 or 2 capsules b.i.d. after meals; **75 mg/50 mg:** 1 tablet daily.

appendix 13
Drug/Food Interactions

A. DRUGS THAT SHOULD BE TAKEN WHILE FASTING

Ampicillin
AzoGantanol/Gantrisin
Bacampicillin
Bethanechol(may experience N&V)
Bisacodyl
Calcium carbonate
Captopril
Carbenicillin
Castor oil
Chloramphenicol
Cyclosporine gel caps only (do not take with fatty meals)
Demeclocycline (avoid high calcium foods/dairy products)
Dicloxacillin
Disopyramide
Digitalis preparations (not with high fiber foods)
Erythromycin base/estolate
Etidronate
Ferrous salts (not with tea, coffee, egg, cereals, fiber, or milk)
Flavoxate
Furosemide
Isoniazid
Isosorbide dinitrate
Ketoprofen (if GI distress occurs, may take with food)
Lansoprazole
Levodopa (not with high protein foods; meals delay absorption and peak plasma concentration; avoid caffeine)
Lisinopril
Lomustil (empty stomach will reduce nausea)
Methotrexate (milk, cream, or yogurt may decrease absorption)
Methyldopa (not with high protein foods; meals delay absorption and peak plasma concentration; avoid caffeine)
Nafcillin (inactivated by stomach acid; absorption variable with/without food)
Nalidixic acid
Naltrexone
Norfloxacin (milk, cream, or yogurt may decrease absorption)
Oxytetracycline (avoid dairy products and foods high in calcium)
Penicillamine (antacids, iron and food decreases absorption)
Penicillin
Phenytoin (if GI distress occurs, may take with food; food effect depends on preparation)
Propantheline
Rifampicin
Sotalol

Sulfamethoxazole
Tetracycline (avoid dairy products and foods high in calcium)
Theophylline (absorption of controlled release varies by preparation)
Thyroid hormone preparations (limit foods containing goitrogens)
Terbutaline sulfate
Trientine (antacids, iron, and food reduces absorption)
Trimethoprim

B. DRUGS THAT SHOULD BE TAKEN WITH FOOD

Buspirone
Carbamazepine (erratic absorption)
Chlorothiazide
Clofazimine
Gemfibrozil
Grisefulvin (high fat meals)
Isotretinoin
Labetatol
Lovastatin
Methenamine
Metoprolol
Nifedipine (grapefruit juice increases bioavailability)
Nitrofurantoin
Oxcarbazepine
Probucol (high fat meals)
Propranolol
Spironolactone
Trazodone
Verapamil SR (absorption varies by manufacturer; too rapid absorption may cause heart block)

C. CONSTIPATING AGENTS

Antacids
Anticholinergic drugs
  Antihistamines
  Anticholinergics
  Phenothiazines
  Tricyclic antidepressants
Corticosteroids
Clonidine
Ganglionic blocking agents
Iron supplements
Laxatives (when abused)
Lithium
MAO Inhibitors
Muscle relaxants
Octreotide
Opiods
Prostaglandin synthesis inhibitors
  NSAIDS

D. DIARRHEAL AGENTS

Adrenergic neuron blockers: reserpine, guanethidine
Antibiotics (especially broad spectrum agents)
Cholinergic agonists and cholinesterase inhibitors
Erythromycin
Osmotic and stimulant laxatives
Metoclopramide
Quinidine

E. TYRAMINE CONTAINING FOODS

Moderate amounts of tyramine:

- Broad beans
- Raspberries
- Banana peel
- Cheese (all except cream cheese and cottage cheese)
- Imitation cheese
- Prepared meats (sausage, chopped liver, pate, salami, mortadella)
- Meat extracts
- Concentrated yeast extracts/Brewer's yeast
- Liquid and powdered protein supplements
- Fermented soy products: fermented bean curd, soya bean paste, miso soup
- Hydrolyzed protein extracts for sauces, soups, gravies
- Fermented cabbage products: sauerkraut, kimchee
- Chianti, vermouth
- Nonalcoholic beers
- Some non-United States brands of beer

Significant amounts of tyramine:

- Avocado
- Yogurt
- Cream from fresh pasteurized milk
- Soy sauce
- Peanuts
- Chocolate
- Red and white wines, port wines
- Distilled spirits

F. FOODS CONTAINING GOITROGENS

- Asparagus
- Brussels sprouts
- Cabbage
- Kale
- Lettuce
- Peas
- Soy beans
- Spinach
- Turnip greens
- Watercress
- Other leafy green vegetables

G. COUMARIN ANTICOAGULANTS AND DIETARY EFFECTS

Consumption of vitamin K enriched foods may counteract the effects of anticoagulants since the drugs act through antagonism of vitamin K. Advise the client on anticoagulants to maintain a steady, consistent intake of vitamin K containing foods. The drug monograph for warfarin clearly lists these foods. Additionally, certain herbal teas (Woodruff, tonka beans, melitot) contain natural coumarins that can potentiate the effects of Coumadin and should be avoided. Large amounts of avocado also potentiate the drug's effects. Brussels sprouts and other cruciferous vegetables increase the catabolism of warfarin thereby decreasing its anticoagulant activities.

H. GENERAL DRUG CLASS RECOMMENDATIONS

Antacids: take 1 hr after or between meals. Avoid dairy foods as the protein in them can increase stomach acid.

Antihistamines: take on an empty stomach to increase effectiveness.

Analgesic/Antipyretic: take on an empty stomach as food may slow the absorption.

NSAIDS: take with food or milk to prevent irritation of the stomach.

Corticosteroids: take with food to decrease stomach upset

Bronchodilators with theophylline: high-fat meals may increase bioavailability while high-carbohydrate meals may decrease it. Food increases absorption of Theo-24 and Uniphyl which may cause increased N&V, headache and irritability.

Diuretics: vary in interactions; some cause loss of potassium, calcium, and magnesium. Avoid salty food and natural black licorice as these increase K and Mg losses. Large doses of vitamin D can elevate blood pressure.

ACE inhibitors: take captopril and moexipril 1 hr before or 2 hrs after meals; food decreases absorption. Avoid high potassium foods as ACE increases K+.

HMG-CoA reductase inhibitors: take lovastatin with the evening meal to enhance absorption.

Anticoagulants: high vitamin K produces blood-clotting substance and may reduce drug effectiveness. Vitamin E >400 IU may prolong clotting time and increase bleeding risk.

Antibiotics: penicillin generally should be taken on an empty stomach; may take with food if GI upset occurs. Do not mix with acidic foods such as coffee, citrus fruits, and tomatoes as the acid interferes with absorption of penicillin, ampicillin, erythromycin and cloxacillin.

Quinolones: Take on an empty stomach 1 hr before or 2 hrs after meals. May take with food for GI upset but avoid calcium containing foods such as milk, yogurt, vitamins/minerals containing iron and antacids because they decrease drug concentrations. Caffeine containing products may lead to excitability and nervousness.

Cephalosporins: take on an empty stomach 1 hr before or 2 hrs after meals. May take with food if GI upset occurs.

Macrolides Take on an empty stomach 1 hr before or 2 hrs after meals. May take with food for GI upset.

Sulfonamides: take on an empty stomach 1 hr before or 2 hrs after meals. May take with food if GI upset occurs.

Tetracyclines: take on an empty stomach 1 hr before or 2 hrs after meals. May take with food but avoid dairy products, antacids, and vitamins containing iron with tetracycline.

Nitroimadazole (metronidazole): avoid alcohol or food prepared with alcohol for at least three days after finishing the medicine. Alcohol may cause nausea, abdominal cramps, vomiting, headaches, and flushing.

Laxatives: avoid dairy foods as calcium can decrease absorption.

MAO inhibitors: have many dietary restrictions, so follow dietary guidelines as prescribed. Foods or alcoholic beverages containing tyramine may cause a fatal increase in BP.

Anti-anxiety agents: caffeine may cause excitability, nervousness, and hyperactivity lessening the anti-anxiety drug effects.

Antidepressant drugs: may be taken with or without food.

Antifungals: avoid taking with dairy products; avoid alcohol.

H_2 blockers: may take with or without regard to food.

appendix 14

Drugs Whose Effects Are Modified by Grapefruit Juice

Increasing numbers of drugs have been identified whose effects are modified by short-term or chronic use of grapefruit juice. The following is a representative list of those drugs, including the mechanism for the altered drug effect. The most frequent result is an increase in plasma levels of the drug, which may increase the risk of side effects.

DRUG	MECHANISM FOR ALTERED EFFECT
Bexarotene	↑ Plasma bexarotene levels R/T ↓ Liver metabolism
Budesonide	↑ Plasma budesonide levels
Buspirone	↑ Peak plasma buspirone levels
Carbamazepine	↑ Peak plasma carbamazepine levels
Cilostazol	↑ Plasma cilostazol levels R/T ↓ Liver metabolism
Cyclosporine	↑ Plasma cyclosporine levels R/T ↓ Liver metabolism
Dofetilide	Possible ↑ dofetilide plasma levels
Erythromycin	↑ Plasma erythromycin levels R/T ↓ Metabolism in the small intestine
Felodipine	↑ Plasma felodipine levels R/T ↓ Liver metabolism
Indinavir	Slight delay in indinavir absorption
Intraconzole	↓ Intraconzole bioavailability R/T inhibition of absorption
Losartan	↓ Liver metabolism to losartan's active form
Lovastatin	↑ Plasma lovastatin levels R/T ↓ Liver metabolism
Methylprednisolone	↑ Plasma methylprednisolone levels R/T ↓ Liver metabolism
Mifepristone	↑ Plasma mifepristone levels R/T ↓ Liver metabolism
Nicardipine	↑ Plasma nicardipine levels R/T ↓ Liver metabolism
Nifedipine	↑ Plasma nifedipine levels R/T ↓ Liver metabolsim
Nislodipine	↑ Plasma nislodipine levels R/T ↓ Liver metabolism
Saquinavir	↑ Plasma saquinavir levels R/T ↓ Liver metabolism
Simvastatin	↑ Plasma simvastatin levels R/T ↓ Liver metabolism
Sirolimus	↑ Plasma sirolimus levels R/T ↓ Liver metabolism
Triazolam	↑ Plasma triazolam levels R/T ↓ Liver metabolsim
Verapamil	↑ Plasma verapamil levels R/T ↓ Liver metabolism

appendix 15

Drugs That Should Not Be Crushed

As a rule of thumb, any sustained release or extended release formulation should never be crushed. Instead, attempt to get a liquid formulation of the product so that it can be administered in that form. Coated products should also not be crushed. They were coated for a specific purpose, e.g., to prevent stomach irritation by the product, to prevent destruction of the product by stomach acid, to prevent an unwanted reaction, or to produce a prolonged or extended effect.

These are some of the drugs that should not be crushed:

Afrinol repetabs
Allerest capsules
Aminodur duratab
Artane sequel
ASA E.C.
ASA enseals
Azulfadine entab
Betaphen-vk
Compazine spansule
Diamox sequel
Donnatol extentab
Drixoral tabs
Ecotrin tabs
E-Mycin tabs
Feosol spansule
Feosol tabs
Ferro Grad-500 tab
Isordil sublingual
Kaon tabs
Nitroglycerin tab
Nitrospan caps
Ornade spanule
Quinaglute duratab
Quinidex extenutab
Slow K tabs
Sudafed SA caps
Teldrin caps
Theo-dur tabs
Trental

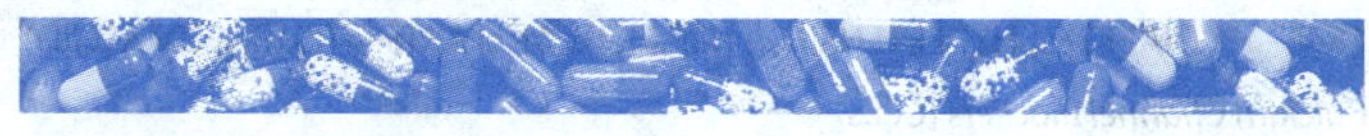

appendix 16

Drugs Commonly Used in the Treatment of Diabetes, Hypertension, Hepatitis, and Arthritis (Rheumatoid)

Drugs Used with Diabetes

Acarbose
Acetohexamide
Chlorpropamide
Glimepiride
Glipizide
Glyburide
Insulin
Metformin
Miglitol
Nateglinide
Proglitazone
Repaglinide
Rosiglitazone
Tolazamide
Tolbutamide

Drugs Used with Hypertension

Beta-Adrenergic Blocking Agents

Acebutolol
Atenolol
Betaxolol
Bisoprolol
Carteolol
Esmolol
Labetolol
Metoprolol
Nadolol
Penbutolol
Pindolol
Propranolol
Sotalol
Timolol

Calcium Channel Blockers (CCBs)

Amlodipine
Bepridil
Diltiazem
Felodipine
Isradipine
Nicardipine
Nifedipine
Nimodipine
Nisoldipine
Verapamil

Diuretics

Loop: bumetanide, ethacrynic acid, furosemide
Potassium sparing: spironolactone, triamterene
Thiazide: hydrochlorothiazide

Angiotensin Converting Enzyme (ACE) Inhibitors

Benazepril
Captopril
Enalapril
Enalaprilat
Fosinopril
Lisinopril
Moexipril
Perindopril
Quinapril
Ramipril
Trandolapril

Angiotensin II Receptor Blockers (ARBS)

Candesartan
Eprosartan
Irbesartan
Losartan
Telmisartan
Valsartan

Other

Clonidine
Diazoxide
Doxazosin
Guanabenz
Guanadrel
Guanethidine
Guanfacine
Hydralazine
Methyldopa
Nitroprusside
Prazosin
Terazosin

Drugs Used to Treat Hepatitis

Interferon alfa-n1 lymphoblastoid; interferon alfa-2b, interferon alfacon-1
Peginterferon alfa-2b
Ribavirin

Drugs Used to Treat Arthritis (Rheumatoid)

Anakinra
Aspirin; choline magnesium trisalicylate (both RA and OA)
Cyclosporine
D-Penicillamine
Etanercept
Glucocorticoids
Gold
Hydroxychloroquine
Infliximab
Leflunomide
Methotrexate
Sulfasalazine
Tylenol (OA)

Nonsteroidal Anti-inflammatory Drugs (NSAIDs)

Celecoxib
Diclofenac
Diflunisal
Etodolac
Fenoprofen
Flurbiprofen
Ibuprofen
Indomethacin
Ketoprofen
Ketorolac
Meclofenamate
Mefenamic acid
Meloxicam
Nabumetone
Naproxen
Oxaprozin
Piroxicam
Rofecoxib
Sulindac
Tolmetin
Valdecoxib

appendix 17

Drug Therapy for Pain Management

PAIN

Pain is a subjective report from the client of what he or she is feeling. It has received a lot of attention since the Joint Commission on Accreditation of Healthcare Organizations mandated that this experience be identified, assessed, and managed. The easiest and most consistent way to evaluate a person's pain is to ask them to rate it on a 0–10 scale (0 being no pain and 10 being the worst possible pain). Have them identify their current pain level and be sure to document it. Some clients may experience a pain level of 5. Always ask them if this is livable or do they need something to help them relieve their pain. If they say it is livable, note that. If they ask for something to relieve it, then start with a low-level pain reliever. Each time they return, evaluate the effectiveness of their pain relief medication. Additionally, assess other modalities that may also relieve pain, e.g., physical therapy, brace, support, ice, heat, positioning.

Mild to Moderate Pain Relievers

Acetaminophen 650 mg po q 4 h
Aspirin 650 mg po q 4 h
Celebrex 200 mg po qd
Choline magnesium trisalicylate (Trilisate, disalcid) 1,000–1,500 mg tid
Diclofenac (Voltaren) 50 mg po tid
Ibuprofen (Motrin, Advil) 400–600 mg po q 6h
Indomethacin (Indocin) 50 mg po tid
Ketoprofen (Orudis) 25–60 mg po q 6–8h
Ketorolac (Toradol) 10 mg po qd 4–6 hr maximum dose 40 mg/day; do not exceed 5 days of IM Toradol
Naproxen (Napsoxyn) 250–550 mg po bid
Sulindac (Clinoril) 200 mg po bid
Valdecoxib
Vioxx 50 mg po qd

Moderate to Severe Pain Relievers

Codeine 15–30 mg po q 6h
Hydrocodone (Vicodin, Loratab) 5–7.5/500mg APAP 1–2 po q 4–6 h up to 8 tablets per day
Meperidine (Demerol) 50 mg/25 mg prometh 1 po q 4–6 h
Oxycodone (OxyContin) 5–40 mg po q 4 h
Oxycodone + ASA (Roxicodone, Aspirin) 5/650 1–2 po q 4–6 hr
Oxycodone + APAP (Percocet) 5mg/500 mg (APAP) 1–2 po q 4–6 h

Propoxyphene (ASA + caffeine) Darvon 65mg/389 mg/324 mg caffeine 1–2 po q 4 h

Propoxyphene +APAP (Darvocet N, Darvocet N-100) 50mg/325-2 po q 4h or 100 mg /650 mg-1po q 4h

Severe Pain Relievers

Fentanyl (Sublimaze)

Fentanyl transdermal patch is absorbed through the skin creating a depot in the upper layer. It offers up to 72 hr of analgesia with steady state achieved in 12–16 hr. Short-acting opioids are generally used to help manage pain that occurs prior to 72 hr (breakthrough pain).

Hydromorphone (Dilaudid) 2 mg IM = 8 mg po duration 3–4 hr

Levorphanol (Levo-dromoran) 2 mg IM = 4 mg po duration 6–8 hr

Meperidine (Demerol) 75–100 mg IM=300 mg po duration 3 hr

Methadone (Dolophine) 10 mg IM=20 mg po duration 6–8 hr

Morphine 10 mg IM/IV/SC = 30 mg po short acting duration 3–4hr (long acting agents last 8–12 hr or 24 hr)

Adjuvant Analgesics

Tricyclic antidepressants: Use for neuropathic pain, insomnia, depression
- Amitriptyline (Elavil)
- Doxepin (Sinequan)
- Imipramine (Tofranil)
- Nortriptyline (Pamelor, Aventyl)

Anticonvulsants: Use for lancinating neuropathic pain
- Carbamazepine (Tegretol)
- Clonazepam (Klonopin)
- Gabapentin (Neurontin)

Other local anesthetics: Use for neuropathic pain
- Mexilitene (Mexitil)

Neuroleptics: Use for refractory neuropathic pain and delirium
- Fluphenazine (Prolixin)
- Haloperidol (Haldol)

Antihistamines: Use for anxiety, nausea
- Hydroxyzine (Vistaril, Atarax)
- Diphenhydramine (Benadryl)

Corticosteroids: Use for infiltration of neuro structures; bone pain
- Dexamethasone (Decadron)

Psychostimulant: Use for reverse opioid induced sedation
- Dextroamphetamine (Dexedrine)
- Methylphenidate (Ritalin)

Drug conversions of oral and parenteral narcotics to transdermal fentanyl

Fentanyl mcg/hr transdermal	Morphine oral mg/d	Morphine IM mg/day	Hydromorphone oral mg/d	Hydromorphone IM mg/day
25	45–134	8–22	5.6–17	1.2–3.4
50	135–224	23–37	17.1–28	3.5–5.6
75	225–314	38–42	28.1–39	5.7–7.9
100	315–404	53–67	39.1–51	8–10
125	405–494	68–82	62.1–73	10.1–12
150	495–584	83–97	—	—
175	585–674	98–112	—	—
200	675–764	113–127	—	—
225	765–854	128–142	—	—
250	855–944	143–157	—	—

275	945–1034	158–172	—	—
300	1035–1124	173–187	—	—

Fentanyl mcg/hr transdermal	Oxycodone oral mg/d	Oxycodone IM mg/d	Levorphanol oral mg/d	Levorphanol IM mg/d
25	22.5–67	12–33	3–8.9	1.6–4.4
50	67.5–112	33.1–56	9–14.9	4.5–7.4
75	112.4–157	56.1–78	15–20.9	7.5–10.4
100	157.5–202	78.1–101	21–26.9	10.5–13.4
125	202.5–247	101.1–123	27–32.9	13.5–16.4
150	247.5–292	123.1–147	33–38.9	16.5–19.4

Fentanyl mcg/hr transdermal	Meperidine oral mg/d	Meperidine IM mg/d	Codeine oral mg/d	Codeine IM mg/d
25	—	60–165	150–447	104–286
50	—	166–278	448–747	287–481
75	—	279–390	748–1047	482–676
100	—	391–503	1048–1347	677–871
125	—	504–615	1348–1647	872–1066
150	—	616–728	1648–1947	1067–1261

Equianalgesic Conversion of Oral Opioids to Morphine Tablets

Drug	Dose/Schedule	Morphine Sulfate Equianalgesic
Hydromorphone	4 mg q 4 h	3 tablets 15 mg q 12h
(Dilaudid)	8 mg q 4 h	3 tablets 30 mg q 12h
	10 mg q 4 h	2 tablets 60 mg q 12h
	25 mg q 4 h	3 tablets 100 mg q 12h
Levorphanol	2 mg q 6 h	2 tablets 15 mg q 12 h
(Levo Dromoran)	4 mg q 6 h	2 tablets 30 mg q 12 h
	6 mg q 4 h	2 tablets 60 mg q 12 h
	14 mg q 4 h	3 tablets 100 mg q 12 h
Meperdine	100 mg q 3 h	2 tablets 15 mg q 12 h
(Demerol)	200 mg q 3 h	2 tablets 30 mg q 12 h
	600 mg q 3 h	2 tablets 60 mg q 12 h
	1000 mg q 3 h	2 tablets 100 mg q 12 h
Methadone	10 mg q 6 h	2 tablets 15 mg q 12 h
(Dolophine)	20 mg q 6 h	2 tablets 30 mg q 1 2 h
	30 mg q 4 h	2 tablets 60 mg q 12 h
	70 mg q 4 h	3 tablets 100 mg q 12 h
Morphine	10 mg q 4 h	2 tablets 15 mg q 12h
(MSIR, Roxanol)	30 mg q 4 h	3 tablets 30 mg q 12h
	80 mg q 4 h	4 tablets 60 mg q 12h
	100 mg q 4 h	3 tablets 100 mg q 12h
Oxycodone	10 mg q 4 h	2 tablets 15 mg q 12 h
(Roxicodone)	20 mg q 4 h	2 tablets 30 mg q 12 h
	40 mg q 4 h	2 tablets 60 mg q 12 h
	100 mg q 4 h	3 tablets 100 mg q 12 h

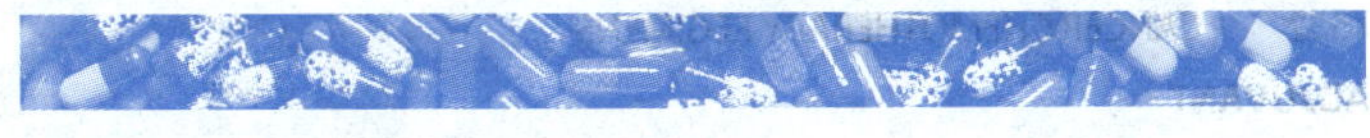

appendix 18

Cancer Chemotherapy Regimens

Approach and management of cancers generally depend on their type, location, size, classification, and cell type; the age and physical condition of the client; the provider's skill, comfort, and experience; as well as what the client requests. The National Cancer Institute (NCI) maintains a record of all clinical trials, ongoing research, references, and treatment guidelines for those who are interested. Its website (http://www.cancer.gov) has a wealth of client and physician/provider resources. It includes an explanation of the types and causes of cancers, the standard therapies, a vocabulary resource, and clinical trials. The site is easy to use and directs you to various areas. NCI may also be contacted by telephone 1-800-4-cancer or 1-800-422-6237.

The American Joint Committee on Cancer (AJCC) has designated staging by the TNM classifications:

PRIMARY TUMOR (T)

Tx: Primary tumor cannot be assessed
T0: No evidence of primary tumor
Tis: Carcinoma in situ
T1: Tumor invades submucosa
T2: Tumor invades muscle
T3: Tumor invades through muscle to surrounding tissue
T4: Tumor directly invades other organs or structures

REGIONAL LYMPH NODES (N)

Ns: Regional lymph nodes cannot be assessed
NO: No regional lymph node metastasis
N1: Metastasis in 1–3 regional lymph nodes
N2: Metastasis in 4 or more regional lymph nodes

DISTANT METASTASIS (M)

Mx: Metastasis cannot be assessed
M0: No distant metastasis
M1: Distant metastasis

RADIATION THERAPY (XRT)

Radiation oncologist uses India ink to tattoo therapy sites

NEOADJUVANT

Chemotherapy prior to other modalities

ADJUVANT

Chemotherapy given after or during therapy with XRT or after surgery

ALL (Acute lymphoblastic leukemia): varies by regimen, age, induction, consolidation

Daunorubicin/Vincristine/Prednisone/L-Asparaginase
ARA-C/Teniposide (VM-26)
Methotrexate/Leukovorin
Etoposide (VP-16)/Cytarabine (ARA-C)/Methotrexate
Total body irradiation (TBI)/Etoposide with allogenic bone marrow transplant

AML (Acute myelogenous leukemia)

ARA-C and Daunorubicin or Mitoxantrone or Idarubicin
Busulfan/Cyclophosphamide or
Cyclophosphamide/Total body irradiation with allogenic bone marrow transplant

Adrenocortical carcinoma

Mitotane

Bladder cancer

Cisplatin/Methotrexate/Vinblastine/Doxorubicin
TUR with fulgration
Intravesical BcG/chemotherapy
Interstitial radiosotope implantation with/without external beam irradiation

Brain tumors

Carmustine/Hydroxurea/Lomustine/Procarbazine

Breast cancer: varies with age, stage, metastasis, and stem cell transplant

CA: Cyclophosphamide and Doxorubicin
Docetaxel and Doxorubicin
CAF: Cyclophosphamide, Doxorubicin, 5-FU
CMF: Cyclophosphamide, Methotrexate, 5-Fluorouracil
AC: Doxorubicin/Cyclophosphamide
Paclitaxel (Taxol)
NFL: Mitoxantrone/5-FU/Leucovorin

Breast cancer, stages I, II, IIIa

Conservative therapy involves lumpectomy, breast irradiation and surgical staging of axilla
Modified radical mastectomy involves removal of the entire breast with level I-II axillary dissection with or without breast reconstruction
Adjuvant XRT post-mastectomy in axillary node + tumors with >4 nodes or extranodal evidence
Stage IV: metastatic disease; Palliative therapy

DIS (ductal carcinoma in situ)

Breast conserving surgery and XRT with or without Tamoxifen
Total mastectomy with or without Tamoxifen

LCIS (lobular carcinoma in situ)

Observation after biopsy
Tamoxifen to decrease incidence of subsequent breast cancers
Bilateral prophylactic total mastectomy without axillary node dissection

Cervical cancer

Irinotecan; Doxorubicin

Colorectal cancer

Depends on staging I–IV; cellular classification, e.g., adenocarcinoma, mucinous

I. Local excision or polypectomy with clear margins
Wide surgical resection and anastomosis

II. Resection, evaluate for clinical trials

III. Surgery
5-FU/Leucovorin x 6 mo
5-FU/Levamisole for 12 mo
Clinical trials

IV. Surgical resection, anastomosis, or bypass/surgical resection of isolated metastasis
Chemotherapy
Clinical trials
XRT to primary tumor to palliate bleeding/obstruction/pain

Endometrial cancer

Depends on cell type, staging I–IV and differentiation of adenocarcinoma G1–G3
Surgery: Hysterectomy, bilateral salpingo-oophorectomy, and node sampling followed by irradiation or
preop intracavity and external beam radiation followed by surgery or
Hydroxyprogesterone, Medroxyprogesterone, and Megestrol acetate or
clinical trials

Gastric cancer

ELF: Etoposide/Leucovorin/5-FU
EAP: VP-16 (Etoposide)/Doxorubicin/Cisplatin
FAMtx: Fluorouracil/Doxorubicin/Methotrexate

Kaposi's sarcoma:
Liposomal Daunorubicin

Lung cancer

Non-small cell (NSCLC)
Surgical resection (segmentectomy or wedge resection)
Endoscopic photodynamic therapy
XRT
Chemotherapy: Cisplatin/Vinblastine/Mitomycin, Cisplatin/Vinorelbine, Cisplatin/Paclitaxel, Cisplatin/Docetaxel, Cisplatin/Gemcitabine, or Carboplatin/Paclitaxel
Clinical trials
Endobronchial laser or brachytherapy to obstructing lesions

Small cell: Depends on classification and staging
  Staging: limited and extensive
  Limited: combination chemotherapy
    EC: Etoposide + Cisplatin + chest XRT
    CCV: Etoposide/Cisplatin/Vincristine/XRT
  Combination chemotherapy with or without PCI (prophylactic cranial irradiation)
External stage:
  Combination therapy with or without PCI
    CAV: Cyclophosphamide/Doxorubicin/Vincristine
    CAE: Cyclophosphamide/Doxorubicin/Etoposide
    EP or EC: Etoposide/Cisplatin or Etoposide/Carboplatin
    ICE: Ifosfamide/Carboplatin/Etoposide

Laryngeal cancer (supraglottis, glottis, subglottis)

  Treatment depends on cell class, location, size, and staging
  XRT; surgery; chemotherapy: Cisplatin/5-FU
Lip/oral cavity
  Surgical excision with STSG (split-thickness skin graft)
  XRT
  Chemotherapy
Oropharyngeal
  Surgery
  XRT
  Chemotherapy: Carboplatin/5-FU
    Pt-FU: Cisplatin/Fluorouracil
    Metastatic MTX: Methotrexate
Melanoma Depends on staging
  Adjuvant: IFN: Interferon Alfa-2b
  Surgical excision or wide excision with clean margins
  LND (lymph node dissection)
  Metastatic INF-DTIC: Interferon Alfa-2B/Dacarbazine
    Pt-DTIC-BCNU-TAM: Cisplatin/Dacarbazine/BCNU/Tamoxifen
  Clinical trials
  Palliative XRT to bone, spinal cord, brain
  Complete resection of all known metastatic disease
  Palliative treatment with Interleukin-2 or Interferon
  Isolated hyperthermic limb perfusions

Ovarian cancer

PAC: Cisplatin/Doxorubicin/Cyclophosphamide
Altretamine
Paclitaxel
Topotecan

Pancreatic cancer

Adenocarcinoma (advanced): Gemcitabine
Metastatic (islet cell): Streptozocin/Doxorubicin

Prostate cancer

Stage I–IV, 95% adenocarcinoma, PSA level, bone scan, and histologic findings
  M1a nonregional lymph nodes
  M1b bone(s)
  M1c other site(s)

Histopathologic grade (G)
Gx: Grade cannot be assessed
G1: Well differentiated (slight anaplasia)
G2: Moderately differentiated (moderate anaplasia)
G3: Poorly differentiated or undifferentiated (marked anaplasia)
Stage I: Careful observation and F/U
Stage II: External beam XRT 4–6 weeks after TUR
Stage III: Radical prostatectomy and PND (prostate node dissection)
Stage IV: Interstitial implantation of radiosotopes: I-125, palladium, iridium
Hormonal manipulation: a. Orchiectomy; b. Leuprolide or other LHRH agonists (Zoladex); c. Estrogen; d. Non-steroidal antiandrogen (Flutamide, Nilutamide, Bicalutamide) or steroidal antiandrogen (Cyproterone acetate)
Chemotherapy: VBL: Vinblastine/Estramustine

Rectal cancer

Classification adeno, muscinous, carcinoid etc.
I: Local excision or polypectomy
II: Full thickness resection by transanal or transcoccygeal route for large lesions not amenable to local excision
III: Endocavity radiation
IV: Local radiation therapy
Chemotherapy: Rectal FU: 5-Fu
Localized anal FU-MMC: 5-FU/Mitomycin and XRT

Sarcomas, soft tissue

MAID: Mesna/Doxorubicin/Ifosfamide/Dacarbazine
Metastatic
CYVADIC: Cyclophosphamide/Vincristine/Doxorubicin/Dacarbazine

REFERENCES

Ignoffo, R. J., Viele, C. S., Damon, L. E., & Venook, A. 1998 Cancer chemotherapy pocket guide. Philadelphia: Lippincott-Raven.
National Cancer Institute, U.S. National Institutes of Health, Bethesda, MD. http://www.cancer.gov

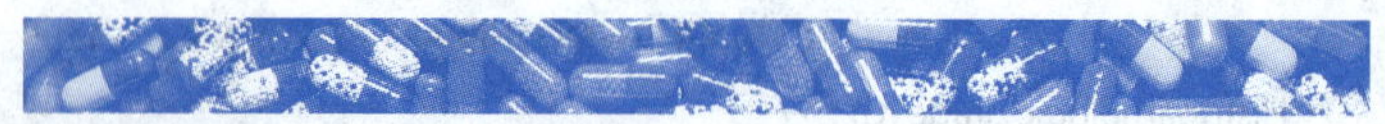

appendix 19

Treatment of Chemotherapy-Induced Emesis

Prevention

Administer antiemetic at least 30 min prior to chemotherapy. With oral agents, give one or two doses at least 2 hr prior to oral treatment.

With severely emetogenic chemotherapy, use 5-HT3 antagonists on each day of chemotherapy. May also include with Dexamethasone if not contraindicated.

With highly emetogenic agents (e.g., Cisplatin), give those that will inhibit emetic stimulus for 24 hr.

Those receiving their first chemotherapy cycle may experience anticipatory nausea and vomiting, so administer anxiolytic agents. May give Lorazepam parenterally or sublingual.

With chemotherapy that may cause delayed emesis, use oral agents (phenothiazines or Metoclopramide) with or without Dexamethasone for 2 or 3 days starting 16 hrs after chemotherapy.

Agents for chemotherapy-induced emesis

Class III Severe

Granisetron 10 mcg/kg IV over 5–15 min q 24 hr, 1 mg po bid on each day of chemotherapy + Dexamethasone 10–20 mg IV 30 min prior to chemotherapy for 1–5 days

Or

Ondansetron 10 mg IV q8h or 24–32 mg IV x 1 for 15 min on each day of chemotherapy + Dexamethasone 10–20 mg IV 30 min prior to chemotherapy for 1–5 days

Class II

Ondansetron 10–20 mg IV over 15–30 min each day of chemotherapy + Dexamethasone 10–20 mg IV 30 min prior to chemotherapy for 1–5 days

Or

Ondansetron 8 mg 3x/day each day of chemotherapy or Granisetron 1 mg po 2x/day for each day of chemotherapy + Dexamethasone

Pediatric Dose

Ondansetron 0.15 mg/kg for 3 doses: first dose starting 30 min. before chemotherapy, second dose 4 hr after first dose, and third dose 8 hr after first dose

Or

Granisetron 10 mcg/kg IV for 15 min every 24 hrs

Plus

Dexamethasone 0.8 mg give in 3 divided doses IV 30 min prior to chemotherapy q 8h for 1–5 days

Delayed Emesis from Chemotherapy (Days 2–5)

Metoclopramide 0.5–1 mg/kg IV/PO q 4 hr x 3 doses

Plus

Dexamethasone 8 mg po bid

Or

Ondansetron 8 mg po bid

Plus

Dexamethasone 8 mg po bid

Or

Prochlorperazine spansules 15 mg po bid plus Dexamethasone 8 mg po bid

REFERENCES

Ignoffo, R. J., Viele, C. S., Damon, L. E., & Venook, A. 1998 Cancer chemotherapy pocket guide. Philadelphia: Lippincott-Raven.

National Cancer Institute, U.S. National Institutes of Health, Bethesda, MD. http://www.cancer.gov

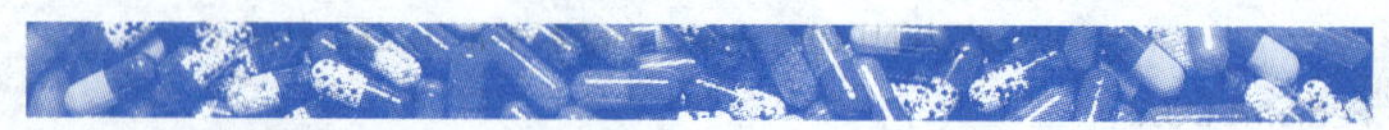

appendix 20

Bioterrorism Agents

Since the September 11, 2001 catastrophe, attention has been focused on the use of biological weapons to create fear in the United States of America. ***Terrorism*** is a term that means the use of fear to intimidate others and to cause economic and political insecurity. Almost any microorganism can be used as a weapon, but most diseases can be treated. The five most dangerous biological warfare threats are anthrax, botulism, pneumonic plague, smallpox, and tularemia.

Anthrax: *Bacillus anthracis*

A. Inhalation

Flu-like S&S (fever, fatigue, muscle aches, SOB, nonproductive cough, headaches), chest pain; 1–2 day improvement then rapid respiratory failure and shock. May develop meningitis.

Incubation: 1–6 days up to 6 weeks; no person-to-person transmission; standard precautions

Dx: CXR evidence of widening mediastinum; sputum C&S

Postexposure prophylaxis: Rx: prophylaxis for 60 days: Doxycycline 100 mg po q 12h or Amoxicillin 500 mg po q8h or Ciprofloxacin 500 mg po q 12h.

Alternative: Ofloxacin 400 mg po q 12h or Levofloxacin 500 mg po q 24 hr; or Gatifloxacin 400 mg po q 24 hr

Treatment: Penicillin G 2–4 MU IV q 4–6h, or Amoxicillin 500 mg IV q 8h, or Ciprofloxacin 400 mg IV q 12 h, or Doxycycline 200 mg IV load, then 100 mg IV q 12h

Alternative Rx: Ofloxacin 400 mg IV q 12h, or Levofloxacin 500 mg IV q 24 hr, or Gatifloxacin 400 mg IV q 24 hr

B. Cutaneous

S&S: Intense itching followed by painless papular lesions, then vesicular lesions, developing into eschar surrounded by edema.

Incubation: 1–12 days. Transmission from person to person by contact with skin lesions may result in cutaneous infection; contact precautions.

Dx: Peripheral blood smear may demonstrate gram + bacilli on unspun smear with sepsis.

Postexposure prophylaxis: Rx: prophylaxis for 60 days: Doxycycline 100 mg po q 12h, or Amoxicillin 500 mg po q8h, or Ciprofloxacin 500 mg po q 12h.

Alternative: Ofloxacin 400 mg po q 12h, or Levofloxacin 500 mg po q 24 hr, or Gatifloxacin 400 mg po q 24 hr

Treatment: Penicillin G 2–4 MU IV q 4–6h, or Amoxicillin 500 mg IV q 8h, or Ciprofloxacin 400 mg IV q 12 h, or Doxycycline 200 mg IV load, then 100 mg IV q 12h

Alternative Rx: Ofloxacin 400 mg IV q 12h, or Levofloxacin 500 mg IV q 24 hr, or Gatifloxacin 400 mg IV q 24 hr

C. Gastrointestinal

S&S: Abdominal pain, nausea and vomiting, severe diarrhea, GI bleeding, and fever

Incubation: 1–7 days; no person-to-person transmission

Dx: Culture blood and stool; standard precautions

Treatment (as long as strains are susceptible): Penicillin G 2–4 MU IV q 4–6h, or Amoxicillin 500 mg IV q 8h, or Ciprofloxacin 400 mg IV q 12 h, or Doxycycline 200 mg IV load, then 100 mg IV q 12h

Alternative Rx (as long as strains are susceptible): Ofloxacin 400 mg IV q 12h, or Levofloxacin 500 mg IV q 24 hr, or Gatifloxacin 400 mg IV q 24 hr

Botulism: *Clostridium botulinum*

S&S: Afebrile, excess mucus in throat, swallowing difficulty, dry mouth and throat, dizziness, then difficulty moving eye, mild pupillary dilation and nystagmus, intermittent ptosis, indistinct speech, unsteady gait, extreme symmetric descending weakness, flaccid paralysis; generally normal mental status.

Incubation time: Inhalation 12–80 hrs; foodborne 12–72 hr; no person-to-person contact; standard precautions

Dx: Lab test available from Centers for Disease Control and Prevention (CDC) or public health department: obtain serum, stool, gastric aspirate, and suspect foods prior to administering antitoxin. Differential diagnosis includes polio, Guillain-Barre, myasthenia, tick paralysis, CVA, meningococcal meningitis.

Postexposure prophylaxis: Pentavalent toxoid (types A, B, C, D, E) 0.5 mL SC may be available as investigational product from U.S. Army Medical Research Institute of Infectious Diseases (USAMRIID).

Treatment: Botulism antitoxins from public health authorities. Supportive care and ventilatory support. Avoid Clindamycin and aminoglycosides.

Pneumonic plague: *Yersinia pestis*

S&S: High fever, cough, hemoptysis, chest pain, N&V, headache. Advanced disease: Purpuric skin lesions, copious watery or purulent sputum production; respiratory failure in 1–6 days.

Incubation: 2–3 days (range 2–6 days); person-to-person transmission by droplet aerosols.

Droplet precautions until 48 hrs of effective ATX therapy

Diagnosis: Presumptive diagnosis may be made by Gram, Wayson, or Wright stain of lymph node aspirates, sputum, or cerebrospinal fluid with Gram negative bacilli with bipolar (safety pin) staining.

Postexposure prophylaxis: Doxycycline 100 mg po q 12h or Ciprofloxacin 50 mg po q 12h

Treatment: Streptomycin 1 gm IM q 12h; or gentamycin 2 mg/kg then 1.0 to 1.7 mg/kg IV q 8 h

Alternative Rx: Doxycycline 200 mg po load, then 100 mg po q 12h or Ciprofloxacin 400 mg IV q 12h

Smallpox: *Variola virus*

S&S: Prodromal period: malaise, fever, rigors, vomiting, headache, and backache. After 2–4 days, skin lesions appear and progress uniformly from macules to papules to vesicles and pustules, mostly on face, neck, palms, soles, and subsequently progress to the trunk.

Incubation: 12–14 days (7–17 days) person-to-person transmission by airborne droplet nuclei or direct contact with skin lesions or secretions until all scabs separate and fall off (3–4 weeks); Practice airborne isolation including N95 mask and contact precautions

Dx: Swab culture of vesicular fluid or scab, sent to BL-4 lab. All lesions similar in appearance and develop synchronously as opposed to chickenpox. Electron microscopy can differentiate variola virus from varicella

Treatment: Early vaccine critical (in less than 4 days). Call CDC for vaccinia. Vaccinia immune globulin in special cases: call USAMRIID at 301-619-2833.

Alternative Rx: Supportive care. Previous vaccination against smallpox does not confer lifelong immunity. May consider Cidofovir.

Tularemia: *Francisella tularensis* bacterium

S&S: flu-like symptoms; one of the most infectious pathogens known. Usually caught from ticks and fleas that have bitten infected rabbits or mice.

Incubation: 3–5 days after exposure. Cannot be spread person to person.

Treatment: If detected early can be treated with antibiotics. Streptomycin is the most effective. The CDC is currently developing a vaccine.

What To Do If Exposed To Any Of These Agents

If exposed, contact your local provider or health department. If you develop severe flu-like symptoms that do not go away after several days, and you have difficulty breathing, severe nausea and/or diarrhea, fever, excessive sweating and abdominal pain, call and report. Without treatment, death may occur in 24–36 hours. The local public health department uses people trained by the CDC to test you for these diseases. They can then provide the antidotes and medical supplies needed to treat you within 12 hours.

A gas mask does not work unless you wear it all the time or have it on at the moment of exposure. A gas mask must be custom-fit for you or you could suffocate. Contamination with bioterrorism agents may present with flu-like symptoms. You are more likely to get the flu than be exposed to bioterrorism agents. You can minimize your risk of the flu by getting the yearly flu vaccine and practicing regular handwashing.

REFERENCES

American Red Cross, http://www.redcross.org

Health Aspects of Biological and Chemical Weapons, World Health Organization, http://www.who.int/emc/deliberate_epi.html

Public Emergency Preparedness and Response, U.S. Centers for Disease Control and Prevention, http://www.bt.cdc.gov

U.S. Federal Emergency Management Agency, http://www.fema.gov

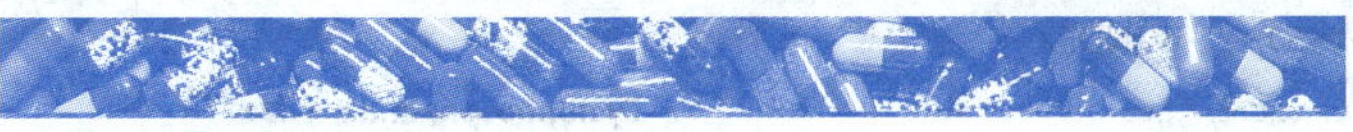

IV Index

Boldface = generic drug name CAPITALS = combination drugs

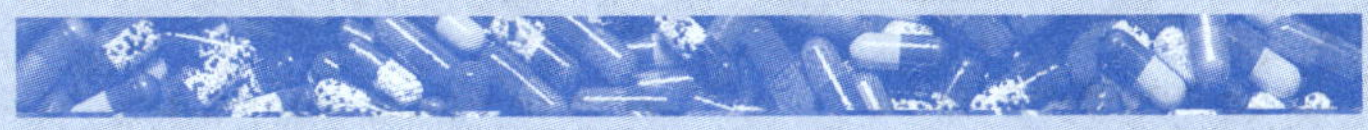

Index

Boldface = generic drug name CAPITALS = combination drugs